Kendig's Disorders of the Respiratory Tract in Children

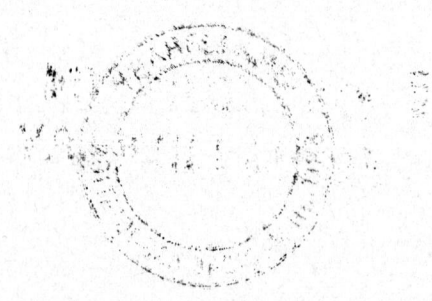

Kendig's Disorders of the Respiratory Tract in Children

NINTH EDITION

Robert William Wilmott, BSc, MB, BS, MD, FRCP (UK)

IMMUNO Professor and Chair
Department of Pediatrics
Saint Louis University
Pediatrician in Chief
SSM Cardinal Glennon Children's Medical Center
St. Louis, Missouri, United States

Robin Deterding, MD

Chief
Pediatric Pulmonary Medicine
Professor of Pediatrics
Department of Pediatrics
University of Colorado
Aurora, Colorado, United States

Albert Li, MBBch, MD, MRCPCH, MRCP(UK), FHKAM(Paeds), FHKCPaed

Assistant Dean (Education)
Faculty of Medicine
Professor of Paediatrics
Prince of Wales Hospital
The Chinese University of Hong Kong
Shatin, Hong Kong

Felix Ratjen, MD, PhD, FRCP(C), FERS

Head
Division of Respiratory Medicine
Program Head
Translational Medicine
Sellers Chair of Cystic Fibrosis
Professor
University of Toronto
Hospital for Sick Children
Toronto, Ontario, Canada

Peter Sly, MBBS, MD, FRACP, DSc

Director
Children's Lung Environment and Asthma Research Group
University of Queensland
Brisbane, Australia

Heather J. Zar, MBBCh, FCPaeds, FRCP (Edinburgh), PhD

Professor and Chair
Department of Paediatrics & Child Health
Director MRC Unit on Child & Adolescent Health
Red Cross War Memorial Children's Hospital
University of Cape Town
Cape Town, South Africa

Andrew Bush, MB BS(Hons), MA, MD, FRCP, FRCPCH, FERS

Professor of Paediatrics and Head of Section
Imperial College London
Professor of Paediatric Respirology
National Heart and Lung Institute
Consultant Paediatric Chest Physician
Royal Brompton Harefield NHS Foundation Trust
London, Great Britain

ELSEVIER

ELSEVIER

1600 John F. Kennedy Blvd.
Ste 1800
Philadelphia, PA 19103-2899

Previous editions copyrighted 2012, 2006, 1998, 1990, 1983, 1977, 1972, and 1967

Library of Congress Cataloging-in-Publication Data

Names: Wilmott, R. W. (Robert W.), editor.
Title: Kendig's disorders of the respiratory tract in children / [edited by] Robert William Wilmott,
    Robin Deterding, Albert Li, Felix Ratjen, Peter Sly, Heather J. Zar, Andrew Bush.
Other titles: Kendig and Chernick's disorders of the respiratory tract in children | Disorders of the
    respiratory tract in children
Description: Ninth edition. | Philadelphia, PA : Elsevier, [2019] | Preceded by: Kendig and Chernick's
    disorders of the respiratory tract in children / [edited by] Robert W. Wilmott ... [et al.]. 8th ed. [edited by]
    Robert W. Wilmott ... [et al.]. c2012. | Includes bibliographical references and index.
Identifiers: LCCN 2017058065 | ISBN 9780323448871 (hardcover : alk. paper)
Subjects: | MESH: Respiratory Tract Diseases | Child | Infant
Classification: LCC RJ431 | NLM WS 280 | DDC 618.92/2–dc23
LC record available at https://lccn.loc.gov/2017058065

Senior Content Strategist: Sarah Barth
Content Development Specialist: Lisa M. Barnes
Publishing Services Manager: Catherine Jackson
Senior Project Manager: Daniel Fitzgerald
Designer: Bridget Hoette

Printed in China.

Last digit is the print number: 9 8 7 6 5 4 3 2 1

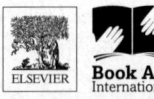

Preface

Welcome to the ninth edition of *Kendig's Disorders of the Respiratory Tract in Children,* which has gone through many changes since the last edition. First, our two senior editors, Dr. Vic Chernick and Dr. Tom Boat, have chosen to hang up their red pens, despite the best efforts of the rest of us to keep them working. A fitting tribute to either of them would take up many, many pages; suffice it to say that they have been giants in our field, and more of us than can be listed here owe them a huge debt. Retire in Peace! We all want to have it on record that the health and high qualities of this volume are in large measure owed to them, while we also acknowledge that they cannot be held responsible for the flaws of their successors.

The editorial team has expanded, and not just because Vic and Tom have left behind two huge pairs of shoes to fill. We wanted to have more global representation on the editorial team, acknowledging that globalization has changed our specialty forever. A child febrile in West Africa can be in England within hours, triggering an Ebola crisis. John Donne reminded us that no man is an island, and today, no island is isolated (even post-Brexit); we have to know about diseases from all around the world if we are to offer the care our children have the right to expect. Furthermore, we can and should learn from each other. Many techniques pioneered in the developed world are less expensive and have been exported to low- and middle-income settings. However, the low- and middle-income countries have exported valuable lessons in the other direction: the focused approach to the millennium development goals, learning from best practice, and new diseases because of new exposures. In the 21st century, learning is a two-way process. We welcome to the editorial team, joining the existing team from the United States, Canada, and Europe, Professors Heather Zar from South Africa, Peter Sly from Australia, and Albert Li from Hong Kong. We believe we have thereby made this edition truly global, with huge clinical relevance all around the world.

In addition to the changes in the editorial team, we have 87 new authors and 8 new chapters, with all the other chapters being completely revised, reorganized, and updated. Our new chapters reflect many developments in pediatric pulmonology.

The era of biologicals is upon us, and we have chapters on molecular therapies for cystic fibrosis and asthma. The importance of interactions with other specialties is reflected in chapters on the principles of mechanical ventilation, respiratory complications of intensive care, and congenital heart disease, as well as pulmonary embolism (no organ is an island, either). Globalization is reflected with a chapter on emerging lung infections, and there are other new chapters on the respiratory complications of Down syndrome and other genetic disorders, as well as hypersensitivity pneumonitis and eosinophilic lung diseases. We have attempted to avoid dishing up the mixture as before, good though it was, in favor of revivifying the book.

The final revivifying theme is the transition from the paper copy of the 20th century to the multimedia and Internet resources of the 21st. There is a rich crop of online resources, in the eBook, including 50 videos, approximately 550 illustrations that can be downloaded for presentations and teaching, and extensive bibliographies with hyperlinks to the original articles.

So we hope you find this ninth edition a worthy successor to its eight forebears. We want to thank our team of authors for their hard and excellent work, and (for the most part!) meeting deadlines, or at least not going too far beyond them. Huge thanks to Elsevier and their whole editorial team, especially Lisa Barnes, for unfailing tolerance of our many sins. To you all belongs the credit for much that we believe is good, and to the editors the blame for any bad things that have slipped through. Special thanks to Bob Wilmott, who has undertaken the monumental task of oversight of the whole volume to iron out unnecessary repetitions and spot overlaps and omissions. We hope that you, the reader, gets as much from studying this book as we have from editing it. Finally, as the ink dries on the blessed words "The End," work starts on the next edition. Please e-mail any of us to let us know what has worked and what has not, what should have been in, and what should never have been allowed to see the light of day, so we can make the 10th edition better yet.

Andrew Bush on the behalf of the editors

Contributors

Robin Abel, BSc, MBBS, PhD, FRCS(Paeds)
Consultant Paediatric Surgeon
Medway Hospital NHS Foundation Trust
United Kingdom

Steven H. Abman, MD
Professor
Department of Pediatrics
University of Colorado Health Sciences Center
Director
Pediatric Heart Lung Center
The Children's Hospital
Aurora, Colorado
United States

Eric Alton, BA Cantab, MBBS, MRCP, MD, MA, FRCP, FMedSCI
Professor of Gene Therapy,
Department of Gene Therapy
National Heart and Lung Institute
Imperial College London
London
United Kingdom

Daniel R. Ambruso, MD
Professor
Department of Pediatrics
University of Colorado
Anschutz Medical Campus
Hematologist
Center for Cancer and Blood Disorders
Children's Hospital Colorado
Aurora, Colorado
United States

William Carl Anderson III, MD
Assistant Professor
Pediatrics, Allergy Section
Children's Hospital Colorado/University of Colorado
Aurora, Colorado
United States

Karthik Balakrishnan, MD, MPH, FAAP, FACS
Consultant
Pediatric Otorhinolaryngology
Quality Improvement Chair
Department of Otorhinolaryngology
Mayo Clinic
Rochester, Minnesota
United States

Ian Michael Balfour-Lynn, BSC, MBBS, MD, FRCP, FRCPCH, FRCS(Ed)
Consultant in Paediatric Respiratory Medicine
Royal Brompton Hospital
London
Great Britain

Anna Bamford, MBBS
Adolescent and Young Adult Medicine Fellow
Department of Adolescent Medicine and Eating Disorders
Princess Margaret Hospital
Perth, Western Australia
Australia

Ronen Bar-Yoseph, MD
Senior Physician
Director of the Pediatric Exercise Center
Pediatric Pulmonary Institute
Ruth Children's Hospital
Rambam Health Care Campus
Haifa
Israel
Visiting Research Scholar
Pediatric Exercise and Genomics Research Center (PERC)
Department of Pediatrics
University of California Irvine
Irvine, California
United States

Erika Berman-Rosenzweig, MD
Director
Pulmonary Hypertension Center
Columbia University Medical Center/New York-
    Presbyterian Hospital
New York, New York
United States

Deepika Bhatla, MD
Associate Professor of Pediatrics
Division of Hematology, Oncology, Bone Marrow
    Transplantation
Saint Louis University
St. Louis, Missouri
United States

Joshua A. Blatter, MD
Department of Pediatrics
Washington University School of Medicine
St. Louis, Missouri
United States

R. Paul Boesch, DO, MS
Assistant Professor
Pediatric Pulmonology
Pediatrics and Adolescent Medicine
Mayo Clinic Children's Center
Rochester, Minnesota
United States

Matias Bruzoni, MD, FACS
Assistant Professor of Surgery
Program Director
Pediatric Surgery Fellowship
Stanford Children's Health
Stanford, California
United States

Andrew Bush, MB BS(Hons), MA, MD, FRCP, FRCPCH, FERS
Professor of Paediatrics and Head of Section
Imperial College London
Professor of Paediatric Respirology
National Heart and Lung Institute
Consultant Paediatric Chest Physician
Royal Brompton Harefield NHS Foundation Trust
London
Great Britain

Michael Bye, MD
Clinical Professor of Pediatrics
Department of Pediatrics
University at Buffalo
Buffalo, New York
United States

Kai Håkon Carlsen, MD, PhD
Professor
Institute of Clinical Medicine
University in Oslo
Professor
Division of Child and Adolescent Medicine
Oslo University Hospital
Oslo
Norway

Anne B. Chang, MBBS, FRACP, MPHTM, PhD, FAAHMS
Division Leader
Department of Child Health
Menzies School of Health Research
Darwin
Australia
Senior Staff Specialist
Respiratory and Sleep Medicine
Queensland Children's Hospital
Institute of Health and Biomedical Innovation
Children's Health Research
Queensland University of Technology
Brisbane
Australia

Stephanie D. Chao, MD
Assistant Professor
Department of Surgery
Division of Pediatric Surgery
Stanford University School of Medicine
Stanford, California
United States

Michelle Chatwin, BSc (Hons), PhD
Consultant Respiratory Physiotherapist
Royal Brompton Hospital
London
Great Britain

Bimal Pankaj Chaudhari, MD, MPH
Clinical Fellow
Department of Pediatrics (Neonatology)
Northwestern University Feinberg School of Medicine
Chicago, Illinois
United States

Lyn Chitty, PhD, MRCOG
Professor of Genetics and Fetal Medicine
UCL Great Ormond Street Institute of Child Health and
    Great Ormond Street NHS Foundation Trust
London
United Kingdom

Nicola Collins, BSc (Hons)
Clinical Lead Physiotherapist Paediatrics
Department of Physiotherapy
Royal Brompton Hospital
London
Great Britain

Dan M. Cooper, MD
Professor
Department of Pediatrics
University of California at Irvine
Irvine, California
United States

Jonathan Corren, MD
Departments of Medicine and Pediatrics
David Geffen School of Medicine at UCLA
Los Angeles, California
United States

Robin T. Cotton, MD, FACS, FRCS(C)
Director
Aerodigestive and Esophageal Center
Pediatric Otolaryngology
Cincinnati Children's Hospital
Professor
Otolaryngology
University of Cincinnati College of Medicine
Cincinnati, Ohio
United States

Andrea Coverstone, MD
Assistant Professor
Division of Allergy, Immunology and Pulmonary Medicine
Department of Pediatrics
Washington University School of Medicine in Saint Louis
St. Louis, Missouri
United States

Suzanne Crowley, DM
Division of Child and Adolescent Medicine
Oslo University Hospital
Oslo
Norway

Steve Cunningham, MBChB, PhD
Professor
Consultant and Honorary Professor in Pediatric
    Respiratory Medicine
Royal Hospital for Sick Children
NHS Lothian and University of Edinburgh
Edinburgh
United Kingdom

Garry R. Cutting, MD
Professor
McKusisk Nathans Institute of Genetic Medicine
Johns Hopkins School of Medicine
Baltimore, Maryland
United States

Dorottya Czovek, MD, PhD
Head of Respiratory Physiology Team
Children's Lung, Environment and Asthma Research
University of Queensland
Postdoctoral Research Fellow
Child Health Research Centre
University of Queensland
South Brisbane, Queensland
Australia

Charles L. Daley, MD
Professor and Head
Divisions of Mycobacterial and Respiratory Infections
National Jewish Health
Denver, Colorado
Professor of Medicine
Division of Pulmonary and Critical Care Medicine and
    Infectious Diseases
University of Colorado, Denver
Aurora, Colorado
United States

Gwyneth Davies, MBChB, MSc, PhD, MRCPCH
NIHR Academic Clinical Lecturer in Paediatrics
UCL Great Ormond Street Institute of Child Health
London
United Kingdom

Jane C. Davies, MB ChB, FRCPCH, MD
Professor of Paediatric Respirology & Experimental
    Medicine
Cystic Fibrosis and Chronic Lung Infection
National Heart and Lung Institute
Imperial College London
London
United Kingdom

Alessandro de Alarcòn, MD, MPH
Associate Professor
Division of Pediatric Otolaryngology—Head and Neck
    Surgery
Cincinnati Children's Hospital Medical Center
Department of Otolaryngology—Head and Neck Surgery
University of Cincinnati College of Medicine
Cincinnati, Ohio
United States

Emily M. DeBoer, MD
Assistant Professor
Department of Pediatrics
University of Colorado and Children's Hospital Colorado
Aurora, Colorado
United States

Marietta Morales De Guzman, MD
Associate Professor
Department of Pediatrics
Baylor College of Medicine
Clinic Chief
Pediatric Rheumatology Center
Texas Children's Hospital
Houston, Texas
United States

Sharon D. Dell, BEng, MD
Professor
Department of Pediatrics
University of Toronto
Staff Pediatric Respirologist
Division of Respiratory Medicine
The Hospital for Sick Children
Senior Associate Scientist
Child Health Evaluative Sciences
The Research Institute
The Hospital for Sick Children
Professor
Institute of Health, Policy, Management and Evaluation
University of Toronto
Toronto, Ontario
Canada

Robin Deterding, MD
Chief
Pediatric Pulmonary Medicine
Professor of Pediatrics
Department of Pediatrics
University of Colorado
Aurora, Colorado
United States

Gail H. Deutsch, MD
Associate Professor of Pathology
Department of Pathology
University of Washington School of Medicine and Seattle
  Children's Hospital
Seattle, Washington
United States

Sunalene Devadason, PhD
Associate Professor
Division of Paediatrics
University of Western Australia
Perth, Western Australia
Australia

William Graham Fox Ditcham, PhD
Research Fellow
University of Western Australia
Perth, Western Australia
Australia

Jill Dorsey, MD, MS
Pediatric Gastroenterology, Hepatology, and Nutrition
Nemours Children's Specialty Care
Jacksonville, Florida
United States

Francine M. Ducharme, MD, MSc
Professor
Departments of Pediatrics and of Social and Preventive
  Medicine
University of Montreal
Montreal, Quebec
Canada

John Engelhardt, PhD
Professor
Department of Anatomy and Cell Biology
University of Iowa
Iowa City, Iowa
United States

Mark L. Everard, MD
Winthrop Professor of Paediatric Respiratory Medicine
Division of Paediatrics
University of Western Australia
Perth, Western Australia
Australia

Leland L. Fan, MD
Professor
Department of Pediatrics
University of Colorado School of Medicine
Aurora, Colorado
United States

Albert Faro, MD
Professor
Department of Pediatrics
Washington University School of Medicine
St. Louis, Missouri
United States

Thomas Ferkol, MD
Alexis Hartman Professor of Pediatrics
Departments of Pediatrics, Cell Biology and Physiology
Washington University School of Medicine
St. Louis, Missouri
United States

Louise Fleming, MB ChB, MRCP, MRCPCH, MD
Clinical Senior Lecturer
National Heart and Lung Institute
Imperial College
Paediatric Respiratory Consultant
Department of Respiratory Pediatrics
Royal Brompton and Harefield NHS Foundation Trust
London
Great Britain

Angela Mary Fonceca, PhD
Research Fellow
University of Western Australia
Perth, Western Australia
Australia

Hammad A. Ganatra, MD
Assistant Professor
Pediatric Critical Care Medicine
University of Illinois College of Medicine
Peoria, Illinois
United States

Amy Michelle Garcia, MD, MS
Assistant Professor
Pediatric Gastroenterology
Oregon Health & Science University
Portland, Oregon
United States

David Gozal, MD, MBA
The Herbert T. Abelson Professor of Pediatrics,
  Neuroscience and Neurobiology
Sections of Pediatric Pulmonology and Sleep Medicine
Pritzker School of Medicine
Biological Sciences Division
The University of Chicago
Chicago, Illinois
United States

Diane Gray, MBChB, FRACP, PhD
Red Cross War Memorial Children's Hospital
University of Cape Town
South Africa

Anne Greenough, MD (Cantab), MB BS, DCH, FRCP, FRCPCH
Professor
Division of Asthma, Allergy and Lung Biology
MRC Centre for Allergica Mechanisms in Asthma
King's College London
London
Great Britain

Uta Griesenbach, PhD
Professor of Molecular Medicine
Department of Gene Therapy
National Heart and Lung Institute
Imperial College London
London
United Kingdom

Jonathan Grigg, MD
Professor of Paediatric Respiratory Medicine
Department of Child Health
Queen Mary University of London
London
Great Britain

James S. Hagood, MD
Professor and Chief
Department of Pediatrics
Division of Respiratory Medicine
University of California, San Diego
La Jolla, California
United States

Jürg Hammer, MD
Professor of Pediatrics
Division of Intensive Care and Pulmonology
University Children's Hospital
Basel
Switzerland

Aaron Hamvas, MD
Professor of Pediatrics
Department Pediatrics/Neonatology
Ann & Robert H. Lurie Children's Hospital/Northwestern
    University
Chicago, Illinois
United States

Jonny Harcourt, MA(Oxon), MBBS(Hons), FRCS
Consultant Paediatric Otolaryngologist
Department of Paediatric Otolaryngology
Chelsea and Westminster Hospital
Consultant Paediatric Otolaryngologist
Department of Paediatric Otolaryngology
Royal Brompton Hospital
London
Great Britain

Pia J. Hauk, MD
Associate Professor of Pediatrics
Pediatric Allergy/Immunology
National Jewish Health
Denver, Colorado
University of Colorado Denver, Anschutz Medical Campus
Aurora, Colorado
United States

Ulrich Heininger, MD
Chair
Pediatric Infectious Diseases
University Children's Hospital
Member
Medical Faculty
University of Basel
Basel
Switzerland

Alexander John Henderson, MD, FRCP, FRCPCH, FRCPEd
Professor of Paediatric Respiratory Medicine
Population Health Sciences
Bristol Medical School
University of Bristol
Bristol
Great Britain

Marianna M. Henry, MD, MPH
Associate Professor of Pediatrics
Division of Pediatric Pulmonology
University of North Carolina at Chapel Hill School of
    Medicine
Attending Physician
University of North Carolina Hospitals
Chapel Hill, North Carolina
United States

Richard J. Hewitt, BSc, DOHNS, FRCS (HNS-ORL)
Consultant Paediatric ENT
Head & Neck and Tracheal Surgeon Great Ormond Street
    Hospital for Children
Honorary Senior Lecturer University College
Director of the UK National Service for Complex Paediatric
    Tracheal Disease
London
United Kingdom

Heather Young Highsmith, MSc, MD
Pediatric Infectious Disease Fellow
Department of Pediatrics
Texas Children's Hospital
Baylor College of Medicine
Houston, Texas
United States

Noah H. Hillman, MD
Associate Professor
Department of Pediatrics
Saint Louis University
St. Louis, Missouri
United States

Heather Ellen Hoch, MD
Assistant Professor
Department of Pediatric Pulmonary
University of Colorado Denver, Anschutz Medical Campus
Denver, Colorado
United States

Jeong S. Hyun, MD
Resident
Department of Surgery
Division of Pediatric Surgery
Stanford University School of Medicine
Stanford, California
United States

Mas Suhaila Isa, MBBS, MRCPCH (UK)
Khoo Teck Puat-National University Children's Medical
  Institute
National University Health System
Singapore

**Adam Jaffé, BSc(Hons), MBBS, MD, FRCPCH, FRCP,
FRACP, FThorSoc**
John Beveridge Professor of Paediatrics/Head of School
School of Women's & Children's Health
UNSW Medicine
Paediatric Respiratory Consultant
Department of Respiratory Medicine
Sydney Children's Hospital
Associate Director of Research
Sydney Children's Hospitals Network, Randwick
Randwick, New South Wales
Australia

Lance C. Jennings, MSc, PhD, MRCPath, FFSc(RCPA)
Clinical Virologist
Canterbury Health Laboratories
Christchurch
New Zealand

Alan H. Jobe, MD, PhD
Professor of Pediatrics
The Perinatal Institute
Cincinnati Children's Hospital Medical Center
Cincinnati, Ohio
United States

Ankur A. Kamdar, MD
Assistant Professor
Department of Pediatrics
McGovern Medical School at University of Texas Health
Houston, Texas
United States

Bhushan Katira, MB, BS, DNB
Clinical-Research Fellow
Paediatric Critical Care & Translational Medicine
Hospital for Sick Children
University of Toronto
Toronto, Ontario
Canada

Brian P. Kavanagh, MB, FRCPC
Professor
Departments of Anesthesia, Physiology & Medicine
University of Toronto Faculty of Medicine
Dr. Geoffrey Barker Chair of Critical Care Medicine
Hospital for Sick Children
Toronto, Ontario
Canada

James Kemp, MD
Professor of Pediatrics
Washington University School of Medicine
Director of Sleep Laboratory
Division of Allergy, Immunology and Pulmonary Medicine
Department of Pediatrics
St. Louis Children's Hospital
Department of Pediatrics
University of Cincinnati College of Medicine
St. Louis, Missouri
United States

Carolyn M. Kercsmar, MS, MD
Director, Asthma Center
Cincinnati Children's Hospital Medical Center
Professor of Pediatrics
Cincinnati, Ohio
United States

Leila Kheirandish-Gozal, MD, MSc
Professor of Pediatrics
Director
Clinical Translational Sleep Research Program
Department of Pediatrics
University of Chicago
Chicago, Illinois
United States

Wilson King, MD
Assistant Professor
Department of Pediatrics
Saint Louis University
St. Louis, Missouri
United States

Paul Kingma, MD, PhD
Associate Professor of Pediatrics
The Perinatal Institute
Cincinnati Fetal Center
Cincinnati Children's Hospital Medical Center
Cincinnati, Ohio
United States

Jennifer Knight-Madden, MBBS, PhD
Director
Sickle Cell Unit
Caribbean Institute of Health Research
University of the West Indies
Kingston
Jamaica

Alan Paul Knutsen, MD
Professor of Pediatrics
Director Allergy & Immunology
Saint Louis University
St. Louis, Missouri
United States

Alik Kornecki, MD
Associate Professor
Department of Pediatric Critical Care
London Health Sciences Centre, Children's Hospital
London, Ontario
Canada

Usha Krishnan, MD, DM
Associate Professor
Department of Pediatrics
Columbia University Medical Center/Children's Hospital of
    New York Presbyterian
New York, New York
United States

Geoffrey Kurland, MD
Division of Pediatric Pulmonary Medicine, Allergy, and
    Immunology
Children's Hospital of Pittsburgh
Pittsburgh, Pennsylvania
United States

Hugh Simon Lam, MBBChir, MD
Associate Professor
Department of Paediatrics
The Chinese University of Hong Kong
Sha Tin, Hong Kong
China

Claire Langston, MD
Professor
Department of Pathology and Pediatrics
Baylor College of Medicine
Pathologist
Department of Pathology
Texas Children's Hospital
Houston, Texas
United States

Ada Lee, MD
Pediatric Pulmonology Section
Department of Pediatrics
Hackensack University Medical Center
Hackensack, New Jersey
United States

Margaret W. Leigh, MD
Professor
Department of Pediatrics
University of North Carolina
Chapel Hill, North Carolina
United States

Daniel Lesser, MD
Associate Professor of Pediatrics
Department of Respiratory Medicine
University California San Diego
Rady Children's Hospital San Diego
San Diego, California
United States

Clare M. Lloyd, PhD
Professor of Respiratory Immunology
National Heart and Lung Institute
Imperial College
London
Great Britain

Anna Maria Mandalakas, MD, PhD
Associate Professor
Pediatrics
Baylor College of Medicine
Houston, Texas
United States

Paulo J.C. Marostica, MD
Division of Pulmonology
Department of Pediatrics
Universidade Federal do Rio Grande do Sul
Porto Alegre
Brazil

Stacey L. Martiniano, MD
Assistant Professor
Department of Pediatrics
Children's Hospital Colorado and University of Colorado
    Denver
Aurora, Colorado
United States

Jennifer Maybee, OTR/L, MA, CCC-SLP
Speech-Language Pathologist
Department of Audiology, Speech and Learning
Children's Hospital Colorado
Aurora, Colorado
United States

Karen M. McDowell, MD
Associate Professor
Division of Pulmonary Medicine
Cincinnati Children's Hospital Medical Center
University of Cincinnati College of Medicine
Cincinnati, Ohio
United States

Peter Michelson, MD, MS
Professor of Pediatrics
Division of Allergy, Immunology and Pulmonary Medicine
Washington University School of Medicine
St. Louis, Missouri
United States

Aaron Samuel Miller, MD, MSPH
Assistant Professor
Department of Pediatrics
Saint Louis University
SSM Cardinal Glennon Children's Medical Center
St. Louis, Missouri
United States

Claire Kane Miller, PhD, MHA
Program Director
Aerodigestive and Esophageal Center
Cincinnati Children's Hospital Medical Center
Field Service Associate Professor-Aff
Department of Otolaryngology, Head & Neck Surgery
University of Cincinnati College of Medicine
Clinical and Research Speech Pathologist
Division of Speech-Language Pathology
Cincinnati Children's Hospital Medical Center
Adjunct Assistant Professor
Communication Sciences and Disorders
University of Cincinnati
Cincinnati, Ohio
United States

Ayesha Mirza, MD, FAAP
Associate Professor
Department of Pediatrics
University of Florida
Jacksonville, Florida
United States

David R. Murdoch, MD, MSc, DTM&H, FRACP, FRCPA, FFSc(RCPA)
Professor, Dean and Head of Campus
University of Otago
Clinical Microbiologist
Department of Microbiology
Canterbury Health Laboratories
Christchurch
New Zealand

Christopher J. L. Newth, MD, FRACP, FRCPC
Professor of Pediatrics
Department of Anesthesiology & Critical Care Medicine
University of Southern California, Children's Hospital Los Angeles
Los Angeles, California
United States

Andrew Gordon Nicholson, DM FRCPath
Consultant Histopathologist
Royal Brompton and Harefield NHS Foundation Trust
Professor
Department of Respiratory Pathology
National Heart and Lung Institute, Imperial College
London
Great Britain

Jerry A. Nick, MD
Professor
Department of Medicine
National Jewish Health
Denver, Colorado
Professor
Department of Medicine
University of Colorado, Denver
Aurora, Colorado
United States

Christina J. Nicolais, MS
Doctoral Student
Department of Psychology
University of Miami
Coral Gables, Florida
United States

Terry L. Noah, MD
Professor of Pediatrics
Division of Pediatric Pulmonology
University of North Carolina at Chapel Hill School of Medicine
Attending Physician
University of North Carolina Hospitals
Chapel Hill, North Carolina
United States

Lawrence M. Nogee, MD
Professor
Eudowood Neonatal Pulmonary Division
Department of Pediatrics
Johns Hopkins University School of Medicine
Baltimore, Maryland
United States

Blakeslee Noyes, MD
Professor of Pediatrics
Department of Pediatrics
St. Louis University School of Medicine
St. Louis, Missouri
United States

Andrew H. Numa, MBBS, FRACP, FCICM
Intensivist and Respirologist
Senior Lecturer
University of New South Wales
Departments of Intensive Care and Respiratory Medicine
Sydney Children's Hospital
Randwick, New South Wales
Australia

Ann-Christine Nyquist, MD, MSPH
Professor
Department of Pediatrics (Infectious Diseases and Epidemiology)
University of Colorado Anschutz Medical Campus and Children's Hospital Colorado
Aurora, Colorado
United States

Hugh O'Brodovich, MD
Professor Emeritus
Department of Pediatrics
Stanford University
Stanford, California
United States

Matthias Ochs, MD
Professor and Chair
Institute of Functional and Applied Anatomy
Hannover Medical School
Hannover
Germany

J. Tod Olin, MD, MSCS
Associate Professor
Director
Pediatric Exercise Tolerance Center
Department of Pediatrics
Division of Pediatric Pulmonology
National Jewish Health
Denver, Colorado
United States

Øystein Olsen, PhD
Consultant Radiologist
Department of Radiology
Great Ormond Street Hospital for Children
NHS Trust
London
Great Britain

Catherine Owens, BSc, MBBS, MRCP, FRCR, FRCP
Department of Radiology
Great Ormond Street Hospital
London
Great Britain

Howard B. Panitch, MD
Professor of Pediatrics
Perelman School of Medicine at the University of
    Pennsylvania
Director
Technology Dependence Center
The Children's Hospital of Philadelphia
Division of Pulmonary Medicine
The Children's Hospital of Philadelphia
Philadelphia, Pennsylvania
United States

Hans Pasterkamp, MD, FRCPC
Department of Pediatrics
University of Manitoba
Winnipeg, Manitoba
Canada

Donald Payne, MBBChir, MD, FRCPCH, FRACP
Associate Professor
Division of Paediatrics
School of Medicine
University of Western Australia
Perth, Western Australia
Australia

Scott Pentiuk, MD, MEd
Associate Professor
Department of Pediatric Gastroenterology, Hepatology, and
    Nutrition
Cincinnati Children's Hospital Medical Center
Cincinnati, Ohio
United States

Jeremy Prager, MD, MBA
Assistant Professor
Department of Otolaryngology
University of Colorado School of Medicine
Assistant Professor
Department of Pediatric Otolaryngology
Children's Hospital Colorado
Aurora, Colorado
United States

Jean-Paul Praud, MD, PhD
Professor
Department of Pediatrics/Respiratory Medicine
University of Sherbrooke
Sherbrooke, Quebec
Canada

Andrew P. Prayle, BMedSci, BMBS, PhD
Child Health, Obstetrics and Gynaecology
The University of Nottingham
Nottingham
Great Britain

Bernadette Prentice, BSc, MB BS, MPH
Department of Respiratory Medicine
Sydney Children's Hospital
School of Women and Children's Health
The University of New South Wales
Randwick, New South Wales
Australia

Philip E. Putnam, MD
Professor of Pediatrics
Division of Gastroenterology, Hepatology, and Nutrition
Cincinnati Children's Hospital Medical Center
Cincinnati, Ohio
United States

Alexandra L. Quittner, PhD
Senior Scientist
Miami Children's Research Institute
Miami, Florida
United States

Shlomit Radom-Aizik, PhD
Executive Director
Pediatric Exercise and Genomics Research Center (PERC)
Department of Pediatrics
School of Medicine
University of California Irvine
Irvine, California
United States

Suchitra Rao, MBBS
Assistant Professor
Department of Pediatrics (Infectious Diseases, Hospital
    Medicine and Epidemiology)
University of Colorado Anschutz Medical Campus and
    Children's Hospital Colorado
Aurora, Colorado
United States

**Mobeen Rathore, MD, CPE, FAAP, FPIDS, FIDSA,
FSHEA, FACPE**
Professor and Director
University of Florida Center for HIV/AIDS Research,
    Education, Service (UF CARES)
Department of Infectious Diseases and Immunology
University of Florida
Wolfson Children's Hospital
Jacksonville, Florida
United States

Gregory J. Redding, MD
Professor
Department of Pediatrics
University of Washington School of Medicine
Chief
Pulmonary and Sleep Medicine Division
Department of Pediatrics
Seattle Children's Hospital
Seattle, Washington
United States

Michael Rutter, BHB, MBChB, FRACS
Professor of Pediatric Otolaryngology
Division of Otolaryngology
Cincinnati Children's Hospital Medical Center
Professor of Pediatric Otolaryngology
Department of Otolaryngology
University of Cincinnati
Cincinnati, Ohio
United States

Estefany Saez-Flores, MS
Doctoral Student
Department of Psychology
University of Miami
Coral Gables, Florida
United States

Sejal Saglani, BSc, MBChB, MD
Professor of Paediatric Respiratory Medicine
National Heart & Lung Institute
Imperial College London
London
Great Britain

Rayfel Schneider, MBBCh
Professor
Department of Paediatrics
University of Toronto
Associate Chair (Education)
Department of Paediatrics
The Hospital for Sick Children
Toronto, Ontario
Canada

Kenneth O. Schowengerdt, Jr., MD
Wieck-Sullivan Professor of Pediatrics
Division Director
Pediatric Cardiology
Saint Louis University School of Medicine
SSM Cardinal Glennon Children's Hospital
St. Louis, Missouri
United States

Marcelo C. Scotta, MD
Division of Infectious Diseases
Department of Pediatrics
Pontifícia Universidade Católica do Rio Grande do Sul
Porto Alegre
Brazil

Thomas Semple, FRCR, MBBS, BSc
Radiology Department
Royal Brompton Hospital
London
Great Britain

Laurie Sherlock, MD
Sections of Neonatology
Department of Pediatrics
University of Colorado Denver, School of Medicine
Children's Hospital Colorado
Aurora, Colorado
United States

Ram N. Singh, MBBS, FRCPC
Associate Professor
Paediatrics
Western University
Director Paediatric Critical Care
Children Hospital
London, Ontario
Canada

Raymond G. Slavin, MD
Professor Emeritus Internal Medicine
Division of Internal Medicine Allergy & Immunology
Saint Louis University
St. Louis, Missouri
United States

Peter Sly, MBBS, MD, FRACP, DSc
Director
Children's Lung Environment and Asthma Research Group
University of Queensland
Brisbane
Australia

Bjarne Smevik, MD
Division of Radiology and Nuclear Medicine
Oslo University Hospital
Oslo
Norway

Keely Garrett Smith, MD
Associate Professor
Department of Pediatrics
McGovern Medical School at University of Texas Health
Houston, Texas
United States

Jonathan Spahr, MD
Division of Pediatric Pulmonary Medicine
Geisinger Medical Center
Danville, Pennsylvania
United States

James M. Stark, MD, PhD
Professor
Department of Pediatrics
McGovern Medical School at University of Texas Health
Houston, Texas
United States

Jeffrey R. Starke, MD
Professor
Department of Pediatrics
Baylor College of Medicine
Houston, Texas
United States

Renato T. Stein, MD
Division of Pulmonology
Department of Pediatrics
Pontifícia Universidade Católica do Rio Grande do Sul
Porto Alegre
Brazil

Paul C. Stillwell, MD
Senior Instructor
Department of Pediatrics (Pulmonary Medicine)
University of Colorado Anschutz Medical Campus and
   Children's Hospital Colorado
Aurora, Colorado
United States

Dennis C. Stokes, MD
Division of Pediatric Pulmonary Medicine
University of Tennessee Health Sciences Center
Memphis, Tennessee
United States

Daniel T. Swarr, MD
Assistant Professor of Pediatrics
Division of Neonatology & Pulmonary Biology
Cincinnati Children's Hospital Medical Center
Cincinnati, Ohio
United States

Stuart Charles Sweet, MD, PhD
W. McKim Marriott Professor of Pediatrics
Department of Pediatrics
Washington University
St. Louis, Missouri
United States

Stanley James Szefler, MD
Director
Pediatrics Asthma Research
Department of Pediatrics
University of Colorado School of Medicine
Research Medical Director
Department of Pediatrics
Children's Hospital Colorado
Aurora, Colorado
United States

Paul Tambyah, MD
National University Health System
Singapore

Christelle Xian-Ting Tan, MBBS (S'pore), MRCPCH (UK), MMed (Paeds)
Khoo Teck Puat-National University Children's Medical
   Institute
National University Health System
Singapore

James Temprano, MD
Allergy & Immunology
Mercy Hospital St. Louis
St. Louis, Missouri
United States

Chad M. Thorson, MD, MSPH
Assistant Professor
Pediatric and Adolescent Surgery
University of Miami
Coral Gables, Florida
United States

Bruce C. Trapnell, MD
F.R. Luther Professor of Medicine and Pediatrics
University of Cincinnati College of Medicine
Translational Pulmonary Science Center
Department of Pediatrics
Cincinnati Children's Hospital Medical Center
Division of Pulmonary, Critical Care and Sleep Medicine
Department of Medicine
University of Cincinnati Medical Center
Cincinnati, Ohio
United States

Brian Michael Varisco, MD
Assistant Professor of Pediatrics
Department of Pediatrics
Cincinnati Children's Hospital Medical Center
Cincinnati, Ohio
United States

Timothy J. Vece, MD
Assistant Professor
Department of Pediatrics
University of North Carolina
Chapel Hill, North Carolina
United States

Harish G. Vyas, DM, FRCP, FRCPCH
Emeritus Professor
Department of Child Health
The University of Nottingham
Nottingham
Great Britain

Ruth Wakeman, MSc, BSc (Hons)
Advanced Practitioner/Physiotherapist
Hospital to Home Service, Paediatrics
Royal Brompton & Harefield NHS Foundation Trust
London
Great Britain

Colin Wallis, MD, MRCP, FRCPCH, FCP, DCH
Consultant Pediatrician
Respiratory Unit
Great Ormond Street Hospital for Children
Senior Lecturer
Department of Respiratory Paediatrics
University of London
London
Great Britain

Jennifer Wambach, MD, MS
Assistant Professor
Department of Pediatrics
Washington University School of Medicine
St. Louis, Missouri
United States

Daniel J. Weiner, MD
Division of Pediatric Pulmonary Medicine, Allergy, and
 Immunology
Children's Hospital of Pittsburgh
Pittsburgh, Pennsylvania
United States

Anja M. Werno, MD, PhD, FRCPA
Medical Director of Microbiology
Canterbury Health Laboratories
Christchurch
New Zealand

Susan E. Wert, PhD
Associate Professor of Pediatrics
University of Cincinnati College of Medicine
Department of Pediatrics
Perinatal Institute
Divisions of Neonatology, Perinatal and Pulmonary
 Biology
Cincinnati Children's Hospital Medical Center
Cincinnati, Ohio
United States

Jeffrey A. Whitsett, MD
Co-Director
Perinatal Institute
Chief
Section of Neonatology, Perinatal and Pulmonary Biology
Professor
UC Department of Pediatrics
Cincinnati Children's Hospital Medical Center
Cincinnati, Ohio
United States

Robert William Wilmott, BSc, MB, BS, MD, FRCP (UK)
IMMUNO Professor and Chair
Department of Pediatrics
Saint Louis University
Pediatrician in Chief
SSM Cardinal Glennon Children's Medical Center
St. Louis, Missouri
United States

Robert E. Wood, PhD, MD
Professor
Departments of Pediatrics & Otolaryngology
Cincinnati Children's Hospital
Cincinnati, Ohio
United States

Christopher Todd Wootten, MD
Assistant Professor
Department of Pediatric Otolaryngology
Vanderbilt University Medical Center
Nashville, Tennessee
United States

Marie Wright, MBChB, MRCPCH
Paediatric Respiratory Registrar
Royal Brompton Hospital
London
Great Britain

Sarah Wright, Grad Dip Phys
Physiotherapist
Department of Physiotherapy
Children's Health Queensland Hospital and Health Service
Brisbane, Queensland
Australia

Rae S. M. Yeung, MD, PhD, FRCPC
Professor
Department of Pediatrics, Immunology and Medical
    Science
University of Toronto
Hak-Ming and Deborah Chiu Chair in Paediatric
    Translational Research
The Hospital for Sick Children
Senior Scientist and Staff Rheumatologist
The Hospital for Sick Children
Toronto, Ontario
Canada

Takeshi Yoshida, MD, PhD
Research Fellow
Keenan Research Centre
Li Ka Shing Knowledge Institute
St. Michael's Hospital
Interdepartmental Division of Critical Care Medicine
University of Toronto
Toronto, Ontario
Canada

Carolyn Young, HDCR
Cardiorespiratory Unit
University College of London
Institute of Child Health
London
Great Britain

Lisa R. Young, MD
Associate Professor of Pediatrics and Medicine
Divisions of Pediatric Pulmonary Medicine and Allergy,
    Pulmonary, and Critical Care Medicine
Vanderbilt University Medical Center
Nashville, Tennessee
United States

**Heather J. Zar, MBBCh, FCPaeds, FRCP (Edinburgh),
PhD**
Professor and Chair
Department of Paediatrics & Child Health
Director MRC Unit on Child & Adolescent Health
Red Cross War Memorial Children's Hospital
University of Cape Town
Cape Town, South Africa

Pamela Leslie Zeitlin, MD, PhD
Professor
Department of Pediatrics
National Jewish Health
Denver, Colorado
United States

David Zielinski, MD, FRCPC, FCCP
Department of Pediatrics
McGill University
Montréal, Quebec
Canada

Contents

Video Contents

General Basic and Clinical Considerations

1 The History and Physical Examination

HANS PASTERKAMP, MD, FRCPC, and DAVID ZIELINSKI, MD, FRCPC, FCCP

In the 21st century, the diagnosis of disease still requires a detailed medical history and a thorough physical examination. For the majority of patients in many areas of the world, additional information from laboratory tests and other data remain rather limited. Modern science and technology have changed the situation considerably in industrialized nations, but we are paying a high price. Cost containment in health care has become essential. Physicians need to be skillful in their history taking and physical examination techniques so they can collect a maximum amount of information before ordering expensive investigations. The relevance of these skills in pediatric respiratory medicine is exemplified by clinical severity scores that are widely used in care maps for asthma, bronchiolitis, and croup, or in scores developed to manage patients suspected to have acute severe respiratory syndromes (e.g., during outbreaks of SARS, H1N1, and other forms of influenza).

The diagnosis of disease in children has to rely on the patient's history and on observations gathered during the physical examination, even more than in older patients. Young children cannot follow instructions and participate in formal physiologic testing, and physicians hesitate before subjecting their pediatric patients to invasive diagnostic procedures. Diseases of the respiratory tract are among the most common in children, and in the majority of cases they can be correctly identified from medical history data and physical findings alone. The following review of the medical history and physical examination in children with respiratory disease includes some observations that were made with the help of modern technology. These technical aids do not lessen the value of subjective perceptions, but rather emphasize how new methods may further our understanding, sharpen our senses, and thereby advance the art of medical diagnosis.

The History

GENERAL PRINCIPLES

The medical history should be taken in an environment with comfortable seating for all, a place for clothing and belongings, and some toys for younger children. Privacy has to be assured, without the usual interruptions by phone calls and other distractions. If possible, the physician should see one child at a time because the presence of young siblings or other children in the room can be distracting. Data that should be recorded at the beginning include the patient's name and address, the parents' or guardians' home and work phone numbers, the name of the referring physician, and information on the kindergarten or school if this is relevant.

In many cases, the history will be given by someone other than the patient, but the physician should still directly ask even young children about their complaints. When asking about the history of the present illness, the physician should encourage a clear and chronological narrative account. Questions should be open-ended, and at intervals the physician should give a verbal summary to confirm and clarify the information. Past medical history and system review are usually obtained by answers to direct questions.

STRUCTURE OF THE PEDIATRIC HISTORY

The physician should note the source of and the reason for referral. On occasion, the referral is made by someone other than the patient or the parents (e.g., a teacher, relative, or friend). The physician should identify the *chief complaint* and the *person most concerned about it*. The *illness at presentation* should be documented in detail regarding onset and duration, the environment and circumstances under which it developed, its manifestations and their treatments, and its impact on the patient and family. Symptoms should be defined by their qualitative and quantitative characteristics as well as by their timing, location, aggravating or alleviating factors, and associated manifestations. Relevant past medical and laboratory data should be included in the documentation of the present illness.

This general approach is also applicable when the emphasis is on a single organ system, such as the respiratory tract. The onset of disease may have been gradual (e.g., with some interstitial lung diseases) or sudden (e.g., with foreign body aspiration). The physician should ask about initial manifestations and who noticed them first. The age at first presentation is important, because respiratory diseases that manifest soon after birth are more likely to have been inherited or to be related to congenital malformations. Depending on the duration of symptoms, the illness will be classified as *acute, subacute, chronic,* or *recurrent.* These definitions are arbitrary, but diseases of less than 3 weeks' duration are generally called *acute;* diseases between 3 weeks' and 3 months' duration are *subacute;* and those that persist longer than 3 months are *chronic.* If symptoms are clearly discontinuous, with documented intervals of well-being, the disease is *recurrent.* This distinction is important because many parents may perceive their child as being chronically ill, not realizing that young normal children may have six to eight upper respiratory infections per year, particularly during the first 2 years if the child is in a daycare setting, or if he or she has older siblings.

Respiratory diseases are often affected by environmental factors. There should be a careful search for seasonal changes in symptoms to uncover possible allergic causes. Exposure to noxious inhaled agents, for example, from industrial pollution or more commonly from indoor pollution by cigarette smoke, can sustain or aggravate a patient's coughing and wheezing. Similarly, a wood-burning stove used for indoor heating may be a contributing factor. The physician should therefore obtain a detailed description of the patient's home environment. Are there household pets (e.g., dogs, cats, or hamsters) or birds (e.g., budgies, pigeons, or parrots)? What plants are in and around the house? Are there animal or vegetable fibers in the bedclothes or in the floor and window coverings (e.g., wool, feathers)? Are there systems in use for air conditioning and humidification? Is mold visible anywhere in the house?

There may be a relationship between respiratory symptoms and daily activities. Exercise is a common trigger factor for coughing and wheezing in many patients with hyperreactive airways. A walk outside in cold air may have similar effects. Diurnal variation of symptoms may be apparent, and attention should be paid to changes that occur at night. These changes may also be related to airway cooling, or they may reflect conditions that are worse in the recumbent position, such as postnasal drip or gastroesophageal reflux (GER). Food intake may bring on symptoms of respiratory distress when food is aspirated or when food allergies are present.

Many children who present with respiratory symptoms are suffering from infection, most often viral. It is important to know whether other family members or people in regular contact with the patient are also affected. When unusual infections are suspected, questions should be asked about recent travel to areas where exotic organisms may have been acquired. Drug abuse by parents or by older patients and high-risk lifestyles may lead the physician to consider the possibility of acquired immunodeficiency syndrome (AIDS).

Descriptions of respiratory disease manifestations may come from the parents or directly from an older child. Common symptoms are fever, cough and sputum production, wheezing or noisy breathing, dyspnea, and chest pain. Most of these are discussed in more detail later in the chapter.

The past medical history will provide an impression of the general health status of the child. First, the birth history should be reviewed, including prenatal, natal, and neonatal events. The physician should inquire about the course of pregnancy, particularly whether the mother and fetus suffered from infections, metabolic disorders, or exposure to noxious agents (e.g., nicotine). The duration of pregnancy, possible multiple births, and circumstances leading to the onset of labor should be noted. Difficult labor and delivery may cause respiratory problems at birth (e.g., asphyxia and meconium aspiration), and the physician should ask about birth weight and Apgar scores. The physician should carefully review the neonatal course because many events during this period may affect the patient's respiratory status in later years. Were there any signs of neonatal respiratory distress (e.g., tachypnea, retractions, and cyanosis)? Treatment with oxygen or endotracheal intubation should be recorded. Some extrathoracic disorders provide valuable clues for diagnosis, such as the presence of eczema in atopic infants or neonatal conjunctivitis in an infant with chlamydia pneumonia, particularly if there was a documented infection of the mother.

Much is learned from a detailed feeding history, which should include the amount, type, and schedule of food intake.

The physician should ask whether the child was fed by breast or bottle. For the newborn and young infant, feeding is a substantial physical exercise and may lead to distress in the presence of respiratory disease, much as climbing stairs does in the older patient. The question of exercise tolerance in an infant is therefore asked by inquiring how long it takes the patient to finish a feed. The caloric intake of infants with respiratory disease is often reduced despite an increased caloric requirement to support the work of breathing. This reduced caloric intake commonly results in a failure to thrive. Older patients with chronic respiratory disease and productive cough may suffer from a continuous exposure of their taste buds to mucopurulent secretions and may quite understandably lose their appetites, but medical treatment (e.g., with certain antibiotics) may have similar effects. Patients with food hypersensitivity may react with bronchospasm or even with interstitial lung disease on exposure to the allergen (e.g., milk). Physical irritation and inflammation occur if food is aspirated into the respiratory tract. This happens frequently in patients with debilitating neurologic diseases and deficient protective reflexes of the upper airways. However, pulmonary aspiration may also occur in neurologically intact children, and their ethnic background, for example, indigenous people of North America, may suggest an increased risk. A history of cough or choking during feeding should alert the physician to the possibility of pulmonary aspiration.

The physical development of children with chronic respiratory diseases may be retarded. Malnutrition in the presence of increased caloric requirements is common, but the effects of some long-term medical treatments (e.g., steroids) should also be considered. Previous measurements of body growth should be obtained and plotted on appropriate charts. Psychosocial development may be affected if chronic lung diseases (e.g., asthma or cystic fibrosis) limit attendance and performance at school or if behavioral problems arise in children and adolescents subjected to chronic therapy. More severely affected patients may also be delayed in their sexual development.

Many diseases of the respiratory tract in children have a genetic component, either with a clear Mendelian mode of inheritance (e.g., autosomal recessive in cystic fibrosis, homozygous deficiency of α_1-antitrypsin, X-linked recessive in chronic granulomatous disease, and autosomal dominant in familial interstitial fibrosis) or with a genetic contribution to the cause. Examples of familial aggregation of respiratory disease are chronic bronchitis and bronchiectasis or familial emphysema in patients with heterozygous α_1-antitrypsin deficiency, in which the susceptibility of the lung to the action of irritants (e.g., cigarette smoke) is increased. A mixed influence of genetic and environmental factors exists in polygenic diseases, such as asthma or allergic rhinitis.

When inquiring about the family history, the physician should review at least two generations on either side. The parents should be asked whether they are related by blood, and information should be obtained about any childhood deaths in the family. The health of the patient's siblings and also of brothers and sisters of both parents should be documented. Particular attention should be paid to histories of asthma, allergies and hay fever, chronic bronchitis, emphysema, tuberculosis, cystic fibrosis, male infertility, and sudden unexpected infant death.

The physician should obtain a detailed report of prior tests and immunizations. Quite often this requires communication with other health care providers. Results of screening examinations (e.g., tuberculin and other skin tests, chest radiographs, and Cystic Fibrosis newborn screening) should be noted. Similarly, childhood illnesses, immunizations, and possible adverse immunization reactions should be documented. If the history is positive for allergic reactions, these have to be confirmed and defined. Previous hospital admissions and their indications should be listed, and the patient's current medications and their efficacy should be documented. If possible, the drug containers and prescriptions should be reviewed. The physician may use the opportunity to discuss the pharmacologic information and the technique of drug administration, particularly with inhaled bronchodilator medications.

One of the most important goals in taking a history is to become more aware of the particular psychological and social situation of the patient. It is impossible to judge current complaints or responses to medical interventions without an individual frame of reference for each patient. The physician should encourage the child and the parents to describe a typical day at home, daycare, kindergarten, or school. This will provide valuable information about the impact of the illness on daily routines, the financial implications, the existing or absent social support structures, and the coping strategies of the family. Compliance with medical treatment is rarely better than 50%, and physicians are generally unable to predict how well their patients follow and adhere to therapeutic regimens. Compliance can improve if the patient and the parents gain a better understanding of the disease and its treatment. It is important to recognize prior experiences that the family may have had with the health care system and to understand individual spiritual, religious, and health beliefs. Particularly in children with chronic respiratory ailments whose symptoms are not being controlled or prevented, the effort and unpleasantness (e.g., of chest physiotherapy) may limit the use of such interventions. The physician should also consider the social stigma associated with visible therapy, especially among peers of the adolescent patient.

A review of organ systems is usually the last part of the history and may actually be completed during the physical examination. Although the emphasis is on the respiratory system, questions about the general status of the child will be about appetite, sleep, level of activity, and prevailing mood. Important findings in the region of the head and neck are nasal obstruction and discharge, ear or sinus infection, conjunctival irritation, sore throat, and swallowing difficulty. The respiratory manifestations of coughing, noisy breathing, wheezing, and cyanosis are discussed in detail at the end of this chapter. Cardiovascular findings may include palpitations and dysrhythmia in hypoxic patients; there may be edema formation and peripheral swelling with cor pulmonale. Effects of respiratory disease on the gastrointestinal tract may appear with cough-induced vomiting and abdominal pain. There may be a direct involvement with diarrhea, cramps, and fatty stools in patients with cystic fibrosis. The physician should ask about hematuria and about skin manifestations, such as eczema or rashes, and about swellings and pain of lymph nodes or joints. Finally, neurologic symptoms (e.g., headache, lightheadedness, or paresthesiae) may be related to respiratory disease and cough paroxysms or hyperventilation.

The Physical Examination

Traditionally, the physical examination is divided into inspection, palpation, percussion, and auscultation. The sequence of these steps may be varied depending on the circumstances, particularly in the assessment of the respiratory tract in children. The classic components of the physical examination and some modern aids and additions are discussed in the following sections.

INSPECTION

Much can be learned from simple observation, particularly during those precious moments of sleep in the young infant or toddler, who when awake can be a challenge even for the skilled examiner. First, the pattern of breathing should be observed. This includes the respiratory rate, rhythm, and effort. The respiratory rate decreases with age and shows its greatest variability in newborns and young infants (Fig. 1.1A). Reference values in hospitalized children, excluding those with respiratory disease, show higher values (see Fig. 1.1B).

The respiratory rate should be counted over at least 1 minute, ideally several times for the calculation of average values. Because respiratory rates differ among sleep states and become even more variable during wakefulness, a note should be made describing the behavioral state of the patient. Observing abdominal movements or listening to breath sounds with the stethoscope placed before the mouth and nose may help in counting respirations in patients with very shallow thoracic excursions.

Longitudinal documentation of the respiratory rate during rest or sleep is important for the follow-up of patients with chronic lung diseases, even more so for those too young for standard pulmonary function tests. Abnormally high breathing frequencies or *tachypnea* can be seen in patients with decreased compliance of the respiratory system and in those with metabolic acidosis. Other causes of tachypnea are fever (~5–7 breaths/min increase per degree above 37°C), anemia, exertion, intoxication (salicylates), anxiety, and psychogenic hyperventilation. The opposite, an abnormally slow respiratory rate or *bradypnea,* can occur in patients with metabolic alkalosis or central nervous system depression. The terms *hyperpnea* and *hypopnea* refer to abnormally deep or shallow respirations. At given respiratory rates, this determination is a subjective clinical judgment and is not easily quantified unless the pattern is obvious, such as the Kussmaul type of breathing in patients with diabetic ketoacidosis.

Significant changes in the rhythm of breathing occur during the first months of life. Respiratory pauses of less than 6 seconds are common in infants younger than 3 months of age. If these pauses occur in groups of three or more that are separated by less than 20 seconds of respiration, the pattern is referred to as *periodic breathing.* This pattern is very common in premature infants after the first days of life and may persist until 44 weeks postconceptional age. In full-term infants, periodic breathing is usually observed between 1 week and 2 months of age and is normally absent by 6 months of age. Apnea with cessation of air flow lasting more than 15 seconds is uncommon and may be accompanied by bradycardia and cyanosis. In preterm infants, a drop in oxygen

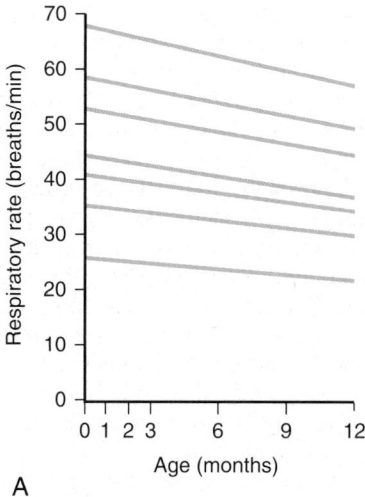

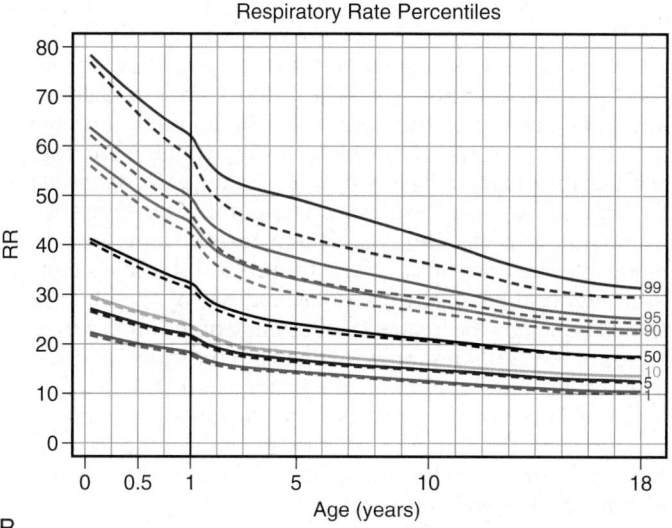

Fig. 1.1 (A) Median and percentile curves for respiratory rates. (B) *Dotted lines* represent sensitivity analysis excluding diseases of the respiratory system. The solid vertical line at 1 year of age represents a change in scale of the x-axis. *RR*, Respiratory rate. ([A] Data from Rusconi F, Castagneto M, Gagliardi L, et al. Reference values for respiratory rate in the first 3 years of life. *Pediatrics*. 1994;94:350. [B] Data from Bonafide CP, Brady PW, Keren R, et al. Development of heart and respiratory rate percentile curves for hospitalized children. *Pediatrics*. 2013;131:e1150.)

and paradoxical respiratory movements. The more negative intrapleural pressure during inspiration against a high airway resistance leads to retraction of the pliable portions of the chest wall, including the intercostal and subcostal tissues and the supraclavicular and suprasternal fossae. Conversely, bulging of intercostal spaces may be seen when pleural pressure becomes greatly positive during a maximally forced expiration. Retractions are more easily visible in the newborn infant, in whom intercostal tissues are thinner and more compliant than in the older child.

Visible contraction of the sternocleidomastoid muscles and indrawing of supraclavicular fossae during inspiration are among the most reliable clinical signs of airway obstruction. In young infants, these muscular contractions may lead to head bobbing, which is best observed when the child rests with the head supported slightly at the suboccipital area. If no other signs of respiratory distress are present in an infant with head bobbing, however, central nervous system disorders, such as third ventricular cysts with hydrocephalus, should be considered. Older patients with chronic airway obstruction and extensive use of accessory muscles may appear to have a short neck because of hunched shoulders. *Orthopnea* exists when the patient is unable to tolerate a recumbent position, for example, with severely increased upper airway resistance and obstruction during sleep.

Flaring of the alae nasi is a sensitive sign of respiratory distress and may be present when inspiration is abnormally short (e.g., under conditions of chest pain). Nasal flaring enlarges the anterior nasal passages and reduces upper and total airway resistance. It may also help to stabilize the upper airways by preventing large negative pharyngeal pressures during inspiration.

The normal movement of chest and abdominal walls is directed outward during inspiration. Inward motion of the chest wall during inspiration is called *paradoxical breathing.* This is seen when the thoracic cage loses its stability and becomes distorted by the action of the diaphragm. Classically, paradoxical breathing with a seesaw type of thoracoabdominal motion is seen in patients with paralysis of the intercostal muscles, but it is also commonly seen in premature and newborn infants who have a very compliant rib cage. Inspiratory indrawing of the lateral chest is known as *Hoover sign* and can be observed in patients with obstructive airway disease. Paradoxical breathing also occurs during sleep in patients with upper airway obstruction. The development of paradoxical breathing in an awake, nonparalyzed patient beyond the newborn period usually indicates respiratory muscle fatigue and impending respiratory failure.

Following inspection of the breathing pattern, the examiner should pay attention to the symmetry of respiratory chest excursions. Unilateral diseases affecting lungs, pleura, chest wall, or diaphragm may all result in asymmetric breathing movements. Trauma to the rib cage may cause fractures and a "flail chest" that shows local paradoxical movement. Pain during respiration usually leads to "splinting" with flexion of the trunk toward and decreased respiratory movements of the affected side. The signs of hemidiaphragmatic paralysis may be subtle. In complete unilateral paralysis, there may be a shift in the epigastric abdominal wall during deep inspiration diagonally toward the side of the lesion and upward. This may be more noticeable in the lateral decubitus position with the paralyzed diaphragm placed up, a position that tends

saturation may be seen up to 7 seconds after a respiratory pause when in room air and up to 9 seconds later when on supplemental oxygen.

Other abnormal patterns include *Cheyne-Stokes breathing,* which occurs as cycles of increasing and decreasing tidal volumes separated by apnea (e.g., in children with congestive heart failure or increased intracranial pressure). *Biot breathing* consists of irregular cycles of respiration at variable tidal volumes interrupted by apnea and is an ominous finding in patients with severe brain damage.

After noting the rate and rhythm of breathing, the physician should look for signs of increased respiratory effort. The older child will be able to communicate the subjective experience of difficult breathing, or *dyspnea.* Objective signs that reflect distressed breathing are chest wall retractions, visible use of accessory muscles and the alae nasi, orthopnea, to accentuate a paradoxical inward epigastric motion on the affected side.

Other methods to augment inspection of chest wall motion use optical markers. In practice, this technique is done by placing both hands on either side of the patient's lateral rib cage with the thumbs along the costal margins. Divergence of the thumbs during expansion of the thorax supposedly aids in the visual perception of the range and symmetry of respiratory movements. This technique is of little use in children. A more accurate method of documenting the vectors of movement at different sites (but one that is not yet practical for bedside evaluation) is to place a grid of optical markers on the chest surface and film their positional changes during respiration relative to a steady reference frame. A similar concept is used in optical studies of chest deformities. Projection of raster lines onto the anterior chest surface allows stereographic measurement of deformities, such as pectus excavatum, and augments the visual image of the surface shape (Fig. 1.2). In practice and without such tools, however, the physician should inspect the chest at different angles of illumination to enhance the visual perception of chest wall deformities. Their location, size, symmetry, and change with respiratory or cardiac movements should be noted.

The physician should measure the dimensions of the chest. Chest size and shape are influenced by ethnic and geographic factors that should be taken into account when measurements are compared with normative data. Andean children who live at high altitudes, for example, have larger chest dimensions relative to stature than children in North America. The chest circumference is usually taken at the mammillary level during midinspiration. In practice, mean readings during inspiration and expiration should be noted (Fig. 1.3A). Premature infants have a greater head circumference than chest circumference, while these measurements are very similar at term (see Fig. 1.3B). Malnutrition can delay the time at which chest circumference begins to exceed head circumference.

Further objective documentation of the chest configuration may include measurements of thoracic depth (antero-posterior [AP] diameter) and width (transverse diameter).

The thoracic index, or the ratio of AP over transverse diameter, is close to unity in infants and decreases during childhood. Measurements should be taken with a caliper at the level of the nipples in upright subjects. Normative values for young children are available but dated (Fig. 1.4). Most of the configurational change of the chest occurs during the first 2 years and is probably influenced by gravitational forces after the upright position becomes common. Disease-related changes in thoracic dimensions occur either as potential causative factors (e.g., the elongated thorax with a stress distribution that favors spontaneous pneumothorax in lanky adolescents, particularly males who increase their thoracic height versus width more than females) or as a secondary event (e.g., the barrel-shaped chest in patients with emphysema and chronic hyperinflation of the lung).

Inspection of the patient should also be directed to the extrathoracic regions. Many observations on the examination of the head and neck provide valuable clues to the physical diagnosis. Bluish coloration of the lower eyelid ("allergic shiners"); a bilateral fold of skin just below the lower eyelid (Dennie lines); and a transverse crease from "allergic salutes," running at the junction of the cartilaginous and bony portion of the nose, may all be found in atopic individuals. The physician should always examine the nose and document bilateral patency by occluding each side while feeling and listening for air flow through the other nostril. Even without a speculum, one can assess the anterior half by raising the nose tip with one thumb and shining a light into the nasal passageways. Color and size of the mucosa should be noted. The frequency of asymptomatic nasal polyps seems to be high. Most polyps arise from the mucosa of the ostia, clefts, and recesses in the ostiomeatal complex and have the appearance of white gelatinous grapes. Easily visible nasal polyps are common in patients with cystic fibrosis. Nasal polyposis may also be familial or associated with allergy, asthma, and aspirin intolerance.

The oropharynx should be inspected for its size and signs of malformation, such as cleft palate, and for signs of obstruction by enlarged tonsils. Evidence of chronic ear infections should be documented, and the areas over frontal and maxillary paranasal sinuses should be tested for tenderness.

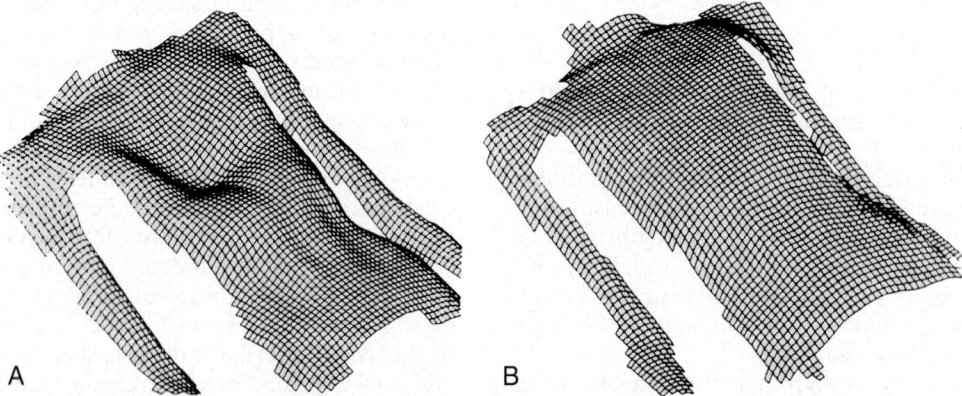

A   B

Fig. 1.2 Optical markers augment the visual perception of chest wall deformities. In this example of rasterstereography, lines are projected onto the anterior thorax, and the surface image is computed as a regular network. The change of the funnel chest deformity before (A) and after surgery (B) is easily appreciated. In practice and at the bedside, the physician should inspect at different angles of illumination to enhance the visual perception of chest wall deformities. (From Hierholzer E, Schier F. Rasterstereography in the measurement and postoperative follow-up of anterior chest wall deformities. *Z Kinderchir*. 1986;41:267-271.)

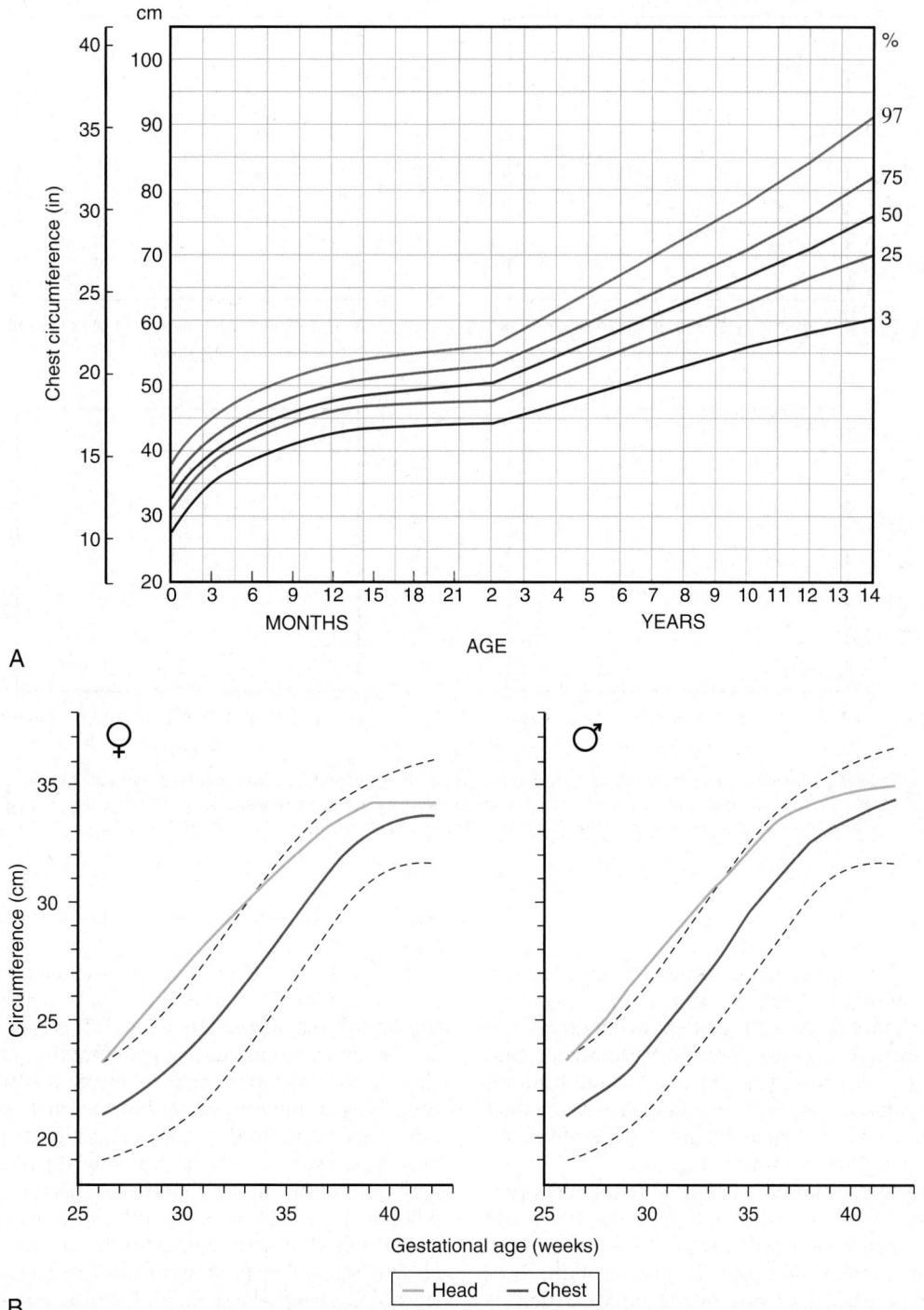

Fig. 1.3 (A) Normal distribution of chest circumference from birth to 14 years. Tape measurements are made at the mammillary level during midinspiration. Before plotting the values on the graph, one should add 1 cm for males and subtract 1 cm for females between 2 and 12 years of age. (B) Normal distribution of chest circumference from 26 to 42 weeks of gestation. The dotted lines indicate the 10th and 90th percentiles, respectively. Note that chest circumference is close to head circumference at term. ([A] From Feingold M, Bossert WH. Normal values for selected physical parameters. An aid to syndrome delineation. *Birth Defects*. 1974;10:14. [B] Data from Britton JR, Britton HL, Jennett R, et al. Weight, length, head and chest circumference at birth in Phoenix, Arizona. *J Reprod Med*. 1993;38:215.)

Inspection of the skin is important and may reveal the eczema of atopy. The finding of a scar that typically develops at the site of a successful bacillus Calmette-Guérin (BCG) vaccination may be relevant. In North American children, these scars are usually found over the left deltoid, but other sites, including buttocks and lower extremities, are also used for BCG inoculation in different parts of the world. Common physical findings such as cyanosis, clubbing, and the cardiovascular signs of pulmonary disease are discussed in more detail at the end of this chapter.

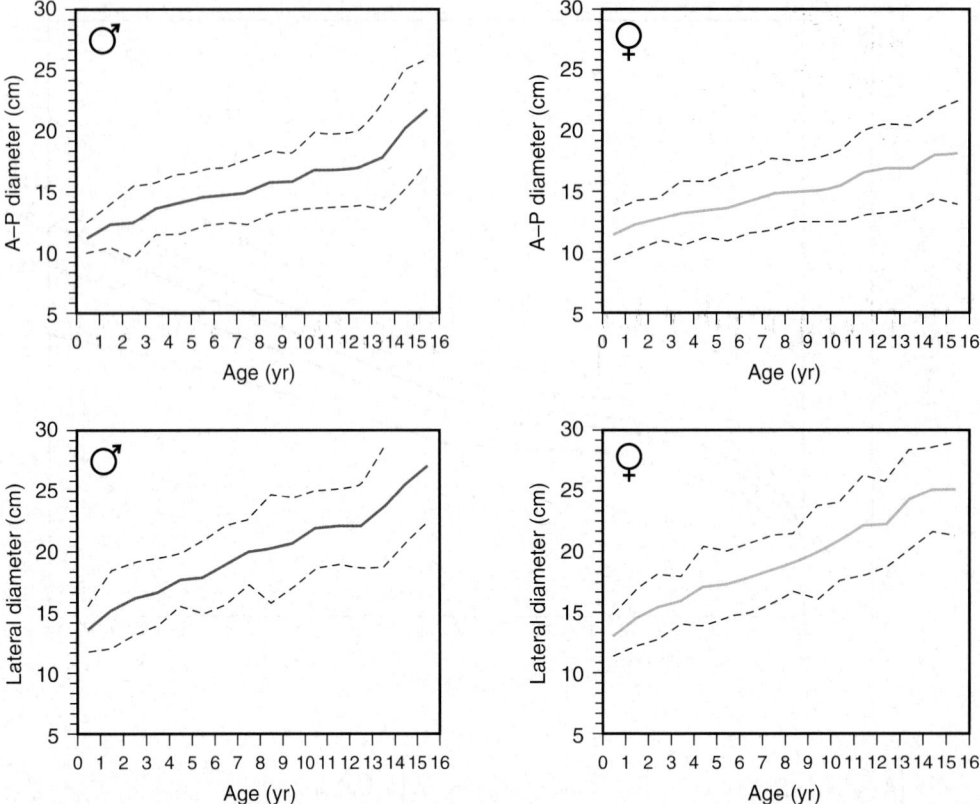

Fig. 1.4 Mean values *(solid line)* ± SD *(dashed lines)* of the normal distribution of anteroposterior (AP) and lateral chest diameters in boys and girls. Caliper measurements are made at the mammillary level during midinspiration. *SD,* Standard deviation. (Data from Lucas WP, Pryor HB. Range and standard deviations of certain physical measurements in healthy children. *J Pediatr.* 1935;6:533-545.)

PALPATION

Palpation follows chest inspection to confirm observed abnormalities, such as swellings and deformations; to identify areas of tenderness or lymph node enlargement; to document the position of the trachea; to assess respiratory excursions; and to detect changes in the transmission of voice sounds through the chest. Chest palpation may offer the first physical contact with the patient, and it is very important for the physician to perform this procedure with warm hands.

Palpation should be done in an orderly sequence. Commonly, one begins with an examination of the head and neck. Cervical lymphadenopathy and tenderness over paranasal sinuses should be noted. Palpation of the oropharynx may be indicated to find malformations such as submucosal clefts or to identify causes of upper airway obstruction. The position of the trachea must be documented in every patient. This is a very important part of the physical chest examination because tracheal deviation most often indicates significant intrathoracic or extrathoracic abnormalities.

In the older child, the tracheal position is assessed by placing the index and ring fingers on both sternal attachments of the sternocleidomastoid muscles. The trachea is then felt between these landmarks with the middle finger on the suprasternal notch. In small children, palpation is done with one index finger sliding gently inward over the suprasternal notch. Looking for asymmetry, the physician should always make sure that the patient is in a straight position, and deformities (e.g., scoliosis) should be taken into account.

A very slight deviation of the trachea toward the right is normal. Marked deviations may indicate a pulling force toward the side of displacement (e.g., atelectasis) or a pushing force on the contralateral side (e.g., pneumothorax). The physician should note whether the displacement is fixed or whether there is a pendular movement of the trachea during inspiration and expiration that may suggest obstruction of a large bronchus. Posterior displacement of the trachea may occur with anterior mediastinal tumors or barrel chest deformities, whereas an easily palpable anteriorly displaced trachea is sometimes seen with mediastinitis. In patients with airway obstruction and respiratory distress, retractions of the suprasternal fossa may be seen, and a "tracheal tug" may be felt by the examiner.

Placing the hands on both sides of the lateral rib cage, the physician should feel for symmetry of chest expansion during regular and deep breathing maneuvers. Slight compression of the chest in the transverse and AP directions may help to localize pain from lesions of the bony structures. Voice-generated vibrations are best felt with the palms of both hands just below the base of the fingers placed over corresponding sites on the right and left hemithorax. Asymmetric transmission usually indicates unilateral intrathoracic abnormalities. The patient is asked to produce low-frequency vibrations of sufficient amplitude by saying "ninety-nine" in a loud voice. In young infants, crying may produce the vibrations that are felt as tactile fremitus over the chest wall.

This fremitus is decreased if an accumulation of air or fluid in the pleural space reduces transmission. Small consolidations of the underlying lung will not diminish the tactile fremitus as long as the airways remain open, whereas collapse of the airways and atelectasis will reduce the transmission of vibratory energy if larger portions of the lung are affected.

PERCUSSION

Percussion is used to set tissues into vibration with an impulsive force so that their mechanical and acoustic response can be studied. If the vibrations are not damped and continue for a significant amount of time, the perceived sound will be resonant or "tympanic," whereas rapid attenuation of the vibrations will lead to a flat or "dull" percussion note. The former occurs when there is a large acoustic mismatch (e.g., tissue overlying an air-filled cavity), whereas the latter occurs when the underlying tissue is similar to the surface tissue and vibratory energy propagates away quickly. Structures that absorb energy when struck by a sound at their natural frequency continue vibrating after the initial sound is gone and are called *resonant*. The fundamental resonance of the thorax depends on body size and is about 125 Hz for adult males, between 150 and 175 Hz for adult females, and between 300 and 400 Hz for small children.

Chest percussion in children is performed by light tapping with the middle finger (the plexor) on the middle or terminal phalanx of the other hand's middle finger (the pleximeter). The pleximeter should be placed firmly but not hard, and care should be taken that other fingers do not touch the chest wall, which may cause artificial damping of the percussion note. Percussion should be gentle, with quick perpendicular movements of the plexor originating from the wrist (Fig. 1.5). The patient should be relaxed during the examination because tension of the chest wall muscles may alter the percussion note. More importantly, chest deformities and scoliosis in particular will have a significant effect on percussion findings.

Symmetric sites over the anterior, lateral, and posterior surface of the chest should be compared in an orderly fashion. As with chest auscultation, findings should be reported with reference to standard external anatomic landmarks (Fig. 1.6). The ribs and vertebral spinous processes are used for horizontal mapping. The level at which the tympanic lung resonance changes to a dull percussion note should be defined over the posterior chest during maximal inspiration and expiration to delineate the lung borders and their respiratory excursions.

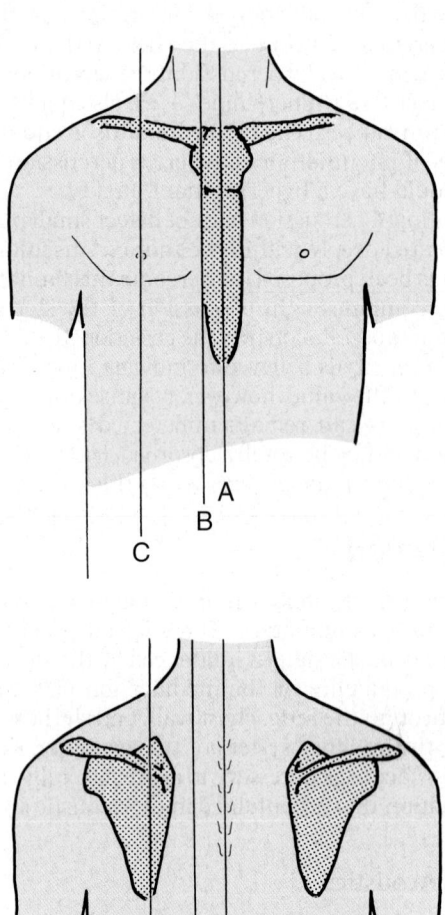

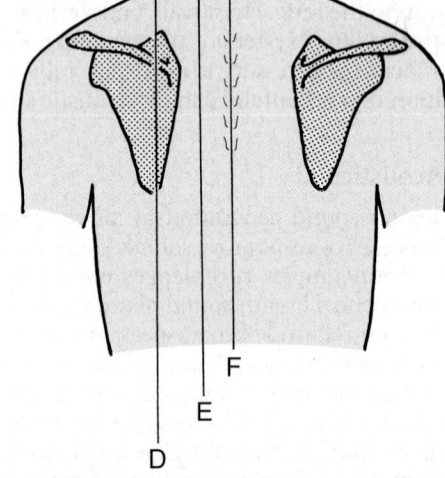

Fig. 1.6 Vertical reference lines of the chest. The center line is indicated anteriorly by the suprasternal notch (A) and posteriorly by the spinous processes (F). The sternal (B) and midclavicular (C) lines over the front, and the scapular (D) and paravertebral (E) lines over the back provide longitudinal landmarks of the thorax. From a lateral view, the midaxillary line is used for orientation. Horizontal reference points are the supraclavicular and infraclavicular fossae, Ludwig angle (junction of the second rib at the sternum), the mammillae (normally at the fourth rib), and the epigastric angle. Posteriorly, the prominent spinous process of the seventh cervical vertebra and the supraspinous and infraspinous fossae of the scapulae provide markers for orientation.

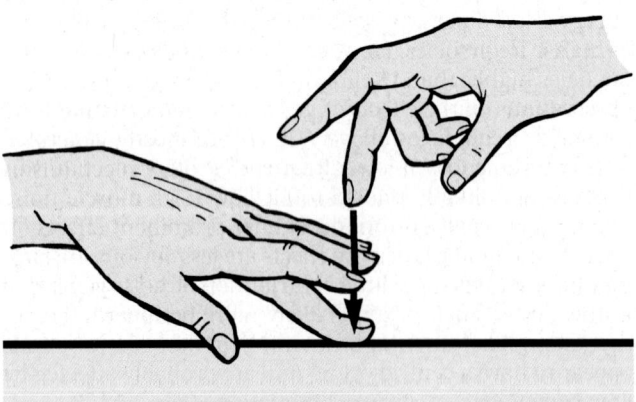

Fig. 1.5 Percussion in children should be done with gentle perpendicular movements from the wrist and tapping of the plexor finger *(right)* on the middle or terminal phalanx of the pleximeter finger *(left)*. The contact area of the pleximeter on the chest should be small, and other fingers should not touch the surface to avoid damping of the vibrations.

Subjective assessment of percussion note differences includes both acoustic and tactile perception. Tympanic, lower-pitched percussion notes mean less-damped vibrations of longer duration, which are felt by the pleximeter finger and heard by the examiner. These resonant sounds can be exaggerated, or hyperresonant, over hyperinflated lungs but also in some otherwise healthy thin individuals. Observer agreement on this sign is relatively poor unless the finding is unilateral.

Dull sounds with higher frequencies correspond to vibrations that die away quickly. Dullness replaces the normal chest percussion note when fluid accumulates in the pleural space or when consolidation occurs in the underlying pulmonary parenchyma close to the chest wall. Similar to the vibrations generated by percussion, the vibrations from the patient's voice ("say 'ninety-nine'") will also not be felt under these circumstances. The tactile fremitus is equally absent over areas of pneumothorax, whereas percussion, as noted above, should have a hyperresonant quality.

Conventional percussion cannot detect small pulmonary lesions located deeply within the thorax. Auscultatory percussion has been proposed to overcome this limitation. This technique combines light percussion of the sternum with simultaneous auscultation over the posterior chest. A decrease in sound intensity is believed to indicate lung disease. The method is of little value, however, because even large intrathoracic lesions can remain undetected since percussion sounds may either be totally absorbed within the lung or may travel as transverse waves along the thoracic bones.

AUSCULTATION

Auscultation is arguably the most important part of the physical chest examination. The subjective perception of respiratory acoustic signs is influenced by the site and mode of sound production; by the modification of sound on its passage through the lung, chest wall, and stethoscope; and, finally, by the auditory system of the examiner. Knowledge about these factors is necessary to appreciate fully the wealth of information that is contained in the acoustic signs of the thorax.

Thoracic Acoustics

Observations on sound generation in airway models and electronic analyses of respiratory sounds suggest a predominant origin from complex turbulences within the central airways. The tracheal breath sound heard above the suprasternal notch is a relatively broad-spectrum noise, ranging in frequency from less than 100 Hz to greater than 2000 Hz. Resonances from the trachea and from supraglottic airways "color" the sound (Fig. 1.7). The lengthening of the trachea with growth during childhood causes lower tracheal resonance frequencies. A dominant source of tracheal breath sounds is turbulence from the jet flow at the glottic aperture. However, narrow segments of the supraglottic passages also contribute to sound generation. There is a very close relationship between air flow and tracheal sound intensity, particularly at high frequencies. In the presence of local narrowing (e.g., in children with subglottic stenosis), flow velocity at the stenotic site is increased, and so is the tracheal sound intensity. Relating tracheal sound levels to air flow measured at the mouth can provide information about

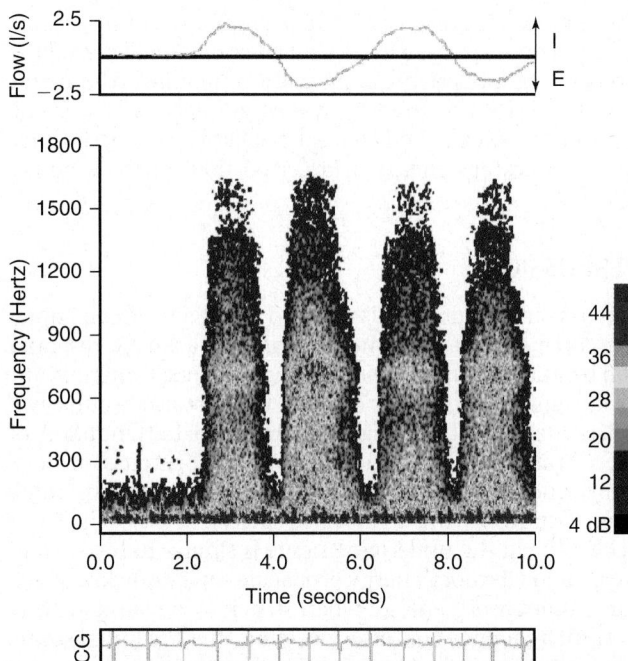

Fig. 1.7 Digital respirosonogram of sounds recorded over the trachea of a healthy young man. Time is on the horizontal axis, frequency is on the vertical axis, and sound intensity is shown on a scale from *red (loud)* over *orange and yellow (medium)* to *green, gray, and black (low)*. Air flow is plotted at the top, with inspiration above and expiration below the zero line. The sonogram illustrates the broad range of tracheal sounds during both inspiration and expiration. There is a distinct pause between the respiratory phases. Expiration is louder than inspiration, and resonance is apparent around 700 Hz. In this example, the subject was holding his breath at the beginning. During this respiratory pause, heart sounds below 200 Hz are easily identified by their temporal relation to the simultaneously recorded electrocardiogram (ECG).

changes during therapy. Auscultation over the trachea will provide some information under these circumstances, but objective acoustic measurements are required for accurate comparisons.

Basic "normal" lung sounds heard at the chest surface are lower in frequency than tracheal sounds because sound energy is lost during passage though the lungs, particularly at higher frequencies. However, lung sounds extend to frequencies higher than traditionally recognized. More recent observations on the effects of gas density indicate that lung sounds at frequencies above 400 Hz are mostly generated by flow turbulence. At lower frequencies, other mechanisms that are not directly related to air flow (e.g., muscle noise and thoracic cavity resonances) have prominent effects on lung sounds, and gas density effects are less obvious. Inspiratory lung sounds show little contribution of noise generated at the glottis. Their origin is likely more peripheral (i.e., in the main and segmental bronchi). Expiratory lung sounds appear to have a central origin and are probably affected by flow convergence at airway bifurcations (Fig. 1.8).

Sound at different frequencies takes different pathways on the passage through the lung. Low-frequency sound waves propagate from central airways through the lung parenchyma to the chest wall. At higher frequencies, the airway walls become effectively more rigid and sound travels further down into the airways before it propagates through lung tissue.

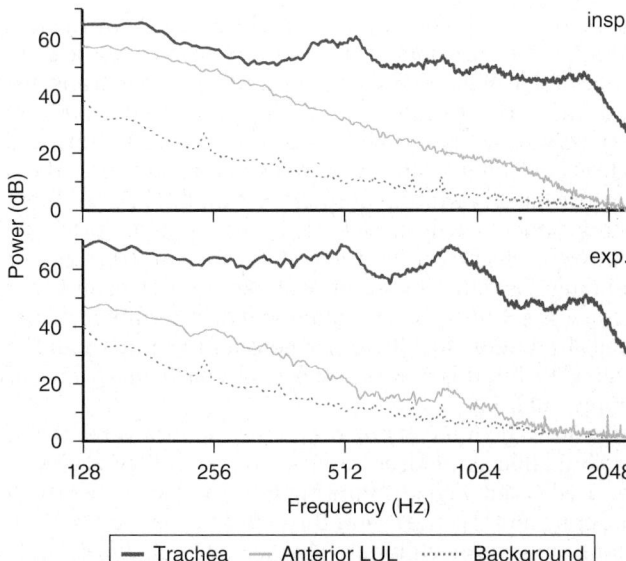

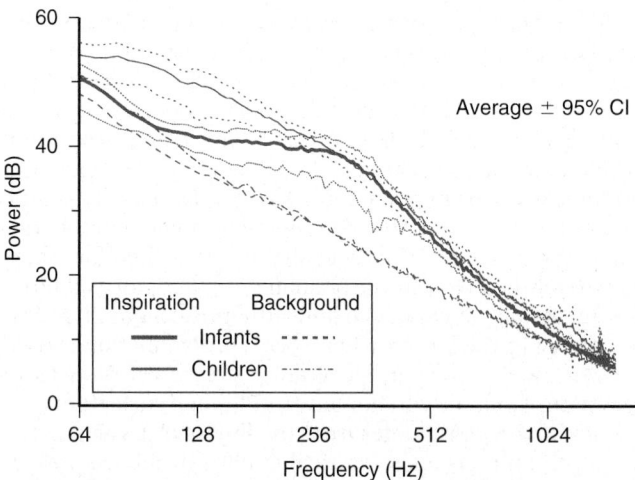

Fig. 1.8 Average spectra of respiratory sounds at air flow of 1.5 ± 0.3 L/s, recorded simultaneously at the suprasternal notch (trachea) and at the second intercostal space in the midclavicular line on the left (anterior left upper lobe [LUL]) of a healthy 12-year-old boy. The average sound spectrum during breath holding at resting end expiration (background) is plotted for comparison. Inspiratory lung sounds are louder than expiratory sounds, while the opposite is true for tracheal sounds. Lung sound intensity is clearly above background at frequencies as high as 1000 Hz. Expiratory lung sounds show some of the same spectral peaks that are present in tracheal sounds.

Fig. 1.9 Average spectra of inspiratory lung sounds, recorded over the posterior basal segment of the right lung in healthy newborn infants ($n = 10$) and children ($n = 9$) at air flows of 15 mL/s per kilogram. The spectra of background noise at resting end expiration are plotted for comparison. Dotted lines mark the 95% confidence intervals (CIs). Note the similarity of spectral slopes in newborn infants and older children at frequencies above 300 Hz and the significantly reduced sound power at lower frequencies in newborns. (Data from Pasterkamp H, Powell RE, Sanchez I. Lung sound spectra at standardized air flow in normal infants, children, and adults. *Am J Respir Crit Care Med.* 1996;154:424-430.)

This information cannot be gathered on subjective auscultation but requires objective acoustic measurements. A trained ear, however, will recognize many of the findings that are related to these mechanisms. For example, lung sounds in healthy children and adults are not necessarily equal at corresponding sites over both lungs. In fact, expiratory sounds are typically louder at the right upper lobe compared with the left side. Similar asymmetry has been recognized when sound is introduced at the mouth and measured at the chest surface. A likely explanation for this asymmetry is the effect on sound propagation by the cardiovascular and mediastinal structures to the left of the trachea. Asymmetry of lung sounds is also noticeable in most healthy subjects during inspiration when one listens over the posterior lower chest. The left side tends to be louder here, probably because of the size and spatial orientation of the larger airways due to the heart.

Objective acoustic measurements have also helped to clarify the difference between lung sounds in newborn infants and in older children. The most obvious divergence occurs in lung sounds at low frequencies where newborn infants have much less intensity. This may be explained by thoracic and airway resonances at higher frequencies in newborn infants and perhaps also by their lower muscle mass. Lung sounds at higher frequencies are similar between newborn infants and older children (Fig. 1.9).

Adventitious respiratory sounds usually indicate respiratory disease. Wheezes are musical, continuous (typically longer than 100 ms) sounds that originate from oscillations in narrowed airways. The frequency of the oscillation depends on the mass and elasticity of the airway wall as well as on local air flow. Widespread narrowing of airways in asthma leads to various pitches, or polyphonic wheezing, whereas a fixed obstruction in a larger airway produces a single wheeze, or monophonic wheezing. Expiratory wheezing is related to flow limitation and can be produced by normal subjects during forced expiratory maneuvers. The situation is less clear for wheezing during inspiration, which is common in asthma but cannot be produced by healthy subjects unless it originates from the larynx (e.g., in vocal cord dysfunction). Very brief and localized inspiratory wheezes may be heard over areas of bronchiectasis.

Crackles are nonmusical, discontinuous (<20 ms duration) lung sounds. Crackle production requires the presence of air-fluid interfaces and occurs either by air movement through secretions or by sudden equalization of gas pressure. Another mechanism may be the release of tissue tension during sudden opening or closing of airways. Crackles are perceived as fine or coarse, depending on the duration and frequency of the brief and dampened vibrations created by these mechanisms. There may be a musical quality to the sound if a short oscillation occurs at the generation site. This has been called a *squawk* and may appear during inspiration, typically in patients with interstitial lung diseases but also in some patients with pneumonia or bronchiectasis. Fine crackles during late inspiration are common in restrictive lung diseases and in the early stages of congestive heart failure, whereas coarse crackles during early inspiration and during expiration are frequently heard in chronic obstructive lung disease. Fine crackles are usually inaudible at the mouth, whereas the coarse crackles of widespread airway obstruction can be transmitted through the large airways and may be heard as clicks with the stethoscope held in front of the patient's open mouth. Some crackles over the anterior chest may occur in normal subjects who were breathing at low lung volumes, but they will disappear after a few deep breaths.

Several other abnormal respiratory sounds are not generated in intrathoracic airways. Pleural rubs originate from mechanical stretching of the pleura, which causes vibration of the chest wall and local pulmonary parenchyma. These sounds can occur during both inspiration and expiration. Their character is like that of creaking leather and is similar in some ways to pulmonary crackles. *Stridor* refers to a more or less musical sound that is produced by oscillations of critically narrowed extrathoracic airways. It is therefore most commonly heard during inspiration. *Grunting* is an expiratory sound, usually low-pitched and with musical qualities. It is produced in the larynx when vocal cord adduction is used to generate positive end-expiratory pressures, such as in premature infants with immature lungs and surfactant deficiency. *Snoring* originates from the flutter of tissues in the pharynx and has a less musical quality. It may be present during both inspiration and expiration.

There may also be cardiorespiratory sounds. These are believed to occur when cardiac movements cause regional flows of air in the surrounding lung. Because of its synchronicity with the heartbeat, this sound may be mistaken for a cardiac murmur. It can be identified by its "vesicular sound" quality and its exaggeration during inspiration and in different body positions.

At the boundary between different tissues, reflection of sound may occur and sound transmission may decrease, depending on the matching or mismatching of the tissue impedances. Many of the acoustic signs of the chest are explained on the basis of impedance matching alone. The stethoscope is basically an impedance transformer that reduces sound reflection at a mismatched interface, namely, body surface to air. Because it is the only part of the sound transmission pathway that can be kept constant, it is best to always use the same stethoscope. The choice of a bell- or a diaphragm-type stethoscope depends on individual preference. Diaphragm chest pieces can be placed more easily and with less pressure on small chests with narrow intercostal spaces. Compared with bell-type stethoscopes, they tend to deemphasize frequencies below 100 Hz. Both the bell-type and the diaphragm stethoscopes show some attenuation at frequencies above 400 Hz.

Technique of Auscultation

Ideally, auscultation of the chest should be performed in a quiet room; however, with pediatric patients the usual setting may be anything but quiet. Fortunately, the human auditory system allows selective evaluation of acoustic signals even when they occur in the presence of much louder surrounding noises. This psychoacoustic phenomenon, known as the "cocktail party effect," at present cannot be reproduced by modern electronic techniques, which is but one of the reasons for the lasting popularity of the stethoscope.

This instrument, the most widely used in clinical medicine since its introduction almost 200 years ago, carries symbolic value for the health care profession, much like a modern staff of Aesculapius. Every child knows that doctors have stethoscopes. The physician should use this to advantage when assessing pediatric patients by encouraging children to listen themselves to their heartbeats and breathing sounds. Even infants may be fascinated as long as the stethoscope is shiny. Ice cold chest pieces, on the other hand, turn off most patients.

The patient should be in a straight position during auscultation because incurvature of the trunk may lead to artificial side differences of sound production and transmission. In newborns and young infants, a straight position may be best achieved when they are supine. Infants and toddlers will often be assessed while their parents hold them on their laps. Beginning auscultation on the back of these young patients will provoke less anxiety than a frontal approach. Older children can be examined in the sitting or standing position. The number of sites over the chest that are assessed during auscultation will be determined by the clinical situation. Ideally, all segments of the lung should be listened to, but this may not be possible, particularly in very young children.

Because the intensity of respiratory sounds is related to air flow, sufficiently deep respirations (with flow >0.5 L/s) are needed for a good sound signal. An older patient will cooperate and breathe deeply through an open mouth. With infants and young children, however, one may have to rely on sounds made during sighs or deep inspirations in between crying. On the other hand, normal breath sounds can mask the presence of some adventitious sounds (e.g., fine crackles of low intensity). Asking the patient to take very slow, deep breaths with less air flow than is needed to generate normal breath sounds can help to unmask these adventitious sounds.

The physician should make note of the lung sound intensity over different areas of the chest in a qualitative way, keeping in mind that this intensity reflects both local sound generation and sound transmission characteristics of the thorax. It is therefore not correct to speak of local "air entry" when one actually refers to local breath sound intensity. Decreased breath sounds, for example, are common in asthma even when normal blood gases indicate that air entry has to be adequate. Obviously, a qualitative distinction between the absence or presence of local breath sounds will be easier than attempts at quantification. Also, when the stethoscope is placed over any given location, it is not known how large an area of the underlying lung is actually being assessed. In adult subjects, moving the chest piece of the stethoscope by 10 cm will position it to receive sound from entirely different lung units, but similar data for children are not available.

Assessment of regional ventilation by thoracic acoustic signs becomes more meaningful when two sites are compared simultaneously. Differential auscultation with special stethoscopes that employ two chest pieces or a single divided chest piece has not become popular in clinical practice. Nevertheless, comparative auscultation is absolutely essential for airway management in the emergency department and intensive care unit for assessment of endotracheal tube position or for identification of the side of a pneumothorax. Listening simultaneously to two homologous sites over both lungs also help to detect local abnormalities. With local airway narrowing, the maximum sound intensity over the affected side may become sufficiently delayed to be perceived as "phase heterophony." In some cases, breath sounds may still be audible over the affected side after inspiratory efforts have ceased. This "post-effort" breath sound is a sign of incomplete airway obstruction.

There are special circumstances in which only the presence or absence of breath sounds is of interest (e.g., during transportation of critically ill patients in noisy vehicles and during resuscitation in the emergency department). Under these conditions, and when a firm attachment of the chest piece is important, a self-adhering stethoscope, based on negative suction pressure within the bell of the chest piece, may be applied. New techniques of adaptive electronic filtering are being used in stethoscopes that are optimized for use in very noisy environments.

Respiratory sounds should be documented according to their location and character. Normal projections of lobar borders to the surface of the chest are shown in Fig. 1.10. These may be distorted by local pulmonary disease, and mapping of respiratory sounds should therefore be done with reference to external anatomic landmarks (see Fig. 1.6). The examiner should be familiar with the segmental structure of the underlying lung.

Respiratory sound characteristics include the intensity (amplitude), pitch (predominant frequency), and timing during the respiratory cycle. Also, sounds will have a particular timbre (character) caused by the presence of resonances and overtones. Unfortunately, the terminology in use for the description of respiratory sounds is still confusing and imprecise. During a symposium on lung sounds in Tokyo in 1985, an attempt was made to achieve a global and uniform nomenclature for breath sounds (Table 1.1). More recently, a Task Force of the European Respiratory Society documented the current use of terminology in Western languages and recommended some modifications. The earlier and current recommendations for classification of adventitious lung sounds are summarized in Table 1.2, which summarizes the mechanisms and sites of generation, acoustic characteristics, and clinical relevance of the major categories of respiratory sounds.

A basic grouping into musical, continuous sounds of long duration and nonmusical, discontinuous sounds of short duration is made, with the former being referred to as *wheezes*

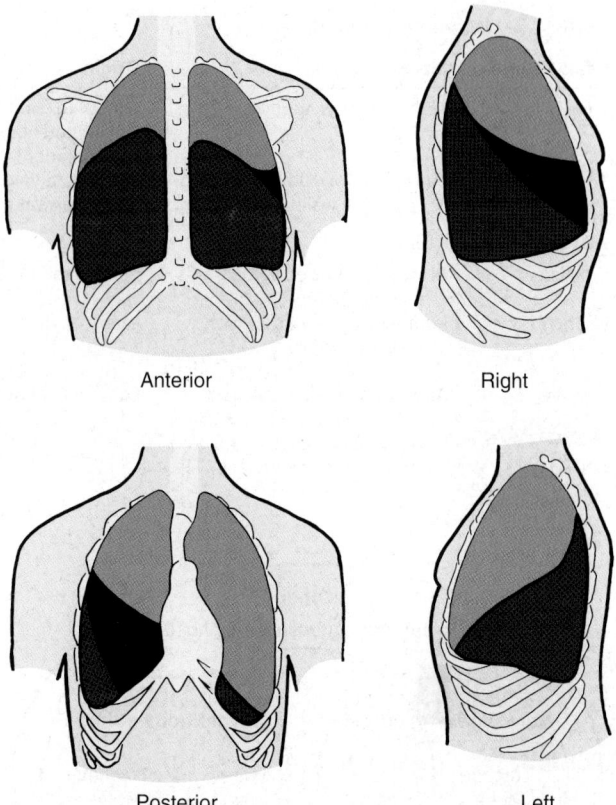

Anterior   Right

Posterior   Left

Fig. 1.10 Projections of the pulmonary lobes on the chest surface. The upper lobes are *pink,* the right-middle lobe is *black,* and the lower lobes are *red.*

Table 1.1   Lung Sound Nomenclature

Discontinuous	English	French	German	Portuguese	Russian	Spanish
Fine (high pitched, low amplitude, short duration)	Fine crackles	*Râles crepitants*	*Feines Rasseln*	*Estertores finos*	мелкопузырчатые влажные хрипы (melkopuzyrchatyye vlazhnyye khripy)	*Estertores finos*
—	—	**Crépitants fins**	**Feinblasige Rasselgeräusche**	**Fervores finos or Crepitações finas**	—	***Crepitantes finos or Estertores finos***
Coarse (low pitched, high amplitude, short duration)	Coarse crackles	*Râles bulleux or sous crepitant*	*Grobes Rasseln*	*Estertores grossos*	влажные хрипы (vlazhnyye khripy)	*Estertores grossos*
—	—	**Gros crépitants**	**Grobblasige**	**Fervores grosseiros**	—	**Crepitantes gruesos**
—	—	—	**Rasselgeräusche**	**or Crepitações grossas**	—	**or Estertores gruesos**
CONTINUOUS						
High pitched	Wheezes	*Râles sibilants*	*Pfeifen*	*Sibilos*	Свистящие хрипы (svistyashchiye khripy)	*Sibilancias*
—	—	**Sifflement or Sibilants**	**Giemen, Pfeifen or Juchzen**	**Sibilos**	—	**Sibilancias**
Low pitched	Rhonchus	*Râles ronflants*	*Brummen*	*Roncos*	Хрипы (khripy)	*Roncus*
—	—	**Râles bronchique or ronchi**	**Brummen**	**Roncos**	—	**Roncus**
—	—	—	—	—	—	—

Modified from Pasterkamp H, Brand PL, Everard M, et al. Towards the standardisation of lung sound nomenclature. *Eur Respir J.* 2016;47:724.

Table 1.2 Respiratory Sounds

Basic Sounds	Mechanisms	Origin	Acoustics	Relevance
Lung	Turbulent flow, vortices, other	Central (expiration), lobar to segmental airways (inspiration)	Low pass filtered noise (<100 to >1000 Hz)	Regional ventilation, airway caliber
Tracheal	Turbulent flow, flow impinging on airway walls	Pharynx, larynx, trachea, large airways	Noise with resonances (<100 to >3000 Hz)	Upper airway configuration
ADVENTITIOUS SOUNDS				
Wheezes	Airway wall flutter, vortex shedding, other	Central and lower airways	Sinusoidal (<100 to >1000 Hz, duration typically >80 ms)	Airway obstruction, flow limitation
Rhonchi	Rupture of fluid films, airway wall vibration	Larger airways	Series of rapidly dampened sinusoids (typically <300 Hz and duration <100 ms)	Secretions, abnormal airway collapsibility
Crackles	Airway wall stress-relaxation	Central and lower airways	Rapidly dampened wave deflections (duration typically <20 ms)	Airway closure, secretions

Modified from Pasterkamp H, Kraman SS, Wodicka GR. State of the art. Respiratory sounds—advances beyond the stethoscope. *Am J Respir Crit Care Med.* 1997;156:974-987.

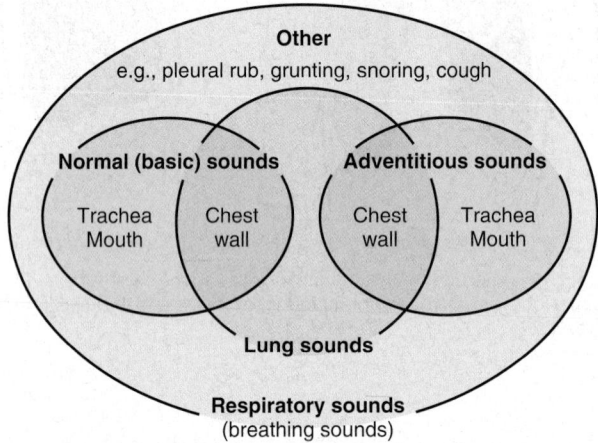

Fig. 1.11 Categories of respiratory sounds. (From Pasterkamp H, H, Brand PL, Everard M, et al. Towards the standardisation of lung sound nomenclature. *Eur Respir J.* 2016;47:724.)

and the latter as *crackles*. Furthermore, musical adventitious sounds or wheezes may be classified as high-pitched or low-pitched. Some use the term *rhonchus* for low-pitched wheezes (<200 Hz), whereas others describe the poorly characterized "secretion sounds," which share musical and nonmusical qualities, as *rhonchi*. Crackles are subclassified as fine or coarse. Basic normal sounds include tracheal and lung sounds. Adventitious sounds may be heard over the chest and sometimes also over the trachea or at the mouth (Fig. 1.11). Other respiratory sounds should be specified, such as pleural rubs, expiratory grunting, and inspiratory stridor. Historical terms such as *rales* should be abandoned, and flowery descriptions such as "raspy" or "blowing" breath sounds should not be used because these adjectives are even less well defined than the suggested terms.

Several auscultatory signs are based on the transmission of voice sounds. Speech sounds have a fundamental note of about 130 Hz in men and 230 Hz in women, with overtones from 400 to 3500 Hz. Vowels are produced when particular pairs of overtones or formants are generated. On passage through the lung, the higher-frequency formants are filtered, and speech heard over the chest becomes a meaningless mumble. With consolidation and transmission of higher-frequency components, however, speech may become intelligible. This occurs with normal speech (bronchophony) and with whispered voice (pectoriloquy). There may be a change in vowels from *e* to *a* over areas of lung consolidation. The acoustic basis for these phenomena is the same as for bronchial breath sounds. The American Thoracic Society and the American College of Chest Physicians recommend the term *egophony* for all of these findings.

TASTE AND SMELL

A complete physical examination extends beyond the perception of vision, hearing, and touch. Olfactory impressions should also be documented, even if they are subtle. Malodorous breath is easily noticed and may, particularly if chronic, indicate infection within the nasal or oral cavity (e.g., paranasal sinusitis), nasal foreign body, or dental abscess. *Extraoral halitosis* may also originate from intrathoracic infections, such as lung abscess or bronchiectasis, and it may also be noted in patients with GER. Nowadays physicians rarely use their taste buds to make a medical diagnosis. One particular disease of the respiratory tract in children, however, lends itself to gustatory diagnosis. Most often the discovery is made by the mother of a patient with cystic fibrosis who notices that the skin of her child tastes abnormally salty.

Common Signs and Symptoms of Chest Disease in Children

There are several common complaints and presentations of children with chest diseases that deserve a more detailed description. In particular, cough and sputum production, noisy breathing, wheezing, cyanosis, digital clubbing, cardiovascular signs, exercise limitation, dyspnea, and chest pain need to be discussed.

COUGH AND SPUTUM

Cough is not an illness by itself, but it is a cardinal manifestation in many chest diseases. Cough is probably the single most common complaint in children presenting to the physician and even in the absence of any underlying chronic lung pathology can cause children and their caregivers significant amounts of distress. The act of coughing is a reflex aimed at removal of mucus and other material from the airways that follows the stimulation of cough or irritant receptors. These receptors are located anywhere between the pharynx and the terminal bronchioles. They send their afferent impulses via branches of the glossopharyngeal and vagus nerves to the cough center in the upper brainstem and pons. The efferent signals travel from the cough center via vagus, phrenic, and spinal motor nerves to the larynx and diaphragm as well as to the muscles of the chest wall, abdomen, and pelvic floor. Cortical influences allow the voluntary initiation or suppression of cough (see Chapter 8).

There are three phases of coughing: (1) deep inspiration; (2) closure of the glottis, relaxation of the diaphragm, and contraction of expiratory muscles; and (3) sudden opening of the glottis. During the second phase, intrathoracic pressures up to 300 mm Hg can be generated and may be transmitted to the vascular and cerebrospinal spaces. Air flow velocity during the third phase is highest in the central airways and may reach three fourths the speed of sound. This speed depends on the sudden opening of the glottis and influences the success of expectoration. Patients with glottic dysfunction and those with tracheostomies may therefore have a less effective cough.

Stimuli that cause coughing may originate centrally, such as in psychogenic cough, or they may be pulmonary, located either in the major airways or in the pulmonary parenchyma. Also, cough can be provoked by nonpulmonary causes, such as irritation of pleura, diaphragm, or pericardium and even through stimulation of Arnold nerve (a branch of the vagus) by wax or foreign bodies in the external ear. Cough is part of the innate defense mechanism, and even a healthy child may cough several times a day. However, this cough should not be bothersome to the child, should disappear when the child is asleep and is frequently not noticed by families or children.

Acute cough is defined as lasting less than 3 weeks, while definitions of chronic cough vary from 4 to 8 weeks duration. The most frequent cause of acute cough is viral respiratory infections and these are usually self-resolving illnesses. In preschool children 50% will have their cough resolve within 10 days and 90% resolve by 25 days. On history there should be a clear viral prodrome associated, and while the symptoms may worsen during the first few days, the cough should be clearly improving with time. Postinfectious cough that lasts >3 weeks may be associated with mycoplasma or pertussis infections especially when there was a history of coughing paroxysms or posttussive emesis. It is important to note that children have on average of five to eight respiratory infections a year. Higher rates may be seen in the very young and in larger households and daycare settings. Children presenting with chronic cough may actually have symptoms from recurrent viral infections. For many parents, these episodes will blend together and they will report their child is "always coughing." Therefore a careful history is particularly important: is there a waxing and waning course of the cough? Is worsening associated with new onset of rhinorrhea? Are there are occasional symptom-free periods, for example, when

the child is away from the daycare during family vacations, or during summer. It is also important to have a complete history to exclude any specific disease pointers.

In assessing chronic cough, the detailed history should define the nature of the cough; whether it is dry, hacking, or brassy; and whether it is productive by sound and appearance. A wet sounding cough is reliably associated with large amounts of secretions on bronchoscopy. In young children, expectoration is unusual, but if observed, the quantity and quality of sputum should be noted. In particular, the physician should inquire about the color and odor of the expectorate and about the presence of blood in the sputum. The yellow-green color of purulent sputum results from the cellular breakdown of leukocytes and the liberation of myeloperoxidase from these cells. This finding indicates the retention of secretions and does not necessarily reflect an acute infection.

The timing of coughing is important, and its relationship to daily routines should be sought. Cough during or after drinking occurs with aspiration. Long-term chronic aspiration, especially in children with neurologic abnormalities, may take the form of silent aspiration. Clinicians should maintain an increased index of suspicion of chronic aspiration in children with neurodevelopmental abnormalities and those with syndromes associated with structural abnormalities, for example, tracheoesophageal fistula or laryngeal-esophageal clefts. Directly observing a feeding in clinic can provide valuable information. A cough that occurs after eating solids only may be associated with esophageal pathology such as eosinophilic esophagitis.

Coughing after a witnessed choking episode is highly suspicious for a retained foreign body aspiration. As foreign body aspirations, especially in preschool children, are often unwitnessed, the clinician should also consider this if there was a sudden onset to the cough or if the onset of cough in a previously healthy preschooler was not associated with signs of an upper respiratory tract infection.

A history of a cough that is progressively worsening or associated with weight loss, night sweats, and fevers may be related to significant infections such as mycobacterium tuberculosis or expanding malignancies compressing the trachea.

A chronic productive cough, especially if it is year-round or early in the morning is typical for bronchiectasis and related diseases such as cystic fibrosis (CF) and primary ciliary dyskinesia (PCD).

A cough with a neonatal onset can be associated with congenital infections, (e.g., chlamydia, especially if it has a staccato nature), with congenital airway or chest malformations (especially if there is an associated wheeze or stridor), and with recurrent aspiration or diseases such as CF and PCD. The latter especially is associated with an early onset of daily cough in the first 6 months of age and neonatal respiratory distress.

Nighttime cough may be related to asthma or to postnasal drip. Cough due to asthma is typically associated with a history of wheezing, with exertional symptoms, an atopic history, or a previous response to asthma medications. Seasonal worsening or coughing on exposure to potential allergens should be documented. In assessing nocturnal cough, the clinician should keep in mind that there is poor correlation between parental report and objective recordings of nocturnal cough. One factor that may influence this is the distance between the child and parents' bedrooms.

Cough that is associated with food regurgitation, throat clearing, supine position, or throat, chest or abdominal pain may be associated with GER. However, it is often the chronic respiratory symptoms that can worsen GER rather than vice versa.

Cough that is honking or loud, brassy and sometimes demonstrative in nature, and that resolves when the child is asleep, can be due to a psychogenic cough. An associated history of psychosocial stressors is important to obtain when considering this diagnosis.

Environmental factors can play an important role in the cause or exacerbation of a cough. The physician should ask about active and passive smoking, keeping in mind that, regrettably, there are quite a few children as young as 8 years of age who smoke regularly.

A detailed diary to note the frequency and timing of cough can be of value. When age appropriate, the patient should be encouraged to maintain the diary with the help of their caregiver as this appears to correlate better with objective measurement of cough.

Technology to record, quantify, and characterize cough is being developed. Some acoustic characteristics of cough are quite specific for certain diseases, such as the sound of a barking seal in viral croup or the whooping noise in pertussis. In patients with chronic cough, the physician should weigh the possible causes in view of their prevalence at different ages (Table 1.3). Also, complications of severe coughing paroxysms, such as pneumothorax, cough syncope, or nonsyncopal neurologic manifestations, should be considered. Regarding the last, the physician should inquire about lightheadedness, headache, visual disturbance, paresthesia, and tremor.

NOISY BREATHING

Quite frequently a child is brought to the physician's attention because of abnormal breathing noises. This noise may be a nonmusical hiss, much like the one produced in normal subjects at increased rates of ventilation, or it may have the musical qualities of stridor and snoring. Also, bubbling and crackling noises may be heard, and the tactile perception may contribute to the impression of a "rattly" chest in these patients.

The physician should focus attention on the noise-generating structures of the extrathoracic airways that are located at points of anatomic narrowing (e.g., the nasal vestibule, the posterior nasal orifices, and the glottis). The most common cause of noisy breathing in toddlers and young children is nasopharyngeal obstruction; in young infants, laryngomalacia is a leading cause. It is uncertain to what degree sounds from large intrathoracic airways contribute to the noise of breathing. Placing the stethoscope within the airstream in front of the mouth, one hears predominantly those sounds that are produced locally in the mouth and larynx. Noisy breathing is a common finding in patients with asthma and bronchitis and does not necessarily reflect intrathoracic airway pathology because the upper airways are also frequently affected in these patients.

To clarify the causes of noisy breathing, the parents or patient should describe their own perceptions of the noise: Does it occur during inspiration, expiration, or both? Is it just an exaggeration of the normal breath sound noise, or does it have musical qualities? Did an episode of choking precede the onset of noisy breathing? Is the abnormal sound more prominent during certain activities, such as exercise? At what times of day or night and in which body positions is it most noticeable? The physician should also inquire about associated cough, sputum production, and dyspnea.

Children may suffer from partial obstruction of the upper airways during sleep; complete obstruction, which is found in adult patients with sleep apnea, is less common. These children snore most nights, whereas normal children's snoring is largely confined to times of upper respiratory tract infection. Usually enlarged adenoids and tonsils cause the breathing disturbance. The physician should inquire about the typical signs and symptoms found in patients with increased work of breathing and abnormal sleep patterns at night (Box 1.1).

In the older child and adolescent, the physician should first inspect the nasal passageways and proceed to an examination of the oropharynx before auscultation of the neck and thorax. The acoustic signs should be checked while the patient breathes first with the mouth open, and then closed. In younger children, examination of the nose and mouth is unpopular and often results in agitation and crying. It is better to start with auscultation before inspection in these children. Noisy breathers should be examined when they are sitting or standing upright and when they are lying down because upper airway geometry is position-dependent and may influence the respiratory sounds. The examiner should also note abnormal crying or speech in the patient, as this may point to laryngeal disease.

WHEEZING

Wheezing is a common respiratory symptom and refers to musical, adventitious lung sounds that are often heard by the patient as well as the physician. When asking the patient or the parents about wheezing, one should keep in mind that the use of lung sound terminology among nonprofessionals is not better standardized than it is among health care providers. The physician should inquire about musical, whistling noises during breathing; audiovisual recordings of wheezy young children may help caregivers

Table 1.3   Causes of Chronic Cough

Infant	Preschool	School Age/ Adolescence
Congenital anomalies	Foreign body	Reactive
Tracheoesophageal fistula	Infections	Asthma
Neurologic impairment	Viral	Postnasal drip
Infections	Mycoplasma	Infections
Viral	Bacterial	Mycoplasma
Chlamydia	Reactive	Irritative
Bacterial (pertussis)	Asthma	Smoking
Cystic fibrosis	Cystic fibrosis	Air pollution
—	Irritative	Psychogenic
—	Passive smoking	—

Data modified from Eigen H. The clinical evaluation of chronic cough. *Pediatr Clin North Am.* 1982;29:67.

to identify abnormal respiratory findings. The video examples show different presentations of two wheezy young children (Videos 1.1 and 1.2).

Most typically, wheezing is associated with hyperreactive airway disease, but any critical narrowing of the airways can produce wheezing. Box 1.2 lists conditions with wheeze and other sounds that may be confused with wheeze. The wheezing that is typical in asthma originates from oscillations of airways at many sites. On auscultation, one hears many different tones simultaneously, which is called *polyphonic wheezing.* Obstruction of a single airway can produce a single monophonic wheeze or, in the obstruction of extrathoracic airways, stridor. Both inspiratory and expiratory wheezes are present in the majority of asthmatic patients. The audible expiratory phase (expirium) is typically prolonged because of wheezing. Objectively measured expiratory time (expiration), however, is rarely prolonged except in very severe airway obstruction. Under these circumstances, air flow is minimal, and thus wheezing is absent. Respiration becomes ominously silent, and the patient may have carbon dioxide retention and cyanosis. In less severe cases, however, the proportion of inspiration and expiration occupied by wheezing correlates to some extent with the degree of air flow obstruction. Objective and reproducible wheeze quantification can be achieved by computer-assisted techniques, but in practice the quantification of wheezing severity is made by subjective assessment at the bedside.

Wheezes are often high-pitched and will therefore attenuate during their passage through lung tissue, particularly if the lungs are hyperinflated. Auscultation over the neck may give a better impression of respiratory sounds and should be included as a part of the routine physical examination. Tracheal auscultation to determine if and when there is wheezing after methacholine inhalation challenge has been advocated instead of spirometry in young children being evaluated for bronchial hyperreactivity. However, wheezing may be absent even if airways become significantly obstructed during bronchial provocation (Fig. 1.12). In our experience, wheezing heard at the chest but not necessarily at the trachea is very suggestive of airway narrowing and hyperresponsiveness. Listening to respiratory sounds over the neck may help to identify patients who are thought to be asthmatic but who generate the wheezing noises solely in the larynx. These are usually older children and adolescents with vocal cord dysfunction.

CYANOSIS

Cyanosis refers to a blue color of the skin and mucous membranes due to excessive concentrations of reduced hemoglobin in capillary blood. The oxygen content of capillary blood is assumed to be midway between that of arterial and that of venous blood. Areas with a high blood flow and a small arteriovenous oxygen difference (e.g., the tongue and mucous membranes) will not become cyanotic as readily as those with a low blood flow and a large arteriovenous oxygen difference (e.g., the skin of cold hands and feet). A distinction is therefore made between peripheral cyanosis (acrocyanosis), which is confined to the skin of the extremities, and central cyanosis, which includes the tongue and mucous membranes. Circumoral cyanosis is not an expression of central cyanosis and is rarely pathologic. The absolute concentration of reduced hemoglobin in the capillaries that is necessary to produce cyanosis is between 4 and 6 g/100 mL of blood. This level is usually present when the concentration of reduced hemoglobin in arterial blood exceeds 3 g/100 mL. Clinical cyanosis will occur at different levels of arterial oxygen saturation, depending on the amount of total hemoglobin (Fig. 1.13).

Physiologically, five mechanisms can cause arterial hemoglobin desaturation in the patient who breathes room air at

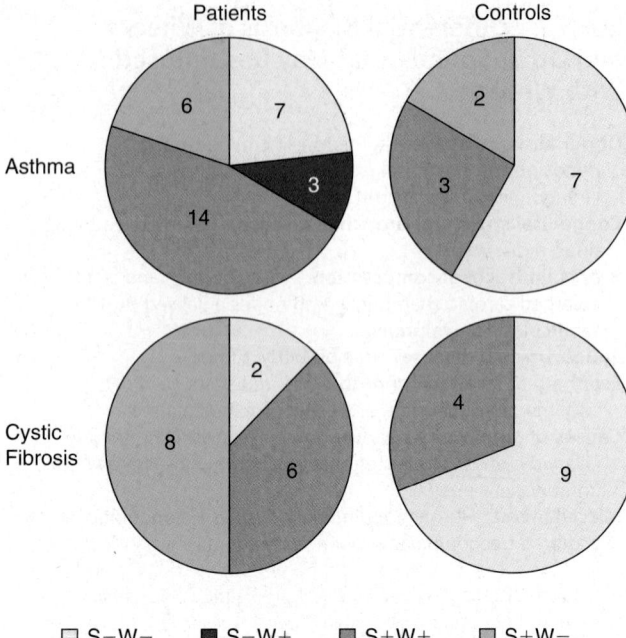

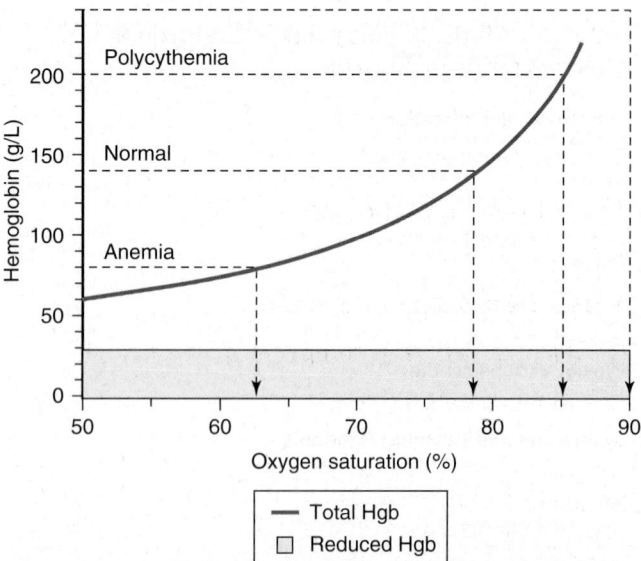

Fig. 1.13 Cyanosis requires at least 30 g/L of reduced hemoglobin (Hgb) in arterial blood or 4–6 g/100 mL in capillary blood. The arterial oxygen saturation (SaO₂) at which cyanosis occurs is dependent on the amount of total Hgb. As illustrated, a child with 30 g/L of Hgb plus 110 g/L of oxyhemoglobin has an SaO₂ of 78%. In the anemic patient (i.e., total Hgb of 80 g/L with Hgb of 30 g/L), SaO₂ will drop much lower (to less than 65% in this example) before cyanosis occurs, whereas in the patient with polycythemia (i.e., total Hgb of 200 g/L), cyanosis appears at a higher SaO₂ (85%).

Fig. 1.12 Summary of findings regarding wheeze as an indicator of significant flow obstruction during methacholine bronchial provocation in children. Negative responses (i.e., less than 20% decline in forced expiratory volume in 1 second at a dose of 8 mg/mL [spirometry] and no wheeze [acoustic monitoring]) are indicated by a minus sign, and positive responses are indicated by a plus sign. Note the low sensitivity of wheeze as an indicator of air flow obstruction, particularly in children with cystic fibrosis. *S*, Spirometry; *W*, wheezing. (Data from Sanchez I, Powell RE, Pasterkamp H. Wheezing and airflow obstruction during methacholine challenge in children with cystic fibrosis and in normal children. *Am Rev Respir Dis.* 1993;147:705, and Sanchez I, Avital A, Wong I, et al: Acoustic vs. spirometric assessment of bronchial responsiveness to methacholine in children. *Pediatr Pulmonol.* 1993;15:28.)

normal altitude: (1) alveolar hypoventilation, (2) diffusion impairment, (3) right-to-left shunting, (4) mismatch of ventilation and perfusion, and (5) inadequate oxygen transport by hemoglobin. Clinically, diffusion impairment is of little importance as a single cause. Imbalance of ventilation and perfusion is by far the most common mechanism and is correctable by administration of 100% oxygen. The physician should therefore look for a change in cyanosis while the patient breathes oxygen.

Observer agreement regarding cyanosis was found to range from poor when assessing acrocyanosis to very good in the evaluation of young children with bronchiolitis. To minimize the variability of this finding, cyanosis is best observed under daylight and with the patient resting in a comfortably warm room. The distribution of cyanosis and the state of peripheral perfusion should be noted. Patients with decreased cardiac output and poor peripheral perfusion can be cyanotic despite normal arterial hemoglobin saturation. Some patients may become cyanotic only during exercise, a common response when restrictive lung disease reduces the pulmonary capillary bed and the transit time of erythrocytes becomes too short for full saturation to occur during episodes of increased cardiac output. Congenital heart disease in infants may lead to differential cyanosis, which affects only the lower part of the body (e.g., in patients with preductal coarctation of the aorta). Less commonly, only the upper part of the body is

cyanotic (e.g., in patients with transposition of the great arteries in association with patent ductus arteriosus, and pulmonary to aortic shunting).

The clinical impression of cyanosis is usually confirmed by an arterial blood gas analysis or, more commonly, by pulse oximetry. Pulse oximetry, however, will not take into account the presence of abnormal hemoglobin. For example, in methemoglobinemia the oxygen-carrying capacity of blood is reduced and patients may appear lavender blue, but pulse oximetry may overestimate oxygen saturation in arterial blood (SaO₂). The blood of newborn infants, conversely, can be well saturated and not cyanotic at lower arterial oxygen tensions because of the different oxygen-binding curve of fetal hemoglobin. In the patient with hypoxemia who does not present with cyanosis (e.g., the anemic patient), the physician has to pay particular attention to other clinical signs and symptoms of hypoxia. These include tachypnea and tachycardia, exertional dyspnea, hypertension, headache, and behavioral changes. With more severe hypoxia, there may be visual disturbance, somnolence, hypotension, and ultimately coma. In addition, the patient may have an elevated level of carbon dioxide. Depending on how rapidly and to what extent the level of carbon dioxide has risen, the clinical signs of hypercarbia will largely reflect vascular dilatation. These signs include flushed, hot hands and feet; bounding pulses; confusion or drowsiness; muscular twitching; engorged retinal veins; and, in the most severe cases, papilledema and coma.

DIGITAL CLUBBING

Digital clubbing refers to a focal enlargement of the connective tissue in the terminal phalanges of fingers and toes, most noticeably on their dorsal surfaces. This sign was first described by Hippocrates, and the term *Hippocratic fingers* is used by some to denote simple digital clubbing. The pathogenesis of clubbing is still not entirely clear. Vascular endothelial growth factor (VEGF) from the continued impaction of shunted megakaryocytes and platelets in the digital vasculature, potentiated by hypoxia, is considered to drive the cellular and stromal changes in clubbing. Enhanced VEGF expression is a common finding in various diseases that are associated with digital clubbing. Aside from VEGF, platelet-derived growth factor may contribute to the stromal changes, including the maturation of new microvessels.

Clubbing of the digits may be idiopathic, acquired, or hereditary. Cystic fibrosis, bronchiectasis, and empyema are the most common pulmonary causes of acquired digital clubbing in children. Clubbing is also seen infrequently in extrinsic allergic vasculitis, pulmonary arteriovenous malformations, bronchiolitis obliterans, sarcoidosis, and chronic asthma. Box 1.3 shows a list of nonpulmonary diseases associated with clubbing. A systemic disorder of bones, joints, and soft tissues known as *hypertrophic osteoarthropathy* (HOA) includes digital clubbing. Abnormal metabolism of prostaglandin E$_2$ has been suggested as the cause of digital clubbing in these patients. In the majority of cases, HOA is associated with bronchogenic carcinoma and other intrathoracic neoplasms, but the pediatrician may see HOA in patients with severe cystic fibrosis or chronic empyema and lung abscess. In addition to clubbing, these patients may have periosteal thickening; symmetric arthritis of ankles, knees, wrists, and elbows; neurovascular changes of hands and feet; and increased thickness of subcutaneous soft tissues in the distal portions of arms and legs. The primary idiopathic or hereditary form of HOA—pachydermoperiostosis—appears with prominent furrowing of the forehead and scalp. Approximately half of the reported cases have a positive family history. Genetic studies suggest an autosomal-dominant inheritance with variable expression and a predilection for males.

Digital clubbing is not only an important indicator of pulmonary disease but also may reflect the progression or resolution of the causative process. Pulmonary abscess and empyema may lead to digital clubbing over the course of only a few weeks. In this case, clubbing will resolve if effective treatment is instituted before connective tissue changes become fixed. Interestingly, even long-standing finger clubbing seems to resolve in patients after successful heart and lung transplantation. In patients with cystic fibrosis, progression of finger clubbing suggests a suboptimal control of chest infections. It is therefore useful to quantify the degree of digital clubbing. Measurements have focused on the hyponychial (Lovibond) angle and on the phalangeal depth ratio (Fig. 1.14). Computerized analysis from digital photographs has provided information on the distribution of the hyponychial angle in healthy subjects and in patients with various diseases. Almost 80% of adult patients with cystic fibrosis have a hyponychial angle greater than 190 degrees, the upper limit of normal.

For routine clinical practice, the sign described by Schamroth, a cardiologist who developed finger clubbing during several attacks of infective endocarditis, is a most useful method of measuring finger clubbing (see Fig. 1.14). Another way is to place a plastic caliper with minimal pressure over the interphalangeal joint. If it is easy to slide the caliper from this joint across the nail fold, the distal phalangeal diameter to interphalangeal diameter ratio must be less than 1, and the patient has no clubbing.

Box 1.3 Nonpulmonary Diseases Associated With Clubbing

Cardiac

Cyanotic congenital heart disease
Subacute bacterial endocarditis
Chronic congestive heart failure

Hematologic

Thalassemia
Congenital methemoglobinemia (rare)

Gastrointestinal

Crohn disease
Ulcerative colitis
Chronic dysentery, sprue
Polyposis coli
Severe gastrointestinal hemorrhage
Small bowel lymphoma
Liver cirrhosis (including α$_1$-antitrypsin deficiency)

Other

Thyroid deficiency (thyroid acropachy)
Chronic pyelonephritis (rare)
Toxic (e.g., arsenic, mercury, beryllium)
Lymphomatoid granulomatosis
Fabry disease
Raynaud disease, scleroderma

Unilateral Clubbing

Vascular disorders (e.g., subclavian arterial aneurysm, brachial arteriovenous fistula)
Subluxation of shoulder
Median nerve injury
Local trauma

CARDIOVASCULAR SIGNS

Pulmonary heart disease, or *cor pulmonale*, is a consequence of acute or chronic pulmonary hypertension and appears as right ventricular enlargement. The progression of chronic cor pulmonale to ultimate right ventricular failure is accompanied by certain physical signs. Initially, the right ventricular systolic pressure and muscle mass increase as pulmonary artery pressure rises. During this stage, cardiac auscultation may be normal or may reveal an increased pulmonary component of the second heart sound, caused by an increase in diastolic pulmonary arterial pressure. The physician should look for a parasternal right ventricular heave. As pulmonary hypertension progresses, there is an increase in right ventricular end-diastolic volume. Dilation of the main pulmonary artery and right ventricular outflow tract lead to systolic pulmonary ejection clicks and murmurs. Diastolic murmurs appear when pulmonary or tricuspid valves or both become insufficient. Third and fourth heart sounds at the left lower sternal border are signs of decreased right ventricular compliance. Most of these right-sided cardiovascular

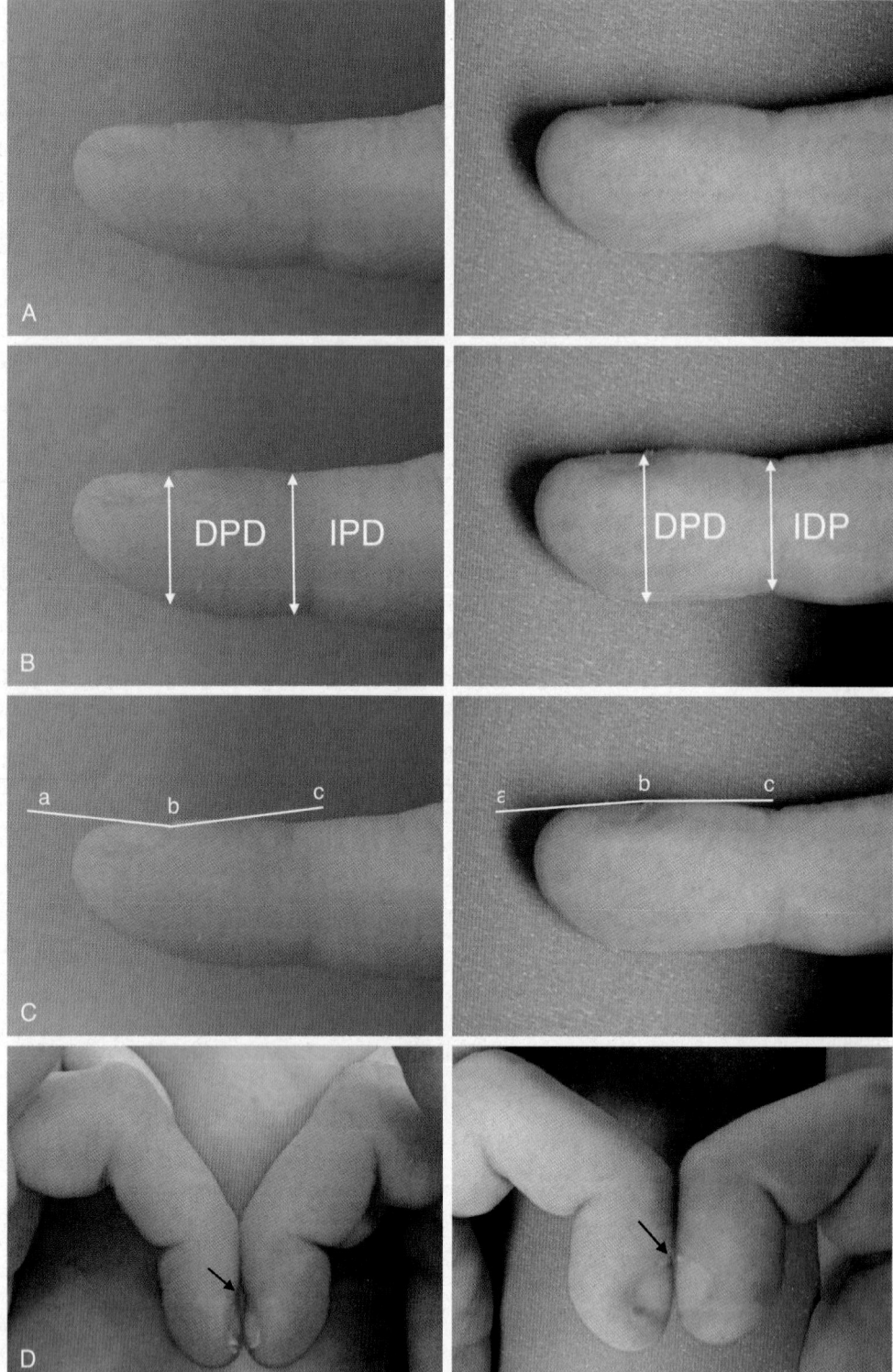

Fig. 1.14 (A) Normal and clubbed finger viewed in profile. (B) The normal finger demonstrates a distal phalangeal finger depth (DPD)/interphalangeal finger depth (IPD) ratio <1. The clubbed finger demonstrates a DPD/IPD ratio >1. (C) The normal finger on the left demonstrates a normal profile (abc) with angle less then 180°. The clubbed finger demonstrates a profile angle >180°. (D) Schamroth sign is demonstrated in the clubbed finger with the loss of diamond shape window in between finger beds that is demonstrated in the normal finger.

findings are accentuated during inspiration, which augments venous return. Finally, cardiac output falls while end-diastolic pressure and volume increase further in the failing right ventricle.

Clinical findings at this stage include hepatic engorgement, jugular venous distention, and peripheral edema. Occasionally, there may be cyanosis and intracardiac right-to-left shunting through a patent foramen ovale. The physician should exclude the possibility of congenital cardiac defects or acquired left-sided heart disease before making the diagnosis of cor pulmonale. Hyperinflation of the lungs should be taken into account as a cause of the attenuation of cardiovascular sounds and the lowering of the subcostal liver margin, which may be misinterpreted as hepatic enlargement.

Complete assessment of the cardiovascular system includes careful auscultation, and palpation of the pulse to detect cardiac arrhythmia. This problem is common in patients with chronic lung disease and may appear as sinus or paroxysmal supraventricular tachycardia, atrial premature contractions, or ventricular ectopic beats. Causes include hypoxemia, acid-base imbalance, and enlargement of the right heart; effects of common drugs such as aminophylline, beta sympathomimetics, or diuretics should not be overlooked.

During quiet spontaneous respiration, there is a phasic variation of arterial blood pressure. The widening of this normal respiratory variation is known as *pulsus paradoxus*. Increased respiratory resistance may exaggerate the normal inspiratory-expiratory difference in left ventricular stroke volume. This is mediated by effects of intrathoracic pressures on ventricular preload. Clinically, pulsus paradoxus is first assessed by palpation of the radial pulse and then it is measured at the brachial artery with a sphygmomanometer as the difference in systolic pressure between inspiration and expiration. The pressure cuff is deflated from above systolic level, and the highest pressure during expiration at which systolic pulse sounds are heard is recorded. Similarly, the highest pressure at which every pulse is just audible throughout inspiration is also noted. In general, a drop of greater than 10 mm Hg during inspiration is taken as clinically significant, but only a severe paradox of greater than 24 mm Hg is a reliable indicator of severe asthma. The poor correlation between pulsus paradoxus and objective measurements of air flow obstruction may be explained by other factors that affect pleural pressure swings (e.g., the degree of pulmonary hyperinflation and the air flow rate). Furthermore, the accurate measurement of pulsus paradoxus is a challenge in tachypneic, tachycardic, and uncooperative young children. A work group of the British Thoracic Society Standards of Care Committee found pulsus paradoxus to be absent in one-third of patients with the most severe obstruction. In contrast to North American practice guidelines, it was therefore recommended that pulsus paradoxus be abandoned as an indicator of severity of asthma attack. In children, wheeze seems to be the clinical parameter of respiratory severity scores that correlates best with pulsus paradoxus, most likely because wheeze requires critical intrathoracic pressures. The application of pulse oximetry to view dynamic changes in the area under the plethysmographic waveform in relation to pulsus paradoxus shows some promise in improving the diagnostic value of this clinical sign.

EXERCISE LIMITATION AND DYSPNEA

Reduced performance on physical exertion is another frequent cause for consultation with a pediatric pulmonologist. Frequently this will be in the context of a child who has difficulty keeping up with his peers and may have many other associated symptoms such as coughing and wheezing.

Dyspnea refers to the subjective perception of difficulty breathing. While there are well-established scoring systems for dyspnea in adult subjects, there are few validated assessment tools for children and adolescents. Pictorial scales may help in documenting and following dyspnea in the young patient (Fig. 1.15).

The most common cause for exertional dyspnea appears to be physiologic limitation. This includes children and adolescents who are deconditioned, have a sedentary lifestyle, and is often associated with obesity. The symptoms typically worsen with increasing exertion and improve rapidly with rest. Although chest pain may be present, cough and wheeze are rarely associated with this. This may also occur in adolescents with normal or above-average cardiovascular conditioning. Often these are motivated children who are unable to keep up with other more "elite" athletes. This can also be seen in children who previously were competing at a high level but on entering adolescence there begins an increasing separation from the elite athletes and other children. They may start to no longer keep up with other children at their level of competition and thereby disappoint not only their own expectations but also those of their parents. Vocal cord dysfunction may be seen in this population as well. Symptoms of stridor and voice changes may be present. However, some children may have symptoms difficult to distinguish from true asthma during these episodes.

Asthma and exercise-induced bronchospasm are a common cause of dyspnea and these are frequently associated with coughing, wheezing, and dyspnea or chest pain. The symptoms may continue to worsen after the child stops the exertion. This can often be the presenting feature of poorly controlled asthma. The more detailed history will elucidate symptoms of persistent asthma, for example, nocturnal coughing or prolonged cough, wheeze with viral illnesses, and an atopic history. There is also evidence that exercise-induced bronchospasm is more common in elite athletes, especially performing endurance and cold weather sports.

Cardiac causes for exertional dyspnea in children are quite rare. A history of congenital or acquired heart disease should raise suspicion. Other cardiac etiologies accounting for dyspnea may include conduction abnormalities, pulmonary hypertension, congestive heart failure, valvular disease, and myocarditis. Associated but nonspecific symptoms may include palpitations, diaphoresis, and severe chest pain.

Exertional limitation can also be seen with chronic lung diseases, for example, cystic fibrosis or bronchopulmonary dysplasia. Airway abnormalities, for example, tracheomalacia or vascular ring abnormalities are also frequently associated with exertional limitation. Finally, children with myopathies and other neuromuscular disorders may have exercise intolerance, not associated with dyspnea, as an early symptom. A careful exploration of triggers leading to the limitation and of other signs of muscle weakness is helpful.

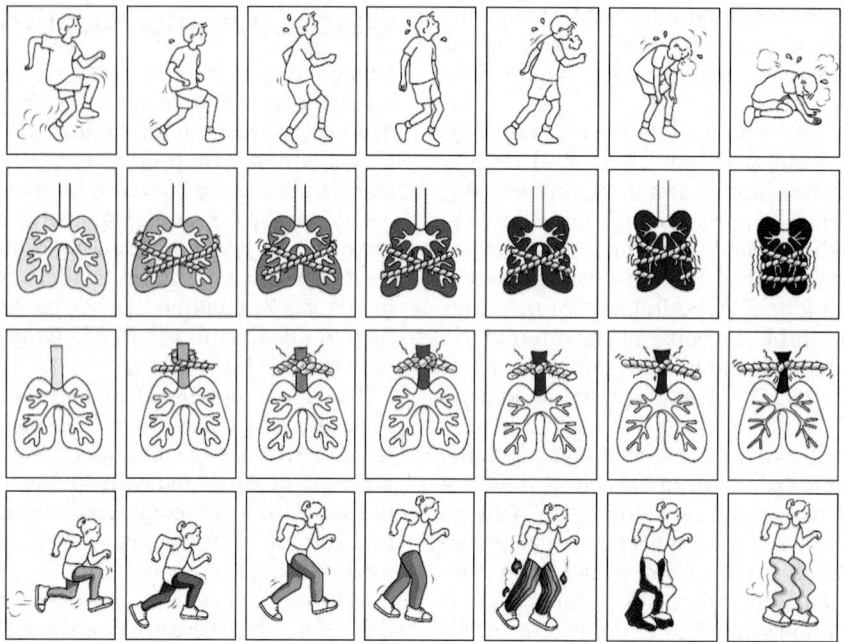

Fig. 1.15 Pictorial scales of perceived breathlessness. These Dalhousie Dyspnea Scales have interval scale characteristics that allow measurements of breathlessness in children more than 8 years old. (McGrath PJ, Pianosi PT, Unruh AM, et al. Dalhousie dyspnea scales: construct and content validity of pictorial scales for measuring dyspnea. *BMC Pediatr.* 2005;5:1)

CHEST PAIN

Chest pain is relatively common in older children and adolescents but may also be present in younger children. The occurrence rate in an emergency department approaches 2.5 per 1000 patient visits, and chest pain accounts for an estimated 650,000 physician visits of patients between 10 and 21 years of age annually in the United States. Chest pain in children is most often benign and self-limited. Typical origins are musculoskeletal problems and idiopathic, dysfunctional, and psychogenic causes (Box 1.4). Younger children have underlying cardiorespiratory problems more frequently, whereas children older than 12 years of age are more likely to have a psychogenic or musculoskeletal cause.

The history is most important in the assessment of these patients who usually have few physical findings and rarely any laboratory data of diagnostic value. The physician should recognize a clinical profile suggestive of psychogenic pain but should also keep in mind that psychogenic and organic causes are not mutually exclusive. A substantial number of patients have a family history of chest pain. Parents of younger children should explain how they know that their child is in pain. It is important to determine whether sleep is affected, because organic pain is more likely than psychogenic pain to awaken the patient or to prevent the child from falling asleep. A close inspection and careful palpation of the chest and abdomen are essential. Common abnormal findings include chest wall tenderness, fever, or both. The physician should use pressure on the stethoscope to elicit local tenderness while the patient is distracted by the auscultation.

In general, the presence of systemic signs such as weight loss, anorexia, or syncopal attacks will direct the attention to organic causes of chest pain in children. Diffuse, deep, substernal, and epigastric pains are likely to be visceral, originating in the thorax if the pain affects dermatomes T1 to T4 and in the diaphragm or abdomen if it affects dermatomes T5 to T8.

The duration of symptoms may be an indicator. Acute, short-lasting pain is more likely to be organic and localized; sharp, and superficial pains suggest an origin in the chest wall. Costochondritis is associated with pain localized to a specific area of the chest that can be reproduced on palpation. There are no associated inflammatory signs and it often follows episodes of severe coughing or chest trauma. Conversely, Tietze syndrome, also known as costochondral junction syndrome, has similar symptoms to costochondritis but is also associated with signs of inflammation such as warmth and redness over the affected joint. It often has a postinfectious etiology. Precordial Catch Syndrome presents with a localized sudden onset that will last several seconds to several minutes followed by complete resolution. It occurs more commonly on the left side. Theorized etiologies include a pinching of the nerve and local muscle spasms. Recent trauma may also lead to chest pain through fractured ribs, muscle bruising, and/or a pneumothorax. Slipping rib syndrome involves irritation of the intercostal nerve slipping under an adjacent floating rib (8th, 9th, and 10th). There is often a history of clicking of the rib. A hooking maneuver in which the physician places his fingers under the lower costal margin at the mid axillary line and lifts anteriorly, reproducing a "click" and the pain, is diagnostic.

Pain that is longer in duration and vague or changing in description is more likely psychogenic in nature. Psychogenic pain may be worse with stressful events and associated symptoms such as headaches and abdominal pains. A detailed social history including family and school situations is important. A history of hyperventilating and/or dizziness of feeling light headed may suggest disordered breathing and/or anxiety disorders.

Box 1.4   Causes of Chest Pain in Children

Thorax

Costochondritis
Tietze syndrome
Muscular disease
Precordial catch
Trauma
Connective tissue disorders
Xiphoid-cartilage syndrome
Rib tip syndrome
Leukemia
Herpes zoster
Breast development or disease (e.g., gynecomastia, mastitis)

Lungs, Pleura, and Diaphragm

Asthma
Cystic fibrosis
Infection (e.g., bronchitis, pneumonia, epidemic pleurodynia)
Inhalation of irritants (e.g., chemical pneumonitis, smoking)
Stitch (associated with exercise)
Foreign body
Pneumothorax
Pleural disease (e.g., pleurisy, effusion)
Diaphragmatic irritation (e.g., subphrenic abscess, gastric distention)
Sickle cell anemia

Cardiovascular System

Structural lesions (e.g., mitral valve prolapse, idiopathic hypertrophic subaortic stenosis [IHSS], coronary disease)
Acquired cardiac disease (e.g., carditis, arteritis, tumor involvement)
Arrhythmia

Esophagus

Gastroesophageal reflux
Foreign body
Achalasia

Vertebral Column

Deformities (e.g., scoliosis)
Vertebral collapse

Psychogenic Causes

Anxiety
Hyperventilation
Unresolved grief
Identification with another person suffering chest pain

Respiratory causes of chest pain are also frequent. Asthma, pneumonia, pleural effusions, and pneumothoraxes can all present with chest pain, although they often have other associated symptoms. Cardiac causes of pain are rare. However, in up to 50% of adolescents seeking medical attention for chest pain, the major worry for the families is a possible cardiac etiology. Pericarditis will be associated with fever and a friction rub. The chest pain is more constant and radiates to the left shoulder and it worsens with deep breathing and lying down. Arrhythmias may be associated with other symptoms such as palpitations, dyspnea, nausea, and fatigue. Cardiac murmurs with or without a midsystolic click may be found in patients with mitral valve prolapse, but this condition is rarely associated with chest pain, at least in children. More commonly, there are noncardiac causes of chest pain in children with mitral valve prolapse (e.g., orthopedic or gastroesophageal disorders).

Pulmonary emboli frequently have a sudden onset of pain and associated dyspnea and tachycardia. However, associated symptoms in children may be minimal even in the presence of a large embolus. A recent history of starting an oral contraceptive should raise the suspicion.

Gastrointestinal causes are also rare causes of chest pain in children. GER with or without esophagitis may produce retrosternal pain and is often associated with eating. Epigastric pain may be indicative of peptic ulcers. Diaphragmatic transmitted pain may also occur from abdominal pathologies such as pancreatitis.

Idiopathic chest pain is a common final diagnosis in many reported prospective and retrospective series in which there is no final diagnosis identified.

Conclusion

In pediatric respiratory medicine, the most common clinical presentation is that of a child who coughs or wheezes, or both. Depending on the geographic location, the information gathered from the history and physical examination will carry different weights in the initial diagnostic approach. Pneumonia kills more children than any other disease. In countries with high morbidity and mortality from lower respiratory tract infections, assessment of children who cough will therefore initially focus on the possibility of pneumonia. A constellation of physical findings—particularly fever, tachypnea and retractions, nasal flaring in infants younger than 1 year of age, and history of poor feeding—increase the likelihood that the child has pneumonia. Any single clinical finding by itself, however, is not useful as a predictor.

Concurrent wheezing is more common in viral than in bacterial infections and a history of preceding similar events and of improvement after bronchodilator inhalation can lead to different first steps in treatment. In most Western countries, the likelihood of bacterial pneumonia in a child who presents with cough with or without wheeze is lower, while asthma or prolonged symptoms after viral infections of the lower respiratory tract are common. Recurrent wheezing is particularly prevalent; up to 40% of children will present with wheezing during their first year of life but less than one-third of these will have asthma when they reach school age. If the parents of a child younger than 3 years of age who only wheezes with colds do not have asthma or eczema and if the child does not have allergic rhinitis, the negative predictive value of this history is close to 90% with regard to having asthma by the age of school entry.

At school age, functional respiratory assessment by spirometry is generally possible. It is therefore surprising that only a minority of children with asthma symptoms will have lung functions tests. It would be comforting if this could be explained by a superiority of history and physical examination to detect abnormalities. However, the physician should recognize limitations of any component in the diagnostic workup. Only then can the value of a detailed history and a skillfully performed physical examination be appreciated.

Suggested Reading

General Reading

Bastir M, Martínez DG, Recheis W, et al. Differential growth and development of the upper and lower human thorax. *PLoS ONE*. 2013;8:e75128.

Benbassat J, Baumal R. Narrative review: should teaching of the respiratory physical examination be restricted only to signs with proven reliability and validity? *J Gen Intern Med*. 2010;25:865.

Bonafide CP, Brady PW, Keren R, et al. Development of heart and respiratory rate percentile curves for hospitalized children. *Pediatrics*. 2013; 131:e1150.

Britton JR, Britton HL, Jennett R, et al. Weight, length, head and chest circumference at birth in Phoenix, Arizona. *J Reprod Med*. 1993;38:215.

Carse EA, Wilkinson AR, Whyte PL, et al. Oxygen and carbon dioxide tensions, breathing and heart rate in normal infants during the first six months of life. *J Dev Physiol*. 1981;3:85.

Chaaban MR, Walsh EM, Woodworth BA. Epidemiology and differential diagnosis of nasal polyps. *Am J Rhinol Allergy*. 2013;27:473.

DeGroodt EG, van Pelt W, Borsboom GJ, et al. Growth of lung and thorax dimensions during the pubertal growth spurt. *Eur Respir J*. 1988;1:102.

Edmonds ZV, Mower WR, Lovato LM, et al. The reliability of vital sign measurements. *Ann Emerg Med*. 2002;39:233.

Feingold M, Bossert WH. Normal values for selected physical parameters. *Birth Defects Orig Artic Ser*. 1974;10:14.

Gadomski AM, Permutt T, Stanton B. Correcting respiratory rate for the presence of fever. *J Clin Epidemiol*. 1994;47:1043.

Gagliardi L, Rusconi F. Respiratory rate and body mass in the first three years of life. The working party on respiratory rate. *Arch Dis Child*. 1997;76:151.

Gilmartin JJ, Gibson GJ. Mechanisms of paradoxical rib cage motion in patients with chronic obstructive pulmonary disease. *Am Rev Respir Dis*. 1986;134:683.

Haight JS, Cole P. The site and function of the nasal valve. *Laryngoscope*. 1983;93:49.

Hierholzer E, Schier F. Rasterstereography in the measurement and postoperative follow-up of anterior chest wall deformities. *Z Kinderchir*. 1986;41:267.

Kerem E, Canny G, Reisman J, et al. Clinical-physiologic correlations in acute asthma of childhood. *Pediatrics*. 1991;87:481.

Lees MH. Cyanosis of the newborn infant. *J Pediatr*. 1970;77:484.

Light JS. Respiratory shift in epigastric abdominal wall—a physical sign seen with complete unilateral paralysis of the diaphragm in infants and children. *J Pediatr*. 1944;24:627.

Margolis P, Gadomski A. Does this infant have pneumonia? *JAMA*. 1998;279:308.

McGee S. *Evidence-Based Physical Diagnosis*. 3rd ed. Elsevier Health Sciences; 2012.

Peters RM, Peters BA, Benirschke SK, et al. Chest dimensions in young adults with spontaneous pneumothorax. *Ann Thorac Surg*. 1978;25:193.

Rambaud-Althaus C, Althaus F, Genton B, et al. Clinical features for diagnosis of pneumonia in children younger than 5 years: a systematic review and meta-analysis. *Lancet Infect Dis*. 2015;15:439.

Staats BA, Bonekat HW, Harris CD, et al. Chest wall motion in sleep apnoea. *Am Rev Respir Dis*. 1984;130:59.

Stinson S. The physical growth of high altitude Bolivian Aymara children. *Am J Phys Anthropol*. 1980;52:377.

Swartz MH. *Textbook of Physical Diagnosis. History and Examination*. 4th ed. Philadelphia: WB Saunders; 2001.

Tangerman A, Winkel E. Extra-oral halitosis: an overview. *J Breath Res*. 2010;4:017003.

Taylor JA, Del Beccaro M, Done S, et al. Establishing clinically relevant standards for tachypnea in febrile children younger than 2 years. *Arch Pediatr Adolesc Med*. 1995;149:283.

Usen S, Webert M. Clinical signs of hypoxaemia in children with acute lower respiratory infection. Indicators of oxygen therapy. *Int J Tuberc Lung Dis*. 2001;5:505.

Warwick WJ, Hansen L. Chest calipers for measurement of the thoracic index. *Clin Pediatr (Phila)*. 1976;15:735.

Watkin SL, Spencer SA, Pryce A, et al. Temporal relationship between pauses in nasal airflow and desaturation in preterm infants. *Pediatr Pulmonol*. 1996;21:171.

Respiratory Sounds

Bohadana A, Izbicki G, Kraman SS. Fundamentals of lung auscultation. *N Engl J Med*. 2014;370:744.

Brockmann PE, Urschitz MS, Schlaud M, et al. Primary snoring in school children: prevalence and neurocognitive impairments. *Sleep Breath*. 2012;16:23.

Falconer A, Oldman C, Helms P. Poor agreement between reported and recorded nocturnal cough in asthma. *Pediatr Pulmonol*. 1993;15: 209.

Gavriely N, Palti Y, Alroy G, et al. Measurement and theory of wheezing breath sounds. *J Appl Physiol*. 1984;57:481.

Hopkins RL. Differential auscultation of the acutely ill patient. *Ann Emerg Med*. 1985;14:589.

Kiyokawa H, Greenberg M, Shirota K, et al. Auditory detection of simulated crackles in breath sounds. *Chest*. 2001;119:1886.

Morrison RB. Post-effort breath sound. *Tex Med*. 1971;67:72.

Pasterkamp H, Kraman SS, Wodicka GR. Respiratory sounds. Advances beyond the stethoscope. *Am J Respir Crit Care Med*. 1997;156:974.

Pasterkamp H, Brand PL, Everard M, et al. Towards the standardisation of lung sound nomenclature. *Eur Respir J*. 2016;47:724.

Yernault JC, Bohadana AB. Chest percussion. *Eur Respir J*. 1995;8:1756.

Pulsus Paradoxus

Arnold DH, Jenkins CA, Hartert TV. Noninvasive assessment of asthma severity using pulse oximeter plethysmograph estimate of pulsus paradoxus physiology. *BMC Pulm Med*. 2010;10:17–24.

Frey B, Freezer N. Diagnostic value and pathophysiologic basis of pulsus paradoxus in infants and children with respiratory disease. *Pediatr Pulmonol*. 2001;31:138.

Pearson MG, Spence DP, Ryland I, et al. Value of pulsus paradoxus in assessing acute severe asthma. British Thoracic Society Standards of Care Committee. *BMJ*. 1993;307:659.

Digital Clubbing

Atkinson S, Fox SB. Vascular endothelial growth factor (VEGF)-A and platelet-derived growth factor (PDGF) play a central role in the pathogenesis of digital clubbing. *J Pathol*. 2004;203:721.

Augarten A, Goldman R, Laufer J, et al. Reversal of digital clubbing after lung transplantation in cystic fibrosis patients. A clue to the pathogenesis of clubbing. *Pediatr Pulmonol*. 2002;34:378.

Coggins KG, Coffman TM, Koller BH. The Hippocratic finger points the blame at PGE2. *Nat Genet*. 2008;40:691.

Husarik D, Vavricka SR, Mark M, et al. Assessment of digital clubbing in medical inpatients by digital photography and computerized analysis. *Swiss Med Wkly*. 2002;132:132.

Martinez-Lavin M. Exploring the cause of the most ancient clinical sign of medicine: finger clubbing. *Semin Arthritis Rheum*. 2007;36:380.

Myers KA, Farquhar DR. Does this patient have clubbing? *JAMA*. 2001;286:341.

Nakamura CT, Ng GY, Paton JY, et al. Correlation between digital clubbing and pulmonary function in cystic fibrosis. *Pediatr Pulmonol*. 2002;33:332.

Schamroth L. Personal experience. *S Afr Med J*. 1976;50:297.

Van Ginderdeuren F, Van Cauwelaert K, Malfroot A. Influence of digital clubbing on oxygen saturation measurements by pulse-oximetry in cystic fibrosis patients. *J Cyst Fibros*. 2006;5:125.

Cough and Wheezing

Altiner A, Wilm S, Däubener W, et al. Sputum colour for diagnosis of a bacterial infection in patients with acute cough. *Scand J Prim Health Care*. 2009;27:70–73.

Bush A, Nagakumar P. Preschool wheezing phenotypes. *EMJ*. 2016;1:93.

Chang AB, Gaffney JT, Eastburn MM, et al. Cough quality in children: a comparison of subjective vs. bronchoscopic findings. *Respir Res*. 2005;6:1.

Chang AB, Robertson CF, van Asperen PP, et al. A cough algorithm for chronic cough in children: a multicenter, randomized controlled study. *Pediatrics*. 2013;131:e1576.

Lalloo UG, Barnes PJ, Chung KF. Pathophysiology and clinical presentations of cough. *J Allergy Clin Immunol*. 1996;98(suppl):91.

Leonardi NA, Spycher BD, Strippoli M-PF, et al. Validation of the Asthma Predictive Index and comparison with simpler clinical prediction rules. *J Allergy Clin Immunol*. 2011;127:1466.

Mountain RD, Sahn SA. Clinical features and outcome in patients with acute asthma presenting with hypercapnia. *Am Rev Respir Dis*. 1988;138:535.

Munyard P, Bush A. How much coughing is normal? *Arch Dis Child*. 1996;74:531.

Pasterkamp H. Acoustic markers of airway responses during inhalation challenge in children. *Pediatr Pulmonol Suppl*. 2004;26:175.

Rempel G, Borton B, Esselmont E, et al. Is aspiration during swallowing more common in Canadian children with indigenous heritage? *Pediatr Pulmonol.* 2011;46:1240.

Shim CS, Williams MH. Relationship of wheezing to the severity of asthma. *Arch Intern Med.* 1983;143:890.

Stern RC, Horwitz SJ, Doershuk CF. Neurologic symptoms during coughing paroxysms in cystic fibrosis. *J Pediatr.* 1988;112:909.

Thompson M, Vodicka TA, Blair PS, et al. Duration of symptoms of respiratory tract infections in children: systematic review. *BMJ.* 2013;347:f7027.

Chest Pain

Owen TR. Chest pain in the adolescent. *Adolesc Med.* 2001;12:95.

Selbst SM, Ruddy R, Clark BJ. Chest pain in children. Follow-up of patients previously reported. *Clin Pediatr (Phila).* 1990;29:374.

Woolf PK, Gewitz MH, Berezin S, et al. Noncardiac chest pain in adolescents and children with mitral valve prolapse. *J Adolesc Health.* 1991;12:247.

Cyanosis

Salyer JW. Neonatal and pediatric pulse oximetry. *Respir Care.* 2003;48:386.

Exercise Limitation and Dyspnea

Del Giacco SR, Firinu D, Bjermer L, et al. Exercise and asthma: an overview. *Eur Clin Respir J.* 2015;2:27984.

Eggink H, Brand P, Reimink R, et al. Clinical scores for dyspnoea severity in children: a prospective validation study. *PLoS ONE.* 2016;11:e0157724.

McGrath PJ, Pianosi PT, Unruh AM, et al. Dalhousie dyspnea scales: construct and content validity of pictorial scales for measuring dyspnea. *BMC Pediatr.* 2005;5:1.

2 *Molecular Determinants of Lung Morphogenesis*

DANIEL T. SWARR, MD, SUSAN E. WERT, PhD, and JEFFREY A. WHITSETT, MD

Introduction

The adult human lung consists of a gas exchange area of approximately 100 m^2 that provides oxygen delivery and carbon dioxide removal required for cellular metabolism. In evolutionary terms, the lung represents a relatively late phylogenetic solution for the efficient gas exchange needed for terrestrial survival of organisms of increasing size, an observation that may account for the similarity of lung structure in vertebrates.[1] The respiratory system consists of mechanical bellows and conducting tubules that bring inhaled gases to a large gas exchange surface that is highly vascularized. Alveolar epithelial cells (AECs) come into close apposition to pulmonary capillaries, providing efficient transport of gases from the alveolar space to the pulmonary circulation. The delivery of external gases to pulmonary tissue necessitates a complex organ system that (1) keeps the airway free of pathogens and debris, (2) maintains humidification of alveolar gases and precise hydration of the epithelial cell surface, (3) reduces collapsing forces inherent at air-liquid interfaces within the air spaces of the lung, and (4) supplies and regulates pulmonary blood flow to exchange oxygen and carbon dioxide efficiently. This chapter provides a framework for understanding the molecular mechanisms that lead to the formation of the mammalian lung, focusing attention to processes contributing to cell proliferation and differentiation involved in organogenesis and postnatal respiratory adaptation. Where possible, the pathogenesis of congenital or postnatal lung disease is considered in the context of the molecular determinants of pulmonary morphogenesis and function.

Organogenesis of the Lung

FORMATION OF THE BASIC BODY PLAN

Events critical to organogenesis of the lung begin with formation of anterior-posterior (A-P), dorsal-ventral, and left-right axes in the early embryo, which, in turn, specifies the basic body plan of each organism. The formation of these axes is determined by genes that control cellular proliferation and differentiation and depends on complex interactions among many cell types. The fundamental principles determining embryonic organization have been elucidated in simpler model organisms (e.g., amphibians, fruit flies, sea urchins, snails, worms, and zebra fish) and applied to increasingly complex organisms (e.g., mouse and human), as the genes determining axial segmentation, organ formation, cellular proliferation and differentiation have been identified. Segmentation and organ formation in the embryo are profoundly influenced by sets of master control genes that include various classes of transcription factors. Critical to formation of the axial body plan are the homeotic, or HOX, genes.[2] HOX genes are arrayed in clearly defined spatial patterns within clusters on several chromosomes. HOX gene expression in the developing embryo is determined in part by the position of the individual genes within these gene clusters, which are aligned along the chromosome in the same order as they are expressed along the A–P axis. Complex organisms have more individual HOX genes within each locus and have more HOX gene loci than simpler organisms. In addition, HOX genes encode nuclear proteins that bind to DNA via a highly conserved homeodomain motif that modulates the transcription of specific sets of target genes. The temporal and spatial expression of these nuclear transcription factors, in turn, control the expression of other HOX genes and their transcriptional targets during morphogenesis and cytodifferentiation.[3,4] Expression of HOX genes influences many downstream genes, such as transcription factors, growth factors, signaling peptides, and cell adhesion molecules,[4] which are critical to the formation of the primitive endoderm from which the respiratory epithelium is derived.[5]

SPECIFICATION OF THE FOREGUT ENDODERM

The primitive endoderm develops very early in the process of embryogenesis, that is, during gastrulation and prior to formation of the intraembryonic mesoderm, ectoderm, and the notochord, which occurs in humans at 3 weeks postconception (WPC).[6] Specification of the definitive endoderm and the primitive foregut requires the activity of a number of nuclear transcription factors that regulate gene expression in the embryo, including forkhead box A2 (FOXA2) (also known as hepatocyte nuclear factor 3-beta, or HNF-3β), GATA-binding protein 6 (GATA6), sex-determining region Y (SRY)-related high mobility group (HMG)-box (SOX) 17 (SOX17), SOX2, β-catenin, retinoic acid receptors (RAR), and members of the T-box family of transcription factors.[7–15] Genetic ablation of these transcription factors disrupts formation of the primitive foregut endoderm and its developmental derivatives, including the trachea and the lung.[11,12,16–20] Some of these transcription factors are also expressed in the respiratory epithelium later in development when they play important roles in the regulation of cell differentiation and organ function.[8,21–25]

LUNG MORPHOGENESIS

Lung morphogenesis is initiated during the embryonic period of fetal development (3–4 WPC in the human) with the formation of a small saccular outgrowth of the ventral wall of

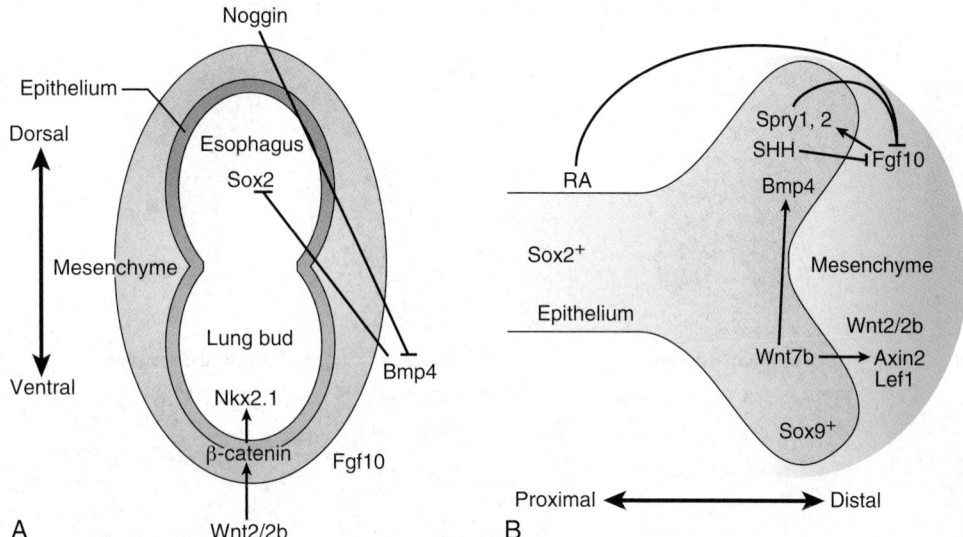

Fig. 2.1 Foregut patterning and lung bud morphogenesis. (A) Prior to outgrowth of the lung bud, the foregut consists of a single undivided tube of epithelium surrounded by mesenchyme *(orange)*. Wnts and fibroblast growth factors (FGFs) secreted by the mesenchyme act to pattern the nascent lung, marked by expression of Nkx2-1 *(green)*. Posteriorly, the future esophagus is marked by Sox2 expression *(blue)* and receives patterning signals from the notochord, such as the bone morphogenic protein (BMP) antagonist Noggin. (B) A complex series of signals involving Wnts, Fgfs, BMPs, and retinoic acid pathways continue to pattern the lung and direct bud outgrowth during the pseudoglandular stage. Fgf10 produced in the distal meso-derm *(green)* acts on the epithelium *(purple)* to promote cell proliferation and morphogenesis. Negative feedback in provided on Fgf10 by retinoic acid (RA), Sprouty-1 and -2 (Spry1,2), and Sonic hedgehog (SHH). Wnt signaling continues to promote growth of both the epithelium and mesenchyme, and interacts with several other signaling pathways, including BMP4.

the foregut endoderm, a process that is induced by expression of WNT2/2b and fibroblast growth factor (FGF) 10, in the adjacent splanchnic mesoderm (Fig. 2.1).[26–28] After the main bronchial tubes form the lung tubules, they undergo branching morphogenesis to create the highly arborized, stereotypical patterns of airway segmentations.[29] This region of the ventral foregut endoderm is delineated by epithelial cells expressing the homeobox gene, NKX2-1 (also known as thyroid tran-scription factor-1 [TTF1]), which is the earliest known marker of the prospective respiratory epithelium.[30] Thereafter, lung development can be subdivided into five distinct periods of morphogenesis based on the morphologic characteristics of the tissue (Table 2.1; Fig. 2.2). While the timing of this process is highly species specific, the anatomic events underlying lung morphogenesis are shared by all mammalian species. Details of human lung development are described in the fol-lowing sections, as well as in several published reviews.[31–37]

The Embryonic Period (3–7 Weeks Postconception)

Relatively undifferentiated epithelial cells of the primitive foregut endoderm form tubules that invade the surrounding splanchnic mesoderm and undergo branching morphogenesis. This process requires highly controlled epithelial cell prolifera-tion and migration to direct dichotomous branching of the respiratory tubules, which form the main-stem, lobar, and segmental bronchi of the primitive lung (see Table 2.1; Fig. 2.2). The respiratory epithelium remains relatively undifferen-tiated and is lined by columnar epithelium during this process. Proximally, the trachea and esophagus also separate into two distinct structures during this period. Experimental removal of mesenchymal tissue from the embryonic endoderm at this time arrests branching morphogenesis, demonstrating the

Table 2.1 Morphogenetic Periods of Human Lung Development

Period	Age (WPC)	Structural Events
Embryonic	3–6	Lung buds; trachea, main stem, lobar, and segmental bronchi; trachea and esophagus separate
Pseudoglandular	6–17	Subsegmental bronchi, terminal bronchioles, and acinar tubules; mucous glands, cartilage, and smooth muscle
Canicular	16–26	Respiratory bronchioles, acinus formation and vascularization; type I and II AEC differentiation
Saccular	26–36	Dilation and subdivision of alveolar saccules, increase of gas-exchange surface area, and surfactant synthesis
Alveolar	36—maturity	Further growth and alveolarization of lung; increase of gas-exchange area and maturation of alveolar capillary network; increased surfactant synthesis

AEC, Alveolar epithelial cells; *WPC,* weeks postconception.

critical role of mesenchyme in the formation of the respira-tory tract.[38] Interactions between epithelial and mesenchymal cells are mediated by a variety of signaling pathways that involve the binding of secreted peptides and extracellular matrix proteins to their respective cell surface receptors, which regulates gene transcription in differentiating lung cells. These epithelial-mesenchymal interactions involve both autocrine and paracrine signaling pathways that are

MAJOR STAGES OF LUNG DEVELOPMENT

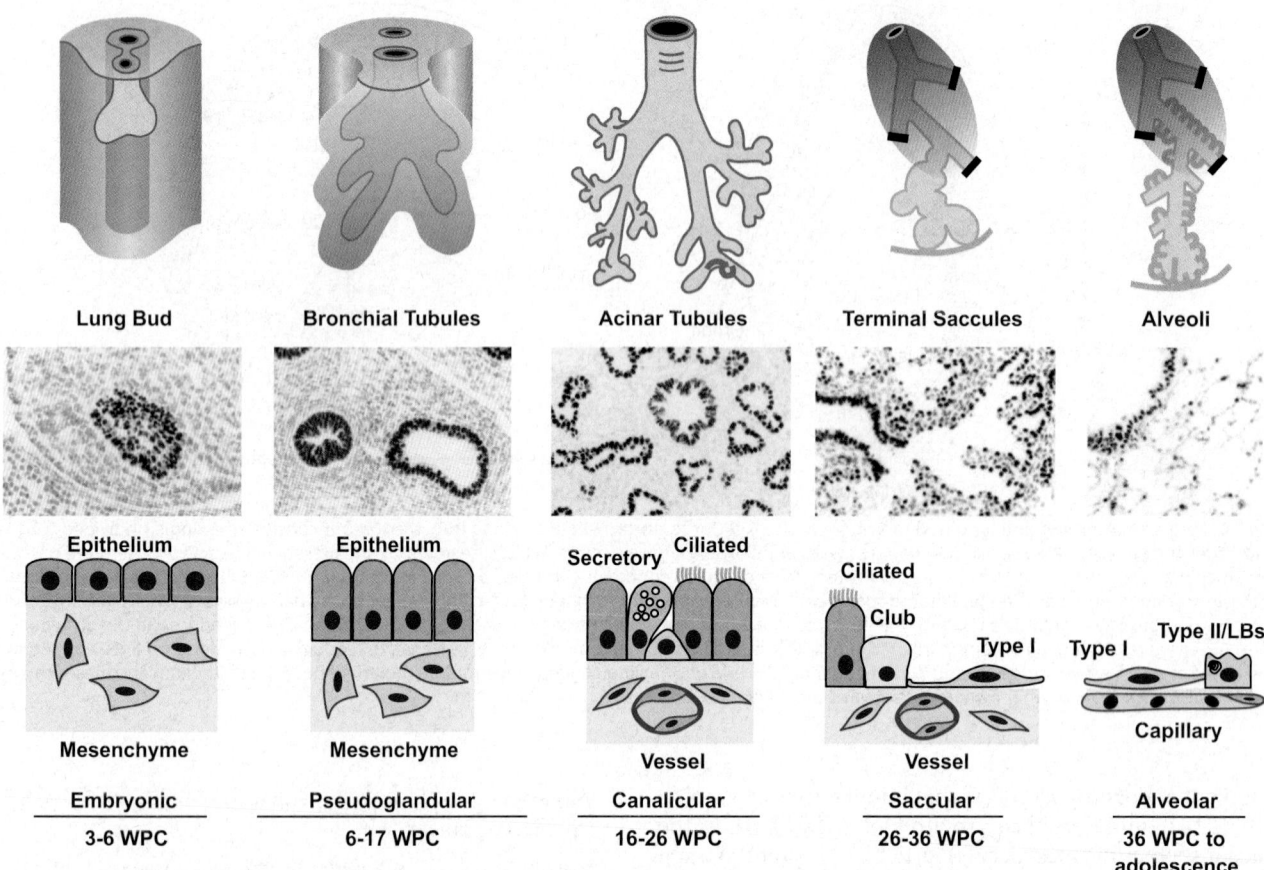

Lung Bud	Bronchial Tubules	Acinar Tubules	Terminal Saccules	Alveoli
Epithelium	Epithelium	Secretory / Ciliated	Ciliated / Club / Type I	Type I / Type II/LBs
Mesenchyme	Mesenchyme	Vessel	Vessel / Capillary	Capillary
Embryonic	Pseudoglandular	Canalicular	Saccular	Alveolar
3-6 WPC	6-17 WPC	16-26 WPC	26-36 WPC	36 WPC to adolescence

Fig. 2.2 Major stages of lung development. Bronchi, bronchioles, and acinar tubules are formed by the process of branching morphogenesis during the pseudoglandular stage of lung development (6–17 WPC). Formation of the capillary bed and dilation/expansion of the acinar structures is initiated during the canalicular stage of lung development (16–26 WPC). Growth and subdivision of the terminal saccules and alveoli continue until early adolescence by septation of the distal respiratory structures to form additional alveoli. Cytodifferentiation of mature bronchial epithelial cells (secretory and ciliated cells) is initiated in the proximal conducting airways during the canalicular stage of lung development, while complete cytodifferentiation in the distal airways (secretory and ciliated cells) and alveoli (type I and type II alveolar epithelial cells [AECs]) takes place later during the saccular (26–36 WPC) and alveolar (36 WPC to adolescence) stages of lung development. The alveolar stage of lung development extends into the postnatal period, during which millions of additional alveoli are formed, and maturation of the microvasculature, or air-blood barrier, takes place, greatly increasing the surface area available for gas exchange.

critical for lung morphogenesis (Fig. 2.3). Paracrine signaling pathways important for initial formation of the lung bud, as well as expansion and branching of the primitive respiratory tubules, include (1) FGF10/FGFR2, (2) sonic hedgehog (SHH/PTCH1), (3) transforming growth factor-beta (TGFβ/TGFβR2), (4) bone morphogenic protein B (BMP4/BMPR1b), (5) retinoic acid (RA/RARα, β, γ), (6) WNT (WNT2/2b, 7b, 5a and R-spondin with their receptors Frizzled and LRP5/6), and (7) the β-catenin signaling pathways.[8,22,23,25,34,38–41] Nuclear transcription factors that are active in the primitive respiratory epithelium during this period include NKX2-1, FOXA2, GATA6, and SOX2. Likewise, transcription factors active in the mesenchyme at this time include (1) the HOX family of transcription factors (HOXA5, B3, B4); (2) the SMAD family of transcription factors (SMAD2, 3, 4), downstream transducers of the TGFβ/BMP signaling pathway; (3) the LEF/TCF family of transcription factors, downstream transducers of β-catenin, (4) the GLI-KRUPPEL family of transcription factors (GLI1, 2, 3), downstream transducers of SHH signaling; (5) the hedgehog-interacting protein, HHIP1, that binds SHH;

and (6) FOXF1, another SHH target. Disruption of many of these transcription factors and signaling pathways in experimental animals causes impaired morphogenesis, resulting in laryngotracheal malformations, tracheoesophageal fistulas, esophageal and tracheal stenosis, esophageal atresia, defects in pulmonary lobe formation, pulmonary hypoplasia, or pulmonary ageneisis.[8,22,23,25,37–41]

Although formation of the larger, more proximal, conducting airways, including segmental and subsegmental bronchi, is completed by 6 WPC, both epithelial and mesenchymal cells of the embryonic lung remain relatively undifferentiated. At this stage, trachea and bronchial tubules lack underlying cartilage, smooth muscle, or nerves; and the pulmonary and bronchial vessels are not well developed. Vascular connections with the right and left atria are established by a common cardiopulmonary vascular progenitor at the end of this period (6–7 WPC), creating the primitive pulmonary vascular bed.[33,42] Human developmental anomalies occurring during this period of morphogenesis include laryngeal, tracheal, esophageal, and bronchial atresia; tracheoesophageal

RECIPROCAL SIGNALING IN LUNG MORPHOGENESIS

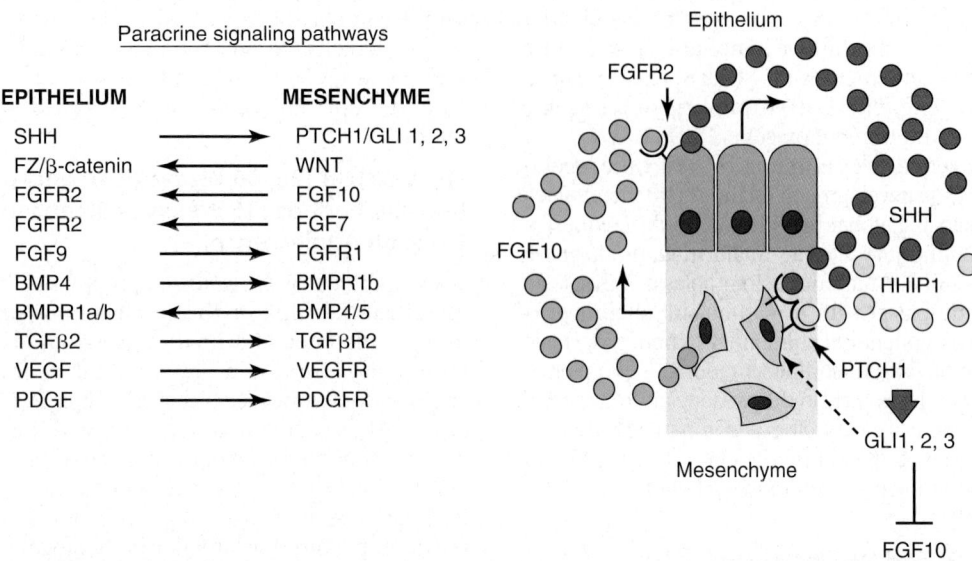

Paracrine signaling pathways

EPITHELIUM		MESENCHYME
SHH	⟶	PTCH1/GLI 1, 2, 3
FZ/β-catenin	⟵	WNT
FGFR2	⟵	FGF10
FGFR2	⟵	FGF7
FGF9	⟶	FGFR1
BMP4	⟶	BMPR1b
BMPR1a/b	⟵	BMP4/5
TGFβ2	⟶	TGFβR2
VEGF	⟶	VEGFR
PDGF	⟶	PDGFR

Fig. 2.3 Examples of reciprocal signaling during lung morphogenesis. Examples of reciprocal signaling during lung morphogenesis. Paracrine and autocrine interactions between the respiratory epithelium and the adjacent mesenchyme are mediated by signaling peptides and their respective receptors, influencing cellular behaviors (e.g., proliferation, migration, apoptosis, extracellular matrix deposition) that are critical to lung formation. For example, fibroblast growth factor (FGF)10 is secreted by mesenchymal cells and binds to its receptor, FGFR2, on the surface of epithelial cells (paracrine signaling). Sonic hedgehog (SHH) is secreted by epithelial cells and binds to its receptor, PTCH1, on mesenchymal cells (paracrine signaling), while HHIP1 is upregulated by SHH in mesenchymal cells, secreted, and binds back to receptors on cells in the mesenchyme (autocrine signaling). Binding of SHH to mesenchymal cells activates the transcription factors, GLI1, GLI2, and GLI3, which, in turn, inhibit the expression of FGF10 (negative feedback loop). In contrast, the binding of HHIP1 to mesenchymal cells attenuates or limits the ability of SHH to inhibit FGF10 signaling. Together, these complex, interacting, signaling pathways control branching morphogenesis of the lung, differentially influencing bronchial tubule elongation (growth), arrest, and subdivision (lateral buds) into new tubules. *BMP,* Bone morphogenic protein; *TGF-β,* transforming growth factor-β; *VEGF,* vascular endothelial growth factor.

and bronchoesophageal fistulas; tracheal and bronchial stenosis; bronchogenic cysts; ectopic lobes; extrapulmonary sequestration; and pulmonary agenesis.[37,43] Some of these congenital anomalies are associated with documented mutations in the genes involved in early lung development, such as GLI3 (tracheoesophageal fistula found in Pallister-Hall syndrome), FGFR2 (various laryngeal, esophageal, tracheal, and pulmonary anomalies found in Pfeiffer, Apert, or Crouzon syndromes), and SOX2 (esophageal atresia and tracheoesophageal fistula found in anophthalmia-esophageal-genital, or AEG, syndrome).[37,43]

The Pseudoglandular Period (6–17 Weeks Postconception)

The pseudoglandular stage is so named because of the distinct glandular appearance of the lung from 6 to 17 WPC. During this period, the lung consists primarily of epithelial tubules surrounded by a relatively thick mesenchyme. Branching of the airways continues with formation of the terminal bronchioles and primitive acinar structures, which is completed by the end of this period (see Table 2.1; Fig. 2.2). During the pseudoglandular period, epithelial cell differentiation is increasingly apparent; and deposition of cellular glycogen and expression of genes expressed selectively in the distal respiratory epithelium are initiated. The surfactant proteins, SFTPB and SFTPC, are first detected in primitive type II AECs at 12–14 weeks of gestation.[44,45] Tracheobronchial glands begin to form in the proximal conducting airways; and the

airway epithelium is increasingly complex, with basal, mucous, ciliated, and nonciliated secretory cells being detected.[35,36] Neuroendocrine cells, often forming clusters of cells, termed *neuroepithelial bodies,* express a variety of neuropeptides and transmitters (e.g., bombesin, calcitonin-related peptide, serotonin, and others) and are increasingly apparent along the bronchial and bronchiolar epithelium.[46–48] Smooth muscle and cartilage are now observed adjacent to the conducting airways,[49] and the pulmonary vascular system develops in close relationship to the bronchial and bronchiolar tubules between 9 and 12 WPC when smooth muscle actin and myosin can be detected in these vascular structures.[33]

During this period, FGF10, BMP4, TGFβ, β-catenin, and the WNT signaling pathways continue to be important for branching morphogenesis, along with several other signaling peptides and growth factors, including members of the (1) FGF family (FGF1, FGF2, FGF7, FGF9, FGF18); (2) TGFβ family, such as the SPROUTYs (SPRY2, SPRY4), which antagonizes and limits FGF10 signaling, and LEFTY/NODAL, which regulates left-right patterning; (3) epithelial growth factor (EGF) and transforming growth factor alpha (TGFα) family, which stimulate cell proliferation and cytodifferentiation; (4) insulin growth factor (IGFI, IGFII) family, which facilitates signaling of other growth factors; (5) platelet derived growth factor (PDGFA, PDGFB) family, whose members are mitogens and chemoattractants for mesenchymal cells; and (6) vascular endothelial growth factor (VEGFA, VEGFC) family, which regulates vascular and lymphatic growth and patterning.[8,22,23,25,34,37,38,40] Many of the nuclear transcription factors that were active during the embryonic period of morphogenesis continue to be important for lung development. Additional transcriptional factors important for specification and differentiation of the primitive lymphatic vessels in the mesenchyme at this time include (1) SOX18, (2) the paired-related homeobox gene, PRX1, (3) the divergent homeobox gene, HEX, and (4) the homeobox gene, PROX1.[34,37]

A variety of congenital defects may arise during the pseudoglandular stage of lung development, including tracheomalacia and bronchomalacia, intralobar bronchopulmonary sequestration, congenital pulmonary airway malformations (formerly cystic adenomatoid malformations), acinar aplasia or dysplasia, alveolar capillary dysplasia with or without misalignment of the pulmonary veins, congenital pulmonary lymphangiectasia, and other pulmonary vascular malformations.[37] The pleuroperitoneal cavity also closes early in the pseudoglandular period. Failure to close the pleural cavity, often accompanied by herniation of the abdominal contents into the chest (congenital diaphragmatic hernia), may cause pulmonary hypoplasia.

The Canalicular Period (16–26 Weeks Postconception)

The canalicular period is characterized by further growth and subdivision of the acinar tubules, rapid expansion of the pulmonary capillary bed, thinning of the pulmonary mesenchyme, and formation of the alveolar-capillary membrane (see Table 2.1; Fig. 2.2). By the end of this period, the terminal bronchioles have divided to form two or more respiratory bronchioles, and each of these has divided into multiple acinar tubules, forming the primitive pulmonary acini. Epithelial cell differentiation becomes increasingly complex and is especially apparent in the distal regions of the lung parenchyma. Bronchiolar cells express differentiated features, such as cilia, and secretory cells synthesize cell-specific secretory proteins, such as mucin and secretoglobin 1A1 (SCGB1A1).[45,50] Cells lining the distal tubules assume cuboidal shapes and express increasing amounts of surfactant phospholipids and the associated surfactant proteins, surfactant protein A (SFTPA), SFTPB, and SFTPC.[44,51] Lamellar bodies, composed of surfactant phospholipids and proteins, are seen in association with rich glycogen stores in the cuboidal pretype II AECs that line the distal acinar tubules.[52] Some cells of the acinar tubules become squamous, acquiring features of typical type I AECs. Capillaries surround the distal acinar tubules and establish contact with the adjacent epithelium to form the primitive alveolar-capillary membrane, which ultimately forms the gas exchange region of the mature lung. By the end of the canalicular period in the human infant (26–28 WPC), gas exchange can be supported after birth, especially when surfactant is provided by administration of exogenous surfactant.[53] Surfactant synthesis and parenchymal thinning can be accelerated by glucocorticoids at this time, which is why they are administered to mothers to prevent respiratory distress syndrome (RDS) after premature birth.[54,55] Abnormalities of lung development that occur during the canalicular period include congenital alveolar dysplasia, alveolar capillary dysplasia, and pulmonary hypoplasia, and the latter is caused by (1) diaphragmatic hernia, (2) compression due to thoracic or abdominal masses, (3) prolonged rupture of membranes causing oligohydramnios, or (5) renal agenesis, in which amniotic fluid production is impaired. While postnatal gas exchange can be supported late in the canalicular stage, infants born during this period generally suffer severe complications related to decreased pulmonary surfactant, which causes RDS and bronchopulmonary dysplasia, and the latter is a complication secondary to the intensive care therapy and increasing survival of very preterm infants.[56,57]

The Saccular (26–36 Weeks Postconception) and Alveolar Periods (36 Weeks Postconception Through Adolescence)

These periods of lung development are characterized by increased thinning of the respiratory epithelium and pulmonary mesenchyme, further growth and expansion of the pulmonary acini, and development of the distal alveolar capillary network (see Table 2.1; Fig. 2.2). Maturation of type II AECs occurs in association with increased synthesis of surfactant phospholipids,[58] the surfactant proteins, SFTPA, SFTPB, and SFTPC,[53,59] and the adenosine triphosphate (ATP)-binding cassette transporter, ABCA3, a phospholipid transporter important for lamellar body biogenesis.[60] Squamous type I AECs line an ever-increasing proportion of the surface area of the distal lung. Adjacent interstitial capillaries become closely associated with the squamous type I AECs, decreasing the diffusion distance for oxygen and carbon dioxide between the alveolar space and capillary bed. Basal laminae of the epithelium and endothelium fuse to form the thin-walled alveolar-capillary membrane; and the interstitial tissue contains increasing amounts of extracellular matrix, including elastin and collagen. Secondary alveolar septa form, which partition the terminal saccules into true alveoli, greatly increasing the surface area of the lung available for gas exchange. In the human lung, the alveolar period begins near the time of birth and continues through the first decade of life, during which time, the lung grows primarily by septation, proliferation, and thinning of the alveolar walls,[61] as well as by elongation and luminal enlargement of the conducting airways. Pulmonary arteries enlarge and elongate in close relationship to the increased growth of the lung.[32] Pulmonary vascular resistance decreases, and considerable remodeling of the pulmonary vasculature and capillary bed continue during the postnatal period.[32] Lung growth remains active until early adolescence, when the entire complement of approximately 300 million alveoli has been formed.[61,62]

Signaling pathways that are critical for growth, differentiation, and maturation of the alveolar epithelium and capillary bed during these periods include the FGF, platelet-derived growth factor (PDGF), vascular endothelial growth factor (VGEF), RA, BMP, WNT, β-catenin, and NOTCH signaling pathways. For example, targeted deletion of the FGF receptors, *Fgfr3* and *Fgfr4*, blocks alveologenesis in mice; likewise, targeted deletion of *Pdgfa* interferes with myofibroblast proliferation and migration, resulting in failure of alveologenesis and postnatal alveolar simplification in mice.[8,22,23,25,34,38,40] Notch2, expressed by type II AECs in the developing lung, induces PDGFA expression, activating platelet-derived growth factor receptor (PDGFR) signaling in alveolar myofibroblast progenitors, which is required for myofibroblast differentiation and normal alveologenesis.[63] Recently, a WNT responsive epithelial cell has been identified that serves as a progenitor for both type I and type II AECs during perinatal alveologenesis.[64]

Nuclear transcription factors found earlier in lung development, that is, FOXA2, NKX2-1, GATA6 and SOX2, continue to be important for maturation of the lung, influencing sacculation, alveolarization, vascularization, and cytodifferentiation of the peripheral lung. Transcription factors associated with cytodifferentiation during these periods include (1) FOXJ1 (ciliated cells), (2) MASH1 (or HASH1) and HES1 (neuroendocrine cells), (3) FOXA3 and SPDEF (mucus cells), (4) ETV5/ERM (type II AECs), and (5) HOPX (type I AECs).[22,65] Morphogenesis and cytodifferentiation are further influenced by additional transcription factors expressed in the developing respiratory epithelium at this time, including (1) several ETS factors (ETV5/ERM, SPDEF, ELF3/5); (2) SOX genes (SOX-9, SOX11, SOX17); (3) nuclear factor of activated T cells/calcineurin-dependent signaling (NFATC); (4) nuclear factor-1 (NF-1); (5) CCAAT/enhancer binding protein alpha (CEBPα); (6) Krüppel-like factor 5 (KLF5); (7) transcription factors, GLI2/GLI3, SMAD3, FOXF1, POD1, and HOX (HOXA5, HOXB2-B5); all of which are expressed in the mesenchyme.[8,22,23,25,40]

Molecular Mechanisms Directing Lung Development

Remarkable advances in our understanding of gene regulatory mechanisms are providing an evermore detailed understanding of the processes by which the genetic code is translated into specific cell types and their organization in organs and tissues. Numerous molecular regulatory mechanisms exist to precisely coordinate cell proliferation, lineage commitment, and subsequent terminal differentiation of over 40 distinct,

but closely intertwined, cell types that form the mature mammalian lung. Although the "blueprints" for organogenesis are encoded in the organism's genomic DNA, this information must be transmitted to cells of the developing lung by transcribing regions of DNA into messenger RNA (mRNA) and then by translating the mRNAs into protein. These cellular proteins, in turn, influence morphologic, metabolic, and proliferative behaviors of cells throughout development. Points of regulation include control over transcriptional RNA expression, mRNA stability, protein translation, and degradation, as well as further refinement in the abundance of mRNAs and proteins synthesized by each specific cell, which ultimately determine its structure and function. At each step in this cascade of information, numerous regulatory mechanisms exist, and many of which are highly interactive with complex feedback and feed-forward loops, as well as built-in redundancies, to assure precise specification of normal developmental patterns (Fig. 2.4).

TRANSCRIPTIONAL MECHANISMS REGULATING GENE EXPRESSION

Transcription Factors and Gene Regulatory Networks

Transcription factors, which are nuclear proteins that bind to specific DNA nucleotide sequences (motifs) in regulatory regions throughout the genome, represent one major mode of transcriptional regulation. The binding of transcriptional factors to the cis-acting elements influences the activity of RNA polymerase II, which binds, in turn, to sequences near the transcription start site of target genes, initiating mRNA

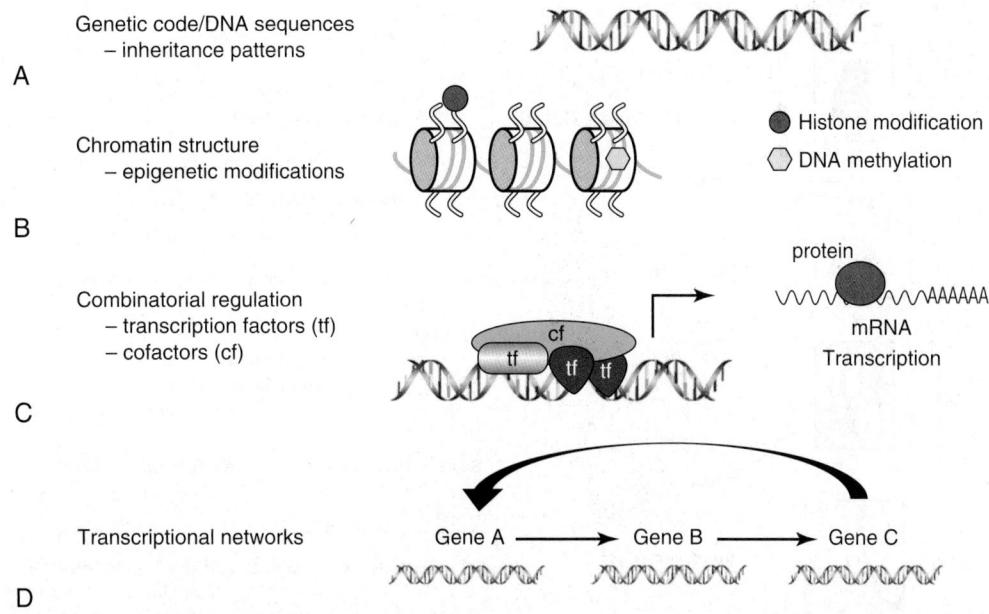

CONTROL OF GENE EXPRESSION

Fig. 2.4 Control of gene expression. Diverse cellular mechanisms regulate varying levels of gene transcription that, in turn, control messenger RNA and protein synthesis governing cell differentiation and function during lung development. Inherited patterns of each individual's genetic code (A) are modified by epigenetic mechanisms that modify chromatin structure through methylation of DNA and/or modification of histone proteins (B). Binding of nuclear transcription factors to specific structural motifs (cis-acting elements) in DNA sequences is modified by associated cofactors and other transcription factors (C). Protein expression is often controlled by transcriptional networks, in which several genes are activated in series to induce or inhibit expression of downstream targets and/or other proteins (D).

synthesis. Transcription factors may recruit additional proteins to the site of binding, modifying various chemical signatures on the DNA or chromatin (e.g., methylation, acetylation) that can continue to influence gene transcription long after the transcription factor itself leaves the region. Numerous families of transcription factors have been identified, and their activities are regulated by a variety of mechanisms, including posttranslational modification and interactions with other proteins or DNA, as well as by their ability to translocate or remain in the nucleus. Due to the large number of individual transcription factors and transcription-binding sites across the genome, these proteins interact combinatorially to form complex gene regulatory networks that direct patterns of gene transcription throughout development.

Although our knowledge of the various factors regulating gene transcription during lung development is still in its infancy, a number of transcription factors and signaling networks that play critical roles in lung morphogenesis have been identified.[8,23,66] A general schematic of important transcriptional regulators of lung epithelial morphogenesis is seen in Figs. 2.5 and 2.6. Lung morphogenesis depends on formation of definitive endoderm, which, in turn, signals from the splanchnic mesenchyme to initiate organogenesis along the foregut, forming thyroid, liver, pancreas, lung, and portions of the gastrointestinal tract.[15,67] FOXA2, a member of the winged helix family of transcription factors, is a "pioneering" transcription factor that is known to play a critical role in committing progenitor cells of the endoderm to form the primitive foregut.[16] Global loss of *Foxa2* in mice results

in catastrophic failure of development at the time of gastrulation. Loss of *Foxa2* at later developmental timepoints, alone or in combination with the related transcription factor *Foxa1*, has revealed its essential role in specification of the pancreas and liver and formation of the lung epithelium,[68–70] and it influences the expression of specific genes in the respiratory epithelium later in development. Conditional deletion of *Foxa2* in the lung epithelium of mice highlights its ongoing role in both the proximal and distal lung epithelium. Conditional loss of *Foxa2* prior to birth resulted in impaired maturation of type II cells, altered regulation of surfactant protein and phospholipid production, and death from RDS after birth.[71] Loss of *Foxa2* after birth caused goblet cell metaplasia, airspace enlargement, and inflammation during the postnatal period.[70] Thus, FOXA2 plays a critical role in specification of foregut endoderm in the early embryo, and it is used again in the perinatal and postnatal period to direct surfactant production, alveolarization, postnatal lung function, and homeostasis (see Fig. 2.5).

The transcription factor NXK2-1 is the earliest known marker of lung formation. This 38-kd nuclear protein contains a homeodomain DNA-binding motif, and it is critical for formation of the lung and for regulation of a number of highly specific gene products produced selectively in the respiratory epithelium. NKX2-1 is also expressed in the thyroid and in specific regions of the developing central nervous system.[30] Ablation of *Nkx2-1* in mice impairs lung morphogenesis, resulting in hypoplastic lungs lined by a poorly differentiated respiratory epithelium and lacking gas exchange

BLUEPRINT FOR LUNG EPITHELIAL CELL DEVELOPMENT

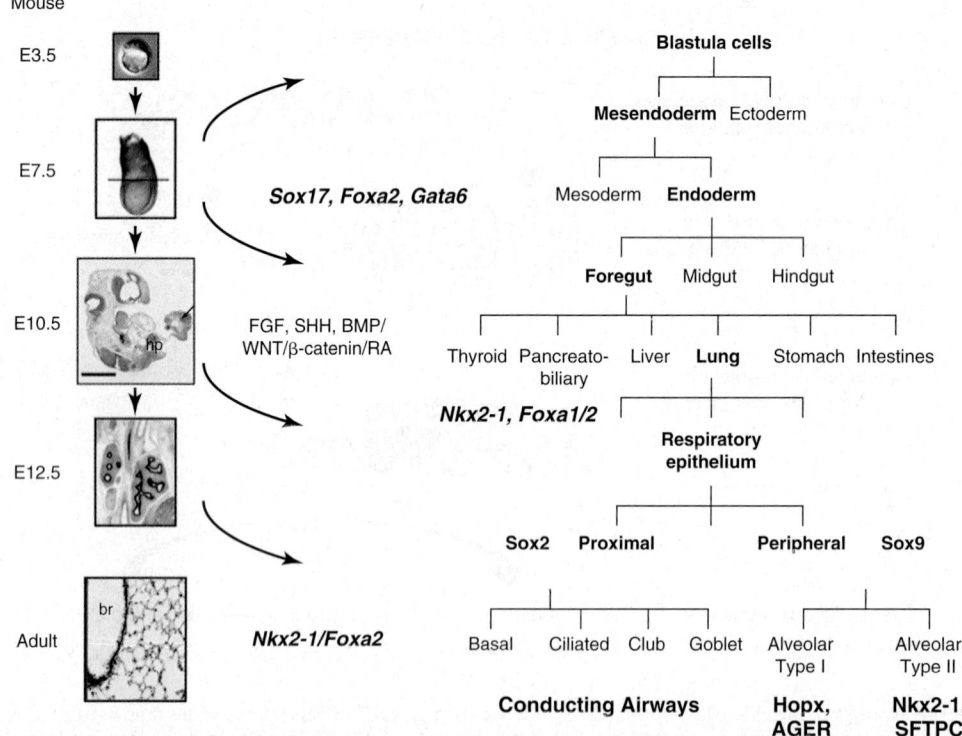

Fig. 2.5 A blueprint for lung epithelial cell development. Cytodifferentiation of the respiratory epithelium is controlled by transcriptional networks of genes that are expressed throughout lung development, in conjunction with autocrine and paracrine signaling pathways that control structural morphogenesis of the lung. Additional transcription factors are induced or repressed later in development and in the adult organ, to influence the differentiation of specific cell types. *BMP*, Bone morphogenic protein; *FGF*, fibroblast growth factor; *SHH*, sonic hedgehog.

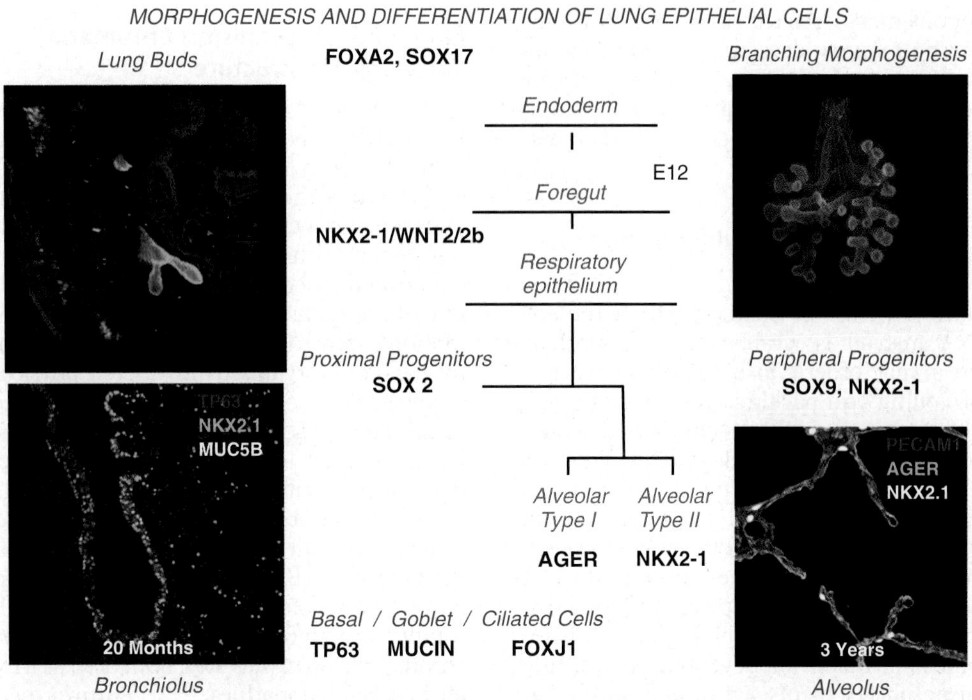

MORPHOGENESIS AND DIFFERENTIATION OF LUNG EPITHELIAL CELLS

Fig. 2.6 Morphogenesis of the conducting and peripheral airway epithelium. The lung bud, visualized by expression of NKX2-1 *(green),* forms from ventral foregut endoderm on embryonic day 9 in the mouse. Endoderm is dependent upon the transcription factors FOXA2 and SOX17. Initiation of lung buds from the foregut endoderm is dependent upon Wnt2/Wnt2b signaling. At E12, bronchial tubes undergo branching morphogenesis marked by NKX2-1 *(green),* while endomucin staining *(red)* identifies endothelial cells. Cells destined to line the conducting airways express SOX2. In contrast, epithelial cells located at the tips of the branches expressing SOX9 and elevated levels of NKX2-1 are progenitors and cells that form the alveoli in the perinatal period. In the human lung, trachea, bronchi, and bronchioles (shown at 20 months of age) are lined primarily by ciliated, basal (stained by TP63), goblet (MUC5B), and other secretory cells, including neuroendocrine cells. In the normal postnatal human lung (shown at 3 years of age), alveoli are lined by squamous, Alveolar Type I that express AGER *(green).* In contrast, cuboidal Alveolar Type II cells express NKX2-1 *(white).* Endothelial cells in alveolar capillaries express PECAM *(red).* The interface between endothelial and alveolar type I cells creates the efficient gas exchange region that facilitates transport of oxygen and carbon dioxide.

areas.[72] Substitution of a mutant *Nkx2-1* gene that lacks phosphorylation sites substantially rescues lung function in the *Nkx2-1* knockout mouse.[73] *Nkx2-1* directly regulates the transcription of numerous downstream targets, including genes involved in surfactant homeostasis, fluid and electrolyte transport, host defense, and vasculogenesis. Just as important, NKX2-1 functions in concert with other transcription factors, including GATA6, the NF-1 family of transcription factors, STAT3, NFAT, FOXA1/FOXA2, and RARs to form a tightly integrated gene regulatory network to direct lung epithelial development and differentiation. For example, NKX2-1 gene transcription itself is modulated by the activity of FOXA2, which binds to the promoter enhancer region of the NKX2-1 gene, thus creating a transcriptional network.[74] The stoichiometry, timing, and distinct combinations of transcription factors, as well as posttranscriptional modification of these transcription factors, are all critical factors in determining the precise transcriptional output at each stage of development (see Fig. 2.5), and our comprehensive understanding of how these signals are integrated on the systems-level is just beginning to emerge.

Cis-Regulatory Networks Controlling Gene Expression

Since the launch of the ENCODE (Encyclopedia of DNA elements) project, it has become increasingly clear that a

significant fraction of the genome outside of protein-coding genes plays a key role in regulating gene expression.[75] Cis-regulatory elements are a key class of regulatory noncoding DNA sequences, which act to regulate the transcription of a neighboring gene (although the distance of the regulated gene may be many megabases away). Promoters and enhancers are examples of cis-regulatory elements and characteristically contain many transcription factor binding motifs, integrating signals derived from the intricate gene regulatory networks described above. Promoter elements are essential for proper assembly of the key machinery necessary to initiate and establish transcription. Enhancers are "canonically defined as short (~100–1000 bp) noncoding DNA sequences that act to drive transcription independent of their relative distance, location, or orientation to their cognate promoter."[76] Consisting of clusters of transcription factor motifs, combinations of transcription factors interact with enhancer elements, recruit additional cofactor protein complexes, and act combinatorially to interact with the promoter of their regulated gene to modulate gene expression. Genome-wide association studies (GWAS) of many common disorders, including lung diseases such as interstitial pulmonary fibrosis, chronic obstructive pulmonary disease, and asthma, demonstrate that many of the genetic variants identified to date, which have been implicated in susceptibility to these diseases, fall within these noncoding regions of the genome.[77–80] Thus, even though our understanding of the location and function of all cis-regulatory elements (referred to as the "cistrome") critical for proper pulmonary development and function remains limited, a deeper understanding of this area of gene regulation will be essential to make progress in understanding the pathogenesis of a wide variety of common pulmonary disorders.

Epigenetic Mechanisms: DNA Methylation and Chromatin State

Genomic DNA does not exist in isolation within the cell, but genomic DNA instead is wrapped around proteins called histones in a very orderly fashion that consists of multiple levels of coiling and packing. Both the efficiency or "tightness" with which chromatin is compacted, as well as numerous associated chemical modifications to either the histone proteins or the DNA itself, are emerging as critical mechanisms by which gene expression is regulated during lung development. Methylation of cytosine at position 5 of the pyrimidine ring (largely on cytosines found in the CpG context) is the best studied of these "epigenetic" modifications, with roles in a large variety of biological processes, including X-chromosome inactivation, genomic imprinting, repression of transposable elements, aging, and cancer.[81] In the context of regulating gene expression, methylation of a promoter region generally acts to repress expression of that gene. The promoters of active genes are typically unmethylated regions, or UMRs, whereas distal regulatory elements such as enhancers often have low levels of methylation, or LMRs.[82] These methylation states have been observed to change dynamically during embryonic stem cell models of development and in organ systems such as the brain.[82–84] Moreover, widespread differences in methylation are observed in a variety of lung diseases such as interstitial pulmonary fibrosis.[85] The precise mechanisms, however, by which DNA methylation directs normal development and subsequent homeostasis of the adult lung remain poorly understood. Over 40 posttranslational modifications to the peptide tails of histones have been described, and they are associated with at least a dozen different chromatin "states."[86] For example, trimethylation of lysine 4 on histone H3 (notated as H3K4me^3) is found on active promoter regions, whereas colocalization of H3K4me^1 and H3K27ac mark active enhancers. Other marks, such as H3K27me^3, are found on regions of silenced heterochromatin. Large-scale efforts such as the ENCODE Project and International Human Epigenome Consortium (IHEC) have generated thousands of datasets to create maps of the cis-regulatory landscape in dozens of tissue- and cell-types.[75,87] It is thought that these various chemical marks act to integrate and retain the directions provided by the binding of transcription factors to chromatin throughout development, helping to "lock-in" specific cell fate decisions and provide cellular memory for these transient, but powerful, developmental cues long after they have passed. Dysregulation of chromatin state has recently been recognized to contribute to a wide variety of human disorders from congenital heart disease to lung adenocarcinoma.[88–91] However, whether these posttranslational modifications of histones are merely associated with various regulatory states or play direct and causal roles in regulation of gene expression is just beginning to be explored, particularly in the context of lung development.[92–97]

Epigenetic Mechanisms: Chromatin Topology/3D Structure

It has long been recognized that many cis-regulatory elements such as enhancers act at great distances, often thousands or even millions of bases-pairs, to regulate the expression of their target genes. Three-dimensional folding of chromatin is essential to mediate these interactions, bringing distant enhancer elements with bound transcription factors and coactivator protein complexes into physical proximity to their target gene promoters.[98,99] Chromatin conformation capture (3C)-based technologies have revealed that the genome is organized into discrete physical domains, called topological-associated domains, or TADs, often forming loops of coregulated genes.[100–103] Other regions of chromatin have been observed to associate with the nuclear membrane (laminin-associated domains or LADs), which typically consist of genes that are silenced or only expressed at low levels, that are thought to help further partition chromatin within the nucleus.[104] Examples of local or global dysregulation of chromatin topology have been reported in human diseases, ranging from blood diseases to Down syndrome, and forced chromatin looping has even been used as a treatment strategy for hemoglobinopathies.[105–107] Future research in this area is likely to have significant implications for our understanding of lung development and pulmonary diseases.

NONTRANSCRIPTIONAL MECHANISMS REGULATING MORPHOGENESIS

Noncoding RNA

With the advent of widespread availability of next-generation sequencing-based analysis of RNA, it has become clear that many regions of the genome (as much as 60%–80%) are transcribed into RNA, even if many of these RNAs do not progress to make a protein.[108,109] The transcripts are called "non-coding RNAs" (ncRNA) and are typically divided into two broad categories based on their size: transcripts greater than 200 bp are referred to as "long non-coding RNAs" (lncRNAs), and their smaller counterparts (<200 bp) are referred to as small ncRNAs. A wide variety of small ncRNAs have been described, including microRNAs (miRNAs), small nuclear RNAs (snRNAs), and Piwi-interacting RNAs (piRNAs). A number of miRNAs have been specifically implicated in lung development, including miR-17-92, miR20a, miR-302-367, miR106a-106b, and miR-34/449.[110–115] For example, loss of the miR-17-92 cluster leads to pulmonary hypoplasia due to decreased cellular proliferation, while overexpression enhances proliferation and differentiation of the lung epithelium. More broadly, loss of the Dicer complex, a key component of the machinery necessary to process longer, immature RNA transcripts (pri- or pre-miRNAs) into their mature miRNA form, results in severe defects in branching morphogenesis, and germline mutations in the DICER gene have been identified in familial cases of the rare pediatric lung malignancy pleuropulmonary blastoma.[116,117] Long noncoding RNAs also exhibit dynamic expression patterns throughout development, and new studies have started to unravel important contributions to lung organogenesis.[118–120] An important subset of lncRNAs appears to be genomically positioned near critical transcription factors, including

Nkx2-1, Foxa2, and *Foxf1*.[119] Loss of the lncRNA, Nanci, adjacent to the transcription factor, *Nkx2-1*, results in a reduction in NKX2-1 expression and recapitulates aspects of the *Nkx2-1* haploinsufficiency phenotype, while loss of the lncRNA, Fendrr, adjacent to *Foxf1* results in a phenotype similar to the human lung developmental disorder alveolar capillary dysplasia.[119,120] Other lncRNAs, such as MALAT1, have been implicated in the pathogenesis of multiple types of malignancy, including lung cancer, but global loss of MALAT1 demonstrated that this lncRNA is not necessary for normal pulmonary development.[121–124] Although individual elements may be dispensable for normal development, it is likely that lncRNAs, similar to miRNAs and many of the other gene regulatory mechanisms discussed earlier, act in highly redundant, coordinated systems to fine-tune gene expression throughout life and will play key roles in response to physiologic stress and disease.

Receptor-Mediated Signal Transduction

Receptor-mediated signaling is well recognized as a fundamental mechanism for transducing extracellular information. Such signals are initiated by the occupancy of membrane-associated receptors capable of transducing additional signals (known as secondary messengers), such as cyclic adenosine monophosphate, calcium, and inositide phosphates, which influence the activity and function of intracellular proteins (e.g., kinases, phosphatases, and proteases). These proteins, in turn, may alter the abundance of transcription factors, the activity of ion channels, or changes in membrane permeability, which subsequently modify cellular behaviors. Receptor-mediated signal transduction, induced by ligand-receptor binding, mediates endocrine, paracrine, and autocrine interactions on which cell differentiation and organogenesis depend. For example, signaling peptides and their receptors, such as FGF, SHH, WNT, BMP, VEGF, PDGF, and NOTCH have been implicated in organogenesis of many organs, including the lung.[8,22,23,25,34,40,63,66]

Gradients of Signaling Molecules and Localization of Receptor Molecules

Chemical gradients within tissues, and their interactions with membrane receptors located at distinct sites within the organ, can provide critical information during organogenesis. Polarized cells have basal, lateral, and apical surfaces with distinct subsets of signaling molecules (receptors) that allow the cell to respond in unique ways to focal concentrations of regulatory molecules. Secreted ligands (e.g., FGFs, TGFβ/ BMPs, WNTs, SHH, and HHIP1) are further influenced by binding of the ligand to basement membranes or to proteoglycans in the extracellular matrix. Spatial information is established by gradients of these signaling molecules and by the presence and abundance of receptors at specific cellular sites. Such systems provide positional information to the cell, which influences its behavior (e.g., shape, movement, proliferation, differentiation, and polarized transport).

EPITHELIAL-MESENCHYMAL INTERACTIONS AND LUNG MORPHOGENESIS

Branching morphogenesis, growth, and differentiation of the respiratory tract depends on precise reciprocal signaling between endodermally derived cells of the lung buds and the surrounding pulmonary mesenchyme. This interdependency depends on autocrine and paracrine interactions that are mediated by a diversity of signaling systems governing cellular behavior.[38,125] Similarly, autocrine and paracrine interactions are known to be involved in cellular responses of the postnatal lung, generating signals that regulate cell proliferation and differentiation necessary for its repair and remodeling following injury. The splanchnic mesenchyme produces a number of signaling peptides critical for migration and proliferation of cells in the lung buds, including FGF10, FGF7, FGF9, BMP5, and WNT 2/2b, which activate receptors found on epithelial cells. In a complementary manner, epithelial cells produce WNT7b, WNT5a, SHH, BMP4, FGF9, VEGF, and PDGF that activate receptors and signaling pathways on target cells in the mesenchyme (see Fig. 2.3).[8,23,25,34]

BRANCHING MORPHOGENESIS, VASCULARIZATION, AND ALVEOLOGENESIS

Three distinct processes, branching, vascularization, and alveologenesis are critical to morphogenesis of the mammalian lung. The major branches of the conducting airways of the human lung are completed by 16 WPC by a process of dichotomous branching, initiated by the bifurcation of the main-stem bronchi early in the embryonic period of lung development. Epithelial-lined tubules of ever-decreasing diameter are formed from the proximal to distal region of the developing lung. The terminal bronchioles divide into two or more respiratory bronchioles, which subdivide further into clusters of acinar tubules and buds at the periphery of the lung. Lung alveologenesis begins in the late canalicular period (16 WPC and thereafter) with expansion of the distal acinar tubules into terminal saccules. Further subdivision of these saccules results in the formation of the adult alveolar ducts and alveoli. During sacculation, a unique pattern of vascular supply forms the capillary network surrounding each terminal saccule, providing an ever-expanding gas exchange area that is completed in adolescence. Both vasculogenesis and angiogenesis contribute to formation of the pulmonary vascular system.[32,34]

The gas-exchange regions of the lung are supplied by the pulmonary arterial system, which originates from the sixth pair of aortic arches. The pulmonary arteries extend into the surrounding mesoderm, where they accompany the developing airways, segmenting with each bronchial subdivision. Ultimately, these arteries anastomose with the pulmonary vascular plexus that is developing in the pulmonary mesenchyme around the peripheral acinar tubules. In contrast, the bronchial vasculature arises from the descending aorta, providing nutrient supply to the conducting airways. The pulmonary veins arise from the left atrium and divide several times before connecting to the pulmonary vascular plexus in the acinar parenchyma, completing the pulmonary circulation.[126] In the adult, these veins are located primarily in the interlobular connective tissue septa that surround each pulmonary lobule.[32,34] Lymphatic vessels form around the bronchi and pulmonary vessels, extending into the interlobular septa and the pleura.[127] Parasympathetic and sympathetic nerve fibers form along the conducting airways and major vascular structures, extending as far as the alveolar ducts.[128] Signaling via SHH, VEGFA, FOXF1, NOTCH, Ephrins, and PDGF plays a significant role in pulmonary vascular development.[8,23,25,34] For example, VEGFA and its receptors (VEGFR1, VEGFR2) are critical factors for vasculogenesis in many tissues. Targeted inactivation of *Vegf* and *Vefgfr1* in mice results in impaired angiogenesis,[129] while overexpression of the VEGFA 164 isoform disrupts pulmonary vascular endothelium in newborn conditional transgenic mice, causing pulmonary hemorrhage.[130] PROX1, a homeodomain transcription factor, is induced in a subset of venous endothelial cells during development and upregulates other lymphatic-specific genes, such as VEGFR3 and LYVE1, which are critical for development of the lymphatic network in the lung.[34] Growth factors important for lymphatic development include VEGFC and its receptor, VEGFR3, as well as the angiopoietins, ANG1 and ANG2, and their receptors, TIE1 and TIE2.[34] Insufficiency or targeted deletion of these factors in mice impairs lymphatic vessel formation.[34,131]

CONTROL OF LUNG PROLIFERATION DURING BRANCHING MORPHOGENESIS

Both *in vitro* and *in vivo* experiments strongly support the concept that the mesenchyme produces signaling peptides and growth factors critical to the formation of respiratory tubules. Dissection of the splanchnic mesenchyme from the lung buds arrests cell proliferation, branching, and differentiation of the pulmonary tubules *in vitro*.[38] Lung growth is influenced by mechanical factors, including the size of the thoracic cavity and by stretch. For example, complete occlusion of the fetal trachea *in utero* enhances lung growth, while drainage of lung liquid or amniotic fluid causes pulmonary hypoplasia.[132,133] Regional control of proliferation is required for the process of branching morphogenesis: division is enhanced at the lateral edges of the growing bud and inhibited at branch points.[134] Precise positional control of cell division is determined by polypeptides derived from the mesenchyme (e.g., growth factors or extracellular matrix molecules) that selectively decrease proliferation at clefts and increase cell proliferation at the edges of the bud. Proliferation in the respiratory tubule is dependent on a number of growth factors, including the FGF family of polypeptides. *In vitro*, FGF1, and FGF7 partially replace the requirement of pulmonary mesenchyme for continued epithelial cell proliferation and budding.[135,136] FGF10 produced by the mesenchyme during lung development binds to and activates a splice variant of FGFR2 (FGFR2IIIb) that is present on respiratory epithelial cells, completing a paracrine loop.[137] Blockade of FGFR2 signaling in the epithelium of the developing lung bud *in vivo*, using a dominant-negative FGF receptor mutant, completely blocked dichotomous branching of all conducting airway segments except the primary bronchi in mice.[138] FGF10 produced at localized regions of mesenchyme near the tips of the lung buds creates a chemoattractant gradient that activates the FGFR2IIIb receptor in epithelial cells of the lung buds, inducing cell migration, differentiation, and proliferation required for branching morphogenesis.[139] Deletion of *Fgf10* or *Fgfr2IIIb* in mice blocked lung bud formation, resulting in pulmonary agenesis.[140,141] Increased expression of FGF10 or FGF7 in the fetal mouse lung caused severe pulmonary lesions with all of the histologic features of cystic

adenomatoid malformations.[142,143] Actions of FGF10 in the mesenchyme are countered by expression of BMP-4 by epithelial cells in the lung buds that together control branching morphogenesis.[144,145] Bidirectional paracrine signaling between mesenchymal and epithelial cells is mediated by a diversity of signaling networks. For example, FGF9, produced primarily by lung mesothelial and epithelial cells, is required for normal growth of the pulmonary mesenchyme.[146] Examples of signaling polypeptides known to influence branching morphogenesis and differentiation of the respiratory tract are listed in Box 2.1.

ROLE OF EXTRACELLULAR MATRIX, CELL ADHESION, AND CELL SHAPE

The pulmonary mesenchyme is relatively loosely packed, and there is little evidence that cell type is specified during the early embryonic period of lung development. However, with advancing gestation, increasing abundance of extracellular matrix molecules, including laminin, fibronectin, collagens, elastin and proteoglycans, is readily detected in the mesenchyme adjacent to the developing epithelial structures.[147–153] Variability in the presence and abundance of various matrix molecules within the mesenchyme influences structural development, cytodifferentiation and cell interactions *in vivo*. *In vitro*, inhibitors of collagen, elastin, and glycosaminoglycan synthesis, as well as antibodies to various extracellular and cell attachment molecules, alter cell proliferation and branching morphogenesis of the embryonic lung. Mesenchymal cells differentiate to form vascular elements (endothelium and smooth muscle) and distinct fibroblastic cells (matrix, myofibroblasts, and lipofibroblasts), which arise from the relatively undifferentiated progenitor cells of the splanchnic mesenchyme. While little is known regarding the factors influencing differentiation of the pulmonary mesenchyme, the development of pulmonary vasculature is dependent on VEGF, while differentiated smooth muscle is dependent upon SHH.[34,144] VEGFA is secreted by respiratory epithelial cells, stimulating pulmonary vasculogenesis via paracrine signaling to receptors that are expressed by progenitor cells in the mesenchyme.[154–157] PDGFA, another growth factor secreted by the respiratory epithelium, influences proliferation and

---

Box 2.1   Examples of Secreted Growth Factors Influencing Lung Morphogenesis and Cell Differentiation

Sonic hedgehog (SHH)
Retinoic Acid (RA)
WNT family members (WNT2/2b, 4, 7b, 5a, and R-spondin)
Fibroblast growth factors (FGF1, FGF7, FGF9, FGF10)
Bone morphogenic proteins (BMP4)
Transforming growth factor-β (TGFβ)
Vascular endothelial growth factor (VEGFA, VEGFC)
Platelet-derived growth factor (PDGFA, PDGFB)
Epidermal/transforming growth factors (EGF/TGFa)
Hepatocyte growth factor (HGF)
Insulin-like growth factors (IGFI, IGF2)
Granulocyte-macrophage colony-stimulating factor (GM-CSF)

differentiation of myofibroblasts in the developing lung by binding to the PDGF alpha receptor, and deletion of *Pdgfa* causes pulmonary malformation in transgenic mice.[158] The organization of both mesenchyme and epithelium is further modulated by cell adhesion molecules of various classes, including the cadherins, integrins, and polypeptides forming cell-cell junctions, which contribute to cellular organization and polarity of various tissues during pulmonary organogenesis. Furthermore, the surrounding extracellular matrix contains adhesion molecules that interact with attachment sites at cell membranes, influencing cell shape and polarity.[150,151] Cell shape is determined, at least in part, by the organization of these cell attachment molecules to the cytoskeleton. Cell shape, polarity, and mobility are further influenced by cytoskeletal proteins that interact with the extracellular matrix, as well as neighboring cells. The planar cell polarity (PCP) pathway and its downstream effector, Rho kinase, are critical for branching morphogenesis *in vivo* through their effects on cytoskeletal remodeling and organization, which influence apical-basal polarity within epithelia.[159,160] Mutations in the genes, *Celsr1* and *Vangl2* that are key components of the PCP pathway, disrupted the actin-myosin cytoskeleton during mouse lung development, resulting in hypoplastic lungs with fewer branches and terminal buds, thickened mesenchyme, and highly disorganized epithelia with narrow or absent lumina.[161]

Cell shape also influences intracellular routing of cellular proteins and secretory products, determining sites of secretion. *In vitro*, epithelial cells grown on intracellular matrix gels at an air-liquid interface form a highly polarized cuboidal epithelium that maintains cell differentiation and polarity of secretions *in vitro*. Changes in cell shape are associated with the loss of differentiated features, such as surfactant protein and lipid synthesis, demonstrating the profound influence of cell shape on gene expression and cell behavior.[162–164]

AUTOCRINE-PARACRINE INTERACTIONS IN LUNG INJURY AND REPAIR

As in lung morphogenesis, autocrine-paracrine signaling plays a critical role in the process of repair following lung injury.[66] The repair processes in the postnatal lung, as in lung morphogenesis, require the precise control of cell proliferation and differentiation and, as such, are likely influenced by many of the signaling molecules and transcriptional mechanisms that mediate lung development. Events involved in lung repair may recapitulate events occurring during development, in which progenitor cells undergo proliferation and terminal differentiation after lung injury. While many of the mechanisms involved in lung repair and development may be shared, it is also clear that fetal and postnatal lung respond in distinct ways to autocrine-paracrine signals. Cells of the postnatal lung have undergone distinct phases of differentiation and may have different proliferative potentials and/or respond in unique ways to the signals evoked by lung injury. For example, after acute or chronic injury, increased production of growth factors or cytokines may influence fibrosis or pulmonary vascular remodeling in neonatal life and be mediated by processes distinct from those occurring during normal lung morphogenesis.[165–170] The role of inflammation and the increasing activity of the immune

system that accompanies postnatal development also distinguishes the pathogenesis of disease in fetal and postnatal lungs.

Development of the Pulmonary Host Defense Systems

MUCOCILIARY CLEARANCE

After birth, the lung is constantly exposed to particles, pathogens, and toxicants that are removed primarily by mucociliary clearance.[171] The human airways are lined by a pseudostratified epithelium, consisting of basal, ciliated, neuroendocrine and various secretory cells (e.g., goblet, Club, and brush cells), that form a robust barrier, control airway hydration and mucociliary escalation, and protect the airway and lung from infection and injury. The critical importance of mucociliary clearance in human physiology is exemplified by the recurrent life threatening infections associated with cystic fibrosis (CF) and primary ciliary dyskinesia (PCD), wherein abnormalities in mucus hydration and in ciliary proteins, respectively, impair airway clearance causing bronchiectasis.[172–174]

INNATE AND ACQUIRED IMMUNITY

Distinct innate and adaptive defense systems mediate various aspects of host responses in the lung (see Chapter 8).[171] During the postnatal period, the numbers and types of immune cells present in the lung expand markedly.[175] Alveolar and tissue macrophages, dendritic cells, innate lymphocytes and classical lymphocytes of various subtypes, polymorphonuclear cells, eosinophils, and mast cells each have distinct roles in host defense. Immune cells mediate acute and chronic inflammatory responses accompanying lung injury or infection. Both the respiratory epithelium and inflammatory cells are capable of releasing and responding to a variety of polypeptides that induce the expression of genes involved in (1) cytoprotection (e.g., antioxidants, heat shock proteins); (2) adhesion, influencing the attraction and binding of inflammatory cells to epithelial and endothelial cells of the lung; (3) cell proliferation, apoptosis and differentiation that follow injury or infection; and (4) innate host defense. Multiple cytokines and chemokines recruit and activate the remarkable diversity of lymphocytes, innate lymphoid, monocytic, and myeloid cells that reside in the lung where they play critical roles in protecting the lung from microbial pathogens, particles, and toxicants.[176,177]

The adaptive immune system includes both antibody and cell-mediated responses to antigenic stimuli. Adaptive immunity depends on the presentation of antigens by macrophages, dendritic cells, or the respiratory epithelium to mononuclear cells, triggering the expansion of immune lymphocytes and initiating antibody production and cytotoxic activity needed to remove infected cells from the lung. The lung contains active lymphocytes (natural killer cells, helper and cytotoxic T cells) that are present within the parenchyma and alveolus. Organized populations of mononuclear cells are also found in the lymphatic system along the conducting airways, termed the *bronchus-associated lymphoid tissue.*

Cytokines and chemokines, including (1) interleukin (IL) 1, or IL1, (2) IL8, (3) tumor necrosis factor-α, or TNFα, (4) regulated on activation, normal T-expressed and secreted protein, or RANTES, (5) granulocyte-macrophage colony-stimulating factor, or GM-CSF, and (6) macrophage inflammatory protein-1α, or MIP-1α, are produced by cells in the lung. They provide proliferation and/or differentiation signals to inflammatory cells that, in turn, amplify these signals by releasing additional cytokines or other inflammatory mediators within the lung.[176] Receptors for some of these signaling molecules have been identified in pulmonary epithelial cells. For example, GM-CSF plays a critical role in surfactant homeostasis. Genetic ablation of GM-CSF or GM-CSF-IL3/5β chain receptor in mice causes alveolar proteinosis associated with macrophage dysfunction and surfactant accumulation.[178–182] Pulmonary alveolar proteinosis in adult human patients is associated with high-affinity autoantibodies against GM-CSF that block receptor activation required for surfactant catabolism by alveolar macrophages.[183,184] Inherited defects in the GM-CSF receptor, including both the GM-CSF receptor alpha and beta chains, have been associated with alveolar proteinosis in children.[183,184] GM-CSF stimulates both differentiation and proliferation of type II AECs, as well as activating alveolar macrophages to increase surfactant catabolism. Thus, GM-CSF acts in an autocrine and paracrine fashion as a growth factor for both the respiratory epithelium and for alveolar macrophages. A number of additional growth factors, including FGFs, EGF, TGFα, PDGF, IGFs, TGFβ and others, are released by lung cells following injury. These polypeptide growth factors likely play a critical role in stimulating proliferation of the respiratory epithelial cells required to repair the injured respiratory epithelium.[170,176] For example, intratracheal administration of FGF7 causes marked proliferation of the adult respiratory epithelium and protects the lung from various injuries.[185]

INNATE DEFENSES

The respiratory epithelium and other lung cells secrete a variety of polypeptides that serve defense functions, including bactericidal polypeptides, lysozyme, defensins, collectins (surfactant proteins, SFTPA and SFTPD), and other polypeptides that enhance macrophage activity involved in the clearance of bacteria and other pathogens. SFTPA and SFTPD, both members of the collectin family of mammalian lectins, are secreted by the respiratory epithelium and bind to pathogenic organisms, enhancing their phagocytosis by alveolar macrophages.[186–189] Polypeptide factors with bactericidal activity, such as lactoferrin, lysozyme, and defensins are produced by pulmonary cells in response to inflammation.[190] Thus, the immune system and accompanying production of chemokines and cytokines serve in an autocrine-paracrine fashion to modulate expression of genes mediating innate and immune-dependent defenses, as well as cell growth, critical for the repair of the parenchyma after injury. Uncontrolled proliferation of stromal cells leads to pulmonary fibrosis just as uncontrolled growth of the respiratory epithelium produces pulmonary adenocarcinoma. Chronic inflammation, whether through inhaled particles, infection, or immune responses, may therefore establish ongoing inflammatory and proliferative cascades that lead to fibrosis and abnormal alveolar remodeling associated with chronic lung disease.[191]

Gene Mutations in Lung Development and Function

Knowledge of the role of specific genes in lung development and function is expanding rapidly, extending our understanding of the role of genetic mutations that cause lung malformation and disease. Mutations in the DNA code may alter the abundance and function of encoded polypeptides, causing changes in cell behavior that lead to lung malformation and dysfunction.

Mutations in NKX2-1 cause neurological symptoms, hypothyroidism, and neonatal RDS followed by development of a chronic interstitial lung disease, the latter caused by disrupted surfactant homeostasis and pulmonary hypoplasia.[192–201] Mutations in SOX9 result in respiratory insufficiency due to severe tracheobronchomalacia in campomelic dwarfism,[202–206] while mutations in SOX2 have been associated with tracheoesophageal fistula, anophthalmia, microphthalmia, and central nervous system defects.[207] Similarly, defects in SHH (for example, GLI3 gene mutations) and FGF (e.g., FGFR2 mutations) signaling have been associated with lung and tracheobronchial malformations in human infants.[208,209] Mutations in the transcription factor, FOXF1, have been causally linked to the lethal congenital malformation, alveolar capillary dysplasia with misalignment of the pulmonary veins.[210,211] Thus, it is increasingly apparent that mutations in genes, or their regulatory elements, that influence transcriptional and signaling networks that control lung morphogenesis cause pulmonary malformations in infants. It is highly likely that allelic diversity in genes influencing lung morphogenesis will impact postnatal lung homeostasis and disease pathogenesis. Findings that SOX2 and NKX2-1 are frequently amplified in adults with squamous and nonsmall cell adenocarcinoma, respectively, links processes controlling morphogenesis with those regulating epithelial cell proliferation and tumorigenesis in the respiratory tract.[212–214]

Postnatally, mutations in various genes critical to lung function, host defense, and inflammation are associated with severe pulmonary disease. Some hereditary disorders affecting lung function include (1) CF, caused by mutations in the cystic fibrosis transmembrane conductance regulator (CFTR) protein[215]; (2) PCD caused by mutations in multiple genes associated with ciliary structure and/or function[173,174]; (3) emphysema, caused by mutations in α₁-antitrypsin[216]; (4) lymphangioleiomyomatosis, caused by mutations in tuberous sclerosis complex 1 and 2 (TSC1/2)[217]; (5) alveolar proteinosis, caused by mutations in the GM-CSF receptor (GMCSFR)[183]; (6) acute respiratory failure in neonates caused by mutations in SFTPB and ABCA3[218]; (7) chronic interstitial lung disease in infants and children caused by mutations in SFTPC, ABCA3, and NKX2-1 genes[53]; (8) chronic interstitial lung disease with progression to pulmonary fibrosis in adults caused by mutations in the SFTPA, SFTPC, ABCA3, and in genes controlling the length of telomeres (TERT, TERC).[53,219] Mutations in signaling systems controlling countless primary immune cell functions lead to pulmonary infections.[220] The severity of disease associated with these monogenetic disorders is often strongly influenced by other inherited genes or environmental factors (e.g., smoking) that ameliorate or exacerbate underlying lung disease. The identification of "modifier genes" and the role of gene dosage in disease susceptibility will be critical in understanding the pathogenesis and clinical course of pulmonary disease in the future.

Summary

The molecular and cellular mechanisms controlling lung morphogenesis and function provide a fundamental basis for understanding the pathogenesis and therapy of pulmonary diseases in children and adults. Future advances in pulmonary medicine will depend on the identification of genes, and their encoded polypeptides, that play critical roles in lung formation and function. Knowledge regarding the complex signaling pathways that govern lung cell behaviors during development and after injury will provide the basis for new diagnostic and therapeutic approaches that will influence clinical outcomes. Diagnosis of pulmonary disease will be facilitated by the identification of new gene mutations that cause abnormalities in lung development and function. Since many of the events underlying lung morphogenesis are likely to be involved in the pathogenesis of lung disease postnatally, elucidation of molecular pathways governing lung development will provide the knowledge needed to understand the cellular and molecular basis of lung diseases. Advances in recombinant DNA technology and the ability to synthesize bioactive polypeptides and to add or delete genes via DNA transfer are also likely to influence the therapy of pulmonary disease in the future.

References

Access the reference list online at ExpertConsult.com.

Suggested Reading

Galambos C, DeMello D. Molecular mechanisms of pulmonary vascular development. *Pediatr Dev Pathol.* 2007;10:1–17.

Long HK, Prescott SL, Wysocka J. Ever-changing landscapes: transcriptional enhancers in development and evolution. *Cell.* 2016;167:1170–1187.

Maeda Y, Dave V, Whitsett JA. Transcriptional control of lung morphogenesis. *Physiol Rev.* 2007;87:219–244.

Morrisey EE, Hogan BLM. Preparing for the first breath of life: genetic and cellular mechanisms in lung development. *Dev Cell.* 2010;18:8–23.

Rankin SA, Zorn AM. Gene regulatory networks governing lung specification. *J Cell Biochem.* 2014;115:1343–1350.

Shannon JM, Hyatt BA. Epithelial-mesenchymal interactions in the developing lung. *Annu Rev Physiol.* 2004;66:625–645.

Smith ZD, Meissner A. DNA methylation: roles in mammalian development. *Nat Rev Genet.* 2013;14:204–220.

Swarr DT, Morrisey EE. Lung endoderm morphogenesis: gasping for form and function. *Annu Rev Cell Dev Biol.* 2015;31:553–573.

Warburton D, El-Hashash A, Carraro G, et al. Lung organogenesis. *Curr Top Dev Biol.* 2010;90:73–158.

Zorn AM, Wells JM. Vertebrate endoderm development and organ formation. *Ann Rev Cell Dev Biol.* 2009;25:221–251.

3 Basic Genetics and Epigenetics of Childhood Lung Disease

JENNIFER WAMBACH, MD, MS, BIMAL PANKAJ CHAUDHARI, MD, MPH, and
AARON HAMVAS, MD

Childhood disease results from the interplay of genetic, environmental, and developmental factors (Fig. 3.1). The rapid development of DNA technologies has permitted the identification of the molecular basis of more than 5500 disorders caused by functional variation in more than 3500 genes (Online Mendelian Inheritance in Man, http://omim.org/statistics/geneMap, accessed June 28, 2016), including more than 100 monogenic lung diseases that contribute to a significant burden of pediatric pulmonary conditions. Cystic fibrosis resulting from disruption of *CFTR* is the most common of these monogenic pulmonary disorders, affecting 1 of 3000 births in Northern European populations.[1] In contrast, asthma is the most common respiratory disease of childhood, affecting more than 300 million individuals worldwide. Although asthma is a heritable disease, multiple candidate genes have been identified, each of which individually explains only a small proportion of this heritability.[2-5]

The availability of high-throughput sequencing has permitted extensive investigation into the "gene" arm of the gene × environment × development interaction, especially for complex traits like asthma, bronchopulmonary dysplasia (BPD), or neonatal respiratory distress syndrome (RDS) where evidence of heritability is present, but for which identified genetic variation explains only a small proportion of disease risk. For example, disparate outcomes of monozygotic twins suggest that genetic factors account for 50%–80% of the risk for BPD[6,7] and approximately 50%–60% of the risk for neonatal RDS,[8,9] but variation in identified genes accounts for only approximately 10% of this risk in RDS.[10] Aside from the fact that only a limited number of genes or individuals have been studied, other sources of this "missing heritability" include environmental and developmental interactions, some of which are epigenetic. BPD, primarily a condition of premature infants, is a classic example of how developmental factors are integral to the mechanisms of disease. An exquisitely coordinated repertoire of genes interacts to form a lung that is structurally and functionally mature to exchange gas once birth occurs, but premature birth at a time when the lung is structurally and functionally immature has the potential to disrupt this cascade of normal development.[11-13] Variation in developmentally expressed genes that are critical for lung maturation can contribute to abnormal lung development after premature birth and lung injury but would otherwise be silent in babies born at term.

Virtually all known mechanisms of genetic or genomic variation can cause pediatric lung diseases. A basic understanding of the types of variation is crucial to appreciating the advantages and limitations to various methods of genetic testing in current clinical use, as well as interpreting a rapidly expanding body of literature on the genetic basis of both monogenic and complex lung disease. Here we review some genetic terminology (Table 3.1) and current strategies for genetic testing, but the reader may also wish to consult several excellent textbooks or review articles for more detail.[14,17] The reader is also referred to the Human Genome Organization (HUGO) guidelines for gene nomenclature (www.genenames.org).

Types of Genetic Variation

Genetic variation comes in many forms, and single nucleotide variants (SNVs), small insertions/deletions (indels), exonic deletions, and trinucleotide repeats have all demonstrated roles in the pathogenesis of lung disease (Fig. 3.2). SNVs are single nucleotide changes in the genome and can occur in coding and noncoding regions. SNVs in coding regions can have relatively little effect on protein function (e.g., no change in amino acid sequence [synonymous] or conservative amino acid substitution), can result in a truncated or nonfunctional protein (e.g., nonsense, frameshift SNVs), or can have intermediate effects (nonconservative missense, splice site, and in-frame indels). SNVs that are present in greater than 1% of the population (minor allele frequency > 0.01) are referred to as single nucleotide polymorphisms (SNPs), and these "common" variants have enabled research methodologies, including genome-wide association studies (GWAS). SNVs present in less than 1% of the population are termed "rare" variants, and, although most are still of modest effect size, they are more likely to have larger effect sizes than SNPs.[18] The term "mutation," often used interchangeably with SNVs and SNPs, has a more negative connotation and may even imply a "disease-causing change," whereas the term "polymorphism" has a more neutral connotation and indicates a more common variant.[19] Indels may affect one or more nucleotides and can be "in-frame," meaning they occur in multiples of three nucleotides and add or delete amino acids in that region without disrupting the remainder of the amino acid sequence, or they can cause a "frameshift," meaning they disrupt the reading frame and all subsequent amino acid sequence. In-frame indels generally result in less disruption to the reading frame, but, as evidenced by the delF508 mutation in *CFTR*, even the deletion of three bases and a single amino acid can be deleterious. Indels that result in addition or deletion of bases that shift the reading frame are frequently pathogenic.

Although the vast majority of monogenic lung disease is caused by SNVs, there are important examples of less common genetic variation causing lung disease. For example, the absence of dozens or hundreds of base pairs encompassing

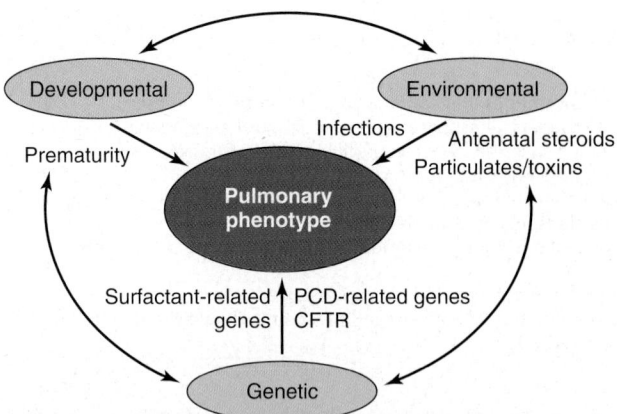

Fig. 3.1 Developmental, environmental, and genetic inputs that interact to result in a pulmonary phenotype and specific examples of each. For example, premature birth increases the risk for neonatal respiratory distress syndrome (RDS) or bronchopulmonary dysplasia, but specific intrauterine exposures, such as infection, or genetic susceptibility may influence the severity of the phenotype. Conversely, antenatal corticosteroids decrease the risk and severity of neonatal RDS for infants born prematurely. The developmental and environmental inputs are partially mediated by epigenetic mechanisms. *PCD,* Primary ciliary dyskinesia.

Original DNA Sequence
Original Amino Acid Sequence

ATG GCT GTG CTC TGG
M A V L W

Synonymous Variant- change in DNA sequence does not change amino acid sequence

ATG GCT GTA CTC TGG
M A V L W

Non-synonymous Variant- change in DNA sequence changes amino acid sequence

ATG GCT GTA CAC TGG
M A V H W

Nonsense Variant- change in DNA sequence results in premature stop codon

ATG GCT GTA CTC TAG
M A V L STOP

Frameshift Variant- deletion/insertion of nucleotide alters reading frame. Frameshift variants can also result in downstream premature stop codons.

ATG GCT AGT GCT CTG G
M A S A L

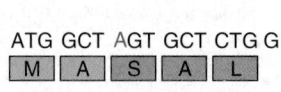

Fig. 3.2 Types of single nucleotide variation. A representative DNA sequence of nucleotide triplets comprising a codon and the corresponding encoded amino acid *(blue box)* is shown at the top. A single nucleotide substitution *(red)* may have no effect on amino acid sequence (synonymous), may change the amino acid sequence (nonsynonymous), or may encode a signal (TAG) to stop transcription prematurely, which typically results in an unstable mRNA and absence of detectable protein. An insertion (or deletion) of a single nucleotide changes the triplet reading frame and changes the subsequent amino acid sequence.

one or more exons (so-called exonic deletions) can cause serious disease. For the pulmonologist the prime examples are Duchenne and Becker muscular dystrophies. Methods for assaying SNVs including Sanger sequencing will not reliably detect exon skipping (see Table 3.3 later in this chapter), and methods such as multiplex ligation-dependent probe amplification (MLPA) must be used when there is high clinical suspicion for these disorders.[20] Disorders such as myotonic dystrophy result from expansion of three nucleotide repeat (so-called trinucleotide repeat) regions in coding regions that result in unstable and abnormal proteins. Methods for

assaying SNVs will not reliably detect trinucleotide repeats, and methods such as polymerase chain reaction (PCR) must be used when there is high clinical suspicion for these disorders.[21]

In addition to single gene variation, copy number variation (deletions, duplications) may occur at the whole chromosome level (e.g., trisomy 13, 18, 21), where pulmonary effects are largely of secondary importance as compared with other organ dysfunction, but also at the microscopic or submicroscopic level, affecting only a portion of a single chromosome or as a translocation involving two or more chromosomes. Autosomal dominant disorders may be caused by deletions, autosomal recessive conditions may be unmasked by deletion of the "normal" allele, and translocations with breakpoints within a given gene may cause similar effects.

Technologies to Identify Genetic Variation

The Human Genome Project, with initial sequencing completed in 2001, has led to the development of multiple technologies of relevance to pediatric lung disease from both clinical and research perspectives.[22] These technologies are being increasingly integrated into clinical medicine, often blurring the lines between clinical diagnostic evaluation and research. Thus it is important to understand both the technologies in current clinical use, as well as those being used on a research basis, to interpret an emerging body of literature and to anticipate the maturation of such technologies for clinical application (see Table 3.2).

Historically, chromosomal or cytogenetic variation was assayed using the classical karyotype or fluorescent in situ hybridization (FISH); however, array-based technologies have become more prevalent in both research and clinical care. Chromosomal microarray (CMA) consists of hundreds of thousands to millions of DNA probes (as oligonucleotides with or without SNPs) spotted onto a solid surface. DNA (or RNA) is hybridized to these probes, and hybridization is measured by a fluorescent reporter. CMA can assess for copy number variation (microdeletions, microduplications, and unbalanced translocations) and (when SNPs are used) regions of excessive homozygosity, suggesting increased risk for recessive or imprinting disorders. Although often used as a first-line tool for genetic analysis, CMA will not detect small changes in the sequence of single genes including point mutations, tiny duplications or deletions within a single gene (e.g., between array probes), or balanced chromosomal rearrangements (translocations, inversions). Microarray can also be used to assess RNA expression as a research tool (e.g., comparing RNA transcripts for an SNV predicted to alter exon-intron splicing).

The International HapMap Project demonstrated that SNPs at different positions in the genome are frequently inherited together, a phenomenon known as linkage disequilibrium.[23,24] Although millions of SNPs were present in the human genome, one could infer, through linkage disequilibrium, many more variants by sequencing only a subset of these "tagSNPs."[25] The use of tagSNPs facilitated the rise of GWAS using arrays that contain up to 2 million previously identified variants.

Table 3.1   Common Genetic Terminology

BASIC TERMINOLOGY

DNA	Double helix–shaped molecule composed of nucleotides that contains code for protein synthesis
Nucleotide	Basic molecules of DNA and RNA composed of sugars, phosphates, and nitrogenous bases: adenine, cytosine, guanine, thymine [A, C, G, T] for DNA; adenine, cytosine, guanine, uracil [A, C, G, U] for RNA
Gene	Sequence of DNA nucleotides that specifies amino acid order for a specific protein
RNA	Typically single-stranded molecule composed of nucleotides that is transcribed from DNA and is essential for protein synthesis (messenger, transfer, and ribosomal RNA [mRNA, tRNA, rRNA])
Exon	The "coding" portion of a gene—the sequence that is transcribed into a messenger RNA for subsequent translation into a protein
Intron	The "noncoding" portion of a gene—important in regulation of gene expression
Complementary DNA (cDNA)	DNA sequence that is derived from reverse transcription of messenger RNA, commonly used to denote the location of a variant within a gene (e.g., c.456 G > T)
Transcription	Process of copying DNA into RNA
Translation	Process of synthesizing protein from RNA
Exome	Portion of the genome formed by the exons or protein coding regions (~1% of human genome)
Genome	Full genetic complement of an individual organism (3 billion base pairs in human)
Genotype	Specific combination of alleles for a particular gene or locus
Phenotype	Observable characteristic of an individual/organism resulting from interaction of genotype with environment
Pleiotropy	One gene affects more than one phenotypic trait
Polygenic trait	More than one gene contributes to a phenotypic trait
Allele	Alternative form of a gene that may occur at a given gene locus
Homozygous	Having two identical alleles at a gene locus
Heterozygous	Having two different alleles at a gene locus
Dominant allele	Gene that is phenotypically expressed whether or not the other allele is identical
Recessive allele	Gene that is phenotypically expressed when the other allele is identical, but whose expression is masked in presence of dominant allele
Haplotype	Group of variants on a single chromosome that are inherited together
LD	Nonrandom assortment of alleles at different genetic loci
TagSNP	Single nucleotide polymorphism in a region of the genome with high linkage disequilibrium that is informative of additional variants at other genomic positions
Recombination	Rearrangement of genetic material resulting from crossing over of chromosomes during meiosis
Germline variant	Variant in DNA sequence transmitted by egg or sperm, presumed to be present in all nucleated cells
Somatic variant	Variant in DNA sequence arising in a specific tissue, presumed to be present in all cells derived from original progenitor cell
Monozygotic twins	Twins resulting from a single zygote (single egg, single sperm) that separates in early development
Dizygotic twins	Twins resulting from two separate zygotes (two eggs, two sperm)

TYPES OF GENETIC VARIATION

SNV	Variation in DNA sequence occurring at a single nucleotide position; variants with a frequency >1% are commonly called SNPs
Synonymous variant	A single nucleotide variant that does not result in a change in the amino acid at that location
Nonsynonymous variant	A single nucleotide variant that results in a change in the amino acid at that location; also called a missense variant
Nonsense variant	Single nucleotide change that results in a premature stop in transcription which results in an unstable messenger RNA that is unable to be translated or, if translated, a truncated and often nonfunctional protein product
CNV	Deletions or amplifications (e.g., duplications, triplications) of chromosomal segments; can arise during meiosis or somatic divisions
Insertion/deletion "indels"	Insertions—extra nucleotides are inserted into the DNA sequence Deletions—nucleotides are deleted from the DNA sequence
In-frame indel	Insertion or deletion of multiples of three nucleotides that add or delete amino acids without disrupting the remainder of the amino acid sequence
Frameshift indel	Insertion or deletion of nucleotides that disrupt the reading frame and the remainder of the amino acid sequence
Mutation	Any variation in the nucleotide sequence of a gene; however, it typically connotes a deleterious effect. All of the aforementioned variants are technically "mutations." The terminology is migrating to the following classification scheme.

VARIANT CLASSIFICATION[16]

Pathogenic	Very strong or strong evidence that a variant is disease causing
Likely pathogenic	Strong to moderate evidence that a variant is disease causing
VUS	DNA changes with too little information known to classify functionality
Likely benign	Strong to supporting evidence that a variant is not disease causing
Benign	Strong evidence that a variant is not disease causing

CNV, Copy number variation; *LD*, linkage disequilibrium; *SNP*, single nucleotide polymorphisms; *SNV*, single nucleotide variant; *VUS*, variant of uncertain significance.
From references 14, 15, and 16.

Table 3.2 Databases for Variant Interpretation

Database	Website
SIFT	http://sift.jcvi.org/
PolyPhen-2	http://genetics.bwh.harvard.edu/pph2/
CADD	http://cadd.gs.washington.edu/
Mutation Taster	http://www.mutationtaster.org/
PMut	http://mmb.pcb.ub.es/PMut/
LRT	http://www.genetics.wustl.edu/jflab/lrt_query.html
GERP	http://mendel.stanford.edu/SidowLab/downloads/gerp/
PhyloP	http://compgen.cshl.edu/phast/help-pages/phyloP.txt
GeneSplicer	http://www.cbcb.umd.edu/software/GeneSplicer/gene_spl.shtml
Annovar	http://annovar.openbioinformatics.org/en/latest/
ClinVar	http://www.ncbi.nlm.nih.gov/clinvar/

The Human Genome Project also fostered significant advancement in sequencing technologies. Classically, sequencing of single genes was done by Sanger sequencing.[26,27] Highly reliable and able to generate reads of greater than 500 base pairs, Sanger sequencing is still used to validate limited numbers of selected variants generated by high-throughput sequencing technologies; however, it does not scale well to sequence multiple genes. "Next-generation" sequencing technologies allow rapid sequencing of hundreds of genes or even whole exomes or genomes simultaneously by combining microarray technology and parallel sequencing of short reads (50–400 base pairs) with computational techniques to align the fragments to a reference sequence.[28–30]

Whole exome sequencing (WES) targets the exonic (protein coding) regions of all approximately 20,000 genes in the genome simultaneously and has become a widely used clinical diagnostic tool to identify rare sequence variants in patients with a phenotype suspected to be due to disruption of a single gene.[15] However, exons comprise only approximately 1% of the genome. Whole genome sequencing (WGS) has therefore emerged as a diagnostic tool and offers several advantages over exome sequencing, including detection of structural variation and variation in nonexonic regulatory, intronic, and intergenic regions. In silico programs to interpret structural and noncoding variation are emerging but lag behind those used for coding variation; currently, genome sequencing is not widely available and is significantly more expensive than exome sequencing.[31,32] Clinical exome and genome sequencing is estimated to identify a causative variant in approximately 25% of trios (affected child plus both parents), but this depends largely on patient selection based on phenotype, family history, and suspected inheritance pattern.[33] Clinical exome and genome sequencing can lead to the identification of previously identified variants or suspected pathogenic variant(s) in a gene *known* to be associated with human disease. Alternatively, exome or genome sequencing may identify suspected pathogenic variants in a gene not previously associated with a human phenotype, in which case additional clinical or laboratory investigation may be needed to establish pathogenicity. Positive results from clinical exome or genome sequencing are highly accurate, but false-negative results can occur, depending on the quality of data from a specific genomic region. In addition, the clinician must consider how well the putative variant(s) explains the patient's phenotype in terms of clinical assessment and interpretation of existing medical literature.[15] In some individuals, more than one candidate gene may be identified or, alternatively, no candidate variants may be identified. Reasons for negative findings include lack of coverage of a genomic region, limitations of variant prediction algorithms, polygenic inheritance, epigenetic mechanisms, or lack of an underlying genetic etiology. Reanalysis of sequence data may be of use as variant prediction algorithms mature, additional patients with similar phenotypes are reported, and the functions of additional genes are characterized.

Interpretation of Genetic Variation

Because each individual has millions of genetic variants, the vast majority of which are functionally insignificant, the principal challenges of sequencing are interpretation, as opposed to sequence generation.[34] For previously described SNVs many databases exist to assist in interpretation or classification, examples of which are listed in Table 3.2. Some programs, such as ANNOVAR, efficiently combine the results of multiple in silico prediction algorithms.[35] However, it should be noted that such databases are not infallible and variant classification is very dynamic (i.e., a variant that might be classified as "benign" or "of unknown significance" might be reclassified with accumulation of additional information). ClinVar provides the most current cataloging of these variants and also allows for conflicting interpretations of the same variant(http://www.ncbi.nlm.nih.gov/clinvar/).[36] Furthermore, because sequencing has the potential of identifying novel variants, both the clinician and the researcher must have a basic understanding of in silico prediction methods and their limitations. Wu and Jiang provide an overview of available tools for this purpose and caution that, although specific algorithms may outperform others under specific conditions, best results are typically obtained by using multiple algorithms and integrating knowledge over all available domains.[37] In addition to in silico prediction algorithms, functional studies and identification of variants in other diseased (or nondiseased) individuals can also aid in variant interpretation. Given the limitations of in silico prediction, there is increasing demand for biologic confirmation of in silico predictions. Although a detailed exploration of the various methods of developing model systems is beyond the scope of this chapter, special attention should be paid to the emerging technology of CRISPR/Cas9, which permits targeted genome editing and is being applied to existing model organisms to test functionality suggested by in silico prediction tools.[38]

If one takes a genomic approach and obtains WES/WGS, many (most) of the genes sequenced and variants that are identified will not have anything to do with the clinical phenotype. Variants in such genes are termed secondary findings and are an area of significant controversy. As the availability of genomic testing spreads and nongeneticist clinicians are able to order such testing, they must be aware of the potential for secondary findings and provide adequate counseling on this possibility.[15] The American College of Medical Genetics has a position statement on secondary findings that can guide clinicians.[39]

When to Consider Clinical Genetic Testing

One approach to obtaining genetic testing for an individual is suggested in Fig. 3.3. First and foremost is clinical suspicion, primarily in cases in which the expression of disease seems out of proportion to what would be typically expected or when there is familial recurrence of an unusual phenotype. For example, severe, refractory RDS in a term or near-term infant should prompt consideration of a surfactant dysfunction disorder; recurrent sinusitis and respiratory infections should prompt consideration of primary ciliary dyskinesia (PCD); familial idiopathic pulmonary fibrosis should prompt consideration of telomerase or surfactant dysfunction.[40–44] As phenotype-associated gene panels continue to be developed, there will be less need for single gene testing and more reliance on panels that permit simultaneous sequencing of tens to hundreds of genes. The results are typically available within several weeks and often will afford the opportunity to intervene clinically.

If the phenotype involves intellectual disability, other structural anomalies, or multiple organ system involvement,

then microarray analysis is the preferred first-line test. Patients who have a suspected genetic disorder despite a nondiagnostic preliminary evaluation as described previously should be considered candidates for WES or WGS. Consultation with clinical geneticists, genetic counselors, and laboratory-based geneticists can assist in selection of the appropriate testing options. The website GeneTests.Org is a useful resource for identifying clinical laboratories that are sequencing specific genes or panels of genes, the testing approaches, and result reporting times (https://www.genetests.org).

Research Study Designs to Attribute Genetic Variation to Disease

A variety of approaches, both from the standpoints of technology platforms for variant identification as well as methods for variant analysis, have been used to identify genetic associations with disease in cohorts of individuals, but there are several key features that are fundamental to any one approach.

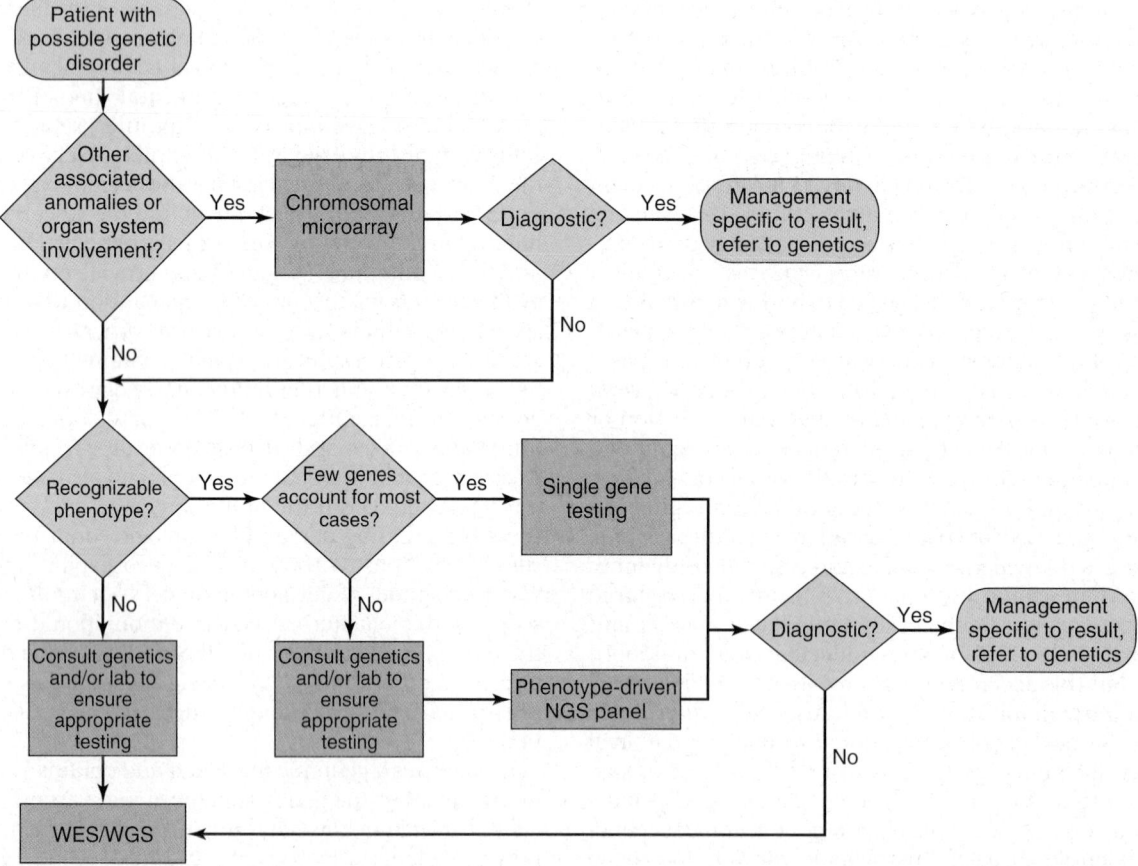

Fig. 3.3 Suggested algorithm for considering genetic testing for an individual with lung disease. Clinical suspicion for a genetic disorder arises when expression of disease seems unusually severe or prolonged or when there is familial recurrence of an unusual phenotype. If the phenotype involves intellectual disability, other structural anomalies or multiple organ system involvement, then microarray analysis is the preferred first-line test. If the phenotype is recognizable or isolated to one organ system, single gene testing or a phenotype-specific gene panel should be considered. Patients who have a suspected genetic disorder despite a nondiagnostic preliminary evaluation should be considered candidates for whole exome or whole genome sequencing. Consultation with clinical geneticists, genetic counselors, and laboratory-based geneticists can assist in selection of the appropriate testing options and interpretation of results. *NGS,* Next-generation sequencing; *WES,* whole exome sequencing; *WGS,* whole genome sequencing.

Table 3.3 Clinical Genetic Testing Methods

Method	Characteristics	Advantages	Disadvantages	References
Karyotype	Microscopic examination of chromosomes: ~5–10 Mb[a] resolution	Speed (initial results within 48 h) Detection of balanced translocations	Low resolution	45
FISH	Microscopic examination of selected locus/loci: ~50–250 kb[a] resolution	Speed (2–3 days) Highly reliable coverage	Identifies copy number only at specified locus/loci	46
Chromosomal Microarray (SNP/Oligo)	Submicroscopic examination of copy number across genome: ~200–500 kb	Well-described coverage across genome Ability to detect copy neutral changes with SNPs (e.g., uniparental disomy, loss of heterozygosity)	Longer turn around (can take 1–3 weeks) Does not detect balanced translocation Identifies copy number variants of unknown significance	45
Sanger Sequencing	Single gene sequencing	Long reads (>500 bp)	Does not scale well for multiple genes	26,29
MLPA	Submicroscopic detection of exon-level gains/losses by PCR-based assay	Reliable detection of exon-level copy number changes	Identifies copy number changes only at specified locus/loci	47
(NGS) Panel	High-throughput, massively parallel sequencing of multiple genes simultaneously	Cost-effective sequencing of 100s of genes simultaneously	Only sequences prespecified genes Variants of unknown significance identified	48
WES	High-throughput, massively parallel sequencing of exons and flanking regions	Cost-effective sequencing of all known coding regions (~1% of genome) for detection of SNVs	Covers only ~1% of genome Variable coverage of specific genes Poor detection of non-SNV changes Short reads (50–400 bp) Variants of unknown significance Incidental findings	15
WGS	High-throughput, massively parallel sequencing across the genome	Cost-effective sequencing of whole genome Detection of structural variants	Large informatics and data storage burden Significant risk of variants of unknown significance being detected Incidental findings	15

[a]*Mb*, Mega basepairs; *kb*, kilo basepairs.
FISH, Fluorescent in situ hybridization; *MLPA*, multiplex ligation-dependent probe amplification; *NGS*, next-generation sequencing; *PCR*, polymerase chain reaction; *SNP*, single nucleotide polymorphisms; *WES*, whole exome sequencing; *WGS*, whole genome sequencing.

First, it is important to remember that most genetic association studies are simply that—associations of variants or genes with a particular phenotype. Identifying the direct mechanism by which a given variant results in a given phenotype requires functional studies, as mentioned previously. Second, understanding the advantages and limitations of the selected genetic testing approach is essential (outlined in Table 3.3), and third, having a statistically robust cohort size that is appropriate for the anticipated volume of data and the analytical approach will optimize the likelihood of detecting a genetic signal, should one exist. Fourth, careful attention must be paid to controlling for population stratification because some genetic variants are more common in some populations than others.

However, the single most important aspect of any genetic association study is defining phenotype. This is particularly challenging for pulmonary diseases because they generally are complex phenotypes, and there are likely to be multiple mechanisms, only some of which are genetic, that result in a single final common constellation of clinical symptoms, such as recurrent wheezing in asthma or need for supplemental oxygen after premature birth for BPD. Also a particular challenge for pulmonary disease is that very few objective, quantitative, minimally or noninvasive biomarkers for disease expression, such as the sweat chloride concentration for cystic fibrosis or nasal nitric oxide for PCD, are available, especially for diseases presenting in the newborn period or infancy. In addition, single gene defects may have pleomorphic

presentations, such as children with pathogenic variants in the ATP-binding cassette member A3 *(ABCA3)* who might present in the neonatal period with severe neonatal respiratory failure or later in childhood with interstitial lung disease (see Chapters 54–57).[49] Alternatively, multiple genes might present with a similar constellation of symptoms, such as with PCD, for which pathogenic variants in more than 30 genes have been identified (Chapter 71).[42] These are just a few examples of phenotypic and genotypic variability that can complicate the search for the causative gene or genes. Thus, the more precisely a phenotype can be defined, the more homogeneous the study cohort can be to perform the appropriate association studies. One approach to increase the likelihood that a phenotype will capture variants of interest is to use an "extremes of phenotype" approach, which compares the individuals with the most severe presentations with the most "normal" controls, with the assumption that the affected individuals will be enriched for highly penetrant variants.[50,51] This approach was successful in using exome sequencing to identify *DCTN4* (dynactin subunit 4) as a modifier for early colonization with *Pseudomonas aeruginosa* in only 91 individuals with cystic fibrosis.[52]

The most traditional study designs to approach gene identification are family-based studies and case-control or cohort studies, thoroughly reviewed by Kosmicki et al.[53] Linkage mapping and family-based studies, which use patterns of allele sharing between individuals concordant for the disease, were the earliest techniques to localize large genomic regions associated with the disease. Traditionally, family-based tests require time-consuming pedigree analysis and recruitment of whole families, preferentially with multiple affected family members. However, with the availability of higher-resolution exome and genome-wide sequencing, a potential disease-causing *de novo* or transmitted variant can be identified using as few individuals as an affected child and parents (trio).[54]

The ability to interrogate regions across the genome using SNP arrays of 500,000 to 2 million known variants led to an expansion of GWAS that were applied to common, complex phenotypes, such as asthma and BPD. This was the application of the "Common Disease, Common Variant" hypothesis suggesting that risk for common diseases such as asthma or BPD is influenced by combinations of disease-predisposing alleles that are common in the population.[55–57] The underlying premise of GWAS is to compare frequencies of common variation across the genome (rather than a single gene) among diseased and healthy individuals for complex diseases. Taken together, GWAS have identified high-frequency variants with only modest associations and with inconsistent results across studies.[58] These variable results demonstrate (1) the challenges of phenotype and population selection, (2) the statistical challenges of assembling cohorts of sufficient size to detect a signal, and (3) the likelihood that these variants or regions are not linked mechanistically to the phenotype. Or if the variants or regions are linked, they explain only a small amount of the heritability and that other factors, including rare variants, gene × gene or gene × environment interactions may account for the missing disease heritability.[59] The National Human Genome Research Institute (NHGRI) and European Bioinformatics Institute (EBI) Catalog of Published Genome-Wide Association Studies provides an archive of more than 2400 published GWASs with more than 20,000 unique SNP-trait associations of $P < 10^{-5}$ (http://www.ebi.ac.uk/gwas/, accessed July 9, 2016).

The major limitation of the GWAS approach is that, because only known variants are interrogated, variant discovery, especially rare variants, is not possible. Sanger sequencing of candidate genes provides the opportunity to identify rare and novel variation in coding and noncoding regions, but it is time consuming, relatively expensive, and is typically used for small numbers of genes and for confirmation of high-throughput sequencing results. Now, exome or genome sequencing approaches are being more commonly applied to identify and incorporate rare variants into studies of complex phenotypes. There are significant limitations to these platforms as well, the major factor being cohort size coupled with the costs of sequencing and most importantly, the computational efforts for analysis of the massive volume of data that has to be reduced to manageable terms.[34] For example, in an exome sequencing study investigating genetic contributions to BPD in 100 infants, more than 55,000 high-confidence, nonsynonymous variants were identified.[60]

Therefore many assumptions that are based on the knowledge of the clinical and genetic epidemiology, hypothesized mechanisms for disease inheritance, and heritability are necessary to permit signals of potentially functional variants to emerge from the much larger group of variants that are likely to be inconsequential. As noted previously, GWAS assume that common variants either directly contribute to disease or tag other causative gene variants. Another approach is to assume that variants contributing to a disease are likely to be under negative selection pressure and are therefore rare. For example, Li et al., identified variants that were unique to a cohort of 100 babies with and without BPD, were not present in publicly available databases, such as ExAC, 1000 Genomes, or EVS (http://exac.broadinstitute.org/; http://www.1000genomes.org/; http://evs.gs.washington.edu/EVS/, respectively), and were postulated to be functional and to contribute to the phenotype.[60] They found more than 500 novel, nonsynonymous variants in more than 400 genes, which is still far too many for functional in vitro studies. Finally, the most agnostic approach is to not make any assumptions about rare versus common variants and include all in the analyses. Methods such as the fast family-based sequence kernel association test (FFB-SKAT) can include both common and rare variants and control for predicted magnitude of effect (relative weight) of each and other covariates, while also incorporating familial transmission.[61–63] Another common approach to further narrow down the variants or genes into more manageable units is to use pathway analysis, in which variants are grouped together into gene networks based on available literature about gene and protein interactions, most of which are derived from studies on cancer tissue.[64] However, these data are only as good as the published models, and many of the genes tend to participate in multiple pathways. The approaches to identify candidate variants and genes that are contributing to the phenotype and to predict the functional consequences of newly identified variants from these massive datasets are rapidly evolving and will become more reliable as new methodologies are developed.

Epigenetics—Terminology and Technology

Epigenetics refers to modifications of the genome or gene expression that do not alter the underlying DNA sequence. For example, mammalian cells have identical DNA sequence, yet they are able to attain and maintain differentiated phenotypes. Because DNA sequence–based strategies do not account for the full heritability of complex traits or diseases, epigenetic mechanisms may contribute to missing disease heritability and are significant components of the "environmental" and "developmental" aspects of the gene × environment × development triad (see Fig. 3.1).[65] Epigenetic modifications are influenced by environmental stimuli, including infection, oxidative stress, and aging/development.[66] The three major types of epigenetic modifications, DNA methylation, histone modifications, and noncoding RNAs, are briefly reviewed here.

DNA methylation refers to the addition of a methyl group to the 5-carbon of the cytosine ring, usually in the context of CpG dinucleotides or islands (Fig. 3.4). Mediated by DNA methyltransferases (DNMTs), this highly stable, covalent modification leads to tight packing of DNA and histones and generally results in transcriptional silencing.[67] Most human gene promoters contain CpG islands and are generally unmethylated in normal cells, although they can become methylated during tissue-specific development.[68] Methylation of promoter regions inhibits gene expression by directly preventing transcription factor binding or indirectly by facilitating

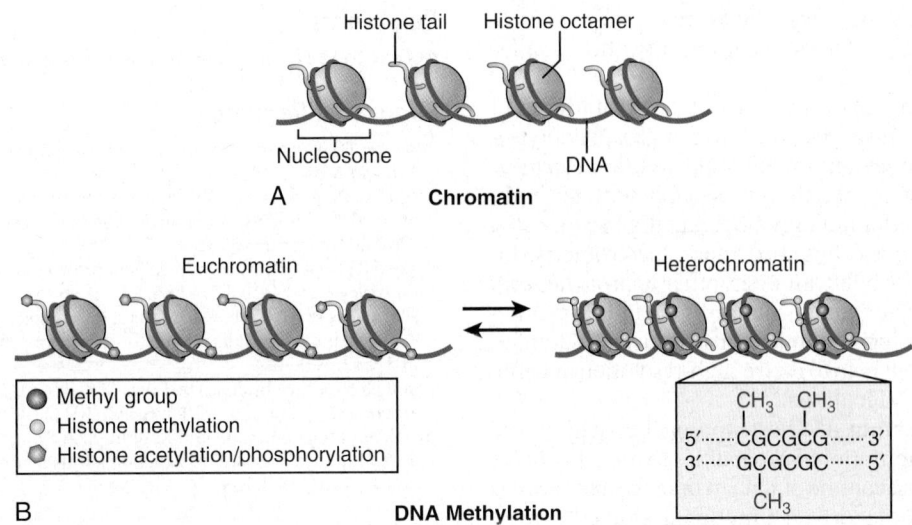

Fig. 3.4 Depiction of epigenetic changes through DNA methylation and histone modification. (A) DNA is wrapped around the nucleosome, which is made up of core histones H2A, H2B, H3, and H4. The free ends of histone tails may undergo posttranslational modifications (e.g., acetylation, phosphorylation, and methylation) that influence the configuration of chromatin. Opened states (euchromatin) allow transcription, whereas closed states (heterochromatin) restrict transcription. (B) Euchromatin is characterized by acetylation and phosphorylation *(purple polygons)*, whereas methylation *(yellow circles)* is more often found at heterochromatin. Specific histone modifications and DNA methylation reciprocally influence each other. For example, histone methylation at H3K9, H3K27, and H4K20 promotes DNA methylation at CpG dinucleotides. This covalent modification results in the transfer of a methyl group *(red circles)* to cytosine residues at gene regulatory regions. Hypermethylation typically results in transcriptional repression, whereas hypomethylation facilitates gene transcription. (Modified with permission from Raabe FJ, Spengler D. Epigenetic risk factors in PTSD and depression. *Front Psychiatry.* 2013. http://dx.doi.org/10.3389/fpsyt.2013.00080 License: https://creativecommons.org/licenses/by/3.0/.)

the binding of methyl-CpG-binding proteins, which then inhibit transcription factor binding.[69] Several studies have identified alterations of DNA methylation patterns among genes important in fibrosis among individuals with idiopathic pulmonary fibrosis.[70,71]

Histones are small, positively charged proteins with an affinity toward negatively charged DNA.[69] In the nucleus, DNA is wrapped around histones and organized into nucleosomes, which condense to form chromatin. Euchromatin is loosely packed and transcriptionally active, whereas heterochromatin is tightly packed and transcriptionally inactive (see Fig. 3.4). Histones are subject to posttranscriptional modifications, including acetylation, methylation, phosphorylation, ubiquitination, and small ubiquitin-like modifier (SUMO)ylation, which result in structural and functional changes that can alter gene transcription, DNA repair and replication, splicing, and chromosome condensation.[72–75] Acetylated and phosphorylated histones typically indicate transcriptionally active states, whereas methylated histones typically indicate repressed/inactive heterochromatin. Changes in histone modifications alter expression of genes important in the pathogenesis of idiopathic pulmonary fibrosis, and inhibition of histone deacetylators has been proposed as a potential therapy for fibrotic lung diseases.[76–79]

In addition to coding RNAs that are translated into proteins, the eukaryotic genome transcribes a large number of noncoding RNAs that are functional molecules that largely regulate gene transcription, posttranscriptional modifications, and translation.[66] Transfer RNA (tRNA) and ribosomal (rRNA) are well-described noncoding RNAs that are essential for protein synthesis. Small (approximately 20–30 nucleotides) noncoding RNAs, including microRNA (miRNA), short interfering RNA (siRNA), and piwi-interacting RNA (piRNA), regulate gene expression through chromatin structure, RNA

processing and stability, and translation. Although siRNAs target specific mRNAs, miRNA can target multiple genes and gene pathways as well as proteins. Decreased expression of a microRNA cluster (miR17–92) required for normal lung growth and development was observed in autopsy specimens from infants with BPD.[80] Long (>200 nucleotides) noncoding RNAs are also thought to play a role in chromatin remodeling, transcription, posttranscriptional processing, intracellular trafficking, and imprinting.[81–83] Disruption of genomic regions encoding long noncoding RNAs that regulate expression of *FOXF1* has been identified among infants with alveolar capillary dysplasia with misalignment of the pulmonary veins.[84]

The contributions of epigenetic modifications to human disease processes are emerging and may account for a portion of disease heritability. Whole genome, high-resolution maps for epigenetic modifications are emerging and comparison of profiles in healthy and diseased individuals and tissues may identify novel disease mechanisms and therapies.[85]

"Multi-Omics" Approaches to Refine Genotype-Phenotype Associations

The availability of high-throughput sequencing has also permitted in-depth identification of microbial elements of the so-called microbiome, including bacteria, viruses, and fungi, that provide important homeostatic functions for the body but also may influence the development of disease.[86] The complex interactions between the microbiome and host immune effector cells are not well understood. In the case of the lung the microbiota may not only modulate local immune regulation, but distant interactions with the gastrointestinal tract may actually be more important in development of local and systemic immunity, the so-called "lung-gut axis."[87,88]

Based on the complexity of assessing contributions of genes, environment, and development to complex phenotypes, it is clear that no single approach is sufficient to determine mechanisms of disease. With the development of high-throughput platforms for not only DNA and RNA sequencing and epigenetic changes, but also mass spectrometry for protein, lipid, and metabolite analysis, other approaches that integrate these multiple "omics" platforms, including genomics, transcriptomics, epigenomics, proteomics, lipidomics, and metabolomics, will help to derive high-resolution, mechanistic phenotype classifications.[89–93]

The key to integrating all these approaches will be the development of computational capabilities to model systems biology and reduce the volume of data to manageable datasets upon which hypothesis-driven functional studies can be developed. However, the ultimate goal will be to tailor therapeutic interventions to the individual's mechanism(s) of disease and anticipated responses to those interventions—"precision medicine."[94] This approach to treating individual patients will require the coordination of basic scientists, bioinformaticians, geneticists, clinicians, and bioethicists to acquire and interpret the data, define treatment, and counsel the family regarding not only the treatment decisions but also the implications of the diagnosis for the entire family.

References

Access the reference list online at ExpertConsult.com.

Suggested Reading

Biesecker LG, Green RC. Diagnostic clinical genome and exome sequencing. *N Engl J Med.* 2014;370:2418–2425.

Green RC, Berg JS, Grody WW, et al. ACMG recommendations for reporting of incidental findings in clinical exome and genome sequencing. *Genet Med.* 2013;15:565–574.

Hagood JS. Beyond the genome: epigenetic mechanisms in lung remodeling. *Physiology.* 2014;29:177–185.

Hall MA, Moore JH, Ritchie MD. Embracing complex associations in common traits: critical considerations for precision medicine. *Trends Genet.* 2016;32:470–484.

Kosmicki JA, Churchhouse CL, Rivas MA, et al. Discovery of rare variants for complex phenotypes. *Hum Genet.* 2016;135:625–634.

Zuk O, Schaffner SF, Samocha K, et al. Searching for missing heritability: designing rare variant association studies. *Proc Natl Acad Sci USA.* 2014;111:E455–E464.

Websites

Human Genome Organization (HUGO): www.genenames.org. Accessed March 14, 2017.

Exome Aggregate Consortium (ExAC): http://exac.broadinstitute.org/. Accessed March 14, 2017.

1000 Genomes: http://www.1000genomes.org. Accessed March 14, 2017.

Exome Variant Server (EVS): http://evs.gs.washington.edu/EVS/. Accessed March 14, 2017.

Online Mendelian Inheritance in Man (OMIM): http://omim.org. Accessed March 14, 2017.

GeneTests.Org: https://genetests.org. Accessed March 14, 2017.

4 Environmental Contributions to Respiratory Disease in Children

PETER SLY, MBBS, MD, FRACP, DSc, and
ANDREW BUSH, MB BS(HONS), MA, MD, FRCP, FRCPCH, FERS

Progress towards meeting the eight United Nations Millennium Development Goals has been accompanied by a substantial change in the global pattern of disease, with a significant shift towards chronic noncommunicable diseases (NCDs). Globally, early childhood deaths have declined, but years lived with disability have increased over the 20 years 1990–2010: cardiovascular disease by 17.7%; chronic respiratory disease by 8.5%; neurologic conditions by 12.2%; diabetes by 30.0%; and mental and behavioral disorders by 5.0%.[1] These trends are continuing with further increases in the global burden of disease related to chronic NCDs reported in the 2013 updates.[2,3] There is increasing recognition that many chronic diseases are initiated in early life.[4] This chapter will review the role that environmental exposures, especially those occurring in early life, play in increasing long-term risk of respiratory disease.

Vulnerability of Children to Adverse Environmental Exposures

In pediatrics the statement that "children are not little adults" is well known and understood. Children are in an active anabolic state as they grow and, as such, have increased requirements for air, water, and food, relative to their body size. This translates into a higher minute ventilation in liters/kg/day, increased maintenance requirements of calories (cal/kg/day) and water (mL/kg/day), especially during infancy and early childhood.[5] In addition, children interact with their environment in ways that adults do not. Young children spend more time on the floor, where the concentration of environmental toxicants is higher. They are also more likely to put hands, feet, and objects into their mouths and noses and to ingest more toxicant-containing dust.[5] Children also have different exposure pathways than adults (Table 4.1). Taken together, these factors result in children receiving a larger dose of toxicants in any given environment than an adult in the same environment.

Transplacental transmission is an exposure pathway that is not always taken fully into account when considering the impact of environmental exposures on increasing long-term disease risk. Previously, there was a view that the placental "barrier" protected the developing fetus from maternal exposures. However, we now know that many xenobiotics pass directly through the placenta[6,7] and that maternal exposure during pregnancy can adversely affect fetal outcomes and increase long-term disease risk. Breast milk is another exposure pathway that is not always considered. Although breast milk is the ideal food for human newborn infants, the milk can contain a variety of environmental toxicants, including persistent organic pollutants, pesticides, heavy metals, plasticizers, and other chemicals[8,9] that can increase disease risk.

Children are likely to be exposed to environmental toxicants in a number of different settings, depending on their age. Infants and young children will be exposed primarily in their home, whereas older children are likely to also be exposed in the local neighborhood, at daycare or school, and in the wider environment. Sources for common environmental exposures within the home are shown in Table 4.2.

In addition to receiving a higher dose of toxicant in any given environment, infants and young children are less able to metabolize and detoxify xenobiotics. Phase I (cytochrome P450 enzymes) and II (antioxidant defense) metabolic enzymes are immature at birth and mature relatively slowly after birth.[5] This is likely to mean that the adverse effect of the increased dose received will be magnified by the young child's inability to handle the toxicant.

Although many organ systems are essentially mature at birth, this is not true for the respiratory, immune, and central nervous systems. Thus these organ systems are vulnerable to both prenatal and postnatal environmental exposures. From the point of respiratory disease the vulnerability of both the respiratory and immune systems is of concern. Although a full description of the developmental profiles of the respiratory and immune systems is beyond the scope of this chapter, a brief overview is warranted. The airway branching tree develops between approximately 6 and 16 weeks' gestation during the pseudoglandular phase of lung development. Thus environmental exposure that influences the structural development of the airways must occur during this window of susceptibility. Maternal exposure to air pollution and maternal smoking during pregnancy are two such exposures. However, environmental exposures occurring after this time, most notably ozone, can result in thicker airways and heightened responsiveness to constrictor stimuli after birth. Alveolar development begins later, at around 24 weeks' gestation and is not complete at birth but continues in the early postnatal period. Although it is not known with certainty when alveolar development stops, the lung is especially vulnerable to environmental exposures occurring during the first 18–24 months of postnatal life.[5] Similarly, both the innate and adaptive arms of the immune system are immature at birth and mature postnatally under the influence of environmental cues.[10] As will be discussed later, delayed maturation of the immune system increases the risk of respiratory infections and asthma.

From a global perspective, socioeconomic factors such as poverty and poor nutrition can magnify the effects of adverse environmental exposures and increase disease risk. Poor nutrition includes both undernutrition resulting in stunting and inappropriate nutrition with high-calorie processed food resulting in obesity. Although this is especially true in low- and middle-income countries, it is also true in high-income countries where social disparities exist.[11–15] Poverty, poor housing, poor nutrition resulting in trace element deficiency, stunting and underweight, excess noise, and emotional/physiologic stress are likely to increase disease risk from a given environmental exposure. Thus in determining with certainty the likely adverse health risk from adverse environmental exposures, one must consider: the developmental stage of the child (prenatal, infant, child, etc.); the social circumstances in which the exposure occurs; and the type and route of exposure. For multiple reasons outlined previously, one cannot extrapolate the risk from, or consequences of, exposures from adults to children.

MECHANISMS UNDERLYING THE INCREASED DISEASE RISK FROM ADVERSE ENVIRONMENTAL EXPOSURES

Epidemiologic studies suggest that a wide variety of environmental exposures in early life can increase long-term disease risk. For example, exposure to traffic-related air pollution has been independently linked to: reduced fetal growth; premature birth; lower lung function at birth; increased respiratory infections; decreased lung function growth during childhood; incident asthma; an increased risk of chronic

obstructive pulmonary disease (COPD); lung cancer; as well as obesity, type 2 diabetes, and cardiovascular disease.[16,17] Other environmental exposures are also related to a wide range of outcomes suggesting that common mechanisms are likely to link such exposures to disease outcomes. Potential mechanisms will be discussed in the next sections.

Individual Susceptibility, Gene by Environmental Interactions, and Epigenetic Mechanisms Contributing to Respiratory Disease in Children

Being exposed to adverse environmental exposures does not, by itself, confer an increased risk of disease. Not all smokers develop lung cancer or COPD; however, some individuals are more susceptible than others. This suggests that individual susceptibility related to genetic variations is likely to be important.

There is increasing evidence that many of the risk factors for respiratory disease have a genetic contribution that may underlie individual susceptibility. Low lung function is a primary risk for both acute respiratory disease in early life and chronic respiratory disease throughout life. Several genetic variations have been associated with low lung function, reduced lung function growth, or accelerated lung function decline.[18–21] Similarly, genetic variations have been associated with an increased susceptibility to lower respiratory infections,[22–24] delayed maturation of the immune system, and early allergic sensitization.[10,25] Genetic variations in the body systems designed to defend against environmental exposures, such as the antioxidant defense system, have also been reported as increasing individual susceptibility to respiratory disease,[26] especially with exposure to traffic-related air pollution.[27] Fig. 4.1 gives a schematic representation of the multiple pathways increasing disease risk in which individual susceptibility related to genetic variation has been reported. These same pathways are also susceptible to environmental exposures, opening the way to environmentally induced epigenetic processes and gene × environment interaction. Although a full description of all of these pathways is beyond the scope of this chapter, several warrant further discussion.

Epigenetic Mechanisms Increasing the Risk of Disease. Despite a clear genetic component to asthma susceptibility— everyone knows that asthma runs in families—the failure

Table 4.1 Exposure Pathways for Environmental Exposures at Different Ages

Pathway	Prenatal	Infant	Child	Adolescent	Adult
Transplacental	√				
Breast milk		√			
Nutritive ingestion		√√√	√√	√	√
Nonnutritive ingestion		√√	√√√	√	√
Inhalation		√√√	√√	√	√
Transdermal		√√√	√√	√	√
Risk-taking behavior			√	√√√	√

Table 4.2 Common Environmental Exposures Encountered in a Home Environment

Toxicant	Matrix	Source	Route of Exposure
Flame retardants	Dust, air, breast milk, food	Furnishings, clothing, electronic equipment	Nutritive and nonnutritive ingestion Inhalation, dermal
Pesticides	Air, dust, breast milk, food and beverages	Pest control sprays, agricultural practices, house and garden insecticides	Nutritive and nonnutritive ingestion Inhalation, dermal
Plastics/plasticizers	Food and beverages, air	Food containers (especially when heated) cosmetics, personal care products	Nutritive ingestion, dermal, inhalation
Combustion-related products (particulates, gaseous pollutants, polyaromatic hydrocarbons)	Air, dust	Cigarettes, candles, mosquito coils, biomass fuel, gas cooking	Inhalation, nonnutritive ingestion, dermal
Volatile organics	Air, dust	Furniture, building materials, glues, carpets, cigarettes, mosquito coils, personal care products	Inhalation, nonnutritive ingestion, dermal
Perfluorinated compounds	Food, water, dust	Teflon-coated cookware, industrial contamination of water	Nutritive and nonnutritive ingestion, inhalation, dermal

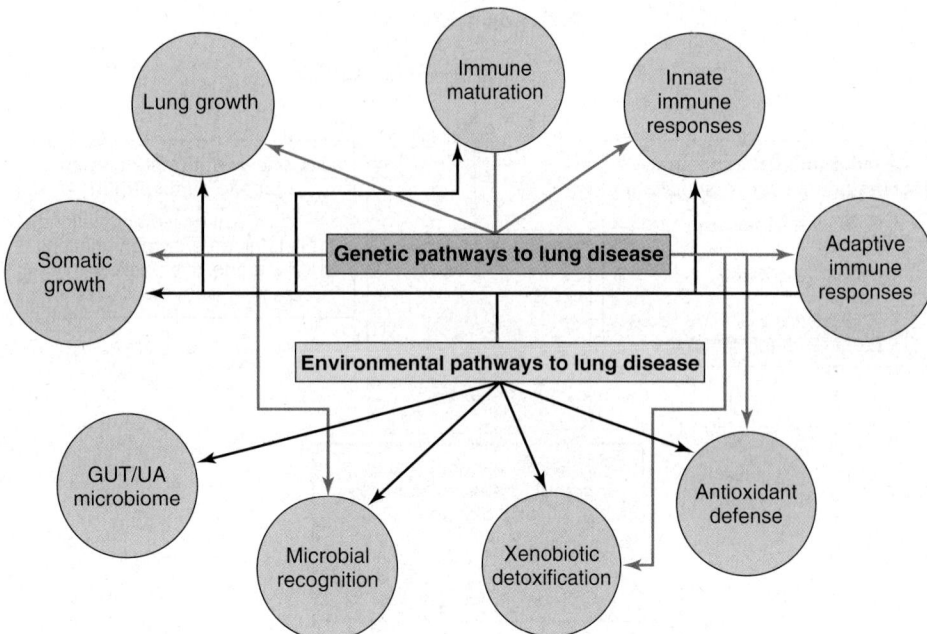

Fig. 4.1 Schematic representation of the multiple potential genetic and environmental pathways that increase respiratory disease risk. *GUT,* Gastrointestinal tract, *UA,* upper airway.

of genetic studies, either candidate gene or genome-wide association studies, to explain more than a fraction of asthma has prompted investigation of other means by which gene variation and dysfunction could be involved.[28] Many have turned to the study of epigenetics and global methylation. Epigenetics refers to the process whereby gene expression and function is altered without altering the DNA sequence of the gene. Several epigenetic mechanisms have been described, including DNA methylation at cytosine-guanine dinucleotide (CpG) residues, posttranslational modification of nuclear histones, and noncoding RNA-mediated gene silencing.[28,29] These changes in gene function can survive cell division and can be heritable,[29] although this is perhaps not as common in mammals as sometimes suggested because global demethylation and germline reprogramming limit transgenerational inheritance of epigenetic marks.[30] DNA methylation changes throughout life,[31] especially in key windows of vulnerability, but much of the epigenome is established during fetal development and provides a mechanism by which prenatal environmental exposures can increase disease risk.[29] Maternal smoking during pregnancy has negative impacts on fetal lung development, immune system development, and somatic growth (as well as on neurodevelopment) that increase the risk of respiratory disease throughout life.[32–34] Although direct data are scarce, epigenetic mechanisms are widely thought to be involved.[28,29,35–37] Third-generation effects in which an increased asthma risk from grand-maternal smoking is passed to grandchildren via mothers exposed in utero is also thought to occur via epigenetic mechanisms.[38] A likely mechanism by which environmental exposures such as tobacco smoke, household air pollution (especially biomass fuel burning), traffic-related pollution, and household chemicals can induce adverse changes in the epigenome that increase disease risk is by causing oxidative stress in the mother during pregnancy, potentially through upregulating expression of proinflammatory genes by histone modification and chromatin remodeling.[35] Individual susceptibility to oxidative stress is increased by genetic variations in antioxidant defense genes.[39–41]

Data showing that maternal factors can influence oocyte development and transfer disease risk to offspring via mitochondrial transfer present another mechanism for environmental exposures to increase disease risk. Mitochondrial transfer from mesenchymal stromal (stem) cells to injured cells has been well established in the lungs.[42,43] More recently, Wu and colleagues[44] have shown that oocytes from obese mice produce heavier fetuses when transferred to lean recipients; direct mitochondrial transfer from oocytes to blastocysts was the proposed mechanism. These data raise the probability that other environmental exposures prior to conception can modify oocytes by mechanisms other than epigenetics and suggest that more attention should be paid to the health of girls and young women to reduce NCDs.

Antioxidant Defense. As outlined previously, antioxidant defense plays a substantial role linking environmental exposures to disease risk. Fig. 4.2 gives a schematic representation of the genetic and epigenetic mechanisms and the environmental exposures increasing disease risk when antioxidant defenses are inadequate.

Microbial Recognition. We are all exposed to microbes and microbial products in our environment. Such exposures are critical for postnatal maturation of the innate and adaptive limbs of the immune system and for decreasing risk of respiratory disease.[45,46] The interplay between resident bacteria and the immune system at times of respiratory viral infections in early life is also likely to have a significant influence on later risk of respiratory disease.[47] Thus genetic and environmental influences on microbial recognition of microorganisms are another potentially critical factor likely to influence disease risk. Fig. 4.3 shows a schematic representation of such interactions.

Allergic Inflammation. Allergic sensitization in early life is a major risk factor for persistent asthma,[25] with the risk of sensitization being altered by genetic and epigenetic

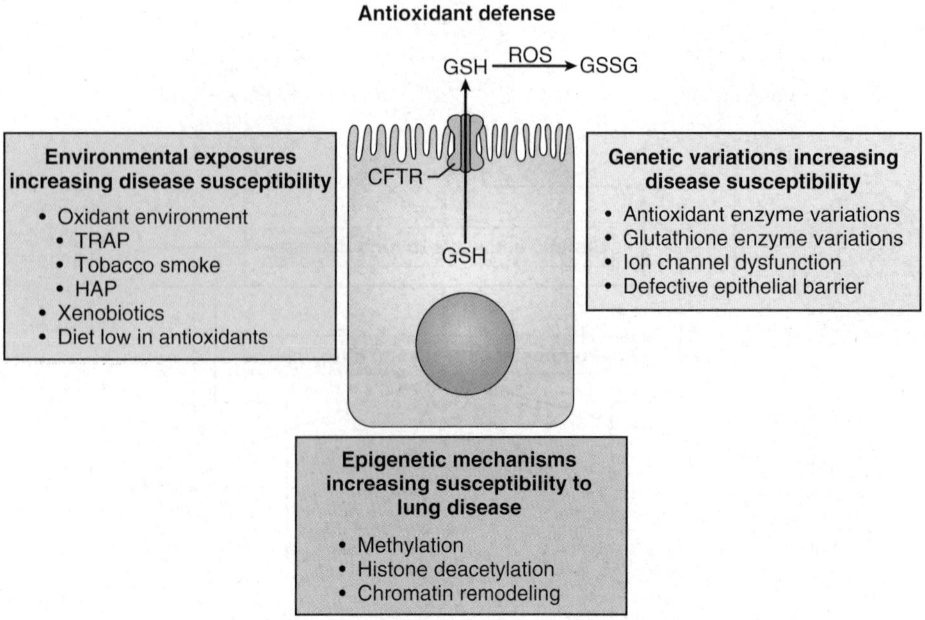

Antioxidant defense

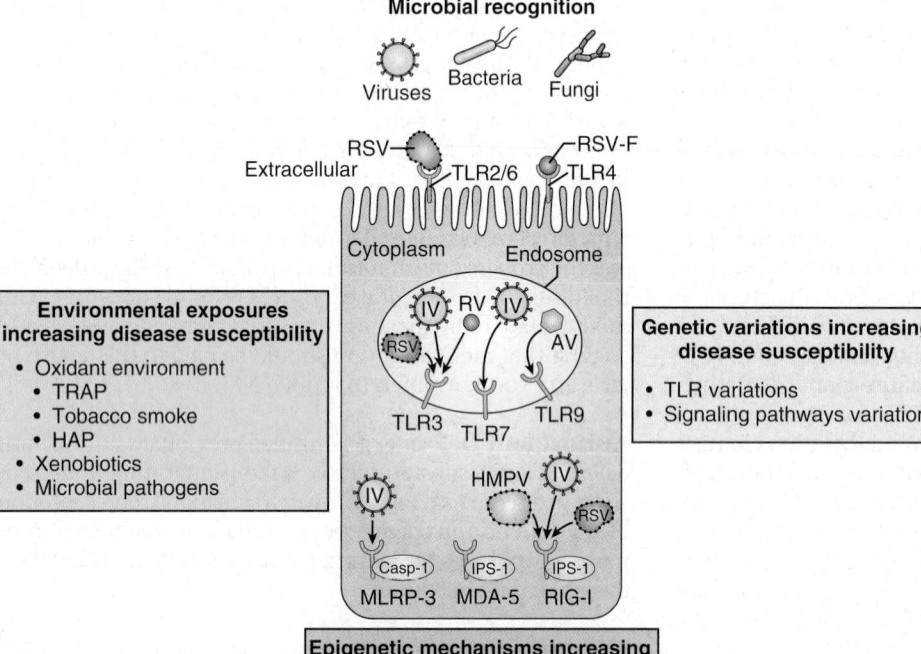

GSH $\xrightarrow{ROS}$ GSSG

CFTR

GSH

Environmental exposures increasing disease susceptibility

- Oxidant environment
  - TRAP
  - Tobacco smoke
  - HAP
- Xenobiotics
- Diet low in antioxidants

Genetic variations increasing disease susceptibility

- Antioxidant enzyme variations
- Glutathione enzyme variations
- Ion channel dysfunction
- Defective epithelial barrier

Epigenetic mechanisms increasing susceptibility to lung disease

- Methylation
- Histone deacetylation
- Chromatin remodeling

Fig. 4.2 Schematic representation of genetic and epigenetic mechanisms that interact with environmental exposures to increase respiratory disease risk via oxidative stress. *CFTR*, Cystic fibrosis transmembrane conductance regulator; *GSSG*, the oxidized form of glutathione; *GSH*, the reduced form of glutathione; *HAP*, household air pollution; *ROS*, reactive oxygen species; *TRAP*, traffic-related air pollution.

Microbial recognition

Viruses   Bacteria   Fungi

RSV   RSV-F
Extracellular   TLR2/6   TLR4

Cytoplasm   Endosome

IV   RV   IV
RSV   AV

TLR3   TLR7   TLR9

IV   HMPV   IV
                  RSV

Casp-1   IPS-1   IPS-1
MLRP-3   MDA-5   RIG-I

Environmental exposures increasing disease susceptibility

- Oxidant environment
  - TRAP
  - Tobacco smoke
  - HAP
- Xenobiotics
- Microbial pathogens

Genetic variations increasing disease susceptibility

- TLR variations
- Signaling pathways variations

Epigenetic mechanisms increasing susceptibility to lung disease

- Methylation
- Histone acetylation
- miRNAs

Fig. 4.3 Schematic representation of genetic and epigenetic mechanisms that interact with microbial recognition to increase respiratory disease risk via oxidative stress. *HAP*, Household air pollution; *HMPV*, human metapneumovirus; *RSV*, respiratory syncytial virus; *RV*, rhinovirus; *TLR*, Toll-like receptor; *TRAP*, traffic-related air pollution.

mechanisms and environmental exposures. In general, low-dose allergen exposure increases the risk of allergic sensitization, whereas high-dose favors the development of immune tolerance and not sensitization,[48] especially in the presence of high concentrations of microbial products.[45,49,50] However, environmental exposures also have the potential to alter genetic responses and modify the risk of allergic sensitization.[51–53] One particular environmental exposure

that has the potential to modify the risk of allergic sensitization is exposure to microbial products, including lipopolysaccharide (LPS). Exposure to microbial-rich animal barn dust during fetal development and early life has been shown to protect against allergic sensitization.[54] However, the protection depends on the level of LPS exposure and genetic variations in the CD14 gene, with the C allele at CD14/-159 increasing the risk of allergic sensitization in the presence

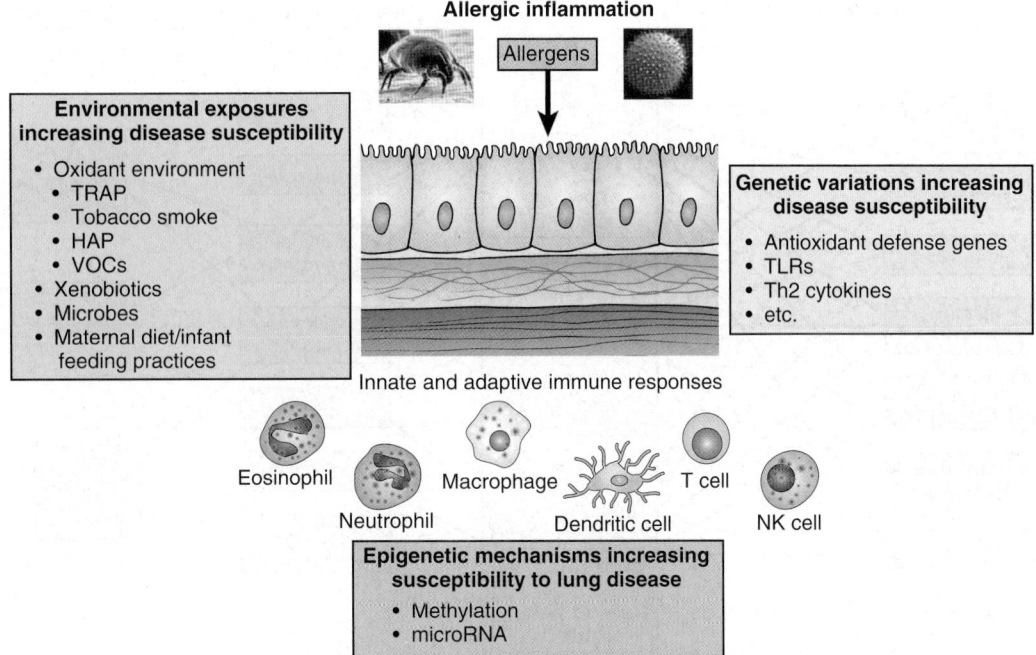

Fig. 4.4 Schematic representation of environmental, genetic, and epigenetic pathways increasing the risk of allergic sensitization. *HAP*, Household air pollution; *NK*, natural killer; *Th2*, type two inflammatory response; *TLR*, Toll-like receptor; *TRAP*, traffic-related air pollution; *VOC*, volatile organic compound.

of low LPS levels and the T allele increasing risk with high levels of LPS.[55] Other genetic variations can also play a role, with the A20 protein, a transcription product of TNFAIP3, in airway epithelial cells mediating LPS-induced attenuation of house dust mite allergen–induced inflammatory responses.[45]

Fig. 4.4 shows a schematic representation of environmental, genetic, and epigenetic factors influencing the risk of allergic sensitization in early life. Whether these pathways increase the risk for other respiratory diseases is less certain, but possible, especially COPD, in which early life exposures do increase risk.[56,57]

Low Lung Function/Reduced Lung Growth, Delayed Immune Maturation, and Somatic Growth Restriction Predisposing to Respiratory Disease

Low lung function is a risk factor for all respiratory diseases, both acute and chronic, throughout all stages of life. The respiratory system is not mature at birth because at least half of the adult complement of alveoli developing postnatally. The lungs are vulnerable to both prenatal and postnatal environmental insults that can limit lung function and lung function growth.[17,56,57] Lung function "tracks" postnatally, meaning that lung function at birth is a major determinant of lung function throughout life[17,56,57]; however, severe respiratory infections and adverse environmental exposures can reduce lung function growth,[27,33,58–62] resulting in a reduction in lung function that should have been gained. Fig. 4.5 shows a schematic representation of the interrelationships between prenatal and postnatal exposures increasing the risk for respiratory diseases in later life.

Prenatal exposures can increase the risk of postnatal respiratory disease by reducing lung function at birth, reducing somatic growth, or delaying immune system maturation during fetal development. Many exposures have more than one effect, possibly by epigenetic alteration of gene function as discussed previously. Maternal smoking during pregnancy increases the risk for all respiratory diseases by causing reduced lung function at birth,[63] low birth weight,[64,65] and delayed immune maturation.[34] Similarly, maternal exposure to higher levels of ambient air pollution has been associated with lower birth weight, reduced lung function, and delayed immune maturation.[16,17,61,66] An increasing range of prenatal environmental exposures are being linked to risk of respiratory disease, especially wheezing in early childhood and persistent asthma. However, for many of these the mechanisms are uncertain and not all studies show strong associations. Further research with both improved exposure assessments and outcome measurements is required.

Common Pathways to Respiratory Diseases

Debate continues about whether the various chronic respiratory diseases are different entities or components of a single disease spectrum.[67] Holt and Sly[68] postulated that atopic asthma, nonatopic asthma, and COPD could be part of a "family tree" of respiratory diseases stemming from a common origin but subject to environmental exposures occurring at different times during postnatal development and with differing frequency and severity. Fig. 4.6 shows a schematic representation of the common susceptibilities and exposures that could lead to atopic asthma, nonatopic asthma, and COPD.

Low lung function at birth and low lung growth during childhood is likely to increase the risk of both acute and chronic respiratory diseases. Low lung function at birth increases the risk of acute respiratory illness (ARI) and pneumonia in early life,[10,57,69] asthma, and COPD.[10,56,61,69,70]

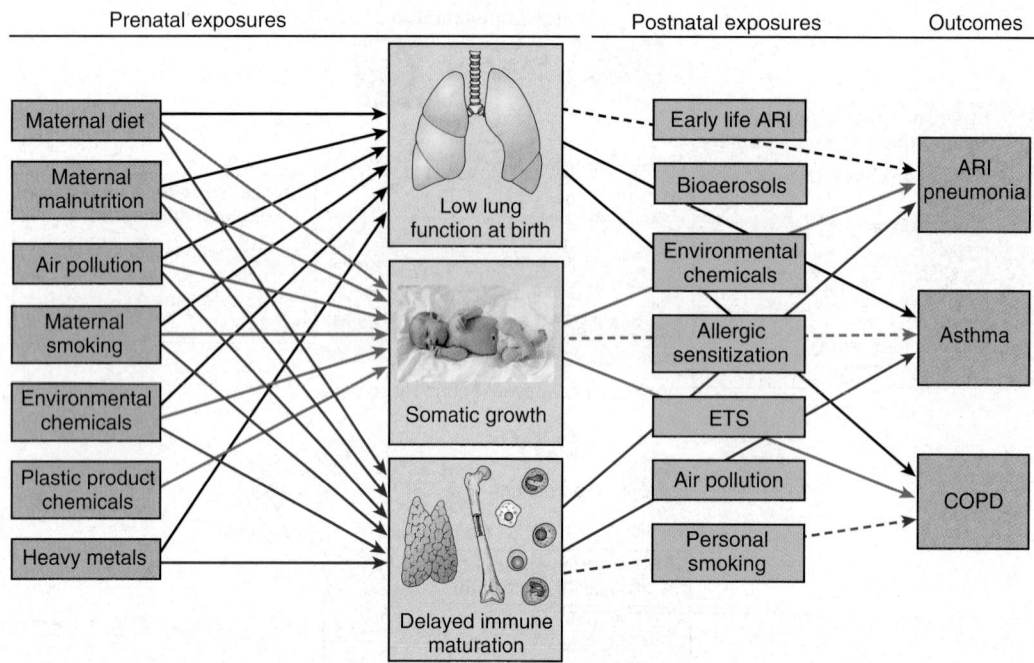

Fig. 4.5 Schematic representation of how environmental exposures increase the risk of respiratory diseases. *ARI,* Acute respiratory infection; *COPD,* chronic obstructive pulmonary disease; *ETS,* environmental tobacco smoke.

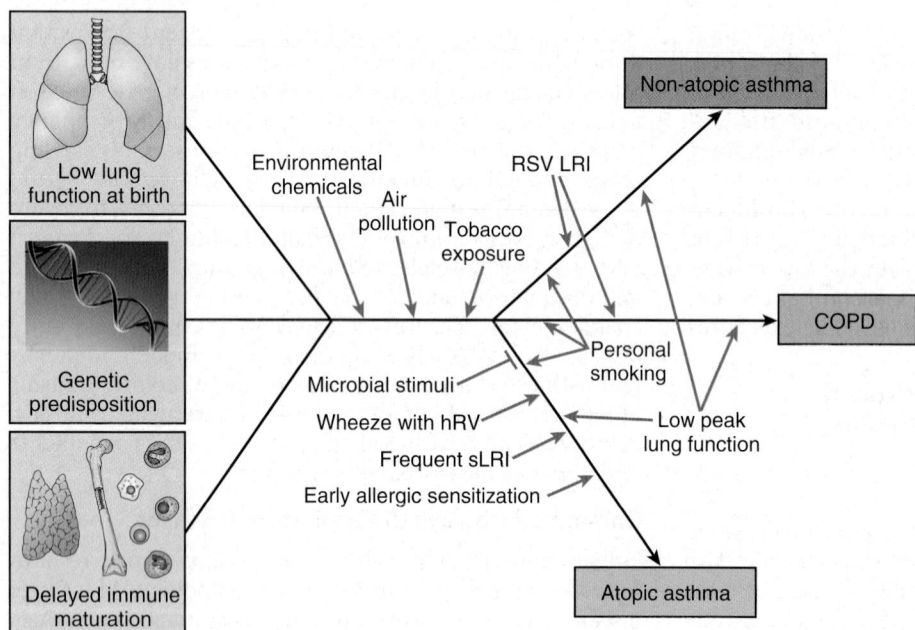

Fig. 4.6 Schematic representation of the "Family Tree" of respiratory diseases. *COPD,* Chronic obstructive pulmonary disease; *hRV,* human rhinovirus; *LRI,* lower respiratory illness; *RSV,* respiratory syncytial virus; *sLRI,* severe lower respiratory illness associated with fever and/or wheeze. (Holt P, Sly P. Non-atopic intrinsic asthma and the 'family tree' of chronic respiratory disease syndromes. *Clin Exp Allergy.* 2009;39:807-811.)

Environmental insults, especially those occurring in the first 2–4 years during the period of rapid lung growth, can decrease lung growth.[12,17,27,33,56,59–61,69–74] Similarly, severe lower respiratory illnesses (sLRIs) and pneumonia in early life can reduce lung growth.[75] Lung function "grows" to reach a peak in early adult life, remains at a plateau for some years, and then begins to decline. Much of the rate of decline is under genetic control but can also be accelerated by smoking and in those exposed to adverse environmental exposures in early life.[76–78] Failure to reach the peak lung function that would be predicted by parental and genetic factors increases the risk of developing respiratory symptoms and COPD in later life. A compilation of data from three large adult cohorts estimated that approximately half of those developing COPD did so because they had a reduced peak lung function and half developed COPD due to an accelerated rate of lung function decline.[70] Thus preventing low lung function at birth and preserving lung function growth during childhood is of the utmost importance in preventing chronic lung disease.

Environmental Contributions to Acute Respiratory Illness and Pneumonia

As outlined in the previous sections, environmental exposures increase the risk of ARI and pneumonia in early life. However, what is less certain is which exposures increase the primary risk (i.e., without which the disease is less likely to occur) as opposed to factors with increase the severity of the disease. To some extent this distinction is artificial but does have implications for disease prevention. Prenatal exposures increasing disease risk may be primary risk factors. These exposures include: maternal smoking during pregnancy,[79] maternal infections, especially HIV[79]; maternal exposures to arsenic[80,81]; and maternal exposure to ambient or household air pollution resulting in lower lung function at birth (see earlier). Exposures that occur both prenatally and postnatally, such as exposure to increased levels of particulate matter in both indoor and ambient environments,[82–85] tobacco smoke exposure,[79,86] poor household ventilation, and overcrowding,[79,84,87] may have primary effects either prenatally or postnatally but may also act to increase illness severity in those young children contracting respiratory viral or bacterial infections. Evidence is increasing that the components of the infant's respiratory microbiome in the upper airway and gastrointestinal system can either increase or decrease risk of ARI, especially at times of respiratory viral infections.[79,84,87] Childhood malnutrition, stunting, and living in poor circumstances are likely to both increase disease risk and severity.[84,85,87–89]

One environmental factor that is frequently overlooked is climate, including humidity, hours of sunshine, temperature, rainfall, and related factors.[90,91] Whether the climate-related factors increase the risk of ARI by increasing viral survival and transmission efficiency or by causing seasonal variations in immunocompetence through nutritional or vitamin D–related pathways is not known.[90–97] However, the influence of global climate change is likely to increase the prevalence and severity of ARI in children.

Environmental Contributions to Asthma

Asthma can be considered to be a developmental disease, where the normal growth and development of the respiratory and immune systems are modified by both genetic and environmental factors that result in altered lung structure and function, increased susceptibility to respiratory infections and allergic sensitization early in life.[10] Both the respiratory and immune systems are vulnerable to adverse environmental exposures occurring both before and after birth. Although most asthma develops in childhood, incident asthma does occur in adults. Thus an understanding of the environmental contributions to asthma across all stages of life is important.

Again, understanding of environmental factors that increase the risk of developing asthma (i.e., asthma inception) is important. The same exposures occurring in a child who already has asthma may also increase the likelihood of having symptoms, increase the severity of symptoms, or trigger acute exacerbations of asthma. An overview of the environmental factors involved in inception or triggering of asthma is shown in Tables 4.3 and 4.4.

Summary

Environmental exposures, especially those occurring during fetal development and in early postnatal life, increase the risk of acute and chronic respiratory diseases. Many of these exposures are avoidable and provide an opportunity to prevent or reduce the burden of respiratory diseases.

Table 4.3 Environmental Exposures Associated With Inception of Asthma at Different Life Stages

	ASTHMA INCEPTION				
	LIFE STAGE OF EXPOSURE				
Exposure	**Preconception**	**Fetal Development**	**Infancy**	**Childhood**	**Adolescence**
Tobacco smoke	Grand maternal smoking imposes risk via maternal oocytes[38]	↓Lung function, ↓Birth weight, ↑BHR,[33,63] delayed immune maturation[34]	↓Lung growth,[65,98–100] ↑ARI[100,101]	↓Lung growth,[58,98,102–105] ↑BHR,[32,33] ↑ARI[58,98,102–105]	↓Lung function, ↑BHR[32,33]
Indoor air pollution	N/S	↓Lung function, ↓Birth weight[106]	↓Lung growth, ↑ARI[12,106–108]	↓Lung growth, ↑ARI[12,106,109]	↓Lung function in girls[110–112]
Ambient air pollution	N/S	↓Lung function[69,113], ↓Birth weight[64]	↓Lung growth, ↑ARI[59,60]	↓Lung growth, ↑ARI[17,27,59,60,69,114,115]	↓Lung function[17,27,59,60,69,114,115]
PCBs	N/S	↓Birth weight[116]	↑ARI[117]	↑ARI[117]	N/S
Bisphenols/phthalates	N/S	↓Birth weight[118]	↑Wheeze[119]	↑Wheeze, ↓Lung function[120]	N/S
Household chemicals	N/S	↓Birth weight[121]	↑Wheeze[121]	↑Wheeze, ↓Lung function[121]	N/S
Bioaerosols	N/S	May be protective[49]	High dose protective, low dose ↑allergy[48]	High dose protective, low dose ↑allergy[48]	N/S

AHR, Airway hyperresponsiveness; *ARI,* acute respiratory infections; *N/S,* not studied; *N/A,* not applicable; *PCBs,* polychlorinated biphenyls.

Table 4.4   Environmental Exposures Associated With Triggering of Asthma at Different Life Stages

			ASTHMA TRIGGERING		
			LIFE STAGE OF EXPOSURE		
Exposure	Preconception	Fetal Development	Infancy	Childhood	Adolescence
Tobacco smoke	N/A	N/A	↑Wheeze, ↑ARI[17,58,102]	↑Wheeze, ↑ARI[17,58,86,102]	↑Wheeze, ↑ARI[17,33]
Indoor air pollution	N/A	N/A	↑Wheeze, ↑ARI[15,122]	↑Wheeze, ↑ARI[15,84,87,102]	↑Wheeze, ↑ARI[12]
Ambient air pollution	N/A	N/A	↑Wheeze, ↑ARI[17,115]	↑Wheeze, ↑ARI, ↑BHR[17,59,115,123–125]	↑Wheeze, ↑ARI, ↑BHR[17,27,59,126]
PCBs	N/A	N/A	↑Wheeze, ↑ARI[117]	↑Wheeze, ↑ARI[117]	N/S
Bisphenols/phthalates	N/A	N/A	N/S	↑Wheeze, ↑BHR[127]	N/S
Household chemicals	N/A	N/A	↑Wheeze[121]	↑Wheeze[121]	N/S
Bioaerosols	N/A	N/A	↑Wheeze[128,129]	↑Wheeze, acute asthma[128,129]	↑Wheeze, acute asthma[128,129]

AHR, Airway hyperresponsiveness; *ARI*, acute respiratory infections; *BHR*, bronchial hyperresponsiveness; *N/S*, not studied; *N/A*, not applicable; *PCBs*, polychlorinated biphenyls.

References

Access the reference list online at ExpertConsult.com.

Suggested Reading

de Planell-Saguer M, Lovinsky-Desir S, Miller RL. Epigenetic regulation: the interface between prenatal and early-life exposure and asthma susceptibility. *Environ Mol Mutagen*. 2014;55(3):231–243.

Duijts L, Reiss IK, Brusselle G, et al. Early origins of chronic obstructive lung diseases across the life course. *Eur J Epidemiol*. 2014;29(12):871–885.

Goldizen FC, Sly PD, Knibbs LD. Respiratory effects of air pollution on children. *Pediatr Pulmonol*. 2015;51(1):94–108.

Heard E, Martienssen RA. Transgenerational epigenetic inheritance: myths and mechanisms. *Cell*. 2014;157(1):95–109.

Heindel JJ, Balbus J, Birnbaum L, et al. Developmental origins of health and disease: integrating environmental influences. *Endocrinology*. 2015;156(10):3416–3421.

Henderson AJ. The child is father of the man: the importance of early life influences on lung development. *Thorax*. 2014;69(11):976–977.

Lange P, Celli B, Agustí A, et al. Lung-function trajectories leading to chronic obstructive pulmonary disease. *New Engl J Med*. 2015;373(2):111–122.

Postma DS, Rabe KF. The asthma–COPD overlap syndrome. *New Engl J Med*. 2015;373(13):1241–1249.

Rigoli L, Briuglia S, Caimmi S, et al. Gene-environment interaction in childhood asthma. *Int J Immunopathol Pharmacol*. 2011;24(4 Suppl): 41–47.

Sly P, Flack F. Susceptibility of children to environmental pollutants. *An NY Acad Sci*. 2008;1140:163–183 (Environmental Challenges in the Pacific Basin).

Suk WA, Ahanchian H, Asante KA, et al. Environmental pollution: an under-recognized threat to children's health, especially in low- and middle-income countries. *Environ Health Perspect*. 2016;124(3):A41–A45.

5 The Surfactant System

PAUL KINGMA, MD, PhD, and ALAN H. JOBE, MD, PhD

Pulmonary surfactant is a complex substance with multiple functions in the microenvironments of the alveoli and small airways.[1] The traditional functions of surfactant are the biophysical activities to keep the lungs open, to decrease the work of breathing, and to prevent alveolar edema. Most of the components of surfactant also contribute to innate host defenses and injury responses of the lung.[2] Surfactant deficiency states occur with prematurity and with severe lung injury syndromes. Recent studies in humans and in mice have defined an expanding number of genetic and metabolic abnormalities that disrupt surfactant and cause lung diseases, which range from lethal respiratory failure at birth to chronic interstitial lung disease in later life.[3] We will summarize those aspects of surfactant biology that are relevant to children.

Surfactant Composition and Metabolism

COMPOSITION

Surfactant recovered from lungs by bronchoalveolar lavage contains about 80% phospholipids, about 8% protein, and about 8% neutral lipids, primarily cholesterol (Fig. 5.1).[4] The phosphatidylcholine species of the phospholipids contribute about 70% by weight to surfactant. The phospholipids in surfactant are unique relative to the lipid composition of lung tissue or other organs. About 50% of the phosphatidylcholine species have two palmitic acids or other saturated fatty acids esterified to the glycerol-phosphorylcholine backbone, resulting in "saturated" phosphatidylcholine, which is the principal surface-active component of surfactant. About 8% of surfactant is the acidic phospholipid phosphatidylglycerol. Surfactant from the immature fetus contains relatively large amounts of phosphatidylinositol, which then decreases as phosphatidylglycerol appears with lung maturity.[5]

Four primary surfactant-associated proteins have been identified: A, B, C, and D.[6,7] Initial analyses of these proteins suggested that the hydrophilic surfactant protein A (SP-A) and surfactant protein D (SP-D) were primarily involved in pulmonary innate immunity, whereas the hydrophobic surfactant protein B (SP-B) and surfactant protein C (SP-C) facilitated surfactant lipid physiology. However, we now know that the surfactant proteins often cross these lines of functional classification.

SP-A and SP-D are members of the collectin family of innate defense proteins. Collectins are defined by four structural domains shared by all family members: a short amino-terminal cross-linking domain, a triple helical collagenous domain, a neck domain, and a carbohydrate recognition domain (CRD).[6–10] Three neck domains combine and facilitate the formation of a collagen-like triple helix that then aggregates to form larger multimers of the collectin trimer. SP-A is a 24-kD monomer that further assembles to a bouquet of six trimers with a molecular size of 650 kD.[11–13] SP-A is encoded by two genes located within a "collectin locus" on the long arm of chromosome 10 that also includes the genes for SP-D and the mannose binding protein.[14] In humans, SP-A synthesis begins during the second trimester of gestation and occurs primarily in the alveolar type II epithelial cells, club cells, and in cells of tracheo-bronchial glands. SP-A is required for the formation of tubular myelin and has several roles in pulmonary host defense.

SP-D is a 43-kD hydrophilic collectin with a monomer structure that is similar to SP-A, although the collagen domain of SP-D is much longer.[13,15] Structural studies demonstrate that SP-D trimers further combine into larger multimeric complexes through N-terminal interactions that are stabilized by N-terminal disulfide bonds.[8,12,16] Although larger, more complex forms have been identified, SP-D exists predominately as a tetramer of trimeric subunits (dodecamer) assembled into a cruciform. SP-D is synthesized by type II cells and by club cells, as well as in other epithelial sites. Like the other surfactant proteins, SP-D expression is developmentally regulated and induced by glucocorticoids and inflammation.[17] In addition to the complex roles of SP-D in pulmonary host defense, SP-D also influences surfactant structure and is required for surfactant reuptake and the regulation of pulmonary surfactant pool sizes.[18,19]

SP-B is a small hydrophobic protein that contributes about 2% to the surfactant mass.[1,6] The SP-B gene is on human chromosome 2 and is expressed in a highly cell-specific manner. The primary translation product is 40 kD, but the protein is clipped in the type II cell to become an 8-kD protein prior to associating with phospholipids during the formation of lamellar bodies. SP-B facilitates the surface absorption of lipids into the expanding alveolar surface film and enhances their stability during the movements of the respiratory cycle. A genetic lack of SP-B causes a loss of normal lamellar bodies in type II cells, a lack of mature SP-C, and the appearance of incompletely processed SP-C in the airspaces.[20]

The SP-C gene is on chromosome 8, and its primary translation product is a 22-kD protein that is processed to an extremely hydrophobic 35 amino acid peptide rich in valine, leucine, and isoleucine.[21] The SP-C gene is expressed in cells lining the developing airways from early gestation. With advancing lung maturation, SP-C gene expression becomes localized only to type II cells. SP-B and SP-C are packaged together into lamellar bodies and function cooperatively to optimize rapid adsorption and spreading of phospholipids. Surfactants prepared by organic solvent extraction of natural surfactants or from lung tissue contain SP-B and SP-C. Such surfactants are similar to natural surfactants when evaluated for *in vitro* surface properties or for function *in vivo*.

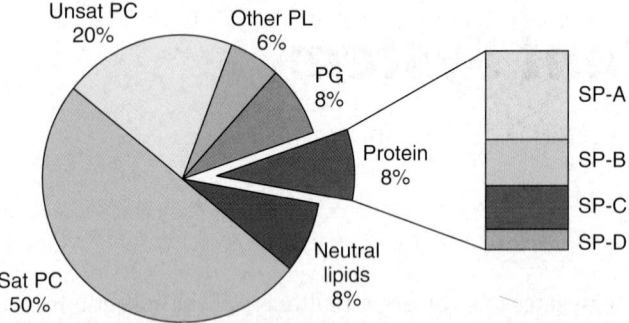

Fig. 5.1 Composition of surfactant. Saturated phosphatidylcholines (PC) are the major components of alveolar surfactant. Minor lipid components include unsaturated PC, phosphotidylglycerol (PG), neutral lipids, and other phospholipids (PL). The proteins contribute about 8% to the weight of surfactant. *SP-A,* Surfactant protein A; *SP-B,* surfactant protein B; *SP-C,* surfactant protein C; *SP-D,* surfactant protein D.

Surfactant Metabolism and Secretion

The synthesis and secretion of surfactant by the type II cell is a complex sequence that results in the release by exocytosis of lamellar bodies to the alveolus.[22] Enzymes within the endoplasmic reticulum (ER) use glucose, phosphate, and fatty acids as substrates for phospholipid synthesis. The details of how the surfactant lipids condense with SP-B and SP-C to form the surfactant lipoprotein complex within lamellar bodies remain obscure. Ultrastructural abnormalities of type II cells with SP-B deficiency and ABCA3 deficiency in full-term infants indicate that these gene products are essential for lamellar body formation.[23] A basal rate of surfactant secretion occurs continuously, and surfactant secretion can be stimulated by β-agonists and purines, or with lung distention and hyperventilation.

The alveolar pool size of surfactant is about 4 mg/kg in the adult human.[24] The lung tissue of the adult human contains much more surfactant, and only about 7% of the surfactant lipids are in the secreted pool. The surfactant pool size per kilogram probably changes little with age after the newborn period. While no estimates exist for the full-term human, full-term animals have alveolar pool sizes of about 100 mg/kg, and this large pool decreases to adult values by about 1 week of age.[25] The alveolar surfactant pool size in the adult (and presumably young child) is small relative to other mammalian species (e.g., about 30 mg/kg in adult sheep), which may make the human lung more susceptible to surfactant deficiency with lung injury. Infants with respiratory distress syndrome (RDS) have alveolar surfactant pool sizes of less than 5 mg/kg.

The kinetics of surfactant metabolism have been extensively studied in adult, term, and preterm animal models.[26] In all species studied to date, including primates, the surfactant component synthesis to secretion interval is relatively long, and the alveolar half-life of newly secreted surfactant is very long, on the order of 6 days in healthy newborn lambs.[27] The surfactant components are recycled back into type II cells, and recycling is more efficient in newborn than adult animals.[28] These observations have been validated by quite extensive studies in preterm and term humans using stable

isotopes to label surfactant precursors or components.[29] A limitation of the studies is the need to have an endotracheal tube in place to allow repetitive sampling of lung fluid. Depending on the labeled precursor, the time from synthesis to peak secretion of new surfactant ranged from 2 to 3 days, and the half-life for clearance was 2 to 4 days in preterm infants. Similar values were measured for term infants. In general, preterm or term infants with lung disease have surfactant with smaller pool sizes, less synthesis and secretion, and shorter half-life values. These measurements include term infants with pneumonia, meconium aspiration syndrome, and congenital diaphragmatic hernia. There are no measurements of surfactant metabolism for older children. In one report in normal adults using sputum samples, peak labeling of surfactant phosphatidylcholine occurred about 2 days after the labeled precursor was given, and the subsequent half-life was about 7 days.[30] These studies demonstrate that the replacement of endogenous surfactant pools is slow, and alveolar pools turn over slowly.

Alveolar Life Cycle of Surfactant

After secretion, surfactant goes through a series of form transitions in the airspace (Fig. 5.2).[22] The lamellar bodies unravel to form the elegant structure called tubular myelin. This lipoprotein array has SP-A at the corners of the lattice and requires at least SP-A, SP-B, and the phospholipids for its unique structure.[31] Tubular myelin and other large surfactant lipoprotein structures are the reservoir in the fluid hypophase for the formation of the surface film within the alveolus and small airways. The hypophase is a very thin fluid layer covering the distal epithelium with a volume of about 0.5 mL/kg body weight that has a surfactant concentration of approximately 10 mg/mL. New surfactant enters the surface film, and "used" surfactant leaves in the form of small vesicles. The surface-active tubular myelin contains SP-A, SP-B, and SP-C, while the biophysically inactive small vesicles that are recycled and catabolized contain very little surfactant protein. The total surfactant pool size is less than the amount of active surfactant because 30% to 50% of the alveolar phospholipids are in catabolic forms in the normal lung. Pulmonary edema and products of lung injury can accelerate form conversion and cause a depletion of the surface-active fraction of surfactant despite normal or high total surfactant pool sizes.[32] Surfactant is catabolized primarily by type II cells and alveolar macrophages. Granulocyte-macrophage colony-stimulating factor deficiency prevents alveolar macrophages from catabolizing surfactant and results in the clinical syndrome of alveolar proteinosis.[33] The important concept is that the alveolar pool of functional surfactant is maintained by dynamic metabolic processes that include secretion, reuptake, and resecretion balanced by catabolism.

Surfactant Function

ALVEOLAR STABILITY

Alveoli are polygonal with flat surfaces and curvatures where the walls of adjacent alveoli intersect. Alveoli are interdependent in that their structure is determined by the shape

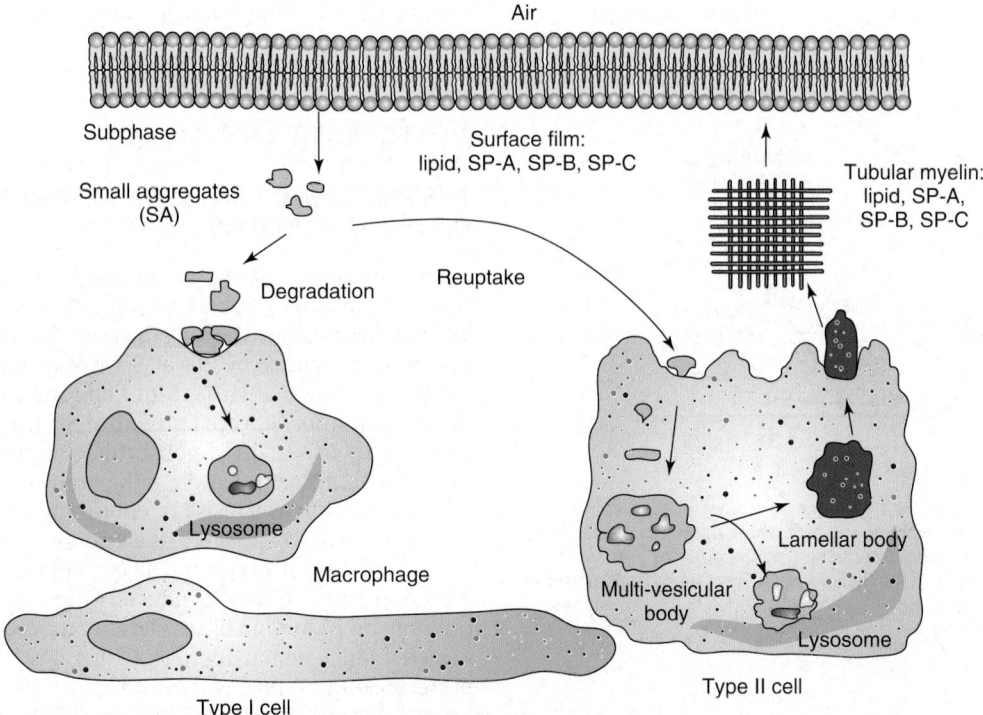

Fig. 5.2 Alveolar life cycle of surfactant. Surfactant is secreted from lamellar bodies in type II cells. In the alveolar fluid lining layer, the surfactant transforms into tubular myelin and other surfactant protein-rich forms, which facilitate surface adsorption. The lipids are catabolized as small vesicular forms by macrophages and type II cells, and are recycled by type II cells. *SP-A,* Surfactant protein A; *SP-B,* surfactant protein B; *SP-C,* surfactant protein C.

and elasticity of neighboring alveolar walls. The forces acting on the pulmonary microstructure are chest wall elasticity, lung tissue elasticity, and surface tensions of the air-fluid interfaces of the small airways and alveoli. Although the surface tension of surfactant decreases with surface area compression and increases with surface area expansion, the surface area of an alveolus changes little with tidal breathing. The low surface tensions resulting from surfactant help to prevent alveolar collapse and keep interstitial fluid from flooding the alveoli. Surfactant also keeps small airways from filling with fluid and thus prevents the potentially ensuing luminal obstruction.[34] If alveoli collapse or fill with fluid, the shape of adjacent alveoli will change, which can result in distortion, overdistention, or collapse. When positive pressure is applied to a surfactant-deficient lung, the more normal alveoli will tend to overexpand, and the alveoli with inadequate surfactant will collapse, generating a nonhomogeneous inflated lung.

Pressure-Volume Curves

The static effects of surfactant on a surfactant-deficient lung are evident from the pressure-volume curve of the preterm lung (Fig. 5.3). Preterm surfactant-deficient rabbit lungs do not begin to inflate until pressures exceed 20 cm H_2O.[35] The pressure needed to open a lung unit is related to the radius of curvature and surface tension of the meniscus of fluid in the airspace leading to the lung unit. The units with larger radii and lower surface tensions will "pop" open first because, with partial expansion, the radius increases and the forces needed to finish opening the unit decrease. Surfactant

decreases the opening pressure from greater than 20 to 15 cm H_2O in this example with preterm rabbit lungs. Because surfactant does not alter airway diameter, the decreased opening pressure results from surface adsorption of the surfactant to the fluid in the airways. The inflation is more uniform as more units open at lower pressures, resulting in less overdistention of the open units.

A particularly important effect of surfactant on the surfactant-deficient lung is the increase in maximal volume at maximal pressure. In this example, maximal volume at 30 cm H_2O is increased over two times with surfactant treatment. Surfactant also stabilizes the lung on deflation. The surfactant-deficient lung collapses at low transpulmonary pressures, whereas the surfactant-treated lung retains about 30% of the lung volume on deflation. This retained volume is similar to the total volume of the surfactant-deficient lung at 30 cm H_2O and demonstrates how surfactant treatments increase the functional residual capacity (FRC) of the lung.

Host Defense Functions of Surfactant

SP-A and SP-D are pattern recognition molecules that bind a variety of polysaccharides, phospholipids, and glycolipids on the surface of bacterial, viral, and fungal pathogens.[6,7] SP-A and SP-D binding forms protein bridges between microbes that induce microbial aggregation and stimulate the recognition, uptake, and clearance of pathogens by host defense cells.[36,37] In addition, SP-A and SP-D binding may have direct antibacterial and antifungal activity by increasing pathogen membrane permeability.[38,39]

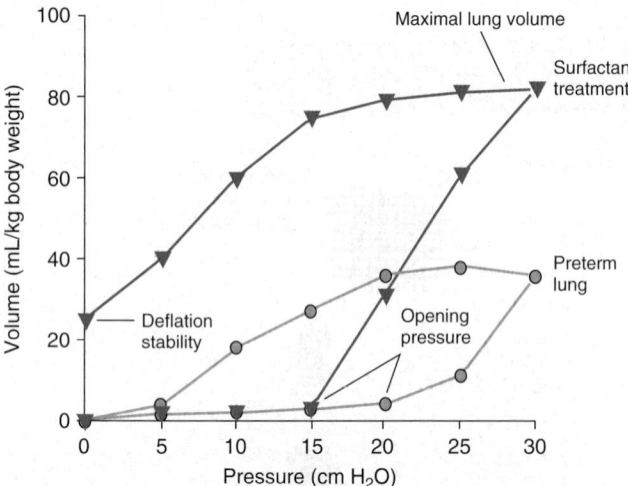

Fig. 5.3 Effect of surfactant treatment on surfactant-deficient lungs. These idealized pressure-volume curves illustrate the effect of surfactant treatment with natural sheep surfactant on the opening pressure, the maximal lung volume, and the deflation stability of lungs from preterm rabbits. (Curves based on data from Rider ED, Jobe AH, Ikegami M, Sun B. Different ventilation strategies alter surfactant responses in preterm rabbits. *J Appl Physiol.* 1992;73:2089-2096.)

Although binding and aggregation of infectious microbes is a critical feature of SP-A and SP-D physiology, these proteins also have more complex roles in host defense.[2] SP-A and SP-D have been implicated in the stimulation and inhibition of several immune pathways. Both SP-A and SP-D bind CD14 and inhibit lipopolysaccharide-induced expression of proinflammatory cytokines through CD14 and toll-like receptor 4.[40–42] SP-A binds toll-like receptor 2 and inhibits proinflammatory cytokine release in response to peptidoglycan.[43] Gardai and colleagues proposed a model by which SP-A and SP-D might stimulate or inhibit inflammation through the competing actions of signal regulating protein α (SIRPα) and calreticulin/CD91.[44] Their model suggests that in the unbound state, the CRDs of SP-A or SP-D inhibit macrophage activation by binding to SIRPα, which inhibits activation of nuclear factor κB (NFκB). In contrast, if the CRDs of SP-A or SP-D are occupied by a microbial ligand, binding to SIRPα is inhibited and instead the collectins bind to the macrophage activating receptor, calreticulin/CD91, which turns on NFκB and subsequently induces proinflammatory mediator release and alveolar macrophage activation. SP-A also may contribute to adaptive immune responses. SP-A inhibits the maturation of dendritic cells in response to potent T cell stimulators and enhances the endocytic ability of dendritic cells.[45] In addition, SP-A downregulates lymphocyte activity and proliferation.[46]

The hydrophobic surfactant proteins SP-B and SP-C may also have host defense functions. Although SP-B can inhibit bacterial growth *in vitro,* overexpression of SP-B or reduced expression of SP-B in the lungs of mice did not alter bacterial clearance, suggesting that SP-B is not involved in innate host defense.[47] However, elevated levels of SP-B in the lungs of endotoxin-exposed mice decreased pulmonary inflammation.[48] Thus, SP-B may contribute to the modulation of inflammation in the injured lung. SP-C binds lipopolysaccharide and blocks the production of tumor necrosis factor-α by macrophages.[49] However, possible roles for SP-C

in bacterial clearance or lung inflammation *in vivo* have not been evaluated.

Surfactant Deficiency

THE PRETERM INFANT WITH RESPIRATORY DISTRESS SYNDROME

RDS in preterm infants is a primary surfactant deficiency that initially does not include lung injury, unless antenatal infection complicates the lung disease.[50] The surfactant system normally is mature by about 35 weeks' gestation, but the early appearance of surfactant and lung maturation is frequent in infants delivered prematurely. Early maturation is thought to occur in response to fetal stress resulting in increased fetal cortisol levels, or by exposure of the fetal lung to inflammation as a result of chorioamnionitis.[38] Maternal treatments with corticosteroids are routinely given to decrease the risk of RDS if preterm delivery before 32 to 34 weeks' gestation is anticipated.[51] Induced lung maturation includes not only an induction of surfactant but also thinning of the mesenchyme, which increases lung gas volumes. Unless preterm infants have early lung maturation, they develop progressive respiratory distress from birth, which is characterized by tachypnea, grunting, increased work of breathing, and cyanosis. Infants who have died of RDS have alveolar pool sizes of surfactant of less than 5 mg/kg. Although this amount is similar to the amount of surfactant recovered from healthy adult humans, surfactant from the preterm infant has decreased function, probably because it contains less of the surfactant proteins, which are critical for biophysical function.[52] The surfactant from the preterm infant also is more susceptible to inactivation by edema fluid, and the preterm lung is easily injured if a stable FRC is not maintained or if the lung is overstretched.

THE INJURED MATURE LUNG

Acute respiratory distress syndrome (ARDS) describes an overwhelming inflammatory reaction within the pulmonary parenchyma leading to global lung dysfunction.[53] ARDS is defined by acute onset, an oxygenation index less than 200, bilateral infiltrates on chest x-ray, and a pulmonary capillary wedge pressure of less than 18 mm Hg, or the absence of clinical evidence for left-sided heart failure. The etiology of ARDS is multifactorial and can occur in association with lung injury secondary to trauma, sepsis, aspiration, pneumonia, massive blood transfusions, or near drowning to name some associations. It is a common disease, affecting approximately 15% to 20% of all patients ventilated in the adult intensive care unit (ICU) and 1% to 4.5% of patients in the pediatric ICU. ARDS has a high mortality rate of 40% to 50%.

Impairment of surfactant with ARDS can result from inhibition, degradation, or decreased production.[32,54–56] The proteinaceous pulmonary edema characteristic of ARDS can inactivate surfactant by dilution and by competition for the interface.[54] Plasma proteins known to inhibit surfactant function include serum albumin, globulin, fibrinogen, and C-reactive protein. In addition to proteins, phospholipases, along with their products, fatty acids, and lipids inhibit surface activity. Epithelial cell injury by inflammatory mediators can decrease surfactant production and contribute to surfactant deficiency. Normally in the lung, about 50% of surfactant is present in the bioactive form that has a high SP-B and SP-C content. In ARDS, small vesicular forms increase, and the pool of active surfactant is depleted.

The phospholipid content is decreased and the phospholipid composition is abnormal in bronchoalveolar lavage fluid (BALF) from patients with ARDS.[57] SP-A, SP-B, and SP-C also are decreased in BALF from patients with ARDS. The surfactant protein levels can remain low for at least 14 days after the onset of ARDS. Changes in surfactant composition, including phospholipids, fatty acids, and proteins, likely represent alveolar type II cell injury with altered metabolism, secretion, or recycling of components. SP-A and SP-B concentrations are also reduced in the lungs of patients at risk for ARDS, even before the onset of clinical lung injury. In contrast, SP-D levels in BALF remain normal, except in a subgroup of patients who later died. Decreased SP-D levels in BALF were 85.7% sensitive and 74% specific in predicting death from ARDS.[58]

GENETIC DEFICIENCIES OF SURFACTANT IN MICE AND HUMANS

Mice with targeted deletion of the *Sftpa* gene *(Sftpa$^{-/-}$)* for SP-A protein survived normally without changes in surfactant composition, function, secretion, and reuptake; however, there was no tubular myelin.[59] Although seemingly normal at baseline, significant defects were detected in pulmonary host defense in SP-A-deficient mice when they were subjected to a microbial challenge. The clearance of group B *Streptococcus, Haemophilus influenzae,* respiratory syncytial virus (RSV), and *Pseudomonas aeruginosa* was delayed in *Sftpa$^{-/-}$* mice, and the recognition and uptake of bacteria by alveolar macrophages were deficient.[60–62] Oxygen radical production and killing of engulfed microorganisms by *Sftpa$^{-/-}$* macrophages were markedly reduced, while markers of lung inflammation were increased following infection in *Sftpa$^{-/-}$* mice.[63]

Despite the considerable innate immune defects that are associated with SP-A deficiency in animal models, we have yet to find a human susceptibility to pulmonary infection that is caused by a *Sftpa* mutation. However, polymorphisms in the human genes for SP-A affecting their function have been identified, and humans with these polymorphisms have increased susceptibility to acquiring infections with RSV and *Mycobacterium tuberculosis.*[64] Analyses suggest that SP-A polymorphisms may also affect infection severity since patients that are homozygous or heterozygous for asparagine at amino acid position 9 are more likely to need intensive care, mechanical ventilation, or longer hospitalization.[55] Although there are no clear associations between *Sftpa* mutation and pulmonary infection, an association has been reported between a rare heterozygous mutation in the *Sftpa* and adult onset interstitial pulmonary fibrosis and lung cancer.[65] It is likely that these mutations cause SP-A misfolding and the trapping of SP-A in the ER, which leads to chronic ER stress and cell injury.[65]

Mice with deletion of the *Sftpd* gene *(Sftpd$^{-/-}$)* for SP-D protein survived normally, but unlike SP-A-deficient mice that had relatively normal lungs at baseline, *Sftpd$^{-/-}$* mice spontaneously developed pulmonary inflammation and airspace enlargement. In addition, *Sftpd$^{-/-}$* mice accumulated

increased numbers of apoptotic macrophages, and enlarged, foamy macrophages that released reactive oxygen species and metalloproteinases.[66,67] When *Sftpd$^{-/-}$* mice were exposed to a microbial challenge, the uptake and clearance of viral pathogens including influenza A and RSV were deficient, whereas the clearance of group B *Streptococcus* and *H. influenzae* were unchanged.[68,69] However, oxygen radical release and production of the proinflammatory mediators were increased in *Sftpd$^{-/-}$* mice when exposed to either viral or bacterial pathogens indicating that SP-D plays an antiinflammatory role in the lung that is independent of the clearance of pathogens.[63,68,69] SP-D deficiency has not been described in humans, but polymorphisms at amino acid position 11 are associated with increased risk of RSV infection.[70]

Gene-targeted mice lacking SP-B, and infants with hereditary SP-B deficiency, demonstrate the critical role of SP-B in surfactant function, homeostasis, and lung function.[71] Targeted disruption of the mouse SP-B gene causes respiratory failure at birth. Despite normal lung structure, the SP-B-deficient mice failed to inflate their lungs postnatally. Type II cells of SP-B-deficient mice had large multivesicular bodies but did not have lamellar bodies, and the proteolytic processing of pro-SP-C (the preprocessed form of SP-C) was disrupted.[6] Infants with SP-B deficiency die from respiratory distress in the early neonatal period with the same anatomic findings.[72] Mutations leading to partial SP-B function have been associated with chronic lung disease in infants. Because SP-B is required for both intracellular and extracellular aspects of surfactant homeostasis, SP-B deficiency has not been treated successfully with surfactant replacement therapy, and survival is dependent on lung transplantation. It is important to note that mice and infants without the adenosine triphosphate-binding cassette transporter A3 (ABCA3) have type II cells without lamellar bodies and the same lethal respiratory failure phenotype as observed in SP-B deficiency.[73]

SP-C-deficient mice survive and have normal surfactant composition and amounts. However, surfactant isolated from the SP-C-deficient mice forms less stable bubbles, demonstrating a role for SP-C in developing and maintaining lipid films.[74] SP-C mutations were recently identified in patients with familial and sporadic interstitial lung disease.[75] *Sftpc* mutations in these patients alter the ability of the protein to fold correctly and result in the retention of SP-C in the ER and the subsequent development of ER stress which, in turn, leads to pulmonary cell injury and death. Histological features of lung disease in these individuals include lungs with a thickened interstitium, infiltration with inflammatory cells and macrophages, fibrosis, and abnormalities of the respiratory epithelium. In isolated reports, infants with respiratory failure from SP-D deficiency have been supported by tracheostomy and chronic mechanical ventilation for years prior to eventual decannulation and survival off ventilator support.[76]

Surfactant Treatment of Surfactant Deficiency

RESPIRATORY DISTRESS SYNDROME

The respiratory morbidities of preterm infants with RDS have strikingly decreased in recent years because of the combined effects of antenatal corticosteroid treatments and more gentle approaches to mechanical ventilation.[77] The original randomized trials of surfactant for RDS evaluated treatments given after the disease was established, generally after 6 hours of age.[78] Other trials evaluated treatment of all high-risk infants soon after birth to prevent RDS. Subsequent trials demonstrated that treatments of the highest-risk infants (generally infants with birth weights less than 1 kg) as soon after birth as convenient and before significant mechanical ventilation will minimize lung injury. However, many very low birth weight infants can be transitioned to air breathing successfully using continuous positive airway pressure (CPAP), and the decision to treat with surfactant can be made after the initial stabilization at birth.[79,80] One advantage of allowing the infant to breathe spontaneously with CPAP used to recruit and maintain FRC, is that hyperventilation and overdistention of the delicate preterm lung by mechanical ventilation can be avoided. Larger infants who develop RDS generally are treated with oxygen and nasal CPAP until the oxygen concentration approaches 40%. Then they are treated with surfactant. Preterm infants will respond to surfactant treatments even if the treatment is delayed for several days.

Full-term infants with severe meconium aspiration or pneumonia also will respond to surfactant treatments with improved oxygenation,[81] and surfactant also can improve lung function in infants with the group B streptococcal sepsis/pneumonia syndrome.[82] Current practice is to treat most infants with severe respiratory failure with surfactant because there are no contraindications.

The surfactants that are commercially available for clinical use in infants are made from organic solvent extracts of animal lungs or alveolar lavages of animal lungs. While there are differences in composition, the clinical results do not demonstrate any compelling differences in clinical responses. All of the commercial surfactants lack SP-A and SP-D, contain SP-C, and have variable amounts of SP-B. Surfactants that contain synthetic peptides or surfactant proteins are being developed for clinical use. Surfactants that contain steroids also are being tested as an approach to decreasing bronchopulmonary dysplasia in infants treated for RDS.[83]

ACUTE RESPIRATORY DISTRESS SYNDROME

ARDS is a significant therapeutic challenge for intensivists despite recent advances in understanding pathophysiology and new treatment modalities. Surfactant content and composition are altered in ARDS, resulting in decreased surface activity, atelectasis, and decreased lung compliance.[54] The injury is generally not uniform throughout the lung,

resulting in overinflation of the more normal lung, and atelectasis and filling of alveolar fluid in other lung regions. The injured lung makes less surfactant, and that surfactant is inhibited by the highly proteinaceous edema and inflammatory fluid, and the fluid-filled alveoli are difficult to recruit to improve ventilation. Multiple animal models of ARDS respond very positively to surfactant treatments when combined with lung recruitment ventilation strategies. Unfortunately, multiple, large, randomized, controlled trials using different surfactants have not shown any benefit for surfactant treatments.[84,85] The experience in adult patients with ARDS differs strikingly from the clinical responses of preterm infants with RDS. Somewhere in between are the clinical responses of term infants with meconium aspiration and pneumonia, who have modest, but consistent clinical improvements that can decrease extracorporeal membrane oxygenation (ECMO) use and save lives.[86] Several small trials and clinical experiences suggested that older infants and children with diseases such as acute RSV pneumonia respond to surfactant treatment. A small trial by Wilson and colleagues demonstrated that for a range of children from 1 to 21 years of age with various causes of ventilator dependent ARDS, surfactant treatments improved oxygenation and decreased mortality.[87] However, a subsequent trial of surfactant for children with lung injury/ARDS was stopped for futility after the enrollment of 110 patients.[88] Although surfactant use decreased hospital days, there was no effect on oxygenation or mortality. A recent meta-analysis of three small trials of surfactant for bronchiolitis in infants showed some benefit, but larger trials will be needed to verify this indication.[89] Future studies could explore the potential for surfactant components for host defense in diseases such as ARDS.

References

Access the reference list online at ExpertConsult.com.

Suggested Reading

Albert RK, Jobe A. Gas exchange in the respiratory distress syndromes. *Compr Physiol.* 2012;2(3):1585–1617.

Han S, Mallampalli RK. The role of surfactant in lung disease and host defense against pulmonary infections. *Ann Am Thorac Soc.* 2015;12(5):765–774.

Kunzmann S, Collins JJ, Kuypers E, et al. Thrown off balance: the effect of antenatal inflammation on the developing lung and immune system. *Am J Obstet Gynecol.* 2013;208(6):429–437.

SUPPORT Study Group of the Eunice Kennedy Shriver NICHD Neonatal Research Network, Finer NN, Carlo WA, et al. Early CPAP versus surfactant in extremely preterm infants. *N Engl J Med.* 2010;362(21):1970–1979.

Whitsett JA, Wert SE, Weaver TE. Diseases of pulmonary surfactant homeostasis. *Annu Rev Pathol.* 2015;10:371–393.

Willson DF, Truwit JD, Conaway MR, et al. The adult calfactant in acute respiratory distress syndrome trial. *Chest.* 2015;148(2):356–364.

6

The Structural and Physiologic Basis of Respiratory Disease

MATTHIAS OCHS, MD, and HUGH O'BRODOVICH, MD

Knowledge of the normal development, structure, and physiologic function of the lungs is required to understand the pathophysiology that is seen in disease. Historically, the understanding of lung function was derived solely from clinical observation and postmortem histologic examination. The development of invasive and noninvasive techniques that were capable of assessing lung structure and function in living subjects greatly improved our understanding of lung physiology on an "organ basis." There has been an explosion of knowledge in cellular and molecular biology, which is covered in detail in other chapters. This chapter will focus on the normal structure of the lung and organ physiology.

Normal Lung Anatomy and Cell Function

Knowledge of normal lung anatomy is one of the basic requirements for understanding lung function in health and disease. Because detailed descriptions of lung anatomy are available elsewhere,[1-3] this section will focus on selected aspects of gross and microscopic anatomy to enable the reader to understand the physiologic changes that occur in congenital and acquired lung disease.

The shape of the lung reveals three faces: the convex costal face opposed to the rib cage, the concave diaphragmatic face resting on the diaphragmatic dome, and the mediastinal face, where the right and left lung are oriented toward each other. The right and left lung are each embedded in a separate pleural cavity and are separated by the mediastinum. Except at the hilum (where airways, vessels, and nerves enter or leave the lung), the lung's outer surface is covered by the visceral pleura, which also extends into the fissures, thereby demarcating the pulmonary lobes (Fig. 6.1).

Airways

The airways are composed of two functional compartments. A proximal conducting zone (the bronchial tree) continuously connects to a distal respiratory zone (the alveolar region), where gas exchange takes place. The basic structure of the airways is already present at birth; therefore, neonates and adults share a common bronchopulmonary anatomy (Figs. 6.2 and 6.3). When airways divide, they do so by dichotomous branching, over an average of 23 generations, although the number of times that branching occurs varies. This airway variability has physiologic implications: different pathways will have different resistances to air flow, and a heterogeneous distribution of gases or inhaled particles may occur. As the bronchi branch and decrease in size, they lose their

cartilage and become bronchioles. Ultimately, a terminal bronchiole opens into the alveoli-containing gas-exchanging area of the lung. In the human, the gas-exchanging area begins with several generations of respiratory bronchioles (i.e., bronchioles with alveoli attached to their wall) that connect to alveolar ducts whose "wall" completely consists of alveolar openings. The most distal alveolar ducts end in blind alveolar sacs. The unit of lung parenchyma distal to a terminal bronchiole (i.e., the unit in which all airways participate in gas exchange) is termed the *acinus* (Fig. 6.4).[4]

The airways are lined with a continuous epithelium that gradually changes from a ciliated pseudostratified columnar epithelium in the bronchi to a ciliated simple cuboidal epithelium in smaller bronchioles near the gas-exchanging units. At the transition into the alveolar region, the epithelium abruptly becomes squamous. At all levels, the epithelium is not made of a single cell type, but rather a mosaic of several cell types: lining cells and secretory cells, often with rarer cells with specialized functions interspersed (Fig. 6.5). Ciliated cells predominate throughout the bronchial and bronchiolar epithelium and are responsible for propelling mucus from the peripheral airways to the pharynx (Fig. 6.6). This mucociliary transport system is an important defense mechanism of the lungs. The mucous layer has two parts, a superficial gel layer with high viscosity and a deeper periciliary layer with a brushlike structure.[5] The cilia form a dense, long carpet on top of the epithelial cells, and their coordinated to-and-fro action propels the gel mucous layer toward the oropharynx. Cilia are a derivative of the centrioles, and there are approximately 200 of them on the apex of each ciliated cell. The cilia are anchored within the cell with a basal body that is oriented in the direction of mucous movement. The shaft of the cilium has a central pair of single tubules that are connected via radial spokes to nine peripheral pairs of tubules. The tip of the cilium has tiny hooklets that probably help grab the gel component of the mucous layer and propel it forward. The cilium has a beat frequency of 12 to 20 Hz and is coordinated both with other cilia on that cell and concurrently with the cilia on adjacent cells to yield a synchronized wave flowing up the airway.[6,7] Primary ciliary dyskinesia (PCD) is a group of disorders that includes Kartagener syndrome and the erroneously named *immotile cilia syndrome.* In PCD, there are defects within the tubules, in their inner or outer dynein arms, or in the radial arms that result in a disorganized movement of the cilia that precludes normal mucociliary transport and results in chronic bronchitis and repeated pneumonias (see Chapter 71). Submucosal glands, which are present in large and small bronchi, are the chief source of airway secretions and contain both serous and mucus cells. Goblet cells are seen in the trachea

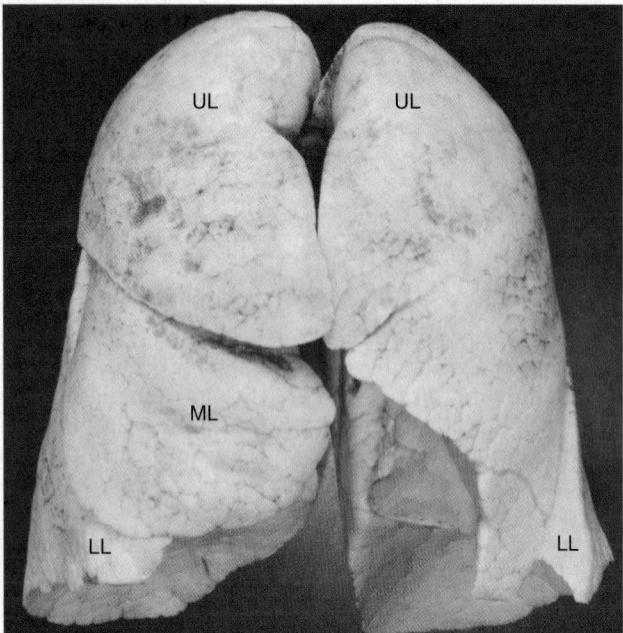

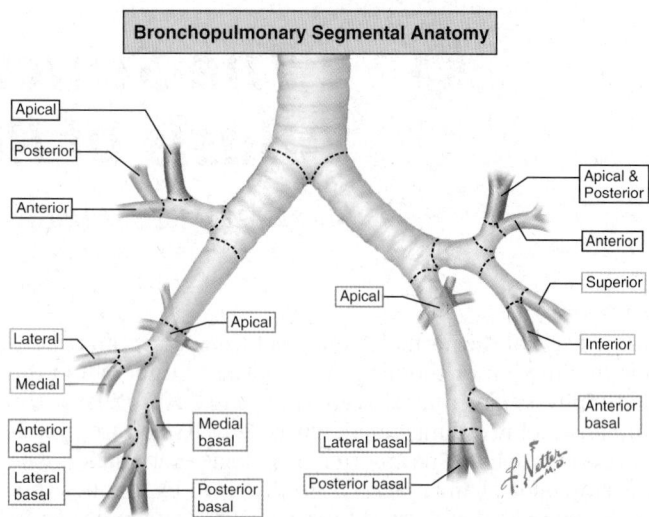

Fig. 6.2 Bronchopulmonary segmental anatomy. (Adapted from figure id #21, Nomenclature of Bronchi: Schema, from Netterimages.com. 2017.)

Fig. 6.1 Dried human lung. The costal and diaphragmatic faces can be seen. The visceral pleura that covers the surface of the lungs extends into the fissures. The oblique fissure separates the upper lobe (UL) and lower lobe (LL) on both sides. The horizontal fissure separates the UL and middle lobe (ML) of the right lung.

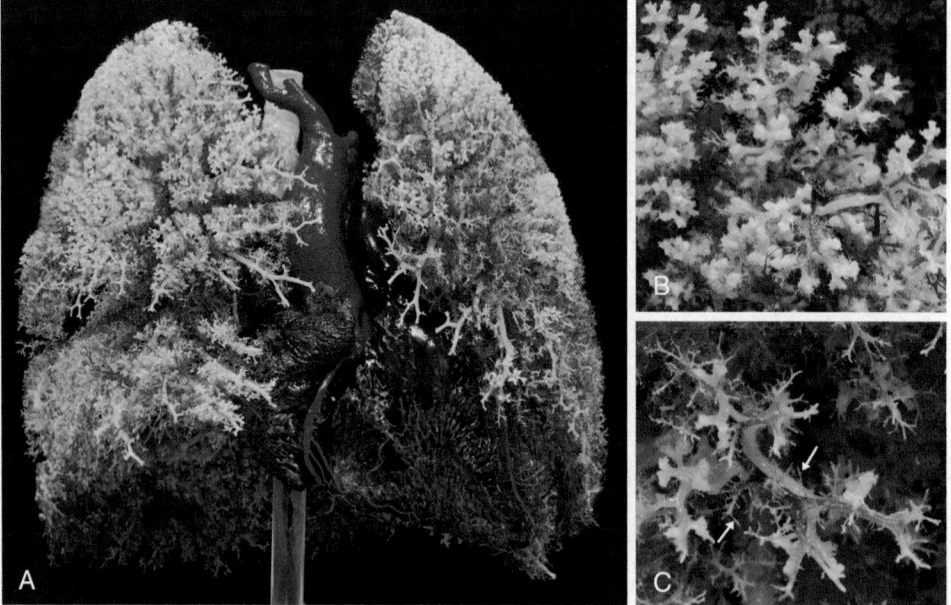

Fig. 6.3 Resin cast of human lung airway and vascular trees. Airways are shown in *yellow,* pulmonary arteries in *blue,* and pulmonary veins in *red.* The chambers of the right heart and the pulmonary trunk *(blue)* as well as coronary arteries originating from the aorta *(red)* can also be seen (A). Higher magnifications show how pulmonary artery branches closely follow the airways, whereas branches of the pulmonary veins lie between bronchoarterial units (B). Small supernumerary arteries *(arrows)* take off at right angles (C).

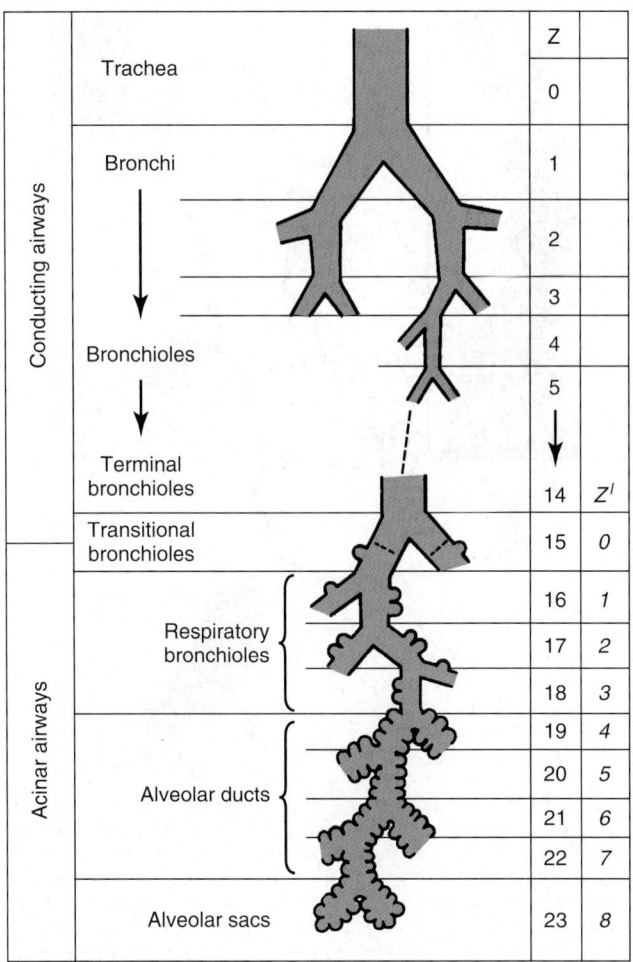

		Z	
Conducting airways	Trachea	0	
	Bronchi	1	
		2	
		3	
	Bronchioles	4	
		5	
	Terminal bronchioles	14	Z^I
Acinar airways	Transitional bronchioles	15	0
	Respiratory bronchioles	16	1
		17	2
		18	3
	Alveolar ducts	19	4
		20	5
		21	6
		22	7
	Alveolar sacs	23	8

Fig. 6.4 Model of airway branching in the human lung over an average of 23 generations. The first 14 generations are purely conducting. Transitional airways lead into acinar airways, which contain alveoli and thus participate in gas exchange. (Modified from Weibel ER. *Morphometry of the Human Lung.* Heidelberg: Springer; 1963. From Ochs M, Weibel ER. Functional design of the human lung for gas exchange. In: Fishman AP, Elias JA, Fishman JA, et al., eds. *Fishman's Pulmonary Diseases and Disorders,* 4th ed. New York: McGraw-Hill; 2008:23-69.)

and bronchi (see Fig. 6.6). They produce mucin, a viscous mixture of acid glycoproteins that contributes to the mucous layer. Submucosal glands and goblet cells can increase in number in disorders such as chronic bronchitis, the result being mucous hypersecretion and increased sputum production. The basal cell, commonly seen within the pseudostratified columnar bronchial epithelium resting on the basement membrane but not reaching the lumen, is undifferentiated and acts as a precursor of ciliated or secretory cells (see Fig. 6.6).[8]

Whereas ciliated cells are still present in smaller bronchioles, goblet cells are gradually replaced by nonciliated bronchiolar epithelial cells (often termed club cells).[9] These cells are characterized by their dome-shaped apex that protrudes into the airway lumen and by secretory granules. Their secretory products, which include the club cell secretory protein (CCSP), add to the bronchiolar lining layer. CCSP is thought to have immunomodulatory functions. In addition, club cells are a site of cytochrome P-450–dependent detoxification of xenobiotics, and they act as progenitor cells for the maintenance of the bronchiolar epithelium.[10]

There are several rarer cell types found within the airways; however, their functional significance is less well understood. The brush cell, which is only rarely found in the human lung, has a dense tuft of broad, short microvilli. It is supposed to "taste" the chemical composition of the airway lining fluid.[11,12] Neuroendocrine cells secrete mediators into subepithelial capillaries. Sometimes these cells are organized in clusters (neuroepithelial bodies) that are thought to have oxygen-sensing functions. Neuroepithelial bodies[13] are found more frequently within the fetal airways or in pediatric disorders characterized by chronic hypoxemia (e.g., bronchopulmonary dysplasia).

Histologically, the remainder of the airway consists of the submucosa, with its network of blood vessels and nerves, and a variable amount of smooth muscle and cartilage. Within the submucosa are mast cells containing vasoactive peptides and amines, cells of the immune system (plasma cells, lymphocytes, and phagocytes), and submucosal glands. In the main stem bronchi, cartilage is present in C-shaped

Fig. 6.5 Schematic representation of wall structure along the airways. The epithelium is reduced from pseudostratified to cuboidal and then to squamous, but it retains its mosaic of lining and secretory cells. Only the trachea and bronchi contain cartilage and submucosal glands. Smooth muscle cells disappear in the alveoli. (From Ochs M, Weibel ER. Functional design of the human lung for gas exchange. In: Fishman AP, Elias JA, Fishman JA, et al., eds. *Fishman's Pulmonary Diseases and Disorders,* 4th ed. New York: McGraw-Hill; 2008:23-69.)

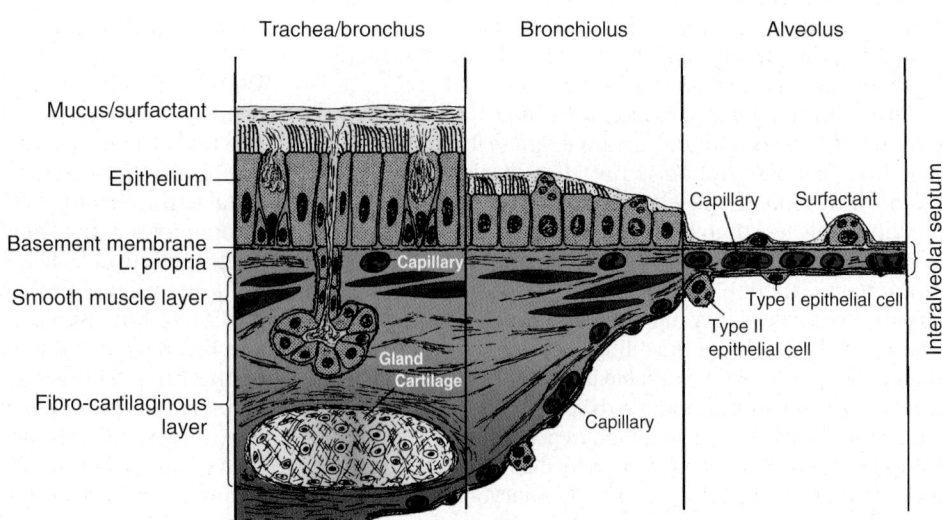

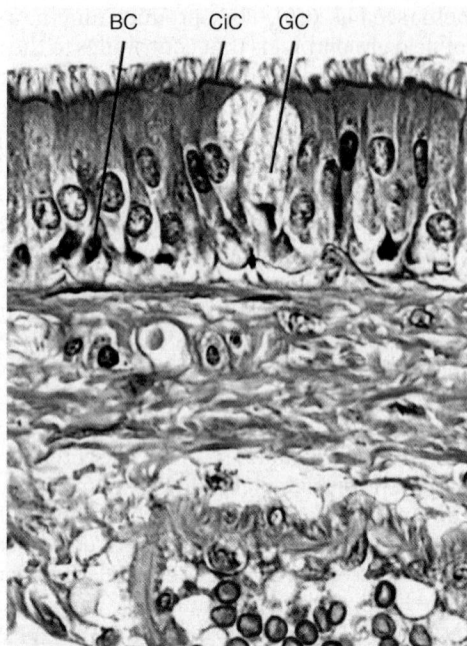

Fig. 6.6 Light micrograph of the bronchial wall. The major cells types of the pseudostratified columnar respiratory epithelium can be seen: ciliated cells (CiC), goblet cells (GC), and basal cells (BC). The mucosa's connective tissue layer (lamina propria), which contains blood vessels, can be seen underneath the epithelium. (Courtesy of G. Bargsten, Hannover.)

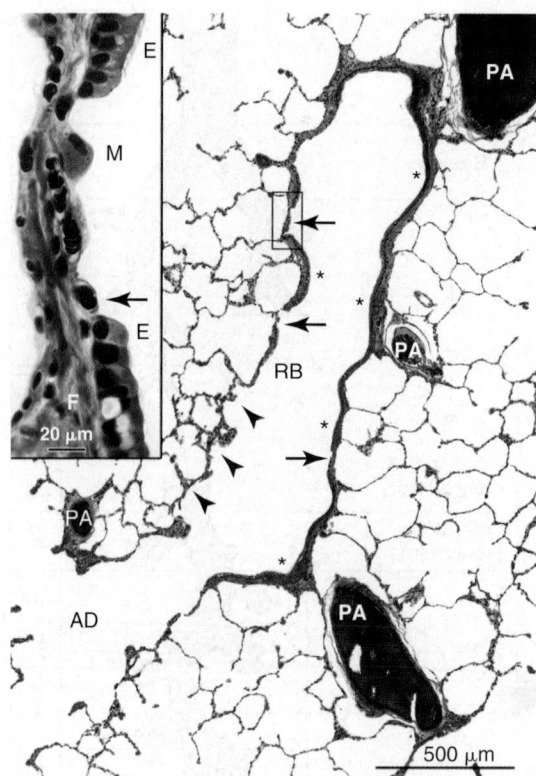

Fig. 6.7 Light micrograph of respiratory bronchiole (RB) from human lung seen extending into alveolar ducts (AD). The wall is lined by typical bronchiolar cuboidal epithelium *(asterisks)*, which is interrupted by respiratory patches *(arrows)* and alveoli proper *(arrowheads)*. Note pulmonary artery branches (PA) following the respiratory bronchiole. *Inset:* Respiratory patch with capillary *(arrow)* and macrophage (M). The cuboidal ciliated epithelium (E) is replaced by thin squamous type I alveolar epithelial cells. Note thick fibrous layer (F) with smooth muscle cells. (From Ochs M, Weibel ER. Functional design of the human lung for gas exchange. In: Fishman AP, Elias JA, Fishman JA, et al., eds. *Fishman's Pulmonary Diseases and Disorders*, 4th ed. New York: McGraw-Hill; 2008: 23-69.)

rings. However, as further branching of bronchi occurs, progressively less cartilage is present as plates. Cartilage adds structural rigidity to the airway and thus plays an important role in maintaining airway patency, especially during expiration. Congenital deficiency of airway cartilage and hence airway instability has been associated with bronchiectasis (Williams-Campbell syndrome) and congenital lobar hyperinflation (previously referred to as *congenital lobar emphysema*).

The smooth muscle content of the airway also varies with its anatomic location. In the largest airways, a muscle bundle connects the two ends of the C-shaped cartilage. As the amount of cartilage decreases, the smooth muscle assumes a helical orientation and gradually becomes thinner, ultimately reaching the alveolar ducts where the smooth muscle cells lie in the alveolar entrance rings. Muscle contraction increases airway rigidity in all airways.

Although it has been widely assumed that the airway muscles of newborn infants are inadequate for bronchoconstriction, this assumption is not correct. Even premature infants have smooth muscle, and although the amount may be statistically less than that seen in adults, it is likely enough to constrict the infant's much more compliant airways. Indeed, pulmonary function test results have demonstrated that airway resistance can be altered with bronchodilating drugs. The belief that infants have little or no smooth muscle in their airways is even less tenable in such disorders as Northway's old bronchopulmonary dysplasia[14] and left-to-right congenital heart disease, in which hypertrophy of the airway smooth muscle has been demonstrated by morphometric measurement. Congenital deficiency of large-airway smooth muscle and elastic fibers is associated with marked dilation of the trachea and bronchi, which promotes retention of airway secretions and ultimately leads to recurrent pulmonary sepsis, a condition known as the Mounier-Kuhn syndrome or tracheobronchomegaly.

Alveolar Region

Within the pulmonary lobule, defined as the smallest unit of lung structure marginated by connective tissue septae, one finds the lungs' region for gas exchange. The terminal respiratory (gas-exchanging) unit consists of the structures distal to the terminal bronchiole: the respiratory bronchioles (bronchioles with alveoli budding from their walls), alveolar ducts, and alveoli (Fig. 6.7).

As mentioned earlier in the chapter, the acinus is the portion of lung parenchyma distal to a terminal bronchiole (see Fig. 6.4). It is the basic functional gas-exchanging unit of the lung. The acinus is approximately 6 to 10 mm in diameter in the adult lung. In the adult lung, these units have a total gas volume of 2000 to 4000 mL and a surface area of about 140 m^2 (Table 6.1),[15] yet all alveoli are within 5 mm of the closest terminal bronchiole. True alveoli are not spherical but more closely resemble hexagons with flat,

Table 6.1 The Human Lung in Numbers

Alveolar number	480 million
Alveolar surface area	140 m²
Capillary volume	210 mL
Air-blood barrier thickness	2 μm

Data from Gehr P, Bachofen M, Weibel ER. The normal lung: ultrastructure and morphometric estimation of diffusion capacity. *Resp Physiol.* 1978;32:121-140; Ochs M, Nyengaard JR, Jung A, et al. The number of alveoli in the human lung. *Am J Respir Crit Care Med.* 2004;169:120-124.

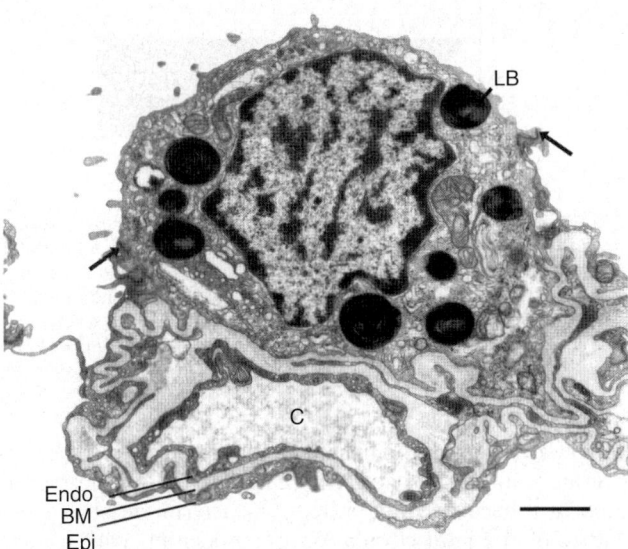

Fig. 6.8 Electron micrograph of a human type II alveolar epithelial cell. The phospholipid-rich surfactant material is stored in lamellar bodies (LB) prior to secretion. On both sides, thin cell extensions of type I alveolar epithelial cells form tight junctions with the type II cell *(arrows)*. A capillary (C) is seen underneath the type II cell. The thin side of the air-blood barrier is trilaminar and consists of the alveolar epithelium (Epi), fused basement membranes (BM) and the capillary endothelium (Endo). Scale bar = 1 μm. (From Ochs M. A brief update on lung stereology. *J Microsc.* 2006;222:188-200.)

Table 6.2 Cellular Characteristics of the Human Lung

Cell Type	Total Cells (%)	Cell Volume (μm³)	Apical Surface Area (μm²)
Epithelium			
Alveolar type I	8	1764	5098
Alveolar type II	16	889	183
Endothelium	30	632	1353
Interstitial	36	637	
Alveolar macrophages	10	2492	

Data from Crapo JD, Barry BE, Gehr P, et al. Cell number and cell characteristics of the normal human lung. *Am Rev Respir Dis.* 1982;125:332-337.

I cells, but because of their cuboidal shape, they occupy only about 5% of the total alveolar surface area (Table 6.2). They are characterized histologically by microvilli and osmophilic inclusions termed *lamellar bodies*, which are storage sites for surfactant components (see Fig. 6.8).[19,20]

The type II alveolar epithelial cell maintains homeostasis within the alveolar space in several ways. First, it is the source of pulmonary surfactant and as such is one index of fetal lung maturity; surfactant decreases the surface tension at the alveolar air-liquid interface. Second, in the postnatal lung, this cell is the precursor of the type I alveolar epithelial cell and thus plays a key role in the normal maintenance of the alveolar epithelium as well as in the repair process following lung injury when progenitor cells from type II alveolar epithelium contribute to alveolar renewal, repair and cancer.[21,22] Third, it is capable of actively transporting ions against an electrochemical gradient and is involved in both fetal lung liquid secretion, in airspace fluid reabsorption at birth, and in the postnatal reabsorption of fluid from the airspace following the development of alveolar pulmonary edema (see the discussion on fetal lung liquid secretion in "The Lung at Birth" later in this chapter). Two pediatric disorders associated with the type II alveolar epithelial cell are (1) its lack of maturity and surfactant secretion in respiratory distress syndrome (RDS) of preterm infants and (2) its decreased lamellar body formation and surfactant secretion in surfactant dysfunction mutations (e.g., in genes encoding surfactant protein B or the lipid transporter ABCA3).

The cell junctions (zonulae occludentes) between type I and type II alveolar epithelial cells are very tight and thus restrict the movement of both macromolecules and small ions (e.g., sodium and chloride) (see Fig. 6.8). This tightness is an essential characteristic of the cells lining the alveolar space; it enables the active transport of ions. Also, these tight junctions provide a margin of safety for patients who are susceptible to pulmonary edema; significant interstitial pulmonary edema can be present without alveolar flooding, thus preserving gas exchange.

There is a thick side and a thin side to the alveolar air-blood barrier. Gas exchange is thought to occur predominantly on the thin side where there are only the thin extensions of type I alveolar epithelial cells, fused basement membranes, and capillary endothelial cells (see Fig. 6.8). Capillaries undergo considerable stress (e.g., during exercise or lung hyperinflation) and must have great tensile strength. This strength is mainly imparted by type IV collagen located in the basement membrane. The thick side of the barrier consists of connective tissue, amorphous ground substance, and

sheetlike surfaces. The average alveolar diameter ranges from 200 to 300 μm. Within the acini, interalveolar holes (termed *pores of Kohn*) are present in alveolar walls. Although they have been thought to provide channels for collateral ventilation, the fact that pores of Kohn are covered with surfactant[16] needs to be taken into consideration. Ultrastructural evidence suggests that they are used by alveolar macrophages to reach neighboring alveoli. In the newborn lung, there are few, if any, pores of Kohn. This might contribute to the fact that relative to adult lung, infant lung is more predisposed to patchy atelectasis.

The alveoli are lined by two types of epithelial cells (Fig. 6.8). Type I alveolar epithelial cells are extremely broad, thin (0.1 to 0.5 μm) cells that in total cover about 95% of the alveolar surface. They are markedly differentiated cells that possess few organelles, and because their cytoplasmic leaflets are so thin, they provide an epithelial barrier for gas exchange that cannot be resolved by routine histology.[17] Recent work has demonstrated that these cells are capable of actively transporting Na⁺ with Cl⁻ and water following, and thus participate in the clearance of airspace fluid (see Chapter 36).[18] Type II epithelial cells are more numerous than type scattered fibroblasts. The thick side, in addition to providing structural support, acts as a site of fluid and solute exchange.[23]

Pulmonary Vascular System

The lung receives blood from both ventricles. In the postnatal lung, the entire right ventricular output enters the lung via the pulmonary arteries, and blood ultimately reaches the gas-exchanging units by one of the pulmonary arterial branching systems. Arterial branches accompany the bronchial tree and divide with it, each branch accompanying the appropriate bronchial division (see Fig. 6.3B). In addition, supernumerary arteries take off at right angles and directly supply the gas-exchanging units (see Fig. 6.3C). The pulmonary capillary bed is the largest vascular bed in the body and covers a surface area of about 120 to 130 m². The network of capillaries is so dense that it may be thought of as a sheet of blood interrupted by small vertical supporting posts. The pulmonary veins that lie at the boundaries between lung units defined by bronchoarterial divisions return blood to the left atrium. By virtue of their larger numbers and thinner walls, the pulmonary veins provide a large reservoir for blood and help maintain a constant left ventricular output in the face of a variable pulmonary arterial flow.

The bronchial arteries (usually three originating directly or indirectly from the aorta, but variable in number)[24,25] provide a source of well-oxygenated systemic blood to the lung's tissues.[26,27] This blood supply nourishes the walls of the bronchi and proximal bronchioles, larger blood vessels, and nerves in addition to perfusing the lymph nodes and most of the visceral pleura. There are numerous communications between the bronchial arterial system and the remainder of the pulmonary vascular bed: a portion of the blood returns to the right atrium via bronchial veins, and a portion drains into the left atrium via pulmonary veins. Although the bronchial arteries normally receive only 1% to 2% of the cardiac output, they hypertrophy in chronically infected lungs, and blood flow may easily increase by more than 10-fold. This is clinically important because virtually all hemoptysis originates from the bronchial vessels in disorders such as cystic fibrosis or other causes of suppurative bronchiectasis.

Histologically, the pulmonary arteries can be classified as elastic, muscular, partially muscular, or nonmuscular. The elastic pulmonary arteries are characterized by elastic fibers embedded in their muscular coat, whereas the smaller muscular arteries have a circular layer of smooth muscle cells bounded by internal and external elastic laminae. As arteries decrease further in size, only a spiral of smooth muscle remains (partially muscular arteries), which ultimately disappears so that vessels still larger than capillaries have no muscle in their walls (nonmuscular arteries). In the adult lung, elastic arteries are greater than 1000 μm in diameter, and muscular arteries are usually in the range of 250 μm. In the pediatric age group, histologic structure is not as easily determined from vessel size. During lung growth, a remodeling of the pulmonary vasculature occurs. Muscularization of the arteries lags behind multiplication of alveoli and appearance of new arteries. Therefore, the patient's age must be considered before histologic structure can be assumed from vessel size within the pulmonary acinus (Fig. 6.9).

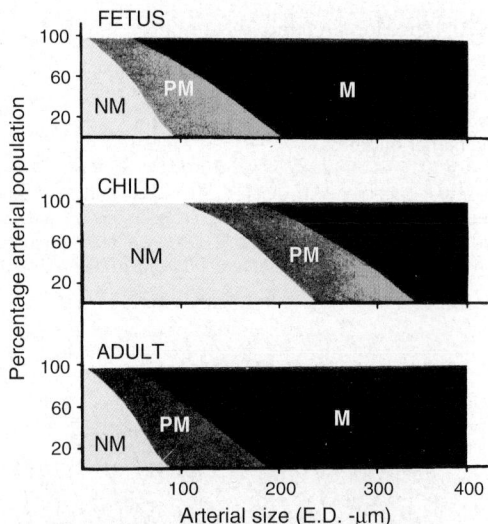

Fig. 6.9 The populations of the three arterial types: muscular (M), partially muscular (PM), and nonmuscular (NM), in the fetus, child, and adult. The distribution of structure in size is similar in the fetus and the adult, whereas during childhood NM and PM structures are found in much larger arteries. *E.D.,* External diameter. (From Reid LM. The pulmonary circulation. Remodeling in growth and disease. *Am Rev Respir Dis.* 1979; 119:531.)

Notably, in the fetus and newborn, the amount of pulmonary arterial smooth muscle is increased. This is functionally important because high pulmonary arterial resistance is a feature of the fetal circulation in association with a large right to left shunt via the ductus arteriosus.

The endothelium of the pulmonary vascular system is continuous and nonfenestrated. It is an intensely active cell layer and is not just serving a passive barrier function. The endothelial cell produces a glycocalyx that interacts with blood-borne substances and blood cellular elements, thereby influencing such homeostatic functions as hemostasis. The endothelium produces von Willebrand factor, which is part of the factor VIII complex and is necessary for normal platelet function. Within endothelial cells, von Willebrand factor is stored in specific granules termed *Weibel-Palade bodies.*[28] Similarly, there are enzymes located on the surface and within the endothelial cell itself that are capable of synthesizing, altering, or degrading blood-borne vasoactive products. The individual cells are separated by gaps of approximately 3.5 nm in radius, which allow the free movement of water and small ions but restrict the movement of proteins. The cells and the basement membrane on which they sit carry different net surface charges, which affect the movement of anionic macromolecules such as proteins and thus affect lung water and solute exchange (see Chapter 36). The capacity of the pulmonary endothelium and its basement membrane to restrict fluid and protein movement is impressive. It has been estimated that in the adult human, the amount of lung lymph flow is only 10 to 20 mL/h despite a total blood flow of 300,000 mL/h.

Lymphatic System

There is an extensive interconnecting network of lymphatic vessels throughout the lung. The major function of this network is to collect the protein and water that has moved out of the pulmonary vascular space and to return it to the circulation, thus maintaining the lung at an appropriate degree of hydration. The lymphatic vessels travel alongside the blood vessels in the loose connective tissue of the pleura and bronchovascular spaces. It is likely that there are no lymphatics within the alveolar wall itself and that juxta-alveolar lymphatics represent the beginning of the pulmonary lymphatic system. Histologically, the lymphatic capillaries consist of thin, irregular endothelial cells that lack a basement membrane. Occasionally, there are large gaps between endothelial cells that allow direct communication with the interstitial space. Larger lymphatic vessels contain smooth muscle in their walls that undergoes rhythmic contraction. This muscular contraction plus the presence of funnel-shaped, monocuspid valves ensures an efficient unidirectional flow of lymph. In addition to helping maintain lung water balance, the lymphatic system is one of the pulmonary defense mechanisms. It aids in removal of particulate matter from the lung, and aggregates of lymph tissue near major airways contribute to the host's immune response.

Innervation of the Lung

The lung is innervated by both components of the autonomic nervous system.[29] Parasympathetic nerves arise from the vagus nerve, and sympathetic nerves are derived from the upper thoracic and cervical ganglia of the sympathetic trunk. These branches congregate around the hila of the lung to form the pulmonary plexus. Myelinated and nonmyelinated fibers then enter the lung tissues and travel along with and innervate the airways and blood vessels. Although the anatomic location of pulmonary nerves has been elucidated, their physiologic role in health and disease is incompletely understood. In general, the airways constrict in response to vagal stimulation and dilate in response to adrenergic stimulation. The postnatal pulmonary vasculature appears to be maximally dilated under normal conditions, and it is difficult to demonstrate any significant physiologic effect of either parasympathetic or sympathetic stimulation. The vascular response, however, is influenced by age and initial vascular tone. For example, in fetal lungs where there is an abundance of pulmonary vascular smooth muscle, vagal stimulation results in significant vasodilation, and sympathetic stimulation results in marked vasoconstriction.

Sensory nerves from the lungs are vagal in origin and arise from slowly and rapidly adapting receptors and from C-fiber receptors. The slowly adapting (stretch) receptors, located in the smooth muscle of the airway, are stimulated by an increase in lung volume or transpulmonary pressure. They induce several physiologic responses including inhibition of inspiration (Hering-Breuer reflex), bronchodilation, increased heart rate, and decreased systemic vascular resistance. The rapidly adapting vagal (irritant) receptors are activated by a wide variety of noxious stimuli, ranging from mechanical stimulation of the airways to anaphylactic reactions within the lung parenchyma. The rapidly adapting receptors induce hyperpnea, cough, and constriction of the airways and larynx. C-fiber receptors are the terminus of nonmyelinated vagal afferents. They include the J receptors that are located near the pulmonary capillaries and are stimulated by pulmonary congestion and edema; they evoke a sensation of dyspnea and induce rapid, shallow breathing along with laryngeal constriction during expiration.

In addition to the sympathetic and parasympathetic nervous systems, humans and several other species have a third nervous system within their lungs. The noncommittal name *nonadrenergic noncholinergic nervous system* has been chosen because its function and properties are not understood. Purines, substance P, and vasoactive intestinal polypeptide have been suggested as possible neurotransmitters for this system.

Interstitium

The interstitium plays several roles in lung function in addition to providing a structural framework that consists of insoluble proteins. The ground substance influences cell growth and differentiation and lung water and solute movement. The cells contained within the interstitial region of the lung not only play individual roles that result from their contractile or synthetic properties, but they also interact with other cells (e.g., the endothelium and epithelium) to alter the basic structure and function of the lung.

A continuous fiber scaffold is present in the interstitium with an axial system (along the airways from the hilum to the alveolar ducts), a peripheral system (along the visceral pleura into interlobular septa), and a septal system (along the alveolar septa) (Fig. 6.10).[30] Most of the interstitial matrix of the lung is composed of type I collagen which, along with the less common collagen subtypes, forms a structural fibrous framework within the lung. Elastin provides elasticity and support to the structures. Both elastin and collagen turn over very slowly under normal conditions. However, rapid remodeling with changes in these proteins sometimes occurs. In diseases such as α_1-antitrypsin deficiency (where neutrophil elastases degrade elastin) and pulmonary fibrosis (where there is increased amounts of collagen), there are marked qualitative and quantitative changes in these proteins. The remainder of the matrix is made up of proteoglycans

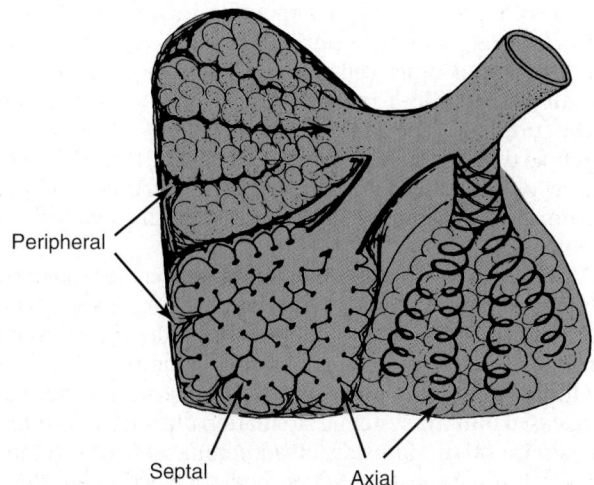

Peripheral

Septal   Axial

Fig. 6.10 Schematic diagram of the fibrous support of the lung. (See text for detail.) (From Weibel ER, Bachofen H. How to stabilize the alveoli. Surfactant or fibers. *News Physiol Sci.* 1987;2:72-75.)

and glycosaminoglycans. These carbohydrate-protein complexes can affect cell proliferation and differentiation in addition to their known effect on cell adhesion and attachment (e.g., laminin) and ability to diminish fluid movement (glycosaminoglycans).

Fibroblasts are capable of synthesizing components of the extracellular matrix (e.g., collagen, elastin, and glycosaminoglycans) and hence contribute significantly to the composition of the lung's interstitial space. They can be found within all of the interstitial regions of the lung, although their apparent structure may change, emphasizing the heterogeneity of this cell population.[31] For example, there are fibroblasts with contractile properties (myofibroblasts), some of which also contain lipid bodies in their cytoplasm (lipofibroblasts), although lipofibroblasts are not a common cell type in the human lung.[32] Similarly, it is likely that morphologically similar fibroblasts are not similar in terms of proliferative capacity and ability to synthesize various types of collagen. Data suggest that fibrotic lung diseases are characterized by the loss of the normal heterogeneous fibroblast population and that there may be a selection for certain clones that promote inappropriate focal collagen deposition within the lung parenchyma.

Smooth muscle cells influence the bronchomotor and vasomotor tone within the conducting airways and blood vessels. They are also seen within the free edge of the alveolar septa together with elastic fibers where they form an alveolar entrance ring that is capable of constricting or dilating. The smooth muscle cells form bundles connected by nexus or gap junctions that enable electrical coupling and synchronous contraction. The pericyte is another contractile interstitial cell that is found embedded in the endothelial basement membrane. It is believed to be a precursor cell that can differentiate into other cell types such as mature vascular smooth muscle cells.

There are a variety of interstitial cells that are concerned with innate and adaptive defense of the lung.[33,34] The interstitial macrophage and the alveolar macrophage are major effectors of the innate immune system, which they manage by ingesting particulate matter and removing it from the lung or by processing proteins or other antigens for presentation to adaptive immune cells. These macrophages are capable of secreting many compounds, including proteases and cytokines (substances capable of modulating the growth and function of other cells). B and T lymphocytes, including subsets such as T-regulatory cells (T-reg), are present in the lung and especially within the bronchus-associated lymphoid tissue (BALT), where they contribute to the humoral and cellular-mediated immune response. Further details on the innate and adaptive immune system are available in Chapter 8.

Although not within the interstitium per se, there are large numbers of intravascular cells such as granulocytes that adhere to the pulmonary endothelium. Indeed, next to the bone marrow and spleen, there are more granulocytes within the lung than in any other organ. These granulocytes can be released into the systemic circulation during such stimuli as exercise or the infusion of adrenalin, and this demargination is responsible for the concomitant blood leukocytosis. These leukocytes are also in a prime location for movement into the lung should an infection or inflammatory stimulus occur. There is much evidence to suggest that the pulmonary

granulocyte contributes to the pulmonary dysfunction seen in acute lung injury or acute RDS. Leukocytes also contain proteases that are thought to play a role in the development of emphysema and in the lung destruction that occurs in cystic fibrosis.

Growth and Development of the Lung

PRENATAL LUNG GROWTH

Lung development has been divided into various stages with names that reflect the respective histological appearance of the lung, the region of the lung that is most obviously developing, or both. The literature quotes different ranges for the different stages of human lung development. This concept is reinforced by the "overlap" between the different stages indicated in Fig. 6.11. However, the available data contrasts with the mouse where at least the airway branching pattern is remarkably stereotypical in that all fetuses develop along the same timeline.[35] It may be that there are inadequate data for the human fetal lung to detect this stereotypical development during the longer gestation or that, as with all developmental profiles, each individual human fetus develops along its own timeline. Prenatal lung growth and development is discussed in greater detail in the literature[36–38] and in Chapter 2.

The embryonic stage is the first stage of human fetal lung development and takes place from approximately 3 to 6 weeks' gestational age (GA). The lung first appears as a ventral outpouching of the primitive gut. The primary bronchi elongate into the mesenchyme and divide into the two main bronchi. Another key event is that the main pulmonary artery arises from the sixth pharyngeal arch. Congenital abnormalities of the lung may occur during this stage (e.g., lung agenesis, tracheobronchial fistula).

The pseudoglandular stage occurs from approximately 6 to 16 weeks' GA. During this period, airway branching continues and the mesenchyme differentiates into cartilage, smooth muscle, and connective tissue around the epithelial tubes. By the end of the pseudoglandular period, all major conducting airways, including the terminal bronchioles, have formed. Arteries are evident alongside the conducting airways, and by the end of the pseudoglandular period, all preacinar arterial branches have formed. Congenital abnormalities of the lung may occur during this stage (e.g., bronchopulmonary sequestration, cystic adenomatoid malformation, and congenital diaphragmatic hernia).

The canalicular stage occurs from approximately 16 to 26 weeks' GA, and during that time, the respiratory bronchioles develop. By the end of this stage, each ends in a *terminal sac* (also termed a *saccule*). The glandular appearance is lost as the interstitium has less connective tissue and the lung develops a rich vascular supply that is closely associated with the respiratory bronchioles.

The saccular stage occurs from approximately 26 to 36 weeks' GA. During this period, significant capillary proliferation and thinning of the epithelium permits close contact between the airspace and the bloodstream, thus enabling gas exchange. Elastic fibers, which will be important in subsequent true alveolar development, begin to be laid down.

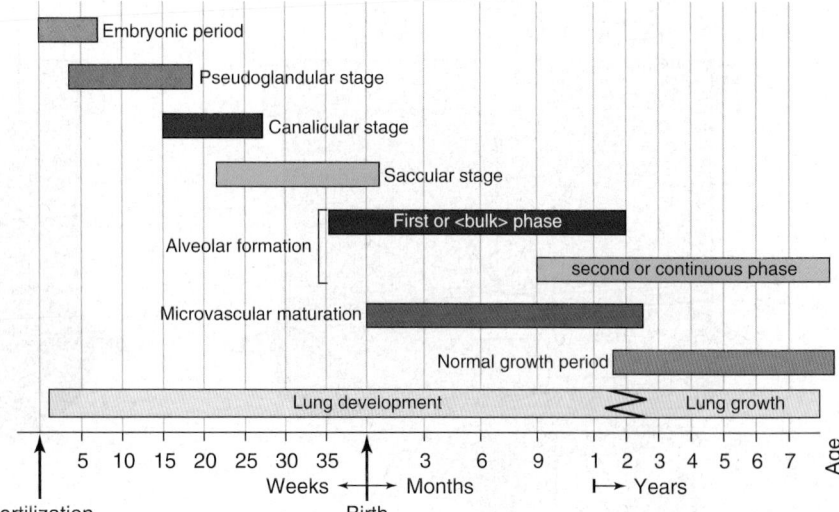

HUMAN FETAL AND POSTNATAL LUNG DEVELOPMENT AND GROWTH

Fig. 6.11 Various stages of lung development. The actual separation of individual stages is not discrete, and it overlaps. (Modified by M. Ochs, Peter Burri and Ewald Weibel from Zeltner TB, Burri PH. The postnatal development and growth of the human lung. II. Morphology. *Respir Physiol.* 1987;67:269-282.)

At this time, cuboidal (type II) and thin (type I) epithelial cells begin to line the airspace.

The alveolar period commences at approximately 36 weeks' GA. Secondary septa form on the walls of the saccules and grow into the lumen forming the walls of true alveoli.

Distention of the lungs' airspaces by fetal lung liquid is essential for normal lung development. This fluid is neither a mere ultrafiltrate of plasma nor aspirated amniotic fluid. Rather it is generated by the epithelium's active secretion of chloride into the developing lung's lumen with sodium and water following passively (Fig. 6.12A). An inadequate amount of fetal lung liquid is associated with lung hypoplasia.

Congenital abnormalities of the lung may occur during the various stages.[38] In addition, factors such as oligohydramnios or decreased fetal breathing may interfere with the development of the distal lung unit, including the development of alveoli. In contrast, if there is obstruction to outflow of tracheal fluid, as occurs in laryngeal atresia, there is pulmonary hyperplasia.

The Lung at Birth

Many dramatic changes must occur in the lungs during the transition from intrauterine to extrauterine life. The lung's epithelium must change from fluid secretion to fluid absorption, the distal lung units must fill with and retain inhaled air, and blood flow must increase approximately 20-fold.

At the time of birth, the lungs contain approximately 30 mL/kg of fetal lung liquid. Approximately ⅓ of this fluid is squeezed out during a vaginal delivery, but all of the fluid remains in the airspaces in an infant born by cesarean section. Thus, fetal lung liquid secretion must either greatly decrease or cease totally, and the fluid must be removed. Catecholamines released during labor can temporarily convert the fetal lung from a fluid-secreting organ to a fluid-absorbing organ[39] by initiating the active transport of sodium by the distal lung epithelium (see Fig. 6.12B). The clearance of fetal lung liquid from the newborn's airspaces takes many hours, and the increase in oxygen tension at the time of birth[40] is one key factor that permanently converts the lung epithelium into a sodium-absorbing mode.

In utero, little blood flows through the lung despite a relatively high perfusion pressure. This is because of the abundance of pulmonary vascular smooth muscle and the vasoconstrictor effect of the low fetal partial pressure of oxygen (PO_2) (<30 mm Hg). Although during the last trimester, concomitant with surfactant production, blood flow increases to 7% of the cardiac output, it is only at birth that marked increases in the capacity and distensibility of the pulmonary vasculature occur. Several mechanisms are responsible for the changes in circulation. Inflation of the lung with air results in mechanical distention of the vessels, and improvement in oxygenation removes hypoxic vasoconstriction. In addition, the increase in partial pressure of oxygen in arterial blood (PaO_2) and changes in flow result in the release of mediators that contribute to the vasoconstriction of the ductus arteriosus[41] and umbilical vessels and dilation of the pulmonary vascular bed. After birth the vessels dilate, which allows the necessary blood flow to the lungs, and the measured wall/lumen ratio decreases. After about 10 days of extrauterine life, the lumina are wider, regardless of the GA of the baby.

Postnatal Lung Growth

Postnatal lung growth continues throughout infancy and childhood and into the adolescent years. Throughout life, the average values of lung lobe weight expressed as a percentage of total lung weight are approximately: right upper lobe 20%, right middle lobe 8%, right lower lobe 25%, left upper lobe 22%, and left lower lobe 25%. Throughout the pediatric years, the tracheal diameter approximately triples, and the airways increase in their cross-sectional diameter (Fig. 6.13). Excised human lung studies suggest that this growth occurs until around 5 years of age and is associated

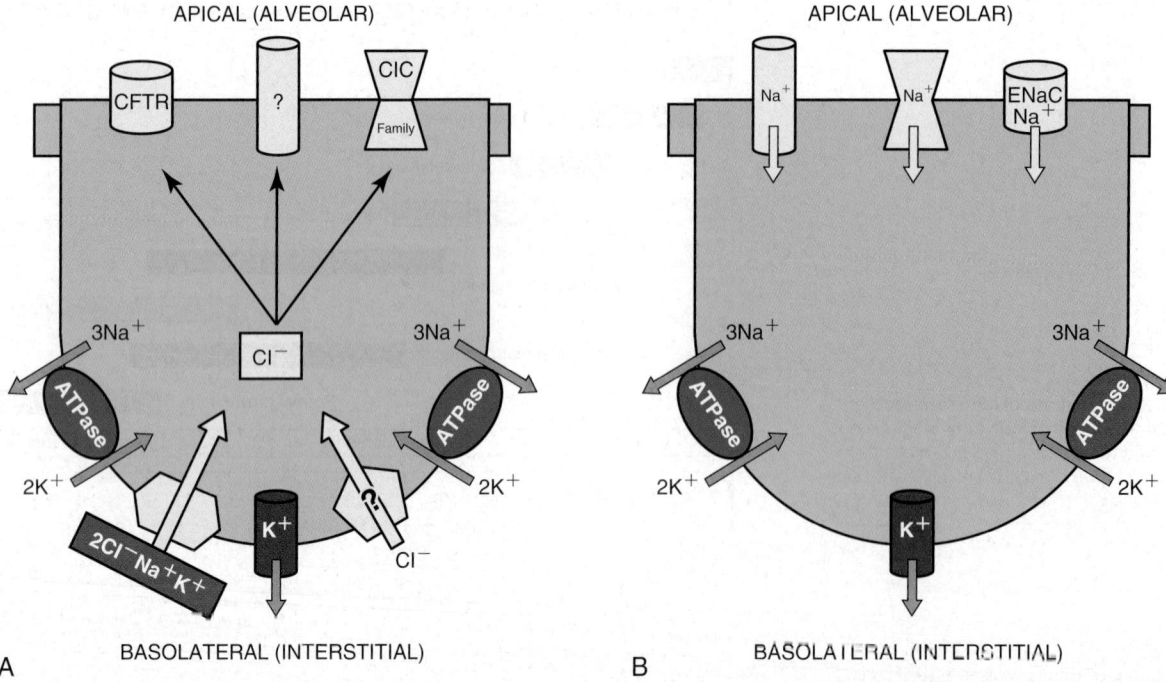

Fig. 6.12 (A) The polarized epithelium lining the fetal lung's lumen actively secretes Cl⁻, with Na⁺ and H₂O following, which creates in the fluid that distends the fetal lung. Cl⁻ enters on the basolateral side through membrane-bound protein transporters and is secreted out the apical membrane through different chloride channels, one of which is the chloride channel encoded by the cystic fibrosis transmembrane regulator (CFTR). The electro-chemical gradient that drives the secretion is created by the basolateral Na⁺/K⁺ ATPase and K⁺ permeant ion channels. (B) The polarized epithelium lining the perinatal and postnatal distal lung actively absorbs Na⁺, with Cl⁻ and H₂O following, which clears the fetal lung liquid that is present at birth. Na⁺ enters the cell down its electrochemical gradient through membrane-bound Na permeant ion channels located on the apical membrane. The basolateral Na⁺/K⁺ ATPase extrudes the intracellular Na⁺ across the basolateral membrane to the interstitial space. The electrochemical gradient that drives the absorption is created by the basolateral Na⁺/K⁺ ATPase and K⁺ permeant ion channels. A recent summary of research on luminal lung liquid and electrolyte transport is available. (From Hughes JMB, Pride NB. Examination of the carbon monoxide diffusing capacity (DLCO) in relation to its KCO and components. *Am J Respir Crit Care Med.* 2012;186:132-139.)

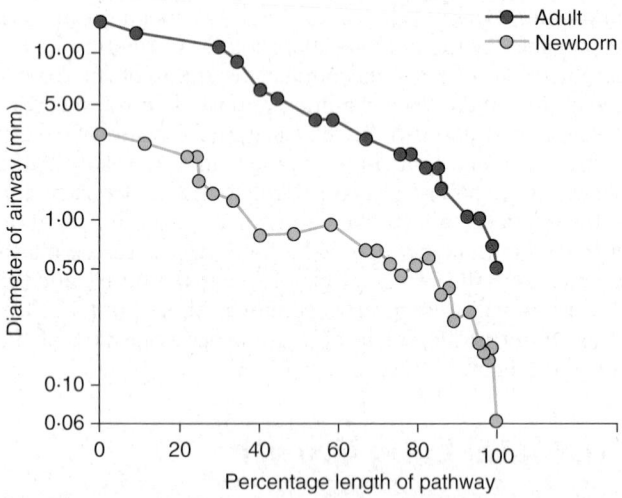

Fig. 6.13 Diameter of the airway at different percentage points along the axial pathway in an adult lung and in the newborn lung. The pathway begins at the trachea, and the distal end of the terminal bronchiole corresponds to the 100% point. (Reproduced from Hislop A, Muir DC, Jacobsen M, et al. Postnatal growth and function of the pre-acinar airways. *Thorax.* 1972;27:265-274.)

with marked changes in the relative conductance of central versus more peripheral airways (Fig. 6.14).

Most postnatal lung growth involves the acinar area. New secondary septa continue to appear on the walls of the saccules and grow into the airspace, thus creating more true alveoli. Alveoli continue to increase in number through segmentation of these primitive alveoli and through transformation of terminal bronchioles into respiratory bronchioles, the latter being a process known as *alveolarization*. Alveolar dimensions and number both increase as the lungs and body grow with the internal surface area of the lung paralleling body mass (~1 to 1.5 m²/kg of body weight). It is agreed that alveoli appear prior to birth, and various studies have suggested that there are approximately 20 to 150 million alveoli at birth. A morphometric study[42] of the lungs of 56 infants and children who died suddenly or after a brief illness indicates that there are approximately 200 to 300 million alveoli by the end of the second year of life, at which time alveolar multiplication slows markedly. After 2 years of age, boys have a larger number of alveoli and alveolar surface area than girls regardless of age and stature. Although recent observations[43,44] suggest that alveolarization continues during adolescence, very few new alveoli develop after 8 years of age.[42] Animal and human case studies suggest that the adult lung can, under certain circumstances, develop a small number of new alveoli.[45-47] After alveolar multiplication stops, further growth of the airspace occurs through an

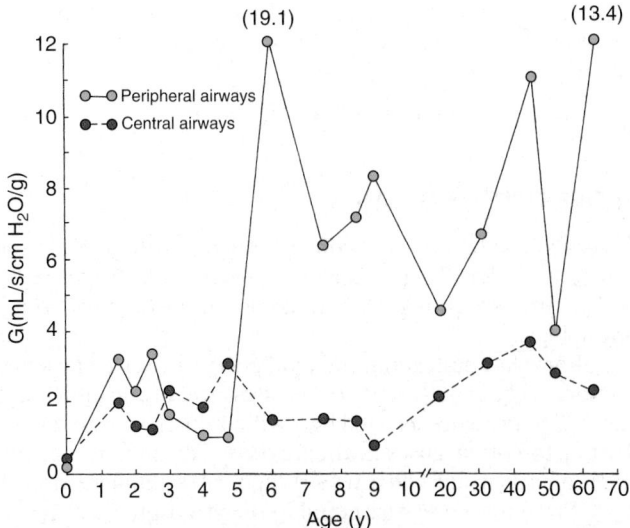

Fig. 6.14 Comparison of peripheral and central airway conductance as a function of age in normal human lungs. The data are corrected for size by expressing the conductance as mL/sec/g of lung and for lung inflation by expressing all data at a transpulmonary pressure of 5 cm H_2O. (Replotted from Hogg JC, Williams J, Richardson JB, et al. Age as a factor in the distribution of lower-airway conductance and in the pathologic anatomy of obstructive lung disease. *N Engl J Med.* 1970;282:1283.)

increase in alveolar dimensions. In the mature adult lung, the final number of alveoli averages 480 million[48] with individual subjects varying from 200 million to 800 million. The final number is related to total lung volume. An individual alveolus is 200 to 300 μm in diameter. As alveolar multiplication occurs, new blood vessels appear within the acinus. This explains the commensurate increase in the single breath diffusing capacity for carbon monoxide (CO) as the lungs grow.[49]

Prenatal (saccular) walls, as well as secondary septa that form postnatally during the alveolar period, contain a double-capillary network. The adult lung, however, contains a single capillary layer interwoven with a sheet of septal connective tissue. The phase of remodeling the septal capillary bilayer into a single layer (microvascular maturation) occurs from early after birth up to the age of about 2 to 3 years.

Healthy children grow along their lung function growth curve[50,51] similar to how children grow along their own height curve. For example, if a healthy child is born with lung volumes at the 10th percentile, he or she will usually maintain this status throughout childhood. It is known that the reference equations for lung function measurements must be adjusted for African-American children, since they have lower lung function for a given height compared to Caucasian children.[52] Indeed, genetic analyses have shown that the forced expiratory flow in 1 second (FEV_1) and forced vital capacity (FVC) are related to the number of ancestral markers related to African ancestry.[53]

When the structure and mechanical behavior of the young infant's and child's respiratory system are compared to those of the mature, but not the elderly, adult, important differences emerge that are likely to influence the pattern of disease. Some of these differences, such as reduced lung recoil, are shared by the infant and elderly and likely influence the pattern of respiratory disease in both populations. The young

lung lacks elastic recoil, because elastin is still being created; as a result, airways are less well supported, and there is greater airway closure; this favors inhomogeneity of gas exchange and the development of patchy atelectasis. The elderly have low lung recoil, because they have lost elastin through the aging process, and there is greater loss of recoil when elastin degradation occurs by mechanisms promoting emphysema. The chest wall is relatively more compliant in the young child and stiffens with increasing age. As a result, the infant can develop paradoxical respiration. Respiratory muscle activation during inspiration can produce inward displacement of the rib cage, contributing to increased respiratory work for a given level of ventilation, particularly during rapid eye movement (REM) sleep. The deformability of the chest wall influences findings on physical examination. Chest wall–abdominal paradox may be normal in the premature infant during REM sleep but not in the older child or adult.

Postnatal lung growth can be impaired by restriction of the lung (e.g., in kyphoscoliosis) or augmented (e.g., in remaining lung post pneumonectomy). Lung capacities and airway flows continue to increase until late adolescence. Once adult life is achieved, then nonsmoking men and women have an annual decline in their FEV_1 of approximately 20 mL/year.[54] The rate of decline during adult life is increased when individuals smoke or have a history of repeated childhood respiratory disorders.

Ventilation and Mechanics of Breathing

The principal function of the lung is to perform gas exchange, that is, to enrich the blood with oxygen and cleanse it of carbon dioxide. An essential feature of normal gas exchange is that the volume and distribution of ventilation are appropriate. Ventilation of the lung depends on the adequacy of the respiratory pump (muscles and chest wall) and the mechanical properties of the airways and gas-exchanging units.

It is traditional and useful to consider mechanical events as belonging to two main categories: the static-elastic properties of the lungs and chest wall and the flow-resistive or dynamic aspects of moving air. Changes in one category may be associated with compensatory changes in the other. Thus, many diseases affect both static and dynamic behavior of the lungs. Often, the principal derangement is in the elastic properties of the tissues or in the dimensions of the airways, and the treatment or alleviation of symptoms depends on distinguishing between them.

Before we discuss the mechanical aspects of lung function and gas exchange, it is important to review several basic physical laws concerning the behavior of gases and also the related abbreviations and symbols that will be used.

Definitions and Symbols

The principal variables for gases are as follows:

V = gas volume
V̇ = volume of gas per unit time

P = pressure
F = fractional concentration in dry gas
R = respiratory exchange ratio, carbon dioxide/oxygen
f = frequency
D_L = diffusing capacity of lung

The designation of which volume or pressure is cited requires a small capital letter after the principal variable. Thus, V_{O_2} = volume of oxygen; P_B = barometric pressure.

I = inspired gas
e = expired gas
a = alveolar gas
t = tidal gas
d = dead space gas
b = barometric pressure

When both location of the gas and its species are to be indicated, the order is V_{IO_2}, which means the volume of inspired oxygen.

STPD = standard temperature, pressure, dry (0° C, 760 mm Hg)
btps = body temperature, pressure, saturated with water vapor
atps = ambient temperature, pressure, saturated with water vapor

The principal designations for blood are as follows:

S = percentage saturation of gas in blood
C = concentration of gas per 100 mL of blood
Q = volume of blood
$\dot{Q}$ = blood flow per minute
a = arterial
$\bar{V}$ = mixed venous
c = capillary

All sites of blood determinations are indicated by lowercase initials. Thus, Pa_{CO_2} = partial pressure of carbon dioxide in arterial blood; $P\bar{V}_{O_2}$ = partial pressure of oxygen in mixed venous blood; and Pa_{O_2} = partial pressure of oxygen in a capillary.

The measurement of pressures can be confusing because pressure can be expressed using different units. For example, atmospheric pressure at sea level can be expressed by many seemingly different, but similar, values: it is important to remember the following:

$$1 \text{ atmosphere} = 100 \text{ kilopascals (kPa)} = 760 \text{ mm Hg}$$
$$= 760 \text{ Torr}$$

The unit Torr is named after Evangelista Torricelli, who discovered the principle of the barometer and used the height of a column of mercury to measure pressures; for general use, one can use the following equation:

$$1 \text{ mm Hg} = 1 \text{ Torr}$$

Both pleural space and ventilator pressures are typically described as cm H_2O, since a water-filled manometer was the initial tool used to measure these pressures; it was very hard to measure these low pressures by looking at only millimeter changes in the height of a column of mercury. Care must be taken when reviewing the literature on pulmonary vascular pressures as they can be expressed in either mm Hg or cm H_2O. The conversion from cm H_2O to mm Hg is as follows:

$$1 \text{ cm } H_2O = 0.736 \text{ mm Hg}$$

PROPERTIES OF GASES

Gases behave as an enormous number of tiny particles in constant motion. Their behavior is governed by the gas laws, which are essential to the understanding of pulmonary physiology.

Dalton's law states that the total pressure exerted by a gas mixture is equal to the sum of the pressures of the individual gases. The pressure exerted by each component is independent of the other gases in the mixture. For instance, at sea level, air saturated with water vapor at a temperature of 37°C has a total pressure equal to the atmospheric or barometric pressure with the partial pressures of the components as follows:

$$P_B = 760 \text{ mm Hg} = P_{H_2O}(47 \text{ mm Hg}) +$$
$$P_{O_2}(149.2 \text{ mm Hg}) + P_{N_2}(563.5 \text{ mm Hg}) +$$
$$P_{CO_2}(0.3 \text{ mm Hg})$$

The gas in alveoli contains 5.6% carbon dioxide, BTPS. If P_B = 760 mm Hg, then,

$$PA_{CO_2} = 0.056(760 - 47) = 40 \text{ mm Hg.}$$

Boyle's law states that at a constant temperature, the volume of any gas varies inversely as the pressure to which the gas is subjected since pressure times volumes is a constant. Because respiratory volume measurements may be made at different barometric pressures, it is important to know the barometric pressure and to convert to standard pressure, which is considered to be 760 mm Hg.

Charles' law states that if the pressure is constant, the volume of a gas increases in direct proportion to the absolute temperature. At absolute zero (−273°C), molecular motion ceases. With increasing temperature, molecular collisions increase so that at constant pressure volume must increase.

In all respiratory calculations, water vapor pressure must be taken into account. The partial pressure of water vapor increases with temperature but is independent of atmospheric pressure. At body temperature (37°C), fully saturated gas has a P_{H_2O} of 47 mm Hg.

Gases may exist in physical solution in a liquid, escape from the liquid, or return to it. At equilibrium, the partial pressure of a gas in a liquid medium exposed to a gas phase is equal in the two phases. Note that in blood, the sum of the partial pressures of all the gases does not necessarily equal atmospheric pressure. For example, in venous blood, P_{O_2} has fallen from the 100 mm Hg of the arterial blood to 40 mm Hg, while partial pressure of carbon dioxide (P_{CO_2}) has changed from 40 to 46 mm Hg. Thus, the sum of the partial pressures of O_2, CO_2, and N_2 in venous blood equals 655 mm Hg. This provides the physiologic reason why patients who experience a pneumothorax can eventually reabsorb their pneumothorax and do so more rapidly if they inhale gases with an $F_iO_2 > 0.21$.

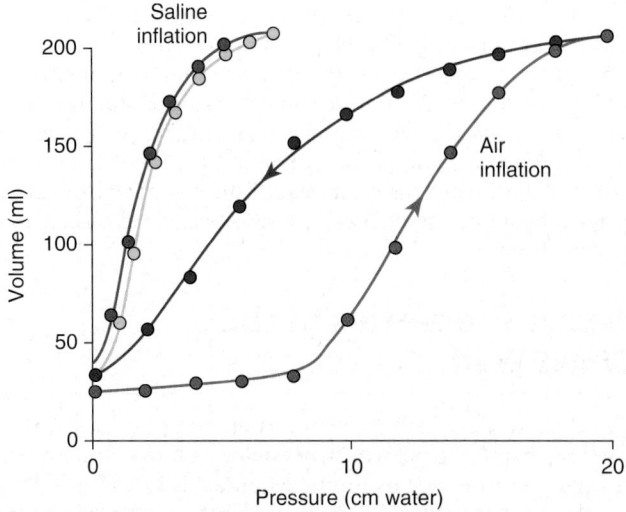

Fig. 6.15 Comparison of pressure-volume curves of air-filled and saline-filled lungs (cat). *Open circles,* inflation, *closed circles,* deflation. Note that the saline-filled lung has a much higher compliance and also much less hysteresis than the air-filled lung. (From West JB. *Respiratory Physiology—The Essentials,* 8th ed. Baltimore: Williams & Wilkins; 2008.)

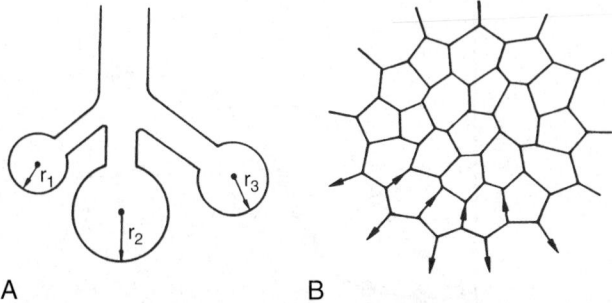

Fig. 6.16 (A) Classic model of the distal lung, in which individual alveoli would be controlled by Laplace's law: P = 2γ/r. Small alveoli would empty into large alveoli. (B) Interdependence model of the lung, in which alveoli share common planar and not spherical walls. Any decrease in the size of one alveolus would be stabilized by the adjacent alveoli. (From Weibel ER, Bachofen H. How to stabilize the alveoli. Surfactant or fibers. *News Physiol Sci.* 1987;2:72-75.)

Elastic Recoil of the Lung

The lung is an elastic structure that tends to decrease its size at all volumes. The elasticity of the lung depends on the structural components, the geometry of the terminal airspaces, and the presence of an air-liquid interface. When a lung is made airless and is then inflated with liquid, the elastic recoil pressure at large volumes is less than half that of a lung inflated to the same volume with air (Fig. 6.15). Thus, the most significant determinant of the elastic properties of the lung is the presence of an air-liquid interface.

The increase of elastic recoil in the presence of an air-liquid interface results from the forces of surface tension. What is surface tension? When molecules are aligned at an air-liquid interface, they lack opposing molecules on one side. The intermolecular attractive forces are then unbalanced, and the resultant force tends to move molecules away from the interface. The effect is to reduce the area of the surface to a minimum. In the lungs, the forces at the air-liquid interface operate to reduce the internal surface area of the lung, and thus they augment elastic recoil. A remarkable property of the material at the alveolar interface, the alveolar lining layer containing pulmonary surfactant, is its ability to achieve a high surface tension at large lung volumes and a low surface tension at low volumes. Surfactant is a phospholipid-protein complex that when compressed forms insoluble, folded-surface films of low surface tension. The ability to achieve a low surface tension at low lung volumes tends to stabilize the airspaces and prevent their closure.

The exact method of lung stabilization and the concomitant role of surfactant in this stabilization can be debated. The classic interpretation is that without surfactant, the smaller alveoli would tend to empty into the larger alveoli in accordance with the Laplace relationship, which relates the pressure across a surface (P) to surface tension (T) and radius (r) of curvature. For a spherical surface, P = 2T/r. The smaller the radius, the greater is the tendency to collapse. The

difficulty with this hypothesis is that the individual lung units are drawn as independent but communicating bubbles or spheres (Fig. 6.16A). This is not representative of structure of the lung because the alveolar walls are planar and not spherical. In addition, the inside wall of one alveolus is the outside wall of the adjacent alveolus. This last explanation has been utilized to develop the interdependence model of lung stability, which indicates that surface and tissue forces interact to maintain the lungs' inherent structure with the fibrous components playing an important role (see Fig. 6.16B).

The elastic recoil of the lung is responsible for the lung's tendency to pull away from the chest wall with the resultant subatmospheric pressure in the pleural space. Lung recoil can therefore be derived from measurement of the pleural pressure when no air flow is occurring and alveolar pressure is zero. (The pressure measurement is taken with the patient holding his or her breath for a brief period with the glottis open.)

The pressure within the esophagus can be used as an index for mean pleural pressure. This is a reasonable assumption as long as there is no paradoxical rib cage movement. However, it is not a reasonable assumption for premature infants, term infants in REM sleep, and older infants with severe lung disease. For these infants, no average pleural pressure exists, and calculations of resistance and compliance will not be accurate using this method. When pleural pressure is estimated with an esophageal balloon, one must be careful to avoid artifacts resulting from the gravitational pressure of the mediastinum. For this reason, these measurements are best performed with the patient in the upright or lateral rather than the supine position. Once a series of pressure measurements has been made during brief breath-holds at different lung volumes, a pressure-volume curve of the lung can be constructed (Fig. 6.17).

Compliance of the Lung

The pressure-volume curve of the lung describes two measurements of the elastic properties of the lung: elastic recoil pressure and lung compliance. Elastic recoil pressure is the pressure generated at a given lung volume, whereas

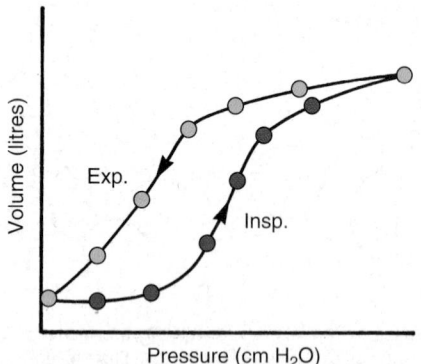

Fig. 6.17 Pressure-volume curve of a normal lung. Pleural pressure and lung volume are simultaneously determined during brief breath-holds. Lung compliance is calculated from data obtained on the expiratory portion of the pressure-volume curve.

compliance is the slope of the pressure-volume curve, or the volume change per unit of pressure:

$$\text{Compliance} = \frac{\Delta \text{volume}}{\Delta \text{pressure}} = \frac{L}{cm\ H_2O}$$

Compliance depends on the initial lung volume from which the change in volume is measured and the ventilatory events immediately preceding the measurement as well as the properties of the lung itself. At large lung volumes, compliance is lower, because the lung is nearer its elastic limit. If the subject has breathed with a fixed tidal volume (V_T) for some minutes, portions of the lung are not participating in ventilation, and compliance may be reduced. A few deep breaths, with return to the initial volume, will increase compliance. Thus, a careful description of associated events is required for correct interpretation of the measurement.

Changes in total lung compliance occur with age for two reasons; the lung's elastic recoil increases during childhood prior to declining during later adult life,[55] and the smaller the subject, the smaller is the change in volume for the same change in pressure. For example, $\Delta V/\Delta P$ is close to 6 mL/cm H_2O in infants, and is 125 to 190 mL/cm H_2O in adults. It is more relevant to a description of the elastic properties of the lung to express the compliance in relation to a unit of lung volume such as the functional residual capacity (FRC). When this is done, the compliance of the lung/FRC, or the specific compliance, changes much less. It is worth reemphasizing that total lung compliance is a function not only of the lung's tissue and surface tension characteristics but also of its volume. This is especially important to remember when compliance has been measured in newborn infants with RDS. The total compliance is a composite of the lung's elastic properties and the number of open lung units. In RDS, sudden changes in total measured compliance (if uncorrected for simultaneously measured lung gas volume) will predominantly, if not exclusively, reflect the opening and closing of individual lung units.

Lung compliance may also be measured during quiet breathing with pressure and volume being recorded at end-inspiration and end-expiration. The resultant value is the dynamic lung compliance. Although dynamic lung compliance does reflect the elastic properties of the normal lung, it is also influenced by the pressure required to move air within the airways. Therefore, dynamic lung compliance increases with increased respiratory rate and with increased airway resistance. Air flow is still occurring within the lung after it has ceased at the mouth, and pleural pressure reflects both the elastic recoil of the lung and the pressure required to overcome the increased airway resistance. Indeed, dynamic lung compliance can be used as a sensitive test of obstructive airway disease.

Elastic Properties of the Chest Wall

The chest wall is also an elastic structure, but in contrast to the lung, it tends to push outward at low volumes and inward at high volumes. For example, when air is introduced into the pleural space: the lung collapses and the chest wall springs outward.

Compliance of the chest wall can be measured by considering the pressure difference between the pleural space or esophagus and the atmosphere, per change in volume. Significant changes in thoracic compliance occur with age (Fig. 6.18). In the range of normal breathing, the thorax of the infant is nearly infinitely compliant. The pressures measured at different lung volumes are about the same across the lung as those measured across lung and thorax together. The functional significance of the high compliance of the neonatal thorax is observed when there is lung disease. The necessarily greater inspiratory effort and more negative pleural pressure can "suck" in the chest wall, resulting in less effective gas exchange and a higher work of breathing.

With advancing age, the thorax becomes relatively stiffer.[56] Changes in volume-pressure relations are profitably considered only if referred to a reliable unit, such as a unit of lung volume or a percentage of total lung capacity (TLC). Considered on a percentage basis, compliance of the thorax decreases with age. It remains unclear how much of this change is contributed by changes in tissue properties (e.g., increasing calcification of ribs and connective tissue changes) and how much is a disproportionate growth of the chest wall relative to the lung.

Lung Volumes

DEFINITION

The partition of commonly used lung volumes can be understood by studying Fig. 6.19. The spirogram on the left represents the volume of air breathed in and out by a normal subject. The first portion of the tracing illustrates normal breathing and is called the tidal volume (V_T). The subject then makes a maximal inspiration followed by a maximum expiration: the volume of expired air is the vital capacity (VC). The volume of air that still remains in the lung after a maximal expiration is the residual volume (RV), whereas the volume of air remaining in the lung after a normal passive expiration with relaxed respiratory muscles is the FRC. The maximum amount of air that a subject can have in the lungs is called the TLC. In healthy young subjects, TLC correlates best with the subject's sitting height.

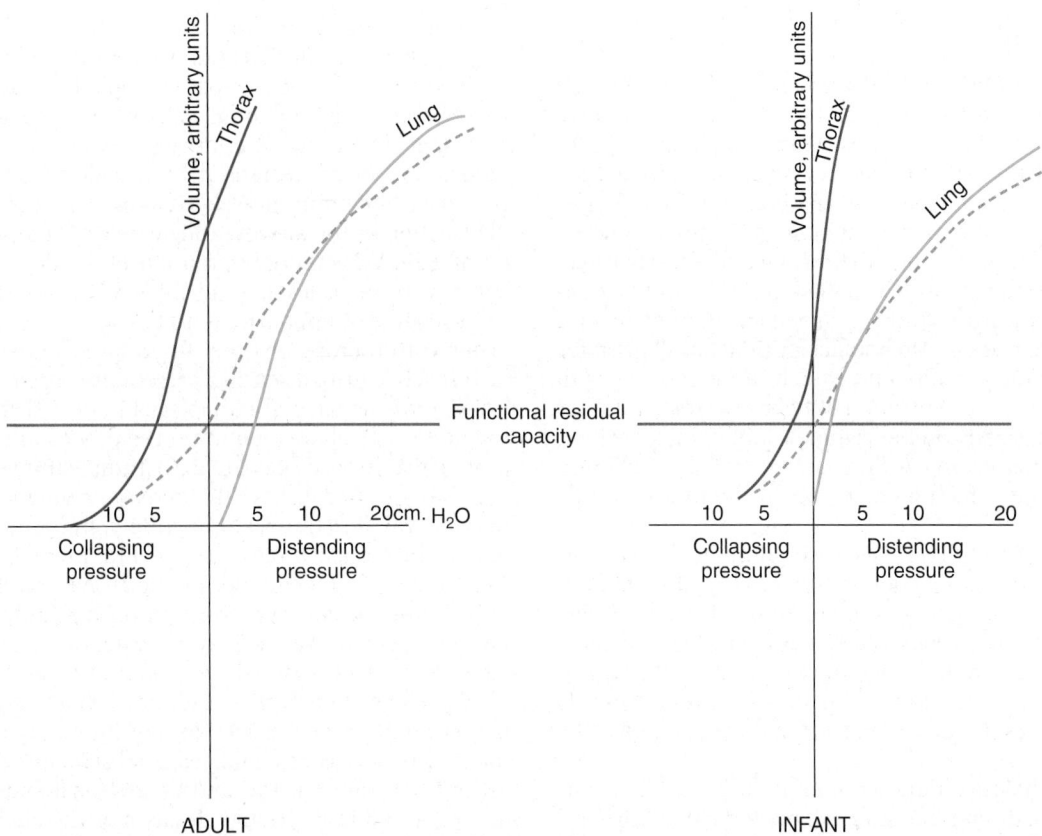

Fig. 6.18 Pressure-volume relations of lungs and thorax in an adult and in an infant. The *dashed line* represents the characteristic of lungs and thorax together. Transpulmonary pressure at the resting portion (functional residual capacity) is less in the infant, and thoracic compliance is greater in the infant.

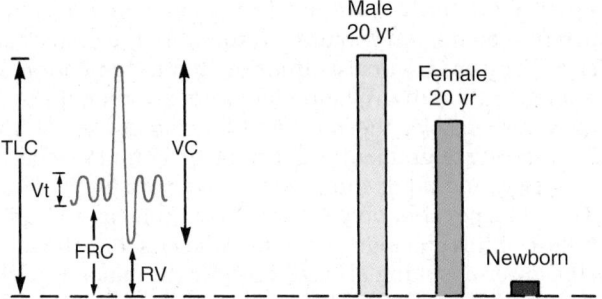

Fig. 6.19 The lung volumes. The spirogram *(left)* demonstrates normal breathing followed by a maximal inspiratory effort and a maximal expiratory effort. *FRC,* Functional residual capacity; *RV,* residual volume; *TLC,* total lung capacity (6.0 L in an average male, 4.2 L in an average female, and 160 mL in an average 3-kg infant; see histograms on right); *VC,* vital capacity; *Vt,* tidal volume.

The volumes and capacities of the lungs are determined by many factors, including muscle strength, static-elastic characteristics of the chest wall and lungs, airway status, and patient age and cooperation. TLC is reached when the force generated by maximal voluntary contraction of the inspiratory muscles equals the inward recoil of the lung and chest wall. FRC occurs when the respiratory muscles are relaxed and no external forces are applied; it is therefore the volume at which the inward recoil of the lung is exactly balanced by the outward recoil of the chest wall (see Fig. 6.18).

Closing volume, the volume at which airways close in dependent regions of the lung, is not routinely measured but is important for our understanding of normal lung function (see: Distribution of Ventilation). Closing volume is graphically illustrated by the atelectasis observed in dependent regions of the infant lung in computed tomography scans of the chest.

In healthy children and young adults, end-expiratory lung volume during tidal volume breathing is equivalent to FRC. This is not the case in infants, who breathe at a lung volume higher than FRC. This higher volume seems to be a sensible solution to the infants' problem of having an airway closing volume that exceeds FRC. An infant maintains the expiratory lung volume higher than FRC by a combination of postinspiratory diaphragmatic activity, laryngeal adduction, and rapid respiratory rate, which minimizes the time for expiration.

The factors determining RV vary with age. In adolescents and young adults, RV occurs when the expiratory muscles cannot compress the chest wall further. In young children and older adults, RV is a function of the patency of small airways and the duration of expiratory effort.

MEASUREMENT

Tidal volume and VC can be determined by measuring the expired volume. The measurement of FRC and RV requires another approach. Because both volumes include the air in the lungs that the patient does not normally exhale, they must be measured indirectly. One method uses the principle of dilution of the unknown volume with a known concentration of a gas that is foreign to the lung and only sparingly absorbed, such as helium. The patient breathes from a container with a known volume and concentration of helium in oxygen-enriched air. After sufficient time has elapsed for the gas in the lung to mix and equilibrate with the gas in the container, the concentration of helium in the container is remeasured. Because initial volume × initial concentration of helium = final volume × final concentration of helium, the final volume, which includes gas in the lungs, can be calculated.

The multiple breath inert gas washout method[57] also can be used to calculate lung volumes such as FRC. In addition, it provides information regarding the lung clearance index (LCI) which is now recognized to be a sensitive indicator of peripheral airway dysfunction. It also has the advantage that it can be performed in uncooperative subjects such as infants and very young children[58] (see Chapters 11 and 12).

Neither the helium dilution nor multiple breath inert gas washout methods can measure gas behind closed airways ("trapped gas") or in regions of the lung that are poorly ventilated. There is, however, a method of measuring total gas volume within the thorax that depends on the change in volume that occurs with compression of the gas when breathing against an obstruction. Practically, this measurement requires the patient to be in a body plethysmograph and to pant against a closed shutter. The change in pressure can be measured in the mouthpiece; the change in volume can be recorded with a spirometer attached to the body plethysmograph:

$$V = P\Delta V/\Delta P$$

This method has the advantage of being able to be repeated several times per minute. It has the disadvantage of including some abdominal gas in the measurement.

There have also been concerns about the validity of the plethysmographic technique in patients with severe obstructive lung disease. This issue has not yet been resolved because the technique has been reported to overestimate the lung volume in adults but underestimate the lung volume in infants with obstructive lung disease.

Interpretation

Similar to body growth percentiles, there is a wide range of normal values for lung volumes. For example, the mean TLC for a child 140 cm tall is 3.2 L; however, the statistical range of normal (mean ± 2 SD) is 1.9 to 4.3 L. This range of normal values, when expressed as percentage predicted, is even greater for younger children or smaller lung volumes (such as RV). Owing to this wide range of normality, care must be exercised in the interpretation of lung volumes. Measurement of lung volumes is of greatest benefit when repeated over several months to assess the progress of a chronic respiratory illness and the efficacy of treatment. Healthy children

grow along their lung function growth curve,[50,51] much like they grow along their growth percentiles.

The VC is one of the most valuable measurements that can be made in a functional assessment, because it is highly reproducible and has a relatively narrow range of normal values. It can be decreased by a wide variety of disease processes, including muscle weakness, loss of lung tissue, obstruction of the airway, and decreased compliance of the chest wall. VC is therefore not a useful tool to discriminate between types of lesions. Its chief role is to assign a value to the degree of impairment and to document changes that occur with therapy or time. To decide whether obstructive or restrictive lung disease is present, it is useful to measure expiratory flow rates (see Chapters 11 and 12) and to observe the pattern of abnormalities in the other lung volumes. In obstructive lung disease (e.g., asthma), the smallest lung volumes are affected first; RV increases owing to abnormally high airway resistance at low lung volumes (air trapping), and as the disease progresses, the FRC increases. Although the increase in FRC (hyperinflation) may rarely be due to loss of lung recoil, the overdistention is usually compensating for partial lower airway obstruction. When the lung volume is increased, intrathoracic airways enlarge, and widespread partial obstruction may be partially relieved by the assumption of a larger resting lung volume. Whereas the TLC is only rarely affected in obstructive disease (e.g., asthma) in children, TLC and VC are the first lung volumes to be affected in restrictive diseases of the chest wall (e.g., kyphoscoliosis) or lung (e.g., pulmonary fibrosis).

Regional Lung Volumes

During normal breathing, different areas of the lung have different regional lung volumes; the upper airspaces are inflated more than the lower airspaces. Because static-elastic properties are fairly constant throughout the lung, these different regional lung volumes result from the gradient of pleural pressure that exists from the top to the bottom of the lung. Although gravitational forces are thought to be largely responsible, the mechanisms responsible for this pleural pressure gradient are incompletely understood. In the erect young adult lung, the pleural pressure is −8 cm H_2O at the apex and only −2 cm H_2O at the base. The significance of this phenomenon is that when a subject breathes in, the lowermost lung units will receive the majority of the inspired air (Fig. 6.20). This is advantageous because the majority of pulmonary blood flow also goes to the base of the lung, and thus, blood flow and ventilation patterns are more closely matched.

Dynamic (Flow-Resistive) Properties of the Lung

GAS FLOW WITHIN AIRWAYS

The respiratory system must perform work to move gas into and out of the lungs. Because air moves into the lungs during inspiration and out of the lungs during expiration, and because the velocity of air flow increases from small airways to large airways, energy must be expended to accelerate the

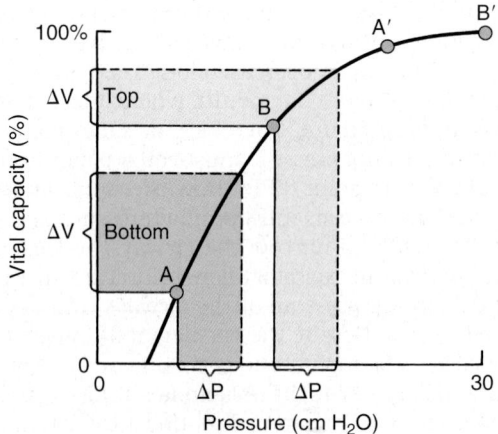

Fig. 6.20 Pressure-volume curve of a normal lung *(heavy solid line)*. At functional residual capacity, distending pressure is less at the bottom than at the top; accordingly, alveoli at the bottom (A) are smaller (i.e., lower percentage regional vital capacity) than those at the top (B). When a given amount of distending pressure (ΔP) is applied to the lung, alveoli at the bottom increase their volume (ΔV) more than alveoli at the top, owing to the varying steepness of the pressure-volume curve. When fully expanded to total lung capacity (100% VC), alveoli at the bottom (A′) are nearly the same size as alveoli at the top (B′), because both points lie on the flat portion of the curve. (From Murray JF. *The Normal Lung*. Philadelphia: Saunders; 1976.)

gas molecules. The respiratory system's resistance to acceleration (inertance) is minimal during quiet breathing and will not be considered further. However, inertance becomes quite significant during very high breathing rates, as occurs in high-frequency ventilation. During quiet breathing, frictional resistance to air flow accounts for one-third of the work performed during quiet breathing. The magnitude of pressure loss due to friction is determined by the pattern of flow. Flow may be laminar (streamlined) or turbulent, and which pattern exists depends on the properties of the gas (viscosity, density), the velocity of air flow, and the radius of the airway. In general, there is laminar flow in the small peripheral airways and turbulent flow in the large central airways.

The laws governing the frictional resistance to flow of gases in tubes apply to pulmonary resistance. The equation for calculating the pressure gradient required to maintain a laminar flow of air through a tube is given by Poiseuille's law:

$$P = \dot{V}\left(\frac{8l\eta}{\pi r^4}\right)$$

where P = pressure, $\dot{V}$ = flow, l = length, r = radius of the tube, and n = the viscosity of the gas. The viscosity of air is 0.000181 poise at 20°C, or only 1% that of water. Because resistance = pressure/flow, it is clear that the most important determinant of resistance in small airways will be the radius of the tube, which is raised to the fourth power in the denominator of the equation.

The pressure required to maintain turbulent flow is influenced by airway diameter and gas density and is proportional to the square of the gas velocity. The effect of gas density on turbulent flow has both therapeutic implications. Children with viral laryngotracheobronchitis have marked narrowing of the subglottic area, which greatly increases the resistance

to air flow. The pressure required to overcome this increased resistance in the large airways, and hence the work of breathing can be decreased by administering a low-density gas mixture (70% helium, 30% oxygen).

MEASUREMENT OF RESISTANCE

Resistance (R) is calculated from the equation:

$$R = \frac{driving\ pressure}{air\ flow}$$

The pressure is measured at the two ends of the system, in the case of the lung, at the mouth and at the alveoli, and the corresponding flow is recorded. Measurement of alveolar pressure presents the greatest problem. Several methods have been used to measure alveolar pressure. The most common method employs a body plethysmograph. The subject sits in an airtight box and breathes through a tube connected to a pneumotachometer, an apparatus that measures air flow. When a shutter occludes the tube and air flow ceases, the mouth pressure is assumed to be equal to the alveolar pressure. Airway resistance can then be calculated because air flow, alveolar pressure, and ambient pressure are known.

Total pulmonary resistance can be measured in infants and children by the forced oscillation technique. This measurement includes airway resistance plus the tissue viscous resistance of the lung and chest wall. Nasal resistance is also included in the measurement if the infant is breathing through the nose. Although there are theoretical objections to this technique, it has several advantages. It does not require a body plethysmograph, estimates of pleural pressure, or patient cooperation, and it can be done quickly enough to be used on ill patients. A sinusoidal pressure applied at the upper airway changes the air flow, and the ratio of pressure change to flow change is used to calculate resistance. When the forced oscillations are applied at the so-called resonant frequency of the lung (believed to be 3 to 5 Hz), it is assumed that the force required to overcome elastic resistance of the lung and the force required to overcome inertance are equal and opposite so that all of the force is dissipated in overcoming flow resistance. This technique has demonstrated that infants with bronchiolitis have about a twofold increase in inspiratory pulmonary resistance and a threefold increase in expiratory resistance.

Several new techniques have been developed that are capable of measuring lung function in infants and young children. Each has its advantages, underlying assumptions, and limitations, and these techniques are discussed in detail in Chapter 11.

SITES OF AIRWAY RESISTANCE

The contribution of the upper airway to total airway resistance is substantial. The average nasal resistance of infants by indirect measurements is nearly half of the total respiratory resistance, as is the case in adults. It is hardly surprising that any compromise of the dimensions of the nasal airways in an infant who is a preferential nose breather will result in retractions and labored breathing. Likewise, even mild edema of the trachea or larynx will impose a significant increase in airway resistance.

In the adult lung, about 80% of the resistance to air flow resides in airways greater than 2 mm in diameter. The vast number of small peripheral airways provides a large cross-sectional area for flow and therefore contributes less than 20% to the airway resistance. Thus, these airways may be the sites of disease that may severely impair ventilation of distal airspaces without appreciably altering the total airway resistance. In the infant lung, however, small peripheral airways may contribute as much as 50% of the total airway resistance, and this proportion does not decrease until about 5 years of age. Thus, the infant and young child are particularly severely affected by diseases that affect the small airways (e.g., bronchiolitis).

FACTORS THAT AFFECT AIRWAY RESISTANCE

Airway resistance is determined by the diameter of the airways, the velocity of air flow, and the physical properties of the gas breathed. The diameter is determined by the balance between the forces tending to narrow the airways and the forces tending to widen them. One of the forces tending to narrow the airways is exerted by the contraction of bronchial smooth muscle. The neural regulation of bronchial smooth muscle tone is mediated by efferent impulses through autonomic nerves. Sympathetic impulses relax the airways, and the parasympathetic impulses constrict them. Bronchi constrict reflexly from irritating inhalants (e.g., sulfur dioxide and some dusts); by arterial hypoxemia and hypercapnia; by embolization of the vessels; by cold; and by some vasoactive mediators (e.g., acetylcholine, histamine, bradykinin, and leukotrienes). They dilate in response to an increase in systemic blood pressure through baroreceptors in the carotid sinus and to beta sympathomimetic agents such as salbutamol (selective $beta_2$ agonist), isoproterenol ($beta_1$ and $beta_2$ agonist), and epinephrine (nonselective alpha and beta agonist). The large airways are probably in tonic contraction in health, because in unanesthetized adults, atropine or isoproterenol will decrease airway resistance.

Airway resistance changes with lung volume but not in a linear manner. Increasing the lung volume to above FRC only minimally decreases airway resistance. In contrast, as lung volume decreases from FRC, resistance rises dramatically and approaches infinity at RV. Although alterations in bronchomotor tone play a role, it is the decrease in lung elastic recoil as lung volume declines that is the predominant mechanism for the change in airway resistance. The recoil of the lung provides a tethering or "guy wire" effect on the airways that tends to increase their diameter. Children of different ages will have different airway resistances owing to the different sizes of their lungs. Therefore, the measurement of airway resistance or its reciprocal (airway conductance) is usually corrected by dividing the airway conductance by the simultaneously measured lung volume. The resultant specific airway conductance is remarkably constant regardless of the subject's age or height.

DYNAMIC AIRWAY COMPRESSION

During a forced expiration, both the pleural and the peribronchial pressures become positive and tend to narrow the airways; forces tending to keep airways open are the intraluminal pressure and the tethering action of the surrounding lung. During active expiration, however, the intraluminal pressure must decrease along the pathway of air flow from the alveoli to the mouth, where it becomes equal to atmospheric pressure. Therefore, at some point in the airway, intraluminal pressure must equal pleural pressure, the equal pressure point (EPP). Downstream from the EPP, pleural pressure exceeds intraluminal pressure and thus is a force that tends to narrow the airways. Indeed, during periods of maximum expiratory flow, pleural pressure exceeds the critical closing pressure of the airways, which become narrowed to slits. Despite the cartilaginous support of the larger airways, the membranous portion of the wall of the trachea and large bronchi invaginates under pressure to occlude the airways. Maximum flow under this circumstance is therefore determined by the resistance of the airways located upstream from the EPP, and the driving pressure is the difference between the alveolar pressure and the pressure at the EPP. In disease states in which there is increased airway resistance, the EPP moves toward the alveoli because of the greater intraluminal pressure drop. Thus, small airways are compressed during forced expiration with severe flow limitation. With the measurement of pressure-flow and flow-volume curves during forced expiration, it is possible to calculate resistance upstream and downstream from the point of critical closure, or EPP. Increasing the lung volume increases the tethering action of the surrounding lung on the airways, and therefore close attention must be paid to the lung volume at which resistance measurements are made during these studies.

WORK OF BREATHING

Work is defined as the force over distance or three-dimensionally as pressure during changes in volume. Thus, the work performed by the respiratory pump is defined by the volume changes of the lungs when the respiratory muscles generate a given pressure. The volume-pressure relationships of the respiratory system depend on properties of the lung and chest wall tissues or the ease with which the airways allow the passage of air. A substantial portion of the pressure generated by the respiratory muscles is applied to produce reversible rearrangements of the structure of the alveolar gas-liquid interface and the fibrous network of the lungs. Another large portion of the effort of the respiratory muscles is directed at producing rearrangements or interactions that are not reversible. The energy spent in such an effort is directly transformed into heat, which is then dissipated into the atmosphere or carried away by the circulating blood. The magnitudes of the work and the pressures derived from these processes generally bear a relationship to the rate of gas flow in and out of the lungs. In this regard, the respiratory system exhibits a resistive behavior for which the driving pressure determines the flow of air. Both the elastic and the resistive components of the work of breathing are usually increased in children with respiratory disease.

Respiratory work normally accounts for about 3% of an individual's total oxygen consumption. This work is increased in various diseases, and establishing a diagnosis and formulating a therapy in these patients is almost always simplified when the clinician distinguishes between conditions that affect primarily the elastic (restrictive respiratory disease) and resistive (obstructive respiratory disease) behaviors of the respiratory system.

Distribution of Ventilation

The distribution of ventilation is influenced by several factors in the normal lung. The pleural pressure gradient results in a greater amount of the tidal volume going to the dependent areas of the lung (see Fig. 6.20). In addition, the rate at which an area of the lung fills and empties is related to both regional airway resistance and compliance. A decrease in an airway's lumen increases the time required for air to reach the alveoli; a region of low compliance receives less ventilation per unit of time than an area with high compliance. The product of resistance and compliance (the "time constant") is approximately the same in health for all ventilatory pathways. The unit of this product is time. Note the following:

$$Resistance = \frac{pressure}{flow} = \frac{cm\ H_2O}{L/sec}$$

and

$$Compliance = \frac{\Delta volume(L)}{\Delta pressure(cm\ H_2O)}$$

The product, then, is a unit of time, analogous to the time constant in an electrical system, which represents the time taken to accomplish 63% of the volume change.

As mentioned earlier in the chapter, peripheral airways contribute little to overall airway resistance after 5 years of age. However, in the presence of small airway disease, some areas of the lung have long-time constants, but those of others are normal. This is particularly evident as the frequency of respiration increases. With increasing frequency, air goes to those areas of the lung with short time constants. These areas then become relatively overdistended, and a greater transpulmonary pressure is required to inspire the same volume of air, because alveoli in these relatively normal areas are reaching their elastic limit. Thus, a decreased dynamic compliance with increasing frequency of respiration has been used as a test of small airway disease and indeed may be the only mechanical abnormality detectable in the early stages of diseases such as emphysema and cystic fibrosis.

Airway closure occurs in dependent areas of the lung at low lung volumes. The lung volume above RV at which closure occurs is called the *closing volume*. In infants, very young children, and older adults, airway closure occurs at FRC and therefore is present during normal tidal breathing.[39] This results in intermittent inadequate ventilation of the respective terminal lung units and leads to abnormal gas exchange, notably to a lower PaO_2 seen in these age groups.

Pulmonary Circulation

PHYSIOLOGIC CLASSIFICATION OF PULMONARY VESSELS

The pulmonary circulation is the only vascular bed to receive the entire cardiac output. This unique characteristic enables the pulmonary vascular bed to perform a wide variety of homeostatic physiologic functions. It provides an enormously large (~120 to 130 m^2) yet extremely thin surface for gas exchange, filters the circulating blood, controls the circulating concentrations of many vasoactive substances, and provides a large surface area for the absorption of lung liquid at birth. The nomenclature of the pulmonary vessels is at times confusing because the anatomic classification of the vessels often does not correspond to their physiologic role.

The anatomic and histologic characteristics of the pulmonary vasculature are described earlier in the chapter. It is important to understand that pulmonary vessels have been classified physiologically as extra-alveolar and alveolar vessels, fluid-exchanging vessels, and gas-exchanging vessels. When the outside of a vessel is exposed to alveolar pressure, it is classified as an alveolar vessel (capillaries within the middle of the alveolar septum), whereas extra-alveolar vessels (arteries, veins, and capillaries at the corner of alveolar septa) are intrapulmonary vessels that are subjected to a more negative pressure resulting from and approximating pleural pressure. The diameter of the extra-alveolar vessels is therefore greatly affected by lung volume, expanding as inspiration occurs. Although extra-alveolar vessels and alveolar vessels are subjected to different mechanical pressures, they are both classified as fluid-exchanging vessels because both leak water and protein and can contribute to the production of pulmonary edema. The anatomic location of gas-exchanging vessels is unclear but is likely limited to the capillaries and smallest arterioles and venules.

Pulmonary Vascular Pressures

The pressure within the pulmonary circulation is remarkably low considering that it receives the entire cardiac output (5 L/min in the adult human). Beginning a few months after birth, pulmonary arterial pressures are constant throughout life, with the average mean pulmonary arterial pressure being 15 mm Hg and the systolic and diastolic pressures being 22 and 8 mm Hg, respectively. The pulmonary venous pressure is minimally higher than the left atrial pressure, which averages 5 mm Hg. The pressure within human lung capillaries is unknown, but work in isolated dog lungs suggests it is 8 to 10 mm Hg, approximately halfway between the mean arterial and venous pressures. These values refer to pressures at the level of the heart in the supine position; because of gravity, pulmonary arterial pressures are near zero at the apex of the upright adult lung and close to 25 mm Hg at the base. Depending on their location, vessels have different pressures on their outside walls. As defined previously, the alveolar vessels are exposed to alveolar pressure, which fluctuates during the respiratory cycle, but will average out close to zero. In contrast, the extra-alveolar vessels are exposed to a negative fluid pressure on their outer walls, estimated to be between −6 and −9 cm H_2O. The pressure on the outside of the pulmonary vessel is not a trivial matter, because the transmural pressure (inside pressure–outside pressure), rather than the intravascular pressure, is the pertinent hydrostatic pressure influencing vascular distention and the transvascular movement of water and protein (see Chapter 36).

Pulmonary Vascular Resistance

The resistance to blood flow through the lungs can be calculated by dividing the pressure across the lungs by the pulmonary blood flow.

$$R = \frac{mean\ PA\ pressure - mean\ LA\ pressure}{pulmonary\ blood\ flow}$$

A decrease in resistance to blood flow can occur only through (1) an increase in the blood vessels' lumenal diameters or (2) an increase in the number of perfused vessels. Each of these will contribute to an increase in the cross-sectional diameter of the pulmonary vascular bed. The diameter of an already open pulmonary vessel can be increased by decreasing the muscular tone of the vessel wall (e.g., with a vasodilating agent) or by increasing the transmural pressure (e.g., through increased pulmonary arterial or left atrial pressure). Previously unperfused pulmonary vessels may be opened up ("recruited") when their transmural pressure exceeds their critical opening pressure. This occurs when intravascular pressures are raised or when a vasodilator has decreased the vessels' critical opening pressure. An increase in cardiac output decreases the calculated pulmonary vascular resistance (PVR). This is important to remember when assessing vasodilating drugs; studies have been performed in which drugs were found to increase cardiac output substantially so that the calculated PVR falls. This decrease in resistance does not ensure that a particular drug has any direct vasodilating action at all, because the entire decrease in PVR may have resulted from its cardiac effects.

The interrelationship between lung volume and PVR is complex and is influenced by pulmonary blood volume, cardiac output, and initial lung volume. The principal reason for this complex relationship is that a change in lung volume has opposite effects on the resistances of the extra-alveolar and alveolar vessels. As the lung is inflated, the radial traction on the extra-alveolar vessels increases their diameter, whereas the same increase in lung volume increases the resistance to flow through the alveolar vessels (which constitutes 35% to 50% of the total PVR). It is reasonable to say, however, that PVR is at its minimum at FRC, and any change in lung volume (increase or decrease) will increase the PVR (Fig. 6.21).

Active changes in PVR can be mediated by neurogenic stimuli, vasoactive compounds, or chemical mediators. The normal adult pulmonary circulation appears to be maximally dilated, since no stimulus has been found that can further dilate the pulmonary vessels. In contrast, the neonatal lung or the vasoconstricted adult lung vasodilates in response to a variety of agents, including nitric oxide, acetylcholine, β-agonist drugs, bradykinin, prostaglandin E, and prostacyclin.

The pulmonary circulation can undergo significant vasoconstriction, which is surprising in view of the paucity of muscle in postnatal lung vessels. Hypoxia is the most common potent pulmonary vasoconstricting agent. Hypoxic vasoconstriction, which occurs when the alveolar P_{O_2} falls below 50 to 60 mm Hg, is a local response independent of neurohumoral stimuli. Although many suggestions have been made, the exact mechanism of hypoxia-induced vasoconstriction is unknown. Acidosis acts synergistically with hypoxia to

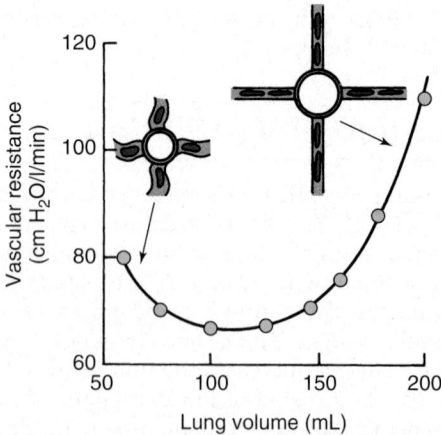

Fig. 6.21 Effect of lung volume on pulmonary vascular resistance when the transmural pressure of the capillaries is held constant. At low lung volumes, resistance is high because the extra-alveolar vessels become narrow. At high volumes, the capillaries are stretched, and their caliber is reduced. (From West JB. *Respiratory Physiology—The Essentials.* Baltimore: Williams & Wilkins; 1974.)

constrict the pulmonary vessels; however, it is unlikely that CO_2 alone has any direct effect on the pulmonary circulation in humans. Stimulation of the pulmonary sympathetic nerves results in a weak vasoconstrictive response in the dog lung but little or no response in the normal human adult pulmonary circulation. Vasoactive substances (e.g., histamine, fibrinopeptides, prostaglandins of the F series, and leukotrienes) are capable of constricting the pulmonary vascular bed. It had been believed that vasoconstriction in the pulmonary circulation took place predominantly, if not exclusively, within the arterial section of the vascular bed. However, it has been demonstrated that other regions of the bed may narrow in response to stimuli. For example, hypoxia can constrict the pulmonary venules of newborn animals and might increase resistance within the capillary bed by inducing constriction of myofibroblasts that are located within the interstitium of the alveolar-capillary membrane. The fetal and neonatal pulmonary circulation contains a large amount of smooth muscle, which enhances the response to vasoconstrictive stimuli.

Distribution of Blood Flow

Blood flow is uneven within the normal lung and is influenced by the vascular branching pattern and gravity that when standing results in more blood flow being directed to the dorsal caudal regions and less to the cephalad regions. Gravitational forces are largely responsible for the increasing flow from apex to base because the intravascular pressure of a given blood vessel is determined by the pulmonary arterial pressure immediately above the pulmonary valve and the blood vessel's vertical distance from the pulmonary valve. Thus, with increasing height above the heart, the pulmonary arterial pressure decreases and less perfusion occurs. The opposite occurs for vessels located in the lung bases, and together these gravitational effects are responsible for a pressure difference of approximately 23 mm Hg between apical and basal pulmonary arteries.

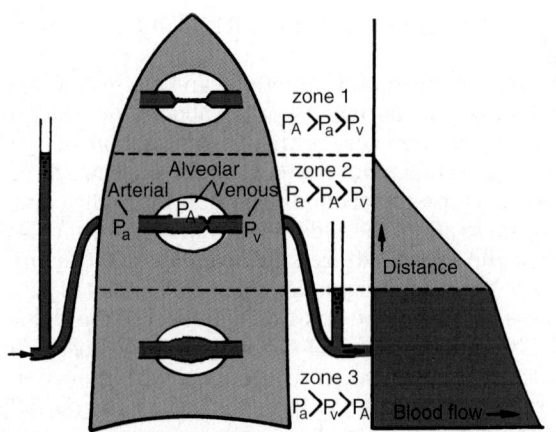

Fig. 6.22 Model to explain the uneven distribution of blood flow in the lung based on the pressures affecting the capillaries. P_a, Pulmonary arterial pressure; P_A, alveolar pressure; P_v, pulmonary venous pressure. (From West JB, Dollery CT, Naimark A. Distribution of blood flow in isolated lung. Relation to vascular and alveolar pressures. *J Appl Physiol*. 1964;19:713.)

These regional differences in lung perfusion are best understood in terms of West's zones of perfusion (Fig. 6.22). West's zone I occurs when mean pulmonary arterial pressure is less than or equal to alveolar pressure, and as a result, no blood flow occurs (except perhaps during systole). Zone I conditions are present in the apices of some upright adults and result in unperfused yet ventilated lung units (alveolar dead space). Moving down from the lung apices, pulmonary arterial pressure becomes greater than alveolar pressure, with the latter being greater than venous pressure. These are zone II conditions, and blood flow is determined by the difference between arterial and alveolar pressures and is not influenced by venous pressure; an appropriate analogy would be that of a vascular "waterfall," in which the flow rate is independent of the height of the falls. In zone III, left atrial pressure exceeds alveolar pressure, and flow is determined in the usual manner (i.e., by the arterial-venous pressure gradient).

Methods of Evaluating the Pulmonary Circulation

The chest radiograph is the most basic noninvasive and nonquantitative tool for determining the possible presence of pulmonary vascular disease. Prominence of the pulmonary outflow tract occurs when the elevated pressure distends the elastic main pulmonary arteries. Vascular markings may be increased or decreased; the former occurs when there is elevated pulmonary blood flow or volume without vascular remodeling, and the latter occurs when there is distal "pruning" of the vessel's image when vascular remodeling has occurred. Computerized axial tomography and magnetic resonance imaging provide greater detail of the right ventricle and pulmonary vessels.

Echocardiography is able not only to assess the structure and function of the right ventricle but also to provide a reasonable estimate of right ventricular pressure by assessing the velocity of the small retrograde flow through the tricuspid valve that frequently occurs in significant pulmonary hypertension. Quantitative assessment of regional pulmonary

blood flow can be made with intravenous injections of macroaggregates of albumin labeled with technetium[99m]. The macroaggregates occlude a very small portion of the pulmonary vascular bed. The amount of regional blood flow can be determined by imaging the lungs with a large field-of-view gamma camera and determining the count rate with a computer. The perfusion lung scintigram can be combined with a ventilation scintigram performed with either a radioactive gas (e.g., xenon 133 or krypton[81m]) or a radiolabeled (^{99m}Tc–diethylenetriamine-pentacetic acid) aerosol that is distributed like a gas.

Regional pulmonary angiography further delineates localized disturbance in blood flow, although the procedure requires cardiac catheterization. Direct measurements of pulmonary artery and pulmonary artery occlusion ("wedge") pressures add further information. Occasionally, drugs can be infused into the pulmonary artery to evaluate the potential reversibility of pulmonary hypertension.

Further details regarding the pathobiology and treatment of pulmonary hypertension are available elsewhere[59,60] and in Chapter 35.

Muscles of Respiration

The importance of the muscles of respiration derives from the fact that these muscles, similar to the myocardium, can fail under abnormal circumstances and can induce or contribute to an impending or existing ventilatory failure.[61]

The principal muscle of respiration is the diaphragm, a thin musculotendinous sheet that separates the thoracic from the abdominal cavity. In adults, its contraction causes descent of its dome and aids in elevation of the lower ribs, the latter referred to as the "bucket handle effect." Some work indicates that the diaphragm has two separate but related functions. The costal part of the diaphragm (largely innervated by C5) acts to stabilize and elevate the lower rib cage during contraction. The vertebral (crural) portion (largely innervated by C3), a much thicker muscle, descends with contraction and is largely responsible for the volume change that occurs.

Three anatomic characteristics of the infant's chest wall and diaphragm lead to decreased diaphragmatic efficiency and a lower fatigue threshold. First, the infant's chest wall is highly compliant[56] so that when there is respiratory disease there is increased work. Second, the diaphragm is less effective as a result of its higher position within the chest and less apposition to the rib cage. Third, the infant's ribs are more horizontal, which lessens the bucket handle effect.[62]

Other skeletal muscles located in the chest or abdominal wall (e.g., the intercostals, scalenes, and abdominal muscles) can play an important role in ventilation. During normal breathing, most of the accessory muscles are silent. However, during abnormal conditions or disease states, these muscles are recruited to stabilize the chest or abdominal wall so that the diaphragm may be more efficient. In addition, it has been demonstrated that the external intercostal muscles contract in acute asthmatic attacks not only during inspiration but also during expiration; this contraction maintains a higher lung volume and hence increases airway diameter. When airways are occluded during inspiration, abdominal muscles contract powerfully during expiration, pushing the abdominal contents and diaphragm toward the thoracic cavity. This action lengthens diaphragmatic fibers and enhances the capability of the diaphragm to generate force during the subsequent inspiration (length-tension curve).

The upper airways must be kept patent during inspiration, and therefore, the pharyngeal wall muscles, genioglossus, and arytenoid muscles are properly considered muscles of respiration. There is an increase in neural output to these muscles immediately before diaphragmatic contraction during inspiration. The newborn also contracts these muscles during expiration to provide an expiratory outflow resistance and thus keeps end-expiratory volume greater than the FRC.

Respiratory muscles, whether the diaphragm, upper airway, intercostal, or abdominal muscles, are not homogeneous muscles in terms of their cellular structure, blood supply, metabolism, and recruitment patterns. Adult mature skeletal muscles have a mixture of fibers, and respiratory muscles are no different. The adult diaphragm, for instance, is made of fast- and slow-twitch fibers. Slow-twitch fibers are oxidative, and fast-twitch fibers are either glycolytic or moderately oxidative. Slow-twitch fibers are fatigue resistant—they are recruited first during a motor act; they generate low tensions; and they usually have a higher capillary/fiber ratio than fast fibers. Fast-twitch fibers can be either fatigue resistant (fast, moderately oxidative) or fast fatiguing (fast glycolytic); they are recruited during motor acts that require large force output. Thus, during normal quiet breathing, it is presumed that only the slow-twitch fibers in the diaphragm are active. In contrast, at the height of an acute attack of croup, asthma, or bronchiolitis during which muscle contractions are strong, both fiber types can be active, with the fast fibers generating the bulk of the force.

Muscle fiber composition, innervation, and metabolism are different in early life. The process of muscle fiber differentiation and interaction with the central nervous system is a continuous process, starting *in utero* and continuing postnatally. For example, slow oxidative fibers increase *in utero* and postnatally, whereas fast glycolytic fibers decrease postnatally. Polyneuronal innervation transforms into one motoneuron = one muscle fiber—the adult type of innervation—postnatally. Whether the young infant's ability to resist muscle fatigue is jeopardized by premature muscle fiber composition, innervation, and metabolism is not known and deserves further investigation.

Respiratory muscle fatigue may arise from central drive fatigue, neural transmission fatigue, contractile fatigue, or a combination of these three phenomena. Many factors predispose respiratory muscles to fatigue. Factors that increase fuel consumption (e.g., increased loads with disease); limit fuel reserves (e.g., malnutrition); alter acid-base homeostasis (e.g., acidosis); modify the oxidative capacity, glycolytic capacity, or both of the muscle (e.g., decreased activity of the muscle and possible atrophy after prolonged artificial ventilation); and decrease the oxygen availability to the muscle (e.g., anemia, low cardiac output states, hypoxemia) all predispose the diaphragm to failure. Reactive oxygen species (free radicals) produced by the contracting diaphragm are also thought to play a role in causing fatigue, particularly in conditions of ischemia/reperfusion and sepsis. In addition, changes in the external milieu of the muscle cell (e.g., low phosphate levels or the presence of certain drugs such as anesthetics) can limit the contractile ability and lead to premature muscle fatigue.

Diaphragmatic muscle function can be assessed clinically by observing the movements of the abdominal wall. During normal inspiration and with the contraction of the diaphragm, the abdominal contents are pushed away from the thorax. Because the abdominal wall is normally compliant during inspiration, the abdominal wall moves out to accommodate the increased pressure from the contracting diaphragm. With diaphragmatic fatigue, weakness, or paralysis, it is possible to observe an inward motion of the abdominal wall. Through the action of other respiratory muscles (intercostals), a drop in pressure occurs in the thorax during inspiration. Because of the "passive" behavior of the fatigued diaphragm, this pressure drop is transmitted to the abdomen; hence, the movement of the abdominal contents toward the thoracic cavity.

The highly compliant chest wall in the newborn infant limits its expansion during inspiration. The chest wall becomes even more unstable during REM sleep, when intercostal muscle activity is inhibited and the rib cage is more prone to distortion. This creates an added load and the potential for diaphragmatic fatigue.

A patient's respiratory muscle strength can be measured using various techniques,[63] all of which are effort dependent. These include maximum inspiratory and expiratory pressures, sniff pressures, and indirectly by maximal cough flows. If the airway is occluded during normal breathing, the infant,[64] child, and adult diaphragm are all capable of generating airway pressures of greater than 100 cm H_2O during a maximal inspiratory effort. In the laboratory, respiratory muscle function can be assessed in more detail (e.g., using electromyographic measurements during repeated stimulation of the phrenic nerve). The measurement of transdiaphragmatic pressure (Pdi) by placing balloon catheters just above (esophageal) and below (gastric) the diaphragm can provide a surrogate measure for muscle strength and susceptibility for fatigue, the time tension index (TTI):

$$TTI = (P_{DI}/P_{DI_{max}}) * (T_I/T_{TOT})$$

P_{DI} = mean transdiaphragmatic pressure
$P_{DI_{max}}$ = maximal transdiaphragmatic pressure
T_I = inspiratory time
T_{TOT} = respiratory cycle time

In adults, when the TTI is less than 0.1, it is unlikely that diaphragmatic fatigue will occur.

A less invasive measure involves measuring inspiratory pressures at the mouth instead of across the diaphragm. In this situation,

$$TTI = (P_{I_{mouth}}/P_{max_{mouth}}) * (T_I/T_{TOT})$$

The caveat for using mouth pressures is that it provides a measurement of force generation during the duty cycle by all respiratory muscles and not just the diaphragm. A TTI > 0.15 has been used to predict unsuccessful extubations in ventilated children.

To consider the main respiratory muscles—the diaphragm and the intercostal muscles—as the only respiratory muscles for breathing is insufficient, especially during stressful conditions or disease states. A number of muscles, such as the alae nasi, pharyngeal wall muscles, genioglossus, posterior cricoarytenoid, and thyroarytenoid, can play major roles in airway patency and hence in ventilatory output. Data indicate that upper airway muscles are strongly recruited during obstructive disease or during inspiratory occlusion, and that blood flow increases considerably to some of them (e.g., genioglossus). How prone these muscles are to fatigue under increased loads is unknown. How different these muscles are in terms of their structure, metabolism, and function in the neonate versus the adult is unclear and needs further research.

Because of the number of muscles involved, their location, and their function, the coordination of respiratory muscles becomes increasingly complex. The motor act of respiration should no longer be viewed as the result of one or two muscles contracting during inspiration and relaxing during expiration. At rest and even more so during disease states, the active coordination of various muscles becomes functionally very important. Defecation, sucking, and talking all involve the activation of several muscles that are shared by the respiratory apparatus for generating adequate ventilation. In some cases, obstructive apneas can actually be the result of muscle incoordination, with the diaphragm contracting when upper airway muscles that normally hold the airway open are relaxed.

Gas Exchange

The vital process of gas exchange occurs in the terminal respiratory unit. The previous sections of this chapter deal with the problems of moving air and blood to and from these gas-exchanging units. This section focuses on the fate of gas once it is introduced into the lungs, how it is transferred from the alveolar space to the bloodstream, and how ventilation and perfusion are matched.

In Fig. 6.23, the partial pressures of oxygen and carbon dioxide are depicted at various stages of the pathway from ambient air to the tissues. Because nitrogen is inert, changes in its partial pressure (P_{N_2}) in the gas phase depend on changes in the partial pressures of oxygen and carbon dioxide, gases

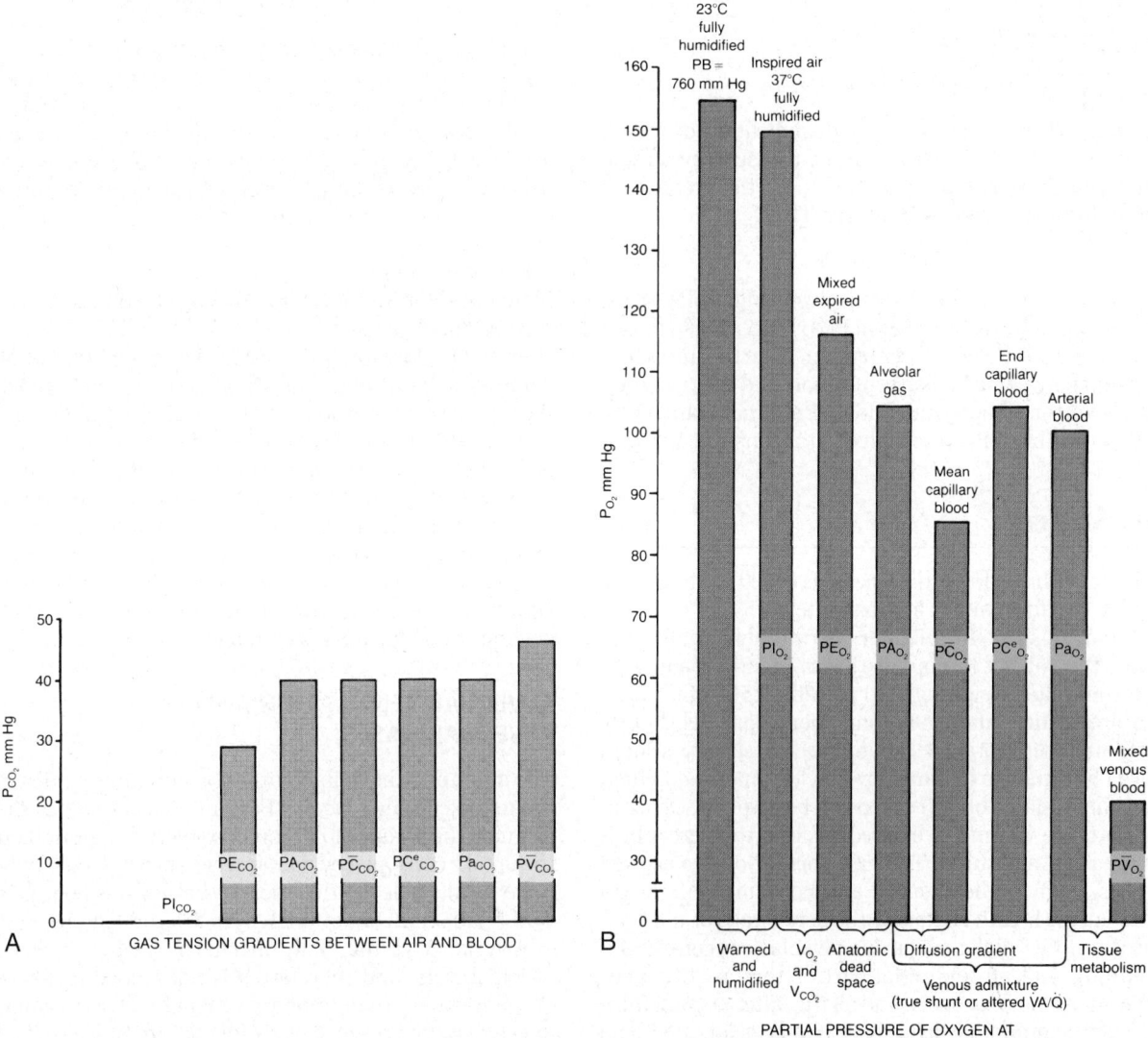

Fig. 6.23 (A) and (B) Partial pressures of oxygen and carbon dioxide in different portions of the airway and blood.

that are utilized and excreted, respectively. In contrast, P_{N_2} in blood and tissue is identical because nitrogen is inert. The rather complex influences of dead space, alveolar ventilation, ventilation-perfusion relationships, and tissue metabolism on the partial pressures of oxygen and carbon dioxide are discussed in some detail, and frequent reference to Fig. 6.23 is useful in clarifying some of the concepts.

Alveolar Ventilation

One component of the V_T is the anatomic dead space, V_D (consisting of the nose, mouth, pharynx, larynx, trachea, bronchi, and bronchioles), where no significant exchange of oxygen and carbon dioxide with blood takes place. The other component of the V_T, V_A, undergoes gas exchange in the alveoli. Alveolar ventilation per minute is measured by the following equation:

$$V_A = V_T - V_D$$

In practice, V_D is difficult to measure, so the alveolar ventilation equation is used. Since all expired CO_2 comes from the alveolar gas,

$$V_{CO_2} = V_A \times \%CO_2/100 \text{ or}$$
$$V_A = V_{CO_2} \times 100/\%CO_2.$$

The $\%CO_2/100$ is the fractional concentration of CO_2 in the alveolar gas (FA_{CO_2}), which can be measure by a rapid CO_2 analyzer. FA_{CO_2} can be converted to partial pressure of CO_2 by multiplying by P_B, 47 mm Hg. Thus,

$$V_A = V_{CO_2}/PA_{CO_2}$$

In normal subjects, the P_{CO_2} in alveolar gas (PA_{CO_2}) is essentially the same as the arterial P_{CO_2} (Pa_{CO_2}), which can be used to determine alveolar ventilation. Note the important relationship between alveolar ventilation and Pa_{CO_2}. When V_A is halved, then Pa_{CO_2} must double at a constant V_{CO_2}; when V_A is doubled, Pa_{CO_2} is halved at a constant V_{CO_2}.

Dead Space

The volume of the conducting airways is called the anatomic dead space (V_{Danat}) and is approximately 25% of each V_T. Anatomic dead space in milliliters is roughly equal to the weight of the subject in pounds (for a 7-pound baby, 7 or 8 mL; for an adult weighing 150 pounds, 150 mL). In the normal premature infant, anatomic dead space is slightly higher than 30%. In practice, anatomic dead space is seldom measured but may be obtained by Fowler's method, which requires that a single breath of oxygen be inspired. On expiration, both the volume of expired gas and the percentage of nitrogen are measured. The first portion of the expired gas comes from the dead space and contains little or no nitrogen. As the breath is expired, the percentage of nitrogen increases until it "plateaus" at the alveolar concentration. By assuming that all the initial part of the breath comes from the anatomic dead space and all the latter portion from the alveoli, the anatomic dead space can be calculated. The same measurements can be made by monitoring the expired carbon dioxide concentration. In practice, anatomic dead

space is difficult to define accurately, because it depends on lung volume (greater at large lung volumes when the airways are more distended) and on body position (smaller in supine position).

Physiologic dead space may be measured by making use of the argument originally developed by Bohr. Since all of the expired CO_2 (FE_{CO_2}) comes from the alveolar gas (FA_{CO_2}) and none from the dead space,

$$V_T \times FE_{CO_2} = V_A \times FA_{CO_2}.$$

And since $V_A = V_T - V_D$, then

$$V_T \times FE_{CO_2} = (V_T - V_D) \times FA_{CO_2}$$

and

$$V_D/V_T \cong FA_{CO_2} - FE_{CO_2}/FA_{CO_2}$$

And since the partial pressure of a gas is proportional to its fractioned concentration (F),

$$V_D/V_T = PA_{CO_2} - PE_{CO_2}/PA_{CO_2} \text{ (Bohr equation)}$$

Or, since alveolar P_{CO_2} and arterial P_{CO_2} are identical in normal subjects,

$$V_D/V_T = Pa_{CO_2} - PE_{CO_2}/Pa_{CO_2}$$

It is now quite clear that V_{Dphys} must be defined according to the gas being measured. Because oxygen is more diffusible in the gas phase than is carbon dioxide, physiologic dead space using oxygen or various inert gases is different from the CO_2 dead space. However, V_{Dphys} measurements using CO_2 are helpful in assessing patients, because they reflect the portion of each breath that participates in gas exchange, particularly with respect to CO_2. An elevated V_{Dphys} indicates that areas of the lung are being underventilated in relation to the amount of blood flowing through the region.

From the foregoing discussion, it is apparent that a V_T value must be chosen that will allow adequate alveolar ventilation. For example, an adult might breathe 60 times per minute with a V_T of 100 mL for a minute ventilation of 6 L. Nevertheless, alveolar ventilation under these circumstances may be inadequate, because the dead space is primarily ventilated. In selecting suitable volumes and rates for patients on respirators, it is useful to approximate normal values and to consider adequate alveolar ventilation rather than total ventilation. A discussion of high-frequency ventilation is beyond the scope of this chapter.

ALVEOLAR VENTILATION AND ALVEOLAR GASES

The amount of alveolar ventilation per minute must be adequate to keep the alveolar P_{O_2} and P_{CO_2} at values that will promote the escape of carbon dioxide from venous blood and the uptake of oxygen by pulmonary capillary blood. In healthy patients at sea level, this means that PA_{O_2} is approximately 105 to 110 mm Hg and PA_{CO_2} is 40 mm Hg (Fig. 6.24).

Arterial P_{O_2} is markedly affected by the presence of right-to-left shunts, and therefore it is not a good measurement of the adequacy of pulmonary ventilation. Pa_{CO_2} is minimally affected in the presence of shunts because $Pv–{CO_2}$ is 46 mm Hg and Pa_{CO_2} is 40 mm Hg. If one third of the cardiac output is shunted, this raises Pa_{CO_2} to only 42 mm Hg. Thus, the

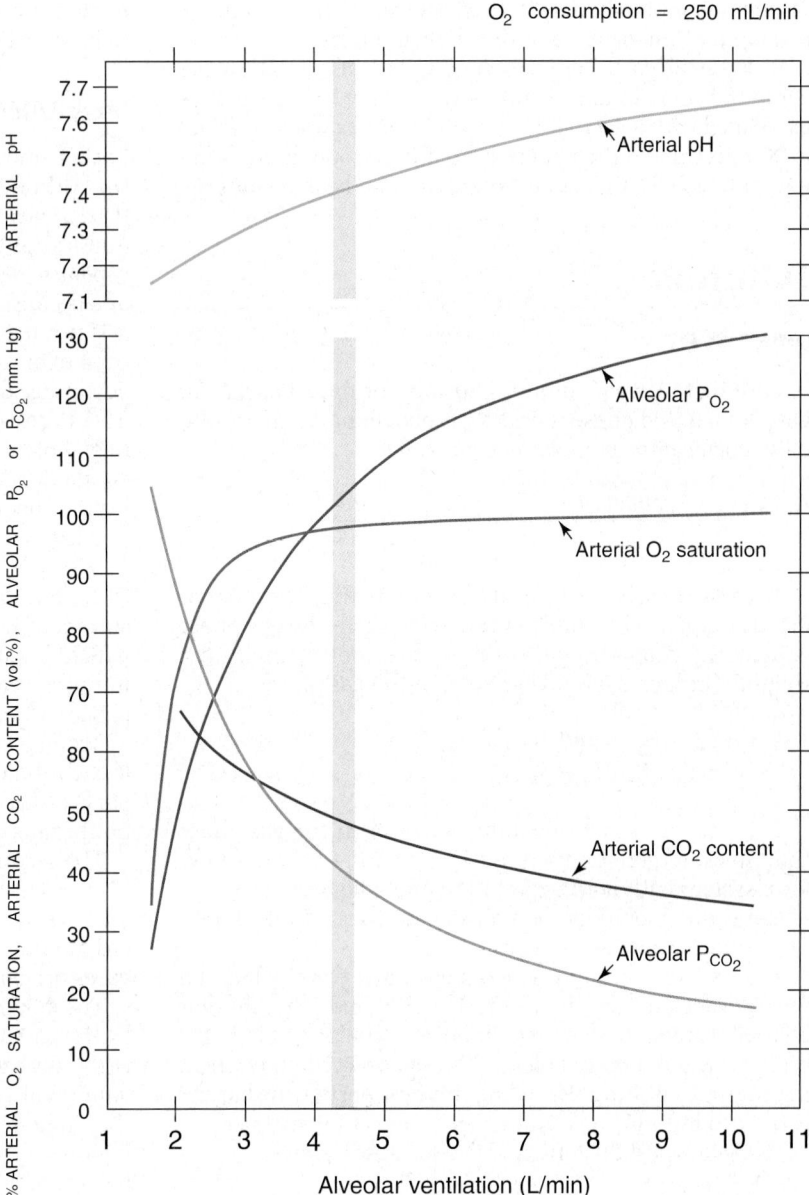

Fig. 6.24 The effect of changing alveolar ventilation on alveolar gas and arterial blood oxygen, carbon dioxide, and pH. (From Comroe Jr JH, Forster RE II, Dubois AB, et al. *The Lung*, 2nd ed. Chicago: Year Book Medical; 1962.)

arterial P_{CO_2} is the optimum measurement of the adequacy of alveolar ventilation. When alveolar ventilation halves, Pa_{CO_2} doubles; when alveolar ventilation doubles, Pa_{CO_2} halves. Hyperventilation is defined as a Pa_{CO_2} less than 35 mm Hg, and hypoventilation as a Pa_{CO_2} greater than 45 mm Hg. Hypoventilation can occur as a result of respiratory center malfunction (e.g., congenital hypoventilation syndrome) or depression (e.g., anesthetics) or when there is profound disease involving the lung, chest wall, or respiratory muscles such that effective alveolar ventilation cannot be maintained. Inspired air has a fraction of inspired oxygen (FI_{O_2}) of 0.2093, and it is "diluted" in the alveoli by the FRC of air containing carbon dioxide and water vapor, so the P_{O_2} in alveolar gas must be less than that of the inspired air (PI_{O_2}; see earlier discussion of Dalton's law). PA_{O_2} must be calculated from the alveolar air equation. When oxygen consumption equals carbon dioxide production, then,

$$PA_{O_2} = PI_{O_2} - PA_{CO_2}$$
$$PI_{O_2} = 0.2093 \times (PB - 47 \text{ mm Hg}) = 150 \text{ mm Hg}$$

If PA_{CO_2} is 40 mm Hg, then PA_{O_2} is 110 mm Hg. Usually, the respiratory exchange ratio (R) is 0.8, or more oxygen is consumed than carbon dioxide eliminated, thereby decreasing PA_{O_2} slightly more than would be expected from the dilution of PA_{CO_2}. To account for changes in R, a useful form of the alveolar air equation for clinical purposes is

$$PA_{O_2} = PI_{O_2} - \frac{PA_{CO_2}}{R}$$

When PA_{CO_2} is 40 and R is 0.8, PA_{O_2} is 100 mm Hg. Note that breathing 40% oxygen raises PA_{O_2} to 235 mm Hg because FI_{O_2} is now 0.40. Note that this equation is less accurate during oxygen breathing when more arduous forms of the alveolar air equation may be used. However, this inaccuracy is seldom of importance in the clinical setting.

Because the partial pressures of alveolar gases must always equal the same total pressure, any increase in one must be associated with a decrease in the other. For example, if Pa_{CO_2} is 80 mm Hg and the patient is breathing room air (assuming an R of 0.8), the highest that PA_{O_2} can be is 50 mm Hg.

Diffusion

PRINCIPLES

According to Henry's law of diffusion, the diffusion rate for gases in a liquid phase is directly proportional to their solubility coefficients. For example, in water,

$$\frac{\text{solubility of } CO_2}{\text{solubility of } O_2} = \frac{0.592}{0.0244} = \frac{24.3}{1}$$

Therefore, carbon dioxide diffuses more than 24 times as fast as oxygen. The diffusion rate of a gas in the gas phase is inversely proportional to the square root of molecular weight (Graham's law). Therefore, in the gas phase,

$$\frac{\text{rate for } CO_2}{\text{rate for } O_2} = 0.85$$

That is, carbon dioxide diffuses slower in the gas phase than does oxygen. Combining Henry's and Graham's laws for a system with both a gas phase and a liquid phase (e.g., alveolus and blood): carbon dioxide diffuses $24.3 \times 0.85 = 20.7$ times as fast as oxygen.

The barriers through which a gas must travel when diffusing from an alveolus to the blood include the alveolar epithelial lining, basement membrane, capillary endothelial lining, plasma, and red blood cell. As observed on electron micrographs of lung tissue, the thinnest part of the barrier is 0.2 μm but may be as much as 3 times this thickness.

Fick's law of diffusion, modified for gases, states:

$$Q/\text{min} = \frac{KS(P_1 - P_2)}{d}$$

The amount of gas (Q) diffusing through a membrane is directly proportional to the surface area available for diffusion (S), the pressure difference of the two gases on either side of the membrane, and a constant (K) that depends on the solubility coefficient of the gas and the characteristics of the particular membrane and liquid used and is inversely proportional to the distance (d) through which the gas has to diffuse. In the lung of a given subject, exact values for K, S, and d are unknown. Therefore, for the lung, Bohr and Krogh suggested "diffusing capacity" (DL). DL is simply the inverse of the total resistance to diffusion and can be expressed as the sum of the individual component resistances:

$$\frac{1}{DL} = \frac{1}{DM} + \frac{1}{\theta Vc}$$

where $1/DM$ is the resistance to diffusion of the gas across the alveolar-capillary membrane, plasma, and red blood cell

membrane; θ is the reaction rate of the gas with hemoglobin (Hb); and Vc is the pulmonary capillary blood volume.

MEASUREMENT

Carbon monoxide and oxygen have been used to measure DL. Although the diffusing capacity of the lung for oxygen (DL_{O_2}) has been measured, the process is both complicated and fraught with technical problems because the average capillary oxygen tension must be determined. For this reason, and because a defect in DL_{O_2} is rarely the cause of hypoxemia, it is not used in the clinical setting. CO, however, has been used extensively in children to test diffusing capacity. The advantage of using CO is its remarkable affinity for Hb, some 210 times that of oxygen; therefore, the capillary P_{CO} is negligible and offers no backpressure for diffusion. To calculate the diffusing capacity of the lungs for CO (DL_{CO}) one need know only the amount of CO taken up per unit time and the PA_{CO}.

Many techniques have been developed to measure the DL_{CO}, but only two are discussed in this chapter. The measurement of steady-state DL_{CO} is performed by having the patient breathe a gas mixture containing 0.1% CO for several minutes. Although this measurement requires only a little patient cooperation, its disadvantage is that the value obtained is strongly influenced by maldistribution of the inspired air; if the inhaled gas mixture is not distributed properly to all parts of the lung, the measured DL_{CO} will be decreased but not because of changes in DM, θ, or Vc.

The second technique, the measurement of single-breath DL_{CO}, is less affected by airway disease. In this test, the subject takes a single large breath (from RV to TLC) of a CO-containing gas mixture. Following a 10-second breath-hold, the expired gases are collected so that PA_{CO} can be determined.

The difference between these two techniques is exemplified by the patient with acute asthma, in whom the steady-state DL_{CO} value will be decreased, whereas the single-breath DL_{CO} value will be normal or increased. Another advantage of the single-breath DL_{CO} method results from the inclusion of helium in the inspired gas. This inert gas allows the DL_{CO} to be corrected for the alveolar volume (VA) in which it was distributed, a measurement known as K_{CO}:

$$K_{CO} = \frac{DL_{CO} \text{ single breath}}{\text{alveolar volume}}$$

The K_{CO} reflects the physiology of the lung[65] and is the most useful parameter for comparing the DL of children of different ages and hence different lung volumes. In addition, the K_{CO} helps differentiate among simple loss of lung units (atelectasis), a decrease in pulmonary blood volume (emphysema), and the (albeit rarely seen) true diffusion defect.

The DL_{CO} increases throughout childhood, is related to lung growth, and correlates best with subject height or body surface area. Clinically, a reduction in DL_{CO} may occur for many reasons, including surgical lung resection, diffuse lung disease (pulmonary fibrosis, cystic fibrosis), and emphysematous destruction of the alveolar-capillary membrane. In addition, anemia may decrease the DL_{CO}, and equations to correct the DL_{CO} for anemia are available. Increases in DL_{CO} rarely occur and usually result from pulmonary vascular engorgement (increased Vc) or pulmonary hemorrhage (e.g., Goodpasture syndrome and idiopathic pulmonary hemosiderosis).

It is important to note that with a nonexercising patient, impaired diffusion of oxygen from the alveolar air to the pulmonary capillary is rarely the cause of a low PaO_2. Diffusion limitation may occur during exercise in patients with interstitial lung disease or in healthy individuals performing extreme exercise. Hypoxemia in pulmonary diseases usually results from alveolar hypoventilation or an imbalance between ventilation and perfusion of lung units. Thus, low $DLCO$ values almost always reflect abnormalities in gas exchange rather than true diffusion defects.

Shunt and Ventilation-Perfusion Relationships

There are four pulmonary causes of arterial hypoxemia. We have already discussed two of these, alveolar hypoventilation and diffusion defects. The remaining two, intrapulmonary shunt and ventilation-perfusion defects, result from abnormalities in the distribution of the ventilation and perfusion of the gas-exchanging units.

Shunt refers to blood that reaches the systemic circulation without coming in direct contact with a ventilated area of the lung. Because this blood is deoxygenated, it lowers the PaO_2. There are several causes of shunt. In normal lungs, a small amount of shunt is present because the Thebesian veins and a portion of the bronchial vascular flow drain into the left side of the heart. Pathologic shunts result when abnormal vascular channels exist, as in cyanotic congenital heart disease or pulmonary arteriovenous fistula. Shunt, however, most commonly occurs in diseased lungs because alveoli are not ventilated but are still being perfused. This condition, known as intrapulmonary shunting, occurs in a variety of lung diseases, including pulmonary edema, atelectasis, and pneumonia.

A characteristic feature of shunt is that the resultant hypoxemia cannot be corrected by breathing pure oxygen, a reasonable consequence because, by definition, shunted blood does not pass ventilated lung units. One caveat is that when patients are placed on high oxygen concentrations, a very small increase in PaO_2 may occur because the blood-perfusing ventilated units will depart those units with higher amounts of dissolved oxygen. The characteristic that shunt is very poorly responsive to breathing pure oxygen can be a useful clinical tool; if PaO_2 is less than 500 mm Hg while the subject is breathing 100% oxygen, a significant shunt is present. If mixed venous (pulmonary arterial) blood is available for measurement (or a mixed venous oxygen concentration is assumed), the amount of shunt can be calculated at any inspired oxygen concentration using the shunt equation:

Amount of oxygen in arterial blood =

amount of oxygen in blood that has

passed through pulmonary capillaries $(\dot{Q}c)+$

amount of oxygen in shunted blood (Qs),

and

Amount of oxygen = content of oxygen per liter (CO_2)
$$\times \text{ blood flow }(\dot{Q}).$$

Therefore,

$$Cao_2 \ \dot{Q}t = CCo_2 \ \dot{Q}c + C\bar{V}o_2 \ \dot{Q}s$$

where $\dot{Q}$ is total blood flow. Since $\dot{Q}c = \dot{Q}t - \dot{Q}s$,

$$Cao_2 \ \dot{Q}t = CCo_2 \ \dot{Q}t - CCo_2 + \dot{Q}s + C\bar{V}o_2 \ \dot{Q}s$$

and

$$\frac{\dot{Q}s}{\dot{Q}t} = \frac{Cco_2 - CaO_2}{Cco_2 - C\bar{V}O_2}$$

where $\dot{Q}s/\dot{Q}t$ is the fraction of the total cardiac output that is shunted.

The average ratio between alveolar ventilation and blood flow (VA/Q) is 0.8, but the ratio even in the normal lung may range from near zero (not ventilated) to infinity (not perfused). Nevertheless, the most common cause of arterial hypoxemia is a result of mismatch of ventilation and perfusion within the lung, which increases the normal scatter of VA/Q values around the mean value. When a lung unit receives inadequate ventilation relative to its blood flow, $PACO_2$ rises (toward the mixed venous value of 46 mm Hg) and PAO_2 falls (toward the mixed venous value of about 40 mm Hg) and the oxygen content of the end-capillary blood falls. When this blood mixes with blood coming from normal VA/Q regions of the lung, the result is a lowering of oxygen concentration and arterial hypoxemia (so-called *shunt-like effect*). In contrast to what occurs in a true shunt, administration of an enriched oxygen mixture will correct the hypoxemia due to ventilation-perfusion mismatch by raising PAO_2 (PN_2 must decrease to keep the sum of the partial pressures of gases equal to PB). The increased PAO_2 results in an increased concentration of oxygen in the pulmonary capillary blood.

Whatever the absolute amount of regional ventilation and perfusion, the lung has intrinsic regularity mechanisms that are directed toward the preservation of normal $\dot{V}A/\dot{Q}$ ratios. When $\dot{V}A/\dot{Q}$ is high, the low carbon dioxide concentration results in local constriction of airways and tends to reduce the amount of ventilation to the area. When $\dot{V}A/\dot{Q}$ is low, the high alveolar carbon dioxide concentration results in local airway dilation and tends to increase ventilation to the area. Furthermore, a low $\dot{V}A/\dot{Q}$ with an associated low alveolar oxygen concentration causes regional pulmonary vasoconstriction and produces a redistribution of blood flow to healthier lung units. These effects on airways and vessels from changing gas tensions tend to preserve a normal $\dot{V}A/\dot{Q}$, but they are limited mechanisms, and derangements are common with pulmonary disease.

Systemic Gas Transport

OXYGEN TRANSPORT

Once oxygen molecules have passed from the alveolus into the pulmonary capillary, they are transported in the blood in two ways. A small proportion of the oxygen exists as dissolved oxygen in the plasma and water of the red blood cell. For 100 mL of whole blood equilibrated with a PO_2 of 100 mm

Hg, 0.3 mL of oxygen is present as dissolved oxygen. If this represented the total oxygen-carrying capacity of blood, cardiac output would have to be greater than 80 L/min to allow 250 mL of oxygen to be consumed per minute. During 100% oxygen breathing, PaO_2 is approximately 650 mm Hg, and 100 mL of blood contains 2.0 mL of dissolved oxygen; a cardiac output of about 12 L/min would be required if no Hb were present and if the tissues could extract all of the oxygen.

Because 1 g of Hb can combine with 1.39 mL of oxygen, between 40 and 70 times more oxygen is carried by Hb than by the plasma, enabling the body to achieve a cardiac output at rest of 5.5 L/min with an oxygen uptake of 250 mL/min.

The potential usefulness of hyperbaric oxygen (i.e., oxygen under very high pressures) for a variety of clinical conditions is because at a pressure of 3 atmospheres (absolute) (PAO_2 of about 1950 mm Hg), approximately 6.0 mL of oxygen is dissolved in 100 mL of whole blood, and this amount can meet the metabolic demands of the tissues under resting conditions even when no Hb is present.

The remarkable oxygen-carrying properties of blood depend not on the solubility of oxygen in plasma but on the unusual properties of Hb. Fig. 6.25 illustrates the oxyhemoglobin dissociation curve, showing that Hb is nearly 95% saturated at a PO_2 of 80 mm Hg. The steep portion of the curve, up to about 50 mm Hg, permits large amounts of oxygen to be released from Hb with small changes in PO_2. Under normal circumstances, 100% oxygen breathing will raise the amount of oxygen carried by the blood by only a small amount, because at a PO_2 of 100 mm Hg, Hb is already 97.5% saturated. Even with air breathing, one is on the flat portion of the curve. The presence of a right-to-left shunt markedly affects PO_2 but may reduce the percentage saturation only

minimally. For example, a 50% shunt with venous blood containing 15 mL of oxygen/100 mL will reduce the oxygen content of 100 mL of blood only from 20 mL to 17.5 mL. The blood is still 88% saturated, but PaO_2 is now 60 mm Hg instead of 100 mm Hg. Thus, the change in oxygen content is linearly related to the amount of right-to-left shunt, but the change in PO_2 is not, because the oxyhemoglobin dissociation curve is S shaped. It is also apparent that at levels greater than 60 mm Hg, PaO_2 is a more sensitive measure of blood oxygenation, because neither percentage saturation nor oxygen content changes as much as PO_2 in this range. However, at PO_2 below about 60 mm Hg, relatively small changes of PO_2 produce large changes in saturation and content, and in this range, the measurement of content may be more reliable than the measurement of PO_2.

The oxyhemoglobin dissociation curve is affected by changes in pH, PCO_2, and temperature. A decrease in pH, an increase in PCO_2 (Bohr effect), or an increase in temperature shifts the curve to the right, particularly in the 20 to 50 mm Hg range. Thus, for a given PO_2, the saturation percentage is less under acidotic or hyperpyrexic conditions. In the tissues, carbon dioxide is added to the blood, and this facilitates the removal of oxygen from the red blood cells. In the pulmonary capillaries, carbon dioxide diffuses out of the blood, facilitating oxygen uptake by Hb. An increase in temperature has an effect similar to that of an increase in PCO_2 and thus facilitates oxygen removal from the blood by the tissues. Note that a patient who is pyrexic with carbon dioxide retention could not have a normal oxygen saturation during air breathing because of the Bohr and temperature effects on the oxyhemoglobin dissociation curve.

The erythrocyte concentration of 2,3-diphosphoglycerate (DPG) plays a major role in shifting oxyhemoglobin

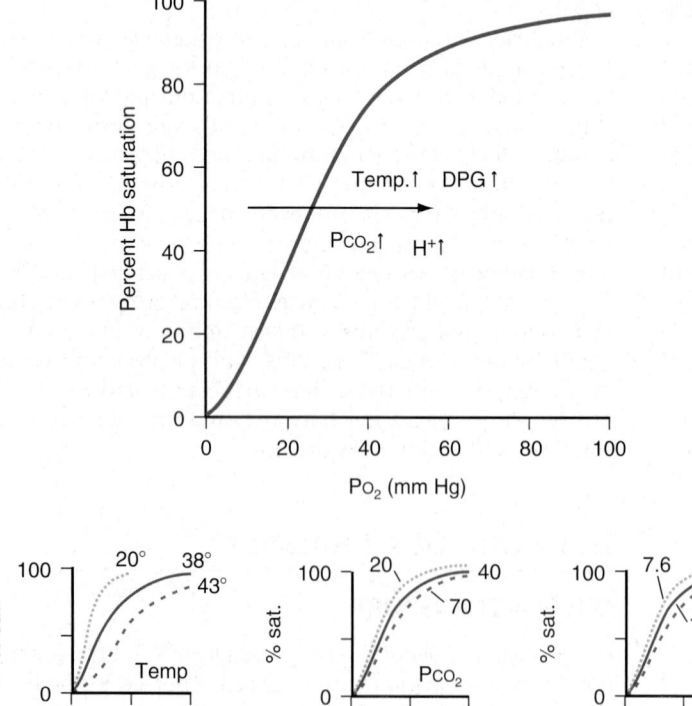

Fig. 6.25 Oxyhemoglobin dissociation curves. The large graph shows a single dissociation curve, applicable when the pH of the blood is 7.40 and temperature is 38°C. The blood oxygen tension and saturation of patients with carbon dioxide retention, acidosis, alkalosis, fever, or hypothermia will not fit this curve because it shifts to the right or left when temperature, pH, or PCO_2 is changed. Effects on the oxyhemoglobin dissociation curve of change in temperature (upper left) and in PCO_2 and pH (lower right) are shown in the smaller graphs. A small change in blood pH occurs regularly in the body (i.e., when mixed venous blood passes through the pulmonary capillaries, PCO_2 decreases from 46 to 40 mm Hg, and pH increases from 7.37 to 7.40). During this time, blood changes from a pH of 7.37 dissociation curve to a pH of 7.40 dissociation curve. Note that increased 2,3-diphosphoglycerate also shifts the curve to the right. (From West JB. *Respiratory Physiology—The Essentials*, 5th ed. Baltimore: Lippincott Williams & Wilkins, 1995.)

dissociation curves. DPG and Hb are present in about equi-molar concentrations in adult human red blood cells. There is strong binding between DPG and the β chain of Hb, and this complex is highly resistant to oxygenation. Shifts of the dissociation curve to the right associated with an increased DPG concentration (e.g., in anemia) facilitate the release of oxygen to the tissues. Because erythrocyte DPG concentration can change within a matter of hours, a regulatory role for DPG in maintaining optimal tissue oxygenation has been suggested.

The fetal oxyhemoglobin dissociation curve is to the left of the adult curve at a similar pH. Thus, at a given PO_2, fetal Hb contains more oxygen than adult Hb. This property ensures that an adequate amount of oxygen will reach fetal tissues, since the fetus *in utero* has a PaO_2 of about 20 to 25 mm Hg in the descending aorta. The different affinity of fetal Hb for oxygen results from its interaction with DPG. Both fetal and adult red blood cells have similar intracellular concentrations of DPG, but fetal Hb, which has a γ chain instead of a β chain, interacts less strongly with this molecule; therefore, the fetal oxyhemoglobin curve is to the left of the adult curve. Fetal Hb disappears from the circulation shortly after birth, and less than 2% is present by a few months of age. Normal fetal development is not dependent on differences in maternal and fetal Hbs, because they are identical in some species.

Abnormal Hbs differ in their oxygen-carrying capacity. For example, Hb M is oxidized by oxygen to methemoglobin, which does not release oxygen to the tissues; a large amount is incompatible with life. The formation of methemoglobin by agents such as nitrates, aniline, sulfonamides, acetanilid, phenylhydrazine, and primaquine may also be life threatening. Congenital deficiency of the enzyme Hb reductase is also associated with large amounts of methemoglobin, and affected patients are cyanotic in room air. Similarly, sulfhemoglobin is unable to transport oxygen. CO has 210 times more affinity for Hb than oxygen, so it is important to note that PO_2 may be normal in CO poisoning but oxygen content will be reduced markedly.

Thus, a variety of factors may affect the position of the oxyhemoglobin dissociation curve. The position of the curve may be described by measuring the PO_2 at which there is 50% saturation, the so-called P_{50}. When the curve is shifted to the left, the P_{50} is low; when the curve is shifted to the right, the P_{50} is elevated. Although the P_{50} is the traditional method of describing the affinity of Hb for oxygen (see Fig. 6.25), a more appropriate clinical measurement is the P_{90}. This is the PaO_2 at which the Hb is 90% saturated and, as outlined in the following section, corresponds to the goal of oxygen therapy (Table 6.3).

ASSESSMENT OF BLOOD OXYGENATION

It is challenging to assess oxygenation at the bedside because the degree of visible cyanosis is influenced by many factors, including the patient's Hb concentration and integrity of peripheral perfusion. Clinical cyanosis reflects the absolute concentration of deoxyhemoglobin (Hb), not the ratio of Hb to oxyhemoglobin (HbO_2). Thus, the presence of anemia makes the clinical detection of a low PaO_2 more difficult, whereas cyanosis may be present in polycythemic patients even though the PaO_2 is only minimally decreased. It has been estimated that cyanosis will be seen when there is

Table 6.3 Effect of Temperature and Acute Respiratory Acidosis and Alkalosis on Hemoglobin Oxygen Affinity

Temperature[a] (°C)		P_{50}	P_{90}
28		16.5	35
32		20.5	44
40		32.0	68
RESPIRATORY ACIDOSIS AND ALKALOSIS[b]			
pH	PCO2	P_{50}	P_{90}
7.56	20	22	48
7.48	30	24.5	52.5
7.40	40	27	58
7.32	50	29.5	63
7.26	60	31	67 P_{50} and P_{90}: PO_2 at which 50% or 90% of the hemoglobin is saturated.

[a]PCO_2 = 40 mm Hg, pH = 7.40.
[b]Temperature = 37°C.
Data from Rebuck AS, Chapman KR. The P_{90} as a clinically relevant landmark on the oxyhemoglobin dissociation curve. *Am Rev Respir Dis.* 1988;137:962-963.

approximately 5 gm/dL of reduced Hb in the capillaries, which correlates with approximately 3 gm/dL in the arterial blood.[66]

HbO_2 can be assessed using oximeters. The pulse oximeter is most commonly used to noninvasively assess a patient's blood oxygenation. The pulse oximeter passes two different wavelengths of light, 660 nm and 940 nm, through the patient's tissues. HbO_2 absorbs the 660-nm wavelength, whereas Hb absorbs the 940-nm wavelength; the oximeter then determines the ratio of HbO_2/(HbO_2 + Hb). The measurement is timed with the pulse of arterial blood and thus facilitates the measurement of an arterial-like Hb saturation value. Although appropriate in the majority of situations, it is important to remember the limitations of a pulse oximeter. It neither detects carboxyhemoglobin (HbCO) nor methemoglobin (metHb), and it will not work well if there is decreased perfusion or the patient has a dyshemoglobinemia. Technical issues, such as skin pigmentation, nail polish or motion artifacts, can also compromise the measurement. The Hb oxygen saturation of a blood sample can be directly analyzed using a co-oximeter, a device that uses multiple wavelengths of light to distinguish HbO_2 from Hb, HbCO, and metHb. The use of a co-oximeter is mandatory when the clinician suspects CO poisoning, as HbCO is pink, or if metHb is suspected.

The PaO_2 of blood can be directly measured using the Clark oxygen electrode within a blood gas analyzer. Usually, the Hb saturation of a blood gas sample is calculated from the PaO_2 using assumptions for various parameters, such as the p50 of the patient's Hb, with correction for the patient's core body temperature.

Normal values for HbO_2 during infancy, as measured by pulse oximetry, and PaO_2 from arterial blood samples, are illustrated in Fig. 6.26.

Today the usual clinical practice is to measure SaO_2 with a pulse oximeter and to estimate $PaCO_2$ by measuring the PCO_2 of either a peripheral venous blood or arterialized blood sample. The latter refers to a blood sample that was obtained after the extremity was warmed and received topical medications to increase capillary blood flow and bring the sample's characteristics closer to those of arteriolar blood. In individuals who have adequate peripheral perfusion, it can be assumed

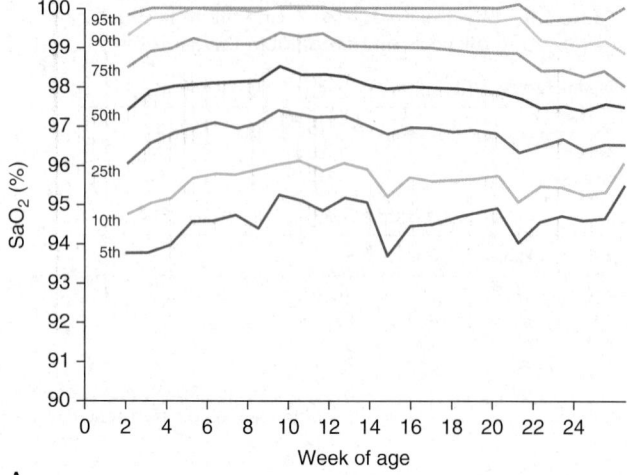

A

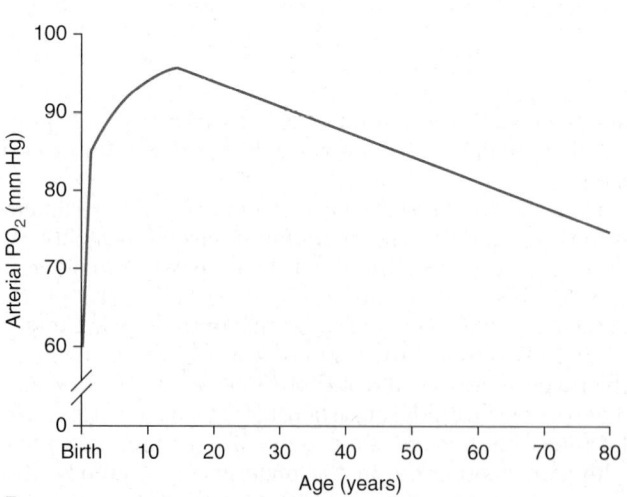

B

Fig. 6.26 (A) Median baseline SaO₂ (SpO₂) for healthy term infants who were studied at each postnatal week from 2 to 25 weeks after birth. Variations in SpO₂ with increasing age were not significant. (B) Arterial PO₂ as a function of age from infancy to 80 years of age. The figure represents the data from numerous studies. (Median baseline SaO₂ reproduced with permission from Hunt CE, Corwin MJ, Lister G, et al. Longitudinal assessment of hemoglobin oxygen saturation in healthy infants during the first 6 months of age. Collaborative Home Infant Monitoring Evaluation (CHIME) Study Group. *J Pediatr.* 1999;135:580-586; Arterial PO₂ reproduced with permission from Murray JF. *The Normal Lung: A Basis for the Diagnosis and Treatment of Pulmonary Disease*, 2nd ed. Philadelphia: Saunders; 1986.)

that the $PaCO_2$ will be 6 mm Hg or less than the peripheral venous CO_2 gas tension ($PvCO_2$). If the estimated $PaCO_2$ is normal, or less than normal, then the clinician can be confident that the patient is not in hypercarbic respiratory failure. However, if the estimated $PaCO_2$ is elevated, then the clinician must obtain an arterial sample to directly measure the $PaCO_2$ because an elevated PCO_2 in an arteriolized capillary or venous sample may indicate decreased peripheral perfusion. The PO_2 and calculated SaO_2 from a venous blood gas should be ignored.

OXYGEN DELIVERY TO TISSUES

The cardiopulmonary unit not only must oxygenate the blood but also must transport oxygen to the systemic tissues in adequate amounts. The total oxygen delivery to the systemic tissues is determined by the PaO_2, the amount of saturated Hb, and the left ventricular output (see the equation that follows). For an average adult with a PaO_2 of 100 mm Hg, a Hb concentration of 15 g/100 mL (97.5% saturation), and a cardiac output (C.O.) of 5 L/min, approximately 1000 mL of oxygen is delivered to systemic tissues each minute. This large delivery of oxygen provides a significant margin of safety because, under normal circumstances, the systemic tissues use only one fourth of the available oxygen; mixed venous PO_2 is 40 mm Hg, and Hb is 73% saturated. Mixed venous blood is by definition the blood within the main pulmonary artery but is often estimated from a central venous line.

The systemic oxygen transport equation is useful to emphasize a therapeutic principle: the three practical ways to improve oxygenation of peripheral tissues are to increase Hb saturation, to increase Hb concentration, and to augment cardiac output.

$$\text{oxygen delivery} = \text{blood oxygen content} \times \text{cardiac output},$$

where

$$\text{blood oxygen content/100 mL} = \text{dissolved oxygen } (0.003 \text{ mL/100 mL blood} \times PaO_2) + \text{oxygen carried by hemoglobin } (1.39 \text{ mL/g} \times \text{gHb/100 mL})$$

Oxygen Therapy

INCREASED INSPIRED MIXTURES

The concentration of oxygen in the inspired air should be increased when tissue oxygenation is inadequate. The response to an increased inspired oxygen concentration depends on which cause of hypoxia is present (Box 6.1). Most of the conditions characterized by hypoxemia respond well to added oxygen. For example, if airway disease results in a 30% decrease in ventilation to an acinus, this can be corrected by an appropriate increase in the concentration of oxygen in the inspired gas. In contrast, patients with shunts will only respond to a minimal degree because the shunted blood does not perfuse alveoli. The slight improvement in PaO_2 and SaO_2 that may be seen when patients with extensive intrapulmonary shunting inhale high concentrations of oxygen results from the additional amount of dissolved oxygen in the blood that perfuses ventilated alveoli. A direct attack on the underlying disorder in anemia, ischemia, and poisonings is clearly indicated; oxygen therapy may be a life-saving measure during the time required to treat the disease.

Oxygen therapy can be utilized to facilitate the removal of other gases loculated in body spaces, such as air in pneumothorax, pneumomediastinum, and ileus. High inspired oxygen mixtures effectively wash out body stores of nitrogen. With air breathing, the blood that perfuses the tissue spaces has an arterial oxygen tension of 100 mm Hg and a venous oxygen tension of 40 mm Hg. With oxygen breathing, although arterial tensions increase to 600 mm Hg, venous

Box 6.1 Four Types of Hypoxia and Some Causes

Hypoxemia (Low P_{O_2} and Low Oxygen Content)

Deficiency of oxygen in the atmosphere
Hypoventilation
Uneven distribution of alveolar gas and/or pulmonary blood flow
Diffusion impairment
Venous-to-arterial shunt

Deficient Hemoglobin (Normal P_{O_2} and Low Oxygen Content)

Anemia
Carbon monoxide poisoning

Ischemic Hypoxia (Normal P_{O_2} and Normal Oxygen Content)

General or localized circulatory insufficiency
Tissue edema
Abnormal tissue demands

Histotoxic Anoxia (Normal P_{O_2} and Normal Oxygen Content)

Poisoning of cellular enzymes so that they cannot use the available oxygen (e.g., cyanide poisoning)

---

oxygen tensions do not increase above 50 to 60 mm Hg because of oxygen consumption and the shape of the dissociation curve. With air breathing, arterial and venous nitrogen tensions are the same, about 570 mm Hg. If the loculated gas were air at atmospheric pressure, the gradient for the movement of nitrogen to the blood would be very small. After nitrogen washout, with oxygen breathing, the lack of high elevation in venous oxygen tension permits movement of both nitrogen and oxygen from the pneumothorax into the blood. The increased pressure differences increase the rate of absorption of loculated air some 5- to 10-fold. This augmented clearance occurs while the extrapulmonary gas is predominately nitrogen.

ADMINISTRATION OF OXYGEN

There are several methods of delivering enriched oxygen gas mixtures to nonintubated patients. Known concentrations of oxygen can be piped into chambers that surround the infant's head, such as an oxygen tent or a head box. Usually, these chambers allow significant leakage of gases, so it is imperative that the O_2 concentration be measured inside the chamber near the patient's face. Another method is to run pure oxygen through nasal prongs or cannulae at specified flow rates. Although this method can be efficacious in improving the Pa_{O_2}, one must remember that it does not provide a constant FI_{O_2} during the breath, nor can the FI_{O_2} be accurately calculated or measured. The reason is that patients will "beat the system," because their inspiratory flow rates exceed the rate at which the pure oxygen is being piped toward their faces. A simple calculation illustrates the point. If a 70-kg man breathes at 30 breaths/min with an inspiratory/expiratory time ratio of 1 : 1, his duration of inspiration will be 1 second. Given a tidal volume of 0.5 L, his average inspiratory flow rate will be 0.5 L/sec or 30 L/min. Given that nasal prongs are usually set at 2 to 6 L/min for the average 70-kg man, it is immediately obvious that his initial portion of inspiration will be 100% oxygen but that the percentage will decrease quickly toward that of room air by the end of inspiration. This pattern is applicable not only to adults but also to younger children. Recently, some intensive care units have been administering very high oxygen flow rates via nasal cannulae to infants and young children; this not only increases the inspired oxygen concentration, but also increases the mean airway pressure.

Thus, although one can "guesstimate" what flow rate of oxygen the patient will require to normalize the blood oxygen tension, the actual FI_{O_2} will vary within and between breaths, especially if the patient changes the depth or pattern of breathing. In practice today in hospitalized children, oxygen flow rate is titrated by measurement of pulse oximetry.

HAZARDS OF HIGH OXYGEN MIXTURES

Hypoxemia in conditions associated with alveolar hypoventilation, such as chronic pulmonary disease and status asthmaticus, may be overcome by enriched oxygen mixtures without concomitant lessening of the hypercapnia. The patient may appear pink but become narcotized under the influence of carbon dioxide retention. In chronic respiratory acidosis, respiration may be maintained chiefly by the hypoxic drive. This is a condition that is rarely seen in pediatric patients but may occur in the terminally ill patient with cystic fibrosis.

With the institution of oxygen therapy, there is usually a small drop in minute ventilation as the hypoxic stimulus to breath is removed by the increase in Pa_{O_2}. Very rarely, a patient with chronic hypercarbic respiratory failure may cease breathing if excessive oxygen is given. It is therefore essential to measure the pH and Pa_{CO_2} in addition to the Pa_{O_2} or saturation in these groups of patients. The goal of oxygen therapy is to give just enough oxygen to return the arterial oxygen saturation to the appropriate amount for the patient. The usual target is 90% in the infant, child, and adult. However, the target saturation may be less in the premature infant who is susceptible to retinopathy of prematurity or higher when there is significant pulmonary hypertension. When there is increased intracranial pressure, the clinician should utilize arterial blood samples to maintain the Pa_{O_2} well above 100 mm Hg to ensure full saturation of Hb and to further increase the oxygen content of blood by augmenting the amount of dissolved oxygen.

Excessive oxygenation of the blood can be dangerous. Human volunteers in pure oxygen at 1 atmosphere experience symptoms in about 24 hours, chiefly substernal pain, and paresthesias. Laboratory animals exposed for longer periods die of pulmonary congestion and edema in 4 to 7 days. The toxicity of oxygen is directly proportional to its partial pressure. Symptoms occur within minutes under hyperbaric conditions and yet are not present after 1 month in pure oxygen at 1/3 atmosphere. Some of the acute effects of oxygen are a slight decrease of minute ventilation and cardiac output and constriction of retinal and cerebral vessels and the ductus arteriosus. Retinal vasoconstriction does not seem to be a significant problem in mature retinas that are fully vascularized. In premature infants, however, the vasoconstriction may lead to ischemia. After the cessation of oxygen therapy, or with maturation of the infant, neovascularization of the retina occurs. The disorderly growth and scarring may cause retinal detachments and fibroplasia, which appears behind the lens; hence, the names retrolental fibroplasia and retinopathy of prematurity.

As the care of premature infants with acute lung disease has improved, the survival rate has increased impressively. Regrettably, many of the survivors have chronic lung disease of prematurity or bronchopulmonary dysplasia (see Chapter 20). At the present time, it is difficult to determine the relative contributions of prematurity, ventilator-induced barotrauma, oxygen toxicity, and the preceding acute lung injury in the evolution of this serious disorder. It does seem prudent, however, to minimize the FIO_2 in these patients, given the damage that occurs in totally normal lungs exposed to very high concentrations of oxygen.

Carbon Dioxide Transport and Acid-Base Balance

BUFFERING AND TRANSPORT

Acids are normally produced in the body at the rates of 15 to 20 moles of carbonic acid and 80 mmol of fixed acids per day. For the cells to maintain their normal metabolic activity, the pH of the environment of the cells must be close to 7.40. The understanding of the regulation of hydrogen ion concentration requires knowledge of the buffering action of the chemical constituents of the blood and of the role of the lungs and kidneys in the excretion of acids from the body.

The most important constituents for acid-base regulation are the sodium bicarbonate and carbonic acid of the plasma, the potassium bicarbonate and carbonic acid of the cells, and Hb.

The concentration of carbonic acid is determined by the PCO_2 and the solubility coefficients of carbon dioxide in plasma and in red blood cell water. Carbonic acid in aqueous solution dissociates as follows:

$$CO_2 + H_2O \leftrightarrow H_2CO_3$$

$$H_2CO_3 \leftrightarrow H + HCO_3^-$$

The law of mass action describes this reaction:

$$\frac{[H^+][HCO_3^-]}{[H_2CO_3]} = K$$

In plasma, K has the value of $10^{-6.1}$. An equivalent form of this equation is

$$pH = pK + \log \frac{[HCO_3^-]}{H_2CO_3}$$

By definition,

$$pH = -\log[H^+]; pK = -\log K = 6.1 \text{ for plasma.}$$

Applied to plasma, in which dissolved carbon dioxide exists at a concentration 1000 times that of carbonic acid, the equation becomes

$$pH = 6.1 + \log \frac{[HCO_3^-]}{0.03\, PCO_2}$$

This form of the equation is known as the Henderson-Hasselbalch equation. A clinically useful form of this equation is as follows:

$$H^+(nmol/L) = 24 \times \frac{PCO_2}{HCO_3^-}$$

Thus, at a normal bicarbonate concentration of 24 mEq/L, when PaO_2 is 40 mm Hg, hydrogen ion concentration is 40 nM.

Just as oxygen has a highly specialized transport mechanism in the blood to ensure adequate delivery to tissues under physiologic conditions, carbon dioxide produced by the tissues has a special transport system to carry it in the blood to the lung where it is expired. The amount of carbon dioxide in blood is related to the PCO_2 in a manner shown in Fig. 6.27. Unlike the relation of oxygen content to PO_2, the relation of carbon dioxide content to PCO_2 is nearly linear; therefore, doubling alveolar ventilation halves $PaCO_2$. Oxygenated Hb shifts the carbon dioxide dissociation curve to the right (Haldane effect) so that there is a lower carbon dioxide content at a given PCO_2. This effect aids in the removal of carbon dioxide from the blood in the lung when venous blood becomes oxygenated. The average arterial carbon dioxide tension ($PaCO_2$) in adults is 40 mm Hg and in infants is closer to 35 mm Hg; venous levels in both are normally 6 mm Hg higher. The small difference between arterial and venous PCO_2 is why the effect of venous admixture on arterial PCO_2 is very small.

Carbon dioxide is transported in the blood in three ways: dissolved in the blood, as bicarbonate, and as carbamino compound. At the tissue level, the processes involved in the uptake of carbon dioxide into the blood are as follows (Fig. 6.28):

1. Carbon dioxide diffuses into the blood from the tissue. Some carbon dioxide is dissolved in the plasma water in physical solution.
2. Carbon dioxide hydrates slowly in the plasma to form a small amount of carbonic acid.
3. Most of the carbon dioxide enters the red blood cells. A small amount is dissolved in the intracellular water. A fraction combines with Hb to form a carbamino compound.
4. Because of the presence of carbonic anhydrase, a larger fraction in the red blood cell hydrates rapidly to form carbonic acid, which dissociates into H^+ plus HCO_3^-.
5. Bicarbonate diffuses into plasma because of the concentration gradient, and Cl^- ions enter the cell to restore electrical neutrality.

Hemoglobin is important in the transport of carbon dioxide because of two properties of the molecule. First, it is a good buffer, permitting blood to take up carbon dioxide with only a small change in pH. Second, Hb is a stronger acid when oxygenated than when reduced; thus, when oxyhemoglobin is reduced, more cations are available to neutralize HCO_3^-. Carbon dioxide exists in two forms in the red blood cell because of this property of Hb: as bicarbonate ion and as hemoglobin carbamate ($HbNHCOO^-$).

$$KHbO_2 + H_2CO_3 \leftrightarrow HHb + O_2 \uparrow + KHCO_3$$

$$KHbO_2NH_2 + CO_2 \leftrightarrow HHb\dot{c}\, NHCOOK + O_2 \uparrow$$

CARBON DIOXIDE DISSOCIATION CURVES FOR WHOLE BLOOD

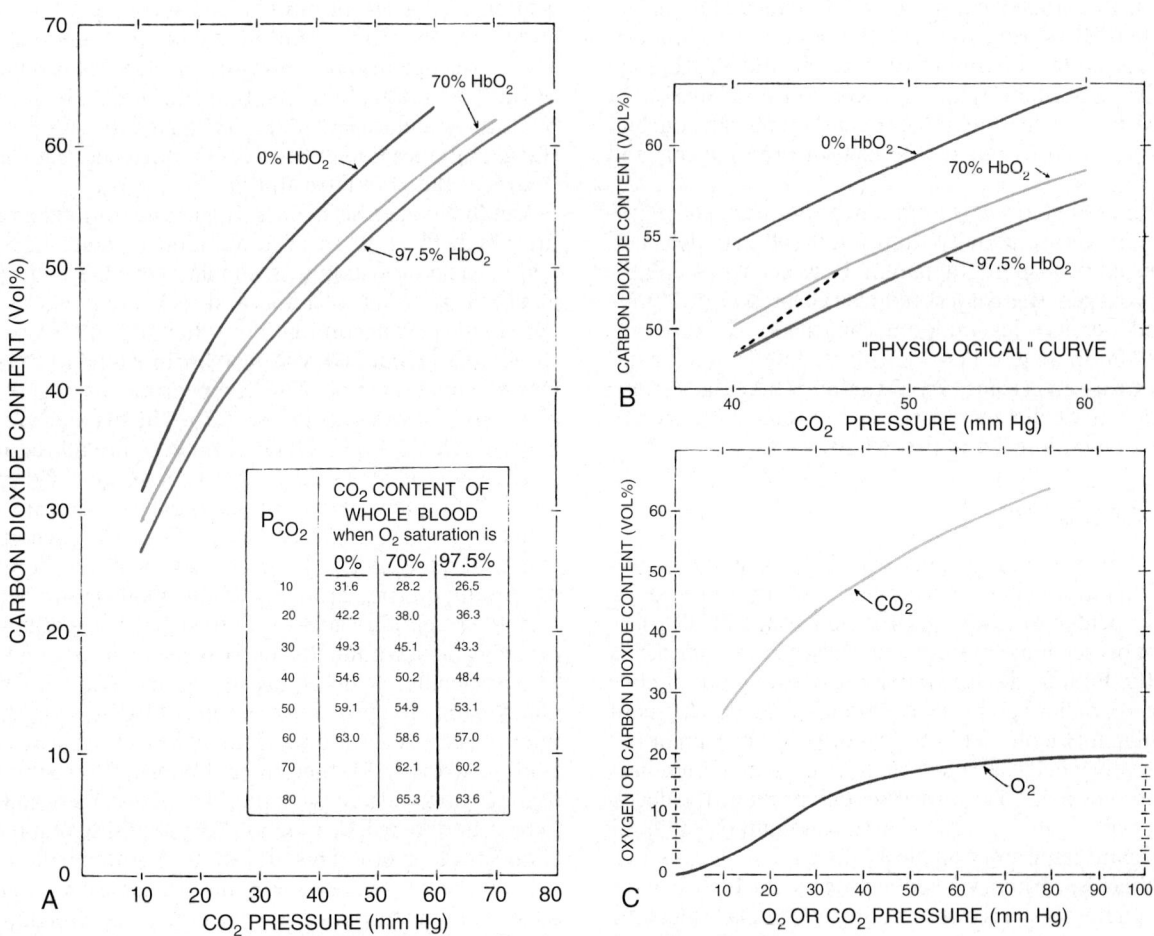

P_{CO_2}	CO₂ CONTENT OF WHOLE BLOOD when O₂ saturation is		
	0%	70%	97.5%
10	31.6	28.2	26.5
20	42.2	38.0	36.3
30	49.3	45.1	43.3
40	54.6	50.2	48.4
50	59.1	54.9	53.1
60	63.0	58.6	57.0
70		62.1	60.2
80		65.3	63.6

Fig. 6.27 Carbon dioxide dissociation curve. The large graph (A) shows the relationship between P_{CO_2} and carbon dioxide content of whole blood; this relationship varies with changes in saturation of hemoglobin with oxygen. Thus, P_{CO_2} of the blood influences oxygen saturation (Bohr effect), and oxygen saturation of the blood influences carbon dioxide content (Haldane effect). The oxygen–carbon dioxide diagram gives the correct figure for both carbon dioxide and oxygen at every P_{O_2} and P_{CO_2}. (B) Greatly magnified portion of the large graph to show the change that occurs as mixed venous blood (70% oxyhemoglobin, P_{CO_2} 40 mm Hg). *Dashed line* is a hypothetical transition between the two curves. (C) Oxygen and carbon dioxide dissociation curves plotted on same scale to show the important point that the oxygen curve has a steep and a flat portion and that the carbon dioxide curve does not. (From Comroe Jr JH. *The Lung*, 2nd ed. Chicago: Year Book Medical; 1963.)

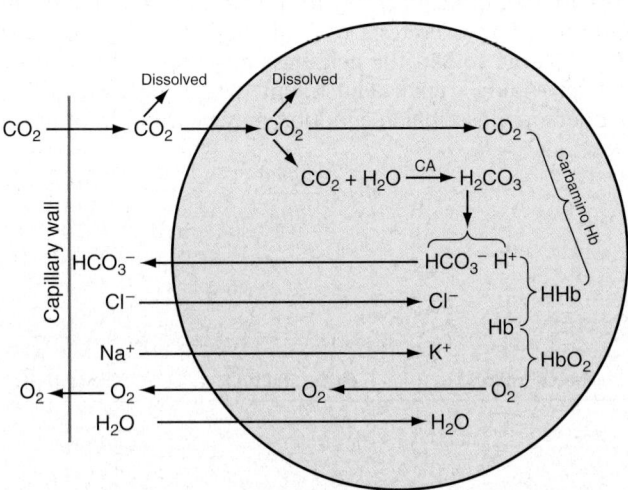

Fig. 6.28 CO₂ transport in blood. (See text for further explanation.)

An enzyme in the red blood cell, carbonic anhydrase, accelerates the reaction $CO_2 + H_2O \leftrightarrow H^+ + HCO_3^-$ some 13,000 times. A concentration gradient between red cell and plasma causes the bicarbonate ion to leave the red cell. Because the red blood cell membrane is relatively impermeable to Na^+ and K^+, the chloride ion and water move into the red cell to restore electrical neutrality (chloride shift or Hamburger shift). Thus, although the larger portion of the buffering occurs within the red cell, the largest amount of carbon dioxide is in the plasma as HCO_3^- (Table 6.4). The shift of chloride and HCO_3^- was previously thought to be passive, that is, to occur by diffusion due to a concentration gradient. It is now known to be an active process dependent on a specific transport protein within the red blood cell membrane. This anion transport occurs rapidly with a half-time of 50 msec.

In the lung, a process the reverse of that just described takes place, because carbon dioxide diffuses out of the blood and into the alveoli. Diffusion of CO_2 is rapid, so the equilibrium between the P_{CO_2} of the pulmonary capillary and that of alveolar air is promptly achieved. About 30% of the CO_2 that is exchanged is given up from hemoglobin carbamate. When Hb is oxygenated in the pulmonary capillary, chloride and water shift out of the red cell, and bicarbonate diffuses in to combine with hydrogen ion to form H_2CO_3, which in turn is dehydrated to form carbon dioxide. Carbon dioxide then diffuses out of the cell into the plasma and alveolar gas.

Although red blood cells from newborn infants have less carbonic anhydrase activity than adult cells, no defect in carbon dioxide transport is apparent. However, when breathing 100% oxygen, there is less reduced Hb present in venous blood, and therefore, less buffering capacity for H^+ is present, leading to an increased P_{CO_2}. This is an important consideration during hyperbaric oxygenation when the venous blood may remain almost completely saturated with oxygen, H^+ is less well buffered, and tissue P_{CO_2} rises.

ACID-BASE BALANCE

To understand acid-base balance within the body, it is important to differentiate between the processes that promote a change in acid–base state and the end result of all these primary and secondary processes. *Acidemia* and *alkalemia* refer to the final acid-base status within the blood (hence the suffix *-emia*). Two processes can promote the development of acidemia: metabolic acidosis (loss of HCO_3^- or gain of H^+) and respiratory acidosis (increase in P_{CO_2}, which increases H^+ via carbonic acid). Two processes can promote the development of alkalemia: metabolic alkalosis (gain of HCO_3^- or loss of H^+) and respiratory alkalosis (decrease in P_{CO_2}). Obviously, if there is a primary acidotic process, the body will try to maintain homeostasis by promoting a secondary alkalotic

process and vice versa. Therefore, to understand the patient's acid-base balance, one must first measure the pH of the blood, and if it is abnormal, determine what primary and secondary (compensatory) processes are involved. This is illustrated in Table 6.5; note, however, that the HCO_3^- shown in Table 6.5 is the standard HCO_3^- (i.e., corrected to a P_{CO_2} of 40 mm Hg; see later section entitled "Difference between Additions of CO_2 to Blood *In Vitro* and *In Vivo*").

Metabolic acidosis occurs in such conditions as diabetes (in which there is an accumulation of keto acids); renal failure, when the kidney is unable to excrete hydrogen ion; diarrhea from loss of base; and tissue hypoxia associated with lactic acid accumulation. When pH falls, respiration is stimulated so that P_{CO_2} will decrease and tend to compensate for the reduction in pH. This compensation is usually incomplete, and pH remains below 7.35. The pH, carbon dioxide content (HCO_3^- P_{CO_2}), HCO_3^-, and P_{CO_2} are all reduced.

Metabolic alkalosis occurs most commonly after excessive loss of HCl due to vomiting (as in pyloric stenosis) or after an excessive citrate or bicarbonate load. The carbon dioxide content is elevated, and the P_{CO_2} will be normal or elevated depending on the chronicity of the alkalosis.

Acute respiratory acidosis is secondary to respiratory insufficiency and accumulation of carbon dioxide within the body. The associated acidosis may be compensated for by renal adjustments that promote retention of HCO_3^-. Compensation may require several days. Patients in chronic respiratory acidosis who receive therapy that improves alveolar ventilation will have a decrease in their Pa_{CO_2}, but their adjustment in bicarbonate will be much slower, resulting in a metabolic alkalosis of several days' duration. A simple rule is that if hypercarbic respiratory failure has occurred over many days, such that compensation has occurred, the clinician should slowly normalize the Pa_{CO_2} to avoid excessive metabolic alkalosis.

Acute respiratory alkalosis (e.g., secondary to fever, psychogenic hyperventilation, or a pontine lesion with meningoencephalitis) is associated with high pH, low P_{CO_2}, and normal bicarbonate level. Renal compensation in time leads to excretion of bicarbonate and return of pH toward normal.

It is important to point out that the lung excretes some 300 mEq/kg of acid per day in the form of carbon dioxide, and the kidney excretes 1 to 2 mEq/kg/day. Thus, the lung plays a large role in the acid-base balance of the body, in fact providing rapid adjustment when necessary. The Henderson-Hasselbalch equation may be thought of as

$$pH \alpha \frac{kidney}{lung}$$

Table 6.4   Carbon Dioxide in the Blood

	ARTERIAL BLOOD		VENOUS BLOOD	
	M M/L BL	**%**	**M M/L BL**	**%**
Total	21.9		24.1	
Plasma dissolved CO_2	0.66	3	0.76	3
HCO_3^-	14.00	64	15.00	63
Cells dissolved CO_2	0.44	2	0.54	2
HCO_3^-	5.7	26	6.1	25
$HbNHCOO^-$	1.2	5	1.8	7

Note: Table gives normal values of various chemical forms of CO_2 in blood with an assumed hematocrit level of 46. Approximately twice as much CO_2 exists in the plasma as in the red blood cells, chiefly as HCO_3^-.

Table 6.5   Blood Measurements in Various Acid-Base Disturbances

	Standard CO_2 (mm Hg)	$PaCO_2$ (mEq/L)	HCO_3^- (mEq/L)	Content pH
Metabolic acidosis	↓	↓	↓	↓
Acute respiratory acidosis	↓	↑	↔	Slight≠
Compensated respiratory acidosis	(↔ or slight ↓)	≠↑	↑≠	↑≠
Metabolic alkalosis	↑≠	Slight↑ ≠	≠↑	↑≠
Acute respiratory alkalosis	≠↑↑	↓	↔	Slight ↓
Compensated respiratory alkalosis	(↔ or slight ↑≠)	↓	↓	↓
Normal values pHα kidney lung	7.35–7.45	35–45	24–26	25–28

DIFFERENCE BETWEEN ADDITIONS OF CO_2 TO BLOOD *IN VITRO* AND *IN VIVO*

An appreciation of the difference between the so-called *in vitro* and *in vivo* CO_2 dissociation curves is necessary to clarify the confusion that has arisen regarding the interpretation of measurements of acid-base balance, particularly during acute respiratory acidosis (acute hypoventilation). When blood *in vitro* is equilibrated with increasing concentrations of CO_2, bicarbonate concentration also increases because of the hydration of carbon dioxide. If, for example, blood with a Pco_2 of 40 mm Hg and a bicarbonate concentration of 24 mEq/L was equilibrated with a Pco_2 of 100 mm Hg, the actual bicarbonate concentration would be measured as 34 mEq/L. In the Astrup nomogram, a correction for this increased bicarbonate due to CO_2 alone is made, and the standard bicarbonate (bicarbonate concentration at Pco_2 of 40 mm Hg) is considered to be 24 mEq/L or a base excess of zero. With this correction, one can readily see that the metabolic (renal) component of acid-base balance is normal. However, confusion has arisen because the *in vitro* correction figures have been incorrectly applied to the situation *in vivo.* Unlike equilibration in the test tube, the additional bicarbonate generated during *in vivo* acute hypercapnia not only is distributed to water in red blood cells and plasma but also equilibrates with the interstitial fluid space; that is, bicarbonate ion equilibrates with extracellular water. If the interstitial fluid represents 70% of extracellular water, then 70% of the additional bicarbonate generated will be distributed to the interstitial fluid. Thus, an arterial sample taken from a patient with an acute elevation of Pco_2 to 100 mm Hg would have an actual bicarbonate concentration of 27 mEq/L. If 10 mEq/L were subtracted according to the *in vitro* correction, the standard bicarbonate would be reported as 17 mEq/L or a base excess of −7, which would indicate the presence of metabolic as well as respiratory acidosis. This conclusion would be incorrect; actually, the bicarbonate concentration *in vivo* is appropriate for the Pco_2. The situation is worse in the newborn infant because of the high hematocrit and large interstitial fluid space. Base excess values of as much as −10 mEq/L (standard bicarbonate 14 mEq/L) may be calculated despite the fact that the *in vivo* bicarbonate concentration is appropriate for the particular Pco_2 and there is no metabolic component to the acidosis. Thus, the appropriate therapy is to increase alveolar ventilation and not to administer bicarbonate.

Tissue Respiration

AEROBIC METABOLISM

The ultimate function of the lung is to provide oxygen to meet the demands of the tissues and to excrete carbon dioxide, a by-product of metabolic activity. Thus, respiratory physiologists have been concerned with the assessment of respiration at the tissue level and the ability of the cardiopulmonary system to meet the metabolic demands of the body.

One method is to measure the amount of oxygen consumed by the body per minute ($\dot{V}o_2$). This is equal to the amount necessary to maintain the life of the cells at rest, plus the amount necessary for oxidative combustion required to maintain a normal body temperature, as well as the amount used for the metabolic demands of work above the resting level. The basal metabolic rate is a summation of many component energy rates of individual organs and tissues and is defined as the amount of energy necessary to maintain the life of the cells at rest under conditions in which there is no additional energy expenditure for temperature regulation or additional work.

In practice, $\dot{V}o_2$ is measured after an overnight fast, the subject lying supine in a room at a comfortable temperature. This "basal" metabolic rate has a wide variability ($\pm 15\%$ of predicted $\dot{V}o_2$). Since absolutely basal conditions are difficult to ensure, the measurement of basal metabolic rate is not widely used at present.

The performance of the cardiopulmonary system can be more adequately assessed and compared with normal measurements under conditions of added work, such as exercise. During exercise, healthy subjects demonstrate an improvement in pulmonary gas exchange, cardiac output, and tissue oxygen extraction. Performance can be increased by physical fitness, and athletes are able to increase their cardiac output by sixfold or sevenfold. In children, the relationship between work capacity, ventilation, and oxygen consumption is the same as that in the adult. The maximal $\dot{V}o_2$ that can be achieved increases throughout childhood, reaches its peak of 50 to 60 mL/min/kg between 10 and 15 years of age, and thereafter declines slowly with age. Different individuals are endowed with different maximal $\dot{V}o_2$ and, although bed rest will significantly decrease $\dot{V}o_2$, even vigorous training only minimally increases an individual's inherent $\dot{V}o_2$.[67]

At the tissue level, the ability of a given cell to receive an adequate oxygen supply depends on the amount of local blood flow, the distance of the cell from the perfusing capillary, and the difference between the partial pressures of oxygen in the capillary and in the cell. The critical mean capillary Po_2 appears to be in the region of 30 mm Hg for children and adults. Exercising muscle has 10–20 times the number of open capillaries as resting muscle does.

The body's response to exercise therefore is complex and depends on the amount of work, the rate at which the workload is increased, and the subject's state of health and degree of physical fitness. A detailed description of the physiologic response to exercise and its use in diagnosing cardiorespiratory disease is beyond the scope of this chapter, but exercise testing is now an important tool in clinical medicine (see Chapter 12).

ANAEROBIC METABOLISM

The adequacy of oxygen supply to the tissues has been assessed by measuring blood lactate, a product of anaerobic metabolism (Embden-Meyerhof pathway). When there is an insufficient oxygen supply to the tissues due to either insufficient blood flow or a decrease in blood oxygen content, lactic acid concentration within the tissues and blood increases. In the blood, this accumulation leads to metabolic acidosis.

During moderate to heavy muscular exercise, cardiac output cannot meet the demands of the muscles, and an oxygen debt is incurred, which is repaid on cessation of exercise. During this period, lactic acid accumulates, and therefore rigorous exercise is often associated with metabolic acidosis.

There is an excellent correlation between the serum lactate level and the oxygen debt. Oxygen debt is not measurable at rest and is difficult to measure during exercise, but the adequacy of tissue oxygenation appears to be accurately reflected in the serum lactate level. In adult humans, blood lactate is less than 1 mEq/L but may increase to 10 to 12 mEq/L during very heavy exercise.

RELATIONSHIP BETWEEN $\dot{V}O_2$ AND $\dot{V}CO_2$

In the normal subject in a steady state, the amount of carbon dioxide excreted by the lung per minute depends on the basal metabolic activity of the cells and the type of substrate being oxidized. The volume of carbon dioxide exhaled divided by the amount of oxygen consumed is known as the respiratory exchange ratio (R). For the body as a whole, the ratio is 1 if primarily carbohydrate is being metabolized, 0.7 if fat, and 0.8 if protein. Normally, the ratio is 0.8 at rest, approximately 1.0 during exercise, and greater than 1 at exhaustion when there is anaerobic metabolism. The respiratory exchange ratio may vary considerably with changes in alveolar ventilation and metabolism and therefore must be measured in the steady state (i.e., with a steady alveolar ventilation and a steady metabolic rate). For an individual organ, the metabolic respiratory quotient ($\dot{R}\dot{Q}$) is nearly constant but may vary from 0.4 to 1.5, depending on the balance of anabolism and catabolism in that organ. Thus, the measurement of R represents the result of many component-metabolizing organs and tissues. After birth, R decreases from nearly 1 to 0.7, indicating a loss of carbohydrate stores; when feeding has started, R approaches 0.8.

With breath-by-breath CO_2 and O_2 concentrations, R can be calculated on a breath-by-breath basis. Using this technique, it is possible to define more precisely the workload at which anaerobic metabolism begins (threshold for anaerobic metabolism). As lactic acid begins to accumulate in the blood, the carbon dioxide dissociation curve shifts to the right, and there is a sudden increase in expired CO_2. R therefore suddenly increases from about 1.0 to above 1.0. It has been shown that the threshold for anaerobic metabolism in both adults and children can be increased by training. This technique is particularly useful in children, because it does not require blood sampling and can be readily applied to cooperative subjects with a variety of pulmonary and cardiac problems.

Regulation of Respiration

The regulation of respiratory rhythm[68] and its control have been extensively studied over the past decades including its abnormalities in diseases such as congenital hypoventilation syndrome[69] caused by Phox2b mutations, sudden infant death syndrome,[70] and sleep disorders.[71,72] A brief discussion is provided later in the chapter, but further details are available in the references cited[70–72] and in Chapters 80 and 81.

The study of the regulation of respiration centers around three main ideas: (1) the generation and maintenance of a respiratory rhythm, (2) the modulation of this rhythm by a number of sensory feedback loops and reflexes, and (3) the recruitment of respiratory muscles that can contract appropriately for gas exchange (Fig. 6.29).

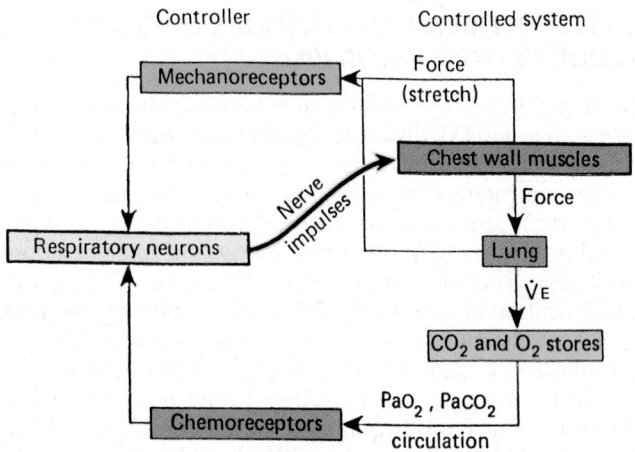

Fig. 6.29 Schematic diagram of the respiratory control system. (From Fishman AP. *Pulmonary Diseases and Disorders*. New York: McGraw-Hill; 1980.)

The central nervous system, particularly the brainstem, has the inherent ability to function as the respiratory "sinus node," or the source of central pattern generation. The pacemaker neurons are located within the brainstem's preBötzinger Complex (preBötC) and are the main source of inspiratory rhythm. Each part of the respiratory cycle is controlled by distinct groups of neurons that interact dynamically with some stimulating, some inhibiting, and others having their effect dependent upon the phase of the respiratory cycle. The overall control of respiratory rhythm is influenced by many factors, including cortical behavioral influences; sleep state; peripheral and central chemoreceptors; and receptors within the lungs, joints, and muscles.

Sensory Feedback System

The respiratory system is endowed with a wealth of afferent pathways to maintain control over several functional variables and adjust them at appropriate times. These pathways inform the central pattern generator about instantaneous changes that take place in, for example, the lungs, the respiratory musculature, the blood (acid-base), and the environment. The terms *sensory* and *afferent* refer not only to peripheral but also to central systems converging on the brainstem respiratory neurons.

Cutaneous or mucocutaneous stimulation of the area innervated by the trigeminal nerve (e.g., the face, nasal mucosa) decreases respiratory frequency and may lead to the generation of respiratory pauses. These respiratory effects become less important with age, their strengths are species-specific, and they depend on the state of consciousness. Because cortical inhibition of the trigeminal afferent impulses is more pronounced during REM sleep, trigeminal stimulation has a greater effect on respiration during quiet (non-REM) sleep.

The laryngeal receptor reflex is probably the most inhibitory reflex on respiration known. Sensory receptors are present in the epithelium of the epiglottis and upper larynx. Introduction into the larynx of small amounts of water or solutions with low concentrations of chloride will result in apnea. The duration and severity of the respiratory changes depend on the behavioral state and are exacerbated by the presence of anesthesia. They are also worse if the subject is anemic, hypoglycemic, or a premature infant. In the unanesthetized subject, the reflex effects are almost purely respiratory and are mediated by the superior laryngeal nerve, which joins the vagal trunk after the nodose ganglion.

Rapidly adapting, slowly adapting, and J receptors (vagal) are present in the tracheobronchial tree and lung interstitial space and were described earlier in this chapter. These play an important role in informing the central nervous system about the status of lung volume, tension across airways, and lung interstitial pressure. Stretch receptors, when stimulated by lung inflation, prolong expiratory duration and delay the start of the next inspiration. J receptors are stimulated by lung edema, and they produce tachypnea with interspersed short periods of respiratory pauses.

O_2 AND CO_2

The respiratory control system also receives information about O_2 and CO_2 tensions from sensory receptors located in specialized neural structures in blood vessels, airways, and the central nervous system.

Central chemoreceptors are located in the ventral lateral medulla, and increases in PCO_2 or H^+ concentration produce an increase in ventilation; conversely, a decrease in PCO_2 or H^+ concentration causes a depression of ventilation. This area is influenced primarily by the acid-base composition of cerebral spinal fluid (CSF), and the delay in ventilatory response to changes in arterial PCO_2 and bicarbonate is due to the time required to change the CSF H^+ concentration. Carbon dioxide, which diffuses into the CSF in a few minutes, has a rapid effect on the central chemoreceptors. Changes in blood bicarbonate are much less rapidly reflected in the CSF (24 to 48 hours). Thus, with acute metabolic acidosis, arterial PCO_2 decreases along with CSF PCO_2. Hyperventilation is produced by the H^+ stimulation of peripheral chemoreceptors, but this stimulus is inadequate to compensate fully for the metabolic acidosis because of inhibition from the decreased H^+ concentration in the CSF. After 24 hours, CSF bicarbonate decreases and restores CSF pH to normal. There is a further decrease in arterial PCO_2, and arterial pH returns toward normal. From these observations, it has been suggested that the control of alveolar ventilation is a function of the central chemoreceptors, which are under the influence of CSF or brain interstitial fluid H^+, acting in association with the peripheral chemoreceptors, which are directly under the influence of the arterial blood.

The peripheral chemoreceptors are found in the human along the structures associated with the branchial arches. Two sets of chemoreceptors appear to be of greatest physiologic importance: (1) the carotid bodies, which are located at the division of the common carotid artery into its internal and external branches, and (2) the aortic bodies, which lie between the ascending aorta and the pulmonary artery. Afferent nerves from the carotid body join the glossopharyngeal (IX) nerve; those from the aortic bodies join the vagosympathetic trunk along with the recurrent laryngeal nerves.

The carotid and aortic bodies are responsive primarily to changes in the PO_2. At rest, they are tonically active, signifying that some ventilatory drive exists even at a PaO_2 of 100 mm Hg. Inhalation of low oxygen mixtures is associated with a significant increase in ventilation when the PaO_2 is less than 60 mm Hg. Potentiation of the hypoxic stimulus is achieved by an increase in $PaCO_2$. The response of the peripheral chemoreceptors to PCO_2 is rapid (within seconds), and ventilation increases monotonically with $PaCO_2$. The rate of the change in $PaCO_2$ may be as important as the change. The peripheral chemoreceptors, also responsive to changes in arterial pH, increase ventilation in association with a decrease of 0.1 pH unit and produce a twofold to threefold increase with a decrease of 0.4 pH unit. A variety of peripheral reflexes are known to influence respiration. Hyperpnea may be produced by stimulation of pain and temperature receptors or mechanoreceptors in limbs. Visceral reflexes (e.g., those that result from distention of gallbladder or traction on the gut) are usually associated with apnea. Afferent impulses from respiratory muscles (e.g., intercostals) may play a role in determining the optimum response of the muscles of ventilation to various respiratory stimuli. In newborn infants, an inspiratory gasp may be elicited by distention of the upper airways. This reflex is mediated by the vagus nerve and is known as the *Head reflex*. It has been suggested that this inspiratory gasp reflex is important in the initial inflation of the lungs at birth.

THE NEWBORN INFANT

A number of studies have demonstrated that the responsiveness to stimuli in newborn infants is different from that of older or mature adult subjects. Although the exact mechanisms for these differences have generally been elusive, the rapid maturational changes that occur in key control systems could serve as the bases for the different responses seen in early life. Similar to adults, infants increase ventilation in response to inspired carbon dioxide, and peripheral chemoreceptors are functional in newborn infants, as demonstrated by a slight decrease in $\dot{V}E$ with 100% oxygen breathing. The effect of hypoxia as a stimulant may differ in the first 12 hours of life; 12% oxygen in the first 12 hours of life fails to stimulate ventilation. In addition, it has been found that the newborn infant will increase ventilation only transiently in response to a hypoxic stimulus; ventilation rapidly falls below baseline. In adults, the increase in ventilation is maintained above basal levels, although it lessens with time.

The mechanisms responsible for this different response to hypoxia in the newborn are not well understood. The biphasic hypoxic response is likely multifactorial and may be due to one or more of the following: (1) reduction in dynamic lung compliance, (2) reduction in chemoreceptor activity during sustained (>1 to 2 min) hypoxia, (3) central neuronal depression due to either an actual drop in excitatory synaptic drive other than carotid input or changes in neuronal membrane properties reducing excitability, and (4) decrease in metabolic rate.

Metabolic Functions of the Lung

The lungs have important nonrespiratory functions, including phagocytosis by alveolar macrophages, filtering of microemboli from blood, biosynthesis of surfactant components, and excretion of volatile substances. An equally important

Table 6.6 Handling of Biologically Active Compounds by the Lung

Metabolized at the endothelial surface without uptake	Bradykinin Angiotensin I Adenine nucleotides
Metabolized by the endothelial cell after uptake	Serotonin Norepinephrine Prostaglandins E and F
Unaffected by passage through the lung	Epinephrine Dopamine Angiotensin II Vasopressin
Released by the lung	Prostaglandins (e.g., prostacyclin) Histamine Kallikrein

nonrespiratory function is the pharmacokinetic function of the pulmonary vascular bed: the release, degradation, and activation of vasoactive substances. The lung is ideally situated for regulating the circulating concentrations of vasoactive substances, because it receives the entire cardiac output and possesses an enormous vascular surface area. As Table 6.6 illustrates, the pulmonary vascular bed not only handles a wide variety of compounds (amines, peptides, lipids), but it also is highly selective in its metabolic activity. For example, norepinephrine is metabolized by the lung, whereas epinephrine, which differs from it only by a methyl group, is unaffected by passage through the pulmonary circulation.

The physiologic consequences of the metabolic functions of the lung can be illustrated by angiotensin-converting enzyme (ACE). A peptidase located on the surface of the endothelial cell, ACE is responsible for the degradation of bradykinin, a potent vasodilator and edematogenic peptide, and for the conversion of angiotensin I to angiotensin II, a potent vasoconstrictor. Angiotensin II production influences systemic blood pressure at all ages but is especially important during the neonatal period, because sympathetic innervation is incompletely developed.

ACKNOWLEDGMENTS

In the previous seven editions of this chapter, the authors have included Mary Ellen Avery, Victor Chernick, Hugh O'Brodovich, Gabriel Haddad, and John West. This chapter has incorporated some information from the late Dr. Mary Ellen Wohl's chapter on Developmental Physiology of the Lung, which appeared in previous editions.

References

Access the reference list online at ExpertConsult.com.

Suggested Reading

Normal Lung Anatomy and Cell Function

Crapo JD, Barry BE, Gehr P, et al. Cell number and cell characteristics of the normal human lung. *Am Rev Respir Dis.* 1982;125:332–337.

Crystal RG, West JB, Weibel ER, et al. *The Lung: Scientific Foundations.* 2nd ed. New York: Lippincott-Raven; 1997.

Gehr P, Bachofen M, Weibel ER. The normal lung: ultrastructure and morphometric estimation of diffusion capacity. *Respir Physiol.* 1978;32:121–140.

Hsia CC, Hyde DM, Weibel ER. Lung structure and the intrinsic challenges of gas exchange. *Comp Physiol.* 2016;6:827–895.

Ochs M, Nyengaard JR, Jung A, et al. The number of alveoli in the human lung. *Am J Respir Crit Care Med.* 2004;169:120–124.

Parent RA. *Comparative Biology of the Normal Lung.* Boca Raton: CRC Press; 1992.

Weibel ER. *The Pathway for Oxygen.* Cambridge: Harvard University Press; 1984.

Weibel ER. Lung cell biology. In: Fishman AP, Macklem PT, Mead J, eds. *The Handbook of Physiology. The Respiratory System.* Baltimore: Williams & Wilkins; 1985:47–91.

Weibel ER. Functional morphology of lung parenchyma. In: Fishman AP, Macklem PT, Mead J, eds. *Handbook of Physiology. The Respiratory System.* Baltimore: Williams & Wilkins; 1986:89–111.

Pulmonary Circulation

Abman SH, Hansmann G, Archer AL, et al. Pediatric pulmonary hypertension. Guidelines from the American Heart Association and American Thoracic Association. *Circulation.* 2015;132:2037–2099.

Stacher E, Graham BB, Hunt JM, et al. Modern age pathology of pulmonary hypertension. *Am J Respir Crit Care Med.* 2012;186:261–272.

Growth and Development of the Lung

Desai TJ, Brownfield DG, Krasnow MA. Alveolar progenitor and stem cells in lung development, renewal and cancer. *Nature.* 2014;507:190–194.

Ochs M, Nyengaard JR, Jung A, et al. The number of alveoli in the human lung. *Am J Respir Crit Care Med.* 2004;169:120–124.

Whitsett JA, Wert SE, Trapnell BC. Genetic disorders influencing lung formation and function at birth. *Hum Mol Genet.* 2004;13(Spec2):R207–R215.

Lung Physiology

West JB, Luks AM. *Respiration Physiology—The Essentials.* 10th ed. Philadelphia: Wolters Kluwer; 2016.

Pulmonary Function Testing

ATS/ERS statement: raised volume forced expirations in infants: guidelines for current practice. *Am J Respir Crit Care Med.* 2005;172:1463–1471.

Beydon N, Davis SD, Lombardi E, et al. An official American Thoracic Society/European Respiratory Society statement: pulmonary function testing in preschool children. *Am J Respir Crit Care Med.* 2007;175:1304–1345.

Loeb JS, Blower WC, Feldstein JF, et al. Acceptability and repeatability of spirometry in children using updated ATS/ERS criteria. *Pediatr Pulmonol.* 2008;43:1020–1024.

Miller MR, Hankinson J, Brusasco V, et al. Standardization of spirometry. *Eur Respir J.* 2005;26:319–338.

Wanger J, Clausen JL, Coates A, et al. Standardization of the measurement of lung volumes. *Eur Respir J.* 2005;26:511–522.

Respiratory Muscle Testing

ATS/ERS Statement on respiratory muscle testing. *Am J Respir Crit Care Med.* 2002;166:518–624.

Control of Breathing

Feldman JL, Del Negro CA. Looking for inspiration: new perspectives on respiratory rhythm. *Nat Rev Neurosci.* 2006;7:232–242.

Fleming PJ, Blair PS, Pease A. Sudden unexpected death in infancy: aetiology, pathophysiology, epidemiology and prevention in 2015. *Arch Dis Child.* 2015;100:984–988.

Marcus CL, Brooks LJ, Draper KA, et al. Diagnosis and management of childhood obstructive sleep apnea syndrome. *Pediatrics.* 2012;130:576–584.

Weese-Mayer DE, Berry-Kravis EM, Ceccherini I, et al. An official ATS clinical policy statement: congenital central hypoventilation syndrome: genetic basis, diagnosis, and management. *Am J Respir Crit Care Med.* 2010;181:626–644.

7 Biology and Assessment of Airway Inflammation

SEJAL SAGLANI, BSc, MBChB, MD, CLARE M. LLOYD, PhD,
and ANDREW BUSH, MB BS(Hons), MA, MD, FRCP, FRCPCH, FERS

Introduction

Inflammation is classically characterized by four cardinal signs: *calor, rubor* (due to vasodilatation), *tumor* (due to plasma exudation and edema), and *dolor* (due to sensitization and activation of sensory nerves. Inflammation is also characterized by infiltration with several types of effector cells, which differ depending on the type of inflammatory process. A normal inflammatory response is essential to allow protection of the body against invasion from external environmental insults such as microorganisms, toxins, and pathogens. Failure of any of the components of the inflammatory response (e.g., neutrophil dysfunction, also known as Job's syndrome) has catastrophic consequences. The inflammatory response not only provides an acute defense against injury (proinflammatory) but is also involved in the healing and restoration of normal function after tissue damage from infection and toxins (regulatory).

Cystic fibrosis (CF) bronchiectasis and persistent bacterial bronchitis are characterized by a neutrophilic pattern of inflammation, driven in part by chronic bacterial infection; and the pathophysiology is covered in more detail in Chapters 49 and 51.

Allergic Inflammation

Allergic inflammation develops following exposure to allergens and is mediated mainly by IgE-dependent mechanisms, resulting in a characteristic pattern of inflammation characterized by eosinophils and mast cells. Details of the development of the allergic inflammatory response, specifically in the context of asthma, are described in Chapter 43. The allergic inflammatory response is unusual, as it develops to innocuous environmental agents such as house dust mite, pollen, and peanut. The development of an allergic inflammatory response is therefore inappropriate and is harmful rather than beneficial, and it results in allergic diseases such as asthma or atopic dermatitis. The inflammatory response seen in allergic diseases is characterized by an infiltration with eosinophils[1] and resembles the inflammatory process in parasitic infections. For some reason, allergens such as house dust mite and pollen proteins activate eosinophilic inflammation, possibly because of their protease activity. Normally, such an inflammatory response would kill the invading parasite (thus preventing the parasite from overwhelming the host) and the process would be self-limiting, but in allergic diseases, the inciting stimulus persists

and the acute inflammatory response turns into chronic inflammation, with structural consequences in the airways and skin.[2,3]

Acute Inflammation

Acute inflammation in the respiratory tract is an immediate defense reaction to inhaled allergens, pathogens, or noxious agents. The structural integrity of the respiratory tract is vital to preventing infection with inhaled microorganisms. Important mechanisms including an intact respiratory epithelium, mucus production, and mucociliary clearance via the action of cilia and cough act to prevent infection with respiratory pathogens. The importance of these mechanisms in host defense is highlighted by high rates of bacterial infection in conditions such as cystic fibrosis and primary ciliary dyskinesia (PCD), which are characterized by abnormal mucociliary function, either as primary or secondary phenomena.

Immune cells such as neutrophils and alveolar macrophages are present in large numbers in the airways and constitute a first line of defense against respiratory pathogens. Macrophages recognize microorganisms via the presence of surface receptors such as toll-like receptors (TLRs) leading to phagocytosis, microbicidal killing, and initiation of immune responses.[4] Components of the bacterial cell wall are recognized by toll-like receptor 4, which is present on macrophages and leads to macrophage activation and phagocytosis. In addition, the membrane protein P2, recognized by toll-like receptor 2 is a specific trigger of macrophage activation, and results in secretion of interleukin 8 (IL-8) and tumor necrosis factor-α (TNF-α) with subsequent recruitment of neutrophils to the site of infection (Fig. 7.1).

Inhalation of an allergen (e.g., house dust mites) activates surface mast cells by an IgE-dependent mechanism. This releases multiple bronchoconstrictor mediators, resulting in rapid contraction of airway smooth muscle and wheezing.[5] These mediators also result in plasma exudation, edema of the airways and recruitment of inflammatory cells from the circulation—particularly eosinophils, neutrophils (transiently), and T-lymphocytes, mainly of the T helper 2 (Th2) type. This accounts for the late response that occurs 4–6 hours after allergen exposure and resolves within 24 hours, which should be regarded as an acute inflammatory reaction. The acute inflammatory response in the respiratory tract is usually accompanied by increased mucus secretion, which is a part of the defense system that protects the delicate mucosal surface of the airways.

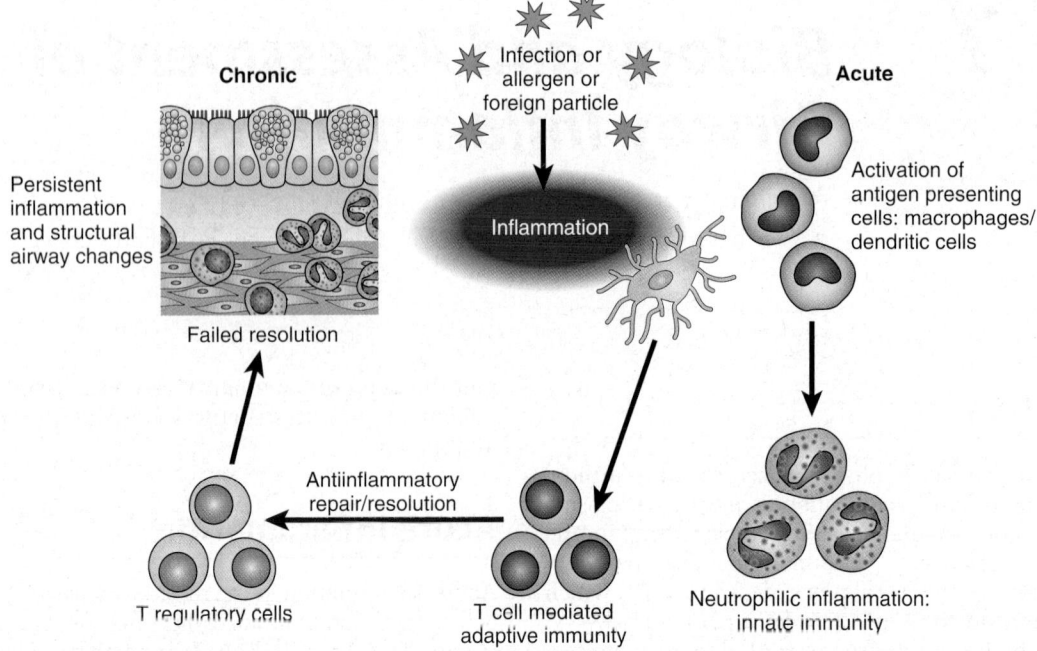

Fig. 7.1 Development of acute and chronic inflammation. Inhaled foreign environmental particles result in the development of an acute inflammatory response by antigen presenting cells (dendritic cells) and innate immune cells such as macrophages. This leads to the induction of an adaptive immune response by conversion of naïve T cells to T helper cells in the lymph nodes. The acute inflammatory response is followed by a process of active repair and resolution; however, if this fails, as is the case in inflammatory diseases, a cycle of sustained chronic inflammation develops resulting in disease pathology.

Chronic Inflammation

The normal consequence of an acute inflammatory process is complete resolution; for example, acute lobar pneumonia due to pneumococcal infection is characterized by a massive influx of neutrophils, with complete resolution and restoration of normal lung structure. However, many airway inflammatory conditions are chronic and result from an exaggerated inflammatory response with failed or inadequate resolution. In certain airway infections such as pulmonary tuberculosis, there may be a prolonged and inappropriate period of acute neutrophilic inflammation, with a failure of development of chronic inflammation that results in pathology.[6] An imbalance between proinflammatory responses and regulatory responses results in pathologic chronic inflammatory airways diseases, and this chronic inflammatory process may persist even in the absence of causal mechanisms (see Fig. 7.1). Examples include occupational asthma in which the pathological process and symptoms continue despite complete avoidance of sensitizing agents and in adult patients with chronic obstructive pulmonary disease who have persistent airway inflammation, even after stopping smoking for many years.

The resolution of inflammation was previously thought to be a passive process, but it is now realized that there are important active control mechanisms. Several potential mechanisms are important in the normal resolution of inflammation. These include IL-10,[7,8] CD200,[9,10] Annexin,[11] lung Kruppel-like factor (LKLF),[12] lipid mediators such as Resolvin E1 (RvE1), Protectin D1 (PD1), and Lipoxin A$_4$ (LXA$_4$), interferon (IFN)-γ, and the IL-23 axis,[13,14] These mediators and regulators will be discussed in more detail in the following paragraphs. The molecular and cellular mechanisms for the persistence of inflammation in the absence of its original causal mechanisms are not fully understood, but they presumably involve some type of long-lived immunologic memory that drives the inflammatory process. Structural cells, such as airway epithelial and airway smooth muscle cells, are also immunologically active and can drive the chronic inflammatory process (see Fig. 7.1). This is a key area of research, as understanding these mechanisms might lead to potentially curative therapies.

STRUCTURAL CHANGES AND REPAIR

A repair process that restores the tissue to normal usually follows the acute inflammatory response. This may involve proliferation of damaged cells (e.g., airway epithelial cells) and fibrosis to heal any breach in the mucosal surface.[15] These repair processes may also become chronic in response to continued inflammation, resulting in "exaggerated" structural changes in the airways that are referred to as *remodeling*.[16] However, the relationship between airway inflammation and remodeling is controversial; the conventional view—that inflammation leads to remodeling—has been challenged by human and animal work, which suggests that they may be parallel processes.[17–19] These structural changes in asthma and CF may result in irreversible narrowing of the airways, with fixed obstruction to air flow. In asthma, several structural changes are found in the airway wall, including increased thickness of the subepithelial basement membrane, an increased amount of airway smooth muscle, and an increased number of blood vessels (angiogenesis) (Fig. 7.2).

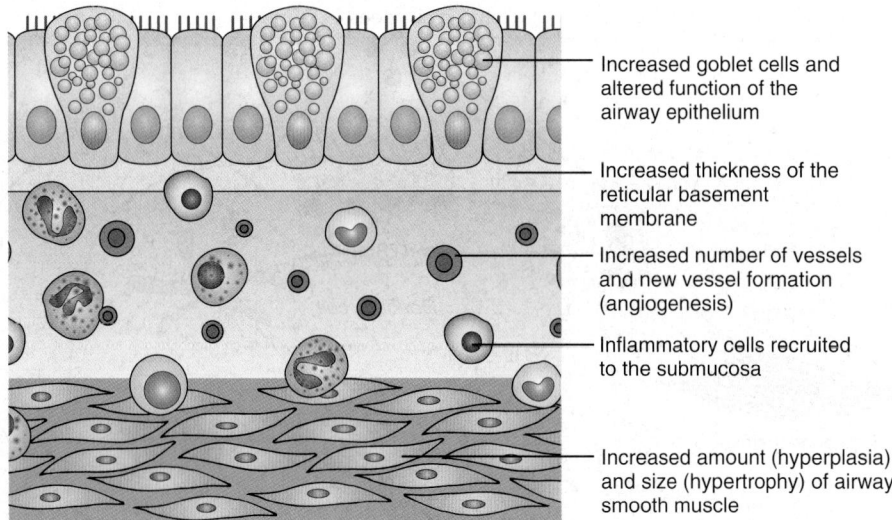

Increased goblet cells and altered function of the airway epithelium

Increased thickness of the reticular basement membrane

Increased number of vessels and new vessel formation (angiogenesis)

Inflammatory cells recruited to the submucosa

Increased amount (hyperplasia) and size (hypertrophy) of airway smooth muscle

Fig. 7.2 Diagram illustrating the airway pathological changes in asthma.

There is much debate about the importance of airway remodeling in asthma, as it is not seen in all patients. It may contribute to airway hyperresponsiveness (AHR) in asthma, but it may also have some beneficial effects in limiting airway closure.[20] Details of each of the structural changes seen in children with asthma and their functional relevance, particularly the role of structural airway cells in mediating inflammation, are provided in Chapter 43.

Inflammatory Cells

Many types of inflammatory cells are involved in airway inflammation, and the functional roles of each cell type and the interrelationship among cells are complex and not completely understood (Fig. 7.3). Chronic inflammatory airways diseases can be divided into those that are predominantly neutrophilic or eosinophilic. Chronic suppurative lung diseases such as CF and PCD demonstrate predominantly neutrophilic inflammation, which may be present even in the absence of detectable infection (at least by conventional culture). This "sterile" inflammation is associated with structural airway damage and is thought to lead to bronchiectasis.[21] Interestingly, in CF, while the predominant inflammatory cell in the airway lumen is the neutrophil (as shown by sputum and bronchoalveolar lavage cytology), T-lymphocytes predominate in the proximal airway wall.[22]

The predominant inflammatory cell pattern seen in children with asthma is eosinophilic since the majority of children have allergic asthma. The same kind of inflammation is seen in bronchial biopsies in children as in adults, which indicates that similar inflammatory mechanisms are likely.[18,23-27] However, inflammatory phenotypes are heterogeneous and may vary between children and over time in the same children.[28] Adults with severe asthma appear to have a predominantly neutrophilic inflammatory profile. In contrast, as a group, children with severe asthma have eosinophilic airway inflammation during stable disease. However, little is known about changes in the airway inflammatory profile in children with asthma during exacerbations, but since most exacerbations are precipitated by infection, it is likely that the patterns

of inflammation change, and this may explain the relative inefficacy of steroids during exacerbations, particularly in children with severe disease. A specific phenotype in which efficacy of steroids can be very variable is preschool wheeze. The inflammatory mechanisms in early wheeze, especially episodic (viral) wheeze, are little studied or understood. It is known that preschool children with severe recurrent wheezing, which is present both during and in between respiratory infections (multiple trigger wheeze), have an airway eosinophilia during stable disease.[18] The pattern of inflammation during acute episodes remains unclear. In addition, the inflammatory pattern seen at bronchoscopy is the same in children with multiple trigger (asthmatic) wheeze, independent of their atopic status.[29] The evidence in episodic (viral) wheeze suggests that the pattern is neutrophilic.[30-33] No single inflammatory cell accounts for the complex pathophysiology of asthma, although some cells predominate in allergic inflammation; and inflammation might vary in different compartments of the lung. In adults with asthma, transbronchial biopsy has shown evidence of very distal inflammation in the absence of proximal airway inflammation; there are no equivalent pediatric studies.[34-36] There is also a dissociation between airway mucosal (wall) and airway luminal inflammatory patterns in asthma.[37]

MAST CELLS

Mast cells are important in initiating the acute bronchoconstrictor responses to allergens[38] and probably to other indirect stimuli such as exercise and hyperventilation (via osmolality or thermal changes). Treatment of asthmatic patients with prednisolone results in a decrease in the number of tryptase-positive mast cells. Furthermore, mast cell tryptase appears to play a role in airway remodeling, as this mast cell product stimulates human lung fibroblast proliferation. Mast cells also secrete cytokines, including IL-4 and eotaxin, which may be involved in maintaining the allergic inflammatory response and the TNF-α.[39] Mast cells are found in increased numbers in airway smooth muscle of asthmatic patients, and this appears to correlate with AHR, suggesting that mast cell mediators may mediate AHR.[40]

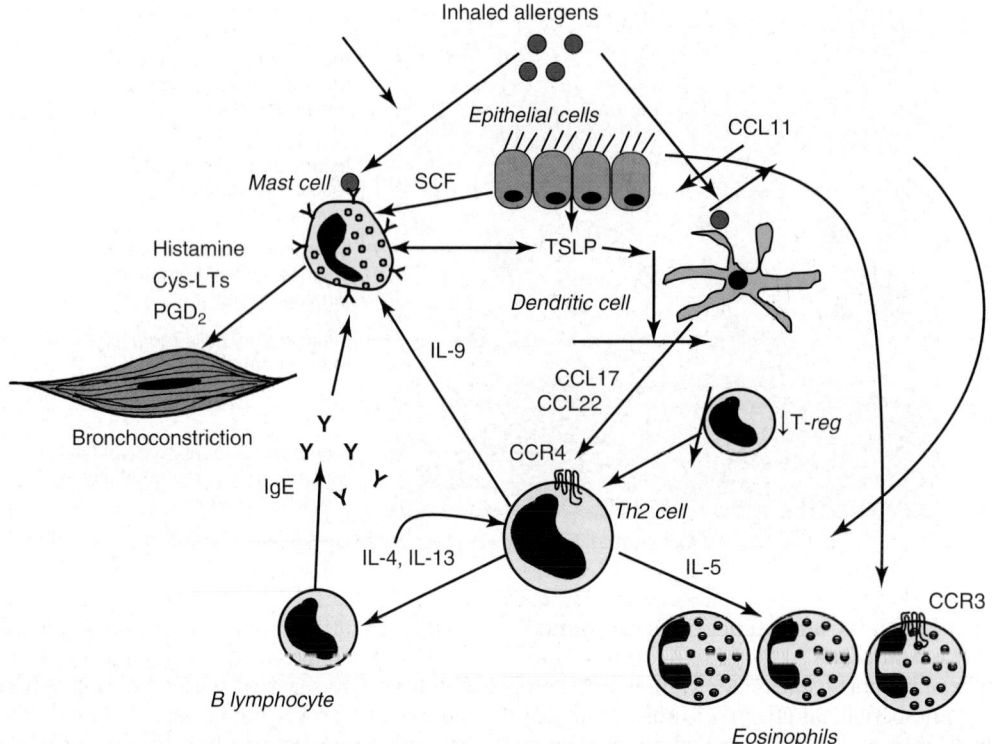

Fig. 7.3 Inflammation in asthma. Inhaled allergens activate sensitized mast cells by cross-linking surface-bound IgE molecules to release several bronchoconstrictor mediators, including cysteinyl-leukotrienes *(cys-LT)* and prostaglandin D_2 *(PGD₂)*. Epithelial cells release stem-cell factor *(SCF)*, which is important for maintaining mucosal mast cells at the airway surface. Allergens are processed by myeloid dendritic cells, which are conditioned by thymic stromal lymphopoietin *(TSLP)* secreted by epithelial cells and mast cells to release the chemokines CC-chemokine ligand 17 *(CCL17)* and *CCL22*, which act on CC-chemokine receptor 4 *(CCR4)* to attract T helper 2 *(Th2)* cells. Th2 cells have a leading role in orchestrating the inflammatory response in allergy through the release of interleukin-4 *(IL-4)* and *IL-13* (which stimulate B cells to synthesize IgE), *IL-5* (which is necessary for eosinophilic inflammation), and *IL-9* (which stimulates mast-cell proliferation). Epithelial cells release *CCL11*, which recruits eosinophils via *CCR3*. Patients with asthma may have a defect in regulatory T cells *(T-reg)*, which may favor further Th2-cell proliferation.

However, mast cells may play less of a role in chronic allergic inflammatory events, and it seems more probable that other cells, such as macrophages, eosinophils, and T-lymphocytes, are important in the chronic inflammatory process and in AHR. Classically, allergens activate mast cells through an IgE-dependent mechanism. The importance of IgE in the pathophysiology of asthma has been underscored by recent clinical studies with humanized anti-IgE antibodies, which inhibit IgE-mediated effects. Anti-IgE therapy is effective in patients, including children, with severe asthma who are not well controlled by high doses of corticosteroids; and it is particularly effective in reducing exacerbations.[41] The relationship between IgE and mast cell degranulation in causing acute allergic responses is discussed in Chapter 43, and the role of omalizumab (anti-IgE monoclonal antibody) in the treatment of severe asthma is discussed in Chapter 48.

MACROPHAGES

The alveolar macrophage (AM) is the most numerous immune cell present within the respiratory tract. Originally thought to be derived from peripheral monocytes, current knowledge of their function is largely based upon studies of macrophages derived from peripheral precursors. Recent evidence, however, suggests that AMs enter the lungs prenatally and proliferate *in situ*,[42–44] suggesting highly specialized functions. It is now apparent that local tissue milieu and regulatory influences

result in macrophages that have very specific phenotypes and functions.[45,46] Bone-marrow derived macrophages have been shown to differentiate to an AM phenotype following pulmonary transplantation, confirming the importance of the local environment in phenotypic development[47]; however, the mechanisms by which this occurs are poorly understood. Airway macrophages are ideally positioned to dictate the innate defense of the airways (Fig. 7.4). Pulmonary macrophage populations are heterogeneous and demonstrate plasticity, owing to variations in origin, tissue residency, and environmental influences. The diversity of pulmonary macrophages facilitates efficient responses to environmental signals and allows rapid alterations in phenotype and in response to a plethora of cytokines and microbial signals.[48] They express a wide range of receptors, which enable them to regulate their local environment by responding to changes within it. These receptors can be activating, such as TLRs to sense pathogens and cytokine receptors for TNF, IL-1, and IFNγ. Alternatively, the receptors may be suppressive, such as CD200, Triggering Receptor Expressed on Myeloid Cells (TREM), and transforming growth factor-β (TGF-β). The receptors enable high level of engagement and interaction with pulmonary epithelial cells. Indeed, this interaction is crucial for maintenance of immune homeostasis within the respiratory tract. Cooperation between the cells facilitates clearance of cellular debris and particulate matter, as well as directing specific immune responses to pathogens.

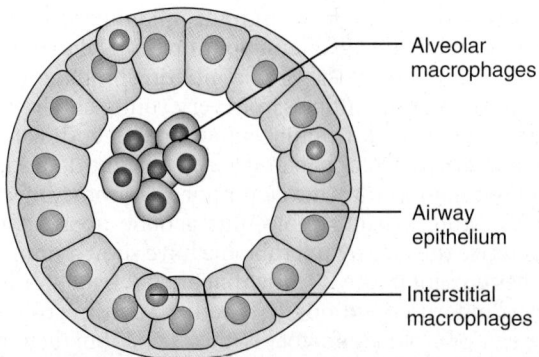

Alveolar
macrophages

Airway
epithelium

Interstitial
macrophages

Fig. 7.4 Interstitial and alveolar macrophages in airway to maintain immune homeostasis. Immune cells are present in the airways and constantly undertaking immune surveillance to ensure homeostasis and on standby to initiate an inflammatory response to foreign particles when needed. Both interstitial *(red)* and alveolar *(blue)* macrophages perform continued immune surveillance in the lungs to maintain immune homeostasis.

Macrophages have the capacity to secrete a large variety of different agents with either proinflammatory or antiinflammatory effects, including cytokines and growth factors, chemotactic factors, lipid mediators, and proteinases. In asthma, macrophages may be activated by allergens via low-affinity IgE receptors (Fcε;RII [Receptor II]). The vast immunologic repertoire of macrophages allows them to produce more than 100 different products, including a large variety of cytokines that may orchestrate the inflammatory response. Macrophages have the capacity to initiate a particular type of inflammatory response via the repertoire of cytokines they release. They may also either increase or decrease inflammation, depending on the activating stimulus. Alveolar macrophages normally have a *suppressive* effect on lymphocyte function, but this may be impaired in asthma after allergen exposure. In patients with asthma, there is a reduced secretion of IL-10 (an antiinflammatory protein secreted by macrophages) in alveolar macrophages. Macrophages may therefore play an important antiinflammatory role by maintaining tolerance within the respiratory tract. There are subtypes of macrophages that perform different inflammatory, antiinflammatory, or phagocytic roles in airway disease; but at present, it is difficult to differentiate these subtypes in the human airway. There is evidence that alveolar macrophages show reduced phagocytosis of apoptotic cells and carbon particles in severe asthma so that inflammation does not resolve.[49,50]

DENDRITIC CELLS

Dendritic cells (DC) are specialized innate antigen presenting cells that have a unique ability to initiate and regulate cell mediated and humoral immune responses. DCs can be defined as any mononuclear phagocyte that can take up antigen, process it for presentation on major histocompatibility complex (MHC)-I or II, migrate to the nearest draining lymph node, and efficiently and effectively activate and polarize naïve T cells.[51] Subsequently, with the aid of costimulatory molecules (e.g., B7.1, B7.2, and CD40), they program the production of allergen-specific T cells. People with genetic defects resulting in a lack of DCs, or mice wherein DCs are experimentally depleted, suffer from severely impaired

adaptive T and B cell responses. DCs reside beneath the pulmonary epithelium in the lung tissue, and are poised to encounter foreign material (allergen), infections, or tissue damage. They are aided by their ability to actively sample antigens in the airways via cellular extensions that protrude through the epithelial tight junctions.[52] Although their numbers are low in the lung, DCs are highly sensitive to their environment, expressing a variety of pattern recognition receptors (PRRs) including TLRs, C-type lectin receptors, and Nodlike receptors (NLRs). Through these receptors, they can sense a wide range of pathogens, microbes, or damage-associated molecules (DAMPs); these include bacterial, viral, fungal and protozoal pathogens, commensals and allergens, particles, and pollutants. Additionally, the pulmonary environment presents some unique features compared to other barrier sites, such as specific surfactants and mucins, which can influence DC activation and function.[53] Importantly, the combination of PRRs can tailor the developing immune response by directly influencing the activation and function of DCs. A number of DC subpopulations have been defined in the lungs including myeloid DCs (mDCs),[54] conventional DCs that initiate T-cell immunity and antibody production, and plasmacytoid DCs (pDCs)[55] that have an important role in antiviral immunity and immune tolerance.[56] DCs induce a T-lymphocyte–mediated immune response and therefore play a critical role in the development of asthma.[57] Increased numbers of mucosal DCs are present in asthma, and they have been identified in endobronchial biopsies, bronchoalveolar lavage, and induced sputum from patients with asthma. Animal studies have demonstrated that myeloid dendritic cells are critical to the development of T helper type 2 (Th2) cells and eosinophilia.

EOSINOPHILS

Eosinophils form an essential part of the innate immune response against parasitic helminths acting through the release of cytotoxic granule proteins. However, airway eosinophilic inflammation is also a central feature in allergic asthma. Allergen inhalation results in a marked increase in eosinophils in bronchoalveolar lavage fluid, and there is a correlation between eosinophil counts in peripheral blood and bronchial lavage in patients who are not receiving steroid treatment. Eosinophils develop from bone marrow precursors and are recruited to the lung via chemokines and cytokines.[58] Eosinophil recruitment initially involves adhesion of eosinophils to vascular endothelial cells in the airway circulation and then is followed by migration into the submucosa and activation. There have been extensive investigations of the role of individual adhesion molecules, cytokines, and mediators in orchestrating these responses. Adhesion of eosinophils involves the expression of specific glycoprotein molecules on the surface of eosinophils (integrins) and expression of such molecules as intercellular adhesion molecule-1 (ICAM-1) on vascular endothelial cells. The adhesion molecule very late antigen-4 (VLA4) expressed on eosinophils, which interacts with vascular cell adhesion molecule-1 (VCAM-1) and IL-4, increases its expression on endothelial cells. Granulocyte macrophage colony stimulating factor (GM-CSF) and IL-5 may be important for the survival of eosinophils in the airways and for "priming" eosinophils to exhibit enhanced responsiveness.

There are multiple mediators involved in the migration of eosinophils from the circulation to the surface of the airway. The most potent and selective agents appear to be chemokines (e.g., CCL5, CC11, CCL13, CCL24, and CCL26), which are expressed by epithelial cells. There appears to be a cooperative interaction between IL-5 and chemokines so that both are necessary for the eosinophilic response in the airway. Once recruited to the airway, eosinophils require the presence of various growth factors, of which GM-CSF and IL-5 appear to be the most important. In the absence of these growth factors, eosinophils undergo programed cell death (apoptosis).

After humanized monoclonal antibody to IL-5 is administered to asthmatic patients, there is a profound and prolonged reduction in circulating eosinophils and eosinophils recruited into the airway following allergen challenge.[59] However, there is no effect on the response to inhaled allergen and no change in lung function. Recent studies with highly selected patients with persistent sputum eosinophilia despite high doses of inhaled corticosteroids have shown a reduction in asthma attacks following treatment with anti-IL-5 antibody therapy.[60,61] The selective response in patients with a persistent eosinophilia underscores the importance of understanding the differing inflammatory processes in subgroups of patients with asthma rather than applying the same strategies to all patients (see Chapter 43).

NEUTROPHILS

In addition to physical barriers, such as the airway epithelium, neutrophils are part of the first line of immune defense. They can be found in the bloodstream, where they have a lifespan of 6–8 hours, and in tissue, where they can survive for up to 7 days.[62] They are the first cells of the immune system to migrate to a site of inflammation, where they play an important role in pathogen elimination and cytokine production. The mechanisms that neutrophils use for host defense include phagocytosis, degranulation, cytokine production, and the recently described production of neutrophil extracellular traps (NETs).[63] NETs were discovered in 1996 as a pathway of cellular death that was different from apoptosis and necrosis.[64] Neutrophil extracellular traps are DNA structures released due to chromatin decondensation and spreading, and they occupy three to five times the volume of condensed chromatin.[65] NETs arise from the release of granular and nuclear contents of neutrophils in the extracellular space in response to different classes of microorganisms, soluble factors, and host molecules.[66] Several proteins adhere to NETs, including histones and components of neutrophil granules with bactericidal activity such as elastase, myeloperoxidase, cathepsin G (CG), and lactoferrin. The detrimental effect of excessive NET release is particularly important to lung diseases, because NETs can expand in the pulmonary alveoli, causing lung injury. Massive NET formation has been reported in pulmonary diseases, including asthma, chronic obstructive pulmonary disease, cystic fibrosis, respiratory syncytial virus bronchiolitis, influenza, bacterial pneumonia, and tuberculosis. Thus, NET formation must be tightly regulated to avoid NET-mediated tissue damage. Recent approaches to target NETs in pulmonary diseases include DNA disintegration with recombinant human DNase, and neutralization of NET proteins with antihistone antibodies and protease inhibitors.

Neutrophils are the predominant inflammatory cells in patients with CF and chronic suppurative lung diseases such as PCD and bronchiectasis. Studies utilizing bronchoscopy to collect lower airway samples from very young children with CF have identified neutrophilic inflammation both with and without cultured bacterial pathogens.[67,68] These data suggest that inflammation may develop prior to chronic infection. However, studies using molecular genetic approaches to characterize the airway microbiome have shown numerous microbes present in the CF lung that are not readily cultured under standard conditions.[69] Whether such microbes are pathogenic or proinflammatory is uncertain,[70] but they can be found in very young children and may also help explain why neutrophilic airway inflammation is present when bacteria are not identified by traditional methods.[71] Nebulized hypertonic saline has been shown to improve mucus clearance in CF and impact positively upon pulmonary exacerbations, but there is also increasing evidence to suggest that hypertonic saline is beneficial through its antiinflammatory properties and its ability to reduce bacterial activity and biofilm formation.[72] The specific mechanisms involved include the downregulation of oxidative burst activity and adhesion molecule expression and the suppression of neutrophil degranulation of proteolytic enzymes. In addition, a potential pathogenic role of neutrophilic inflammation in both CF and non-CF bronchiectasis has been shown by interventional studies that have demonstrated improved lung function with the use of antiinflammatory agents such as the macrolide azithromycin, although the exact mechanisms of benefit of macrolides is unclear.[73-75]

In contrast to CF and non-CF bronchiectasis, the numbers and function of airway neutrophils in asthma remains uncertain. Although they are reported to be increased in severe asthma in adults, numbers in the airway lumen and lung parenchyma are not elevated in children with severe asthma.[76,77] However, a sub-group of children have increased intraepithelial neutrophils. Intriguingly, these patients have better lung function and asthma control, suggesting the neutrophils may be protective rather than pathogenic. The functional role of neutrophils in asthma has been further questioned by interventional studies that have shown little/no benefit of the antiinflammatory macrolide azithromycin either during infective exacerbations[78] or to prevent exacerbations.[79] Putative causes for airway neutrophilia in asthma are corticosteroid therapy, which inhibits neutrophil apoptosis, chronic infection with atypical organisms such as Chlamydia or Mycoplasma, exposure to passive smoking and other environmental pollutants, and gastroesophageal reflux and aspiration. However, it is still not clear whether neutrophils play a pathophysiologic role in the disease.

T-LYMPHOCYTES

T-lymphocytes play a very important role in coordinating the inflammatory response in asthma[80] through the release of specific patterns of cytokines, resulting in the recruitment and survival of eosinophils and in the maintenance of mast cells in the airways.[81] T-lymphocytes are coded to express a distinctive pattern of cytokines, which are similar to that described in the murine T helper 2 (Th2) type of T-lymphocytes, which characteristically express IL-4, IL-5, IL-9, and IL-13 (Fig. 7.5; see also Fig. 7.3). This programming of T-lymphocytes

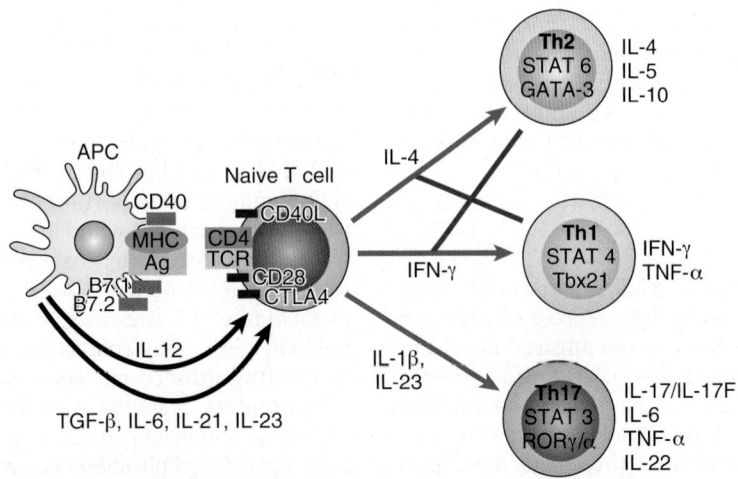

Fig. 7.5 T cell differentiation and cytokine production in pulmonary adaptive immunity following antigen presentation. The pulmonary antigen presenting cell *(APC)*, or dendritic cell, presents antigen via MHC class II to the naïve T cell, and under the influence of the cytokines that have been secreted, the naïve T cell is converted to a T helper cell, which secretes further cytokines. In allergy, these are IL-4, IL-5, and IL-13 from Th2 cells; in infection, Th1 cells secrete IFN-γ and TNF-α; and in both allergy and infection, Th17 cells secrete IL-6, IL-17, or IL-22. *CTLA4*, Cytotoxic T-lymphocyte-associated protein 4; *IL*, interleukin; *IFN*, interferon; *MHC*, major histocompatibility complex; *TCR*, T cell receptor; *TGF*, transforming growth factor; *TNF*, tumor necrosis factor.

is presumably due to antigen-presenting cells, such as dendritic cells, which may migrate from the epithelium to regional lymph nodes or interact with lymphocytes resident in the airway mucosa. The naïve immune system is skewed to express the Th2 phenotype; data now indicate that children with atopy are more likely to retain this skewed phenotype than normal children. There is some evidence that early infections or exposure to endotoxins might promote Th1-mediated responses to predominate and that a lack of infection or a clean environment in childhood may favor Th2 cell expression and thus atopic diseases.[82] Indeed, the balance between Th1 cells and Th2 cells is thought to be determined by locally released cytokines, such as IL-12, which tip the balance in favor of Th1 cells, or IL-4 and IL-13, which favor the emergence of Th2 cells. There is accumulating evidence that a population of tissue resident memory cells (Trm) are long lived within the lung and facilitate development of T-cell responses upon reencounter with allergen. Although these Trm ensure efficient clearance of viruses, they may exacerbate allergic inflammation.[83] Regulatory T cells (Tregs) suppress the immune response through the secretion of inhibitory cytokines (e.g., IL-10 and TGF-β) (see Fig. 7.3, Chapter 43) and play an important role in immune regulation with suppression of Th1 responses; there is some evidence that Treg function may be defective in asthmatic patients.[84] Details of lymphoid cell responses in children with asthma, including the role of Th17 cells, T regulatory cells and the recently described innate lymphoid cells are discussed in Chapter 43.

Patients with CF are known to have an imbalance in the composition of lymphocytic inflammation as well as the presence of neutrophilia. Interestingly, the neutrophilia seems confined to the airway lumen, while the infiltrate in the airway wall in children with CF is predominantly lymphocytic,[85] specifically being composed of IL-17+ CD4+ (Th17) cells and gamma delta T cells.[86] A Th2/Th17 skewed inflammatory response has been associated with increased risk for *Pseudomonas aeruginosa* infection.[87] Moreover, the numbers of regulatory T cells (CD4+CD25+FoxP3+) in peripheral blood

are reduced in patients with CF with chronic *P. aeruginosa* infection and the reduction correlates with impaired lung function,[88] suggesting immune manipulation of Tregs to try and dampen proinflammatory responses might be a therapeutic strategy in patients with established CF lung disease.

INNATE LYMPHOID CELLS

Innate lymphoid cells (ILCs) are classified into three groups based on their transcription factors and cytokine production patterns, which mirror helper T-cell subsets. Unlike T cells and B cells, ILCs do not have antigen receptors. They respond to innate factors released by the bronchial epithelium, such as cytokines and alarmins, including IL-33, IL-25, and thymic stromal lymphopoietin (TSLP). ILCs produce multiple proinflammatory and immunoregulatory cytokines for the induction and regulation of inflammation.[89] These cells are specifically produced at mucosal surfaces and thus are important in airway inflammation. The role of ILCs, and more specifically type 2 ILCs, in the pathogenesis of allergic airways diseases has been extensively investigated over the last decade,[90] and the evidence for their involvement in pediatric severe asthma has been discussed in Chapter 43. However, the role of ILCs in infectious and nonallergic airway inflammatory diseases remains largely unknown. Specifically, the role of ILC1 cells, which produce IFNγ and may be important in viral infections and ILC3 cells, which produce IL-17 and may be important in suppurative lung disease such as cystic fibrosis, are unknown.

B-LYMPHOCYTES

In allergic diseases, B-lymphocytes secrete IgE, and the factors regulating IgE secretion are now much better understood.[91] IL-4 is crucial in switching B cells to IgE production, and CD40 on T cells is an important accessory molecule that signals through interaction with CD40-ligand on B cells. There is increasing evidence for local production of IgE, even in patients with intrinsic asthma.[92,93] For example, a recent clinical trial has shown treatment of adult patients with nonatopic asthma with the anti-IgE antibody omalizumab reduced bronchial mucosal IgE+ mast cells and improved lung function despite withdrawal of conventional therapy.[94]

BASOPHILS

Functionally, basophils are closely related to mast cells. Both cell types express the high-affinity IgE receptor (FcεRI) and rapidly release preformed mediators from intracellular stores upon IgE-mediated activation. However, in contrast to mast cells, basophils mature in the bone marrow and have a lifespan of only 2–3 days.[95] The exact role and importance of basophils in asthma is uncertain, as these cells have been difficult to detect by immunocytochemistry and most studies investigating the mechanistic role of these cells are limited to experimental murine models. However, it appears that basophils have both proinflammatory and antiinflammatory actions. They recruit effector cells such as Th2 cells, ILC2s, eosinophils, and inflammatory macrophages to the site of inflammation; and they are also able to limit inflammation by release of amphiregulin, induction of alternative activation of macrophages, and orchestration of an antiinflammatory Th2 milieu.[96] Using a basophil-specific marker, a slight increase in basophils has been documented in the airways of asthmatic patients, with an increased number after allergen challenge. However, these cells are far outnumbered by eosinophils (approximately 10:1), and their functional role is unknown.[97] There is also an increase in the numbers of basophils, as well as mast cells, in induced sputum after allergen challenge.

Structural Cells as Sources of Mediators

Structural cells of the airways, including epithelial cells, endothelial cells, fibroblasts, and even airway smooth muscle cells,[98] may be an important source of inflammatory mediators, such as cytokines and lipid mediators in asthma and CF. Indeed, because structural cells far outnumber inflammatory cells in the airway, they may become the major source of mediators driving chronic airway inflammation. Epithelial cells play a key role as immunologically active cells in translating inhaled environmental signals into an airway inflammatory response and they are at the center of the inception and propagation of immune responses in asthma (Fig. 7.6).[99–101] Epithelial cells may also play an important role in CF by driving the neutrophilic inflammatory response through the release of CXCL1 and CXCL8. Airway epithelial cells may also be important in driving the structural changes that occur in chronic airway inflammation through the release of growth factors.[102] Epithelial cell integrity might also be an important factor in denying allergens exposure to the immune system, and an increasing number of asthma susceptibility genes are expressed in the airway epithelium.[103–105] The critical role of the airway epithelium in orchestrating the pathophysiology of asthma has been discussed in detail in Chapter 43.

Inflammatory Mediators

Many different mediators have been implicated in asthma, and they may have a variety of effects on the airway, which

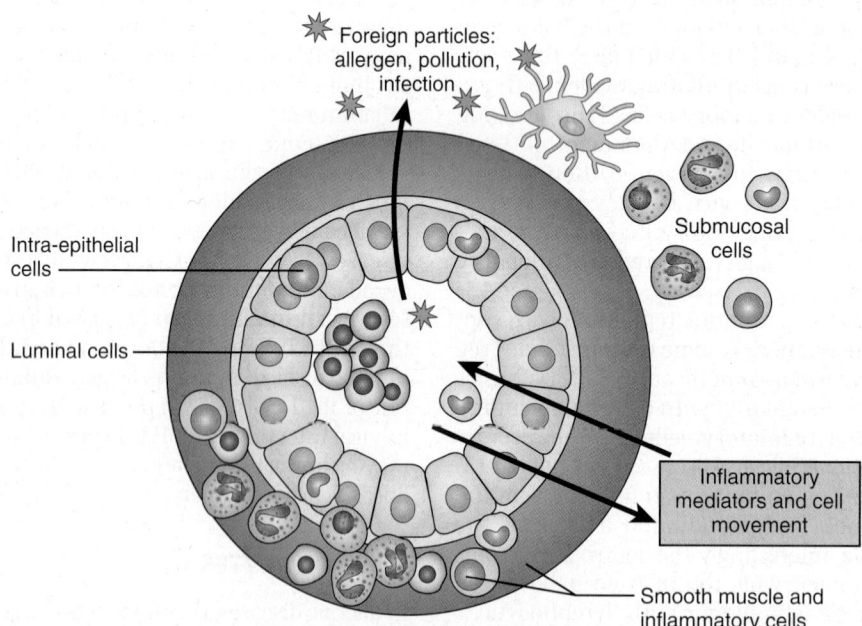

Fig. 7.6 The airway epithelium at the center of the immune response in asthma. The airway epithelium forms both a barrier to prevent the entry of foreign particles and is immunologically active. There is continued movement of immune cells through the epithelium that allows detection of foreign particles and the development of an appropriate immune response in health. However, in asthma, the barrier becomes "leaky" and particles move from the lumen through to the submucosa with the induction of a type 2 inflammatory response and secretion of mediators and a parallel impact on the submucosal structural cells such as the airway smooth muscle, which also actively secretes inflammatory cytokines.

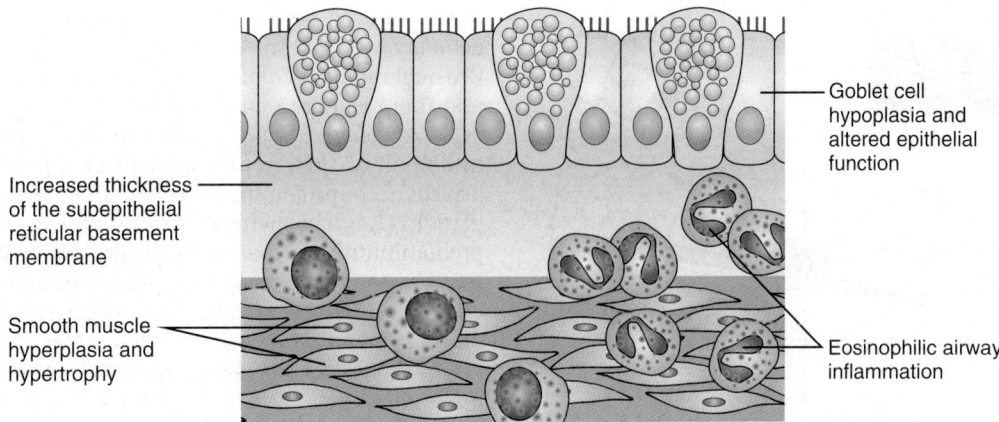

Fig. 7.7 The characteristic features of the airway pathology of asthma: inflammation and remodeling.

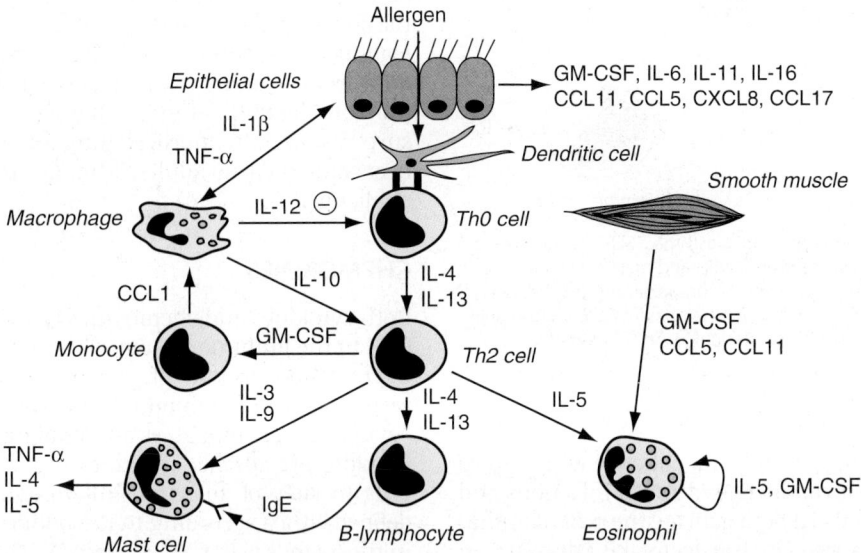

Fig. 7.8 The cytokine network in asthma. Many inflammatory cytokines are released from inflammatory and structural cells in the airway and orchestrate and perpetuate the inflammatory response. *CCL*, Chemokine; *IgE*, immunoglobulin E; *IL*, interleukin; *Th0*, T helper 0; *Th2*, T helper 2; *TNF*, tumor necrosis factor.

accounts for all the pathological features of asthma (Fig. 7.7).[106] Although less is known about the mediators of CF,[107] it is becoming clear that they differ from those implicated in asthma. Because each mediator has many effects, the role of individual mediators in the pathophysiology of airway inflammatory disease is not yet clear. The multiplicity and redundancy of effects of mediators make it unlikely that preventing the synthesis or action of a *single* mediator will have a major impact in the therapy of these diseases. However, some mediators may play a more important role if they are upstream in the inflammatory process. The effects of single mediators can only be evaluated with specific receptor antagonists or mediator synthesis inhibitors.

CYTOKINES

Cytokines play a significant role in orchestrating the type of inflammatory response seen in airways diseases (Fig. 7.8; see also Fig. 7.3).[108] Many cytokines currently form the target for the development of new asthma therapies.[109] Multiple

inflammatory cells (macrophages, mast cells, eosinophils, and lymphoid cells) and airway structural cells are capable of synthesizing and releasing cytokines. While inflammatory mediators such as histamine and leukotrienes may be important in the acute and subacute inflammatory responses and in exacerbations of asthma, it is likely that cytokines play a dominant role in maintaining chronic inflammation in airway diseases. The cytokines that appear to be of importance in asthma include the type 2, or Th2 cytokines that are secreted by T-lymphocytes and innate lymphoid cells. These include IL-4, IL-5, and IL-13. Details of the cellular source, functional role, and potential of these cytokines as therapeutic targets in asthma are summarized in Chapter 43. Other proinflammatory cytokines (e.g., IL-1β, IL-6, TNF-α, and GM-CSF) are released from a variety of cells, including macrophages, epithelial cells, T helper 1, and T helper 17 cells (see Fig. 7.8), and may be important in amplifying the inflammatory response. TNF-α may be an amplifying mediator in asthma and is produced in increased amounts in airways of patients with severe asthma. However, blocking TNF-α with a potent

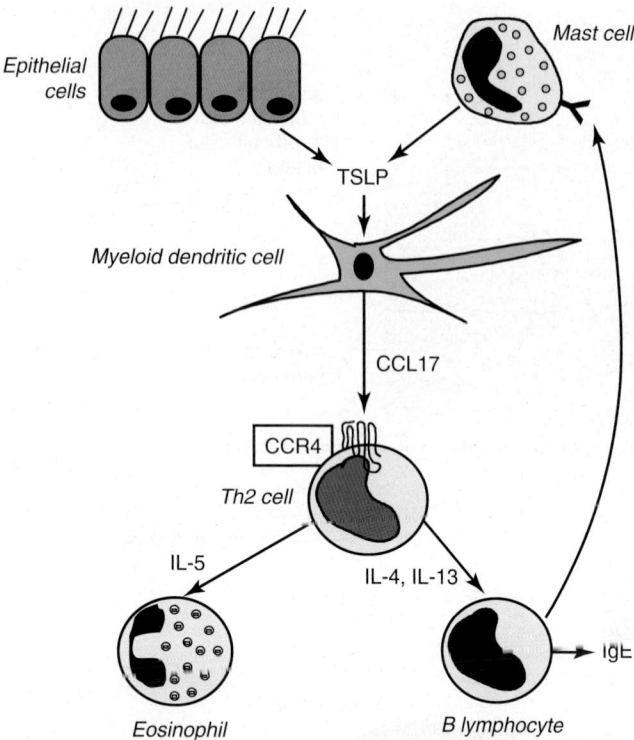

Fig. 7.9 Thymic stromal lymphopoietin in asthma. TSLP is an upstream cytokine produced by airway epithelial cells and mast cells in asthma that acts on immature dendritic cells to mature and release CCL17, which attracts Th2 cells via CCR4. *CCL,* Chemokine; *CCR,* chemokine receptor; *IgE,* immunoglobulin E; *IL,* interleukin; *Th2,* T helper 2.

antibody had no clinical benefit in patients with severe asthma, and it also led to an increased risk of infections and cancers.[110] TNF-α and IL-1β both activate the proinflammatory transcription factors—nuclear factor-κB (NF-κB) and activator protein-1 (AP-1)—which then switch on many inflammatory genes in the asthmatic airway.

Thymic stromal lymphopoietin (TSLP) shows a marked increase in expression in airway epithelium and mast cells of asthmatic patients.[111] TSLP appears to play a key role in programing airway dendritic cells to release CCL17 and CCL22 to attract Th2 cells (Fig. 7.9).[112] A clinical trial of an anti-TSLP antibody in adults with mild allergic asthma showed reduced bronchoconstriction and reduced airway eosinophilic inflammation after an acute allergen challenge in the patients who received the active drug,[113] suggesting that this may be a novel target following an acute allergen induced exacerbation of asthma, but this was a small trial that requires further confirmation.

LIPID MEDIATORS

The cysteinyl-leukotrienes, LTC_4, LTD_4, and LTE_4, are potent constrictors of human airways and may also increase AHR. Leukotriene antagonists have some bronchodilator and anti-inflammatory effects but are much less effective than inhaled corticosteroids in the management of childhood asthma.[114] Platelet-activating factor (PAF) is a potent inflammatory mediator that mimics many of the features of asthma, including eosinophil recruitment and activation and induction of

AHR; yet even potent PAF antagonists, such as dominant, do not control asthma symptoms, at least in chronic asthma. Prostaglandins (PG) have potent effects on airway function, and there is increased expression of the inducible form of cyclooxygenase (COX-2) in asthmatic airways; however, inhibition of their synthesis with COX inhibitors, such as aspirin or ibuprofen, has no effect in most patients. Prostaglandin D_2 is a bronchoconstrictor prostaglandin produced predominantly by mast cells; it also activates a novel chemoattractant receptor termed *chemoattractant receptor of Th2 cells* (CRTh2) or *DP_2-receptor*, which is expressed on Th2 cells and eosinophils and mediates chemotaxis of these cell types. It may provide a link between mast cell activation and allergic inflammation. Several oral CRTh2/DP_2 antagonists are now in clinical development.[115]

Lipid mediators are also crucial for the resolution of inflammation. Resolvins and protectins are a relatively newly described class of lipids that are thought to be important for the down regulation and resolution of inflammation, thereby leading to restitution of immune homeostasis. Mechanistic data from experimental models show that resolvins can promote clearance of inflammatory cells after allergen exposure, resulting in improved lung function.[14] They have also been described in adult asthmatic patients after allergen challenge.[116]

CHEMOKINES

Both cytokines and chemokines are small proteins made by cells in the immune system. They are important in the production and growth of immune cells and in regulating responses to inflammation and wound healing. The term "cytokines" encompasses all signaling molecules while chemokines are specific cytokines that function by attracting cells to sites of infection/inflammation. Chemokines are defined either according to the pattern of cysteine residues in the ligands (CC, CXC, C, and CX3C) or their function and pattern of expression (homeostatic and inflammatory chemokines).[117] Many chemokines are involved in the recruitment of inflammatory cells to the airways.[34] Over 50 different chemokines are now recognized, and they activate more than 20 different surface receptors. Chemokine receptors belong to the seven-transmembrane receptor superfamily of G-protein–coupled receptors; this makes it possible to find small molecule inhibitors, which has not been possible for classical cytokine receptors.[118] Some chemokine receptors appear to be selective for single chemokines, whereas others are promiscuous and mediate the effects of several related chemokines. Chemokines appear to act in sequence in determining the final inflammatory response, and so inhibitors may be more or less effective depending on the kinetics of the response. T-cell migration in response to G-protein coupled receptor (GPCR)-coupled chemokine receptors plays a prominent role in navigating distinct T-cell subsets at different stages of the immune response to their intended destinations at sites of infection and inflammation (Fig. 7.10).

Several chemokines, including CCL5, CC11, CCL13, CCL24, and CCL26, activate a common receptor on eosinophils termed *CCR3*. Increased expression in the airways of asthmatic patients is correlated with increased AHR. CCR4 chemokines are selectively expressed on Th2 cells and are activated by the CCL17 and CCL22 chemokines. Epithelial cells of patients

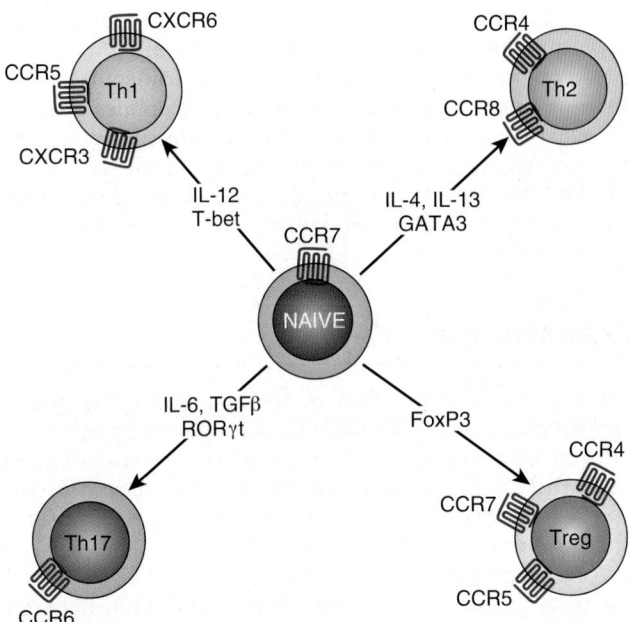

Fig. 7.10 Chemokine and cytokine interactions on T lymphocytes. Chemokine receptors are g-protein coupled receptors (GPCR) that span the cell membrane of T lymphocytes, and binding of cytokines to these receptors defines the functional phenotype of the T lymphocyte subset. *CCR*, Chemokine receptor; *IL*, interleukin; *TGF*, transforming growth factor.

with asthma express CCL22, which may then recruit Th2 cells, resulting in coordinated eosinophilic inflammation.

CXC chemokines are involved in the recruitment of neutrophils. CXCL1 and CXCL8 play an important role in neutrophilic inflammation in severe asthma and CF.

OXIDATIVE STRESS

As in all inflammatory diseases, there is increased oxidative stress associated with pulmonary inflammation, as activated inflammatory cells, such as macrophages, neutrophils, and eosinophils, produce reactive oxygen species. Evidence for increased oxidative stress in asthma and CF is provided by the increased concentrations of 8-isoprostane (a product of oxidized arachidonic acid) in exhaled breath condensates and increased ethane (a product of oxidative lipid peroxidation) in exhaled breath of asthmatic patients.[119,120] Increased oxidative stress is correlated with disease severity and may amplify the inflammatory response and reduce responsiveness to corticosteroids, particularly in severe disease and during exacerbations.

NITRIC OXIDE

Nitric oxide (NO) is generated from various resident and inflammatory cells in the human airway when L-arginine undergoes the process of oxidation by one of three NO synthase (NOS) isoenzymes: endothelial NOS, inducible NOS, and neuronal NOS. The physiologic roles that NO has in the respiratory system are numerous and include neurotransmission, vasodilatation, bronchodilation, and immune augmentation. At the onset of an asthma attack, an enhanced production of NO strongly correlates with increased inducible NOS activity,

whereas endothelial NOS and neuronal NOS primarily regulate normal metabolic functions in the central and peripheral airways.[121] During allergic inflammatory responses, NO and superoxide form peroxynitrite, which has deleterious effects in the respiratory tract. The inducible form of NOS (iNOS) shows increased expression, particularly in the airway epithelial cells and macrophages of asthmatic airways. Although the role of NO in the asthmatic airway is not fully understood, the levels of NO are often increased in asthma.[122] This elevation is thought, in part, to reflect increased inducible NOS activity in the airways. Although the cellular source of NO within the lung is not known, inferences based on mathematical models suggest that it is the large airways that are the source of NO; in severe asthma, there is evidence that small airways also produce it.[123] Extended NO analysis is a promising tool in different diseases such as asthma where NO metabolism is altered. One single exhalation cannot give insight to the NO production in the whole respiratory system; the use of multiple exhalation flows has therefore been used to give the alveolar levels (C(A)NO), the airway wall concentration (C(aw)NO), and the diffusion rate of NO (D(aw)NO).[124] Low levels of bronchial NO flux (J'(aw)NO) are seen in cystic fibrosis, PCD and in smoking subjects. However, more studies are needed to evaluate the clinical usefulness of the extended NO analysis; this has been done in systemic sclerosis where a cutoff value has been identified, predicting pulmonary function deterioration.[125,126]

GROWTH FACTORS

Many growth factors are released from inflammatory and structural cells in airway diseases; these may play a critical role in the structural changes that occur in chronic inflammation, including fibrosis, airway smooth muscle thickening, angiogenesis, and mucous hyperplasia. While the role of individual mediators is not yet established, there is evidence for increased expression of TGF-β (a mediator associated with fibrosis), vascular-endothelial growth factor (a mediator associated with angiogenesis), and epidermal growth factor (a mediator that induces mucous hyperplasia and expression of mucin genes) (Fig. 7.11). A key pathological component of asthma is airway remodeling, and it is likely that several growth factors are important in mediating the development of these structural changes; however, to date, there are no specific therapeutics that target airway remodeling.

Neural Mechanisms

Neural mechanisms may play an important role in the inflammatory response of airways. Neural reflexes may be activated by inflammatory signals, resulting in reflex bronchoconstriction; and airway nerves may release neurotransmitters, particularly neuropeptides, that have inflammatory effects.[127] There is a close interaction between nerves and inflammatory cells in allergic inflammation, as inflammatory mediators activate and modulate neurotransmission, whereas neurotransmitters may modulate the allergic inflammatory response. Inflammatory mediators may act on various prejunctional receptors on airway nerves to modulate the release of neurotransmitters. Inflammatory mediators also activate sensory nerves, resulting in reflex cholinergic bronchoconstriction or release of inflammatory neuropeptides (Fig. 7.12). There is particular interest in the role of neural mechanisms in animal models and human disease caused by respiratory syncytial virus.[128–130]

Inflammatory products may also sensitize sensory nerve endings in the airway epithelium so that the nerves become hyperalgesic. Hyperalgesia and pain *(dolor)* are cardinal signs of inflammation; and in the asthmatic airway, hyperalgesia may mediate cough and chest tightness, which are characteristic symptoms of asthma. The precise mechanisms are not yet certain, but mediators such as prostaglandins, certain cytokines, and neurotrophins may be important. Neurotrophins, which are released by various cell types in peripheral tissues, may cause proliferation and sensitization of airway sensory nerves.[131] Neurotrophins, such as nerve growth factor (NGF), may be released from inflammatory and structural cells in asthmatic airways and then stimulate the increased synthesis of neuropeptides (e.g., substance P [SP]) in airway sensory nerves, as well as sensitizing nerve endings in the airways. NGF released from human airway epithelial cells after exposure to inflammatory stimuli may play an important role in mediating AHR in asthma.

Airway nerves may also release neurotransmitters that have inflammatory effects. Thus, neuropeptides such as SP, neurokinin A, and calcitonin-gene–related peptide may be released from sensitized inflammatory nerves in the airways, increasing and extending the ongoing inflammatory response in asthma and other types of chronic airway inflammation.[132]

Transcription Factors

The chronic inflammation of asthma and CF is due to increased expression of multiple inflammatory proteins (i.e., cytokines, enzymes, receptors, adhesion molecules). In many cases, these inflammatory proteins are induced by transcription factors, DNA binding factors that increase the transcription of selected target genes (Fig. 7.13). One transcription factor that may play a critical role in asthma is NF-κB, which can be activated in asthmatic airways, particularly in epithelial cells and macrophages. NF-κB regulates the expression of several key genes that are overexpressed in asthmatic and CF airways, including proinflammatory cytokines (IL-1β, TNF-α, GM-CSF), chemokines (IL-8, Regulated on Activation, Normal T Cell Expressed and Secreted [RANTES], macrophage inflammatory protein [MIP]-1α, eotaxin), adhesion molecules (ICAM-1, VCAM-1), and inflammatory enzymes (cyclooxygenase-2, iNOS).[133] Many other transcription factors are involved in the abnormal expression of inflammatory genes in asthma, and there is growing evidence that there may be a common mechanism that involves activation of coactivator molecules at the start site of transcription of these genes. They are activated by transcription factors that induce acetylation of core histones around which DNA is wound in the chromosome. Local unwinding of DNA opens the chromatin structure and allows RNA polymerase and other transcription factors to bind, thus switching on gene transcription.[134]

Transcription factors play a critical role in determining the balance between Th1 and Th2 cells. The transcription factor GATA-3 determines the differentiation of Th2 cells and the expression of Th2 cytokines, and it shows increased expression in asthmatic patients.[135] Increasing numbers of therapeutics that target specific transcription factors are

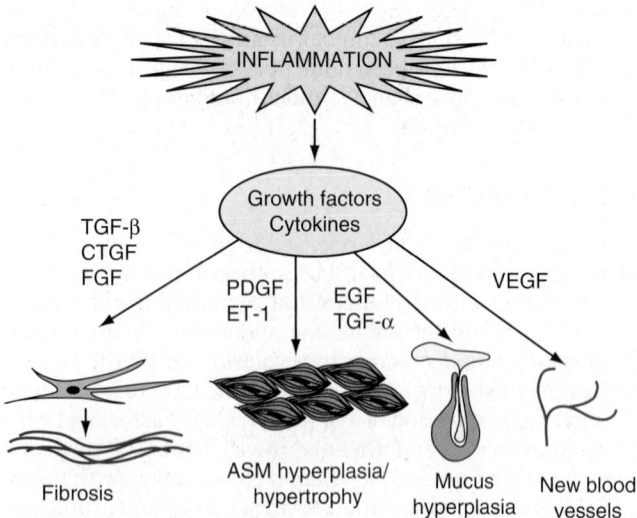

Fig. 7.11 Growth factors and airway structural changes in asthma. *CTGF,* Connective tissue growth factor; *EGF,* epidermal growth factor; *ET,* endothelin; *FGF,* fibroblast growth factor; *PDGF,* platelet-derived growth factor; *TGF,* transforming growth factor; *VEGF,* vascular-endothelial growth factor.

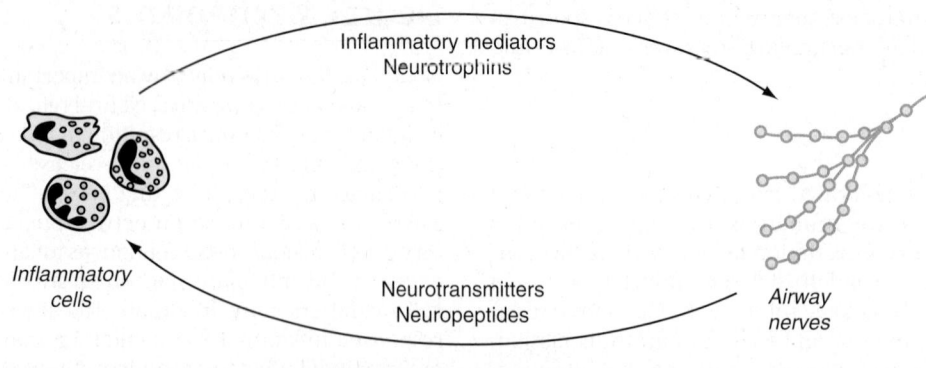

Fig. 7.12 Two-way interaction between inflammation and neural control of the airways.

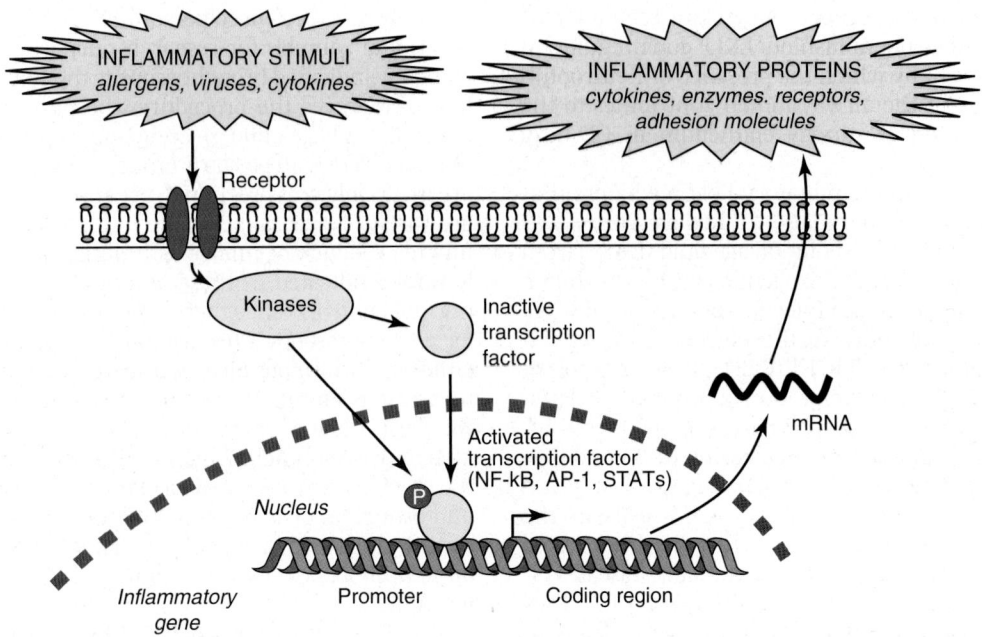

Fig. 7.13 Proinflammatory transcription factors in asthma. Transcription factors play a key role in amplifying and perpetuating the inflammatory response in asthma. Transcription factors, including nuclear factor kappa-B (*NF-κB*), activator protein-1 (*AP*-1), and signal transduction-activated transcription factors *(STATs)*, are activated by inflammatory stimuli and increase the expression of multiple inflammatory genes.

being developed, especially for asthma since these factors are upstream of the cytokines released from T helper cells. However, as they are intracellular factors, they cannot be targeted by antibodies. GATA-3 is considered the master regulator of type 2 immunity and therefore an ideal target for asthma. Development of a GATA-3-specific DNAzyme, a molecule class that combines the specificity of antisense molecules with an inherent RNA-cleaving enzymatic activity, has recently moved from preclinical development toward a proof-of-concept clinical study.[136] The differentiation of Th1 cells is regulated by the transcription factor T-bet, and the differentiation of Th17 cells is regulated by Ror-γT.[137,138]

Antiinflammatory Mechanisms

Although most emphasis has been placed on inflammatory mechanisms, there may be important antiinflammatory mechanisms that may be defective in asthma, resulting in increased inflammatory responses in the airways.[139] Endogenous cortisol may be important as a regulator of the allergic inflammatory response, and nocturnal exacerbation of asthma may be related to the circadian fall in plasma cortisol. The blockade of endogenous cortisol secretion by metyrapone results in an increase in the late response to allergen in the skin. Cortisol is converted to the inactive cortisone metabolite by the enzyme 11β-hydroxysteroid dehydrogenase, which is expressed in airway tissues. The molecular apparatus that underpins circadian variations, controlled by so called 'clock' genes, has recently been characterized. Clock genes control circadian rhythms both centrally, in the brain and peripherally, within every organ of the body. It has therefore been proposed that the peripheral lung clock and the peripheral immune clock might relate to both the pathogenesis and treatment of asthma.[140]

Various cytokines have antiinflammatory actions. IL-1 receptor antagonist (IL-1RA) inhibits the binding of IL-1 to its receptors and therefore has a potential antiinflammatory capability in asthma, and it is reported to be effective in an animal model of asthma. IL-12 and IFN-γ enhance Th1 cells and inhibit Th2 cells. IL-12 promotes the differentiation and thus the suppression of Th2 cells, resulting in a reduction in eosinophilic inflammation, and its expression may be reduced in asthmatic airways.

IL-10, which was originally described as cytokine synthesis inhibitory factor, inhibits the expression of multiple inflammatory cytokines (TNF-α, IL-1β, GM-CSF) and chemokines, as well as inflammatory enzymes (iNOS, COX-2). There is evidence that IL-10 secretion and gene transcription are defective in macrophages and monocytes from asthmatic patients; this may lead to enhancement of inflammatory effects in asthma and may be a determinant of asthma severity.[141] IL-10 secretion is lower in monocytes from patients with severe asthma compared to mild asthma, and there is an association between haplotypes associated with decreased production and severe asthma.

Another family of molecules of potential interest is the lung Kruppel-like transcription factor (LKLF) family of proteins. LKLF plays a pivotal role in maintenance of T-lymphocyte quiescence,[12] which this is of interest in view of our recent findings of increased T cells in the CF airway.[142] A recent manuscript showed that LKLF suppresses *P. aeruginosa*–induced activation of NF-κB and subsequent IL-8 release from airway cells, but, in turn, its expression was inhibited by the proinflammatory cytokine TNF-α.[12] There was evidence that LKLF is abundantly present in normal small airway human tissue sections, but the signal lessens as inflammation worsens, and the presence of activated human neutrophils "switches off" LKLF in airway epithelial cells. This suggests a counter-inflammatory role for LKLF in airway epithelium and provides evidence for cytokine regulation of LKLF in a TNF-α–dependent fashion. LKLF downregulation may be a mechanism by which the presence of neutrophil-secreted cytokines in the airway lumen contributes to the continuous activation of airway epithelium in CF lung disease.

Lipoxins (LX) are antiinflammatory lipid mediators that modulate neutrophilic inflammation.[13] Reduced LXA$_4$ was first described in broncho-alveolar lavage fluid (BALF) from CF patients; in a mouse model, exogenous LXA$_4$ was shown to abrogate inflammation and infection and reduce disease severity.[143] Recent studies have further elucidated the regulation of this mediator.[14] Resolvin E1 (RvE1), which is a potent inhibitor of neutrophil transmigration across epithelial and endothelial barriers, has been shown to promote the resolution of airway inflammation by suppressing IL-23 and IL-6 production in the lung. This is of particular interest, given that IL-23 promotes the survival of T$_H$-17 cells in the airway.[144] These cells secrete IL-17A, which has been linked to the pathogenesis of a number of inflammatory diseases,[145] and has been found in BALF from children with CF.[146] Furthermore, administration of antibodies to IFN-γ leads to increased BALF leukocytosis, which was abrogated by coadministration of RvE.[147] So far, there is little, if any, evidence for a role of this axis in CF or other pediatric inflammatory lung diseases.

The docosohexanoic acid prostaglandin D (PD)1-derived mediator is one of the arachidonic acid–derived family of mediators that terminates inflammation, along with LXA$_4$ and its epimer aspirin-triggered LXA$_4$, and RvE1 (see earlier, derived from eicosopentanoic acid). A murine peritonitis model was used to demonstrate that inhibition of COX-2 or lipoxygenases leads to a defect of resolution of inflammation, which could be rescued by RvE1, PD1, or an aspirin-triggered LPX$_4$ analog.[148] No airway data have been reported, but this is another potential mechanism of resolution of inflammation that merits further investigation.

Other mediators may also have antiinflammatory and immunosuppressive effects. PGE$_2$ has inhibitory effects on macrophages, epithelial cells, and eosinophils; and exogenous PGE$_2$ inhibits allergen-induced airway responses. In addition, its endogenous generation may account for the refractory period after exercise challenge. However, it is unlikely that endogenous PGE$_2$ is important in most asthmatics, since nonselective COX-2 inhibitors only worsen asthma in a minority of patients (aspirin-induced asthma). Several other lipid mediators, including lipoxins, resolvins, and protectins, promote resolution of inflammation and may be reduced in asthma patients.[116]

Direct Measurements of Airway Inflammation

There are far fewer bronchoscopic studies in children than in adults. This in part relates to ethics; any invasive procedure must be clinically indicated and of direct benefit to the individual child. Neither parents nor children can consent to an invasive procedure that is of no direct benefit to the child. It has been shown that bronchoscopy, bronchoalveolar lavage, and endobronchial biopsy are safe in school-aged children with severe asthma, preschool children with severe wheezing, and children of all ages with cystic fibrosis when performed

carefully by experienced personnel.[149–152] It is ethical to take additional samples for research purposes at the time of a clinically indicated bronchoscopy if the Institutional Review Board approves the procedure, the parents give informed consent, and the child gives age-appropriate assent.[153] The main problem with pediatric bronchoscopic studies is that they are invariably cross-sectional, because serial bronchoscopies are rarely, if ever, appropriate in children. Other problems include the lack of milder asthmatics, since bronchoscopy is rarely indicated in these children, and the lack of true normal controls, since there is no nonrespiratory indication for a bronchoscopy. This last issue is addressed by studying children with upper airway disease; hemoptysis, for which no cause is found; or chronic cough unrelated to asthma. However, none of these controls is completely suitable. An alternative approach, which is also completely ethical with the previous caveats, is to do a blind nonbronchoscopic lavage and bronchial brushings in children who are intubated for routine pediatric surgery.[154,155] This is the only way that large numbers of normal or mildly asthmatic children can be studied.

There are several advantages of lower airway samples that are obtained directly by bronchoscopy: ability to obtain endobronchial biopsies (Fig. 7.14), which are the only way of assessing airway wall structural changes; no current samples obtained noninvasively, or even nonbronchoscopically will allow an assessment of remodeling. This is important, as it is increasingly recognized that the structural airway cells such as smooth muscle, vessels, and collagen have key immunological as well as functional roles in airways diseases. In addition, we know that the pattern of inflammation in the airway wall may be very different to that in the airway lumen, and importantly, the specific pattern of inflammation within airway wall structures may have functional implications. Examples of this are the presence of mast cells within airway smooth muscle as a characteristic feature of AHR in asthma[156] and the presence of neutrophils in the epithelium as a subphenotype of severe childhood asthma.[77] However, nonbronchoscopic sampling does offer the opportunity to obtain

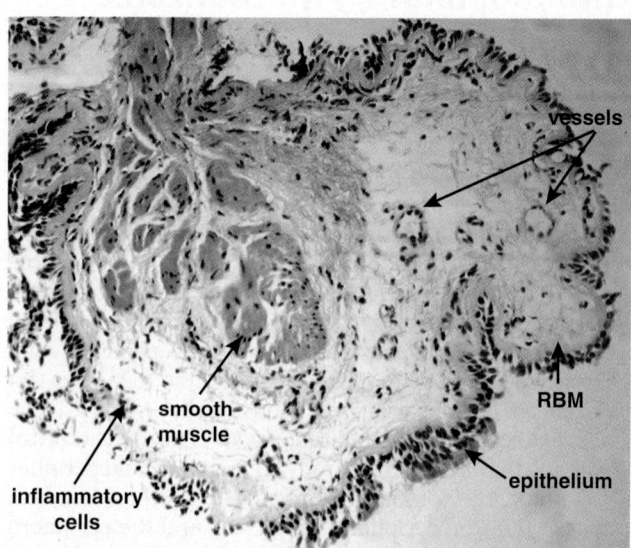

Fig. 7.14 Endobronchial biopsy from a child with asthma stained with hematoxylin and eosin. *RBM*, Reticular basement membrane.

Traditional culture methods

Novel 'lung on a chip' methods incorporating microfluidic chanber, endothelial cells and inflammatory cells

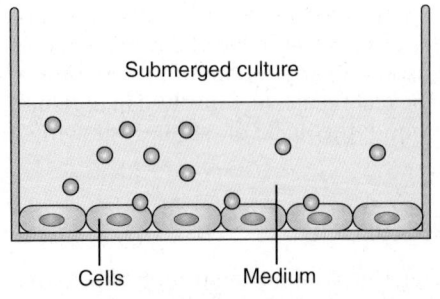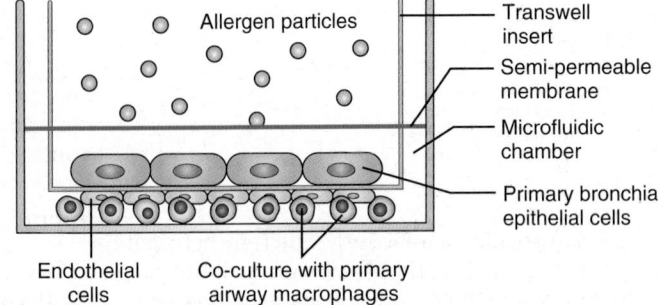

Fig. 7.15 Complex epithelial *in vitro* culture techniques to allow optimal assessments of airway cell function. The culture of cells at an air-liquid interface and the addition of a microfluidic chamber allow dynamic movement to mimic blood flow, and the addition of inflammatory cells with epithelial cells allows optimal reflection of the dynamics of the airways and an opportunity to investigate mechanisms in vitro.

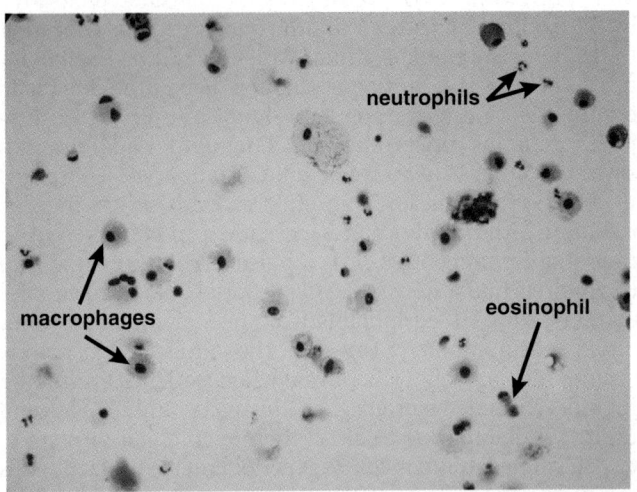

Fig. 7.16 Broncho-alveolar lavage fluid cytospin showing airway luminal leukocytes.

epithelial cells that can be cultured in vitro and stimulated with allergen, infection, or pollutants to investigate altered function in disease compared to controls. More recently, complex and realistic cultures that have an interface with basal endothelial cells, an apical airway lumen, and cocultures with leukocytes, representing a "lung on a chip" have been developed; and these represent significant advances for investigation of "in vivo" responses more closely using "in vitro" techniques (Fig. 7.15).[157–160]

In addition to a difference between inflammatory cell patterns in the airway wall and airway lumen, it is known that inflammation may be very different in the upper compared to the lower airways, and upper airway samples (which can be obtained noninvasively) do not reflect the lower airways. Therefore bronchoalveolar lavage samples are important, as they can be used to obtain both inflammatory cells, which can be phenotyped and quantified using cytology (Fig. 7.16) or flow cytometry, and the supernatants can be used to measure inflammatory cytokines. However, there has always been a question relating to the reliability of mediators measured in broncho-alveolar lavage (BAL) because of the variability that may be introduced by dilution of the lavage fluid.

An important advance in this area has been the recent introduction of techniques to sample the mucosal lining fluid of the airways directly using absorptive materials, such as a synthetic absorptive matrix.[161] This technique allows the collection of concentrated mucosal lining fluid and, using multiplex cytokine assays that allow the measurement of up to 20 cytokines from a small volume, enables a detailed characterization of airway inflammatory mediators.[162]

This novel technique has been used to collect samples of the nasal mucosal lining fluid in infants to detect inflammatory mediators and has been used to collect bronchial mucosal lining fluid from adult patients with asthma, but it has not yet been used to compare inflammatory mediators from the upper and lower airways from the same patients. This information would be very helpful in determining the utility of nasal mucosal lining fluid as a surrogate for lower airway inflammation, with the advantage of being able to collect samples longitudinally from the same patient.

Noninvasive Assessment of Airway Inflammation

Inflammation plays a key role in the pathophysiology of airway diseases, and suppression of this inflammation is a major aim of therapy. This implies that the degree of inflammation should be assessed during clinical management,[163] while physiologic measurements, such as spirometry, only reflect inflammation indirectly. Furthermore, spirometry is a notoriously poor asthma endpoint in children,[164–166] and treatment with bronchodilators makes changes difficult to interpret. Direct measurement of inflammation by bronchial biopsy or bronchoalveolar lavage is valuable in research studies, but it is clearly inappropriate for routine assessment and for repeated measurements, especially in children. This means that less invasive procedures for assessing airway inflammation need to be devised.

The characteristics of the ideal "inflammometer" are shown in Table 7.1. Unfortunately, no such instrument exists. There are two broad reasons for wishing to measure airway inflammation: to study the mechanisms of disease and as a clinical tool to monitor treatment in an individual. Unfortunately, the two are frequently confused. The finding that levels of

Table 7.1   Characteristics of the Ideal "Inflammometer"

Cheap
Easy to maintain and calibrate
Completely noninvasive
Easy to use, no cooperation needed
Directly measures all relevant aspects of inflammation
Provides rapid availability of answers
Evidence of beneficial clinical outcomes
Provides reliable longitudinal assessments

a mediator are statistically significantly different between groups may lead to valuable pathophysiologic insights, but if the overlap between asthma and normal groups is considerable, measuring the mediator is likely to be of little value as a monitoring tool in clinical practice. This is illustrated by measurements of exhaled and nasal NO in PCD; exhaled nasal NO is lower in PCD than in normal groups, but the overlap means that it cannot be used as a diagnostic tool; on the other hand, a low nasal NO almost completely differentiated PCD from normal.[167] Biomarkers for asthma have been identified from a variety of sources, including airway, exhaled breath, and blood. Biomarkers from exhaled breath include fractional exhaled NO, and the measurement of which can help identify patients most likely to benefit from inhaled corticosteroids and targeted antiimmunoglobulin E therapy. Biomarkers measured in blood are relatively noninvasive and technically more straightforward than those measured from exhaled breath or directly from the airway.[168] The use of biomarkers can therefore potentially help to identify patients and avoid inappropriate therapies; if used correctly, it may allow the development of an individualized approach to treatment.

INDUCED SPUTUM

Sputum may be induced by nebulized hypertonic saline (3.5% or 7%) for analysis of inflammatory cells and mediators. This technique has been applied successfully to children; however, it is difficult to use in clinical practice, and up to 25% of children do not produce a useable sample.[169] However, sputum induction can be performed safely in children with severe asthma.[170] More recently, the technique has been adapted for use in younger, preschool children. Although sputum induction can be performed safely and repeatedly in preschool children, the samples can only reliably be used to assess airway infection and not inflammation.[171] In addition, the procedure can be uncomfortable and requires significant technical expertise in terms of reliable processing and analysis. Sputum induction has proven to be a useful research technique in investigating airway inflammation in children. Initially, samples were assessed by simple cytology, but more recently, it has been shown that detailed inflammatory phenotyping can be undertaken using flow cytometry, and even rare populations such as innate lymphoid cells can be quantified.[172] Sputum measures proximal luminal inflammation but relates poorly to airway wall pathology and distal inflammatory changes. One study showed that the absence of eosinophils in induced sputum was predictive of a successful taper of inhaled steroids.[173] Another study[174] showed that a strategy of adjusting treatment to try to normalize induced sputum eosinophils measured every 3 months in

children with severe asthma was not beneficial compared with a standard strategy. In addition, a *post hoc* analysis showed a reduction in exacerbations in the month immediately following the measurement.[174] Currently, there is insufficient evidence to recommend the routine use of induced sputum to assess airway inflammation in clinical practice because of the technical issues involved in obtaining samples in children and the lack of studies showing improved outcome.[175]

PERIPHERAL BLOOD

The increasing use of monoclonal antibodies to treat patients with eosinophilic asthma, specifically, anti-IL-5 antibody has shown the potential of peripheral blood eosinophils as a noninvasive surrogate for airway inflammation. However, this has only been shown convincingly in adult studies, since clinical trials with the antibody have only been undertaken in adult patients. However, it is apparent, that a blood eosinophil count $>0.3 \times 10^9$ eosinophils/L is considered elevated in the context of asthma and has been used as a marker to define eosinophilic asthma, which would be eligible for a trial of anti-IL-5 antibody therapy. The cutoff for blood eosinophils that corresponds to significant airway eosinophilia remains uncertain in school-aged children with severe asthma. When airway inflammation was compared to blood eosinophil levels in children with severe therapy resistant asthma who had been shown to be adherent to their maintenance high-dose inhaled steroids, the majority of children had a normal age-appropriate blood eosinophil count ($<0.1 \times 10^9$ eosinophils/L) despite having a persistent airway eosinophilia.[176] However, the cutoff for high blood eosinophils is likely to be lower when patients are taking high dose inhaled steroids, and this value and its potential utility as a biomarker to direct therapy in children is yet to be determined. It is possible that peripheral blood eosinophils are more useful as a noninvasive biomarker to guide the utility of inhaled steroids in preschool children with wheeze in whom there is a good correlation between BAL and blood eosinophils.[171] In addition, a recent clinical trial showed that phenotyping with aeroallergen sensitization and blood eosinophils is useful for guiding treatment selection in preschool wheeze.[177]

EXHALED GASES

There has been considerable progress in the measurement of exhaled gases that may reflect the inflammatory process in the airways.[178] This technique is technically simple and is feasible, even in young children; and repeated measurements are possible and achievable in patients with severe disease.

Exhaled Nitric Oxide

The most progress has been made with NO, which can be detected in exhaled breath by chemiluminescence analyzers. The concentration of NO is increased in the exhaled breath of children (including infants) with asthma and decreases with inhaled corticosteroid therapy.[179] Recent evidence indicates that FeNO identifies T-helper cell type 2 (Th2)–mediated airway inflammation with a high positive and negative predictive value for identifying corticosteroid responsive airway inflammation.[180] In addition, using multiple flows, it is possible to partition exhaled NO into central and peripheral fractions; and this provides information about inflammation in central and peripheral airways.[181] Exhaled NO is correlated with other markers of inflammation such as eosinophils in induced sputum and AHR in children; however, the relationship is not a particularly close one. The correlation between NO and airway eosinophilia is closest in steroid-naïve children (the group in whom it is least likely to be useful). Longitudinal studies[174] show that even in the same individual, the relationship between NO and sputum eosinophilia varies over time, with a high NO sometimes seen with a normal sputum eosinophil count, and vice versa.

There is some evidence that NO measurement may be useful in pediatric asthma. It may predict exacerbations in pollen-sensitive asthma[182] and may be helpful in supporting a diagnosis in steroid naïve patients. Two recent studies showed no evidence of benefit in adding exhaled NO to standard monitoring.[183,184] This probably indicates that, if basic management is optimized, most children respond so well to low to moderate doses of asthma therapy that there is little opportunity to demonstrate additional benefit with NO measurements. Disappointingly, to date, there are no convincing data to show clinical utility of exhaled NO in guiding management of children with asthma.[185] It is apparent that exhaled NO is a steroid sensitive marker with potential clinical utility to demonstrate adherence to maintenance therapy. The exhaled NO suppression test demonstrated the distinction between adherent and nonadherent patients following a period of directly observed therapy.[186] Nonadherent patients had a greater reduction in exhaled NO after a period of directly observed therapy compared to patients who were adherent. Exhaled NO is paradoxically reduced in CF, which may reflect the high degree of oxidative stress and generation of superoxide anions that combine avidly with NO to form peroxynitrite, and high concentrations of which are detectable in CF airways. It is also reduced in PCD, which is generally characterized by a less severe airway disease than CF; and the mechanism of this reduction, and how it fits with the relative severity of airway disease, is still being studied.

Other Exhaled Gases

There are other exhaled volatile markers of inflammation, but these are less well characterized than NO. Exhaled carbon monoxide (CO) reflects the activation of heme oxygenase-1, an enzyme induced by stress. Concentrations of CO are increased in asthmatic children and children with CF; however, there is a large degree of overlap with values in normal children, and environmental factors interfere with the measurements, so it is less useful than exhaled NO. Ethane is formed by lipid peroxidation in response to oxidative stress, and levels are increased in asthma and CF, but this technique requires complex measurements by gas-chromatography/mass spectrometry (GC/MS), so it is not practical in clinical studies.[187,188] Breathomics incorporates the multidimensional molecular analysis of exhaled breath by combining analysis of exhaled breath with GC/MS with electronic noses (e-noses) and metabolomics of exhaled breath condensate (EBC). The latter is a noninvasive technique that provides information on the composition of airway lining fluid, generally by high-resolution nuclear magnetic resonance (NMR) spectroscopy or MS methods.[189] Exhaled breath contains multiple

hydrocarbons, and there is emerging evidence that these show different patterns in different diseases, reflecting the different components of inflammation; so each disease may have a unique "breathogram."[190,191] There are no studies to indicate that these measurements are useful in the clinical management of children.[175] An electronic nose (e-nose) is an artificial sensor system that consists of an array of chemical sensors for detection of volatile organic compound profiles (breathprints) and an algorithm for pattern recognition. They are handheld, portable devices that provide immediate results.[192] E-noses may discriminate between patients with different respiratory disease, including asthma, chronic obstructive pulmonary disease (COPD), and lung cancer, and healthy control subjects; e-nose breathprints are also associated with airway inflammation activity.[192] The pattern of volatile organic compounds has been shown to identify the presence of airway bacterial colonization in clinically stable patients with COPD.[193]

Exhaled Breath Condensate

Exhaled breath condensate (EBC) is formed through condensation of cooled exhaled breath and has been analyzed for a variety of mediators, including hydrogen peroxide, lipid mediators, purines, and cytokines.[194,195] Measurement of pH has shown differences between diseases,[196] but it is difficult to interpret these data because the hydrogen ion concentration differences seem unphysiological and do not correlate with direct measurements of airway surface pH at bronchoscopy.[197] Differences in the patterns of mediators are found between asthma and CF, reflecting the different inflammatory mediators in the respiratory tract. Exhaled 8-isoprostane is a useful measurement of oxidative stress, with increased concentrations in severe asthma and CF. The concentrations of mediators in EBC are low; therefore sensitive assays are needed and great attention must be paid to the collection procedure and the avoidance of salivary contamination. Innovative approaches in the future will include metabolomic analysis, in which multiple metabolites are monitored, giving unique patterns for each disease.[198] The term *metabolomics* refers to the quantitative analysis of sets of small compounds from biological samples with molecular masses less than 1 kDa that usually require sophisticated instrumentation. The practical success of clinical metabolomics hinges on a few key issues such as the ability to capture a readily available biofluid that can be analyzed to identify metabolite biomarkers with the required sensitivity and specificity in a cost-effective manner in a clinical setting.[199] A systematic review of adults with asthma has shown that concentrations of exhaled hydrogen ions, NO products, hydrogen peroxide, and 8-isoprostanes were generally elevated and corresponded to lower lung function tests in adults with asthma compared to healthy subjects, but longitudinal studies, using standardized analytical techniques for EBC collection, are required before the tool can be used reliably.[200] EBC has never been shown to be a useful clinical tool in pediatric chest disease. A thorough review of the utility of breath biomarkers in pediatric airway diseases has shown several volatile organic compounds in exhaled breath with the potential to distinguish affected patients from healthy controls and to monitor treatment responses.[201] However, the lack of standardization of collection methods and analytical techniques hampers the introduction of these techniques to clinical practice. The measurement of metabolomic profiles may have important advantages over single markers, but this remains at very early stages. Furthermore, there is a lack of longitudinal studies and external validation to reveal whether exhaled breath and EBC analysis have benefit in the diagnostic process and follow-up of children with respiratory diseases. In conclusion, the use of volatile organic compounds and biomarkers in EBC for evaluation of inflammatory airway diseases in children remains a research tool, but it is not validated for clinical use.[201]

Is AHR an Inflammatory Surrogate?

The first adult study to suggest that something more than standard monitoring improved asthma outcomes used AHR measurement over a 2-year period and demonstrated that a strategy aimed at normalizing AHR led to a greater use of inhaled corticosteroid and improved asthma outcomes.[202] There is one such pediatric study, which showed minor evidence of benefit using an AHR strategy.[203] This is not likely to be a clinically useful strategy; the measurements are time-consuming, and there are only loose relationships between inflammation and AHR[204] and between changes in AHR and changes in inflammation.[205,206]

Other Potential Indirect Inflammatory Markers

There have been studies of blood and urine levels of various eosinophil proteins, but there is no evidence that their routine measurement in clinical practice is useful. Elevations in these proteins may be due to an extrapulmonary atopic disease, such as eczema or rhinoconjunctivitis, leading to a lack of specificity.

Is There a Role for Assessing Inflammation in Pediatric Respiratory Disease?

Despite a profusion of research papers, no single set of guidelines has made an evidence-based recommendation that inflammometry should be a routine clinical tool.[207] This may be due in part to a false perception that measurement of an inflammatory marker will mean perfect sensitivity and specificity, with no need to make any other measurement. It is interesting to compare the expectations of inflammatory markers compared to what spirometry has delivered. No one would suggest abandoning spirometry, a routine measurement in every good asthma clinic, but spirometry is rarely diagnostic of asthma, correlates poorly with disease severity, and is a poor endpoint in clinical trials. It is likely that, as with spirometry, measurement of airway inflammation will find a role as part of the assessment process.

There is no gold-standard diagnostic test for asthma. Many different physiologic measurements of airway caliber and responsiveness can be made; in general, they have poor sensitivity but reasonable specificity for the diagnosis. Most

clinicians would take the view that the more such tests are performed and the more that are negative, the more critically an alternative diagnosis should be sought. It may be that measurements of airway inflammation should be used in the same way.

In terms of monitoring asthma, it is clear that if the basics are right, most asthmatic children respond well to low-dose medications, and there is not likely to be a role for assessments of inflammation. Whether such assessments have a role in severe asthma is discussed in Chapter 46. However, just as reports of severe symptoms of asthma in conjunction with no evidence of AHR should lead to a suspicion of over reporting, perhaps the same will be true for those with reports of severe symptoms and no evidence of inflammation.

In summary, currently, there is no evidence that measurement of airway inflammation should be used routinely. There are hints of a possible role in the future, perhaps if it can be shown in children, as well as adults, that there are patients with discordance between inflammation and symptoms. Disappointingly, much more work is needed to determine which inflammatory markers should be measured, and in which children.

Therapeutic Implications

Inflammation is a key feature of asthma and CF, so antiinflammatory treatments should play an important role in therapy. Inhaled corticosteroids have become the first-line therapy for asthma in children, as low doses are usually sufficient to control asthma. However, in severe asthma, there is cellular and molecular resistance to the antiinflammatory effects of corticosteroids.[208] The inflammation in CF is also corticosteroid-resistant, and adverse effects have resulted from antiinflammatory therapy. Better understanding of the inflammatory mechanisms involved in severe asthma, and CF should lead to more effective therapies in the future.[209]

Conclusion

Airway inflammation is a critical component of many chronic airway diseases in children. The inflammatory response involves many different inflammatory cells that are recruited to and activated in the airways. Each of these cells releases multiple mediators, which then exert effects on the airway wall. In asthma, the major effects are bronchoconstriction, whereas in CF, the predominant response is mucus hypersecretion and airway wall destruction, ultimately leading to respiratory failure. Among the multiple mediators of inflammation, cytokines play an important role in orchestrating the inflammatory response and amplifying and perpetuating inflammation, whereas chemokines play a key role in selective recruitment of inflammatory cells to the airway. The molecular basis of inflammation is now understood better, with increased expression of multiple inflammatory genes, which are regulated by transcription factors. Endogenous antiinflammatory mechanisms counteract these effects, and there is some evidence that the mechanisms are defective in asthma, allowing inflammation to become more severe or to persist longer. This complex inflammatory process should be monitored in the management of airway disease, and there are several noninvasive approaches, including exhaled NO, and minimally invasive approaches such as sputum induction and assessment of the mucosal lining fluid, that look promising. Corticosteroids are highly effective in suppressing inflammation in asthma, but they are poorly effective in severe asthma and are ineffective in CF as the result of several corticosteroid-resistance mechanisms. Novel therapeutics that target the molecular mechanisms mediating inflammation in specific airway diseases should be pursued to allow effective reduction of proinflammatory pathways and promotion of regulatory or homeostatic pathways.

References

Access the reference list online at ExpertConsult.com.

8 Lung Defenses: Intrinsic, Innate, and Adaptive

KEELY GARRETT SMITH, MD, ANKUR A. KAMDAR, MD, and
JAMES M. STARK, MD, PhD

Intrinsic Lung Defenses

Intrinsic defenses arise from the very structure of the conducting airways and the lung surfaces. The anatomy of the airways and airflow properties of the lung remove particles due to impaction or settling. Once they interact with the airway surface, these particles can elicit reflexes to remove them from the airway (sneezing or cough).

AERODYNAMIC FILTERING

The anatomy of the upper and lower airways contributes to the defense of the lungs against infection. The nose provides the initial filtration and humidification of inspired air because of its structure and surface area. Very large particles are filtered by the nasal hairs, and particles larger than 10 μm impact on the surfaces of the turbinates and septum.[1] Impaction is facilitated by the inertia of large particles that have a high linear velocity and do not easily change direction to follow air flow. The tonsils and adenoids are strategically located to deal with larger soluble particles by specific local defenses. If the tonsils and adenoids are markedly enlarged, nasal resistance increases. This potentially results in mouth breathing, bypassing the nasal anatomic defenses. Edema of the turbinates from viral infections or allergies may produce similar effects. Hydrophilic particles are enlarged by humidification of the inspired air, and this facilitates their impaction in the upper airways.

Particles between 2 and 10 μm are removed from the air flow by impaction on the walls of the branching airways beyond the nose, and by sedimentation. Sedimentation occurs because the increasing cross-sectional area of the conducting airways leads to a decrease in the linear air flow velocity such that gravitational forces may act on the particles. Smaller particles (as small as 0.2 μm) may not sediment at all and are exhaled. Particles in the size range of 0.2 to 2 μm generally penetrate the airways and can be deposited in the alveoli.[2] Aerosol devices and metered-dose inhalers use particle size to direct deposition of the medication to different levels of the airway. Deposition of particles can trigger local inflammatory responses in the lung and airway reflexes.

HUMIDIFICATION

Warming and humidification begins at the nose and continues distally. Ultimately, inspired air is warmed to body temperature (37°C) and 100% relative humidity. Adequate hydration of airway mucus is essential to its proper functioning. The upper airway receives some humidity from convection of warm, humidified alveolar gas. During exhalation, the temperature drops and condensation forms on the upper airways, keeping their surfaces wet. At the isothermal saturation boundary (the point where air becomes body temperature) air is at 100% relative humidity that remains constant as it continues to move distally. This point typically occurs below the carina and will shift, depending on ambient temperature, humidity, and volume and rate of air exchange. It will also shift distally when the upper airway is bypassed, such as by tracheostomy. It never drops to the level of the respiratory bronchioles, so that at functional residual capacity (FRC), inspired gas is at body temperature and 100% humidity in the normal airway.[3]

AIRWAY REFLEXES

Sneezing, bronchoconstriction, and coughing are airway reflexes that act as nonspecific host defenses. Sneezing is a forceful expulsion of air that is triggered by receptors in the nose and nasopharynx and is effective in clearing the upper pharynx and nose. The mechanisms are similar to coughing (http://thekidshouldseethis.com/post/85595081892). Bronchoconstriction may prevent entry of particles into the distal airways by decreasing airway caliber and redirecting air flow away from the irritated airways. However, it also leads to increased pulmonary resistance, decreasing air velocity in the peripheral airways, and thus, increasing the likelihood of sedimentation. Coughing is a forceful expulsion of air from the lungs that is under both voluntary and involuntary control (https://curiosity.com/paths/cough-grosser-than-sneeze-curiosity-worlds-dirtiest-man-discovery/#cough-grosser-than-sneeze-curiosity-worlds-dirtiest-man-discovery). There are at least nine sensory receptors in the bronchopulmonary system located within the epithelium of the pharynx, larynx, trachea, and the bifurcations of the major bronchi. At least five of these are involved in the cough reflex, including the unmyelinated C fibers and the myelinated irritant receptors containing substance P and calcitonin-gene–related peptide (CGRP).[4] These receptors can be stimulated by inflammatory mediators, chemical irritants, osmotic stimuli, and mechanical stimulation. Stimulation of respiratory afferents results in cognitive awareness of breathing and the urge to cough. The transient receptor potential (TRP) class of ion channels expressed on sensory neurons have recently been implicated in perception of noxious stimuli that lead to cough.[5] The reflex of cough is initiated by stimulation of afferent fibers leading to the vagus nerve that connect to the cough center in the medulla oblongata and conscious awareness in the suprapontine brain. Efferent fibers transmit stimuli along the vagus nerve and spinal cord to the larynx, diaphragm, chest wall, and abdominal muscles to produce cough.

After the cough, a feedback loop occurs to determine if the cough relieved the stimulation to cough. The cognitive urge to cough is an integration of respiratory afferents, respiratory motor system, affective state, attention, learning, and experience.[6]

THE MECHANICS OF COUGH AND ABNORMALITIES IN THE COUGH REFLEX

Six phases of cough create high air flow velocities that produce the shear forces required to clear mucus from the airway walls and to promote its expulsion through the larynx.[7]

1. *Irritation phase*—cough triggered by stimulation of the irritant receptors in the tracheobronchial tree
2. *Inspiratory phase*—initiated by a deep breath, which is usually 1.5 to 2 times the tidal volume. Air enters the airway distal to secretions. The length-tension relationships of the respiratory muscles are increased and optimized for contraction, elastic recoil potential increases, and the bronchi dilate.
3. *Glottic closure*—necessary to build pressure for subsequent phases of cough
4. *Compression phase*—begins with closure of the larynx and is followed by contraction of the intercostal muscles and abdominal musculature, which rapidly leads to increased intrathoracic pressure (up to $300 \text{ cm } H_2O$ or more in normal adults). This phase is fast, lasting approximately 200 msec.
5. *Expulsive phase*—initiated when the glottis opens and high air flows are achieved. Following the glottic opening, the airways may collapse by as much as 80% in tracheal cross-sectional area, which further increases the velocity of exhaled gas (approaching 25,000 cm/sec the speed of sound) shearing mucus from the airway walls. The cough may be interrupted by a series of glottic closures, each with its own compressive and expulsive phases. These "spikes" in flow (flow transients) can improve cough effectiveness by increasing the shear forces. In patients with significant tracheomalacia, the equal pressure point may be quite proximal and limit cough effectiveness. Efforts to move this point distally (e.g., positive expiratory pressure device at the mouth) improve cough effectiveness.
6. *Relaxation phase*—characterized by a decrease in intrathoracic pressure associated with relaxation of the intercostal and abdominal muscles.

Abnormalities of the cough mechanism can result in an ineffective cough. Cough receptors are not present in the alveoli or lung parenchyma, and therefore coughing can be absent in children with extensive alveolar disease or consolidation. A decrease in the sensitivity of the cough center occurs in obtunded patients and individuals under the influence of opiates. The efferent nerves can be affected by poliomyelitis or infantile botulism. The muscular force needed to generate the cough can be decreased by neuromuscular diseases such as spinal muscular atrophy or muscular dystrophy. Laryngeal disorders such as vocal cord paralysis or the presence of a tracheostomy tube prevent laryngeal closure so that the cough can lose its explosive quality. The use of cough-assist devices may be useful in enhancing airway clearance.[8,9]

Innate Lung Defenses

Innate immunity provides immediate defense against a wide variety of pathogens or noxious substances without previous exposure to them. Innate immunity can remove infectious agents from the airway by binding and trapping them for removal (mucus and mucociliary clearance). Several PRRs recognize conserved patterns of molecular structures on pathogens (pathogen associated molecular patterns, PAMPs). Engagement of PRRs can activate cascades of intracellular signals producing inflammatory cytokines and chemokines that recruit and activate effector cells. Innate PRRs and receptor proteins facilitate cellular adhesion, and activation of soluble bactericidal factors such as complement. Secreted proteins contribute to innate lung defenses (e.g., the collectins and antibiotic proteins). There are resident innate immune cells that function as "first responders" to infection (dendritic cells [DC], macrophages, and mast cells). These "first responders" not only fight infection, but also produce mediators that recruit "early responders" from the circulation. These defenses protect the lung before adaptive immune processes can develop.

MUCUS AND AIRWAY SURFACE LIQUID

Mucus and mucociliary clearance are essential components of innate mechanical defenses in the lungs. Airway mucus is a complex network of mucins, electrolytes, enzymes, and protein defenses that immobilize, destroy, and remove noxious particles, foreign bodies, and invading microorganisms from the airway. It is the first line of innate defense in the lung.[10,11]

The airways between the larynx and the respiratory bronchioles are lined by ciliated columnar epithelium and covered by an airway surface liquid (ASL) layer that is 5 to 100 μm thick. Mucus provides several important airway defense functions: It (1) provides a covering sheet that entraps particulate matter and microorganisms; (2) is a movable medium that can be propelled by cilia (the tips of cilia drive the mucus gel layer toward the oropharynx); (3) provides a waterproofing layer that acts to reduce fluid loss through the airways; (4) detoxifies noxious inhaled irritants; and (5) transports essential secreted substances such as enzymes, defensins, collectins, antiproteases, and immunoglobulins (discussed later).

ASL consists of two distinct layers: the low-viscosity periciliary gel layer (PCL) adjacent to the epithelial surface, and the mucus layer that floats on the PCL. The viscoelastic mucus layer is composed of secreted mucus glycoproteins (termed mucins) in addition to several secreted products. These mucins have high molecular weight, are long (0.5 to 20 μm), and are highly glycosylated and branched. MUC5AC and MUC5B are the major mucins in the mucus layer. Studies in gene knockout mice demonstrate that MUC5AC and MUC5B play distinct and important roles in airway homeostasis. The PCL is made up of the tethered surface mucins (MUC1 [MUCIN 1, cell surface associated], MUC4 [MUCIN 4, cell surface associated], MUC16 [MUCIN 16, cell surface associated], MUC20 [MUCIN 20, cell surface associated]) and is approximately the height of the cilia (7 μm). These tethered mucins provide a brushlike network that prevents penetration of inhaled particles and organisms to the epithelial surface. The PCL layer is crucial because it provides a low-viscosity fluid in which the cilia can beat rapidly (8 to 20 Hz), moving the more viscous mucus layer over it and shielding the epithelial surface from the substances trapped in the overlying mucus layer. The diversity of the carbohydrate side chains of the mucin macromolecules provides a library of carbohydrate sequences that can bind to an enormous repertoire of particles that land on the mucus layer.[10–12]

The properties of this mucin gel are the product of the mucin and water contents, concentrations of monovalent and divalent ions, and the pH of the ASL. The water content of ASL is controlled by regulating levels of ion transport in the PCL layer via chloride channels (cystic fibrosis transmembrane conductance regulator [CFTR] and a calcium-activated [alternative] chloride channel), and the epithelial sodium channel (ENaC).[11,13] These channels control Na^+ reabsorption and Cl^- secretion by the respiratory epithelial cell via energy dependent mechanisms, with passive movement of water across the epithelial membrane in response to ion transport. There is active sensing of the mucus depth and viscosity by the underlying epithelium through cilia interaction with the overlying mucus. Increase in the "strain" on ciliary movement is transmitted through the cilial shaft, resulting in release of adenosine triphosphate (ATP) from the epithelial cell. The extracellular ATP activates purinoreceptors that inhibit sodium reabsorption through ENAC and accelerate Cl^- secretion through CFTR and the calcium activated channel, resulting in a net fluid secretion onto the airway surface.[11] The mucin concentration in the PCL is greater than that of the mucus layer, resulting in a higher osmotic pressure in the PCL (~ 500 Pa) compared to that of the mucus layer (~ 100 Pa). This difference in osmotic pressures makes the overlying mucus layer a "reservoir" for fluid in the airway and helps maintain the depth of the PCL layer.[11] Inflammation can result in the deposition of large macromolecules such as DNA and polymerized actin from white cells, proteoglycans, biofilms, and other combinations of bacteria and inflammatory cells that can significantly increase the viscosity of the mucus. This increased viscosity of the overlying mucus layer increases its osmotic pressure, resulting in the equilibration of the osmotic pressures of the mucus and PCL layers and potential depletion of the PCL, eventually resulting in in the "collapse" of the ASL and loss of normal ciliary function.

Ciliary beat frequency and the effectiveness of the ciliary beat are the primary determinants of the mucus clearance rate. Ciliary motion is broken down into two steps: a unidirectional power stroke that sweeps forward and a recovery phase in which the cilia bend backward and extend to their starting position. Ciliary movement occurs within the same plane so that the movement is forward and backward without any lateral movement.[14] Cilia also impart a vertical motion within the mucus layer, mixing particles, bacteria, and other pathogens into the mucus and facilitating their clearance. The lubricating effect of the mucous layer on the surface of the PCL allows the cilia to propel the overlying mucus layer with ease.

DISORDERS OF THE MUCOCILIARY SYSTEM

Primary ciliary dyskinesia (PCD) is a genetic disease associated with defective ciliary structure and function, with resultant chronic oto-sino-pulmonary disease, male infertility, and (in about half of patients) *situs inversus.* Cilia are complex structures composed of a highly organized array of microtubules and accessory elements, including inner and outer dynein arms, radial spokes, and nexin links (see Chapter 71). Disruption of this structural organization has been associated with ciliary immotility or dysmotility. Measurements of mucociliary clearance in patients with PCD have revealed no basal, cilia-dependent mucus clearance, although cough-dependent clearance is nearly normal. These patients maintain a nearly normal mucus clearance rate by increasing the dependence on cough. As a result, these patients exhibit milder airway disease than seen in cystic fibrosis (CF) and typically live into middle age and beyond. However, bronchiectasis and obstructive airway disease may occur in preschool children.

CF results from mutations in the respiratory epithelial inducible chloride channel (CFTR; see Chapters 49 to 53). In people with CF, mucus transport appears to be significantly altered by depletion of ASL and pH and electrolyte alterations that result from mutations in CFTR. Resulting defects in Na^+ and Cl^- transport result in volume depletion on the airway surfaces which, in turn, depletes the PCL, disrupts normal ciliary activity, and inhibits mucociliary clearance.[13]

ADHESION PROTEINS

Adhesion and migration of circulating inflammatory cells (or their progenitors) are integral to cell recruitment and activation response to injury (Fig. 8.1).[15,16] Three major families of adhesion molecules participate in these processes in the lung: the immunoglobulin superfamily, the integrins, and the selectins.

The immunoglobulin superfamily is a group of polypeptide genes characterized by the presence of one or more regions homologous to the basic structural unit of the immunoglobulin gene. Immunoglobulins and the T cell receptors (TCRs) are the only members of this family that undergo somatic diversification for antigen recognition (adaptive immunity). Several members of this family are required for cell-cell adhesion and migration of leukocytes from the vascular space into the airway.[17,18] Moreover, they are required for adaptive immune responses (antigen presentation to T cells by DC and macrophages).

The integrins are a diverse family of molecules that are involved in cell-substrate or cell-cell interactions. The integrins are composed of two noncovalently associated polypeptide chains (α and β). In humans, there are 18 α and 8 β subunits that form 24 different heterodimers.[19] Subgroups of this family are defined by common, shared $\beta 1$ chains. $\beta 1$ integrins function primarily by interacting with matrix components (collagen, laminin, fibronectin). Very Late Antigen 4 (VLA4, $\alpha 4\beta 1$) is expressed by lymphocytes and monocytes. The $\beta 2$ integrins (heterodimers of CD11 and CD18) are expressed almost exclusively on leukocytes and mediate cell-cell adhesion.[16] Upon binding their extracellular ligands, integrins transmit signals that regulate various cellular functions (see Fig. 8.1).[16] Integrins are critical for maintaining endothelial integrity, repair of damaged cells, and regulation of cell differentiation and proliferation.[19] The importance of the $\beta 2$ integrins in leukocyte recruitment is demonstrated in patients with leukocyte adhesion deficiency type 1 (LAD1),

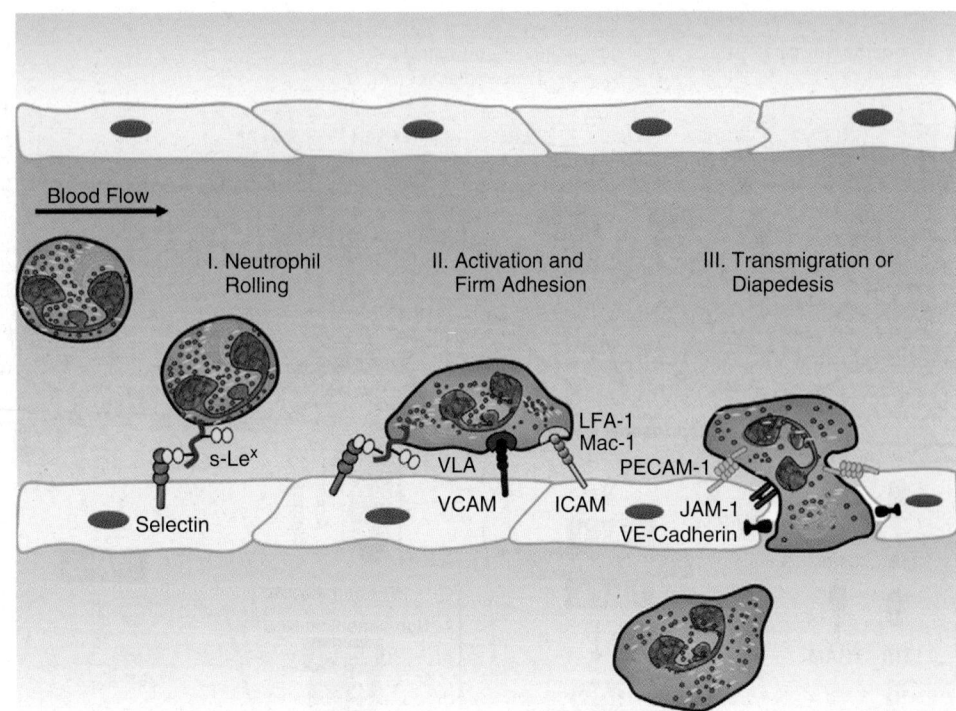

Fig. 8.1 Schematic process of neutrophil adhesion and transendothelial migration. In response to inflammatory stimuli, adhesion molecules such as selectins are upregulated on endothelial cells and neutrophils, and neutrophils roll along the vascular endothelial wall through selectin-mediated weak interactions (I). This is followed by firm adhesion of neutrophils to endothelium through binding of integrins (LFA-1, CD11a/CD18; Mac-1, CD11b/CD18; p150,95) on the neutrophil surface to ICAM-1 or VCAM-1 on the endothelial cell surface through VLA-4 (II). Subsequently, neutrophils transmigrate through the microvascular endothelium via a process involving complex interactions with endothelial cell-cell junction molecules, including VE-cadherin, JAM-1s, and PECAM-1 (III). (Reprinted with permission from Yuan SY, Shen Q, Rigor RR, Wu MH. Neutrophil transmigration, focal adhesion kinase and endothelial barrier function. *Microvasc Res.* 2012;83[1]:82-88.)

as characterized by recurrent bacterial skin and soft-tissue infections, diminished pus formation, and impaired wound healing.[20]

Selectins are glycoproteins rich in O-linked and N-linked carbohydrates that mediate adhesion between leukocytes and vascular endothelium (see Fig. 8.1).[21] The N-terminal ends of these molecules function as calcium-dependent carbohydrate lectin molecules.[16] Three selectins have been identified: E-selectin (ELAM-1 [endothelial leukocyte adhesion molecule-1]), P-selectin, and L-selectin (LECAM-1 [leukocyte-endothelial cell adhesion molecule]). E-selectin is expressed on endothelial cells following stimulation by cytokines (such as IL-1 or tumor necrosis factor-α) and supports neutrophil adhesion. L-selectin is expressed on all leukocytes and is shed following adhesion to endothelial cells. P-selectin mediates cellular adhesion of neutrophils and monocytes to activated platelets and endothelial cells.

PATTERN-RECOGNITION RECEPTORS IN LUNG INNATE IMMUNITY

The innate immune system utilizes a wide repertoire of conserved membrane-associated or soluble PRRs able to identify pathogens or cellular injury and initiate host defenses. These include the Toll-like receptors (TLR), nucleotide-binding leucine-rich repeat (LRR) containing receptors (NLR), retinoic acid-inducible gene 1 (RIG-1)-like receptors (RLR), C-type lectins (CTLs), and absent-in-melanoma (AIM)-like receptors (ALR). This pattern recognition receptor (PRR) recognizes patterns of sugars, ribonucleic acid (RNA), and deoxyribonucleic acid (DNA) as PAMPs that function as danger-associated molecular patterns (DAMPs). Through interactions with various cellular signaling cascades, they initiate and modulate inflammation, detect metabolic changes in the cell or cell death, and develop adaptive immune responses.

Toll-Like Receptors

The TLRs are a highly conserved family of membrane-associated PRR that have been identified in plants, insects (drosophila), and animals (mouse, human). They have two functional regions. The extracellular domain recognizes an array of microbial components: sugars, proteins, lipids, DNA motifs, and double-stranded RNA. The intracellular region contains a Toll/IL-1 receptor (TIR) domain that provides an intracellular scaffold interacting with a number of "adapter" proteins to initiate and integrate signaling cascades that result in cellular activation and the production of several cytokines and chemokines (Fig. 8.2).[22] Ten TLRs have been described in humans, and they are expressed by cell types involved in both innate immune defenses (such as macrophages, neutrophils, and airway epithelial cells) and adaptive immunity (macrophages, DC and lymphocytes). Ligands have been identified for all but TLR10 (see Fig. 8.2). The TLRs can be located in the plasma membrane (TLR1, TLR2, TLR4, TLR 5, TLR6, and TLR10) or intracellularly (TLR3, TLR7, TLR8, TLR9; see Fig. 8.2). The TLR proteins can associate as homodimers or as heterodimers of different TLR proteins thereby extending the target repertoire. The TLRs can also utilize a variety of coreceptor molecules. For example, TLR2 and TLR4 interact with MD-2 (soluble extracellular protein) and CD14 in binding to LPS. Several other PRR can cooperate with TLR in response to pathogens.[23,24]

The TIR domains of the TLR interact with intracellular adaptor proteins (MYD88 or TIR-domain-containing adapter-inducing interferon-β [TRIF]+TRAM), resulting in activation of transcription factors that lead to the expression of cytokines or interferons (see Fig. 8.2).[25] In addition, activation of TLR has been implicated in the upregulation of microbial killing mechanisms such as production of nitric oxide (NO). TLR signaling in DC drive T cell differentiation into T-helper type 1 (Th1) or T-helper type 2 (Th2) phenotypes. Thus,

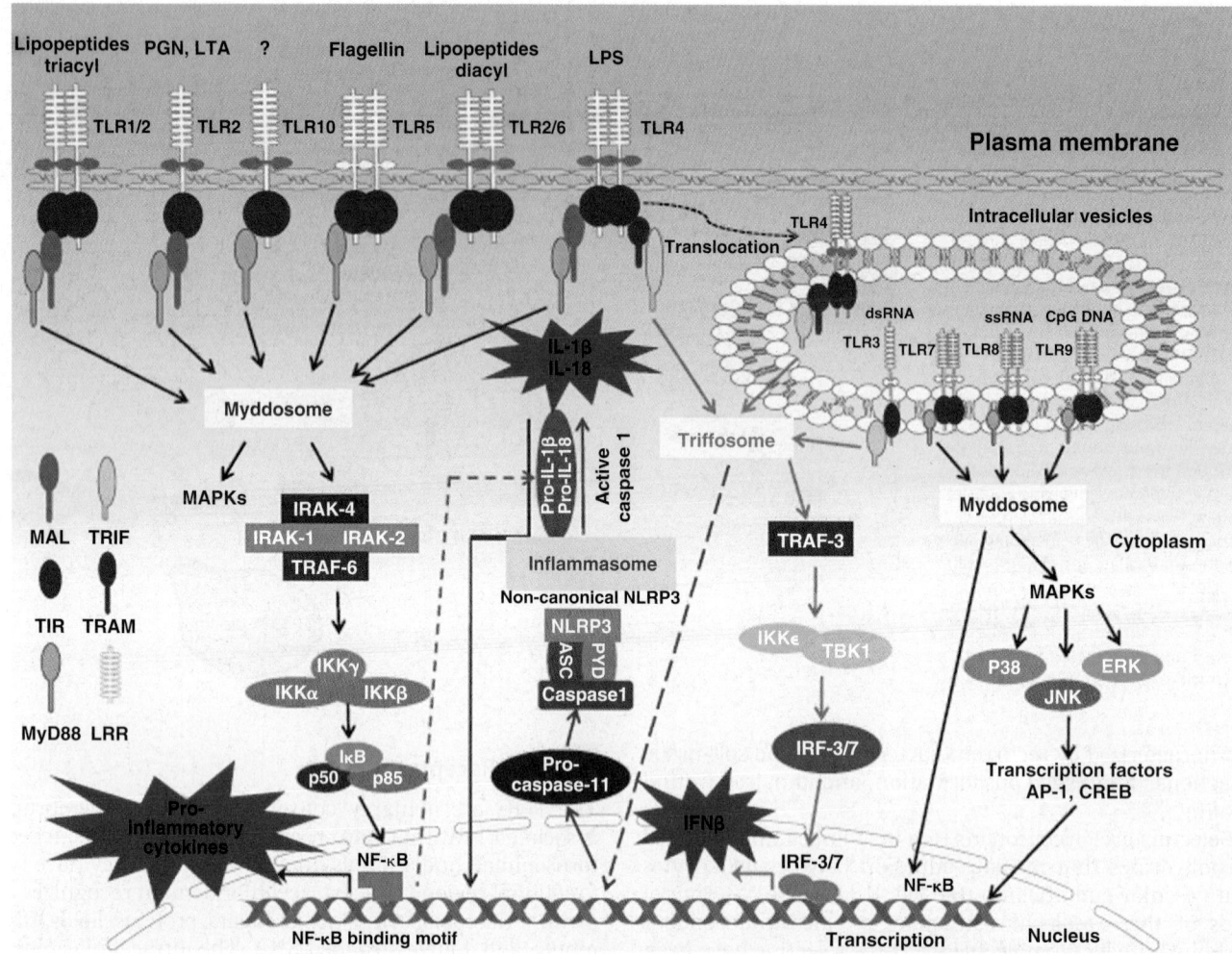

Fig. 8.2 Toll-like receptor (TLR) pathways: receptors, ligands, and signaling. All TLR contain the extracellular tandem repeats of leucine-rich regions (LRR) that are responsible for the binding to different ligands. The cytoplasmic Toll/interleukin (IL)-1 receptor domain (TIR) interacts with adaptors including MyD88, MAL, TRIF, and TRAM. Ligand binding triggers the dimerization of surface TLR, followed by the assembly of "Myddosome" complexes that activate MAPK or NF-κB signaling, which, in turn, induce transcriptionally the production of proinflammatory cytokines. Intracellular TLR or internalized TLR4 dimers initiate the assembly of "Triffosome" complexes for subsequent activation of interferon (IFN)-regulatory factors (IRF). TLR are also involved in the priming and activation of inflammasomes that promote the proteolytic cleavage and activation of inflammatory cytokines. *AP-1*, Activator protein 1; *CREB*, cAMP response element-binding protein; *ERK*, extracellular signal-regulated kinase; *IFN*, interferon; *IKK*, nuclear factor kappa-B kinase subunit; *IL*, interleukin; *IRAK4*, IL-1 receptor-associated kinase 4; *IRF*, IFN-regulatory factor; *JNK*, c-Jun N-terminal kinase; *LPS*, lipopolysaccharide; *LTA*, lipoteichoic acid; *MyD88*, myeloid differentiation primary response gene; *MAL*, MyD88-adaptor-like protein; *MAPK*, mitogen-activated protein kinases; *NF*, nuclear factor; *NF-κB*, transcription factor nuclear factor kappa-light chain-enhancer of activated B cells; *NLRP3*, NOD-, LRR-, and pyrin domain-containing 3; *PDN*, peptidoglycan; *ss/dsRNA*, single/double-stranded RNA; *TBK1*, TRAF family member-associated NF-κB activator-binding kinase 1; *TRAF*, tumor necrosis factor receptor-associated factor; *TRAM*, TRIF-related adaptor molecule; *TRIF*, TIR domain-containing adaptor protein inducing interferon-β. (Reprinted with permission from Wang Y, Song E, Bai B, Vanhoutte PM. Toll-like receptors mediating vascular malfunction: Lessons from receptor subtypes. *Pharmacol Ther.* 2016;158:91-100.)

TLR activation interfaces both innate and adaptive immune responses.[23,24]

C-Type Lectin Receptors

CTL receptors are membrane associated PRR that can bind either carbohydrate and noncarbohydrate (lipid or protein) ligands through a conserved CTL-like domain. They are expressed primarily on myeloid cells where they function in antifungal immunity.[26]

Nodlike Receptors

The nodlike receptors (NLR) are a family of cytosolic PRR that participates in cellular inflammatory responses, apoptosis

(programmed cell death), formation of phagosomes, and transcriptional activation of major histocompatibility complex proteins (MHC). These proteins are expressed in many cell types, including immune cells and epithelial cells. There are 22 members of the NLR family in humans.[27,28] Their general structure includes a central nucleotide-binding oligomerization (NOD) domain and a C-terminal LRR domain. The N-terminal effector region varies between the different proteins, resulting in activation of diverse downstream signaling pathways. The NLR receptors participate in signal transduction, autophagy, transcriptional activation, and inflammasome assembly (see Fig. 8.2). NOD1 and NOD2 activate Rip2 kinase, leading to activation of NFκB. The

NOD-like receptor pyrin domain (NLRP) family can lead to the assembly of inflammasomes, which consist of one or two NLRs, an adapter molecule ASC (inflammasome adaptor protein apoptosis-associated speck-like protein containing CARD), and caspase 1, that participate in caspase-1-mediated cell death and post translational production of mature IL-1β and related cytokines (including IL-18; see Fig. 8.2).[25] NOD2 interacts with bacteria at the cell entry site and initiates autophagosome formation. CIITA (class II, MHC, transactivator) and NLRC5 (NLR family, CARD Domain Containing 5) are transactivators of the MHC in the nucleus.[27]

RIG-Like Receptors

RIG-like receptors (RLRs) are cytoplasmic RNA helicases that recognize nonself RNA motifs. RIG-1 binds to 5′ tri and diphosphates present on short double stranded (ds) RNA, whereas MDA5 binds to long dsRNA molecules. Both helicases signal through the downstream adaptor MAVS (mitochondrial antiviral signaling) activating the IRF3/7-dependent production of type 1 interferons and NFκB-mediated production of proinflammatory cytokines.[29]

Absent-in-Melanoma-Like Receptors

ALRs are a small group of PRR that can interact with ASC to form inflammasomes activating caspase 1 resulting in production of IL-1 and IL-18 (see Fig. 8.2). These PRR interact with both bacterial and viral derived dsDNA and are located in both the cytoplasm and nucleus.[30]

SOLUBLE EXTRACELLULAR PATTERN-RECOGNITION PROTEINS

The soluble extracellular pattern-recognition proteins can be transfer from the bloodstream (complement, mannose binding lectin [MBL]) or secreted directly into the airway epithelium (surfactant proteins A and D) and provide innate defenses in the lung by carbohydrate recognition domains (CRDs). Several members of the collectins and ficolins activate complement.

Complement

Complement proteins play an important role in lung defenses. Complement components arrive in the lung both by extravasation due to vascular injury and leak and by local production by the respiratory epithelium and macrophages.[31] Complement activation occurs by three pathways (classical, lectin or alternative) and contributes to host defense through several mechanisms:

- opsonization by deposition of complement components on the pathogen surface
- activation of phagocytic cells by the local release of chemotactic agents (e.g., C5a)
- lysis of pathogens through the activation of the late components C5, C6, C7, C8, and C9
- generation of anaphylatoxins (C3a and C5a) that cause the release of vasoactive mediators from mast cells
- generation of C3b and C4 on cell surfaces that bind to receptors on phagocytic cells.[31]

Complement deficiency is associated with recurrent infections, glomerulonephritis, or collagen vascular diseases such as systemic lupus erythematosus.[32]

Collectins

The collectins are a family of collagenous, calcium-dependent (C-type) lectins, including MBL (mannose-binding lectin) and surfactant-associated proteins A and D (SP-A and SP-D, respectively). They have a key role as a first line of innate defense against invading microorganisms in the airway. Both SP-A and SP-D are secreted into the air spaces by alveolar type II cells and nonciliated bronchiolar cells. Selective binding of collectins to specific complex carbohydrates is mediated by the CRD and requires calcium. Human SP-A is assembled as heterotrimers or homotrimers of two genetically different chain types and forms hexamers of these trimeric subunits ($6 \times 3 = 18$ chains). SP-D is assembled as homotrimers that form tetramers ($4 \times 3 = 12$ chains).[33] This arrangement of subunits increases the binding affinity and specificity: multiple CRD domains can simultaneously bind to different ligands on a single polysaccharide chain, increasing the binding avidity of the complex. SP-A and SP-D interact with a variety of gram-negative and gram-positive organisms, fungi, and viruses including respiratory syncytial virus (RSV), Influenza A virus, and cytomegalovirus (CMV). Lung collectins can lead to opsonization through activation of complement and deposition of C3 (MBL) or can directly opsonize microorganisms (SP-A and SP-D), leading to phagocytosis and pathogen killing. SP-A binds to LPS and interacts with CD14 and TLR4, suggesting a role for SP-A in LPS-mediated cell responses. MBL is produced in the liver but is found in the lung at sites of inflammation. MBL is a serum protein, although small amounts of this protein have been found in lung secretions.

The ficolins are lectin recognition molecules that are structurally and functionally homologous to MBL. Three ficolins have been described. Ficolin-1 (M-ficolin) is expressed in the lung, monocytes, and spleen. Ficolin-2 (L-ficolin) is a serum protein expressed in the liver. Ficolin 3 (H-ficolin) is expressed in liver but also by bronchial and type II alveolar epithelial cells. They share the collagenous structure of MBL, but the CRD of MBL is replaced by a fibrinogen-like domain. They assemble in large multimeric structures of several hundred kilodaltons and recognize molecular patterns such as acetylated compounds and sugars. Similar to MBL, they activate complement through the lectin pathway.[34]

Antimicrobial Peptides

Several intrinsic microbiocidal and microbiostatic proteins are found in human respiratory secretions, including lysozyme, lactoferrin, secretory leukoprotease inhibitor (SLPI), and neutrophil and epithelial defensins.

Lysozyme is the one of the most abundant antimicrobial proteins in the airways with concentrations estimated at 0.1 to 1 mg/mL, which is sufficient to kill important pulmonary pathogens such as *S. aureus* and *P. aeruginosa*. Lysozyme damages the walls of bacteria and fungi by hydrolyzing β1–4 glycosidic bonds between N-acetylmuramic acid and N-acetylglucosamine, structural components of bacterial peptidoglycan and fungal chitin. In humans, lysozyme is secreted predominantly by the serous cells of submucosal glands in the conducting airways, and, to a lesser extent, by airway epithelial cells and alveolar macrophages (AM). It is also a component of both phagocytic and secretory granules of neutrophils.[35]

Lactoferrin is present in tears, saliva, and bronchial secretions. It is present in ASL at concentrations similar to lysozyme (0.1 to 1 mg/mL). It is produced by the submucosal glands and neutrophils and has activity against both gram-positive and gram-negative bacteria and *Candida* species. The antimicrobial actions of lactoferrin results from iron chelation (iron is required by many bacteria for optimal growth) or from destabilization of bacterial membranes.[36]

SLPI and elafin were originally described as protease inhibitors. They have subsequently been shown to have a wider range of biologic activities.[37] SLPI is an 11.9-kDA protein about 10-fold less abundant than lysozyme and lactoferrin in ASL. The N-terminal domain has modest activity against both gram-positive and gram-negative organisms. The C-terminal domain is an effective inhibitor of neutrophil elastase, cathepsin G, trypsin, chymotrypsin, tryptase, and chymase. Elafin/Trappin-2 is a 9.9-kDA protein that has a narrower spectrum of protease inhibition (only inhibiting neutrophil elastase and proteinase 3). In addition, the protease inhibitors exhibit antiinflammatory effects on NFκB activity and antimicrobial activity against a number of organisms, including *Staphylococcus aureus* and *Pseudomonas aeruginosa*. SLPI may also play a role in adaptive immunity through maintenance of mucosal tolerance.[37]

Human defensins are antimicrobial peptides (3 to 5 kDa) found in BAL fluid from noninflamed lungs at a concentration of about 100 ng/mL, but at increased levels in inflamed airways. Four human alpha defensins, (human neutrophil defensins 1-4, human neutrophil peptide [HNP]-1, HNP-2, HNP-3, and HNP-4) are found in neutrophil azurophilic granules. Four beta-defensin molecules have been described (hBD-1, hBD-2, hBD-3, and hBD-4). hBD1 is expressed constitutively by epithelial cells, while hBD2 to hBD4 are inducible. In addition to their antimicrobial effects, defensins help recruit inflammatory cells and promote both innate and adaptive immune responses.[38]

Cathelicidins are peptides produced by neutrophils and respiratory epithelial cells that have functions similar to those of defensins.[38] The human cathelicidin (LL-37) displays LPS-binding activity and broad-spectrum microbiocidal activity.

CELLULAR DEFENSES: AT THE CROSSROADS OF INNATE AND ADAPTIVE IMMUNITY

Our knowledge of the cellular constituents in the lung, their activation state, and their function has been considerably augmented by the flexible fiberoptic bronchoscopy and biopsy. Using bronchoalveolar lavage (BAL), the normal cellular constituents of the airway and alveolar space have been measured in both adults and children. In normal subjects, macrophages are the major cellular component of BAL, making up 81% to 95% of the cells; the remaining cells are lymphocytes, neutrophils, and eosinophils. The BAL cell number and percent composition vary greatly in disease states.[39] Data obtained from BAL and biopsy studies provide direct evidence of the role of inflammatory cells, adhesion molecules, and cellular mediators in humans, confirming findings in cell culture and animal studies.

The Respiratory Epithelium

The respiratory epithelium is a functional interface between the pathogen and the innate or adaptive immune responses,

making it a pivotal structure in respiratory physiology and pathology.[40] The respiratory epithelium participates in lung immunity in many different ways. The epithelium provides physical barrier to infection, lining the respiratory tract from the nose to the alveoli with a wide range of cell types.[41] Ciliated epithelial cells are important in propelling mucus up the airway, thereby removing particulate material. Ciliated cells line the respiratory tract down to the level of the respiratory bronchiole. Tracheobronchial glands and goblet cells are important sources of airway mucus, which serves to nonspecifically trap particulates. The respiratory epithelium also functions in the regulation of water and ion movement into the airway mucus.[40] It secretes SP-A and SP-D, lysozyme, lactoferrin, and antimicrobial peptides (β-defensins and cathelicidins),[42] and releases reactive oxygen and nitrogen species to kill invading pathogens.[43] The respiratory epithelium can produce a number of bioactive cytokines that recruit and activate inflammatory cells in the lung (interferon [IFN]-α, IFN-γ, IL-1, TNF-α, IL-8, RANTES [Regulated on Activation, Normal T Cell Expressed and Secreted]). The respiratory epithelium influences adaptive immunity through cytokine release: fostering a Th2-like response through release of IL-25, IL-33, and TSLP (thymic stromal lymphopoietin). The epithelium promotes recruitment and activation of DC and lymphocytes (CCL20) and mast cells (stem cell factor [SCF], IL-33, TSLP release). The respiratory epithelium also acts as its own reservoir for injury repair. Finally, the epithelium promotes remodeling through release of transforming growth factor-beta (TGF-β). It is therefore a key modulator of lung defense, lung injury, and repair.[40,43]

Resident Cell Defenses: At the Interface of Innate and Adaptive Immunity

Three major groups of inflammatory cells reside primarily within the lung parenchyma itself: DC, macrophages, and mast cells. The cells (particularly the macrophages and DC) are capable of migration; however, they reside primarily within the lung itself. Other inflammatory cells are recruited from the circulation in their mature form (neutrophils, eosinophils, and lymphocytes) and become activated in the lung. The pulmonary DC and macrophages participate in both innate and adaptive immune responses in the lung.[44]

Dendritic Cells. DC are the primary resident antigen-presenting cells in the lung and airway.[44] Activation of DC in response to innate stimuli is essential to initiate the adaptive response to antigens. In these processes, the phenotype and function of DC play an important role in initiating adaptive immune responses (tolerance, memory, and polarized Th1 and Th2 differentiation). Antigen presentation to T cells is actively and tightly regulated *in vivo* by soluble factors produced by mature tissue macrophages. Therefore, the phenotype of the DC, the response to innate stimuli and cytokines produced by macrophages, and the lung microenvironment play important roles in determining host adaptive responses.[45]

In humans, three different subsets of DC (2 "myeloid" and one "plasmacytoid") have been described: mDC1 (expressing BDCA1/CD1c), mDC2 (BDCA3/CD141), and pDC (BDCA2/CD123). The origin of human DC is not completely understood, but they appear to arise from common granulocyte/

macrophage and multilymphoid progenitors in the bone marrow.[44] DCs have a rapid half-life in the conducting airways (about 2 days), whereas more distal lung DCs have a slower turnover rate. mDC1 cells have been associated with induction of CD8+ and CD4+ Th1 responses, whereas mDC2 cells are associated with CD4+Th2 and Th17 responses, although there is some overlap.[45,46] pDC have been ascribed an antiviral role, although in the steady state, their main role appears to be induction of tolerance.[45] mDC are associated with the airways and appear to "sample" the airway by extending dendrites through the airway epithelial layer. pDC locate mainly in the alveolar interstitium. However, they have the ability to migrate to inflammatory foci, where they can take up and process antigen, migrate through the lymphatics to the draining lymph nodes, and associate with T cell–rich areas to initiate adaptive immune responses.

Macrophages. The pulmonary macrophages are central regulators of airway inflammation. They exhibit mobility, phagocytosis, receptor expression for signal recognition, and production and release of a number of bioactive mediators. In the lung, they are capable of scavenging particulates, removing macromolecules, killing microorganisms, recruiting and activating other inflammatory cells, maintaining and repairing injured tissue, removing apoptotic cells, and modulating normal lung physiology.[45,47,48] Many of these functions are "turned off" in the resting state but are upregulated with macrophage activation. Therefore, regulation of macrophage activation and turnover is important in determining pulmonary health or disease.[47,48] Macrophages can cooperate with other cell types (DC, neutrophils, lymphocytes, fibroblasts) by direct cell–cell interactions and by cytokine signals to orchestrate development of cell-mediated immunity and humoral immunity.[44,47] (https://www.youtube.com/watch?v=LwLYGTS_3EI). Macrophages are more abundant in the distal respiratory tract, particularly the alveolus, than in the tracheobronchial tree. The macrophage population is usually constant in size, but this is the result of a dynamic steady state of cellular recruitment, cell division, and cell turnover. At least two types of macrophages reside in the lungs: interstitial macrophages (IM) and AM. The macrophages populating the airways above the alveolus are thought to arise from those in the alveolus. IM are in the interstitial space between alveolae where they interact with DC and interstitial lymphocytes. They promote tolerance and prevent Th2 mediated airway inflammation. The IM are thought to be derived from circulating precursor peripheral blood cells of the monocyte/macrophage lineage.[44]

AM, along with the epithelium, are the first line of defense against infection. They are mobile, traveling between the alveoli and sampling the alveolar surface.[47,49] They are phagocytic and express numerous PRR that trigger expression of cytokines, chemokines, and other reactive products (lipids, reactive oxygen, and nitrogen species) that are crucial in control of infection through the innate immune system and balance of proinflammatory and antiinflammatory pathways in the lung. The AM are classified according to their activation status as M1 or M2. M1 macrophages (also termed classically activated macrophages) respond to IFN-γ, LPS, and TNFα to produce proinflammatory cytokines leading to the destruction of intracellular pathogens and promoting a Th1 environment. M2 (alternatively activated macrophages) are characterized by their participation in Th2 responses. The switch to M1 or M2 phenotype is associated with the specific transcriptional response to the local microenvironment.

AM are thought to arise from yolk sac macrophages or fetal liver monocytes that enter the lung during embryonic development and colonize the alveoli in the first days after birth. AM mature under the influence of local production of CSF-2 (GM-CSF). This population of early progenitors populates the lung and self-maintains throughout the host's lifetime.[44,48] Under inflammatory conditions, some AM may arise from mononuclear cells, but these more resemble the IM in function. The turnover time for AM has been calculated to be 21 to 28 days in animal models. At the end of this time, they exit from the lungs up the mucociliary escalator, although the mechanisms for this efflux are still unknown.

AM produce a number of reactive oxygen metabolites and nitrogen metabolites and a large diverse array of enzymes (acid hydrolases, neutral hydrolases, and lysozymes) capable of killing bacteria. AM also produce cytokines and chemotactic factors that play a central role in phagocyte recruitment and activation, wound healing, fibrosis, and modulation of actions of other innate and adaptive immune responses in the lung.[47,48]

Mast Cells. Mast cells are the major effector cells of allergic reactions. They are distributed in tissues throughout the body in close proximity to blood vessels and do not circulate in the blood. It has been postulated that they play roles in host defense against parasites, wound healing, immunoregulation, and tumor angiogenesis. Mast cells originate in the bone marrow from granulocyte and monocyte pluripotent CD34+ and CD117+ stem cells. Homing to specific tissues is driven by active local recruitment. Growth and survival of mast cells requires stem cell factor (SCF) production by structural cells (epithelial cells, fibroblasts, endothelial cells, smooth muscle cells). SCF promotes proliferation and differentiation, chemotaxis, and suppression of apoptosis that promotes mast cell growth, recruitment, and survival.[50] Mature differentiated mast cells are capable of proliferation. Therefore, tissue-specific increases in mast cell numbers can occur by either recruitment or local proliferation.

Mast cells can express a wide variety of receptors that allow them to detect intracellular and extracellular signals and interact with other inflammatory cells and with the extracellular matrix. Ligand binding and activation of the FcεRI results in release of a number of bioactive products responsible for allergic reactions.

Mast cells participate in antigen presentation and interactions with other immune cells via costimulatory molecules or secreted products that can enhance or suppress the development of innate or adaptive immune functions.[50,51] There is strong evidence that mast cells play significant roles in atopic and nonatopic asthma, pulmonary fibrosis, pulmonary hypertension, and may contribute to acute respiratory distress syndrome (ARDS). Persistent activation of mast cells can also exacerbate Th2-dependent or autoimmune disorders.[50,51]

Recruited Cellular Defenses

All recruited pulmonary inflammatory cells are initially derived from bone marrow precursors and arrive from the pulmonary circulation in their mature, active forms. In the process of recruitment, these cells move from a "quiescent" resting state to a state in which they are fully "activated" or "primed" for further cellular activities.

Neutrophils. Neutrophils are characterized by their multilobed nucleus and distinctive cytoplasmic granules that contain an arsenal of enzymes and proteins. Neutrophils constitute about half the circulating white blood cell population, and their primary function is phagocytosis and killing of invading pathogens. In order for the neutrophil to accomplish this, it must respond to signals in the area of injury, adhere and transmigrate through the vascular endothelium, migrate to the area of infection, recognize the pathogen, phagocytose, and kill it. Interruption of any of these steps will leave the host susceptible to infections. Patients with leukocyte adherence deficiency (LAD) are unable to recruit neutrophils into sites of inflammation, and, as a result, they sustain recurrent, life-threatening infections. In chronic granulomatous disease (CGD), the neutrophils lack components of the nicotinamide adenine dinucleotide phosphate hydrogen (NADPH) oxidase system, and affected neutrophils that have engulfed organisms cannot efficiently kill them. The processes of neutrophil recruitment and activation, followed by neutrophil removal (cell death, or apoptosis) after the resolution of the infectious process or injury, are closely regulated at several levels. Disruption of these regulatory processes can lead to acute or ongoing lung injury.[52]

Neutrophils are short-lived cells; their life span from stem cell differentiation to removal in the tissues is 12 to 14 days. CD34+ myeloid progenitor cells in the bone marrow produce myeloblasts, which then differentiate through several recognizable morphologic stages into mature, nondividing polymorphonuclear neutrophils. It normally takes about 14 days for the neutrophil precursor to mature and be released into the blood.[53] Once in the circulation, neutrophil half-life is quite short (~6 to 7 hours). The pulmonary capillary bed is unique in its ability to "concentrate" neutrophils. The term *margination* has been proposed to describe this increased concentration of neutrophils in noninflamed lungs. Margination is proposed to result from discordance between the diameter of neutrophils (6 to 8 μm) and the capillary segments (2 to 15 μm), increasing the pulmonary capillary transit time. This is postulated to allow neutrophils time to sense and respond to the presence of inflammatory processes.[53] In response to inflammatory stimuli, neutrophils accumulate in preparation for migration (see Fig. 8.1). In much of the systemic circulation, neutrophil sequestration occurs in postcapillary venules in the form of rolling and is mediated by selectins. In the pulmonary capillary, inflammatory mediators alter the mechanical properties of the neutrophils, resulting in changes in deformability and "stiffening" that reduces the neutrophil deformability, lengthens the capillary transit time, or stops the movement of the neutrophil altogether at the sites of inflammation.[53] Once sequestration has occurred, the neutrophils can adhere via selectin or CD11/CD18-intercellular adhesion molecule-1 (ICAM-1) and migrate across the vascular endothelium (see Fig. 8.1). During migration into the lung, the neutrophils become activated, resulting in a change in surface receptors compared to blood neutrophils.[54] The migration and activation of neutrophils requires a number of products of the endothelium, epithelium, and AM including IL-1β, TNF-α,

IL-6, IL-8/KC, macrophage inflammatory protein (MIP)-1α, MIP-1β, MIP-2, CCL2, G-CSF, and LTB4. Once the neutrophil has migrated into the tissue, its primary purpose is to recognize, ingest, and destroy pathogens.

Similar to the resident innate cellular defenses, neutrophils express numerous PRR and respond by production of reactive oxygen species and secretion of azurophilic granule contents (myeloperoxidase, elastase, defensins), specific granule contents (lactoferrin, cathelicidins), gelatinase granule contents (lysozyme) and the formation of neutrophil extracellular traps (NETs).[49,55] NETs are weblike structures composed of dsDNA, histones, antimicrobial peptides, and proteases ejected by neutrophils to ensnare microbes in a sticky matrix of extracellular chromatin and antimicrobial peptides, making the microbes more vulnerable to phagocytosis and clearance.[56] (https://www.youtube.com/watch?v=TIFmtnSdolM). Overexuberant neutrophil activity can contribute to ARDS and to tissue destruction in autoimmune diseases.[55,56] There are data supporting a role for neutrophils in wound healing and homeostasis.[57]

Eosinophils. Eosinophils are usually the second largest group of granulocytic cells in the circulation. They can be morphologically distinguished from neutrophils by their ability to be stained by negatively charged dyes, such as eosin. They are 8 μm in diameter and typically have two nuclear lobes. Eosinophils arise from bone marrow precursor cells under the influence of a number of cytokines including IL-3, IL-4, IL-5, IL-14, and GM-CSF. IL-4 and IL-13 stimulate IgE production and promote eosinophil recruitment by increasing expression of eotaxin and endothelial cell vascular cell adhesion molecule 1 (VCAM1). IL-5 mediates eosinophil production and egress from the bone marrow, eosinophil activation, and survival.[58] The migration of eosinophils from the bone marrow takes about 3.5 days after DNA synthesis has completed. In the blood, the half-time of an eosinophil is ~18 hours. Similar to neutrophils, there appears to be a marginated pool of eosinophils, which are in dynamic equilibrium with the circulating pool. Eosinophils marginate and emigrate into the tissues through postcapillary venules. Eosinophils, but not neutrophils, adhere to the ligand vascular cell adhesion molecule (VCAM)-1 on the endothelial surface and once adherent, can be attracted by a specific array of chemotactic agents into the lung. Eosinophils express the receptor CCR3 that binds eosinophil specific chemokines including eotaxin (CCL11) eotaxin-2, monocyte chemoattractant protein (MCP)-3, MCP-4, and RANTES (CCL5). Eosinophil recruitment into the lungs occurs under the influence of Th2 mediated inflammation. Once present in the lungs, eosinophils degranulate and release a number of granular components including major basic protein (MBP), eosinophil peroxidase (EPO), eosinophil cationic protein (ECP), and eosinophil-derived neurotoxin (EDN); as well as cytokines and chemokines. Some of these cytokines promote eosinophil survival and activation. In addition, eosinophils can undergo extracellular trap cell death (ETosis) and release extracellular traps similar to those released by neutrophils. The eosinophil traps bind eosinophil granules as intact structures, unlike the traps formed by neutrophils.[59] Collectively, these eosinophil products have potent activity that implicates the eosinophil in the control of parasitic diseases. However, these proteins also have activities that are associated with the pathogenesis of a number of pulmonary disorders. Asthma is by far and away the most common eosinophil-associated lung disease in children. The pathophysiology of asthma results from contributions from a number of inflammatory cells including eosinophils, mast cells, neutrophils, and T lymphocytes.[58] In addition to asthma, eosinophils contribute to the development of a number of eosinophilic pneumonias (see Chapter 65). These can be roughly divided into primary eosinophilic pneumonias (eosinophilic granulomatosis with polyangiitis, idiopathic acute eosinophilic pneumonia, idiopathic chronic eosinophilic pneumonia) and secondary pneumonias (pneumonia in response to parasitic worms, allergic bronchopulmonary aspergillosis, drug reactions).[60]

Innate Lymphocytes: Innate Lymphocyte Cells and Natural Killer Cells. Over the past decade, there has been strong interest in newly described subsets of lymphocytes referred to as innate lymphocyte cells (ILCs). There are currently three groups of ILC (ILC1, 2, 3) characterized by cytokine products and transcription requirements for maturation. They display a wide variety of effector functions that contribute to defense against pathogens, to lymph node development, and to tissue remodeling. Given the ongoing research to further characterize ILCs, a full discussion is beyond the scope of this chapter, and the focus will be directed to NK cells, which comprise part of the ILC1 subset.

Natural killer (NK) cells are large granular lymphocytes that are key players in early immunity along with other cells involved in the innate immune system, including neutrophils, monocytes, and mast cells. At first, they were recognized in having cytotoxicity against tumor cells and virus-infected cells. Over the past four decades, their role has been well established in a variety of functions, including cytokine production and interaction with other immune cells to promote immune system homeostasis.[61] Although they were traditionally considered part of the innate immunity, there is a significant amount of evidence to support NK cells having a role in adaptive immunity (below). NK cells have been shown to respond to their local environment by indirectly modulating T cell effector and antigen presenting cell function, and forming immunologic memory, which are hallmarks of adaptive immunity.

Derived from the bone marrow, NK cells are characterized by CD56. Peripheral NK cells can be further divided into two subsets; CD56^{bright} and CD56^{dim}. CD56^{bright}, which are more predominant in serum, are known to be more responsive to soluble factors, while CD56^{dim}, which are more abundant in tissue, respond better to cell surface ligands.[62] NK cells lack a TCR/CD3 complex, and represent approximately 2% to 18% of the total lymphocyte population circulating in the blood. NK cells can initiate natural cytotoxicity via release of perforin and granzyme granules. Perforin results in pore formation on the target cell, which allows entrance of granzyme that induces apoptosis. In addition, their effector functions (enhancing cytotoxicity, inducing cytokine secretion, modulating immune homeostasis) are largely exerted by the wide and diverse number of activating and inhibitory receptors expressed on the NK cell surface. Binding of antibody to CD16 (FcγR III) on the NK cell surface induces antibody-dependent cell-mediated cytotoxicity. The natural killer cell receptors (NCR), can bind to a stressed cell, caused by infection or cellular damage. These stressed cells express ligands that the NK cell can bind to and subsequently induce cell lysis. There are several receptors that bind proinflammatory cytokines, which stimulate NK cells to respond to infection, proliferate, and promote further cytokine secretion.

Inhibitory receptors will downregulate NK cell function. Killer cell immunoglobulin like receptors (KIR) are MHC class I inhibitory receptors, and when bound to self MHC molecules, they ensure tolerance to self, preventing damage to healthy cells.

Recently, there has been a better understanding of the tissue bound NK cells, particularly in the mucosa, including uterus, and lung. These "nonconventional" NK cells are unique NK cells with varying phenotypic properties. With their proximity to the epithelia, they express unique receptors to enhance protection against the external environment as well as to provide homeostasis to prevent an exuberant inflammatory response.[62–66]

Adaptive Lung Defenses

Most pathogens gain entry to the lung across mucosal surfaces. An important aspect of inflammatory and immune responses to the entry of respiratory pathogens is the ability to mount an appropriate, regulated immune response that can clear the infection rapidly and efficiently but not expose the surrounding tissues or the whole host to chronic inflammation. Innate immunity provides the first level of protection. Adaptive or specific immunity provides specific responses to antigens during acute infection and provides specific immune memory that protects in the event of reexposure. A number of cell types contribute to airway mucosal defense, as discussed earlier in the chapter. As part of the mucosal surface from the nasal airway to the conducting airways, the bronchial-associated lymphoid tissue (BALT) functions in the development of adaptive lung defense. The BALT is made up of intraepithelial lymphocytes, macrophages, DC, NK, and natural killer T cells (NKT) cells that recognize foreign substances, invading organisms or their exoproducts, and products of cell injury using their receptor systems. The DC or macrophages interact with lymphocytes to create the cellular immune responses, or to signal antibody production. These cells migrate to local lymph nodes, tonsils, or adenoids; process antigens; generate cytokines; and generate the adaptive immune responses. While extensive reviews of humoral (B cell mediated) and cellular (T cell mediated) immunity, antigen presentation, and cellular activation are well beyond the scope of this chapter, we will briefly discuss the roles of humoral and cellular immunity with respect to lung defense.

BRIDGING THE ADAPTIVE AND INNATE DEFENSES

NKT cells are heterogeneous group of T cells that express a unique set of cellular receptors. They owe their name due to the coexpression of receptors typically found on NK and conventional T cells that likely contribute to their activation and regulation. NKT cells are characterized by Cd1 restriction. Cd1 is a MHC class I like molecule that presents lipid antigens as opposed to peptides. Activation of the NKT cells subsequently leads to rapid release of Th1 or Th2 cytokines.

NKT cells function primarily to provide protective immunity against a variety of pathogens, regulate autoimmunity, and support natural immunity against tumor development.

Invariant natural killer T (iNKT) cells are a subset of NKT cells that express an invariant TCRα chain and a limited TCRβ chain. By recognizing foreign lipid antigens via CD1d restriction, they can contribute to defense against pathogens in a quick manner. After activation, they rapidly secrete cytokines and chemokines, including IFNγ, IL-4, and IL-17, to stimulate immune cells downstream. After their rapid innate effector functions, they can perform adaptive functions as well via activation of antigen-presenting cell (APC). The APC, in turn, upregulate expression of lipid antigens recognized by the iNKT cells, which bind to the APC. The iNKT cells are then stimulated to secrete cytokines that activate NK cells, leading to enhanced antigen presentation to MHC-restricted T cells. Thus, iNKT cells are felt to play an important role in "bridging" the adaptive and innate immune systems.[67]

γδ T lymphocytes are innate T lymphocyte populations that express the γδ TCR with limited diversity. They make up approximately 0.5% to 5% of all circulating T cells. Yet in the epithelial and mucosal tissue, they make up a significant portion of the T cell population. In humans, the Vγ9Vδ2 TCR is utilized by the majority of peripheral γδ T cells. These cells recognize small organic phosphate antigens (phospho-antigens) from microbes, which are produced by a number of intracellular pathogens, such as *M. tuberculosis*. The heterogeneity of the γδ TCR is not as diverse as αβ T cells due to the relative lower number of V (variable) γ and Vδ genes. In contrast to αβ T cells, they are not MHC restricted and can be activated by protein and nonprotein antigens. The population expands significantly in protozoan infections (e.g., malaria and toxoplasmosis) and mycobacterial infections. Downstream, activated γδ T cells can influence T cell effector function, as well as B cell activation, providing the boost to the adaptive immune response. Subsequent differential expression of IFNγ, IL-4, and IL-17 influences the development of Th1, Th2, and Th17 responses, respectively.[67–69]

T LYMPHOCYTES AND LUNG DEFENSE

Several types of T (thymus derived) lymphocytes (T cells) contribute to lung immunity and tissue pathology. All mature T cells express a unique TCR, with the majority made up of an α and β chain (αβ), while others are composed of a γδ chain. The αβT cells make up ~95% of the T cells peripherally, although the γδ T cells can reach up to 50% in mucosa, suggesting a stronger role in lung defense. Almost all αβT cells are CD4(+) or CD8 (+). CD4(+) T cells are known as T helper (Th) cells, while CD8(+) T cells are termed cytotoxic/suppressor cells. CD4(+) T cells recognize antigens presented via the MHC class II antigen, and they provide effector function primarily by the release of cytokines. Initially, two subsets of T cells, of Th1 and Th2 were identified, characterized by their cytokine profiles, IFNγ and IL-4, respectfully, as the driver for the Th functions. IL-12 induces the Th1 pathway, and IL-4 activates the Th2 pathway. In general, the Th1 pathway helps regulate cellular immunity and Th2 pathway produces cytokines to activate mast cells and eosinophils and stimulate B cell production of immunoglobulin. Th2 cytokine network (IL-4, IL-5, IL-10, and IL-13) has been well established in the model of understanding the pathophysiology of asthma, increased production of mucus and fibrosis. Over the past decade, several other Th subsets have been identified, including the Th17 and Treg (regulatory T cell) subsets. The Th17 subset is characterized by secretion of IL-17, which plays a significant role in host defense against extracellular bacteria, autoimmunity, and asthma. Over expression of IL-17 has been associated with collagen deposition and airway inflammation. It has been identified as a potentiator at the local level that induces bronchial fibroblasts to release proinflammatory cytokines and increase airway responsiveness. It can also recruit neutrophils to the site of airway inflammation, which may contribute to the pathophysiology of steroid-resistant asthma.

Treg cells are a subset of CD4 (+) T cells which is characterized by the CD25 receptor along with coexpression of CD45. They regulate T cell effector functions via the transcriptional regulator Foxp3. Mutations in the Foxp3 subsequently lead to autoimmunity and uncontrolled lymphoproliferation. Treg cells also play a strong role in the pathogenesis of asthma. They produce IL-10, and TGF-β, which are inhibitory cytokines that help dampen the inflammatory response and downregulate airway remodeling. They also block the Th2 response, which suggests a balance of these systems in the setting of allergy and asthma.

In response to peptides presented by the MHC class I molecules, CD8(+) T cells function in target cell toxicity. CD8(+) T cell toxicity is mediated by the release of perforin and granzyme, and Fas-FasL interaction, in a similar fashion to NK cell cytotoxicity. CD8(+) cells reinforce viral defenses by rendering adjacent cells resistant to infection, presumably by the release of interferons. T cell responses are tightly regulated. Whereas responses are necessary to eliminate pathogens, uncontrolled responses can cause autoimmune inflammatory diseases.[70]

B LYMPHOCYTES

B (bone marrow derived) cells play a critical role in the maintenance of health largely by mediating host defense against infections and by generating a robust vaccine response. The mechanisms behind this include production of high affinity, isotype-switched antibodies, as well as regulated interaction with T cells, to stimulate T cell differentiation, activation, and formation of memory cells. The initial development of a B cell occurs in the bone marrow with subsequent maturation in the periphery in the lymphoid tissue (i.e., lymph nodes, spleen). During the maturation process, the pro-B cell undergoes V(D)J recombination to produce a vast array of B cell receptors (BCR). This subsequently leads to the expression of surface IgM BCR on an immature B cell, which leaves the bone marrow for further development in the spleen. Testing for autoreactivity occurs at multiple checkpoints, via clonal deletion, anergy, and receptor editing/revision. Activation and further differentiation of the naïve B cell (mature B cells that have not been exposed to antigen) then occurs in the peripheral lymphoid tissue. Protein antigens are considered T cell–dependent antigens, as they cannot activate B cells without T cell assistance. The antigen is bound by the BCR, endocytosed, processed, and with a small peptide, presented to the cell surface via the MHC class II receptor, which is recognized by the Th cells. They activate and release cytokines that drive maturation of B cells into plasma cells, which secrete a "class switched" antibody. More importantly, the activated T cell also exposes the CD40 ligand and binds to the B cell receptor, CD40 Receptor. With this process, the B cell undergoes somatic hypermutation and isotype class switching to develop high affinity antibodies, a process which occurs in the germinal centers of secondary lymphoid follicles. The organization of these structures provides an immune microenvironment that maximizes the generation of antibody responses by bringing all relevant cell types into close contact for cell-cell signaling. Polysaccharide antigens, considered to be T cell independent antigens, can activate B cells without assistance from T cells. Examples of T cell–independent antigens include polysaccharides and polymerized flagellin, which provide numerous repeating epitopes. T cell–independent antigens do not induce the formation of germinal centers and therefore cannot induce the generation of memory B cells or somatic hypermutation that results in the production of high-affinity antibodies. The extent of class switching from IgM to other classes of antibodies is also severely limited in the absence of Th cell–generated cytokines.[71,72]

HUMORAL IMMUNITY

Depending on the stage of development of the B lymphocyte, different immunoglobulin isotypes are produced. Prior to antigenic stimulation, the "naïve" B lymphocyte expresses IgM (and IgD) on its surface. Early in the antigenic response, IgM, IgG3, and IgG1 are produced by B lymphocytes. In the chronic response, the predominant isotypes produced are IgG2 and IgG4. In addition, IgA is important in the mucosal immune response.

Immunoglobulin A

Secretory immunoglobulin A (IgA) is the predominant immunoglobulin isotype present in mucosal surfaces. Secretory IgA is composed of two IgA molecules (dimeric IgA), a joining protein (J chain), and a secretory component (SC). The dimeric IgA-J chain complex is produced by B lymphocytes in the submucosal tissues. The SC is produced by mucosal epithelial cells and acts as a receptor for dimeric IgA. After IgA binds to the SC, the entire complex undergoes transcytosis and is transported to the apical surface of the cell, where the secretory IgA complex is released into the mucosal environment. The SC protects the secretory IgA complex from proteases present in the mucosal environment. Secretory IgA serves several functions, including neutralization of viruses and exotoxin, enhancement of lactoferrin and lactoperoxidase activities, and inhibition of microbial growth. Because dimeric IgA is able to bind two antigens simultaneously, it is capable of forming large antigen-antibody complexes. In this manner, IgA neutralizes microbes and facilitates their removal by mucociliary clearance, inhibits microbial binding to epithelial cells, and inhibits uptake of potential allergens.

Selective IgA deficiency is defined as less than 7 mg/dL with normal values of IgM and IgG in patients 4 years old or greater. It is the most common primary immunodeficiency. The threshold of 4 years of age is used to avoid premature diagnosis of IgA deficiency, which may be transient in younger children due to delayed maturation of IgA production. Approximately 85% to 90% of patients with selective IgA deficiency are asymptomatic. Symptomatic individuals present with various manifestations including recurrent sinusitis, otitis media, pharyngitis, bronchitis, pneumonia, chronic diarrhea, and autoimmune syndromes. Patients with selective IgA deficiency are treated symptomatically for respiratory, gastrointestinal, and allergic problems. Since most preparations of intravenous immunoglobulin (IVIg) contain IgA, its use increases the risk of anaphylaxis if the recipient has anti-IgA antibodies. Transfusion of blood products presents a similar problem for these individuals. In patients with IgA deficiency and a history of anaphylaxis to IVIg products, it is recommended to consider an IVIg preparation with low IgA content or subcutaneous immunoglobulin.[73–75]

Immunoglobulin G

Immunoglobulin G (IgG) is the most abundant antibody isotype in serum. It makes up 80% of the serum antibody levels and is the only one that can cross the placenta. It activates the complement cascade through the classical pathway. All IgG subclasses are found at the mucosal barriers at significant levels, and in some points, total mucosal IgG is the most abundant isotype, compared to secretary IgA amounts, such as in bronchoalveolar fluids. Mucosal IgG reaches the mucosal surface either being produced locally by mucosal plasma cells, or systemically, by the neonatal Fc Receptor (FcRn). There are four subclasses of IgG (IgG 1 to 4) numbered by their amount in the serum and with differences based on the antigenic differences in structure of the heavy chain. However, in terms of effector functions, IgG3 has the highest effector capacity. IgG1 and IgG3 respond to protein antigens. They are T-dependent antigens; IgG2 and IgG4 respond to polysaccharide antigens, which are T-independent antigens. IgG functions by opsonizing microbes for phagocytosis and killing, activating the complement cascade, and neutralizing many bacterial endotoxins and viruses. Selective IgG deficiency is associated with upper respiratory tract infections.

Common variable immunodeficiency (CVID) is defined as significantly low levels of IgG in addition to one of isotypes IgA or IgM and poor vaccine response after test vaccination. The clinical phenotype is heterogeneous and is associated with recurrent otitis media, sinusitis, bronchitis, and pneumonia along with multiple autoimmune features and malignancy. Recurrence of airway infections may result in chronic airway injury with bronchiectasis. The combination of altered opsonic activity and bronchiectasis results in chronic colonization with respiratory pathogens such as *Pseudomonas aeruginosa*.

In patients suspected of IgG deficiency, quantification of IgG subclasses should be performed in addition to measurement of the antibody response to polysaccharide vaccines (*Streptococcus pneumoniae, Haemophilus influenzae*). IgG-deficient patients with recurrent respiratory tract infections often benefit from prophylactic antibiotics, immunoglobulin replacement, and the use of airway clearance techniques. X-linked agammaglobulinemia is characterized by low levels of all antibody isotypes due to a mutation in the Bruton's tyrosine kinase gene, which leads to a block in maturation of the B cell. Children with this disease uniformly develop chronic airway infection and lung dysfunction unless treated aggressively with supportive measures and immunoglobulin replacement.[76,77]

Immunoglobulin E

Of the five antibody isotypes, serum immunoglobulin E (IgE) has the lowest concentration in humans due to the high affinity of mast cells for IgE. While other immunoglobulins require an antigen/antibody complex to bind to the cell bound Fc receptor (FcR), IgE does not require an antibody to bind to the FcR. IgE serves to protect via mast cell degranulation, which induces multiple functions, such as sneezing, coughing, emesis, and diarrhea, to expel pathogens (largely helminth parasites). It also can induce an antibody-dependent, cell-mediated cytotoxic response against helminthes. It binds to the parasites, and eosinophils then bind to the opsonized organisms via the IgE FcR. Eosinophils are then stimulated to release granular contents, resulting in lysis of the parasite. IgE also has a pathologic, central role in hypersensitivity reactions in response to benign allergens (antigens).

The hyper IgE syndromes (HIES) are characterized by elevated IgE levels, recurrent skin infections, eczema, and pulmonary infections. Many genetic defects have been identified, and the best elucidated are the mutations in the signal transducer and activator of transcription 3 (STAT3) gene, which is an autosomal dominant disease; mutations/deletions in dedicator of cytokinesis 8 (DOCK8); and tyrosine kinase 2 (TYK2) with the last two inherited as autosomal recessive defects. In STAT3 HIES, mucocutaneous candidiasis, sino-pulmonary infections with development of bronchiectasis and pneumatoceles, and associated facial and bone abnormalities are noted. In patients with DOCK8, sino-pulmonary infections are common, but pneumatoceles have not been described. Treatment relies on supportive measures, including IVIg, although there is a growing body of evidence to suggest hematopoietic stem cell transplant is beneficial for those with DOCK8 mutations. Isolated IgE deficiency has not been reported.[78,79]

Immunoglobulin M

Immunoglobulin M is the first antibody isotype to be synthesized, and it is the first antibody produced in response to a foreign antigen. It is mostly found in the bloodstream, although mucosal IgM has been noted in physiologic amounts. It has been hypothesized that it provides a level of protection in those patients with selective IgA deficiency who are asymptomatic.

IgM gains access to the airway by exudation or by active secretion via the SC. IgM is capable of agglutinating bacteria and activating the complement cascade, with a greater efficiency compared to IgG due to an increased number of binding sites.

Both selective IgM deficiency and hyper-IgM have been highly associated with recurrent upper and lower respiratory infections. In selective IgM deficiency, the genetics is not well known, although it has been hypothesized that there is a functional defect in B cell differentiation prior to the secretion of IgM. Recurrent sino-pulmonary infection is the most common manifestation, up to 65% in one cohort.[80]

Hyper IgM syndromes are a group of disorders defined by a class switching defect involving the CD40 ligand/CD40 signaling pathway. The loss of this signaling leads to impairment of isotype switching and is characterized by an elevated IgM level with normal levels of IgG, IgA, and IgE. Clinical manifestations depend on the type of specific defect. Defects at the CD40 ligand or CD40 interrupt the costimulatory cross talk between CD 4+ T cells and B cells. In patients with defects in CD40 ligand (inherited as an X-linked disease, X-HIGM), patients can develop recurrent sino-pulmonary infections, including opportunistic infections such as *Pneumocystis jiroveci*, within the first 2 years of life. Data from international registries document that 81% of patients with X-HIGM develop pneumonia, with 65% of these being Pneumocystis jirovecii pneumonia (PJP).[81]

Role of Programmed Cell Death and "Clearing the Garbage" in Lung Homeostasis

During the course of lung development, growth, and injury repair, cells must be replaced in orderly processes controlling the breakdown and turnover of internal contents (autophagy), cell death (apoptosis, necroptosis, ETosis), and removal of dead or dying cells (efferocytosis) to help preserve lung structure and function and prevent lung injury. In acute lung injury (ALI) and chronic lung diseases (such as CF), there is evidence that disordered programmed cell death and removal of dead cells result in ongoing inflammation and lung injury. While detailed description of these processes is beyond the scope of this chapter, a brief description of their role in lung homeostasis and repair is provided here.

Autophagy is an evolutionarily conserved process present in virtually all eukaryotic cells. It is responsible for regenerating metabolic precursors and clearing subcellular debris, thereby maintaining cellular homeostasis. Autophagy involves the sequestration of regions of the cytosol or organelles within double-membrane–bound compartments and the delivery of these compartments to the lysosome for degradation. Autophagy is important in the "recycling" of cell components for reuse in a starvation state and is a key component of innate immunity: leading to the elimination of intracellular pathogens and processing antigens for presentation to lymphocytes. Impaired autophagy can result in accumulation of materials in the cell, leading to cell and tissue dysfunction. It is a highly regulated process that can be divided into three stages: initiation, execution, and maturation.[82,83] Initiation of autophagy is regulated by target of rapamycin (TOR) kinase that functions as an inhibitor or by alternative pathways that require activation of trimeric G proteins and class III phosphoinositide 3-kinases. Execution of autophagy involves conjugation pathways and complex formation that require autophagy gene (Atg) products. The maturation step involves fusion of these complexes with endosomal vesicles containing lysosome-associated membrane proteins (LAMP1 and LAMP2). These structures fuse with the lysosomes and acquire cathepsins and acid phosphatases to form autolysosomes.[82,83]

Apoptosis is one form of programmed cell death. Morphologically, apoptosis is characterized by nuclear shrinkage and formation of apoptotic bodies, keeping the cell membranes intact. Apoptotic cells are characterized by caspase activation, DNA fragmentation, and externalization of phosphatidyl serine onto the cell surface in a process dependent on caspase 3 activation. Seven of the 13 distinct human caspase genes are suggested to participate in apoptosis as initiator caspases (caspase-2, caspase-8, caspase-9, and caspase-10) or effector caspases (caspase-3, caspase-6, and caspase-7) that cleave a wide array of proteins that contribute to the structural or bioenergetic integrity of the cell (https://www.youtube.com/watch?v=9KTDz-ZisZ0). The initiator caspases can be activated by a series of polyprotein complexes, and each is activated in response to particular death signals. Apoptosis can occur through convergent extrinsic or intrinsic pathways. The *extrinsic pathway* involves cell surface death receptors belonging to the tumor necrosis factor-receptor (TNF-R) family (including TNF-R1, Fas/CD95, Death Receptor 3 [DR3], DR4, DR5, and DR6). These receptors are characterized by an intracellular death domain (DD) that transmits the apoptotic signal and leads to the formation of a complex of the death receptor, adaptor protein, and procaspase 8 (called the *death inducing signaling complex*), which leads to the autoproteolytic cleavage of procaspase 8 to caspase 8. The intrinsic pathway is induced by the stimulation of the mitochondrial membrane and translocation of the bcl2 family of proteins within the mitochondrial membrane, altering mitochondrial membrane permeability. This increased permeability results in the release of cytochrome c and other factors into the cytoplasm, where they recruit a caspase adaptor molecule (APAF1) and the apoptosis initiator enzyme procaspase 9. Cytochrome c, APAF1, procaspase 9, and ATP form a complex called the *apoptosome*, and procaspase 9 becomes activated to caspase 9. At this point, both intrinsic and extrinsic pathways converge into a common pathway, leading to activation of executioner caspases 3, 6, and 7.[84,85]

Efferocytosis is the process of removal of apoptotic cells. This process is different from complement-induced or Fcγ-induced phagocytosis in that it involves both "professional phagocytes" (macrophages and DC) and other cell types (epithelial cells and fibroblasts).[86] Apoptotic cells are recognized by membrane alterations (the "eat me" signals) that include externalization of phosphatidylserine and calreticulin onto the cell surface. CD31 (platelet-endothelial cell adhesion molecule-1) functions as a co-ligand that enhances attachment and engagement of the "eat-me" signals. An array of receptors has been shown to be associated with efferocytosis, including the low-density lipoprotein receptor-related protein (LRP, CD91), Mer receptor tyrosine kinase, αvβ3 integrins, scavenger receptors, CF44, CD14, and complement receptors 3 and 4.[87] Receptor binding results in cell activation and engulfment of the apoptotic target cell. Efferocytosis results

in the removal of apoptotic cells before their membranes become permeable, thereby preventing release of toxic intracellular contents.[87]

During late stages of cell death, soluble components are released that serve as "find me" signals. Soluble innate PRR can contribute to the identification of the "eat me" signals on the apoptotic cell surface, bind to them, and serve to bridge the apoptotic cell with phagocytes, promoting efferocytosis, thereby limiting inflammation.[87] Impaired efferocytosis plays a role in CF and asthma.[86]

Summary

The lung is continuously exposed to potential pathogens. The multilayered defenses provided by the intrinsic, innate, and adaptive systems protect the lung from invasion, limit inflammation, and repair lung injury. Although there is considerable overlap in the activities of these defenses, defects can result in recurrent infection, persistent inflammation, and lung injury.

References

Access the reference list online at ExpertConsult.com.

Suggested Reading

Brubaker SW, Bonham KS, Zanoni I, et al. Innate immune pattern recognition: a cell biological perspective. *Annu Rev Immunol.* 2015;33:257–290.

Byrne AJ, Mathie SA, Gregory LG, et al. Pulmonary macrophages: key players in the innate defence of the airways. *Thorax.* 2015;70(12):1189–1196.

Hallstrand TS, Hackett TL, Altemeier WA, et al. Airway epithelial regulation of pulmonary immune homeostasis and inflammation. *Clin Immunol.* 2014;151(1):1–15.

Man SM, Kanneganti TD. Converging roles of caspases in inflammasome activation, cell death and innate immunity. *Nat Rev Immunol.* 2016; 16(1):7–21.

McCool FD. Global physiology and pathophysiology of cough: ACCP evidence-based clinical practice guidelines. *Chest.* 2006;129(1 suppl):48S–53S.

O'Neill LA, Golenbock D, Bowie AG. The history of Toll-like receptors—redefining innate immunity. *Nat Rev Immunol.* 2013;13(6):453–460.

Szondy Z, Garabuczi É, Joós G, et al. Impaired clearance of apoptotic cells in chronic inflammatory diseases: therapeutic implications. *Front Immunol.* 2014;5:354.

Vestweber D. How leukocytes cross the vascular endothelium. *Nat Rev Immunol.* 2015;15(11):692–704.

Williams AE, Chambers RC. The mercurial nature of neutrophils: still an enigma in ARDS? *Am J Physiol Lung Cell Mol Physiol.* 2014; 306(3):L217–L230.

9 Bronchoscopy and Bronchoalveolar Lavage in Pediatric Patients

ROBERT E. WOOD, PhD, MD

Visualization of the interior of the body is often the most effective and efficient way to evaluate a patient's problem. As an old Chinese proverb says, "A picture is worth a thousand words." Advances in endoscopic techniques and instrumentation have greatly enhanced the pulmonary specialist's ability to visualize the interior of the respiratory tract. This in turn has led to improvements in diagnosis and treatment.

Bronchoscopy—the visual examination of the airways—is usually performed for diagnostic purposes but is also useful for certain therapeutic maneuvers. Bronchoscopy may be performed with either rigid or flexible (fiberoptic) instruments depending on the particular needs of the patient and the skills and instrumentation available to the bronchoscopist. In general, most things that can be done with a rigid bronchoscope can be done with a flexible instrument and *vice versa*. However, there are some notable exceptions. For example, a rigid instrument cannot be passed around a curve into the apices of the lungs or very far into the peripheral bronchi, while a flexible instrument is quite unsuited for removal of aspirated foreign bodies from the lungs of children. For the most effective care of pediatric patients, both rigid and flexible instruments must be available, and there must be practitioners trained in the use of each type of instrument (although not necessarily the same person). In many patients, the combined use of both instruments may yield the most optimal result.

In addition to visualization, bronchoscopes also provide an effective means to obtain specimens from the lungs and airways. Tissue samples may be obtained by biopsy forceps, secretions can be aspirated from the airways, and bronchoalveolar lavage (BAL) yields samples of the fluid resident on the surfaces of the alveoli and distal airways. Bronchoscopy is primarily a clinical tool but is increasingly being used for investigational purposes as well. Although pediatric patients present special challenges (technical as well as ethical) to the investigative use of bronchoscopy, age alone is no contraindication to the use of bronchoscopy for research.[1]

Bronchoscopy involves the examination of at least part of the upper airway as well as the trachea and bronchi; this is especially true with (and an advantage of) flexible instruments. Rigid bronchoscopes are generally passed through the patient's mouth, while flexible bronchoscopes are generally passed through the patient's nose. Bronchoscopes may also be used to examine just the upper airway, although the high incidence of concurrent upper and lower airway lesions[2-4] makes it wise to examine both upper and lower airways unless there is a good reason not to do so.

Instrumentation

RIGID BRONCHOSCOPES

The rigid ("open tube") bronchoscope consists of a metal tube of appropriate diameter and length that is passed into the trachea and through which the operator may look and the patient may breathe. The instrument is not a *simple* metal tube; it is equipped to deliver anesthetic gasses and light to the distal tip.

The large open channel, through which instruments may be passed, is one of the major advantages of rigid bronchoscopes. However, visualization is challenging, especially when passing an instrument (such as a biopsy forceps). A major advance in bronchoscopic technique came with the development of the glass rod telescope.[5] This device yields exceptionally fine optical performance, and various instruments such as biopsy and grasping forceps have been designed specifically to work with the telescopes. Rigid bronchoscopes have holes in the side along the distal tip to allow ventilation of the contralateral lung when the bronchoscope is advanced into one main-stem bronchus.

The rigid bronchoscope must be an appropriate size for the patient. Therefore, a variety of instruments must be available to the pediatric bronchoscopist ranging in diameters from 3 to 7 mm or larger and in length from 20 to 50 cm. There must be a full range of telescope lengths and diameters for the different bronchoscopes. In addition, glass rod telescopes may be made with a prism on the distal end to facilitate observation of the upper lobes (typically, 30, 70, or even 120 degrees).

Likewise, the auxiliary instruments (e.g., biopsy or grasping forceps) must match the telescopes and/or bronchoscopes. A large variety of forceps and other devices has been devised for specialized purposes. Perhaps the most valuable are the "optical forceps," which are matched with a glass rod telescope and allow the bronchoscopist to operate the forceps under close and direct visualization.

The nomenclature of bronchoscope sizes can be confusing. In general, rigid instruments are defined by the diameter of the largest instrument that will pass through the bronchoscope, while flexible bronchoscopes are defined by their outer diameter. For example, a 3.5-mm flexible bronchoscope will easily pass through a "3.5-mm" rigid bronchoscope.

FLEXIBLE BRONCHOSCOPES

The flexible bronchoscope is essentially a solid instrument composed of thousands of glass fibers that carry the light for illumination and the image. The tip of the instrument can be deflected to guide it into the desired path or location. Most flexible bronchoscopes have a small suction channel through which secretions may be aspirated, fluids may be delivered to the airways, or small flexible instruments may be passed.

The typical pediatric flexible bronchoscopes in use today are 2.8 mm in diameter and with a suction channel approximately 1.2 mm in diameter. Smaller instruments (2.2 mm) have no suction channel, and therefore have somewhat limited utility when there are secretions or blood in the airways; they also cannot be used to obtain diagnostic specimens. Larger instruments, ranging from 4.2 to 6.3 mm in diameter, are used in adults. These instruments have suction channels ranging from 2.0 to 3.2 mm in diameter.

In contrast to the rigid bronchoscope, through which the patient breathes (either spontaneously or by positive pressure); the flexible bronchoscope forces the patient to breathe around the instrument. Therefore, the instrument must be small enough not only to fit into the airway but also to allow the patient to breathe. Most infants as large as 1.5 kg can breathe spontaneously around the 2.8-mm bronchoscope, but great care must be taken to ensure the adequacy of ventilation during procedures.

Flexible bronchoscopes are quite limited in their capacity to accommodate instruments. The most common instruments used with flexible bronchoscopes are flexible biopsy forceps and cytology or microbiology brushes. Small grasping forceps and folding retrieval baskets are also available but have limited usefulness, especially in pediatric patients. Suctioning is done directly with the bronchoscope rather than by passing a device through the channel, as is the case with rigid bronchoscopes.

Flexible bronchoscopes are limited in their optical performance by the number of glass fibers, which conduct the image. While larger, adult-size instruments now mostly utilize a video chip at the working tip (and thus generate an image of much higher resolution), pediatric instruments, because of their small diameter, continue to rely on glass fibers to transmit the image. While the images obtained by flexible instruments are quite satisfactory for most clinical purposes, the glass rod telescopes and video scopes provide much greater resolution and image quality.

CARE AND MAINTENANCE OF BRONCHOSCOPES

Bronchoscopy is not a *sterile* procedure, since the instruments pass through a nonsterile area (the nose or mouth). However, bronchoscopes and associated instruments must be cleaned and sterilized before use in a patient.[6] Transmission of infectious agents from patient to patient due to inadequate cleaning or sterilization procedures has been well documented.[7,8] In general, bronchoscopic equipment should be cleaned as soon as possible after use, as dried blood or mucus is much more difficult to remove and will prevent adequate sterilization by any method.[9] At a minimum, the instruments should be flushed with water immediately after use and, if possible, soaked in an enzymatic detergent until formal cleaning can be done.

Rigid bronchoscopes are cleaned by vigorous brushing with detergent, followed by rinsing; they may be sterilized by steam autoclaving. Glass rod telescopes (unless specially marked) may not be exposed to steam, however, and must be sterilized with ethylene oxide or with liquid agents such as glutaraldehyde or peracetic acid.[10]

Flexible bronchoscopes are cleaned by careful scrubbing of the exterior with a soft cloth and enzymatic detergent. The suction channel must be cleaned by multiple passes of an appropriate cleaning brush. Thorough rinsing is followed by high-level disinfection[9,10] (with glutaraldehyde or peracetic acid) or sterilization (with ethylene oxide). Flexible bronchoscopes will melt in a steam autoclave...

The lenses of rigid telescopes and flexible bronchoscopes must be carefully scrubbed and polished with a soft cloth during cleaning. Otherwise, small amounts of protein left on the lens will accumulate over time, making the image progressively less satisfactory. Flexible bronchoscopes and glass rod telescopes are made of glass and are fragile (not to mention expensive). They must never be dropped and must not be subjected to forces that will cause breakage. Flexible bronchoscopes should never be passed through a patient's mouth unless protected by a rigid bite block, since an endotracheal tube will not protect the bronchoscope from severe damage by teeth. The care with which instruments are cleaned and handled must match the care with which they are utilized in the patient's airway. Individuals responsible for cleaning and preparing the instruments must be well trained and supervised.

Techniques for Bronchoscopy

FACILITIES FOR BRONCHOSCOPY

It is important that bronchoscopy be performed in a suitable venue. Because of the need for general anesthesia, rigid bronchoscopy is almost always performed in an operating room. The relative ease with which flexible bronchoscopy can be done makes it tempting to use the instrument in unconventional places such as at the bedside or in an emergency room. However, while there are clearly circumstances in which such practice is justified, bronchoscopy is a serious procedure with the potential for lethal complications and should be performed only by physicians who are well trained, with the necessary cognitive and technical skills, and with full preparation for all contingencies. Therefore, a fully equipped and staffed endoscopy suite or operating room is the most appropriate venue. With suitable preparation, bronchoscopy (rigid or flexible) can be performed at the bedside in an intensive care unit, but this may still place the bronchoscopist at a disadvantage in terms of access to equipment and supplies in the event of difficulties. If bronchoscopy is performed in an intensive care unit, the bronchoscopist must take along everything that will possibly be needed and have it readily at hand.

RIGID BRONCHOSCOPY

The appropriate rigid bronchoscope (length and diameter) is chosen for the patient. Under a satisfactory level of anesthesia, the patient is positioned supine with the shoulders supported and the head slightly extended. The larynx is exposed with a laryngoscope and the tip of the bronchoscope is gently advanced through the glottis and into the trachea. With the proximal end of the bronchoscope closed with a lens cap or with a telescope in place, the side port is attached to the anesthesia circuit, and the patient can be ventilated with positive pressure.

The bronchoscope is manipulated to visualize the tracheal and bronchial anatomy; the head and neck may be turned to help direct the bronchoscope into the right or left main bronchi. Telescopes greatly facilitate inspection and can be used in conjunction with a video camera. Angulated telescopes make it much easier to visualize the upper lobe segments. The telescope must be removed and cleaned if the lens becomes covered with secretions; suctioning is performed with a suction pipe or a suction catheter. During these times, ventilation is momentarily interrupted. It is also possible to work for extended periods with an open proximal end while maintaining ventilation with a Venturi jet injector.

When instrumentation is required, such as for the removal of a foreign body, the instruments may be passed through the open channel of the bronchoscope. Unfortunately, this significantly impairs the view of the operative site, as the instruments obstruct the line of vision. Optical forceps, which incorporate the glass rod telescope and allow direct visualization of the operative site, is the preferred instrument for biopsy and for foreign body extraction. Very small flexible forceps can also be passed through a side arm and alongside the telescope, but the tips of these instruments may be difficult to control.

In our practice, at Cincinnati Children's Hospital, the vast majority of rigid bronchoscopic procedures (including foreign body removal) are performed using only the glass rod telescopes; the open tube sheath is employed in special circumstances. This technique requires that the patient breathe spontaneously, so anesthetic technique is critical, but it is much easier to evaluate airway dynamics. Because the overall size of the instruments is smaller, mechanical complications are less frequent.

FLEXIBLE BRONCHOSCOPY

Most diagnostic procedures in pediatric patients can be performed with the standard 2.8 mm or 3.5-mm pediatric flexible instruments. In older children, a small "adult" instrument may be used (especially if a larger suction channel is needed); while in very small infants, it may be appropriate to use a 2.2-mm ultrathin bronchoscope. The patient is properly prepared for the procedure and positioned supine with the head and neck in a neutral position. It is also possible to perform flexible bronchoscopy in a sitting or some other position in special circumstances.

Flexible bronchoscopes are usually inserted transnasally. This avoids the potential for the patient to bite (and thus destroy) the instrument and also affords a view of the nasal and nasopharyngeal anatomy. Another advantage of this approach is that the bronchoscope does not contact the tongue; the tongue is a very powerful muscle and can readily move the bronchoscope in ways contrary to the intent of the bronchoscopist. A flexible bronchoscope may also be inserted orally if desired, always with a suitable bite block, even with the patient under general anesthesia, or through an artificial airway such as an endotracheal tube (with a

Table 9.1 Artificial Airways and Flexible Bronchoscopes Used in Pediatric Patients

Instrument Diameter (mm)	Smallest Tube That Can Be Used (mm)[a]	Smallest Tube for Assisted Ventilation (mm)	Smallest Tube for Spontaneous Ventilation (mm)
2.2	2.5	3.0	3.5
2.8	3.0 (not recommended)	3.5	4.0
3.5	4.5	5.0	5.5
4.2	5.0	5.5	6.5
4.9	5.5	6.0	7.0

[a]For intubation only.

bite block), a tracheostomy tube or a laryngeal mask airway (LMA).

The tip of the flexible bronchoscope can be flexed or extended in a single plane; movement to one side or another is accomplished by rotation. The instrument is directed to the site of interest by advancing the shaft while controlling the angulation and rotation at the tip. This combination of three simultaneous movements requires good hand-eye coordination on the part of the bronchoscopist. In contrast to glass rod telescopes, the image rotates as the instrument is rotated; this may produce disorientation on the part of operators unaccustomed to using flexible instruments. As the instrument is advanced through the airway, secretions may be removed by suctioning, and topical anesthetic can be applied, also through the suction channel.

The patient must be able to breathe around the instrument; most infants 3 kg or larger can breathe satisfactorily around the 3.5-mm pediatric flexible bronchoscope (infants larger than about 1.5 kg can usually breathe around the 2.8 mm instrument). Smaller infants will not be able to do so, and their procedures must be performed with an ultrathin instrument or with an apneic technique. If the patient is intubated, the bronchoscope must be small enough to readily pass through the tube (Table 9.1).

Flexible bronchoscopes are much smaller than rigid instruments (although the glass rod telescopes, if used alone, are equally small) and can be advanced much farther into the distal airways. Depending on the instrument used and the size of the patient, airways as small as 2 mm and as far as 14 to 16 generations from the carina may be inspected.

The instruments that can be passed through a flexible bronchoscope are quite limited, because of the small diameter of the suction channel (1.2 mm in pediatric instruments, 2.0 to 3.2 mm in "adult" instruments). Cup or "alligator" biopsy forceps, brushes, grasping forceps, expandable basket retrieval devices, balloon catheters (for dilation of stenoses), monopolar electrodes, and laser fibers are the most common such instruments.

Anesthesia for Bronchoscopy

Safe and effective bronchoscopy requires that the patient be comfortable and reasonably still during the procedure. Adequate oxygenation and ventilation must be maintained, and the patient must be carefully and continuously monitored.

These criteria can be met with either general anesthesia (administered by an anesthesiologist) or with sedation (usually performed by the intravenous administration of a narcotic and/or a benzodiazepine,[11] and administered by the bronchoscopist or sedation nurse) depending on the individual child's situation and the procedure planned. Sedation and general anesthesia are merely points on a continuum between the fully awake state and surgical anesthesia; it matters little how the desired, safe state is achieved. Deep sedation and light "general anesthesia" are virtually indistinguishable. An advantage of general anesthesia is that an anesthesiologist takes full responsibility for monitoring the patient. Current practice guidelines for sedation[12] mandate the presence of a trained individual whose sole responsibility is to monitor the patient, although this person does not have to be an anesthesiologist. Our current practice at Cincinnati Children's Hospital is to utilize an anesthesiologist, and the child is sedated with general anesthetic agents (inhaled or given intravenously) to a point that maintains spontaneous breathing but ensures safe comfort. A significant advantage of using "general anesthetic" agents for sedation is rapid induction and relatively rapid emergence, as well as the ability to quickly change the degree of sedation (and therefore respiratory effort) during the procedure.

Sedation and anesthesia diminish or abolish protective reflexes. To reduce the risk for aspiration of gastric contents, patients should be given nothing by mouth for several hours prior to the procedure. Clear liquids may be given up to 2 hours before the procedure. It is prudent to aspirate the stomach with a catheter before proceeding with the bronchoscopy. Young infants may become dehydrated or hypoglycemic if kept NPO for too long, and intravenous fluid may be necessary prior to a procedure.

When general anesthesia is utilized for diagnostic bronchoscopy, careful attention must be given to airway dynamics. If the patient does not breathe spontaneously, then the usual airway dynamics are reversed—airway pressure during inspiration exceeds that during expiration. This may result in diagnostic confusion in patients with tracheomalacia and/or bronchomalacia. During therapeutic procedures, deeper anesthesia and positive-pressure ventilation are often utilized.

Flexible bronchoscopes are small enough that the patient can usually breathe around them. Spontaneous breathing is the rule for most flexible procedures. Oxygen can be supplied through an oral airway or a mask. Many practitioners routinely utilize an LMA; this, while providing a secure airway, requires deeper sedation, eliminates the ability to evaluate the anatomy and dynamics of the upper airway, and may mask tracheomalacia or bronchomalacia. It is therefore not recommended as a routine practice.

Sedation, similar to general anesthesia, may be produced by a variety of agents and techniques. Important principles of sedation include careful preparation of the patient, the use of fractional doses of relatively short acting agents with titration of total dose to the needed effect, appropriate monitoring before, during, and after the procedure, and careful selection of agents.

Sedative/anesthetic agents have a variety of physiologic effects in addition to reducing the level of consciousness. The most important of these is depression of respiratory drive, and this effect may last longer than the sedation.

Children who have undergone sedation for procedures may be at greater risk after the procedure is completed than during the procedure itself, as there is no longer the stimulation of the procedure, and staff awareness and alertness may be diminished. Effective monitoring must be continued until all the effects of sedation have resolved.

Pharmacologic agents to reverse the effect of narcotics and benzodiazepines are available, and some physicians have utilized these agents routinely at the completion of procedures. This is not necessarily a good idea, however, as their effect is considerably shorter than the respiratory depression induced by the sedative agents. Furthermore, patients awakened abruptly from sedation are often disturbed and may become combative. Monitoring must be continued regardless of whether a reversal agent has been given; indeed, it may be argued that monitoring must be continued longer after reversal than without it. On the other hand, such agents should always be readily available in the event of serious respiratory depression.

Sedation—no matter how administered—involves more than giving drugs. Children are often very responsive to suggestion—whether positive or negative, whether intentional or inadvertent. Simple distraction or more formal methods of focusing attention on something other than the procedure[13,14] may be surprisingly effective in children, especially in the 3- to 8-year age group. Even infants respond to tone of voice and the atmosphere around them. Careful preparation of the child and the parents, focusing on positive aspects and creating positive expectations can be powerful adjuncts to chemical sedation. On the other hand, negative suggestions can make even the most powerful drugs less effective. A screaming, upset child will require much higher doses of virtually any agent to achieve effective sedation, and that child's recovery will be prolonged. For this reason, presedation with oral drugs such as midazolam and careful attention to atmosphere and language can often facilitate deeper sedation with minimal doses of other agents.

Airway management during bronchoscopy can be a challenge. The anesthesiologist must understand the goals of the procedure and enable the bronchoscopist to accurately evaluate not only the anatomy, but also the dynamics of the upper and lower airways. During evaluation of the upper airway, it is best to have a native airway with no devices or support, as in many pediatric patients, the diagnostic finding of most interest is dynamic obstruction of the upper airway. Once this has been evaluated, an oral airway can be placed to secure the upper airway, and oxygen and anesthetic gas can be delivered through an endotracheal tube inserted into the oral airway (Fig. 9.1). After the tracheal and bronchial dynamics have been evaluated, then if necessary, the bronchoscope can be removed and an LMA or endotracheal tube can be used for the remainder of the procedure.

Indications for Diagnostic Bronchoscopy

It is difficult to categorize the indications for diagnostic bronchoscopy without a great deal of overlap. In a given situation, there is often more than one indication for bronchoscopy (for example, a child with recurrent pneumonia may also be suspected of aspiration). In general, however, one may utilize a bronchoscope to define airway anatomy and airway dynamics, and to obtain specimens for further diagnostic study. The diagnostic result of a particular procedure may include anatomic findings, definition of airway dynamics, and the results of microbiologic and/or microscopic evaluation of specimens obtained during the procedure. Bronchoscopy performed for diagnostic purposes may also have therapeutic benefit, such as the removal of a mucus plug causing atelectasis.

It should be noted that there is often great value in a normal bronchoscopic examination; the definitive exclusion of suspected problems (such as foreign body aspiration, for example) may be as important as a specific diagnostic finding. Bronchoscopy (rather than simple laryngoscopy) is often performed in patients in whom the suspected lesion is in the upper airway. Since effective laryngoscopy in children usually

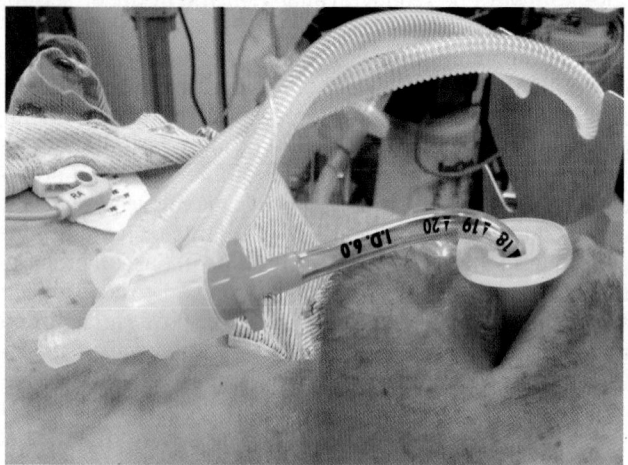

Fig. 9.1 Oral airway for delivery of oxygen and anesthetic gas during flexible bronchoscopy.

requires sedation and laryngeal anesthesia, it adds very little to the risk of the procedure to continue the examination into the lower airways. Unsuspected lesions in the lower airways are not uncommonly found,[3,15] even in patients in whom significant pathology, explaining the patient's symptoms, is seen at or above the glottis.[2]

Airway obstruction is one of the most common general indications for diagnostic bronchoscopy, and may involve the upper or lower airways or both. The extent of anatomic obstruction, especially fixed obstruction in the subglottic space, is often much greater than would be suspected from clinical examination. If a patient is stridulous during the examination, the vibrating structures causing the noise will *always* be visible, if one is looking in the right place.

Imaging techniques, such as CT or MRI scans, can yield considerable diagnostic information about the lungs and airways. In some cases, such techniques may make bronchoscopy unnecessary. However, imaging studies are quite limited and cannot provide specimens or (in most cases) adequately define abnormal airway dynamics. In general, radiologic studies should be performed prior to bronchoscopy, as it may be important to direct the focus of the bronchoscopy (e.g., BAL site) to a specific region of the lungs. In general, there is only one indication for diagnostic bronchoscopy—there is information in the lungs or airways necessary to the care of the patient, which is best obtained by bronchoscopy (Table 9.2).

Care must be taken to ensure that airway dynamics are not altered by positive-pressure ventilation, which will often prevent dynamic airway collapse. The depth of sedation may also influence airway dynamics; if the patient is too deeply sedated, abnormal dynamics may not be visible, as they are dependent on the transmural pressure gradients generated by breathing.

The choice between rigid and flexible instruments should be made with some care if there is a choice available. In

Table 9.2 Indications for Diagnostic Bronchoscopy

Indication	Rigid Instruments	Flexible Instruments
Stridor	May alter airway dynamics	Preferred
Persistent wheeze (not responsive, or poorly responsive to bronchodilator therapy)		Preferred
Atelectasis (persistent, recurrent, or massive)	May be needed to remove airway obstruction	
Localized hyperinflation		Preferred
Pneumonia		Preferred (much better to obtain BAL specimens)
▪ Recurrent		
▪ Persistent		
▪ Patients unable to produce sputum		
▪ Atypical or in unusual circumstances (e.g., immunocompromised patients)		
Hemoptysis	May be best if there is brisk bleeding	Preferred to evaluate distal airways
Foreign body aspiration	Mandatory for removal of foreign bodies	May be useful to examine for the possibility of foreign body; rarely useful for removal
▪ Known		
▪ Suspected		
Cough (persistent)		Preferred
Suspected aspiration	Preferred to evaluate posterior larynx and cervical trachea	Preferred to obtain BAL
Evaluation of patients with tracheostomies	Preferred to evaluate posterior larynx and subglottic space	Preferred to evaluate tube position and airway dynamics
Suspected mass or tumor	Preferred for laryngeal or tracheal lesions	Preferred for lesions in distal airways
Suspected airway anomalies		
Complications of artificial airways		

BAL, Bronchoalveolar lavage.

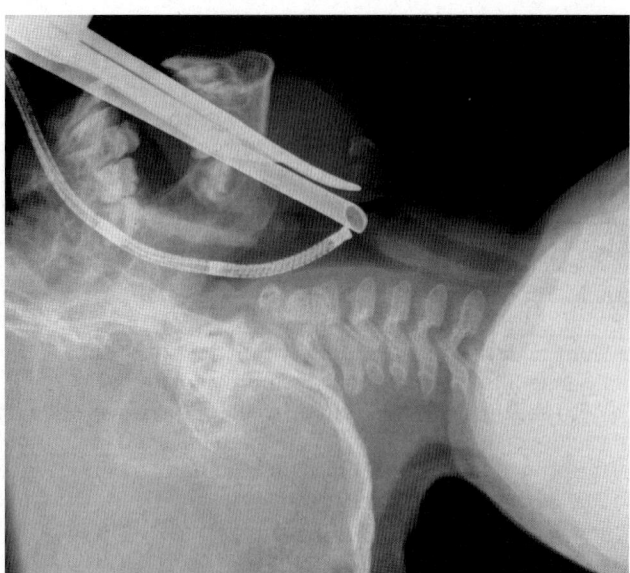

Fig. 9.2 The rigid bronchoscope approaches the larynx directly, with mandibular lift. The flexible instrument approaches the larynx from behind, making it difficult to evaluate the subglottic space and posterior cervical trachea.

Box 9.1   Indications for Bronchoalveolar Lavage

Diagnosis of suspected infection	Pulmonary hemorrhage
Evaluation for aspiration	Alveolar proteinosis
Pulmonary infiltrates	Pulmonary histiocytosis
Dyspnea	Aspiration
Hypoxia	Lung transplant
Tachypnea	Hypereosinophilic lung
Recurrent pulmonary infiltrates	diseases
Persistent pulmonary infiltrates	Therapeutic removal of
Interstitial infiltrates	materials
Diffuse alveolar inflammation	

many patients, the *combined* use of *both* rigid and flexible instruments can add immeasurably to the value of the procedures. Rigid instruments often distort the airway, while at the same time allowing better visualization of anatomic details. This is especially true in the larynx and upper trachea. Rigid instruments lift the mandible and hyoid but allow for a much better view of the posterior aspects of the larynx and cervical trachea. Flexible instruments produce little or no anatomic distortion (they follow the natural curvature of the airway), but they approach the larynx *from behind* and are therefore less capable of viewing details of the posterior aspects of the larynx, subglottic space, and cervical trachea (Fig. 9.2).

Contraindications to Bronchoscopy

Bronchoscopy should not be performed in the absence of a suitable indication or appropriate equipment and personnel skilled in its use. Otherwise, there are no absolute contraindications to bronchoscopy. However, if the same diagnostic information can be obtained by a less expensive, less invasive, or potentially less dangerous technique, then bronchoscopy is not indicated.

Relative contraindications to bronchoscopy include any factor that will increase the risk. Specific risk factors should be treated and if possible alleviated prior to bronchoscopy. Cardiovascular instability, bleeding diatheses (thrombocytopenia or hypoprothrombinemia), severe bronchospasm, and hypoxemia are primary examples. Some conditions that increase the risk are themselves indications for bronchoscopy, such as severe airway obstruction. In these cases, the procedure is performed with both diagnostic and therapeutic intent and can be lifesaving. Appropriate modifications must be made in the techniques chosen for anesthesia and monitoring when there are additional risk factors.

Bronchoalveolar Lavage

There is more to bronchoscopic diagnosis than meets the eye. BAL[16,17] yields a specimen that can give representative data from the distal airways and alveolar surfaces and has become one of the more important aspects of diagnostic bronchoscopy. BAL may be defined as the instillation into and recovery from the distal airways of a volume of saline sufficient to ensure that the fluid returned contains at least some fluid that was originally present on the alveolar surface. Both soluble and cellular constituents of the alveolar (and small airway) surface fluid are contained in the effluent. This epithelial surface fluid is diluted to an unknown but significant degree by the saline used in its collection. Therefore, the concentrations of substances measured in the BAL fluid do not give an accurate estimate of the concentration at the epithelial surface. Various methods have been employed to derive a reasonable measure of the dilution,[18] although none are free of problems since the epithelial fluid is not static. There is constant flux of fluid and soluble constituents across the epithelial surface, and the duration and volume of the fluid employed for lavage may have substantial impact on the concentration of substances in the effluent.[19] Fortunately, for clinical purposes, and especially in pediatric patients, the information in most cases need not be quantitative. The primary value of BAL is to obtain a specimen from the distal airways that is relatively representative, and which can yield information about infectious and/or inflammatory processes. However, the interpretation of BAL data is rarely totally free of ambiguities.

INDICATIONS FOR BRONCHOALVEOLAR LAVAGE

BAL is performed primarily for diagnostic purposes, although it can also be performed for therapeutic reasons. The main indications are listed in Box 9.1. BAL may be indicated for the diagnosis of infectious processes when a sputum specimen cannot be obtained or when the results from sputum analysis are equivocal. In immunocompetent individuals, this may include the infant or young child with cystic fibrosis with pulmonary symptoms requiring therapy. These children may be unable to produce sputum spontaneously, and cultures from the upper airway may either yield no pathogens when the bronchi are infected or yield pathogens when the lungs are sterile. In immunocompromised individuals with pulmonary infiltrates, the diagnosis of potential infections is often impossible except by BAL.[20,21] In either immunocompetent or immunocompromised individuals, BAL may help to distinguish infectious from noninfectious processes in the child with radiographic abnormalities. In general, however, if a satisfactory sputum specimen can be obtained, bronchoscopy solely to obtain cultures from the distal airways is not indicated as a primary approach. It may, however, be indicated when therapy geared towards suspected pathogens based on a sputum sample fails to provide therapeutic response. BAL should ideally be performed before antimicrobial therapy is started, but BAL may still be informative if there is a lack of clinical response or clinical deterioration.

BAL is often helpful to distinguish infectious from noninfectious processes, such as alveolar hemorrhage (which may occur without frank hemoptysis), pulmonary alveolar proteinosis, histiocytosis, or interstitial lung diseases. BAL is also indicated in the evaluation of patients with suspected aspiration, both to obtain microbiologic specimens to guide antibiotic therapy and to obtain evidence of the aspiration. Although a specific exogenous marker is not available, the presence of significant numbers of macrophages heavily laden with lipid[22] is a strong correlate of aspiration. "Soft" markers for aspiration of oral secretions include large numbers of oropharyngeal flora and squamous epithelial cells. In patients who have undergone lung transplant, BAL is often used in conjunction with transbronchial biopsy (TBBX) to distinguish rejection from infection.[23] BAL alone, however, is not sufficient to establish a diagnosis of rejection in these patients.

In addition to diagnostic indications, BAL is occasionally indicated for the therapeutic removal of materials from the airway. This may include the removal of mucus plugs or blood clots, the removal of bronchial casts in plastic bronchitis, or whole lung lavage as a therapy in pulmonary alveolar proteinosis. Additionally, BAL may be therapeutic for the removal of foreign lipoid material from the lungs.

TECHNIQUES FOR BRONCHOALVEOLAR LAVAGE

BAL is most conveniently performed during flexible bronchoscopy. Care must be taken to avoid contamination of the lower airway specimen with upper airway secretions during passage of the bronchoscope through the upper airway (or by aspiration following topical laryngeal anesthesia). For routine procedures, it is helpful to gently suction away excessive nasal and oral secretions before inserting the bronchoscope and to flush oxygen through the suction channel (flow ca 2 L/min) while passing the bronchoscope through the upper airway. Excessive volumes of topical anesthetic should be avoided. In a supine patient, there is a 30-degree downhill slope from larynx to carina, and as soon as the larynx is anesthetized, oral secretions may begin to flow towards the carina. For this reason, suction should not be performed through the bronchoscope until the tip of the instrument is deep within the lungs. It is helpful to preselect the BAL site and to perform the BAL as soon after entering the trachea as possible to minimize the chance of aspirating significant volumes of oral secretions into the specimen. In immunocompromised patients or those in whom it is vital to minimize ambiguity in the results, it is useful to electively intubate the patient and pass the flexible bronchoscope through the

endotracheal tube or to use a laryngeal mask. The upper airway can be examined later after removing the endotracheal tube. In children who already have a tracheostomy tube in place, performing BAL through the tracheostomy tube prior to examining the upper airway may lead to less contamination.

After the bronchoscope has been introduced into the lower airway, it should be gently wedged into the selected bronchus. Site selection is based on clinical, bronchoscopic, or radiographic findings. If there is diffuse disease, however, it is advantageous to wedge the bronchoscope into the lingula or right middle lobe bronchus (although in suspected aspiration, dependent bronchi may be more appropriate).

With the bronchoscope gently wedged into the bronchus, sterile normal saline is instilled through the suction channel of the bronchoscope and immediately withdrawn. Enough air should be instilled after each aliquot to ensure clearance of the saline from the suction channel. The volume of the channel can be as high as 2 mL in bronchoscopes with larger suction channels. The fluid may be withdrawn by hand suction with a syringe, or may be aspirated into a trap. Although enough suction must be applied to overcome the resistance of the channel in the bronchoscope; too much negative pressure will cause the bronchus to collapse, preventing efflux of fluid and possibly causing trauma to the airway mucosa. Fluid return may also be impaired if the patient is not breathing spontaneously. In some patients, almost any amount of negative pressure will result in collapse of the bronchus, and fluid return may be challenging. In such situations, it may be necessary to instill additional volumes of saline to recover a representative specimen. The suction port at the tip of a flexible bronchus is offset from the optical axis of the instrument so that if the bronchus into which the instrument is wedged is centered in the image, the suction port may be partially occluded by the bronchial wall. Positioning the bronchoscope so that the image of the bronchus is off center may improve fluid return.

Some centers utilize saline that has been warmed to body temperature (37°C) (supposedly to minimize bronchospasm and increase return), although with small volume BAL, there is little risk, and room temperature saline may be safely used. There is no consensus as to the number and volume of aliquots that should be used in BAL. In adult patients, it is common to utilize three aliquots of 100 mL or five aliquots of 50 mL. In children, various protocols have been used. Some bronchoscopists use a standard volume of 10 to 20 mL in 2 to 4 aliquots regardless of body weight and age; others adjust the volume to the patient's FRC based on weight or adjust the volume based on weight using 3 mL/kg divided into three aliquots with a maximum of 20 mL per aliquot.[24] Given the great variability in alveolar surface area being sampled based on the child's size, the size of the bronchoscope, and the location of the wedge, no BAL technique is truly capable of standardization. Smaller bronchoscopes will pass further into the distal airways before wedging, and each bronchial division cuts the lung volume that is sampled by at least half. For clinical purposes, the precise volume is probably of little relevance, as the primary application in children is the detection of infectious agents and examination of the cellular constituents. There should be reasonable uniformity in technique within a given institution. For clinical research, consistent protocols may be helpful, but no technique will ensure that the dilution of specimens is truly uniform.

Generally, 40% to 60% of the instilled fluid will be recovered, and the remainder of the fluid will be absorbed over a few hours. The first aliquot returned is relatively enriched in fluid from the surface of the conducting airways and may have a higher percentage of neutrophils.[25] Some bronchoscopists therefore separate out this first aliquot for culture rather than pooling it with subsequent aliquots, although the bronchial surface fluid will be washed into the alveolar spaces by each aliquot, therefore "contaminating" the subsequent aliquots with bronchial contents. For routine purposes, the small differences in content from one aliquot to the next do not warrant different handling.

Performing a BAL usually prolongs the bronchoscopic procedure by 1 to 3 minutes, minimally increasing the risks of hypoxia or hypercarbia, but is well tolerated by most patients, even those who are critically ill. If a patient is thrombocytopenic, BAL could theoretically increase the risk of bleeding, but can be performed relatively safely in children with platelet counts greater than 20,000 platelets/mL.[26] Some children do develop transient fever after BAL, especially if their airways were significantly inflamed, but this is almost always transient and self-limited. A theoretical risk of spreading infection and causing iatrogenic pneumonia exists,[7] but is rarely proven. The most problematic complication of BAL is not obtaining the correct information by not preparing for and adequately performing the procedure, or by failing to perform the appropriate analysis of the specimen.

An extension of BAL is whole lung ("bronchopulmonary") lavage that is used therapeutically in individuals with pulmonary alveolar proteinosis. Alveolar proteinosis is less common in children than adults, and special techniques may be required for whole lung lavage.[27] Whole lung lavage can be performed with partial cardiopulmonary bypass or by sequential single lung lavage. In children with pulmonary alveolar proteinosis, multiple whole lung lavages are usually needed over a prolonged period (years) so that the use of bypass is quite problematic. I have successfully performed sequential (single) whole lung lavage on infants as small as 3.5 kg.[28]

Another special technique is nonbronchoscopic BAL.[29] This involves blindly placing a catheter through an endotracheal or tracheostomy tube into a distal "wedged" position, instilling normal saline and then withdrawing that saline into a trap or syringe. The suction catheter should have only one hole at the end. This is truly a blind procedure and will likely only yield useful results in diffuse lung disease. Some groups have advocated use of this technique routinely in neonates intubated with small endotracheal tubes. However, the wide availability of a 2.8 mm flexible bronchoscope that can be used through endotracheal tubes as small as 3.5 mm has significantly decreased the need for nonbronchoscopic procedures.

PROCESSING OF BRONCHOALVEOLAR LAVAGE SPECIMENS

BAL fluid should be processed promptly. Some centers keep the sample at 4°C prior to processing to maintain cell viability,[16] although this is most important if the sample will not be promptly transported to or processed by the laboratory and is not generally necessary. The sample should routinely be processed for microbiology and cytological studies. Some research protocols call for filtering of the BAL fluid prior to processing (to remove mucus plugs, etc.). However, this procedure may alter the diagnostic value of the specimen, as cells and microorganisms may adhere to the filter, and there may be important information hidden within mucus plugs. The bronchoscopist should organize a routine technique for processing with the institutional laboratory service; pediatric specimens require different processing and interpretation than do specimens from adult patients.

Microbiologic studies are performed according to the clinical indications for the procedure. Because of the potential for contamination of BAL specimens by secretions from the oropharynx, semiquantitative culture techniques may help in the interpretation of results. Large numbers of "oral flora" may indicate contamination of the specimen with oral secretions (or may be a reflection of aspiration of oral secretions prior to the procedure). In addition to cultures, other techniques such as special stains or PCR may help to identify pathogens; the bronchoscopist should consult with the laboratory to determine what analyses may be available and the specific requirements for specimen volume and handling.

The basic cytological analysis of a BAL specimen involves a cellular differential, which can be performed with simple stains such as Wright's or Giemsa. The specimen is centrifuged onto a slide; most centers perform cytospins at 250 to 500 × g for 5 to 10 minutes. Special stains are performed according to the clinical indications (e.g., lipid or iron stains and methenamine-silver stains). Differential cell counts are more useful than total cell counts, because of the variable dilution of the specimen. A hypocellular specimen (defined either by cell count or observation of the stained slides) may indicate an inadequate specimen, and the data from such specimens should be interpreted with caution. Flow cytometry can be done for special indications.

Although all BAL samples should routinely be processed for microbiologic studies and cytology, there is wide variability in practice as to the specific tests that are considered routine. This variability stems from differences in patient population, in institutional capabilities and preferences, and in advancing technologies. Box 9.2 lists some potential analyses for BAL fluid.

INTERPRETATION OF BRONCHOALVEOLAR LAVAGE FINDINGS

Interpretation of BAL findings must be undertaken with the knowledge that both technique and disease state play a large role in results. For instance, wedging more proximally increases both cell number and percentage of neutrophils. Small volumes sample mainly the airway. BAL samples the bronchial and alveolar surfaces and does not necessarily reflect parenchymal processes. In general, cell numbers in normal children will range between 100,000 and 250,000 cells/mL. Normal BAL fluid contains less than 5% neutrophils (usually 1% to 2%).[30,31] Patients with an active bacterial infection may have up to 95% neutrophils, and rarely less than 25%. Patients with bacterial infection often have bacterial forms visible in the cytoplasm of neutrophils recovered in BAL[32]; this may be a useful measure to differentiate between infection and contamination of the specimen with

Box 9.2   Potential Bronchoalveolar Lavage Assays

Microbiologic studies	Viruses
Gram stain	Cytological studies
Cultures	Total cell count
Bacterial (quantitative)	Stains for differential cytology
Viral	Giemsa, Wright's, H&E
Fungal	Flow cytometry
Mycobacterial	Trypan blue exclusion for cell
Anaerobic	viability
Stains	Lymphocyte subsets
Gomori-Grocott	Special Stains
(methenamine-silver stain)	Lipid Stains
Ziehl-Neelsen (AFB)	Oil Red O
Immunoassays	Sudan IV
Chlamydia	Iron Stain
Mycoplasma	Prussian Blue
Legionella	PAP Stains (Alveolar
Fungi	proteinosis)
Viruses	Periodic Acid Schiff
PCR	Electron Microscopy
Viruses	Noncellular components
Chlamydia	Surfactant proteins
Mycoplasma	Cytokines
In situ	

oral secretions. Increased neutrophils can also be seen in chronic inflammatory states associated with aspiration or cystic fibrosis, in ARDS, in alveolitis, in scleroderma, and even in asthma. Normally, 80% to 90% of the nonepithelial cells in BAL are alveolar macrophages. Lymphocytes are the next most common cell type, comprising 5% to 10% of the BAL cells in normal children. Although increased percentages of lymphocytes are not diagnostic of any specific disease, increased numbers are seen in interstitial lung disease such as hypersensitivity pneumonitis or sarcoidosis and mycobacterial infection. Eosinophils are rare in normal subjects (0% to 1%); significant numbers suggest an allergic state, eosinophilic pneumonia, parasitic infection, interstitial lung disease, drug-induced lung disease, *Pneumocystis jirovecii* infection, or a foreign body reaction. Very high numbers are seen in eosinophilic pneumonia. Epithelial cells are common in BAL fluid but are not counted in the differential. Squamous cells from the upper airway, often covered in oral bacteria, and ciliated columnar cells from the lower airway can also be seen.

Opinions vary as to what number of bacteria constitutes adequate evidence of infection, and the variable dilution of BAL specimens adds to the uncertainty. In general, for common bacterial species such as *Staphylococcus aureus*, *Haemophilus influenzae*, and *Streptococcus pneumoniae*, concentrations of more than 100,000 organisms/mL of BAL fluid, in association with significant numbers of neutrophils, are adequate evidence of infection. In the absence of neutrophils (except in neutropenic patients), bacteria are more likely to represent contamination than infection. Numbers of bacteria more than 500,000 organisms/mL are common in clear-cut bacterial infection, as is the finding of intracellular bacteria. However, the interpretation is not always straightforward, especially if significant numbers of "oral flora" are also recovered. In pediatric patients, it is possible to obtain BAL specimens that are sterile, but the majority

will have at least some oral flora even if there are no pathogens. In immunocompromised patients, the finding of pathogens that are not normally in the lung may be diagnostic, regardless of numbers. *P. jirovecii*, *Mycobacterium tuberculosis*, *Legionella pneumophila*, Nocardia, Histoplasma, Blastomyces, Mycoplasma, influenza virus, and respiratory syncytial virus would therefore be true pathogens; whereas Herpes simplex virus, CMV, Aspergillus, atypical mycobacteria, bacteria and Candida may not be pathogens but merely contaminants or colonizing agents.

Viruses can be grown from BAL fluid but may take weeks, limiting the utility of this assay. Using PCR to detect viruses can speed diagnosis and may be more sensitive. Another indication of viral infection is the finding of viral cytopathic effect on stains of cytospins. Fungi can be seen on stain as well as grown in culture. Distinguishing contamination or colonization from true infection can be difficult, however. Mycobacteria must be cultured on special medium and may take up to 8 weeks to grow. With significant infection, the AFB smear may be positive as well. Newer molecular methods such as nucleic acid probes or DNA amplification can speed detection.

A Gomori-Grocott (methenamine-silver) stain helps in the detection of fungi, especially for *P. jirovecii*, for which it can be diagnostic. Periodic Acid Schiff (PAS) staining is used to characterize the diffuse proteinaceous material in pulmonary alveolar proteinosis. The lamellar bodies defining the material as surfactant can be seen on electron microscopy. Prussian blue stains detect iron in macrophages from pulmonary hemorrhages or hemosiderosis. Macrophages become positive for iron staining about 50 hours after bleeding occurs, not immediately. If no further bleeding occurs, iron will clear in 12 to 14 days from the airways and in 2 to 4 weeks from the parenchyma. It can be normal to have up to 3% of macrophages staining positive for iron.

Lipid stains (Oil Red O or Sudan IV) are used to detect lipid-laden macrophages in an attemptto diagnose aspiration of food (from swallowing or gastroesophageal reflux). Although this technique is plagued by a lack of sensitivity and specificity,[33] the use of a "lipid index"[22] may increase the utility of the test. A positive lipid stain does not reveal the source of the lipid (aspiration vs. endogenous sources). Also, lipid stains may not identify children who aspirate oral secretions but who are not being fed orally.

RESEARCH APPLICATIONS OF BRONCHOALVEOLAR LAVAGE

A widely untapped arena for BAL is its use in clinical, translational, and basic science research. In recent years, many new assays for detection of inflammatory markers, for the function of bronchoalveolar cells, and for the detection of a wide array of noncellular BAL components have been developed. Some of these are used sporadically in clinical assays, such as the determination of lymphocyte subpopulations and the identification of surfactant proteins, but most are used strictly for research purposes. One of the limitations of such assays is the lack of control data, as normal children do not ordinarily undergo flexible bronchoscopy with BAL. Development of collaborations and specimen banks may help define the normal population, allowing research to proceed more rapidly.

Diagnostic Techniques Other Than Bronchoalveolar Lavage

BIOPSY

Mucosal samples can be obtained by direct biopsy. However, in practical terms, the only location from which a specimen can be readily obtained is from the carina; the biopsy forceps must contact the airway wall at a near-perpendicular angle. The very small forceps capable of passing through the 1.2 mm suction channel of pediatric bronchoscopes are usually inadequate for this purpose.

Endobronchial lesions (granulation tissue, tumors) can be readily biopsied under direct visual control. The forceps are advanced to the lesion, opened, pressed into the surface of the lesion, and then closed. Bleeding may result, and care must be taken to avoid biopsy of obviously vascular lesions. Topical application of a vasoconstrictor such as oxymetazoline can help control bleeding.

Biopsy of lesions adjacent to the trachea or central bronchi is possible, utilizing transbronchial needle aspiration (TBNA). The operator must be absolutely certain that the "lesion" being biopsied is not vascular; a contrasted CT scan and/or endobronchial ultrasound can be essential to safe conduct of TBNA. TBNA is a very uncommon procedure in pediatric patients, and if it is felt to be necessary, the pediatric bronchoscopist would be wise to consult with an adult interventional bronchoscopist.

TBBX is often used in adult patients in the evaluation of diffuse lung diseases or suspected malignancy. Forceps are advanced through the bronchoscope and into a peripheral site, as guided by fluoroscopy. There is a substantial risk of brisk hemorrhage, as well as pneumothorax. TBBX is rarely if ever indicated in pediatric patients, other than lung transplant recipients, in whom it is important to evaluate for rejection. The specimens are very small, and for most non-transplant pediatric patients, a thoracoscopic biopsy is more likely to yield a diagnosis.

BRONCHIAL BRUSHING

A cytology brush can be used to obtain a large number of epithelial cells from the bronchial mucosa. In pediatric patients, this is most often performed for evaluation of ciliary motility and ultrastructure. The brush is passed through the bronchoscope, the mucosa is gently abraded with the brush, and then the brush is retracted to the tip of the bronchoscope, which is then withdrawn from the airway (this is best done through an endotracheal tube or LMA). The brush is then advanced and cut, delivering the brush and specimen into a suitable container. If the brush is pulled through the suction channel of the bronchoscope, most of the specimen may be lost.

Brushes are also used to obtain specimens for microbiologic diagnosis. One potential advantage of bronchoscopy is that specimens can be obtained from the lower airways without contamination by mouth flora. Unfortunately, however, there is a significant risk of such contamination by passage of the bronchoscope through the nose or mouth on the way to the distal airways. Specimens obtained by simple aspiration through the bronchoscope often show evidence of oral flora.

To surmount this problem, a protected microbiology specimen brush has been developed[34]; this brush is protected by two concentric sheaths; the outer sheath is plugged with wax to prevent secretions in the bronchoscope channel from contaminating the brush. This specimen collection system functions very well to avoid contamination of the brush specimen by secretions present in the suction channel of the bronchoscope. Unfortunately, however, it does not guarantee freedom from contamination by upper airway flora. If during the preparation for the procedure and insertion of the bronchoscope any oral secretions are aspirated into the trachea and bronchi (which is an almost universal occurrence), then the site from which the specimen is collected will be contaminated, and it makes relatively little difference what technique is used to obtain the specimen. Topical laryngeal anesthesia almost always results in contamination of the trachea and at least central bronchi to some extent with oral flora. Protected specimen brushes are not small enough to use through pediatric bronchoscopes.

VISUAL ANALYSIS

The optical properties of bronchoscopes (both rigid and flexible) are such that it is extremely difficult to gauge the size of an object in view unless there is another object of known size at precisely the same distance from the tip of the scope.[35] One can estimate *relative* size, but not *absolute* size; it is not uncommon to gain the impression that the subglottic space is normal by visual examination only to find that the patient's airway will not accept a normal size endotracheal tube.

It is often possible to visualize the movement of mucus, bubbles, or debris across the mucosal surface by mucociliary transport. Normal mucociliary transport is approximately 10 mm/min, and thus readily visible in real time. These observations should be done on the anterior tracheal wall, since there will often be a flow of oral secretions along the posterior wall. If the selected marker can be seen to move across one or more tracheal rings, then one can be confident that mucociliary transport is normal. The inability to observe movement, however, does not establish a diagnosis of ciliary dysfunction (PCD), as there are many factors that influence mucociliary transport function other than ciliary beat/ultrastructure (see Chapter 71).

Therapeutic Bronchoscopy

Therapeutic indications for bronchoscopy in infants and children primarily involve the restoration of airway patency. While the majority of such applications will involve the use of a rigid bronchoscope, considerable therapeutic benefit can often be achieved with flexible instruments as well. Therapeutic bronchoscopy is indicated when it is the best way to achieve the desired therapeutic goals. There are many techniques loosely referred to as "interventional" techniques that are used in adults, but they are much less applicable to pediatric patients. In large part this is due to the different pathologic entities encountered in the pediatric airways, but it is also due to the small size of the pediatric airways.

The *removal of foreign bodies* is one of the more common therapeutic applications of bronchoscopy in children. It is also one of the more difficult and potentially dangerous bronchoscopic procedures in children. Only under the most unusual circumstances should foreign body removal be attempted with a flexible bronchoscope. The devices that can be passed through a flexible instrument and used for foreign body retrieval are rudimentary at best, and airway management is difficult. Small, peripherally located foreign bodies may best be reached with a flexible bronchoscope but may yet be difficult to remove. Passage of a Fogarty catheter beyond the foreign body, subsequent inflation of the catheter's balloon, and gentle retraction of the catheter may help move the foreign body to a more central location from which it may be more easily recovered. Care must be taken to avoid pushing the foreign body to a more distal position.

When the foreign body is a manufactured object and can be identified beforehand, it is helpful to practice on a duplicate object to ensure that the forceps chosen will secure a firm grasp of the object. There is a great variety of forceps available for use with different types of foreign bodies. Foreign body extraction may be complicated by the presence of inspissated secretions or granulation tissue. Foreign bodies such as nuts, which may fragment, may be present in multiple sites, and a very thorough examination of all bronchi should be made after removing any foreign body. In rare circumstances, such as a straight pin lodged in the periphery of the lung, a flexible bronchoscope may be the only suitable instrument.

Mucus plugs or blood clots in the airways causing atelectasis will usually yield to endoscopic treatment. Localized trauma from endotracheal suctioning is a common cause of mucus plugs. Children with small (usually organic) foreign bodies, cystic fibrosis, asthma, allergic bronchopulmonary aspergillosis, or pneumonia may also develop central mucus plugs. In some cases, the plugs must be removed with forceps, much as though they were a foreign body. Most mucus plugs, however, will yield to suctioning through a flexible bronchoscope. By touching the tip of the flexible bronchoscope to the proximal surface of the mucus plug and applying constant suction while withdrawing the instrument, plugs much larger than the diameter of the suction channel can often be removed, even if in pieces. Because mucus plugs and clots extend into distal bronchial branches, they have "roots" that often make extraction challenging and time-consuming. Local lavage with saline or a mucolytic agent (dornase alfa) can also be helpful to dislodge a mucus plug. In older patients, it may be feasible to extract large clots or mucus plugs with a cryoprobe.

Tracheal or bronchial stenosis can sometimes be effectively managed endoscopically, especially if the stenosis is short; longer lesions are usually best dealt with surgically. A very narrow, membranous stenosis may be dilated with the bronchoscope or a small endotracheal tube, for acute relief, and then managed more definitively by other means. In general, the most effective technique for dilation is the application of radial force through an angioplasty catheter. These devices are less than 2 mm in diameter, can be passed through the (adult) bronchoscope working channel, and then inflated to high pressure (as much as 20 atmospheres) to a defined diameter. Care must be taken in selection of the appropriate catheter (err on the side of caution), as rupture of the airway is a potential complication.

A relatively short stenosis due to dense scar tissue can also be treated by laser. While a laser is intuitively attractive, it is also potentially a very dangerous tool. Vaporization of tissue produces steam, which can cook surrounding normal tissues. Exuberant use of the laser can also lead to more scarring as the lesion heals; it is good practice to limit laser excision of a circumferential lesion to three points, leaving untreated tissue between the lased areas (as appropriate, the untreated areas can be handled at a subsequent procedure). Furthermore, if the laser beam penetrates the target tissue, there is nothing to stop it from affecting tissue distally with potentially catastrophic consequences. Therefore, great caution must be exercised in the endoscopic use of any laser such as using the lowest workable power setting, short, intermittent bursts, and careful visual control of the effect. In benign lesions, it may be preferable to merely desiccate the target tissue, rather than vaporize it, allowing the treated tissue to slough over the next few days to weeks. The use of a laser in the airways always requires a follow-up evaluation, and possibly repeated treatments. The use of a laser can also be combined with balloon dilation.

Lasers that are useful in the pediatric airways include the blue light lasers (KTP, argon) and CO_2. The blue light lasers offer good hemostasis and can be used through very small fibers (as small as 0.3 mm diameter), which can be inserted through the suction channel of pediatric bronchoscopes and precisely positioned. The fibers are relatively stiff, however, and the tip of the instrument cannot be deflected to a sharp angle, thus limiting the sites that can be reached with the laser. The CO_2 laser is generally used without a fiber, and is primarily used in the upper airway, perhaps to the midtrachea. Other lasers are available, and their use depends on institutional factors as well as patient needs.

Mass lesions in the airways can often be dealt with effectively with a bronchoscope. Granulation tissue is the most common such lesion and may result from foreign bodies, mycobacterial infection, or mechanical trauma associated with artificial airways. Less commonly, tumor masses may be found in children, usually a hemangioma or a bronchial carcinoid tumor.

Benign mass lesions can be resected, if appropriate, with forceps, an endoscopic cautery electrode, or a laser. The operator must be alert to the potential for hemorrhage with vascular lesions such as hemangiomas or carcinoid tumors; biopsy (or forceps removal) of such lesions is rarely a bright idea. Malignant lesions, or lesions that extend through the bronchial wall, are usually best dealt with surgically rather than endoscopically, although endoscopic resection may be employed for temporary relief of obstruction in selected cases. In general, the use of endobronchial forceps is easier with rigid bronchoscopes; in addition, there is better potential for control of bleeding, and the forceps are larger and more readily manipulated than the small, flexible instruments that can be used with flexible bronchoscopes. Laser applications may utilize either rigid or flexible instruments. A monopolar cautery electrode as small as 3Fr can be passed through the suction channel of a pediatric bronchoscope and used to directly destroy endobronchial lesions such as granulation tissue or papillomata. Advantages of this technique include the ability to fully flex the tip of the bronchoscope, thus accessing lesions in the upper lobes, and the fact that the effect is limited to the tissue in direct contact with the tip of the electrode. However, as with a laser, care must be taken to limit collateral damage by using the lowest effective power and short, repeated applications.

There is a variety of *stents* that may be placed to ensure airway patency under certain conditions. However, none of these devices are truly appropriate for pediatric patients, and there is little experience with such devices in children, especially young infants. Great caution should be taken when considering stenting in pediatric patients. Stents are associated with numerous problems, such as mucus retention, formation of granulation tissue, and migration of the stent. In growing children, a stent will have to be replaced periodically; otherwise, the child will develop an iatrogenic stenosis. However, if the stent has become embedded in the airway mucosa, it may be extremely difficult to remove safely.[36] Nevertheless, in highly selected patients, stenting may be the only way to achieve and maintain airway patency. The US Food and Drug Administration, which approves medical devices, strongly cautions against using expandable metal stents in benign conditions (which includes almost all potential pediatric applications).[37]

Alveolar filling disorders such as alveolar proteinosis or lipid aspiration are treated by bronchopulmonary lavage. While this may be accomplished, after a fashion, directly through a bronchoscope, it is more effective to utilize large volumes of saline and to lavage relatively large areas of the lung at one time. In adults, a double-lumen endotracheal tube is used; this is not feasible in patients younger than approximately 10 years, as the smallest double lumen endotracheal tube is 26 Fr (the patient's larynx must accept a 6.5 mm endotracheal tube, which is approximately 8.5 mm in outer diameter). A flexible bronchoscope can be used to position a single-lumen cuffed endobronchial catheter through which an entire lung can be lavaged with large volumes, while ventilation is maintained with a nasopharyngeal tube.[28]

Flexible bronchoscopes are valuable in the management of tracheostomy and endotracheal tubes. Problems with tube positioning or tube patency can be resolved quickly with a flexible instrument.

Bronchoscopy can be useful in the management of *intractable air leaks*. A systematic search for the bronchus leading to the air leak can be made with a Fogarty catheter, which is inflated in a bronchus while observing the air leak from the chest tube (this requires that there be an active leak during the evaluation). When the site of the leak is defined, fibrin glue or Gelfoam can be packed into the bronchus leading to the site of the air leak. In older patients, a one-way valve can be placed in the bronchus leading to the leak and removed after the lung has healed.[38] More proximal leaks, as from the stump of a resected bronchus, can be treated directly by application of tissue adhesive.[39]

Bronchoscopic intubation is a technique that facilitates difficult or complicated intubations and should almost always be successful if the right instruments are available and the operator is skilled in their use. A flexible bronchoscope is passed through a suitable endotracheal tube. The bronchoscope is then passed into the trachea (usually through the nose, but an oral approach may be used instead). With the tip of the bronchoscope held just above the carina, the endotracheal tube is advanced over the flexible bronchoscope until its tip is seen through the bronchoscope. The bronchoscope must be held so that its shaft is straight while the endotracheal tube is advanced over it; otherwise, damage to the bronchoscope (or bronchi) may result. The bronchoscope is withdrawn, the patient is ventilated, and then the bronchoscope is again inserted to verify the position of the endotracheal tube and to ensure that the anatomy and patency of the distal airways are adequate.

A skilled bronchoscopist should be able to accomplish a bronchoscopic intubation in 30 seconds or less. When bronchoscopic intubation is required, there must be a plan to achieve safe extubation—if the patient fails extubation, a flexible bronchoscope may be urgently needed to restore a safe and effective airway.

Complications of Bronchoscopy

Other than death of the patient, the most serious complication of a bronchoscopy is to have performed the procedure and obtained the wrong (or no) answer or the wrong (or inadequate) therapeutic result. Every procedure has potential for complications ranging from trivial to lethal. Bronchoscopy is no exception, although reported lethal complications of bronchoscopy in pediatric patients are rare. The risk of complications is a function of inherent risk factors in the patient (e.g., disease state, severity of disease, and age), the procedure performed, the skill and experience of the bronchoscopist and the bronchoscopy team, and the patient's preparation for the procedure.

In general, the risk is greater with rigid bronchoscopy than with flexible bronchoscopy. This is because foreign body extraction is perhaps the most challenging, difficult, and risky bronchoscopic procedure commonly performed in pediatric patients and is always done with a rigid instrument. In addition, the relatively large diameter and rigid nature of the rigid bronchoscope make it more likely to traumatize the mucosa of the subglottic space or airways. However, flexible bronchoscopy is not immune to serious complications, and at least one death has been reported in association with a flexible bronchoscopy in a pediatric patient.[40] Disaster lurks around the corner for the unwise or unwary.

Mechanical complications of bronchoscopy result from direct trauma to the airway. Pneumothorax or pneumomediastinum, mucosal edema, and hemorrhage are most common. Such complications are more likely when auxiliary instruments such as biopsy forceps are used. The greatest risk is incurred during the extraction of foreign bodies and in the performance of TBBX. The risk of mechanical complications can be reduced by careful selection of instruments and procedures. Epistaxis is common in thrombocytopenic patients; consideration should be given to passing the flexible bronchoscope via an orotracheal tube instead of transnasally. Since most such patients are also immunosuppressed, this practice will also reduce the risk of contamination of the BAL specimen (and the lower airways) with oral secretions and flora. Patients with large adenoids often develop epistaxis when a nasopharyngeal tube is passed to facilitate ventilation during the procedure; NP tubes should only be placed after examination of the nasopharyngeal airway.

When a flexible bronchoscope is passed through an endotracheal tube, there is the potential for the development of inadvertent PEEP. It is easy to force air through the tube around the bronchoscope, but exhalation is passive, and if the expiratory resistance is high, intrapulmonary pressure may increase to the point of impairing pulmonary perfusion or producing a pneumothorax.

Physiologic complications of bronchoscopy include hypoxia, hypercapnia, hypotension, laryngospasm, bronchospasm, cardiac arrhythmias, and aspiration. There is a constant risk of hypoventilation during bronchoscopy due to anesthesia or to airway obstruction, and smaller patients are at greater risk of airway obstruction. All bronchoscopes (rigid as well as flexible) produce some degree of airway obstruction. Vagal stimulation due to inadequate topical anesthesia or catecholamine release due to inadequate sedation/anesthesia may result in cardiac arrhythmias. Laryngospasm or bronchospasm are usually due to inadequate topical anesthesia. Seizures can result from lidocaine toxicity. The risk of physiologic complications can be reduced by careful attention to patient preparation as well as anesthetic and monitoring techniques.

Bacteriologic complications of bronchoscopy include the introduction of infectious agents into the lungs from the patient's own upper airway or from another patient if the instruments are not adequately cleaned and sterilized. Infection in one part of a patient's lung can be spread to other areas. Although the risk appears to be low, it is possible that bacterial endocarditis could result in susceptible patients following bronchoscopy; appropriate antibiotic prophylaxis should be considered for the patient at high risk. However, if a BAL specimen is to be obtained for culture, the prophylactic antibiotics should not be administered until after the BAL specimen is obtained. Bronchoscopy can also result in spread of infectious agents from the patient to the personnel performing the procedure, so precautions should be taken to protect personnel. Older patients known to have cavitary tuberculosis, for example, represent very high risk to the bronchoscopy team, and bronchoscopy should in most cases be delayed until appropriate therapy has been given for a sufficient time to greatly reduce this risk.

There are also *cognitive risks of bronchoscopy:* the failure to obtain useful information or making the wrong diagnosis. Even failure to perform bronchoscopy when it is the best or only way to obtain information necessary for the patient's care could be considered an error or complication. The bronchoscopist must be aware of the many pitfalls that await the unwary.[41] Video recording the procedure allows later review of the observations, and sometimes leads to a revision of the diagnosis. Serious consideration should be given to recording all procedures, to augment teaching, consultative reports, and even research data acquisition.

Cognitive risks are reduced by adequate training and experience on the part of the bronchoscopist and support staff. There is no simple guideline as to the requirements for training of a bronchoscopist; obviously, inherent aptitude varies greatly from individual to individual. The bronchoscopist must develop both manual skills and an effective knowledge of anatomy, pathology, indications for bronchoscopy, and techniques for anesthesia/sedation to safely and effectively perform procedures. A formal, comprehensive training program should be a prerequisite, but there is no substitute for good judgment and experience. Most authorities suggest that a minimum of 50 to 100 procedures performed with a suitable mentor are required before an individual should be certified to do bronchoscopy independently.[42,43]

Complications of bronchoscopy may include more than adverse effects on the patient or personnel. Failure to utilize a bite block when a flexible bronchoscope is passed through a patient's mouth, for example, can result in destruction of the instrument. Flexible bronchoscopes currently cost more than $27,000 (USD), and smaller bronchoscopes are more fragile. Flexible bronchoscopes are often damaged during passage through endotracheal tubes, and biopsy forceps can also perforate the suction channel, thus decommissioning the instrument.

Economic Aspects of Bronchoscopy

Bronchoscopy is not a simple, inexpensive procedure. Total cost will depend on institutional factors as well as the nature and extent of the procedure performed. Specific costs include support for equipment and procedure rooms, consumable supplies, laboratory charges for processing of diagnostic specimens, monitoring of the sedated patient before and after the procedure, record keeping, support of ancillary staff, and professional fees. When general anesthesia is used instead of sedation performed by the bronchoscopist, costs are generally higher, but this should not be a significant factor in decision making if the services of an anesthesiologist significantly enhance the safety of the patient. In large part because of the need for general anesthesia, rigid bronchoscopy may be more expensive than flexible,[44] but again, the decision as to choice of technique should be made on the basis of the patient's medical needs.

Although definitive studies of cost-effectiveness in pediatric practice have not been reported, bronchoscopy is often a cost-saving procedure. For example, the early identification of a specific infectious agent in the immunocompromised patient with pneumonia can mean that more expensive, multiple antimicrobial therapies can be avoided (thus also reducing potential risk of complications of such treatment). Young patients with cystic fibrosis admitted to hospital for intensive therapy are not infrequently discovered at bronchoscopy to have no evidence of bacterial infection; evidence may be found instead for other causes of the persisting symptoms (such as gastroesophageal reflux with microaspiration). The definitive identification of causes of pulmonary symptoms such as stridor can reduce "doctor shopping" and multiple expensive diagnostic evaluations. The cost associated with missed diagnoses (when bronchoscopy is not performed) may be enormous.

"We dance around the patient, and suppose... but the bronchoscope sees into the patient, and knows" (with apologies to Robert Frost—"The secret").

References

Access the reference list online at ExpertConsult.com.

Suggested Reading

Cote CJ, Wilson S, American Academy of Pediatrics, American Academy of Pediatric Dentistry. Guidelines for monitoring and management of pediatric patients before, during, and after sedation for diagnostic and therapeutic procedures: update 2016. *Pediatrics.* 2016;138:pii:e20161212.

de Blic J, Midulla F, Barbato A, et al. Bronchoalveolar lavage in children. ERS Task Force on bronchoalveolar lavage in children. European Respiratory Society. *Eur Respir J.* 2000;15:217–231.

Wood RE. Spelunking in the pediatric airways: explorations with the flexible fiberoptic bronchoscope. *Pediatr Clin North Am.* 1984;31:785–799.

10 *Diagnostic Imaging of the Respiratory Tract*

THOMAS SEMPLE, FRCR, MBBS, BSc, CAROLYN YOUNG, HDCR, ØYSTEIN OLSEN, PhD, and CATHERINE OWENS, BSc, MBBS, MRCP, FRCR, FRCP

Pediatric chest radiology is a complex subject, and the clinical sections of this book cover a full understanding of all relevant pathologies with which it aids diagnosis. This chapter gives a brief overview of the imaging modalities used to help achieve an accurate and timely diagnosis, thus enabling prompt treatment of the many varied pathologic entities encountered within the pediatric thorax. The dedicated reader may wish to consult more specialized and comprehensive texts.[1-3]

The utility of imaging modalities is often uncertain because of (1) an increasing number of available techniques; and (2) the presence of numerous rare disease entities in children. Nevertheless, modern clinical practice is highly dependent on radiology.

We will discuss areas of specific concern within the pediatric age group, in particular: (1) radiation protection; (2) technical challenges (e.g., motion and breathing artifacts); (3) developing anatomy and pathophysiology (see Chapters 2 and 6); and (4) different interpretation of images compared with images obtained in adults (to a certain degree).

Plain Radiography

The plain chest radiograph remains the basis for the evaluation of the chest in childhood. In the neonate, satisfactory images can be obtained in incubators using modern mobile x-ray apparatus. The baby lies on the cassette, and the detector is exposed. Although one can automate triggering of the exposure, an experienced radiographer will usually be able to judge the end of inspiration. An adequate inspiration occurs with the right hemidiaphragm at the level of the eighth rib posteriorly. Films in expiration frequently show varying degrees of opacification of the lung fields, with apparent enlargement of the heart. Films should be well collimated, with the baby positioned as straight as possible. Lordotic films should be avoided, especially if the size of the heart is of particular interest. Monitoring equipment should be removed to the extent that is clinically safe. Digital/computed radiography is particularly useful in intensive care, and the facility of data manipulation (e.g., edge enhancement) can improve the visualization of support apparatus, such as tubes and lines.

Children older than 5 years of age can usually cooperate sufficiently to stand for a posteroanterior film in the same way as adults. In younger children, some form of chest stand is needed in which an assistant, preferably the caregiver, can hold the child in front of a cassette while standing behind a suspended protective lead apron. With proper collimation, the dose to both child and caregiver is small, and this position allows straighter positioning of the child than a position to the side. The difference between a posteroanterior projection and an anteroposterior projection in the small child is usually negligible. A high-kilovoltage technique, with added filtration and the use of a grid, allows evaluation of the trachea and major bronchi, which is important in stridor.

Specific Features of the Chest Radiograph in Children

THE THYMUS

The normal thymus (Fig. 10.1) is a frequent cause of widening of the anterior mediastinum during the first years of life. The lateral margin often shows an undulation, the thymic wave, which corresponds to the indentations of the ribs on the inner surface of the thoracic cage. Particularly on the right, the thymus may have a triangular, sail-like configuration. The thymus may involute in times of stress, and steroids can induce a decrease in size. At times, the differentiation of a physiologic thymus from pathology in the anterior mediastinum can be difficult. Ultrasound examination will usually differentiate cystic lesions from the homogeneous normal thymic tissue (see ultrasound section later in this chapter). Occasionally, the normal thymus can act as a significant space-occupying structure in the superior mediastinum, and in such cases, differentiation may be helped by either ultrasound or magnetic resonance imaging (MRI), which shows a homogeneous echogenicity/signal within a normal thymus. On MRI, a normal thymus has an intermediate signal on T2-weighted images (similar to the spleen and lymph nodes) and shows minimal uniform enhancement on T1-weighted images after intravenous contrast medium injection (Fig. 10.2).

THE CARDIOTHORACIC RATIO

In toddlers, the cardiothoracic ratio can at times exceed 0.5, and care should be exercised in overdiagnosis of cardiomegaly, particularly if the film may be expiratory.

KINK OF THE TRACHEA TO THE RIGHT

Kinking of the trachea to the right is a frequent feature of a chest film taken at less than full inspiration. This is a physiologic buckling and does not suggest a mass lesion.

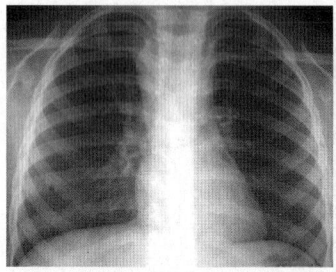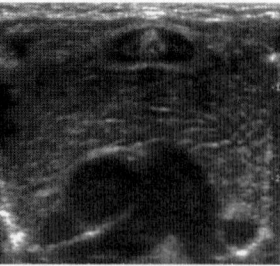

Fig. 10.1 Chest radiograph demonstrating slight widening of the superior mediastinum. Corresponding ultrasound demonstrates normal thymic tissue. (Image courtesy of P. Tomà.)

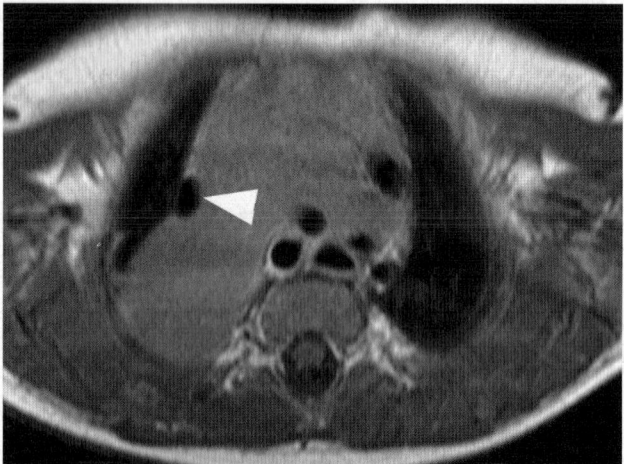

Fig. 10.2 Chest radiograph *(not shown)* in a 3-month-old child showed an unusual upper mediastinal contour. Magnetic resonance imaging (T1-weighted spin echo after intravenous injection of gadolinium chelate) shows a normal signal and no abnormal contrast enhancement from a normal but large thymus, extending posterior to the right brachiocephalic vein *(arrowhead)*. There is no sign of vascular or airway compression.

SOFT TISSUE

Soft tissue may be prominent in children, and the anterior axillary fold that crosses the chest wall can mimic pneumothorax. Similarly, skin folds can cast confusing shadows at times. Braids (plaits) of hair over the upper chest can mimic pulmonary infiltrations in the upper lobes.

PLEURAL FLUID

Whereas in adults an early sign of pleural effusion is blunting of the costophrenic angles, in children it is more common to see lateral separation of the lung from the chest wall, with reasonable preservation of the clarity of the costophrenic angles and accentuation of the interlobar fissures. In the supine position, an apical rim of soft tissue density is seen, and if a moderate to large unilateral effusion is present, the affected hemithorax has a diffuse increase in density, with preservation of vascular markings simulating ground-glass parenchymal opacification. This is due to pleural fluid collecting in the dorsal (dependent) pleural space.

Systematic Review of the Chest Radiograph

Without a systematic analytical approach to the pediatric chest radiograph, the possibility of missing relevant radiologic information is high. To combat this, knowledge of the various pitfalls in interpretation, anatomic variants, and pathologic processes relevant to the specific age group are vital. This is particularly important when there is one very conspicuous abnormal imaging finding, which can result in the cessation of more intense scrutiny of the remainder of the film. Therefore, an image review should follow a strict systematic order, including checking the putative identity of the radiograph, and should include the following.

GENERAL DEGREE OF LUNG INFLATION

Flattening of the diaphragm or diaphragmatic domes below the level of the eighth posterior ribs, elongation of the mediastinum, and widening of the intercostal spaces are all signs of pulmonary overinflation. Intercostal bulging of the pleura or lung parenchyma may be a sign of excessive ventilator pressures in an intubated child.

Generalized pulmonary underinflation is usually due to radiographic exposure during expiration, but it may be a real finding confirming small lung volumes (as in cases of respiratory distress syndrome [RDS] of the newborn, in which the lung parenchyma is noncompliant, or in bilateral pulmonary hypoplasia) or associated with lobar collapse.

One should also consider elevation of the diaphragm, with consequential lung compression due to bowel distention, pneumoperitoneum, or the presence of a large abdominal mass. Hence, the periphery of the radiograph (e.g., the area under the diaphragm) should always be carefully and routinely inspected as part of a systematic review.

ASYMMETRICAL LUNG VOLUME

In the absence of a pneumothorax, mediastinal shift toward a lung with uniformly increased density compared with the contralateral lung is a sign of differential inflation of the two lungs. This may be caused by overinflation of the more lucent lung (e.g., due to a ball-valve mechanism in the central airways), in which case the ipsilateral hemidiaphragm would be flattened (Fig. 10.3).

Alternatively, it may be caused by volume loss in the denser lung, in which case the diaphragm of the denser hemithorax would be elevated. This may be a sign of unilateral pulmonary hypoplasia, aplasia, or agenesis (Figs. 10.4–10.6), in which case the mediastinum is shifted toward the hemithorax containing the small lung, and ipsilateral elevation of the hemidiaphragm is seen. Combined overinflation of one lung and volume loss of the other can sometimes be seen secondary to mass lesions that affect the central airways (Fig. 10.7).

Other causes of asymmetrical lung volumes include diaphragmatic paresis/paralysis and a large abdominal mass lesion that causes elevation of the ipsilateral hemidiaphragm. The diaphragm may also be apparently elevated secondary to a subpulmonic fluid collection. In congenital diaphragmatic hernia, the multicystic appearance of bowel contents may or may not be obvious within the thorax (Fig. 10.8). If seen,

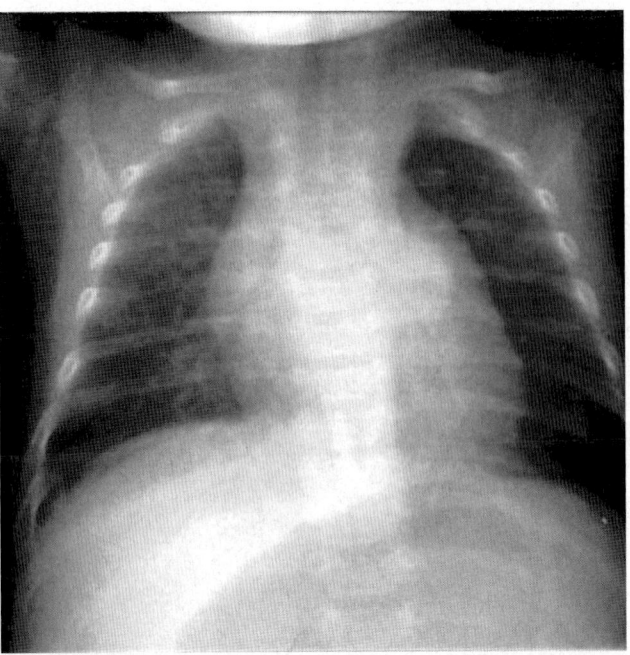

Fig. 10.3 Chest radiograph in a young child shows a semicircular left convex distortion of the left mediastinal outline due to a bronchogenic cyst and secondary overinflation of the left lower lobe.

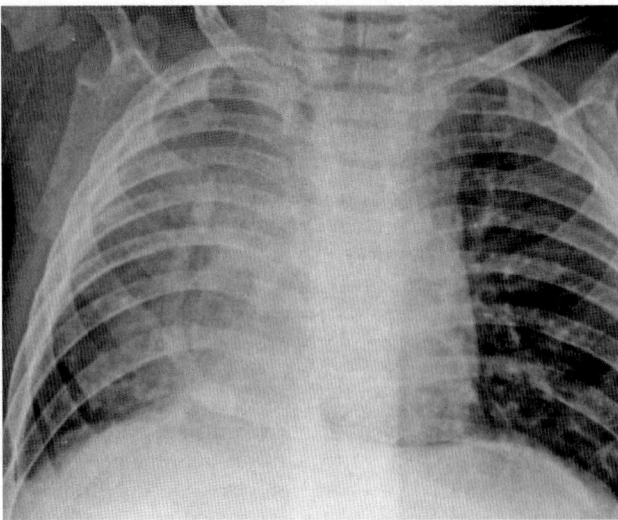

Fig. 10.5 Chest radiograph shows a hypoplastic right lung with an abnormal vascular structure running toward the diaphragmatic level medially. This represents systemic venous drainage of the right lung. The shape of the abnormal vein resembles a Turkish scimitar (bowed sword); hence, the denotation scimitar syndrome (see Figs. 10.44 and 10.46).

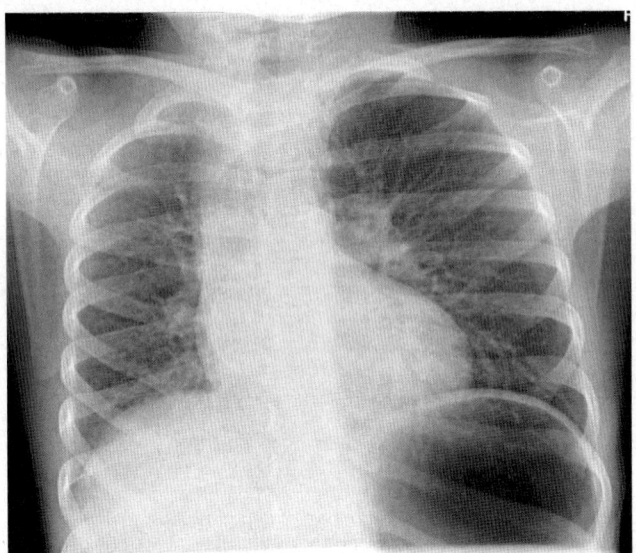

Fig. 10.4 In a 10-year-old girl who presented with shortness of breath, this chest radiograph shows a small right hemithorax (rib crowding, diaphragmatic elevation, compensatory large left lung), but no lung opacification. This was later diagnosed as an interrupted right pulmonary artery (see Figs. 10.45 and 10.70).

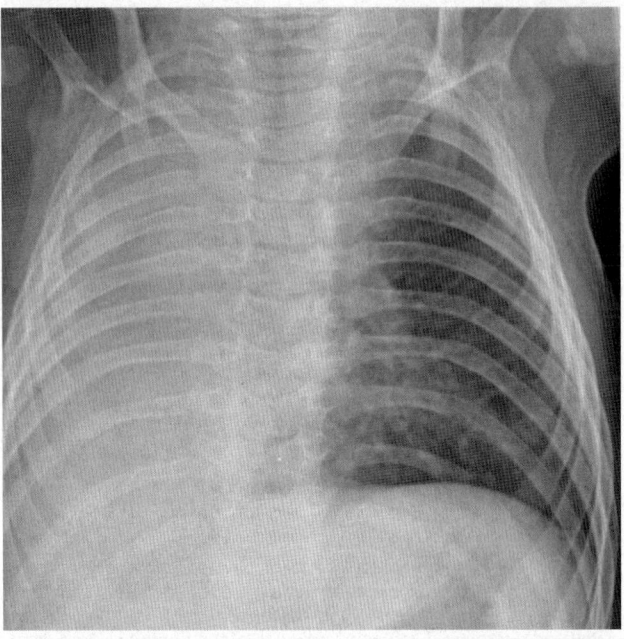

Fig. 10.6 The right hemithorax is opacified by the mediastinal structures that are shifted to the right. However, there is no overexpansion of the left lung or pleura. On computed tomography, the right lung was absent (see Fig. 10.47).

it may sometimes be difficult to distinguish from congenital cystic adenomatoid malformation (Table 10.1).

LOBAR OVERINFLATION

Lobar overinflation may have a similar appearance to whole-lung overinflation. However, there is usually evidence of lobar confinement because one can identify the lobar outline as it herniates across the midline, and the remaining ipsilateral

pulmonary lobes show compressive atelectasis or collapse (Fig. 10.9). The left-upper, right-middle, or left-lower lobe is usually affected by congenital lobar overinflation (congenital lobar emphysema). A lateral radiograph may be helpful in deciding which lobe is involved, although computed tomography (CT) of the chest is required in most cases to clarify the anatomy and to identify a potential underlying causative abnormality. This could be an extrinsic lesion causing partial bronchial compression (e.g., a mediastinal bronchogenic cyst) or a mass within the bronchial lumen causing a ball-valve effect (e.g., endobronchial granuloma or adenoma).

MEDIASTINAL DISTORTION

Mediastinal distortion may occur secondary to a mediastinal mass. Therefore, the normal outline of the mediastinum should always be reviewed. On the left, this normally constitutes the thymus, aortic arch, pulmonary outflow tract, pulmonary hilum, and left heart border; on the right, it constitutes the thymus, azygos vein, hilum, and the right heart border. In young children, the outline of the superior structures may be obscured by a normal thymus (discussed earlier), but this should never obscure the posterior paraspinal lines as the thymus lies in the anterior mediastinum. Distortion of the airways (e.g., narrowing, deviation, or splaying of the main bronchi) suggests extrinsic mass effect or functional/structural abnormalities of the airways (Fig. 10.10).

Mass lesions disrupting the paraspinal lines or involving the apices of the chest are most likely localized in the posterior

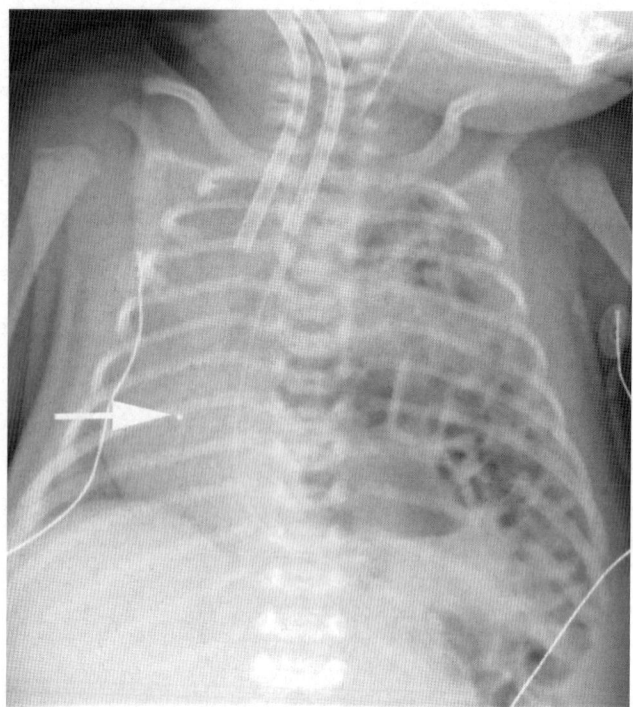

Fig. 10.8 An infant with antenatally diagnosed left congenital diaphragmatic hernia. Chest radiograph shows disruption of the lateral left diaphragmatic outline, bowel in the left hemithorax, and mediastinal shift to the right. Note venous-arterial extracorporeal membrane oxygenation with a metal marker on the tip of the venous cannula *(arrow)*. The endotracheal tube is too high.

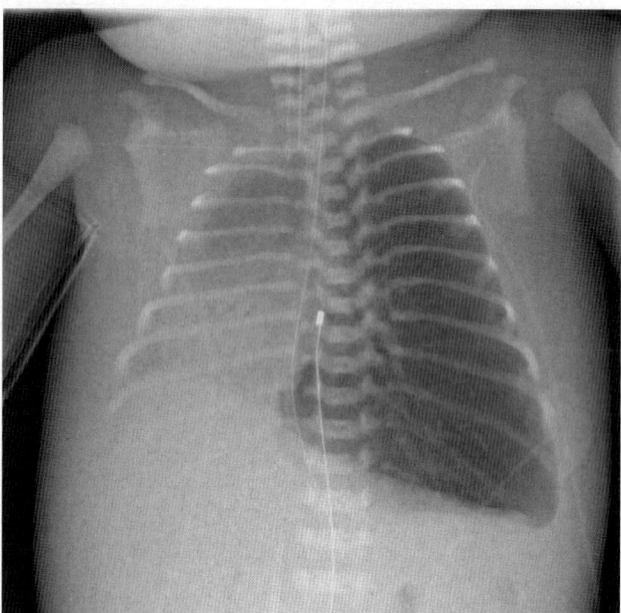

Fig. 10.7 Chest radiograph of a neonate with respiratory distress syndrome shows an overexpanded left lung (inverted left hemidiaphragm, intercostal bulging of the left lung) as well as a small right hemithorax (elevated right hemidiaphragm, crowding of the right ribs). Both were secondary to a central bronchogenic cyst (see Fig. 10.43), although this is not apparent on the chest x-ray, but is seen subsequently on computed tomography scan.

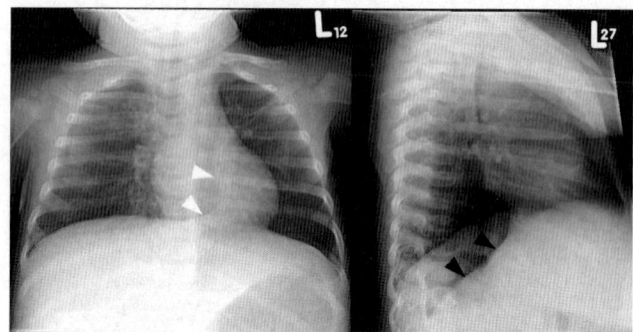

Fig. 10.9 The lateral view is not part of a routine chest radiograph. In this case, the anteroposterior view shows probable lobar overexpansion of the right lung *(white arrowheads)*, but it is not clear which lobe is involved. The lateral view is helpful, showing depression of the posterior diaphragm *(black arrowheads)* and thereby clarifying right lower lobe involvement, which is uncommon in lobar overinflation (congenital lobar emphysema).

Table 10.1   Differential Diagnoses in Asymmetrical Lung Volume

	Increased Ipsilateral Density	Decreased Ipsilateral Density	Normal Density
Small lung	Atelectasis Central airway obstruction Congenital venolobar syndrome Diaphragmatic elevation/paresis	Swyer-James syndrome (Macleod syndrome)	Hypoplasia Interrupted pulmonary artery
Large lung		Primary/secondary congenital overinflation Central airway obstruction with ball-valve effect	

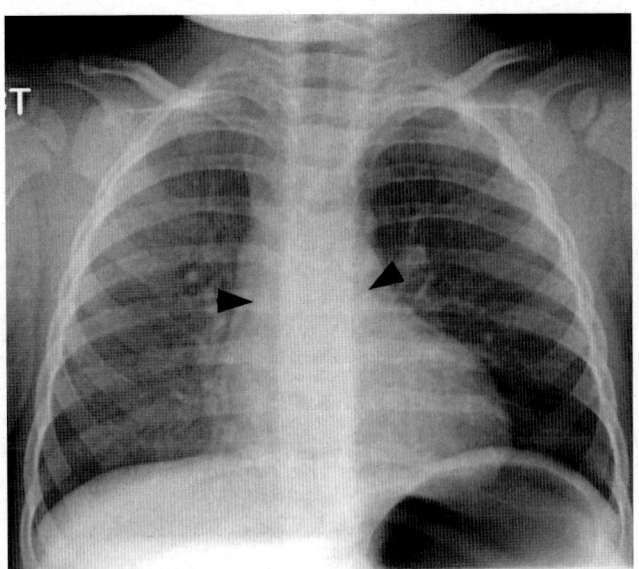

Fig. 10.10 A 2-year-old boy presents with pyrexia. Chest radiograph shows displacement of the left main and lower lobe bronchi by a subcarinal mass *(between arrowheads)* and associated increased transradiency of the left lung due to air trapping. The mass was later proven to be lymphadenopathy caused by *Mycobacterium avium-intracellulare*.

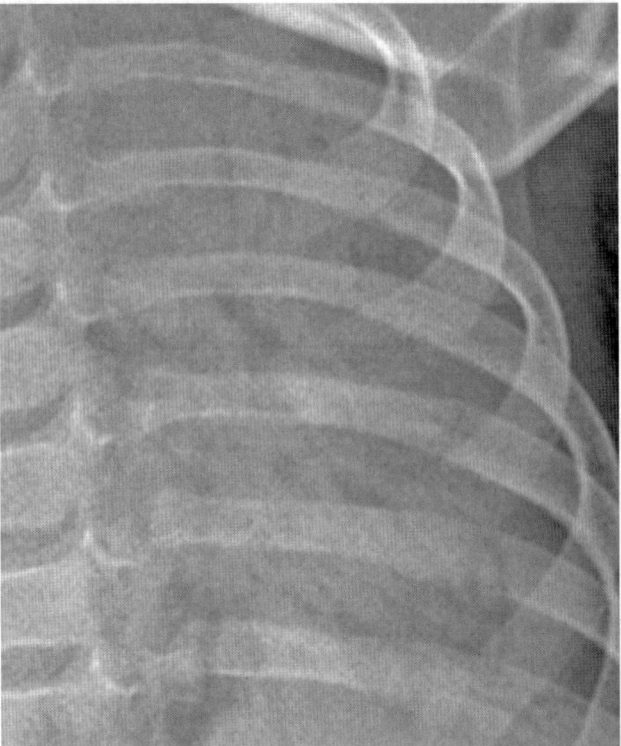

Fig. 10.11 Consolidation. The lung parenchyma is opacified with obvious air bronchograms, but there are no vascular markings.

mediastinum, and the list of differential diagnostic possibilities includes congenital abnormalities (lateral meningocele, neurenteric cyst, duplication cyst), neoplasm (neurogenic tumor), and infection (spondylodiscitis). Rib or vertebral body erosion suggests an aggressive lesion, such as infection or malignancy (e.g., neuroblastoma).

Any abnormal appearance of the thymus (discussed earlier), such as inappropriate size or shape or evidence of associated airway compression, suggests an anterior mediastinal mass lesion. Diagnostic differentials include rebound thymic hyperplasia, germ cell tumor, T cell lymphoma, and thymoma.

Any other mass lesion in the mediastinum usually originates from the middle mediastinum. In the young child, the diagnosis is likely to be a congenital abnormality (e.g., bronchogenic cyst). In the older child, the diagnosis is likely to be enlarged lymph nodes, which may be reactive or due to malignant disease (lymphoproliferative disease, which is rarely metastatic); sarcoidosis (rare, usually paratracheal); or idiopathic hyperplasia.

Lung atelectasis (discussed earlier) should be considered when there is loss of the upper mediastinal outline, even without apparent lung opacification.

HILAR EXPANSION

Unlike in adults, where bronchogenic carcinoma is a common cause of hilar adenopathy, in children, hilar enlargement is often secondary to acute infection. However, prominent hila may also be seen due to enlargement of the pulmonary arteries and, in infants, due to a bronchogenic cyst (see Fig. 10.3). Distinguishing vascular from nodal enlargement can be difficult, but pulmonary arterial enlargement should result in a concave lateral hilar outline, whereas soft tissue masses are said to cause a convex lateral hilar margin, with a noticeable increase in soft tissue density at the enlarged hilum.

False impressions of hilar enlargement occur when the child is rotated on the film cassette: a hilum that is pointing away from the detector becomes more distinct from the heart shadow and consequently appears more prominent. A repeat exposure may be necessary in difficult inconclusive cases, and CT/MRI may be performed if there is doubt.

Peribronchial markings should not be prominent in children, unlike in adults. More distinct markings in the perihilar regions, particularly with coexisting general overinflation, often represent bronchial inflammation (e.g., asthma or infection). Other conditions included in the differential diagnosis will be discussed in the section on high-resolution computed tomography (HRCT). Patchy perihilar opacification, with air bronchograms, is usually due to radiographic summation of peribronchial thickening, but may be difficult to distinguish from airspace opacification (consolidation).

LUNG OPACITIES

The plain radiograph usually allows distinction between *atelectasis*, which is defined as parenchymal opacification with loss of volume, and *consolidation*, which is opacification without volume loss and with the outline of gas-filled bronchi (air bronchograms) (Fig. 10.11). Opacities in the lungs can be localized according to the neighboring structure, which is obscured (silhouette sign). Loss of the upper mediastinal outline is consequent on upper lobe opacification; loss of the heart borders is caused by right middle lobe or lingular opacification; and loss of diaphragmatic definition is caused by lower lobe pathology.

There are several important signs of volume loss. First, the entire hemithorax may appear shrunken, with ipsilateral

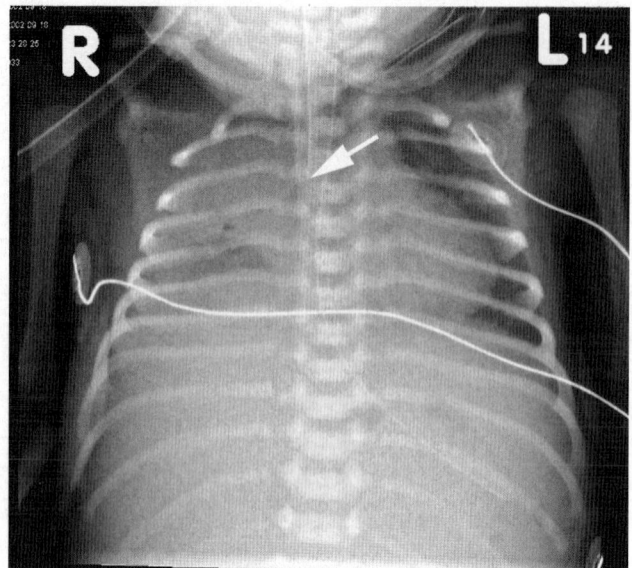

Fig. 10.12 The tip of the endotracheal tube is in the proximal right main stem bronchus *(arrow)*. There is associated atelectasis of the right upper lobe (loss of definition of the right upper mediastinal border, opacification of the right upper hemithorax, elevation of the right hemidiaphragm, and crowding of the right ribs).

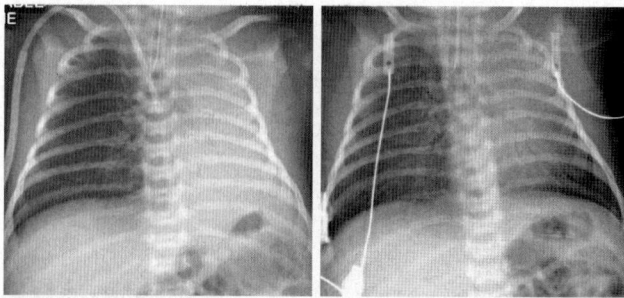

Fig. 10.13 A neonate in the intensive care unit with increasing oxygen requirement. The chest radiograph *(left)* shows loss of the left cardiomediastinal and diaphragmatic outlines, opacification of the left hemithorax without air bronchograms, and mediastinal shift to the left. These findings strongly suggest left lung collapse, and, at bronchoscopy, a mucous plug was removed from the left main stem bronchus. Immediately afterward *(right)*, there is considerably improved aeration of the left lower lobe (diaphragm now seen), but persistent collapse of the left upper lobe (persisting mediastinal blurring and shift).

mediastinal shift, diaphragmatic elevation, and crowding of the ribs. Second, adjacent noncollapsed lung may show compensatory overinflation and appear hyperlucent due to dilution of vascular shadows. Third, the hilum may be displaced, either cranially or caudally, toward the atelectasis (Fig. 10.12).

It is important to recognize these signs, even with no apparent lung opacity, particularly in upper lobe atelectasis, where the affected segments, or the whole lobe, may be collapsed against the mediastinum and therefore difficult to identify.

The clinical and radiographic history of atelectasis may give important clues as to the causative pathology. Acute atelectasis may be caused by a dislodged endotracheal tube, an aspirated foreign body, or mucous plugging (Fig. 10.13) and may therefore require further nonradiologic investigation and intervention. Chronic atelectasis is more likely caused by extrinsic airway obstruction (e.g., bronchogenic cyst, mediastinal lymphadenopathy, neoplasms) or chronic infection (e.g., tuberculosis) and may therefore warrant CT/MRI. In a febrile infant with respiratory distress and multifocal segmental atelectasis that changes location over the course of hours, one may suspect infection with respiratory syncytial virus, causing bronchiolitis.

Consolidation has many causes, as in adults, and is due to any process that replaces air in the terminal airspaces with fluid, mucus, or cellular material. The clinical history, the distribution of abnormality, and the presence of associated calcification, lymphadenopathy, or pleural effusion may assist in deduction of the specific cause (Figs. 10.14 and 10.15). Typically, pulmonary edema causes bilateral patchy consolidation in a perihilar distribution as well as pleural fluid (discussed earlier), although there may be lateral predominance.

Ground-glass change, a description initially confined to HRCT, is also used now to describe radiographic lung opacification with partial preservation of vascular markings, with or without air bronchograms (Fig. 10.16). This sign

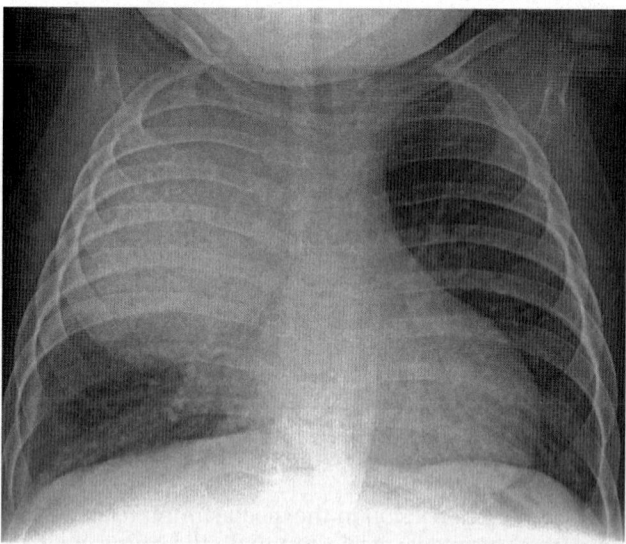

Fig. 10.14 In a 1-year-old girl with a cough, the chest radiograph shows a calcified mass in the right upper and mid zones. Also seen is pleural fluid, which was caused by infection with *Mycobacterium tuberculosis*.

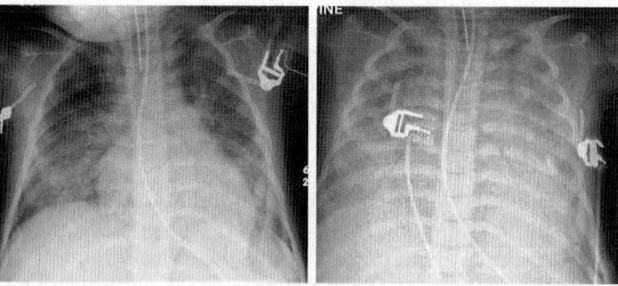

Fig. 10.15 A 3-year-old boy who was treated in the intensive care unit after a traffic accident had increasing difficulty with oxygenation. A chest radiograph on admission *(left)* shows patchy areas of consolidation. Hemorrhagic fluids returned via the endotracheal tube. The second day *(right)*, there was almost complete whiteout of both lungs, with air bronchograms and loss of the cardiomediastinal and diaphragmatic outlines. The findings confirm extensive pulmonary hemorrhage.

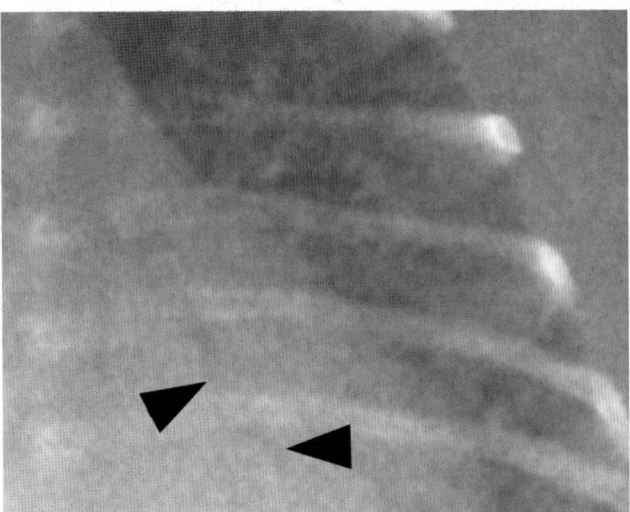

Fig. 10.16 Ground-glass change. There is moderately increased opacity of the lung with air bronchograms *(arrowheads)*, but preservation of vascular markings.

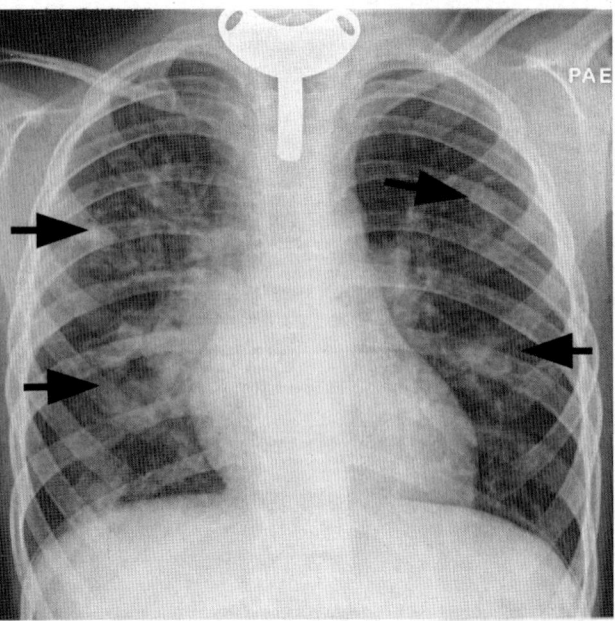

Fig. 10.18 In a 13-year-old boy with a tracheostomy tube because of laryngeal papillomatosis, the chest radiograph shows multiple nodular processes, some of which are cavitating, caused by parenchymal dissemination of the papillomatosis *(arrows;* see Fig. 10.48).

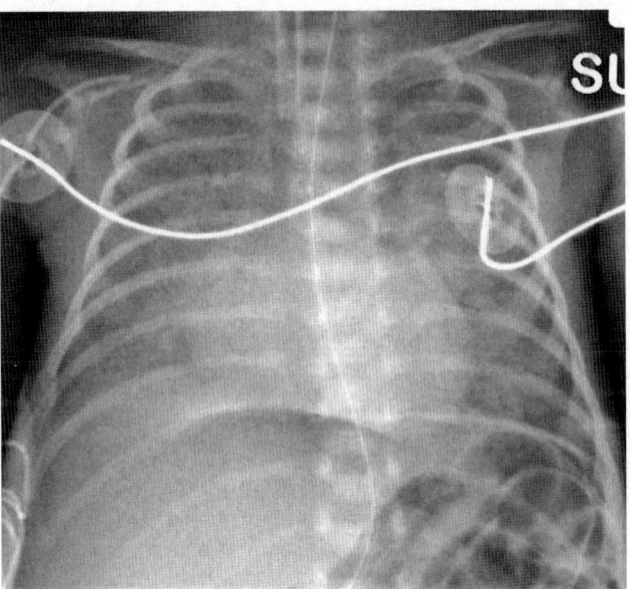

Fig. 10.17 In a 3-week-old infant born at 32 weeks' gestation, on ventilator support, there is bilateral diffuse ground-glass change (opacification, blurring of the cardiomediastinal and diaphragmatic outlines, preserved vascular markings), in keeping with respiratory distress syndrome. Note the lucency overlying the liver, outlining the right hemidiaphragm as well as the bowel wall in the upper left quadrant. This is diagnostic of pneumoperitoneum. The child had bowel perforation secondary to necrotizing enterocolitis.

vessels in consolidated lung tissue as opposed to pleural collections (see ultrasound section later in this chapter).

FOCAL AND MULTIFOCAL LUNG DENSITIES

Focal and multifocal lung densities often require additional CT/MRI for their definitive underlying cause to be elucidated, except in cases with clear clinical evidence of infectious pneumonia. In children, pneumonic consolidation often has a more distinct, rounded appearance (round pneumonia), which should be recognized and followed with plain radiographs only. In equivocal cases, CT/MRI is necessary for further characterization of the lesion. Differential diagnosis of a solitary parenchymal lesion includes congenital malformation, such as sequestration (usually in the posterobasal left lower lobe), microcystic congenital cystic adenomatoid malformation, and vascular malformation. A lung abscess may have no apparent gas-fluid level.

Multifocal lesions may represent infectious processes (e.g., fungus, tuberculosis, papillomatosis, or septic emboli) (Fig. 10.18), granulomatous disease, Langerhans cell histiocytosis, other inflammatory disease (Figs. 10.19 and 10.20), diffuse interstitial lung disease (Fig. 10.21), or metastases (e.g., nephroblastoma, hepatoblastoma, malignant germ cell tumor, sarcoma).

Some lung lesions tend to be predominantly cystic in radiographic terms (containing a gas-filled cavity). Pneumatoceles usually follow pneumonia, which is classically caused by infection with *Staphylococcus aureus*, and occasionally by *Klebsiella*.

Multifocal, multicystic parenchymal lesions may be congenital cystic adenomatoid malformation, Langerhans cell histiocytosis nodules at the cavitating stage, granulomatosis with polyangiitis, disseminated laryngeal papillomatosis (see Fig. 10.18), or necrotizing vasculitis (see Fig. 10.20).

is nonspecific and may be caused by interstitial or partial airspace opacification processes. In the neonatal setting, it is often used in the description of RDS (Fig. 10.17), and is usually combined with generally decreased lung volumes. Pleural fluid may give a similar appearance (discussed earlier). Where there is continued clinical doubt, an ultrasound can prove useful in differentiating pleural fluid from peripheral consolidation, demonstrating the presence of ultrasonographic air-bronchograms and normal arborization of pulmonary

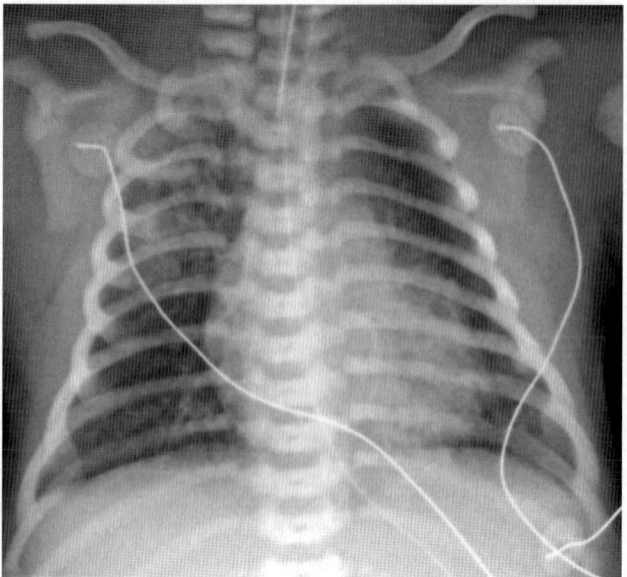

Fig. 10.19 Radiograph of a male neonate shows patchy consolidation in the right upper zone and behind the heart on the left, with overinflated lungs. This picture is commonly seen in meconium aspiration.

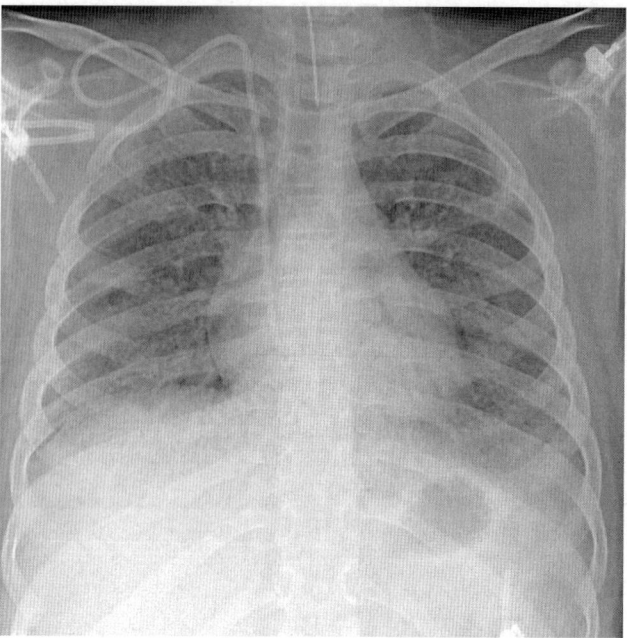

Fig. 10.21 A 4-year-old boy undergoing chemotherapy had acute respiratory failure. Chest radiograph shows globally increased density of both lungs in a granular pattern, with preservation of vascular markings. This was due to diffuse interstitial pneumonitis caused by bleomycin (see Fig. 10.52).

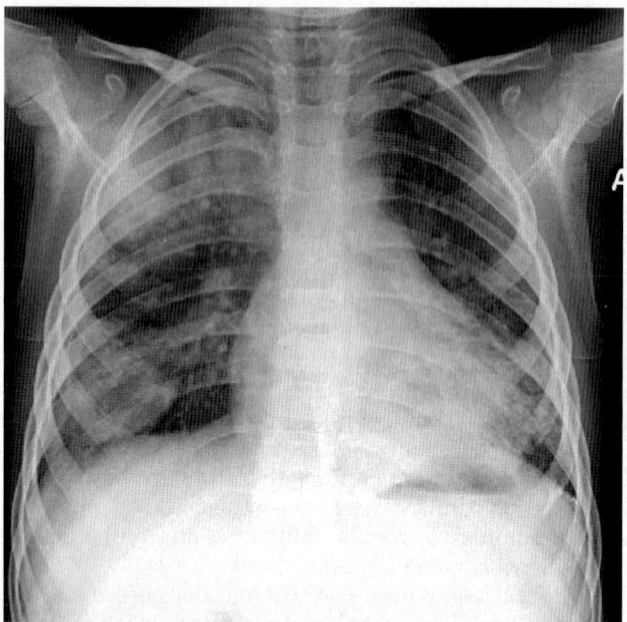

Fig. 10.20 A 6-year-old boy presented with difficulty breathing. Inflammatory markers were increased. The chest radiograph shows areas of opacification in the right upper and mid zones, and the left mid zone, which represent vasculitic lesions (see Fig. 10.60). On plain film, this is indistinguishable from multifocal pneumonia.

cases, this may be difficult to distinguish radiologically from ventilator-induced central bronchial dilation. There are rare reported cases of apparent spontaneous pulmonary interstitial emphysema in term babies who have never been ventilated. The differential diagnosis includes congenital or acquired cystic lung disease.

LUNG ABSCESS

A lung abscess is a cavitated lesion that normally contains both fluid and gas. The consequent gas-fluid level is easily recognized, but it may be missed if the x-ray beam is not tangential (i.e., horizontal) to the gas-fluid interface. With a diverging beam, the fluid level appears more blurred and meniscoid (Fig. 10.25).

DIFFUSE INTERSTITIAL LUNG DISEASE

We will discuss diffuse interstitial lung disease in more detail later in the chapter in the section on HRCT. More advanced interstitial processes may be appreciated radiographically as peribronchial thickening, ground-glass change, septal lines, or interstitial nodules (Fig. 10.26; see also Fig. 10.21).

PNEUMOTHORAX

In young children, the appearance of a pneumothorax differs from the typical adult appearance. The variation is due to differences in lung parenchymal elasticity. In children, there is often no peripheral lucent zone on supine radiographs, which is the typical appearance in adults, because in the child, gas collects anteriorly in the anterior pleural reflection

PULMONARY INTERSTITIAL EMPHYSEMA

Pulmonary interstitial emphysema is a complication that occurs when high ventilator pressures are used to ventilate stiff lungs. It appears as lacelike lucencies in a linear pattern radiating from the pulmonary hilum to the surface of the lung, and it may be further complicated by pneumothorax or pneumomediastinum (Fig. 10.22–10.24). In some

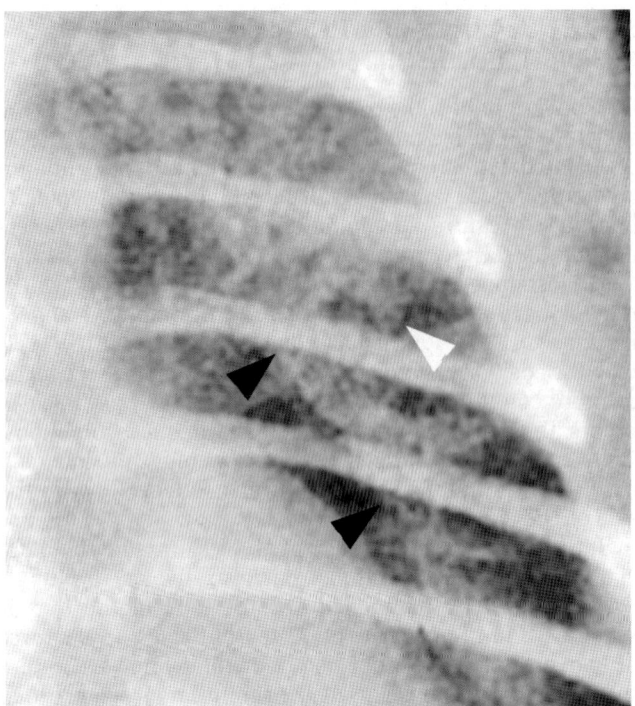

Fig. 10.22 Detail from a chest radiograph in an infant after long-standing ventilatory support shows monotonous tubular lucencies *(white arrowhead)* suggestive of pulmonary interstitial emphysema. The mediastinal border is seen very crisply, with a medial lung edge *(black arrowheads)* due to anterior pneumothorax.

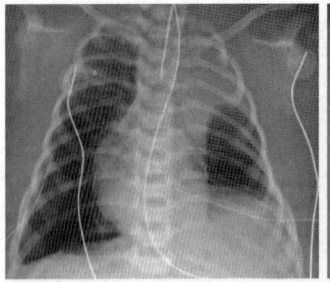
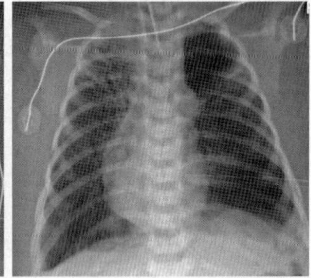

Fig. 10.24 A 6-week-old girl was ventilated with high-pressure settings (chest radiographs show a flattened diaphragm and splayed ribs). After an acute exacerbation *(left)*, the radiograph showed collapse of the left upper lobe (opacification without air bronchograms, increased interlobar fissure, and elevated diaphragm). The next day *(right)*, the left upper lobe had reexpanded, but a left pneumothorax is seen. Linear bubbly lucencies can be seen from the hila to the lung edges, suggesting pulmonary interstitial emphysema.

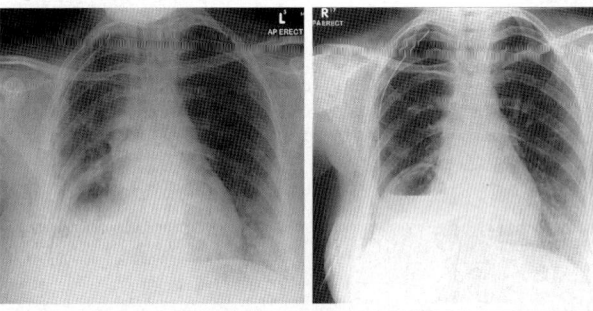

Fig. 10.25 Two chest radiographs obtained in the same patient on the same day. The right is a true erect exposure showing the gas-fluid level of an abscess within the right lung, whereas the left is semierect and does not show the gas-fluid level of the abscess.

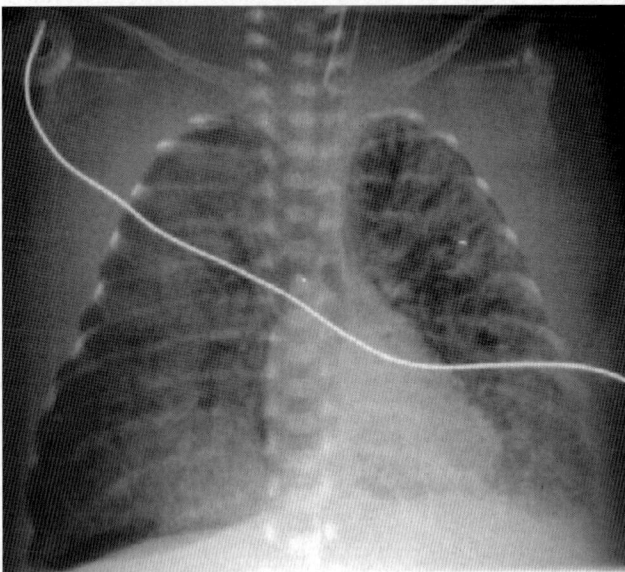

Fig. 10.23 A 6-week-old girl born at 30 weeks' gestation was very difficult to ventilate. Chest radiograph shows overexpanded lungs that are seen bulging out intercostally, with the diaphragm flattened. Concurrently, there is increased opacification of the lungs, which is presumed to be due to respiratory distress syndrome. Linearly arranged bubbly lucencies can be seen radiating from the hila, suggesting pulmonary interstitial emphysema secondary to high-pressure ventilation. There is also a pneumothorax seen at the base of the right lung.

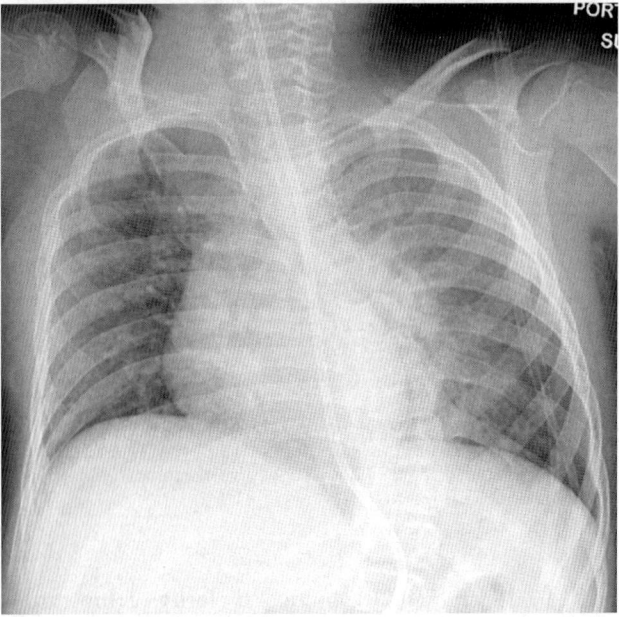

Fig. 10.26 Chest radiograph of a 9-year-old girl with gastroesophageal reflux and chronic aspiration shows bilateral perihilar bronchial wall thickening, particularly in the upper zones (see Fig. 10.59). The apparent rotation is caused by scoliosis.

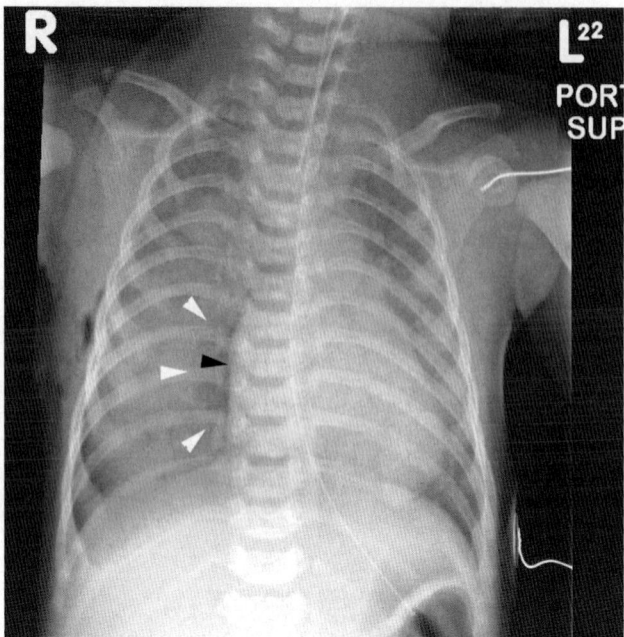

Fig. 10.27 An anterior pneumothorax as seen typically in infants. The *white arrowheads* show the lateral boundary of the lucency. The gas adjacent to the right heart border causes a crisp outline *(black arrowhead)*.

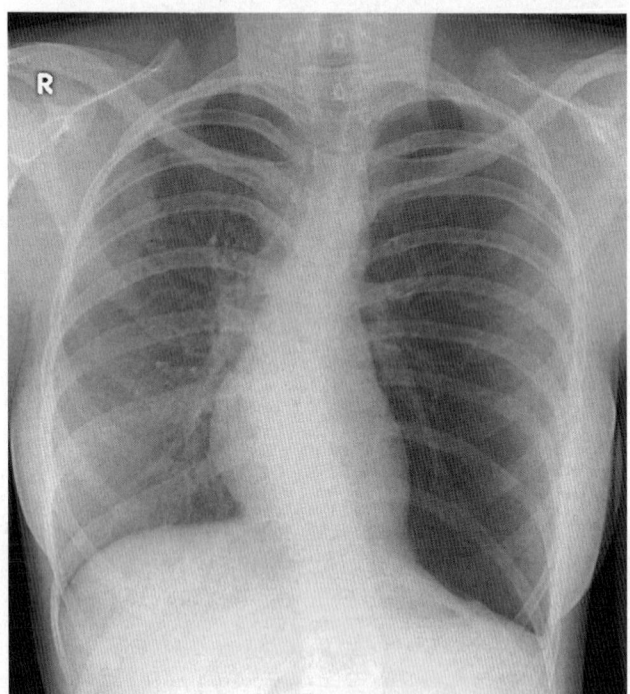

Fig. 10.28 Chest radiograph of a 12-year-old girl shows a hyperlucent left hemothorax, inversion of the left hemidiaphragm, and a very crisp cardiodiaphragmatic outline. This is suggestive of anterior tension pneumothorax. Scoliosis is noted.

(Figs. 10.27 and 10.28). Increased clarity of the cardiac outline may be the only finding, and it should be assessed carefully. If there is clinically significant doubt, a lateral shoot-through or decubitus x-ray should be performed. These are more sensitive for detecting small-volume pneumothoraces.

SKELETAL ABNORMALITIES ASSOCIATED WITH RESPIRATORY DISORDERS

On conventional radiographs, undermineralization of the skeleton can be diagnosed confidently only in severe cases. Associated with prematurity, this metabolic bone condition is commonly seen in infants with idiopathic RDS. Bone mineral loss is also a feature of a multitude of constitutional disorders and may be seen secondary to systemic corticosteroid therapy.

Scoliosis may be caused by vertebral abnormalities, which may be part of the VATER (Vertebral, Anorectal, Tracheo-Esophageal, Renal/Radial malformations) or VACTERL (VATER with the addition of cardiovascular malformations) sequences, or more commonly, may be caused by neuromuscular disorders. In addition, it may be secondary to chest conditions, such as hypoplastic lung, atelectasis, or empyema, in which case the resultant spinal curvature is concave toward the side of the abnormality.

Both focal and multifocal osseous lesions may be associated findings in conditions that also involve the lungs. Well-defined lytic ("punched out") lesions in the ribs or scapulae and the collapse of vertebral bodies are features of Langerhans cell histiocytosis. More ill-defined lesions are seen in primary neoplasms (e.g., primitive neuroectodermal tumors [PNET], previously known as Ewing/Askin tumor), lymphoma, infection (e.g., tuberculosis), or infection associated with chronic granulomatous disease. Erosion of posterior rib elements, with splaying, is seen with thoracic paraspinal neuroblastoma.

Fluoroscopic Techniques

Limitation of radiation exposure is vital in childhood, but a quick fluoroscopic screening examination of the chest (using pulsed rather than continuous fluoroscopy) can prove extremely useful, particularly when evaluating differing lung radiolucencies in suspected foreign body aspiration and in chronic stridor.[4] With obstructive overinflation, the affected lung will show little volume change with respiration, and the mediastinum will swing contralaterally on expiration. Fluoroscopic lateral views also may be valuable for dynamic evaluation of tracheomalacia, where the trachea may be seen to collapse during expiration.

Barium swallow is still the primary study in patients with a suspected vascular ring, which abnormally indents the contrast column in the esophagus. This test may also be valuable for assessing extrinsic masses. Tracheoesophageal fistula and large laryngeal clefts can be excluded with a good-quality single-contrast study when a water-soluble contrast medium with a high iodine concentration is delivered under pressure via a nasal tube to the esophagus. The child is kept prone and screened with a horizontal beam to facilitate visualization of contrast leakage into the trachea or bronchi.

Thin-section CT has almost eliminated the need for bronchography in children; however, the technique is still used in functional studies for assessing the dynamics of intermittent airway obstruction (Fig. 10.29 and Video 10.1). With this technique, the mucosa of the trachea and the first to third generations of bronchi are coated with water-soluble contrast medium, which is instilled with a repeated small-bolus technique via a fine tube at the subglottic level in the intubated child.[5]

There is also a limited role for fluoroscopy in diaphragmatic assessment, although ultrasound assessment is preferred, with some authors suggesting M-mode imaging as a useful adjunct (Videos 10.6 and 10.7).

Computed Tomography

CT is an invaluable technique in many pediatric chest diseases.[6] However, it is vital to assess the diagnostic benefit versus the potential radiation risk to the patient. CT is currently the most sensitive way of imaging the lungs due to its high spatial resolution. High-speed scanning allows for superb depiction of even small vessels after delivery of an intravenous bolus of iodinated contrast medium. In the child younger than 5 years of age, sedation or general anesthesia may be required, although recently this need has been

significantly reduced with the introduction of state of the art multidetector row (MDCT) and dual-source CT scanners allowing much faster acquisition times, thus reducing the effect of respiratory, cardiac, and patient motion (Fig. 10.30).

Traditional noncontiguous (interrupted/interspaced) HRCT has largely been superseded by high pitch spiral CT (Fig. 10.31).

Isotropic Computed Tomography

Modern MDCT scanners, with increasing number of detector rows (currently up to 320 simultaneous sections per tube rotation) and sub-second tube rotation speeds, have further enhanced performance, delivering faster scan time (improved temporal resolution) with a wider scan range. When this is combined with the use of smaller detector elements (down to 0.5 mm), this enables acquisition of isotropic volumetric datasets (where the slice thickness is equal to the pixel dimensions), resulting in improved spatial resolution in the cranio-caudal/longitudinal axis and reduced partial volume artifacts. It is now possible to acquire high-resolution thoracic

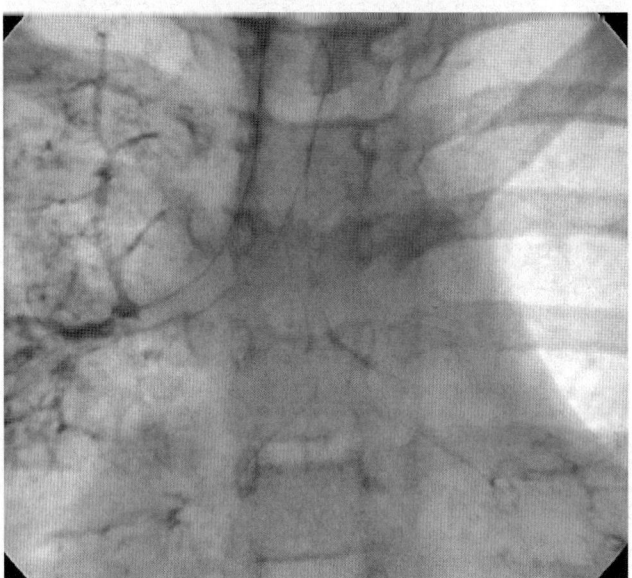

Fig. 10.29 Bronchogram in a girl with stridor shows a long stenosis of the distal trachea, with an abnormal origin of the right upper lobe bronchus from the trachea (see Figs. 10.35 and 10.36). (Image courtesy of Dr. D. Roebuck.)

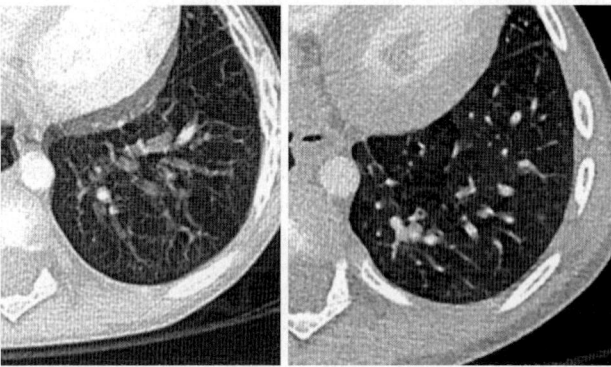

Fig. 10.30 CT sections demonstrating the effect of increased pitch and higher temporal resolution scanning on a state-of-the-art scanner. The image on the *left* (pitch = 1) on an older scanner with lower temporal resolution demonstrates respiratory and cardiac motion artifact. These are eliminated by high-pitch, high temporal resolution scanning (pitch = 3.2) on a current state-of-the-art scanner, demonstrating focal air trapping in the medial left lower lobe (image on the *right*).

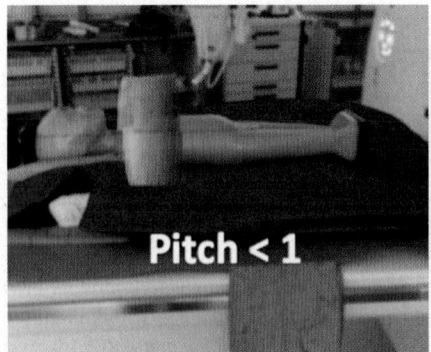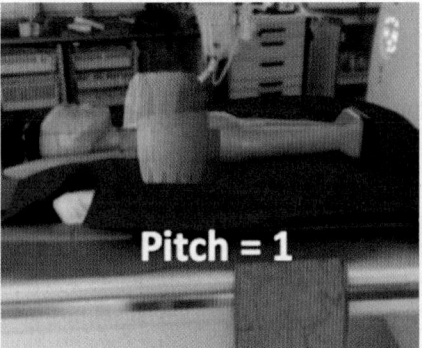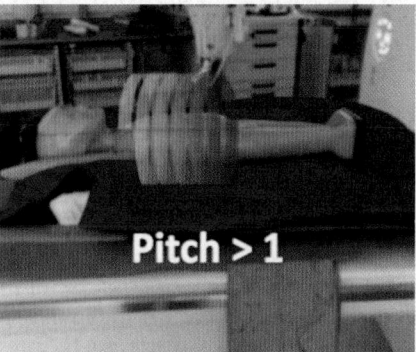

Fig. 10.31 Explanation of computed tomography pitch. Pitch is the relationship of beam width and gantry rotation speed to rate of table movement. A pitch of less than 1 provides overlapping sections with duplicated data; a pitch of more than 1 contains gaps in which data must be interpolated, but reduces scan time and therefore motion artifact.

CT in spiral mode in children, without breath holding and with minimal respiratory, cardiac, and patient motion artifact, with a reduced reliance on sedation and general anesthesia.

Isotropic imaging necessitates the reconstruction of overlapping thin sections that are susceptible to image noise. To overcome this, using postprocessing software, the data are manipulated into arbitrary cross-sectional planes and presented as two-dimensional or three-dimensional displays that have the same partial resolution as that of the original acquired dataset. The ability to view volumetric data in any plane enhances the interpretation and assessment of the bronchial tree and cardiovascular system. It is crucial in defining pulmonary nodules, and it allows better differentiation between organ interfaces parallel to the scan plane (e.g., the horizontal fissure) to aid diagnostic accuracy.

These benefits have dramatically expanded the application of CT in the evaluation of cardiovascular and airway diseases. MDCT is now commonly used in place of conventional angiography because the images are acquired more safely, without the need for arterial puncture, and often, given the very rapid acquisition times (2–8 seconds), without the need for general anesthesia or sedation. The additional benefit over angiography is that superb anatomic images of the mediastinum and lung parenchyma are acquired in the same data set, without additional radiation. The overall radiation dose in MDCT is significantly lower than that in conventional angiography. Thus, MDCT can aid in the diagnosis of pulmonary embolus, arteriovenous malformation, aneurysm, and dissection. However, unlike MDCT, conventional angiography has the advantage of allowing therapeutic intervention in the same procedure. Images of the airway acquired simultaneously can ascertain the presence of airway stenosis and narrowing as well as show the causes of possible extrinsic compression.

Data Processing

Depending on the clinical application, the acquired volumetric data can be reformatted and displayed as a two-dimensional image using multiplanar reconstruction (MPR) and multiplanar volume reconstructions, known as maximum intensity projections (MIP) or minimum intensity projections (MinIP). The techniques used to display three-dimensional images include volume-rendering technique (VRT) and perspective rendering (e.g., virtual bronchoscopy [VB]).

MULTIPLANAR RECONSTRUCTION

MPRs are two-dimensional tomographic sections manipulated by the operator into an arbitrary imaging plane (i.e., the coronal, sagittal, or arbitrary angulated planes) or into a single tomographic curved plane along the axis of a structure of interest (e.g., a bronchus or a tortuous vessel).[7,8] Slice thickness of the MPR is operator-dependent, and increasing the thickness will improve the signal-to-noise ratio. MPR enhances the perception of the image, provides additional diagnostic value in demonstrating the presence of small focal lesions (e.g., defining the vertical extent of a bronchial stenosis) (Fig. 10.32), and is often used in the presurgical assessment of vascular rings and the tracheobronchial tree.[9]

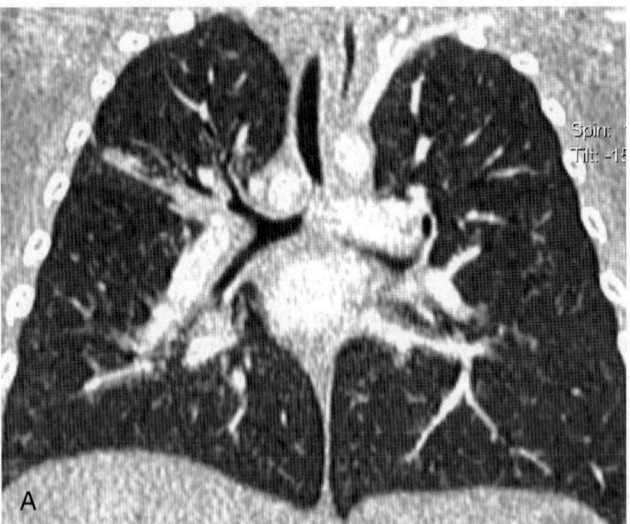

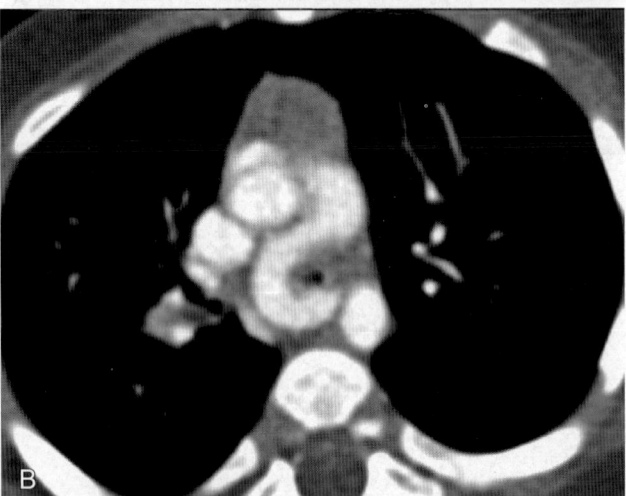

Fig. 10.32 Coronal multiplanar reconstruction (MPR) (A) and axial maximum intensity projection (B) images in a 5-month-old child presenting with stridor. There is tracheal stenosis caused by the presence of a pulmonary sling with almost complete occlusion of the distal trachea with marked narrowing of the left main bronchus (LMB) origin related to the aberrant left pulmonary artery, which has an anomalous origin from the right pulmonary artery, passing behind the trachea and in front of the esophagus. Cartilaginous rings were not identified in this examination. The coronal MPR image (A) has been postprocessed on a high-resolution (bony) algorithm more suitable for viewing lung parenchyma but giving a more "noisy" (i.e., grainy) image.

MULTIPLANAR VOLUME RECONSTRUCTIONS: MAXIMUM INTENSITY PROJECTION AND MINIMUM INTENSITY PROJECTION

MIP is a rendering tool used to extract contrast-enhanced anatomic structures of higher attenuation values than adjacent structures, as in CT angiography (Fig. 10.33 and Video 10.1). The data are displayed in volume slabs to avoid obstruction from overlying vessels or bony structures. These thicker slabs are useful in depicting the peripheral airway, detecting and localizing micronodular or microtubular patterns, and analyzing mild forms of uneven attenuation of the lungs.[10] On the other hand, MinIP displays structures with the lowest attenuation values used in demonstrating the

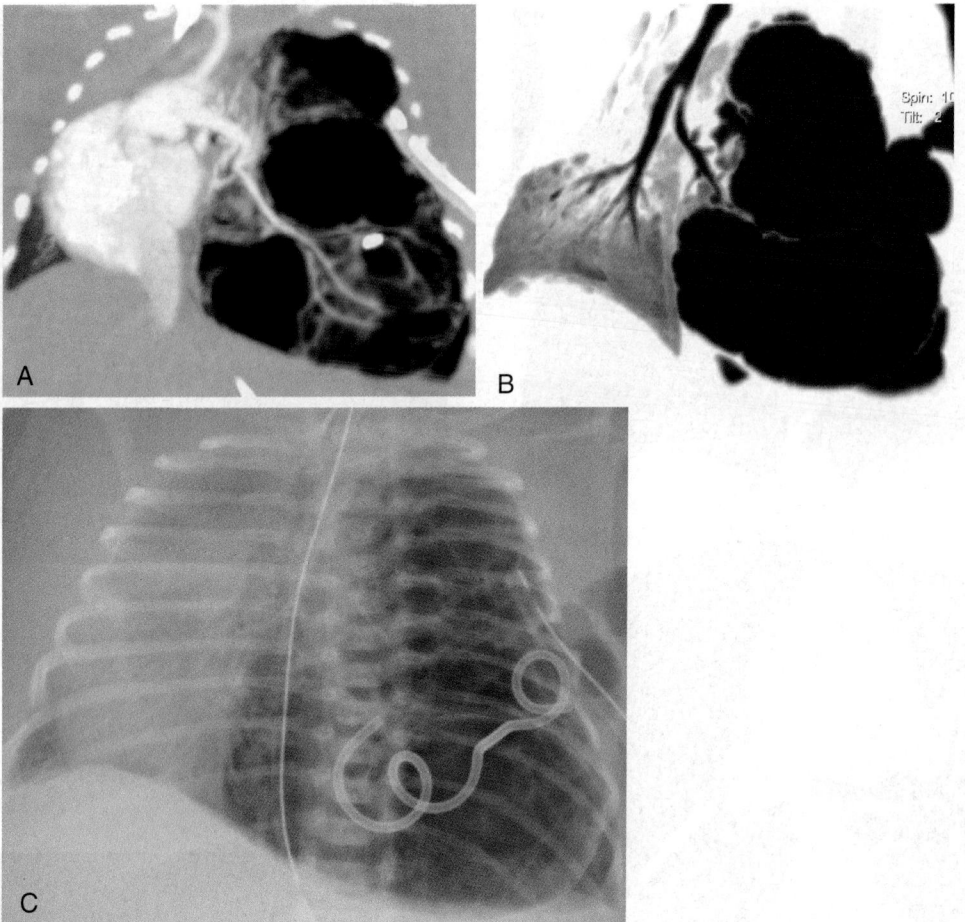

Fig. 10.33 Multiloculated air-filled cystic mass in a 4-day-old neonate with an antenatally diagnosed congenital thoracic malformation treated with antenatal drainage; see catheter on chest x-ray (C). (A) Maximum intensity projection image, where data with maximum intensity (contrast) is aggregated thus enhancing the blood supply. A branch pulmonary artery can be seen supplying the left lower lobe. (B) Minimum intensity projections, where data with lowest intensity (air) is combined to highlight the tracheobronchial tree emphasizing the very dilated cystic acinar units in the lung parenchyma and the abnormal ptosed and narrowed LMB. The chest radiography in (C) shows the enlarged hyperlucent left lung with herniation across the midline causing compression and shift of the mediastinum and right lung (which is atelectatic). Note the coiled left intrathoracic pigtail drain that was placed antenatally.

central airway and air trapping in the lungs (Fig. 10.34 and Video 10.2).

VOLUME-RENDERING TECHNIQUE

VRT is a processing technique (used for interpreting CT angiography, CT bronchoscopy, and orthopedic imaging datasets) that utilizes all acquired volumetric data without being subject to information loss. This is in order to display an image in a three-dimensional format so that the image can be further manipulated and viewed in different orientations (Fig. 10.35).

VRTs are used to depict structural and vascular anatomy (Fig. 10.36) and their relationship to adjacent structures, and to displaying structures that course parallel or oblique to the transverse plane (and also those that develop or extend into multiple planes).[7,8] Applying a transparency filter highlights the tracheobronchial tree, which, in turn, better illustrates short focal areas of narrowing, the craniocaudal length of a tracheobronchial stenosis, and other tracheobronchial anomalies. The mediastinal vasculature is best displayed as color-coded opacifications used for evaluating complex congenital cardiovascular anomalies (Video 10.4).

VIRTUAL BRONCHOSCOPY

VB is a perspective surface-rendering technique that takes advantage of the natural contrast between the airway and the surrounding tissues,[9] mimicking a bronchoscopic view of the intraluminal surface of the air-containing tracheobronchial tree (Fig. 10.37 and Video 10.5). VB provides an additional viewing dimension; the operator can navigate along the lumen of the airway, where bronchial surfaces can be visualized, and even across obstructions that an endoscope cannot traverse.[7,11] This technique is used when bronchoscopy is contraindicated or when tracheal stenosis cannot be otherwise evaluated.[12] Although dynamic VB can technically be used, virtual bronchography is more valuable.

Further Advanced Postprocessing

Postprocessing software packages are beginning to include more advanced tools allowing further data extraction. While many of these techniques remain to be validated against established measurements, especially in children, they hold promise for future areas of research and clinical practice. Examples include automated segmentation algorithms

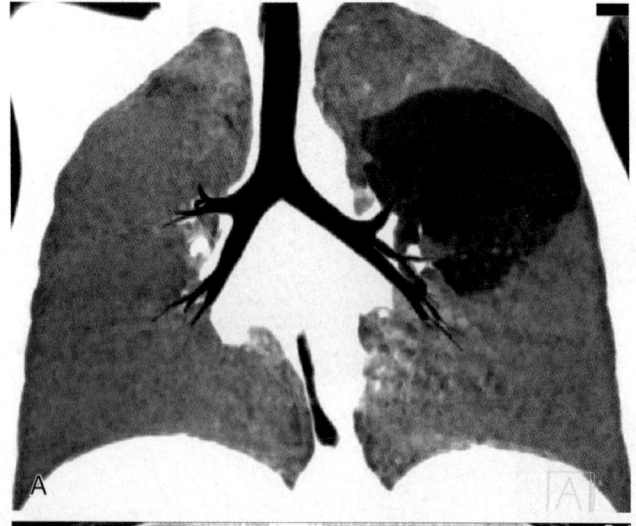

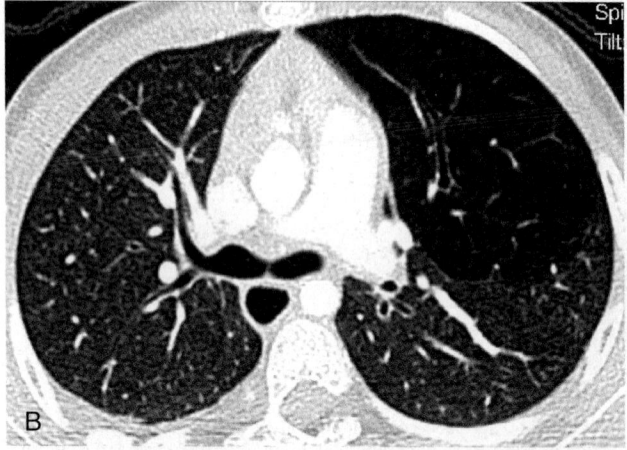

Fig. 10.34 A 5-year-old child with segmental left upper lobe (LUL) over-inflation. The coronal thin minimum intensity projections (A) shows a well-defined anterior segmental area of regional air trapping in relation to segmental overinflation. A thin axial section (B) shows the lung parenchyma anatomy in the most favorable setting. Note the clarity of the definition of the bronchial wall and adjacent pulmonary artery branch within the hyperlucent segment of the LUL.

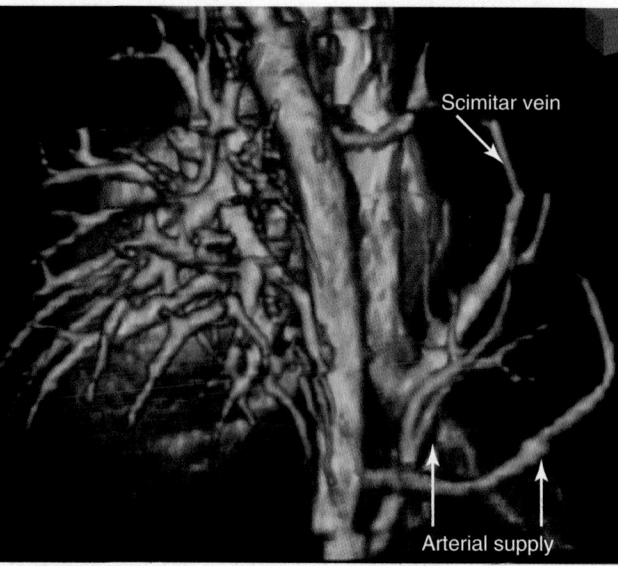

Fig. 10.36 Volume-rendering technique image of a 4-year-old child. A scimitar vein is seen joining the supra-hepatic portion of the inferior vena cava (IVC) inferior to the right atrium. The systemic artery arises from the descending aorta and supplies the right lung.

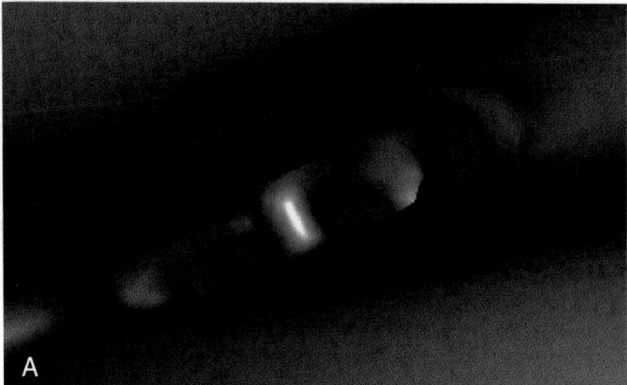

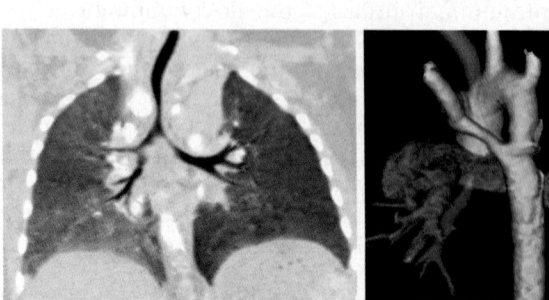

Fig. 10.35. Coronal minimum intensity projections computed tomography image and volume-rendering technique (viewed from a posterior perspective) demonstrating a double aortic arch, with a dominant right arch, forming a vascular ring with resultant tracheal compression. There is also compression of the main bronchi at the level of the pulmonary arteries. Note the particularly tight left bronchial compression with decreased attenuation in the left lung consistent with air trapping.

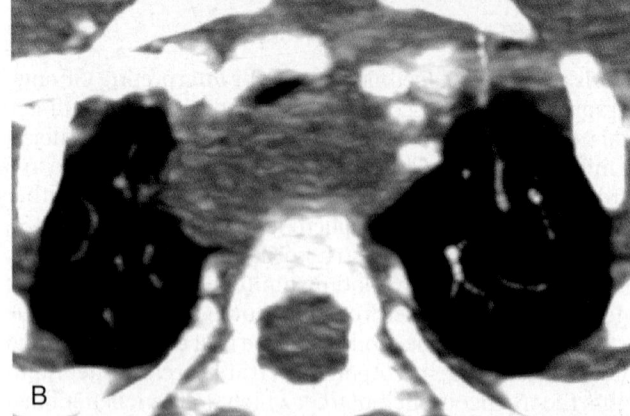

Fig. 10.37 This 2-year-old child presented with tracheal stenosis. The virtual bronchoscopy (A) demonstrates a dramatic anteroposterior (AP) narrowing of the trachea at the level of the carina, which is compressed by an enlarged esophagus posteriorly (diagnosed as achalasia of the esophageal cardia on barium study), as seen in (B).

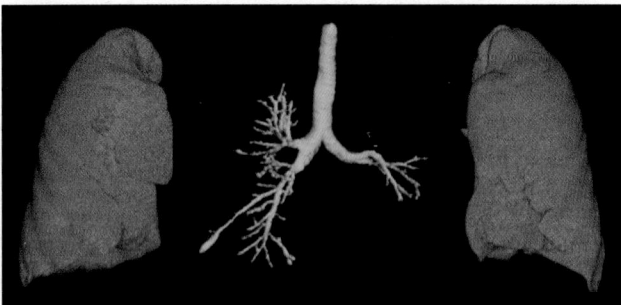

Fig. 10.38 Automated segmentation—automatically segmented lung and airway volumes allowing quantification structural volume—for example, lung volume measurement prior to transplantation and potential quantification of bronchiectasis in cystic fibrosis.

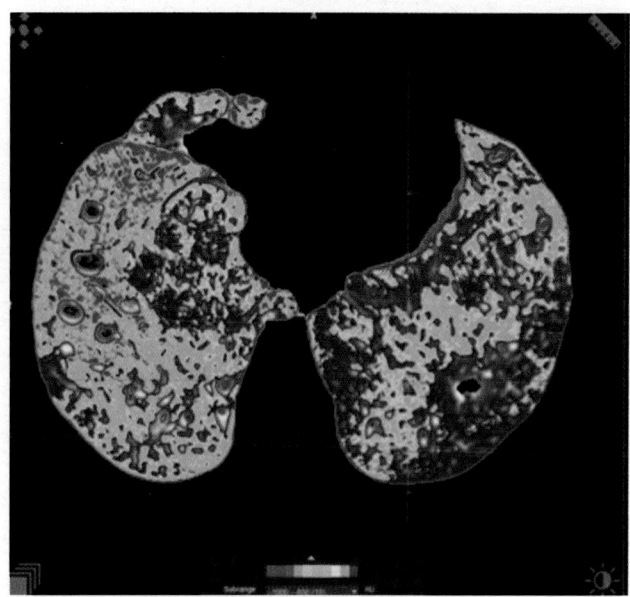

Fig. 10.40 Low attenuation map image through the lung bases of a patient with cystic fibrosis. Note the air-trapping (in *blue*) around the dilated, thick-walled, air-fluid level containing bronchi. This technique allows the calculation of the total volume of lung of each attenuation value range, thus providing a potential marker of the extent of air-trapping.

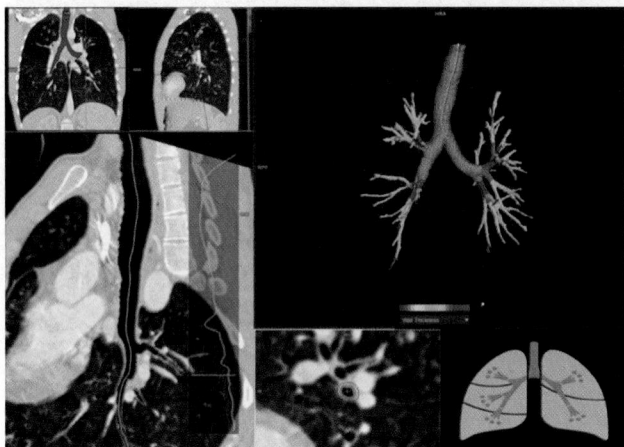

Fig. 10.39 Automated airway wall thickening measurement (measured between the *green* and *red circles* with thickness represented by a color scale in the three-dimensional reconstruction on the *top right*). Images produced using Syngo.Via, Siemens

allowing the measurement of lung volumes, low attenuation mapping potentially enabling quantification of regions of air-trapping, and automated methods of quantification of airway thickening and bronchiectasis (Figs. 10.38–10.40).

Review of Findings

The interpretation of findings requires a systematic review of all anatomic structures and areas, including those shown in Table 10.2 and Figs. 10.41–10.50.

Axial depiction of pulmonary parenchymal anatomy and abnormalities with spiral CT is slightly inferior to that depicted with traditional interspaced HRCT. On the other hand, the spiral scan covers the whole volume of the lungs with no gaps and is therefore more sensitive for demonstrating small solitary lesions, such as small metastases or fungal lesions.

CT performs poorly in differentiating between pleural effusion and empyema.[13] Pleural thickening and enhancement are often present in reactive effusions. Plain radiography, followed by ultrasound, is the investigation of choice because ultrasound has the ability to visualize the fibrinous septations of an infectious process (see Fig. 10.49).

Table 10.2 Main Review Areas for Spiral Computed Tomography of the Chest

Structure/Area	Abnormalities
Airways	Extrinsic compression (see Figs. 10.41 and 10.42)
	Caliber change
Vessels	Vascular rings
	Aberrant vessels
Anterior mediastinum	Thymic enlargement, nodularity, heterogeneous enhancement
Middle mediastinum	Enlarged lymph nodes
	Bronchopulmonary foregut malformations (see Fig. 10.43)
	Cardiac abnormalities
Posterior mediastinum	Benign lesions: Duplication cyst, meningocele, ganglioneuroma, abscess, extramedullary hematopoiesis
	Malignant lesions: Neuroblastoma
Hila	Enlarged lymph nodes
Lung parenchyma	Lung/lobar aplasia, agenesis, hypoplasia, overinflation (see Figs. 10.44–10.47)
	Focal lesions: Nodules, consolidation, atelectasis (see Fig. 10.48)
Pleura	Transudate, exudates, pus, hemorrhage, lymph (see Fig. 10.50)
Chest wall and spine	Osseous or soft-tissue lesions: Infection, benign and malignant tumors
	Abnormal configuration: Scoliosis, pectus deformities
Upper abdomen	Lesions of the liver, spleen, adrenal glands, and upper poles of kidneys
	Retroperitoneal, peritoneal, and abdominal wall lesions

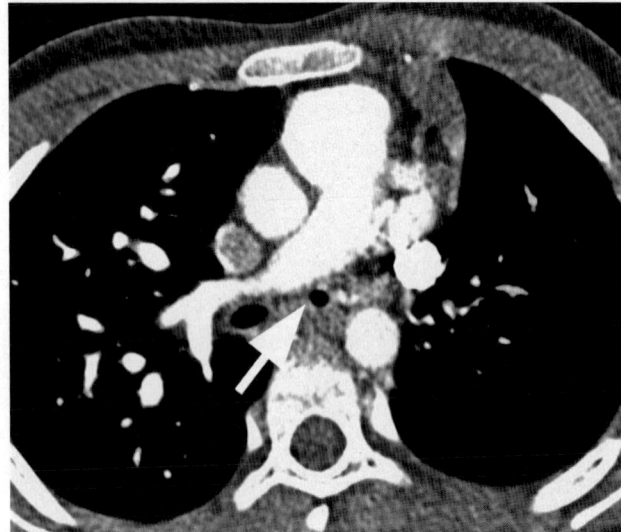

Fig. 10.41 On arterial phase computed tomography of the same girl as in Fig. 10.29, there is narrowing of the left main bronchus *(arrow)* where it passes between the right pulmonary artery and the descending aorta, which was found to represent an intrinsic defect due to complete cartilaginous rings.

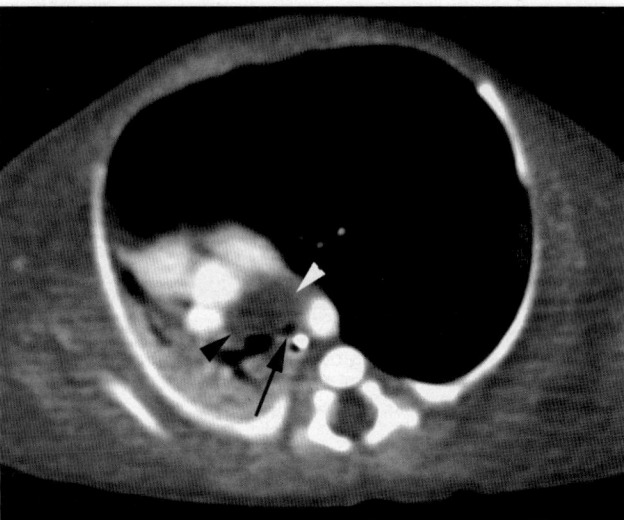

Fig. 10.43 Contrast-enhanced spiral computed tomography shows a precarinal bronchogenic cyst *(arrowheads)*, with associated narrowing of the left main stem bronchus *(arrow)*, a hyperinflated left lung, and a collapsed right lung (see Fig. 10.7).

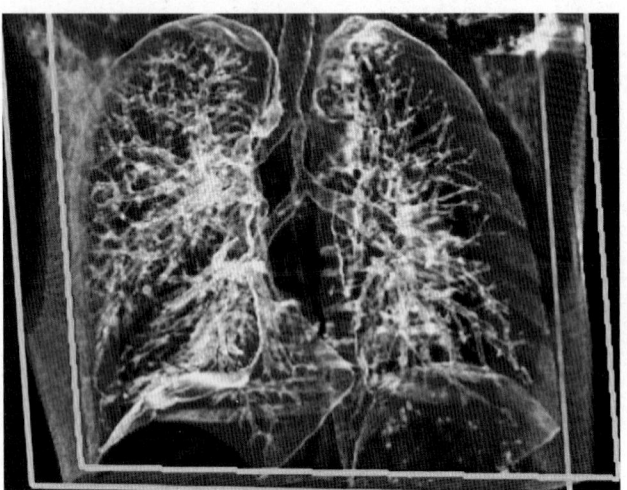

Fig. 10.42 Volume-rendering of computed tomography volume data in the same child as in Figs. 10.29 and 10.41 shows the anatomy of both the central and peripheral airways, with distal tracheal stenosis.

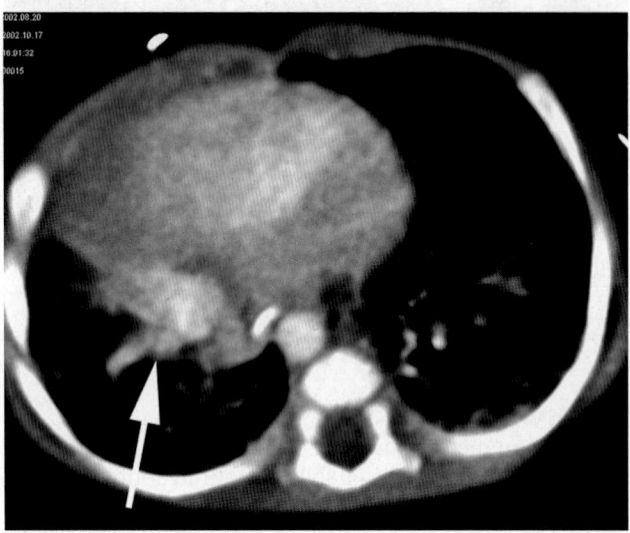

Fig. 10.44 Contrast-enhanced spiral computed tomography shows systemic venous drainage of the hypoplastic right lung into the right atrium *(arrow; see Figs. 10.5 and 10.46).*

However, CT is useful in distinguishing between empyema and lung abscess. Empyema shows a wide pleural base (see Fig. 10.50), whereas a lung abscess is usually seen partially separated from the pleura, with a wedge of lung on either side in the imaging plane.

Pitfalls

Technical factors may confound interpretation. Some artifacts may impede detection of significant lesions. In young children, there is invariably some degree of dependent lung opacification. This is often further exacerbated when general anesthesia or sedation is employed. When the distinction between atelectatic lung and nodular change is difficult, it may be helpful to repeat a few slices of the scan with the child in the prone position. Streak artifacts may be seen, which are caused by high-concentration contrast medium in the innominate vein at the site of delivery. This may degrade the imaging of structures in the upper mediastinum. The addition of a "saline chaser" to contrast injections, via a high-pressure pump, has been employed to reduce this phenomenon. The peridiaphragmatic areas also can be difficult to assess, as soft tissue lesions can be difficult to distinguish from the diaphragm in the transaxial plane. Therefore, whenever possible, multiplanar reconstructions in the coronal and sagittal planes should be reviewed.

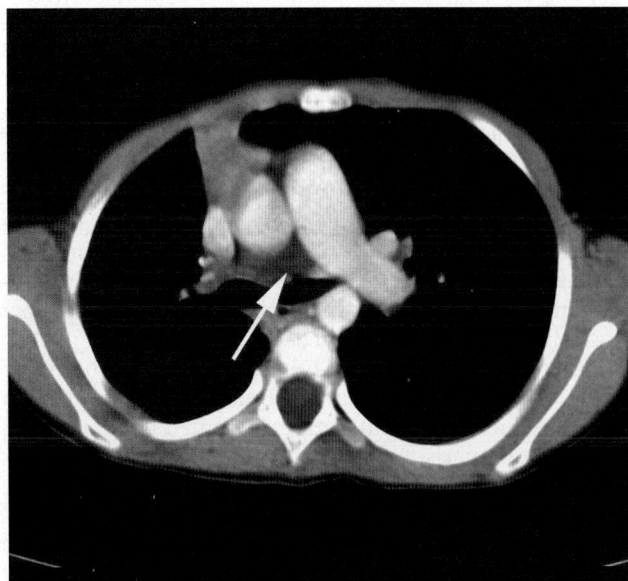

Fig. 10.45 Contrast-enhanced computed tomography through the mediastinum shows a small right lung and no enhancement in the normal site of the right pulmonary artery *(arrow)*. Because the right pulmonary artery is absent, the right lung must receive a systemic supply; however, the collaterals cannot be seen (see Figs. 10.4 and 10.70).

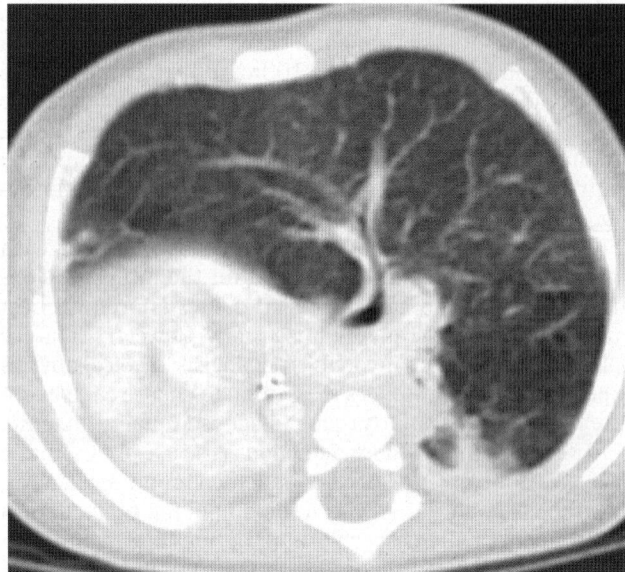

Fig. 10.47 Contrast-enhanced computed tomography shows agenesis of the right lung and compensatory increased volume of the left lung, which appears structurally normal (see Fig. 10.6).

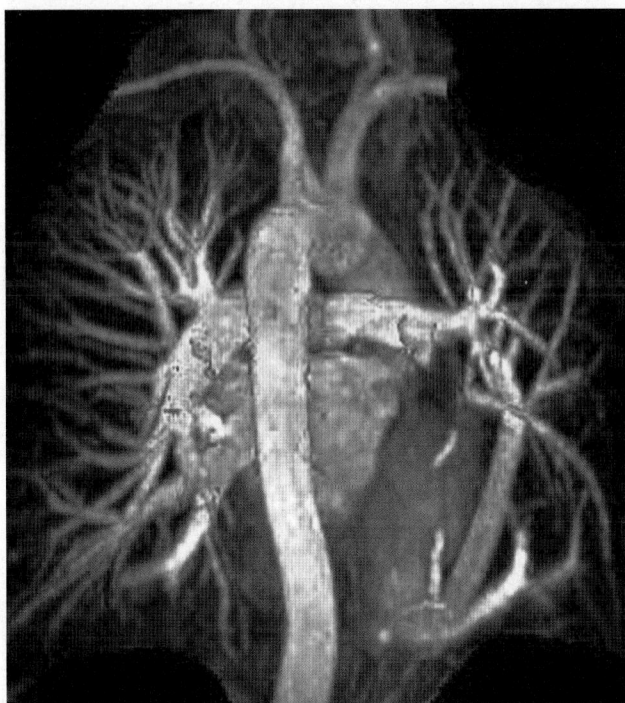

Fig. 10.46 Three-dimensional magnetic resonance imaging scan shows the infra-atrial drainage of a scimitar vein *(arrow*, posterior view; see Fig. 10.5 and 10.44).

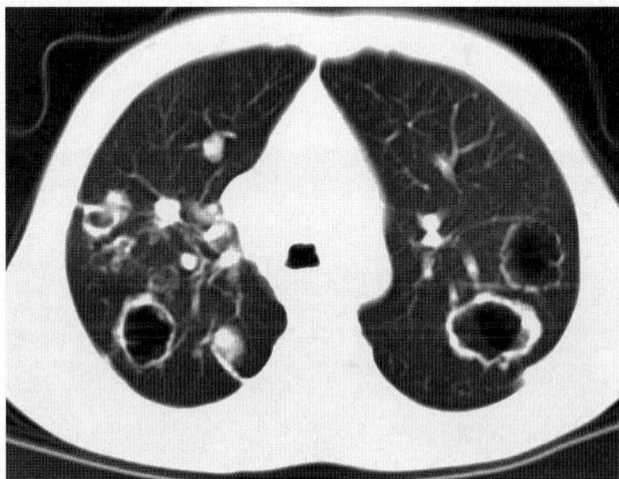

Fig. 10.48 Chest computed tomography of an 8-year-old girl with laryngotracheal papillomatosis shows multiple peripheral nodules and cavities with posterior dominance, in keeping with pulmonary dissemination (see Fig. 10.17).

Radiation Dose

Radiation dose considerations are particularly important in pediatric imaging. CT delivers the largest radiation burden of all diagnostic imaging modalities except for a limited number of nuclear medicine tests. Therefore its indications should be carefully considered and the scan protocol optimized to produce sufficiently diagnostic images while keeping the radiation dose as low as reasonably achievable.[15,16]

Pediatric scanning parameters should be optimized and adjusted according to patient size, based on body weight, diameter, or the region of interest. Reducing the tube current (mA) and/or tube potential (kV) will reduce the radiation

Some artifacts mimic pathology. Tachypnea or motion will inevitably blur the final image, and this phenomenon is easily confused with ground-glass change. Apparent (pseudo) bronchiectasis in the lingula and right middle lobe may sometimes be simulated by cardiac motion in which a single airway branch is represented twice in the image.

dose; this is because the dose is directly proportional to the tube current and is exponentially related to kVp, so that a reduction in kV from 120 to 100 can further reduce the dose by 30%–70%.[17,18] In fact, it is preferable (in angiographic chest CT imaging) to use a lower kV as it enhances the CT attenuation of iodinated contrast, thus increasing the contrast-to-noise ratio in the perfused structures and improving overall image quality while minimizing dose.

It is widely accepted that dose reduction is associated with an increase in image noise. Air within the lungs provides high contrast with adjacent soft tissue, affording chest imaging a higher tolerance of image noise. However, a regular optimization program involving radiologists, medical physics experts, and radiographers is essential to ensure each exposure remains sufficient to produce diagnostic quality imaging.

Another method of dose reduction is the use of automatic exposure control (AEC) that is now a common application in MDCT. The aim of AEC is to modulate the tube current according to patient-specific attenuation that ultimately reduces dose without degrading image quality.[19] However, this technique still requires adjustment of parameters to patient size to ensure dose optimization. Three basic methods of tube current modulations are used in AEC, with different manufacturers adopting a different methodology, or a combination of the three that includes: (1) patient-size modulation, (2) z-axis modulation, and (3) rotational or angular modulation.

Scanner detector configuration and use of beam-shaping filters also affect dose efficiency. Scanners that use a matrix array detector configuration (equal width of all detector rows) are less dose-efficient than those using adaptive array detectors (outer rows wider than inner rows), with greater beam utilization and reduced penumbra.

Depending on the collimation (e.g., slice thickness of 0.6 or 1.2 mm with a 64-slice scanner), tube current, and longitudinal length of the scan, the absorbed dose varies in equivalence to between 25 and 50 chest radiographs for a 2-month-old infant. In pediatric applications, the tube current should be substantially reduced, and image quality usually can be dropped (lower signal-to-noise ratio) without loss of relevant diagnostic information. Data from a recent audit of CT dose at our institution are presented in Tables 10.3 and 10.4. Comparison of computed tomography (CT) doses (volume CT dose index [CTDIvol], dose length product [DLP], and whole body effective dose) from CT thorax examinations with intravenous contrast on older (see Table 10.3) and newer (see Table 10.4) dual-source CT scanners from the same manufacturer (Siemens, Erlangen, Germany). The newer dual-source scanner is capable of high-pitch, high temporal resolution imaging compared to the previous dual-source machine with lower pitch and temporal resolution capabilities.

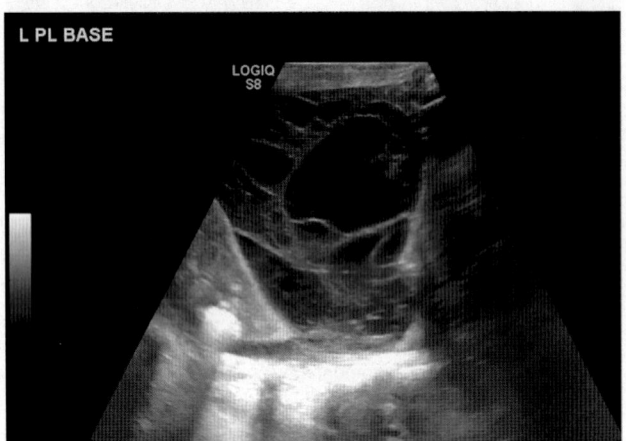

Fig. 10.49. Ultrasound image demonstrating an extensively septated pleural collection (empyema) with collapse and consolidation of the underlying lower lobe, which contains an echogenic round focus posteriorly, possibly representing gas within a pulmonary abscess cavity.

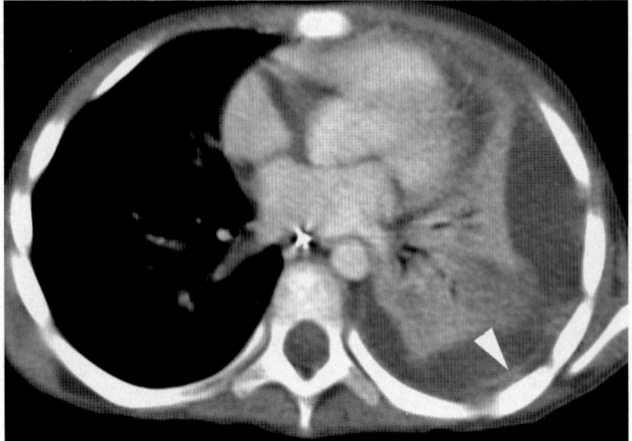

Fig. 10.50 Contrast-enhanced computed tomography (CT) confirms the ultrasound finding of consolidated lung (note air bronchograms) and pleural fluid. There is mild pleural thickening and enhancement that is nonspecific (arrowhead). CT did not show calcification. Acid-fast bacilli were cultured from the pleural fluid. This case shows the currently nonspecific role of CT in the imaging of pleural fluid (see Fig. 10.51).

Table 10.3   Computed Tomography Thorax With Contrast—Siemens Definition Ds 2014

Weight Group	<5 kg	5–<15 kg	15–<30 kg	30–<50 kg	50–<80 kg	>80 kg
Mean weight (kg)	3.5	11	21	38	58.1	108
Mean DLP (mGy.cm)	12.5	22	44.5	98.5	155	256
Mean CTDIvol (mGy)	0.89	1.3	2.05	4.07	5.2	9.8
Mean scan length (cm)	10.1	13.5	17.9	21.9	25.7	22.5
Mean effective dose (mSv)	**1.4**	**1.4**	**1.9**	**2.1**	**4.4**	**5.7**

CTDIvol, Volume CT dose index; DLP, dose length product.

Table 10.4　Computed Tomography Thorax With Contrast—Siemens Definition Force 2015

Weight Group	<5 kg	5–<15 kg	15–<30 kg	30–<50 kg	50–<80 kg	>80 kg
Mean weight (kg)	3.5	10	20	37.4	60	91.7
Mean DLP (mGy.cm)	4.2	10	19	37	72.7	115
Mean CTDIvol (mGy)	0.27	0.52	0.86	1.38	2.55	4.33
Mean scan length (cm)	10.8	15.6	20.1	24.3	26.7	22.7
Mean effective dose (mSv)	**0.6**	**0.6**	**0.92**	**1.6**	**1.49**	**1.95**

CTDIvol, Volume CT dose index; *DLP,* dose length product.

High-Resolution Computed Tomography

HRCT is the modality of choice in suspected interstitial lung disease. It allows a detailed structural assessment of secondary pulmonary lobules and intrapulmonary interstitium, thereby aiding the diagnostic workup. HRCT usually allows a confident radiologic diagnosis in cases of alveolar proteinosis, pulmonary lymphangiectasia, and idiopathic pulmonary hemosiderosis.[20] It can be used to guide lung biopsy and thoracoscopic procedures, targeting areas of active disease. HRCT allows early detection of diffuse pulmonary parenchymal disease to the level of the secondary pulmonary lobule, and is useful in the characterization of opportunistic infection in the immunocompromised patient. Serial imaging may be useful in monitoring disease activity.

The recommended technique in children with diffuse pulmonary disease includes high-pitch spiral CT from the lung apices to the lung bases, reconstructed to 1 mm sections using a high spatial resolution reconstruction kernel. If possible, in cooperative children (>5 years), CT slices should be obtained at full inspiration to diminish vascular crowding, particularly in the dependent areas of the lung, where atelectasis is more common in children than in adults. In certain circumstances three extra slices through the lung apices, mid-zones, and bases are added to the scan protocol in an expiratory phase for looking at small airways disease. In infants and small children unable to follow breathing instructions, lateral decubitus positioning can be employed with the dependent lung relatively expiratory due to gravity.

Knowledge of the anatomic basis for HRCT is a prerequisite for understanding abnormal features. Supplying arterial and bronchiolar branches pass in the core of the secondary pulmonary lobule, and draining veins and lymphatics in the connective tissue between lobules—the interlobular septa. The subpleural interstitium connects to the interlobular septa, constituting the peripheral fiber system. The bronchovascular interstitium extends centripetally from the hila.

Controlled Ventilation Technique

A method for noninvasive controlled ventilation in sedated children may be particularly useful in HRCT. Positive pressure is applied at a facemask, and the pressure applied adjusted by changing the setting of a pressure pop-off valve. Respiratory pauses are induced by means of a step increase in ventilation combined with rapid lung inflation at a pressure of 25 cm water, given synchronously with spontaneous tidal

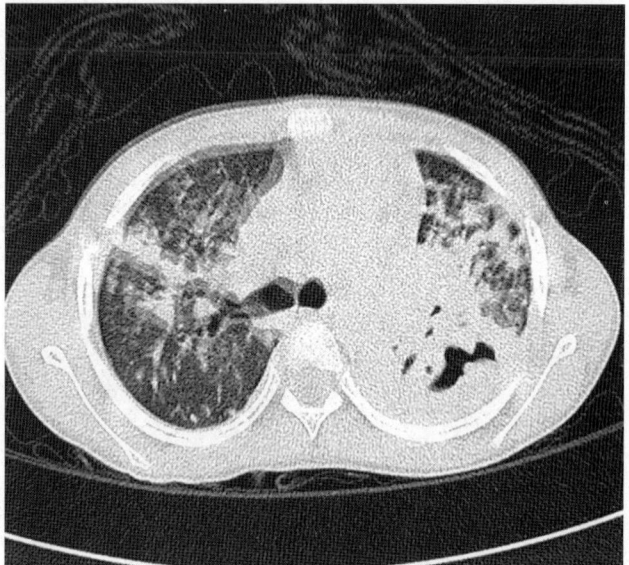

Fig. 10.51 High-resolution computed tomography at a higher level in the same child as in Fig. 10.50 additionally shows cavitation within the left upper lobe consolidation. This was later proven to be due to *Mycobacterium tuberculosis.* Abundant motion artifacts are noted.

inspiration. Lung inflations are repeated approximately three to six times until a respiratory pause occurs. Inspiratory or expiratory scans then can be acquired with minimized motion artifact.[21] However, it should be noted that the advent of high-pitch spiral scanning has largely eliminated the requirement for controlled ventilation techniques outside of research studies employing postprocessing techniques that are dependent on strict standardization of image acquisition protocols.

Interpretation

Interpretation of HRCT images is based on the presence and distribution of certain findings (e.g., septal thickening, ground-glass change, nodular change), which may represent a variety of histopathologic processes.

REGIONAL OR GENERALIZED INCREASED DENSITY

Consolidation (Fig. 10.51) and atelectasis may appear alike on plain radiographs, as discussed earlier. On HRCT, subsegmental atelectasis may be recognized by the traction it exerts on adjacent bronchi (traction bronchiectasis).

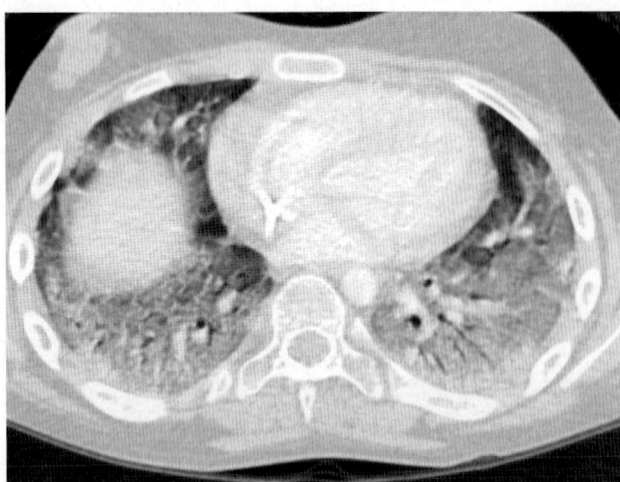

Fig. 10.52 High-resolution computed tomography in a 4-year-old child undergoing chemotherapy shows widespread ground-glass change whose cause cannot be determined. However, in this setting, it is suggestive of drug-induced pneumonitis—in this case, probably bleomycin (see Fig. 10.21).

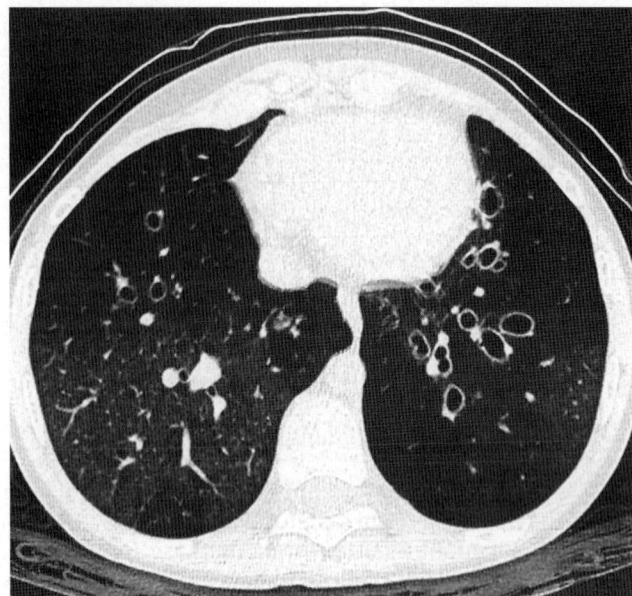

Fig. 10.54 High-resolution computed tomography slice shows bronchial dilation with mild bronchial wall thickening (large airway disease), as well as almost globally hypoattenuating lung parenchyma and associated hypovascularity (small airway disease) in a 9-year-old boy with bronchiectasis.

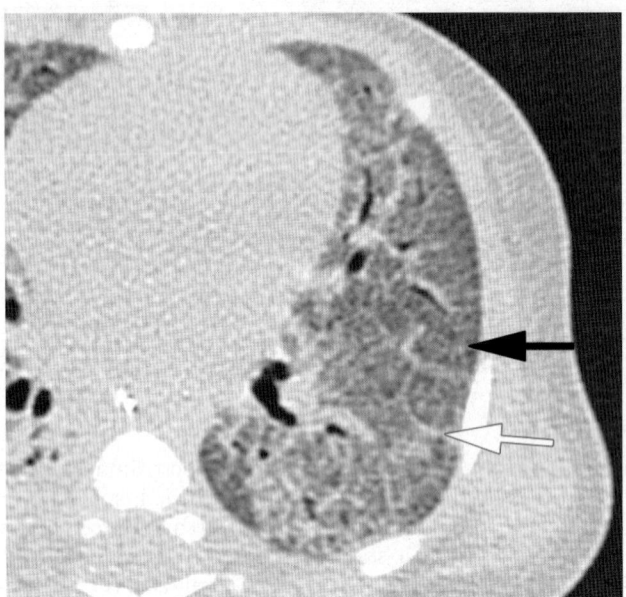

Fig. 10.53 Detail from high-resolution computed tomography in a 3-month-old boy with neonatal onset of childhood interstitial lung disease (ChILD) shows homogeneous ground-glass change, interlobular septal thickening *(white arrow)*, and discrete centrilobular nodules *(black arrow)*.

Ground-glass change is increased pulmonary attenuation, with preservation of vascular markings (Figs. 10.52 and 10.53). This may be due to partial airspace filling or may represent dense intralobular septal thickening that is too subtle to be resolved due to the inherent resolution of the HRCT scanner. Thus, the concept of partial volume effect comes into play when HRCT images show hazy opacification resembling airspace opacification when the abnormality lies in the interstitium.

Lung attenuation differs substantially between full inspiration and expiration. Diffuse, global ground-glass change may therefore be difficult to distinguish from a normal expiratory phase in the lungs. The posterior tracheal membrane is a helpful indicator because it is posteriorly convex on inspiration and horizontal or slightly anteriorly convex on expiration.

REGIONAL OR GENERALIZED DECREASED DENSITY

Circulating blood accounts for most of the normal parenchymal radiopacity. Consequently, decreased radiodensity is most commonly caused by abnormally reduced perfusion due to reflex vasoconstriction in small airway disease. This can be regional (mosaic attenuation) or global (Fig. 10.54).

Differentiation between mosaic attenuation and regional ground-glass change is often difficult. In this case, acquisition of expiratory scans to document air trapping associated with small airway disease can be useful (Figs. 10.55 and 10.56). As described above, in uncooperative children, if breathing cannot be controlled voluntarily (normally younger than 5 years of age), a few slices can be acquired in alternating decubitus positions. The dependent lung simulates expiration as the dependent hemithorax is splinted and its motion restricted, causing underaeration of the dependent lung and relative hyperaeration of the nondependent lung, effectively providing an expiratory view of the dependent lung and an inspiratory view of the nondependent lung.[22]

This is useful in practice for the detection of air trapping in the dependent lung. In small airway disease, the contrast between underperfused and more normal tissue increases on expiration due to air trapping, enforcing the mosaic appearance.

SEPTAL THICKENING

Intralobular interstitial thickening appears as fine weblike outlines, representing abnormal thickening of the lobular

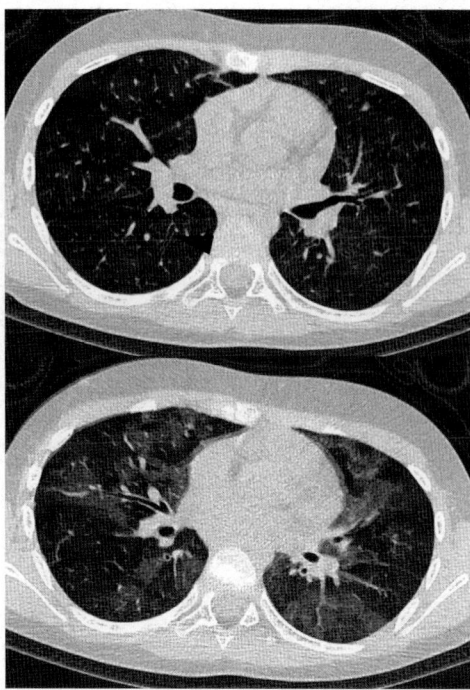

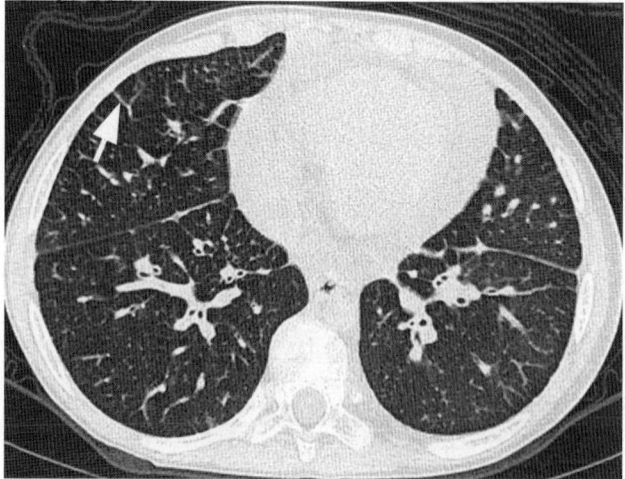

Fig. 10.57 In a 13-year-old boy with known enteric lymphangiectasia, high-resolution computed tomography shows thickening of the oblique fissures, interlobular septal thickening *(arrow)*, and peribronchovascular thickening. This suggests mild pulmonary involvement.

Fig. 10.55 In an 11-year-old girl who received a bone marrow transplant, on inspiration *(top)*; there are global attenuation differences seen in a mosaic pattern, as well as bronchial dilation *(arrowhead)*. The mosaic pattern is accentuated on expiration *(bottom)*, suggesting air trapping within low-attenuating segments.

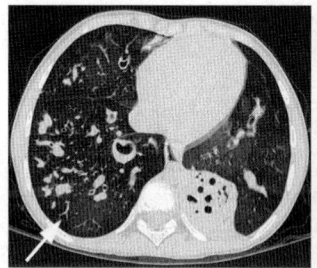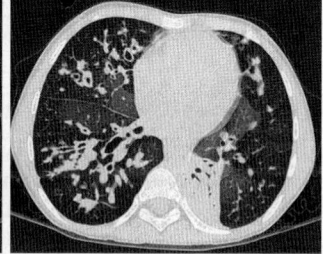

Fig. 10.56 High-resolution computed tomography in an adolescent girl with end-stage cystic fibrosis shows mosaic attenuation, dilation, and wall thickening of the bronchi; mucus within the bronchi; and terminal branches with tree-in-bud sign *(arrow)*. On expiration *(right)*, there is accentuation of the mosaic pattern, confirming small airway obstruction.

connective tissue or lobular bronchovascular interstitium due to inflammation or edema. If it is coarser, it resembles ground-glass change (discussed earlier).

Interlobular septal thickening is best appreciated in the subpleural lung, where it outlines the secondary pulmonary lobules. It may be the result of interstitial edema, hemorrhage, fibrosis, cellular infiltration, or lymphangiectasia (Fig. 10.57; see also Fig. 10.53). Diseases that affect the peripheral acini of two adjacent lobules may give the same appearance.

Peribronchovascular thickening is prominence of the bronchial walls or pulmonary arteries, usually with conspicuous centrilobular arteries. In the more extreme forms, this is caused by cellular infiltration (tends to appear nodular) or edema (smooth).

Interlobular septal thickening superimposed on ground-glass change is termed the *crazy paving pattern*, which is most commonly seen in childhood-type pulmonary alveolar proteinosis.

NODULES

Random nodules are small infiltrates with no predominant anatomic association, typically seen in hematogenously spread disease (e.g., metastatic disease, miliary tuberculosis). Centrilobular nodules are nodular densities located centrally within secondary pulmonary lobules and are therefore equally spaced. They represent small infiltrates associated with bronchioles and alveolar ducts (e.g., infection, hypersensitivity pneumonitis). Centrilobular nodules (Fig. 10.58; see also Fig. 10.53) may coexist with peribronchial inflammation and impaction of fluid, cells, or mucus in the centrilobular bronchioles (see Fig. 10.56). The nodular branching patterns cause the characteristic tree-in-bud finding. This is a sign in infectious bronchitis/bronchiolitis, bronchiectasis, and tuberculosis. Perilymphatic nodules are small infiltrates associated with the visceral pleura, interlobular septa, and bronchovascular bundles (e.g., sarcoidosis).

BRONCHIAL CHANGE

Bronchiectasis is dilation of the bronchus. The commonly used cutoff point for normal/abnormal equals the diameter of the adjacent artery. In early phases of cystic fibrosis, small airway disease represented by mosaic attenuation may be the only finding evident on HRCT. With advancing disease, the typical pattern is seen: bronchial dilation accompanied by bronchial wall thickening, mucus impaction, and architectural distortion (see Fig. 10.56). Bronchial dilation with minimal bronchial wall change and coexisting severe small airway disease usually points toward constrictive obliterative bronchiolitis (see Fig. 10.54). Bronchial wall thickening without dilation, often with patchy consolidation, is often seen in chronic aspiration (Fig. 10.59). It is sometimes difficult to distinguish between bronchial distention secondary to high ventilator pressure and genuine

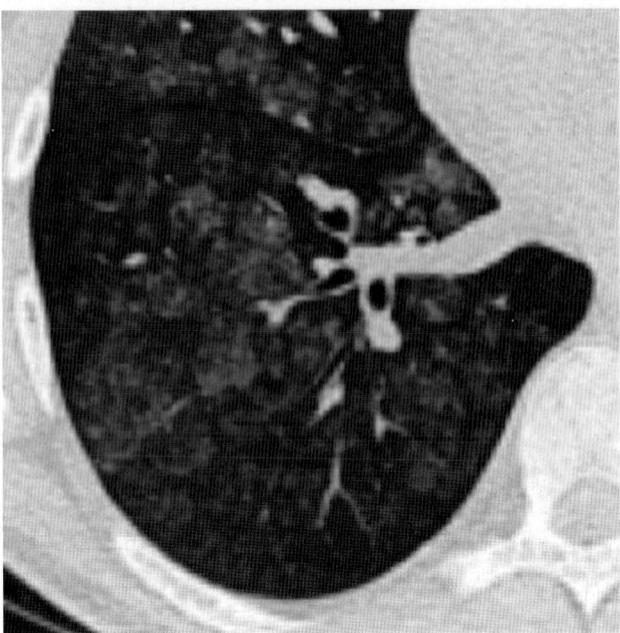

Fig. 10.58 In a 12-year-old girl with anemia and intermittent hemoptysis, high-resolution computed tomography shows centrilobular ground-glass nodules suggestive of idiopathic pulmonary hemosiderosis.

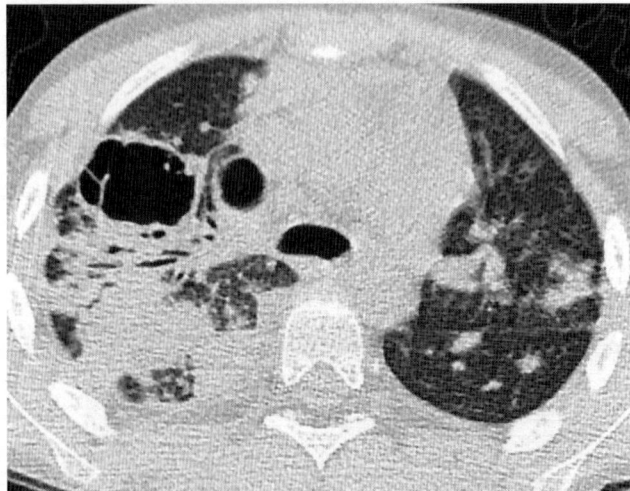

Fig. 10.60 High-resolution computed tomography shows architectural distortion with large nodular change, air cyst, traction bronchiectasis, and pleural thickening in the right lung, and nodular change in the left. Histopathology verified nonspecific necrotizing vasculitis (see Fig. 10.20).

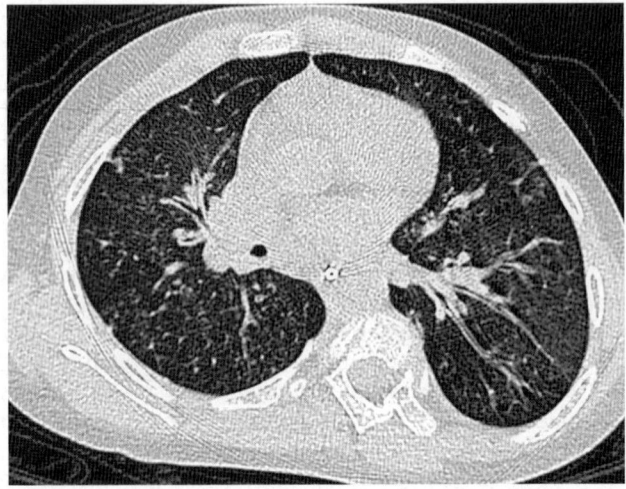

Fig. 10.59 High-resolution computed tomography confirms bronchial wall thickening and shows small foci of subpleural interlobular septal thickening in a 9-year-old girl with gastroesophageal reflux and chronic aspiration (see Fig. 10.26).

bronchial dilation. There is much controversy regarding reversibility of bronchiectasis, so serial imaging is the gold standard for irreversibility (i.e., fixed dilatation and wall thickening).

A paper by Gaillard and colleagues[23] advised caution with diagnosing "bronchiectasis," as reversibility of radiologic findings can be seen in children. They suggest that serial imaging is required to confirm irreversibility before using the term *bronchiectasis* in children. They add that, as diagnostic criteria are derived from adult studies that have not

been validated in children, cautious interpretation be made of CT findings. Their study included 22 children over a 6-year period, who had at least two lung CT scans, with a median scan interval of 21 months (range 2–43 months). Bronchial dilation resolved completely in 6 children, and there was improvement in another 8 patients. Hence, labeling children with an irreversible lifelong condition requires caution on the part of the radiologist.

ARCHITECTURAL DISTORTION

Fibrosis and altered elasticity of the tissues permanently alters the structure of the lung parenchyma. This is seen as reduced parenchymal attenuation, cysts, deviation of vessels, bronchi and interlobular septa, and traction bronchiectasis (see Fig. 10.56). Cyst formation may also be caused by cystic resolution of pneumonia, forming a pneumatocele, or necrotic change of a preexisting parenchymal nodule (e.g., degeneration of granulomatous change in Langerhans cell histiocytosis, vasculitis, or granulomatosis with angiitis) (Fig. 10.60). Seen in end-stage disease, honeycombing is the result of clusters of thick-walled air cysts, representing structurally distorted, dilated respiratory bronchioles lined by fibrotic tissues, collapsed alveoli, and vessels.

Angiography

In noncardiac chest pathology, angiography is most commonly used for mediastinal vasculature and cystic congenital lung malformations. Magnetic resonance angiography is a useful noninvasive technique with no radiation burden.

Interventional techniques, such as embolization of bronchial arteries, are performed in cases of severe hemorrhage/hemoptysis in cystic fibrosis. Therapeutic embolization of feeding vessels to intralobar or extralobar sequestrations or to pulmonary arteriovenous malformations can be performed using metallic coils, thereby avoiding thoracotomy.

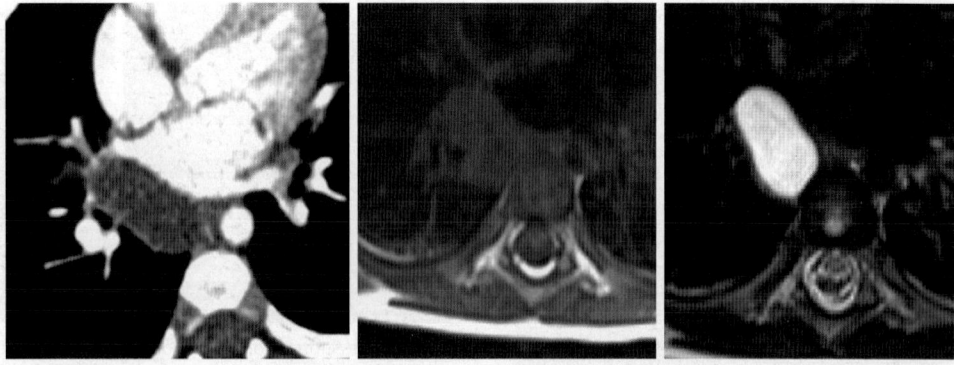

Fig. 10.61 Axial computed tomography demonstrating a low attenuation lesion inferior to the right hilum. T1- and T2-weighted magnetic resonance imaging images demonstrating low T1 signal and high T2 signal in keeping with fluid, further suggesting the diagnosis of mediastinal bronchogenic cyst.

Magnetic Resonance Imaging

Nonionizing radiation techniques should always be considered in pediatrics, and MRI is a highly desirable diagnostic tool for use in children, although drawbacks include the increased use of sedation or general anesthesia to accommodate the prolonged scan times and resultant susceptibility to movement artifact.

The multiplanar imaging capabilities of electrocardiogram-gated MRI and magnetic resonance angiography make these important methods for evaluating cardiac lesions; anomalies of the mediastinal vessels; and masses, such as bronchopulmonary foregut malformations, chest wall masses, bone marrow infiltrations, tracheobronchial abnormalities, and neurogenic masses (Fig. 10.61).

The multiplanar capability of MRI, combined with its superb soft-tissue contrast resolution, allow for diagnosis that is more specific. Ongoing refinements, with improved gating techniques and shorter scan times, are under continuous development and continue to enhance the role of MRI in evaluating the pulmonary hila, lung parenchyma, heart, and diaphragm.

Although MRI is well established in cardiac imaging, experience with lung MRI is still limited. The main technical problems are: (1) low proton density in the lungs—hence a very weak signal return (echo) from the lung parenchyma; and (2) pulse and motion artifacts from the heart, great vessels, and respiration, causing significant image degradation.

MRI achieves tissue contrast first by adjusting the train of excitation, refocusing radiofrequency pulses, and switching magnetic field gradients. A T1-weighted MRI sequence takes advantage of the relatively fast realignment with the main magnetic field of fat molecules, so that fat appears bright on the acquired images. Such images are generally useful for studying anatomy. T2-weighted MRI sequences play on the relatively slow realignment of water molecules with the main magnetic field. Because water appears bright on these images, they are particularly helpful in detecting fluid collections and edema. These fundamental MRI techniques provide good depiction of structural pulmonary changes in cystic fibrosis.[24]

A second facility for creating image contrast, or enhancing inherent tissue imaging contrast, is the administration of intravenous MRI contrast medium, which is usually gadolinium chelate. This is typically combined with a T1-weighted

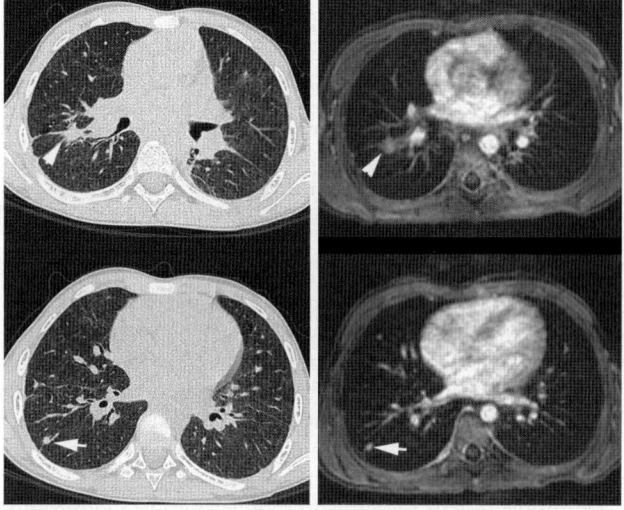

Fig. 10.62 In a 12-year-old boy with chronic granulomatous disease, high-resolution computed tomography *(left)* and contrast-enhanced three-dimensional gradient echo magnetic resonance imaging *(right)* acquired on the same day, show corresponding findings of spiculated, enhancing lesions near the right hilum *(arrowheads)* and subpleurally in the right lower lobe *(arrows)*.

pulse sequence and gives superb images of vascular structures, and potentially even the most peripheral vessels. Additionally, contrast media are useful for detecting vascular enhancement in inflammatory or neoplastic lesions (Figs. 10.62 and 10.63).

Ultrafast pulse sequences with three-dimensional acquisition of volumetric MRI data are diagnostically promising and can be implemented on most modern scanners. Although the diagnostic accuracy is still largely unknown, MRI potentially may be used for imaging parenchymal lung lesions,[25] and high accuracy compared with CT has been demonstrated for nodules of 3 mm or larger in size.[26] Recent headway has been made utilizing respiratory-gated ultrashort echotime MRI sequences with radial reconstruction, allowing fast and quiet imaging with a spatial resolution far closer to that of CT than previously possible (0.86 mm³).[27] While these techniques show promise in the setting of larger focal lung lesions and established bronchiectasis, particularly in cystic fibrosis, the spatial resolution is still not yet sufficient to replace CT in the context of more subtle disease, such as the mosaic

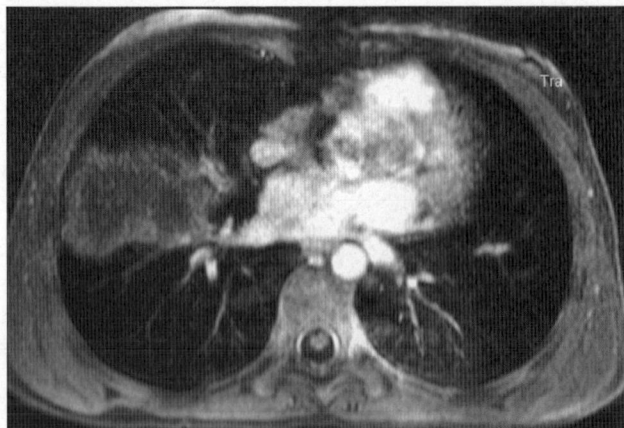

Fig. 10.63 A 12-year-old boy who received a heart-lung transplant had a right-sided density on chest radiographs. Magnetic resonance imaging (T1-weighted gradient echo, breath-hold, gadolinium-enhanced) shows an enhancing mass lesion in close relation to the right oblique fissure. Histopathologically, this was diagnosed as (posttransplant) lympho-proliferative disease.

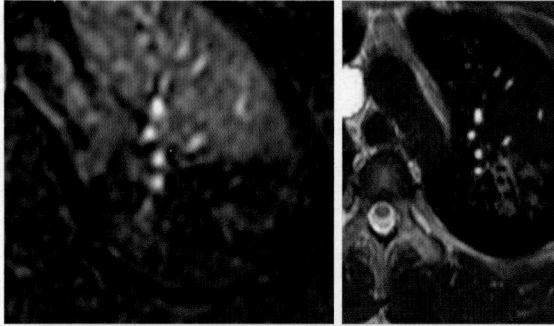

Fig. 10.64 Subtraction perfusion image (fat suppressed T1 volume interpolated breath-hold examination [VIBE] precontrast subtracted from postcontrast) and fusion image (previous image superimposed in red over the T2 turbospin echo image to better demonstrate underlying anatomy) in a cystic fibrosis patient demonstrates thick-walled bronchi in the left upper lobe associated with a regional hypoperfusion.

attenuation demonstrated by CT in constrictive obliterative bronchiolitis and in early CF lung disease.

Currently, more promising MRI techniques offer functional measures of lung disease.

Breathing hyperpolarized helium allows the detection of a signal from within the airspaces, offering ventilation maps similar to those obtained via nuclear medicine studies. Unfortunately, the necessary equipment is expensive and the gas has a short half-life. As a result, this technique is not readily available in most imaging centers. Less expensive methods of gas imaging utilizing inhaled fluorinated gases or pure oxygen show great future clinical potential.[28]

Quantification of regional pulmonary perfusion is promising in the assessment of small airway disease. This can be achieved with time-resolved measurements, following an intravenous bolus of gadolinium. Although not widely used, the technique is available on most modern MRI systems, and there is good agreement with functional tests (Fig. 10.64).[29]

A noncontrast technique—arterial spin labeling—is promising, judging by early feasibility studies.[30] Its potential advantage is that no injection is required and measurements may be repeated as necessary. A combined noncontrast ventilation/perfusion technique utilizing Fourier decomposition has also been described.[31] Roles for diffusion-weighted imaging in the assessment of inflammatory and neoplastic disease are also rapidly emerging.

Endobronchial Ultrasonography

A paper published by Steinfort and colleagues[32] advocates that endobronchial ultrasound (EBUS) should be used in pediatric patients. The technique of endoscopic ultrasound has been used for the gastrointestinal tract for many years and has significantly advanced bronchoscopic techniques in adult respiratory medicine. In adults, the use of image guidance with ultrasound allows more accurate localization and sampling of peripheral pulmonary lesions, as well as mediastinal and hilar masses. This results in a greater diagnostic yield with reduced procedural complication rates in clinical practice, so it would appear that EBUS performance

characteristics in adult populations are equivalent to surgical procedures that were previously considered the gold standard. Moreover, when compared to surgical approaches, there has been a dramatic reduction in morbidity and mortality among adult patients requiring invasive diagnostic procedures.

Steinfort and colleagues illustrate and advocate the various types of EBUS in clinical use, the methods of usage, and the clinical indications for each procedure, highlighting the potential role for EBUS in pediatric pulmonology.[32] Radial probe EBUS is used in the investigation of peripheral lung lesions (e.g., suspected invasive pulmonary aspergillosis) and could be adopted in children to achieve accurate biopsy of such lesions.

Linear probe EBUS allows a minimally invasive biopsy of mediastinal and hilar lesions. It has potentially greater performance characteristics than current biopsy techniques, with no significant complications reported to date. It may be useful in the diagnosis of lymphoma, or neurogenic tumors, and many other diseases resulting in mediastinal or hilar lymphadenopathy.

Certainly EBUS is a minimally invasive technique allowing tissue sampling of peripheral lung lesions, or mediastinal/hilar masses, with high diagnostic accuracy, and a significantly lower morbidity and mortality than alternative approaches. Hence, the indications for and the usage of EBUS in pediatric patients appear to be promising and will surely increase in the future.

Optical coherence tomography is a further promising bronchoscopic imaging technique allowing detailed imaging of the airway wall to a depth of 2–4 mm at a resolution of 1–15 µm. The technique involves the interpretation of backscattered, near-infrared frequency light from a diode at the tip of an endobronchial probe, similar in principle to ultrasound, using light instead of sound. Additionally, rotation of the probe enables the formation of three-dimensional image data.[33] Numerous uses have been investigated in pulmonary medicine, including the investigation of tracheal stenosis and real-time dynamic evaluation of tracheobronchomalacia.[34]

Ultrasonography

There has been controversy within the recent literature surrounding the possible uses of ultrasound within pediatric lung parenchyma. Ultrasound has a well-established role in the investigation of many thoracic diseases, in differentiating simple pleural effusion from complex (loculated, septated) empyema or densely consolidated peripheral lung parenchyma (Fig. 10.65) and its real-time dynamic imaging in assessment of differential organ motion, such as diaphragmatic and laryngeal movement in phrenic and recurrent laryngeal nerve palsies, respectively (Videos 10.7 and 10.8). Color flow Doppler imaging allows functional assessment of vascularity and can aid identification of systemic feeding vessels in pulmonary sequestration (Fig. 10.66). Suggested roles for ultrasound in noncardiac thoracic investigation can be found in Box 10.1. Further example images and videos can be found in the online supplement (Box 10.2).

There are recent publications suggesting a role for ultrasound in the bedside assessment of the lung parenchyma, suggesting its use as a replacement for chest radiography. This has led to some confusion as various physical artifacts have been cited as implying the presence (or indeed absence) of intrathoracic lung parenchymal pathology. "A lines" refer to horizontal reflections of the lung edge resulting from an aerated subpleural lung. "B lines" refer to vertical bright lines resulting from ring-down artifact from isolated gas bubbles within extravascular fluid, suggesting pathology. However, these signs are not specific for a given pathology (Fig. 10.67).[35]

The "lung point" sign—that is, the presence of a transition from darker, more transonic lung towards the apices to brighter lung inferiorly—has been associated with transient tachypnea of the newborn, with the suggestion that more nonresorbed fluid in the dependent lung causes an increase in "B lines" (Fig. 10.68). The lungs of premature neonates with idiopathic respiratory distress syndrome (iRDS) have been found to produce particularly bright B lines, which become coarser with the onset of more chronic lung disease (Fig. 10.69).

While there is no doubt that ultrasound is capable of demonstrating pulmonary parenchymal disease, its significant limitations should be understood. While the above changes consistent with iRDS can be demonstrated, the diagnosis

---

Box 10.1 Suggested Roles for Ultrasound Within Pediatric Respiratory Medicine

Peripheral increased opacification—pleural effusion vs. consolidation (see Fig. 10.49 vs. Fig. 10.65)
Pleural fluid—simple effusion (transudate) vs. empyema or hemothorax (see Fig. 10.49)

Chest Wall Lesions

Widened mediastinum—mass lesions, prominent thymus, etc.
Thymus—focal abnormalities, presence or absence; e.g., DiGeorge syndrome (see Fig. 10.1)
Diaphragm—phrenic nerve palsy, hernia, eventration (see Video 10.7)
Larynx—recurrent laryngeal nerve palsy (see Video 10.8)
Sequestration—presence of infradiaphragmatic systemic "feeding" vessel (see Fig. 10.66)
To guide intervention—aspiration, drainage, and biopsy (pleural, peripheral parenchymal, and mediastinal)

Box 10.2 Online Material

CT Postprocessing

Maximum intensity projection (MIP)—increasing slab thickness (see Video 10.1)
Minimum intensity projection (MinIP)—increasing slab thickness (see Video 10.2)
Narrowing the window width to accentuate mosaic attenuation (see Video 10.3)
Volume rendering technique (VRT)—double aortic arch with tracheal narrowing (see Video 10.4)
Virtual bronchoscopy (see Video 10.5)

Techniques

Fluoroscopic diaphragm assessment in phrenic nerve palsy (see Video 10.6)
Ultrasound assessment in phrenic nerve palsy (see Video 10.7)
Laryngeal ultrasound (see Video 10.8)
Ultrasound of the normal thymus (transverse section) (see Video 10.9)
Ultrasound of pulmonary consolidation (see Video 10.10)
Bronchogram in extrinsic airway compression (see Video 10.11)

Cases

Bronchial atresia (see Video 10.12)
Constrictive obliterative bronchiolitis following mycoplasma pneumonia (see Video 10.13)

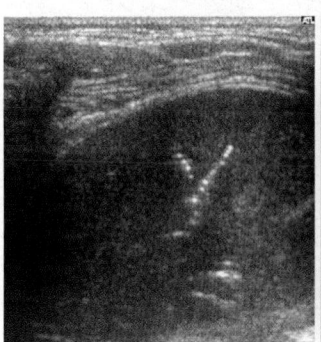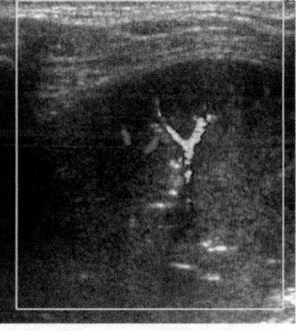

Fig. 10.65 Ultrasound images of pulmonary consolidation. B mode image *(left)* demonstrating a bright air bronchogram in a densely consolidated lobe. Addition of color flow imaging *(right)* demonstrates flow in the adjacent accompanying pulmonary artery *(red)* demonstrating their relationship to the bronchial tree. Pulmonary venous *(blue)* branches are also shown. (Image courtesy of P Tomà.)

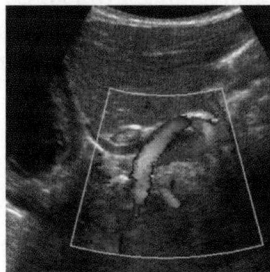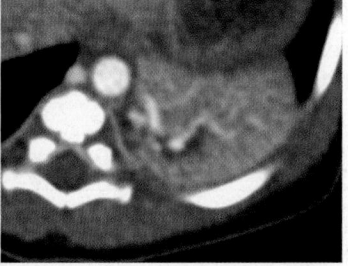

Fig. 10.66 Color flow ultrasound image *(left image)* demonstrating a large collateral vessel from the abdominal aorta, passing superiorly to supply the left basal extralobar sequestration demonstrated on computed tomography *(right image)*. (Image courtesy of P Tomà.)

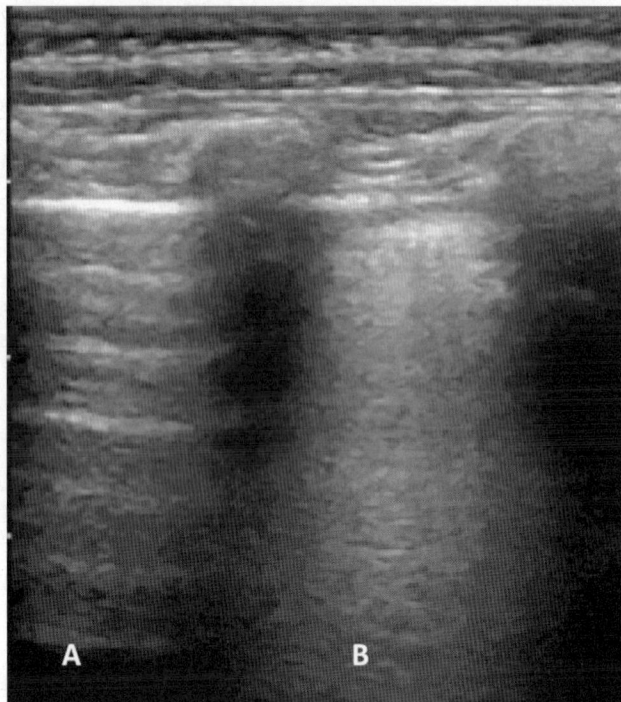

Fig. 10.67 "A lines"—horizontal bright reflections of the pleural surface—indicate that the subpleural lung is aerated. "B lines"—vertical bright lines—"ring-down" artifact from isolated gas bubbles within extravascular fluid. (Image courtesy of P Tomà.)

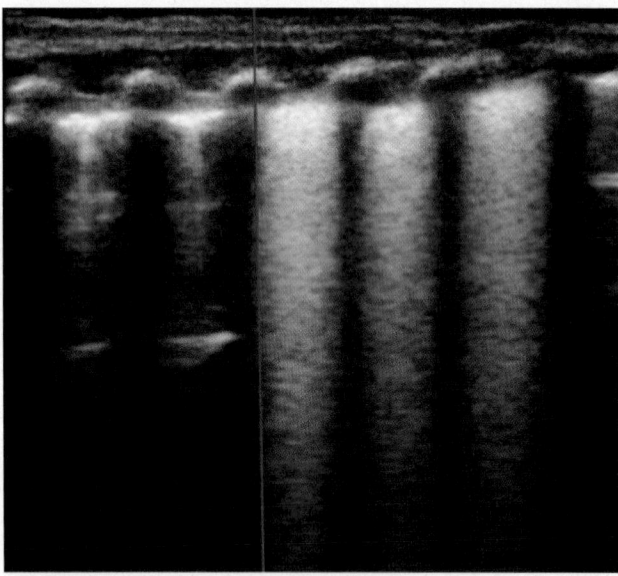

Fig. 10.68 The "lung point" sign. The transition from darker apical lung (to the left of the *red line*) to brighter lung at the bases (to the right of the *red line*) is suggestive of transient tachypnea of the newborn (TTN). (Image courtesy of P Tomà.)

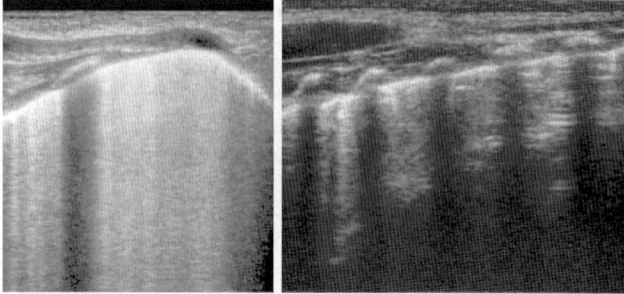

Fig. 10.69 Ultrasound images of a premature neonate with idiopathic respiratory distress syndrome. At day 0, bright B-lines are demonstrated *(left image)*. By day 5 *(right image)*, the appearance is more coarse and heterogeneous. (Image courtesy of P Tomà.)

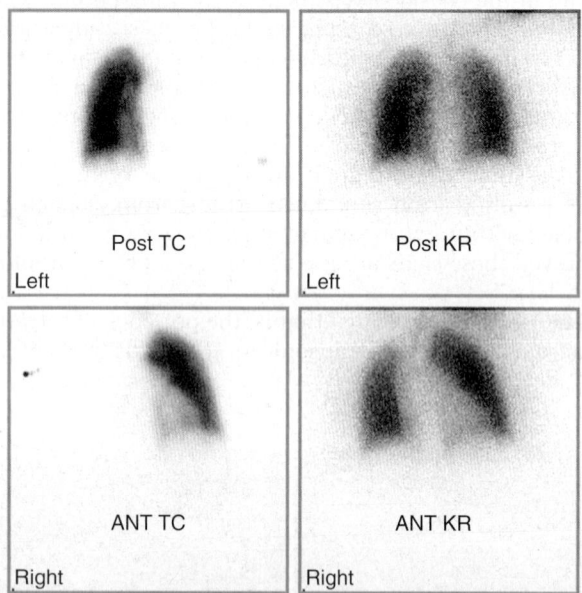

Fig. 10.70 A ventilation/perfusion isotope study in a patient with absent right pulmonary artery on computed tomography confirms interrupted pulmonary arterial supply to the right lung *(left panel)*. The hypoplastic right lung has preserved ventilation *(right panel;* see Figs. 10.4 and 10.45). *KR,* Inhaled krypton ventilation images; *TC,* intravenous 99m technetium microaggregated albumin (MAA) perfusion images.

infection, which does not subtend the pleural surface, will not be appreciated, and any related mediastinal lymphadenopathy will be overlooked. However, lung ultrasound has played a role in the research-based frequent follow-up of pneumonic consolidation in resource-poor areas, as utilized in the Drakenstein Child Heath Study.[36]

The chest radiograph remains the first modality of choice within pediatric chest imaging, with the other modalities reserved for further, more specific questions, directed by the preceding radiograph.

Radionuclide Imaging

Nuclear medicine techniques are used to help delineate cardiac function, right-to-left pulmonary arteriovenous malformations, pulmonary embolism, inflammatory lung disease, and lung ventilation/perfusion (Fig. 10.70). While nuclear medicine has been the main tool for functional assessment of the

can be made clinically with no imaging at all, and ultrasound cannot adequately demonstrate the complications (particularly the clinically significant air leaks: pulmonary interstitial emphysema, pneumopericardium, etc.) and the positions of the numerous support tubes and lines that are so readily demonstrated via chest radiography. Peripheral pneumonic consolidation is readily identified, but more deep-seated heart and lung, the technique is gradually being replaced by CT for assessment of pulmonary embolism and small airway disease, and by MRI for combined assessment of cardiac morphology and function.

Positron emission tomography (PET) is a promising modality. It uses biologically interesting radionuclides (e.g., fluorine 18, carbon 11, oxygen 15, nitrogen 13) to mark biochemical substrates (e.g., glucose). PET is therefore a modality for metabolic rather than structural studies, and in patients with malignant disease, PET uses the relatively high glucose metabolism in malignant cells for imaging. Combined with CT, or more recently MRI, anatomic and functional data can be fused into one image. The clinical efficacy of the technique is being explored, but the modality shows particular strength in oncologic imaging, both at diagnosis and in the follow-up of metabolic response to treatment.

Conclusion

The approaches to radiologic evaluation of the child cannot be extrapolated from adult imaging. Particular awareness of the issues of radiation protection, anatomy and physiology, and the range of pediatric disorders is crucial. As with every test, the key is first to pose a focused question and then to select the best way of answering it, usually in consultation with expert colleagues. In general, chest radiography gives the first overall assessment of the presence or absence of disease, with the other modalities used to provide further more detailed information: CT for fine detail of the lung parenchyma; ultrasound for the definition of pleural pathology; and, more recently, MRI for functional information and more gross structural disease.

References
Access the reference list online at ExpertConsult.com.

Suggested Reading
Frush DP, Donnelly LF, Rosen NS. Computed tomography and radiation risks. What pediatric health care providers should know. *Pediatrics.* 2003;112:951–957.

Garcia-Peña P, Guillerman RP. *Pediatric Chest Imaging.* Berlin Heidelberg: Springer-Verlag; 2014.

Owens CM, Gillard JH. *Grainger & Allison's Diagnostic Radiology: Paediatric Imaging.* 6th ed. London: Elsevier; 2016.

Puderbach M, Eichinger M, Gahr J, et al. Proton MRI appearance of cystic fibrosis: comparison to CT. *Eur Radiol.* 2007;17:716–724.

Siegel MJ. *Pediatric Body CT.* Philadelphia: Lippincott Williams & Wilkins; 1999.

Siegel MJ, Schmidt B, Bradley D, et al. Radiation dose and image quality in pediatric CT: effect of technical factors and phantom size and shape. *Radiology.* 2004;233:515–522.

11 *Pulmonary Function Tests in Infants and Children*

DOROTTYA CZOVEK, MD, PhD

Introduction

The childhood years represent a very important period of lung growth and development, during which the respiratory system is exceptionally vulnerable to any insult. Measuring lung function in infants and young children presents significant and particular challenges. An ideal lung function test for clinical use should: (1) be easy and quick to perform for both the children and testers even in a busy outpatient setting; (2) have standard operating procedures, guidelines and robust healthy reference data available; (3) discriminate between healthy children and those with respiratory disease with high specificity and sensitivity; (4) be feasible at any age for longitudinal follow-up of individuals with lung disease; and (5) be cheap and widely available to fulfill health care equality.

While the indications, methodology, and interpretation of lung function testing in children above 6 years of age is similar to those in adults, infants and preschool-age children require special technical and safety considerations (these will be discussed below). However, staff with a special attitude, understanding, patience, and love for the children are essential: child-friendly personnel is one of the main determinants of the success of any lung function test in young children.

INDICATIONS AND SPECIAL CONSIDERATIONS FOR PULMONARY FUNCTION TESTS IN INFANTS

Lung function can be measured as early as in the first days of life in infants for both clinical and research purposes. Correctly performed lung function tests during infancy can provide information on lung growth and development, disease status, and progression, and can aid the clinicians in decision making. Most of the lung function tests were originally developed for adults and later modified for the special requirements of infants and young children (e.g., plethysmography and multiple breath washout [MBW]), while others have been designed specifically for infant testing (e.g., single occlusion technique [SOT]). Although commercial devices and validated guidelines are often available, infant lung function testing is not always part of the routine practice of pediatric respiratory laboratories. This is most probably due to the special technical and personal requirements that are essential for successful lung function testing during infancy.

Technical and Staff Requirements

Since all of the lung function tests are performed during quiet sleep or sedation, the appropriate location of the infant testing room is very important for the success of the test. In laboratories where lung function testing is performed routinely as part of the clinical care, the infant study room should be isolated from those for preschool- and school-age children. The room containing the lung function devices and consumables has to be comfortable and large enough to accommodate two examiners, one or two parents (and sometimes siblings), and equipped with everything that is necessary for changing and settling the infant.

Since the visit can take as long as 3 or 4 hours, the procedures and their duration (either clinical or research study visit) should be discussed in detail with the parents prior to the appointment. It is important to consider that many of the mothers may be still breastfeeding at the time of the measurement; therefore privacy has to be provided to the parents, if necessary.

Resuscitation equipment has to be available in the room and, for safety and technical reasons, two skilled examiners have to be present at the time of the testing. If the test is performed during sedation (see later) heart rate and oxygen saturation should be monitored continuously.

Infant lung function testing is technically challenging; therefore the examiners have to be properly trained. They should be able to recognize any technical problems (such as software problems, leak in the system during the test), and it is desirable that they have a basic understanding of respiratory physiology. Since the test is time consuming, there is usually no opportunity to repeat it (especially when performed for research); therefore the real-time quality control (i.e., whether the test fulfills all quality criteria) and interpretation (i.e., whether the results are physiologically meaningful) of the test are crucial.

The infant lung function devices vary in their size and the consumables required. Since the tidal flow and volume during infancy are relatively small, maximum reduction of the dead space is a very important requirement in all lung function equipment. To avoid rebreathing of CO_2, most of the devices employ a bias flow (usually with medical air, but sometimes with oxygen or special gas mixtures).

In spontaneously breathing infants, all of the lung function tests are done through a facemask in the supine position (Fig. 11.1), which introduces the most common source of error in infant testing: the leak around the mask. Any leak invalidates all infant lung function tests; therefore the size of the facemask always has to be selected carefully and its position checked before and throughout the test. Furthermore, the facemask increases the equipment dead space, and its volume should always be taken into account for corrections. However, mask volume correction is not straightforward as one cannot always predict how much of the mask is occupied by the infant's face, raising the possibility of overcorrection for mask volume. Unsedated babies sometimes do

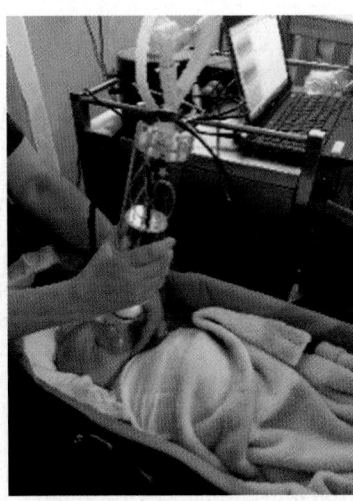

Fig. 11.1 Infant lung function test using the forced oscillation technique.

not tolerate the facemask and wake up every time when the mask is positioned on their face; this is less frequent under sedation.

In unsedated infants, the natural variability of the breathing pattern is significant, especially during rapid eye movement (REM) sleep. Previous studies have shown that during REM sleep breathing frequency is increased[1] and functional residual capacity (FRC) is unstable; therefore if the lung function test is undertaken without sedation, lung function should be measured during deep, non-REM sleep (whenever possible). Non-REM sleep can be recognized by observation of the baby, and a pulse oximeter can sometimes help to detect stable, regular heart rate (as heart rate is usually irregular and fast during REM sleep). Note: monitoring of oxygen saturation is mandatory when infants are sedated for lung function testing and optional for studies conducted during natural sleep. The sleep of preterm babies and neonates is usually superficial, and it is not always possible to differentiate between REM and non-REM sleep phases. Therefore a lung function test in preterm infants and newborns cannot always be undertaken in one sitting and sometimes requires two or three sessions. If more than one lung function test is performed in an infant, the tests that require tidal breathing should be undertaken first while the tests that require a controlled maneuver and may affect the respiratory status (e.g., rapid thoracoabdominal compression [RTC]) should be performed at the end of the visit.

Notes on the time and duration of the tests, and replacement of the facemask between measurements should always be recorded as well as the behavior of the infant (i.e., expiratory noise, snoring, sighs). These comments are useful for the correct interpretation of any infant lung function test.

Lung Function Test in Sedated Infants

Although some lung function tests (typically the ones that require quiet tidal breathing) can be performed in unsedated babies sometimes as late as 1 year of age,[2] there are tests that are difficult or impossible to perform without sedation. Sedation for lung function testing has become less common and has to be considered carefully for either clinical or

research purposes. If lung function is measured as part of the clinical care in an infant with ongoing respiratory problems, sedation is more accepted and tolerated by the parents. Collection of reference data in healthy infants can therefore be challenging, although it is required for the meaningful interpretation of any lung function measure in children with respiratory disease. Nowadays, many human research ethics committees hesitate to approve the sedation of healthy children or even children with respiratory disease for research purposes. Sedation is also contraindicated in neonates and preterm babies with immature respiratory control or any disorders that affect the neural system of the infant. Sedation affects the breathing pattern and the FRC of the infants; therefore data collected in unsedated and sedated babies with the same technique cannot be compared directly. However, it has been shown that the sedation has no effect on the activation of the Hering-Breuer reflex[3]; therefore it can be used safely in techniques such as the SOT or the low-frequency forced oscillation technique (LFOT).

Independently of the purpose of the sedation (i.e., clinical or research test), the exact process and the possible side effects always have to be discussed in details with the parents. It is important to note that even in sedated babies it can take from 15 to 90 minutes to reach quiet sleep that is necessary for the test. Chloral hydrate in an oral dose of 50–100 mg/kg is most frequently used for sedation and usually allows 30–45 minutes for the examiner to perform the lung function test(s). Side effects are extremely rare; however, parents always have to be provided with a phone number to call if they have any concerns after the visit, and they should also be advised not to leave the child unattended during the first few hours.

INDICATIONS AND SPECIAL CONSIDERATIONS FOR PULMONARY FUNCTION TESTS IN CHILDREN

Children older than 2 years of age cannot be sedated for a lung function test; however, their cooperation during the preschool years is limited: they are rarely able to perform complex respiratory maneuvers that are required for lung function tests routinely used in older children and adults. Furthermore, the anatomical and physiological differences in the respiratory system between young children and adults make the interpretation of lung function measures originally developed in adults less straightforward and sometimes meaningless. Common interests of clinicians and researchers have resulted in the development of novel lung function methods and modifications of previously available techniques; therefore nowadays more than half of the children at 3 years of age and 80% of the children between 4 and 6 years of age are able to perform acceptable lung function tests. Similar to adults, spirometry is the most frequently used lung function test in children above 6 years of age, while tests that only require tidal breathing are more favorable in preschool-age children.

Technical and Staff Requirements

A child-friendly environment (Fig. 11.2) with engaged and friendly respiratory technicians or researchers is one of the most important key points for successful lung function testing in preschool-age children. Since children have a short

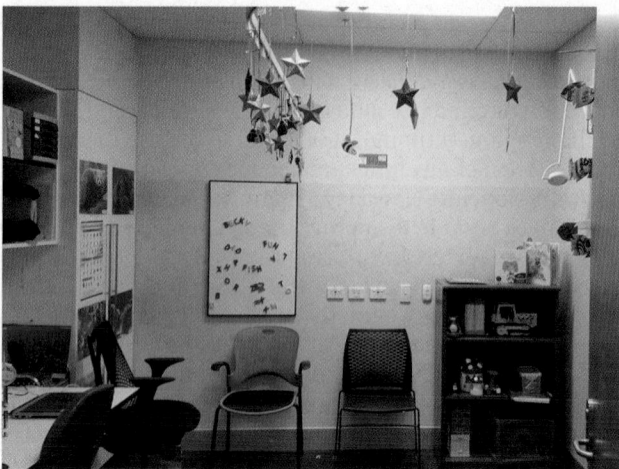

Fig. 11.2 Lung function testing room designed for preschool-aged children. (Child Health Research Centre, Brisbane, Australia.)

attention span, their engagement throughout the test is crucial and sometimes challenging. The examiner should understand and respect the personality (and the current mood) of the child and should recognize which children will be able to (or will not be able to) perform the lung function test after some encouragement (if the child does not even want to stand on the scale, it is usually a bad sign). In a clinical setting, especially in children with chronic respiratory disease, attempts should always be made to perform the appropriate lung function test(s) even if the failure is predictable. This will make the child comfortable and familiar with the test and can be considered as training for the next occasion. Giving the mouthpiece and nose clip to the child to play with at home can be a useful introduction and may increase testing success on the next visit.

It is always important to take the time and explain the test to the child in understandable language and even involve them in the preparation of the test (e.g., to connect the mouthpiece to the device). Young children can cope with the test better if it is separated into small steps and they have to complete one step at a time. Continuous positive feedback is very important and all the attention of the examiner should be focused on the child throughout the visit. For safety reasons, children should never be left unattended in the respiratory laboratory. Preschool-aged children are very open-minded and creative, they are always ready for some play and magic; therefore (if the examiner is prepared) the visit can be great fun.

Since clinicians are rarely present during the lung function test, technicians should provide them with written or verbal comments on the test when the results are presented. Comments on effort (in spirometry), posture, leak, etc., should always be recorded and taken into account for the interpretation. Bronchoprovocation tests are hardly ever done in children younger than 5 years of age; however, the response to bronchodilator is frequently assessed in both clinical and research settings. The bronchodilator test, its interpretation, and clinical utility will be discussed as a part of the detailed description of the lung function methods later in this chapter (see *Measurements of Forced Expiration* and *Measurements of Respiratory Resistance and Compliance*). Bronchoprovocation tests in children above 5 years of age are discussed in detail

in Chapter 12 and therefore will not be included in this chapter.

As a part of the lung function test, information that is expected to influence the interpretation of the lung function results should always be collected, including date of birth, height, weight, sex, environmental data, and relevant medical and family history. The interpretation of the lung function data in adolescents is further complicated by the hormonal changes and their effects on lung growth. Healthy reference values, appropriate for both the measured population and the lung function device, therefore need to be selected carefully. Ideally, the results are presented in terms of *z-scores*, which take into account both the measured and predicted values as well as the test variability within the population. Reference values collected in multicenter studies are especially useful as they can prove the robustness of the technique in different research and clinical environments. The examiner always needs to investigate the relevance of the reference data and the results should be reported accordingly.

Manufacturers and local distributors should be aware of any specific requirements that are necessary for the clinical testing of infants and young children (i.e., dead space reduction, appropriate calibration device, facemask and filter, etc.) and always provide the users with in-depth training and relevant guidelines. This is especially important when a novel lung function method is introduced for clinical use to respiratory technicians and physicians who are not familiar with the requirements of the test and interpretation of data. The proper introduction of a novel method requires a high level of flexibility from the manufacturer and strong collaboration between researchers and clinicians to ensure the collection of reliable data and meaningful interpretation of the results in a clinical situation.

Measurement of Lung Volumes

Summary

- The measurement of lung volumes is crucial for the interpretation of lung function
- Functional residual capacity is the only lung volume that can be measured at any age
- Vital capacity and its subdivisions can only be measured in cooperative children with spirometry
- Total lung capacity and residual volume can be determined from the spirometric measures if FRC is known

The measurement of lung volumes in infants and children is crucial for the interpretation of the measures of lung mechanics (resistance and compliance), respiratory flows, and ventilation inhomogeneity, and can provide information on lung growth and development. There are two techniques that were originally developed for adults and later modified for infants and young children: *body plethysmography* and the *gas dilution technique.* While in cooperative, older children, a wide range of lung volumes can be determined, infants are not able, and preschool-age children have limited ability to perform complex respiratory maneuvers, therefore, only FRC (the volume of the gas present in the lungs at the end of a tidal expiration) can be determined reliably in the early years of life. The underlying assumptions of the measurement of FRC with plethysmography (FRC_p) or gas dilution technique (FRC_g) are different and therefore they require different devices and techniques; both methods have advantages and limitations over the other. Plethysmography estimates all gas compartments in the lungs irrespectively of whether or not they communicate with the airway opening, whereas in the gas dilution measurements only the communicating compartments are measured. In healthy individuals, the difference between FRC_p and FRC_g is minimal; however, this can be significant in the presence of air trapping when FRC_g can be underestimated. In the recent years, measurement of FRC_g with the MBW technique has become popular as it does not require sedation during infancy and it is more feasible in young children than plethysmography.

WHOLE BODY PLETHYSMOGRAPHY

Summary

- Measurement of thoracic gas volume (including nonventilating areas)
- Commercial devices are available for both infants and children
- Mainly used in infants and cooperative older children as preschool-age children rarely tolerate the measurement
- Results are unreliable in the presence of severe airway obstruction (FRC is overestimated)
- Has become less common in infants and preschool-age children with the commercialization of MBW
- Frequently used in children above 6 years of age

The plethysmographic measurement of thoracic gas volume was first described in 1956 by DuBois and his colleagues[4]; however, the idea of performing respiratory efforts against a closed airway to measure lung volumes has been known since 1882.[5] Unlike the gas dilution technique, plethysmography measures the total thoracic gas volume, including the air that is not communicating directly with the airway opening. Commercial devices with normative values are available; therefore plethysmography has been used in both clinical and research environments during infancy.[6-8] Since sedation is usually required for the test in younger children, plethysmographic measurement of FRC has become less frequent in pediatric lung function laboratories. Despite the few studies that reported FRC_p in preschool-age children,[9] its use is highly limited below 6 years of age and no robust reference data are available for young children. In research studies, reference values calculated for school-age children have been extrapolated to those between 3 and 6 years of age; this method does not meet criteria for predicting lung function in preschool-age children and cannot be used in clinical practice.

Physiological Principles and Assumptions

The measurement of FRC_p is based on Boyle's law, which describes the relationship between volume and pressure of a given amount of gas within a closed system, that is, in the thorax. The assumption is that if the temperature is constant within the system (isothermal conditions) the compression/decompression of the gas (decrease/increase in volume) will change the pressure, so that the product of pressure (P) and volume (V) is constant *(k)* at any moment:

$$PV = k$$

During an (inspiratory) breathing effort against a closed airway, the changes in P from P_1 to P_2 (ΔP) can be measured, and the simultaneous expansion of the intrathoracic gas ($\Delta V = V_2 - V_1$) results in an opposite change in the gas volume in the plethysmograph box (V_{box}), that is,

$$\Delta V_{box} = -\Delta V$$

Thus, knowing ΔV and from the relative changes in alveolar pressure as measured by P_1 at the airway opening, preocclusion lung volume V_1 can be calculated as

$$V_1 = -P_1(\Delta V/\Delta P)$$

ΔV can be measured in the body box in which the subject is enclosed, in different ways: (1) as a volume displacement sensed by a closed-circuit spirometer (volume displacement plethysmograph), (2) via the pressure changes in the closed box (pressure plethysmograph), and (3) by integration of the flow across the box wall (flow plethysmograph).[10] This latter type including correction for the residual pressure in the box (pressure corrected flow plethysmograph) is the most commonly used equipment for measurement of intrathoracic gas volume.

In the actual measurement of thoracic gas volume, the patient is seated (or the infant placed, Fig. 11.3) in a tightly closed chamber where the changes in the mouth pressure and volume of the chamber are measured over different conditions. At the beginning of the test, tidal breathing is recorded. At this time, the volume of the gas in the chest is unknown while the alveolar pressure is equal to the atmospheric pressure when there is no airflow (i.e., end of expiration or inspiration). Once the end-expiratory level (EEL) is stable, the airways are occluded with a shutter and the patient generates respiratory efforts against a closed airway. In this new condition, mouth pressure is expected to equilibrate quickly with alveolar pressure (this equilibrium can be delayed in lung heterogeneity[11-13]; see also below concerning the limitations of the technique). From the pressure changes at the mouth and the changes in the volume of the airtight chamber, intrathoracic gas volume can be calculated, as described above. In infants, it is best to occlude the airways at the end of inspiration as it is less uncomfortable and more tolerable for the infant. If the occlusion appears at end inspiration, tidal volume (V_T) has to be extracted from the total gas volume when FRC_p is calculated.[14]

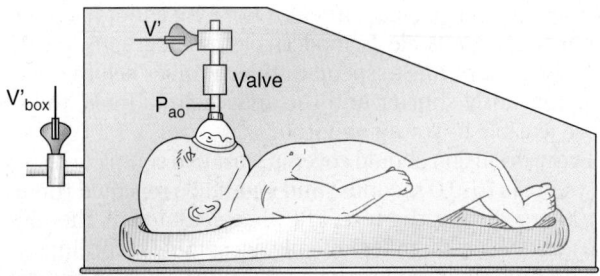

Fig. 11.3 Schematic arrangement of the infant plethysmograph designed for the measurements of functional residual capacity (FRC) and specific airway resistance (sR_{aw}). Flows V' and V'_{box} are measured with pneumotachographs at the airway opening and through the plethysmograph box wall, respectively, for the estimation of sR_{aw}. The valve is closed against breathing efforts during the measurement of FRC.

Since the volume of the plethysmograph is relatively large in children and adults, they are asked to pant during the test with a frequency of approximately 60 breaths/min (1 Hz). This controlled breathing frequency helps the equilibrium of the alveolar and mouth pressures, keeps the glottic aperture open, minimizes the thermal drift, and so improves the quality of the test.[10] However, it is important to note that panting does not reflect the normal conditions within the respiratory system during tidal breathing. In infants, the volume of the chamber can be kept relatively small; therefore tidal breathing is adequate to ensure the quality of the test.

The feasibility of the test in infants depends on the sleep state (usually under sedation) and the stability of the EEL.[6] In preschool-aged children, the feasibility is limited as they do not tolerate the closed chamber and panting against a closed airway. In the studies where FRC_p was measured in children between 3 and 7 years of age, the measurements were preceded by a long training session both outside and inside of the chamber (i.e., breathing through the mouthpiece and then mouthpiece occluded, supporting their cheeks, etc.). With this method, the test was successful in nearly 70% of the children.[9] In older children, the success rate is similar to that in adults.

Quality Control, Acceptability Criteria, and Limitations

The installation of the equipment has to be planned carefully as both the infant and child plethysmographs are bulky and not portable. For infants, extra room for the adjustment of the facemask and rapid access to the infant has to be allowed for.

Even if the test appears successful, many factors can influence the quality of the measurement and the interpretation of the results. All plethysmographs require precise calibration on the day of the test, which can be time-consuming. Accuracy also has to be checked at least monthly (usually with a lung model or biological control). Prior to the test, the equipment has to be turned on to allow a sufficient warm-up period. The calibration procedure is equipment-dependent; therefore, the instructions of the manufacturer have to be followed step by step. Once the patient is comfortable inside the plethysmograph, the door is closed for a few minutes to stabilize the thermal conditions. Both the calibration and patient preparation (sedation in infants, training in preschool-age children) are time consuming and require patience from both the technicians and parents (and children). If the time allowed for thermal adjustment is not long enough the measurement is unreliable. In modern plethysmographs, the time that the patient has to spend in the chamber before the test is significantly shorter and this may help to make the test more feasible in young children.

Every occlusion should cover at least two complete respiratory efforts (6–10 seconds) and should be repeated three to five times during the test. FRC_p is calculated as the mean (SD) of at least three technically acceptable recordings.

The time required for the equilibrium between the pressures at the airway opening and the alveolar system is highly influenced by the resistance and compliance of the upper airways. Usually, a firm support of the cheeks of the patient with the palms is sufficient to decrease the compliance of the cheeks and adequately measure FRC. In the presence of

a severe obstruction, transmission of changes in the alveolar pressure may become too slow to reach equilibrium. In this case the change in airway-opening pressure, ΔP will underestimate the change in alveolar pressure and hence FRC will be overestimated.[12] Since infants are preferential nasal breathers, cheek support is not required for the test; however, after the placement of the facemask the system always has to be checked for leaks.

The steps necessary to ensure the quality of the test are equipment dependent and include high-quality pressure transducers and linear pneumotachographs (in the flow plethysmograph), carefully performed calibration, the measurement of biological controls, sufficient warm-up times, and correction of thermal drift. The general recommendations for standardization of the technique have been published, and specific recommendations for infant measurements are also available (see *Suggested Reading*).

Spirometric Measurements of Lung Volumes in Cooperative Children

Once FRC is known, other physiologically and clinically important lung volumes can be measured with a simple spirometer and TLC and RV calculated (Fig. 11.4). The complex respiratory maneuver starts with tidal breathing wearing a noseclip. After a few breaths, the child is instructed to take a deep breath to the maximum inspiratory level and perform a maximum expiration thereafter, and finish with tidal breathing. The volume between the maximal inspiratory and expiratory levels is called vital capacity (VC). Following a maximal expiration there is always an air volume in the lungs that cannot be actively exhaled; this is called the residual volume (RV). TLC is therefore the air volume that the lungs contain at maximum inspiration, i.e., VC+RV. TLC and its subdivisions and their definitions are shown in Fig. 11.4. FRC, TLC, and RV have clinical relevance and therefore they are the most frequently reported lung volumes in older children and adults.

GAS DILUTION TECHNIQUE

Summary

- Measurement of FRC_g with closed-circuit Helium dilution or MBW technique
- FRC_g only represents the ventilated lung parts that are in communication with the airway
- This test is more popular than plethysmography as it is relatively easy to perform in unsedated infants and preschool-age children
- It is less commonly used in children above 6 years of age who are able to cooperate with the plethysmographic and spirometric measurements of lung volumes
- Commercial devices are available for both infants and children
- Main limitation is the underestimation of FRC in severe airway obstruction

The measurement of FRC with the gas dilution technique has been employed widely in infants and young children as it only requires tidal breathing. Until recently, closed-circuit helium (He) dilution was the most frequently performed test, while nowadays (since commercial devices for MBW test have

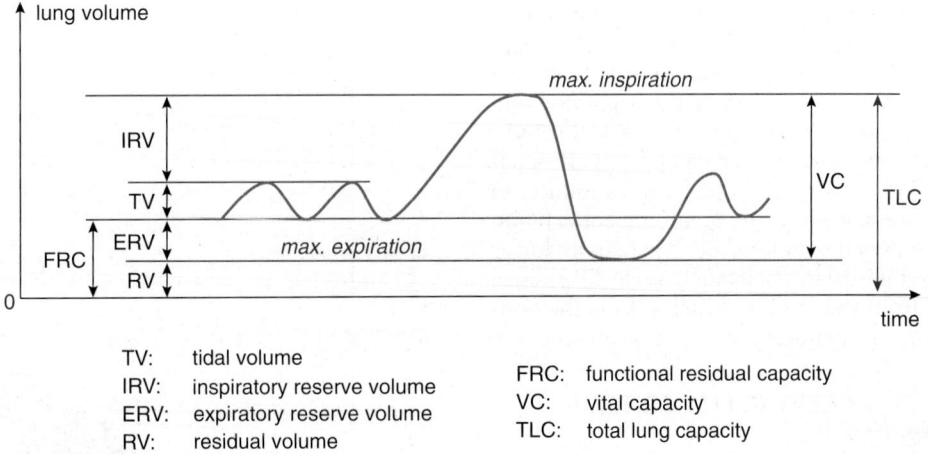

TV: tidal volume
IRV: inspiratory reserve volume
ERV: expiratory reserve volume
RV: residual volume

FRC: functional residual capacity
VC: vital capacity
TLC: total lung capacity

Fig. 11.4 Lung Volumes and Capacities: The spirogram demonstrates normal breathing followed by a maximal inspiratory effort to TLC and a maximal expiratory effort to RV. The sum of 2 or more volumes is defined as a "capacity."

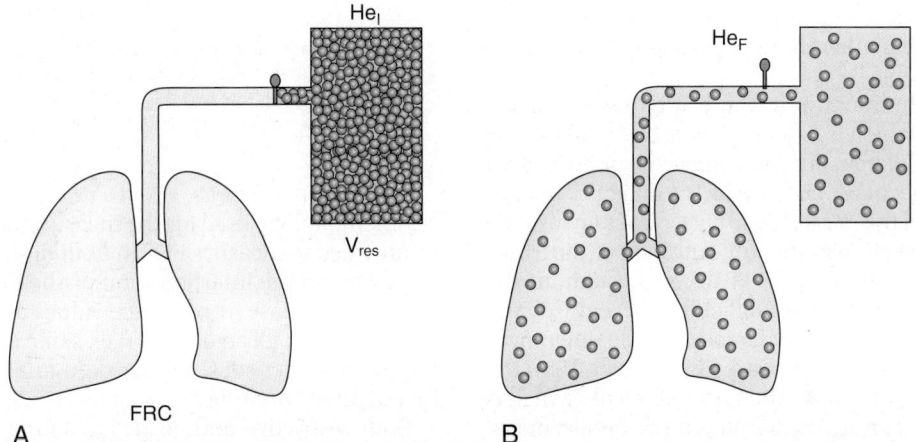

Fig. 11.5 Schematics of the helium dilution technique. (A) Lung and reservoir filled with air and a mixture of helium (He), respectively. (B) Equilibration of He in the respiratory system and the reservoir. *FRC,* Functional residual capacity; *He_F,* final He concentration; *He_I,* initial He concentration; *V_{res},* volume of the reservoir $He_F = He_I \times V_{res}/(V_{res} + FRC)$. See text for details.

been introduced), MBW has become more popular in both infants and preschool-aged children.

Physiological Principles and Assumptions

The use of He to determine lung volumes was first introduced in 1941.[15] Since then, the gas analyzer systems have improved significantly; however, the concept of the test and the method of the measurement have remained nearly unchanged.[10] The basic assumption of the method is that the patient with an unknown lung volume breathes from a reservoir of known volume containing He in a known concentration (usually is around 15%). If the circuit is closed, lung volume equilibrates with He (as indicated by less than 0.02% fluctuation in the He concentration for at least 15 seconds) resulting in a decrease in the He concentration (Fig. 11.5). Since He does not transfer through the alveolar membrane to and from the circulation, the final amount of the He is the same as the initial amount (but distributed in a higher volume):

$$He_I \times V_{reservoir} = He_F \times (V_{reservoir} + FRC_g)$$

where He_I is the initial and He_F is the final concentration of He that is measured with a gas analyzer. The correction for the deadspace volume (facemask or mouthpiece and the switching valve) and the BTPS (body temperature, pressure, saturated) adjustment of the results are crucial for the calculation of FRC_g. The circuit has to be leak free; therefore O_2 has to be continuously added to the system while CO_2 is being absorbed throughout the test.

With the commercialization of MBW, the parallel measurements of FRC_g and ventilation inhomogeneity have become more popular in both preschool-age children and infants. The details of the MBW technique are discussed in the *Measurements of Gas Mixing* part of this chapter. Briefly, N_2 washout with pure O_2 is the most common MBW test in preschool-age children. N_2 is already present in the lungs in a concentration of about 80%, which is decreasing with every breath that the child takes of pure O_2. The concentration of N_2 as well as the tidal flow is recorded throughout the test. (In the commercial devices, the concentration of N_2 is measured indirectly: the level of CO_2 and O_2 are detected in the exhaled air and the quantity of N_2 is calculated secondarily.) FRC_g is calculated as the product of the net volume of the inert gas exhaled during the test and the difference between the end tidal N_2 concentration at the beginning and at the end of the test, assuming that FRC was stable throughout the test. FRC can also be calculated for each breath separately. SF_6 is frequently used as a tracer gas in infants to avoid the effect of pure oxygen on the breathing pattern and respiratory mechanics. The value of FRC_g is usually lower when extrinsic tracer gases are used (such as He, SF_6), since N_2 is also excreted from the tissues, which affects the concentration of N_2 within the lungs.[16]

QUALITY CONTROL, ACCEPTABILITY CRITERIA, AND LIMITATIONS

The quality control, the acceptability, and the limitations of the MBW test are discussed in the *Measurement of Gas Mixing* part later in this chapter.

Generally, the main acceptability criteria of the different gas dilution tests are independent of the test gas, and it is always desirable to have at least three recordings with FRC_g within 25% from each other; however, two tests within 10% may also be acceptable.

Similarly to plethysmography, the test requires a stable breathing pattern, which is difficult to achieve in unsedated infants and young children. Further complications are caused by the use of the facemask because of the difficulty in controlling leaks around the mask. While bigger leaks are usually identifiable by a quick drop in the concentration of the tracer gas during the washout phase of MBW or throughout the He dilution test, small leaks are difficult to recognize, and the risk of reporting false data increases. If the differences in FRC_g between successive tests are bigger than 25%, the examiner should always check the system for leak, which is usually resolvable with the replacement of the facemask. Real-time quality control is therefore of utmost importance during the gas dilution test.

Although the gas dilution tests are relatively easy to perform, FRC_g only reflects the parts of the lungs that are ventilated and communicating directly with the airway opening. Therefore true FRC can be underestimated with lung disease; this remains one of the main limitations of the technique.

INTERPRETATION OF LUNG VOLUMES IN INFANTS AND YOUNG CHILDREN

Longitudinal measurement of lung volumes in healthy subjects provides information on lung development and growth; however, this is not necessarily true in children with lung disease. In healthy children, FRC correlates with height (Fig. 11.6)[17] and weight, and it is frequently reported as a normalized value for body weight (mL/kg), especially during infancy. Despite the unstable end-expiratory lung volume (EELV) in neonates and infants, the relationship between body weight and FRC is relatively strong in early life. It is a common observation that there is a difference between plethysmographic and gas dilution estimates of FRC, although this difference becomes relatively smaller with growth in healthy children.[18] Since the normative values reported in older infants and young children are highly influenced by the device and

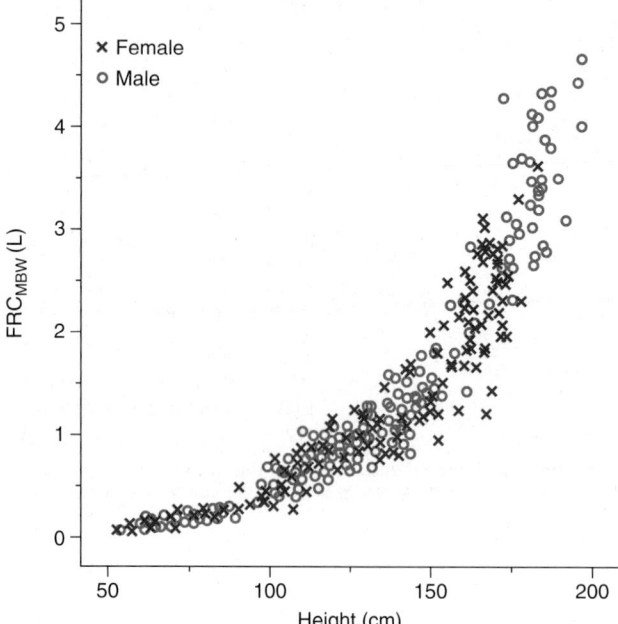

Fig. 11.6 Relationship between functional residual capacity (FRC) measured by multiple-breath washout (MBW) and body size. (Lum S, Stocks J, Stanojevic S, et al. Age and height dependence of lung clearance index and functional residual capacity. *Eur Respir J.* 2013;41(6):1371-1377.)

the methodology used for the measurement of FRC, it is recommended to measure FRC in *healthy* subjects in each laboratory to aid the interpretation of the FRC data in children with lung disease. If reference values are available, the relevance of that given dataset (i.e., same device, similar population characteristics, similar data analysis, etc.) has to be investigated carefully.

Both restrictive and obstructive lung diseases affect the value of FRC directly; however, this effect can be distorted because of the different limitations of the measurement technique.[6] FRC can be underestimated with the gas dilution technique in the presence of air trapping[18,19]—or overestimated if FRC is measured with the plethysmographic method in severe airway obstruction.[12]

One of the most common reasons for low FRC during infancy is surfactant deficiency in preterm babies (respiratory distress syndrome), which results in atelectasis with low lung volumes and low respiratory compliance.[20] In studies on bronchopulmonary dysplasia (BPD) low FRC has been reported during infancy[19-21] (in most of the studies FRC has normalized later in life). Lung volumes can also be diminished in conditions that affect the chest wall such as muscular disease or chest wall deformations and in congenital diaphragmatic hernia.[22] Some of the autoimmune diseases cause restrictive pattern in the lungs resulting in lower FRC, RV, and TLC with a marked decrease in diffusion capacity of carbon monoxide (DLCO, see also in the DLCO part of this chapter).[22a–22d]

Airway obstruction is the most common mechanism underlying the changes in FRC in both infants and young children.[19,21,23] Depending on the severity of the obstruction, dynamic hyperinflation may result in increased FRC and can be detected with both the plethysmography and the gas dilution technique. In contrast, closure of the peripheral airways and the consequent air trapping during expiration does not modify the FRC_p, whereas trapped air is not included in the value of FRC_g (see explanation above). Bronchiectasis-related increase in FRC, RV, and TLC are often present in older children with CF or primary ciliary dyskinesia (PCD), and the increase correlates with the extent of the bronchiectasis and air trapping on the chest CT.

The measurement of FRC is fundamental for the understanding and interpretation of respiratory mechanics; however, it is important to note that FRC is unstable in infants and also highly variable in preschool-age children; therefore the interpretation of a low or high FRC without other measures of lung function has limited clinical value.

The knowledge of FRC is particularly important in the plethysmographic measurement of airway resistance, which is commonly reported as sR_{aw} (R_{aw} normalized for the FRC); this will be discussed in the *Measurement of Respiratory Resistance and Compliance* part later in this chapter.

Measurement of Diffusing Capacity of Carbon Monoxide

Summary

- It is called transfer factor of carbon monoxide (T_{LCO}) in Europe and diffusing capacity (DLCO) in the United States
- It provides information on the rate at which the oxygen is transferred via passive diffusion from the lungs to the circulation
- The diffusion across the alveolar-capillary interface can be impaired by both structural and functional changes of the alveoli or the capillaries
- Except for a few research studies in infants, the measurement of diffusion is only performed in cooperative, older children
- New measurement guidelines using rapidly responding gas analyzers (RGA) and robust reference values for the Caucasian population (over 5 years of age) have recently been published. Commercial devices are available

As a very important part of gas exchange, oxygen has to transfer from the alveoli to the capillaries. Oxygen travels through the alveolar-capillary barrier via passive diffusion and the rate is highly determined by structural and functional properties of this system. However, oxygen transfer through the lungs cannot be determined directly.

PHYSIOLOGICAL PRINCIPLES AND ASSUMPTIONS

Carbon monoxide (CO) is a gas perfectly designed to measure diffusion from the lungs to the circulation. As there is no CO in the blood (except in heavy smokers), even at low concentrations, CO transfers from the alveoli to the capillaries driven by the pressure difference between the partial pressure of CO in the alveoli (P_{ACO}) and the capillaries (P_{aCO}). CO has an enormous ability to bind with hemoglobin (hb) in the vessels, and hb becomes fully saturated even at very low partial pressures. During this transport, the partial pressure of CO changes in the blood to only a minimal degree. Therefore diffusion is the only limiting factor for CO uptake into

the blood and CO has been used to assess diffusion for many decades.

The rate of transfer of carbon monoxide from the alveoli to the pulmonary capillaries is a strong indicator of the efficiency of gas exchange in the lung. This recognition resulted in the development of a new lung function method. Although the measurement of diffusion via CO intake was introduced over 100 years ago,[23a] it was first standardized for clinical testing in the late 1950s.[23b] DLCO is an indicator of all the main determinants of diffusion such as the area and thickness of the alveolar-capillary barrier and the diffusion constant of the measured gas. It can be defined as the conductance of CO from the inspired gas from the alveolar space to the hb-binding sites within the capillaries. Since all the technical details of the measurement method have been published in-depth recently (see *Suggested Reading*),[23c] only the main principles and interpretation of the test are summarized in this chapter.

During the test, after a few tidal breaths, the child is asked to exhale to RV. According to the recently published recommendations, the expiration time can be as long as 12 s. Because of their smaller lung volumes it is easy for children to empty the lungs over 12 s, even in the presence of severe obstruction. Then, the child is instructed to take a deep, quick breath of a gas mixture containing 0.3% CO, a tracer gas (usually 10% He or 0.3% neon), 21% oxygen and the balance as nitrogen. It is assumed that CO reaches the alveolar space instantly and the alveolar concentration of CO changes rapidly by mixing with the gas volume in the lungs (i.e., RV). The volume of CO in the lungs will be a product of the alveolar volume (V_A) and the fractional concentration of the CO in the alveolar space (F_{ACO}). The volume of the inspired gas should be close to VC (between 90% and 95%). A suboptimal inspiration (i.e., less than 85% of VC) affects the alveolar volume significantly and hence the DLCO values (see below). Since the assumption of the test is that CO reaches the lungs instantaneously, rapid inspiration is an important acceptability criterion in the measurements of DLCO. Once the child reaches full inspiration, the breath should be held for about 10 s. The proper breath-hold is one of the most difficult parts of the measurement of DLCO. Since both increased and decreased blood flow and alveolar surface area affect diffusion, the breath-hold needs to be voluntary and without effort. Müeller and Valsalva maneuvers should therefore be avoided (see below).[23d] Following the breath-hold, the child should exhale immediately with a smooth, relaxed expiration. During the maneuver, modern RGA systems can provide continuous monitoring of the concentrations of CO and the tracer gas as well as the volume over time. However, the analysis of the gas is often performed the same "classical" way as in the older systems. The unit of DLCO is traditionally $ml.min^{-1}.mmHg^{-1}$ in the United States, while in Europe the SI unit is preferable ($mmol.min^{-1}.kPa^{-1}$). Changes in both the structure and function of the alveolar-capillary interface can alter the diffusion of CO, making the interpretation of the results less straightforward.

QUALITY CONTROL, ACCEPTABILITY CRITERIA, AND LIMITATIONS

The technical details of the measurement setting, gas analyzers and quality control criteria are discussed in detail in the newest guideline and they are outside of the scope of this chapter. Once children can cooperate with the respiratory maneuver necessary for the test, the measurement is quick and easy to perform. In small children, when the VC is less than 1.5–2.l, cooperation is not the only limitation; the measurement can be invalid because of the small volumes and technical modifications should be considered.

Physiological increases or decreases in DLCO and conditions that influence the diffusing capacity that are unrelated to the respiratory system make the interpretation of the results difficult. This remains the main limitation of the test and is discussed in detail below.

INTERPRETATION OF DLCO

The largest set of reference values for DLCO has been established for the Caucasian population from 4 to 91 years of age.[23e] This dataset includes the recently published children-specific reference values (ref Kopman 2011, Kim 2012).[23f,23g] When body weight-adjusted dead space correction was applied to the data, the between site differences in the pediatric values were minimized. The main predictors of DLCO were age, height, and sex and z-scores were created for both males and females. Between 4 and 18 years of age, the absolute value of DLCO increases steeply, while DLCO decreases after 30 years of age. Therefore, DLCO should always be reported as z-scores, using the new Global Lung Function Initiative (GLI) equations in Caucasian children. A physiologically relevant change in DLCO was defined as 0.5 z-score or 10% relative change (around 0.3–0.8 mmol.ml^{-1}.kPa^{-1}, which is equal to 0.9–2.4 ml.min^{-1}.mmHg^{-1}). Lower limit of normal (LLN) is frequently used to define abnormal lung function and has been defined as below the 5th percentile of the dataset. Since increased DLCO values usually have limited clinically relevance, and the increase is often physiological, an upper limit of normal (ULN) was not established. Adjusting for hb levels had no significant effect on the z-scores, but hb concentration should be considered, especially in patients with anemia. Recommendations for altitude-correction have also been established.[23c,23e]

Physiologically, there are factors that affect the value of DLCO and they can complicate interpretation of the test. One of these factors is increased pulmonary blood flow, which can increase the value of DLCO. This occurs in exercise, via the recruitment of new pulmonary capillaries. In patients with lung fibrosis, the exercise-dependent increase in DLCO is usually missing and this characteristic feature of lung fibrosis can aid the diagnosis. Increased intrathoracic pressure, such as the Müeller maneuver, increases the alveolar surface and hence DLCO; therefore it is important that the child should hold their breath with minimal effort during the test. Hormonal changes in women can also affect the measurement; DLCO is greatest just before menses with high intrasubject variability, while girls in their prepuberty are able to produce a more stable DLCO with minimal variation. The lowest value of DLCO is measured on the third day of menses.[23h]

Cigarette smoke can decrease DLCO due to the increase in the COhb in the blood, which increases the back pressure of CO.[23i] Therefore a smoking history should always be collected from older children and, in the case of regular smoking, they should be asked to refrain prior to the test. Other nonpulmonary diseases can also influence the diffusing capacity. Increased (e.g., polycythemia) or decreased (e.g., anemia) hb levels can either increase or decrease DLCO, respectively. Left-to right cardiac shunts also increase the blood flow and hence DLCO.

Uneven distribution of ventilation-perfusion in the lungs can reduce DLCO. Since CO only reaches the areas of the lungs where there is ventilation, alveolar volume and hence DLCO can be underestimated in severe airway obstruction. When lung emptying becomes nonhomogeneous, the discrimination between the conductive and alveolar gas can be altered and the sample one takes might not be reflective of the alveolar gas compartment. Since diffusion of CO only happens in areas of the lungs where there are both ventilation and perfusion, if perfusion is diminished in an area it can decrease the global value of DLCO. This can be the case with pulmonary emboli or pulmonary hypertension. However, it is well established that when perfusion is limited in a part of the lungs, perfusion can increase in other parts to maintain normal gas exchange. This is why in pneumonectomy (when the cardiac output flows through a single lung and new capillaries are recruited) DLCO does not decrease to 50% of the original value.

DLCO is most informative in interstitial lung disease (independently of the mechanism of fibrosis) and measurement of CO diffusion is one of the most common tests in this patient group. DLCO has also been shown to be useful in lupus erythematosus, scleroderma, sarcoidosis, and other lung disease that affect the alveoli such as alveolar proteinosis. DLCO can be elevated in obstructive lung disease, keeping in mind the limitations regarding severe obstruction as discussed above.

Measurement of Forced Expiration

Measurement of flow and volume during forced expiration from total lung capacity (TLC) is the most frequently used lung function test in clinical practice in both children and adults. After proper training, 50%–80% of preschool-aged children are able to perform acceptable spirometry, but interpretation of the forced expiratory measures is less straightforward than in adults. To further extend the measurement of forced expiration, two techniques have been developed specifically for the use in infants. Since infants are not able to perform a forced expiratory maneuver, flow-volume curve can only be obtained by rapidly applying pressure around the infant's chest and abdomen with an inflatable jacket during tidal breathing (rapid thoracoabdominal compression [RTC]) or after inflation of the lungs to TLC (raised volume RTC: RV-RTC). These tests still remain the most commonly performed lung function techniques in infants in a clinical setting.

The underlying physiological principles apply for both the infant techniques and the conventional spirometry; therefore they will be discussed together.

PHYSIOLOGICAL PRINCIPLES AND ASSUMPTIONS

The basic finding underlying clinical use of the forced expiratory flow volume curve was established in the 1950s when transpulmonary pressure and flow were measured in parallel

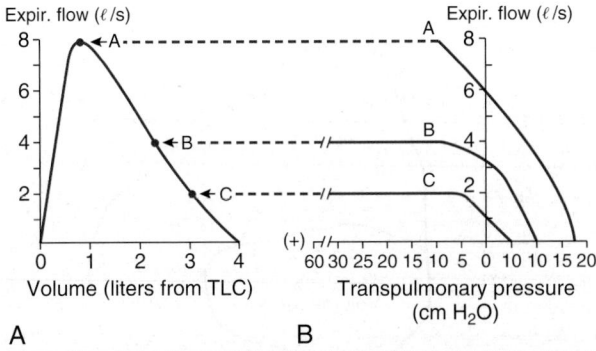

Fig. 11.7 Three isovolume pressure-flow curves from normal subject are shown in panel B. Curves A–C were measured at volumes of 0.8, 2.3, and 3.0 L, respectively, from total lung capacity (TLC). Transpulmonary pressure is the difference between pleural (estimated by esophageal balloon) and mouth pressures. Panel A is flow-volume plot for same subject. Maximal expiratory flows are plotted vs. their corresponding volumes as points (0) A–C and define maximal expiratory flow-volume curve *(solid line)*. See text for details. (Hyatt R. Expiratory flow limitation. *J Appl Physiol Respir Environ Exerc Physiol.* 1983;55:1-8.)

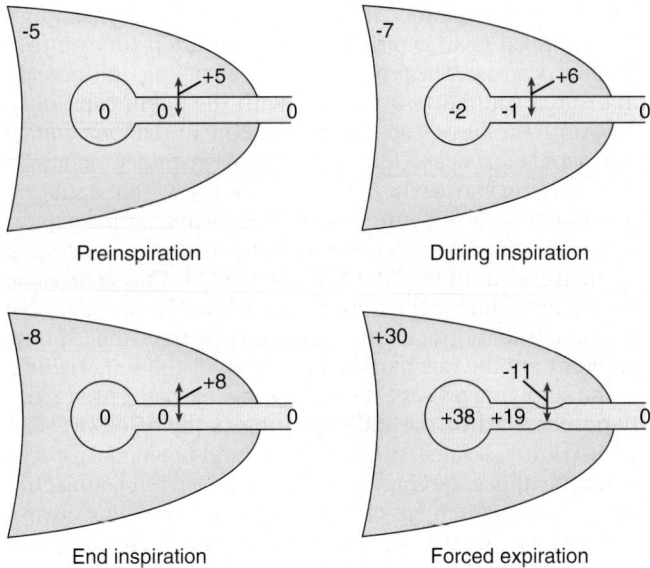

Fig. 11.8 Scheme showing why airways are compressed during forced expiration. Note that the pressure difference across the airway is holding it open, except during forced expiration. (West JB. *Respiratory Physiology the Essentials.* 8th ed. Philadelphia: Wolters Kluwer Health/Lippincott Williams & Wilkins; 2008.)

at isovolumic conditions in adults.[24] Subjects were sitting in a plethysmograph while an esophageal balloon was employed to detect the transpulmonary pressure continuously, and they were asked to breathe at a given lung volume with increasing effort. While at high lung volume the flow increased easily with the driving pressure, at low lung volumes flow could not increase any further even if the transpulmonary pressure increased (Fig. 11.7). This phenomenon is called flow limitation. Following this observation it did not take long to realize that forced flow-volume curves and hence flow limitation can be achieved during forced expiration across a wide range of lung volume (from TLC to RV) without the need to measure transpulmonary pressure.[25] The maintenance of flow limitation is fundamental to the interpretation of forced expiration and this can be difficult at very high and at low lung volumes. Most adults and older children can achieve and maintain flow limitation in the mid-range of lung volumes and this determines the clinical application of spirometry.

When the expiratory muscles are maximally activated at a high lung volume, the pleural pressure is suddenly raised and this rise is transmitted to the alveoli. However, this pressure rise also changes the transmural pressure of the bronchi and tries to decrease their lumen (Fig. 11.8). Thus, both emptying the lung and obstructing the pathway to the airway opening are driven by the same (maximum) expiratory effort. The two opposing processes determine a dynamic equilibrium resulting in flow limitation. If the airways were rigid, the decrease of expiratory flow would occur gradually because of the loss of force that can be generated by the muscles at decreasing lung volumes. The additional drop in flow is the result of the collapsibility of the airways (or certain segments). Flow limitation occurs when, at a given lung volume, the increase in transpulmonary pressure cannot increase the flow any further. Expiratory flow becomes highly turbulent and passes the narrowed airway segment at a very high velocity. The relationship between the flow and volume during a forced expiratory maneuver shows a characteristic shape in healthy subjects (Fig. 11.9A). At the very beginning of

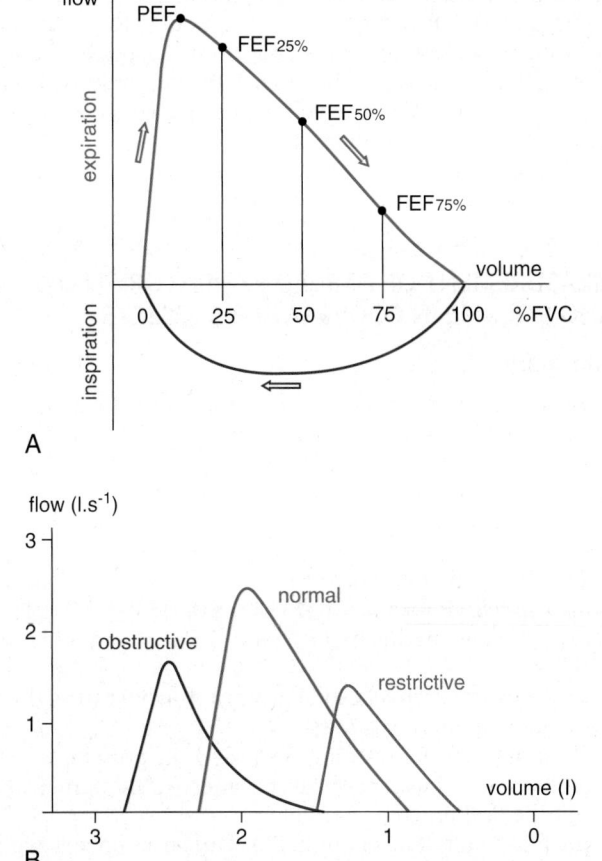

Fig. 11.9 Schematic illustrations of the flow-volume curve. (A) Normal curve with the expiratory limb shown in *green* and the inspiratory limb in *red*. (B) Typical obstructive *(red)*, normal *(green)*, and restrictive *(blue)* patterns. *%FVC,* % Forced vital capacity exhaled; $FEF_{25\%}$, $FEF_{50\%}$, and $FEF_{75\%}$, forced expiratory flow at 25%, 50%, and 75% of forced vital capacity; *PEF,* peak expiratory flow.

the maximum expiration the airflow fast reaches its maximum value (called peak expiratory flow) and then turns into a gradual decrease. The progress of lung emptying (the increase in expired volume) is associated with the fall in expiratory flow until the latter stops on reaching the RV. This *association between flow and volume* during the forced expiratory maneuver is very strong and can be highly reproducible within a subject, provided the starting lung volume and the maximum expiratory effort are consistently maintained in the successive maneuvers. Intuitively, the key issues are (1) how collapsible are the bronchial segments, (2) where is the most collapsible segment (the "choke point") in the airway tree, and (3) how different are the mechanical properties of the lung regions in the emptying process. Indeed, the diverse patterns of emptying observed in the different lung pathologies (see Fig. 11.9A) are associated with these structural-functional aspects. Since the lung emptying happens much faster in young children, the measurement of forced expiration does not always provide meaningful clinical information even if the maneuver was performed correctly.[26] Narrowing of airways due to inflammation, mucus production, bronchoconstriction, and airway wall remodeling potentiate the bronchi for the flow limitation to occur at relatively high lung volumes, and loss of the tethering forces in an emphysematous lung facilitates airway collapse. This means that the expiratory flow drops faster with expiratory volume, the flow-volume diagram becomes concave, and the lung emptying is delayed (Figs. 11.9A and 11.10). Several indices derived from the maximum expiratory flow-volume curve have been suggested for characterization of the types and degrees of flow limitation (Fig. 11.9B), among which the volume expired in the first time segment (FEV_t), for example, in the 1st second (FEV_1), is the most commonly measured index (see also in the *Interpretation and Clinical Application* below).

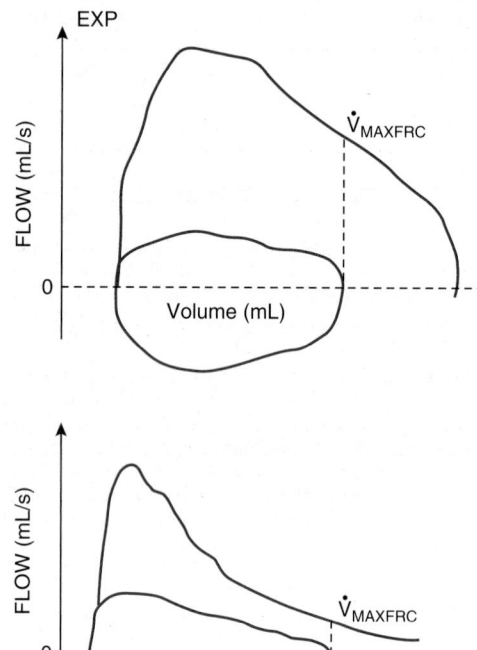

Fig. 11.10 Partial expiratory flow volume curves measured with the Rapid Thoracoabdominal Compression technique. Smaller inner curve represents tidal breathing, and larger curve represents maximal expiratory flow generated by rapid compression technique. Maximal expiratory flow at functional residual capacity ($V'_{max,FRC}$) is indicated by dashed line. Difference between tidal breathing and maximal expiratory flow represents expiratory flow reserve. (A) Normal control infant has convex to linear maximal expiratory flow volume curve, with large expiratory flow reserve. (B) Infant with bronchopulmonary dysplasia has concave flow volume curve, with decreased expiratory flow reserve and V'_{maxFRC}, compared with A. (Tepper RS, Morgan WJ, Cota K, et al. Expiratory flow limitation in infants with bronchopulmonary dysplasia. *J Pediatr.* 1986;109(6):1040-1046.)

MEASUREMENT OF FORCED EXPIRATORY FLOW AND VOLUME IN COOPERATIVE SUBJECTS

Summary

- Spirometry remains the most common lung function test both in children and adults
- Flow is measured during forced expiration from TLC to RV and a flow-volume curve is constructed
- Success rate is above 85% in children older than 6 years of age
- The main outcome measures reported in older children are: forced vital capacity (FVC), FEV_1, FEV_1/FVC, forced expired flow between 25% and 75% of expired FVC (FEF_{25-75}).
- In young children, acceptability criteria differ from those in older children or adults
- With appropriate training 50%–80% of preschool-aged children are able to perform spirometry although FEV_1 is not the best outcome variable
- If expiration is long enough, FEV_t can be acceptable while forced vital capacity (FVC) and consequently FEF_{25-75} and flows at fixed lung volumes may not be valid in preschool-age children
- Clinical usefulness of the forced expiratory flow and volume variables remains controversial in young individuals with lung disease

Spirometry is the most commonly used lung function method in cooperative children (usually above 6 years of age) and it remains very popular amongst clinicians. The interpretation of the forced expiratory flow-volume curve in children during the teenage years is very similar to that in adults. In the last two decades it has also become evident that children below 6 years of age are able to perform acceptable spirometry after appropriate training.[26-34] Although forced expiratory maneuvers are feasible, the acceptability criteria and the interpretation of the flow and volume measures are different from those in older children and adults. Later in this chapter, the age-specific limitations, quality criteria, and interpretation of the measures derived from the flow-volume curve will be discussed.

Quality Control, Acceptability Criteria, and Limitations

The criteria for acceptable spirometry are less strict than those in adults; therefore the subjective impression of the technician becomes exceptionally important. The success of the test depends on the effort of the child who has to be continuously instructed and encouraged throughout the maneuvers. If the effort was insufficient, the test is invalid. The "emptying of the lungs" happens much faster in young children than in adults, and the termination of the test differs between individuals. For a valid test, older children and adults are required to exhale at least for 6 s, to accurately determine FVC. This is called the plateau phase of the flow-volume curve, during which the volume is not changing anymore with time. In preschool-aged children a 3-s-long plateau can be accepted; however, young children can usually empty their lungs quicker than 3 s. The technician should be able to recognize whether the child reached RV or finished the expiration too early (so-called premature termination). Premature termination occurs if the expiration is stopped at a flow greater than 10% of the peak flow. Premature termination is the most common reason of unsuccessful test in children, which can be improved with training. In young children FEVt can still be acceptable if they reached RV earlier than 3 s, while FVC should be reported with caution. Artefacts (e.g., cough) are usually recognizable by observation of the flow-volume curve.

The exclusion criteria and the data reporting are fairly consistent in older children, they vary between centers in preschoolers. Three acceptable measurements are desirable; however, the recommendations are flexible on this question.[27] In special cases it should be considered that clinically meaningful information can sometimes be gained from a single successful maneuver. Highest values for FVC and FEV$_t$ should be reported, even if they do not belong to the same maneuver. The reproducibility of spirometry in preschool-age children has not been assessed systematically, and this fact contributes to the limited clinical value of spirometry in young individuals (see also the *Assessment of Bronchodilator Response* below).

Prediction equations for spirometry measures have recently been published in the framework of collaboration between 33 countries (Global Lung Function Initiative),[35] which was established to standardize spirometry worldwide. Age-appropriate lower limits of normal are also available.

MEASUREMENT OF FORCED EXPIRATORY FLOW AND VOLUME IN INFANTS

Summary

- The most common clinical lung function tests during infancy
- Flow-volume curve can be measured at both FRC (RTC) and in an extended range of lung volumes (RV-RTC)
- Commercial devices and reference values are available
- Maximum flow at FRC (RTC) and FVC, FEV$_{0.4/0.5}$, and FEV$_{0.5}$/FVC (RV-RTC) can be reported
- Flow limitation in the intrathoracic airways can be detected with minimal influence of the nasal pathway
- Main drawbacks are the sedation and the controversies in the interpretation of the results

Both RTC and RT-RVC were developed for infant use to extend the knowledge of normal lung growth and development, to aid the diagnosis of acute and chronic pulmonary lung disease, and to allow the longitudinal follow-up of lung function from infancy through adulthood. Recommendations and guidelines are available for both techniques (see *Suggested Reading*).

Rapid Thoracoabdominal Compression and Raised Volume-Rapid Thoracoabdominal Compression

With RTC, a partial flow-volume curve can be recorded, and the main outcome variable reported is the maximum flow at FRC ($V'_{max,FRC}$, see Fig. 11.10). Although this technique had great clinical promise when first introduced, it has been increasingly criticized, especially after the introduction of the RV-RTC.[36-38] The advantage of the partial flow-volume curve analysis during tidal breathing over RV-RTC is the lack of the unpredictable and variable effects of the lung inflation on the airways.

Infants are usually sedated for the test. They breathe through a pneumotachograph or ultrasonic flow meter that is attached to a facemask. Flow is continuously monitored during the test and volume is calculated by integration of the flow signal. Following the placement of the jacket around the chest and upper abdomen, tidal breathing is recorded for ~30 seconds. Signals of airway-opening pressure, jacket pressure, volume, and flow are displayed real time. A stable EELV is required for at least three consecutive breaths prior to the maneuver; a criterion that is difficult to meet in infants because of their highly variable FRC. Once a stable EELV has been recorded, the jacket is inflated at the end of inspiration with a nonstandardized pressure (30-40 cm H$_2$O, different for each device and center) and the flow at the airway opening is recorded during the maneuver. The test is repeated with increasing the inflation pressure stepwise (5 or 10 cm H$_2$O) until flow limitation can be demonstrated. The pressure required for the development of flow limitation varies between subjects and it is expected to be significantly lower in children with lung disease (flow limitation develops easier), while in some healthy children pressures as high as 120 cm H$_2$O can be insufficient to evoke flow limitation. It also varies between individuals how much pressure is transmitted to the pleural space from the jacket via the chest wall[39]; therefore comparing the jacket pressure between individuals as the main outcome variable is meaningless. The test finishes when maximum flow has been achieved and no further increase in flow is detected despite the increasing pressure. Similarly to spirometry, the best values of $V'_{max,FRC}$ are reported instead of the average of all the values. Results are sometimes corrected for lung volume ($V'_{max,FRC}$/FRC).

Studies employing an esophageal catheter during RTC have shown that infants can inspire before the end of the maneuver and the chest wall muscle activity can decrease both the intrathoracic pressure and chest wall compliance, resulting in a decreased transpulmonary pressure.[39] It was also shown that if the RTC maneuver was preceded by deep lung inflations, the inspiratory drive of the infant was inhibited.[40] This recognition led to the invention of a new lung function technique: the RV-RTC. This technique is very similar to RTC; however, in RV-RTC the facemask is attached to a T-piece connector (or valves in the modern automatized systems), which contains a valve to separate inspiration and expiration (Fig. 11.11). By occluding the expiratory side of the T-piece, the airway-opening pressure increases until the target pressure (usually 30 cm H$_2$O but may differ between centers) is achieved, where activation of the stretch receptors in the lungs results in the relaxation of the respiratory muscles; this is called the *Hering-Breuer reflex* (see also in

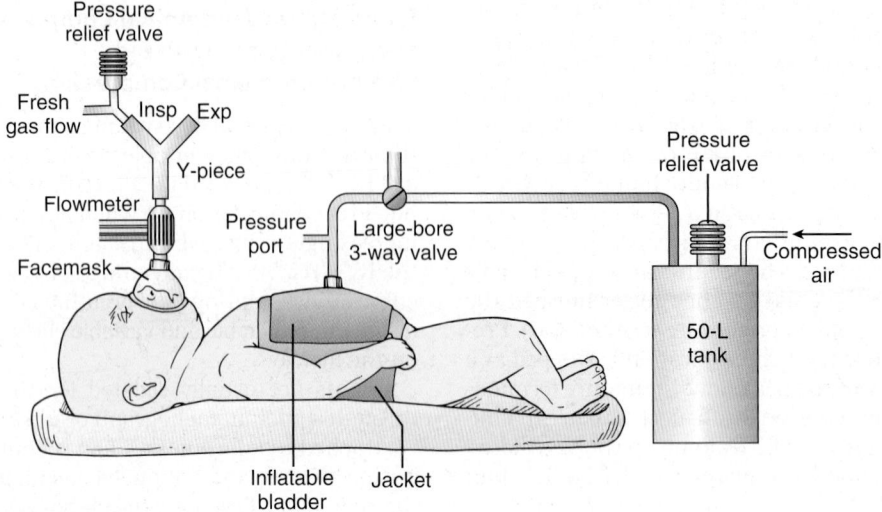

Fig. 11.11 Schematic illustration of equipment used for the Raised Volume Rapid Thoracoabdominal Compression maneuver. *Exp,* Expiratory; *Insp,* inspiratory. (American Thoracic Society; European Respiratory Society. ATS/ERS statement: raised volume forced expirations in infants. Guidelines for current practice. *Am J Respir Crit Care Med.* 2005;172:1463-1471.)

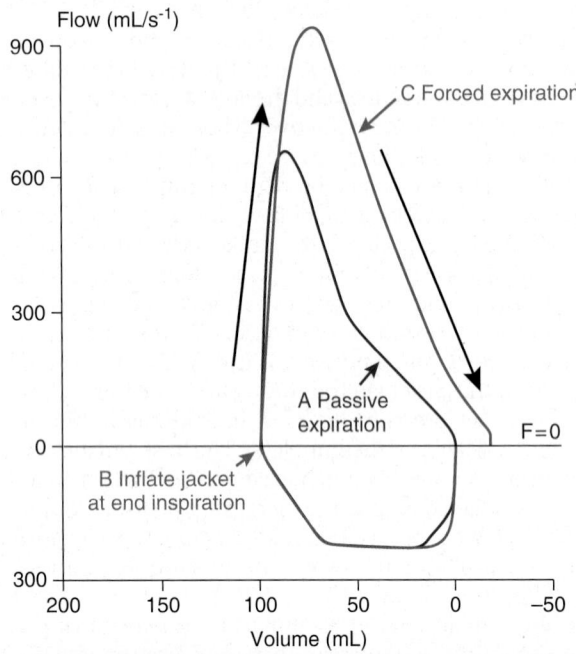

Fig. 11.12 Forced expiratory flow-volume curved measured with raised volume rapid thoracoabdominal compression technique. (American Thoracic Society; European Respiratory Society. ATS/ERS statement: raised volume forced expirations in infants. Guidelines for current practice. *Am J Respir Crit Care Med.* 2005;172:1463-1471.)

the *Single Occlusion Technique* later in this chapter). At the target pressure the valve opens, which allows the infant to exhale passively. In some centers, cricoid pressure is applied during inflation to prevent the entry of the gas in the stomach. The benefits of this technique, however, have not been addressed systematically and they have been questioned in some studies.[41,42] The inflation/passive expiration is repeated three to five times and then at the next inflation rapid compression is performed (Fig. 11.12). The variables derived from this maneuver are similar to those measured with spirometry

in cooperative subjects. In most of the centers where RV-RTC is performed routinely, the measurement of partial flow-volume curve is undertaken first to record $V'_{max,FRC}$ (the measurement of $V'_{max,FRC}$ with RV-RTC is not reliable as the lung inflations can change EELV) and to establish the ideal jacket pressure for the rapid compression in RV-RTC.

Quality Control, Acceptability Criteria, and Limitations

Once the infant is ready for the lung function test (either RTC or RV-RTC), a jacket matching the infant's size should be selected carefully. The infant is then wrapped in the jacket to cover as much of the chest and the upper abdomen as possible; however, the jacket should not interfere with the breathing of the baby. If the jacket pressure is other than zero, or if it is changing during tidal breathing, then the jacket is too tight.

Following the 30-second tidal breathing recording, a short occlusion should be applied to check the system for leaks. If there is a drop in the airway-opening pressure during the occlusion it indicates an insufficient seal around the facemask, while if flow is detected in the system it suggests a leak through the occlusion valve (or T-piece in RV-RTC). As in other lung function tests, the correct placement of the mask is crucial. Leaks are more frequently present during the inflation phase of RV-RTC when the airway-opening pressure increases. In contrast, pressing the facemask too hard might result in the occlusion of the upper airways (and underestimation of the measured flow).

Artefacts are frequently present during the test. The compression-decompression of the chest might activate muscle and respiratory reflexes, resulting in muscle constriction and sometimes glottic closure during the test. The latter is easily recognizable by the observation of the flow-volume curve. Respiratory reflexes (e.g., early inspiration) can also interfere with the measurements. Negative effort dependence, with decreasing expiratory flows and a concave flow-volume curve, can be seen if the jacket pressure is too high, leading

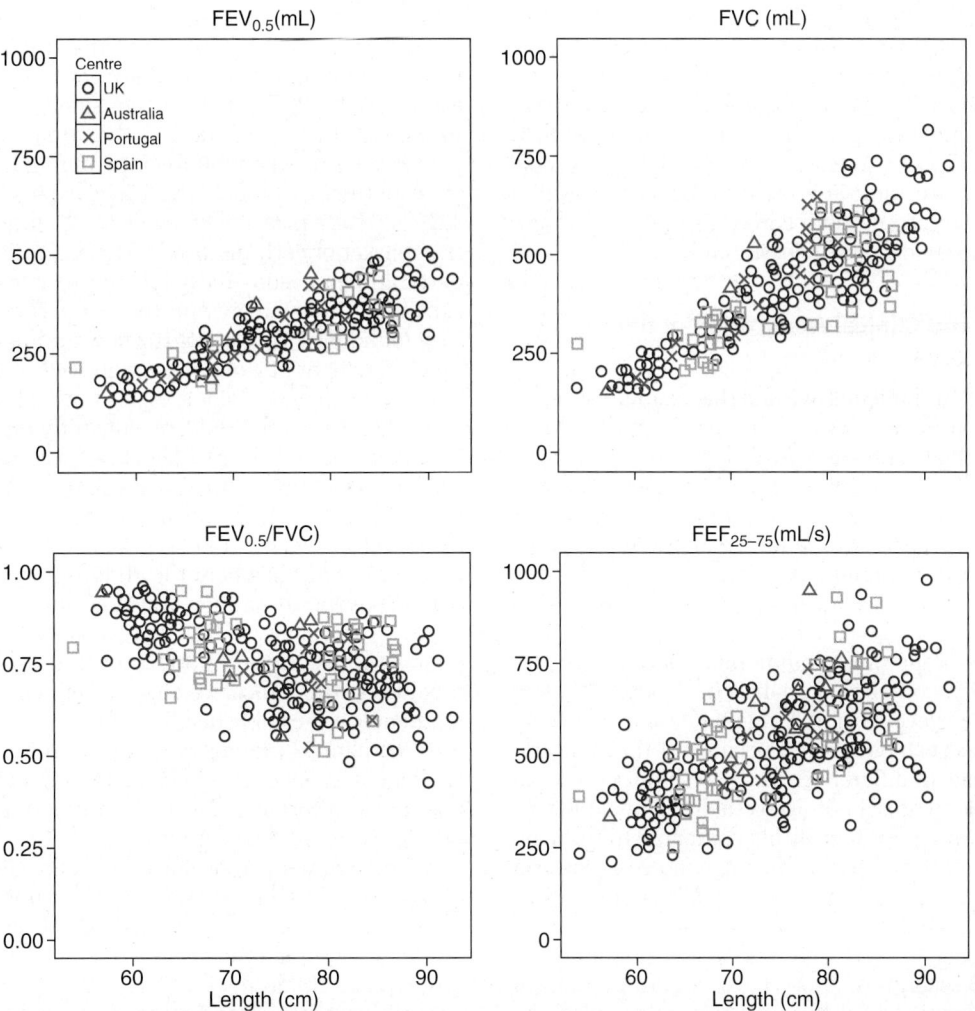

Fig. 11.13 Forced expiratory flow volume (FEFV) measured with the raised volume rapid thoracoabdominal compression technique using commercial equipment in four different centers (United Kingdom, Spain, Portugal, and Australia). (Lum S, Bountziouka V, Wade A, et al. New reference ranges for interpreting forced expiratory manoeuvres in infants and implications for clinical interpretation: a multicentre collaboration. *Thorax.* 2016;71(3):276-283.)

to external compression of the chest wall and large intrathoracic airways.

Normative values are available for both techniques, and device-specific reference values have been published recently for RV-RTC (Fig. 11.13).[43] Z-scores have also been calculated for a mainly Caucasian population. If z-scores are not relevant for the measured population, absolute values should be reported instead of the percent predicted values. Values of forced expiratory flows and volumes measured with RTC and RV-RTC show a markedly nonlinear relationship with body length and weight and a linear relationship with age during infancy.[44] Interestingly, forced expiratory flows are generally higher in girls than boys.[44]

If multiple lung function tests are performed in the same infant, RTC or RV-RTC should be performed as the last tests, because these radical pressure changes may influence the baseline respiratory mechanics and measurements of ventilation inhomogeneity. It has recently been published that the inflation/compression maneuvers necessary for RV-RTC affect the value of lung clearance index (LCI) measured with MBW (LCI is lower after the maneuver).[45] However, if the most relevant clinical (or research) question is related to the forced expiratory variables, it always has to be considered

that the time of the proper sedation (30–45 minutes) might not be sufficient to undertake multiple lung function tests. In this case (RV-) RTC may need to be prioritized.

Rapid Thoracoabdominal Compression-Specific Considerations

Once acceptable flow-volume curves are detected, the best value for $V'_{max,FRC}$ should be reported and it is desirable if it is within 10% from the second highest value. From the three best measurements the coefficient of variation (COV: 100[SD/mean]) can be calculated. The values of COV are usually higher than 10%, which is likely to be explained by the changes in the absolute lung volume between measurements (even if EELV was reproducible within one test).

Raised Volume-Rapid Thoracoabdominal Compression-Specific Considerations

The jacket pressure has to be selected carefully, since if the jacket pressure is not high enough, it will decrease the value of FEV_t (while it may not affect FVC); if the jacket pressure is too high, it can cause airway obstruction.

The test is technically acceptable if the relaxation is complete and it lasts until RV is reached. This is easily recognizable by visual observation of the flow-volume curves. A test meets the quality criteria if it is artifact-free (no closure, no inspiratory effort, etc.) and if the peak flow is achieved before 10% of the volume is expired. At least two technically acceptable maneuvers with FVC (and FEV_t) within 10% are required for a meaningful interpretation. Forced expiratory volumes and flows are reported from the best maneuver.

Interpretation and Clinical Application of the Flow-Volume Curve

Independently of the patient's age and the technique used to assess forced expiratory flows or volumes, the flow-volume and the volume-time curves should always be observed carefully. This is crucial for the correct interpretation of the test. The interpreter should be able to recognize if the maneuver was not performed correctly, be aware of the presence of artefacts, and—if the examiner is experienced enough—the shape of the curve can provide unique clinical information (Fig. 11.9A).

While $V'_{max,FRC}$ is the most commonly reported measure of the RTC, various outcome variables have been obtained from RV-RTC. The relevance of FEV_1 in infants and preschool-aged children has been questioned because of the anatomical and physiological differences in the respiratory system between infants and preschool-aged children and adults. In infants, the airways are relatively big compared to the lung volumes; therefore the emptying during a forced expiration happens much faster (the lungs are basically "empty" after the first second). Therefore the most commonly reported variable is the $FEV_{0.5}$,[43,44] which reflects the expired volume over the first 0.5 seconds of a forced expiration. In preterm infants and neonates, $FEV_{0.4}$ has also been introduced.[46,47] In preschool-age children it is still undecided which variable should be reported from the flow-volume curve. Although FEV_1 has been commonly used in both clinical practice and research studies,[26,30–32,34] FEV_1 has proven insensitive for airway obstruction in children below 6 years of age.[26,48] As a consequence, reporting the FEV values either for 0.5 or 0.75 seconds has become more popular over the last years.[28,29,33,48,49] In older children, FEV_1 is the most commonly reported measure of lung function and has been used worldwide to aid the diagnosis or to track the progress of lung disease. Healthy subjects are able to empty about 80%–90% of their FVC in the 1st second of a forced expiration. In the presence of airway obstruction, flow limitation appears at higher lung volume delaying expiration. A normal or increased FVC with a decreased FEV_1 and hence an FEV_1/FVC ratio below 80% (or −1.64 z-score) suggests airway obstruction. In contrast, diminished FVC and FEV_1 with a normal (i.e., >80%) FEV_1/FVC ratio usually reflect restrictive lung disease (if the forced expiratory maneuver was performed correctly). FEV_1/FVC has been reported as a more sensitive indicator of early lung disease than FEV_1 alone.[49a] The ratio of FEV_t to FVC as a measure of airway obstruction offers very limited clinical potential in children below 6 years of age. As discussed above, this is most probably due to the anatomical and physiological differences in the respiratory system between children and adults and hence an invalid FVC. It is important to note that the FEV_t values,

whichever t is selected for the analysis, cannot be directly compared between infants and older children. Additionally, when longitudinal measurements of forced expiratory flow are interpreted, it has to be considered that infants were measured during sedation in the supine position and the measurements were obtained through a facemask.

From the measures of the forced expiry flow, FEF_{25-75} was suggested as a measure of small airway function and a sensitive marker of early disease.[49b] This value is read as the slope of the line connecting the points between 25% and 75% of the expired FVC and it represents the mid-portion of forced expiratory maneuver. This site of the flow limitation is assumed to reflect small airway obstruction; however, the usefulness of FEF_{25-75} is still under debate especially in children. It is highly variable in children, and a recent study reported that FEV_1/FVC was more sensitive to detect early disease in both CF and asthma in children above 6 years of age.[49a] The other popular measure of flow during forced expiration is the maximum or peak expiratory flow (PEF). This can even be measured with a peak flow meter where the child is instructed to take the biggest possible inspiration and blow out as quick and hard as they can. Variabilty in PEF was suggested as an indicator of poor asthma control[49c] and hence this test is still frequently included in the clinical management of children. However, it is still not well-established how much this information adds into the clinical management of an individual. The device is cheap and once the child learns the technique it is easy and quick to perform daily even at home. The best of 3 or 5 attempts should be recorded.

In children with cystic fibrosis (CF) the clinical application of spirometry is controversial.[28,29,30,50] It has been shown that structural lung disease begins in early life and can be seen on a chest computed tomography (CT) scan in preschool- and school-aged children with CF while their spirometry results are still normal.[50] Despite this fact, spirometry is used in most studies of CF, and forced expiratory flow and volume measures are still the main outcome measures in clinical trials. It has been recognized in recent years that other lung function tests (e.g., MBW) might be more useful in detecting abnormalities of the respiratory system in early CF.[51–53] Despite these controversies, spirometry is considered the standard test for monitoring lung disease in CF to detect changes in lung function or response to treatment. FEV_1 is traditionally included in the evaluation protocols for lung transplantations in CF-related terminal lung disease: an FEV_1 value below 30% predicted is one of the indications to be placed on a lung transplant waiting list.[53a,53b] Following lung transplantation, repeated spirometry is the only lung function test that is routinely performed to diagnose chronic allograft dysfunction, even if it does not seem to be the most sensitive test to detect bronchiolitis obliterans.[53c] In contrast, the RV-RTC method has provided meaningful clinical information on flow limitation in infants with CF.[36,54–57] Since newborn screening of CF is routinely performed in many countries worldwide, the need for a sensitive lung function test that detects early lung disease, does not require sedation, and can be undertaken easily and safely in young children is high.

In young wheezy and asthmatic children, significantly lower values of $FEV_{0.5}$ and $FEV_{0.75}$ have been reported compared to those in healthy children; however, it is unclear how informative the spirometry is in the clinical management of an individual. It is likely that the test is more useful in "older" preschoolers (i.e., 5 and 6 years of age) and school-age children, and their longitudinal follow-up with spirometry provides important information on the progression of their lung disease. The correct interpretation of abnormal lung function in older children can confirm the diagnosis of asthma. These indices include (1) a low FEV_1 (below -1.64 z-score), (2) a low FEV_1/FVC (below -1.64 z-score), and (3) an exaggerated variability in PEF (morning-to-evening more than 20%). Children do not always have airflow limitation on the day of the test and their lung function is often normal when measured with the spirometry between two exacerbations. Therefore it is worthwhile to perform BDR or bronchoprovocation test: a positive BDR (see below) or a confirmed bronchial hyperresponsiveness (see Chapter 12) can support the diagnosis of asthma. It has recently been suggested that different obstruction phenotypes defined with spirometry are related to different risk of poor asthma outcomes such as exacerbation or medication use in children.[57a] In poorly controlled or severe asthma, deep inspiration and forced expiration per se can induce bronchospasm and worsen lung function. This is rarely seen in children and when it is present it is difficult to produce reproducible flow-volume curves. Decreasing FEV_1 with each maneuver can be a sign of severe asthma and should be interpreted accordingly. It is important to note here that spirometry can be very difficult and tiring to perform for children with severe lung disease and alternative tests should be considered. Interestingly, it has been suggested that variables derived from the forced expiratory flow-volume curve during infancy (both during tidal breathing and following lung inflation) not only discriminate between health and disease, but also that the early presence of flow limitation predicts lung disease later in life[47,58,59] Attempts have also been made to assess bronchial hyperresponsiveness in wheezy infants[60–63]; however, it remains unclear whether it adds any value to the clinical management of individuals.

In research studies, variables derived from the spirometry are the most commonly used outcome measures in clinical trials, studies on lung growth and development, and classification of wheezy and asthmatic children.

THE ASSESSMENT OF BRONCHODILATOR RESPONSE

The assessment of the response to albuterol is one of the most frequently performed tests in both clinical practice and research studies. The main limitation of the measurement of bronchodilator response (BDR) in infants and preschool-age children is the high intrasubject variability of the forced expiratory flow-volume curves, which makes the characterization of the bronchodilator-related changes in lung function difficult. Since the forced flow-volume curve is highly reproducible in older children, this problem is far less significant.

In infants, the therapeutic use of albuterol was questioned for a long time because of the lack of objective and sensitive lung function techniques in early life. Since RTC is able to detect flow limitation, it had great promise in the assessment of diagnostic or therapeutic drug interventions. Unfortunately, these tests have revealed the most important clinical limitation of the test: the uncontrollable changes in the absolute lung volume following an intervention. A stable EELV is

required for the proper interpretation of the results; however, this is difficult to achieve in infants. Although EELV equals FRC (where the lung and chest wall recoils are equal but opposite in sign, also called equilibrium volume) in a quietly breathing adult, this assumption is not always fulfilled in infants, especially in the presence of lung disease. Therefore EELV may change after the administration of albuterol and the flow-volume curves are obtained on different absolute lung volumes before and after albuterol. Since flow is measured at "FRC," it may appear—misleadingly—that the bronchodilator treatment had no beneficial effect (or even had an inverse effect)[64–66]; however, most probably only the lung volume changed and consequently the maximum flow at FRC decreased. This is a well-documented limitation of the RTC and explains the controversies in the interpretation of BDR when measured with this technique.

Flow-volume curves obtained with the RV-RTC have been shown to be more reproducible and hence more useful in the detection of BDR (Fig. 11.14).[67–69] When the two techniques were compared in the same infants, no changes were detected with RTC in children with acute viral bronchiolitis, while more than half of the children had a positive response to albuterol when assessed with RV-RTC.[67] When changes in individuals were analyzed, $V'_{max,FRC}$ was unchanged or decreased in all of the subjects. The fact that previous studies have reported both positive and negative BDR during infancy precluded the establishment of the optimal response to albuterol that differentiates health and disease with the highest specificity and sensitivity for any of the variables.

Positive BDR as assessed with the spirometry is usually defined as $\geq 12\%$ and/or 200 mL improvement in FEV_1 in older children, but this is not appropriate in children younger than 6 years of age. A positive BDR assessed when the child is symptom-free can strengthen the diagnosis of asthma. On the basis of the limited data available in preschool-age children on BDR and spirometry, $FEV_{0.75}$ has been suggested to have the biggest potential to detect positive BDR in children between 3 and 6 years of age.[33,49,70] In a relatively small population of 43 asthmatic and 22 healthy children, 14% improvement in $FEV_{0.75}$ was defined as a positive response.[49] A more recent study on a much larger population of healthy ($n = 431$) and asthmatic ($n = 289$) children has suggested that 11% increase in $FEV_{0.75}$ was 51% sensitive and 88% specific to detect altered lung function in asthmatic children.[33]

Measurement of Resistance and Compliance

Resistance and compliance are the most important mechanical properties of the respiratory system. The measurement of respiratory resistance is the most frequently chosen alternative lung function test in clinical practice in preschool-age children who are not able to do spirometry. The resistance of the airways is highly dependent on the airway caliber; therefore the measurement of resistance can be informative in both obstructive and restrictive lung diseases. Resistance describes the relationship between pressure (P) and flow (V'), and combines the determinants of energy dissipation in the airways and the respiratory tissues. Compliance describes

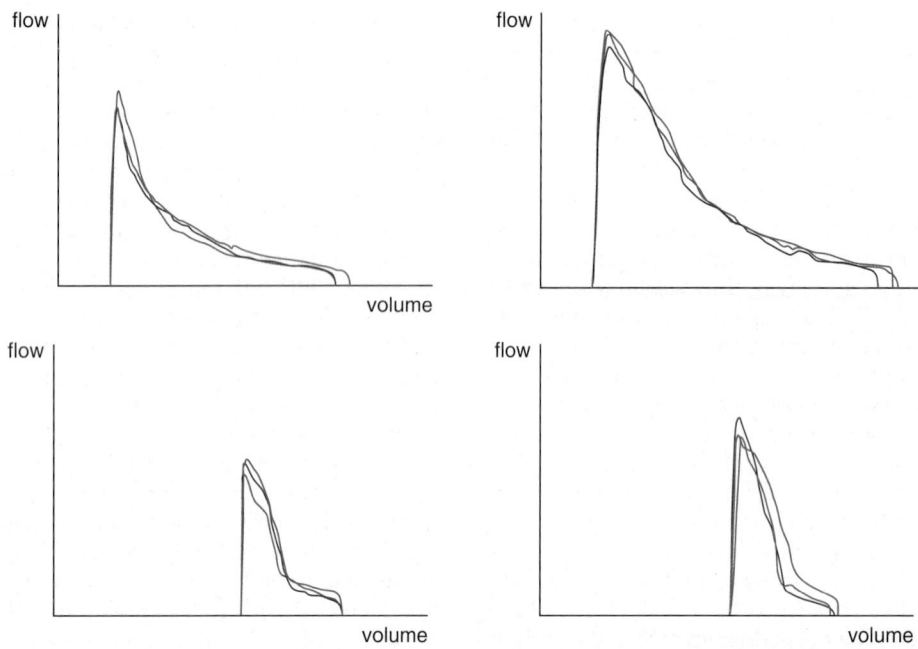

Fig. 11.14 Changes in the flow-volume curves after the administration of albuterol in infants. Reproducibility: Three prebronchodilator *(left)* and three postbronchodilator *(right)* flow–volume curves from an infant are superimposed for the raised volume rapid thoracoabdominal compression technique *(top)* and for the RTC technique *(bottom)*. (Modl M, Eber E, Weinhandl E, et al. Assessment of bronchodilator responsiveness in infants with bronchiolitis. A comparison of the tidal and the raised volume rapid thoracoabdominal compression technique. *Am J Respir Crit Care Med.* 2000;161(3 Pt 1):763-768.)

the relationship between P and volume (V), and characterizes the ability of the tissues to expand in response to distending pressure and to store elastic energy. Both resistance and compliance depend on (1) the range of deformation of the respiratory system and (2) the rate (frequency) of the deformation. These factors make the comparison of measurements with different techniques difficult.

Several techniques are available for the measurement of resistance and compliance in infants and preschool-age children both during dynamic and quasi-static conditions. Although the techniques differ in their measurement principles and outcome measures, the feasibility in different patient groups, and the level of cooperation required, the main physiological assumptions of the measurement and interpretation of resistance and compliance apply to all of these techniques; therefore they will be discussed together below.

PHYSIOLOGICAL PRINCIPLES AND ASSUMPTIONS

Breathing is accomplished by the rhythmic action of the respiratory muscles, which create forces to overcome the opposing elastic and viscous forces of the lungs and also other structures involved in the respiratory movements, including the muscles themselves. Knowledge on the mechanical properties of the lungs and chest wall is important not only for the assessment of the work needed to maintain breathing but also because significant alterations in elastance and resistance may occur as a result of pathological processes. In infancy and childhood, it is also important to know whether the values of mechanical parameters observed in a subject are in accordance with those predicted for the particular stage of lung development.

The respiratory muscles are responsible for the tidal expansion of a passive system (i.e., lungs and upper airways), and therefore they have to overcome a pressure (the so-called transpulmonary pressure, P_{tp}) that arises from the elastic, resistive, and inertial forces of the lungs during tidal breathing. In general, we can describe this pressure as

$$P_{tp} = P_{0,L} + P_{el,L} + P_{res,L} + P_{i,L}$$

where $P_{0,L}$ is a constant corresponding to the recoil pressure in the lungs at the end of expiration (the static balance between the inward recoil of the lungs and outward recoil of the chest wall); $P_{el,L}$ is the pressure required to distend the elastic structures while $P_{res,L}$ is required to overcome the frictional forces of the lungs. Increase in any of these components leads to an elevated P_{tp} and consequently increases the work of breathing, which is one of the most common symptoms of a severe respiratory disorder. $P_{i,L}$ is the pressure necessary to accelerate and decelerate the gas columns in the large airways; while the contribution of $P_{i,L}$ is relatively insignificant during quiet breathing, it can be increased at high breathing frequencies contributing to the elevation of the work of breathing accomplished by the respiratory muscles. The above equation can thus be written as

$$P_{tp} = P_{0,L} + E_L \times V + R_L \times V' + I_L \times V'',$$

where E_L, R_L, and I_L, respectively, denote the elastance, resistance, and inertance of the lungs. We note that, in general, these mechanical parameters are not simple coefficients but are functions of V, V', and acceleration (V''). For example, R_L depends on the actual lung volume and also the flow itself as airway resistance increases at higher V' values due to turbulences. Still, the above "equation of motion" of the lungs is often considered as a linear model of pulmonary mechanics.

In the routine clinical practice, P_{tp} cannot be measured easily in children, since it is semi-invasive and requires the placement of a pressure (balloon) transducer in the esophagus. Therefore pulmonary resistance, elastance, and inertance are not calculated directly in children in a clinical setting (except in mechanically ventilated children[71]; however, respiratory mechanics measured in the intensive care unit are out of the scope of this chapter).

When an external driving pressure is applied (e.g., during mechanical ventilation or when forced oscillations are employed to measure respiratory mechanics), the driving pressure that has to overcome the resistive, elastic, and inertial forces of the total respiratory system including the chest wall compartment is higher than P_{tp} and called transrespiratory pressure (P_{rs}):

$$P_{rs} = P_{0.rs} + E_{rs} \times V + R_{rs} \times V' + I_{rs} \times V''$$

where E_{rs}, R_{rs}, and I_{rs} reflect the elastance, resistance, and inertance of both the lungs and the chest wall (Fig. 11.15), respectively, and $P_{0.rs}$ is a constant (e.g., it can be a positive end-expiratory pressure [PEEP] level in mechanical ventilation but in most measurements the setting is zero).

INTERPRETATION OF RESISTANCE AND COMPLIANCE

Summary

- Respiratory resistance and compliance are the most important mechanical properties of the respiratory system, and they describe the relationships between pressure, flow, and volume
- The values of resistance and compliance depend on the measurement method; therefore values obtained with different tests are not directly comparable
- Respiratory resistance (R_{rs}) is the sum of the lung resistance (R_L) and the resistance of the chest wall (R_{cw}). The components of R_L are the airway resistance (R_{aw}) and lung tissue resistance ($R_{ti,L}$)
- The relative contribution of the airways, tissue, and chest wall resistance to the total resistance varies with age and between respiratory conditions
- Respiratory compliance is the reciprocal of the respiratory elastance (E_{rs}), which is the sum of the lung elastance (E_L) and the chest wall elastance (E_{cw})

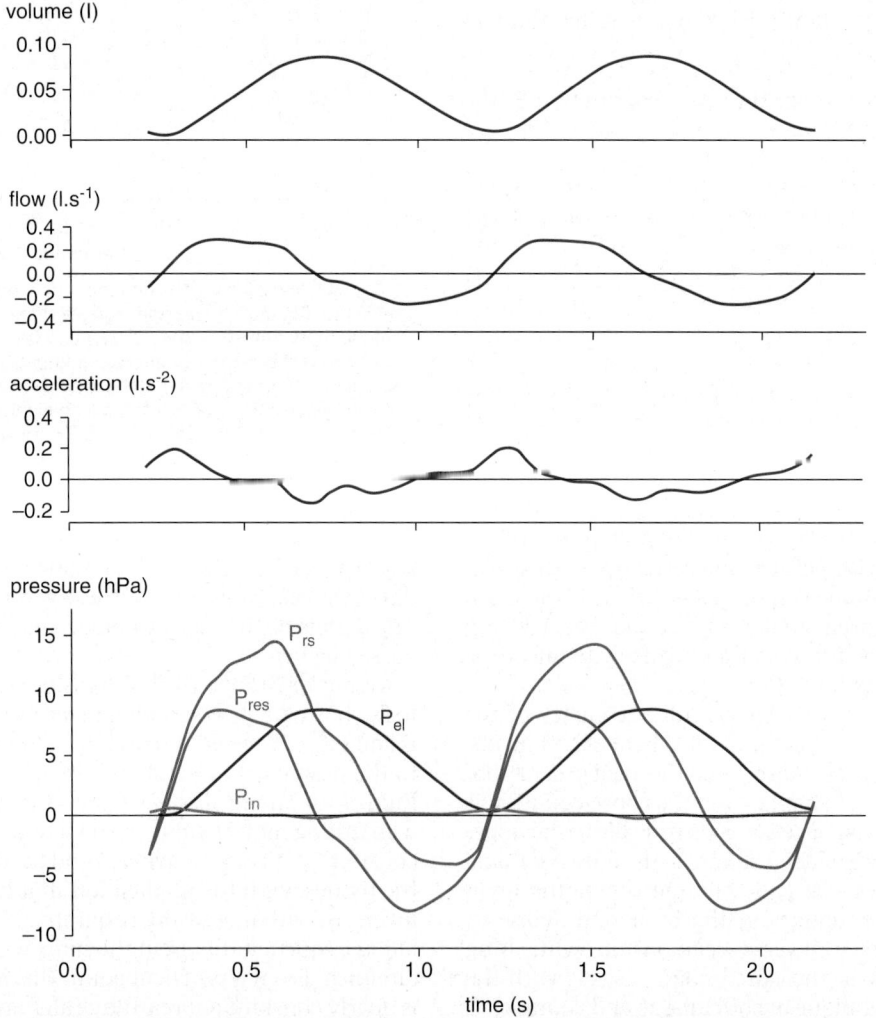

Fig. 11.15 Equation of motion of the respiratory system. Signals of volume, flow, and acceleration during sleep in an infant, illustrating the general equation of motion of the respiratory system. The pressure necessary to maintain breathing (P_{rs}, *black line*) is the sum of elastic (P_{el}, *red line*), resistive (P_{res}, *blue line*), and inertial (P_{in}, *green line*) components, which are proportional to volume, flow, and acceleration, respectively. During tidal breathing the contribution of P_{in} is negligible (even in an infant) and P_{rs} is mainly determined by P_{el} and P_{res}.

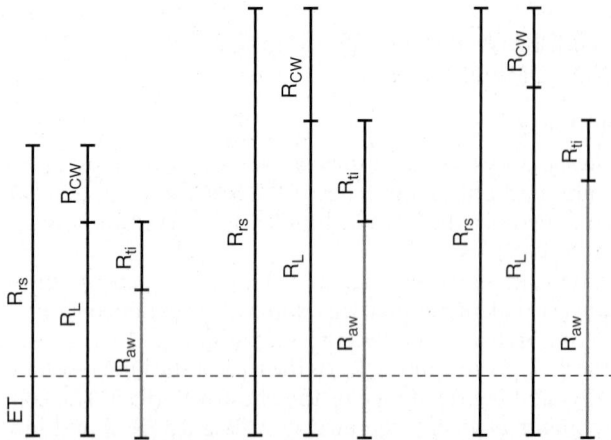

Fig. 11.16 Schematic contribution of the lung (R_L) and chest wall resistance (R_{cw}) to the total respiratory system resistance (R_{rs}) in health *(left)*, restrictive *(middle)*, and obstructive *(right)* lung disease. Please note that the relative contribution of the extrathoracic airways (ET) is the most significant in healthy subjects. R_{aw}, Airway resistance; R_{ti}, tissue resistance.

- E_{rs} is mainly determined by E_L in infants and preschool-age children as the chest wall is much softer than in adults

Total respiratory resistance (R_{rs}) is a combination of the resistance of the chest wall and the lungs (including the extrathoracic airways, Fig. 11.16). One of the main components of R_{rs} is the airway resistance (R_{aw}), which is the main interest of clinicians, and it is defined as the ratio of the pressure drop across the airway tree (P_{aw}) to the resulting airflow (V'):

$$R_{aw} = P_{aw}/V'$$

Ideally, R_{aw} depends only on the geometry of the airway tree and the viscosity of the resident gas. R_{aw} shows a very strong inverse relationship with the airway radius, r ($R\sim 1/r^4$), which (theoretically) means a 16-fold increase in resistance if the airway caliber decreased to 50% of its original value (since the airway tree is a complex system of airways from different sizes with parallel and serial units, this relationship is less straightforward in reality). This is the main reason why the measurement of resistance has become very popular in respiratory disorders that are likely to affect the airway caliber (e.g., asthma, CF).

However, it is known that the irregular geometry of the airways and high flows lead to the development of turbulence where P_{aw} increases faster than V', and the ideal proportionality between P_{aw} and V' changes and the above equation is not true anymore. Turbulence develops typically in the upper airways because of the sudden changes in the cross-sectional area, such as in the nasal pathway and the glottic area. Additionally, via the changes in the bronchial diameter, R_{aw} exhibits a marked inverse relationship with lung volume. R_{aw} can only be measured noninvasively with the plethysmographic technique in both infants and young children in whom the alveolar pressure can be estimated from the volume changes within the box (see details below). Since FRC is hardly ever measured in preschool-age children (see also in the *Measurement of Lung Volumes* part of this chapter),

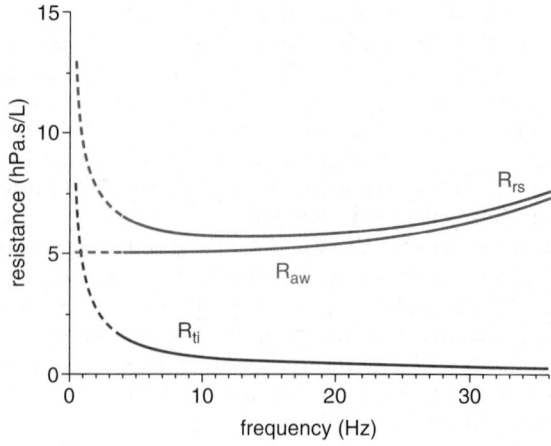

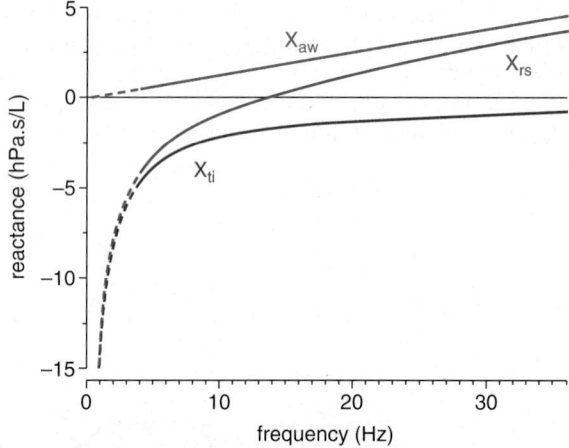

Fig. 11.17 Illustration of the frequency dependence of total respiratory resistance (R_{rs}, *top*) and reactance (X_{rs}, *bottom*), and their corresponding components from the airways (aw) and respiratory tissues (ti). Solid lines depict the frequency interval of impedance available from measurements during normal breathing; broken lines indicate the courses of low-frequency impedance measurable only during apnea. Note the zero-crossing of X_{rs} (the resonant frequency) where the elastic and inertial forces are equal in magnitude.

sR_{aw} (specific R_{aw}, which is the product of R_{aw} and FRC, without directly measuring either of these variables) can be obtained. The details of the measurement and its limitations are discussed below.

Tissue resistance (R_{ti}) is another significant contributor to R_{rs}; however, its description in terms of classical mechanics is limited.[72] As recent research has shown, R_{ti} is closely linked to the elastic behavior of the tissues, in the sense that the ratio of the energy dissipated and stored in the tissues during a breathing movement (i.e., the tissue hysteresivity) is fairly constant.[73,74] This is a general and fundamental property of the tissues, with the implication that R_{ti} decreases, roughly inversely, with increasing respiratory rate or external oscillation frequency, that is, in the same way as the elastic forces diminish. From a practical point, this means that while R_{aw} is nearly constant at breathing rates and up to 10–20 Hz of external oscillations, R_{ti} contributes equally to R_{rs} during spontaneous breathing but rapidly disappears above 3–5 Hz (Fig. 11.17; see also below in the discussion of *Forced Oscillation Technique*). This fact has often been overlooked both when interpreting R_{rs} obtained with different techniques as a measure of airway resistance and assuming R_{ti} as a constant, frequency-independent resistance. R_{rs} can be obtained from the measurement of respiratory impedance (Z_{rs}) with the forced oscillation technique (FOT) and with the single-breath occlusion technique (SOT); while the FOT employs oscillation frequencies well above the tidal breathing rate (>4 Hz), the latter estimates R_{rs} over a passive expiration from end-inspiration; therefore the contribution of R_{ti} to R_{rs} is more significant when measured with the SOT. Resistance values obtained with the interrupter technique (R_{int}) are also influenced by the tissues as a result of the involvement of the stress relaxation in the measurement of airway-opening pressure (see below).

Elastance (E) expresses the relationship between changes in distending pressure (ΔP_{el}) and the corresponding volume (ΔV) as

$$E = \Delta P_{el}/\Delta V$$

E is the reciprocal of compliance ($C = 1/E = \Delta V/\Delta P_{el}$), which is perhaps more commonly reported to characterize the elastic properties of the respiratory system. The elastance of the total respiratory system, E_{rs} is the sum of that of the pulmonary (L) and chest wall (cw) components (Fig. 11.18):

$$E_{rs} = E_L + E_{cw} = (1/C_L) + (1/C_{cw})$$

In newborns and infants who have very compliant chest wall structures, E_{rs} is practically determined by the lungs, whereas it is nearly equally contributed by the pulmonary and chest wall compartments at adulthood. Similarly to the resistances, the values of E vary with lung volume: E_L is the lowest when measured at medium lung volumes (i.e., between FRC and FRC+VT) and increases both toward RV and TLC, whereas E_{cw} increases only at low lung volumes (Figs. 11.18 and 11.19). The volume dependences of each compartment have more or less known structural determinants. The stiffening of the lungs at high volumes is due to the recruitment of the collagen fibers in the parenchymal matrix, whereas at low lung volumes the alveolar configuration and surfactant

distribution become suboptimal. The increasing stiffness of the chest wall at low volumes is primarily the consequence of the restriction of the rib cage. Therefore values of E or C are dependent on the level(s) of inflation of the respiratory system, at which the measurements are made. Of course, the measure most relevant to normal breathing is the reading of ΔP_{el} and ΔV between the endpoints of tidal breathing, that is, the FRC and FRC+V_T; these estimations utilize two points on the nonlinear P-V curve (see Fig. 11.19) and are denoted "chord" compliance (C_{chord}) or elastance (E_{chord}). Estimation of C_{chord} is either confined to the lungs and requires measurement of esophageal pressure or it is estimated for the total respiratory system during mechanical ventilation, an application outside the scope of the present chapter. Nevertheless, the value of C derived from the SOT measurements

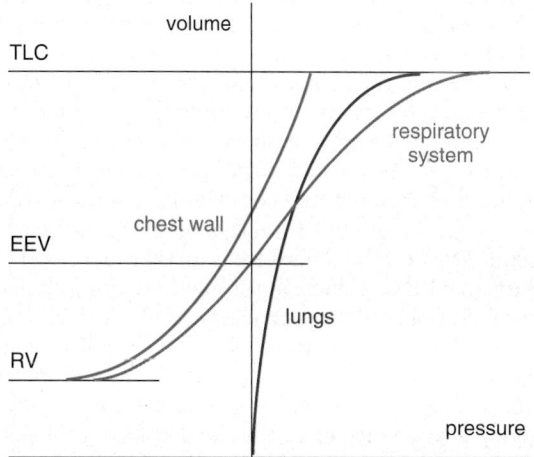

Fig. 11.18 The pressure-volume relationship of the respiratory system as added up by the pulmonary and chest wall components. Note the decrease in slope at low volumes (near residual volume, RV) and high volumes (approaching total lung capacity, TLC) caused by the nonlinearity of the chest wall and the lungs, respectively. The highest slope (maximal compliance) is observed in the normal breathing range, that is, just above elastic equilibrium volume (EEV).

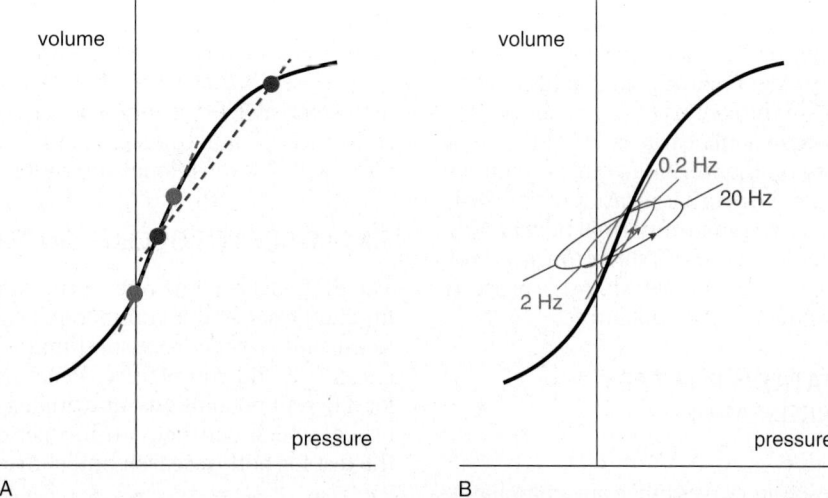

Fig. 11.19 Estimation of chord compliance. (A) Effect of the nonlinearity of the pressure-volume curve of the respiratory system on the estimation of chord compliance. The highest compliance is obtained in the tidal breathing range (slope between *blue symbols*); at higher volume levels *(red symbols)* compliance is reduced significantly (slope between *red symbols*). (B) Frequency dependence of dynamic compliance. From slow breathing *(green loop)* through panting *(blue loop)* to fast external oscillation *(red loop)* dynamic compliance falls steeply because of lung tissue viscoelasticity.

(see below) is also based on two-point readings and can be considered as a chord estimate.

Similarly to the resistance measures, the estimates of compliance are also dependent on the rate of changes in the respiratory system. The term "static compliance" (C_{st}) is commonly associated with any change that is slower than the normal breathing and is therefore often misused. The only correct use of C_{st} is in connection with the weighted spirometer technique, where added weights to the bell of a closed spirometer result in stepwise changes in P_{rs} and lung volume, and these steps can last for minutes and cover many breaths. Compliance values based on the SOT are determined from a passive expiration to atmospheric pressure following an end-inspiratory airway occlusion. The readings of P and V are taken at both ends of the (relaxed) expiration and are just a fragment of a second apart; accordingly, they reflect the compliant behavior on a much shorter time scale. Finally, the FOT measurements that cover the frequency range from a few Hz to 40–50 Hz reveal the combined effects of elasticity of the tissues and the inertial behavior of the large airways, the former dominating at the lower frequencies and the latter being the main determinant above the resonance frequency (see Fig. 11.17). As a result of the dependence of the elastic properties on frequency, the compliance determined by the FOT is ~5–10 times lower than that observed at the breathing frequency, and the difference is further increased in the comparison with C_{st} values. In the low-frequency implementation of FOT (LFOT), frequencies as low as 0.5–1 Hz are employed during apneic intervals,[75] the compliance values derived from the impedance spectra represent more the dynamic compliance relevant to spontaneous breathing. The frequency dependence of C, that is, the decrease in C with frequency is augmented in the case of inhomogeneous obstruction of the lungs.[76]

In summary, it is important to emphasize that the measures of both resistance and compliance are fundamentally determined by the measurement technique because of the two main underlying properties of respiratory mechanics: the nonlinearity and the frequency dependence. *Nonlinearity* means that higher flows increase resistance because of changes in the airway flow profile and the development of turbulent flow (especially in the central airways). A particularly serious form of nonlinear behavior is the flow limitation, which may occur during tidal breathing in collapsible segments of the airway tree. In the context of the elastic properties of the respiratory system, nonlinearity refers to the value of compliance depending on the working point or segment of the pressure-volume curve where it is measured: the "best" compliance is measured in the range of normal tidal breathing and the respiratory system becomes stiffer towards both large and low lung volumes. *Frequency dependence* is a property that applies to both resistance and compliance

GENERAL CONSIDERATIONS FOR THE MEASUREMENT OF RESISTANCE AND COMPLIANCE

The measurements of respiratory resistance and compliance are usually performed during tidal breathing. In both infants and children the upper airways should always be free and open; therefore the position of the child needs to be checked carefully during the test. When the measurement is done

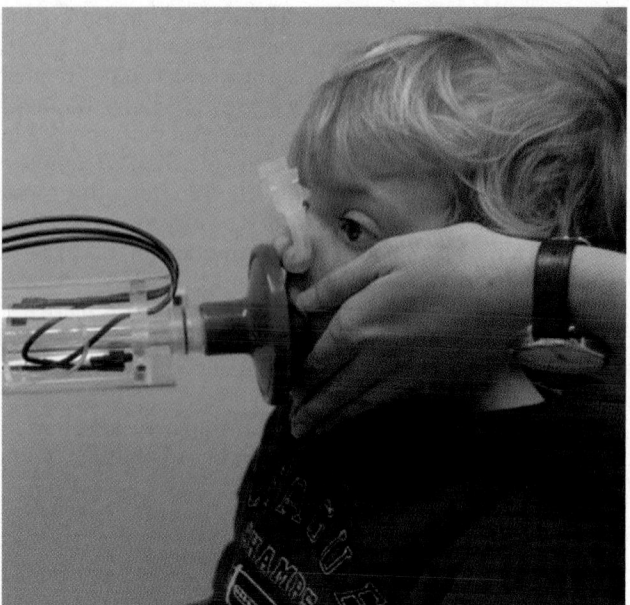

Fig. 11.20 Measurement of respiratory resistance and compliance with a forced oscillation technique in a 3-year-old child. Nose clip is worn during the test and cheeks are also firmly supported by a staff member.

via a mouthpiece in children, the cheeks and the floor of the mouth are supported firmly to minimize the upper airway shunt. To avoid nasal breathing, a nose clip must be worn during the test (Fig. 11.20).

The main limitation of the measurement of resistance in spontaneously breathing children and adults is the involvement of the upper airways (i.e., extrathoracic airways), which makes it nearly impossible to assess the intrathoracic airways objectively. Furthermore, the breathing pattern is naturally variable in children (e.g., unstable FRC, frequent expiratory braking, etc.), which can increase the values of resistance even in healthy children. These factors contribute to the wide range of reference data for a given height in healthy preschool-age children (Fig. 11.21) resulting in a limited clinical utility of respiratory resistance in individuals (see also below).

The involvement of the upper airways and their contribution to the total resistance is even more significant in infants who are preferential nasal breathers. The narrow nasal pathways are responsible for as much as 25%–50% of the respiratory resistance[77,78] and this significant contribution of the upper airways might mask small alterations within the lungs.

SINGLE-BREATH OCCLUSION TECHNIQUE

The SOT has become one of the most popular infant lung function tests, as it is commercially available, relatively easy to use and provides robust estimates of the total respiratory resistance and compliance. Reference values are available for different populations, and guidelines have also been published, which can help an inexperienced user to establish the test for both research and clinical studies.

Summary

- Commercial devices and reference values are available
- In infants, interruption of spontaneous breathing evokes reflex relaxation of respiratory muscles

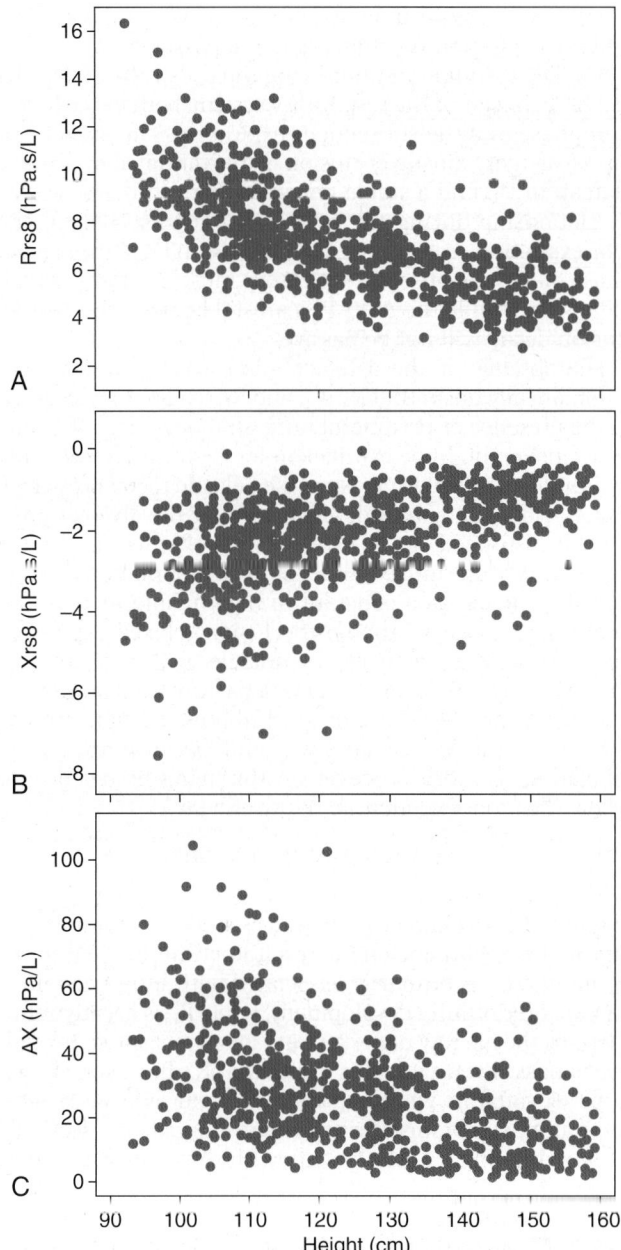

Fig. 11.21 Baseline respiratory resistance at 8 Hz (Rrs8) (A), reactance at 8 Hz (Xrs8) (B), and area under the reactance curve (AX) between 6 Hz and the resonant frequency (C) against height in healthy children measured in two centers in Australia and Italy. Note the wide range of reference values for a given height. (Calogero C, Simpson SJ, Lombardi E, et al. Respiratory impedance and bronchodilator responsiveness in healthy children aged 2-13 years. *Pediatr Pulmonol.* 2013;48(7):707-715.)

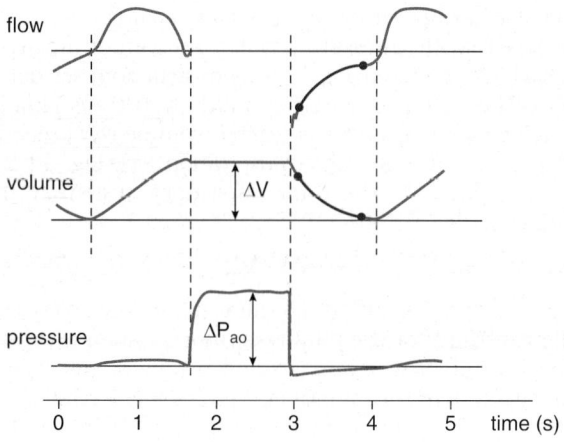

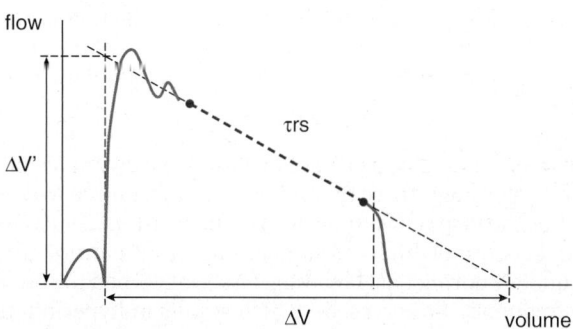

Fig. 11.22 Schematics of the single-breath occlusion measurement (SOT). Top: The airway is occluded at end inspiration, evoking the Hering-Breuer reflex apnea. From the developing airway-opening pressure (ΔP_{ao}) and the volume exhaled in the subsequent relaxed expiration (ΔV), the total respiratory compliance (C_{rs}) is calculated. Bottom: In the middle of the expiration phase (between the blue dots), the flow-volume relationship is closely linear, and the slope $\Delta V/\Delta V'$ gives the time constant of the respiratory system (τrs). Respiratory resistance (R_{rs}) is then calculated as ($R_{rs} = \tau rs/C_{rs}$).

- Compliance of the respiratory system (C_{rs}) is estimated from occlusion pressure and the passively expired volume recorded subsequently
- Flow-volume relationship during relaxed expiration yields the time constant of the total respiratory system (τ_{rs}) to enable estimation of the resistance as $R_{rs} = \tau_{rs}/C_{rs}$
- Limitations in airway obstruction and where full relaxation is not achieved

The SOT offers a simultaneous assessment of the resistance and compliance of the *passive* respiratory system during interruption of spontaneous breathing in the expiratory phase. In infants, the occlusion evokes the Hering-Breuer lung inflation reflex via mediation of stretch receptors (see also *Lung function in Sedated Infants,* earlier in this chapter), which inhibits inspiratory effort and leads to an apnea and, following the release of occlusion, a passive expiration. While the apneic condition is difficult to achieve in adults and older children, the Hering-Breuer lung inflation reflex can be evoked in neonates and infants for the measurement of lung function with the SOT[79] or LFOT (see below).[75] The duration of the reflex relaxation of the respiratory muscles decreases with age; however, it can still be evoked during sedation in young children.[80]

During the measurement procedure, tidal breathing is recorded with a flow meter through the facemask for at least 30 seconds or until a stable breathing pattern is achieved. Interruption is accomplished with closing a valve at the airway opening, usually at end inspiration or at various phases of expiration. If the Hering-Breuer reflex is active, the respiratory system relaxes against the valve and the developing increase in airway-opening pressure (ΔP_{ao}) will represent the change in the elastic pressure belonging to the volume change (ΔV) above the relaxation volume (V_r) (Fig. 11.22). During the occlusion, the equilibration of P_{ao}

to the alveolar pressure is indicated by a plateau in P_{ao} (we note here that the pressure equilibrium cannot always be achieved in the presence of airway obstruction; see details below). The occlusion is released after a 100-ms plateau, and a flowmeter records the expired volume (ΔV) reached until the next uninterrupted inspiration (see Fig. 11.22). The compliance of the total respiratory system (C_{rs}) is estimated as[81]:

$$C_{rs} = \Delta V / \Delta P_{ao}$$

From the same occlusion-reopening maneuver, an estimate of the resistance of the total respiratory system (R_{rs}), that is, the sum of airway and tissue resistances, can also be obtained. From the linear part of the V' versus V relationship (see Fig. 11.22), the time constant (τ_{rs}) of the respiratory system can be obtained during a passive expiration. The τ_{rs} is by definition the time that required for the lung volume to decrease passively by 63% in an exponential manner. The time of this decrease will depend on the mechanics of the respiratory system, that is, R_{rs} and C_{rs} the following way:

$$\tau_{rs} = R_{rs} \times C_{rs}$$

Therefore R_{rs} can be calculated from the estimates of C_{rs} and τ_{rs}. Normally, three time constants are required to empty 95% of the inspired volume. If the time constant is increased (e.g., because of high resistance), the lungs cannot empty adequately during tidal breathing (especially when the breathing frequency is increased), which results in hyperinflation of the lungs. In contrast, if the time constant is shorter (e.g., because of low compliance), atelectasis can occur during tidal breathing. This latter can often be seen in preterm babies with BPD or respiratory distress syndrome.

Since in neonates and young infants FRC is maintained actively above V_r, a single reading of $\Delta V / \Delta P_{ao}$ can lead to underestimations of C_{rs},[82] and this error will in turn lead to false high values of R_{rs} calculated using the same τ_{rs}. Occlusions performed in separate breaths at different phases of expiration (multiple occlusion technique: MOT) provide a set of $\Delta V / \Delta P_{ao}$ values, and regression on these points establishes a more correct estimate of C_{rs}.

Quality Control, Acceptability Criteria, and Limitations

Similarly to all the other infant lung function tests, the most common failure of the measurement is a leak around the facemask. The leak can be recognized by a continuing slow decay in P_{ao} (while a sudden decrease in P_{ao} more likely indicates inspiratory muscle activity). Therefore V, V', and P_{ao} should be continuously monitored throughout the test and the V' versus V curves should be displayed real time for quality control purposes.

The test requires a stable EEL, which can be difficult to achieve in young infants (especially when unsedated). Before each occlusion at least 5 breaths should be recorded for the calculation of EEL. Similarly, following the occlusion, EEL should be calculated as an average of 3–4 normal breathing cycles (this might take time after the occlusion; therefore the first few breaths right after the opening of the valve should be excluded from such calculation). The occlusion maneuver is valid if the preocclusion and postocclusion EEL values do not differ more than 1 mL/kg. C_{rs} and R_{rs} are calculated from

at least 5 occlusion maneuvers where EEL remains stable and the expiration is artifact-free and passive.

The key assumption underlying the use of the SOT is the passive behavior of the respiratory system, both in the occlusion phase and the subsequent expiration. The absence of muscle activity during occlusion is substantiated by a stable plateau in P_{ao} and a stable linear segment in the V' versus V relationship during the expiration (at least 40% of the total expiration, see Fig. 11.22). A late rise in P_{ao} in the plateau phase marks the onset of expiratory muscle activity, which means that while the $\Delta V / \Delta P_{ao}$ can still be read, the postocclusion decay will not be passive.

The absence of the artefacts discussed above does not automatically mean that the C_{rs} and R_{rs} readings are correct. In the presence of peripheral lung inhomogeneity, the time of occlusion might be insufficient for P_{ao} to equilibrate fully to a uniform alveolar pressure (i.e., elastic recoil pressure), which will lead to an underestimation of the alveolar pressure. It also needs to be stressed that the SOT and MOT methods rely on simple biomechanical assumptions. While C_{rs} can be taken as a constant in healthy infants within a tidal range above V_r, the postocclusion relaxed expiration may not follow a strictly exponential decay if R_{rs} is not constant during the tidal expiration. Departure from a constant R_{rs} may occur in the case of marked pressure-flow nonlinearities in the upper airways, and because the stress relaxation/recovery processes in the living tissues do not follow the monoexponential decay either.

Potential Clinical Applications in Infants

With the above-mentioned methodological limitations kept in mind, the SOT can be employed as a relatively simple and informative technique on the respiratory mechanical status in infancy. C_{rs} is primarily associated with lung size and is an indicator of lung development, while R_{rs} is greatly influenced by the narrow upper airways when measured through a facemask. Even with this limitation, R_{rs} has been shown to be elevated in wheezing infants[83] and associated with respiratory symptoms during human rhinovirus infection[84] while exhibiting no relationship with respiratory problems later in life. R_{rs} was also increased in late preterms compared to term infants.[85,86]

Low C_{rs} at birth was shown to predict wheeze during the first 5 years of life[83] and related to the development of asthma later in life.[83,87] Infants with BPD have reduced C_{rs} values[88]; however, the interpretation of low C_{rs} values in small infants warrants caution. It has been reported that somatic growth is a very strong confounding factor in C_{rs}[86]; therefore the normalization of the C_{rs} measures to body size is recommended. This also explains the importance of the measurement of FRC in the interpretation of respiratory mechanics.

MEASUREMENT OF INTERRUPTER RESISTANCE

The measurement of the respiratory resistance during a short interruption of the tidal flow was first described in the late 1920s. Nowadays, commercial devices and age-specific recommendations are available and healthy reference values with z-scores have also been established.[89] The technique is highly feasible in young children (similarly to the FOT and sR_{aw} test) as it only requires tidal breathing; therefore it is easy and quick to perform. Since portable devices are also available, it can also be employed in field work.

Summary

- Measurement of interrupter resistance (R_{int}) during tidal breathing via short occlusions of the flow either during inspiration or expiration
- Highly feasible in children
- R_{int} is calculated from the mouth pressure during the interruption and the flow right before the interruption
- Reference values for both inspiratory and expiratory R_{int} values, commercial devices, and recommendations are available
- Main limitation is the underestimation of airway resistance in the presence of severe airway obstruction

It was first described in 1927 that if at any point of the breathing cycle the airway opening is briefly occluded, then V' falls immediately to zero while the P_{ao} rapidly increases to a new level during the occlusion.[90] It has also been established that the magnitude of this rapid pressure change depends on the difference between the alveolar and mouth pressure immediately before the occlusion. These findings have led to the development of a lung function technique that is highly feasible in spontaneously breathing young children and provides an estimate of resistance.

The principle of the technique is a brief occlusion of the tidal flow (usually peak flow) that is not recognizable by the child (~100 ms), but sufficient enough to reach equilibrium between the mouth pressure (P_{mo}) and the alveolar pressure. The interrupter resistance (R_{int}) is then calculated as

$$R_{int} = P_{mo}/V'$$

where P_{mo} is the mouth pressure during the occlusion while V' is the tidal flow measured before the occlusion. During the short occlusion, the plateau that indicates the equilibrium is reached in a typical manner (Fig. 11.23). First, P_{mo} is immediately and rapidly increasing as a result of the pressure difference due to the airway resistance at the time of the occlusion (P_{init}). In reality, this rapid change is not constant and involves several rapid oscillations due to the air movement in the respiratory system (see Fig. 11.23). This makes the measurement of P_{init} technically challenging. This short initial phase of rapid increase is followed by a slow elevation in the pressure that reflects the stress adaptation of the viscoelastic tissue and the gas redistribution between the peripheral lung units (this phenomenon of the gas movement between parallel units of the lung is called *pendelluft*). The third phase of the pressure change following the occlusion is a plateau of the pressure, which represents the elastic recoil pressure of the respiratory system. Various methods have been suggested to calculate the fast initial resistive pressure drop (i.e., P_{init}). The most commonly applied method is the linear back-extrapolation of the pressure by using the two-point method: P_{mo} at 70 ms and 30 ms to either 15 ms or 0 ms after the interruption (see Fig. 11.23). This means that the obtained value of P_{init} is not only dependent on the resistive pressure drop but is also influenced by the viscoelastic properties of the respiratory system (i.e., R_{int} does not equal to R_{aw}).

In the commercial devices, the occlusion is automatically triggered usually at either the inspiratory or expiratory peak

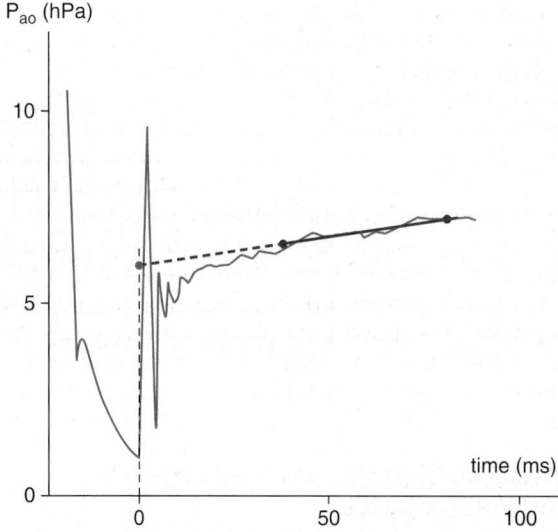

Fig. 11.23 Measurement of the airway-opening pressure (P_{ao}) with the interrupter technique. Following the brief occlusion (0 ms), P_{ao} is rapidly increasing with characteristic oscillations (see the text for details). The initial pressure that represents all the Newtonian resistive pressure in the respiratory system is obtained with linear back-extrapolation *(solid and dashed red line)* between 30 and 70 ms *(red symbols)* to 0 ms *(blue symbol)*.

flow. Findings on expiratory and inspiratory R_{int} values in preschool-age children are inconsistent, as some studies reported higher R_{int} during expiration[91,92] while others have found no difference.[89,93,94] Nevertheless, the timing of the occlusion always has to be reported and comparisons with data collected in other centers should always be made carefully.

Quality Control, Acceptability Criteria, and Limitations

For an acceptable R_{int} test, a minimum of 5–10 interruptions should be made and the average of at least 5 technically acceptable measurements is reported. A measurement is considered technically acceptable if there is no leak around the mouthpiece (as indicated by the decrease in P_{mo} following the initial rapid increase) and there are no obvious artefacts such as vocalization, coughing, or swallowing. Although the brief occlusion is not recognizable by the patient, the fast closing of the shutter makes a noise, which can disturb the child. Time should be allowed for the child to become familiar with the device and the measurement method.

Similarly to the plethysmography and the SOT, the main limitation of the R_{int} technique is related to moderate or severe airway obstruction and inhomogeneity in the lung periphery. If heterogeneity is present, the equilibrium might not be achieved during the interruption; therefore P_{init} is underestimated. The effect of the cheek support has also been investigated, and there was no difference between R_{int} values measured in the same children with and without the cheek support.[89,94] However, these studies only included healthy children in whom the compliant upper airways are not expected to have a huge influence on the equilibrium between the mouth and the alveolar pressures. This may not be the case in the presence of severe airway obstruction, as upper airway shunting can delay pressure equilibration significantly; therefore it is highly recommended to apply cheek support during the measurement of R_{int} in young children.

The clinical usefulness of R_{int} has been investigated in asthmatic children at both baseline and following bronchodilators.[94a,95–97] A decrease of 35% in R_{int} was defined as clinically significant,[96,97] and this cut-off was also validated against spirometry in young children.[98] R_{int} has also been suggested as a potential outcome measure for a clinical trial in young asthmatic children.[99] Findings on R_{int} in CF are controversial.[100–102] Recently, R_{int} was suggested as a feasible measure of diminished lung function in pre-term infants compared to those born term[102a]; however, this technique in infants needs more research.

PLETHYSMOGRAPHIC MEASUREMENT OF AIRWAY RESISTANCE

Summary

- R_{aw} in older children and adults is measured during a two-step procedure and calculated from the FRC and specific R_{aw} ($sR_{aw} = FRC \times R_{aw}$)
- In young children, FRC cannot be measured reliably; therefore sR_{aw} reflects R_{aw} at a given FRC without actually knowing either R_{aw} or FRC
- Since the technique has been adopted for young children (i.e., special mouthpiece, the possible presence of an adult in the box, etc.) it has become highly feasible in preschool-age children
- Commercial devices, healthy reference data, and measurement guidelines are available
- Changes in sR_{aw} values can reflect changes in R_{aw} or FRC or both—this remains the main limitation of the technique

Airway resistance has a strong inverse relationship with lung volume; therefore knowledge of the FRC is very useful in the interpretation of R_{aw}. The product of FRC and R_{aw} is called specific airway resistance (sR_{aw}), which can be measured with the plethysmographic technique in young children.[103] During growth, FRC is increasing while R_{aw} is decreasing; therefore sR_{aw} remains relatively constant during early life and its value is more or less independent of height, weight, and sex. The classical measurement of R_{aw} with the plethysmographic method requires two steps in older children and adults: (1) the measurement of FRC during brief occlusions, and (2) the measurement of sR_{aw}. R_{aw} is then calculated as sR_{aw}/FRC. The reliable measurement of FRC is very difficult in young children (see also in the *Measurement of Lung Volume* part of this chapter); therefore sR_{aw} can be obtained without actually knowing R_{aw} and FRC separately. An abnormal sR_{aw} can therefore be a consequence of changes either in FRC or R_{aw} (or both) and its value cannot tell which one of these components is abnormal. This remains one of the main limitations of the technique in preschool-age children. R_{aw} is only sporadically reported in children and it is far less frequently used in older children than sR_{aw}. Although the measurement is also possible in infants, there are numerous technical limitations, and the interpretation of sR_{aw} data in nasally breathing infants remains unclear. These are the main reasons why this method has not been used frequently in infants and its application is limited to a few centers worldwide. Therefore we will limit our discussion to the measurement of sR_{aw} in children.

Before the measurement, every detail of the procedure should be explained to the child to avoid any unexpected stress and discomfort during the test. Once the child is seated into the plethysmograph chamber, the door should be closed for at least 1 minute before the first measurement to minimize the thermal drift. If the child is hesitant to enter or stay in the closed chamber, one of the parents or a technician can join the child. During the test, the child has to wear a nose clip, and the cheeks should be firmly supported to avoid upper airway shunting (see above). A mouthpiece or facemask with a modified mouth tube is connected to a pneumotachograph, and the tidal flow is monitored until a stable breathing pattern is established. The principle of the plethysmographic estimation of sR_{aw} is the indirect measurement of the alveolar pressure through the changes in the box pressure or volume (ΔV_{box}) during tidal breathing. sR_{aw} is calculated from the changes in the flow at the airway opening ($\Delta V'$) and ΔV_{box} as

$$sR_{aw} = (\Delta V_{box}/\Delta V') \times (P_{amb} - P_{H_2O}),$$

where P_{amb} is ambient pressure and P_{H_2O} is the pressure of the water vapor at body temperature; hence $P_{amb} - P_{H_2O}$ is the approximate pressure of the compressible thoracic gas. In the earlier plethysmograph models, the BTPS conditions were achieved by the rebreathing technique, while in the new, commercial devices the correction is accomplished electronically. This is one of the reasons why reference data collected with home-built and commercially available devices are not comparable.[104] Since the first publications, the sR_{aw} test has undergone many modifications, standardization for measurement in young children and reference data from a multicenter study published for children between 2 and 11 years of age (see *Suggested Reading*).

Quality Control, Acceptability Criteria, and Limitations

The feasibility of the test has improved significantly with the introduction of specifically designed facemasks and with the possibility of an adult accompanying the child in the box. These improvements have made the measurements of sR_{aw} successful in more than half of 2-year-olds and in more than two-thirds of the children at 3 years of age.[105] The success rate of the measurement of R_{aw} in older children is similar to that of spirometry in the same population. It seems however that the test is still not standardized appropriately in children.[105a] If an adult is present in the box during the test, they should be instructed to take a deep breath and have a constant, slow (~20 seconds) expiration while the child's lung function is being recorded.[104] The constant drift caused by the long expiration can be compensated automatically in most of the commercial devices. Importantly, the volume displacement caused by the adult person must be corrected by using an approximate volume based on the body weight. In devices with electronic BTPS correction, it is ideal if the child is breathing at a frequency between 30 and 45; however, this is not always easy to achieve. This is one of the limitations that was introduced during the procedure of simplification and automatization of the technique. Furthermore, it has been shown that the electronic BTPS correction might result in a systematic overestimation of sR_{aw}.[104] This also explains why data collected with custom-built equipment using a heated rebreathing system are not comparable with the reference data obtained with commercial devices. The frequency of panting also varies between centers, which further limits the generalizability of sR_{aw}.[105a]

The simultaneous recording of the changes in the tidal V' against the changes in V_{box} (the so-called specific resistive loops, Fig. 11.24) and their observation provide the examiner with important information on the quality and reliability of the test. Obvious artefacts such as coughing, swallowing, and breath holds can easily be recognized real time. A test is acceptable if five artifact-free loops have been recorded. The outcome variable presented depends on the reading of these loops (see the different readings on Fig. 11.24); however, the most commonly reported variable is sR_{awtot}, which reflects the relationship between V' and the maximum change in V_{box}. Note here that since the breathing pattern is highly variable in young children, this is reflected in the variable V' vs. V_{box} loops obtained during tidal breathing. This is responsible for the relatively high within-subject variability of sR_{aw} values, especially when sR_{awtot} is reported (see Fig. 11.24).

Since sR_{aw} is a product of FRC and R_{aw} without knowing their values separately, it mainly reflects the relationship between lung volume and resistance. Nevertheless, sR_{aw} has been employed in research studies in young children with asthma or CF.[102,106] sR_{aw} was increased in children with parental atopy[107] and was able to discriminate between persistent and late-onset wheeze phenotypes.[108] sR_{aw} has also been useful to assess the response to both bronchodilator[103,109] and constrictor[110,111] agents in asthmatic children. Based on these reports, 25%[103]–42%[109] decrease (bronchodilation) or increase (challenge test) should be considered as clinically significant changes; however, both the clinical and physiological interpretation of these findings requires caution.

FORCED OSCILLATION TECHNIQUE

Summary

- Measurement of respiratory resistance (R_{rs}) and reactance (X_{rs}) during tidal breathing

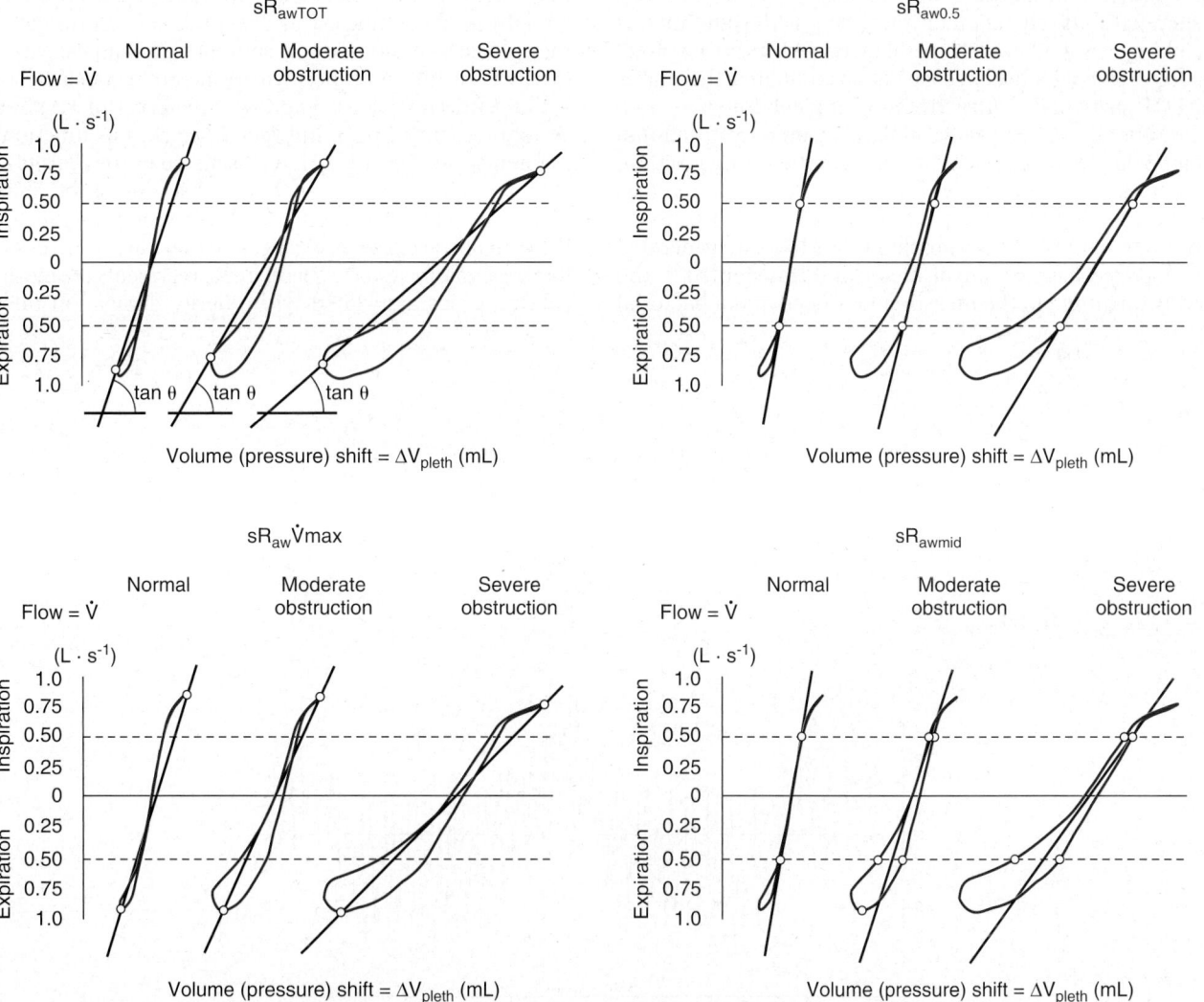

Fig. 11.24 Specific resistive flow-volume loops obtained with the plethysmographic method in children. An illustration of how different estimates of sR_{aw} may be calculated from the specific resistance loop, depending on how various parameter lines are applied on the loop and the slope of such lines. (Bisgaard H, Nielsen KG. Plethysmographic measurements of specific airway resistance in young children. *Chest.* 2005;128(1):355–362.)

- Commercial devices and reference values in children are available
- R_{rs} reflects the resistance of the airways and the tissues, while X_{rs} is determined by the elasticity of tissues and the inertance of the central airway gas
- The conventional estimates of R_{rs} and X_{rs} have limited diagnostic value in individuals
- Within-breath tracking of R_{rs} and X_{rs} at a single frequency reveals different airway dynamics in health and disease

Similarly to the MBW technique, FOT has its renaissance with an in-depth development in the recent years. This includes the introduction of novel methods in both preschool-aged children and infants, and new aspects of interpretation of the data. Therefore in this chapter both MBW and FOT receive a special focus to summarize the current knowledge on these techniques.

The basic principle of the FOT is the application of an external pressure (or flow) signal superimposed on spontaneous breathing (Fig. 11.25), and the measurement of the flow (or pressure) response of the respiratory system.[27,74,112] The oscillatory signals are specifically designed to measure the resistive and elastic characteristics of the respiratory system without relying on or interfering with spontaneous breathing. Since no special breathing maneuvers are involved, the requirement for patient cooperation is minimal; this makes the FOT particularly attractive in young children.[27]

Preschool-aged and older children (similarly to adults) breathe tidally through a mouthpiece in the sitting position, wearing a nose clip and with their cheeks supported (see Fig. 11.20). Single-frequency sinusoids or multiple-frequency composite signals of small amplitude (<2 hPa) are generated by a loudspeaker or a linear motor and transmitted to the airway opening via the measurement head and a bacterial

filter. A breathing tube provides a pathway for normal breathing. The input impedance of the respiratory system (Z_{rs}) is determined from the relationship between the airway-opening pressure (P_{ao}) and the resulting flow (V') at all oscillation frequencies. An alternative device measuring Z_{rs} is the wave tube[113] whose inlet (P_1) and outlet (P_2) pressures are used in the computation of Z_{rs} (Fig. 11.26).

While FOT is one of the most popular tests in clinical lung function laboratories in preschool-aged children, its adaptation to infants has been limited to research settings; therefore only the principles of the infant FOT test are summarized here. Similarly to the other infant lung function tests, Z_{rs} is measured in the supine position through a facemask in spontaneously breathing infants during natural sleep (see Fig. 11.1), during which time several Z_{rs} measurements of 30–60 seconds recording time can be collected. Once the baby is asleep, the test should not take longer than 15 minutes. The success rate of the infant FOT test is reported to be between 60% and 90%,[114,115] and mainly determined by the time available for waiting until the infant falls asleep.

Main Outcome Measures and Their Interpretation

In children, the FOT measurements can be accomplished in a relatively short time (10–20 seconds per recordings), and they provide a multitude of respiratory mechanical data; this is why their interpretation warrants much consideration.

Conventionally, Z_{rs} is expressed in terms of respiratory system resistance (R_{rs}) and reactance (X_{rs}) as functions of frequency (see Fig. 11.17). As discussed in the *Physiological Principles of the Respiratory Mechanics* section of this chapter, the forced oscillatory signal as the driving pressure equals the sum of the resistive, elastic, and inertial pressures of the total respiratory system. Therefore R_{rs} represents the mechanical properties associated with energy dissipation (airway

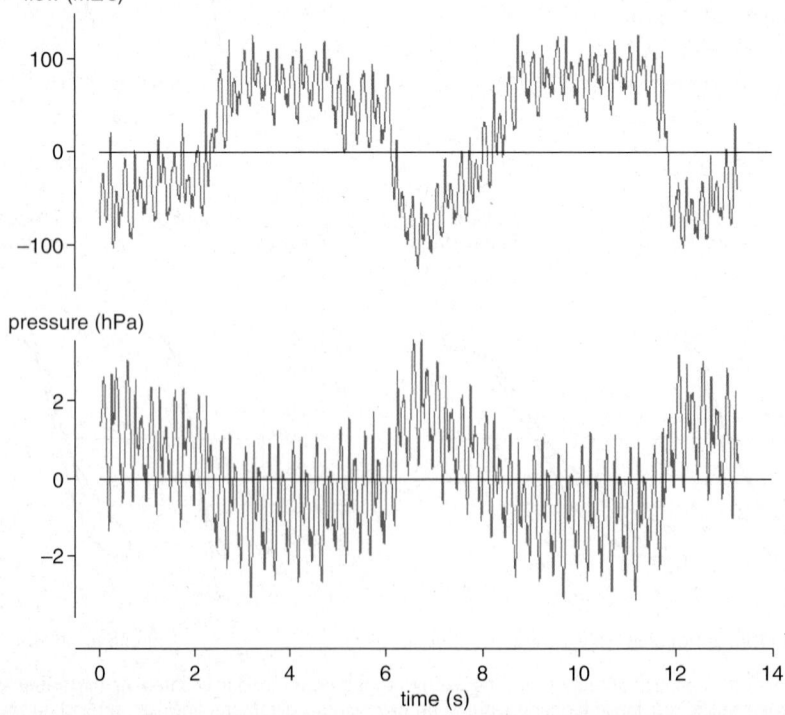

Fig. 11.25 Superposition of the forced oscillatory and spontaneous breathing signals in a child.

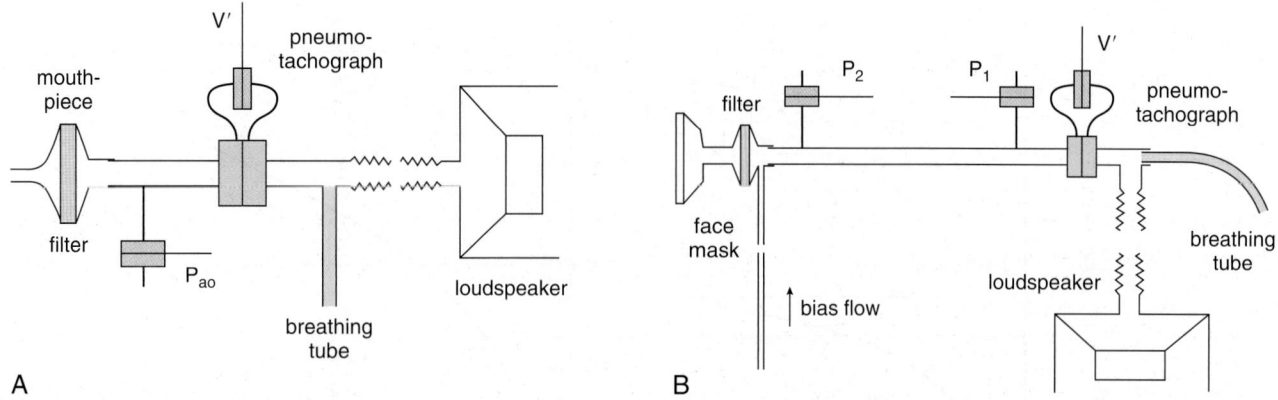

Fig. 11.26 Schematics of forced oscillatory setups. (A) A conventional arrangement for the estimation of respiratory impedance based on the signals of flow (V′) and airway-opening pressure (P_{ao}). (B) A wave-tube setup for measurement of the high impedances in infants, which are computed on the basis of the inlet (P_1) and outlet (P_2) pressures, as well as the geometrical and material properties of a cylindrical tube. Loudspeakers deliver the computer-generated oscillatory signals; breathing tubes impose low resistance against spontaneous breathing.

resistance, R_{aw} and tissue resistance, R_{ti}), while X_{rs} is a sum of two opposing energy-storing components: the elastance of the pulmonary and chest wall tissues (E_{rs}; the reciprocal of total respiratory compliance, C_{rs}) and the inertance (I_{rs}) determined primarily by the accelerated gas column in the large airways. Both R_{rs} and X_{rs} exhibit characteristic frequency dependence in both healthy children and adults. As shown in a schematic diagram in Fig. 11.17, at low frequencies X_{rs} follows the course of the tissue reactance, X_{ti}, which changes roughly inversely with frequency, and approaches the linear increase of the inertial reactance (X_{in}) dominating at higher frequencies. The point where the two reactances are equal in magnitude (i.e., $|X_{ti}| = |X_{in}|$) but opposite in sign is called resonant frequency (f_{res}).

R_{rs} is relatively constant in the range 10–20 Hz in infants and children and exhibits an elevation toward both low and high frequencies. Of more physiological significance is the low-frequency behavior of R_{rs}, where the marked frequency-dependent change is caused by the contribution of R_{ti} which in turn mirrors the change of X_{ti} (see Fig. 11.17). At normal breathing rates, the contributions of R_{aw} and R_{ti} to R_{rs} are comparable, while X_{rs} is basically determined by X_{ti}; however, this low-frequency region can be explored only in the absence of breathing activity by the LFOT.[75,116] During spontaneous breathing in young children and infants, the relatively high breathing frequency interferes with the oscillation signal; therefore reliable values of R_{rs} and X_{rs} cannot be obtained at frequencies lower than 4, 6 (older children, preschoolers) or 8 Hz (infants).

Conventionally, Z_{rs} is obtained from a number of averaged recordings, each covering several breaths; thus R_{rs} and X_{rs} represent mean values from the whole breathing cycle. The most commonly reported variables of a FOT measurement are the average values at low frequencies (i.e., R_{rs} or X_{rs} at 6 or 8 Hz). f_{res} and the area between X_{rs} curve and x-axis (AX) are important outcome measures that provide information on the global characteristic of the X_{rs} curve. Unfortunately, as a result of the low lung compliance in the early years, f_{res} is not always reached in the measured frequency range in preschool-age children (Fig. 11.27). In the presence of respiratory disease, this delayed course of X_{rs} below the AX can be more significant (see below). AX is theoretically

calculated between the lowest measured frequency and f_{res}; however, some devices still display AX values when f_{res} is not achieved in the measured frequency range. Therefore the AX values reported in young children should always be treated with caution. An increased AX and f_{res}, however, are useful outcome measures in older children, reflecting inhomogeneous constriction of the peripheral airways.[74]

In the frequency range that can be covered with FOT during normal breathing there is an interval where R_{rs} is relatively independent of frequency, and which covers the transition of X_{rs} from the dominance of elastance to that of the inertance. In this range, Z_{rs} can be described by a simple resistance (R)–inertance (I)–compliance (C) model.[117,118] However, departure from this ideal frequency, dependence of Z_{rs} may occur for several reasons that introduce a negative frequency dependence of R_{rs} and/or a retarded negative course in X_{rs}: (1) involvement of R_{ti} at lower frequencies; (2) insufficient support of the cheeks, that is, the upper airway artifact[119]; (3) other airway wall shunts proximal to an elevated bronchial resistance[120]; and (4) peripheral inhomogeneities, that is, lung units with different time constants.[121] R_{rs} at the upper frequency part (>20 Hz) can be a measure of the resistance of the large proximal airways, whereas the higher values of resistance at less than 10 Hz reflect the involvement of the mechanisms (1)–(4) listed above. It is therefore a simplistic and wrong approach when the low-frequency R_{rs} is regarded as the simple sum of the central and peripheral resistances.

While most of the lung function outcome measures are easy to understand and put in a physiological context, the concept and the interpretation of the reactance remains one of the most difficult tasks in respiratory mechanics. As discussed previously, X_{rs} is far more complex than a variable that reflects the tissue elasticity. Nevertheless, the future direction of the conventional application of the FOT might include the (re-)introduction of the R-I-C model fitting in infants and preschool-age children.[121a] Compliance obtained from this model fitting might be a term easily embraced by researchers and clinicians. Since neither f_{res} nor AX can be obtained reliably in preschool-age children, compliance can be a robust descriptor of the whole reactance curve (as it is obtained from all the measured reactance values) instead

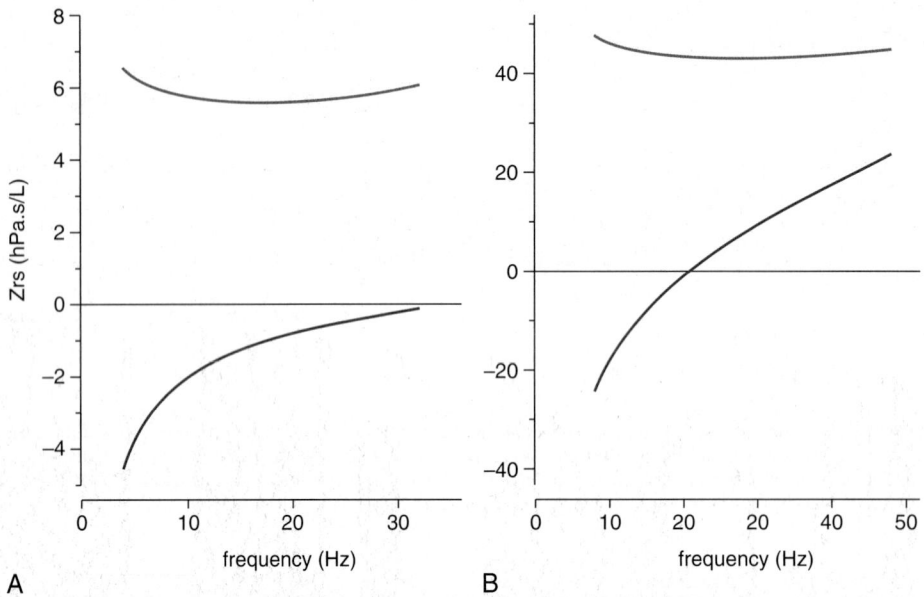

Fig. 11.27 Schematic illustration of impedance (Zrs) curves in terms of resistance *(blue lines)* and reactance *(red lines)*, measured in a healthy 4-year-old child (A) and a healthy newborn infant (B), using different scales in Zrs. Note the lack of resonant frequency in the measured frequency range (4–32 Hz) in the 4-year-old child and the steep rise in reactance, due to the inclusion of the nasal pathways, in the infant.

of reporting X_{rs} at a single frequency. However, once the R-I-C model becomes obviously inconsistent with the measured Z_{rs} data (as in severe impairments in respiratory mechanics), the derived parameters lose physiological relevance. It is also important to note here that while the concept of compliance is easy to deal with, the values of C derived from Z_{rs} remain affected by the same factors that influence reactance; therefore a low compliance value will not always reflect decreased lung elasticity. Finally, as mentioned earlier in this chapter, the values of C determined by the FOT are not comparable numerically with that of the C_{rs} obtained at breathing frequencies (e.g., with SOT) or during static conditions (i.e., weighted spirometer technique).

Since infants are preferential nasal breathers, the measured Z_{rs} includes the impedance of the narrow upper airways, which makes the inference to the resistance of the lower respiratory system difficult. This is one of the main reasons why C_{rs} measured with the FOT has been reported as a potentially useful outcome measure over R_{rs}.[114] The effect of the nasal pathway is also obvious on the X_{rs} curve as the inertance of the respiratory system is much more significant in nasal breathers than when Z_{rs} is measured through the mouth. This explains the relatively low f_{res} in infants (see Fig. 11.27) despite their low lung compliance.

The main limitation of the FOT in preschool-age children is the wide range of healthy reference data for a given height (see Fig. 11.21), which explains why the current FOT studies have shown limited clinical potential in individuals. To overcome this problem, novel aspects of the methodology have been suggested and new outcome variables have also been introduced.[122] The biggest dataset in preschool-aged Caucasian children has recently been published and z-scores (including those for R and C) were created for this very unique population.[121a]

Intensive investigation has focused on the measurement and interpretation of the dynamic changes of respiratory mechanics during the breathing cycle.[122–125] The most important point of the new concept is that instead of considering the average values of R_{rs} and X_{rs} over several breaths and their frequency dependence, a fast single-frequency signal is employed to track the within-breath fluctuations of R_{rs} and X_{rs}. The analysis of R_{rs} and X_{rs} in different phases of the breathing cycle and their changes with tidal flow and volume can provide us with unique information on respiratory mechanics.

Quality Control, Acceptability Criteria, and Limitations

The calibration of the FOT device is exceptionally critical, and the proper concept of the calibration is not always embraced by the manufacturers. The calibration requires a device with known impedance that should be appropriate for the largest Z_{rs} values expected in the measured population. Since Z_{rs} is much higher in children than in healthy adults, a calibration device with a minimum impedance of 15 hPa.s/L should be used (we note here that the impedance of an adult with chronic obstructive pulmonary disease [COPD] can sometimes reach a Z_{rs} as high as 30 hPa.s/L; therefore a low-impedance calibration device is not recommended for adults either). In infants, Z_{rs} is 4–5 times higher than in preschool-age children, and the calibration of the infant setup requires a calibration device with a Z_{rs} of at least 80 hPa.s/L. Currently, only the wave-tube FOT setting[115] proves accurate enough to measure Z_{rs} in these extreme ranges.

As a part of the calibration, the impedance of the bacterial filter and the mouthpiece should be extracted from the measured Z_{rs}. In addition to the resistance of the filter, the shunting effect of the mouthpiece gas compliance can also be significant in young children with lung disease; therefore its correction requires a comprehensive approach. The method of mouthpiece correction differs between manufacturers, and it is not known for the users; this might contribute to the fact that reference values collected with different devices are not always comparable.

In children, at least three technically acceptable recordings of Z_{rs} must be obtained. The recording time varies between commercial devices but usually takes at least 15 seconds and should cover at least 3–5 tidal breathing cycles. A recording can be considered artifact-free if there is no leak around the mouthpiece, and no vocalization, cough, or swallowing occurs during the test. Temporary increases in P_{ao} and decreases in V' indicate epochs of upper airway closure. The artifact that is the most difficult to recognize is the small leak around the mouthpiece; this may be detected via increases in R_{rs} and X_{rs} at the lowest frequencies (Fig. 11.28). Recently, automatized artefact-detection system has been proposed[125a]: its usefulness in the everyday practice, particularly in children requires further research. Although the breathing pattern has a high natural variability in children, it is ideal if both the breathing frequency and tidal volume values are in the normal range for the child's age.

The assessment of the reliability of the Z_{rs} data is important. Although the commercial devices report coherence values and set acceptance limits for Z_{rs} based on them, the coherence values are dependent on their calculation that varies between manufacturers and is usually not transparent to the users. Importantly, coherence has been shown unreliable in the presence of nonlinearities (an inherent property of the respiratory system during breathing) and multifrequency oscillations typically used in the FOT devices.[126] Therefore the interpretation of these values in young children requires caution and cannot be considered as the main acceptability criteria of a test. Inspection of large measurement sets indicates that a high coherence value in young children does not always belong to an acceptable test, while low coherence does not always reflect poor quality. In young children, the reproducibility of the Z_{rs} spectra is far more important, and the measurement can be considered acceptable if: (1) it is artifact free, (2) the values and the shape of the impedance curves are appropriate for the age (and disease status) of the child, and (3) the Z_{rs} spectra are reproducible if the R_{rs} and X_{rs} values are within a 10% range of the Z_{rs} magnitude at the lowest frequencies measured. As in spirometry, experienced technicians or clinicians can also obtain useful information from the observation of the Z_{rs} versus frequency diagrams (frequency dependence of R_{rs} and X_{rs}, repeatability, etc.).

Potential Clinical Applications in Children

Findings on the clinical utility of the FOT in respiratory disease are controversial. In children with CF, FOT is able to detect the early lung disease[127]; however, it has been shown recently that the alterations in the outcome measures of FOT seem to be independent of the clinical symptoms, presence of inflammation, and structural abnormalities.[128] Furthermore, in older children R_{rs} has failed to discriminate between healthy children and those with CF[102,129,130] even when FEV_1 was decreased.[102,130] These findings suggest that the mean value of R_{rs} is unlikely to be sensitive for peripheral airway obstruction. In infants with CF, resistance has shown a relationship with pulmonary inflammation[131] when measured with the LFOT.

Follow-up studies on infants with neonatal chronic lung disease have reported increased R_{rs} and more negative X_{rs} during the preschool-[132] and school-age years.[133,134]

Similarly to CF, the diagnostic power of the conventional estimates of R_{rs} and X_{rs} in young individuals with recurrent wheeze and asthma appears to be highly limited. R_{rs} and X_{rs} were able to discriminate between children with different types of wheeze and healthy children (although rather statistical than clinical significance was reported),[135] while other studies with smaller sample size have not found such difference.[136,137] Z_{rs} measures have also been investigated in response to both bronchodilator[136,138–141] and bronchoconstrictor[142,143] agents, and the clinically significant (relative) changes in R_{rs} at 6, 8, and 10 Hz have been established between 32% and 40%.

It has been reported in various research and clinical settings that FOT is a highly feasible lung function test in young

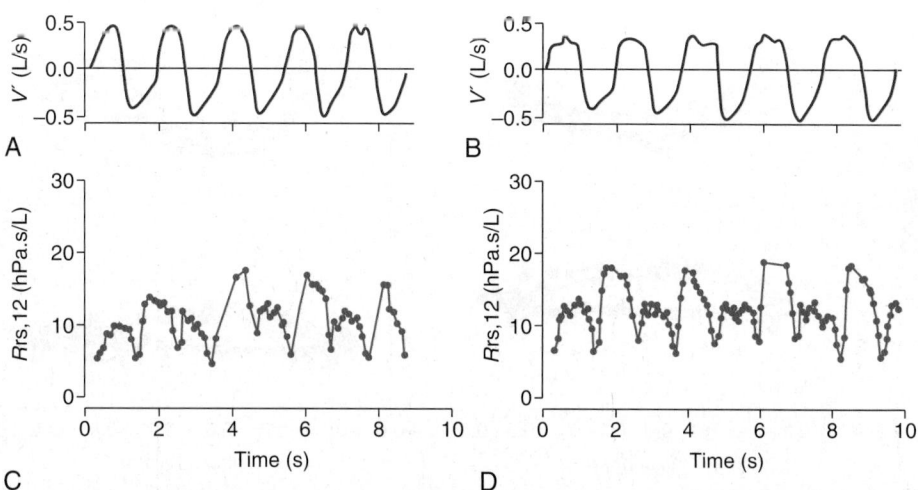

Fig. 11.28 Representative time courses of: (A and B) tidal flow (V') and (C and D) respiratory resistance (R_{rs}) at 12 (R_{rs},12) and 20 Hz (R_{rs},20) at baseline. Flow values are negative during expiration. Both R_{rs},12 and R_{rs},20 show periodic within-breath fluctuations. Most of the R_{rs} variation is reflected in the absolute value of the tidal flow. (Marchal F, Loos N, Monin P, et al. Methacholine-induced volume dependence of respiratory resistance in preschool children. *Eur Respir J.* 1999;14(5):1167-1174.)

children as young as 2 years of age. Despite the great feasibility, FOT has been suggested to have limited clinical potential in the clinical management of individuals with lung disease. This is most probably due to the combination of a number of factors that affect R_{rs} during tidal breathing in both healthy children and those with lung disease.[122,144]

Studies employing a single-frequency signal have revealed that R_{rs} shows a characteristic fluctuation throughout the breathing cycle (Fig. 11.29): it has its minimum at the transitions between inspiration and expiration, while it is increasing with both inspiratory and expiratory flows, reaching its maximum value at the peak expiratory flow.[122,123,145] With this faster signal (usually 10 or 12 Hz in young children), the inspiratory and expiratory R_{rs} (and X_{rs}) values are easy to separate. Inspiratory resistance was found to correlate better with R_{aw} (measured with plethysmography) than expiratory resistance,[145] and this is likely to be explained by the

narrowing of the glottic aperture during expiration. The clinical value of the separate assessment of inspiratory and expiratory X_{rs} values remains unclear in children (while it is extremely useful in adults with COPD). The option of the use of a single-frequency signal and the separation of inspiration and expiration is now available in some of the commercial devices.

A recent study has also suggested that if the within-breath changes of R_{rs} are tracked over many breathing cycles, phases can be identified where the values of R_{rs} are the least affected by the variable breathing pattern of young children. Reading R_{rs} at the end-expiration and at end-inspiration (i.e., where tidal flow is zero and R_{rs} is at its minimum) may provide a better estimate of the airway caliber and reveal the volume-related changes in R_{rs} (see Fig. 11.28). Indeed, the difference between end-expiratory and end-inspiratory R_{rs} values has been shown to be a sensitive and specific indicator of airway

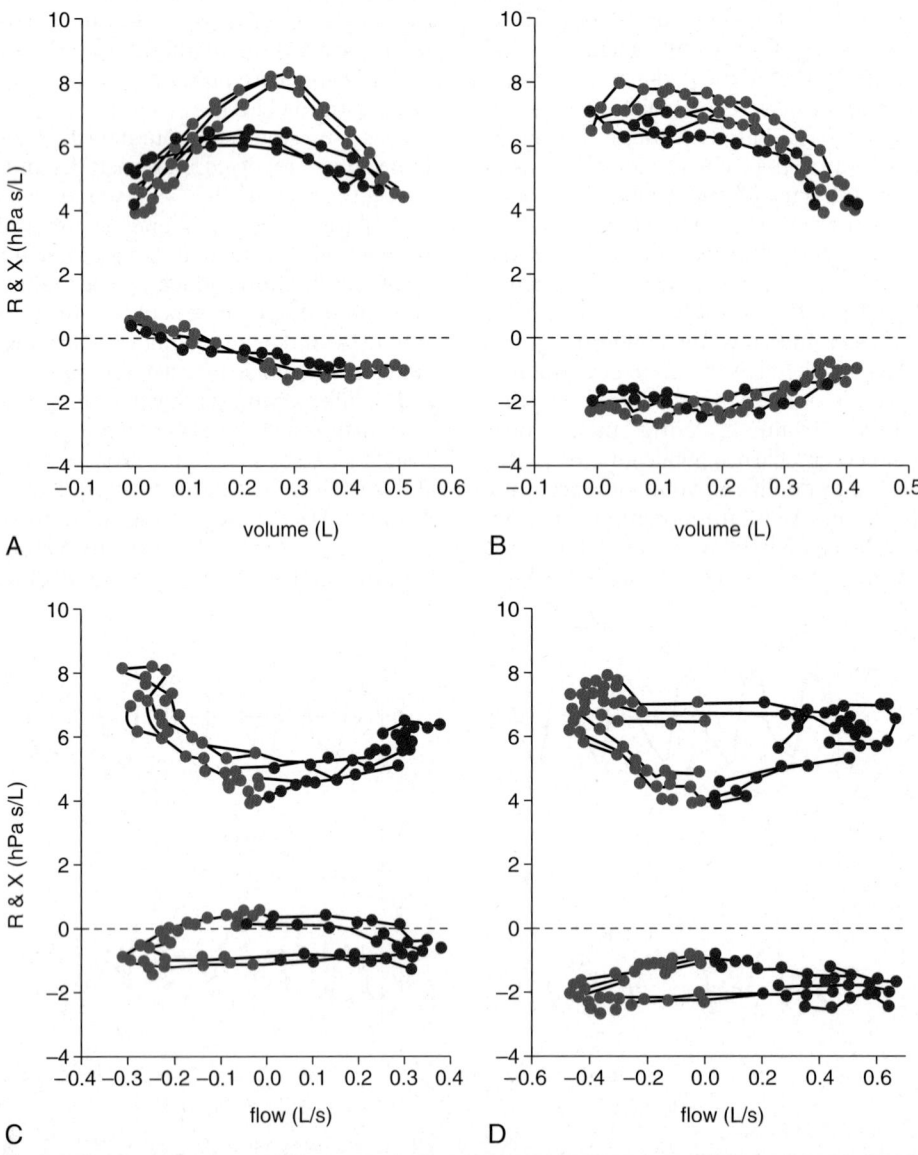

Fig. 11.29 Tidal changes with volume (A and B) and flow (D and C) in resistance (R, *top*) and reactance (X, *bottom*) during inspiration *(open circles)* and expiration *(closed circles)* in a healthy subject (A and C) and in a child with acute airway obstruction (B and D). Note the elevated end-expiratory resistance (B, "0" volume) and the increased hysteresis (D) in the presence of airway obstruction. (Czovek D, Shackleton C, Hantos Z, et al. Tidal changes in respiratory resistance are sensitive indicators of airway obstruction in children. *Thorax.* 2016;71(10):907-915.)

obstruction in children with both acute and recurrent wheeze.[122]

Although these novel approaches of the FOT have a great clinical promise, their validation requires multicenter collaboration that can carefully assess the clinical utility of the within-breath FOT in different patient groups and different settings. Nevertheless, robust reference values for the new intra-breath Zrs measures are in press, which will improve the clinical utility of this technique in the detection of lung disease in young children.

Measurement of Gas Mixing

Detection of ventilation inhomogeneity with a noninvasive lung function test has been of primary interest to researchers and respiratory physicians for many decades. Two methods have been developed for this purpose: the single breath washout (SBW) and MBW techniques. Similarly to spirometry, SBW requires high cooperation from the subject to perform a well-coordinated, complete TLC maneuver for the assessment of the gas-mixing capacity of the lungs over a wide range of lung volumes. Since the use of SBW is not feasible in infants and young children, we will restrict to discussing the MBW technique in this chapter.

MULTIPLE BREATH WASHOUT TECHNIQUE

Summary

- Measurement of FRC and LCI in tidally breathing subjects
- Commercial devices are available for both infants and children
- Data collected with different devices, gases, and analytic methods are not comparable
- Main limitations are the inconsistent methodology and the time required for the test
- Clinical potential in CF

MBW has been a focus for clinical research studies in both infants and young children in recent years, as its application requires only tidal breathing and it provides unique information on the overall ventilation inhomogeneity in the lungs. Although the physiological background and importance of the measurement of "uneven ventilation" via the gas-mixing ability of the respiratory system were already described in the 1940s[146] (see also the *Measurement of Lung Volumes* part of this chapter), its precise assessment has required technical development and a high level of computerization. Nowadays, different commercial devices specifically designed for infants and preschool-aged children are available; however, the method of measurement, the software algorithms, and the outcome measures vary between these devices. To aid the general application of MBW in patients with lung disease, an ERS/ATS consensus statement was published in 2013 (see *Suggested Reading*). There has also been a great effort to modify and standardize the technique for the special needs of infant and preschool-aged children. Despite the intensive research on the clinical utility of the MBW in children (with more than 80 peer-reviewed articles published on this topic only between 2013 and 2017) and its promising clinical potential, it is still far more frequently used in research settings than the everyday clinical practice.

Physiological Principles and Assumptions

The main principle of MBW is the continuous measurement of the changes in the exhaled concentration of an inert gas simultaneously with the tidal flow over many breathing cycles in spontaneously breathing subjects. Various gas mixtures can be used for the MBW test; however, the measured gas has to fulfill the following criteria: it has to be safe to inhale and should not transfer through the alveolar wall into and from the circulation and tissues. In other words, the aim is to measure the alveolar ventilation independently of the influence of circulation and diffusion. The cheapest and the most widely used method is the N_2 washout technique, since N_2 can be considered as an intrinsic inert gas in the respiratory system. However, it is well documented that N_2 is also excreted into the lungs from the tissues, which can be responsible for as much as 1% of the total N_2 concentration in the respiratory system. Although different correction methods for the tissue N_2 have been suggested,[146a] complete solution of this problem requires further research. Additionally, pure oxygen (which is used to wash the N_2 out of the respiratory system) affects the breathing pattern in infants; therefore the N_2 washout technique cannot be used in this age group. The most commonly used test gas in infants is sulfur hexafluoride (SF_6, delivered into a closed circuit via bias flow in a concentration of either 4% or 5%) with 21% O_2 balanced with N_2. SF_6 has many advantages over N_2 being an extrinsic inert gas (i.e., not present in the human body), the detection of the changes in the alveolar concentration of SF_6 is technically easier and provides more reliable and precise results. However, SF_6 is expensive, not registered for human use in many countries, and was also recognized as an "extremely potent greenhouse gas."

Since N_2 is already present in the respiratory system (intrinsic inert gas), no wash-in phase is required for the N_2 MBW technique, which makes the protocol shorter compared to other gases (e.g., He, SF_6). At the beginning of the test, the alveolar concentration of N_2 can be considered to be 80%. Before the washout phase begins, the patient is breathing room air from an open circuit (Fig. 11.30) while the concentration of N_2 and the tidal flow are being recorded. Once the breathing pattern is stable and at least 5 steady-state breathing cycles are recorded as baseline, the circuit is switched to pure oxygen (closed circuit) at the end of the last breathing cycle of the wash-in phase. This step is crucial for the correct calculation of FRC (for details of the calculation of FRC from gas mixing, see the part *Measurement of Lung Volumes* of this chapter). This can be particularly challenging in children because of their high breathing frequency (especially when unwell), and therefore the test requires an experienced examiner. The basic assumption of MBW is that the known end-expiratory concentration of the test gas (in this case N_2) will be diluted with every breath that the subject takes from the test gas-free gas mixture (in the case pure O_2) during the washout phase. The alveolar concentration of the test gas is thus decreasing with each breath during the washout phase, and the test finishes when the concentration of the test gas has decreased below 1/40 of its original alveolar concentration. In healthy lungs with homogenous ventilation, this dilution to 1/40 will happen

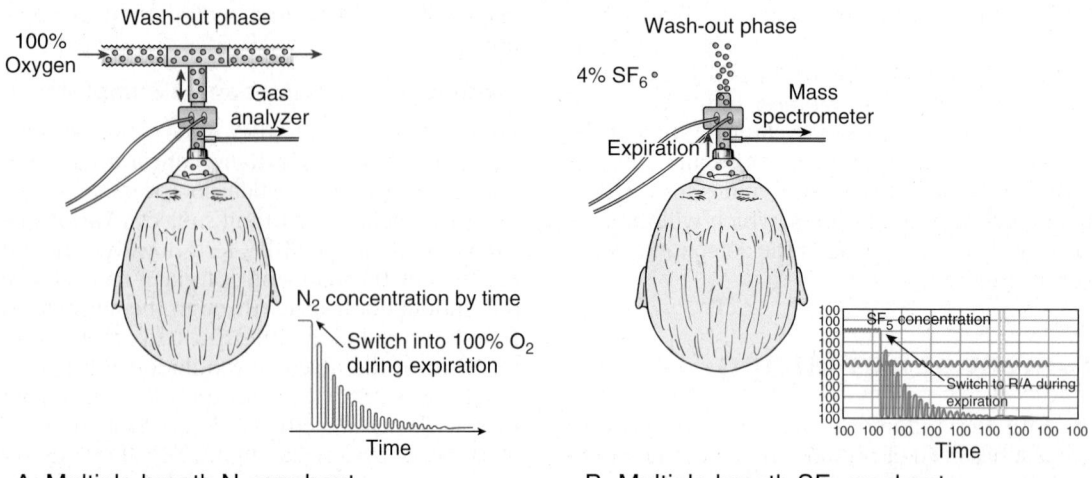

Fig. 11.30 Schematic representation of two washout phase tests using the two techniques. (A) N_2-based setup. During the N_2 washout, 100% oxygen is delivered using a bias flow. The blue tracing shows the decay in the N_2 signal during expiration. (B) Extrinsic gas, SF_6-based setup. The green tracing shows the decay in the SF_6 concentration during the washout-phase. *R/A*, Room air. (Subbarao P, Milla C, Aurora P, et al. Multiple-breath washout as a lung function test in cystic fibrosis. a cystic fibrosis foundation workshop report. *Ann Am Thorac Soc.* 2015;12(6):932-939.)

faster (i.e., fewer breaths are required to clear the test gas from the lungs) than in the presence of lung disease where the parallel lung units have different time constants—this is the simple assumption underlying the potential clinical use of MBW.

In infants, the washout precedes a long wash-in phase, lasting until the concentration of SF_6 (which is 0% before the test) is equilibrated in the lungs as indicated by the same inspiratory and expiratory concentrations (4% or 5%) of SF_6 (see Fig. 11.30). The washout phase starts when the expiratory concentration of SF_6 is stable for at least 5 consecutive breaths. When washout begins, the circuit is opened to room air (open circuit) and the decreasing concentration of SF_6 is detected continuously. The test ends when the concentration of SF_6 falls below 1/40 of its original concentration for at least 3 consecutive breaths.

Main Outcome Measures of Multiple Breath Washout

During the MBW test, the concentration of the test gas and the tidal flow are continuously recorded. The inspiratory and expiratory volumes are calculated with the integration of the flow signal. The calculation of FRC, one of the main outcome measures, has been discussed in detail earlier in this chapter (see *Measurement of Lung Volumes*).

Many attempts have been made to properly quantify the washout phase of the test. Historically, N_2 dilution was measured in healthy subjects and patients with emphysema when researchers recognized that after a few minutes of breathing pure O_2, N_2 nearly disappeared from the exhaled gas in healthy subjects while N_2 concentration was still high in patients with emphysema.[146] Therefore the time that was required to decrease the N_2 concentration to 2% of its original alveolar concentration was used as the main outcome variable.[147] However, it was realized early that the time of the measurement not only depends on the heterogeneity of the ventilation but also on the minute ventilation of the subject (i.e., higher breathing frequency or tidal volume result in faster washout

of the test gas, Fig. 11.31). To standardize the test and minimize the effect of the breathing pattern on the reading of the test, the term "turnover" (TO) was introduced. One turnover is the cumulative expiratory volume which is equivalent to the subject's FRC. The number or turnovers that are required to decrease the concentration of the tracer gas to 1/40 of its initial concentration—called the LCI[148]—is the most commonly reported outcome measure to date. LCI is calculated as the cumulative expired volume (CEV) normalized by FRC ($LCI = CEV/FRC$). The value of LCI indicates the overall lung ventilation homogeneity at the point when the test gas is cleared from the lungs. LCI is expected to be increased (i.e., more TOs are needed to clear the gas from the lungs) in respiratory diseases where the ventilation inhomogeneity is increased. According to the guidelines, LCI is read at the end of expiration of the first of three consecutive breathing cycles where the concentration of the tracer gas remains below 1/40.

Although LCI is the most commonly used variable in pediatric clinical research studies, it has some limitations that can be important especially in young children with lung disease. LCI is affected by changes in the breathing pattern during the test, and it sometimes takes too long to reach the target concentration. While LCI reflects the general ventilation inhomogeneity, alternative outcome measures have been introduced to facilitate identifying the parts of the lungs that are mainly responsible for the uneven ventilation and describing the underlying mechanisms.

In 1975, Saidel and his colleagues proposed a novel analysis for the washout curve that takes the entire curve into account by analyzing the shape and well-defined parts of the *normalized end-tidal tracer gas concentration (Cnet) vs the number of turnovers* curve.[149] This is the moment analysis, which is less influenced by the changes in the breathing pattern during the test and which makes it potentially useful in pediatric patients (Fig. 11.32). Despite all these advantages of the moment ratios, they are still rarely reported, since their clinical interpretation is difficult, while LCI appears to be more straightforward for researchers and clinicians. The area under

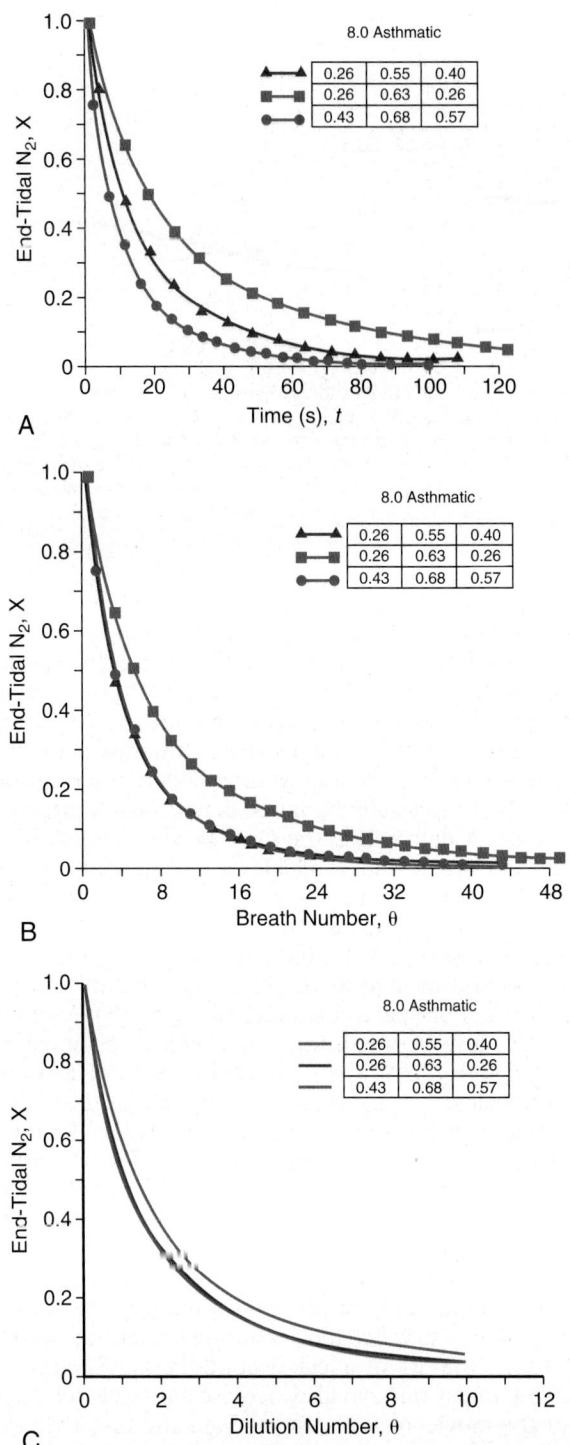

▲	0.26	0.55	0.40
■	0.26	0.63	0.26
●	0.43	0.68	0.57

Fig. 11.31 Reproducibility of the washout curve. Data from three washout runs performed with a variety of breathing patterns by an asthmatic (BG). Washout curve is graphed with ordinate variable normalized end-tidal nitrogen fraction, X, and abscissa variable: A: time (seconds), t; B: breath number, θ; C: dilution number, η. Dilution number (so called the turnover in the newest terminology) is the least affected by the variable breathing frequency and tidal volume as indicated by the reproducibility of the washout curves within the same subject (C). (Saidel GM, Salmon RB, Chester EH. Moment analysis of multibreath lung washout. *J Appl Physiol.* 1975;38(2):328-334.)

the curve represents the zero*th* moment (M0), the first moment (M1) is calculated as *Cnet*TO*, and the second moment (M2) is equal to *Cnet*TO²*. This calculation of M1 and M2 results in weighted values of area segments of the curve with M1 reflecting the center of the curve while M2 is more influenced by the tail regions (i.e., the TOs at low concentrations). The relationships between these moments have been studied and M1/M0 (first moment ratio) was found to represent mainly the mean, nonuniform alveolar flow distribution while M2/M0 (second moment ratio) accounts more of the lung regions that empty late during the washout. Moment ratios are generally calculated for all the TOs (starting from the first breath of the washout and finishing with the first breath of 3 consecutive breath below a concentration of 1/40).

An alternative way to analyze the shape of the washout curve is the phase III slope (S_{III}) analysis (Fig. 11.33), which can be done for each breath during the washout phase. The two main outcome measures of the S_{III} analysis are S_{cond} and S_{acin}. In theory, S_{cond} reflects the contribution of the conductive airways while S_{acin} represents the contribution of the acinar airways to the global ventilation inhomogeneity.[150] The analysis of S_{III} was originally developed in studies on adults where tidal volume was maintained at a certain level throughout the test. However, it has apparent limitations in small children: if tidal volume does not exceed a certain limit, S_{III} cannot be identified, and a variable tidal volume also affects the S_{III} analysis, making the interpretation of these variables difficult or misleading.[151] While sometimes S_{cond} and S_{acin} can be calculated in preschool-age children, the high breathing frequency and low tidal volumes make it impossible to identify and hence analyze the S_{III} during infancy. The analysis of S_{cond} and S_{acin} has been proven useful in older children in situations when alveolar compartment and the conducting airways need to be assessed separately.[151a,151b] The clinical significance of outcome measures other than LCI requires further evidence.

FEASIBILITY IN OLDER CHILDREN

Quality Control, Acceptability Criteria, and Limitations

The proper installation of the MBW device is crucial for the test. Since the test requires gas cylinders or wall gas, the portability of the device is largely limited and this has to be considered at the time of installation. This factor makes the bedside use of the test difficult or sometimes impossible. Furthermore, commercial devices and SF₆ cylinders are expensive; therefore MBW is not widely available at the moment for infant studies.

There are special requirements of the settings in infants and preschool-age children that the examiner has to address before recording the first test. Since the calculations of FRC and LCI are strongly dependent on the dead space, minimization of the dead space is an absolute must for the test in young children.[152,153] Additionally, the volume of the dead space compared to the tidal volume is relatively higher in infants and young children than in older children or adults; therefore settings using a mass spectrometer as a gas analyzer are preferable: the equipment dead space is smaller and it detects the gas concentration reliably even when the tidal

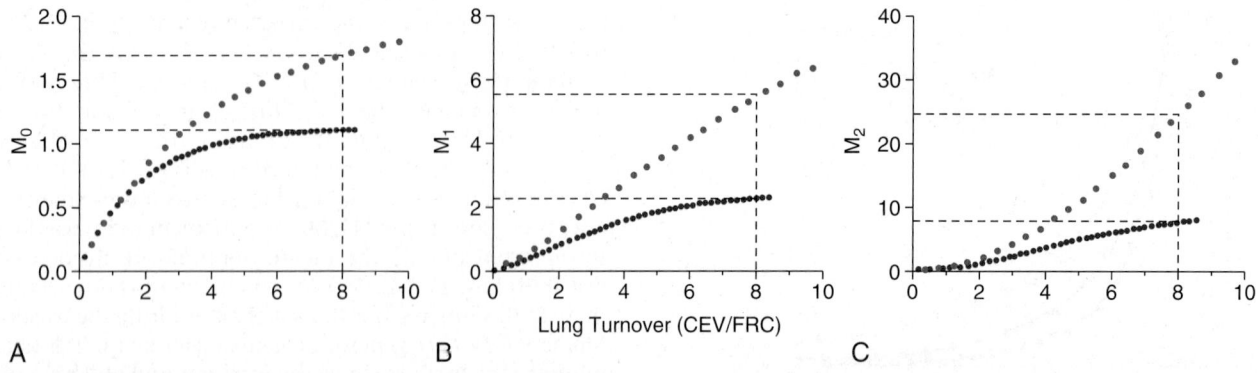

Fig. 11.32 Illustration of concept of moments. Graph shows moments derived from multiple breath washout (SF$_6$) in term infant *(red circles)* and preterm (gestational age, 28 weeks) infant with chronic lung disease of infancy at 38 weeks postmenstrual age *(blue circles)*. *Dotted lines* indicate values for moments at eight lung turnovers (TO). (A) 0th moment (M0), obtained from area under normalized tracer concentration vs. TO graph. (B) First moment (M1) derived from area under curve described by A. (C) Second moment (M2) derived from area under curve described by B. As moment number increases, there is increased weighting toward end of washout trace. *CEV,* Cumulative expired tidal volume; *FRC,* functional residual capacity. (Pillow JJ, Frerichs I, Stocks J. Lung function tests in neonates and infants with chronic lung disease: global and regional ventilation inhomogeneity. *Pediatr Pulmonol.* 2006;41(2):105-121.)

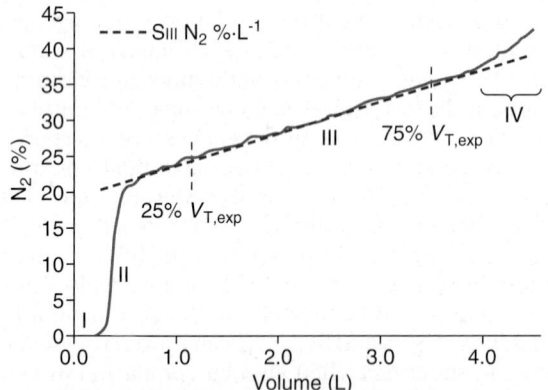

Fig. 11.33 Example of a typical single-breath washout (SBW) trace and the explanation of the phases of the washout curve within-a-breath. Nitrogen gas (N$_2$) expirogram showing calculation of phase III slope (SIII) in a vital capacity SBW test in a 60-year-old smoker. SIII is calculated between 25% and 75% of the expired volume, to avoid the contribution of phase IV. The four phases of the expirogram are also demonstrated: phase I (absolute dead space), phase II (bronchial phase), phase III (alveolar phase), and phase IV (fast rising phase at end of expiration). Closing volume (CV) is the expired volume (L) from the start of the upward deflection where phase IV starts, to the end of the breath. If residual volume (RV) is known, closing capacity (CC) can be calculated: CC = CV + RV. VT, exp: expired tidal volume. (Robinson PD, Latzin P, Verbanck S, et al. Consensus statement for inert gas washout measurement using multiple- and single-breath tests. *Eur Respir J.* 2013;41(3):507-522.)

volume is small. Nevertheless, the new generation of ultrasonic flow meters offers a reasonable alternative to the mass spectrometers and therefore has become widely used in the measurement of MBW.

The calibration of any of the commercial devices requires detailed and age-specific standard operating procedures. Each step of the calibration procedure is crucial for the quality and reliability of the test; therefore it should be performed before each test occasion by experienced examiners.

The time of the measurement varies between individuals and it depends on age, breathing pattern, and disease; however, despite the faster breathing frequency the test is particularly time consuming in infants and young children.

The time required for the test is one of the most important key points of MBW, since this will determine the feasibility of the test in young children in a clinical setting. Generally, three reproducible recordings (FRC within 25% in the three tests) are accepted as a complete test. This is usually difficult to achieve in infants and young children for multiple reasons.[154] In unsedated infants, is not always possible to collect all the data within the same sleeping period. At this stage, there are no data available on how the different sleep states affect the results of the test. Additionally, the lack of sedation increases the natural variability of the breathing pattern, which makes it more difficult to fulfill the acceptability criteria in infants. In preschool-age children, their limited attention span makes it challenging to record three acceptable tests in one sitting. It has recently been reported that although MBW was successful in 82% of asthmatic children below 7 years of age,[155] only 15% of the children were able to complete the three trials necessary for a valid test within 20 minutes. Even if the acceptability criteria were modified to two trials, 40% of the children were not able to complete the test within 20 minutes. Success rate was reported to increase significantly with age.[155a] In older children, success rate between 70% and 91% was achieved.[155b] To relax the children and divert their attention from the test, they are usually allowed to watch movies during the testing; however, it increases the risk of a leak around the mouthpiece, and their respiratory rate can also increase if they get too excited about the movie, or it also invalidates the test if they are making noises (e.g., singing) during the test; therefore the movie has to be selected wisely.

Many attempts have been made to decrease the length of the measurements and hence increase the feasibility of the test in young children.[156] New end points of the test have been suggested and examined, such as increasing the end-concentration level of the test gas from 1/40 to 1/20 or stopping the test after a certain number of turnovers such as 6. However, it was shown that these modifications might not influence the specificity of the test (i.e., the discrimination between healthy and diseased study groups remained unchanged) but decrease the sensitivity (i.e., the small differences such as the effect of a treatment disappeared).[156]

Also, reading LCI at an end-tidal concentration of 5% (instead of 2.5%) did not increase the success rate significantly in children and young adults.[155b] In has also been suggested that two measurements can be accepted if they are reproducible (FRC within 10%) as this was shown to have minimal or no effect on the results of the test.

To further increase the feasibility of the test in preschool-age children, a facemask can be used during the test; however, the effect of the different surfaces (of the mouthpiece and the facemask) on the outcome measures of MBW has not been established yet. The use of facemask increases the dead space by a variable amount and it should be corrected for as much as possible in the settings. When a facemask is used, it may be difficult to establish whether the child is breathing through the nose or the mouth. It has also been suggested that the pathway of the breathing (nasal vs. oral) can affect the number of turnovers required for the washout; hence it affects the value of LCI.

One of the main limitations of MBW is the requirement of a stable breathing pattern, which is difficult to achieve in both infants and preschool-age children. Since the calculation of the main outcome measure, LCI, is calculated based on the assumption of a stable FRC and tidal volume throughout the test, any variability in the breathing pattern can make the results of the test unreliable. Furthermore, sighs are frequently present as part of the normal breathing pattern in infants, which can invalidate the test especially if they occur during the washout phase. In this case a new test should be considered.

Further limitations of MBW are the effects of different gases, measurement methods, and algorithms of data analysis that vary not only between commercial devices but also between different hardware and software versions of one given device.[157] The data collected with different gases or with different equipment are not comparable and only reference data collected with the same device, gas, and method can be used for any comparison. This also makes the interpretation of longitudinal studies difficult, as the results from an SF_6 washout in infants cannot be directly compared with that from a N_2 washout in the same children later in life. Different software algorithms (e.g., the reading of the results at the end of expiration or inspiration, the end-point of the test) also change the results of the test[157]; therefore the standardization of the test is of utmost importance. An ATS/ERS working group has been established to review these issues and standardize the test in preschool-age children. Infant and preschool-age specific acceptability criteria would significantly improve the clinical utility of MBW.

Potential Clinical Applications in Infants and Children

Since, theoretically, MBW can be performed during tidal breathing in any age group, its application has great potential in the follow-up of chronic respiratory disorders, or early detection of lung disease, that are expected to influence the gas mixing capacity of the respiratory system.

In research studies that aimed to investigate the respiratory health in early life, MBW was performed in both spontaneously breathing and ventilated infants, and most of these studies have focused on the effect of preterm birth on ventilation inhomogeneity (Figs. 11.32 and 11.34).[158–163] As a

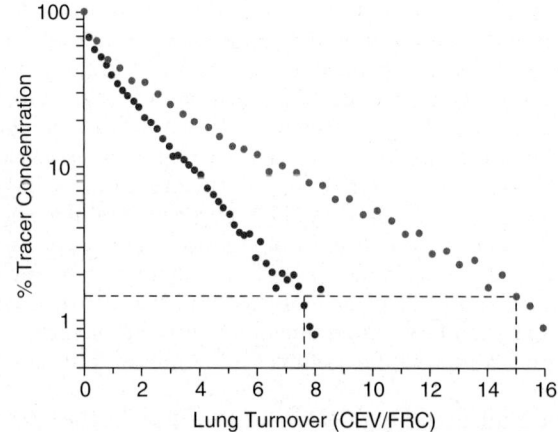

Fig. 11.34 Tracer concentration as function of lung turnover: Representative graphs of fall in normalized tracer concentration during MBWSF6 washout in term infant *(red circle)* and preterm infant (28 w PMA) at 10 weeks of postnatal age *(blue circle)*, demonstrating prolonged tail associated with increased ventilation inhomogeneity. *Dotted lines* show number of turnovers required to reduce tracer gas to 2% of initial tracer concentration (equivalent to lung clearance index, LCI). *CEV,* Cumulative expired volume; *FRC,* functional residual capacity. (Pillow JJ, Frerichs I, Stocks J. Lung function tests in neonates and infants with chronic lung disease: global and regional ventilation inhomogeneity. *Pediatr Pulmonol.* 2006;41(2):105-121.)

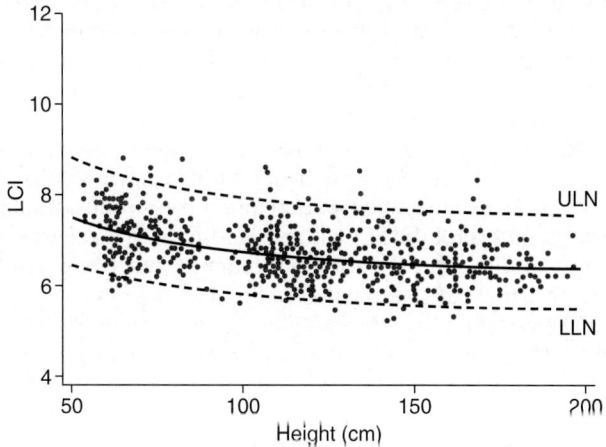

Fig. 11.35 Lung clearance index (LCI) from infancy to 19 years of age. The solid line denotes the predicted (50th centile) LCI for height and the dashed lines denote the upper limit of normal (ULN; 97.5th centile) and lower limit of normal (LLN; 2.5th centile). (Lum S, Stocks J, Stanojevic S, et al. Age and height dependence of lung clearance index and functional residual capacity. *Eur Respir J.* 2013;41(6):1371-1377.)

summary of these studies, preterm babies had reduced ventilation homogeneity[158–163] which improved after the administration of surfactant.[162,163] In healthy neonates and young infants, the degree of ventilation inhomogeneity (i.e., the value of LCI) is highly dependent on the age when LCI is measured, and this makes the evaluation of these tests more difficult. Generally, LCI shows an age-dependent decrease in the first 2 years of life with the highest being in the first days of life (Fig. 11.35),[17] and after the toddler years, the value of LCI plateaus throughout life (until elderly when it starts to increase again). It warrants further investigation whether the age-dependence of LCI in the early years reflects less homogeneous ventilation in infancy, lung development with ongoing alveolarization, or merely the switch between primarily nasal and oral breathing. Note here that although LCI seems to be independent of age, height, and sex between 2 years of age and adulthood, most of the other outcome measures are strongly affected by age. Therefore—similarly to other lung function tests—z-scores should be established for both infants and children, and the presentation of raw data at any age group should be reviewed carefully. Short- and long-term reproducibility of LCI has recently been established and 15% change in LCI was defined as clinically relevant change in preschool-aged children.[163a] In infants and older children reproducibility also requires further research to improve the usefulness of LCI to track respiratory disease.

The clinical utility of MBW in infants is further limited due to the variability of indices reported in the literature, which can be explained by the home- or custom-made devices used exclusively until very recently. The data reported in these studies are therefore not comparable; hopefully this problem will disappear with the introduction of commercially available devices, standard operating procedures, and large datasets from healthy subjects.

The interpretation of "normal" or "high" LCI values also requires careful consideration, as it has been shown that a normal LCI value does not always reflect a lack of ventilation inhomogeneity, especially in infants. Since MBW only measures the ventilation of the lung units that are in direct communication with the airway opening at the time of the measurement, if there is atelectasis or hyperinflation with air trapping, LCI can still be normal. It is also important to note that in many research studies infants have been sedated for the MBW test, which can also cause atelectasis and air trapping during the test and, hence, false negative results on ventilation inhomogeneity. Therefore it is of utmost importance to interpret the LCI values together with measures of lung volume, clinical data, and imaging (whenever available). Normal LCI values with low FRC can reflect atelectasis, while a normal LCI with high FRC can be a result of airway obstruction with hyperinflation. Although MBW has been shown to have some potential in the detection of airway obstruction, to date no evidence supports the clinical use of this technique in recurrent wheezers or young asthmatics.

One of the main clinical potentials of MBW in both infants and preschool-age children is the early detection of respiratory abnormalities related to CF. Several research studies and clinical observations have suggested that preschool-age children with CF have normal spirometry even when structural alterations in their lungs are already present on the CT scan.[50] The assessment of these early alterations and their longitudinal changes with a technique that does not involve radiation would be of utmost importance for pediatric respiratory physicians. Although early intervention would significantly improve the life expectancy and quality of life of children with CF, it remains difficult to find an objective, sensitive, and specific outcome measure that might be suitable to assess the response to therapeutic interventions. Recent studies have reported promising results in both preschool- and school-age children with CF (Fig. 11.36),[106,164–169] and some of these results were further validated with imaging techniques.[165–168] Therefore LCI was suggested as a potential outcome measure for clinical trials of therapies for CF in young children[51,170] and the first studies have already been

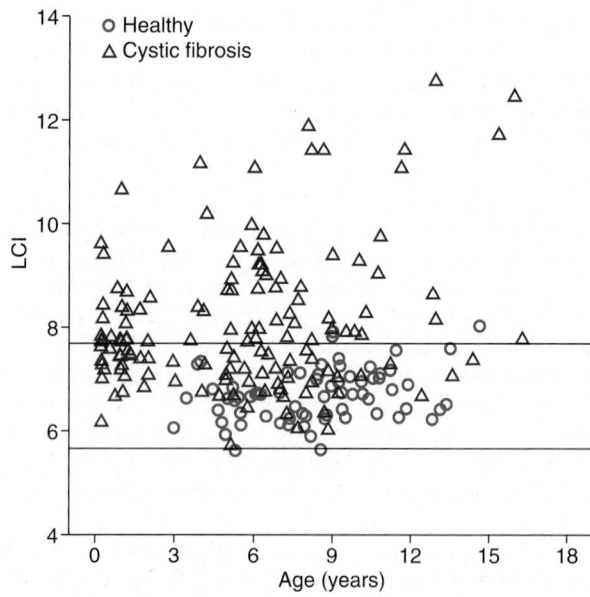

Fig. 11.36 Lung clearance index (LCI) plotted against age for healthy control children (*circles*) and children with cystic fibrosis (*triangles*). Horizontal lines indicate the upper (7.7) and lower (5.7) limits of normal for LCI. (Ramsey KA, Rosenow T, Turkovic L, et al. Lung Clearance Index and structural lung disease on computed tomography in early cystic fibrosis. *Am J Respir Crit Care Med.* 2016;193(1):60-67.)

set up worldwide. Unfortunately, the results remain less straightforward in infants, since LCI is less discriminative between healthy infants and those with CF, and its value seems to be insensitive to early structural abnormalities detected on the CT scan.[165]

Although MBW shows great potential in the detection and longitudinal follow-up of early lung disease, as a consequence of the discussed limitations in infants and preschool-age children, the technique requires further validation and standardization before it is introduced into everyday clinical practice.

References

Access the reference list online at ExpertConsult.com.

Suggested Reading

American Thoracic Society; European Respiratory Society. ATS/ERS statement: raised volume forced expirations in infants. Guidelines for Current Practice. *Am J Respir Crit Care Med.* 2005;172:1463–1471.

Bates JH, Irvin CG, Farré R, et al. Oscillation mechanics of the respiratory system. *Compr Physiol.* 2011;1:1233–1272.

Beydon N, Davis SD, Lombardi E, et al. An official American Thoracic Society/European Respiratory Society statement: pulmonary function testing in preschool children. *Am J Respir Crit Care Med.* 2007;175:1304–1345.

Bisgaard H, Nielsen KG. Plethysmographic measurements of specific airway resistance in young children. *Chest.* 2005;128:355–362.

Busi LE, Restuccia S, Tourres R, et al. Assessing bronchodilator response in preschool children using spirometry. *Thorax.* 2017;72(4):367–372.

Calogero C, Simpson SJ, Lombardi E, et al. Respiratory impedance and bronchodilator responsiveness in healthy children aged 2–13 years. *Pediatr Pulmonol.* 2013;48:707–715.

Cournand A, Baldwin ED, Darling RC, et al. Studies on intrapulmonary mixture of gases. IV. The significance of the pulmonary emptying rate and a simplified open circuit measurement of residual air. *J Clin Invest.* 1941;20:681–689.

Czövek D, Shackleton C, Hantos Z, et al. Tidal changes in respiratory resistance are sensitive indicators of airway obstruction in children. *Thorax.* 2016;71:907–915.

DuBois AB, Botelho SY, Comroe JH. A rapid plethysmographic method for measuring thoracic gas volume: a comparison with a nitrogen washout method for measuring functional residual capacity in normal subjects. *J Clin Invest*. 1956;35:322–326.

DuBois AB, Brody AW, Lewis DH, et al. Oscillation mechanics of lungs and chest in man. *J Appl Physiol*. 1956;8:587–594.

Frey U, Stocks J, Coates A, et al. Specifications for equipment used for infant pulmonary function testing. ERS/ATS task force on standards for infant respiratory function testing. European Respiratory Society/American Thoracic Society. *Eur Respir J*. 2000;16:731–740.

Gappa M, Colin AA, Goetz I, et al. Passive respiratory mechanics: the occlusion technique. *Eur Respir J*. 2001;17:141–148.

Graham BL, Brusasco V, Burgos F, et al. 2017 ERS/ATS standards for single-breath carbon monoxide uptake in the lung. *Eur Respir J*. 2017;49:1600016.

Kirkby J, Stanojevic S, Welsh L, et al. Reference equations for specific airway resistance in children: the Asthma UK initiative. *Eur Respir J*. 2010; 36:622–629.

Lowe L, Murray CS, Custovic A, et al. Specific airway resistance in 3-year-old children: a prospective cohort study. *Lancet*. 2002;359:1904–1908.

Lum S, Bountziouka V, Wade A, et al. New reference ranges for interpreting forced expiratory manoeuvres in infants and implications for clinical interpretation: a multicentre collaboration. *Thorax*. 2016;71:276–283.

Lum S, Stocks J, Stanojevic S, et al. Age and height dependence of lung clearance index and functional residual capacity. *Eur Respir J*. 2013; 41:1371–1377.

Mele L, Sly PD, Calogero C, et al. Assessment and validation of bronchodilation using the interrupter technique in preschool children. *Pediatr Pulmonol*. 2010;45:633–638.

Merkus PJ, Stocks J, Beydon N, et al. Reference ranges for interrupter resistance technique: the Asthma UK Initiative. *Eur Respir J*. 2010;36:157–163.

Ramsey KA, Rosenow T, Turkovic L, et al. Lung clearance index and structural lung disease on computed tomography in early cystic fibrosis. *Am J Respir Crit Care Med*. 2016;193:60–67.

Robinson PD, Latzin P, Verbanck S, et al. Consensus statement for inert gas washout measurement using multiple- and single-breath tests. *Eur Respir J*. 2013;41:507–522.

Rosenfeld M, Allen J, Arets BH, et al. An official American Thoracic Society workshop report: optimal lung function tests for monitoring cystic fibrosis, bronchopulmonary dysplasia, and recurrent wheezing in children less than 6 years of age. *Ann Am Thorac Soc*. 2013;10:S1–S11.

Sly PD, Tepper R, Henschenet M, et al. Tidal forced expirations. *Eur Respir J*. 2000;16:741–748.

Stanojevic S, Graham BL, Cooper BG, et al. Official ERS technical standards: Global Lung Function Initiative reference values for the carbon monoxide transfer factor for Caucasians. *Eur Respir J*. 2017;50:1700010.

Stocks J, Godfrey S, Beardsmore C, et al. Plethysmographic measurements of lung volume and airway resistance. *Eur Respir J*. 2001;17:302–312.

Subbarao P, Milla C, Aurora P, et al. Multiple-breath washout as a lung function test in cystic fibrosis: a cystic fibrosis foundation workshop report. *Ann Am Thorac Soc*. 2015;12:932–939.

van der Gugten AC, Uiterwaal CSPM, van Putte-Katier N, et al. Reduced neonatal lung function and wheezing illnesses during the first 5 years of life. *Eur Respir J*. 2013;42:107–115.

Vilozni D, Efrati O, Hakim F, et al. FRC measurements using body plethysmography in young children. *Pediatr Pulmonol*. 2009;44:885–891.

12 Exercise and Lung Function in Child Health and Disease

DAN M. COOPER, MD, RONEN BAR-YOSEPH, MD, J. TOD OLIN, MD, MSCS, and
SHLOMIT RADOM-AIZIK, PhD

The Biological Importance of Physical Activity in the Growing Child

Exercise in children and adolescents is not merely play, but is an essential component of growth and development.[1–3] Children are among the most spontaneously physically active human beings.[4] It is not surprising that habitual physical activity (HPA) is a major determinant of health across the lifespan and health-related quality of life in both healthy children and in children with chronic diseases.[5–8] Despite this essential biologic role for HPA, children have not been spared the relentless reduction in levels of physical activity (PA) that is creating a crisis in health care in our nation and throughout the world.[9] Recognition of the enormous morbidity and cost of physical inactivity-related diseases, such as atherosclerosis, type 2 diabetes, and osteoporosis,[10–12] along with the deleterious consequences of physical inactivity and deconditioning in pediatric respiratory diseases like asthma and cystic fibrosis (CF), has spurred new policy initiatives targeting preventive medicine early in life. The concept of pediatric origins of adult health and disease is gaining scientific merit (e.g., chronic obstructive pulmonary disease [COPD]),[13–17] highlighting the need to transform existing notions of how to evaluate health in a growing child. A physically inactive child may have no symptoms of disease, but evidence of deterioration in vascular health may already be present.[18–20] As we move into the era of population health management and precision medicine,[21] the notion of what it means to be a healthy child must change and include robust metrics of physical fitness.

As noted, the deleterious health effects of physical inactivity and poor fitness are exacerbated in children with chronic disease and/or disabilities[22–27] or with environmental-lifestyle conditions like obesity.[28] Children with previously fatal diseases or conditions (e.g., CF, prematurity, acute lymphocytic leukemia) are living longer due to remarkable advances in research and care, but are often unable to achieve levels of PA and fitness associated with health benefits in otherwise healthy children.[27,29–31] Not surprisingly, the *healthspan* (the period of life free from serious chronic diseases and disability[32]) of children with chronic diseases is threatened not only by the underlying disease but by the compounding effects of insufficient PA and sedentary behavior.[33–37] Increasing PA and fitness is feasible, but has proven quite challenging to implement in a systematic manner.[38] Once a pattern of physical inactivity and a sedentary lifestyle is established, a vicious cycle ensues (Fig. 12.1), in which constraints on PA harm immediate health and contribute to lifelong health impairment ranging from cardiovascular and metabolic disease to osteoporosis.[1,39–43] Exactly what constitutes ideal physical fitness in a child with a chronic condition remains unknown. Finding beneficial levels of PA in children with chronic disease or disability is challenging because the optimal range of exercise is much narrower than in a healthy child (Fig. 12.2).

Change in policy and practice, and the resources necessary to achieve such change, must increasingly be fueled by translational scientific evidence.[44] Despite the broad recognition that many children in the United States (and throughout the world) no longer engage in healthy levels of PA,[45] defining what the level of optimal PA should be remains quite vague. For example, in a recent study of 182, 9–11-year-olds, Füssenich and coworkers[46] noted, *"there were no differences between CCVR [composite cardiovascular risk score] of children who undertook 60 min MVPA [moderate to vigorous physical activity] per day in accordance with WHO recommendations, and those who did not. This implies that current recommendations may be an underestimation of the PA [physical activity] necessary to reduce clustered CVD risk. A gender difference between the CVD risk in active and inactive children raises the possibility that gender specific guidelines may be needed, although much work is needed to determine if these differences are a result of gender specific responses to PA or sex differences in PA level.... Taken together these findings suggest that in order to reduce CVD risk, the current guidelines should be updated...."*

From the Playground to the Bench to the Physician's Office

INTEGRATING LABORATORY CARDIOPULMONARY EXERCISE TESTING AND FIELD ASSESSMENTS OF PHYSICAL FITNESS

Although it might seem intuitive that physically active children and adolescents score well in cardiopulmonary exercise testing (CPET), quantifying the mechanistic relationship between these two components of physical fitness and activity in children and adolescents has proven to be challenging. Only weak correlations between HPA and CPET are consistently found[47,48]; HPA and CPET are not interchangeable physical fitness–associated biomarkers. Traditional CPET focuses on measuring maximal efforts, but as we and others have shown, high-intensity PA occurs relatively infrequently in real lives of children and adolescents[49–51]; thus, even high levels of HPA may not be evident in traditional CPET. Until recently, there has been little standardization of the methodologies used to assess HPA in children, which include a myriad of tools and technologies such as questionnaires, activity logs, HR monitoring, and wearable accelerometers.[52–57] Most practicing primary care child health care providers perceive the overall levels of and participation in daily HPA as a more important indicator of child health than the results of CPET *per se* (if only because formal education in exercise physiology and CPET is lacking in medical school[58] or most residency programs).

Schools and communities are currently investing substantial resources in physical fitness assessments in children; such tests are **mandated** in 46 of 50 states in the fifth, seventh, and ninth grades. In California, testing is done *"to help students in starting life-long habits of regular physical activity."*[59] The school-based tests typically used are the 20 m shuttle run or the mile run. The raw data from these tests are entered into standardized equations to estimate maximal oxygen uptake ($\dot{V}O_{2max}$), but none of the data become part of the child's medical record.

WHAT CAN WE LEARN FROM CARDIOPULMONARY EXERCISE TESTING (Fig. 12.3)

Consider, for example, the important acts of fleeing from a predator or, in more modern terms, running to avoid an oncoming car. When sudden and large increases in metabolic demand are imposed by PA, the whole organism can

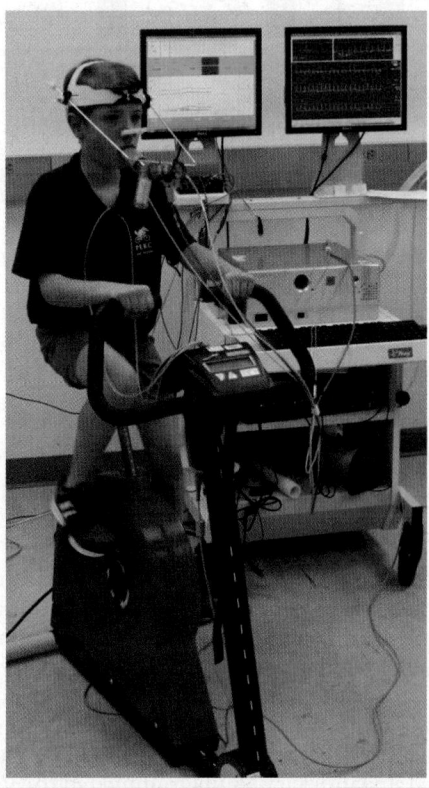

Fig. 12.3 Eight-year-old boy performing a cardiopulmonary exercise testing in a laboratory setting. Note the cycle ergometer that is designated for young children. Nose clip and mouth piece enable accurate gas exchange measurement during the exercise test.

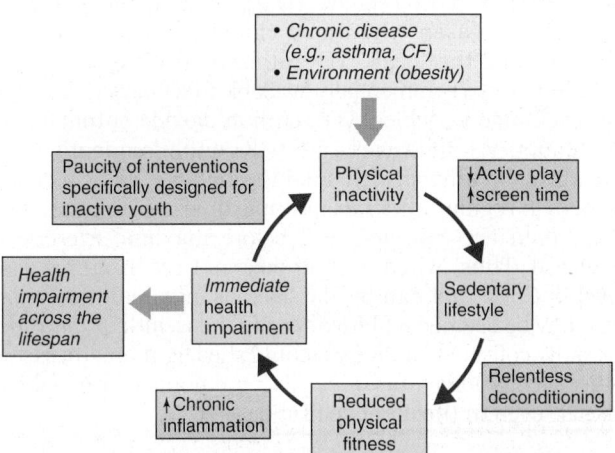

Fig. 12.1 Physical inactivity in childhood, be it imposed by environmental factors or chronic diseases or conditions, leads to a vicious cycle that impairs health across the lifespan. *CF,* Cystic fibrosis.

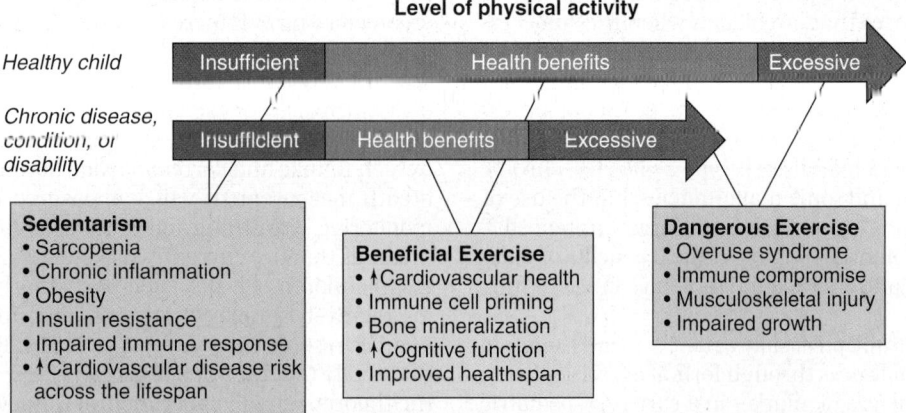

Fig. 12.2 Health benefits of exercise are determined, in part, by the energy expenditure associated with physical activity. Both too much (excessive) and too little (sedentarism) exercise can impair health. As shown, the range of healthy exercise is narrower in the child with chronic disease or disability. Formal cardiopulmonary exercise testing and field assessments of physical activity can be translated into a well-informed "exercise prescription" for the child with respiratory, cardiovascular, or metabolic diseases. The prescription must specify the mode, frequency, duration, and intensity of exercise that can benefit health during critical periods of growth.

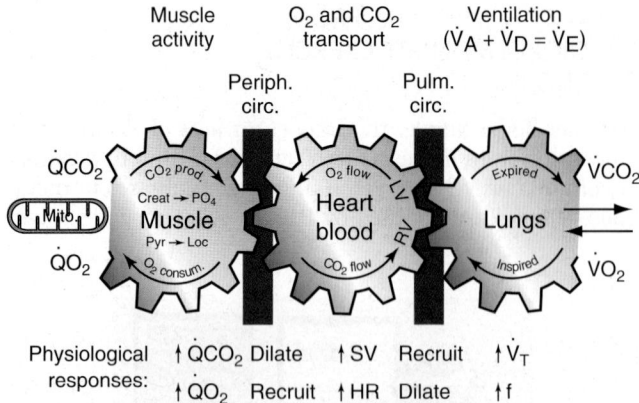

Fig. 12.4 Wasserman gears. The physiologic mechanisms that link respiration at the cellular and whole-body levels made famous by Karlman Wasserman in this depiction of interlocking gears. *HR,* Heart rate; *SV,* stroke volume.

successfully function only by means of an integrated response among several organ systems. At the very onset of exercise, before there has been sufficient time for an in increase in environmental oxygen uptake, the healthy human must have sufficient stores of oxygen, high-energy phosphates, nonaerobic metabolic capability, and supplies of substrate to perform significant amounts of PA. As exercise proceeds, cardiac output increases and blood flow is diverted to the working muscles without compromising the critical flow of oxygen and glucose to the brain.

Ventilation and pulmonary blood flow must increase to precisely match the energy demand of the working muscles so that homeostasis for $PaCO_2$ and pH are maintained. There must be sufficient increase in substrate availability (glucose, fat, protein) but without depleting the peripheral blood glucose stores. And finally, the heat produced during exercise must be dissipated so that homeostasis for body temperature is maintained. In summary, as diagrammed in the late 1960s by Wasserman and coworkers,[60] events at the cell are closely linked to events at the heart and lungs (Fig. 12.4).

Physical fitness and exercise biomarkers are promising "disease-agnostic" tools for a remarkably wide range of health conditions, ranging from asthma in children to COPD in the elderly.[61–64] Exercise testing provides insight into integrated physiological responses that are hidden when the subject is at rest. Despite this promise, exercise-related outcome variables are used far more commonly in the research laboratory than in clinical trials or clinical practice. Poor fitness and low PA are major causes of morbidity and mortality from obesity, cardiovascular disease, type 2 diabetes, chronic respiratory diseases, and some malignancies, but the use of exercise biomarkers in clinical trials is still largely untapped.[65] Consequently, the potential tangible clinical benefits of exercise as a diagnostic and therapeutic tool have failed to fully materialize.

Children are naturally physically active,[66,67] and therefore quantifying physical fitness through formal exercise testing is increasingly useful as a biomarker in a variety of pediatric conditions such as congenital heart disease, sickle cell anemia, athletic training, and cerebral palsy.[68–72] Physiological parameters obtained at maximal or peak exercise (most notably, maximal oxygen uptake-$\dot{V}O_{2max}$ or peak $\dot{V}O_2$) remain the most widely used type of exercise laboratory test in pediatric

clinical trials and research. As outlined below, true plateaus or reductions in oxygen uptake despite increasing work rate (WR), the hallmark of $\dot{V}O_{2max}$, occur only in a minority of children. CPET is minimally invasive, rendering it suitable for studies in children. CPET is typically performed with cycle ergometers or treadmills, in which the work input increases progressively until the child reaches the limit of his or her tolerance.

Maximal exercise tests are, by definition, highly dependent on the willingness of each child to continue exercise at relatively high WRs when dyspnea, muscle fatigue, and other stress sensations are commonly experienced. Not surprisingly, the "cheerleading" abilities of the laboratory personnel contribute to the achievement of a true maximal response in CPET. Despite its proven clinical and research utility, $\dot{V}O_{2max}$, as noted, only occurs in a minority of exercise tests even in otherwise healthy children and maybe less so in children with chronic disease or disability. For example, in a recent large study of children and adolescents (mean age 12.3 years old) who had undergone the Fontan correction for congenital heart disease during childhood, only 166 of 411 patients (40%) achieved an acceptable $\dot{V}O_{2max}$ using current criteria.[73] This is one reason why many clinicians and researchers choose to use the "peak" $\dot{V}O_2$ rather than $\dot{V}O_{2max}$.

Most modern commercially available CPET devices measure gas exchange variables ($\dot{V}O_2$, carbon dioxide output-$\dot{V}CO_2$, ventilation-$\dot{V}_E$) and heart rate (HR) quite frequently (e.g., breath-by-breath or with mixing chamber gas collection devices in regular intervals multiple times per minute), and these data are collected well before maximal exercise is achieved. Thus, when a child does not reach an exercise level in CPET that can be classified as maximal, the whole test may be deemed a failure despite the wealth of data successfully collected. Such data could shed light on fitness and other specific indicators of cardiac, pulmonary, or metabolic disease even in the absence of a true $\dot{V}O_{2max}$.

Physiologic Response to Progressive Exercise Testing

A ramp protocol is often used in CPET in adults and children, and is so named because exercise is performed on a cycle ergometer and WR increases linearly in a ramp-type pattern until the participant reaches the limit of his or her tolerance (Fig. 12.5). Gas exchange is typically measured with the use of mouthpieces or facemasks and the many technological advances made over the past several decades in assessing oxygen uptake and carbon dioxide output permit breath-by-breath measurement. HR is measured using standardized monitoring. Armstrong and Fawkner summarized noninvasive methods that are currently used to assess exercise biomarkers in children.[74] It has been particularly useful in developing relatively simple equations to describe the gas exchange and HR responses to the progressive WR exercise protocols that typify CPET. Whipp and coworkers[75] elegantly outlined the theoretical and experimental framework that predicted and demonstrated the largely linear response of $\dot{V}O_2$ to the steady increase in WR during ramp exercise protocols. Their model assumed a system with first-order linear dynamics, an assumption that is accurate for low-intensity exercise. A number of studies have attempted to determine the value

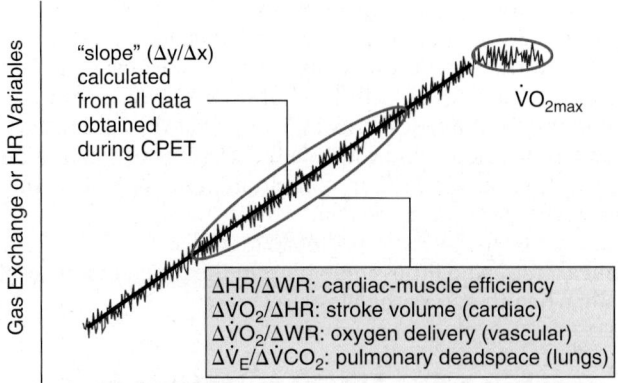

Fig. 12.5 A schematic generalization of the determination of slopes of key cardiopulmonary exercise testing (CPET) variables from a ramp-type, cycle ergometry, progressive exercise protocol. The classic CPET metric, peak or $\dot{V}O_{2max}$ is shown as the plateau at the end of the test. Unlike the peak $\dot{V}O_2$ or $\dot{V}O_{2max}$, which rely on a relatively small set of data obtained during very heavy exercise, the slopes are derived from a much larger set of data obtained throughout the exercise protocol. As shown, the slopes can serve as noninvasive biomarkers of health and disease providing insights and biomarkers of respiratory and cardiovascular physiology. *HR*, Heart rate.

of τ (the time constant for the first-order linear equation) for gas exchange and HR variables in children.[76,77] Factors such as maturational status and the presence of disease and obesity appear to play a role.[26,78] After the initial minutes of the ramp test, $\dot{V}O_2$ approaches a linear increase as the ramp progresses. We do recognize that system dynamics become more complex when exercise is performed at high intensities.[79]

The anaerobic threshold (AT, also referred to as the "lactate threshold") indicates the point at which excess lactic acid production leads to increases in circulating lactate concentrations and acidosis. Although the mechanism of the AT is not completely clear, one possibility is that at some point during exercise, oxygen supply to the working muscles is inadequate and anaerobic metabolism is necessary to supply the energy requirements of physical work. The AT can be measured directly from blood samples taken during exercise. The onset of anaerobic metabolism is affected by such factors as anemia and the presence of peripheral vascular disease. The ramp protocol and breath-by-breath analysis of gas exchange allow a noninvasive measurement of the ventilatory threshold (a synonym for AT when gas exchange data is used) and $\dot{V}O_{2max}$ in a single exercise test.[75,80] Measuring the AT in children is a potential biomarker of both respiratory and cardiovascular disease,[81] first, because the test is noninvasive, and second, because the protocol is both brief and stimulating to the young child whose sense of competition is high but whose attention span is low. Additional work is needed to examine the maturation of the kinetics of CPET variables during growth and maturation.

The dynamic relationships among gas exchange and HR variables during progressive CPET are promising tools for evaluating fitness in healthy children or in children with chronic disease and disability.[82] The relationship between $\dot{V}_E$ and $\dot{V}CO_2$ is given by a modification of the alveolar gas equation:

$$\dot{V}_E = [863 \times PaCO_2^{-1} \times (1 - V_D/V_T)^{-1}] \times \dot{V}CO_2$$

where $\dot{V}_E$ is ventilation, $\dot{V}CO_2$ is CO_2 production, $PaCO_2$ is arterial CO_2 tension, and V_D/V_T is deadspace to tidal volume ratio. As can be seen, the factors affecting the relationship between $\dot{V}_E$ and $\dot{V}CO_2$ will be the $PaCO_2$ and the V_D/V_T. The equation implies that as the regulated level of PCO_2 decreases, more ventilation will be required for a given increase in $\dot{V}CO_2$.

Because ventilation and CO_2 production during exercise are determined in large measure by muscle mass (highly related to body mass), $\Delta\dot{V}_E/\Delta\dot{V}CO_2$ should be a body-size–independent CPET variable. However, others and we have noted a weak but significant correlation between $\Delta\dot{V}_E/\Delta\dot{V}CO_2$ and both total body mass (TBM) and lean body mass (LBM). As has been described in greater detail earlier,[83] analysis of the alveolar gas equation indicates that $\Delta\dot{V}_E/\Delta\dot{V}CO_2$ is determined by ventilatory factors such as physiological deadspace, CO_2 storage capacity, and the $PaCO_2$ set point (the concentration of CO_2 that is homeostatically maintained despite changes in CO_2 production). Maturation of each of these factors is reflected by the higher values of the slope in younger children compared with adolescents.[83]

$\Delta\dot{V}_E/\Delta\dot{V}CO_2$ is abnormal in children with chronic lung diseases like CF, in which ventilatory deadspace is known to be increased,[27] and was recently found to be an independent predictor of mortality in adult patients with chronic obstructive pulmonary disease undergoing surgery for nonsmall-cell lung cancer.[84] Thus, analysis of $\Delta\dot{V}_E/\Delta\dot{V}CO_2$ in children with chronic lung diseases may provide specific information about lung function not readily determined from maximal exercise values alone.

The Challenge of Scaling Cardiopulmonary Exercise Testing to Body Mass in Children and Adolescents and the Special Case of Obesity

Physical fitness and PA are essential components in both the diagnosis and treatment of the overweight and obese child and adolescent.[85–87] Despite this, evidence-based guidelines do not yet exist on how best to assess and track physical fitness in this population. Recently, Hansen and coworkers[88] reviewed a number of studies focused on assessing fitness from CPET in obese adolescents. They were unable to find consensus among these studies, and reached the following conclusion: *"Whether cardiopulmonary anomalies during maximal exercise testing would occur in obese adolescents remains uncertain. Studies are therefore warranted to examine the cardiopulmonary response during maximal exercise testing in obese adolescents."*

Measuring fitness in children (whether normal weight, overweight, or obese) is complicated because muscle and fat mass and hormonal regulation of metabolism and growth change rapidly in children and adolescents.[89–91] Consequently, any physiological variable derived from CPET must be scaled to some index of body size and maturational status. In the obese child, useful scaling of CPET variables is further confounded because body fat (virtually metabolically inactive during exercise) may obscure the effect of the metabolically active muscle tissue when CPET is normalized to body mass.

As noted, maximal exercise tests are highly dependent on the willingness of each child to continue exercise at relatively high WRs. In some cases, investigators purposefully do not exhort obese children during progressive exercise testing. For example, Salvadego and coworkers[92] studied exercise in a group of obese, otherwise healthy adolescents and stopped exercise when the participant achieved a HR of 180 bpm. The authors noted, *"A true maximal test was not performed to avoid the cardiovascular risks associated with maximal exercise in obese subjects."* Further, several studies suggest that obese children and adolescents perceive high-intensity exercise differently than normal-weight controls.[93,94] It is not surprising that the plateau in oxygen uptake, the classical physiologic proof that $\dot{V}O_{2max}$ had been reached, is found in relatively small proportions of normal-weight or obese children and adolescents.[95]

The data from our earlier study of CPET slopes in children and adolescents with body mass index (BMI) below the 85th percentile showed that many of these variables, like peak or maximal $\dot{V}O_2$, were highly correlated with muscle mass.[82] We recently found that both CPET submaximal values and peak $\dot{V}O_2$ were lower in high-BMI adolescents (BMI >95th percentile). We observed this deficiency even after referencing CPET values to LBM. The mechanisms for reduced both peak *and* submaximal CPET results are not entirely clear. Obese children may not push themselves as hard as normal-weight children in the high-intensity range of exercise that typifies peak or maximal $\dot{V}O_2$. Shim and coworkers[94] in obese children with asthma and Marinov and coworkers[96] in otherwise healthy obese children, for example, noted greater sense of breathlessness at high WRs than in normal-BMI children. Salvadego and coworkers[97] showed in a recent elegant study that obese adolescents improved their rate of perceived exertion during high-intensity exercise by reducing the work of breathing (using Heliox).

Development of Physiological Responses to Exercise in Children and Adolescents and Predicting Cardiopulmonary Health Across the Lifespan

With respect to exercise and PA, children are not simply miniature adults.[98] When normalized to body size, strength is lower in children,[99] as is the magnitude of the physiologic response to chronic exercise training (both resistance and aerobic).[100,101] Children use relatively more oxygen than adults for high-intensity exercise.[102] Gas exchange and HR response kinetics are also different in children (Fig. 12.6),[83,103–106] as are metabolic responses such as lactate concentrations,[107] high-energy intramuscular phosphate dynamics (using ^{31}P-MR spectroscopy[108]), and CO_2 storage capacity.[109] Recent work on the genomic responses to exercise in children shows differences in the pattern of leukocyte gene expression between early- and late-pubertal girls.[110] The mechanisms that link the distinct processes of growth and adaptation to exercise are largely unknown.

A number of pioneering, thoughtfully designed, long-term studies now confirm that cardiovascular disease risk factors begin in youth, track into symptomatic atherosclerosis in adulthood, and are, fortunately, modifiable (e.g., the Muscatine Study,[111] the Young Finns Study,[112] the Bogalusa Heart Study,[113] the CARDIA study,[114] and Pathobiological Determinants of Atherosclerosis in Youth [PDAY][115]). Efforts to develop childhood- and youth-based preventive interventions focused on diet and PA, in combination or separately, have not met expectations. Similar work is needed to determine the long-term effects of pediatric lung disease and the role that exercise and fitness may have in the trajectory of respiratory health across the lifespan.

Searching for Normal Values in Pediatric Cardiopulmonary Exercise Testing

Resources are needed and in many cases have been mobilized to support the development of drugs and devices focused specifically on children.[116,117] Clinical investigators are increasingly aware of regulatory incentives to perform clinical trials on drugs used specifically for childhood diseases, rather than relying on adult studies. Moreover, clinical researchers understand that effective clinical trials focused on childhood disease must be accompanied by improved laboratory reference standards developed for children.

In a comprehensive review, Shaw and coworkers[118] outlined the challenges facing the development of laboratory reference values in pediatrics. Although focused primarily on blood biomarkers, the following summary provides a relevant framework for establishing normative values in pediatric CPET:

Reliable and accurate reference intervals for laboratory analyses are integral for correct interpretation of clinical laboratory test results and therefore for appropriate clinical decision making. Ideally, reference intervals should be established based on a healthy population and stratified for key covariates including age, gender, and ethnicity. However, establishing reference intervals can be challenging as it requires the collection of large numbers of samples from healthy individuals. This challenge is further augmented in pediatrics, where dynamic changes due to child growth and development markedly affect circulating levels of disease biomarkers.

Mounting literature suggests that fitness (assessed as peak $\dot{V}O_2$) can help predict morbidity and mortality in children.[119] Therefore the development of robust reference values for CPET will serve as a powerful tool in the clinician's ability to (1) identify children in whom the "exercise prescription" might be most beneficial, and (2) assess the success of exercise interventions across the child health spectrum. Of equal importance is the larger public health question of the degree to which fitness and PA levels are decreasing in children and adolescents in the United States and throughout the world and the extent to which these serious threats to health across the lifespan[120] are related to environmental, socioeconomic, and genetic/epigenetic factors. Absent the development of robust CPET normal values, we cannot answer these critically important questions. However, reference values that may be helpful for CPET in children are available.[80,82,121,122]

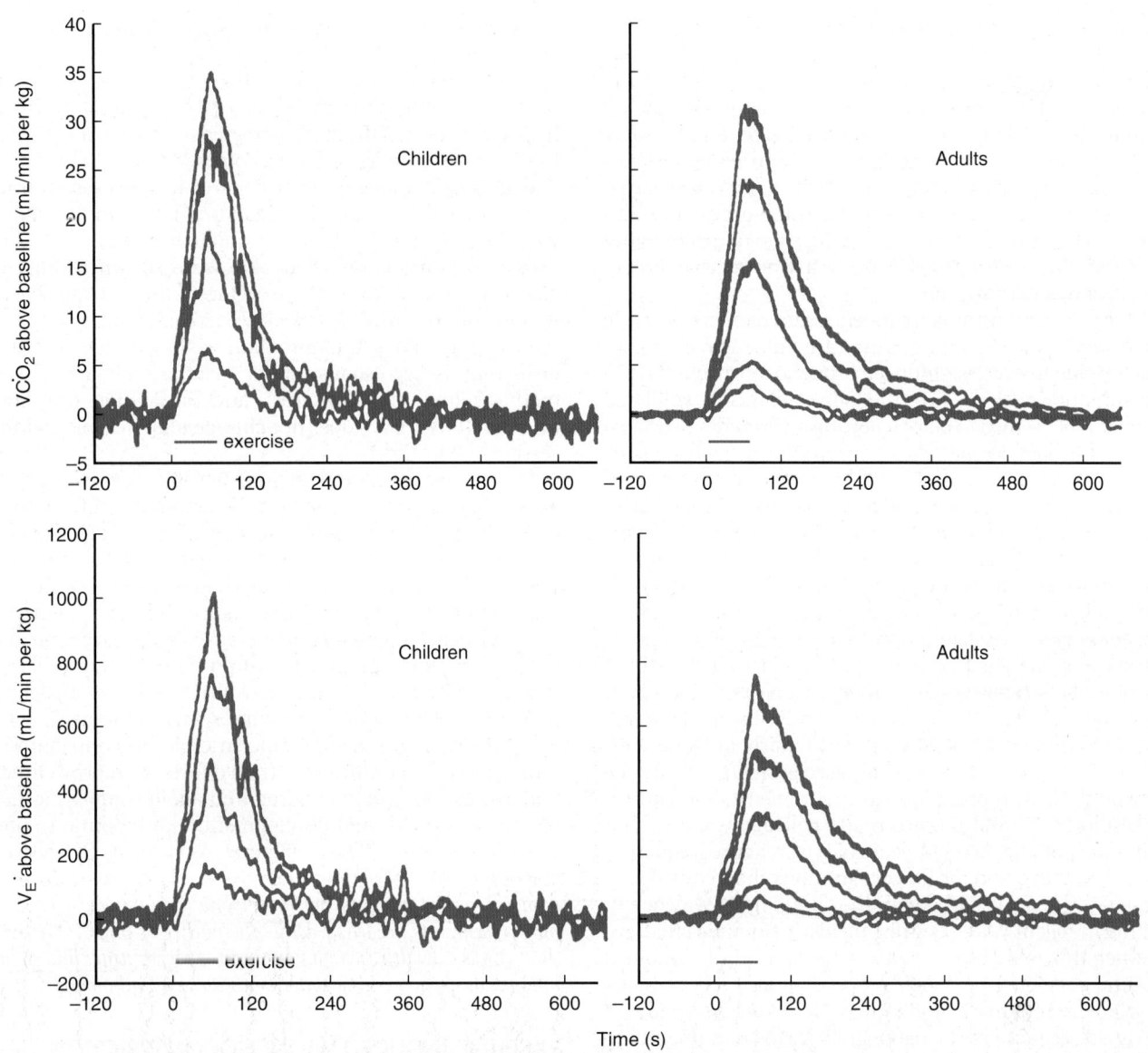

Fig. 12.6 Examples of differences in physiologic responses to exercise between children and adults. V̇CO₂ and V̇E responses to just 1-min of exercise reveal substantial differences at increasing work intensity (50% of the anaerobic or lactate threshold [AT], 80% of the AT, 75%max, 100%max, and 125%max where maximal exercise (max) was determined from a ramp test previously performed). For both V̇CO₂ *(top panel)* and V̇E, the recovery times were substantially faster in the children compared with the adults. (From Armon Y, Cooper DM, Zanconato S. Maturation of ventilatory responses to 1-minute exercise. *Pediatr Res* 1991;29(4 pt 1):362-368.)

Asthma and Exercise

THE ROLE OF EXERCISE AND PHYSICAL ACTIVITY IN ASTHMA

Despite much recent progress in understanding asthma pathophysiology and the development of new therapies, the health care use associated with asthma and the disruptions it causes to family and community life have not decreased substantially.[123] From the 1990s to the 2000s, asthma prevalence was reported to plateau or even decrease in high-income countries while, in many cases, asthma symptoms became more common.[124,125] At the same time, many low- to middle-income countries with large populations showed increases in prevalence, suggesting that the overall world burden is

increasing and nonexpensive strategies are needed to cope with the challenge.[124] Similar to patterns observed in asthma prevalence, children experience higher rates of incident asthma than adults and younger children have higher rates as compared with older children.[126]

The link between PA and asthma is strong, but remains enigmatic. PA is a "double-edged sword" for the child with asthma. On the one hand, PA and exercise is a common trigger of bronchoconstriction, occurring in as many as 90% of asthmatic children and 45% of children with allergic rhinitis.[127–129] Exercise-induced bronchospasm inhibits the ability of affected children to participate normally and perform optimally in physical activities,[128] and it is recognized as an indicator of risk for urgent medical visits.[130] On the other hand, exercise and fitness training seem to benefit asthma control and severity in many children with asthma.[131–134] As succinctly stated by Lucas and Platts-Mills,[135] "It is our belief that an exercise prescription should be part of the treatment for all cases of asthma. The real question is whether prolonged physical activity and, in particular, outdoor play of children play a role in prophylaxis against persistent wheezing. If so, the decrease in physical activity might have played a major role in recent increases in asthma prevalence and severity. The move from traditional lifestyle to urban living can be seen as the progressive loss of a lung-specific protective effect against asthma."

Critical exercise-asthma treatment issues remain enigmatic and poorly studied, ranging from rare but tragic instances of death due to exercise-induced bronchoconstriction (EIB) in asthmatic youth[136–138] to the lack of clinically validated paradigms of "return to play" following an exercise-associated asthma attack.[139] Despite the accepted clinical goal of ensuring that children with asthma fully participate in all types of exercise, physical fitness and participation in PA have been shown to be impaired in children with asthma.[140–144] Participation in school PE among children with asthma is reported to be reduced by as much as 40%,[145,146] and only 1% of adolescents with asthma and 6% of their teachers gave the correct answer on how to prevent exercise-induced asthma, emphasizing the challenge.[147] Children with asthma were less fit (10% lower $\dot{V}O_{2max}$) than their peers.[144] Moreover, Conn and coworkers[148] discovered excessive use of electronic media in children with asthma, particularly in those with activity limitation. Studies using accelerometers (a device worn on the body that can measure movement) show equivocal results,[133,149] and Lovstrom and colleagues found that asthmatic patients (10–34 years old) were more frequently physically active and for longer durations than controls.[150] These latter reports can add to the changing prevalence in asthma in recent years. For the inactive asthmatic children, whether this is a result from the perception of disability, parental restrictions,[151] or from poorly managed exercise-associated symptoms is not known. Nevertheless, whatever the causes, reduced participation in PA is an ominous finding in a child with asthma.

There are emerging data, which suggest that exercise is beneficial for asthma in terms of disease control and pathogenesis. A growing number of animal studies (such as those by Pastva and coworkers[152] and Hewitt and coworkers[153]) examined how brief exercise and exercise-training modulated subsequent lung inflammatory responses to ovalbumin (OVA) challenge in OVA-sensitized rats. An intriguing finding from Kodesh and coworkers showed that rats sensitized to OVA were subsequently more susceptible to bronchoconstriction following exercise, a nonspecific challenge.[154] These studies demonstrated a generally moderating effect of exercise on subsequent lung inflammatory responses to acute allergen and exercise challenges, specifically by decreasing nuclear factor κB (NF-κB) nuclear translocation and IκB-α phosphorylation, thereby diminishing key proinflammatory (and possible neuroadrenergic) control pathways. Aerobic training reduced leukocyte activation, reversed airway remodeling, and airway inflammation. Specifically it reversed OVA-induced eosinophil and macrophage airway migration and decreased expression of Th2 cytokines (IL-4, IL-5, IL-13), eotaxin, RANTES, chemokines (CCL5, CCL10), adhesion molecules (VCAM-1, ICAM-1), reactive oxygen and nitrogen species (GP91phox and 3-nitrotyrosine), inducible nitric oxide synthase (iNOS), and NF-κB. It also increased the expression of the antiinflammatory cytokine (IL-10).[155,156] Repeated bouts of moderate-intensity aerobic exercise improve airway hyperresponsiveness (AHR) in OVA-treated mice via a mechanism that involves β_2-adrenergic receptors.[157]

In children, studies of the benefits of PA and exercise training have yielded similar results. Lung function in children who are more physically active tend to be higher.[143] Aerobic training programs (8–16 weeks) were shown to improve disease control (Asthma Control Questionnaire) and severity (daily doses of inhaled steroids), exercise capacity ($\dot{V}O_{2max}$), reduce pulmonary inflammation (exhaled NO), decrease bronchial hyperresponsiveness (exercise challenge test/methacholine challenge test), and medication use. Lung function (FEV_1, FVC) does not change after aerobic training sessions.[131,133,158,159]

Most training sessions include aerobic exercise, and the effect of resistance training on the asthmatic child is yet to be evaluated. Bonsignore and coworkers concluded that exercise training in combination with antiinflammatory therapy might synergize to attenuate airway response to methacholine challenge in asthmatic children.[159] Furthermore, physical inactivity and increased sedentary time were found to predict childhood asthma directly and indirectly (obesity induced).[141,160] Uncontrolled asthma is associated with reduced fitness and daytime spent in intensive activity.[144] Poorly controlled asthma in children contributes to lung disease in adulthood[17]; thus efforts to improve fitness and asthma control in children and adolescents, a "critical period" of growth and development,[161] are bound to have effects on health that last a lifetime. As noted by Ploeger and coworkers,[162] "To optimize exercise prescriptions and recommendations for patients with a chronic inflammatory disease, more research is needed to define the nature of physical activity that confers health benefits without exacerbating underlying inflammatory stress associated with disease pathology."

EXERCISE-INDUCED BRONCHOCONSTRICTION

Exercise-related respiratory symptoms are underdiagnosed and undertreated in many cases and may reflect an isolated clinical condition or uncontrolled underlying asthma.[128] EIB is the acute transient airway narrowing during or after exercise.[163] EIB is defined by the American Thoracic Society (ATS) as percent fall in FEV_1 from the preexercise level of >10%–15%, with responses graded as mild, moderate, or severe (10%–25%, 25%–50%, and >50%, respectively).[163] This grading was based on measured values before the widespread use of inhaled steroids; and currently when a child performs an exercise challenge test, FEV_1 fall of ≥30% can be graded as "severe." The upper limit of postexercise fall in FEV_1 (mean ± 2 SD) in normal children was found to be 6%–8%[164] and higher values for percent fall in FEV_1 (13%–15%) have been recommended for diagnosing EIB. Protocols developed by a pioneer in the field, Simon Godfrey, suggest a threshold of FEV_1 of ≥13%.[165,166] This threshold was recommended also for preschool children.[167] Other laboratories use a threshold of FEV_1 fall of >15% from baseline when testing children to increase sensitivity of the test.[163] Fonseca-Guedes found that FEF25%–75% (postexercise fall >26%) may add to the sensitivity of the test, mainly in children with mild asthma.[168]

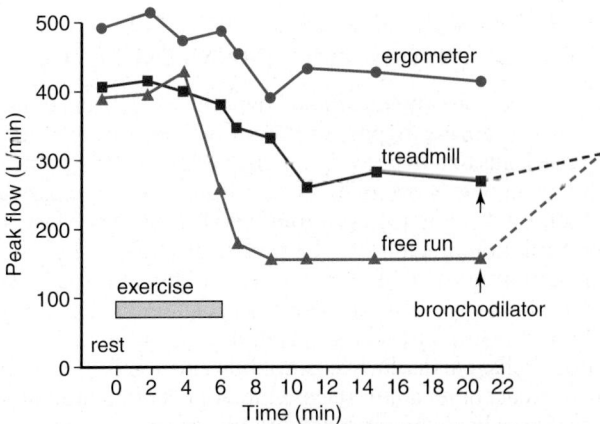

Fig. 12.7 Response to three types of exercise tests in a healthy 15-year-old boy. Reduction in peak flow was greatest in the field test (free run), less with treadmill testing, and least with the cycle ergometer. (From Anderson SD, Connolly NM, Godfrey S. Comparison of bronchoconstriction induced by cycling and running. *Thorax* 1971;26:396-401.)

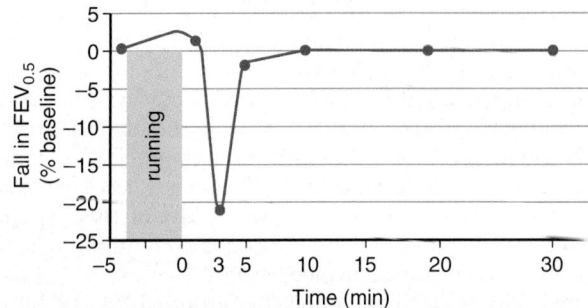

Fig. 12.8 Exercise-induced bronchoconstriction in preschool children: a representative diagram of the changes in $FEV_{0.5}$ (as a percentage of baseline values) during an exercise challenge test on a treadmill performed by a preschool child. (From Vilozni D, Bentur L, Efrati O, et al. Exercise challenge test in 3- to 6-year-old asthmatic children. *Chest* 2007;132:497-503.)

Symptoms of EIB typically begin after 5–10 minutes of vigorous exercise, peak a few minutes after stopping physical exertion, and usually last for 30–90 minutes.[163] Symptoms may include shortness of breath, dyspnea, chest tightness, coughing, wheezing, decreased performance, increased fatigue, chest pain, and chest tightness.[127,169] In children, the exertional symptoms can be less profound and may include a combination of symptoms.

Obese asthmatic children have a greater exercise-induced fall in FEV_1 and a slower recovery from EIB than nonobese asthmatic children, which can limit their participation in physical and sporting activities with peers. Dietary-induced weight loss in overweight and obese asthmatic children leads to significant reduction in severity of EIB and improvement of the quality of life.[170]

EXERCISE CHALLENGE TEST

An exercise challenge test is usually performed on a treadmill or a cycle ergometer. Most children are more used to walking or running than to cycling, and exercise complaints often appear during running (such as when playing tag, dodge ball, or soccer) (Fig. 12.7).[171] Therefore running is the preferred exercise in children, and can be standardized using a treadmill.[172] ATS and ERS[163,172] guidelines for EIB testing involves a rapid increase in exercise intensity over approximately 2–4 minutes to achieve a high level of ventilation while breathing dry air (<10 mg H_2O/L). It should be noted that in adults, breathing dry air enhances EIB and is associated with circulating biomarkers of epithelial damage.[173] The test is performed with a nose clip in place while running or cycling at a load sufficient to raise the HR to ~90% of predicted maximum (predicted maximum HR = 220-age in years) or ventilation to reach ≥17.5–21 times FEV_1 (the two most important determinants of EIB are the sustained high level ventilation reached and the water content of the air inspired). Once this level of exercise is attained, the subject should continue exercise at that high level for an additional 4–6 minutes for a total time of 6–8 minutes. These targets are achieved more rapidly with running than cycling. Pulmonary

function tests should be measured 5 minutes before the exercise and repeated 1, 3, 5, 10, 15, 20, 30 minutes postexercise; the percent fall in FEV_1 compared to baseline is recorded. Nebulized albuterol (salbutamol) or an albuterol inhaler + spacer should be prepared before the exercise test as some children may respond with a severe asthmatic attack. In our lab 200–400 μg albuterol (2–4 puffs of 100 μg) or 0.5 mL of Salbutamol nebulized solution is given to any child immediately after the last pulmonary function test (PFT) done to treat and/or evaluate responsiveness.

It is important to note that the recovery from EIB differs in children compared to adults and in younger compared with older children. For example, Vilozni and coworkers elegantly showed that in very young children (3–6 years old) PFTs should be performed several times during the first 5 minutes after the run due to a very short-lived nadir 2–3 minutes postexercise and that $FEV_{0.5}$ describes the bronchoconstriction event better than the traditional FEV_1 (Fig. 12.8).[167] Hofstra and coworkers[174] demonstrated that 7–10-year-olds with EIB improved FEV_1 by a mean of 1.60%/min following the challenge, but improvement in 11–12 year-olds was significantly prolonged (0.54%/min). In a group of adolescents, 50% with a positive EIB test showed a maximum postexercise decline at 15 or 30 minutes after exercise cessation[175] and previous reports support this finding.[176] These observations should be taken into account when measuring PFTs after the exercise challenge and when symptoms or complaints indicate a high suspicion of asthma, it is reasonable to measure lung function very early (1–2 minutes postexercise) or late (30 minutes postexercise). Our standard test for demonstrating EIB is either a 6–8-minute run on a treadmill at a speed of 3–5 mph with a slope of 10% or, alternatively, cycle ergometer exercise calculated to achieve about 70% of the child's predicted $\dot{V}O_{2max}$. This will result in an oxygen consumption of about 60%–80% of $\dot{V}O_{2max}$ and a HR of 170–180 beats/min.[177,178]

Pretest

Children should avoid PA for at least 4 hours before exercise testing because otherwise they may show an attenuated response due to refractoriness following vigorous repeated exercise. The mechanisms underlying the refractory period are not fully understood but may be due to depletion of catecholamines, prostaglandin release, degranulation of mast cell mediators, and cooling of the airways.[179–181] Medications that can influence the pulmonary response to exercise should be stopped prior to the test: 6 and 12 hours for short- and long-acting beta-adrenergic drugs, respectively; 8 hours for anticholinergic drugs; and 24 hours for cromolyn sodium,[178] leukotriene receptor antagonist (montelukast)[182,183] and nonsteroidal antiinflammatory medications. Recent exposure to inhaled allergens may alter the severity of the response to exercise challenge.[163,179,180,184] Caffeine-containing drinks or food should also be avoided before the test.[185] Inhaled corticosteroids (ICS) are often discontinued 24–48 hours prior to testing, but it is not yet entirely clear whether or not ICS inhibit EIB in the testing context.[181,186] Baseline pulmonary function (FEV_1) should be at least 65% of the predicted value.[178] Abrupt cessation of the test or an audible complaint on the part of the patient is suggestive of an alternate diagnosis of deconditioning, upper airway dysfunction, or cardiopulmonary disorders.[187–189] Some studies have shown a higher incidence of EIB in girls while others did not show a sex difference.[175,190]

The diagnosis of asthma in preschool children may be difficult, as these children typically cannot perform reliable spirometric measurement of lung function. Phenomena of wheezing and prolonged expiration appearing and disappearing within 5 minutes after exercise have been described in a group of 3–6-year-old asthmatic children and may have an important clinical application in defining EIB in early childhood, in the absence of spirometry.[167] There are promising new approaches including digitized assessment of recorded breath sounds that may prove useful in years to come in assessing EIB in younger children, a difficult age group to study.[191]

EXERCISE AND OTHER TESTS FOR BRONCHIAL REACTIVITY

Bronchial hyperreactivity to methacholine (MCH) or histamine is a characteristic feature of asthma but is also present in patients with other types of chronic obstructive lung diseases.[164] Positive MCH results showed significantly higher sensitivity and higher positive predictive value in the diagnosis of asthma in children with *postexercise symptoms* than did exercise challenge tests.[164,192] Free-running and sport-specific exercise challenges have been suggested to increase the specificity and sensitivity of exercise challenge test (ECT) in children and young athletes.[193,194] For example, bronchoconstriction associated with a field test (e.g., free run, 6-minute run on a 100 m flat grassed track with nose clip on and continuous heart monitoring) increased the specificity of ECT in children (8–11 years old) for diagnosing asthma, recent wheezing, or atopy to 95%. The sensitivity and specificity were comparable to histamine challenge test.[193] Although field tests may increase ECT sensitivity and specificity, such challenges performed outside the laboratory are difficult to control in terms of exercise intensity and standardizing environmental conditions.[195]

In asthmatic children the severity of EIB may be influenced by the severity of asthma[196] and by preexposure to allergens.[184] Moreover, the severity, duration, and type of exercise may influence the severity of EIB. Running, as compared to swimming under the same inspired air conditions and work intensity, will result in much more EIB.[197]

THE MECHANISM OF EXERCISE-INDUCED BRONCHOCONSTRICTION REMAINS ENIGMATIC

In the widely accepted osmolar hypothesis, dehydration of the airway during hyperventilation of inspired air during exercise leads to a hyperosmolar environment. This environment promotes movement of the water from the airway epithelium, leading to degranulation of mast cells. Mast cell degranulation precipitates the release of mediators such as transglutaminase, which preferentially activates the leukotriene pathway, histamine, and prostaglandin. Release of cellular recruitment factors promotes an influx of inflammatory cells, particularly eosinophils and T cells. The combined impact of mediator releases and influx of inflammatory cells causes bronchoconstriction and inflammation.[189]

There have been extensive studies of the effect of climate on EIB. Breathing warm and humid air during exercise attenuates EIB, but not inevitably,[198] while breathing dry and cold air increases its severity.[199,200] Facial cooling combined with either cold or warm air inhalation causes the greatest EIB, as compared with the isolated challenge with cold air inhalation, a possible vagal effect.[201] Respiratory heat loss (RHL) from the airway mucosa during exercise was suggested by Deal and his colleagues[200] as the trigger for bronchoconstriction, and they showed that exercise and hyperventilation with similar RHL will result in similar bronchoconstriction. Anderson and coworkers showed that epithelial injury in the airways arising from breathing poorly conditioned air at high flows for long periods of time or high volumes with airway hyperemia can obstruct the airway (the "vascular theory").[202]

RHL cannot entirely account for the triggering stimulus for EIB. First, both patients with known asthma and nonaffected controls develop the same degree of RHL during exercise,[203] yet only the patients tend to have EIB. This suggests additional mechanisms that render asthmatics more susceptible (a "second hit" phenomenon). Moreover, as noted, some asthmatic patients will develop EIB while breathing warm humid air at body temperature and humidity, which will not result in RHL.[204] Also, Noviski and his colleagues[205] exercised a group of asthmatic children at two levels of exercise while the respiratory heat and water loss was kept constant by altering the inspired air conditions. They found that the harder exercise with a mean $\dot{V}O_2$ of approximately 1.6 times greater than $\dot{V}O_2$ of the less strenuous exercise resulted in EIB which was greater by almost 1.7 times.

Exercise has been demonstrated to be a vigorous stimulant of the stress/inflammatory immune system[206–209] involving increased levels of circulating IL-6, intracellular adhesion molecules, and increased circulating immune cells, many of which are involved in the pathophysiology of bronchoconstriction.[210] Indeed, given the robust stress/inflammatory response in healthy children along with the increased number of inflammatory cells in the circulation, one might wonder why not all children wheeze when they exercise. Mediator release from circulating leukocytes and/or the airway mast cells was suggested as the intermediary pathway involved in EIB. Leukotrienes C_4, D_4, and E_4 were found in induced sputum and exhaled breath condensate of asthmatic patients with EIB associated with greater desquamation of epithelial cells into the airway lumen.[189] The neutrophil is emerging as a key player early on triggering bronchospasm.[154,211]

Preexercise treatment with antagonists of neutrophil-related mediators reduced the severity of EIB and in some reports even prevented EIB refractoriness.[179,212] There is increasing research focused on novel pharmacological agents that would specifically inhibit neutrophil migration and function that may eventually prove to be of benefit in asthma.[213]

AIR QUALITY, EXERCISE, AND ASTHMA

As noted by McConnell and coworkers,[214] "Incidence of new diagnoses of asthma is associated with heavy exercise in communities with high concentrations of ozone, thus, air pollution and outdoor exercise could contribute to the development of asthma in children." Competition or training at areas close to busy roadways, or in indoor ice arenas or chlorinated swimming pools, harbors a risk for acute and chronic airway disorders from high pollutant exposure.[215]

EXERCISE-INDUCED BRONCHOCONSTRICTION IN NONASTHMATICS

In recent years, an increasing number of nonasthmatic children (e.g., no asthma diagnosis by a physician and/or negative methacholine/Histamine challenge test) are diagnosed with positive ECT with or without exercise complaints. Up to 50% of Olympic athletes, 29% of adolescent athletes, and 15% of the general pediatric population were reported to have this diagnosis.[175,189,216,217] Most of the data were collected from control children participating in asthma and exercise studies in which they found to have positive ECT or from athletes with/without exercise complaints.

The mechanism suggested for the bronchial responsiveness in nonasthmatic children and athletes is not completely clear but seems to be strongly related to high ventilation rates in cold-dry air; time duration of the exercise challenge may be less important.[218] Other possible mechanisms were suggested in specific circumstances (e.g., ice rink athlete exposure to high-emission pollutants from fossil-fueled ice resurfacing machines, swimmers exposure to chlorine).[195] Airway inflammation was suggested to be involved but the reports are controversial. Some studies reported that nonasthmatic EIB positive athletes have neutrophil-dominant or mixed-type sputum compared to asthmatic EIB-positive patients who have eosinophil dominant inflammation,[219] while other studies on airway inflammation in nonasthmatic EIB-positive athletes have found sputum eosinophilia in a higher percentage compared to asthmatics.[194] Haby and coworkers reported that more than 50% of children with a positive free running exercise challenge had a negative histamine challenge test and concluded that mediators other than histamine may be more important in BHR to exercise or that an additional, nonmast cell mechanism may be involved in BHR to exercise.[193]

In light of the high percentage of exercise complaints in athletes, it was suggested that there may be a different reference range for the drop in FEV_1 in elite athletes compared with the general population.[219] One study compared sport/environment specific field-based exercise challenge (cold weather athletes) to a lab-based ECT and concluded that only a 7% drop in FEV_1 after treadmill exercise challenge in the laboratory is sufficient to make the diagnosis of EIB compared with a greater drop in FEV_1 (e.g., 15%) in a sports-specific setting.[194]

Hallstrand and coworkers studied 256 adolescents participating in organized sports and diagnosed EIB in 9.4% of them. The screening history identified people with symptoms or a previous diagnosis suggestive of EIB in 39.5% of the participants, but only a third of these persons actually had EIB. Among adolescents with a negative review of symptoms of asthma or EIB, 7.8% had EIB. Among adolescents with no previous diagnosis of asthma, allergic rhinitis, or EIB, 7.2% had EIB diagnosed by exercise challenge. Children who screened negative on all questions about symptoms or history of asthma, EIB, and allergic rhinitis accounted for 45.8% of the adolescents with EIB. The authors concluded that "EIB occurs frequently in adolescent athletes, and screening by physical examination and medical history does not accurately detect it."[220] Other studies reported similar findings in athletes.[221]

EXERCISE, ASTHMA, AND BRONCHOCONSTRICTION: TREATMENT CONSIDERATIONS

The approach to treatment of EIB mainly depends on a preliminary assessment of the isolated clinical condition or uncontrolled underlying asthma with more exercise focused recommendations for the nonasthmatic children and a broader approach including appropriate controller medications for chronic asthma. Therapy should result in optimal control of exercise-induced symptoms during HPA and exercise, and allow unrestricted participation in sports activity in children and athletes.[222] Both nonpharmacological and pharmacological treatment should be discussed in the management plan (Fig. 12.9).[189]

Nonpharmacological Approaches

HPA[135,141] and aerobic training[131,159] should be encouraged for treatment and prophylaxis of EIB. Children tend to play in short exercise bouts (up to 1–2 minutes),[50,51] and repeated exercise bouts may increase the threshold for triggering bronchospasm and decrease EIB response.[223] Swimming is less likely to trigger EIB than running.[223] Recommendations should include 1 hour of moderate-vigorous exercise per day and to be as active as possible the rest of the time. Preexercise warm-up is recommended for all patients to attenuate the fall in FEV_1 postexercise. Similar results were found whether high-intensity interval or variable intensity warm-up exercise was performed.[163,181] Screen time was found to correlate with activity limitation in children with asthma.[224] Daily screen time should be limited to no more than 2 hours/day and children should be as active as possible during that period.

There is evidence to support a beneficial role for diet in mitigating EIB as well. The most salient example of this is the rare but life-threatening phenomenon of exercise-induced anaphylaxis, which occurs when an individual with a food allergy (often unknown to the patient) engages in exercise several hours following a meal with the offending dietary element.[225] It has been postulated that the mechanism for exercise-induced anaphylaxis in this instance results from the exercise-associated release (perhaps, by catecholamines) into the peripheral circulation of immune cells in the spleen and GALT (gut associated lymphoid tissue) that were locally

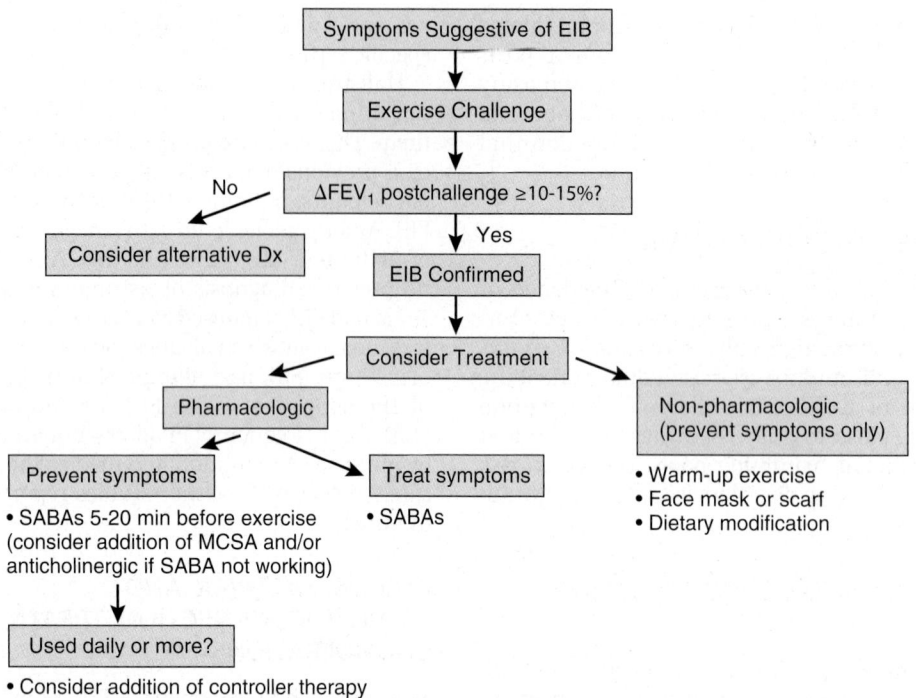

Fig. 12.9 ATS algorithm for diagnosis and treatment of exercise-induced bronchoconstriction. *EIB,* Exercise-induced bronchoconstriction; *ICS,* inhaled corticosteroid; *LABA,* long acting β₂-agonist; *LTRA,* leukotriene receptor antagonist; *MCSA,* mast cell stabilizing agent; *SABA,* short-acting β₂-agonist. (From Parsons JP, Hallstrand TS, Mastronarde JG, et al. An official American Thoracic Society clinical practice guideline: exercise-induced bronchoconstriction. *Am J Respir Crit Care Med* 2013;187:1016-1027.)

activated by the ingestion of the food allergen prior to the exercise bout.

Increased intake of natural foods, particularly fresh fruit, vegetables, and oily fish, and decreased salt consumption are the most promising strategies to improve pulmonary function to below the clinical threshold for the diagnosis of EIB.[226] High doses of caffeine (6–9 mg/kg) were shown to provide a significant protective effect against EIB (no significant difference from preexercise β₂-agonist alone) in a group of adolescent-young adults.[163,227] Reduction in susceptibility to EIB is yet another reason that overweight and obese children should be encouraged to modify dietary intake to gradually decrease body weight.[228] Lower levels of vitamin D are associated with increased reactivity to exercise,[229] and more studies are needed to evaluate the role of vitamin D in EIB management. Ascorbic acid (vitamin C) supplementation may provide a protective effect against exercise-induced airway narrowing. A 50% reduction in the postexercise FEV₁ drop and EIB-related symptoms were reported in small groups of adolescent–young adult asthmatic subjects[185,230]; other studies did not find strong correlation between vitamin C and self-reported wheezing.[231] A Cochrane analysis concluded that evidence is not available to provide a robust assessment on the use of vitamin C in the management of asthma or EIB.[232]

Wearing a mask or scarf in cold weather for those with cold weather–EIB offers considerable protection against bronchospasm induced by cold air.[163,189,233] In young adults, combining a β₂-agonist with a face mask prevented EIB and was superior to treatment with β₂-agonist or a face mask alone.[233] Breathing through the nose to humidify and warm the inhaled air is suggested to decrease the amount of thermal and moisture loss during exercise.[234]

Pharmacological Approaches

Prophylactic intermittent treatment (10–15 minutes preexercise) with short-acting bronchodilators is the most commonly used treatment for EIB. β₂-agonists, both short-acting β₂-agonist (SABA) and long-acting β₂-agonist (LABA), when administered preexercise in a single dose, are effective and safe in preventing the symptoms of EIB. Longer-term administration of inhaled β₂-agonists induces tolerance and lacks sufficient safety data and is not recommended as a single therapy.[163,235] A daily administration of a leukotriene receptor antagonist to ameliorate EIB is also recommended.[163] A single-dose of montelukast was shown to attenuate EIB 1–24 hours after consumption,[183,236] although it is less effective than β₂-agonists (albuterol) for prevention of EIB in children with asthma.[159] Tolerance to the protective effect of β₂-agonist does not develop with regular use of montelukast and if breakthrough EIB occurs, a β₂-agonist can be used effectively as rescue medication. Montelukast treatment added to aerobic training in asthmatic children may exert beneficial effects on BHR.[159]

For daily or frequent EIB complaints, daily administration of an ICS is recommended. It may take 2–4 weeks after the initiation of therapy to see maximal improvement. Administration of ICS only before exercise ("as needed") is not recommended.[222] EIB is one of the earliest signs of chronic asthma and one of the last symptoms to disappear upon treatment with ICS (Fig. 12.10).[237] In a double-blind, randomized, placebo-controlled trial, intranasal corticosteroid (fluticasone furoate) reduced EIB in asthmatic children with allergic rhinitis.[238] If EIB symptoms are not controlled with regular use of ICS, a LABA or montelukast is recommended.[222]

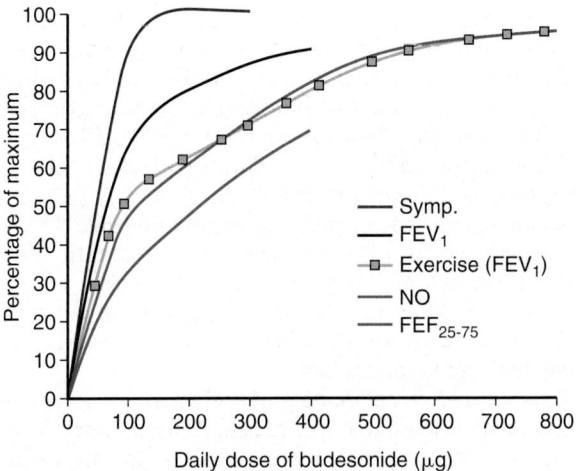

Fig. 12.10 Response of various outcome parameters of asthma severity with increasing doses of inhaled budesonide. *Exercise (FEV₁),* The fall in FEV₁ on exercise; *FEF₂₅₋₇₅,* forced expiratory flow between 25% and 75% of forced vital capacity; *NO,* nitric oxide concentration in expired air; *symp.,* both morning and evening asthma symptoms. (From Anderson SD. Single-dose agents in the prevention of exercise-induced asthma: a descriptive review. *Treat Respir Med* 2004;3(6):365-379.)

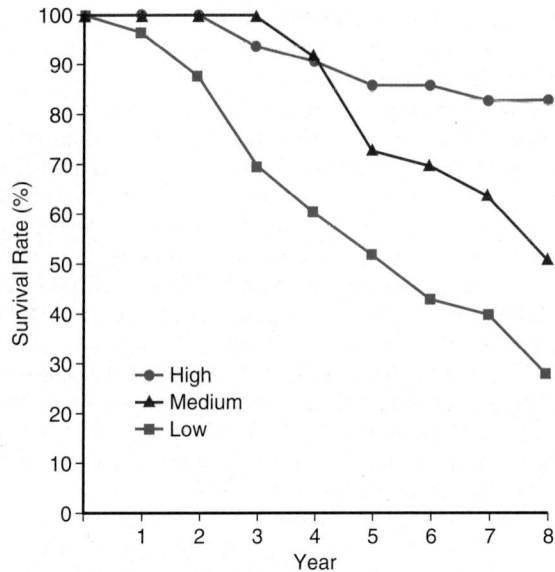

Fig. 12.11 Survival among 109 cystic fibrosis patients (mean age 17 years old) according to fitness levels (peak V̇O₂). (From Nixon PA, Orenstein DM, Kelsey SF, Doershuk CF. The prognostic value of exercise testing in patients with cystic fibrosis. *NEJM* 1992;327:1785-1788.)

A multimodal treatment concept including physical training and medical treatment with an inhaled steroid for 7 days resulted in a decrease in airway hyperresponsiveness to exercise in children (13.5 ± 2.7 [SD] years). Adding montelukast to the treatment protocol resulted in a further decrease in airway hyperresponsiveness.[239] Chronic treatment with a combination of inhaled corticosteroid and LABA (fluticasone propionate/salmeterol) was shown to provide superior protection compared with an inhaled corticosteroid alone (fluticasone propionate) in protecting against EIB in children with persistent asthma.[240] To date, most of the treatment recommendations are the same between EIB positive asthmatic and EIB positive nonasthmatics. Specific irritants (e.g., cold weather, pollutants, chlorine) should be avoided if possible. It was reported that athletes with positive EIB may compete successfully at the international level despite their symptoms.[189,194]

Physical Activity, Exercise and Cystic Fibrosis

Recommendations for PA are already part of regular outpatient care offered to most CF patients, sparked by the groundbreaking study of Nixon and coworkers in the New England Journal of Medicine.[241] HPA should be considered as a "vital sign" for health in children and is a key factor for mental health and social life in health and chronic conditions. CF patients are less active than their healthy peers even in those with good lung function, and overall PA declines with age, similar to healthy populations.[241–243] High activity levels in CF patients (12–40 years old) have been linked to improved exercise capacity[243–245] and exercise prescriptions that detailed specific ways to increase HPA improved exercise capacity as well.[244] An increase in HPA was associated with a slower rate of decline in FEV₁ in pediatric CF patients (7–17 years old).[246,247] Physical inactivity is a factor significantly contributing to skeletal muscle force in adults with CF.[248]

Duration and intensity of daily PA were positively correlated with bone mineral density (BMD) in adolescents and adults with CF and shown to be predictors of BMD Z score.[243]

Gender differences have been reported in habitual activity of CF patients. Girls were less active, but only after the onset of puberty, and pancreatic insufficiency had an impact on measures of fitness and habitual activity that was greatest in late pubertal females.[247,249] A recent statement by the Exercise Working Group European CF Society emphasized the importance of monitoring HPA. It recommended that "activity monitors such as SenseWear or ActiGraph offer informed choices to facilitate a comprehensive assessment of physical activity, and should as a minimum report on dimensions of physical activity including energy expenditure, step count and time spent in different intensities and sedentary time."[242]

Pediatric CF patients were shown to have decreased exercise capacity[27,250]; girls have lower values than boys,[251] and early pubertal have higher values than adolescents.[252] Most CF patients present an annual deterioration in peak V̇O₂ (2.1 mL/min/kg per year), and risk factors for deterioration were adolescence, high IgG levels, chronic infection with *P. aeruginosa*, FEV₁ < 80%, and rapid rate of FEV₁ deterioration.[252,253] Exercise capacity (peak V̇O₂) has been negatively related to morbidity (rate of hospitalization, total IgG levels, chronic infection with *Pseudomonas aeruginosa*),[252,254] quality of life,[255] and mortality[241] in CF patients (Fig. 12.11). Pianosi and coworkers studied 28 CF patients (8–17 years old) with CF who performed annual pulmonary function and maximal exercise tests over a 5-year period to determine FEV₁ and peak V̇O₂, the magnitude of their change over time, and survival over the subsequent 7–8 years. Peak V̇O₂ fell during the observation period in 70% of the patients, with a mean annual decline of 2.1 mL/min per kg. Initial peak V̇O₂ was not predictive of rate of decline or mortality, but rate of decline and final peak V̇O₂ of the series were significant predictors. Patients with peak V̇O₂ less than 32 mL/min per kg exhibited a dramatic increase in mortality, in contrast to those whose peak $\dot{V}O_2$ exceeded 45 mL/min per kg, none of whom died. The first, last, and rate of decline in FEV_1 over time were all significant predictors of mortality.[254]

Besides $\dot{V}O_{2max}$ or peak $\dot{V}O_2$, additional submaximal gas exchange measurements (e.g., $\dot{V}_E/\dot{V}CO_2$-slope and $\Delta\dot{V}O_2/\Delta HR$-slope) that do not rely on achievement of maximal effort have a diagnostic potential that is important, especially in children with chronic conditions as CF. As shown in healthy children,[256] slopes can predict maximal values with very good correlations and should be used more often in exercise testing of pediatric CF patients. For example, a model consisting of BMI, $FEV_1\%$ predicted, and $\dot{V}_E/\dot{V}O_2$ was found to be a strong predictor of mortality rate in adolescents with CF[257] or delayed $\dot{V}O_2$ response time, and $\Delta\dot{V}O_2/\Delta WR$ was suggested to be useful to detect impairment in oxygen transport and oxygen utilization in young patients with CF.[258] $\dot{V}_E/\dot{V}CO_2$, as a marker of ventilation response, was shown to better determine exercise limitation in mild-to-moderate lung disease.[259] Other submaximal tests have been described for evaluating exercise capacity in CF such as the 3-minute step test; HR during and after a 3-minute step test may reflect $\dot{V}O_2$ peak in children with CF.[260]

Several factors might contribute to the reduction in exercise capacity in CF:

1. *Peripheral (muscle) limitation:* Several mechanisms provide some insight that muscle mass and muscle metabolism contribute to exercise intolerance in CF. A defect in sarcoplasmic reticulum CFTR Cl channels could alter the electrochemical gradient, causing dysregulation of Ca homeostasis, essential to excitation-contraction coupling and leading to exercise intolerance and muscle weakness.[261] In another study, impairment in oxygen transport and oxygen utilization by the muscles was described in addition to exercise limitation that was significant just for peak $\dot{V}O_2$ normalized for fat free mass (FFM).[258]

2. *Respiratory limitation:* Peak $\dot{V}O_2$ is correlated with FEV_1 during childhood in CF patients.[253,262] Exercise limitation is not primarily limited by respiratory factors in young patients and in mild CF lung disease (peak $\dot{V}O_2$ remains stable or rises slightly over time in younger patients), while it shows a downward trend in older children with CF, particularly once FEV_1 falls below 80% predicted.[262,263] Exercise limitation in adult CF patients is largely dependent on the magnitude of the ventilatory response (reduced or absent breathing reserve and $\dot{V}_E/\dot{V}CO_2$) in patients with mild-to-moderate lung disease, and on FEV_1 in patients with severe lung disease.[259] In children, Bongers and coworkers found exaggerated, but adequate, ventilatory response to exercise for $\dot{V}CO_2$ and higher ventilatory demand during submaximal exercise in CF patients with mild-to-moderate airway obstruction.[264] For some exercise-derived parameters it is suggested to use a disease-specific approach. For example, maximal voluntary ventilation (MVV) may be determined directly or indirectly from pulmonary function data, using the functions MVV = (FEV_1) × 35. In CF patients, MVV is expressed as MVV = 27.7 × (FEV_1) + 8.8 × Pred(FEV_1) ($R^2 = 0.98$, $P < .05$).[265]

3. *Genotype:* The class of CFTR mutation correlates with aerobic capacity and peak anaerobic power. Patients with mutations causing defective CFTR production or processing (class I or II) had a significantly lower peak aerobic capacity than those with a mutation conferring defective regulation of CFTR (class III). The peak anaerobic power in subjects with mutations inducing decreased CFTR conduction (class IV) or CFTR mRNA (class V) were significantly higher than children with class I, II, or III mutations.[266] Two studies failed to show any association between genotype or polymorphism and peak $\dot{V}O_2$.[252,267] The presence of CFTR at the sarcoplasmic reticulum of skeletal muscle of CF patients may partly explain genotype/phenotype differences in exercise capacity of patients.[261] However, the relationship between genotype and exercise capacity remains unclear.

4. *Training and deconditioning:* Aerobic training has been repeatedly shown to improve peak aerobic capacity (peak $\dot{V}O_2$),[244,268] and increases in exercise capacity result in significantly improved lung function and habitual activity.[269] Anaerobic training has measurable effects on aerobic performance, anaerobic performance, and health-related quality of life in children with CF.[270] Resistance training was shown to increase strength, exercise capacity, and work capacity.[271] The beneficial effects of exercise and training in CF patients could be partially explained by blockage of amiloride-sensitive sodium conductance in the respiratory epithelium in response to moderate-intensity exercise. The inhibition of luminal sodium conductance could increase water content of the mucus in the CF lung during exercise.[272]

Responsiveness to exercise training is similar in CF patients and in healthy untrained people regardless of disease severity. Higher improvements in exercise parameters were noted in subjects with lower initial fitness levels.[273] Training programs mainly include a combination of aerobic exercise and resistance and have been reported to have very high adherence (>95%) for 6–8 week sessions[274,275] and 85% for year sessions.[271] This combination may offer multiple important advantages such as improvement in exercise capacity, quality of life (aerobic training), better weight gain (total mass, as well as % fat and fat-free mass), lung function, and leg strength (resistance training).[268,271,275] Short-term (8 weeks) combined aerobic and resistance training program performed in a hospital setting induces significant benefits in the cardiorespiratory fitness and muscle strength of children with CF.[274]

A relatively new training strategy in health and chronic conditions is the high-intensity interval training (HIIT). HIIT includes short (e.g., 10–30 seconds) high-intensity exercise bouts with rest periods in between (e.g., 60–120 seconds). The total amount of work is usually less than a constant aerobic session and total time of training is shorter. A relative short period of HIIT (6 weeks) for a patient with CF with a ventilatory limitation resulted in peak $\dot{V}O_2$ and peak workload increased by 19% and 16%, respectively; there was a rise in peak ventilation by 50% (50–75 L/min), with an increase in both breathing depth and respiratory rate. HIIT should be considered as one of the potential training regimens due to its effectiveness and efficiency, especially in CF patients with a ventilatory limitation and a high treatment burden.[276] Training using interactive gaming consoles represents high-intensity exercise for children and young adults with CF and may be a suitable alternative to conventional exercise modalities.[277] Female patients had lower exercise tolerance than males. Pulmonary function, respiratory rate, and tidal volume did not differ between sexes. Male and female patients, irrespective of disease severity, utilized similar proportions of their ventilatory capacity at exhaustion.[251] Physical exercise in low-inflammation/infection status (e.g., at a young age) should be encouraged. It was reported that chronic systemic inflammation and infection (high total IgG levels and *P. aeruginosa* colonization) leads to negative effects on skeletal muscles, preventing skeletal muscle tissue from improving with regular physical exercise.[252]

It is noteworthy that despite causing significant acute bronchodilation, inhaled albuterol did not improve maximal exercise performance in ventilatory-limited CF adults, adding to the body of literature that fails to show any clinical benefit of SABAs in CF subjects.[278] Further study is needed to better understand the role of SABAs in CF patients.

Safety

Exercise testing and training is safe in patients with CF. A survey study was conducted in Germany and 78/107 CF centers caring for 4208 patients responded with 256 patients answering a web-based survey. No serious adverse events were reported for 713 exercise tests. With in-hospital training, the yearly incidence of exercise-related serious adverse events such as pneumothorax, cardiac arrhythmia, injury, or hypoglycemia was less than 1% each.[279]

In summary, a recent Cochrane review regarding exercise training in CF including young children and young adults concluded as follows: "Although improvements are not consistent between studies and ranged from no effects to clearly positive effects, the most consistent effects of the heterogeneous exercise training modalities and durations were found for maximal aerobic exercise capacity with unclear effects on FEV$_1$ and health-related quality of life. ... Exercise training is already part of regular outpatient care offered to most people with cystic fibrosis, and since there is some evidence for beneficial effects on aerobic fitness and no negative side effects exist, there is no reason to actively discourage this."[280]

Recommendations

Exercise prescription should be personalized to each patient. In mild-to-moderate CF lung disease, the current guidelines for PA for healthy children (one hour of moderate-vigorous intensity exercise per day) should be the basis for exercise advice in CF patients. With increasing disease severity, a more considered approach to exercise programs is required, incorporating more interval-type training with frequent reevaluation.[281]

Physical Activity, Exercise, and Lung Disease of Prematurity

Despite remarkable improvements in survivorship of prematurely born babies, the incidence of lung disease and other developmental abnormalities remains a considerable challenge for pediatricians.[282] Results from studies reporting PA levels in children born premature are controversial. A recent study[283] showed a small difference in objectively measured moderate to vigorous PA (MVPA by accelerometry) in 7-year-old children born less than 32 weeks' gestation. Proulx and

coworkers reported that 80% of adolescents (16.1 ± 2.5 years old, born ≤29 weeks gestation) did not meet MVPA guidelines (using accelerometry). Risk factors for inactivity were older age, female gender, additional health problems, and marked movement difficulties.[284] However, other studies have not shown the same effect on children and adolescents (8–18 years old).[285,286] Physically fit individuals lose the association between birth weight and metabolic disease, and the association between low birth weight and metabolic syndrome is accentuated in unfit individuals. PA intervention studies indicate that most cardiometabolic risk factors respond to exercise in a protective manner, independent of birth weight.[287]

EXERCISE CAPACITY

Extremely preterm (gestational age of <25 weeks) birth and early preterm (gestational age of <32 weeks) birth were associated with a significant reduction in peak $\dot{V}O_2$ in school-aged children (8–11 years old) compared to full-term controls. These findings were not explained by differences in physical cardiopulmonary factors, or activity levels, but were best predicted by lean body mass. Ventilation did not limit exercise performance, although it appears that breathing during exercise is regulated differently in prematurely born children compared to term-born children and may reflect a long-term pathophysiological impact of EP birth. Postnatal corticosteroids had no effect on aerobic fitness or HPA.[286,288,289] Clemm and coworkers reported contrary findings. Children 10 and 17 years old born preterm (<28 weeks of gestational age) achieved normal exercise capacity, and their response to physical training was comparable to peers born at term. Neonatal BPD and current FEV$_1$ were unrelated to exercise capacity.[290]

In young adults born with a gestational age of less than 32 weeks, a birth weight less than 1500 g, or both factors, preterm birth was associated with lower FEV$_1$, peak WR and AT, but no differences were found in peak $\dot{V}O_2$, and breathing reserve compared to a full-term control group. Again, there were no significant differences in lung function and exercise parameters between preterms with and without BPD. Exercise-induced arterial hypoxemia was not found to contribute to the reduction in aerobic exercise capacity. Severe dyspnea and leg discomfort associated with critical constraints on tidal volume expansion may lead to reduced exercise capacity despite differences in expiratory flow limitation and BPD history, similar to patients with chronic obstructive pulmonary disease.[291–294] Submaximal tests are frequently used in the pediatric population to estimate exercise capacity. No difference was found in submaximal exercise capacity (six-minute walking distance) between school-age subjects (born mean 27 weeks of gestational age) with and without a diagnosis of bronchopulmonary dysplasia (BPD) and controls.[295] However, Tsopanoglou reported that children born prematurely with very low birth weight (<1500 g, mean 30 weeks of gestational age), especially those who had BPD, demonstrated limited functional capacity during submaximal exercise (6-minute walking distance).[296]

In conclusion, PA and exercise, as recommended for healthy children, should be recommended for children who survive prematurity. Potential exercise and health benefits could be achieved by increasing PA levels and exercise training.

Exercise at Altitude in Child Health

The environment plays a key factor in determining a child's exercise performance and limitations.

Worldwide, it is estimated that >140 million people live at a high altitude (HA), defined as greater than 2500 m (8200 ft.), and millions are visiting HA areas for short periods every year.[297] HA environments pose a number of unique physiological challenges to the child's body, such as lower ambient temperatures, reduced humidity, and lower barometric pressures. To understand the effect of these changes, the "alveolar air equation" can be used:

$$P_AO_2 = P_IO_2 - (P_ACO_2/R)$$

where:

- P_AO_2 = Alveolar pressure of oxygen.
- P_IO_2 = Partial pressure of oxygen inhaled = F_IO_2 X (PB-P_{H2O}).
- F_IO_2 = The fraction of oxygen in the inspired gas.
- PB = Barometric Pressure.
- P_{H2O} = Partial pressure of water vapor (at body temperature of 37°C).
- P_ACO_2 = Alveolar pressure of carbon dioxide = ~40 mmHg (usually kept in a narrow range).
- R (Respiratory Exchange Ratio) = $\dot{V}CO_2/\dot{V}O_2$ (O_2 uptake/CO_2 exhaled) ~0.8 at rest (>0.8 during intense exercise).

At sea level (at rest): P_IO_2 = 0.2093 × (760−47) = 150 mmHg and P_AO_2 = 150 − (40/0.8) = 100 mmHg.

At HA (at rest): P_IO_2 decreases because of the decrease in PB while F_IO_2 and P_{H2O} stays constant. P_AO_2 decreases respectively and P_aO_2 as well. For example, at La-Paz, Bolivia (at rest), altitude of ~3700 m, PB = 490 $_{mmHg}$ → P_IO_2 = 0.2093 × (490−47) = 93 $_{mmHg}$ and P_AO_2 = 93 − (40/0.8) = 43 $_{mmHg}$ (correlates to SpO_2 = ~80%). P_AO_2 decreases as does P_aO_2 leading to decreased SpO_2 (oxygen saturation as percent). The reduced saturation is accompanied by a robust ventilatory response that can lead to true hyperventilation (reduced P_ACO_2, P_aCO_2, and pH). Not surprisingly, exercise performance at altitude is initially reduced.[298,299] The lower value of P_aCO_2 can cause respiratory alkalosis and shifting of the oxyhemoglobin dissociation curve to the left which, paradoxically, might exacerbate the decreased SpO_2. These effects, however, are partially compensated for by the increased $\dot{V}_E$ with accompanying elevations in P_AO_2, P_aO_2. The net effect is a higher SpO_2 than might be expected for a certain P_aO_2. These are normal physiologic acute responses to HA, and most individuals note a sensation of breathlessness.[300] Acclimatization does occur over time, but our understanding of these mechanisms in children is, at best, incomplete.[301,302]

In children, Major and coworkers reported a mean SpO_2 of 87% for adolescent children (16–19 years old) at 3450 m.[303] Children exposed acutely to HA are more sensitive to hypobaric hypoxia than their parents and decrease SpO_2 to lower levels.[304,305] Sushi and coworkers conducted a systemic review and reported SpO_2 of 0–5-year-olds at greater than 2500 m measured in several studies. The SpO_2 depended on the altitude and ranged from 93% at 2600 m to 88% at 4000 m.[306] From their extensive review of the literature in children, Subhi and coworkers concluded, *"Above altitudes of 2500 m, giving oxygen for SpO_2 less than 90% may be too liberal for facilities with limited oxygen supplies. There is evidence that for altitudes greater than 2500 m a threshold of SpO_2 of 85% can be used to identify children most in need of oxygen. A balance needs to be achieved between using accurate altitude-specific definitions of hypoxemia, and ensuring simple and safe indications for oxygen that can be taught to and used by health workers."*

When reviewing the effect of HA on exercise performance it was shown that $\dot{V}O_{2max}$ is decreased by ~20% when comparing near sea level (~450 m) to 3500 m in young children and adolescents[304] and up to 45% when young adults ascend from sea level to 5260 m.[307] The same effect continues as the adolescents exercise at increasing altitudes (3700–4300 m).[308] Moderate altitude also decreased significantly 3000 m race results in young adults (sea level vs. 2100 m).[299]

Two main mechanisms are involved in the reduction of exercise performance: (1) arterial oxyhemoglobin saturation (SaO_2) during maximal exercise and (2) the ratio of lung diffusing capacity to $\dot{V}O_{2max}$.[299] During exercise at HA the capillary transient time of the red blood cell at the alveoli is shorter and the time to complete diffusion is reduced. The ventilatory response is no longer sufficient to prevent arterial oxygen desaturation with exercise (as in most cases at sea level), and the result is a further decrease in PaO_2 and SpO_2, and the extent of the decrease is dependent upon the exercise intensity.[303,304,309]

Another possible limiting mechanism could be changes in the peripheral muscle. Calbet and colleagues studied young adults exercising at sea level and after 9 weeks at 5260 m and concluded that the major limiting factor to muscle performance at HA was oxygen delivery and not intrinsic peripheral factors.[307] Several studies have confirmed a strong positive relationship between maximal oxygen uptake ($\dot{V}O_{2max}$) at sea level and the magnitude of the decline in $\dot{V}O_{2max}$ at altitude in young adults (the more "fit" on sea level the higher the decline in $\dot{V}O_{2max}$ at altitude).[299,310,311] Chen and coworkers showed that exposure to HA from birth to adolescence resulted in a higher SpO_2 at peak $\dot{V}O_2$ and a greater aerobic exercise performance compared to adolescents acclimatized to HA. This may reflect adaptation to life at HA.[308] Cardiorespiratory adaptation to altitude seems to be at least partly hereditary.[304]

High Altitude and Children With Chronic Lung Disease

The data regarding the effect of HA on chronic conditions in children is scarce.

Asthma

Environmental factors play an important role on disease symptoms and pathophysiologic mechanisms. Acute exposure to cold air and exercise are considered important inducers of asthma exacerbations.[128,312] Golan et al.[312] examined asthma exacerbation in 147 young adults engaging in HA trekking. In this study 60% of the subjects had an asthma attack, and two independent risk factors for attacks during travel were determined: frequent use (>3 times weekly) of inhaled bronchodilators before travel, and participation in intense physical exertion during treks. When both risk factors were present, the risk for an asthma attack was 5.5-fold. It was concluded that therapy should be intensified to achieve better disease control and uncontrolled patients should be discouraged from participating in intense HA trekking. Patients should consider the use of short-acting β_2 agonists or antileukotrienes.[313]

Seys and coworkers studied a group of 18 asthmatic adults climbing the Aconcagua mountain (6965 m, Argentina) and concluded that "exposure to environmental conditions at high altitude (hypoxia, exercise, cold) was associated with a moderate loss of asthma control, increased airway obstruction and neutrophilic airway inflammation. The cold temperature is probably the most important contributing factor as 24-hour cold exposure by itself induced similar effects"[314] and protection of the mouth and nose was recommended (e.g., with a scarf) during rest and exercise.[313]

Chronic exposure to HA could have beneficial effects. Droma and coworkers studied 3196 children 13–14-years-old Tibetan highland residents (3658 m above sea level) who participated in written and video questionnaire investigations (ISAAC Phase III program), and the prevalence of asthma, allergic rhinoconjunctivitis, and eczema over the past 12 months was found to be the lowest among the centers that performed ISAAC worldwide.[315] Rijssenbeek-Nouwens and coworkers reviewed the long-term effect of HA as a treatment for asthma for children and concluded that HA has beneficial effects in patients with severe refractory asthma on symptoms, lung function, and oral corticosteroid requirement, irrespective of atopic status. The suggested mechanisms were decreased levels of mite allergens, pollens, fungal spores, and air pollution in the dry air, as well as high exposure to UV light with immunomodulatory and antiinflammatory effects.[316]

Cystic Fibrosis

We could find only one published study regarding CF children and exercise at HA. Blau and coworkers looked at the effects of an intensive 4-week summer camp at an altitude of 1500 m on 13 CF patients (9–25 years old, mean FEV_1 predicted = 75%). The exercise during the camp was mainly done during physiotherapy and by climbing mountains. Full assessment was done at sea level before and after the camp. At sea level, as well as at the camp, rest SpO_2 were in the normal range and during intense exercise lowered to 94% at sea level (no training effect) and 89% at 1500 m. There was a significant training effect on $\dot{V}O_2$ and AT. FEV_1 did not improve, but minute ventilation and maximal minute ventilation did, and it was concluded that this could be respiratory muscle training effect.[317] CF patients with obstructive airways disease are at significant risk for decreased SpO_2 during exercise. Ryujin and coworkers studied 50 CF patients (15–50 years old, mean FEV_1 predicted = 54%) and evaluated oxygen saturation during maximal exercise (cycle ergometer ramp test) at moderate altitude (1500 m). Percent predicted FEV_1 and FEV_1/FVC ratio most highly correlated with arterial oxyhemoglobin saturation at peak exercise. $\dot{V}O_{2max}$ was measured at 1500 m but comparison to sea level values was not reported.[318]

Lung function in 36 adults with CF (19–47 years old, FEV_1 = 66%) at sea level and after 7 hours at HA (2650 m) was assessed before and after mild exercise (5 minutes of cycling at a work load of 30 watt). Pulmonary function test improved significantly from sea level, and mild exercise led to pronounced hypoxemia in almost two-thirds of all patients, without relevant symptoms.[319] Predictive equations for hypoxia in CF patients during exposure to HA are available.[320] CF patients are at increased risk to develop HA pulmonary edema (HAPE) upon fast ascending to HA and exercising.[300]

Few studies have addressed the dilemma of low cabin pressure during air travel in children with chronic lung disease. During commercial air travel the cabin pressure is reduced to that found at an altitude of 1800–2450 m, corresponding to a P_IO_2 ~125 mm Hg and P_AO_2 ~65 mm Hg.[321] Buchdahl and coworkers evaluated 87 children with CF (7–19 years old), preflight (hypoxic chamber) and during flight, and concluded that preflight spirometry was a better predictor of desaturation during flight than preflight hypoxic challenge.[322] Thews and coworkers investigated 10 moderate CF patients (age 19–35-years-old, FEV_1 = 55% predicted) and 27 healthy control subjects in a hypoxic chamber where the ambient pressure was reduced to that found at 2000 and 3000 m and reported that pulmonary function tests (FEV_1, FVC) did not change significantly while they slightly improved in the control group. At each ambient pressure the SpO_2 in the control subjects was 3%–4% higher than in the CF patients, with SpO_2 for all subjects higher than 80% (risk level for complications during commercial flights).[321]

Bronchopulmonary Dysplasia

One case report was found regarding BPD and exercise at HA. Lovering and coworkers reported a 27-year-old male with a history of BPD (FEV_1 = 66.5% predicted, normal FVC and DLCO, $\dot{V}O_{2max}$ = 41.4 mL/kg per minute, 92% predicted) and a case of HAPE.[300] Significant changes in gas exchange were observed at maximal hypoxic exercise (incremental cycle ergometer test while breathing F_IO_2 = 0.12). $\dot{V}O_{2max}$ was reduced ~50% to 21.9 mL/kg per minute and PaO_2 decreased from 67.8 mm Hg (normoxic exercise) to 29.9 mm Hg (hypoxic exercise). These findings suggest higher susceptibility of subjects with a history of BPD to hypoxemia[323] and HAPE.[300]

Exercise and Laryngeal Obstruction

Exercise-induced laryngeal obstruction (E-ILO) is the preferred term based on a recent international multispecialty consensus document, describing the condition in which glottic or supraglottic structures inappropriately obstruct the larynx during exercise, "causing breathing problems."[324] This condition was formerly known under the umbrella terms of *vocal cord dysfunction* and *paradoxical vocal fold motion*, and was first described in the modern literature in 1983.[325] It was recognized as a cause of adolescent exertional dyspnea in 1984 and later famously described as a cause of "choking during athletic activities."[326,327]

E-ILO is important to the pediatric pulmonologist for its combination of prevalence and impact. It is estimated to affect roughly 5% of the adolescent population.[328] Its impact was first characterized in terms of its identification as an entity distinct from asthma. When clinicians made this diagnosis, it became possible to decrease the cost and side effects associated with inappropriate treatment with asthma medication.[329] A second domain of impact is quantified in terms of the symptom burden experienced by patients, as patients with E-ILO are not able to exercise comfortably and may

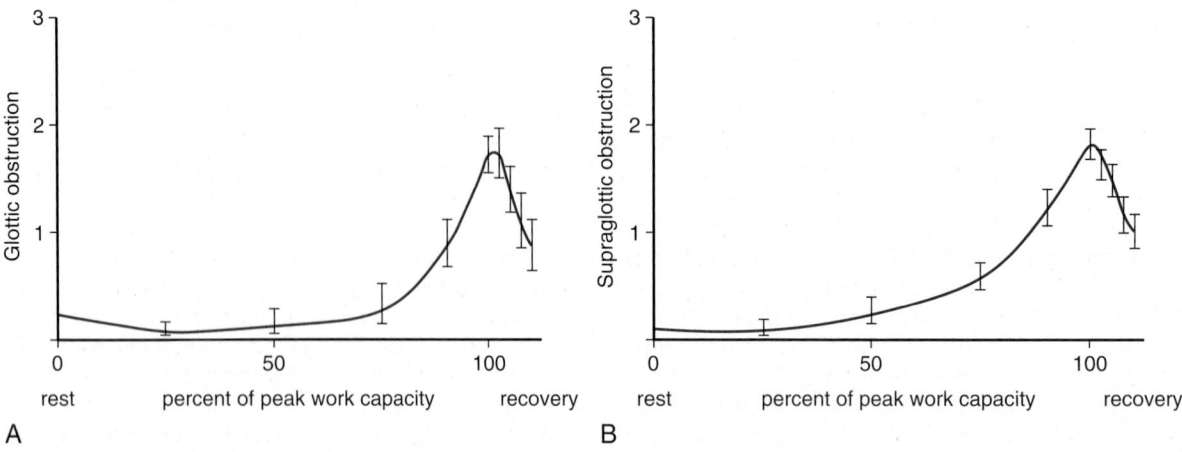

Fig. 12.12 Laryngeal obstruction across a symptom limited incremental exercise test and recovery period in subjects with moderate/severe inspiratory glottic adduction observed during continuous exercise laryngoscopy. Plots A and B represent glottic and supraglottic obstruction, respectively. Confidence intervals surround estimates, which were based on Roksund's scoring scale. At submaximal exercise, obstruction at both levels is minimal, at peak exercise is not complete, and rapidly resolves during recovery. (Modified figure reproduced with permission Olin JT, Clary MS, Fan EM, et al. Continuous laryngoscopy quantitates laryngeal behaviour in exercise and recovery. *Eur Respir J* 2016;48:1192-1200.)

potentially change exercise habits.[330] The impact of E-ILO in terms of perturbations of exercise physiology variables has not been described to date.

Currently, the mechanism of E-ILO is unclear, although many hypotheses exist. The roles of upper airway size, epithelial integrity, tissue pliability, tissue tone, tissue reactivity, neural plasticity, and neurophysiological coupling with the lower airways have been pondered, but are unclear.[331,332] Behavioral traits of affected patients may also contribute in undefined ways.[333,334]

Patients with E-ILO generally present with a chief complaint of exertional dyspnea. Historical clues to the diagnosis may include a description of breathing as noisy, frightening, and distressing to observers. The time course of symptoms is distinct from asthma and localized to short durations that are generally associated with very high WRs. The condition typically does not respond to albuterol.[327] The history can also overlap with the history of the prototypical patient with asthma, in part because the condition can coexist with asthma.

Diagnostic procedures and criteria have not been standardized within or across specialties. In practice and in the literature, a variety of methods have been used to diagnose E-ILO, including documentation of a characteristic history, noninvasive techniques, resting laryngoscopy, postexercise laryngoscopy, preexercise and postexercise laryngoscopy, and continuous laryngoscopy during exercise (CLE).[335–339]

CLE, a procedure in which a flexible laryngoscope is mounted in place during high-intensity exercise challenges, has been advocated as the diagnostic method of choice because glottic and supraglottic behavior varies across rest, incremental exercise, and recovery. It is now clear that, even during periods of maximal symptomatology at peak work capacity, observed maximal laryngeal obstruction is not synonymous with complete inspiratory glottic or supraglottic obstruction (Video 12.1). The resolution of laryngeal obstruction during recovery is rapid (starting in <30 seconds), precluding representative assessment by postexercise laryngoscopy (Fig. 12.12).[340]

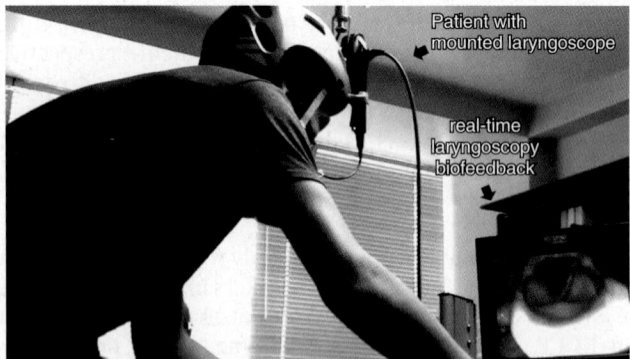

Fig. 12.13 A 15-year-old male with refractory exercise-induced laryngeal obstruction performs therapeutic laryngoscopy during exercise. (From Olin JT, Deardorff EH, Fan EM, et al. Therapeutic laryngoscopy during exercise: a novel non-surgical therapy for refractory EILO. Pediatr Pulmonol 2017;52(6):813-819.)

There is noted variability in the therapeutic modalities used to treat E-ILO. Therapies that have been promoted include medical intervention (with anticholinergic agents and treatment of associated conditions),[341] surgical interventions (which minimize supraglottic obstruction),[342] and behavioral interventions (including respiratory retraining, voice therapy, biofeedback, hypnosis, and cognitive behavioral therapy).[325,329] Recently, therapeutic laryngoscopy during exercise, an innovative procedure designed to treat E-ILO by harnessing visual laryngeal biofeedback during exercise, was also described (Fig. 12.13).[343] In 2016, high-quality clinical trials designed to evaluate the relative effectiveness of different therapeutic techniques have not been performed.

Research into E-ILO is in its infancy, in part due to the lack of field tests and simple diagnostic tests. Notable gaps in the literature include our poor understanding of disease mechanism, disease phenotypes, and the relative effectiveness of various therapeutic modalities. Moving forward, these are critical areas that must be understood to improve care of these patients.

Toward the Future: Exercise in the Age of Omics

Pediatric pulmonologists are keenly interested in the impact of respiratory disease during childhood on lung health across the lifespan. Developmental biologists, pediatricians, and other child health care specialists have long suspected that exercise during infancy, childhood, and adolescence is not merely play, but is essential for healthy growth and development. The pattern and intensity of PA during key stages of growth and development can provide the organism with mechanical and other thermodynamic inputs, essential information that could optimally adapt the growing child to his or her specific environment. Precisely how the molecular transducers of PA interact with the molecular transducers of normal growth and development remains poorly understood. But recent advances in "omics," namely genomics and epigenetics, metabolomics, and proteomics, now provide exciting approaches and tools that can be used for the first time to address this gap.

Exciting preliminary data and pioneering publications from a variety of investigators are beginning to identify the effect of brief exercise on gene and microRNA expression of these cells (Fig. 12.14). Several specific mechanisms have been identified in child health that link exercise and innate immune cell function with disease prevention and clinical outcomes.[65,344–348]

Many of the genomic and epigenetic pathways identified in leukocytes of children and adults are related to growth and repair, and prevention of diseases such as asthma, cancer, and atherosclerosis.[349,350] Advanced use of techniques such as flow cytometry has stimulated research into the effect of acute and chronic exercise on leukocyte function (summarized recently by Gjevestad and coworkers[351]). These studies include the impact of exercise on mitochondrial function[352] and oxidative stress,[353,354] each of which has been implicated as an essential component of the molecular transduction of PA in other tissues such as skeletal muscle.[355–357]

The sequencing of the human genome (completed in 2003 by the Human Genome Project) launched a new era of discovery in human biology. Technologies such as microarrays and sequencing permitted investigators to interrogate the expression of the whole human genome and to identify specific genes, or interacting pathways of genes, that could play a role in health and disease. More recently, these techniques have been used to explore an intriguing aspect of transcription mechanisms, namely the timing of gene expression across the lifespan.[358]

Epidemiological studies suggest that the early-life environment can affect epigenetic regulation of specific genes and make an important contribution to disease risk factors later in life. For example, exposure to famine in utero is associated with altered methylation status of genes related to the cardiometabolic disease (CMD) phenotype in elderly individuals.

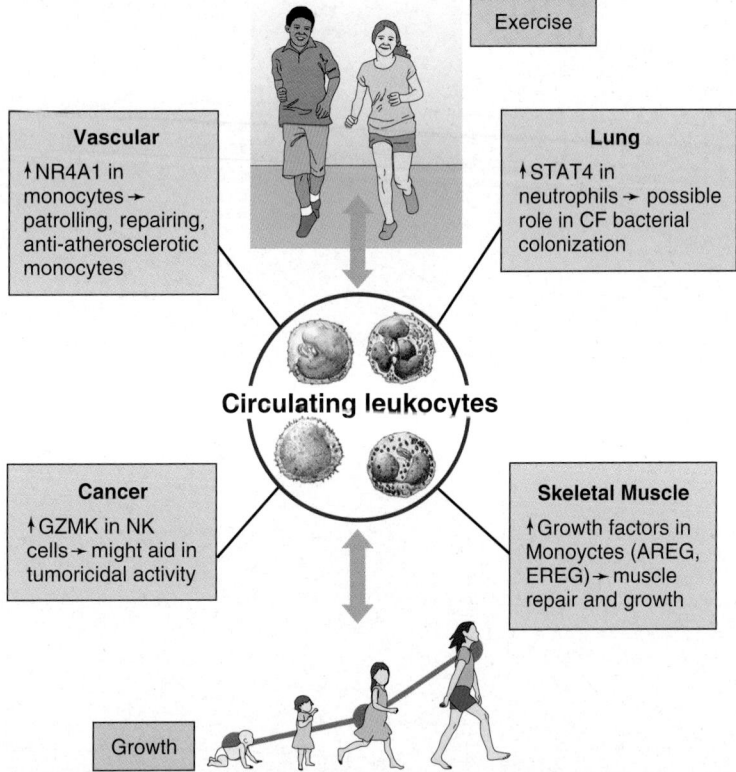

Fig. 12.14 Examples of gene expression changes in circulating leukocytes following brief exercise. These data reveal intriguing mechanistic links between physical activity and health. We hypothesize that these effects are influenced by growth and maturational status. *AREG*, EGF-like growth factor Amphiregulin; *CF*, cystic fibrosis; *EREG*, EGF-like growth factor Epiregulin; *NK*, natural killer. (Data from Radom-Aizik S, Zaldivar Jr. FP, Haddad F, Cooper DM. Impact of brief exercise on circulating monocyte gene and microRNA expression: implications for atherosclerotic vascular disease. *Brain Behav Immun* 2014;39:121-129; Radom-Aizik S, Zaldivar Jr. F, Leu SY, Galassetti P, Cooper DM. Effects of 30 min of aerobic exercise on gene expression in human neutrophils. *J Appl Physiol* 2008;104:236-243; and Radom-Aizik S, Zaldivar FP, Haddad F, Cooper DM. Impact of brief exercise on peripheral blood NK cell gene and microRNA expression in young adults. *J Appl Physiol* 2013;114:628-636.)

Furthermore, methylation of the retinoid-x-receptor-a in umbilical cord predicted greater than 25% of the variation in age- and sex-adjusted fat mass in children at 6 and 9 years old. Such findings imply that epigenetic changes that are induced by environmental exposures early in life can persist beyond the period of challenge. Alisch and coworkers investigated pediatric age-associated DNA methylation changes in peripheral blood mononuclear cells (PBMCs) of 398 healthy males (3–17 years old) and reported 2078 loci that exhibit age-associated DNA methylation differences.[359]

Human beings no longer live in the ecological niche into which they evolved. Survival for our hunter-gatherer human ancestors depended on a remarkably efficient integration of neuromotor, cardiovascular, and respiratory systems. Being "fit" meant the capability to quickly escape predation and the ability to expend just enough energy to access food while remaining in net-positive energy balance. Modern, more sedentary humans are facing the ominous fact that absent repeated bouts of exercise (each a sizeable physiological challenge to cellular homeostasis), fitness dissipates and the risk of serious disease is increased. Exercise activates a complex set of mechanisms that can affect a panoply of tissues ranging from mitochondria to bone. The molecular transducers of exercise in large measure prepare the organism to better deal with the thermodynamic, oxidative, and inflammatory stress of physical work.

The immediate implications and long-term consequences of insufficient PA are particularly concerning for child health. Childhood is a "critical period of growth and development" in which environmentally modifiable mechanisms (likely involving epigenetic reprogramming), can shape health across the lifespan. In the context of child health, the information gained from omics mapping of exercise responses can transform health policy that promotes optimal exercise in communities, schools, and in individual families, and begin to mitigate the current epidemic of childhood obesity. This approach will also impact an equally challenging and looming health problem—namely the role of exercise in children with chronic disease and disability. As medicine has advanced in recent years, there is an increasingly large population of child survivors of previously often fatal diseases and conditions (e.g., prematurity, CF, sickle cell anemia, childhood malignancies, and congenital heart disease). These conditions inevitably limit the child's ability to engage in exercise, and a better biologic definition of "healthy" exercise will pave the way for more precise and effective exercise prescriptions for the child or adolescent with chronic disease and disability.

References

Access the reference list online at ExpertConsult.com.

13 Integrating Patient-Reported Outcomes Into Research and Clinical Practice

ALEXANDRA L. QUITTNER, PhD, CHRISTINA J. NICOLAIS, MS, and
ESTEFANY SAEZ-FLORES, MS

Patient-centered care is based on a collaborative relationship between the patient and health care professional, in which the patient's perceptions, beliefs, and preferences are taken into account.[1,2] This provides an opportunity to develop a culture of collaboration in which patients can be actively engaged in decision-making.[3] One effective, standardized method of including the patient and family perspective on both clinical care and daily functioning is the use of patient-reported outcomes (PROs).[4] PROs are developed using patient input and are designed to systematically measure the frequency and impact of the disease on daily functioning, thus capturing the patient's "voice." In 2009, the US Food and Drug Administration (FDA) recognized the importance of PROs for evaluating the efficacy of new medications and laid out a framework for PRO development.[5,6] This guidance reflects a profound change in the process of regulatory approval of new medications and outcomes research.[7] This chapter focuses on the reliability, validity, and utility of PROs for children with respiratory diseases in the context of both research and clinical practice.

Definition of a Patient-Reported Outcome

A PRO is any measure of a patient's health status that reflects how he/she functions, feels, or survives, as reported by the patient him/herself.[3] Health-related quality of life (HRQoL) measures are one type of PRO that include "profiles" of functioning across several domains (e.g., respiratory symptoms, physical functioning, treatment burden).[4,5] These instruments measure aspects of functioning that are known only to the patient, including his/her symptoms, behaviors, and daily functioning. PROs can be used for several purposes: (1) as primary or secondary outcomes in clinical trials of new medications and treatments (including behavioral interventions), (2) to characterize the course of the disease and its progression, (3) to assess the effects of a disease on multiple aspects of patient functioning, and (4) to develop individualized treatment plans.[8–11]

To date, 27% of registered clinical trials include a PRO as either a primary or secondary endpoint.[12] This has nearly doubled from 14% in 2009[13] and is expected to increase as new PROs are developed.[14,15] This trend has been attributed to the movement toward collaborative care, as well as the complexities and burdens of treating and managing chronic conditions. In the period from 2006 to 2010, 17% of new drugs approved by the FDA used a PRO as a primary endpoint.[16] In 2009, Aztreonam for Inhalation was approved on the basis of a PRO (Cystic Fibrosis Questionnaire-Revised Respiratory [CFQ-R] Symptom Scale).[17] This was the first time a respiratory drug was approved using a PRO as the primary endpoint, highlighting the importance of the patient's perspective.[18]

Development and Utilization of Patient-Reported Outcomes

To utilize a PRO in a drug registration trial, it must be developed using patient and stakeholder input and meet strict psychometric criteria (e.g., reliability, validity, responsivity). A conceptual framework links the relevant concepts identified by qualitative data to the label claim (e.g., improvement in respiratory symptoms). This claim must also be hypothesized and tested, followed by calculation of several types of reliability and validity (Table 13.1). PROs must be sensitive to change on both an individual and group level.

To interpret the magnitude of this change, several qualitative and statistical methods have been developed. The minimal important difference (MID) score establishes the smallest, clinically meaningful, change that a patient can reliably detect.[19–21] The MID can be established using a visual analog scale, which asks the patient to indicate the amount of change he/she has experienced (i.e., anchor-based method). The MID can also be determined using statistical methods, such as calculation of $\frac{1}{2}$ standard deviation (SD) of change or 1 standard error of measurement. These analyses are bolstered by triangulating these values to establish the MID for a particular scale. A new term, the *clinically important difference* (CID), can also be used to identify clinically relevant changes in scores between two treatment groups.[22] This should be followed by a response distribution curve mapping individual changes for the two groups; ideally, there should be maximal separation between these curves.

Health-Related Quality of Life Measures

HRQoL measures are one of the most frequently used types of PROs first characterized by the World Health Organization's 1946 definition of health, which was "a state of complete physical, mental, and social well-being, and not merely the absence of disease or infirmity."[23] HRQoL measures are multidimensional, profile instruments focusing on several aspects of daily functioning. Typically, HRQoL

Table 13.1 Psychometric Criteria for a Patient-Reported Outcome

Measurement Property	Definition
CONSTRUCT VALIDITY	
▪ Content or face validity	▪ Extent to which items and response options are relevant and measure the domain
▪ Convergent validity	▪ PRO correlates with health-related variables in expected directions and with related measures
▪ Divergent validity	▪ Scores on disparate measures are not correlated (e.g., digestive symptoms and lung function)
▪ Discriminant validity	▪ Instrument distinguishes between groups sharing common characteristics (e.g., healthy vs. unhealthy)
▪ Responsivity	▪ Ability of PRO to detect change in predicted direction or no change when patient is stable
INTERPRETABILITY	
▪ MCID or the MID	▪ Smallest difference that can be reliably detected by patients and has clinical meaning
RELIABILITY	
▪ Internal consistency	▪ Whether items in a domain are intercorrelated, as evidenced by an internal consistency statistic (e.g., coefficient α)
▪ Interrater reliability	▪ Agreement between child and parent proxy on the construct or rating choices
▪ Test-retest	▪ Stability of patient report over time when no change has occurred in the measured concept

MCID, Minimal clinically important difference; *MID,* minimal important difference; *PRO,* patient-reported outcome.

Reprinted with permission of the American Thoracic Society. Copyright © 2017 American Thoracic Society.

Cite: Goss CH, Quittner AL/2007/Patient-reported outcomes in cystic fibrosis/Proc Am Thorac Soc/4/378-286.

Proceedings of the American Thoracic Society is an official journal of the American Thoracic Society.

measures evaluate four core domains: (1) disease state and physical symptoms, (2) functional status (e.g., performing daily activities), (3) psychological and emotional functioning, and (4) social functioning. Patient's scores are likely to differ across different domains of functioning and, thus, a total score should not be calculated. HRQoL instruments can track the natural progression of a disease, evaluate responsivity to pharmacological or behavioral interventions, and facilitate shared medical decision-making. For example, if a patient starts a new treatment for asthma, an HRQoL measure can assess its effectiveness in reducing asthma symptoms, such as wheezing. The tool can also be used to evaluate whether this new treatment is burdensome if this domain is measured.[4,24]

HRQoL instruments can be either generic or disease-specific. Generic measures are composed of general items that are relevant to populations with and without a chronic illness. Examples include the Pediatric Quality of Life Inventory,[25] the Child Health and Illness Profile,[26] and the Youth Quality of Life Instrument.[27] Generic HRQoL measures can be utilized across patient populations to compare the impact of a disease on different patient groups or to perform cost utility analyses (e.g., EuroQol-Five Dimensions Questionnaire [EQ-5D]).[28]

However, these measures are not specific to the symptoms experienced by patients with a particular illness; therefore, they are less sensitive to their effects on daily functioning and are not acceptable to test the efficacy of new medications.[29]

In contrast, disease-specific instruments are designed to assess the unique symptoms and challenges of a particular patient population. For example, a hallmark symptom of cystic fibrosis (CF) is excess mucus production. This symptom would not appear on a generic measure or one focused on a different respiratory condition, such as asthma. Thus, inclusion of items that are most relevant to a specific condition leads to greater sensitivity to treatment effects and is more informative for clinical care. This is the rationale for using disease-specific instruments for the purposes of drug registration trials.[30]

Developmental Considerations

Developing HRQoL measures for children poses unique challenges, ranging from differences in reading ability to the shifting importance of peers, school, and parents over the course of development. Comprehension and the ability to respond to items require several cognitive skills, such as focused attention, receptive and expressive language, and a conceptual understanding of the illness. All of these skills emerge gradually and at different points across development. Furthermore, the relevance and importance of a given domain is likely to change over the course of childhood and adolescence.[4] For example, social functioning is integral to adolescents' overall quality of life but is less relevant for preschoolers. Thus measures created within a developmental age group are more valid than measures downwardly extended from adult instruments. This ensures that the most relevant areas of functioning are measured in a developmentally appropriate way for a particular age group.[31]

HRQoL measures for children must undergo rigorous testing to ensure that individuals in the target age understand the vocabulary and concepts contained in the questionnaire. Research shows that children between 2 and 6 years have a more limited understanding of medical terms and concepts.[32] Children in this age group are able to report on observable areas of health, such as symptoms and levels of pain, using a pictorial format. They may, however, have more difficulty reporting on their emotional and social functioning.[33] By school age, children demonstrate a better understanding of the interplay between their health status and daily functioning. In fact, several studies have found that school-age children are able to provide reliable reports of their symptoms and functioning.[31–33]

Changes in cognitive and attentional capacity across development underscore the importance of response options and mode of administration when eliciting information from children. PROs can be administered electronically (computer, tablet), accompanied by colorful, animated pictures to increase understanding and attention.[9,15,34] Alternatively, to reduce errors based on reading difficulties and distractibility, measures can be administered to young children by an interviewer. For preschoolers, the CFQ-R Preschool version is administered by an interviewer using pictures to represent the items and rating scale options. In addition, because young children tend to select response options at endpoints rather than using

Do you cough up mucus or phlegm or spit?

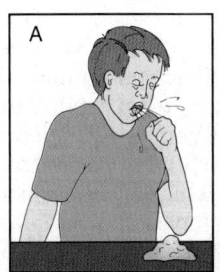 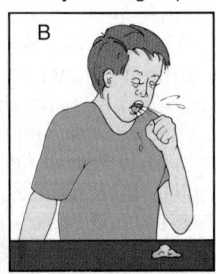 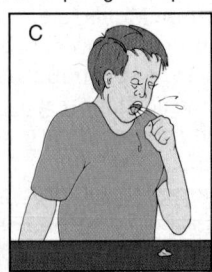 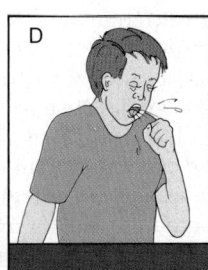

Fig. 13.1 (A–D) Example of CFQ-R response choices for the preschool version. The interviewer asks "Do you cough up mucus or phlegm or spit?" Children are asked to first choose between the extreme choices (1 and 4) and then to discriminate between the extreme and less extreme choice (e.g., 1 and 2, "Do you think you cough up very, very much phlegm, or a bit of phlegm?").

the full range of responses, a forced choice format is a useful alternative. Research shows that children as young as 3 years old can make forced choices. To make it more interactional and rewarding, we also use concrete rewards, such as stickers, to maintain their focus (Fig. 13.1).

Use of Proxy-Respondents

Parents or other caregivers can also complete HRQoL measures for young children to provide a different perspective.[35] Parent reports tend to correlate better with child reports for observable phenomena, such as physical functioning and symptom frequency (e.g., climbing stairs, coughing), but more poorly for emotional and social functioning (e.g., sadness).[36] Findings have suggested that children endorse more emotional distress, somatic complaints, and physical difficulties than their parents.[37] Thus, proxy measures cannot typically be substituted for patient reports. However, proxy respondents may be particularly useful for infants, patients with severe disease, or those with significant cognitive limitations.[38] In addition, differences between respondents may inform the focus of a clinic visit, medical decision-making, and health care utilization. Although proxy measures for health care providers have been developed, their validity is limited, because providers spend less time with their patients and observe them across fewer contexts.

Clinical Utility

Use of HRQoL measures in routine practice facilitates systematic, efficient collection of information about patients' ratings of their daily functioning. These data serve several purposes: (1) promoting communication between the patient and provider, (2) identifying frequently overlooked problems (e.g., school functioning), (3) monitoring disease progression and treatment burden, and (4) tailoring interventions to key aspects of a patient's daily life.[4,39] Thus both quality of life and health outcomes may improve as a result of integrating information from these instruments into routine care. Enhanced communication and monitoring symptoms are the best established benefits of this integration.[40,41]

First, HRQoL measures can provide a systematic way to facilitate discussions between patients and providers. Depending on the patient, he/she may report some symptoms (i.e., frequent cough), but disclose others only when directly asked

(e.g., fatigue or absences from school or work).[42] Research shows that both patients and physicians find these assessments helpful in identifying patient concerns, which has important implications for health outcomes.[41] Numerous studies have found that discussions of both physical and psychosocial issues during medical visits lead to improved treatment adherence, higher patient satisfaction, and fewer symptoms.[43,44]

A second benefit is the identification of frequently overlooked symptoms and problems that are important to the patient (e.g., depression, treatment burden).[45,46] This is particularly critical in the management of chronic respiratory diseases, because multiple domains of functioning are affected typically and treatment regimens are both time- and energy-intensive.[47–49] For example, patients with CF may spend 2 to 4 hours each day completing prescribed treatments, leading to social isolation and depression.[45,49] In addition, physiological measures, such as lung function and nutritional status, correlate modestly with HRQoL measures that assess symptom frequency, physical functioning, daily activities, or emotional functioning.[17,50] Thus, HRQoL data may alert providers to these critical issues, which are not captured by traditional medical assessments. Note that most of this research has been conducted with adults, highlighting a need for research in pediatric populations.

When given at regular intervals, HRQoL measures can monitor disease course, both in terms of natural progression and response to drug or behavioral interventions. Monitoring disease progression can lead to early identification of new concerns (e.g., weight loss) or ongoing challenges (e.g., increased fatigue). In addition, HRQoL assessment can measure the patient's responsivity to a new treatment. Because these instruments are multidimensional, they allow for differentiation of the benefits of a new medication (e.g., improvement in respiratory symptoms) from its side effects (e.g., increased treatment burden).[40] It is also possible that patients with the same lung function score may report very different levels of functioning in physical, social, or emotional domains.

HRQoL feedback can be used by providers to inform their treatment decisions and ensure that they are patient-centered, considering the individual's perceptions of their treatments, how they affect daily functioning, and their priorities.[40] HRQoL feedback has been shown to impact clinical decision-making in CF patients listed for lung transplant,[51] arthritis, epilepsy, and cancer.[52] Furthermore, if data are collected systematically on HRQoL instruments and included in national and international registries, trends identified in these data can be used to (1) predict health outcomes for individuals (e.g., lung function decline, number of exacerbations), (2) predict an individual's response to a new treatment, (3) conduct comparative effectiveness studies of similar medications (e.g., inhaled antibiotics), and (4) identify which treatments are most likely to maximize benefits and minimize costs.[53]

Studies testing the feasibility of integrating HRQoL and physiologic measures in routine care for respiratory disorders are just beginning but demonstrate considerable promise.[54,55] For example, adult patients with CF are using home spirometers that are linked to their pulmonary center along with daily symptom diaries.[54] Utilizing HRQoL and medical measures together may allow the CF team to identify early signs of an exacerbation, prompting a prescription for antibiotics or a visit to the clinic. A study by Santana and colleagues demonstrated that administration of HRQoL measures was feasible in a lung transplant clinic and did not prolong clinic visits.[56] Results also demonstrated improved communication between patients and health care providers and better patient management (e.g., medication changes). Furthermore, preliminary findings in pediatric and adult asthma clinics indicated that patients and providers were satisfied with implementation of an electronic quality of life (e-QOL) questionnaire about asthma during their routine visits.[57] The feasibility of routine assessment of quality of life is improving given technological advances (e.g., web- and computer-based applications) that increase the efficiency of measure completion and scoring.[39,58,59]

Summary

In summary, as the medical community transitions toward a patient-centered model of care, PROs will become a central mechanism for improving patient-provider communication, measuring health outcomes in chronic respiratory conditions, obtaining regulatory approval for new medications, and informing clinical decision-making. To move the field forward, we need to develop and utilize HRQoL instruments that are disease-specific and demonstrate good psychometric properties (e.g., reliability, validity). The following section reviews the strengths and limitations of disease-specific HRQoL measures for several pediatric respiratory disorders (i.e., aerodigestive disorders, asthma, bronchopulmonary dysplasia, CF, primary ciliary dyskinesia, and sleep apnea). Based on this information, we have recommended the best instrument for each condition.

Review of Disease-Specific Respiratory Health-Related Quality of Life Measures

AERODIGESTIVE DISORDERS

Vocal Cord Dysfunction

To date, four HRQoL measures for vocal cord dysfunction have been developed for pediatric populations. Three of these measures are completed by parents, and one offers both parent and child versions. All of them are brief with minimal respondent burden (Table 13.2). Additionally, these instruments

demonstrate good test-retest reliability and discriminant and convergent validity. However, internal consistency for the pVHI has not been reported. Most of these measures are limited by their reliance on parents or caregivers as informants and thus, they do not capture the patient perspective. The pediatric voice symptom questionnaire (PVSQ) has both child and parent proxy versions, and the child version utilizes pictorial responses, which enables patients who have different verbal abilities to complete the measure. Unfortunately, none of the instruments have established MIDs, and additional research on responsiveness is needed. Finally, the pediatric voice outcome survey (PVOS) lacks good psychometric properties and consists of only four items, which provides little information across domains.

Recommendation. Based on these findings, we recommend the PVSQ, because it has child and parent versions with age-appropriate pictorial responses and strong psychometric properties.

Feeding/Swallowing and Velopharyngeal Insufficiency

Currently Feeding/Swallowing Disorders and Velopharyngeal Insufficiency each have only one PRO measure. The VPI effects on life outcomes (VELO) includes both patient and parent versions, strong internal consistency, and good construct, convergent, and discriminant validity. The VELO has good test-retest reliability for the parent version, but this has not been evaluated for the child version.

The Feeding/swallowing impact survey (FS-IS) is the only published PRO for feeding/swallowing disorders. It is brief, has good internal consistency for the domain and total scores, and demonstrates good construct and discriminant validity. No child-report version of the measure is currently available.

Recommendation. Based on their strong psychometric properties, both the VELO and the FS-IS are recommended for use with their respective populations. However, the FS-IS has no MID, and a child report version is needed.

ASTHMA

There are currently 13 disease-specific HRQoL measures for children with asthma. While most of these measures demonstrate good internal consistency and test-retest reliability, they vary in their clinical utility and responsiveness to change (Table 13.3). Specifically, only the pediatric asthma quality of life questionnaire (PAQLQ) has an established MID, enhancing its clinical utility in assessing meaningful change to pharmacological or behavioral interventions. These measures vary with respect to informant type, age range, and practical utility (e.g., language translations, respondent burden). While several measures have corresponding child and parent versions, few include self-report versions for children under 5. Translations into multiple languages exist for three measures (childhood asthma questionnaires [CAQ], DISABKIDS-Asthma Module, and PAQLQ).

The majority of asthma measures have at least one limitation in terms of reliability, validity, sensitivity, responsivity, or clinical utility. With the exception of the PAQLQ, all measures lack an established MID, leaving clinicians and

Table 13.2 Health-Related Quality of Life for Children With Aerodigestive Disorders

Measure	Number of Items and Domains	Age Range and Respondent	Psychometrics: Reliability	Psychometrics: Validity
AERODIGESTIVE DISORDERS				
pVHI[60–62]	Number of items = 23 Domains (3): Functional, physical, emotional Total and visual analog scale	4–21 years Parent only	Test–Retest = .77–.95 *No internal consistency reported*	▪ Discriminates between healthy children and those prelaryngotracheal or postlaryngotracheal reconstruction ▪ Discriminates between children with benign vocal cord pathologies and other airway conditions
PVOS[63,64]	Number of items = 4	2–18 years Parent only	α = .69–.86 by age Test-retest = .89	▪ Discriminates between patients with and without tracheotomies (P = .004) ▪ Discriminates between patients before and after adenoidectomy ▪ Does not discriminate between healthy children and those with paradoxical vocal fold dysfunction
PVR-QOL[65]	Number of items = 10 Domains (2): Social-emotional, physical-functional	2–18 years Parent only	α = .96 Test-retest = .80	▪ Correlates with the PVOS (r = .70) ▪ Responsive to change in 9 patients with adenoidectomy (P < .001) ▪ Discriminates between healthy children and those with vocal fold paralysis, vocal nodules, or paradoxical vocal fold dysfunction
aPVSQ[66]	Number of items = 19	5–13 years Child & parent versions Child version includes pictorial answer choices	α = .88 (child) α = .82 (parent) Test-Retest = .88 (child) Test-Retest = .76 (parent)	▪ Discriminates between healthy children and those with dysphonia
aFS-IS[67]	Number of items = 18 Domains (3): Daily activities, worry, feeding difficulties	Parents/caregivers of children with feeding/swallowing disorders	Total score α = .89; daily activities α = .88, worries α = .85, feeding difficulties α = .85	▪ Three subscales and total score correlated with PedsQL Family Impact Module ▪ Discriminates between children with and without a feeding tube on completion of daily activities
aVELO[68–70]	Number of items = 23 (patient), 26 (parent) Domains (6): Speech limitation, swallowing, situational difficulty, emotional impact, perception by others, caregiver impact	5–17 years Patient- and parent-report	Parent α = .96, Patient α = .95 all domains α > .70 Test-retest: Parent ICC > .6 for total score and domains	▪ Factor analysis yields four-factor solution with some domains loading onto the same factor ▪ Parent- and patient-report significantly correlated with the PedsQL4.0 (r = .73) ▪ Discriminates between patients with and without velopharyngeal insufficiency ▪ Responsive to treatment ▪ Established MCID

FS-IS, Feeding/swallowing impact survey; *ICC*, intraclass correlation coefficient; *MCID*, minimal clinically important difference; *pVHI*, pediatric voice handicap index; *PVOS*, pediatric voice outcome survey; *PVR-QOL*, pediatric voice-related quality of life; *PVSQ*, pediatric voice symptom questionnaire; *VELO*, VPI effects on life outcomes instrument.
aDenotes the recommended measures.
Adapted with permission from Quittner AL, Modi A, Cruz I. Systematic review of health-related quality of life measures for children with respiratory conditions. *Paediatr Respir Rev.* 2008;9(3):220–232.

researchers with little guidance on how to interpret what changes in these scores mean. Respondent burden is a limitation of several measures (AMA [About My Asthma], TACQOL-Asthma [TNO-AZL Questionnaires for Children's Health-Related Quality of Life for Asthma], and LAQ [Life Activities Questionnaire for Childhood Asthma]). Thus, because of the time they take to complete, they are less feasible for use in routine care. In addition, the AMA only provides a total score, which limits providers' ability to isolate problem areas. Furthermore, for those measures with child and parent proxy versions, cross-informant agreement is rarely reported. Finally, additional self-report measures are needed for children under age 5.

Recommendation. To date, the PAQLQ is the most widely used asthma instrument. Several studies have demonstrated the PAQLQ's reliability and validity, and it is the only

disease-specific asthma measure that has an established MID. The PAQLQ is responsive to both pharmacological and behavioral interventions, and has been translated into over 30 languages. The corresponding parent-proxy measure (Pediatric Asthma Caregiver's Quality of Life Questionnaire) and the computerized/web-based administration options add to the utility of this instrument. The miniPAQLQ, a validated version of the questionnaire with 13 items instead of 23, and a pictorial version for children ages 5 to 7 are also available.

CYSTIC FIBROSIS

Five measures are available to assess HRQoL in children and adolescents with CF (Table 13.4). All of these are profile measures that assess respiratory symptoms and other domains of functioning. Only the Questions on Life Satisfaction–Cystic

Table 13.3 Health-Related Quality of Life Measures for Children With Asthma

Measure	Number of Items and Domains	Age Range and Respondent	Psychometrics: Reliability	Psychometrics: Validity
ASTHMA				
AMA[71]	Number of items = 55 Domains: Total score only	6–12 years Child No parent version	α = .93 Test-retest = .57	■ Moderately correlates with the PAQLQ ■ Responsive to a week-long asthma day camp
AAQOL[72,73]	Number of items = 32 Domains (6): Symptoms, medication, physical activities, emotion, social interaction, and positive effects	12–17 years Child No parent version	α = .70–.93 Test-retest = .76–.90	■ High correlation with PAQLQ (r = .81) ■ Weak to moderate correlation with patient-rated symptom severity, number of hospitalizations, severity of coughing, and severity of wheezing (r's = .25–.65)
ARQOLS[74]	Number of items = 35 Domains (5): Restriction of social life, physical disturbances, limitations in physical activity, daily inconveniences in managing the disease, and emotional distress	6–13 years Child No parent version	α = .81–.96	■ Responsive to pharmacological intervention
CAQ[75,76]	CAQ-A—Number of items=14 Domains (2): QOL and distress CAQ-B—Number of items=22 Domains (4): Active QOL, passive QOL, severity, and distress CAQ-C—Number of items=31 Domains (5): Active QOL, passive QOL, severity, distress, and reactivity	4–7 years Child (CAQ-A) 8–11 years Child (CAQ-B) 12–16 years Child (CAQ-C) No parent version	α = .60–.63 (CAQ-A) α = .57–.84 (CAQ-B) α = .50–.80 (CAQ-C) Test-retest (Pearson Coefficient) = .59–.63 (CAQ-A); .73–.75 (CAQ-B); .73–.84 (CAQ-C) Test-retest (ICC) = .59–.63 (CAQ-A); .72–.75 (CAQ-B); .68–.84 (CAQ-C)	■ Discriminates between asthmatic and nonasthmatic children ■ Correlates with parent ratings of asthma severity
CHSA[77]	Child Version—Number of items = 25 Domains (3): Physical health, child activities, and emotional health Parent Version—Number of items = 48 Domains (5): Physical health, activity (child), activity (family), emotional health (child), and emotional health (family)	7–16 years Child 5–12 years Parent	α = .74–.81 (child) Test-retest = .88–.91 α = .81–.92 (parent) Test-retest = .60–.85 *No cross-informant reliability reported*	■ Correlates with parent reports of their children's health status, and treatment burden as measured by the Asthma Symptom Day-14 (ASD-14) ■ Parent version correlates with disease severity as measured by symptom activity (e.g., number of days wheezing, coughing, tightness of chest) and medication use (e.g., number of times child used inhaler, nebulizer, bronchodilator)
DISABKIDS—Asthma Module[78,79]	Number of items = 37 Generic domains (6): Medication, emotion, social inclusion, social exclusion, limitation, and treatment Number of items = 11 Asthma-specific domains (2): Impact (consists of limitations and symptoms) and worry	"Smileys" version for children ages 4–7 years child 8–14 years child	α = .86–.92 (generic) α = .83–.84 (asthma module) Test-retest = .42–.53	■ Correlates with symptoms (cough), frequency of doctor visits, and use of inhaled medications ■ Discriminates between levels of disease severity ■ Linked to International Classification of Functioning, Health and Disability (ICF)
HAY[80]	Number of items = 32 Generic Domains (4): Physical activities, cognitive activities, social activities, and physical complaints Number of items = 40 Asthma-Specific Domains (4): Asthma symptoms, emotions related to asthma, self-concept, and self-management	8–12 years Child No parent version	α = .71–.83 (generic) α = .61–.81 (asthma module) Test-retest = within-subject SD for differences between first and second measurement differed significantly on "self-management," "physical activities," and "social activities"	■ Discriminates between healthy and asthmatic children in terms of physical and social activities ■ Correlates with the Child Attitude Toward Illness Scale ■ Responsive to illness severity over time

Table 13.3 Health-Related Quality of Life Measures for Children With Asthma—cont'd

Measure	Number of Items and Domains	Age Range and Respondent	Psychometrics: Reliability	Psychometrics: Validity
ITG-CASF[81,82]	Number of items = 8 Domains (3): Daytime symptoms, nighttime symptoms, & functional limitations	2–17 years Parent only	$\alpha = .84–.92$ *No test-retest reliability reported*	■ Correlates with asthma severity ($P = .002$), dyspnea ($P = .03$), and emergency room visits ■ Correlates with the number of days of school missed or limited activities for the child ($r = -.45$) and parent ($r = -.25$) ■ Responsive to illness severity over time
LAQ[83]	Number of items = 71 Domains (7): Physical, work, outdoor, emotions and emotional behavior, home care, eating and drinking, and miscellaneous	5–17 years Child No parent version	$\alpha = .97$ Test-retest = .76	■ Not reported
[a]PAQLQ[84–86]	Number of items = 23 Domains (3): Activity limitations, symptoms, and emotional function	7–17 years Child *Pictorial version for ages 5–7 in development*	Test-retest (ICC) = .84–.95 Cross informant r = .61 *No internal consistency reported*	■ Discriminates between levels of disease severity ■ Established MID (0.5 on a 7 point scale) ■ Converges with issues from asthma focus groups conducted by independent investigators ■ Responsive to pharmacological and behavioral interventions ■ Used in clinical trials
[a]Pediatric Asthma Caregiver's Quality of Life Questionnaire[87–88]	Number of items = 13 Domains (2): Activity limitations and emotional function	7–17 years Parent	Test-retest (ICC) = .80–.85 *No internal consistency or cross-informant reliability reported*	■ Discriminates between levels of disease severity ■ Established MID (0.5 on a 7-point scale) ■ Responsive to pharmacological intervention ■ Used in clinical trials
PedsQL-Asthma Module[89]	Number of items = 23 Generic Domains (4): Physical functioning, emotional functioning, social functioning, school functioning Number of items = 28 Asthma-Specific Domains (4): Asthma symptoms, treatment problems, worry, communication	5–18 years Child 2–18 years Parent	$\alpha = .74–.90$ (child) $\alpha = .77–.91$ (parent) $\alpha = .58–.85$ (child) $\alpha = .82–.91$ (parent) Parent-Child agreement (ICC) = .29–.87 *No test-retest reliability reported*	■ Discriminates between healthy children and children with asthma ■ Correlates with the PAQLQ ■ Responsive to an evidence-based asthma management intervention (N = 10)
TACQOL Asthma[30]	Number of items = 68 Domains (5): Complaints (spontaneous asthma symptoms), situations (that provoke symptoms), treatment (visits to doctors), medication (use of), and emotions (negative emotions)	8–16 years Child Parent	$\alpha = .60–.85$ (child) $\alpha = .64–.82$ (parent) Parent-Child agreement (ICC) = .64–.76 *No test-retest reliability reported*	■ Discriminates between levels of disease severity, except in the complaint domain ■ Responsive to a behavioral intervention to promote medication adherence ■ Correlates with the PAQLQ

AAQOL, Adolescent asthma quality of life questionnaire; *AMA*, about my asthma; *ARQOLS*, asthma-related quality of life scale; *CAQ*, childhood asthma questionnaires; *CHSA*, children's health survey for asthma; *HAY*, how are you?; *ICC*, intraclass correlation coefficient; *ITG-CASF*, integrated therapeutics group child asthma short form; *LAQ*, life activities questionnaire for childhood asthma; *MID*, minimal important difference; *PAQLQ*, pediatric asthma quality of life questionnaire; *QOL*, quality of life; *SD*, standard deviation; *TACQOL*, TNO-AZL Questionnaires for Children's Health-Related Quality of Life.
[a]Denotes the recommended measures.
Adapted with permission from Quittner AL, Modi A, Cruz I. Systematic review of health-related quality of life measures for children with respiratory conditions. *Paediatr Respir Rev.* 2008;9(3):220–232.

Fibrosis (FLZM-CF) and Cystic Fibrosis Questionnaire–Revised (CFQ-R) measure digestive symptoms and a new version of the CFQ-R includes Sinus Symptoms. Although all measures demonstrate good reliability, validity has only been established for the FLZM-CF, CFQol, and CFQ-R. Responsiveness to pharmacological and/or behavioral interventions has been established for most measures, and they

all discriminate between levels of disease severity and stable versus exacerbation events. The CFQ-R has been translated into 36 languages and is the only instrument with child and parent proxy versions.

Despite good reliability and validity, some weaknesses were noted. The FLZM-CF only has 1 item per scale, limiting its ability to reflect more complex constructs (e.g., treatment

Table 13.4   Health-Related Quality of Life Measures for Children With Cystic Fibrosis

Measure	Number of Items and Domains	Age Range and Respondent	Psychometrics: Reliability	Psychometrics: Validity
CYSTIC FIBROSIS				
CFRSD[91,92]	Number of items = 16 Domains (3): Respiratory symptoms, emotional impact, activity impact	12+Child No parent version	α =.72–.87 Test-retest = .71–.91	▪ Differentiates between ill and well states ▪ Responsiveness is currently being evaluated as part of several clinical trials
CFQoL[93]	Number of items = 52 Domains (9): Physical, social, treatment issues, chest symptoms, emotional responses, concerns for future, interpersonal relationships, body image, and career	14 through adulthood No parent version	α = .72–.92 Test-retest > .80; .74 for treatment issues	▪ Discriminates between levels of disease severity ▪ Sensitivity to change following intravenous antibiotics, as measured by FEV_1 and BMI ▪ Correlates with total Short-Form Health Survey (SF-36) scores (r's = .64–.74)
[a]CFQ-R[94–96]	Child Version—Number of items = 35 Domains (8): Physical, emotional state, social, body image, eating, treatment burden, respiratory, and digestion Adolescent/Adult Version Number of items = 50 Domains (12): Physical, emotional state, social, body image, eating, treatment burden, respiratory, digestion, role, vitality, health perceptions, and weight Parent Version—Number of items = 44 Domains (11): Physical, emotional state, body image, eating, treatment burden, respiratory, digestion, vitality, school, and weight	6–13 Child 14 through adulthood Adolescent 6–13 Parent *Pictorial version for children 3–6 in development*	α = .34–.73 (child); .55–.94 (adolescent); .58–.90 (parent) Test-retest =.45–.90 (teen/adult) Parent-child agreement = .27–.57	▪ Teen/adult version correlates with SF-36 ▪ Child version correlates with PedsQL ▪ Discriminates between healthy children and children with CF ▪ Discriminates between levels of disease severity ▪ Correlates with FEV_1, BMI, height, and weight ▪ Establishes 4-point MID on Respiratory Scale ▪ Sensitivity to change following treatment with IV antibiotics ▪ Used in many Phase III clinical trials as a primary endpoint ▪ Used as primary endpoint for approval of a new antibiotic
DISABKIDS—Cystic Fibrosis Module[97]	Number of items = 37 Generic domains (6): Medication, emotion, social inclusion, social exclusion, limitation, and treatment Number of items = 10 CF-specific domains (2): Impact (consists of limitations and symptoms), treatment	"Smileys" version for children ages 4–7 Child 8–16 Child	α =.80–.85 *No test-retest reliability reported*	▪ Distinguishes between clinician-rated illness severity
FLZM-CF[98]	Number of items = 9 Domains (9): Breathing difficulties/coughing, abdominal pain/digestive trouble, eating, sleep, routine therapy, adherence to daily therapy, significance for others, understanding, and free from disadvantage	12–17 Child 16 through adulthood Adolescent No parent version	α = .80 Test-retest = .69	▪ Child version correlates with KIDSCREEN ▪ Discriminates between healthy children and children with CF ▪ Adolescent/adult version correlates with FEV_1 and amount of time spent doing treatments ▪ Discriminates between mild, moderate, and severe disease severity ▪ Responsive to change after inpatient rehabilitation and following pulmonary exacerbations

BMI, Body mass index; *CFQoL*, cystic fibrosis quality of life questionnaire; *CFQ-R*, cystic fibrosis questionnaire—revised; *CFRSD*, CF respiratory symptom diary; *FEV₁*, forced expiratory volume in one second; *FLZM-CF*, questions on life satisfaction—cystic fibrosis, *MID*, minimal important difference.
[a]Denotes the recommended measure.
Adapted with permission from Quittner AL, Modi A, Cruz I. Systematic review of health-related quality of life measures for children with respiratory conditions. *Paediatr Respir Rev.* 2008;9(3):220–232.

adherence). Additionally, this measure has a 4-week recall period, which is quite long and may increase error.[99] The cystic fibrosis respiratory symptom diary (CFRSD) focuses on respiratory symptoms that are relevant to pulmonary exacerbations rather than using a multidimensional framework. Additionally, an MID value has only been established for the CFQ-R, thus increasing its clinical utility compared to other measures. The CFQ-R has been downwardly extended to children ages 3 to 6 years using pictures with an accompanying parent proxy version (see Fig. 13.1).[14] The CFQ-R Parent Preschool Proxy measure for children under 6 years of age has also demonstrated good construct validity and internal consistency. In contrast, the CFQol, FLZM-CF, and CFRSD measures do not extend below the age of 12.

Recommendation. The CFQ-R is the most widely used, well-established, instrument for CF and is recommended for both clinical and research purposes.[17] The CFQ-R covers the widest age range (ages 3 through adulthood). Advantages of the CFQ-R include its availability in more than 36 languages, an established MID of four points for the Respiratory Symptom scale, with an e-PRO version and computerized administration and scoring. Furthermore, CFQ-R scores have been found to correlate with health outcomes, including forced expiratory volume in one second (FEV_1)% predicted, body mass index (BMI) percentile, frequency of exacerbations, and improvements following lung transplantation. Sensitivity to change has been established for the CFQ-R in several clinical trials.[100–102] In fact, the Respiratory Symptom scale was used as a primary endpoint in the drug registration trial for aztreonam lysine for inhalation (AZLI).[18]

SLEEP-RELATED BREATHING DISORDERS

Two measures are available to assess HRQoL in children with sleep-related breathing disorders (Table 13.5). Both instruments rely on parent-proxy reports of sleep disturbances, physical symptoms, and emotional functioning. These instruments extend down to children as young as 6 months and

demonstrate adequate psychometric properties. Although both measures can detect postsurgical change, only the obstructive sleep apnea-18 (OSA-18) has an established MID. Despite these strengths, limitations exist with respect to utility and informant type. The OSA-18 uses a 1-month recall period, increasing the potential for recall bias and error. Furthermore, the obstructive sleep disorders-6 (OSD-6) utilizes only one item per scale, which limits its ability to assess more complex constructs. Finally, both measures rely solely on parent or caregiver report, highlighting the need to develop patient-report instruments.

Recommendation. The OSA-18 is recommended due to the established MID. However, more research on the internal consistency of this measure is warranted.

PRIMARY CILIARY DYSKINESIA

Just recently, the first disease-specific HRQoL measures for primary ciliary dyskinesia (PCD) were developed. This is a rare, difficult to diagnose chronic respiratory condition and, thus, we utilized a collaborative approach to recruit patients and parents in North American (i.e., United States and Canada) and Europe. We developed four versions of the Quality of Life-PCD instruments (QOL-child, parent-proxy, adolescent and adult).[15,105] Although PCD shares some commonalities with CF, there are also important differences. For example, children with PCD often develop hearing problems due to chronic otitis media, which can lead to challenges at school (i.e., Individual Education Plans) and with peer relationships. In contrast, they are not pancreatic insufficient and therefore do not have the growth and digestive issues that are common among pediatric patients with CF.

All of these measures were developed using the FDA Guidance,[5] beginning with focus groups with stakeholders (e.g., pulmonologists, ear, nose, and throat (ENT) specialists, patients/parents), followed by open-ended interviews, content analysis, and cognitive testing of the draft instruments.[15,105] We developed a school-age measure for children ages 6 to

Table 13.5 Health-Related Quality of Life Measures for Children With Sleep-Related Breathing Disorders

Measure	Number of Items and Domains	Age Range and Respondent	Psychometrics: Reliability	Psychometrics: Validity
SLEEP-RELATED BREATHING DISORDERS				
[a]OSA-18[103]	Number of items-18 Domains (5): Sleep disturbance, physical symptoms, emotional distress, daytime functioning, and caregiver concerns	6 months–12 years Parent Only	Item-total correlations = .38–.86 Test-retest > .70 *No internal consistency reported*	■ Discriminates between mild, moderate, and severe sleep apnea ■ Correlates with the OSD-6 and with Brouillette score ■ Correlates with the number of hourly apneic episodes, the number of hypopneic events, adenoid size ■ Responsive to change after surgery ■ Established MID
OSD-6[104]	Number of items=6 Domains (6): Physical suffering, sleep disturbance, speech and swallowing difficulties, emotional distress, activity limitation, and level of concern	6 months–12 years Parent only	α = .80 across items Test-retest = .69–.86	■ Responsive to change after adenotonsillectomy ■ Correlates moderately with physician estimates of child's QOL ■ Correlates with a global sleep-related QOL rating

MID, Minimal important difference; *OSA-18,* obstructive sleep apnea-18; *OSD-6,* obstructive sleep disorders-6 survey.
[a]Denotes the recommended measure.
Adapted with permission from Quittner AL, Modi A, Cruz I. Systematic review of health-related quality of life measures for children with respiratory conditions. *Paediatr Respir Rev.* 2008;9(3):220–232.

12 years, a parent-proxy measure for this age group, an adolescent measure for ages 13 to 17 years, and an adult version for those 18 years or older. The school-age version is a "speaking questionnaire" in which the computer/tablet asks the questions aurally with accompanying pictures. All measures take less than 10 minutes to complete and all have been developed and validated for electronic patient-reported outcomes (ePRO) administration; platforms including internet, tablet, and phone administration.

The preliminary measures for school-age children include 37 items, the parent proxy has 41 items, and the adolescent measure has 43 items. We are now performing international, psychometric validation studies of these measures and plan to reduce the number of items on each questionnaire once we have analyzed the items in relation to their scales. Generally, the domains represented on the pediatric measures, depending on respondent, include Respiratory Symptoms, Physical Functioning, Emotional Functioning, Treatment Burden, Ears & Hearing, Sinus Symptoms, Social and Role Functioning, Vitality, Health Perceptions, and School Functioning. Preliminary psychometric testing in the UK and North America indicate that these measures have good reliability (both internal consistency and test-rest reliability) and strong content, convergent and divergent validity (with the St. George's Respiratory Questionnaire [SGRQ] and the Sino-nasal Outcome Test [SNOT]). All versions of the QOL-PCD have now been translated into German, Danish, Dutch, Spanish, and Arabic. Further translations are planned.

There is an urgent, unmet clinical need for FDA/European Medicines Agency (EMA) approved medications for PCD, and given that it is unlikely that lung function will be a sensitive indicator of improvement in this population, the use of HRQoL measures as a primary or secondary endpoint is critical for clinical trials of new medications. The QOL-PCD measures have been designed to meet this need. In addition, these measures can be used to better understand this complex, rare disease including its course and progression, predictors of exacerbation, and long-term functioning.

Recommendation. To date, the newly developed QOL-PCD measures are the only disease-specific HRQoL measures to be developed. PCD is extremely rare and, thus, we developed these measures in both North America and Europe. Their preliminary development and psychometric properties indicate they will become the "gold standard" for this population. We are in the process of translating these measures into multiple languages and they will be utilized soon to evaluate the benefits of a new medication for PCD.

Conclusions and Future Directions

The shift in medicine toward a patient-centered model of care is consistent with the PRO guidance established by the FDA and guidelines written by the EMA.[6] The FDA Guidance outlines the steps needed for PRO development and highlights the importance of including the patient perspective in the evaluation of new pharmacological interventions. HRQoL instruments are one of the most commonly used types of PROs and provide a more comprehensive assessment of functioning across several domains (i.e., symptoms, physical, emotional and social functioning, treatment burden). This information is useful for both research and clinical purposes. These measures can improve patient-provider communication and care, track progression of disease and health outcomes, evaluate the efficacy of new pharmacological or behavioral interventions, and inform decision-making.

Several well-established HRQoL instruments exist for aerodigestive disorders, asthma, CF, bronchopulmonary dysplasia, primary ciliary dyskinesia, and sleep-related breathing disorders. There is a need to develop disease-specific HRQoL measures for other pediatric respiratory disorders, such as interstitial lung disease, lung cancer, and ventilator dependency. Previous research has utilized generic measures for these disorders.

In conclusion, HRQoL measures provide unique information on patient symptoms, level of functioning, and response to treatment. Inclusion of these instruments has been shown to facilitate patient-provider communication, detect problematic areas of functioning, and enhance shared decision-making. As technology advances, these instruments can be administered electronically on tablets, smart phones, or computers, which facilitates data entry and immediate scoring. Thus, use of these instruments is increasing in both clinical and research domains. Integration of HRQoL measures into clinical care is a critical step in promoting patient-centered care and quality of life.

References

Access the reference list online at ExpertConsult.com.

Suggested Reading

Committee for Medicinal Products for Human Use. European Medicines Agency. *Reflection Paper on the Regulatory Guidance for the Use of Health-Related Quality of Life (HRQL) Measures in the Evaluation of medicinal Products.* London: EMA; 2005.

PROMIS Dynamics tools to Measure Health Outcomes from the Patient Perspective [Internet]. [Place unknown]: National Institutes of Health; 2015. Available from: http://www.nihpromis.org/sitemap. Cited May 27, 2016.

Quality of Life Resource [Internet]. New York: American Thoracic Society; 2007. Available from: http://qol.thoracic.org/. Cited May 27, 2016.

Snyder CF, Aaronson NK, Choucair AK, et al. Implementing patient-reported outcomes assessment in clinical practice: a review of the options and considerations. *Qual Life Res.* 2012;21(8):1305–1314.

US Food and Drug Administration. Guidance for industry. Patient-reported outcome measures: use in medical product development to support labeling claims; 2009. Available from: www.fda.gov/downloads/Drugs/Guidances/UCM193282.pdf.

14 Transition From Pediatric to Adult Care

ANNA BAMFORD, MBBS, and DONALD PAYNE, MBBChir, MD, FRCPCH, FRACP

Introduction

Children and adolescents with chronic respiratory disease become adults with chronic respiratory disease. As a result of ongoing improvements in health care, this is now increasingly the norm rather than the exception. Therefore professionals who look after children and adolescents with chronic illness have a responsibility to consider how their patients' health care needs will continue to be met as they become adults. This chapter discusses the background to transition from pediatric to adult health care and provides a practical approach to assist health professionals, administrators, patients, and families to plan and negotiate the process.

What Is Transition?

Transition, as defined by the Society for Adolescent Health and Medicine in the United States, is a "purposeful, planned process that addresses the medical, psychosocial and educational/vocational needs of adolescents and young adults with chronic physical and medical conditions as they move from child-centered to adult-oriented health care systems."[1] There is a wide range of chronic pediatric respiratory disorders that persist through adolescence into adulthood (Box 14.1). For some conditions, such as cystic fibrosis, models of transition are already relatively well established, with the existence of recognized specialist adult centers and clear pathways to facilitate the move from pediatric to adult care.[2–5] For other, rarer (e.g., primary ciliary dyskinesia) or more heterogeneous conditions (e.g., bronchiectasis), transition models are less well established.[6–8] Finally, there is an increasingly large cohort of adolescents and young adults growing up with respiratory disorders (e.g., chronic lung disease associated with extreme prematurity, muscular dystrophy, or ventilator-dependent airway malacia) with which adult health professionals may have had little or no clinical experience and minimal training.[9–11] These young adults may have associated co-morbidities, (e.g., significant neurologic disease or cognitive impairment) that present an additional challenge to ensuring a successful transition.

Why Is Transition Important?

Before outlining some of the practical steps involved in developing a transition plan, it is important to consider why the process needs to be addressed at all. Why should patients and families, who have developed a trusting and collaborative relationship with their health care providers over many years, have to leave this behind and develop a completely new set of relationships? There are a number of aspects to this question. These include acknowledging the process of adolescent development, the emerging health care needs and patterns of morbidity in adulthood, the differences between pediatric and adult models of care, and the views of patients and their carers.[12–14]

UNDERSTANDING ADOLESCENT DEVELOPMENT

For adolescents and young adults with a chronic respiratory disorder, the transition from pediatric to adult health care is just one of a number of transitions they will encounter. Adolescence refers to the developmental stage between childhood dependence and adult independence. During this time, individuals begin to establish their own identity and self-image and take on adult roles (Box 14.2).[15] Key tasks that adolescents and young adults usually complete include developing independence from parents or caregivers, forming relationships outside the family, and providing for themselves financially. Significant transitions during this period include leaving school and joining the workforce or enrolling in higher education, moving away from the parental home, and possibly becoming parents themselves. Health professionals who work with adolescents and young adults need to acknowledge and understand this process of adolescent development, and recognize that the transition from pediatric to adult health care occurs within the wider context of a more general transition from childhood to adulthood.

Seen within this context of increasing independence and autonomy, transition to adult care thus sends a powerful message to young people with chronic illness that they have a future and that they are expected to participate in and contribute to society as adults, which the majority of young people with chronic illnesses go on to do.[16,17] Remaining within the pediatric health care system may give the impression that living life as an adult is unlikely to be achievable. With increasing age and maturity, many young people become increasingly uncomfortable being cared for in a child-centered setting. A danger of not addressing the transition to adult care is that they may become lost to follow-up when they decide for themselves that they have outgrown their pediatrician.

It is also important to be aware that some young adults with chronic illness (e.g., those with muscular dystrophy, severe neurologic impairment, or who are ventilator dependent) will never be able to attain the same degree of independence as that achieved by their healthy peers. However, this does not mean that these young adults should be looked after within a pediatric model of care indefinitely. There are

Box 14.1 Pediatric Respiratory Disorders That May Persist Into Adulthood

- Cystic fibrosis
- Asthma
- Primary ciliary dyskinesia
- Other causes of bronchiectasis (e.g., immunodeficiency, postinfectious)
- Interstitial lung disease
- Chronic lung disease of prematurity
- Obliterative bronchiolitis
- Neuromuscular disorders (e.g., muscular dystrophy)
- Tracheomalacia/bronchomalacia
- Lung transplant recipients

Box 14.2 Tasks of Adolescence

- Separate from parents
- Develop a coherent sense of self
- Come to terms with physical self
- Come to terms with sexual self
- Develop mature altruistic relationships
- Develop financial independence

many ways to acknowledge a young person's development into adulthood (seeing them on their own, discussing age-appropriate topics, providing them with opportunities to be involved in decision making), even if their physical independence is limited. These issues are discussed in more detail later in the chapter. For young adults who are physically dependent on others for providing aspects of their care, one obvious example of emerging adulthood can be seen when this assistance is no longer provided by parents but by other adults (e.g., friends or partners).

ADULT HEALTH CARE NEEDS AND PATTERNS OF MORBIDITY

Pediatricians are trained to deal with children and, increasingly, with adolescents.[18] However, few are trained to provide care for adults. In the same way as pediatricians recognize that it is inappropriate for adult-trained physicians to manage young children, it also becomes increasingly inappropriate for pediatricians to continue to care for their patients once they have completed the tasks of adolescence and are living their lives as adults. While pediatricians may feel relatively confident and competent managing certain disease-specific aspects of respiratory disorders, such as asthma or bronchiectasis, more general areas of adult health care (e.g., sexual and reproductive health, cardiovascular problems, or liaison with employers) are likely to be less well managed. There are some clinics (e.g., for cystic fibrosis) in which the same team provides care for children, adolescents, and adults. However, in the interest of optimal health care, it is important that whatever model is employed, professionals who manage adults with chronic respiratory disease receive adequate training in general adult health issues. Adult-trained physicians may be more likely to address issues, such as fertility, teratogenicity of treatments, and the importance of genetic counseling, which pediatric physicians may not be as comfortable discussing.[19,20]

DIFFERENCES BETWEEN PEDIATRIC AND ADULT MODELS OF CARE

Logistical and financial considerations also come into play when considering transition. Pediatric and adolescent medical departments are not designed or funded to provide care for adults. Budgets are limited, and staffing, equipment, and hospital systems are designed to provide high-quality and developmentally appropriate care for infants, children, and adolescents rather than adults. Therefore at some point, a decision must be made to transfer adolescents and young adults with chronic illness to a unit that can provide developmentally appropriate care.

Traditionally, the adult model expects patients to take responsibility for their own care. If they do not attend for regular outpatient review, they are less likely to be contacted and followed up than if they are being managed within a pediatric setting. A challenge for adult physicians is to recognize and understand that adolescents and young adults are still developing and that they may continue to need a greater degree of involvement by the health care team, at least for the first few years after transfer.

WHAT IS THE EVIDENCE BASE FOR TRANSITION?

Over time, a number of principles regarding the transition process have been developed, which have gained widespread consensus.[21-25] A number of studies have highlighted problems associated with unsuccessful transition from pediatric to adult care, in different subspecialty areas. These include unexpected transplant rejection following transfer to adult care in young adults who had received renal or liver transplants in childhood,[26,27] and the deaths of young adults with congenital heart disease who were cared for by clinicians lacking specific training in the management of these conditions.[28] The absence of an appropriately trained adult team is a significant barrier to successful transition, as discussed later in the chapter. Less extreme consequences of unsuccessful transition to adult care include the loss of young adult patients to follow-up, frequent missed appointments, and deterioration in disease control.[29-31] For young people with chronic respiratory disease, there is a very real possibility that lack of regular contact and follow-up with the medical team over a number of years can result in a major and potentially irreversible deterioration in lung function and quality of life.[32]

The evidence base for particular transition programs is small. What evidence there is suggests that having planned transition activities for chronic disease is preferable to none at all, with improvements in adult clinic attendance, disease control, and fewer complications when there are pathways in place. Cole et al. (2015) implemented a transition service for young people with inflammatory bowel disease, which resulted in decreased admissions and need for surgery, and improved adherence to medication and clinic attendance following transfer to adult health care, compared with those who did not go through the program.[33] In young people with type 1 diabetes, establishing a formal transition pathway has been shown to improve adult clinic attendance, HbA1c measures, and patient and carer satisfaction.[34,35] In chronic respiratory disease, the most substantial evidence relates to the transition of young people with cystic fibrosis. Progressing through a transition program, or at least the introduction of the adult team prior to transfer, has been shown to reduce patient and parent concern regarding transition to an adult service.[36-38] Gravelle and colleagues evaluated three components of their transition program—a clinical pathway, a joint pediatric and adult pregraduation workshop for patients, and a readiness for transition scale delivered to young people about to graduate from pediatric services. The combination of these interventions led to improved identification of deficits in patient knowledge and improved patient understanding of the adult care system and confidence for transition.[39] In terms of disease outcomes, one study found that young people appropriately transferred to adult care had a less rapid decline in lung function, compared with disease severity–matched patients who remained in pediatric care centers.[40] Duguépéroux and colleagues have described outcomes for young adults with cystic fibrosis 1 year after transfer to an adult center and demonstrated that the clinical status of the patients transferred remained stable, with an increase in the mean number of outpatient attendances in the year after transfer to the adult center, compared to the year before.[41]

Transition: A Practical Approach

Transition refers to the process of preparing adolescents and young adults for the move to the adult health care system and to an adult health team. It is widely acknowledged that this is a continuous process leading to the single event of transfer of care. The transition process needs to be planned in advance and begin early. While there are certain elements of transition that are disease-specific, there are many aspects that are generic to all chronic illness. Russell Viner, a leading advocate for adolescent and young adult health in the United Kingdom, has summarized the approach to transition as follows[42]:

- Prepare young people and their families well in advance for moving from pediatric to adult services
- Ensure that they have the necessary skill set to survive and thrive there
- Prepare and nurture adult services to receive them
- Listen to young people's views

PREPARING YOUNG PEOPLE FOR TRANSITION

Preparing young people and their families for transition involves discussing the process with them early. Some suggest making transition a topic of discussion from the moment of diagnosis. In practice, this may prove difficult, given the amount of information that families have to take in at the time of diagnosis of a chronic illness. However, the prospect of transition to adult care is an issue that needs to be brought up in any discussion of long-term prognosis—a subject that usually arises in conversations at an early stage. For older children and adolescents, there is no "right" time to start increasing the focus on transition. However, the consensus is that the emphasis on transition should increase as children enter adolescence, often at the same time as they move from primary to secondary school. Transition is one aspect of the wider process of providing developmentally appropriate health care for adolescents. Health professionals can employ certain practical strategies to help promote healthy adolescent development and prepare adolescents for their subsequent move to adult care. These strategies include the following:

- Seeing adolescents on their own, separate from their parents, for part of the consultation
- Emphasizing the importance of confidentiality
- Discussing their understanding of their illness and actively promoting self-management
- Addressing general adolescent health issues, in addition to those related to their specific condition

Seeing adolescents alone for part of the consultation is a visible way of demonstrating to them and their families that adolescence is a time of developing independence. It conveys a message to the whole family that it is appropriate for the adolescent to begin to take increasing responsibility for his or her own health.[43] A major advantage of seeing adolescents alone is that it increases the chance that they will talk. Asking questions about school, friends, and activities shows an interest in the adolescent as an individual, rather than in his or her disease. This allows time for a rapport to develop and provides an opportunity to see how the young person's illness fits in with the rest of his or her life—in particular, whether or not the adolescent sees his or her condition and its treatment as a priority.

Box 14.3 shows the Home, Education, Eating, Activities, Drugs, Sexuality, Suicide, Safety (HEEADSSS) framework, used widely around the world, which is a helpful guide for clinicians to use when interviewing adolescents.[44] HEEADSSS begins with relatively unthreatening questions about home, school, and activities. These have the dual purpose of gathering information and allowing time to develop rapport. However, difficulties in these areas (e.g., prolonged school absence, no hobbies or interests) may be a reflection of poor disease control or other underlying problems, such as anxiety or depression. As discussed later in the chapter, mental health problems and health risk behaviors, such as smoking, alcohol, and other drug use, are common in adolescents with chronic illness and always need to be considered.[45-47] It is essential that such a risk and protective health screen is used at the outset of adolescence and is continually revisited and updated.

ESTABLISHING CONFIDENTIALITY

When seeing adolescents on their own, it is essential to explain at the outset that the conversation will remain confidential and that, while you may have to consult with colleagues, information will not be discussed with parents, without the adolescent's permission. The limits of confidentiality must also be made explicit. The disclosure of any activity that puts the young person at serious risk of significant harm (such as suicidal thoughts or physical/sexual abuse) cannot remain confidential. Neither can the disclosure of activities that put others at risk. If adolescents are assured of some degree of confidentiality, they are more likely to speak frankly.[48] In practice, this increases the chances of being able to address issues that can have a major impact on disease control (e.g., treatment adherence, smoking, and anxiety), thus opening up the real possibility of providing effective health care.[49]

Box 14.3   The HEEADSSS Framework

H Home

- Where do you live? Who lives with you?
- What are relationships like at home?
- Who would you talk to if you had a problem?

E Education (or Employment)

- Which school do you go to? Which year are you in?
- Which subjects do you enjoy? What are you good at?
- Who do you spend time with at school? What are the teachers like?
- Is your school a safe place?

E Eating

- Does your weight or body shape cause you any stress?
- Has there been any change in your weight recently?

A Activities

- What do you enjoy doing outside of school?
- Are you in any clubs or sports teams?
- Who do you meet up with at weekends?
- Do you see your friends mostly in person or catch up online?
- Some young people tell me they spend a lot of time online. What sort of things do you use the internet for?
- How many hours per day do you spend using screens (computer/television/phone)?

D Drugs

- Do any of your friends or family smoke cigarettes or drink alcohol? How about you?
- How much do you smoke/drink? Every day? On weekends?
- Have you ever tried marijuana or other drugs not prescribed to you?

S Sexuality

- Are you interested in boys, girls, or both? Are you not yet sure?
- Have any of your relationships been sexual relationships?
- What do you understand by the term "safer sex"?

S Suicide

- Do you feel stressed or more anxious than you would prefer to feel?
- Do you have any trouble with your sleep pattern?
- How would you describe your mood? Do you ever get really down?
- Some people who feel really down often feel like hurting themselves or even killing themselves. Have you ever felt like that?
- Have you ever tried to hurt yourself?

S Safety

- Is there any violence at your home or school? Do you feel safe at home?
- Have you ever met (or planned to meet) with anyone whom you first encountered online?
- Have you ever been seriously injured? How? How about anyone else you know?

From Klein D, Goldenring J, Adelman W. HEEADSSS 3.0: the psychosocial interview for adolescents updated for a new century fueled by media. *Contemp Pediatr.* 2014:31:16-28.

ACTIVELY PROMOTING SELF-MANAGEMENT

Self-management of chronic disease is a major focus of adult programs. Pediatricians can assist in helping adolescents to develop self-management skills through the gradual process of increasing the focus on the adolescent, rather than their parents, during each consultation. As mentioned earlier in the chapter, this is helped by seeing adolescents on their own. Discussions should focus on the understanding of their illness, their priorities and goals, the reasons for and the effects of adhering to a specific treatment regimen, and ways to minimize the impact of the illness on their day-to-day life. Over time, other practical issues can be discussed. These include how to book or reschedule an appointment, obtaining prescriptions and knowledge of any fees payable, whom to contact in an emergency, and how to get to the adult clinic (e.g., public transport, parking). These are issues common to all chronic illnesses and, when addressed, can help to reduce the anxiety around the eventual transfer of care to an adult center.[38] To assist in this process, many transition programs have developed checklists that patients and professionals can use to track each individual's progress through adolescence and identify issues that may need to be addressed at specific times. An example is shown in Box 14.4, and others are available on the transition websites listed in the Suggested Reading at the end of the chapter.[22,23] There is new evidence for the use of other technology to encourage self-management and assist with transition, such as scheduled mobile phone text messages, web-based programs, or online contact with transition mentors.[50–52]

ADDRESSING GENERAL ADOLESCENT HEALTH ISSUES

Health professionals who work with adolescents need to acknowledge and understand the process of adolescent development and be aware of both the impact of emerging adolescent behaviors on disease management, as well as the effect of a chronic respiratory disorder on normal adolescent development.[53,54] Regular appointments and hospital admissions, time off school, limitation of normal activities, and reduced ability to interact with peers can inhibit an adolescent's path toward independence. Parents may also find it difficult to let go. Therefore it is important that health professionals monitor their patients' progress through adolescence and identify problems when they arise.

Certain features of adolescence, such as engaging in exploratory behaviors (e.g., smoking, drug use) and challenging authority (e.g., reluctance to adhere to a regular treatment regimen, nonattendance at appointments), may lead to poor disease control.[45] The available data suggest that adolescents with chronic illness are just as likely, or even more likely, to engage in health-risk behaviors as their healthy peers.[45–47,55] The effects of certain behaviors, such as smoking, on health outcomes are more pronounced in adolescents with chronic respiratory disease than in those without.[43,56] Adolescents with chronic illness are more likely to suffer from anxiety and depression, which may also have a considerable impact on health outcomes and on a young person's ability to manage their illness.[57,58] Health professionals need to develop confidence in discussing health-risk behaviors and mental health problems with their adolescent patients and be able to offer

Box 14.4   Transition Readiness: Sample Checklist for a Young Person Aged 15 to 16 Years

Independence

Sees health professional alone for some of the consultation
Understands about confidentiality (and its limits)
Feels comfortable asking questions during the consultation

Awareness of Transition and Transfer

Understands that transfer to the adult center will occur within the next 2 to 3 years
Understands some of the differences between pediatric and adult health care
Knows which adult center he or she will be going to and where it is

Self-Management

Understands his or her medical condition and can explain it to a friend
Understands his or her treatment regimen (what the treatments do, why they are important, and the side effects)
Able to administer own medication/treatment
Able to discuss any difficulties with adherence to treatment
Knows whom to contact in an emergency
Beginning to know how to make appointments, obtain new prescriptions

General Adolescent Health

Able to discuss body image, healthy eating, exercise
Has discussed sexual health/fertility with his or her doctor
Has discussed alcohol, smoking, and other drug use—impact on their health
Able to discuss mood (anxiety, depression)
Able to identify support systems outside the family and how to access psychological support if required

Educational and Vocational Planning

Has discussed school, plans for the future
Able to discuss any difficulties at school (attendance, bullying, subject difficulties)

---

support along with access to more specialized services (e.g., clinical psychology or psychiatry) when appropriate. In support of this approach, a study in primary care involving adolescents 11–16 years of age demonstrated that adolescents had more positive perceptions of their primary care physician when sensitive issues, such as drugs, sex and mental health, were discussed.[59] The adolescents studied were also more likely to take an active role in their treatment if the consultation included the discussion of these types of sensitive topics.[59]

Providing this level of care for adolescent patients requires that systems be organized to facilitate the process, such as scheduling longer appointment times for young people. This has significant implications for the provision of appropriate resources. However, taking a long-term view, the argument for providing intensive input during adolescence and young adulthood is that this will lead to improved health outcomes and reduce the potential for unscheduled emergency visits and hospital admissions, which account for the majority of the health care costs associated with chronic illness.

PREPARING ADULT SERVICES TO RECEIVE YOUNG PEOPLE WITH CHRONIC RESPIRATORY DISORDERS

A successful transition requires there to be an adult service that is willing and able to receive young people with chronic illness and to provide high-quality care. For cystic fibrosis, the existence of specialist adult centers is well established, and the models of transition are those to which other subspecialties often look for guidance. Transition programs for asthma, a much more common condition than cystic fibrosis, are less well established, probably because most young adults with persistent asthma do not require the same level of specialist, multidisciplinary input as young adults with cystic fibrosis.[60] However, for children and adolescents with severe or treatment-resistant asthma, transition and transfer to a specialist adult center will be required.[61]

For young adults with rarer conditions, the challenge for pediatric health professionals is to identify suitable colleagues in the adult system that have the skills and training to provide ongoing care. The absence of suitable providers is one of the reasons why some patients may remain under the care of the pediatric team indefinitely. For example, the increasing number of young people dependent on ventilatory support now reaching adulthood creates a challenge for their transition.[62] In the longer term, one of the many roles for pediatricians to play is that of advocate for the provision of suitable training programs for adult physicians. Adolescent medicine is an accredited specialty in the United States, Canada, and, most recently, Australasia.[63] Good communication, collaboration, and respect between pediatric and adult units are essential. Depending on the availability of services and personnel, different models of transition and transfer may develop. One option is the establishment of a regular joint clinic for adolescents and young adults, involving both pediatric and adult teams, which may be based either at one center or the other, or rotate between the two. Another model is for patients to have one or two appointments at the adult center while still being seen at the pediatric center prior to the eventual final transfer of care to the adult center. With this type of arrangement, it is important to make clear who should be the first port of call in an emergency. There is no evidence that any one model is superior to another, and, in practice, the model developed will depend on a variety of factors. These include the number of patients to be transitioned and the availability of appropriately trained staff, funding, and clinic space. More important than the precise model of transitional care employed is the need for all health professionals who work with adolescents and young adults to recognize and understand the process of adolescent development and to incorporate this into their day-to-day practice.

LISTENING TO YOUNG PEOPLE'S VIEWS

It is vital to involve adolescents and young adults in the transition process.[42] Transition is often an unsatisfactory experience for young people, as well as for their parents or carers. Often they report that the process is uncoordinated, complicated, and anxiety provoking, and that they feel lost and unprepared for moving to an adult service, particularly if the move is sudden.[12,64] On the other hand, young people do appreciate the relative independence and increased responsibility expected of them in the adult service if supported appropriately.[12] Engaging with young people to develop or improve processes means ensuring that they not only participate actively in their own individual transition and transfer to adult care but also that they can contribute to effective planning and implementation of the wider program of transition.[65] The Royal College of Paediatrics and Child Health in the United Kingdom has published guidelines to promote the participation of children and young people in the planning of health services.[66] Transition programs are much more likely to be successful if they incorporate the views and ideas of the young people they are designed to support, and it has been shown that feeling less involved in their health care results in poorer disease outcomes in adolescents and young adults.[67]

Providing a suitable environment, considering both the physical space characteristics and the staff attitude and values, is also important.[68] Too often, young people report that they feel like they do not belong in either pediatric or adult care, with the pediatric setting feeling paternalistic and too controlling, and the adult service overwhelming, impersonal, and unwelcoming.[69] It is essential to engage with young people in the design and style of clinical areas as well as how the service operates. This is likely to increase the chances of them remaining engaged in their own health care.[66] Simple measures can be very effective, such as considering the color scheme of the clinic area, the furniture, and the reading material available (e.g., age-appropriate magazines and health promotional literature).

Barriers to Transition

In addition to the participation of adolescents and young adults in the process, successful transition requires health professionals to advocate continually for the needs of this group and for the provision of adequate services. As mentioned earlier in the chapter, a major barrier to successful transition is the absence of appropriately trained health professionals within the adult health care system.[28] Where adult services are lacking, pediatricians need to provide training for their adult colleagues, while adult health professionals need to acknowledge and embrace the need to provide a clinical service for the increasing number of young adults with chronic respiratory disorders who will be moving to adult care. This process also needs the support of the health service administrators and politicians who control the funding. Above all, it requires a shift in attitude and culture of all concerned in order to recognize and understand the importance of adolescent and young adult health.[70]

Where adult services do exist, mutual trust and respect between the pediatric and adult centers is important; a lack of these qualities may hamper transition. Guidelines for transition recommend that a nominated individual is identified who is responsible for the overall transition process (a transition lead or coordinator).[23] This role may be performed by any member of the health care team. The coordinator should ensure that all aspects of the process have been considered and follow up on any difficulties encountered. One of the coordinator's roles should be to facilitate communication between the pediatric and adult centers and to provide a written summary of the young person's condition in advance of the transfer date. Financial considerations and health insurance coverage are also key issues.[60] With increasing age, the rules regarding eligibility for certain services and allowances may change. For example, financial support or equipment, which is provided during childhood and adolescence, may not be available indefinitely. These issues need to be anticipated well in advance.

Summary

Transition from pediatric to adult care is one aspect of the wider provision of health services for adolescents and young adults. An understanding of the health issues affecting this group along with specific training in adolescent and young adult health is essential for all health professionals. The number of young adults with chronic respiratory disorders of childhood is only going to increase, as will the range of specific disorders that adult physicians will need to be competent to manage. For pediatric and adult respiratory physicians, the clinical landscape is changing. The challenge is there to be met.

References

Access the reference list online at ExpertConsult.com.

Suggested Reading

Agency for Clinical Innovation and Trapeze, the Sydney Children's Hospitals Network. Key principles for transition of young people from paediatric to adult health care. Available at: http://www.aci.health.nsw.gov.au/__data/assets/pdf_file/0011/251696/Key_Principles_for_Transition.pdf.

Boyle MP, Farukhi Z, Nosky ML. Strategies for improving transition to adult cystic fibrosis care, based on patient and parent views. *Pediatr Pulmonol.* 2001;32:428–436.

Klein D, Goldenring J, Adelman W. HEEADSSS 3.0: the psychosocial interview for adolescents updated for a new century fueled by media. *Contemp Pediatr.* 2014:31:16–28.

National Institute for Health and Care Excellence (NICE). Transition from children's to adults' services for young people using health or social care services. Available at: https://www.nice.org.uk/guidance/ng43

Rosen DS, Blum RW, Britto M, et al. Transition to adult health care for adolescents and young adults with chronic conditions: position paper of the Society for Adolescent Medicine. *J Adolesc Health.* 2003;33:309–311.

Royal Children's Hospital, Melbourne, Australia. Transition to adult health services. Available at: http://www.rch.org.au/transition; Accessed September 26, 2010.

Sawyer S, Drew S, Duncan R. Adolescents with chronic disease—the double whammy. *Aust Fam Physician.* 2007;36:622–627.

Tuchman LK, Schwartz LA, Sawicki GS, et al. Cystic fibrosis and transition to adult medical care. *Pediatrics.* 2010;125:566–573.

Viner RM. Transition of care from paediatric to adult services: one part of improved health services for adolescents. *Arch Dis Child.* 2008;93:160–163.

15 Long-Term Consequences of Childhood Respiratory Disease

ANDREW BUSH, MB BS(Hons), MA, MD, FRCP, FRCPCH, FERS, and
PETER SLY, MBBS, MD, FRACP, DSc

Introduction

For too long, pediatricians and adult respiratory physicians have operated within developmental silos to the detriment of both and, more importantly, to the detriment of children. There are four reasons why better interactions between pediatricians and adult chest physicians are crucial for lung health. First, early life, pregnancy, and even preconception factors impact adult lung function and health; second, new chest diseases are coming to adult chest clinics as a result of advances in pediatric respiratory care, the classical disease being the survivors of prematurity; and third, children with diseases conventionally the province of the pediatrician (e.g., cystic fibrosis [CF], Duchenne muscular dystrophy) are now surviving into adult life, and pediatricians need to educate their adult colleagues about these new issues. Finally, adult physicians have very large cohorts from which we can learn in pediatrics; for example, the increased risk of respiratory infections in adults treated with inhaled corticosteroids (ICS) sounds a warning note in pediatric practice.[1-4]

An illustration of the danger of working in silos is the first figure in the classical Fletcher and Peto paper[5] showing the trajectories to chronic obstructive pulmonary disease (COPD), which could be called the "Star Trek" figure, the adult beamed down with a normal forced expired volume in the first second (FEV_1), with no concept that early life was of any relevance or even existed. In fairness, their second figure did acknowledge the possibility of failure to reach the full potential of lung development, but even today, we suspect that this is mere lip service for many.

Two recent papers have shown how interactions between pediatric and adult studies can build understanding of pathophysiology. The adult study finally nailed that COPD is a disease set up in childhood and that adult factors divorced from an understanding of pediatric risk factors are irrelevant; specifically, smoking is neither necessary nor sufficient for the development of COPD. A large study combining three adult cohorts[6] defined two pathways to COPD, contributing equally to the burden of the disease: normal spirometry at age 40 years, with accelerated decline thereafter, and low FEV_1 at 40 years with a normal rate of decline. Of those not attaining the normal plateau (determined before adult life, see below) 26% developed COPD at follow-up, whereas if a normal plateau was reached, the risk was 7%. Neither from this nor any of the other four major studies reporting decline in lung function[6-9] over time was there any consistent adult factor identified that was associated with accelerated decline. The pediatric paper was a follow-up of the Childhood Asthma Management Program (CAMP) asthma study participants,[10] in whom annual prebronchodilator and postbronchodilator spirometry was performed into the third decade of life.

Roughly equal proportions had a normal growth pattern and normal rate of decline, a normal growth pattern with accelerated decline, reduced growth with normal rate of decline, and both reduced growth and reduced rate of decline, interestingly a category not found in the COPD paper. Clearly, more follow-up data is needed to be sure this is a true decline rather than a transient dip in growth. This discrepancy may be related to the fact that the COPD study recruited all comers, and this last trajectory may have been missed because there were insufficient asthmatics; in other words, this last trajectory may only be seen in asthmatics, which hypothesis requires further confirmation.

Further underscoring the importance of pediatric factors in adult lung disease, a European study[11] identified five markers of childhood disadvantage (maternal asthma and smoking, paternal asthma, and childhood asthma and severe respiratory infections), which in combination were associated with worse adult FEV_1, a steeper rate of decline in FEV_1, and increased COPD risk, at least as strong a signal as smoking. The conclusion is stark and unavoidable; if COPD is to be prevented, it is too late to start thinking about this in adult life.

Part of the difficulty of understanding the developmental perspective of adult diseases is that recall of childhood events by adults is notoriously unreliable; in one study, the incidence of pertussis and pneumonia (two fairly major pediatric respiratory illnesses!) was recorded prospectively.[12] False positive and negative recall was very common (Table 15.1), and the message is that retrospective recall may not be reliable. Similarly, so-called newly diagnosed asthma at age 22 years in 49 of 161 asthmatics diagnosed at all ages in the Tucson study was predicted by bronchial hyperresponsiveness and low lung function at age 6 years.[13] Even the limited information that can be recalled is often not sought; in one survey, very few adult physicians asked about early life events.[14]

There are, however, important caveats when assessing the role of potential risk factors for long-term adverse outcomes; probable pathways are shown in Box 15.1. Most often, it is not possible to untangle these possibilities, especially in the context of multiple interlinked exposures (e.g., increased risk of smoking, increased pollution exposure, living where there is a lot of neighborhood violence, reduced rate of breastfeeding all linked to low socioeconomic status [SES]). It is impossible to consider the long-term consequences of childhood disease without considering the long-term consequences of those factors underlying disease, some of which are discussed in more detail in earlier chapters in this book. However, the mantra that association does not prove causation should always be remembered. Causation can be demonstrated by intervention studies, or the likelihood bolstered by demonstration of biological plausibility by laboratory studies.

Table 15.1 High Prevalence of False Positive and False Negative Recall in Adult Life of Childhood Pneumonia and Pertussis

	Pneumonia	Pertussis
Prospective parental report in first 7 years of life	N = 195	N = 215
True retrospective recall in adulthood	106/193, (55%)	77/215 (36%)
False retrospective recall in adulthood	53/159 (33%)	74/151 (49%)

Johnston ID, Strachan DP, Anderson HR. Effect of pneumonia and whooping cough in childhood on adult lung function. *N Engl J Med.* 1998;338:581-587.

Box 15.1   Pitfalls in Ascertaining Causation Between Exposure and Outcome

- The exposure is causative of the disease (disease would not happen without the exposure)
- An exposure may be causative of disease, but it is masked by other effects, for example, the interactions between cigarette smoke and glutathione transferase polymorphisms
- The underlying cause of being exposed is itself the reason for the association and not the exposure itself
- The exposure makes the disease manifestation worse but is not actually causative
- Treatment of the consequences of the exposure, but not the exposure itself, causes the disease
- An unknown underlying factor causes both the exposure and the disease; a good example of this is antibiotic prescription to infants, as discussed in more detail below
- The exposure is merely a marker for an unknown underlying exposure factor that causes the disease
- Berkson's bias (a selection bias leading to hospital cases and controls in a case control study to be systematically different because the combination of risk exposure and occurrence of disease increases the likelihood of hospital admission). In other words, the harder you look in a selected population, the more you will find.

New diseases and the more prolonged survival of children with "childhood" diseases make cross-developmental interactions ever more important. Survivors of preterm birth have fixed and variable airflow obstruction,[15–18] but no evidence of eosinophilic airway inflammation[19,20] and are not helped by ICS.[21] It is essential that adult physicians understand this is different from atopic asthma (and probably also COPD later in life) and needs different approaches. The increased longevity in CF has led to the importance of reduced bone mineral density and insulin deficiency being appreciated, which has in turn meant that pediatricians diagnose and treat these complications early. The next challenge will be the high prevalence of colonic malignancy[22] and whether any childhood management strategies can reduce this risk.

How the Lung Develops in Health and Disease

Knowledge of normal lung development is essential if the long-term consequences of disease are to be understood.

This is covered in detail elsewhere, so is only briefly summarized here. Interestingly, there is increasing evidence of adverse, preconception, transgenerational effects on the fetus. Thus, two studies have suggested that grandmaternal smoking increases the risk of her daughters' children having asthma even if the daughters themselves never smoked.[23,24] This has been attributed to epigenetic mechanisms, but it is not easy to reconcile this explanation with the mammalian germline reprograming that removes epigenetic signatures immediately after fertilization.[25] The effect is not accounted for by the increased risk of asthma in the daughters of smoking mothers. Clearly, more work is needed to understand the mechanisms of these transgenerational effects and to determine if other adverse insults such as pollution may have the same effect.

NORMAL ANTENATAL LUNG DEVELOPMENT

This is described in more detail in Chapter 2. The embryonic phase lasts from 0 to 7 weeks of gestation, and the primitive lung buds are outpouchings from the primordial gut. An anterior diverticulum appears at 4 weeks, the diverticulum bifurcates at 5 weeks, and lobes and segments become delineated thereafter. The main pulmonary arteries develop during this time, and blood vessel development follows the airways. From an early stage, there is phasic airway contraction and relaxation that are thought to be important in growth factor release. During the pseudoglandular phase, from 6 to 17 weeks, all generations of airways and their accompanying vessels are laid down, the latter by vasculogenesis (*de novo* blood vessel formation); thereafter airways increase in size but not number. From 16 to 26 weeks is the canalicular phase, during which time, the acinar structures form, surfactant synthesis in type 2 cells becomes apparent, and the respiratory barrier thins. True alveoli and their accompanying blood vessels first appear in the saccular phase from 26 to 35 weeks; the vessels develop by angiogenesis (outsprouting from existing vessels) and the alveoli develop by secondary septation. The details of the molecular pathways and genetic control of these processes are beyond the scope of this chapter; the reader is referred to recent reviews and manuscripts.[26–28] Important in this scheme is that adverse influences on airway branching are active in the first trimester and those active on airway caliber in the second and third trimester of pregnancy; and anything that interferes with the normal airway branching pattern will by definition adversely impact on the final alveolar numbers.

ADVERSE EFFECTS ACROSS THE LIFE COURSE: INTRODUCTION

Although it is convenient to separate adverse influences into discrete developmental blocks such as antenatal, childhood, and adult life, this is to some extent artificial, since environment across the developmental stages is closely linked. A recent study attempted to take a more holistic look, spanning pregnancy and infancy. They reported that in adjusted analyses, there was a dose-dependent increased risk of subsequent asthma with maternal urinary tract infection and maternal and infant antibiotic use and a decreased risk if there were more older siblings at home.[29] Delivery by Caesarean section increased the risk of subsequent asthma. The greater the number of risk factors, the greater the risk of asthma.

However, these are all associations and are discussed in more detail below.

ADVERSE EFFECTS OPERATING ANTENATALLY

There are four main mechanisms whereby antenatal insults may impact on long-term outcomes, both disease in childhood and subsequent adverse effects in adult life. These are by leading to abnormal lung structure by causing abnormal immunological function and indirectly by causing either or both low birth weight and prematurity. The fourth mechanism, fetal programming, has been much less studied in humans, but there is evidence that early and discrete adverse exposures in animals prime adulthood responses to allergens and infections.[30,31] A challenging human study showed that adult survivors of primary pulmonary hypertension of the newborn had much greater hypoxic pulmonary hypertensive responses than controls.[32] It is of course impossible to be certain whether this relates to fetal programing or different developmental manifestations of some unknown underlying condition.

Tobacco and Nicotine Exposure

These are the most studied adverse influences. Structural changes have been most studied in animal models; of note, nicotine itself is damaging, calling into question the safety of e-cigarettes, nicotine patches, and nicotine chewing gum during pregnancy. Either may be safer than cigarettes, but this is unproven, and they certainly cannot be considered harmless.

Nicotine exposure in pregnancy has been shown to lead to airway remodeling, with increased deposition of type 1 and 3 collagen, airway lengthening and narrowing, airway wall thickening, and loss of alveolar tethering points leading to airway instability.[33–35] The airway wall may be thickened postnatally.[36] There is also increased MUC5AC expression in bronchial epithelial cells.[37] The postnatal functional readout of these structural changes is airway hyperresponsiveness (AHR) even in the absence of allergen exposure.[34] This is of particular importance, since three cohort studies[38–41] have shown that AHR in the newborn period, long before there is any evidence of airway infection or inflammation,[42] is associated with long-term adverse respiratory outcomes. Children of mothers who smoke are more likely to have asthma, and more likely to smoke themselves, thus perpetuating the cycles of avoidable damage to the lungs.[43] Finally, tobacco exposure may lead to premature emphysema,[44] with reduction of secondary septation and enlargement and simplification of alveoli; the relative contributions to this worrying effect of antenatal and postnatal smoke exposure have not been determined. Tobacco exposure of pregnant women is associated with a number of alterations in cord blood, including an increased responsiveness to allergens of cord blood mononuclear cells, abnormal Toll-like receptor function, and abnormal cytokine responses with a readout of increased viral wheeze in the first year of life.[45–48] The effect of maternal smoking on infant atopy is controversial with some finding no effect at all.[49] However, recently[50] an association between maternal smoking and food allergy and also with atopic dermatitis[51] has been reported, and a recent meta-analysis confirmed an association with atopy.[52] The mechanism may be via reduction in cord blood regulatory

T cells (Tregs).[53] Finally, that active smoking is associated with prematurity and low birth weight has long been known; new data also shows that reduction of passive smoke exposure leads to reductions in preterm delivery.[54]

Antenatal Effects of Pollution

There is increasingly compelling evidence that exposure of pregnant mothers to environmental pollution may adversely impact the fetus. In a study from Spain, the developmental residential exposure to benzene and nitrogen dioxide was related to spirometry at age 4.5 years in 624 children. There was a dose-dependent reduction in spirometry with increasing exposure levels in pregnancy but no other time point. This was worse for allergic children and those of low SES.[55] In another study of 736 North American children, mostly ethnic minorities, but also mostly nonsmokers, there was an association between $PM_{2.5}$ exposure levels between 16 and 25 weeks of gestation and the development of early childhood asthma; however, this result only appeared in boys.[56] It is likely that there will be adverse effects on the fetus of maternal biomass fuel exposure during pregnancy, but this has yet to be determined.

Maternal Malnutrition and Obesity

It is a shameful commentary on the human condition that maternal malnutrition is still an issue in the 21st century. The best-known long-term data are from the Dutch famine lasting 5 to 6 months at the end of the Nazi occupation in the Second World War.[57] Famine exposure in the first and second trimester of pregnancy was associated with wheezing, but not airflow obstruction or increased atopic sensitization at follow-up in adult life; wheezing remained significant after adjusting for relevant confounders, and wheezing was independent of birth weight in this group (famine-born babies were on average 250 g lighter, a fairly small effect). An important follow-up paper demonstrated that not merely was there more wheezing illness at age 50, but also more coronary heart disease, hyperlipidemia, altered clotting, and obesity after early gestational exposure to famine.[58] Microalbuminuria and decreased glucose tolerance were reported in those exposed to famine in late gestation.

Maternal obesity is likely to become ever more common. Prepregnancy obesity is associated with early wheeze and asthma in the offspring.[59–62] There is no doubt that pregnancy obesity (which is of course closely linked with prepregnancy obesity) increases the risk of obstetric complications, but is also associated with wheeze in infancy and childhood. In a cohort study in which more than 38,000 mother-baby pairs were identified, maternal obesity in pregnancy was also associated with wheeze in the first 18 months of life in the baby[63]; this was confirmed by a pooled analysis of more than 85,000 mother-child pairs.[64] Risk increased linearly with body mass index, and the risk was not mediated via obstetric complications, prematurity or low birth weight. In another study of more than 6000 mother child pairs, prescription of inhaled bronchodilators in the first 4 years of life was associated with prepregnancy obesity.[65]

Antenatal Effects of Acetaminophen?

There is ongoing controversy about whether acetaminophen given to mothers in pregnancy or to infants postnatally is associated with the development of asthma.[66,67] A recent murine model in which acetaminophen was given using various regimens to pregnant mice, lactating mice, and mouse pups, alone or in any combination, and no effect could be shown on the development of murine allergic airways disease.[68] A recent birth cohort study showed an association between acetaminophen use in both the first and last trimesters of pregnancy and subsequent wheeze in the offspring. However, this disappeared when adjusted for confounding factors, and there was no association between acetaminophen use for noninfectious reasons and subsequent wheeze.[69] However, given there are other available antipyretic and analgesic medicines such as ibuprofen (the safety of which has not been challenged), it would seem prudent to avoid acetaminophen in pregnancy and childhood.

Maternal Hypertension?

Maternal hypertension in pregnancy has also been associated with an increased risk of wheeze,[70,71] although this has recently been challenged in the Avon Longitudinal Study of Parents and Children (ALSPAC) study.[72] They found that maternal hypertension before pregnancy, but not gestational hypertension, was associated with subsequent childhood wheeze, but even this association needs replication.

Maternal Antibiotic Use?

Antibiotic prescription in pregnancy has been associated with subsequent wheeze,[73–75] and certainly in a murine model, antibiotic use in pregnancy affects adaptive antiviral immune responses via alterations in the pup's microbiome.[76] However, a recent birth cohort study has clarified the association. Maternal use of antibiotics in the first trimester was not associated with wheeze; in the last trimester, there was an association with wheeze, and this remained, albeit weakly, when adjusted for confounding factors. Genitourinary infection in pregnancy increased the risk of subsequent wheeze in the offspring, irrespective of antibiotic treatment. No mechanisms for these possible associations were defined.[77]

Maternal Stress in Asthma—A Developing Field

There is increasing evidence that maternal stress (in the very broadest sense) is important in disease outcomes, in particular, asthma. There are extra pitfalls in determining this relationship (Box 15.2).

The interaction between maternal atopy and wheeze was studied in 653 families.[78] Stress was defined as negative life events during pregnancy and in the first and second years postpartum. Mothers were asked about the presence of wheeze in the babies quarterly. Maternal stress was a risk factor for wheeze, but only in nonatopic mothers. This was taken forward in a second, more mechanistic study in 557 families.[79] Prenatal maternal stress was defined as any of financial hardship, difficult life circumstances, community violence, and poor neighborhood housing. Cord blood mononuclear cells were incubated with several stimuli of the innate and adaptive responses. There were greater interleukin (IL)-8 and tumour necrosis factor (TNF)-α responses to infection-based, and a higher IL-13 and reduced IFN-γ to house dust mite (HDM) stimuli (T_H2 polarization), but there was no explanation of the detailed mechanisms. However, there is at least one possible way in which altered responses to infection may impact longer-term outcomes, namely via upper airway bacterial colonization. The first Copenhagen

Prospective Studies on Asthma in Childhood (COPSAC) Study reported on 321 infants who had hypopharyngeal cultures performed at 1 month of age, which these were infants of atopic mothers.[80] Twenty-one percent colonized with one or more of *Staph aureus, Moraxella catarrhalis, Strep pneumonia, Haemophilus influenzae*, and when followed up, they had worse wheeze outcomes, both in terms of percentage with any wheeze, and percentage with persistent wheeze. However, it should be emphasized that maternal stress was not measured in the COPSAC study.

A further study reported conflicting interactions between atopy and maternal stress.[81] The investigators approached 989 women, of whom 488 (<50%) were actually studied. They used the Crisis in Family Systems-Revised (CRISYS-R) questionnaire (which has 11 domains that were summarized to account for stress in multiple domains). They performed prenatal environmental HDM sampling and measured cord blood immunoglobulin E (IgE). They reported that maternal stress was associated with higher cord blood IgE; confusingly, for atopic mothers, the strongest association was in the high HDM exposure group, whereas in the nonatopic mothers, the reverse was found, the strongest association being in the low HDM group. These findings are difficult to explain, although supportive of an association between maternal stress and atopic outcomes.

Even more intriguing was a study looking at early life events in the mother herself long before pregnancy.[82] The investigators defined the mother's SES in childhood, age up to 10 years, by whether she lived in a home owned by her family. They recorded potential pregnancy effects, including sociodemographics, exposure to violence or trauma, financial status, and exposure to allergens and traffic pollution. Postnatally, they recorded reported wheeze every 3 months. They reported that lower maternal SES was associated with higher cord blood IgE and more infant wheeze. They also reported direct effects, namely cumulative maternal adversity was independently associated with cord blood IgE; and indirect effects, operating through adult SES, cumulative stress, and pollution. They proposed a complex model integrating all these findings, but it has to be said that mechanistically there are no answers and the model must be said at this time to be hypothesis generating not definitive.

In summary, maternal stress is clearly *associated* with altered cytokine responses (T_H2 and innate immune responses to infection) in the baby. There is also a readout with increased reports of wheeze in the offspring, but the weaknesses of relying on parental reports of wheeze have been highlighted elsewhere.[83–86] The pathways are clearly complex and ill-understood, although the interactions between stress and atopy are important. However, we are a long way from proving causation, since so many factors cosegregate with stress.

LONG-TERM EFFECTS OF EVENTS DURING DELIVERY

Caesarean section delivery is *associated* with an increased risk of atopic disorders in the baby[87,88] probably mediated via an effect on the fetal microbiome.[89] Especially if at least one parent is allergic, children delivered by Caesarean section are more likely to have asthma at 8 years of age, and children of nonallergic parents are more likely to be sensitized.[90] Since there are no randomized controlled trials of Caesarean section delivery, it is not clear if the reported asthma prevalence changes are related to Caesarean delivery itself or to the reason Caesarean delivery was undertaken.

A further factor to be considered is changes in the way newborns (including term newborns) are resuscitated.[91] Many babies require a brief period of resuscitation immediately after birth and thereafter remain well and are not reevaluated. Resuscitation policies have become less aggressive, with intubation and hyperoxic gas mixtures given after a delay, and there is evidence in animals that this may be less damaging to the newborn lung.[92] The long-term sequelae of newborn resuscitation have not been considered outside the setting of prematurity, but the long-term effects of these changes are worth at least considering.

The Canadian CHILD (Canadian Healthy Infant Longitudinal Development national population-based birth cohort [www.canadianchildstudy.ca]) study has also reported on the interactions between mode of delivery, the use of intrapartum antibiotics, and subsequent breast-feeding on the fecal microbiome in infancy.[93,94] Intrapartum antibiotics for whatever indication (Group B streptococcal prophylaxis, prolonged rupture of membranes, and elective or emergency Caesarean section) led to alterations in the fecal microbiome at 3 months of age and these persisted in babies delivered by Caesarean section to a year of age, particularly if the Caesarean section was an emergency and the infant was not breast-fed. The development and importance of the early life microbiome is discussed in more detail below.

BIRTH WEIGHT AND GESTATIONAL AGE

The long-term consequences of extreme prematurity are considered later; here we discuss the effects of modest decrements in birth weight and gestational age, and some of which have hitherto been thought to be in the "normal" range. A meta-analysis has demonstrated that low birth weight of whatever underlying cause is associated with subsequent asthma across the life course.[95] There is a linear relationship between birth weight (adjusted for all known relevant maternal factors) and spirometry both at the peak in the early twenties and at age 45 to 50 years.[96] Tobacco smoking causes preterm delivery and importantly the risk is reduced by tobacco legislation[54]; it is obviously of the first importance to focus particularly on factors that are remediable, such as smoking and pollution, rather than those that are not, such as maternal atopy. Modest degrees of prematurity (up to 37 weeks gestation) are associated with impaired spirometry in the late teenage years[97] and increased prescription of asthma medications in childhood.[98–100] Low birth weight of itself is a risk factor for subsequent asthma.[101] There may be a differential effect of low birth weight in babies who are small (SGA), as opposed to appropriate (AGA), weight for gestation age; at age 20 to 22, spirometry was strongly predicted by birth weight in the SGA, but not the AGA, group.[102]

NORMAL POSTNATAL LUNG GROWTH

Most is known about airway growth and the Global Lung Initiative has provided the best all-age spirometry data. These show a steady rise in lung function from the preschool years to a plateau between ages 20 and 25 years and then a steady decline.[103] If these figures are back-extrapolated to birth cohort studies that have used either the rapid thoraco-abdominal compression technique (RTC) or the raised volume RTC (RVRTC), which is more closely relates to spirometry in children and adults, it is clear that there are three key issues that are needed to ensure lifelong airway health (Box 15.3)

We have learned important lessons from birth cohort studies. There is no study that has extended over the entire life course, and so we rely on a series of overlapping cohorts,[104–107] reviewed in.[108] Although there are some discrepancies, the general message is that lung function at age 4 to 6 years is determined by lung function and AHR soon after birth, and thereafter tracks; hence decrements at age 4 to 6 are reflected in adult lung function, at least to age 50. There may be further deterioration over the life course, but no improvements. This has obvious implications for adult disease.

Understanding AHR and its long-term consequences requires a developmental perspective. Three groups have measured neonatal AHR and all showed significant relationships with long-term respiratory outcomes, albeit slightly different.[38–41] COPSAC[41] showed that 40% of airway obstruction at age 7 was determined antenatally and 60% postnatally

---

Box 15.3   Three Key Stages for Lung Health

- Normal lung function as shown by RVRTC/RTC at birth (genes and antenatal factors)
- Normal lung growth in the first two decades of life (genes, postnatal and antenatal factors)
- Normal rate of decline, from the fourth decade of life (genes, antenatal and postnatal factors; minimal contribution from adult life effects)

RTC, Rapid thoraco-abdominal compression technique; *RVRTC*, raised volume rapid thoraco-abdominal squeeze technique.

and that AHR in the newborn period was the strongest predictor of asthma at age 7. Neonatal AHR is clearly not related to airway inflammation[42] or previous infection, and must be determined by anatomical factors; thus, in small airways, resistance increases more for a given proportionate radius change. Although AHR and lung function at birth are said to be independent risk factors for childhood lung function, abnormal anatomy is likely to be the root cause of both. Finally, a study of AHR from birth to adult life showed that the relationship in adulthood between AHR and asthma was established before 6 years of age.[109]

There is much less known regarding developmental changes in lung volumes. They probably increase through childhood, with at least one study suggesting a phase of accelerated growth during puberty,[110] and more marked in boys than girls, reflecting changes in the dimensions of the thoracic cavity.

Alveolar development is a controversial subject. Conventionally, this has been described as being a largely postnatal phenomenon with a rapid phase in the first 2 years of life, while there is some neo-alveolarization until about age 8 years, at which point, alveoli increase only in size and not number. This has been challenged by some controversial studies in which hyperpolarized Helium (He^3) has been used to infer alveolar size from observation of path lengths after inhalation.[111,112] These studies have suggested that neo-alveolarization continues throughout somatic growth, which is supported by direct morphometric measurements in primates.[113] If this is the case, the implications are two-fold; first, there is greater scope for recovery from adverse neonatal events than we thought; and second, the period of vulnerability of the growing alveoli extends further than we previously considered. These are both particularly important in the context of preterm delivery and adverse environmental exposures.

ADVERSE IMPACTS ON LUNG GROWTH AND RELATIONSHIP TO DISEASE OUTCOMES

As with neonatal adverse influences, the postnatal interactions between adverse effects and their consequences are complex. Included in this are the ways whereby an adverse influence causes long-term respiratory morbidity by leading to obesity, which obviously of itself causes substantial respiratory morbidity. Another example is wheezing and asthma, which are associated with adverse long-term effects, but have magnified effects by acute exacerbations of wheeze or "lung attacks" (below).

Effects of Nutrition on the Life Course of Lung Development

The single most easily modifiable trait that may impact on long-term outcomes is breast-feeding. The general health merits of breast-feeding are too well known to recapitulate here. Whether breast-feeding protects against asthma and wheeze is controversial; a meta-analysis showed benefit in the first 2 years of life, with diminishing effects thereafter[114]; however, a recent birth cohort study did not confirm any protective effect at age 7 years.[115] Breast-feeding is also associated with a reduced risk of snoring and sleep-disordered breathing,[116] and likely, but not certainly, protects against

obesity. Early and rapid weight gain may be associated with poorer lung growth in addition to the effects of low birth weight and SGA.[117] However, paradoxically, greater weight gain (but almost certainly not obesity) in later childhood may be associated with better spirometry.[118] The multiple respiratory adverse effects of childhood obesity including a number of phenotypes of wheeze, deconditioning, and obstructive sleep apnea are well known. There is mounting evidence that the origins of later obesity are antenatal and in the first 2 years of life. In a systematic review, 282 publications were identified, from which high maternal prepregnancy body mass index, prenatal tobacco exposure, excessive maternal weight gain in pregnancy, high birth weight, and greater weight gain were implicated as risk factors for childhood obesity.[119] There was less strong evidence (fewer studies) implicating gestational diabetes, child care attendance, poor maternal-infant bonding, low SES, reduction in infant sleep time, inappropriate formula feeding, introduction of solid foods before 4 months of age, and infant antibiotic exposure. Clearly many of these risk factors are interlinked, such as low SES, smoking, and low rates of breast-feeding.

Passive and Active Exposure to Tobacco Smoke

The effects of passive smoking were described in a series of meta-analyses,[120-126] which have been recently updated.[43] Passive smoke exposure is associated with an increased risk of sudden infant death syndrome, more and more severe childhood upper and lower respiratory infections, and more childhood wheeze. Finally, maternal smoking and the child taking up smoking (which is more likely if the parents smoke) have additive effects on the child's lung function.[127]

Environmental Pollution

Globally, the most significant antenatal exposure is indoor exposure to biomass fuels. In a study from Guatemala,[128] a subset of children whose families had been randomized to receive a chimney stove to reduce indoor pollution either at birth or at 18 months of age underwent spirometry at around 5 years of age. Later stove introduction was associated with a statistically significant reduction in peak flow growth and a large but not statistically significant decrement in FEV_1.

There is a large amount of literature on the adverse respiratory effects of ambient pollution. Lung growth over time is adversely affected by pollution,[129,130] meaning that the normal plateau of lung development will not be reached, putting the child at risk of later COPD. Furthermore, pollution interacts with respiratory infection to increase the prevalence and worsen attacks of preschool wheeze and asthma[131,132] with the adverse long-term results described below. Encouragingly, legislation to reduce air pollution is also temporally associated with improved lung growth in children, identifying outdoor as well as indoor pollution as something that can and should be dealt with to preserve long-term lung health.[133]

Asthma, Atopy, and Acute Attacks of Wheeze

Three factors reflecting long-term consequences of childhood asthma and wheeze emerge from the literature: (1) the importance of different temporal patterns of wheeze[134,135]; (2) the significance of different patterns of atopic sensitization[136]; and (3) the crucial importance of attacks of wheeze, or better "lung attacks."[137,138] These last have been the subject of attention in other contexts (as follows) including CF[139–141] and primary ciliary dyskinesia.[142] It has been suggested that these are so important that the rather feeble word "exacerbation," implying a mere temporary and reversible inconvenience, should be replaced by the more forceful "lung attack" to reflect the long-term adverse effects of these episodes in many airway diseases.[143,144]

In terms of wheeze patterns, the birth cohort studies have confirmed the shrewd observations of our forebears that all wheeze is not the same, and 4 to 6 patterns or phenotypes can be discerned,[145–147] which are broadly reproducible across the cohorts, and associated with particular gene expression patterns.[148] Broadly, there are early wheezing periods in the first 0 to 4 years of life and persistent and late onset wheeze phenotypes leading to symptoms into mid-childhood. The cohorts with more sophisticated epidemiological classifications have yet to reach late adulthood, so the long-term consequences can only be inferred. An alternative, and more clinically useful, time-honored classification, recently endorsed by the European Respiratory Society, is into "wheezy bronchitis"/episodic viral wheeze (symptoms only during viral upper respiratory tract infections) and asthma/multiple trigger wheeze, in which additionally there are symptoms between infections, with typical asthma triggers such as exercise and allergen exposure.[134,135] The Aberdeen cohort, which used just this classification, has been followed into the seventh decade and showed that both groups were associated with COPD, but neither were associated with an accelerated decline in spirometry[10]; hence, failure of normal lung growth in childhood was the cause of COPD in adult life. In this context, it is worrying that one-third of children with relatively mild asthma in the CAMP study had impaired growth in spirometry irrespective of whether they were prescribed ICS.[11,149] This is one more indication of the disconnect between airway inflammation and airway remodeling, which was presumably the cause of impaired growth.

We have also come to realize that all atopies are not equal, and approaches such as the quantification of atopy and determining the temporal patterns of sensitization lead to delineation of subgroups of atopy of different significance. The Manchester cohort used a machine learning approach to define patterns of atopy, and this approach identified early multiple atopic sensitization and persistent wheeze as being the only combination of wheeze and atopic phenotypes that predicted progressive airflow obstruction measured by specific airway resistance.[136,137] Additionally, attacks of wheeze worsened the progression of airflow obstruction.

Lung attacks have been specified as important in the evolution of lung function in two contexts: the first is the Manchester birth cohort study[137]; and the second is in a *post hoc* analysis of the Inhaled Steroid Treatment as Regular Therapy in Early Asthma (START) trial[138] in which asthma lung attacks were shown to be associated with a long-term effect on airway obstruction; in this case, the effect was abrogated by treatment with ICS.

Finally, the Melbourne study has shown that people with asthma that remits and normal subjects have the same spirometry in the sixth decade of life, whereas asthma that does not remit (even if not severe at recruitment) is associated with decrements in lung function across the life course.[150] Risk factors identified for persistence were severe childhood asthma, female gender, and childhood hay fever.

Stress and Its Outcomes

A number of manuscripts link childhood psychological stress with asthma attacks; but as in other areas, associations are described, and there are no intervention trials to prove that psychological intervention is beneficial. In the most significant prospective longitudinal follow-up study, 113 children were approached and 90 participated.[151] They filled in the Psychological Assessment of Childhood Experiences (PACE) questionnaire at baseline, 9, and 18 months and undertook home peak flow monitoring. Acute, severe stresses were defined as a death or divorce in the family, while chronic stresses were chronic physical or mental illness in family, substance abuse, family discord, school-related stress (bullying), and poor living conditions. They found that female gender, higher baseline severity, frequent previous attacks, and (unsurprisingly) the autumn to winter season were all associated with more attacks. Although this is expected, these positive controls add value to the study by demonstrating adequate power to show real associations. They reported that social class and chronic stress were not associated with acute attacks. Severe acute events, with or without high chronic stress, however, did increase the risk of new asthma attacks. There were quite complex time-relationships between stress and asthma attacks. If there was no background chronic stress, there was a time lag of around 2 weeks before the increased risk of acute attacks, which was manifested in the subsequent 4 weeks.[152] If the child suffered from acute on chronic stress, there was an almost immediate increased risk of asthma attacks. In other work, detailed analysis revealed a biphasic risk pattern with early and late periods of vulnerability.

The effects of positive life events have also been studied.[153] "Acute" positive events were defined as receiving valued presents, joining clubs (new activities and friends), and winning prizes. "Long-term" positive events included being a member of a sports team and having a hobby. The group had low to medium chronic stress levels, but not high chronic stress. They found that positives could reverse the risk of an acute stressful event, but the presence or absence of long-term positives did not affect attack risk.

Finally, a horrifying paper from Brazil studied the effects of violence on asthma attacks.[154] A total of 1232 parents/guardians were surveyed, and, appallingly, more than three-quarters had been exposed to violence. Children exposed to violence were more likely to report asthma (International Study of Asthma and Allergies in Childhood [ISAAC]; 28.4% vs. 16.4%), and if violence was maximal, the odds ratio for asthma was 1.94, with 95% confidence intervals of 1.12 to 3.36. Of course, one cannot exclude that what was being reported by the children was hyperventilation or panic attacks, triggered in part by traumatic events.

Another approach is to look at new cases (incident) of asthma rather than exacerbations of a preexisting disease. One group conducted a postal survey of 16,681 males and females, aged 20 to 54, to determine the presence of stressful life events and determined the onset of asthma from national registries.[155] There were 192 cases of incident asthma, which were associated with acute stress; the worst were illness of family member, marital problems, divorce or separation, and conflict with a supervisor. Again, whether they were reporting true asthma or dysfunctional breathing could not be determined.

Antibiotics?

This literature clearly shows the importance of not confounding causation and association. Many papers show an association; a recent study in more than 900 babies followed to age 11 years obtained data on prescription of antibiotics, wheeze prevalence, and asthma attacks.[156] Peripheral blood mononuclear cell responses to rhinovirus and respiratory syncytial virus, and *H. influenzae* and *Streptococcus pneumoniae* were assessed at 11 years, and genotyping for polymorphisms at the 17q21 locus was performed. The expected association of wheeze and asthma with antibiotic prescription was noted, but the children who were prescribed antibiotics were in fact significantly different from those who were not both in terms of immunological responses to viruses but not bacteria and 17q21 polymorphisms. Hence, the association between wheeze and antibiotic prescription is likely related to confounding factors and not causative.

Early Viral Infections

Acute viral infections are important causes of early respiratory morbidity due to bronchiolitis and wheeze, but whether viruses cause asthma to develop in an infant who would otherwise not go on to the disease or are a marker for an asthma propensity is controversial. It should be noted that these are not mutually exclusive. Cord blood studies (above) show that the host immune system may be programmed before birth such that the baby has a propensity to viral wheeze. Another study demonstrated impairment of respiratory function prior to the development of bronchiolitis, and this decrement tracked into mid-childhood.[157] Respiratory syncytial virus has been most studied; infection with this virus in infancy is universal, but whether severe infection causes asthma is controversial.[158,159] Recently, rhinovirus infection has been shown to be more strongly associated with subsequent asthma than respiratory syncytial virus, although association and causation are not the same.[29] Probably, allergic sensitization precedes viral wheezing,[160] and it is likely that sensitization rather than viral infections is important in pushing the trajectory of the child into school-age asthma, although this is by no means certain.

Microbiome

The lower airway is not sterile as was once believed based on conventional culture techniques. Molecular techniques, which detect a hundred-fold more bacteria, have shown that the airway has abundant flora.[161] Furthermore, alteration in the normal lower airway flora may skew immune development,[162,163] and interactions between allergen and the microbiome influence the body's immune responses.[164,165] Early nasopharyngeal bacterial colonization of human infants is associated with altered early immune responses,[166] and a greater prevalence of subsequent wheezing[167] and worse respiratory infections.[168] It is likely that early upper airway colonization with pathogens is a sign of an underlying mucosal immune defect, but this is still unproven. By contrast, environmental bacterial and fungal diversity is associated with a reduced risk of asthma.[169] The long-term effects of an abnormal early microbiome on lung aging are currently unknown, but the influences on asthma risk mean that the early microbiome will at least have an indirect effect on outcomes.

THE AGING LUNG

There are a large number of studies of lung aging, including population based and in those with established COPD. As discussed above, no single factor operative in adult life emerges as associated with accelerated decline in lung function; either no factors are identified, or they are not replicated. The Evaluation of COPD Longitudinally to Predict Surrogate Endpoints (ECLIPSE) study showed there was accelerated decline in current smokers, patients with a bronchodilator response, and patients with emphysema[6]; the Body Mass Index, Airflow Obstruction, Dyspnea and Exercise Capacity Index (BODE) study[7] by contrast reported higher rates of decline in those with a higher basal metabolic index and a higher starting FEV_1. A study in adults with severe asthma showed that an elevation in exhaled nitric oxide, especially in those with $FEV_1 \geq 80\%$, was predictive of accelerated decline in lung function.[170] The likely pathological basis of this is an abnormal airway inflammatory response, elevation of CD8 and CD4 T cells in baseline bronchial mucosal biopsies and CD8, CD3, and granzyme B at follow-up.[171]

LUNG DEVELOPMENT: MORE THAN JUST AIRWAYS

Much less is known about alveolar as opposed to airway growth, and it is mostly in the context of prematurity and its treatment. Neonatal hyperoxia, systemic steroids, and nicotine all impair neoalveolarization via effects on secondary septation in animals.[172–174] Human He^3 data[175] suggest that maternal smoking in pregnancy, as well as affecting the airway, may increase alveolar size and reduce their numbers leading to premature "emphysema." Since it is nicotine that is implicated in both processes, the safety of e-cigarettes is called into question.[176] There may be the alveolar equivalent of catch-up growth based on cross-sectional studies; there are no longitudinal neonatal data with extension into childhood and adult life. Carbon monoxide transfer (DL_{CO}) is a surrogate for the size of the alveolar-capillary membrane, and one group demonstrated that this was normal at rest and on exercise in adult life.[177] He^3 data in preterm survivors in adolescence showed that alveolar size was normal,[112] implying catch-up growth, but there were no measurements in the newborn period. Nitrogen washout can be used to partition gas mixing abnormalities into airway (S_{cond}) and alveolar (S_{acin}) components.[178,179] Preterm survivors in childhood had as expected an abnormal S_{cond} compared with controls, but S_{acin} was normal, implying alveolarization had normalized (but again, there were no neonatal data).[180] However, if in fact many alveoli had been completely destroyed, S_{acin} would still be normal. However, taken together, there is suggestive evidence that alveolarization continues for longer and with more potential for catch-up growth than previously thought. Certainly, lungs apparently destroyed by necrotizing pneumonia usually recover completely,[181] so there is certainly potential for catch-up. Intriguingly, being reared in hypoxic conditions at altitude appears to stimulate alveolarization but has no effect on airway function[182]; this raises the hitherto unexplored question as to whether keeping preterm survivors very well oxygenated is as beneficial as we currently think.

SUMMARY: WHAT HAVE WE LEARNED ABOUT THE IMPORTANCE OF ANTENATAL AND CHILDHOOD FACTORS?

We have summarized factors across the developmental spectrum that clearly either lead to either or both of impaired lung function at birth and impaired lung growth in childhood leading to a failure to reach the normal adult plateau. There are clearly important genetic effects and gene by environment interactions discussed elsewhere in this book (see Chapters 3 and 4).

It is very clear that asthma and many if not most childhood wheezing syndromes, including atopic asthma, are not mere childhood inconveniences to be outgrown but have long-term consequences in terms of premature airflow obstruction and thus early onset of respiratory disability. The exact importance of multiple factors operative in an individual may not be possible to dissect, but the importance of a focus on antenatal and early childhood factors is indisputable. The combined effect of these adverse influences and their childhood consequences is to lead to an increased risk of adult COPD (below). However, what is also clear is that the rate of lung aging must be largely dependent on genetic and childhood factors. The inescapable conclusion is that if adult COPD is to be prevented, then efforts to do this must be focused in childhood.

The End-Stage—Chronic Obstructive Pulmonary Disease

Damage to an airway can only manifest by premature onset of airway obstruction, just as the end stage of insults to the kidney is an elevation in serum creatinine. Thus, to define a disease (COPD) by a fixed ratio (FEV_1/FVC) of <70% is as imprecise as calling a raised serum creatinine a disease and is almost incomprehensible to most pediatricians. Furthermore, as age increases, more and more people have a ratio in the "COPD" range, and in young children, FEV_1/FVC of 75% is very abnormal[183]; so using a fixed ratio across the developmental spectrum is akin to defining short stature as being 120 cm tall without knowing the age of the patient! The best life course study from Melbourne has a number of important lessons.[150] First, the risk of adult "COPD" is 30-fold greater in those with severe asthma, a signal far outweighing that of smoking. Second, those with COPD fail to reach the normal spirometric plateau but undergo lung aging at the same rate. Finally, those given an adult diagnosis of COPD were those with the most abnormal spirometry at age 10 years. This paper should surely kill the concept of a disease diagnosed by a ratio stone dead (but probably it will not!); premature airflow obstruction does not happen when an arbitrary fixed threshold is crossed but happens across the life-course. Therefore, either adult "COPD" therapeutic strategies such as ICS, antimuscarinics, and long-acting β-2 agonists should be applied across the life course irrespective of the etiology of the airflow obstruction rather than waiting for a fixed and arbitrary line to be crossed; or more logically, dissect airway disease into components such as inflammation, infection, and fixed and variable obstruction, as discussed in Chapter 46, and deploy treatment against such treatable traits as are present.

Long-Term Consequences of Specific Diseases

PREMATURITY, INCLUDING EARLY-TERM DELIVERY

Despite there being a large amount of literature on the long-term consequences of prematurity, many adult physicians are not aware of the problem and do not even make early life events part of the clinical history.[184] The literature can only briefly be summarized here. The possible reasons for adverse effects of prematurity are complex (Box 15.4).

The resuscitation and treatment strategies used for premature babies have changed and are likely to develop further. Modern ventilator strategies (high rate, low pressures), for example, may lead to very different sequelae compared to older methods (lower rate, higher pressures). Long-term survivors have tended to have airway disease and obstruction, whereas the smaller, more preterm survivors of neonatal intensive care in the 21st century have alveolar hypoplasia.

It is also important to note that even babies delivered at early term (37 to 38 weeks gestation) have respiratory morbidity in mid-childhood, as discussed above. The implication is that early delivery *per se* is deleterious, and so improvements in neonatal intensive care will not take away the problems of prematurity; consequently, there is a much larger pool of at-risk children than may have been thought.

Summarizing the literature, survivors of preterm delivery have increased respiratory symptoms and morbidity going into adult life; they have fixed and variable airflow obstruction, but without evidence of eosinophilic airway inflammation; and they have alveolar hypoplasia and structural parenchymal damage. Additionally, they may have impaired exercise performance, abnormal control of breathing, and pulmonary hypertension. Most survivors of preterm delivery have, however, been lost to medical follow-up and are living active lives in the community. It is likely but not proven that many of them will be being treated inappropriately for "asthma" with ICS because of symptoms and abnormal physiology, again emphasizing the need to deconstruct airway disease into its components.

> **Box 15.4 Adverse Factors Interacting With Prematurity**
>
> - The effects of prematurity itself
> - The effects of treatment of prematurity (especially supplemental oxygen, barotrauma and systemic corticosteroids; Caesarean section delivery
> - The effects of the underlying cause of premature delivery, such as maternal smoking or hypertension
> - The effects of low birth weight independent of prematurity (including small vs. appropriate for gestational age)
> - Genetic effects: 258 genes have been associated with BPD[185]
> - The effect of programming by events at a critical time period (DOHAD)
> - The indirect effect of premature delivery on the baby, operating through the mother, such as maternal stress

There have been no really long-term studies following these survivors into late adult life, and in any case, such studies are likely not relevant to modern survivors. It is likely, however, that they will not reach a normal plateau of spirometry, and thus will be at high risk of "COPD." There is no information about whether there is an accelerated rate of decline in this group. It will be really important that these people have their airway disease evaluated critically; it is hard to believe that the survivor of prematurity who has never had airway eosinophilia should be treated the same way as a lifelong smoker or a severely atopic asthmatic just because all three have an FEV_1/FVC ratio <70%.

IMPLICATIONS FOR SPECIFIC DISEASES SUCH AS CYSTIC FIBROSIS AND PRIMARY CILIARY DYSKINESIA

The general focus on these inflammatory airways diseases is to treat disease specific manifestations, especially airway infection and inflammation, the latter of which may be (but is not inevitably) damaging in its own right; and of course this is very important. However, there is no evidence or biological plausibility that because the child has one of these diseases they are exempt from the early adverse events (e.g., maternal smoking) on the airway and alveoli as discussed above. The inevitable conclusion is that, no matter how excellently (say) a CF clinic delivers multidisciplinary care, outcomes will be less good if general childhood lung health is neglected. This is one powerful argument for newborn screening for CF, although even this will preclude addressing antenatal factors. It is more worrying for conditions such as primary ciliary dyskinesia that are diagnosed symptomatically, often very late. This highlights the importance of diagnostic alertness to, for example, unexplained neonatal respiratory distress, so early intervention is possible.

The other important implication is the importance of lung attacks as more than just a temporary inconvenience. So in patients with CF, and in one small study of primary ciliary dyskinesia, around 30% of patients did not recover lung function despite treatment with intravenous antibiotics.[140] CF lung attacks have also been shown to be associated with a greater subsequent rate of decline in spirometry and a greater risk of death or lung transplantation at follow-up.

Summary and Conclusions

This chapter has discussed the transgenerational, antenatal and early childhood factors that affect lung development across the life course. The consequences of these adverse influences may be direct or secondary to an intermediate disease state such as prematurity and obesity. Many of these adverse effects cannot be remedied; we cannot stop atopic women bearing children, for example! There are two important take-home messages. The first is that we must identify and focus on what is preventable. This means legislation to protect vulnerable lungs against tobacco and nicotine (cigarettes and e-cigarettes), and traffic pollution; the institution of affordable and practical measures to minimize or eliminate exposure to biomass fuel; and being sure that due weight is given to the longer-term consequences of Caesarean section by women and obstetricians when planning delivery. The second is to convince the community, especially adult thoracic physicians, to see that many lung diseases would disappear if our vulnerable fetuses, babies, and infants were better protected from the consequences of adult behavior.

References
Access the reference list online at ExpertConsult.com.

16 Drug Administration by Inhalation in Children

ANGELA MARY FONCECA, PhD, WILLIAM GRAHAM FOX DITCHAM, PhD, MARK L. EVERARD, MD, and SUNALENE DEVADASON, PhD

Aerosol therapy is the cornerstone of treatment for many respiratory disorders in children. For those with asthma, the use of inhaled β-agonists and corticosteroids has formed the basis of optimal therapy for many decades, while inhaled antibiotics are increasingly being used to treat patients with cystic fibrosis and other forms of bacterial bronchitis (with or without bronchiectasis). The inhaled route has the advantage of more rapid onset of action for β-agonists; reduced systemic exposure for a given therapeutic effect for a range of drugs including corticosteroids, β-agonists, and antibiotics, and it also permits the use of certain drugs such as tobramycin, which are not readily absorbed by the enteral route. The improved therapeutic index of inhaled therapy as compared with oral therapy for the treatment of pulmonary disease is of course relative and systemic side effects do occur with high doses. For example, significant adrenal suppression can result from the use of high doses of inhaled corticosteroids (ICS), this being more likely when doses in excess of licensed doses are used.

While a great deal of research has gone into the development of devices that enable more efficient delivery of drugs to the lung, the commercial inhalers that are most widely used, particularly for children, are largely based on technologies that are more than 60 years old. These systems include pressurized metered dose inhalers (pMDIs), which may be used with or without an attached spacer or holding chamber. Few patients can use pMDIs optimally without spacers or holding chambers, which may be valved or unvalved. Spacers have the advantage of removing much of the upper airways' deposition of drug, which helps reduce local side effects. Thus, spacers should be used by anyone prescribed an ICS in a pMDI. Dry powder inhalers (DPIs) are currently dependent on a forceful inhalation to aerosolize the drug and hence are not suitable for preschool children. However, they do represent a valuable class of delivery system both for the treatment of asthma and, increasingly, for the delivery of antibiotics. Traditional jet nebulizers, whose basic design goes back many decades, are being used less frequently while devices such as vibrating mesh nebulizers, which are quiet and provide more rapid delivery of drug, are being used increasingly for antibiotic therapy.

Advantages and Disadvantages of Aerosols for Drug Delivery

Inhaled aerosolized drugs enable more direct access to the respiratory and cardiovascular systems (Table 16.1), which both include lung perivascular tissues. Aerosol drug delivery is most commonly used in children for the treatment of respiratory conditions such as asthma, cystic fibrosis, croup, and bronchopulmonary dysplasia. An inhaled entry route provides relatively unhindered access to actively exchanging capillary beds in the lungs. This ensures more rapid onset of drug action within the target organ compared with other administration methods such as oral (swallowed solid or liquid doses) and subcutaneous or intramuscular injection routes. Therefore a lower dose is needed for an equivalent effect[1] and aerosol delivery has the advantage of reducing systemic side effects.

Devices used for aerosol drug delivery vary in design, which can be tailored for application or dose. However, instructions for use and optimal inhalation techniques vary greatly depending on device type, which can lead to confusion and misuse if patients are prescribed multiple devices for different drugs. Hence, to achieve optimal benefits, instructions for using a device are best achieved when given through personal professional guidance. Consistency of dosing can be an issue as this is affected by many factors including tissue and systemic absorption and airway obstruction as well as training and ability of the patient to perform the required inhalation technique. In addition, the patient's cognitive ability to use the device and anatomical factors specific to the patient's age or disease condition may affect the efficacy of drug delivery.

A good understanding of the principles that determine aerosol particle deposition within the lungs enables health professionals to assess the best drug-device "fit" for patients of different ages and disease conditions.

There is a wide range of types of aerosol delivery systems and formulations currently in use or in development; the focus of this chapter will be on aerosol delivery systems and therapeutic applications currently in use in children.

What Is a Therapeutic Aerosol?

Aerosols are considered to be biphasic as they contain a gaseous and a particulate phase, which in practice equates to a gas in which solid and/or liquid particles are suspended.[2] The "gas" in which the aerosol is carried may be independently generated as part of the device itself (e.g., nebulizers using ambient air, medical air, or oxygen; pMDIs using hydrofluoroalkane [HFA] propellants). Alternatively, devices may require the patient's inspiratory air flow to disperse and "pull" the aerosol into the lungs (e.g., most DPIs currently used). The particulate phase consists of the therapeutic agent, generally in combination with additive compounds. Solid aerosols may consist purely of the therapeutic agent (e.g., Turbuhaler) or may contain a carrier (e.g., Accuhaler). Liquid aerosols

Table 16.1 Advantages and Disadvantages of Drug Administration by Inhalation Compared With Oral or Parenteral Administration

Advantages	Disadvantages
Improved therapeutic index compared with systemic administration (reduced incidence of systemic side effects for a given therapeutic effect)	The more portable metered dose devices (pressurized metered dose inhalers used alone, and dry powder inhalers) require specific inhalation techniques for optimal delivery
More rapid onset of action for bronchodilators	Correct use of current portable devices is not intuitive; repeated training in optimal use is often essential
Ability to administer drugs to the lungs that are not effective via the oral route due to poor gastrointestinal absorption or hepatic first pass elimination	Drug delivery is impaired in diseased regions of the lungs resulting in more central and heterogeneous distribution as lung disease progresses

Table 16.2 Determinants of Aerosol Deposition

Device and Formulation-Related Factors	Patient-Related Factors
Particle size	Age
Particle velocity	Inspiratory flow rate
Hygroscopic properties	Breathing pattern (inspiratory volume, rate)
Drug viscosity and surface tension	Nasal versus mouth breathing
Suspension versus solution	Anatomy (upper and lower airways)
	Disease severity
	Physical and cognitive ability
	Adherence, contrivance

may be solutions or suspensions; in either case, the solubility of the drug (whether in saline or propellant) will affect the aerosol characteristics. In addition, for solutions, the drug concentration and viscosity may be an important factor. The aerosol generation method of the device and the drug formulation in combination will affect the type of aerosol created and the efficiency with which the aerosol deposits in the lungs.

Principles of Aerosol Delivery

In general, the higher the proportion of drug that can bypass the upper airways and deposit in the lung, the greater the therapeutic response obtained from a given label or nominal dose. Some factors that affect this therapeutic efficacy are listed in Table 16.2; of these, the particle size of the aerosol and the velocity at which it is generated and inhaled are two key determinants.

Mathematical modeling and deposition studies have shown particles with a mass median aerosol diameter (MMAD) of greater than 5–10 µm are likely to be removed in the upper airways (by way of comparison a red blood cell has a diameter of ~7 µm). The proportion of particles within this range penetrating into the lower airways is in large part dependent on the inspiratory flow. The slower the inspiratory flow the

greater chance particles have to follow the inspiratory flow rather than impact in the upper airways. More particles will reach the lower airways if inhalation is via the mouth rather than the nose. Particles less than 1 µm are generally exhaled as their inertia and settling velocities are very low, though particles in the nano-micron range do deposit with increasing efficiency by bypassing the upper airways and depositing through Brownian motion. (A 1 µm particle carries 1000 less drug mass than a 10 µm particle.) Within the so call "respirable range" (roughly 1–7 µm) the pattern of distribution varies with finer aerosols tending to deposit more peripherally and the coarser ones tending to deposit in the conducting airways.[3–5] The pattern of deposition in an individual subject is influenced by particle size (affecting the likelihood of depositing through impaction or sedimentation, inspiratory flow (affecting the likelihood of impaction in upper and central airways) breath holding (influencing the deposition by sedimentation distally), as well as airway geometry, which can be influenced by age, natural variation, and disease.

Currently available commercial inhalers are primarily designed to generate heterodisperse or polydisperse aerosols (Fig. 16.1), with a mixture of particle sizes within a given "respirable" range, to ensure deposition in the different regions of the lung and, in part, to compensation for variability in patient use of the devices. Regional differences in drug deposition within the lung affect local responses and thereby treatment efficacy.[6,7]

The most important consideration with aerosolized drugs is to maximize drug deposition in the required areas of the respiratory tract. Three main factors govern this: inertial impaction, gravitational sedimentation, and diffusion. In addition, the electrostatic charge on both the aerosol and the respiratory mucosa may affect drug deposition.[8–10]

Drug formulations for aerosol therapy consist of either aqueous solutions or suspensions. Solutions are a mixture of two or more components forming a homogenous molecular dispersion in a single-phase system. Suspensions consist of a dispersed system where insoluble solid particles are dispersed in a liquid medium.[11,12] Colloidal suspensions are made up of solid particles less than 1 µm in diameter, whereas coarse suspensions contain solid particles greater than 1 µm in diameter. Wetting agents are usually required for the dispersion of solid particles in suspension and generally consist of surfactants, which may make up 0.05%–0.5% of the drug suspension.[11,12]

PHYSICAL PRINCIPLES AFFECTING AEROSOL DELIVERY AND DEPOSITION

Particle Size

There are many factors that can affect the site and amount of aerosolized drug depositing in a patient's airways (see Table 16.2); the aerosolized particle size is one of the key determinants.[13] Particles less than 3 µm will deposit in the lower and smaller airways, whereas particles greater than 5 µm generally deposit in the oropharynx or upper airways.[14] Therefore minimizing the particle size of aerosolized drugs is essential for targeted deposition in the smaller airways. Due to the proportional cubic increase in volume of drug that can be carried with unit increase in the diameter of the

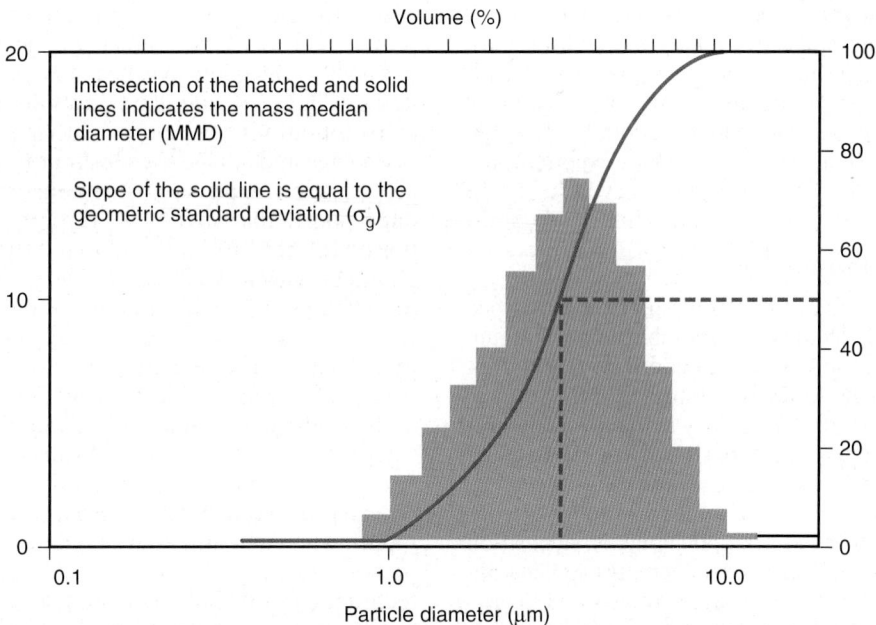

Fig. 16.1 The particle size distribution of a medical aerosol generator that has been measured by laser diffraction. Each bar to the histogram represents a size band of particles (the height of the bar represents the percentage of the sample within that band). The scale on the left is used to read the histogram; the scale on the right is used to read the cumulative plot represented by the solid line going through the histogram. The particle size that corresponds to 50% on the cumulative curve is the MMD—in this case 3.3 μm. The slope of the line at the 50% point corresponds to the geometric standard deviation.

particles, larger particles carry a much greater volume of drug. However, aerosols that contain a large proportion of particles greater than 15 μm in diameter will deliver most of the drug available for inhalation to the oropharynx. This results in little therapeutic effect and increased systemic exposure. Measurement of particle size is complicated by variability in the shape of aerosolized droplets, which may be irregular rather than strictly spherical. For this reason, particles of different shapes that behave in a similar manner (aerodynamically) are grouped together and visualized as spherical droplets with a common diameter, known as the aerodynamic diameter and geometric standard deviation (GSD). This is defined as the diameter of a sphere of unit density with the same terminal sedimentation velocity in air as the particle or droplet in question,[8] and is usually determined by the mass of the droplet. Most forms of aerosol therapy generate droplets of varying sizes known as polydisperse aerosol droplets, as opposed to monodisperse particles, which are characterized by uniformly sized particles of the same aerodynamic diameter. Polydisperse aerosols are further characterized by half of the aerosol mass having an aerodynamic diameter below the mass median aerodynamic diameter (MMAD), and half with diameters greater than the MMAD.[14] Overall, this means lung deposition for a highly polydisperse aerosol with an MMAD of 3 μm would be much lower than that for a monodisperse aerosol of the same diameter, whereas the reverse would be the case if the MMAD was greater than 5 μm.[15]

Optimizing the delivery of inhaled aerosols to patient populations is most important when drugs such as corticosteroids are being administered, especially in the pediatric age group. Ideally, drug delivery to the airways should be maximized, with minimal oropharyngeal and gastric deposition.

Inertial Impaction

The way in which a particle travels in an airstream depends on momentum, which is determined by mass and velocity. High velocity ensures continued movement in a particular direction due to inertia despite obstacles or bends. However, these may cause the direction of air flow to change as when particles approach a surface such as the back of the throat or a bifurcation of the airways. Importantly, inhaled particles may not follow the direction of air flow, and instead may impact on the surface. Therefore particles with a higher momentum, such as larger particles or those with a higher velocity are more likely to impact in the oropharynx or the larger airways. Hence inertial impaction has a greater effect on larger particles (>3 μm),[10] and in areas where the velocity of inhaled particles is greatest; such as the oropharynx and upper airways.

Gravitational Sedimentation

All particles will settle under gravity. Particles will accelerate to a steady terminal velocity when gravitational force is balanced by the resistance of air through which it is traveling, which is aided by breath holding.

Larger particles become filtered out by the upper airways and, as the velocity of these decreases, impaction is most likely to occur in the oropharynx, meaning particles greater than 15 μm are unlikely to enter the trachea.[15] Even for particles less than 15 μm, further deposition of the larger particles will occur at airway bifurcations.[16,17]

Particles less than 3 μm are unlikely to be affected by inertial impaction in the upper airways; therefore sedimentation due to gravity is the most important mechanism for deposition of these particles in the smaller airways. Within the less than 3 μm size range, the effect of sedimentation is greatest on the larger particles (>0.5 μm)[16,17] that have escaped deposition due to initial inertial impaction. Breath holding after inhalation of the aerosolized particles helps deposition in the airways due to sedimentation.[16,17] The rate of deposition though sedimentation reduces exponentially over time and as a generalization there is very little benefit to be gained from breath holds of greater than 10 seconds.

Brownian Motion/Diffusion

Particles less than 0.5 μm are small enough to be perturbed by surrounding gas molecules. This bombardment (impaction with gas particles) can interrupt intended particle routes, which will move particles towards the surface of the respiratory tract, with the observed diffusivity being inversely proportional to the diameter of the particle.[8] For particles of 0.1–1 μm, deposition by sedimentation and diffusion is very slow but below this size (which includes a number of constituents of tobacco smoke) the efficiency of deposition through the effects of Brownian motion increases significantly, which is one of the reasons there are significant concerns regarding the increasing use of nanoparticles in manufacturing processes.[13]

Electrostatic Attraction

Deposition may occur due to attraction between charged particles in the inhaled aerosol and an induced charge on the mucosa of the respiratory tract.[8] The extent to which this factor affects drug delivery and deposition has not been investigated in detail. The drug and other components of the formulation, device materials, and the generation of the aerosol from the device itself, can all affect the electrostatic charge of an emitted aerosol particle.

PATIENT-RELATED VARIABLES

Quite apart from the device and drug formulation related factors, patient related variables can markedly change the effective dose of aerosolized drug received by patients (see Table 16.2). These factors include anatomical and physiological variation between subjects as well as disease severity and distribution. However, the most important patient variable is their ability to use the device, both effectively and consistently, which is influenced in part by the quality of training provided.

As noted above, airway obstruction due to structural disease as in progressive bronchiectasis, bronchoconstriction as in asthma, or intraluminal mucus all contribute to more central deposition with hot spots in regions of flow limitation and distal areas of little or no drug delivery. For asthma, this is of relatively little consequence as the ICS lead to progressive improvement and improved homogeneity of deposition while β-agonists given in the face of diffuse constriction when the patient is symptomatic are probably redistributed to more peripheral regions of the lungs via the bronchial circulation. In progressive disease such as CF, the effectiveness of inhaled therapy is increasingly compromised as progressively less drug reaches the more diseased areas.

Age

In some respects, the greatest challenges for using inhaled therapy result from cognitive and physical limitations at each end of the life course. For children, the period from birth to primary school is one of great change in physical and cognitive ability, which impacts their ability to use inhalers initially designed for use by adults. Conventional jet nebulizers with constant output can be used with standard tidal breathing at any age and can be used by infants and toddlers but they are relatively expensive, time consuming, inefficient, and often poorly tolerated by very young children (due to the noise and need to have a closely fitting mask). A holding chamber with a facemask can very effectively deliver drug to the lungs proving the infant/young child is not upset and will tolerate a closely fitting mask. Crying or screaming results in little or no drug reaching the lungs due to impaction in the upper airways, while if the mask is not closely fitting the patient inhales entrained air mainly rather than aerosol.

By their third birthday, most subjects are able to learn the "panting" technique with a mouthpiece, in which they take repeated inspiratory and expiratory breaths through their mouth when inhaling from a holding chamber. By 5–7 years of age, most will be able to master the optimal inhalation technique from a holding chamber with a slow inspiratory breath over 4–5 seconds followed by a 10-second breath hold or the rapid forceful inhalation required to optimally aerosolize drug from DPIs.

In terms of drug delivered, the absolute dose delivered to the lungs tends to increase over early life. For nebulized therapy, drug delivery probably reaches a maximal in the early preschool years as the inspiratory flow exceeds the flow of the nebulizer and the increased tidal volume consists of entrained air. However, drug delivery on a weight corrected basis is likely to be influenced by the device. The absolute dose delivered from a DPI with a reasonably steep dose to lung flow dependency curve may continue to increase into the teen years. However, the dose delivered per kilogram may be relatively constant for DPIs that are less flow dependent. The absolute dose delivered from a pMDI holding chamber combination may be fairly constant across age but the dose per kilogram will fall from the primary school ages as the child grows.

Regimen and Device Compliance

Compliance with an optimal treatment regimen is commonly poor in all therapeutic areas resulting in suboptimal health outcomes. That is patients frequently miss multiple doses for a variety of reasons. The situation with inhaled therapy is compounded by the need to use prescribed inhalation techniques with many studies indicating that the majority of patients, physicians, and pharmacists are unable to use devices optimally. Hence, for inhaled therapy, true adherence to a recommended treatment regime is the product of regimen compliance × device compliance (is the device used at all) × (is the device used effectively).

If the device is not taken out of the drawer the inhaler technique is irrelevant, but true adherence can still be zero if the patient attempts to take the treatment in line with the prescribed pattern of use but the patient is unable to use the device effectively. Reasons for being unable to use the device (lack of competence) include lack of adequate instruction compounded by lack of reinforcement while for others ineffectual use is due to ignoring what they know and using it efficiently (contrivance—contriving to use it inefficiently), such as the patient who demonstrates a perfect technique with a pMDI spacer but who "knows" he does not need to use the spacer and simply fires it into their mouth while taking a rapid inspiration.

The importance of true compliance can be illustrated if one considers "difficult asthma." In general, certainly in pediatrics, there are only three causes for difficult asthma in the vast majority of patients.

1. A misdiagnosis of symptoms being attributable to another condition all together, such as bacterial bronchitis.
2. Asthma and a comorbidity such as a persistent bacterial bronchitis (often secondary to poor control) or an intercurrent pertussis infection.
3. Ineffective drug delivery, which may be due to poor regime compliance or device compliance (due to lack of competence or contrivance).

For those who require regular therapy because of ongoing symptoms or significant exacerbations, the evidence suggests that adherence probably needs to exceed 80%—that is of a potential 14 doses a week (twice daily dosing) the patient should not miss more than 3 doses.[17a] Fewer than 20% of subjects who require this intensity of treatment appear to reach this threshold for a wide variety of reasons such as fear of side effects, concerns regarding development of "dependency," and financial considerations. "Drug holidays" are frequently observed in clinical trials suggesting that patients are testing to determine whether medication is still required. However, the most commonly reported cause is simply forgetting to take the medication. Failure to develop a routine that deals with the need to take the medication regularly and with consistency is a common factor amongst those with poor compliance. Unfortunately, lack of explanation regarding the rational for adhering to regular medication and confusing messages from different health care professionals compound the problem. Until health care professionals are able to do the simple things well this situation is likely to persist.

Evidence suggests that competence and contrivance can both be addressed with effective education by healthcare professionals, but these messages need to be repeated and reinforced. Education has, in general, little or no impact on behavior in the vast majority of patients unless considerable resources are invested and to date, the most effective interventions appear to be monitoring with feedback. Studies that provide patients with feedback regarding their behavior have consistently shown improved adherence and studies that are more recent have started to demonstrate clinically important improvements resulting from the improved adherence. It seems likely that more devices will have data loggers incorporated or will be provided with an add-on data logger that can provide real time feedback. Improved data provides for more open and honest discussion between physician and patient.

Assessment Techniques

Aerosol drug formulations and devices need to be assessed in combination because the formulation can greatly affect the type of aerosol emitted from a given device. These evaluations may be purely in vitro assessments of aerosol generation and efficiency of aerosol delivery, or in vivo measurements of drug delivery to the patient and deposition within the lungs. In general, these aerosol-specific assessments are conducted as part of the development and initial assessment of the performance of an inhaler, prior to conducting larger scale trials of clinical outcomes in different patient groups.

AEROSOL GENERATION

Assessment of aerosol characteristics with in vitro techniques consists of the measurement of those characteristics of the aerosol that have a major effect on drug delivery to the lungs. The efficacy of drug delivery from the aerosol generated by a particular device is largely dependent on two factors:

1. The range of particle sizes present in the aerosol cloud, termed the *particle size distribution*.
2. The total output of drug.

The size distribution of the particles or droplets making up a therapeutic aerosol can be described in three ways: the frequency of occurrence of particle volumes, masses, or counts. The description of the aerosol cloud can then be expressed as, respectively, the volume median diameter (VMD), the mass median diameter (MMD), and the count median diameter (CMD). These diameters are those above and below which, respectively, half the volume of the aerosol, half the mass of the aerosol, and half the number of particles in the aerosol reside. The VMD and the MMD will be identical if all the particles comprising the aerosol have the same density, as is normally the case when a drug in solution is nebulized. As the amount of drug contained within a droplet or particle is defined by the volume of the particle, and this is related to the cube of the radius of the particle, the CMD is not useful in assessing the likelihood of successful drug delivery from a therapeutic aerosol, as one droplet 5 µm in diameter will contain 1000 times as much drug as one droplet 0.5 µm in diameter and therapeutic aerosols are generally polydisperse, consisting of particles with a range of diameters. The particles may also be irregular in shape and differ in density, which will alter their behavior when entrained in an air flow. The aerodynamic behavior of a particle is best described by its aerodynamic diameter, that is, the diameter of a spherical particle of unit density that behaves in the same way when entrained in a defined air flow. Measurement of the MMAD, of an aerosol by inertial impaction, helps to describe and predict the behavior in an air flow of a polydisperse aerosol consisting of particles of different shapes and densities. The extent to which the aerosol is polydisperse is defined by the GSD (σ_g), the ratio of the particle diameter below which 84.3% of the mass is contained to that below which 50% is contained. The larger the GSD, the more polydisperse the aerosol. Most inhaler devices produce aerosols consisting of large numbers of small particles with progressively fewer larger particles, within the range of approximately 1–10 µm MAD.

All of these factors can be greatly affected by the way in which the inhaler is stored and used. Optimizing the particle size distribution and output from an inhaler by careful formulation, and good storage and use practice, will maximize the amount of drug available for inhalation by the patient.

Particle Size Distribution

There are two main methods of assessing the particle size distribution from a given aerosol: inertial impaction and laser diffraction. Inertial impaction measures the actual drug content within particles of a precalibrated size range while laser diffraction measures particle size by volume. For most drug solutions and for dry powders consisting only of the drug compound, we may assume that the drug is evenly distributed through the aerosol droplet or particle.

Inertial Impaction. The generated aerosol is drawn by an entraining air flow (defined and calibrated for each device) through the impaction device, which consists of a series of stages. Each stage acts as a low pass filter, where "larger" particles, above the defined aerodynamic diameter cut-off for that stage, impact and are retained, while "smaller" particles remain entrained in the air flow to move further through the device. At each consecutive stage, remaining particles above the cut-off aerodynamic diameter of that stage are retained, while particles of smaller aerodynamic diameter remain entrained until they reach the final stage, which consists of an absolute filter to remove very small particles that have not impacted further up the series of stages.

There is a wide variety of impaction devices available. Cascade impactors collect particles in discrete size ranges that impact on a series of solid stages, sometimes coated with grease to trap the impacting particles and prevent them from bouncing off the stage, to be reentrained and drawn on to a lower stage. Liquid impingers have a layer of solvent on each stage (except the absolute filter), which performs the same function. Each impaction device may be made up of a different number of stages. The greater the number of stages, the greater is the resolution in the characterization of the particle size distribution of a particular aerosol. The particle size cut-offs for the stages in each impaction device are calibrated for a particular entraining air flow, which may also affect the characteristics of the aerosol. Particles reaching the lower stages of inertial impactors (with particle size ranges of around 1–5 µm) are often referred to as "respirable"

particles, though the amounts of drug captured on these stages tend to be a significant overestimate of the proportion of drug emitted from the inhalation device that would reach the lungs of patients.[18,19] An example of two impaction devices, a multistage cascade impactor and the Next Generation Impactor (Copley, UK), are shown in Fig. 16.2.

Once the aerosol dose has been drawn through the device, the air flow is stopped and the surface of each stage is washed separately to remove impacted particles. The amount of drug retained on each stage is assayed, usually using high performance liquid chromatography or ultraviolet spectrophotometry. The sum of the amount of drug deposited on these stages provides the total drug output of the device tested. The components of the inhalation system, such as the pMDI actuator or the nebulizer body, may also be washed to measure the amount of drug retained by the device and not administered to the patient. Using this method, an assessment can be made of the amount of drug contained within each fraction of the total range of particle sizes contained within the generated aerosol, and hence a prediction can be made of the amount of drug that will reach the target area within the lungs. Any changes in particle size distribution and total drug output in the aerosol generated by an inhaler under different conditions, or with changes in formulation can also be assessed.

The particle size distribution is given in discrete ranges, not the continuous spectrum of sizes actually generated by the device being tested, which is a disadvantage of inertial impaction techniques. Hence, direct comparisons between different impaction devices are not easy, especially if they are calibrated for different entraining air flows.

Laser Diffraction. Measurement of particle sizes using laser diffraction involves passing the aerosol through a laser beam, resulting in light scattering (Fraunhofer diffraction) by the edges of the aerosolized particles. The scattered light passes

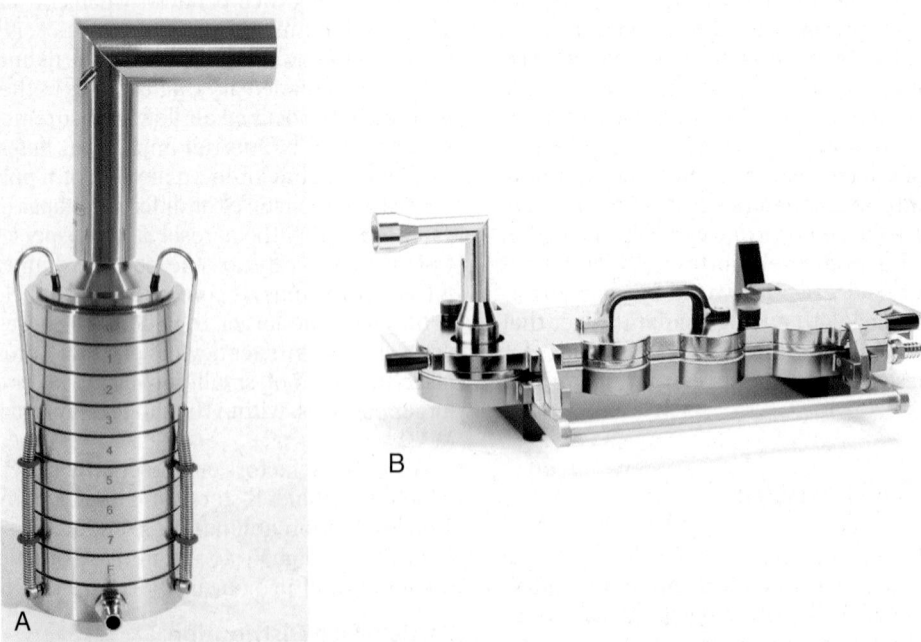

Fig. 16.2 Examples of two most widely used impaction devices for measurement of particle size of aerosol drug-device combinations for regulatory approvals. (A) The Andersen Cascade Impactor and (B) the Next Generation Impactor. (From Copley Scientific Limited, http://www.copleyscientific.com/.)

through a lens that focuses the rays onto a series of detectors. The angle of diffraction is inversely proportional to the droplet size.[20] This information is used to calculate the numbers of aerosolized particles at any volume in the aerosol. This method only measures particle volumes (VMD) and not the actual amount of drug present. For aerosols generated from a solution of a drug, as produced by a nebulizer, the total volume of the combined droplets of any given size is proportional to the amount of drug contained within those droplets, and so may be useful in predicting therapeutic efficiency. For aerosols where the drug is contained within particles suspended in the aerosol, the particles may be larger than the smallest droplets, and so droplets in this range would contain no drug.

Measurement of particle size distributions using either of the techniques described above is complicated by a number of factors. Particle size distributions can vary greatly with the conditions of testing, such as inhalation flows through impaction devices, and driving gas flows through nebulizers.[21] Changes in particle sizes once an aerosol has been generated can also occur due to factors such as hygroscopic growth, which is dependent on humidity and the composition of the aerosolized particles,[22] and evaporation of the more volatile components of a drug suspension.

Total Drug Output

The total amount of drug contained in a dose of aerosol generated by an inhalation system can be measured by delivering the aerosol through a low resistance filter, and assaying for the amount of drug deposited on the filter. Another method is measurement of the weight of the inhalation device before and after aerosol generation, but this method usually greatly overestimates aerosol output due to high levels of evaporation.[23] Total drug output, as well as the particle size distribution, can be determined using impaction devices, if the masses of drug in each size fraction are added together. This is not possible using laser diffraction techniques.

Factors other than particle size and output can also play an important role in the assessment of an inhalation system. In the case of nebulizers, the time taken to deliver the aerosolized drug is also important, especially in the pediatric age range. Factors such as driving gas flows through the nebulizer or inhalational flows through pMDIs, spacers, and DPIs can significantly affect all the parameters mentioned above.

DELIVERY

In vitro studies under carefully controlled laboratory conditions are used to assess the aerosol generated by a particular device, giving relatively reproducible results. While these techniques provide useful information on optimizing aerosol generation, drug delivery from these same aerosol generation devices, to patients in a clinical situation, can still be extremely variable, largely due to variation in the patient's inhalation technique.

Filter studies can be used to assess aerosolized drug delivery to patients using different inhalation systems and inhalation techniques. For these studies, a low resistance filter is placed between the inhaler and the patient's mouth. When the device is actuated and the patient inhales, the amount of drug that would normally be inhaled by the patient is deposited on the filter. This equates to the "total body dose" that would have

been administered to the patient. The filter can then be washed, and the amount of drug deposited can be assayed. This method is noninvasive, since the patients do not inhale any drug, and the performance of the inhaler can be assessed by measuring the "total body dose" delivered to the patient over a range of patients' breathing patterns. The approach provides some idea of the variability that inevitably occurs in the clinical use of these inhalers especially in children.[24] It does not however provide any information on the particle size distribution of the delivered aerosol, which can be influenced by inspiratory flow when using a nebulizer or dry powder inhaler, and gives no information about the pattern of deposition of the drug in the lung, mouth, throat, esophagus, and stomach that would have occurred if the filter was not present. To obtain information about where the inhaled drug deposits in the body, deposition scintigraphy by imaging following inhalation of a radioisotope labeled aerosol may be utilized.

IN VIVO DEPOSITION

Deposition scintigraphy is an imaging modality, which enables the investigator to visualize the in vivo distribution of drug within the patient's body. Two-dimensional (2-D) planar scintigraphy, three-dimensional (3-D) single photon emission computed tomography (SPECT), and positron emission tomography (PET) may all be utilized[25]; however planar scintigraphy involves the lowest radiation exposure and is generally the method utilized in children. The data obtained from scintigraphy studies takes into account both the drug-device delivery characteristics and the effect of the patients' inhalation techniques in determining the amount and distribution of aerosolized drug depositing within the body.[26–28] The drug is labeled with a low level of a radioisotope and gamma scintigraphy is used to quantify the deposition of the label in the lungs after inhalation by the patient. These tests are necessary to ensure that the aerosolized drug produced by an inhaler is reaching the target site, and the number of such studies should be minimized by only performing them with optimal delivery systems. Hence, initial assessments of any new inhaler should be carried out using in vitro and filter studies.

The most common radioisotope used for aerosol deposition studies is technetium (Tc^{99m}), a gamma emitter that has a short half-life of 6 hours. The half-life in the lungs is much shorter than this, about 15–20 minutes, as the isotope is rapidly cleared from the lungs. Mouth and throat deposition can be reduced by the use of a spacer with radiolabeled pMDIs, as well as mouth washing and gargling after inhalation of the radiolabeled aerosol.

Useful results can be obtained from images obtained after administration of a very low amount of activity (for planar scintigraphy) (Fig. 16.3), comparable to the radiation exposure received during a 12 hour plane flight, or from two to four weeks of exposure to natural background radiation.

Studies to observe the deposition patterns obtained when using nebulizers generally involve adding the required amount of radioisotope to give detectable deposition to saline or a drug solution in the nebulizer bowl.[29,30] Labeling of drugs in metered dose inhalers (both pMDIs and DPIs) is more difficult, and requires stringent validation of the labeling technique to ensure radioactivity comigrates with the administered

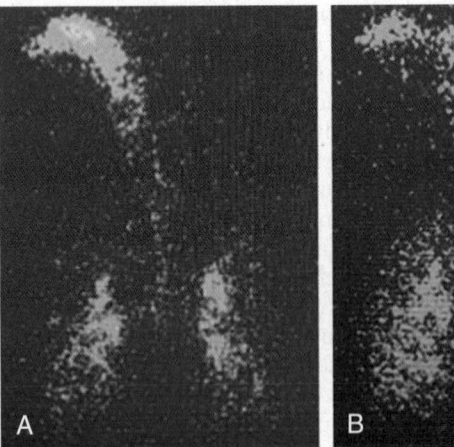

Fig. 16.3 Examples of gamma scintigraphic images of an 15 year old asthmatic patient, obtained after inhalation of a radiolabeled aerosol from a pMDI, used (A) without a spacer and (B) with a spacer. The images capture the distribution of the label, Tc^{99m} only, hence it is critical that the radiolabeling method is carefully validated to ensure that the label "follows" the drug when aerosolized, prior to use in patients. The validation method utilizes the measurement of the aerosol particle size distribution using impaction devices, such as those shown in Fig. 16.2. Note the higher oropharyngeal deposition when the pMDI was used without a spacer.

drug, and hence is a good proxy for it, prior to administration to patients.

There are a number of techniques for labeling drugs in pMDIs,[31–33] most of which are based on the original method of Kohler.[34] The success of each labeling method depends on the drug formulation being used.[6] The labeling technique for drugs administered as a dry powder, used in inhalers such as the Turbuhaler, involves drying of the radiolabel onto the surface of the drug particles.[18,35]

To ensure that the radiolabel detected by scintigraphy is indicative of where drug has deposited in vivo, the effect of radiolabeling on the commercial aerosol must be minimal, and this and the comigration of radiolabel and drug must be confirmed in vitro.[36] In order to do this, firstly, the particle size distribution of the aerosolized drug in the commercial formulation is compared to that of the same drug formulation following radiolabeling. The second step is to ensure that the radioisotope also comigrates with the drug in this formulation. This is done by comparing the particle size distribution from assay of both the drug, and the radiolabel activity in the labeled formulation, by cascade impaction of the radiolabeled aerosol, and measurement of the activity in each fraction, followed by assay of the drug in each fraction when radioactivity has decayed to undetectable levels. More stringent guidelines for the validation of radiolabeled inhalers including limits for the comparison of the commercial to the radiolabeled inhaler have been published following consultation with a committee of international experts.[37,38] Following these guidelines is necessary to ensure that results from measuring the deposition of the radiolabel are a good proxy for the distribution pattern of the drug.

Using deposition studies, the proportion of the inhaled drug deposited in the airways, as well as oropharyngeal and gastric deposition, can be imaged using gamma scintigraphy to detect the radiolabel as a proxy for the drug. Attenuation of the gamma rays by body tissues is accounted for by

calculating the attenuation of the counts obtained from a planar flood source by the body of the subject prior to inhalation of the radiolabeled aerosol. A measure of the penetration of the administered activity, and by association the drug, to the peripheral airways is made by calculating the amount of drug deposited centrally in a defined region of interest on the image, and comparing this to the total deposition seen in the same lung image.

Although the risk to the subjects from inhaling radiolabeled aerosols is low, there is still a risk associated with any exposure to radioactive materials, and the number of patients subjected to this form of testing should be minimized.[39] Preliminary noninvasive testing is still required for many drug formulations to characterize the type of aerosol generated by the delivery systems.

Aerosol Devices

The three broad groups of devices used for inhalation therapy are

1. pMDIs
   These may be patient actuated (frequently prescribed with a holding chamber to address some of the problems that are inherent with this type of device) or breath actuated.
   Conventionally these have contained suspension-based formulations but some of the HFA formulations are solution based. To date it is has not been shown that there are any inherent advantages of one type of formulation over the other.
2. DPIs
   These may be single or multidose devices and vary in their flow dependence (the extent to which changes in inspiratory flow affect the efficacy of drug dispersal). While debated, there is again no clear benefit attributable to those devices that have a high or low flow dependency providing the patient can generate flow sufficient to reach the minimum desirable flow. All current devices are dependent on the patient to provide the energy to aerosolize the drug (though a patient independent device was briefly marketed during the past decade for the delivery of inhaled insulin).
3. Nebulizers
   These generate a "wet" aerosol usually from a solution formulation and include conventional jet nebulizers, ultrasonic and, increasingly vibrating mesh devices.

PRESSURIZED METERED DOSE INHALERS

pMDIs have long been the most widely used form of asthma therapy in adults and older children, and are now the method of choice in infants and children under 5 years old (Fig. 16.4), when used in combination with an appropriate small volume spacer and, if required in young children, a well-fitting facemask.[27] pMDI canisters contain the drug, in suspension or solution in a propellant with surfactants, under high pressure (300–500 kPa, 40–70 p.s.i.). Chlorofluorocarbons (CFCs) were used as propellants in pMDIs, but these have now been replaced with HFAs, which are less destructive to the ozone layer. More than 99% of the dose from a typical inhaler consists of propellant, and so this must be nontoxic

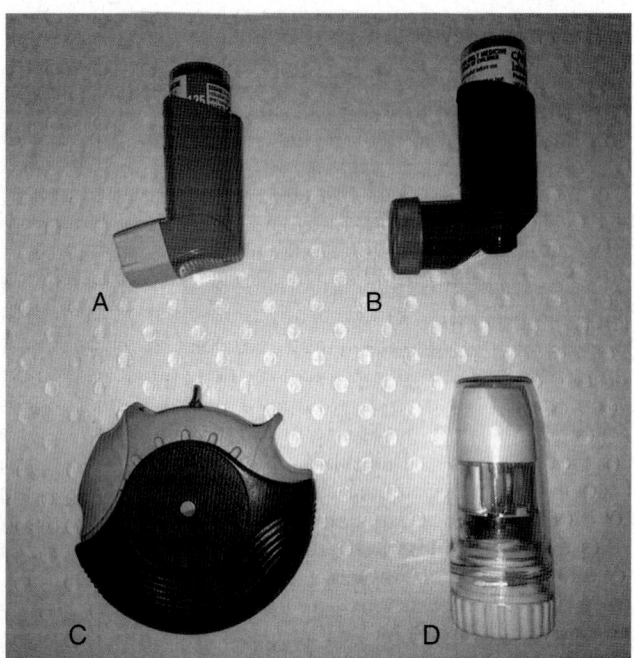

Fig. 16.4 Examples of two types of pressurized metered dose inhalers (A, B) and two DPI types—the Accuhaler or Diskus (C), and the Turbuhaler (D).

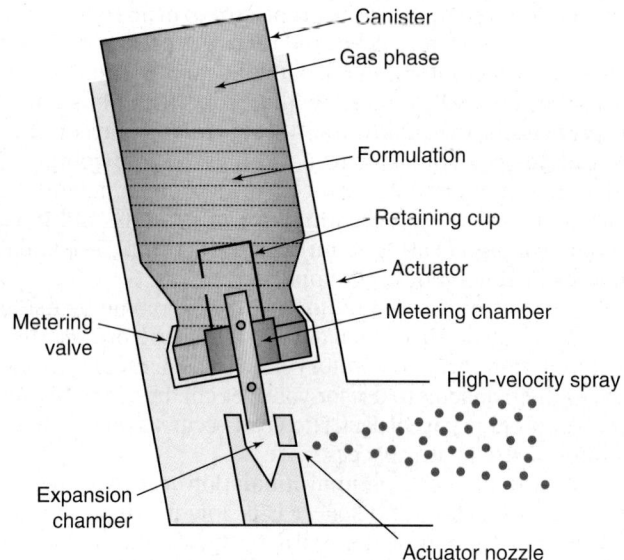

Fig. 16.5 Schematic of a pMDI.

to the patient, as well as fulfilling the other requirements: having a low boiling point, a high vapor pressure, and a density close to that of the drug to be delivered.[40] Aerosols generated by pMDIs using HFA propellants in the formulation have very different properties, which sometimes increase the efficacy of these formulations. HFA propellants can be used to radically alter the particle size distribution of drug formulations, particularly from corticosteroid inhalers.[41] Some formulations have changed from a suspension to a solution of the drug, and MMADs can be decreased to as low as 1 µm. The character of the emitted plume is different, being warmer and softer, and this can decrease unwanted deposition in the mouth and throat due to lower particle velocities on activation. Lung deposition patterns detected in radiolabel deposition studies have been shown to be greatly altered by changes in the particle size distribution of inhaled aerosols.[30] Surfactants such as phospholipids or oleic acid are included in the formulation to increase bioavailability of the administered drug by decreasing the surface tension of the fluid lining the airways. Low concentrations of ethanol are sometime included to modify droplet surface tension and thus modify particle size distribution of the generated aerosol.

Prior to actuation of the pMDI, the dose, still under high pressure, is contained within the metering chamber (Fig. 16.5). For drugs that are not in solution, the canister must be shaken immediately prior to actuation to resuspend the drug particles uniformly in the propellant. When the valve is opened to the atmosphere, the propellant expands and the suspension in the metering chamber is expelled at high velocities, up to 30 m/s. Initially, the particles are very large, up to 20 µm in diameter, but rapid evaporation of the volatile propellants reduces their size. This initial high velocity in conjunction with the larger particle sizes results in a sizeable proportion of particles impacting in the mouth and throat

before the propellant evaporates, both decreasing the number of particles available for inhalation and deposition in the lungs and increasing the local oropharyngeal exposure and, potentially, the systemic dose. As mentioned above, some formulations using HFAs as propellants decrease oropharyngeal deposition due to the softer plume and smaller MMAD of aerosols generated from pMDIs using this propellant.

Patient-dependent problems, such as difficulty in coordinating actuation and inhalation, are common with the use of pMDIs.[42] For inexpensive drugs such as bronchodilators, which are mostly given in supramaximal doses and have few, relatively mild systemic side effects, this is of little importance. However, for drugs such as corticosteroids, it is critical to reduce local and systemic side effects (particularly in the pediatric age group) and to maximize lung deposition for several reasons: achieving the maintenance dosage is important, side effects such as oral candidiasis and hoarseness can occur with repeated oropharyngeal deposition, and these drugs are generally more expensive. Device-based problems include variation in the administered dose. An increase in drug concentration can occur following multiple actuations without shaking with the canister held in the inhalation orientation whereas a decrease in drug dose can occur if the metering valve is refilled with propellant alone, as drug settles out leaving only propellant to fill the metering chamber. Use of pMDIs at very low temperatures can reduce the vapor pressure above the propellant and thus decrease the efficiency of plume generation upon actuation, as well as decreasing the propensity of the initial large propellant droplets to evaporate to a size more conducive to penetration to the lungs, depositing instead in the mouth and throat. Inhalers using HFA as a propellant are less prone to ambient temperature related problems,[43] although this may not be the case for all HFA inhaler formulations.[44]

Patient dependent problems can be reduced by the use of spacers, also termed *holding chambers* or *extension devices*.[45] These are generally made of plastic (although a metal spacer is available). The pMDI actuator is inserted into an opening at one end and aerosol inhaled through a mouthpiece or facemask with a one-way inspiratory valve at the other end.

As there is more time for the propellant to evaporate before entering the mouth or nose, and there is a greater distance between the actuator and the patient's mouth, smaller particles are eventually inhaled, with a reduction of impaction of particles in the mouth and throat. Infant spacers have been developed for use with a facemask. These contain a separate expiratory valve, which allows younger patients in particular to use tidal breathing for inhalation, and have smaller volumes (150–250 ml) that only require 5–10 tidal breaths by the infant to be emptied.

The problem of coordination can be overcome by using breath-actuated pMDIs, such as the Autohaler. However, they require a minimum inspiratory flow to be actuated, which makes them difficult to use for younger children, and higher levels of oropharyngeal deposition can occur, as these devices cannot be used with spacers.

The recommended optimal inhalation technique when using a pMDI without a spacer is a slow maximal inhalation with actuation of the pMDI as the slow inhalation is commenced. The pMDI is held between the teeth and with the lips sealed around the mouthpiece. The inhalation is followed by 10 second breath hold to increase sedimentation of particles.[46,47] An open mouth technique where the pMDI is held 2–3 cm from the open mouth and actuated at the start of the inhalation may help to reduce oropharyngeal deposition as the plume has a chance to slow and particles to decrease in size by evaporation before entering the mouth. This reduces the ballistic impaction of particles in the upper airway. The slow inhalation and resulting low air flow can reduce inertial impaction of large particles. As infants and young children are unable to perform this maneuver, they inhale aerosols by tidal breathing through a spacer. The use of spacers is essential in this age group even for delivery of bronchodilators.

Drugs for the treatment of asthma such as bronchodilators, corticosteroids, and sodium cromoglycate, are often delivered by pMDIs, particularly in younger children.

As noted previously, calculating the most appropriate device for use with a pMDI/spacer is not easy. Currently, adult doses of inhaled asthma medication are being given to infants and young children. This practice may mean that children are receiving a much higher dose for their size than adults. On the other hand, differences in inhalation patterns and tidal volumes could mean that the dose delivered to young children will be size corrected. There is some evidence that lung deposition in children under 5 years of age using a pMDI with a small volume spacer is only about 2% of the nominal dose,[48] whereas in a 70 kg adult it may be up to 20% of the nominal dose, giving similar dose rates per kilogram of body weight.

There is an extensive body of literature on the optimal use of pMDIs and their accessory devices.[49–53] Factors such as temperature,[54] altitude,[55] and storage conditions[56] can affect the performance of pMDIs, while the aerosol output from spacers is greatly affected by factors such as multiple actuations,[57,58] spacer volume and valve design,[57,59] and time delays between actuation and inhalation.[60] Static electricity buildup on the spacer wall can result in the loss of up to 50% of an aerosol dose, but this can be minimized by using a charged detergent to clean the spacer. The extent of practical application of this knowledge is still unclear.[61,62] Static is not a problem with metal spacers.[57]

DRY POWDER INHALERS

There are many advantages to DPIs, including their portability, the lack of a requirement for coordinated actuation and inhalation, and the relative simplicity of construction of some types.

DPIs are used to deliver a similar range of drugs as pMDIs. The aerosols generated by these devices consist of solid drug particles and carrier, dispersed in air. The DPIs most commonly used commercially are breath-driven, and so do not require coordination of actuation and inhalation as pMDIs do. DPIs generally require a mid-high peak inspiratory flow (PIF) to deaggregate and suspend the drug particles into the air flow. Small particles less than 5 μm in diameter, produced by milling or spray drying, tend to clump together due to electrostatic forces, and exhibit poor flow characteristics. Inclusion of an excipient such as lactose in the formulation can loosely bind these small respirable drug particles to larger carrier particles of about 30–60 μm diameter, which exhibit much better flow characteristics, allowing a forceful inhalation to draw the drug and excipient through a turbulence-inducing device, which deaggregates the drug from the excipient as the dose is suspended in air. The smaller drug particles are then free to be drawn down to the lungs, while the larger excipient particles impact in the mouth and throat. Increased inspiratory effort generating higher PIFs will optimize the particle size of the drug output. Although high PIFs generally increase the impaction of particles in the oropharynx, this effect is offset by the much reduced drug particle size range due to more effective deaggregation. Flows less than the minimum required to deaggregate the drug and excipient will lead to poor pulmonary deposition. Children, especially those who are unwell, are often not capable of producing sufficient flow to successfully deaggregate the powder and, in addition, the total volume of the inspiration may not be sufficient to draw powder deep into the lungs to the therapeutic site of action. DPIs are not recommended for young children under five years of age.

Variable drug delivery associated with the use of DPIs can arise in several ways. These include inadvertently tilting the device so that the powder falls out, or exhaling through the device, thus blowing out the powder prior to inhalation.

Two of the most widely used DPI types are the Accuhaler (or Diskus) and Turbuhaler. The Accuhaler (see Fig. 16.4) utilizes individual doses of drug combined with lactose as a carrier, sealed in blisters on a medication disk. Each blister is pierced within the device just before inhalation. The Diskus delivers a fairly uniform drug dose with patient inspiratory flows between 30–90 L/min.[63] The Accuhaler is also a lower resistance device, so it may be easier for children to achieve the required inspiratory flows.

The Turbuhaler (see Fig. 16.4) is a reservoir device where the drug is stored in the form of spheronized, micronized particles, which do not require a carrier. The metered dose is dispensed from the reservoir into the dosing chamber at the base of the channel, through which the drug will be inhaled, by twisting the base of the device. As the drug is inhaled, the spheronized drug particles are broken up into smaller "respirable" particles, as they are pulled through the spiral disaggregation channels in the mouthpiece. The greater the PIF generated by the patient, the smaller the overall particle size range of the aerosol produced by the device.[64–66]

The output of this type of device is affected by many factors, which have also been studied in detail.[67,68] One important recommendation is that the peak inspiratory flow should be achieved by the patient as early as possible in the inspiratory maneuver, as this markedly reduces the particle size of the deaggregated drug, which is likely to increase the amount of drug reaching the lungs.[69]

Patients must be able to generate flows of at least 30 L/min while using the Turbuhaler to achieve a good clinical response[70] but flows of 60 L/min are considered optimal.[63] While it is a high resistance device, making it more difficult for patients to achieve the required flows, children greater than 6 years of age have been shown to be able to use it optimally with appropriate training.[71] Lung deposition does not appear to increase with flows greater than 60 L/min. Young children (younger than 5 or 6 years of age) are generally unable to use this device optimally since (a) their inhalation technique is not reliable (they may blow into the device rather than inhaling) and (b) they may not be able to consistently generate the required peak inspiratory flow. Infants are obviously unable to use this device.[72]

In adults, when used optimally, lung deposition using this device[18,19] is higher than that of other DPIs[33] and nebulizers,[73,74] and similar to optimal values using a spacer in conjunction with a pMDI.[75]

NEBULIZERS

Nebulizers can be used to deliver a wide range of drugs, in both solution and suspension formulation (i.e., a single nebulizer unit can be used to deliver multiple drugs). Metered dose inhalers (pressurized and dry powder), on the other hand, are specific for a drug-device combination and involve a high cost during the R&D phase and, in the postdevelopment phase, testing is required to obtain regulatory approval.

Hence, aerosolized drugs for diseases such as cystic fibrosis are most often delivered via nebulizer.

However, it is now recognized that because of the large variability in delivery from different nebulizer types, safety and efficacy testing (particularly of new drugs) needs to take into account the specific drug-nebulizer combination being used. For example, the product literature for Pulmozyme (dornase alpha) includes a list of recommended nebulizers, and specifies the compressors to be used with each of the recommended jet nebulizers.

Nebulizers may not be ideal devices to generate a therapeutically effective aerosol from a novel drug formulation. This could lead to overdosing or underdosing of the lung as nebulizer performance can vary widely when used to aerosolize a drug either not intended to be delivered in an aerosolized form, or designed to be used in a different nebulizer. Off-label use of drug and/or delivery devices with a failure to match the drug to the delivery device can lead to problems.

Drugs such as antibiotics (tobramycin) used in the treatment of *Pseudomonas spp.* lung infections have comparatively high MICs and the large volumes required to achieve a therapeutic concentration at the site of action preclude their use as a pMDI formulation. More potent drugs such as those used in the treatment of asthma require far less total dose; hence the widespread use of pMDI formulations for asthma. Thus nebulizers generating a "wet" aerosol are the device of choice for many drugs.[76]

Jet nebulizers have been used for many years for the treatment of respiratory disease (Fig. 16.6). Drug formulations for jet nebulizers are generally aqueous solutions, although some drugs are dispensed in the form of suspensions (corticosteroids) or viscous solutions (antibiotics). The simplest of the nebulizer designs is the T-piece jet nebulizer (Fig. 16.7). An aerosol is generated by passing air flow through a Venturi in the nebulizer bowl. This forms a low-pressure

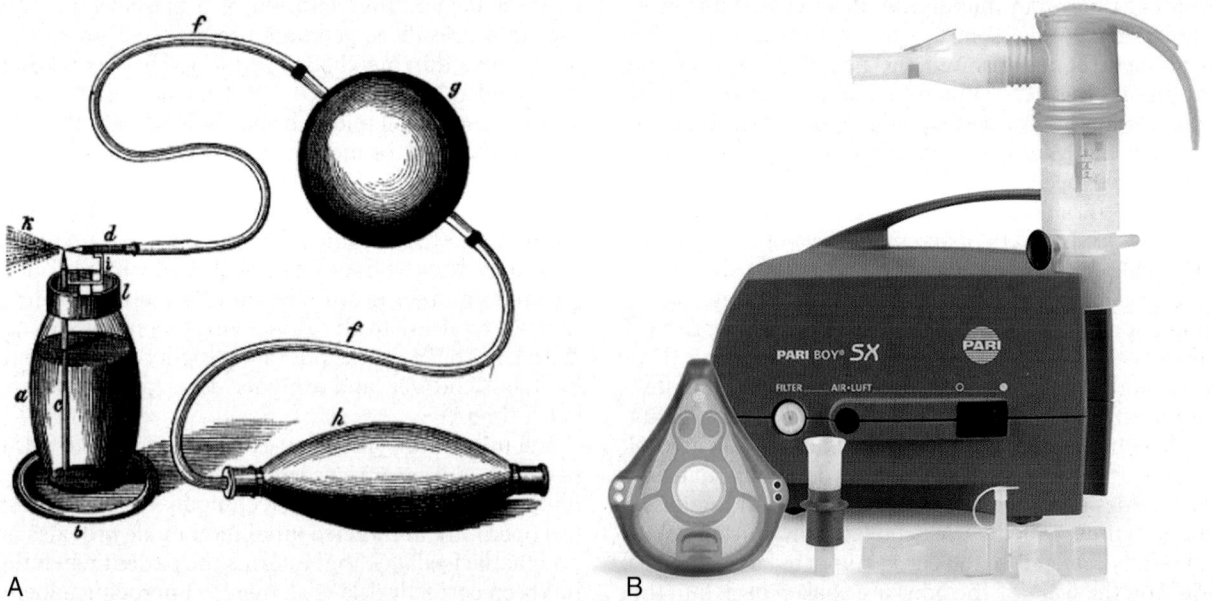

A   B

Fig. 16.6 Jet nebulizers old and new: An example of one of the very early jet nebulizers (A, Bergson's apparatus with the foot bellows) and an entrainment or breath-enhanced nebulizer and compressor currently in widespread use, the LC Sprint with the PARI Boy SX compressor (B). ([A] Reused from Beatson G. Practical papers on the materials of the antiseptic method of treatment, vol. III, on spray producers. In: Coats J, ed: History of the Origin and Progress of Spray Producers, Glasgow Medical Journal, edited for the West of Scotland Medical Association, July to December 1880, Vol. XIV. Glasgow: Alex and Macdougall, 1880, pp 461-484, 463. [B] From PARI Respiratory Equipment, Inc. https://www.pari.com/us-en/products/nebulizers/.)

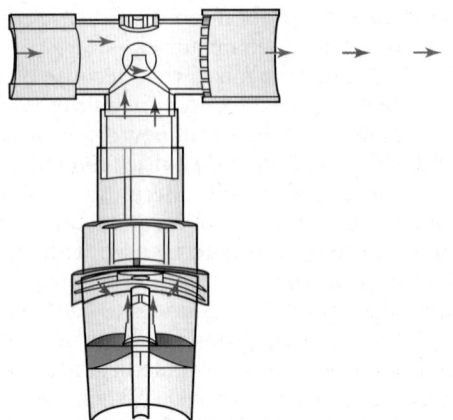

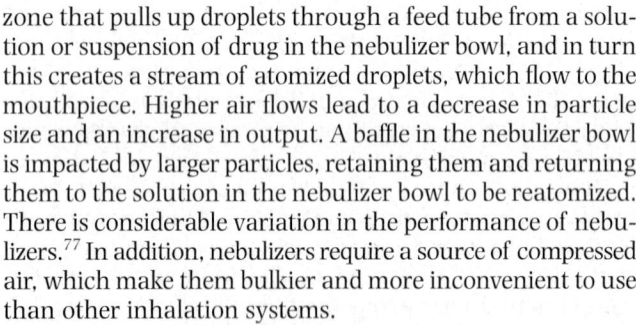

Fig. 16.7 A schematic of a T-piece jet nebulizer. Air under high pressure passes through a small hole as it expands, and the negative pressure generated sucks the drug solution or suspension up the feeding tube, where it is atomized. The atomized drug either impacts on the baffle, returns for renebulization, or leaves the nebulizer.

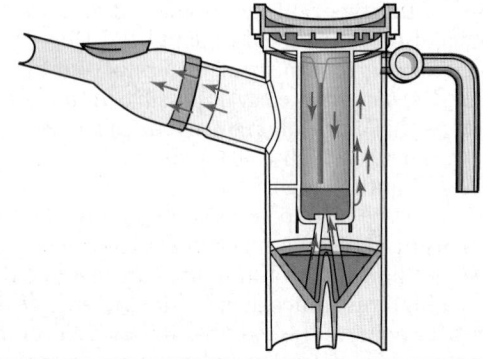

Fig. 16.8 A schematic of an entrainment or breath-enhanced nebulizer. A vent at the top of the nebulizer opens when the patient breathes in, thus allowing extra air to be entrained through the device. This extra air carries with it more aerosol than would normally have been deposited within the device and renebulized. Drug delivery is increased, as proportionately more drug is inhaled during inspiration than is lost during the expiratory phase when the valve at the top of the nebulizer closes.

zone that pulls up droplets through a feed tube from a solution or suspension of drug in the nebulizer bowl, and in turn this creates a stream of atomized droplets, which flow to the mouthpiece. Higher air flows lead to a decrease in particle size and an increase in output. A baffle in the nebulizer bowl is impacted by larger particles, retaining them and returning them to the solution in the nebulizer bowl to be reatomized. There is considerable variation in the performance of nebulizers.[77] In addition, nebulizers require a source of compressed air, which make them bulkier and more inconvenient to use than other inhalation systems.

Another solution to increase total drug delivery and improve deposition was the storage of aerosol generated during expiration in a holding chamber.[73,78,79] These solutions proved inconvenient for widespread use, increasing nebulization times and making the delivery systems even more bulky and cumbersome.

Entrainment of air through the nebulizer bowl as the patient inhales has been shown to increase aerosol output during inspiration.[80] The development of nebulizers utilizing this principle (entrainment or breath-enhanced nebulizers) (Fig. 16.8) have been shown to result in increased deposition.[81] These "entrainment" jet nebulizers are now commonly used for long-term delivery of aerosol medications for diseases such as cystic fibrosis (see Fig. 16.6). Fig. 16.9 shows the increase in colistin delivery resulting from the use of an entrainment nebulizer compared with a standard T-piece jet nebulizer.

The duration of nebulization ranges from 5 to 20 minutes, depending on the type of nebulizer and the volume of drug formulation in the nebulizer bowl.[82] Generation of an aerosol with a smaller particle size distribution is desirable, but using a nebulizer designed to do this can result in an increased nebulization time. Tapping the nebulizer bowl during nebulization results in increased total drug output as larger droplets deposited on the walls of the bowl are shaken back into the main volume of drug solution, but this also increases the nebulization times.[83] The "dead volume" of jet nebulizers containing the residual drug solution that cannot be nebulized also results in wastage of drug. Any evaporation of the solution in the nebulizer bowl during nebulization means

that the concentration of drug in the dead volume is higher than that in the aerosol generated.[83] If saline is used to dilute the nebulization solution, drug wastage can be reduced at the expense of increased nebulization times.

Children usually inhale the aerosols generated by these nebulizers using tidal breathing, although some reports suggest that deep inspirations, either with or without breath holding, would give better results.[84–86] Administration via a face mask that allows nasal inhalation, or a nasal mask, has been shown to greatly reduce lung deposition,[87] since the nose is much more efficient than the mouth in filtering out any particles with a diameter greater than 1 μm.

A further development in nebulizer technology is the vibrating mesh nebulizer, also now commonly used for long-term nebulizer therapy. These were developed in the early 2000s. In these devices the vibration of a piezoelectric crystal is not used directly to generate the aerosol, but rather used to vibrate a thin metal plate perforated by several thousand laser-drilled holes (Fig. 16.10). One side of the plate is in contact with the liquid to be aerosolized, and the vibration forces this liquid through the holes, generating a mist of tiny droplets. By altering the pore size of the mesh, the device can be tailored for use with drug solutions of different viscosities, and the output rate changed. Mesh nebulizers are powered either by mains electricity or by battery, are more portable than jet nebulizers, and they are silent in operation, in contrast to the rather noisy compressors used to drive jet nebulizers. Output rate is higher than that attained by a jet nebulizer, and a higher dose can be attained in a short time.[88]

Nebulizers can also be used to provide feedback to the patient to indicate when correct use has been achieved and to reinforce optimal inhalation technique. The I-neb (Respironics) operating in targeted inhalation mode provides audible and tactile feedback that informs the patient when the dose has been correctly delivered, thereby improving adherence.[89]

Refinements of standard jet and vibrating mesh nebulizers are aimed at both increasing lung deposition rates of drug, and reducing waste of the drug during expiration, as conventionally, the aerosol is continuously generated. This is important when treating children, as compliance with instructions on how to breathe can be reinforced by active feedback from the device being used. Breath activated nebulizers detect the patient's inspiratory flow and only release aerosol when the flow is sufficient to open a valve (AeroEclipse, Trudell Medical International, Ontario, Canada). Breath-controlled nebulizer compressors, such as the Akita (Activaero, Gemunden, Germany), monitor the child's breathing pattern and only generate aerosol during the phase of the respiratory cycle when inspiratory flows are conducive to drawing the aerosol into the lungs (Fig. 16.11). The duration of the inspiratory flow on triggering can be set, to encourage

slow and deep breathing by feedback from the device.[90] A refinement of this is adaptive aerosol delivery, where the device such as the I-neb (Respironics) "learns" the child's breathing pattern and tailors the release of the dose to match the individual breathing pattern.[91] These enhancements of the aerosol delivery process decrease the wastage of drug, which is increasingly important with expensive new peptide and recombinant protein drugs, as well as improving targeting of the inhaled drug to the site of action, by only introducing aerosol into the inhaled air flow when the flow rate is optimal to target the desired region of the lung region with the particle size being generated.

Ultrasonic nebulizers generate aerosols using the vibration of a piezoelectric crystal, which is transferred to the drug solution. The solution breaks up into droplets at the surface, and the resulting aerosol drawn out of the device by the patient's inhalation, or pushed out by an air flow through the device generated by a small compressor.[92] Ultrasonic nebulizers are not suitable for suspensions (corticosteroids) or viscous solutions (antibiotics) since very little drug is carried in the aerosolized particles,[80] and hence they have a more limited application than mesh nebulizers. Droplet sizes tend to be larger with ultrasonic nebulizers than with jet nebulizers.

Small volume liquid inhalers such as the Respimat (Boehringer Ingelheim, Ingelheim, Germany) are devices that use a spring to provide the energy to nebulize a small-metered volume of liquid, analogous to the metered dose produced by actuation of a pMDI. The energy in the spring is used to push a small volume of drug solution through a Venturi, generating a soft wet aerosol plume of about one second duration. The slow generation decreases the requirement for accurate coordination of actuation and inhalation, making it easier to use than a pMDI. Efficiency of drug delivery to the lungs is high, up to 40% of the nominal dose. However, the volume of liquid nebulized is only 15 µl, making it only suitable for drugs with high potency and low dosage mass.[93]

DEVICES FOR USE IN MECHANICALLY VENTILATED PATIENTS

Delivery of aerosols to patients who are mechanically ventilated presents numerous challenges. Many factors conspire

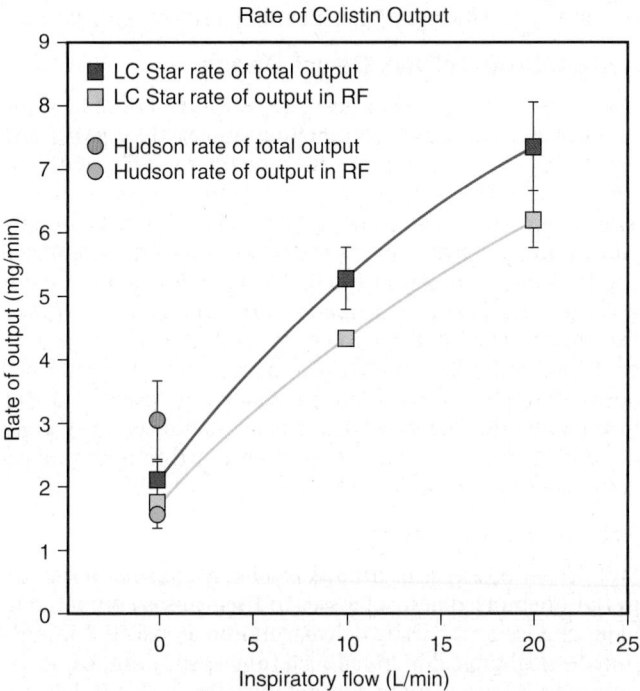

Fig. 16.9 The rate of output of colistin from an unvented (Hudson Updraft II) and a breath-enhanced (PARI LC Star) nebulizer in relation to entrained flow. The breath-enhanced nebulizer dramatically increases the rate of output (both total and that in the respirable fraction), whereas the inspiratory flow (entrained flow plus nebulizer driving flow) has no effect on the unvented nebulizer. *RF,* Respirable fraction. (Modified from Katz SL, Ho SL, Coates AL. Nebulizer choice for treatment of cystic fibrosis patients with inhaled colistin. *Chest.* 2001;119:250-255.)

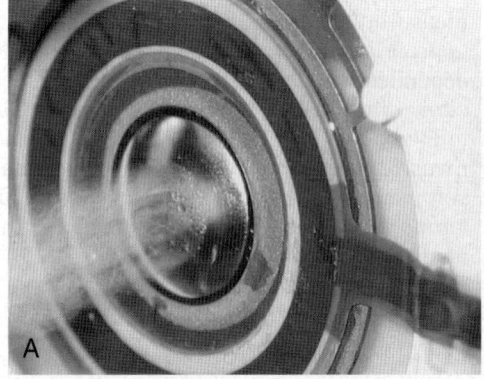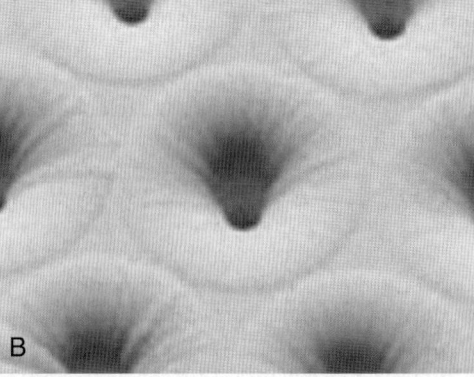

Fig. 16.10 Examples of the vibrating perforated-membrane technology used in mesh nebulizers. (A) The aerosol generator from a Pari eFlow device shows the aerosol being generated from the "mesh," which is driven by the surrounding piezo element. (B) A magnified view of a perforated membrane used in Aerogen nebulizers is shown.

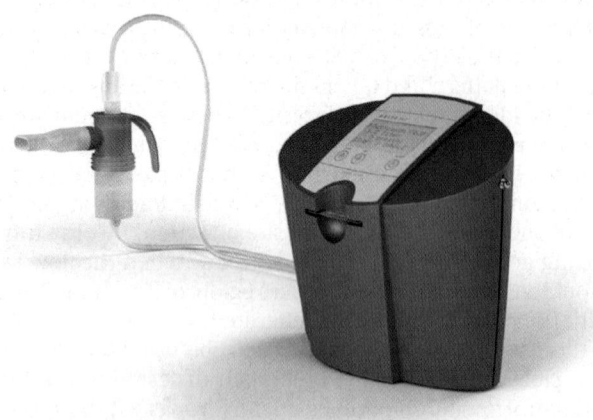

Fig. 16.11 The device is breath-actuated and it guides the patient to inhale with a pre-set inspiratory flow rate and inhalation time to ensure precise and targeted drug delivery to the child's lungs. (From Vectura plc Group, http://www.akita-jet.de/en/.)

to decrease the efficiency of drug delivery to mechanically ventilated patients, such as timing of actuation of the pMDI in relation to ventilator air flow, placement of the in-line adaptor or spacer in the circuit, heat and humidity of the air flow in the ventilator circuit, and density of the inhaled gas[94] A recent international survey of intensive care physicians concluded that optimal administration of aerosols generated by pMDIs or nebulizers was rare.[95] T-piece jet nebulizers often used to administer aerosolized drugs to noninvasively mechanically ventilated patients are notoriously inefficient and deliver less than 10% of the nominal dose to the lungs.[29,73,74] Reasons for this include large deadspace volumes and wastage of aerosol during expiration.[59,96] To overcome this problem, nebulizers were developed with interrupters[8,97] and dosimeters[80] so that aerosol is only generated during inspiration.

Invasively ventilated pediatric patients under anesthesia who suffer a bronchospasm during surgery require prompt administration of a bronchodilator. In-line pMDI actuators are often poorly designed, leading to breakage of the pMDI valve stem on actuation, and in-line spacers with too large a volume can take too long for adequate clearance by pediatric tidal breathing patterns. Often the route of administration of choice is to actuate a pMDI directly into the end of the endotracheal tube (ETT), but this requires breaking into the ventilator circuit and problems can occur due to changes in the design of the pMDI and actuator.[98] A nebulizer can be inserted into the circuit ready to be used if required.[99] Furthermore, drug can bind to the plastic of the ETT, leading to little or no drug reaching the lungs when an aerosol is delivered either via an in-line adaptor in the circuit, or by breaking into the circuit and administering drug directly into the connector. Many actuations of the pMDI are required to achieve bronchodilation, and the drug has to be administered during the ongoing surgical procedure. Devices such as the Microjet,[100] which generate the aerosol at the tip of the ETT, present a possible solution.

Dosage Considerations

CALCULATING DOSE

Despite large losses of emitted dose observed across devices, aerosol drug delivery remains the mainstay of respiratory care. Research and development continues to increase the efficiency of aerosol delivery systems. The early T-piece jet nebulizers delivered less than 10% of the drugs to the lungs. Lung deposition with current inhaler devices can be as high as 50%–60% when optimally used, even in children.[26,101] Improved drug deposition and dosage has resulted from a range of factors, including drug delivery device design and use of different formulations, including ratio of propellant.[102]

Aerosol Drug-Delivery Device Design

The oropharynx is the largest site of inhaled dose loss due to adsorption because of impaction observed for pMDI and DPIs. This can be as high as 80% of the total loss with the remaining 20% lost to mouthpieces and poor technique.[102] The addition of holding (spacer) devices and good technique can improve delivery by as much as 5%–10%. Nebulized drug delivery is mostly lost to the surrounding environment and therefore it requires a greater starting dose.[102] Few studies exist to compare all three major types of devices in order to create a standardized matrix to ensure equivalent prescribed doses. A single study comparing a starting dose of 5 mg of bronchodilator delivered using a jet nebulizer to 400 µg delivered via pMDI and DPI to severe asthmatics showed comparable increases in FEV1.[103]

Patient Considerations

Smaller air passages of infants is a likely cause of large (up to half) nebulized aerosol losses in their noses compared to older children.[29,104] Drug delivery in noncooperative infants may be negligible due to reduced time spent inhaling, or by maintaining inadequate contact with facemask or delivery device; demonstrating the importance of patient cooperation in efficient drug delivery.[9,59,67] For these reasons, it is also clear that smaller breath size is not the only cause of lower aerosol drug dosage. It is likely that infants and young children receive much the same dose from a given device, when size-corrected using either body weight, lung volume, or airway surface area.[105–108]

Estimating dose for children is not easy given size variation within age groups, and clinical responses are not a reliable measure that can be used in this age group to determine appropriate dose.[9,109,110] As noted before, delivery is highly dependent on device, highlighting consideration of device choice with respect to its use in a particular age group and individual capability. In particular, it is difficult to find noninvasive clinical measures or outcomes that can be used in very young children, and are sensitive enough to detect differences in therapeutic efficacy when comparing different devices or dosage regimes.[111]

MINIMIZING SYSTEMIC DOSE FROM INHALED DRUGS

Inhalation via the mouth to avoid nasal absorption of drugs[104] and avoiding swallowing for delivery systems with high oropharyngeal deposition will both minimize systemic absorption. Mouth washing can be also be used to help reduce ingestion of drugs from the oropharynx. This is especially important for drugs such as fluticasone where any swallowed drug is not likely to reach the systemic circulation; first pass metabolism to an inactive metabolite is almost complete.[112]

Advice and Training for Parents

ROLE OF THE CLINICIAN/THERAPIST

There are many inhalation devices currently available to be prescribed for use, and great variability in devices approved for use in different parts of the world. Well-developed national and local guidelines and training programs for health professionals are important in ensuring that patients are prescribed the best available devices and formulations for their ages and disease conditions, and trained adequately in their optimal use. Despite training, surveys have shown diverging practices between health care centers for using and testing efficacy for inhaled treatments.[113] This demonstrates the confusion that arises due to the lack of consistency concerning advice around inhaled treatment devices from trained therapists and prescribers.

ROLE OF THE PARENT

Lack of cooperation is to be expected in this young age group and poses the main problem to adequate aerosol delivery observed. While several techniques can be successfully used, the degree of success largely depends on the advice given to parent. Positive, understanding advice results in higher success rates, while a negative attitude on the part of the person giving advice can make failure a self-fulfilling prophecy. There is currently no reliable data on this important aspect of aerosol therapy; however, these issues may explain the relatively lower use of pMDI with spacers and higher use of nebulizers in some regions. Nebulizers are generally thought to be better tolerated by infants, but again, data in this area are sparse.

Progress Toward the Ideal Delivery System

Future research into providing an ideal delivery system for use in infants and young children could take several approaches. For pMDI-based systems, the development of low emission velocity breath-actuated devices designed for use at lower inspiratory flows and lung volumes would be more suited for use in younger children than the current commercial breath-actuated devices. The more recent use of low or antistatic plastics, and better-designed valves resulting in improved drug delivery from small volume spacers could possibly lead to the future development of smaller, single unit pMDI-spacer devices that are more portable and easier to use.

Dry powder systems are being developed to achieve better deaggregation of the powder into fine particles at low air flows to allow slow inhalation of the powder. The advent of engineered particles such as PulmoSpheres (Novartis), which are hollow porous particles with low surface energy, has led to the development of DPIs that achieve good lung penetration and deposition at low inspiratory flows, as the low density of the large particles make them behave in a similar manner to smaller, more dense particles in an air flow.[114-116] Nonbreath driven DPI systems, which do not require the patient to achieve a given optimal inspiratory flow for effective use of the device, are also being developed.

A device that produces a continuous aerosol of dry powder in an airstream analogous to a nebulizer has been developed to deliver surfactant to premature infants[117] and has achieved concentrations of aerosolized surfactant of up to 12 g/m^3 at a flow of 0.84 L/min and particles sizes of 3–3.5 μm. It is designed as a platform for the administration of many drugs that require high total therapeutic doses with slow delivery rates.

A recently developed device, the tPAD (**t**rans-Nasal **P**ulmonary **A**erosol **D**elivery), has been shown to be suitable for administration of extra fine aerosols via a cannula and nasal prongs over extended periods, up to 8 hours, at low flows. A comparable dosage of hypertonic saline to the lungs to that from a conventional jet nebulizer was achieved in healthy subjects.[118] The hands-free design makes it suitable for administration of drugs to children, who can continue activities while receiving their medication, or potentially while sleeping.

Intrapulmonary generation of aerosols is one potential method to avoid the problems of low inspiratory flow rates and small breath volumes leading to poor drug deposition in the lungs of small children and infants. A device known as the Microjet has been developed, where the aerosol is generated at or near to the target site, by intrapulmonary aerosolization within an endotracheal tube.[100] This instrument is designed to administer aerosolized surfactant to infants with respiratory distress syndrome.

References

Access the reference list online at ExpertConsult.com.

Suggested Reading

Dal Negro RW. Dry powder inhalers and the right things to remember: a concept review. *Multidiscip Respir Med.* 2015;10(1):13.

Everard ML. Role of inhaler competence and contrivance in "difficult asthma. *Paediatr Respir Rev.* 2003;4(2):135–142.

Everard ML. Regimen and device compliance: key factors in determining therapeutic outcomes. *J Aerosol Med.* 2006;19(1):67–73.

Goralski JL, Davis SD. Breathing easier: addressing the challenges of aerosolizing medications to infants and preschoolers. *Respir Med.* 2014; 108(8):1069–1074.

Laube BL, Janssens HM, de Jongh FH, et al. What the pulmonary specialist should know about the new inhalation therapies. *Eur Respir J.* 2011; 37(6):1308–1331.

Roche N, Dekhuijzen PN. The evolution of pressurized metered-dose inhalers from early to modern devices. *J Aerosol Med Pulm Drug Deliv.* 2016; 29(4):311–327.

17 Physical Therapies in Pediatric Respiratory Disease

SARAH WRIGHT, Grad Dip Phys, RUTH WAKEMAN, MSc, BSc (Hons), NICOLA COLLINS, BSc (Hons), and MICHELLE CHATWIN, BSc (Hons), PhD

Pediatric cardiorespiratory physical therapy (physiotherapy) management spans the spectrum of care from specialist advice to nonpharmacologic interventions for patients with a variety of respiratory conditions. Physiotherapists are an essential part of the multidisciplinary team and physiotherapy is administered from birth to the time of transition to adult services across the continuum of care settings. To provide optimal care, the therapist will clearly identify the indicators for intervention and balance these against the possible risks. Physiotherapy is not a prescribed procedure; the frequency and dosage of therapy is continually adapted and modified in response to identified outcomes and targeted goals.[1,2]

Treating children can be difficult, and the physiotherapist must be responsive to individual needs and have the technical and nontechnical knowledge, skills and attributes to meet these challenges.

General Principles of Physiotherapy

Physiotherapy often focuses on treating or alleviating generic problems that are amenable to intervention rather than being disease-specific (Fig. 17.1). In some instances, however, interventions are selected based upon the underlying disease process (e.g., primary ciliary dyskinesia [PCD] versus cystic fibrosis [CF]), whereby the elements of the mucociliary escalator affected by the disease process may differ (predominantly ciliary dysfunction versus altered sputum rheology). The pediatric respiratory physiotherapist/therapist will perform a wide variety of roles. The professionals and their training vary internationally. In the United Kingdom, physiotherapists are able to treat patients without a referral from a medical doctor and are therefore independent practitioners. Prior to pediatric physiotherapy, informed consent from caregivers and age-appropriate assent from the child are obtained.

The respiratory physiotherapist/therapist needs physiologic knowledge and practical skills to perform a competent respiratory assessment of the child. From this assessment, problems responsive to physiotherapy are identified and treatment strategies are recommended and implemented. Physiotherapists may also assess the reaction to inhaled pharmacologic agents (e.g., bronchodilator response and nebulized antimicrobial bronchoconstriction trials; Chapter 16), provide education in inhaler and nebulizer techniques, and advise on the optimal timing of inhaled medications with respect to sessions of respiratory physiotherapy. They can also assess

the need for home oxygen therapy by performing exercise testing with oximetry.[3] Physiotherapists may also help to identify potential causes of respiratory problems (e.g., gastroesophageal reflux [GER] during airway clearance). These issues can then be escalated to be reevaluated by the medical team. If it is felt that pulmonary secretions are a result of aspiration secondary to uncoordinated swallowing, a speech and language assessment is warranted (see section "Aerodigestive Disease").

The timing of physiotherapy treatments can be important; for example, airway clearance should be timed before feeds or delayed for a sufficient time after feeds to avoid vomiting and aspiration. Likewise, physiotherapy should be timed around analgesia when clinically necessary.

Role of Physiotherapy in Pediatric Respiratory Disease

Physical therapies are essential in the removal of excess bronchopulmonary secretions and maintaining and improving exercise capacity. Physical therapy can support ventilation using high-flow nasal cannulas (HFNCs), continuous positive airway pressure (CPAP) or noninvasive ventilation (NIV). Physical therapy should include postural education where appropriate; it can be used to prevent, correct, or improve postural problems, such as kyphosis in CF patients (Fig. 17.2). Postural education can also be helpful in musculoskeletal dysfunction, in children with contractures that inhibit function, or in children with pain that limits range of motion, mobility, and ability to breathe normally. Poor posture leads to tightening of the respiratory muscles, which can lead to chest wall deformity and contribute to a decline in pulmonary function. It is therefore essential that patients with chronic lung disease have a postural assessment and treatment of any musculoskeletal disorders identified, including core muscle imbalance.

Specifically in neuromuscular disease (NMD), physical therapy is essential to maintain ambulation or facilitate standing, where possible, to improve lung function. Optimizing the maturing musculoskeletal and neuromuscular systems of a child with CF may play an important role in the long-term outcome of the child's mental and physical state.[4] It is essential to ask children with chronic lung disease about urinary and fecal incontinence in a private and empathetic setting; reluctance to cough may stem from fear of incontinence. Physical therapies should be directed toward managing this problem.[5,6]

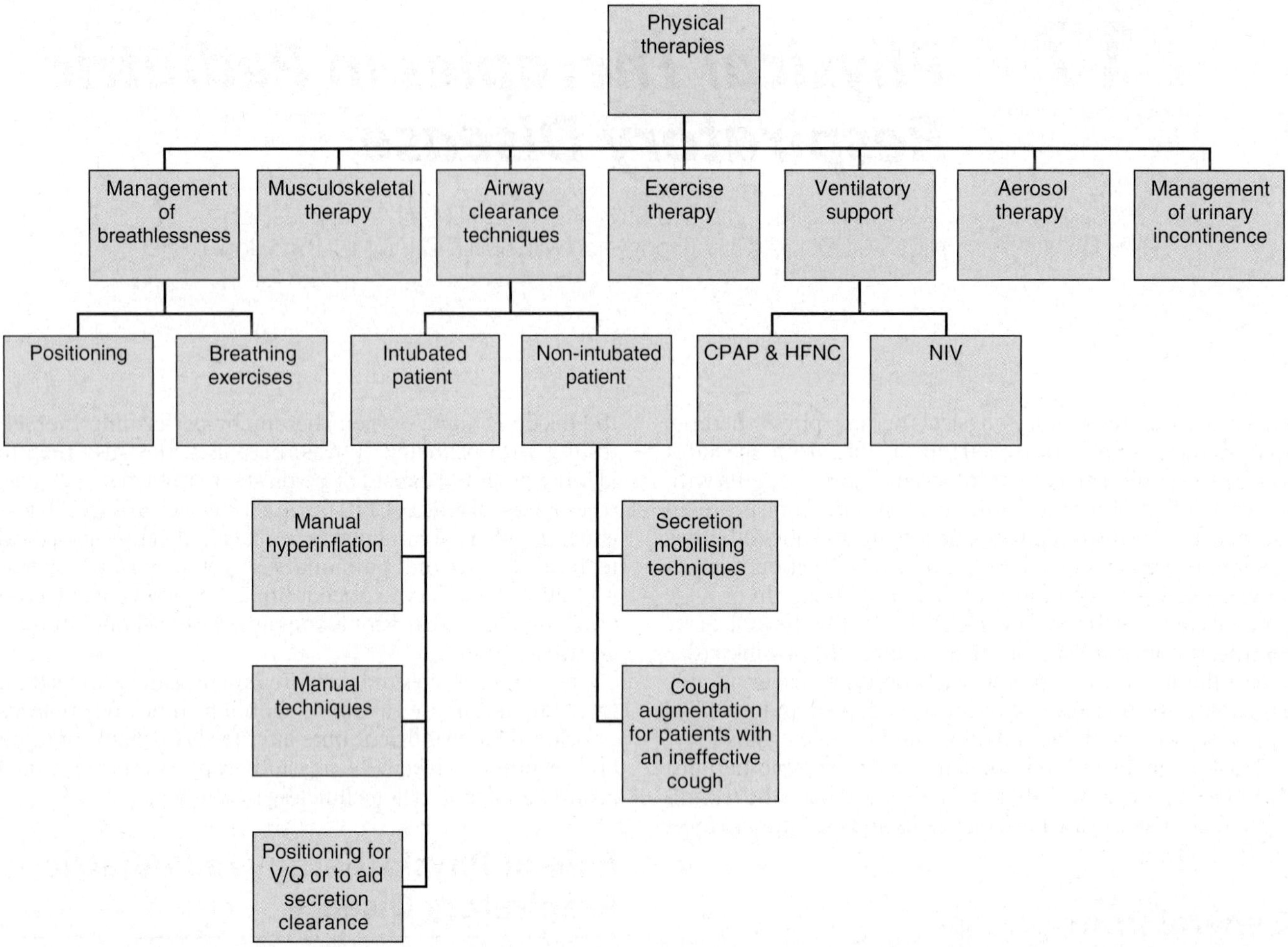

```
                              ┌──────────────┐
                              │   Physical   │
                              │  therapies   │
                              └──────┬───────┘
```

| Management of breathlessness | Musculoskeletal therapy | Airway clearance techniques | Exercise therapy | Ventilatory support | Aerosol therapy | Management of urinary incontinence |

| Positioning | Breathing exercises | | Intubated patient | Non-intubated patient | | CPAP & HFNC | NIV | | | |

| Manual hyperinflation | | Secretion mobilising techniques |

| Manual techniques | | Cough augmentation for patients with an ineffective cough |

| Positioning for V/Q or to aid secretion clearance |

Fig. 17.1 The physical therapies that can be offered to a child with respiratory disease are shown. *CPAP,* Continuous positive airway pressure; *NIV,* noninvasive ventilation; *V/Q,* ventilation perfusion.

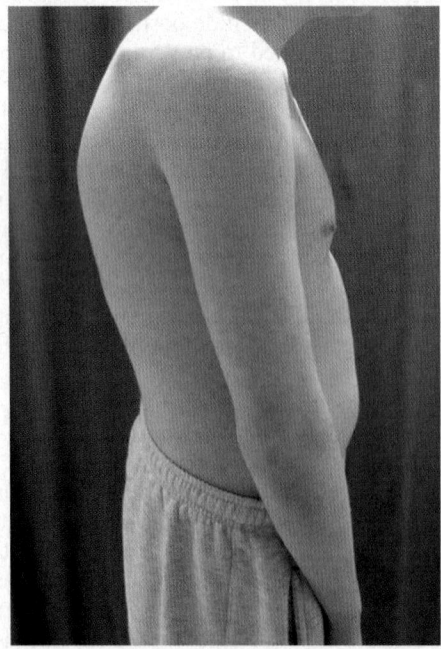

Fig. 17.2 The onset of kyphosis in a male patient with cystic fibrosis.

Respiratory Physiotherapy in Specific Conditions

CYSTIC FIBROSIS AND NONCYSTIC FIBROSIS BRONCHIECTASIS (INCLUDING PRIMARY CILIARY DYSKINESIA)

Airway Clearance

Treatment options for airway clearance depend on the child's age and ability to participate in treatment. There is a wide variety of airway clearance techniques (ACTs; Figs. 17.3–17.5). There is no single best technique, so the therapist should not assume that the findings all apply to non-CF bronchiectasis.[2,7–12]

The technique should be tailored to the individual, and choice is dependent on efficacy, simplicity of use, and cost.[1,2] A good starting point is with the technique that is simplest to use and that impinges least on the patient's life.[13] The term *airway clearance* describes a number of different treatment modalities that aim to enhance the clearance of bronchopulmonary secretions.[14] Through clinical reasoning, the therapist decides the aim of treatment and how to address

Text continued on p. 279

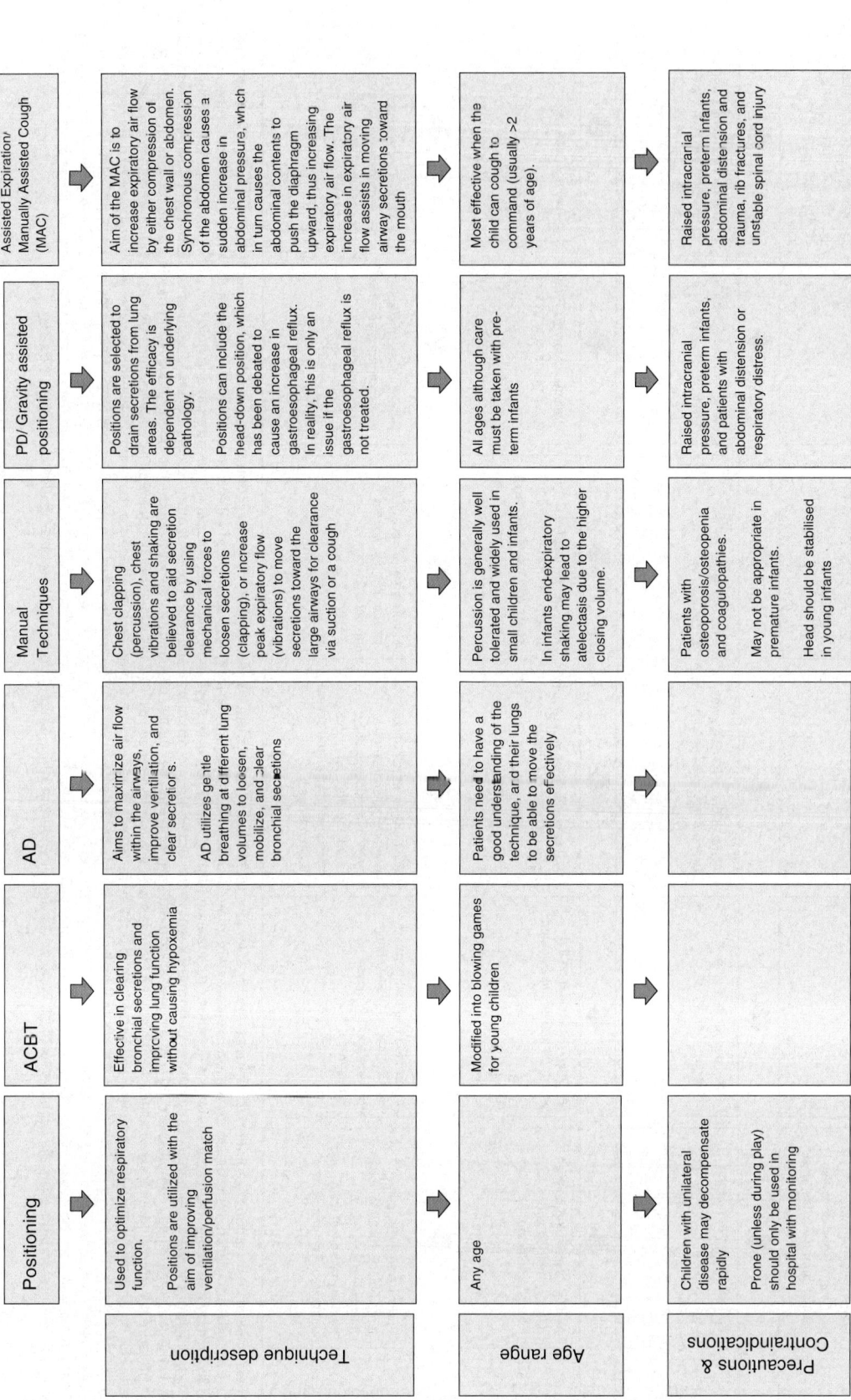

	Positioning	ACBT	AD	Manual Techniques	PD/Gravity assisted positioning	Assisted Expiration/Manually Assisted Cough (MAC)
Technique description	Used to optimize respiratory function. Positions are utilized with the aim of improving ventilation/perfusion match	Effective in clearing bronchial secretions and improving lung function without causing hypoxemia	Aims to maximize air flow within the airways, improve ventilation, and clear secretions. AD utilizes gentle breathing at different lung volumes to loosen, mobilize, and clear bronchial secretions	Chest clapping (percussion), chest vibrations and shaking are believed to aid secretion clearance by using mechanical forces to loosen secretions (clapping), or increase peak expiratory flow (vibrations) to move secretions toward the large airways for clearance via suction or a cough	Positions are selected to drain secretions from lung areas. The efficacy is dependent on underlying pathology. Positions can include the head-down position, which has been debated to cause an increase in gastroesophageal reflux. In reality, this is only an issue if the gastroesophageal reflux is not treated.	Aim of the MAC is to increase expiratory air flow by either compression of the chest wall or abdomen. Synchronous compression of the abdomen causes a sudden increase in abdominal pressure, which in turn causes the abdominal contents to push the diaphragm upward, thus increasing expiratory air flow. The increase in expiratory air flow assists in moving airway secretions toward the mouth
Age range	Any age	Modified into blowing games for young children	Patients need to have a good understanding of the technique, and their lungs to be able to move the secretions effectively	Percussion is generally well tolerated and widely used in small children and infants. In infants end-expiratory shaking may lead to atelectasis due to the higher closing volume.	All ages although care must be taken with preterm infants.	Most effective when the child can cough to command (usually >2 years of age).
Precautions & Contraindications	Children with unilateral disease may decompensate rapidly. Prone (unless during play) should only be used in hospital with monitoring			Patients with osteoporosis/osteopenia and coagulopathies. May not be appropriate in premature infants. Head should be stabilised in young infants	Raised intracranial pressure, preterm infants, and patients with abdominal distension or respiratory distress.	Raised intracranial pressure, preterm infants, abdominal distension and trauma, rib fractures, and unstable spinal cord injury

Fig. 17.3 Airway clearance techniques requiring no equipment. Active cycle of breathing techniques: The technique consists of (1) breathing control (BC), which is a resting period of gentle relaxed breathing at the patient's own rate and depth; (2) thoracic expansion exercises, which are 3–5 deep breaths emphasizing inspiration; and (3) forced expiration technique (or "huff"), which combines 1–2 forced expirations followed by a period of BC. The technique is flexible and can be performed in any position. Autogenic drainage (AD): The patient breathes in and holds his or her breath for 2–4 seconds (the hold facilitates equal filling of the lung segments). Expiration is performed keeping the upper airways open (as if sighing). The expiratory force is balanced so that the expiratory flow reaches the highest rate possible without causing airway compression. This cycle is repeated at different lung volumes while collecting secretions from the peripheral airways and moving them toward the mouth. Intermittent positive pressure breathing: Makes include Alpha 200 (Air Liquide Medical Systems, France), NiPPY Clearway (B&D Electromedical, Warwickshire, United Kingdom). Positive expiratory pressure (PEP): Usually PEP consists of a mask with a one-way valve to which expiratory resistance is added. A manometer is inserted into the circuit between the valve and resistance to monitor the pressure, which should be 10–20 cm H₂O during midexpiration. The child usually sits with his or her elbows on a table and breathes through the mask for 6–10 breaths with a slightly active expiration. Makes include PEP Mask (Astratech, Stonehouse, Gloucestershire, United Kingdom), TheraPEP (Smiths Medical, Watford, United Kingdom), Pari PEP (PARI GmbH, Germany). Oscillatory PEP: Positions during use may vary slightly depending on the device type. Often patients will perform 4–8 deep breaths followed by a forced expiration. Makes include the Flutter device (Clement Clarke International Limited, Harlow, Essex, United Kingdom), the Acapella (Henleys Medical, Welwyn Garden City, Hertfordshire, United Kingdom), Aerobika (Trudell Medical Int, Canada). Mechanical in-sufflation/exsufflation (MI-E): The weaker the child the higher the requirement will be for high insufflation and exsufflation pressures. In children, an insufflation time of less than 1 second is required for equilibration of insuf-flation pressure and alveolar pressure. Longer exsufflation times do not significantly alter expiratory flows. Higher insufflation and exsufflation pressures both increase expiratory flows, but greater exsufflation pressure had more substantial impact on expiratory flows (not) Cough Assist (Philips Respironics, Andover, Massachusetts) NiPPY Clearway, Pegaso (Dimla-Italia, Bologna, Italy; HFCWO—Makes include Vest (Hill-Rom, St Paul, Minnesota) or Smart Vest (Electromed, New Prague, Minnesota); Intrapulmonary percussive ventilation—Makes include IMPULSATOR—F00012, IPV1C—F00001-C, IPV2C—F00002-C. (Percussionaire Corporation, United States of America), IMP II (Breas, Sweden), Metaneb (Hill-ROM St. Paul, Minnesota). Manual hyperinflation: Patients receive normal tidal volumes coupled with an increased tidal volume using a 500-mL infant bag (or a 1-L bag for older children). A manometer is applied to the circuit to monitor pressures. As a general guide, manual hyperinflation ventila-tion pressures should not exceed 10 cm H₂O above the ventilator pressure. Flow rates of gas should be adjusted according to the child: 4 L/min for infants, increasing to 8 L/min for children. (From Striegl AM, Redding GJ, Diblasi R, Crotwell D, Salyer J, Carter ER. Use of a lung model to assess mechanical in-exsufflator therapy in infants with tracheostomy. *Pediatr Pulmonol*. 2011;46(3):211–217.)

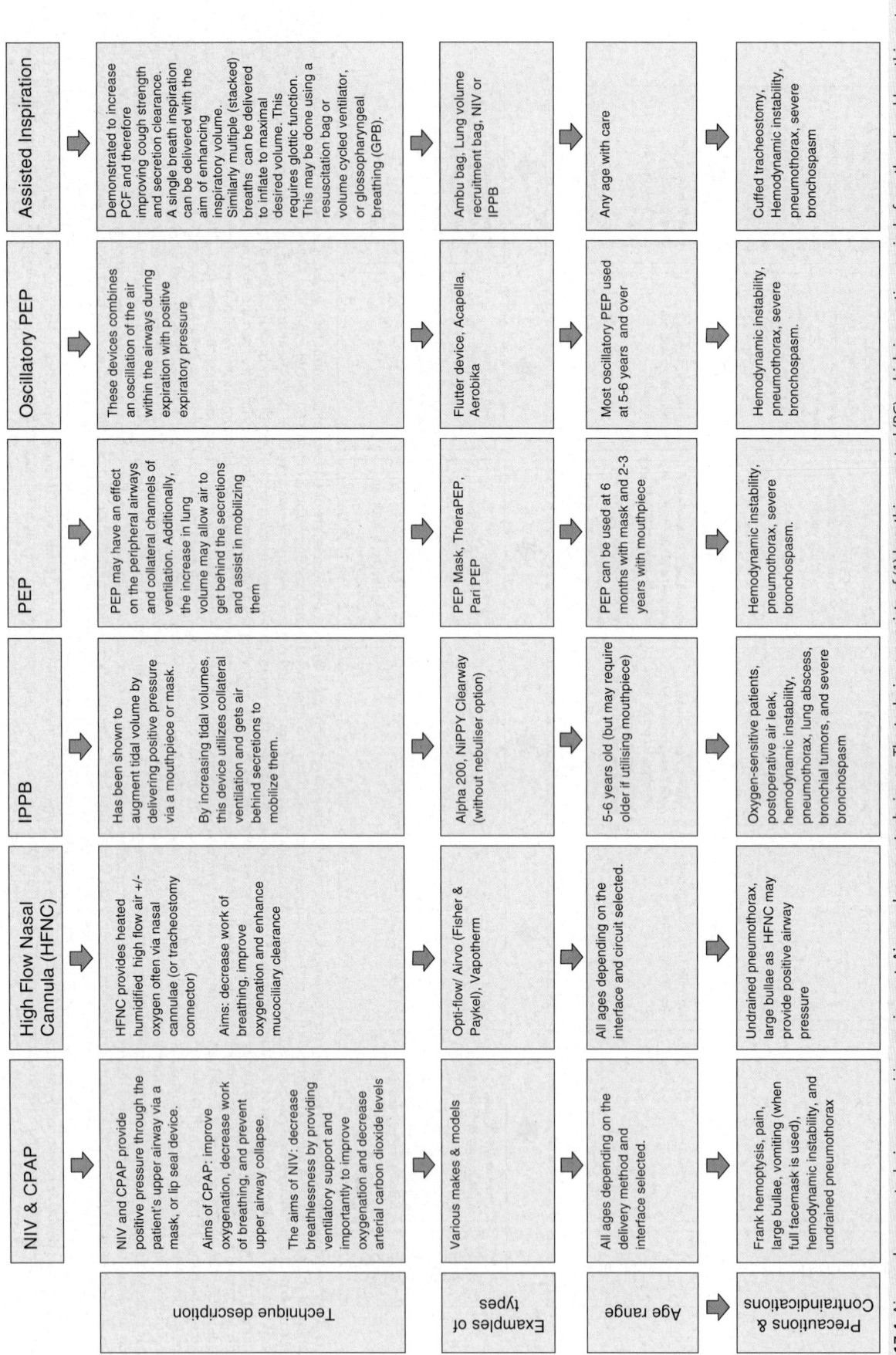

Fig. 17.4 Airway clearance techniques requiring equipment. Airway clearance techniques: The technique consists of ((1) breathing control (BC), which is a resting period of gentle relaxed breathing at the patient's own rate and depth; (2) thoracic expansion exercises, which are 3–5 deep breaths emphasizing inspiration; and (3) forced expiration technique (or "huff"), which combines 1–2 forced expirations followed by a period of BC. The technique is flexible and can be performed in any position; Autogenic drainage: The patient breathes in and holds his or her breath for 2–4 seconds (the hold facilitates equal filling of the lung segments). Expiration is performed keeping the upper airways open (as if sighing). The expiratory force is balanced, so that the expiratory flow reaches the highest rate possible without causing airway compression. This cycle is repeated at different lung volumes while collecting secretions from the peripheral airways and moving them toward the mouth. Intermittent positive pressure breathing (IPPB): Makes include Alpha 200 (Air Liquide Medical Systems, France), NiPPY Clearway (B&D Electromedical, Warwickshire, United Kingdom); Positive expiratory pressure (PEP)—Usually PEP consists of a mask with a one-way valve to which expiratory resistance is added. A manometer is inserted into the circuit between the valve and resistance to monitor the pressure, which should be 10–20 cm H_2O during midexpiration. The child usually sits with his or her elbows on a table and breathes through the mask for 6–10 breaths with a slightly active expiration. Positions during use may vary slightly depending on the device type. Often patients will perform 4–8 deep breaths followed by a forced expiration. Makes include PEP Mask (Astratech, Stonehouse, Gloucestershire, United Kingdom); TheraPEP (Smiths Medical, Watford, United Kingdom), Pari PEP (PARI GmbH, Germany); Oscillatory PEP. Positions during use may vary slightly depending on the device type. Makes include the Flutter device (Clement Clarke International Limited, Harlow, Essex, United Kingdom), the Acapella (Henleys Medical, Welwyn Garden City, Hertfordshire, United Kingdom), Aerobika (Trudell Medical Int, Canada).

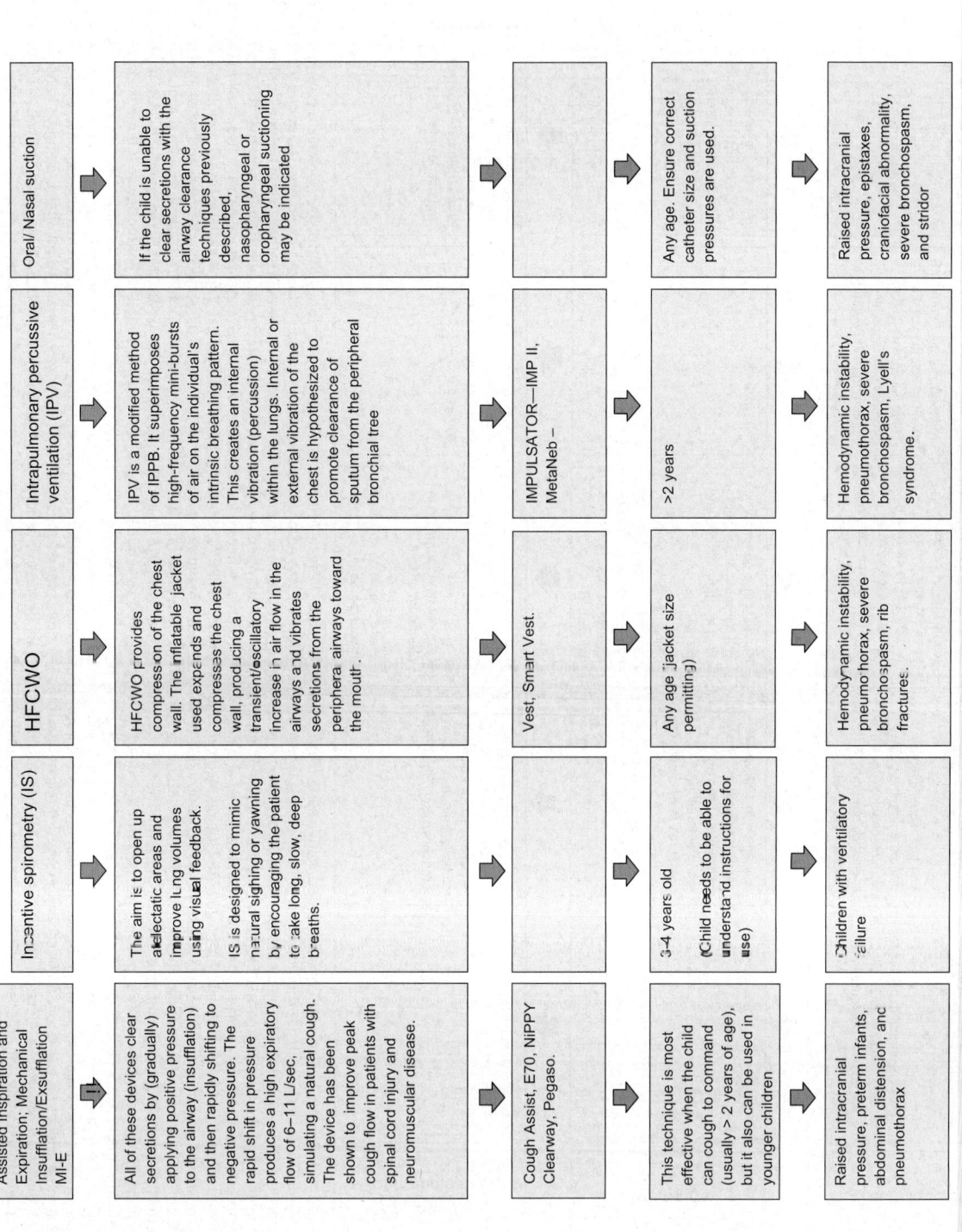

Fig. 17.4, cont'd Mechanical insufflation/exsufflation (MI-E): The weaker the child the higher the requirement will be for high insufflation and exsufflation pressures. In children, an insufflation time of more than 1 second is required for equilibration of insufflation pressure and alveolar pressure. Longer exsufflation times do not significantly alter expiratory flows. Higher insufflation and exsufflation pressures both increase expiratory flows, but greater exsufflation pressure had more substantial impact on expiratory flows (1) Cough Assist (Philips Respironics, Andover, Massachusetts) NiPPY Clearway, Pegaso (Dimla-Italia, Bologna, Italy); High frequency chest wall oscillation—Makes include Vest (Hill-Rom, St Paul, Minnesota) or Smart Vest (Electromed, New Prague, Minnesota); Intrapulmonary percussive ventilation (IPV)—Makes include IMPULSATOR—F00012, IPV1C—F00001-C, IPV2C—F00002-C. (Percussionaire Corporation, United States of America). IMP II (Breas, Sweden), Vietaneb (Hill-ROM St. Paul, Minnesota). Manual hyperinflation—Patients receive normal tidal volumes coupled with an increased tidal volume using a 500 mL infant bag (or a 1-L bag for older children). A manometer is applied to the circuit to monitor pressures. As a general guide, manual hyperinflation ventilation pressures should not exceed 10 cm H₂O above the ventilator pressure. Flow rates of gas should be adjusted according to the child: 4 L/min for infants, increasing to 8 L/min for children. *CPAP,* Continuous positive airway pressure; *HFCWO,* high frequency chest wall oscillation; *NI-V,* noninvasive ventilation. (From Striegl AM, Redding GJ, Diblasi R, Crotwell D, Salyer J, Carter ER. Use of a lung model to assess mechanical in-exsufflator therapy in infants with tracheostomy. *Pediatr Pulmonol.* 2011;46(3):211-217.)

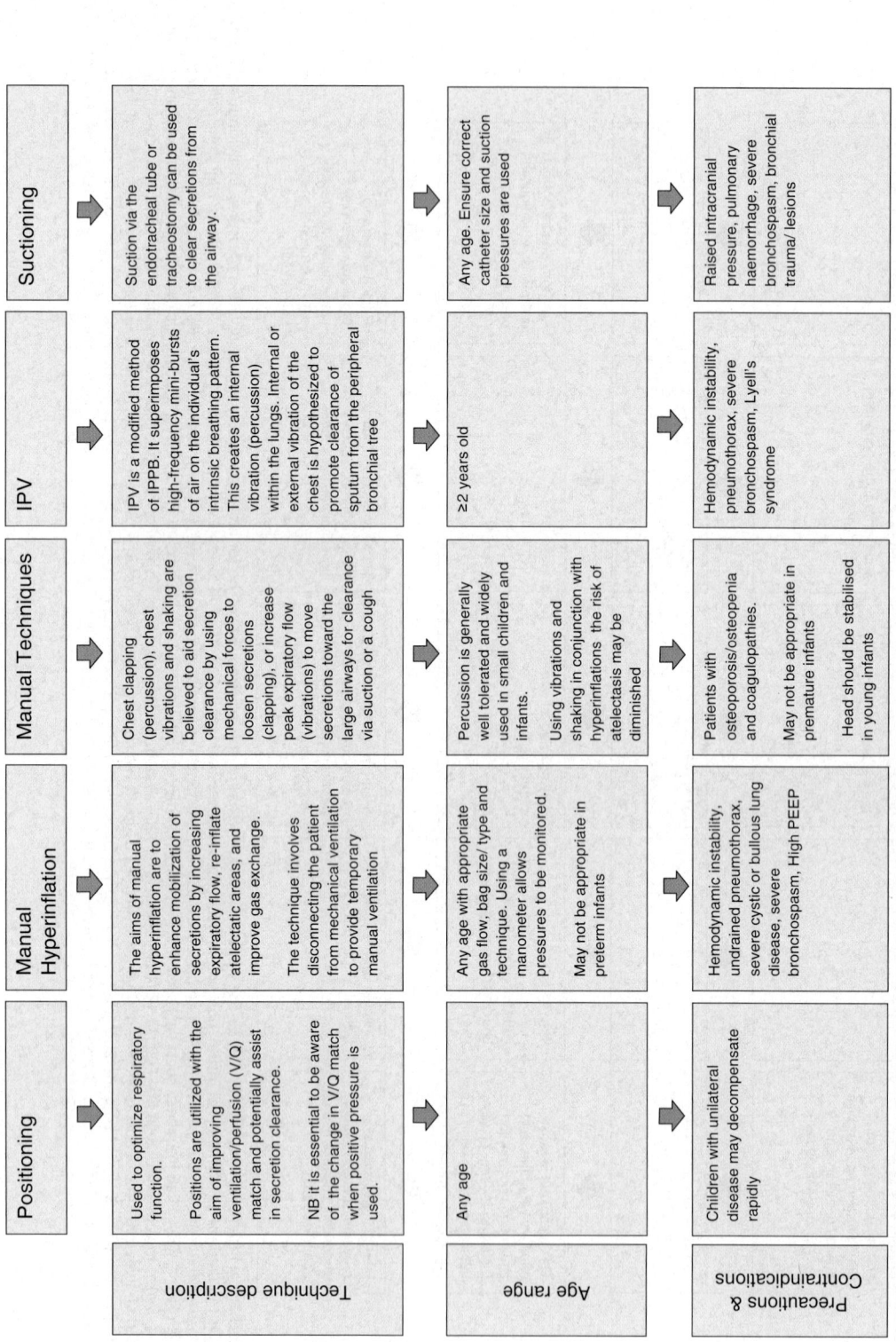

Fig. 17.5 Airway clearance techniques when the patient is intubated. Active cycle of breathing techniques: The technique consists of (1) breathing control (BC), which is a resting period of gentle relaxed breathing at the patient's own rate and depth; (2) thoracic expansion exercises, which are 3–5 deep breaths emphasizing inspiration; and (3) forced expiration technique (or "huff"), which combines 1–2 forced expirations followed by a period of BC. The technique is flexible and can be performed in any position. Autogenic drainage: The patient breathes in and holds his or her breath for 2–4 seconds (the hold facilitates equal filling of the lung segments). Expiration is performed keeping the upper airways open (as if sighing). The expiratory force is balanced so that the expiratory flow reaches the highest rate possible without causing airway compression. This cycle is repeated at different lung volumes while collecting secretions from the peripheral airways and moving them toward the mouth. Intermittent positive pressure breathing: Makes include Alpha 200 (Air Liquide Medical Systems, France), NiPPY Clearway (B&D Electromedical, Warwickshire, United Kingdom). Positive expiratory pressure (PEP): Usually PEP consists of a mask with a one-way valve to which expiratory resistance is added. A manometer is inserted into the circuit between the valve and resistance to monitor the pressure, which should be 10–20 cm H₂O during midexpiration. The child usually sits with his or her elbows on a table and breathes through the mask for 6–10 breaths with a slightly active expiration. Makes include PEP Mask (Astratech, Stonehouse, Gloucestershire, United Kingdom), TheraPEP (Smiths Medical, Watford, United Kingdom), Pari PEP (PARI GmbH, Germany). Oscillatory PEP: Positions during use may vary slightly depending on the device type. Often patients will perform 4–8 deep breaths followed by a forced expiration. Makes include the Flutter device (Clement Clarke International Limited, Harlow, Essex, United Kingdom), the Acapella (Henleys Medical, Welwyn Garden City, Hertfordshire, United Kingdom), Aerobika (Trudell Medical Int, Canada). Mechanical insufflation/exsufflation: The weaker the child the higher the requirement will be for high insufflation and exsufflation pressures. In children, an insufflation time of less than 1 second is required for equilibration of insufflation pressure and alveolar pressure. Longer exsufflation times do not significantly alter expiratory flows. Higher insufflation and exsufflation pressures both increase expiratory flows, but greater exsufflation pressure had more substantial impact on expiratory flows (1) Cough Assist (Philips Respironics, Andover, Massachusetts) NiPPY Clearway, Pegaso (Dimla-Italia, Bologna, Italy); HFCWO—Makes include Vest (Hill-Rom, St Paul, Minnesota) or Smart Vest (Electromed, New Prague, Minnesota); Intrapulmonary percussive ventilation—Makes include IMPULSATOR—F00012,IPV1C—F00001-C, IPV2C—F00002-C. (Percussionaire Corporation, United States of America), IMP II (Breas, Sweden), Metaneb (Hill-ROM St. Paul, Minnesota). Manual hyperinflation: Patients receive normal tidal volumes coupled with an increased tidal volume using a 500-mL infant bag (or a 1-L bag for older children). A manometer is applied to the circuit to monitor pressures. As a general guide, manual hyperinflation ventilation pressures should not exceed 10 cm H₂O above the ventilator pressure. Flow rates of gas should be adjusted according to the child: 4 L/min for infants, increasing to 8 L/min for children. *IPV*, Intrapulmonary percussive ventilation; *V/Q*, ventilation perfusion. (From Striegl AM, Redding GJ, Diblasi R, Crotwell D, Salyer J, Carter ER. Use of a lung model to assess mechanical in-exsufflator therapy in infants with tracheostomy. *Pediatr Pulmonol.* 2011;46(3):211-217.)

the specific issue (or issues). Lannefors and colleagues clearly identified the following four stages of airway clearance; they are the cornerstones to decision making.[15]

1. To get air behind mucus so as to open up the airways
2. To loosen/unstick the secretions from the small airways (Video 17.1)
3. To mobilize the secretions through the smaller airways to the larger airways
4. To clear the secretions from the central airways

The age and adherence of the individual and caregivers as well as disease severity will affect the modalities introduced and in what combination. In the infant, manual techniques[16] (Figs. 17.6–17.8), positioning,[17] infant positive expiratory pressure (PEP[18]; Fig. 17.9), and assisted autogenic drainage (AAD)[19] are used. PEP and AAD focus on enhancing changes in air flow and ensuring the move from "passive" techniques to a more dynamic approach. The use of movement is encouraged from an early age, as it is not only more effective but also more realistic in the younger age group (Video 17.2).

As the child grows older and can become an active participant in therapy, the emphasis will change. The therapist can incorporate techniques that augment volume and introduce the concept of a change in expiratory flow; in many cases, this is a forced expiration.[20] Forced expiration or "huffing" is integral to many techniques and utilizes the theory of the equal pressure point to move mucus to the larger airways.[21] It is also a valuable assessment tool for children, as chest palpation during a "huff" can often be abnormal, with crackles being palpable, even when there are no abnormalities on auscultation. In young children, forced expiration will start as blowing games and then become a more formal component of ACT.

With the child's increasing ability to participate, the active cycle of breathing techniques (ACBT[17,22]; Fig. 17.10) can be taught and may be used in postural drainage (PD) positions (see Figs. 17.3–17.5). Physiotherapy may consist of modified PD targeting the area of lung affected or rotating through different areas to ensure that the lung fields are clear.[16] Other techniques such as autogenic drainage (AD; Fig. 17.11) also can be considered.[23] In addition, many adjuncts are available, with PEP (Figs. 17.12 and 17.13)[24] or oscillatory PEP (Figs. 17.14 and 17.15)[25,26] commonly used to facilitate clearance and to help move the child toward independence if appropriate. PEP has been shown to reduce exacerbations significantly more than other ACTs.[12] However, different

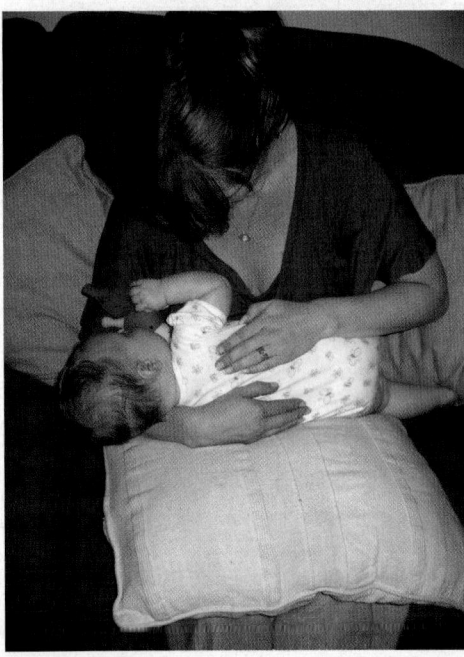

Fig. 17.7 Infant with cystic fibrosis in side-lying position for physiotherapy.

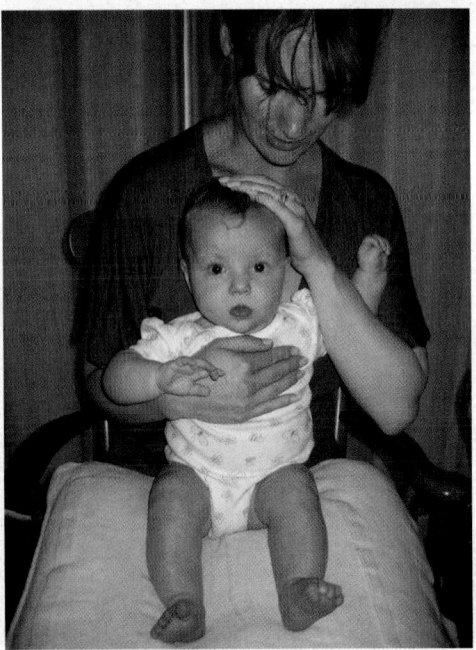

Fig. 17.6 Percussion to the anterior chest for an infant with cystic fibrosis.

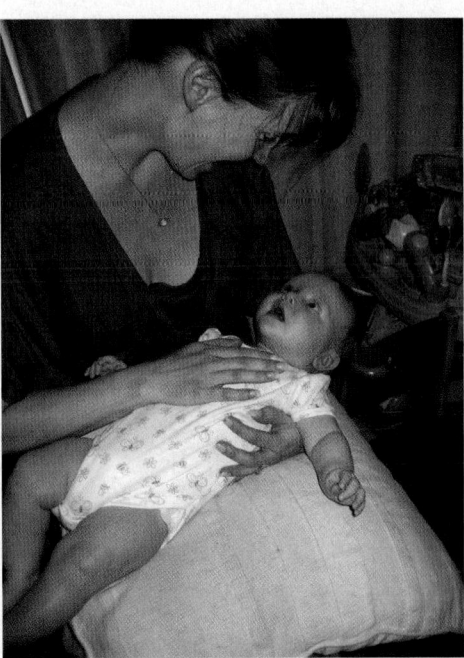

Fig. 17.8 Infant with cystic fibrosis in supine position for physiotherapy.

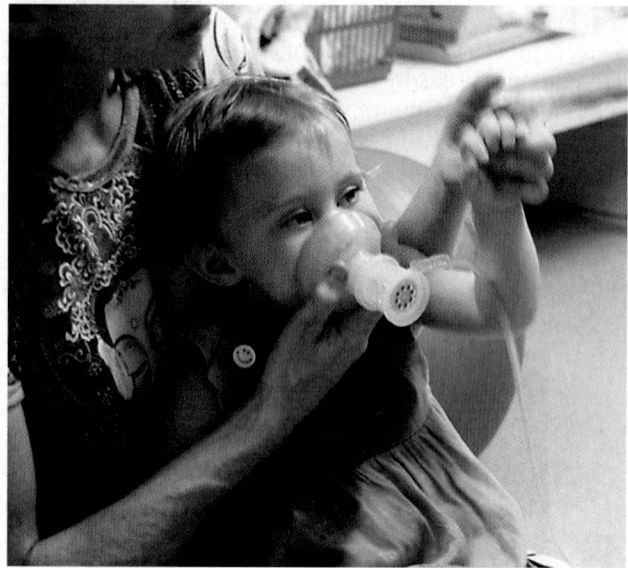

Fig. 17.9 Toddler with cystic fibrosis using mask positive expiratory pressure.

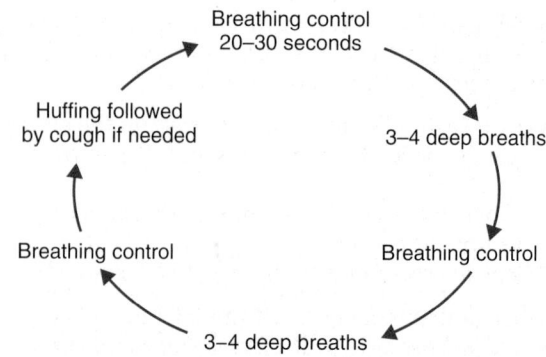

Fig. 17.10 Active cycle of breathing technique.

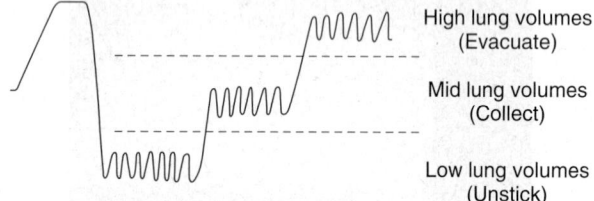

Fig. 17.11 Lung volumes for autogenic drainage.

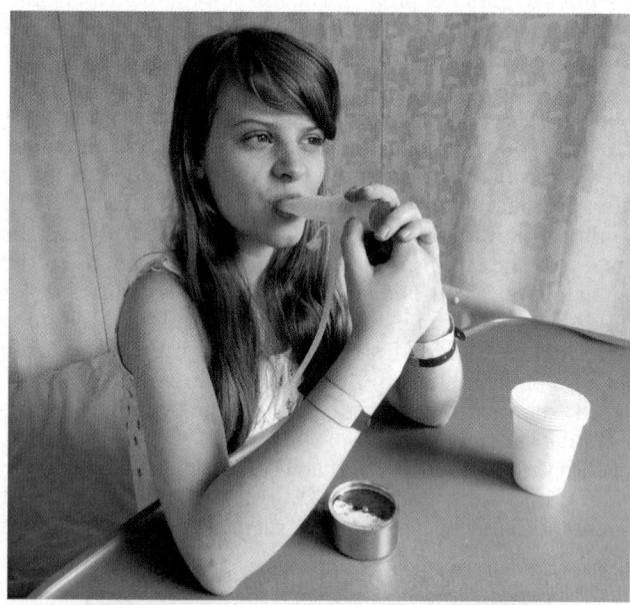

Fig. 17.12 Girl with cystic fibrosis using PEP (*Pari PEP* [PARI GmbH, Germany]) via a mouthpiece. *PEP,* Positive expiratory pressure.

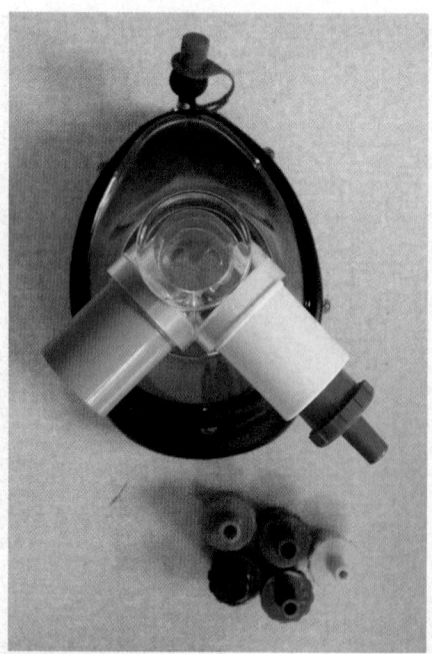

Fig. 17.13 Mask positive expiratory pressure—Astra PEP (Astratech, Stonehouse, UK).

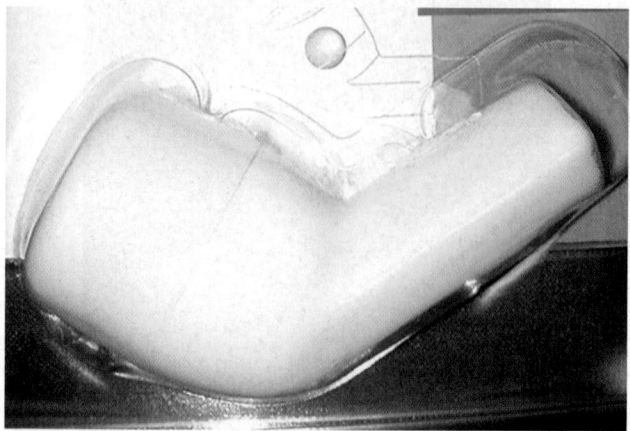

Fig. 17.14 Oscillatory positive expiratory pressure—Flutter (Clement Clark International, UK).

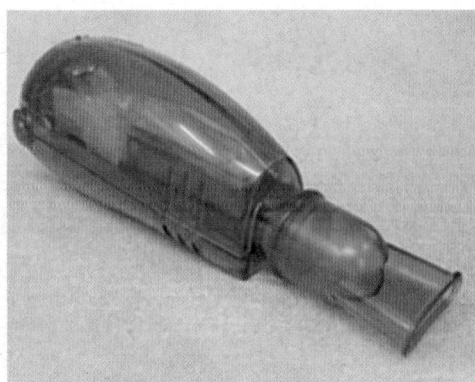

Fig. 17.15 Oscillatory positive expiratory pressure—Acapella.

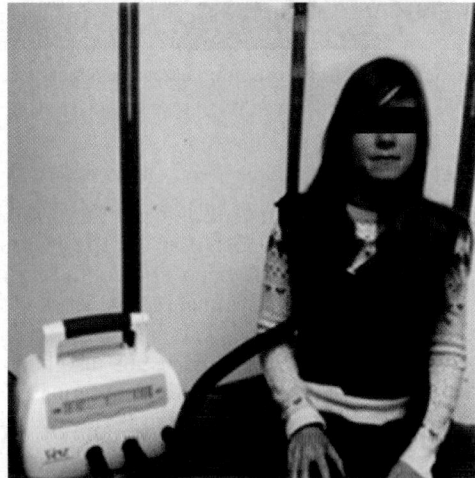

Fig. 17.16 High-frequency chest wall oscillation.

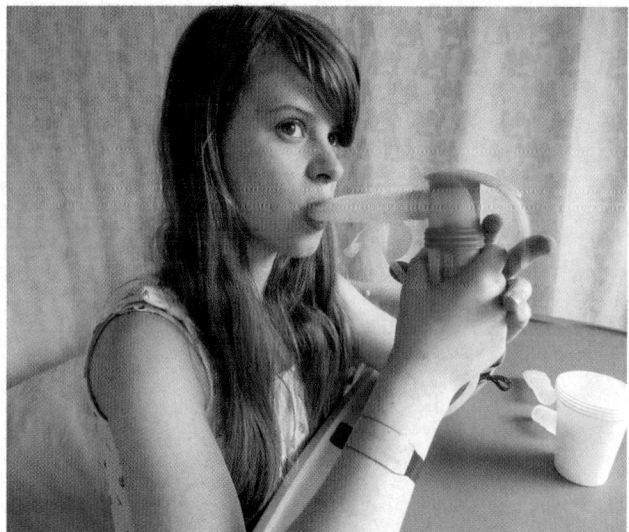

Fig. 17.17 Girl with cystic fibrosis using positive expiratory pressure in combination with nebulized hypertonic saline.

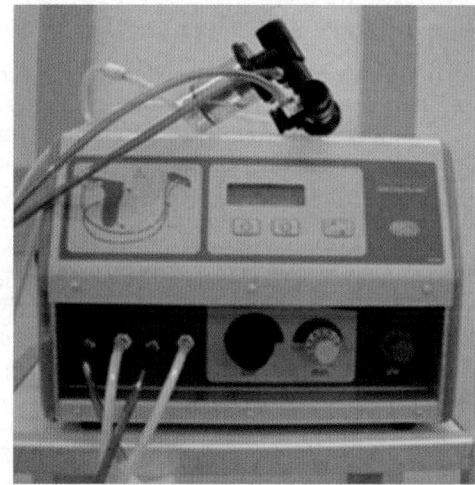

Fig. 17.18 Intrapulmonary percussive ventilation.

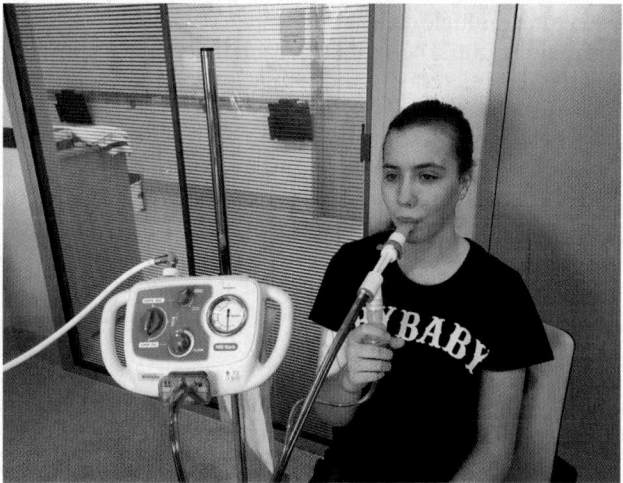

Fig. 17.19 The MetaNeb® System (Hill-ROM, St. Paul, Minnesota).

physiotherapy techniques and devices may be more or less effective at varying times (e.g., stable state and during an exacerbation) and in different individuals. CF registry data from 2011 found that oscillating PEP and "huffing" were the most commonly used techniques in the United Kingdom and that PD and high-frequency chest wall oscillation (HFCWO; Fig. 17.16) were the least common.[27] Several of these adjuncts can be used in combination with inhaled medications (e.g., hypertonic saline; Fig. 17.17) or in conjunction with exercise.

HFCWO (see Figs. 17.3–17.5) is widely used across North America. Although evidence indicates that it may be less effective than other therapies,[28,29] including one study showing significantly greater pulmonary exacerbations in patients using HFCWO compared with PEP,[30] it can still be considered for specific individuals or used in combination with other ACTs. One other device that may be of benefit is intrapulmonary percussive ventilation (IPV; Fig. 17.18 and 17.19). Previous studies have investigated sputum mobilization in CF patients by comparing the use of IPV to other modes of airway clearance (e.g., PD and percussion, HFCWO, and oscillatory PEP).[31–33] These studies have shown IPV to be as effective as the other methods of airway clearance in sputum mobilization.

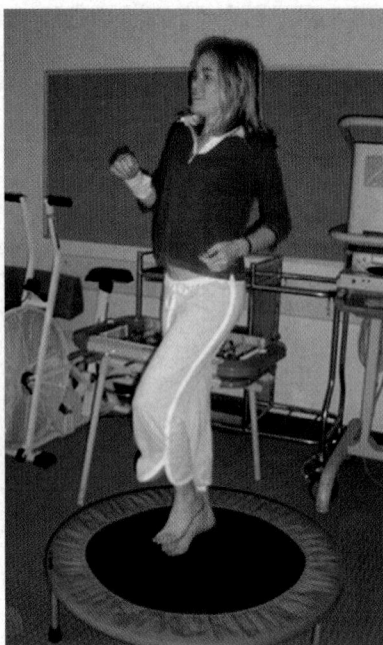

Fig. 17.20 Teenager with cystic fibrosis exercising on a "trampet."

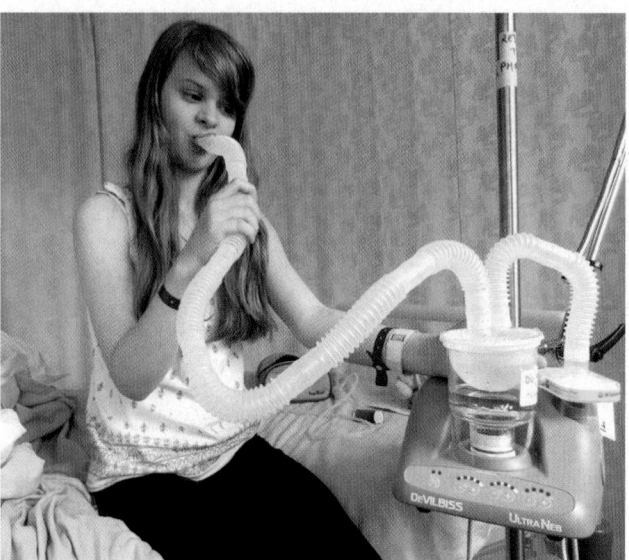

Fig. 17.21 Girl with cystic fibrosis using ultrasonic nebulizer for saline inhalation.

Exercise has many benefits for people with CF and bronchiectasis: improving cardiovascular fitness, bone mineral density, and quality of life (Fig. 17.20). In CF it has been shown to slow the rate of pulmonary function decline[34] and may increase survival independent of FEV_1.[35] Exercise has also been shown to have an additive effect on sputum production, and it improves oxygen saturation in adolescents and adults with CF when used before airway clearance.[36] In fact, Dwyer and coworkers[37] have shown that exercising on a treadmill increases expiratory air flow and moves sputum from peripheral lung regions, but this must be combined with "huffing" to be an effective method of airway clearance.

Regular review of ACT is advised to ensure continuing effectiveness and adherence with therapy; appropriate adjustments to treatment can be made as necessary.[38,39] It is vital to monitor adherence, as, for example, poor adherence in bronchiectasis has been shown to affect important health outcomes including pulmonary exacerbations.[40] The most effective technique may not be the optimal strategy for the individual; multiple contributing factors must be considered. The regimen must be specific to each individual's changing needs and preferences, and as patients grow older, their understanding of the need for the treatment and of its goals must be clear. ACTs have been shown to have short-term effects on mucus transport, but the long-term effects are less clear.[41] There is debate worldwide regarding the introduction of ACT prior to diagnosis of bronchiectasis. There is consensus on the symptomatic patient, where response to treatment is evident; however, there is less agreement on the asymptomatic patient.[14] Chest physiotherapy does not have to be routinely performed unless the underlying diagnosis affects the normal mechanisms of airway clearance. In CF, there is evidence that inflammation, infection, abnormal lung function and ventilation inhomogeneity are present early in life.[42] In addition, for CF or PCD, it seems unethical to wait for airway damage to occur, as the child will thus never have normal mucociliary clearance.[43]

Ventilatory Support

As the disease progresses, use of devices that provide some inspiratory ventilatory support may be the treatment of choice. The use of NIV has been shown to significantly improve ease of sputum clearance, reduce work of breathing,[44] facilitate inspiration and correct respiratory failure; it is widely used in the adult setting. It has also been shown to significantly increase FEV_1 and reduce fatigue in CF adults hospitalized with an acute exacerbation.[45] However, a review of its use in CF children[46] demonstrated a need for more evidence and protocols to identify indications for this age group.

Inhalation Therapies

Effective treatment in this group of patients might have to be supported by inhaled therapies (Fig. 17.21) such as bronchodilators; mucoactive agents such as hypertonic saline, dry powder mannitol (Bronchitol, licensed for over 6 years in Australia and 18 years in Europe) and deoxyribonuclease (RhDNase); antimicrobials, and, where indicated, oxygen therapy.[47–49] The timing of inhalation therapy around airway clearance is important (Fig. 17.22). For example, bronchodilators and mucokinetics should be given before or during ACT to prepare the airways.[50] RhDNase can be administered before (minimum 30 minutes) or after ACT to suit the individual, although in children with well-preserved lung function FEF_{25} was improved if RhDNase was given prior to ACT.[51] If RhDNase is given before ACT, it should be a longer time interval than immediately before ACT; in children it may be given before bed.[52] Antimicrobials and inhaled steroids should be administered following ACT.

Complications and Implications for Physical Therapy

The relationship between ACT (particularly gravity-assisted positions) and GER remains unclear.[53,54] Physiotherapists must be aware of the possible risks with treatment and modify their therapies accordingly; thus the decision should not be

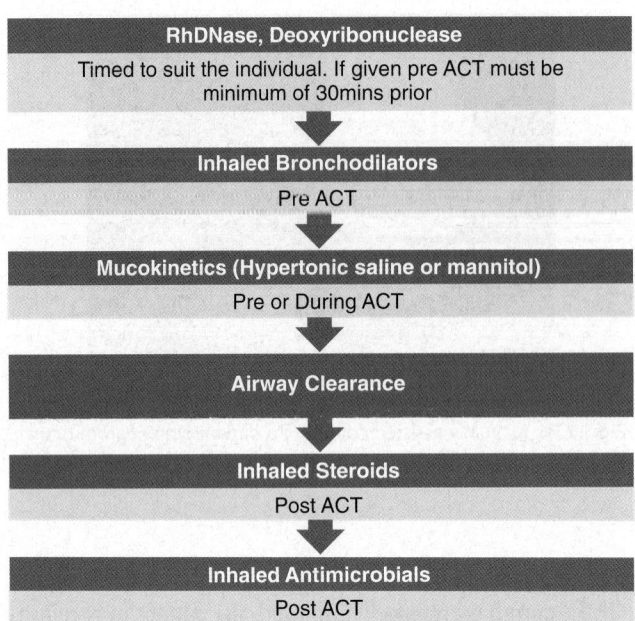

Fig. 17.22 The timing of inhaled therapies around physiotherapy. The algorithm is individualized to the patient and will not necessarily take all of the inhaled therapies listed. *ACT,* Airway clearance technique.

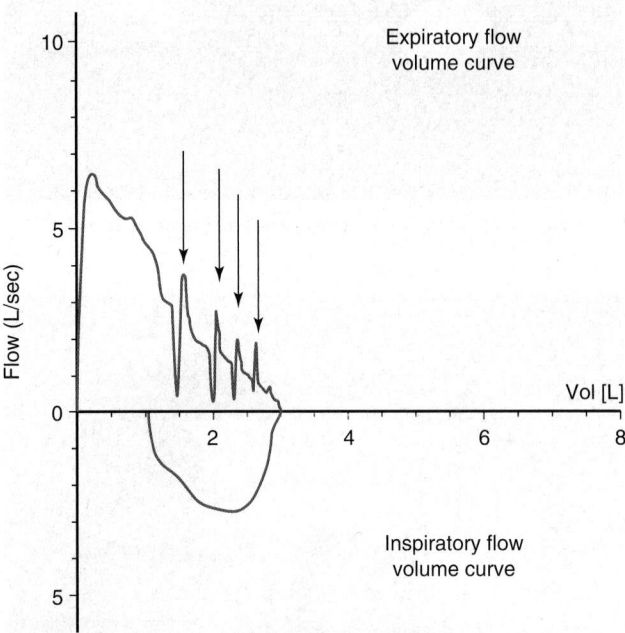

Fig. 17.23 A series of cough spikes is superimposed on the maximal expiratory flow. Cough flow spikes are highlighted *(arrows)*.

on whether gravity will induce reflux but whether it is necessary to tip at all. Few therapists would tip a 4-week-old asymptomatic CF infant, but in a 1-year-old child with PCD that is at risk of developing acute large airway mucus impaction and lobar changes, PD may well form part of the treatment.

As mentioned, the impact of musculoskeletal issues including posture, incontinence,[55] and pain should be assessed and managed appropriately, including limiting muscle imbalance and strength training to improve the mechanics of breathing and overall well-being.[56] In addition, with the increasing longevity of patients and comorbidities such as diabetes, osteopenia will have to be considered by the therapist and management modified responsively. Often the combination of treatments can be beneficial; for example, ACT using PEP while the patient is on a therapy ball, utilizing core muscle strengthening can provide enhancements as well as reduce treatment time.

RESPIRATORY MUSCLE WEAKNESS

Neuromuscular Disease

The ability to clear bronchopulmonary secretions is essential to prevent sputum retention and associated complications, including lower respiratory tract infection. An effective cough is a vital mechanism to protect against respiratory tract infections, which are the commonest causes of hospital admission in patients with respiratory muscle weakness from NMD.[57] An intact afferent and efferent pathway is required for an effective cough. Reduced airway sensation will fail to elicit a cough in response to a noxious stimulus. Diseases of the nerves (upper or lower motor neuron), neuromuscular junction, or muscles may impair the efferent pathway.

The act of coughing involves the following three main components[58]:

1. Deep inspiration up to 85%–90% of total lung capacity
2. Glottic closure, which requires intact bulbar function so a rapid closure of the glottis occurs for approximately 0.2 seconds
3. Effective contraction of the expiratory muscles (abdominal and intercostal) to generate intrapleural pressures of more than 190 cm H_2O.

If one or more of these three components is impaired, the cough will be less effective[59] and the individual may be unable to produce the transient flow spikes essential for an effective cough (Fig. 17.23).[60] Cough strength can be measured by peak cough flow (PCF). PCF is the result of an explosive decompression that generates a flow rate as high as 360–944 L/min in children older than 12 years of age.[61] It is important not to quote adult PCF threshold values for children younger than 12 years of age and to use the appropriate quartile reference value.[61] Physical therapies involve the assessment of cough efficacy by formally evaluating the inspiratory, glottic and expiratory components of the cough along with audibility and measuring PCF with a peak flow meter attached to a face mask.

Poponick and coworkers[62] demonstrated that acute viral illness was associated with a reduction in vital capacity (VC) due to reduced inspiratory and expiratory respiratory muscle strength (by 10%–15% of baseline values). This reduction in

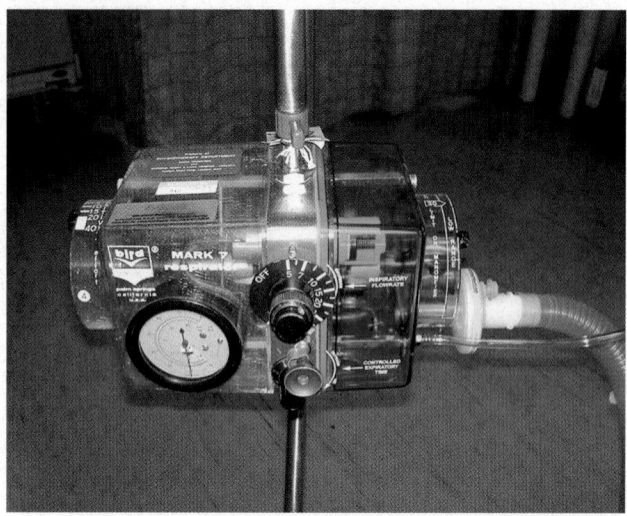

Fig. 17.24 Intermittent positive pressure breathing device.

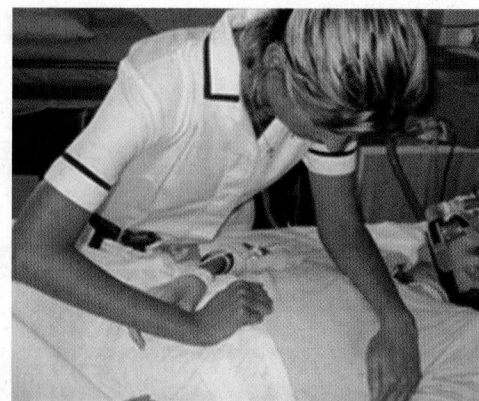

Fig. 17.26 Manually assisted cough for a patient with neuromuscular disease.

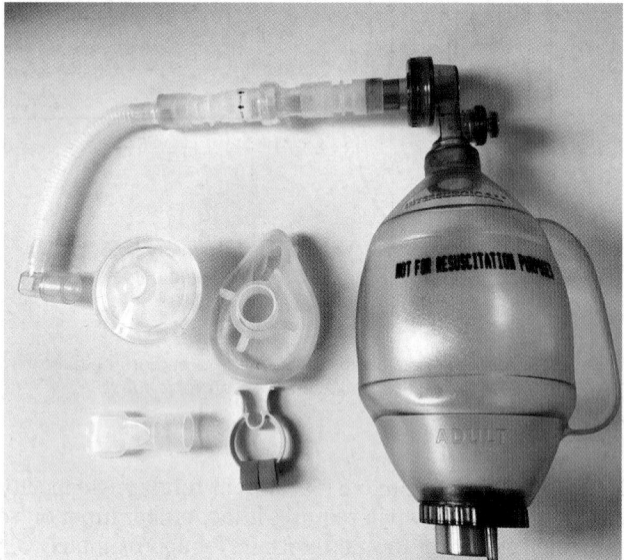

Fig. 17.25 Lung volume recruitment bag (Intersurgical, Wokingham, England, UK) for the use in assisted inspirations.

inspiratory and expiratory muscle strength will also cause a decline in PCF, possibly to the critical level where the child is unable to clear secretions alone or with his or her normal assisted cough technique. Assisted cough techniques should be targeted to whichever component of the cough is reduced and may consist of assisted inspiration: single breaths (inspiration with expiration between) given with an Ambu bag or an intermittent positive pressure breathing (IPPB) device (Fig. 17.24).[63] They may also consist of stacked breaths (no breath out between inspirations) performed with an Ambu bag (Fig. 17.25), a lung volume recruitment bag, volume-cycled NIV,[64] or glossopharyngeal breathing (GPB).[65] Assisted cough techniques may also be applied during expiration, as with a manually assisted cough (Fig. 17.26; see also Figs. 17.3–17.5). If there is both inspiratory and expiratory muscle weakness, then a combination of assisted inspiration and expiration techniques should be utilized. These techniques have been shown to increase PCF either alone or in combination.[66–69]

If the cough is extremely impaired, the patient may require mechanical insufflation/exsufflation (MI-E) (Fig. 17.27).[70,71] This procedure clears secretions by gradually applying a positive pressure to the airway (insufflation) and then rapidly shifting to negative pressure (exsufflation). The rapid shift in pressure produces a high expiratory flow, simulating a natural cough. In pediatric patients with NMD, MI-E has been provided as part of a protocol in patients with a PE_{max} of 20 cm H_2O or less.[72] MI-E has also been shown to expedite secretion removal[73] and prevent intubation.[74] A combination of NIV and MI-E in spinal muscular atrophy type I has been associated with increased life expectancy when compared with the untreated natural history in observational studies.[75–78]

NIV (Fig. 17.28) may also have a role in preventing chest wall deformity in NMD.[78,79] Physical therapies that consist of secretion-mobilizing techniques in NMD may need to provide ventilator support. Such options include IPV (see Figs. 17.3–17.5),[80–82] a modified ACBT (adjusting the patients NIV settings), or HFCWO[83] on NIV where indicated (see Figs. 17.3–17.5). Patients who use NIV should not be taken off their ventilator for physiotherapy or transferred to CPAP. Some patients with NMD are provided with NIV to decrease their work of breathing and augment tidal volumes to enhance ACT. The ACBT can be modified by using NIV to provide deep breaths that mobilize secretions with or without manual techniques, followed by an assisted cough technique.

Outcome is improved when children with NMD are treated with an oximetry-driven protocol when they are unwell to avoid intubation or in preparation for extubation.[84] The protocol consists of carrying out cough augmentation techniques when the oxygen saturations decline below 95% on room air or on NIV without supplementary oxygen therapy. The rationale is that patients have atelectasis with secretion retention and treatment is required to reverse the process; this has been shown to increase survival in patients with NMD. Performing cough augmentation when the patient's oxygen saturation has declined below 95% has contributed to successful extubation and prevented the need for intubation in this patient group.[57,75,78,85]

Currently there is no evidence base for the use of respiratory muscle training in this patient group.[84]

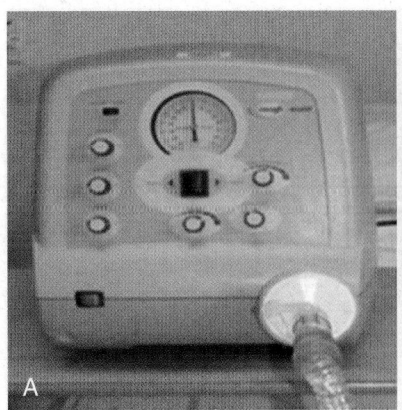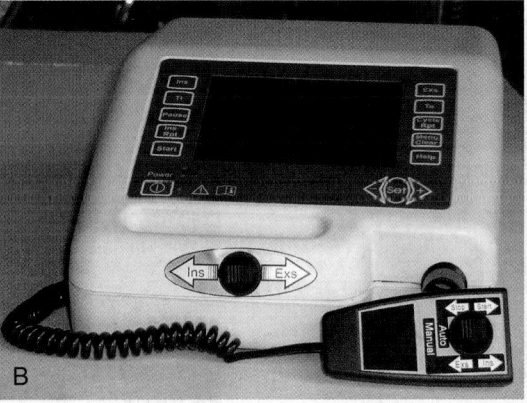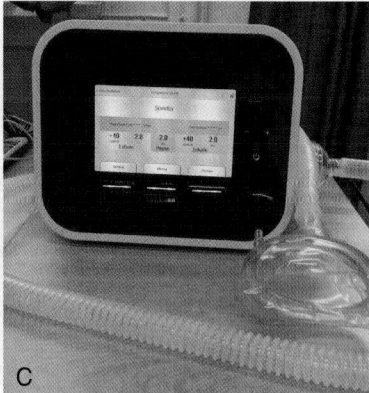

Fig. 17.27 Cough assist device.

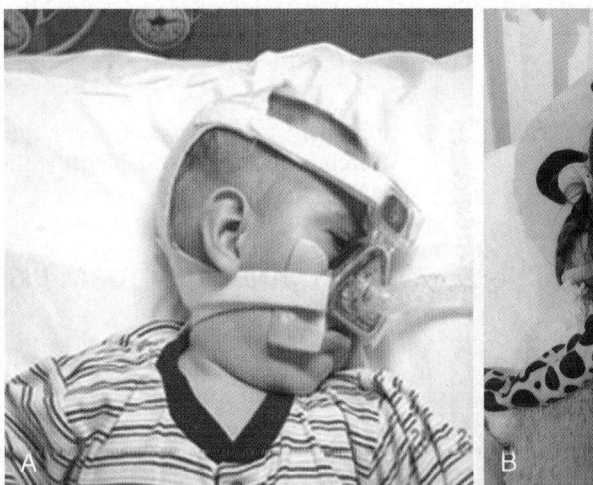

Fig. 17.28 Child with noninvasive ventilation via nasal mask.

Spinal Cord Injury

Physical therapies should be appropriate to the level of the spinal cord injury. Cervical spinal cord injuries may require ventilator support in the form of NIV or, in higher spinal cord injuries, tracheostomy with intermittent positive pressure ventilation (TIPPV). Patients may need to be taught lung volume recruitment maneuvers in the form of assisted inspirations (see section "Neuromuscular Disease" and Figs. 17.3–17.5) to promote chest wall stretching,[86] along with lung growth and development. For injuries that included the thoracic spine, MAC should be taught (see Chapter 72 and Figs. 17.3–17.5).[87] Patients who are significantly weak are likely to benefit from MI-E either via a mask or tracheostomy; this has been reported to be less uncomfortable than suctioning.[88] Abdominal binders may also be required to minimize the effect of postural hypotension and aid in respiration.[89,90]

SURGICAL AND CRITICAL CARE

Preoperative and Postoperative Management

Routine preoperative therapy is not indicated[91]; however, it may be desirable to teach physical therapies to high-risk children prior to surgery—for example, patients with coexisting respiratory conditions that may predispose to postoperative respiratory atelectasis and infection or patients with reduced mobility.

Exercise therapy is an essential part of postoperative care, and endurance training has a favorable influence on pulmonary function in patients after surgical correction of scoliosis.[92] Other postoperative physical therapies differ depending on the patient's status. Breathing exercises such as ACBT may be appropriate (or blowing games in younger children) if secretion retention is an issue. Incentive spirometry should not be used routinely[93] or if the child is mobilizing sufficiently; however, in isolated cases it can give visual feedback and encourage the child to take deeper breaths in an attempt to resolve atelectasis.[94] If there is a significant amount of atelectasis with a decline in oxygen saturation, a step up to HFNC,[95] CPAP or NIV may be necessary. IPPB (Bird Mark 7, Viasys Health Care, Bilthoven, The Netherlands)[96] may be of benefit for older children with sputum retention (see Fig. 17.24).[63,97]

Critical Care

The physiotherapist is an integral part of the intensive care team, the indicators for intervention must be clearly defined and possible adverse events to these recognized. In the

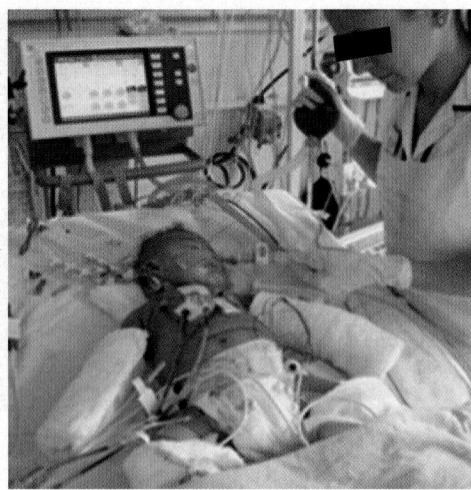

Fig. 17.29 Physiotherapy (manual hyperinflation and manual techniques) being performed on a intubated and ventilated infant.

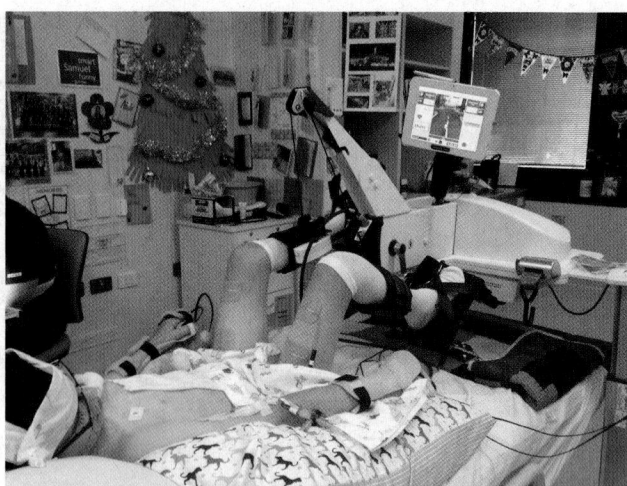

Fig. 17.31 Functional electrical stimulation being used to assist rehabilitation for the lower limbs.

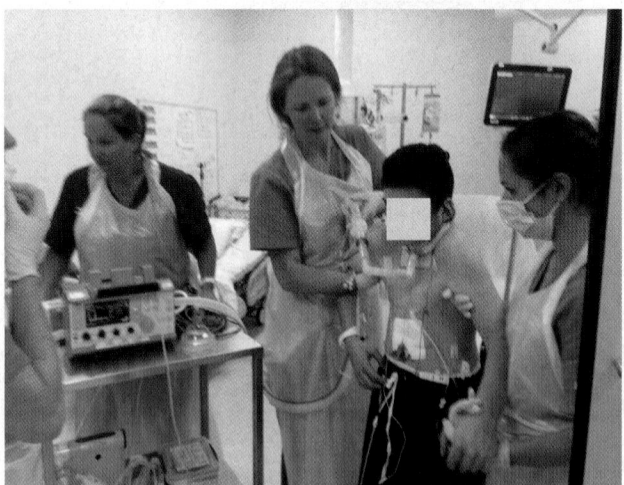

Fig. 17.30 Mobilizing a young man on the intensive care while ventilated via a tracheostomy.

intubated child, ACTs are often used in combination for greater efficacy and appropriate anticipatory strategies put in place prior to treatment (e.g., preoxygenation, sedation). In addition to manual techniques and positioning, manual hyperinflation (MHI) may be indicated when areas of focal atelectasis or retained secretions are identified, with greater expiratory to inspiratory flow bias critical to the maneuver (Fig. 17.29, Video 17.3).[98] The roles of ventilator hyperinflations (VHIs) and the intrapercussive ventilator are currently under investigation.

The focus in pediatric critical care is now directed toward early rehabilitation, even prior to extubation where possible (Fig. 17.30), as it has been shown to reduce ventilator days, length of stay and delirium and to increase muscle strength.[99] Recommendations in "at risk" adults also include the use of continuous passive motion (CPM) and electronic muscle simulation (EMS) daily (Fig. 17.31).[100] For some patients, inspiratory muscle training can facilitate weaning.[101] In the pediatric arena, there is evidence supporting a similar

approach[102,103]; advocacy from the therapist is critical to overcome barriers and identify the children who would benefit.

AIRWAY AND STRUCTURAL DISORDERS

Asthma

A crucial part of physical therapy management of asthma is education of the child and parents, in particular the need for regular exercise when the child stable.[104] It is important to ensure ongoing adherence to prescribed medication (see Chapters 45 and 46). Physiotherapy includes advice on exercise that is specific to age and severity. In some children, breathing retraining using a reduced volume and/or frequency with relaxation can reduce symptoms and therefore improve quality of life. Several groups advocate specific techniques, but it is important to stress that these techniques are adjunctive to medication and are not replacement therapy. Routine airway clearance is rarely indicated in asthmatic patients, and it is important to remain aware that ACTs may exacerbate bronchospasm.

Breathing Pattern Disorders

This is a particularly challenging area. It is important that the child undergo a full assessment prior to referral for physical therapies to rule out organic disorders (e.g., croup) and neurologic disorders (e.g., Rett syndrome). A careful history should be taken to investigate when symptoms are present. If the child is symptom-free during sleep, this may help to refine the diagnosis. If the child is suffering from a psychogenic disorder or other abnormal breathing patterns (e.g., hyperventilation syndrome and sighing dyspnea), then physiologic input will have benefit to identify triggers and provide advice on how to cope with them. Breathing reeducation is essential in this group of children and adolescents. Breathing retraining, which incorporates reduced respiratory rate and/or tidal volume, is a first-line treatment for hyperventilation syndrome with or without concurrent asthma. Identification of precipitating factors (e.g., sighing) and other triggers is important.

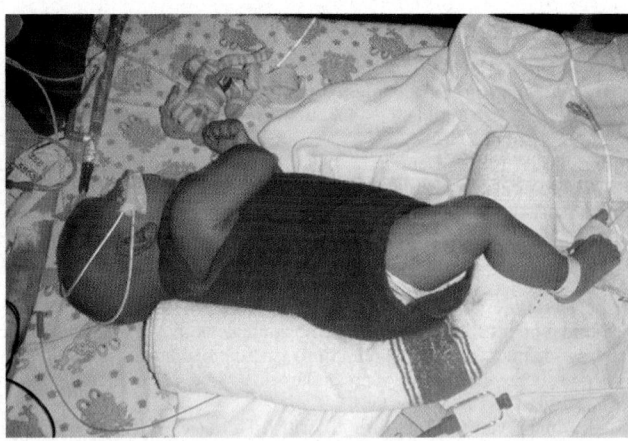

Fig. 17.32 Positioning of an infant with chronic neonatal lung disease.

Chest Wall Disorders

Physical therapies in chest wall disease are aimed at maximizing lung function. This includes pulmonary rehabilitation,[105] manual musculoskeletal therapies for postural pain, and initiation of NIV in the hypercapnic patient[106] along with postoperative rehabilitation after corrective surgery.

Airway Structural Disorders

With the increased diagnosis of tracheomalacia and bronchomalacia via bronchoscopy, physiotherapists are building evidence for the use of PEP.[107] It is hypothesized that in children with some structural abnormalities, PEP can increase airway stabilization and enhance cough expiratory flow.[108] It is well known that children with airway malacia are prone to recurrent respiratory infections,[109] and further research is needed on the role of physiotherapy.

Interstitial Lung Disease

There is little published evidence on physiotherapy for interstitial lung disease. Studies in adult patients have shown an improvement with exercise training in patients with this disease.[110–112] Adult patients with more advanced disease may benefit from ambulatory oxygen therapy and breathlessness management. Physical therapies for this condition include positioning to ease breathlessness. Given the very different spectrum of interstitial lung diseases in children (Fig. 17.32 and Section 6: Interstitial Lung Disease, of this book), recommendations based on adults should only be adopted with extreme caution and a detailed individualized assessment is essential.

Conditions Not Generally Amenable to Physiotherapy

ACUTE LARYNGOTRACHEOBRONCHITIS (CROUP)

Physical therapies are usually contraindicated in the spontaneously ventilating child with croup. However, other techniques may be indicated if the child is intubated and mechanically ventilated and secretions cannot be cleared by suction airway clearance alone.

PERTUSSIS

Any physical therapies during the acute phase of pertussis can precipitate paroxysmal cough and its complications. If the child is mechanically ventilated, paralyzed, and sedated and there are issues with retained secretions, ACTs may be of benefit (see Figs. 17.3–17.5). In the child with persistent lobar collapse and in whom the paroxysmal cough phase has ended, appropriate ACTs can be taught.

INHALED FOREIGN BODY

Physical therapy is not indicated to remove the foreign body. These children require bronchoscopic removal of the material, usually with a rigid bronchoscope. After bronchoscopic removal, PD, manual techniques, and breathing exercises may be necessary to clear excess secretions that have accumulated in the obstructed airway behind the foreign body.

PULMONARY EDEMA

ACTs are not indicated for pulmonary edema; however in some situations CPAP or NIV may be an appropriate strategy to help children with significant work of breathing while waiting for diuresis or other medical strategies to take effect.

LOBAR PNEUMONIA AND EMPYEMA

There is little evidence to support chest physiotherapy to treat lobar pneumonia[113,114] or empyema.[115] The pathophysiology of both conditions indicates that physiotherapy will not be effective in the acute stages or even during the resolution phase when secretions can appear in the airways; previously healthy children have the capability to clear these independently, with particular focus on mobilization. However, specific ACTs may be required in children with conditions that alter muscle tone (e.g., cerebral palsy), mobility/muscle strength (e.g., neuromuscular conditions), or mucociliary clearance (e.g., bronchiectasis).

BRONCHIOLITIS

Physical therapy is counterproductive during the acute stage of bronchiolitis. Mechanically ventilated infants will need careful assessment and may benefit from ACTs if there is retention of secretions. Chest physiotherapy has not been shown to reduce length of hospital stay, oxygen requirements or clinical severity score[116]; intervention should be based on specific focal signs or comorbidities. In these cases, physiotherapy may need to be modified to reduce the impact on the infant's work of breathing and should be continually reassessed.

In children with normal lung defense mechanisms and function, chest physiotherapy is very unlikely to be of benefit for acute respiratory disorders. However, lack of evidence does not mean that this should be extrapolated to all children. It is imperative that the therapist be able to assess the patient and liaise with the medical team regarding the necessity of intervention so that appropriate treatment is provided.[117]

Summary

Physical therapy is well established as part of the management of many respiratory conditions, in particular for children requiring mechanical ventilation and those with chronic disorders such as bronchiectasis or neuromuscular conditions. Over the past few decades, the profession has evolved, and a wide variety of techniques and modalities is available with a growing evidence base. Fundamentally the key to effective physiotherapy is identifying the physiologic issue, deciding whether physiotherapy strategies can assist, and identifying outcomes that can be measured. The latter must include both positive and negative effects so the therapist can assess the risk and take an informed approach to patient care. Integral to all of this are the therapeutic skills required in communication and engagement with the child and family to ensure an optimal outcome in the ever-changing face of the presentation.

Acknowledgments

Ruth Wakeman, Nicola Collins, and Michelle Chatwin were supported by the NIHR Respiratory Disease Biomedical Research Unit at the Royal Brompton and Harefield NHS Foundation Trust and Imperial College London.

Video contributions thanks to Cameron Greenland, Christine Wilson, and Children's Health Queensland Hospital and Health Service.

References

Access the reference list online at ExpertConsult.com.

Suggested Reading

Balfour-Lynn IM, Field DJ, Gringras P, et al. Paediatric Section of the Home Oxygen Guideline Development Group of the BTS Standards of Care Committee. BTS guidelines for home oxygen in children. *Thorax.* 2009;64(suppl 2):ii1–ii26.

Button BM, Wilson C, Dentice R, et al. Physiotherapy for cystic fibrosis in Australia and New Zealand: a clinical practice guideline. *Respirology.* 2016;21(4):656–667.

Chatwin M, Bush A, Simonds AK. Outcome of goal-directed non-invasive ventilation and mechanical insufflation/exsufflation in spinal muscular atrophy type I. *Arch Dis Child.* 2011;96:426–432.

Cystic Fibrosis Foundation, Borowitz D, Parad RB, et al. Cystic Fibrosis Foundation practice guidelines for the management of infants with cystic fibrosis transmembrane conductance regulator-related metabolic syndrome during the first two years of life and beyond. *J Pediatr.* 2009;155(6 suppl):S106–S116.

Hull J, Aniapravan R, Chan E, et al. British Thoracic Society guideline for respiratory management of children with neuromuscular weakness. *Thorax.* 2012;67(suppl 1):i1–i40.

Niggemann B. How to diagnose psychogenic and functional breathing disorders in children and adolescents. *Pediatr Allergy Immunol.* 2010; 21:895–899.

Prasad S, Main E, Dodd M, et al. Association of Chartered Physiotherapists. Finding consensus on the physiotherapy management of asymptomatic infants with cystic fibrosis. *Pediatr Pulmonol.* 2008;43:236–244.

Pryor JA, Prasad SA, eds. Physiotherapy techniques. In: *Physiotherapy for Respiratory and Cardiac Problems.* Vol. 1. 4th ed. Edinburgh: Elsevier Limited; 2008:632.

Simonds AK, ed. *ERS Practical Handbook of Noninvasive Ventilation.* Sheffield, UK: European Respiratory Society; 2015.

Wright SE, Kelly K. Cardiopulmonary acute paediatric physiotherapy. www.sdc.qld.edu.au/courses/151.

18 Congenital Lung Disease

ANDREW BUSH, MB BS(Hons), MA, MD, FRCP, FRCPCH, FERS, ROBIN ABEL, BSc, MBBS, PhD, FRCS(Paeds), LYN CHITTY, PhD, MRCOG, JONNY HARCOURT, MA(Oxon), MBBS(Hons), FRCS, RICHARD J. HEWITT, BSc, DOHNS, FRCS (HNS-ORL), and ANDREW GORDON NICHOLSON, DM FRCPath

Introduction

The increased skill and widespread application of antenatal ultrasound and more recently antenatal magnetic resonance imaging (MRI) not only has allowed precise early diagnosis of many congenital malformations, but also has brought new problems. UK National Screening Committee guidelines recommend that all women be offered a detailed fetal anomaly scan at around 20 weeks' gestation to confirm the gestational age and examine the fetal anatomy in detail according to standards dictated by the Fetal Anomaly Screening Programme.[1] Many parents are now faced with having to decide what to do for a baby affected by one of many different abnormalities, some of which would have previously escaped detection. The natural history of many of these malformations is unknown, and so health professionals can have difficulty offering accurate information to parents faced with the unexpected diagnosis of an abnormality in their baby. The diagnosis of fetal lung lesions is one good example. Early reports published in the 1980s described a poor outcome for fetuses with lung masses detected in the second trimester. However, these studies were biased by a high incidence of intervention, including termination of pregnancy. With increasing use of antenatal ultrasound and the detection of many less obvious lesions, it has become clear that, if conservative management is followed, many may disappear or regress considerably by term. Indeed, as we will demonstrate in this chapter, the outcome for such fetuses is generally very good, and the dilemma now is whether to pursue conservative or surgical management in an asymptomatic infant. Further confusion arises as to how these malformations should be described. The nomenclature of congenital lung disease was never very clear, with terms such as sequestrated segment, cystic adenomatoid malformation, hypoplastic lung, and malinosculation being used to describe abnormalities that often overlap. Now, however, they are used inconsistently before and after birth. For example, congenital cystic adenomatoid malformation (CCAM), subsequently renamed as congenital pulmonary airway malformation (CPAM),[2] is used by perinatologists to describe a lesion that may well disappear before birth, but is used postnatally to describe an abnormality that may require lobectomy. CPAMs may have a pulmonary arterial supply or be supplied like a sequestration from systemic arteries, and histologic features of these lesions may overlap. Furthermore, overlap lesions, containing features of two or even three pathological entities, are common.[3–5] MRI now delineates the blood supply of antenatal malformations with increasing precision, although the ability to acquire sophisticated images is not necessarily the best indication for so doing. New treatment options, such as fetal surgery and even fetal interventional bronchoscopy, and

postnatal embolization of feeding vessels, are available; however, the exact place of novel interventions is unclear. A complete reappraisal of the diagnosis, investigation, and management of congenital lung disease is thus timely. A complete review of congenital lung disease might also include a few disorders that are acquired in utero, such as congenital pneumonias (discussed in Chapter 19), but this chapter is limited to the stricter definition of developmental disorders. There is overlap with the developmental components of pediatric interstitial lung disease, and these are described in detail in Chapters 54 and 57.

Clinical Approach

To clarify dialogue among various professionals (obstetricians, perinatologists, pediatric surgeons, pathologists, pediatricians), it is suggested that these principles be followed[6]:

1. What is actually seen should be described without indulgence in embryologic speculation, which may later be proved wrong. Clinical descriptions should not include assumptions of pathology, since the same clinical appearance (e.g., a multicystic mass) may have different pathologic etiologies (see examples previously). Indeed, specific antenatal diagnoses often have to be revised after postnatal excision of the lesion[7]
2. The description should be in common language, discarding Latin.
3. The lung and associated organs should be approached in a systematic manner, because abnormalities are often multiple and associated lesions will be missed unless carefully sought.
4. Pathologic descriptions should describe what is actually seen (epithelial and mesenchymal elements), which may then be related to a diagnostic category (CPAM). However, even distinguished pathologists disagree over the classification of excised specimens, underscoring that clinicans seeing greyscale images are most unlikely to get it right.[2,8]

DESCRIBE WHAT IS ACTUALLY SEEN

The recommendation to describe what is actually seen should be followed by the clinician both before and after birth. In principle, antenatal ultrasound abnormalities should be described using such terms as increased echogenicity with large, small, or multiple cysts rather than as "CPAM," which is, and remains, a histological diagnosis. The presence or absence of abnormal feeding vessels should be defined using imaging appropriate to developmental stage (i.e., antenatal or postnatal). Other features, such as mediastinal shift, should also be described. In the postnatal period, a radiographic abnormality should be described as solid or cystic. If cystic, the cysts are either single or multiple, and the uniformity and thickness of the walls should be described. They may be filled with air, or partially or completely with fluid; moreover, their size should be recorded. Postnatally, an air–fluid level suggests that the abnormality is ventilated, albeit with a long time constant. If the lesion has been excised, the pathologist should describe the tissues found (epithelial, mesenchymal) and the contents of any cysts that may be present, thus giving a simple description of what is seen under the microscope. Only then is it relevant to make a pathologic diagnosis, such as one of the various histologic types of CPAM (see subsequent sections). Any classification system that is to be robust cannot be based on embryologic speculation.

USE CLEAR TERMS

Many terms are ambiguous and are best avoided. For example, hypoplastic lung could be taken as meaning a lung that is small but otherwise normal, or small because the underlying structure is abnormal; the term congenital small lung (CSL, which is what is actually seen) avoids such ambiguity. The use of the term emphysema as in congenital lobar emphysema is another source of confusion, since it implies lung destruction, whereas in at least some variants (e.g., polyalveolar lobe) there may be too many, not too few, alveoli. What is actually seen is a congenital large hyperlucent lobe (CLHL), which is the term that should be used in clinical practice. Throughout this chapter, unwarranted established terms will be given in parentheses after our proposed nomenclature; for the convenience of the reader, the new terms will be spelled out in full, with the abbreviated form being given in parentheses. A summary comparison of old and our current nomenclature is provided in Table 18.1.

USE A SYSTEMATIC APPROACH

The lung can be considered to be formed from six "trees": bronchial, arterial (systemic and pulmonary), venous (systemic and pulmonary), and lymphatic. There are no known congenital abnormalities of bronchial venous drainage, so in practice, only five trees have to be considered. There are three other areas wherein malformations may affect the

Table 18.1 Comparison of New and Old Terms Used to Describe the Clinical, but Not Pathological, Appearances of Congenital Lung Malformations

New Nomenclature	Old Terms Superseded
CLHL	Congenital lobar emphysema Polyalveolar lobe
CTM	Cystic adenomatoid malformation (Type 0–4 pathologically) Sequestration (intrapulmonary and extrapulmonary) Bronchogenic cyst Reduplication cyst Foregut cyst
CSL	Pulmonary hypoplasia
Absent lung, absent trachea	Agenesis of lung, tracheal aplasia
Absent bronchus	Bronchial atresia

CLHL, Congenital large hyperlucent lobe; *CSL,* congenital small lung; *CTM,* congenital thoracic malformation.

respiratory system and that should also be assessed. These are (1) the heart and great vessels; (2) the chest wall, including the respiratory neuromuscular apparatus; and (3) the abdomen. Finally, the possibility of multisystem disease (e.g., tuberous sclerosis) should be considered. Each patient suspected of having a congenital lung malformation should be systematically evaluated along these lines, if important coexistent abnormalities are not to be missed. The importance of a systematic approach to treatment, with an appropriate evaluation of all trees and associated systems before embarking on treatment, cannot be overstated.

KEEP CLINICAL AND PATHOLOGIC DESCRIPTIONS SEPARATE

This is an extension of the principle of describing what is seen. Black-and-white images on a scan are unlikely to be pathognomonic of a single histologic entity. It is more logical to describe the clinical appearances and construct a pathologic differential diagnosis. Only after excision of the lesion can the pathologist make an appropriate diagnosis from examination of the excised specimen.

The Size of the Problem: Epidemiology of Congenital Malformations of the Lung

There is a paucity of high-quality, population-based, epidemiological studies. The requirement for a high-quality study to be performed is for all women in a large population to have access to diagnostic quality, mid-trimester ultrasound scans, which are properly interpreted by experienced radiologists. The European Surveillance of Congenital Anomalies (EUROCAT) is the largest network of population-based registers for the epidemiological surveillance of congenital anomalies including congenital thoracic malformations (CTMs). Current EUROCAT data (2008–2012) reported a prevalence of cystic adenomatoid malformation of 1.05 (95% confidence intervals 0.96–1.15) per 10,000 pregnancies (which included live births, fetal deaths, and terminations of pregnancy), an increasing trend over 4 consecutive years.[9] There was one cluster of cases in Emilia Romagna between mid-April 2010 and the end of February 2011, consisting of 12 cases when 3.65 cases would be expected ($P = .014$). The cause could not be found, and no reason determined further to investigate this cluster. Reported prevalence was 2.55 (2.40–2.71) for esophageal atresia with or without tracheo-esophageal fistula (TEF), a slight increase over time[9] and 2.81 (2.65–2.97) for diaphragmatic hernia.[10] EUROCAT prevalence data, although the best currently available must be treated with caution because the database captures less than 30% of all European data.

Antenatal Diagnosis and Management of Congenital Lung Disease

The age-related clinical presentations of congenital lung disease are summarized in Table 18.2. Postnatal aspects are

Table 18.2 Presentation of Congenital Lung Disease by Age

Age	Presenting Feature
Antenatal	Intrathoracic mass
	Pleural effusion
	Fetal hydrops
	Oligohydramnios or polyhydramnios
	Other associated abnormalities discovered
Newborn period	Respiratory distress
	Stridor
	Bubbly secretions in mouth, not able to swallow
	Failure to pass nasogastric tube
	Unable to establish an airway
	Cardiac failure
	Chance finding
	Cyanosis in a well baby
	Poor respiratory effort
Later childhood/ adulthood	Recurrent infection (including tuberculosis, aspergillus)
	Hemoptysis, hemothorax
	Bronchiectasis, bronchopleural fistula
	Steroid resistant airway obstruction
	Cardiac failure
	Malignant transformation
	Cyanosis
	Coughing on drinking
	Chance finding of mass or hyperlucent area on chest x-ray
	Air embolism (rare)

Table 18.3 The Differential Diagnosis of Fetal Intrathoracic Lesions

Solid Lesions	Cystic Lesions
Microcystic adenomatoid malformation	Macrocystic adenomatoid malformation
Pulmonary sequestration	Congenital diaphragmatic hernia
Right-sided diaphragmatic hernia	Bronchogenic cyst
Tracheal/laryngeal atresia	Mediastinal encephalocele
Rhabdomyoma	Pleural and pericardial effusions
Mediastinal teratoma	

described subsequently in this chapter, as are the important abnormalities encountered, which are described in terms of the branching trees comprising the lung.

ANTENATAL PRESENTATION

Antenatal presentation is usually associated with an abnormality detected at the time of a routine fetal anomaly scan as described in detail later. However, abnormalities of amniotic fluid volume may also be associated with underlying pulmonary pathology. This may be secondary, as in bilateral CSL (pulmonary hypoplasia) associated with both early-onset oligohydramnios for whatever reason (bilateral renal dysplasia/agenesis, first- or early second-trimester rupture of the membranes, etc.), or polyhydramnios associated with conditions, such as the Pena-Shokeir phenotype or antenatal onset of severe spinal muscular atrophy, wherein severe neuromuscular disease prevents normal respiratory movements and lung development; another possibility is compression of the fetal esophagus by a mass, preventing normal swallowing of amniotic fluid. In other situations there is a primary pulmonary anomaly (e.g., tracheoesophageal fistula or laryngeal/tracheal agenesis) that causes the polyhydramnios. Other presentations include short limbs in those skeletal dysplasias associated with bilateral CSL secondary to small chests and short ribs (e.g., Jeune's asphyxiating thoracic dystrophy), or talipes and polyhydramnios in congenital myotonic dystrophy.

WHAT CAN WE DIAGNOSE AND WHEN?

Fetal lung abnormalities are increasingly detected prenatally as a result of advances in ultrasound imaging, which improves the diagnosis, and because fetal anomaly scanning is now

routinely offered to many women in the developed world. A fetal lung lesion is suspected either when a mass (cystic or solid) is identified in the thorax or because of mediastinal shift (Tables 18.3 and 18.4). The opportunity to identify an intrathoracic anomaly in the antenatal period permits further investigation and occasionally offers the potential for intra-uterine therapy. It also identifies fetuses that may benefit from delivery in a center offering tertiary-level neonatal support and the option of early postnatal surgical intervention. Many of these lesions can be detected around 20 weeks' gestation, but for some, in particular diaphragmatic hernias and pleural effusions, late presentation is well recognized. Such lesions may not be detected until an incidental scan in the third trimester is undertaken, or, indeed, until after birth when the neonate or infant presents clinically. It must also be recognized that a sonographic diagnosis can only describe the macroscopic nature of the lesion, and a definitive diagnosis for many anomalies must await definitive radiologic or histologic diagnosis after birth. Many reported studies are seriously limited, because they base conclusions solely on prenatal ultrasound or postnatal imaging, which is often limited to plain radiology. While advances in technology have improved antenatal diagnosis of lesions that may benefit from early postnatal intervention, many of the abnormalities detected appear to resolve spontaneously or are clinically silent. The pediatrician is frequently faced with a new dilemma: how to manage a healthy infant with a lesion that would not have been brought to medical attention were it not for antenatal imaging. What is the natural history of some of these lesions; do they require intervention, or are they benign variants? This section will present an overview of the antenatal diagnosis and management of the more common types of congenital intrathoracic abnormalities. Postnatal management of the abnormalities is discussed in subsequent sections. A summary approach to counseling mothers whose fetus has a cystic or solid CTM is given in Box 18.1, and discussed in more detail below. The enormous anxiety that is caused by uncertainty, even when the malformation probably has a good prognosis, should be acknowledged.[11,12]

In addition to fetal ultrasound, in recent years there has been an increasing use of fetal MRI to define pathology, detected with ultrasound. There are reports of its use for the delineation and evolution of fetal cystic masses,[13–15] but how much MRI adds to the ultrasound diagnosis remains to be demonstrated.[16] It may be more sensitive to small lesions than ultrasound, but it is arguable whether detection of tiny abnormalities really matters. It has been shown to be superior to screening ultrasound for the diagnosis of congenital high airway obstruction syndrome (CHAOS) when it changed the diagnosis in 70%, but in 9 of these 10 cases, the MRI

Table 18.4   Summary of Cohort of Patients With Cystic Lung Lesions Seen at University College London Hospital in 12 Years

Ultrasound Findings	Total[a]	Liveborn	Postnatal Management Surgical Emergency	Surgical Elective	Conservative	ToP[c]	Perinatal Death[d]	Postnatal Diagnosis[b] CCAML	No Evidence of Pathology	PS	Other	No Diagnosis	LTFO/ WFI
Macrocystic	40	35	7	5	22	2	0	28	2	0	6	4	1/2
Microcystic	47	39	5	3	23	4	3	22	6	5	11	3	1/0
Mediastinal shift	55	44	11	11	23	6	2	33	5	3	13	5	1/2
Hydrops	14	7	4	0	3	5	2	6	0	1	7	0	0
Intrauterine therapy	9	9	4	0	5	0	0	6	0	0	3	0	0
Apparent resolution in utero	19	19	1	4	12	0	0	15	2	0	1	1	0
Total cases seen	87	74	12	8	46	6	3	50	8	5	17	7	2/2

[a]Total cases in cohort.
[b]Some cases with conservative management do not have a definitive diagnosis.
[c]Pregnancies were terminated for the following reasons: 45,XO with pulmonary lymphangiectasia, severe hydrops, congenital pulmonary lymphangiectasia, Fraser syndrome (2 cases), Fraser syndrome, and extra lobar sequestration.
[d]Perinatal deaths were secondary to Fraser syndrome, severe hydrops, and pulmonary sequestration with hydrops.
Others included: congenital diaphragmatic hernia (3), pulmonary lymphangiectasia (2), Fraser syndrome (3), eventration of the left diaphragm, teratoma, congenital intradiaphragm cystic lung abnormality, Sturge Weber syndrome, intraabdominal calcification, echogenic mass below abdomen, unclassified abnormal lung, neuroblastoma, and Peter's syndrome with pulmonary hypoplasia.
CCAML, Cystic adenomatoid malformation of the lung; *LTFO*, lost to follow-up/WFI, waiting for information (in some cases details of outcome are awaited or the pregnancy is ongoing); *PS*, pulmonary sequestration; *ToP*, termination of pregnancy.
From Bush A, Hogg J, Chitty LS. Cystic lung lesions—prenatal diagnosis and management. *Prenat Diagn*. 2008;28:604-611.

Box 18.1   Suggested Summary Approach to Counseling a Mother Whose Fetus Has an Antenatal Diagnosis of Congenital Thoracic Malformation

The majority of CTMs will increase in size to the end of the second trimester, then regress

Antenatal intervention is very rarely required

Although apparent complete regression of the mass as pregnancy progresses has been reported, many babies are shown postnatally to have persistent abnormalities

Most babies are asymptomatic in the newborn period, and any treatment decisions can be made electively

CTM, Congenital thoracic malformation.

---

diagnosis was concordant with the referral center ultrasound findings.[17] However, it may be useful to accurately determine the level of airway obstruction in this condition.[18] MRI may also be of use to determine the location of feeding vessels in fetuses with pulmonary sequestration,[19] but further comparison with ultrasound-based methods is required before we can say whether it adds significantly to Doppler-based methods. The role of MRI to determine lung volumes in fetuses with congenital diaphragmatic hernia (CDH) or lung masses has been evaluated[20] and may ultimately prove superior to other ultrasound-based methods (see later). Finally, virtual bronchoscopy can be undertaken with fetal MRI.[21,22]

Specific Diagnoses: Congenital Diaphragmatic Hernia

The prenatal incidence of CDH is around 1 in 2000. There is a wide variety of abnormalities associated with CDH including aneuploidy, in particular Trisomy 18 and 13, genetic syndromes and structural abnormalities. Many of these will result in a stillbirth or termination of pregnancy, so isolated CDH is much more common in neonates. Anomalies associated with this condition include neural tube defects, such as myelomeningocele, cardiac defects, and midline anomalies, such as cleft lip and palate. Genetic syndromes, such as Fryns syndrome, can account for up to 10% of cases in some series. The herniation of abdominal contents into the chest inhibits normal lung development resulting in pulmonary hypoplasia, which, in isolated lesions, is the main cause of death.

The diagnosis of a left-sided CDH is usually first suspected when a mediastinal shift is observed and abdominal viscera are seen within the fetal thorax (Fig. 18.1). The most useful clue is usually the identification of a cystic structure (the stomach) in the chest together with absence of an intra-abdominal stomach. The observation of peristalsis in the chest can also be a useful clue as loops of bowel may be difficult to distinguish from other cystic lesions. Occasionally it is possible to observe paradoxical movement of the viscera in the chest with fetal breathing movements. Once alert to the possible diagnosis, careful radiological examination of the fetus in the coronal and parasagittal planes will show the diaphragmatic defect. Right-sided CDH are more difficult to recognize as it is usually just the liver that is herniated, and this is of similar echogenicity to lung tissue. Often the only clue is mediastinal shift, and this may not be apparent at the time of a routine anomaly scan unless the degree of shift is great. Sometimes the diagnosis is made when a scan is performed in the third trimester because of polyhydramnios resulting from the presence of herniated abdominal contents in the chest, which prevents normal swallowing movements and results in late onset of increased amniotic fluid.

The overall prognosis for fetuses with CDH is poor with the major causes of death being pulmonary hypoplasia and/

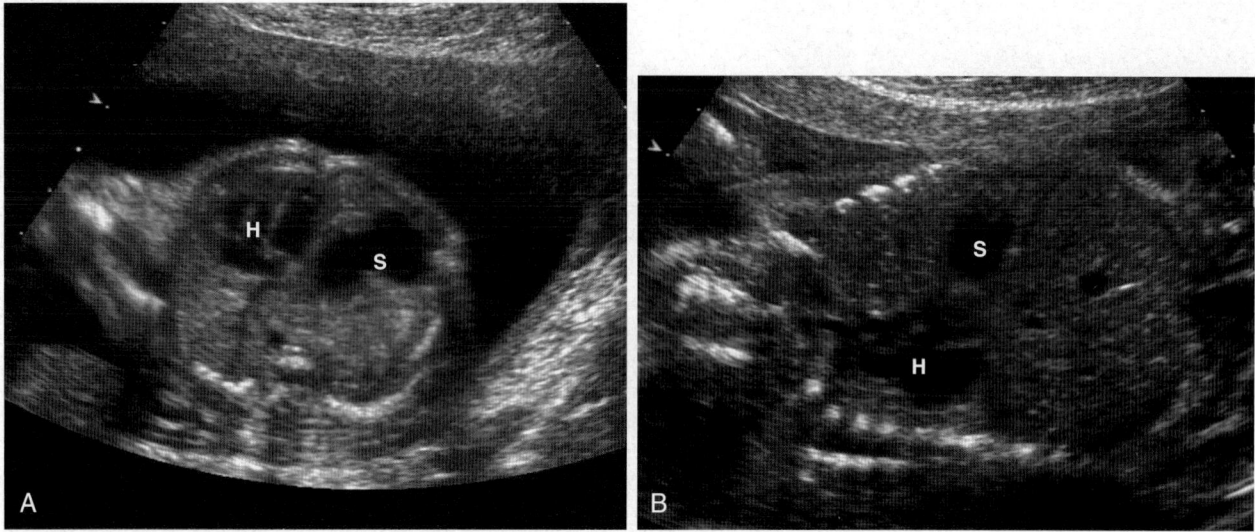

Fig. 18.1 Transverse view through the thorax at 20 weeks' gestation in a fetus with a diaphragmatic hernia. (A) The stomach (S) is seen displacing the heart (H) to the right. In the longitudinal plane (B), no diaphragm can be seen and the stomach is in the chest.

Table 18.5   Outcomes of Congenital Diaphragmatic Hernia

Authors	Number	Chromosome Abnormality, n (%)		Overall Survival (%)	Survival at <24 Weeks (%)	Survival at >24 Weeks (%)	Survival in Isolated Cases (%)
Thorpe-Beeston et al., 1989[351]	36	11	31	25			60
Adzick et al., 1989[352]	38	6	16	24	0	38	38
Sharland et al., 1992[353]	55	2	4	27	26	40	28
Manni et al., 1994[354]	28	3	11	14	0	100	30
Bollman et al., 1995[355]	33	6	18	18			44
Dommergues et al., 1996[356]	135	14	10	19			30
Howe et al., 1996[357]	48	13	34	27	24	30	50
Geary et al., 1998[358]	34	5	15	18	31	33	38
Bahlmann et al., 1999[26]	19	1	7				
Betremieux et al. 2002[359]	31	4	13	38			60
Garne et al., 2002[360]	187	20	11	71			
Laudy et al., 2003[361,a]	26	0	0	50			
Dott et al., 2003[362]	249	18	7	19/54[c]			
Hendrick et al., 2004[363,b]	22	0	0	70			
Bouchghoul et al., 2015[367]	377			61			Only isolated analyzed
Akinkuotu et al., 2016[368]	176	28	16	74			
Coughlin et al., 2016[369]	61			38			Only isolated analyzed
Total	941	103	13	32/35	16	48	42

[a]Only isolated left-sided CDH cases were included in study.
[b]Only right CDH were included in study.
[c]Overall survival has increased during the period of the study from 19% (1968–1971) to 54% (1996–1999).
Where there are no figures for the survival, data were not given in the publication.
CDH, Congenital diaphragmatic hernia.

or the associated abnormalities. The time of diagnosis is related to outcome with those diagnosed early faring the worst. Lung size, expressed as lung-to-head ratio (LHR) or the observed-to-expected LHR measured by ultrasound[23] and the observed-to-expected total lung volume as measured by MRI and liver herniation are reasonable predictors of neonatal outcome.[24] However, they are not good predictors of other poor outcomes, such as pulmonary hypertension.[25] Other poor prognostic indicators include evidence of liver within the chest and cardiac disproportion before 24 weeks. Isolated left-sided hernias, an intraabdominal stomach, and diagnosis after 24 weeks are favorable prognostic factors. Survival in these cases is now more than 60% (Table 18.5).[26]

Following the prenatal diagnosis of CDH, management should include a detailed search for other anomalies and fetal karyotyping. Expert fetal echocardiography is indicated as examination of the heart is complicated by distortion of intrathoracic contents. Consultation with a pediatric surgeon should be offered and, given the variable prognosis both in terms of perinatal mortality and morbidity, termination of pregnancy is an option that should be discussed. Intrauterine surgery has been performed for CDH. In principle, the airway is occluded and the continued secretion of lung liquid beyond the obstruction leads to expansion of the lung. Early studies involved an open procedure including hysterotomy, which is demanding and carries significant maternal risks,

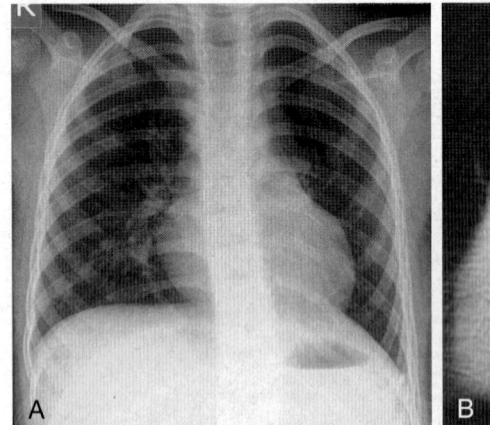
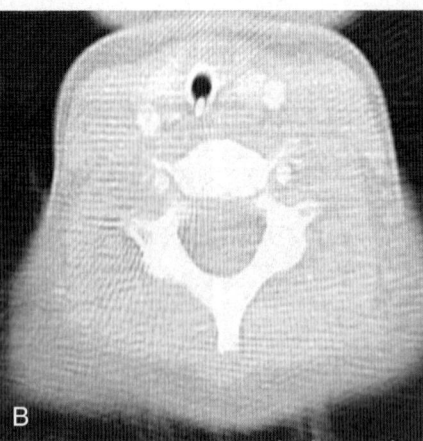
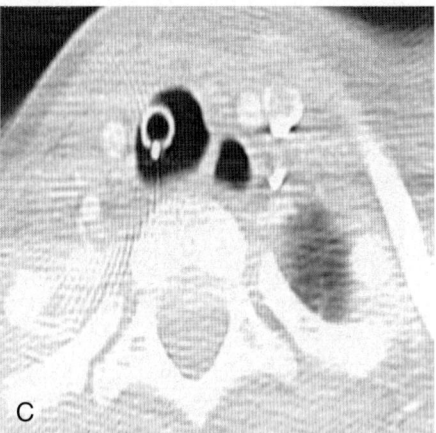

Fig. 18.2 (A) Plain chest radiograph of an infant treated in utero with FETO. Note the huge trachea. (B) High-resolution computed tomography showing the infant has been intubated with an endotracheal tube, which fits snugly in the cervical trachea. (C) The intrathoracic trachea is hugely dilated.

including complications in future pregnancies, as well as the possibility of precipitating preterm labor. Furthermore, although there was some apparent improvement in outcome following in-utero surgery, there has been no well-designed, randomized, controlled trial, so it is not possible to objectively assess the benefits and costs.[27] More recently, fetal endoscopic tracheal occlusion (FETO) using a variety of methods has been used and is currently the only approach used clinically.[28] The currently favored method for FETO is using an inflatable balloon that is placed in the trachea endoscopically. Compared to historical controls in large series, FETO does seem to improve neonatal survival, with preterm labor being the most common complication of pregnancy,[29] and many infants develop tracheomalacia or tracheomegaly (Fig. 18.2).[30] There is now an international randomized controlled trial of FETO in progress. These results are needed, together with long-term follow-up of children who underwent *in utero* therapy, before the true value of this procedure can be accurately evaluated.

Delivery of any ongoing pregnancy should be planned in a center with neonatal intensive care and pediatric surgical facilities. In the event of fetal or perinatal death, a postmortem examination is recommended. This should include a genetic opinion in order to facilitate an accurate diagnosis of any possible underlying syndrome, which may confer an increased risk of recurrence in future pregnancies.

CTM SUBSEQUENTLY DIAGNOSED POSTNATALLY AS CPAM

Antenatal Diagnosis and Prognosis

CPAM is traditionally classified according to histological and clinical findings; however, sonographic classification is best achieved by considering them as either macrocystic (Fig. 18.3) or microcystic (Fig. 18.4).[8] The main differential diagnosis to consider with a macrocystic CPAM is diaphragmatic hernia. Differentiating features are described above. However, in a series of 87 fetuses seen in the Fetal Medicine Unit at University College London Hospitals (UCLH) with a prenatal diagnosis of CPAM, two in fact had a diaphragmatic hernia and one an eventration of the diaphragm (see Table 18.4). In those with a diaphragmatic hernia, the correct diagnosis

was made prenatally after serial scanning. In the patient with an eventration, the correct diagnosis was made only on postnatal imaging.[31] Most CPAMs occur in isolation, although other abnormalities, including bronchopulmonary sequestration and CDH, have been reported to occur in association with CPAM as they have a broad range of extrapulmonary malformations, including renal and cardiac anomalies.[32,33] Indeed, differentiation of these lesions histologically can be challenging as many have a mixed etiology.[2-5] Aneuploidy is not a recognized association.

In general, the prognosis for a fetus with a CPAM is good with only a small number going on to develop hydrops, which is a poor prognostic sign, particularly if it is evident at the initial presentation in the second trimester.[31] Traditionally, both polyhydramnios and mediastinal shift were considered poor prognostic indicators, but data that are more recent suggest that these may be less reliable. Accurate prediction of outcome for prenatally diagnosed lesions can be difficult following a single scan because they can change in size significantly during pregnancy with the majority reducing in size and many appearing to disappear spontaneously. Some may increase in size until around 26 weeks' gestation before reducing in size, while others appear to resolve on sonography.[34] Spontaneous resolution of features, such as hydrops or mediastinal shift, which are usually associated with poor prognosis,[35] has been observed. Various attempts have been made to predict outcome using models that include cyst volumes,[36] but the varied course of these lesions means that serial scans are required to detect those lesions that progress in size or display adverse prognostic features that may warrant consideration of intervention. The Kings College London group has reported on 67 fetuses with an antenatally diagnosed congenital lung malformation.[37] A total of 64 were born alive, and 42 underwent postnatal surgery (see later). Surgery was performed in 45% of lesions showing late gestation "resolution." Although there was some correlation between the antenatal appearances and the need for surgery, this was not usefully predictive for an individual, and the need for operation was judged on the postnatal features of clinical need. In a case series of 119 neonates with an antenatal diagnosis, and who were followed up to the age of 5–16 years, and were cared for at Great Ormond Street Hospital (GOSH),[38] only 8 (6.7%) were symptomatic and required

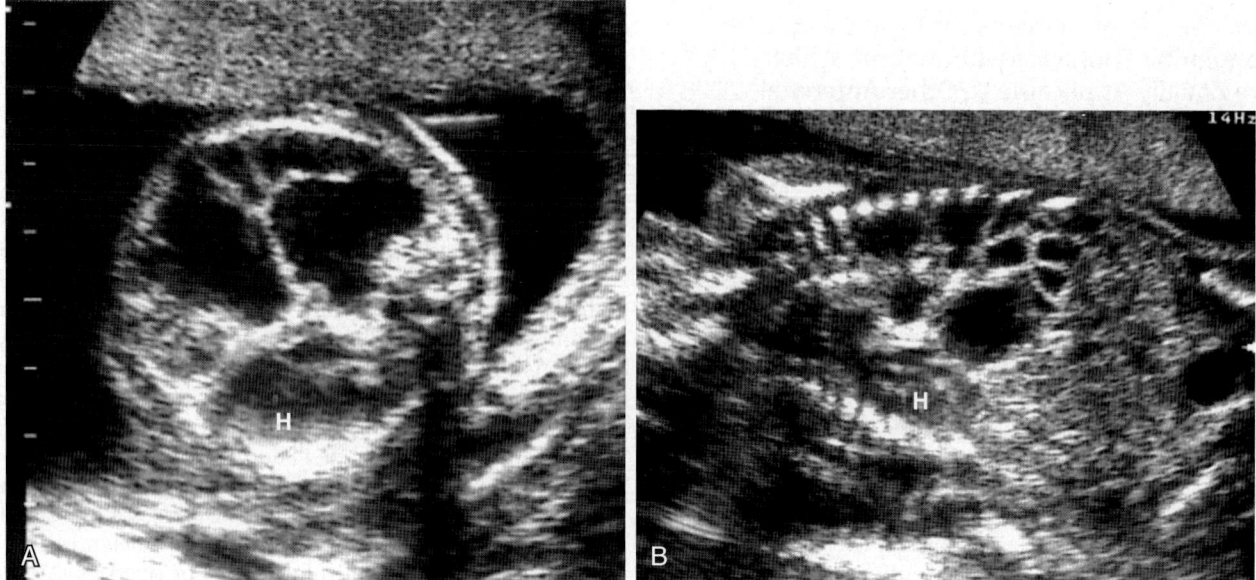

Fig. 18.3 Axial (A) and longitudinal (B) view through the fetus thorax in a fetus referred at 21 weeks' gestation with skin edema and increased liquor. The heart (H) can be seen displaced to the left, and the whole chest appears to be full of abnormal lung tissue. In the longitudinal view the diaphragm is displaced downwards by the abnormally expanded lung tissue. The large cysts were aspirated and pleuro-amniotic shunts inserted, following which the skin edema resolved. The pregnancy continued to term; respiratory support was required at birth with surgery in the neonatal period. The child is now alive and well at school age.

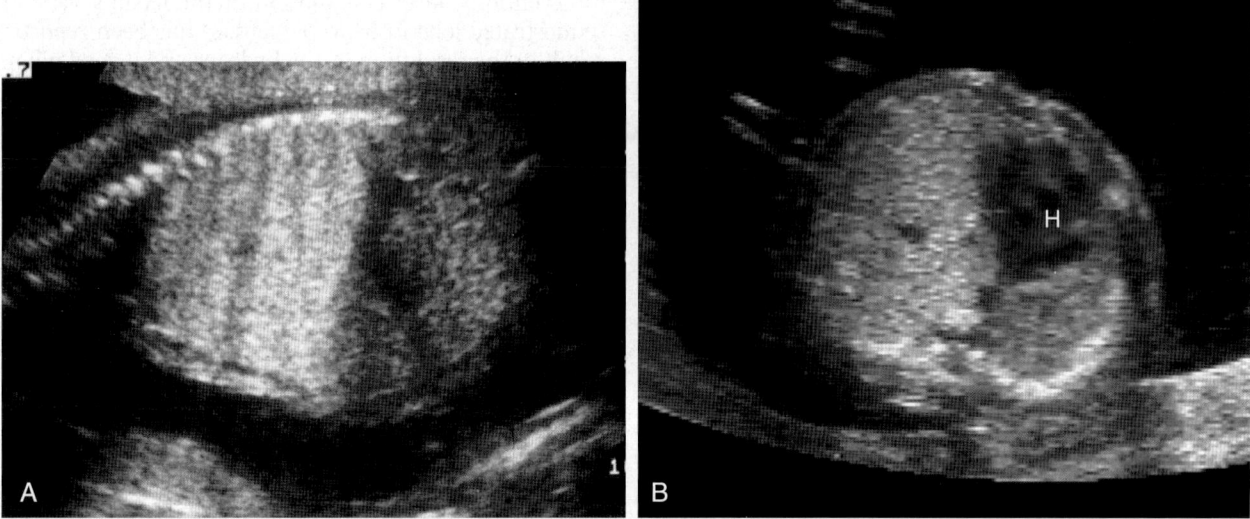

Fig. 18.4 (A) Parasagittal view through the chest at 21 weeks' gestation showing the echogenic wedge-shaped left lower lung behind the chest in a fetus with a microcystic lesion. In the axial view of the fetal chest (B), the abnormal lung can be seen causing marked mediastinal shift with the heart (H) lying in the right chest. The mediastinal shift resolved as pregnancy progressed, and the baby was well at birth. Postnatal imaging confirmed the presence of the lesion, and a conservative management policy was followed.

emergency surgery during the neonatal period. This is in keeping with another large case series from the University of Southampton of 72 neonates with a prenatal diagnosis of congenital lung malformation, where only one required emergency surgery.[39] The use of elective surgery remains controversial[40] as indicated by the lower rate of surgery overall (43%) in the GOSH cohort where surgery was usually only performed on clinical grounds compared with the Kings series, and these data demonstrate the varying approach to management. Table 18.4 shows the type of cystic lung lesion, other sonographic findings, diagnosis, and outcome for the

UCLH cohort.[31] In all cases, early consultation with neonatal and pediatric surgical staff is helpful for parents.

Antenatal Treatment Options

There is very little agreement on definitions, even for something as basic as fetal hydrops, and only a limited evidence base as to the antenatal options for treatment. There have been no randomized, controlled trials,[41] so small case series are the only basis for decision making. Most would agree that an expectant approach is best, reserving treatment for hydropic fetuses, or perhaps in the rare case with a rapidly

---

Box 18.2   Requirements for Fetal Surgery for Congenital Thoracic Malformation, Which Are Equally Applicable to Other Antenatal Interventions

A CTM causing hydrops or preventing acceptable fetal lung development

Singleton fetus with no other important abnormality

Serial assessment to ensure the CTM really requires fetal surgery, and is salvageable

Family counseled and agree to treatment and long-term follow up

Multidisciplinary team agree on a treatment plan

Access to high level obstetric and neonatal care, and bioethical and psychosocial consultation

CTM, Congenital thoracic malformation.

---

expanding lesion in the last trimester. Even in large units, the performance of invasive interventions is unusual.[37] The least aggressive intervention is the administration of betamethasone to the mother for which there is limited reported experience.[42–46] In a case series of nine patients who had not responded to a single dose, repeat doses led to stabilization (*n* = 4), improvement (*n* = 3) or had no effect and the lesion progressed, necessitating antenatal surgery, both of whom died, as did one other baby.[44] Obstetric complications in the mother were common, mandating careful follow-up. Long-standing requirements for fetal surgery are shown in Box 18.2,[47] and these are surely applicable to any antenatal intervention for a CTM. However, intrauterine surgery is increasingly performed for a widening spectrum of diagnoses,[48] including CTMs.[49,50] Where there are single or multiple large cysts (see Fig. 18.3) with associated hydrops or polyhydramnios, in-utero decompression by thoracentesis or the insertion of a shunt has led to improvement.[51,52] Intrauterine surgery to remove these lesions has been reported, but has been very rarely undertaken due to the associated fetal mortality and maternal morbidity.[51] In one small series, the outcomes of shunting were good, and decompressing a single cyst was sufficient to cause the mass to collapse; it was suggested that shunting might be indicated early, before hydrops develops, in high-risk lesions.[53] Other surgical options include fetal sclerotherapy[49,54,55] and radiofrequency ablation. However, fetal death has resulted from this last technique.[36] Percutaneous laser ablation, guiding the beam into the fetal thorax via a fine needle placed under ultrasound control may be aimed at vascular or "interstitial" ablation.[56] The results were best for babies with a postnatal sequestration (87.5% survival) rather than CPAM (28.6%), and the immediate results were better with vascular ablation. It is concerning that marked postnatal chest deformity has been associated with fetal shunt insertion. Finally, there are case reports of interventional fetal bronchoscopy to treat congenital lesions with a poor prognosis[57,58]; as always, it is difficult to assess such reports, and this intervention must be considered highly experimental until more data become available.

Where a lesion has persisted, or increased in size, and mediastinal shift persists in the third trimester, delivery in a center with neonatal intensive care and surgical facilities is indicated. In all cases there should be careful postnatal follow-up, with computed tomography (CT) being offered to all.

There are many examples of lesions that apparently involuted completely in utero being present when examined by CT after birth.

CONGENITAL THORACIC MALFORMATION SUBSEQUENTLY DIAGNOSED PATHOLOGICALLY AS BRONCHOPULMONARY SEQUESTRATION

In the fetus a sequestered lobe of lung is most often identified as a mass of uncertain origin in the chest or subdiaphragmatic area. Prenatally it is not possible to make a definitive diagnosis unless an independent blood supply is demonstrated using Doppler ultrasound, although it should be noted that a CPAM might also have an aortic blood supply. The sequestrated lobe usually appears as an echogenic mass in the chest (Fig. 18.5) or abdomen (Fig. 18.6). It can be associated with hydrops, mediastinal shift, and polyhydramnios (see Fig. 18.5). The outcome for fetuses with bronchopulmonary sequestration is generally good when presentation is uncomplicated by pleural effusions or hydrops. As such, the prenatal management of fetuses with lesions suspected to be a sequestration is similar for those with a suspected CPAM; therefore, serial scanning should be undertaken and the fetus should be delivered in a tertiary unit if there is significant mediastinal shift in the third trimester. Spontaneous improvement in utero is frequently reported. In a review of the literature describing neonatal outcomes after in-utero interventions, laser coagulation of the feeding vessel to a sequestrated lobe in hydropic fetuses has been reported to result in the resolution of the hydrops and a good neonatal outcome in several cases.[59]

PRESENTATION OF CONGENITAL THORACIC MALFORMATIONS IN THE IMMEDIATE POSTNATAL PERIOD

Postnatal presentations of many abnormalities of course overlap; in summary, presentation is with immediate neonatal respiratory distress; the delayed development of symptoms or a complication of a known or previously undiagnosed abnormality; or the child may have an asymptomatic lesion for which active management may or may not be indicated.

The differential diagnosis of acute unexpected respiratory distress in a term newborn extends well beyond congenital lung disease to include conditions such as congenital infections, interstitial lung disease, pneumothorax, cardiac disease, and primary ciliary dyskinesia. If a congenital lung abnormality has been identified antenatally, the diagnosis of the cause of the respiratory distress is likely obvious. Not all lesions are detected prenatally, although with increasing use and improvements in technology and sonographic skills, postnatal presentation is becoming less common. Late detection may particularly be an issue in diaphragmatic hernias, some of which do not present with sonographic findings until after the time of the routine anomaly scan, or, indeed, well after birth. Respiratory distress in the absence of major airway disease may be due to disorders of the lung parenchyma. These include a large cystic or solid CTM, the presence of unilateral or bilateral small lungs, and congenital pleural effusion or lymphatic disorder. The differential diagnosis of a cystic abnormality detected postnatally, but not antenatally, includes cysts secondary to infection[60] or pulmonary

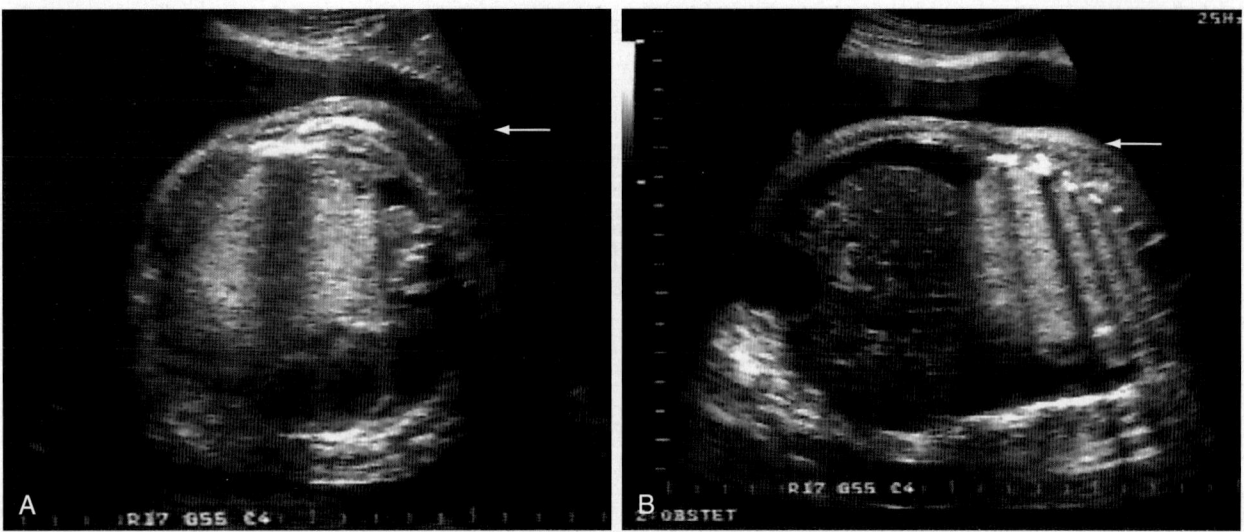

Fig. 18.5 Axial (A) and longitudinal (B) view through the thorax of a fetus that presented at 34 weeks' gestation with hydrops and polyhydramnios. The large echogenic mass can be seen occupying most of the chest. There is a significant rim of ascitic fluid seen in the abdomen as well as pleural effusions in the chest. Preterm labor ensued after amniodrainage. Resuscitation failed and a postmortem demonstrated a sequestrated lobe with associated pulmonary hypoplasia.

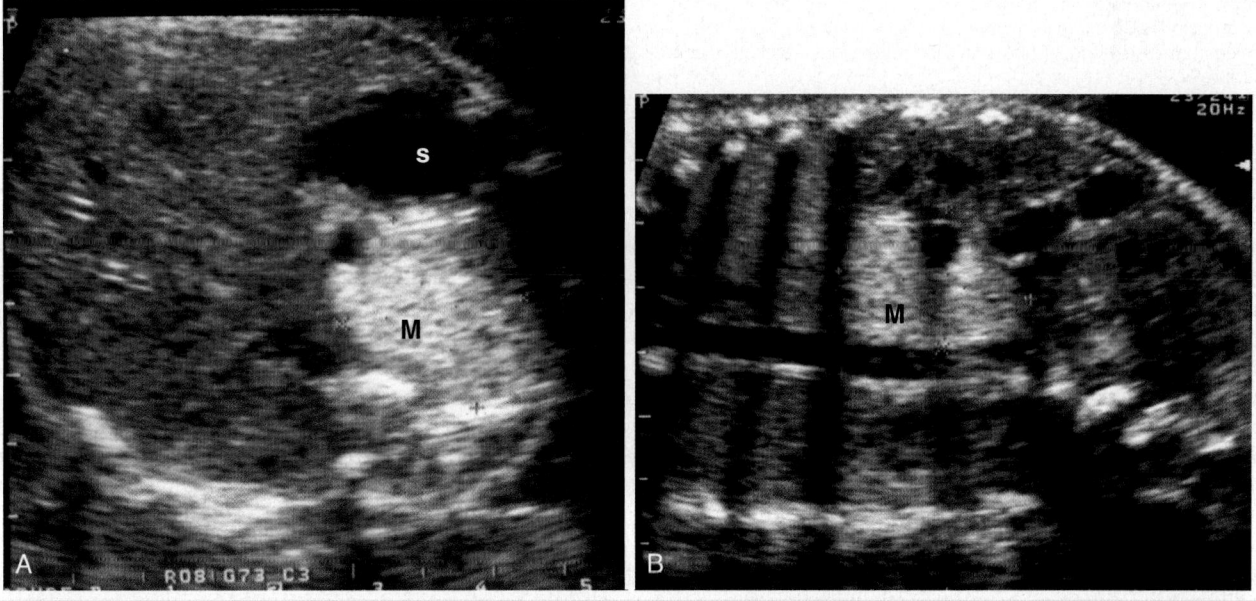

Fig. 18.6 Axial (A) and longitudinal (B) view through the abdomen of a fetus at 22 weeks' gestation. Note the echogenic mass (M) related to the diaphragm lying behind the stomach (S). An ultrasound-guided needle biopsy after birth confirmed this to be a pulmonary sequestration. This subsequently resolved spontaneously in early childhood.

interstitial emphysema,[61] which may present in localized form even in a term baby who has not been ventilated.

The management of CTMs after the immediate postnatal period, both asymptomatic and those that have become symptomatic after a latent period of as long as many years, is discussed below. The King's College Hospital group (see earlier)[37] actually performed surgery in 45% of lesions showing late-gestation "resolution." Although there was some correlation between the antenatal appearances and the need for surgery, this was not usefully predictive for an individual, and the need for an operation was judged on postnatal features rather than clinical need. In general, the approach to the postnatal management of neonates with

prenatally diagnosed cystic lung lesions is very variable. There are those who feel that all lesions should be surgically removed, and others who favor a more conservative approach (Table 18.6). At UCLH, we have seen 110 fetuses with cystic lung lesions in the last 15 years, of whom 100 are alive, 20 having had surgery. This is a much lower proportion than in the King's series and demonstrates the varying approach to management. In all cases, early consultation with neonatal and pediatric surgical staff is helpful for parents. The issues of postnatal management are discussed in more detail below. Where a lesion has persisted or increased in size and mediastinal shift persists in the third trimester, delivery in a center with neonatal intensive care and surgical facilities should

Table 18.6   Reported Outcomes and Postnatal Management in Recent Series of Cystic Lung Lesions

	Total	Resolved in Utero	Alive	Other Diagnosis	ToP	IUD/PND	Postnatal Management		
							Surgery Emergency	Elective	Conservative
Kunisaki 2007[370,a]	12	0	9	5	0	3[b]	4	5	0
Illanes 2005[371]	48	22 (5)	39	5	3 (1[b])	6[b]	0	23	6 (+5 LTFU)
Pumberger 2003[372]	35	11 (6)	29	3	4	2	4	17	2
Laberge 2001[373]	48	23 regressed	36	4	7	5	Not reported	Not reported	Not reported
De Santis 2000[374]	17	3	14	0	2	2	4		6 (+2 LTFU)
Miller 1996[375]	17	0	12	0	3	2	12		0
Sauvat 2003[376,c]	29	4 (4)	29	0	0	0	3	14	12
Davenport 2004[37]	67	8 (1)	64	7	1	4	42		12 (+10 LTFU)
Lacy 1999[38]	23	9 (4)	19	5	4	1	5		13
Calvert 2007[62]	19	0	19	0	5	2	3	13	3
UCLH[31]	110	11 (9)	100	12	7	3	12	8	46 (+17 postnatal diagnosis awaited & 4 LTFU)
Ehrenberg-Buchner, 2013[377]	64	0	61 (2 lost to follow-up)	3	0	1	7	Not stated	Not stated
Ruchonnet-Metrailler, 2014[378]	89	0	87	9	0	2	5	Not stated	Not stated
Kunisaki 2015[379]	100	17	99	1	0	1	11	Not stated	Not stated

[a]Only large lesions.
[b]Only severe hydrops.
[c]Only reports antenatally diagnosed cases who were asymptomatic.
Numbers in parentheses refer to cases with no signs on postnatal imaging either. Other diagnoses include CDH, tracheal atresia, etc.
CDH, Congenital diaphragmatic hernia; *IUD/PND*, intrauterine or perinatal death; *LTFU*, lost to follow-up; *ToP*, termination of pregnancy.
Modified from Bush, Hogg J, Chitty LS. Cystic lung lesions—prenatal diagnosis and management. *Prenat Diagn*. 2008;28:604-611, with permission from Wiley Blackwell.

be considered. In all cases, careful postnatal follow-up should be undertaken, with CT being offered to all, even if the lesion has apparently disappeared completely antenatally; chest x-ray (CXR) is only 61% sensitive to the presence of lesions on high-resolution computed tomography (HRCT).[62] Lesions that have apparently involuted completely in utero are well documented to still be present when examined by CT after birth.

Vascular abnormalities may present at this time. One such group are aortopulmonary collaterals supplying either a CSL or a CTM. These act hemodynamically as systemic arteriovenous malformations and cause high-output heart failure. Abnormalities of venous drainage, such as "scimitar" syndrome (hemianomalous pulmonary venous drainage to the inferior caval vein), may also present as heart failure or enter the differential diagnosis of pulmonary hypertension in the newborn period. Other vascular problems that may present at this time include alveolar-capillary dysplasia (discussed in Chapter 54) and pulmonary arteriovenous malformation (PAVM), which may present as cyanosis in a well infant (not with heart failure, unless there is an associated systemic, usually cerebral, arteriovenous malformation). The presentations of congenital lung disease after the postnatal period, and the issues around prophylactic surgery, are discussed in more detail below.

Specific Diagnoses: Upper Respiratory Tract Atresias

Laryngeal or tracheal atresia are rare malformations that may be isolated or found in association with other abnormalities or genetic syndromes, the most common of which

is Fraser syndrome.[63] The diagnosis of laryngeal or tracheal obstruction should be suspected when enlarged, uniformly hyperechogenic lungs are seen on ultrasound (Fig. 18.7). Other sonographic features include cardiac and mediastinal compression, flattening or convexity of the diaphragms, hydrops, and polyhydramnios. A dilated, fluid-filled upper trachea can also be seen in tracheal atresia (Fig. 18.8). The differential diagnosis of laryngeal or tracheal atresia includes subglottic stenosis (SGS) and bilateral microcystic CCAM. When associated with Fraser syndrome, there may be renal anomalies, syndactyly of fingers and toes, and cryptophthalmos. The prognosis is invariably poor, and the option of termination of pregnancy should be discussed. Parents should also have the opportunity to discuss the prognosis with a pediatric surgeon, and, if the pregnancy is continued, delivery should be planned in a unit with neonatal intensive care and pediatric surgical facilities. Prenatal analysis of chorionic villi or amniocytes using exome sequencing may help reveal any underlying genetic etiology, which will aid prenatal counseling.[64] Rarely, antenatal tracheostomy has been reported, although this may precipitate fetal distress and preterm delivery.[65] Ex utero intrapartum treatment (EXIT procedure) has been reported (below).

Specific Postnatal Problems: Congenital Abnormalities of the Upper Airway

This section will detail the variety of different congenital abnormalities that involve the upper airway and will deal with clinical problems involving the larynx and trachea.

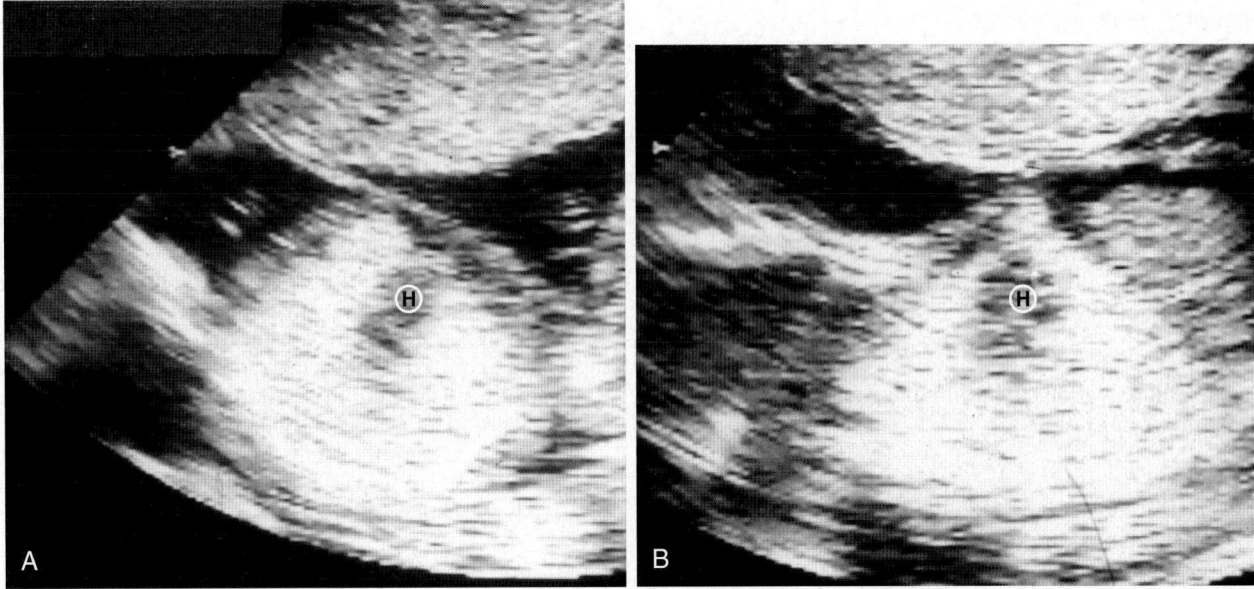

Fig. 18.7 Axial (A) and longitudinal (B) view the thorax of a fetus at 19 weeks' gestation with tracheal agenesis. The lungs are completely bright and can be seen compressing the heart (H) in (A). In the longitudinal plane, the diaphragms are displaced downwards by the expanded lung issue.

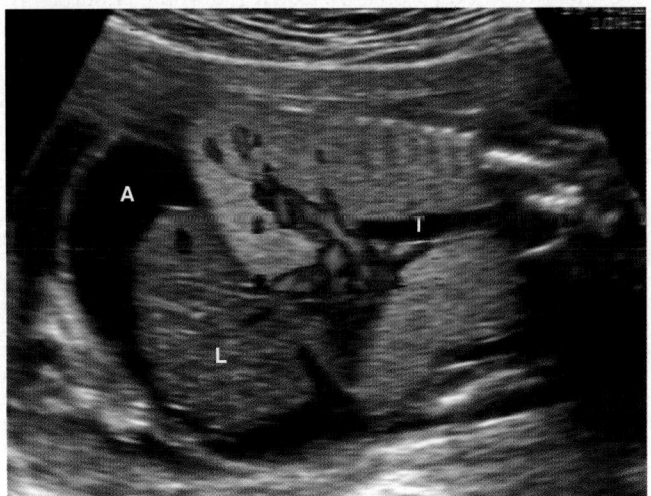

Fig. 18.8 Longitudinal view of a fetus with tracheal agenesis. The heart can be seen highlighted by the color Doppler with the abnormally dilated trachea (T) seen as a fluid-filled structure in the mediastinum. The lungs bulge downwards into the ascites (A) in the abdominal cavity in which the liver (L) can be seen.

Table 18.7 Congenital Conditions Above the Larynx and Trachea Causing Neonatal Airway Obstruction

INTRINSIC	
Nose	Atresia (absence); e.g., arhinia
	Choanal atresia (complete obstruction)
	Piriform aperture stenosis (narrowing)
	Severe craniofacial abnormalities; e.g., hemifacial microsomia (Goldenhar syndrome) and the mid-facial syndromes (e.g., Apert or Crouzon syndrome)
Oral Cavity and Oropharynx	Macroglossia; e.g., Pierre-Robin sequence
	Retrognathia; e.g., Treacher-Collins syndrome
EXTRINSIC	
Viscero-cranial and Neck masses	Lymphatic malformations; e.g., cystic hygroma
	Vascular malformations; e.g., arterio-venous malformation
	Vascular tumors; e.g., capillary hemangiomas
	Encephaloceles

Though this section will not cover the complete spectrum of congenital disorders that can cause respiratory disorders in neonates, the pediatric otolaryngologist will be experienced in dealing with airway problems due to congenital abnormalities involving the whole airway from the anterior nares to the bronchi. The abnormalities may be intrinsic or extrinsic to the airway and be single or multiple. The spectrum of disorders is detailed in Tables 18.7 and 18.8.

These abnormalities may present with immediate respiratory distress at delivery but may equally be more subtle in their clinical symptoms and signs. Airway abnormalities should be considered in the presence of an abnormal cry, weak or husky voice, or recurrent crouplike episodes.

Difficulties with feeding may also be a feature of airway abnormalities, such as laryngomalacia or laryngeal cleft. In these situations, there may be recurrent episodes of aspiration with feeding (laryngeal cleft) or respiratory distress and gastroesophageal reflux (laryngomalacia)

This text aims to offers a practical guide to the management of airway obstruction. This initial section describes a comprehensive assessment of a child presenting with stridor in the office-based scenario moving onto management of this child, including descriptions of common elective procedural-based assessments. The subsequent sections augment the discussion of airway management with consideration of the acutely unwell child presenting in the emergency room and the increasingly common scenario we are faced with in the hospital setting concerning children with intubation/extubation difficulties. As always, the appropriate assessment

Table 18.8 Congenital Abnormalities of the Larynx and Trachea

Larynx	Laryngeal atresia and webs
	Laryngeal cleft
	Laryngomalacia
	Vocal cord paralysis
	Saccular cysts and laryngoceles
	Subglottic hemangiomas
	Congenital subglottic stenosis
Trachea	Tracheomalacia
	Congenital tracheal stenosis
	(complete tracheal rings)

of pediatric airway problems commences with clinical history taking and examination.

STRIDOR

Quite often the most important feature in the history is the time of onset and character of stridor. Stridor present since birth most indicates a congenital pathology, such as laryngeal webs or bilateral vocal cord paralysis, whereas a more gradual onset of symptoms over days/weeks to months points to diagnoses such as laryngomalacia, subglottic hemangiomas, or cysts. An acute onset of symptoms, accompanied by corroborating factors in the history, can lead towards diagnosing foreign body aspiration and inflammatory or infectious conditions as the etiological factor (see Chapter 23). The characteristics of the stridor itself can also be a diagnostic aid: inspiratory suggests glottic pathology (and that in the immediate supraglottis); biphasic subglottic or extra thoracic trachea pathology; and expiratory intrathoracic, trachea, and bronchial pathology. Another diagnostic indicator of stridor is its character. Stridor of a constant nature indicates a fixed lesion pathology as opposed to the intermittent symptoms of conditions such as laryngomalacia.

VOICE/CRY

In addition to stridor there are other laryngeal symptoms that should be taken into consideration such as the voice/cry and cough. These symptoms particularly implicate glottis level pathology, either structural (webs, papilloma) or functional (vocal cord paralysis).

COUGH

Cough itself can be associated with other factors in the history, such as its relation to upper respiratory tract infections (URTIs) and croup. If there is a history of recurrent or prolonged croup, consideration should be given to the need to diagnose an underlying airway stenosis or inhaled and retained foreign body, or subglottic hemangioma. Cough can also be related to aspiration events related to feeds where, with the aid of swallowing, assessment of the presence of vocal cord palsy, laryngeal cleft, or TEF may need to be investigated.

CYANOSIS

Episodes of cyanosis certainly indicate severe respiratory difficulty and can be due to several causes, but they are often associated with tracheal disease, including external compression due to the presence of a vascular ring.

NEONATAL INTUBATION

Perhaps one of the most important factors in the history should be that pertaining to the birth history and, more specifically, neonatal intubation. Respiratory difficulty at birth and the need and duration of intubation and ventilation should lower the threshold for proceeding to diagnostic microlaryngobronchoscopy (MLB) in those children with an otherwise less concerning symptomatic history. Subglottic cysts and acquired stenosis are often an endoscopic finding in these cases. The premature infant is therefore often in this high-risk group for airway pathology. Additionally, this patient subgroup is also more likely to have undergone cardiac surgery, which can be associated with upper airway pathology, such as recurrent laryngeal nerve palsy.

OTHER COMORBIDITIES

These should also be sought in the history as these can be associated with particular pathologies. Many of the craniofacial syndromes are associated with airway difficulties that are often multilevel problems. Down syndrome children are known to have difficulties due to macroglossia and congenital SGS. There are also several conditions that can be associated with hypotonia, such as cerebral palsy, leading to airway difficulties.

Examination of a Child Presenting in the Clinic Setting

This starts with appropriate exposure and inspection to allow an overall assessment to be made about the severity of respiratory distress as well as diagnostic clues to the underlying pathology. The presence and nature of stridor can indicate the level of likely airway pathology as previously discussed. Chest wall movement, the use of accessory muscles, tracheal tug, sternal recession and subcostal or intercostal recession, nasal flaring and head bobbing, the voice/cry, the presence of cutaneous hemangiomas, and any dysmorphic features should be given careful consideration. In particular, craniofacial abnormalities are likely to impact on the airway, and the most common ones include macroglossia and retrognathia. The oral cavity should always be inspected as part of the airway assessment and, in addition to tongue and mandibular features, tonsillar pathology (size) should also be taken into consideration. Obstructive airway problems, such as these at the oropharyngeal level, lead to stertor and, therefore, can be distinguished from those causes of stridor at a more distal level. The nasal airway also should be assessed for patency to exclude choanal atresia.

Fiberoptic nasoendoscopy (FNE) should be performed where possible to complete an airway assessment in the office/clinic setting. With parental cooperation, this can be achieved in infants and in the older child, but it may be more challenging in the 2- to 5-year-old age group where restraint is often not practical. Topical nasal preparations of local anesthetic combined with decongestant can be used to aid the

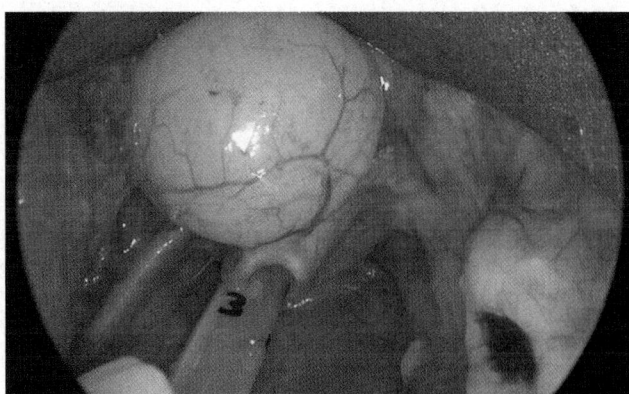

Fig. 18.9 A large vallecular cyst seen on fiberoptic nasoendoscopy. It was subsequently excised at microlaryngobronchoscopy.

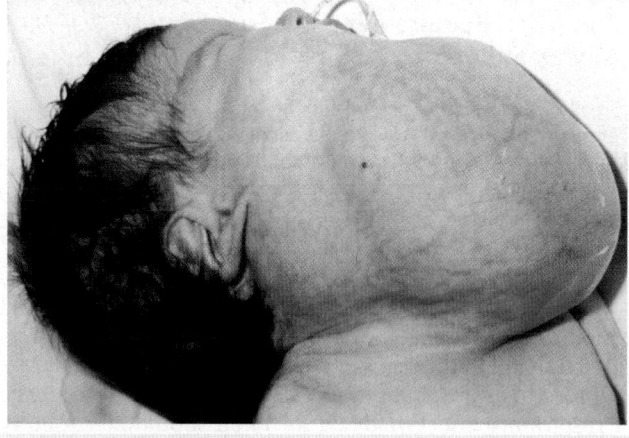

Fig. 18.10 Severe neonatal upper airway obstruction due to cystic hygroma. (Picture reproduced courtesy of Mr. C.M. Bailey.)

examination with the fiberoptic scope; this is often used in the older child, but is often omitted in the examination of the infant. FNE is particularly useful to assess nasal anatomy and pathology down to the glottic level with conditions such as choanal atresia and laryngomalacia readily diagnosed with this technique. It can also identify other supraglottic pathology, such as vallecular cysts, and such information can be beneficial in planning airway assessment under general anesthetic (Fig. 18.9). However, it is unsuitable to evaluate pathology at a more distal level to the glottis.

Definitive assessment of the airway is by means of a diagnostic MLB performed under general anesthetic. This technique allows for a full structural and dynamic assessment of the upper airway from nares to bronchi. Increasingly, MLB techniques have developed to allow treatment as well as diagnosis in conditions previously considered only to be amenable to open airway surgery. Successful MLB relies on good collaboration between the surgical and anesthetic teams. The technique requires an anaesthetized but spontaneously ventilating patient with a nasal prong and gas/air mix or with titrated total intravenous anesthesia (TIVA). The larynx is sprayed with a local anesthetic solution to reduce the depth of anesthesia required to allow instrumentation of the larynx; however, this may exaggerate the appearances of laryngomalacia.[66] The patient should be positioned with a head ring and shoulder roll to achieve the optimal position for airway endoscopy. Diagnostic MLB can be performed successfully with an anesthetic straight or curved blade laryngoscope and a zero-degree Hopkins rod of the appropriate size, usually 4 mm. This simple technique with minimal instrumentation allows the main subsites to be visualized without major irritability to the airway. If required, suspension MLB can then be performed using one of the many laryngoscopes that are available. This technique is preferred for treatment purposes when a two-handed approach is required. The ventilating bronchoscope should always be available. Once the airway subsites have been assessed, the cricoarytenoid joints are palpated for fixation and interarytenoid area for a laryngeal cleft, any stenosis present is sized with an endotracheal (ET) tube and, finally, a dynamic assessment should be made checking for vocal cord movement in addition to any supraglottic prolapse due to laryngomalacia.

The Emergent/Marginal Airway and Difficult Intubations

DEFINITION

The *Emergent Airway* is that transition point at which a patient's oxygen saturation becomes difficult or impossible to maintain above 90% during an intubation or procedure.

Assessment of a neonate presenting in an emergency with airway difficulty is often an unnerving situation for all concerned. It is important to have a clear and methodical plan to implement in these circumstances to aid prompt diagnosis and appropriate intervention. The history is again important and should aim to cover those points discussed in the previous section. Immediate examination in the delivery room may provide an obvious diagnosis by the pediatric staff, such as a major craniofacial abnormality, but severe airway problems, such as congenital tracheal stenosis, may have no external physical signs.

Accordingly, it is not unusual for children to be stabilized by the attending pediatric team before a definitive diagnosis is made. This might include intubation of the child; the use of oral airways in the case of nasal obstruction (e.g., choanal atresia); nursing the child prone in cases of oral/oropharyngeal obstruction (e.g., in Pierre-Robin sequence); and the use of a nasopharyngeal airway (NPA) if the obstruction is not easily relieved. If intubation is extremely difficult, it may be appropriate to consider immediate tracheostomy to avoid the risk of the ET tube becoming dislodged and failure to reintubate. This might be considered with a large cystic hygroma (Fig. 18.10). If the anatomy of the neck is very abnormal, it may be useful to pass a rigid bronchoscope to allow ventilation and act as a marker for the trachea within the distorted anatomy of the neck.

As outlined above, a child who has chronic or episodic stridor may be examined with a flexible endoscope to assess the upper airway and diagnose supraglottic pathology. The requirements for this procedure to be performed safely are given in Box 18.3.

Box 18.3   Requirements for Safe Upper Airway Endoscopy

Small diameter endoscope (ideally 1.8 mm)
Access to pediatric resuscitation equipment and personnel, especially skilled pediatric anesthesiology
Stable neonate (minimal oxygen or air pressure support)

Examination of the child in this situation is often performed concurrently, as rapid assessment is required. The principle of assessment in this "emergency" should principally address the need to establish an immediate safe airway. The degree of respiratory effort made by the child should be carefully observed, and signs such as an opisthotonic posture with severe recession prompt urgency. Pulse oximetry can be very useful in this situation but not relied upon, as decompensation can be rapid with reduced oxygen saturations being a late sign; in particular, if the child is breathing oxygen-enriched mixtures, severe hypercapnia can be masked. Often a child that is quietening in terms of their respiratory effort could be tiring and deteriorating rather than improving.

General assessment of signs of toxicity should also be made and these include measures of temperature, heart rate, and capillary refill. These signs can be determined by inspection of the patient alone with minimal contact. In an emergent airway, a more probing examination can lead to a rapid deterioration in symptoms and this should be avoided in an uncontrolled environment.

Attempts should be made to further evaluate such a child in a relatively more controlled theatre environment with a senior anesthetist and ear-nose-throat (ENT) surgeon present to assess and secure the airway as deemed appropriate. Several measures can be employed to manage an emergent airway that can lead to adequate control of the symptoms or at least to provide a holding measure whilst deploying the appropriate teams to manage the situation definitively. These include oxygen, nebulized adrenaline, Heliox, and steroids. If an infective etiology is suspected, a diagnostic MLB may not be necessary and, in fact, is often contraindicated in severe cases, such as acute epiglottitis.

The aim should be to stabilize the airway with either medical treatment that can include oxygenation, steroids, and antibiotics, or to secure the airway with intubation, often by the anesthetists with an ENT surgeon merely on standby in case of difficulty. Techniques for a difficult intubation include the use of the ventilating bronchoscope or intubation with an ET tube placed over a 2.7 mm Hopkins rod. These techniques are perhaps used less often by ENT surgeons due to the advances in airway adjuncts for our anesthetic colleagues. Equipment, such as video glidascopes, can improve the grade of view at laryngoscopy facilitating intubation. Fiberoptic intubation is also more commonplace but very difficult in the neonate.

Again, if intubation is not possible, the option of a surgical airway must be considered. The situation is still controlled if ventilation can still be achieved by either the bag and mask technique or a laryngeal mask airway (LMA). An NPA should be considered if the level of obstruction is at the nasal or oropharyngeal level. Similarly, distal disease may require positive airway pressure support.

Extubation Difficulties/Failed Extubation

Once successful intubation has been achieved, it is hoped that a child can be successfully extubated with a view to further elective treatment or investigation as necessary. This is certainly the situation in cases of infective etiologies. However, those with underlying structural abnormalities represent a far more challenging situation and may require more immediate management as often intubation can lead to an irritation and worsening of the structural component. In fact, there are an increasing number of cases with difficulties in extubation, and this correlates with the number of premature infants with prolonged periods of intubation and ventilation.

Unfortunately, difficulty with extubation often leads to cases of multiple reintubations that can lead to further airway trauma, particularly to the very fragile neonatal subglottic mucosa.[67] Successful extubation relies upon optimal respiratory function, including a patent airway and sufficient respiratory drive and neuromuscular function. Therefore, in the very premature, the preferential management may require the neonate to remain ventilated for a prolonged period allowing lung function to improve. A period of expectant intubation can also minimize the problems that occur with repeated attempts at intubation following failed extubation. This period of "laryngeal rest" is often overlooked as a management option. In these cases, when extubation is finally planned, a 24- to 48-hour period of corticosteroid cover and aggressive management of gastro esophageal/laryngopharyngeal reflux is beneficial prior to extubation.

If there is a failed attempt at extubation, it is important to determine the symptoms and signs leading up to reintubation. Any accounts of stridor should suggest the likelihood of airway pathology although it may not be necessary to investigate this immediately if successful extubation can be achieved with the more conservative measures described above. However, if there is a recurrent problem, MLB should be performed to diagnose and plan the management of any underlying structural airway pathologies. For example, seal flipper granulations or subglottic cysts can be identified and removed to relieve any airway obstruction (Fig. 18.11). The caliber of the subglottis can also be assessed, and most importantly an early and evolving sub glottis stenosis can be treated (Fig. 18.12). If there are continued difficulties with failed extubation relating to ventilation issues or continued and significant airway pathology, a tracheostomy may be required in this period. If a tracheostomy is performed, it is important to monitor these cases so that any changes in the clinical situation can be monitored and the option of decannulation entertained.

Congenital Abnormalities of the Larynx

LARYNGOMALACIA

Laryngomalacia is a dynamic condition and is the most common cause of stridor in infants (Fig. 18.13). It occurs due to collapse of the relatively immature cartilaginous supraglottic structures, which has been postulated due to an incoordination of the laryngeal muscles due to neuromuscular immaturity. This leads to a mistiming of laryngeal movements and tends to cause indrawing and lengthening of the supraglottic structures. However, laryngomalacia may just be a structural variation.[68,69]

This functional collapse can be related to specific structural features:

1. The aryepiglottic folds are short and vertical, curling the epiglottis into an omega shape.

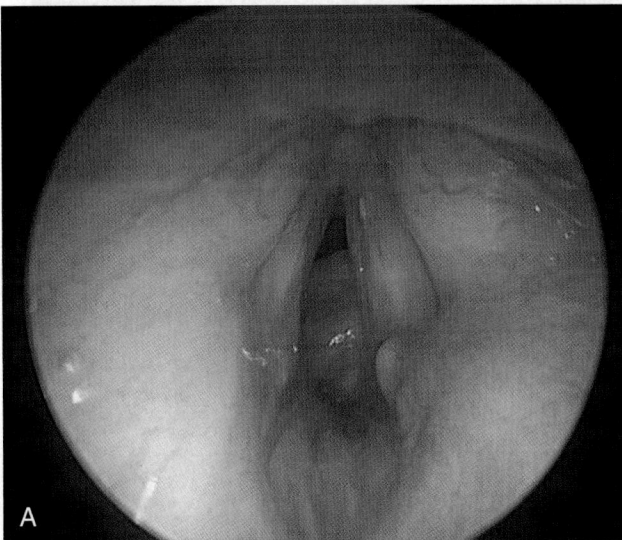

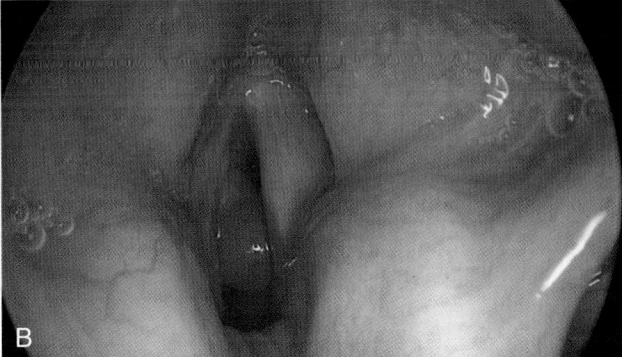

Fig. 18.11 (A and B) Two examples of sublottic cysts secondary to intubation.

2. Prominent cuneiform and corniculate cartilages lie over the arytenoid cartilages, which prolapse into the airway.
3. A loose, redundant mucosal covering of the aryepiglottic fold prolapses into the airway.

There is a high concomitant incidence of gastroesophageal reflux in infants with laryngomalacia, presumably because of the more negative intrathoracic pressures necessary to overcome inspiratory obstruction.[70] Conversely, children with significant reflux may also exhibit pathological changes similar to laryngomalacia, especially enlargement and swelling of the arytenoid cartilages.

Presentation

Laryngomalacia is most often managed without involvement of ENT surgeons in its mildest form with infants presenting to the primary care physician or pediatrician with stridor, but are otherwise well. The stridor is often not present at birth, but occurs during the first few weeks of life as it is postulated that inspiratory flow rates may not be adequate initially to generate airway noise. Symptoms are rarely present beyond the age of 2 years.

The prolapse of supraglottic structures produces an inspiratory stridor that is most evident when the infant is supine, or during feeding or crying; also, it has a characteristically high-pitched nature. Severe cases present with failure to thrive with infants falling off the growth centiles. Some children with laryngomalacia can have obstructive sleep apnea (OSA) associated with the condition and may require a detailed sleep history.

In most cases, diagnosis can be made on clinical grounds alone. As this is a dynamic condition, awake FNE can confirm the diagnosis. Cases that are moderate to severe or those with atypical features in the history may require MLB to rule out synchronous airway lesions and/or provide surgical therapeutic intervention. A sleep study may be indicated in those cases with a strong history of OSA.

Often the management is conservative with observation and reassurance until the symptoms subside with age. Serial plotting on a growth chart can be a useful tool in assessing satisfactory progress. Infants with reflux can be trialed on antireflux treatments. Surgical intervention, most commonly an aryepiglottoplasty/supraglottoplasty, is usually only required if there is concern about failure to thrive, or severe respiratory compromise/cyanotic spells, or, in cases of an

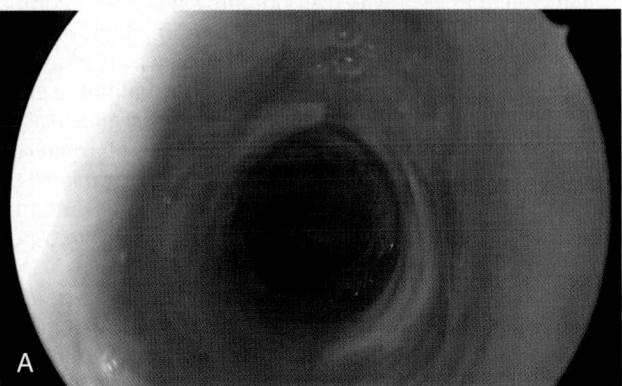

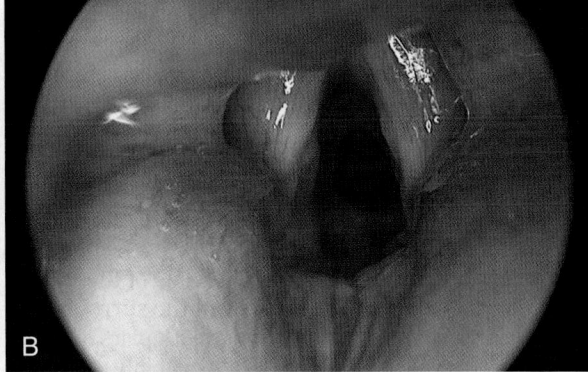

Fig. 18.12 Intubation injury (A) removal of the endotracheal tube at microlaryngobronchoscopy reveals blanching of the subglottic mucosa. (B) Damage to this fragile area subsequently leads to an acquired subglottic stenosis.

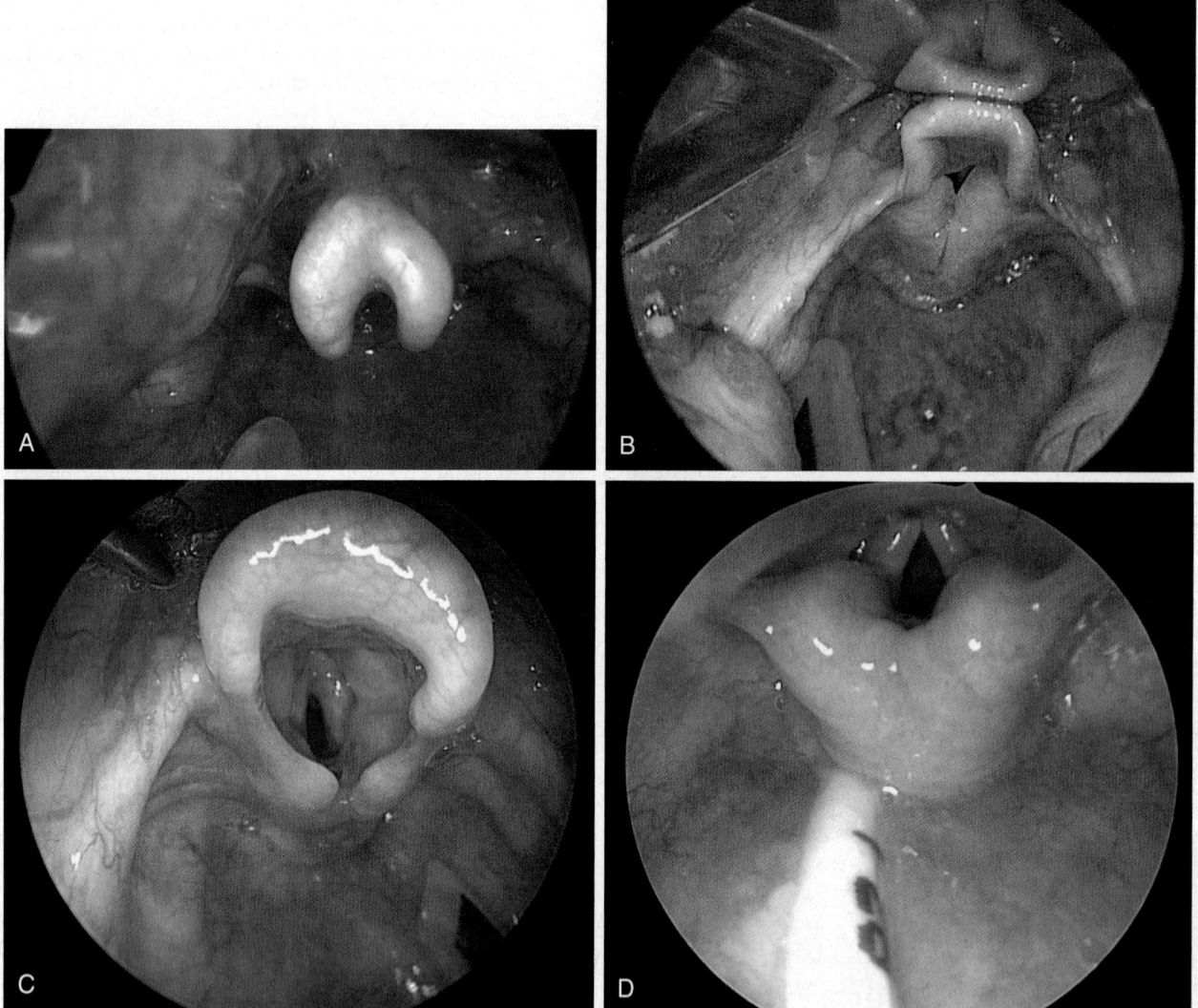

Fig. 18.13 Appearances of laryngomalacia at microlaryngobronchoscopy. (A) Typical omega-shaped epiglottis. (B) Posterior view of collapsing laryngeal inlet. (C) Shortened aryepiglottic folds. (D) prominent arytenoid cartilages.

atypical history and an unclear diagnosis.[71] There are serious potential complications of excessive removal of the supra-glottic tissues including stenosis and aspiration. To avoid this, the surgery should be as limited as possible. However, surgery is very successful in controlling severe airway obstruction, but less so if there is concomitant neurological etiology; for example, cerebral palsy. Feeding problems often improve but still may be significant in a minority of patients.[72] Long-term consequences of severe laryngomalacia include exercise-induced laryngeal obstruction,[73] which may be diagnosed during direct laryngoscopy on exercise.[74,75]

LARYNGEAL ATRESIA AND WEBS

The larynx develops from the endodermal lining of the cranial end of the laryngotracheal tube and from the surrounding mesenchyme derived from the fourth and sixth pairs of bran-chial arches. The epithelium proliferates rapidly, and this leads to an occlusion of the laryngeal lumen, which recan-nalizes by the tenth week of gestation. Failure to reestablish

a complete lumen leads either to a laryngeal web or, in extreme cases, to complete atresia.

Laryngeal Atresia

Laryngeal atresia was traditionally said to be incompatible with life, but with the advent of prenatal diagnosis there is the possibility of planned immediate airway treatment. This type of anomaly and similar gross abnormalities (e.g., laryn-geal cysts) have been given the label of *congenital high airway obstruction syndrome (CHAOS).*[76] CHAOS is characterized by ultrasound findings of large echo genic lungs, a dilated airway distal to the obstruction, inverted diaphragms, and massive ascites. The early prenatal diagnosis provides two possible choices for airway intervention as follows:

1. *Ex utero intrapartum treatment (EXIT).* The principle of this management is to allow the infant's oxygenation to be maintained by the uteroplacental circulation for as long as possible. This can be prolonged by anesthetic treatment to produce uterine relaxation, though this relaxation must

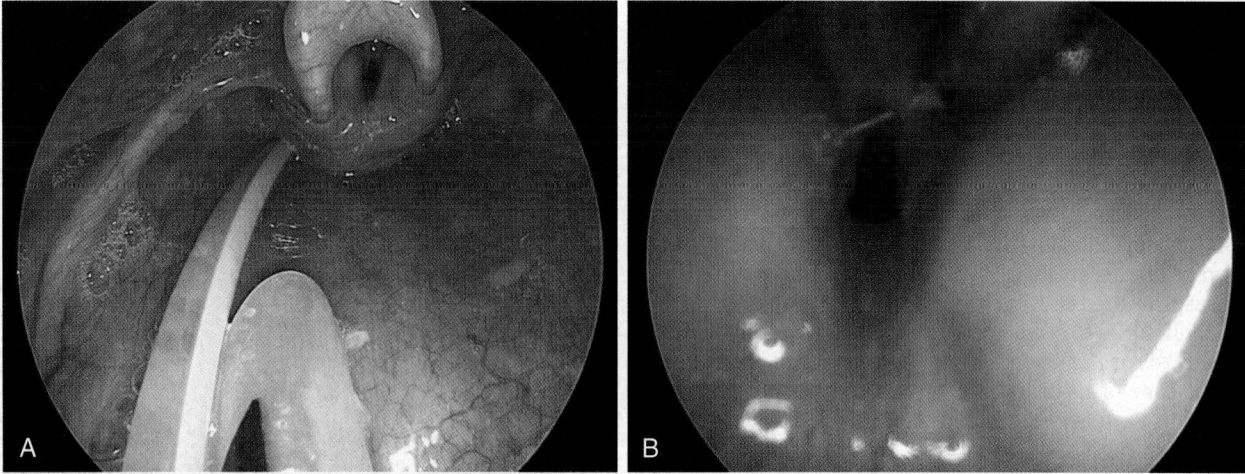

Fig. 18.14 Laryngeal web seen at microlaryngobronchoscopy before (A) and after (B) treatment.

be reversed just before the cord is clamped to prevent uterine atony and excessive maternal bleeding. The hysterotomy is ultrasound-controlled to prevent damage to the placenta. Limited exposure of the fetus also helps in maintaining the uterine volume and fetal temperature.[77]

2. *Fetal Intervention*. It has proved technically possible to introduce a tracheostomy while still *in utero* (above)

Laryngeal Webs

Laryngeal webs are a rare congenital anomaly (Fig. 18.14). They result from a failure of recanalization of the laryngotracheal tube during the third month of gestation and similarly can result in varying degrees of laryngeal webs. The most common site at which these develop is the anterior commissure, although webbing can be present in the posterior interarytenoid area, subglottic, or supraglottic regions. Key diagnostic points are to delineate any subglottic disease as well as any underlying congenital diagnosis, such as velocardiofacial syndrome (chromosome 22q11.2 deletion[78]).

Cohen's classification system subdivides laryngeal webs into four types:

Type I: An anterior web involving 35% of the glottis or less. The vocal cords are visible through these thin webs.
Type II: An anterior web involving 35%–50% of the glottis, which may be thin or thick, with extension into the subglottis. The vocal cords are usually visible within the web.
Type III: An anterior web involving 50%–70% of the glottis, typically with a thick anterior portion and extension into the subglottis.
Type IV: 75%–90% of the glottis is involved by a uniformly thick web, which extends into the subglottic larynx. The individual vocal cords are not identifiable and may be fused together. There may be an associated abnormality of the anterior cricoid cartilage.

As anterior laryngeal involvement is the most common site, hoarseness is the most common presentation. This is certainly most likely with a thin anterior laryngeal web although a thicker lesion can result in aphonia. If the web is extensive and involves the subglottis, respiratory compromise may be evident (Fig. 18.15). The rarer posterior inter

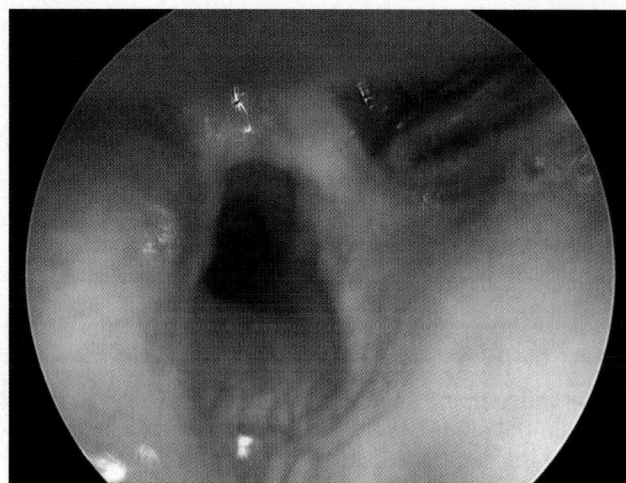

Fig. 18.15 Microlaryngobronchoscopy picture of an anterior glottic web and associated grade 3 subglottic stenosis.

arytenoid webs can present with stridor secondary to the inability to abduct the vocal cords. Flexible nasoendoscopy can diagnose a laryngeal web but on its own is insufficient to evaluate the extent of the lesion or plan any treatment. Formal endoscopic evaluation by way of an MLB allows for the character and true extent of the lesion to be determined.

The management of a laryngeal web may simply be conservative with voice therapy support. Much of the concern regarding surgery relates to the possibility of web reformation and resultant scarring. The rare, thin anterior laryngeal webs may be endoscopically divided and dilated to good effect. More complex, thicker, or larger webs may require an endoscopic or an open approach. Endoscopic approaches involve wedge resection, suturing of the cut edges, placement of stents, mitomycin C topical application, or local flap reconstructions. Open approaches require laryngofissure and anterior cartilage graft placement. In most cases of complex webbing, revision procedures are commonplace and a tracheostomy is inevitable.[79]

Laryngeal Cleft

These congenital anomalies arise from incomplete development of the posterior cricoid lamina and trachea-esophageal septum. The midline defect can be of varying length and this tends to correspond to the severity. Laryngeal clefts are associated with trachea-esophageal fistulas in 25% of cases. They are also associated with many syndromes including Opitz-Frias and Pallister-Hall.[76–78] The length of the cleft corresponds to the severity of symptoms. The main symptom itself is aspiration, but this can be a simple cough with some feeding difficulties to severe cases of frank aspiration coupled with cyanosis or respiratory distress. In children presenting with a history of aspiration, there should be a high index of suspicion for a laryngeal cleft.

Diagnosis and classification of a laryngeal cleft is made at MLB (Video 18.1). The interarytenoid area must be carefully visualized and palpated for the presence of a cleft. There are several classification systems for laryngeal clefts, but perhaps the most commonly used and simplest is as follows:

Type 1—interarytenoid cleft down to and including the vocal cords
Type 2—extension into cricoid cartilage
Type 3—extension through cricoid into cervical trachea
Type 4—extension into intrathoracic trachea

Contrast studies, such as barium swallow and video fluoroscopy, will demonstrate a cleft and the aspiration. The severity of symptoms and the cleft itself will determine the treatment with surgical repair of laryngeal clefts reserved for symptomatic children:

Type 1 Clefts

Conservative management of interarytenoid clefts should be the initial choice, with swallowing therapy particularly aimed at thickening feeds to prevent aspiration. If this fails, endoscopic repair is advocated.[79] Through a laryngoscope, the mucosa is cut from the inner margins of the cleft, which are then sutured together (Fig. 18.16).

Management of Type 2 and 3 Clefts

Some smaller Type 2 clefts may be easily closed with an endoscopic technique,[79] but for more extensive defects there are difficulties of access and instrumentation and late breakdown of the repair.[79,80] Open procedures are advocated for Type 3 clefts and usually involve an anterior approach, as this avoids damage to the recurrent laryngeal nerves. A vertical laryngo-fissure is performed and the cleft is closed with either direct suturing with consideration of an interposition of a fascial graft. A tracheostomy may be necessary if prolonged postoperative ventilation is anticipated, but with shorter clefts 7–10 days of postoperative intubation may suffice to stent the surgical segment.[81]

Management of Type 4 Clefts

Type 4 clefts include two very different prognostic outcomes from surgical repair.[82] The total group carries a 50% mortality but in cases where there is no carinal structure; that is, a true carinal cleft, there are no reported survivors from surgical reconstruction. Where there is an intact carina repair the thoracic segment via sternotomy or thoracotomy with

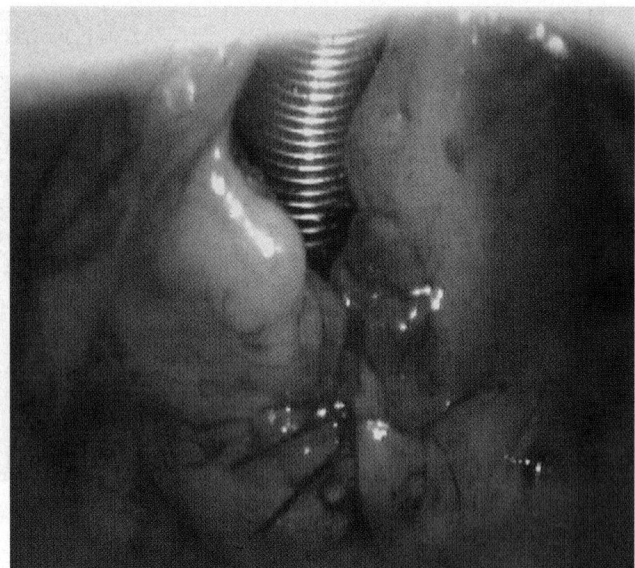

Fig. 18.16 Endoscopic repair of laryngeal cleft type 1.

or without the use of cardiopulmonary bypass is very difficult. If the tracheoesophageal folds are very basic, it may be necessary to close off the esophageal sphincters and to use the whole of the undivided foregut as the airway. Because treatment entails significant morbidity and mortality, the decision on whether to operate should be based upon the associated comorbidity and fully informed parental choice.[83] These children will need continued input from the speech and language therapy service in the postoperative period.

Vocal Cord Paralysis

Vocal cord palsy is the second commonest congenital anomaly of the larynx and can be bilateral or unilateral. Unilateral lesions are more common on the left, due to the longer course of the recurrent laryngeal nerve, and generally due to a nonfunctioning peripheral nerve. Other causes of unilateral palsy include peripheral nerve pathology, mediastinal lesions, such as tumors, vascular malformations, or thoracic surgery. Bilateral palsies are associated with lesions of the central nervous system, including Arnold-Chiari malformation, hydrocephalus, meningoceles, and myasthenia gravis. Birth trauma is often the cause for transient cord palsies, and these can be bilateral or unilateral.[84,85]

Vocal cord palsy can vary tremendously in its presentation as the functional impairment can vary from minor feeding difficulties and voice issues to severe respiratory distress that may warrant tracheostomy. Classically, there is inspiratory stridor and a weak cry, and this is the usual case with unilateral palsies. In older children dysphonia and exertional dyspnea may be the presenting symptoms. In cases of bilateral vocal cord palsy, stridor associated with respiratory distress is the predominant feature, and the presentation can be at a birth.

Awake FNE allows for dynamic assessment of the vocal cords and often clinches the diagnosis. Naturally, the procedure can be technically difficult in some cases, but with experience this can often be managed and lead to a clear diagnosis. Video recording of the procedure can prove invaluable in difficult cases. Ultrasonography of the vocal cords is relatively noninvasive and growing in popularity. With continued experience, the sensitivity and specificity of this technique is likely to improve. Other radiological modalities imaging the full length of the recurrent laryngeal nerve, specifically MRI, should be arranged to exclude intracranial causes and CT scanning to exclude compressive causes in the neck or thorax. Laryngeal electromyography is not commonly employed but may be useful in monitoring function and recovery. MLB should be performed in these patients which can additionally confirm the diagnosis as it includes dynamic assessment but it allows for other pathologies to be excluded, particularly cricoarytenoid joint fixation and posterior glottic stenosis.

Unilateral cord palsy can usually be managed conservatively, although speech and language therapy input is often vital to combat issues related to voice and feeding. Bilateral cord palsy can present with neonatal airway distress requiring intubation followed by tracheostomy. However, if the child is carefully monitored, tracheostomy may be avoided in 50% of cases.[86] Underlying causes should be treated to allow for resolution of the paralysis. Idiopathic cases certainly exhibit resolution in about 70% of cases, and this can be as late as a decade on from diagnosis. Tracheostomy decannulation can be achieved following resolution of the paralysis, but it is also often sought when the paralysis is likely to be permanent. Any surgical intervention to aid decannulation must take into consideration the possible adverse effects on laryngeal function related to voice, airway, and aspiration risk. The techniques that can be considered to aid decannulation include cordotomy, arytenoidectomy, and suture lateralization.[87] Open or endoscopic posterior laryngeal grafting techniques have also been employed, as have laryngeal reinnervation procedures.

SACCULAR CYSTS AND LARYNGOCELES

The saccule is a blind ending structure that opens into the laryngeal ventricle, the lateral space between the true and false vocal cord. It runs in an anterior-superior direction and is usually of modest size in the normal larynx. It is lined by pseudostratified columnar epithelium and contains serous and mucous glands. A laryngocele is an abnormally enlarged laryngeal saccule and is air-filled. The condition is a rare congenital abnormality but may produce significant airway obstruction. It may be entirely within the confines of the larynx or extend into the neck via the thyrohyoid membrane. If the lesion is small, it may be excised using an endoscopic approach. Alternatively, an open operation may be necessary for larger lesions, with the possible need for a prior tracheostomy to ensure an adequate airway postoperatively.

Saccular cysts are mucous filled and are found in the false vocal cord or aryepiglottic fold (Fig. 18.17). They are presumed to arise from a part of the saccule that has become sealed off from its outlet into the ventricle. They may be massive and cause immediate and severe airway obstruction. Standard endoscopic therapy is aspiration and marsupialization with scissors or laser. There is a high rate of recurrence, and open resection may eventually become necessary.[88]

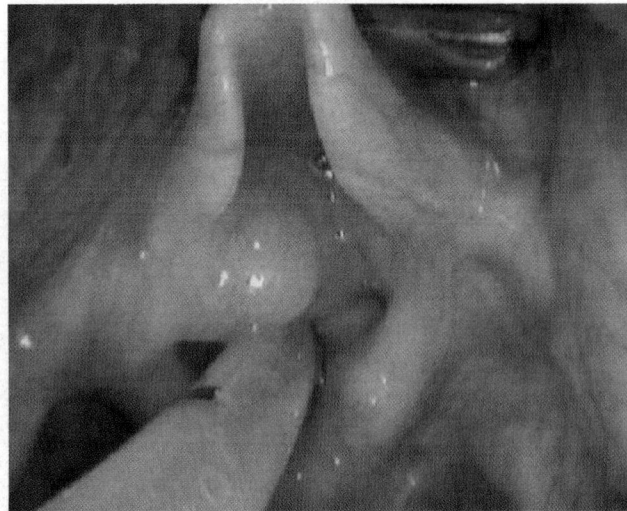

Fig. 18.17 Congenital saccular cyst of aryepiglottic fold.

HEMANGIOMAS—SUBGLOTTIC AND TRACHEAL

Infantile hemangiomas are benign vascular tumors and account for 1%–2% of all congenital anomalies of the larynx. Similar to cutaneous hemangiomas, they have a natural history, which includes a phase of rapid growth and proliferation followed by phases of involution. They can occur at all sites in the airway but are rare; the subglottis is the most common subsite. They usually present with symptomatic airway obstruction in the first 3 months of life, and this condition manifests itself more commonly in females than males, at a ratio of 2:1.

Infants with subglottic hemangiomas present with stridor that is not characteristically present at birth. As the lesion grows, symptoms ensue and typically the child presents with biphasic stridor around the age of 6 weeks. Symptoms can deteriorate as the lesion grows in size and this can occur up until the age of 2 years when the lesion then reduces in size, as seen in many cases of cutaneous hemangiomas. Presentation may mimic croup, and, since the lesion transiently regresses with dexamethasone treatment, the diagnosis may be missed until there have been recurrent bouts of airway obstruction.[89] Infants with subglottic hemangiomas are likely to have a cutaneous lesion in 50% of cases. The need for treatment arises due to the growth of the subglottic lesion in a confined space, which inevitably gives rise to airway compromise.[90]

Again, the gold standard for diagnosis is MLB. This allows for exclusion of other pathologies as well as direct visualization of the lesion. Photo-documentation of the lesion allows subsequent MLBs to determine the response to treatment. The lesion is most often seen as a solitary entity posteriorly in the subglottis, although multiple lesions can occur and rarely, these can be located at the mid-tracheal level. The lesion itself appears as a soft, compressible, red mass. The neurocutaneous disorder, PHACES syndrome (posterior fossa brain malformations, hemangiomas, cardiac anomalies and coarctation of the aorta, and eye anomalies with or without sternal clefts) should be considered and ruled out in cases of subglottic hemangioma.[90–92]

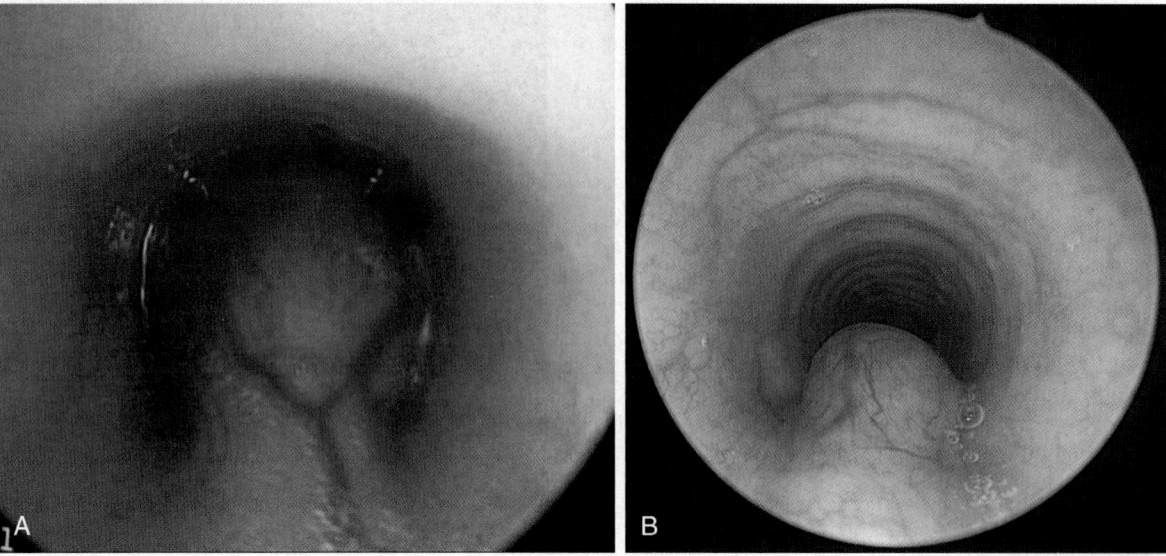

Fig. 18.18 (A and B) Case of tracheal hemangioma prepropranolol and postpropranolol therapy (pictures 2 weeks apart).

In 2008, the treatment of hemangiomas was revolutionized by the serendipitous discovery of propranolol therapy.[93–95] Previous treatments had included systemic and topical steroids and surgical excision; these options are now secondary with propranolol therapy being the first-line treatment option. However, treatment with propranolol is protracted and needs careful monitoring for side effects, and dosages need to be adjusted over the treatment period, which can typically vary from 12 to 18 months, although it can be longer in some cases. Responses, as determined by MLB findings and symptoms, can be seen within a few days of commencing treatment (Fig. 18.18). A minority of patients does not show any improvement with propranolol therapy and may require traditional interventions, such as open or endoscopic debulking or resection of the lesion.

Congenital SGS

This is a relatively common congenital anomaly of, and the second most common cause of, stridor in infants.[96,97] The underlying pathophysiology of congenital SGS involves incomplete recanalization of the laryngotracheal tube during the third month of gestation. This can lead to varying degrees of stenosis, complete laryngeal atresia being the extreme form. There are two main types of congenital SGS. Membranous SGS is the result of circumferential submucosal hypertrophy with excess fibrous connective tissue and mucus glands. This type is the most common and milder form. Cartilaginous congenital SGS results from a deformity of the cricoid cartilage or entrapment of the first tracheal ring within the cricoid. The cartilage usually narrows laterally, but may also develop generalized thickening or growth of the anterior or posterior laminae.

Congenital SGS may not manifest itself until the first few months of life, typically when a child develops an acute inflammatory process/illness. Naturally, a severe stenosis may result in symptoms from birth. The stridor associated with SGS is characteristically biphasic in nature, and this may be present with varying degrees of respiratory compromise. In an acute illness, when the congenital narrowing is further compromised by an overlying inflammatory process, the presentation is typically that of a child presenting with laryngotracheobronchitis or croup. An underlying SGS should be suspected in all cases of recurrent or refractory croup. An additional scenario in which this condition should be suspected is one of difficulty in intubation or extubation in an otherwise asymptomatic child. Children with Down syndrome may also have an underlying congenital SGS.

The gold standard for diagnosis and classification of SGS is by MLB. Formal endoscopic examination of the airway allows for the diagnosis to be made and for other abnormalities to be excluded. The dimensions of the stenosis (length and diameter) can be assessed during endoscopy, and this is vital for any consideration of surgical repair. The lumen diameter can be assessed by passing appropriate-sized ET tubes—the largest tube that demonstrates a leak at normal ventilation pressures—and determining the degree of obstruction according to the Cotton-Meyer grading system:

Grade I: 0%–50% obstruction
Grade II: 51%–70% obstruction
Grade III: 71%–99% obstruction
Grade IV: No detectable lumen

Surgical correction, when indicated, takes the form of

1. Cricoid split, with our without interposition cartilage graft.
2. Laryngotracheal reconstruction (LTR). Rib cartilage is used to hold open a vertical slit in the cricoid and upper trachea, either in the anterior wall alone, or as separate anterior and posterior grafts.
3. Cricotracheal resection (CTR). The stenotic segment is excised with direct anastomosis of the airway. This is technically difficult when the stenosis involves the vocal cords.

A single-stage procedure is ideal (though not possible in all cases). Postoperatively, the child is intubated for 7–10 days prior to a trial of extubation. Airway reconstruction has been shown to have good outcomes, even in the presence

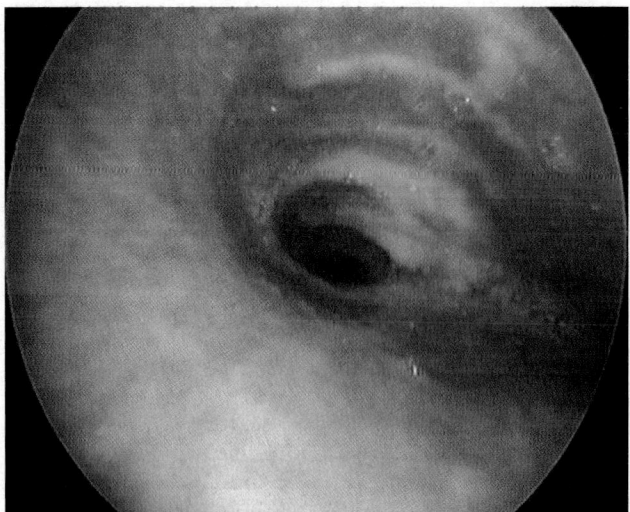

Fig. 18.19 Tracheomalacia, which was acquired secondary to cardiac surgery.

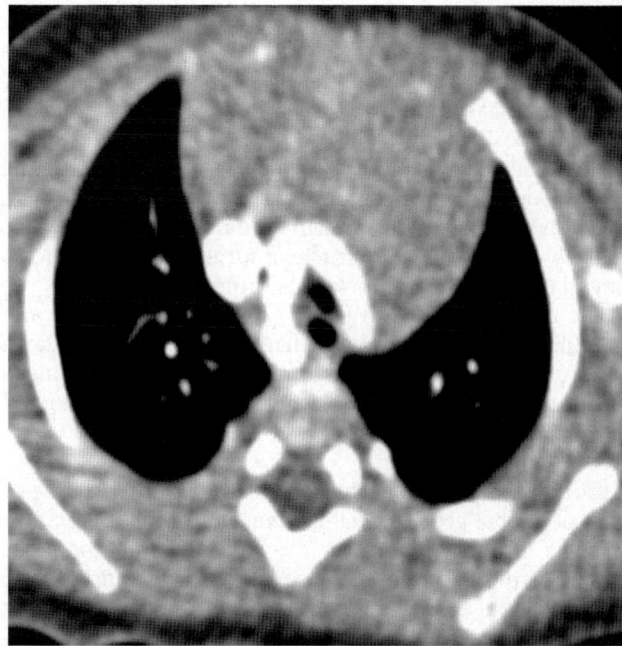

Fig. 18.20 Double aortic arch demonstrated on computed tomography angiography, compressing the trachea.

of concomitant anomalies.[98–100] Balloon dilatation has also been described.[101]

Congenital Abnormalities of the Trachea

TRACHEOMALACIA

Tracheomalacia is an abnormal collapse of the trachea during the respiratory cycle due to localized or generalized weakness of the tracheal wall (Fig. 18.19).[94,95] Microscopically, specimens show an increase in the ratio of muscle to cartilage. It is sub-divided into primary or secondary, though either form can be congenital. In primary tracheomalacia, there is an intrinsic abnormality of the tracheal wall, whereas in secondary cases there is extrinsic compression. In congenital cases, this is usually in association with cardiovascular abnormalities including the following (these are discussed in more detail in Chapter 39[102,103]):

1. *Double aortic arch*—surrounds the trachea, producing a concentric compression (Fig. 18.20)
2. *Anomalous innominate artery*—compresses the right anterior trachea
3. *Pulmonary artery sling*—compresses the lower trachea and the right and left main bronchi (Fig. 18.21)

Congenital tracheomalacia may be associated with bronchomalacia, particularly in more generalized cases. It also may be found with other tracheal abnormalities, such as TEF or laryngeal cleft. Although they may coexist, there is no connection with laryngomalacia.

The clinical manifestations of the condition are very variable, and it is often a diagnosis that can only be reliably made by endoscopy. There is likely to be stridor, which is usually expiratory as the obstruction is predominantly intrathoracic. There are usually recurrent acute episodes of stridor and dyspnea, during which the child may become cyanosed and moribund ("dying spells"). This may be precipitated by severe

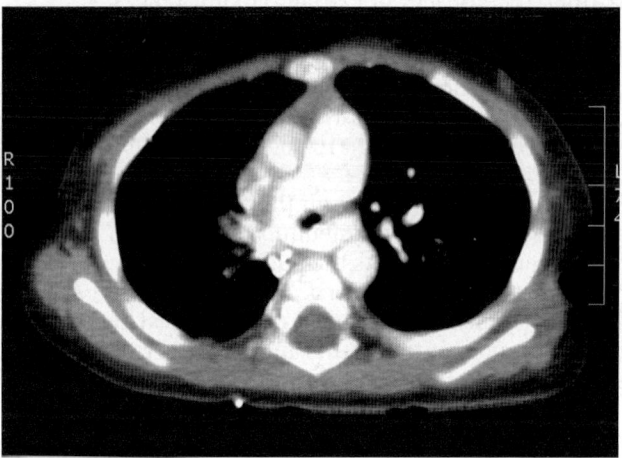

Fig. 18.21 Computed tomography angiogram showing left pulmonary artery taking origin from the right pulmonary artery, thus compressing the airway: a pulmonary artery sling.

crying, coughing, or even feeding. The symptoms are usually apparent in the immediate neonatal period, but may deteriorate in the first and second year of life, in an almost stepwise manner.

Diagnosis is generally by endoscopy and subsequent tracheobronchography (Video 18.2). The pediatric airway is very elastic and may collapse during forceful inspiration and certainly during coughing fits. The membranous part of the trachea also tends to bulge forward, giving the impression of a narrow airway. During endoscopy, it is important that the child be adequately anesthetized to avoid coughing while there is still spontaneous respiration. There is no generally accepted definition of the degree of collapse that can be taken as abnormal, but it seems reasonable to suggest that more than 25% reduction of the lumen is a significant finding and that greater than 50% is likely to be symptomatic. As well as overdiagnosis, it is possible to miss the condition if the trachea is splinted by the bronchoscope or if there is excessive positive end-pressure applied by the anesthetist through the sidearm of the instrument. The procedure should involve a detailed laryngoscopy to screen for a laryngeal cleft, and active vocal cord movements should be confirmed, particularly if there has been tracheal surgery for a TEF or cardiovascular surgery for a vascular anomaly.

The diagnosis may be made (and later confirmed and quantified by bronchoscopy) with multiple detector CT scans; however, the radiation dose is significant, but can be reduced with variation of the expiratory phase of the investigation.[104]

Treatment

Although the condition may progress in the first couple of years of life, it is generally self-limiting, and, if mild, it requires no active treatment. However, the patient's family should be taught cardiopulmonary resuscitation, particularly if the acute episodes are severe, and they can be provided with a facemask and ventilation bag. There may be associated recurrent respiratory infections, and training in home chest physiotherapy may need to be provided. In more severe cases, active treatment might be considered, though many of the choices have severe potential complications and should only be utilized in the face of extreme circumstances:

Surgery for Abnormal Vasculature. This may relieve the compression, though once the tracheal wall has become weakened from external pulsatile pressure, it may not immediately recover following the removal of the anomalous vessel.

Aortopexy. A suture through the adventitial lining of the aortic arch and the periosteum of the sternum is used to pull the arch forward. As the anterior tracheal wall is intimately connected to the aortic arch with fascial tissue, it is also towed forward, thus widening the tracheal lumen. There may be a failure of the suture, and there is a risk of damage to the aortic arch itself. This procedure can be performed via a thoracoscopic approach, which has the potential of reducing operative morbidity.[105,106]

Tracheostomy. This is very effective for short-segment tracheomalacia, but is unsatisfactory when the distal trachea is involved. The tube tip should pass through the segment to stent it; custom-made tubes can be manufactured to optimize the length. However, with a distal segment, the tube tip may pass into the right main bronchus on neck flexion and may not adequately stent the tracheomalacia segment on neck extension.

Nasal or Tracheostomy Continuous Positive Airway Pressure. A pneumatic splint of the segment can be achieved with continuous positive airway pressure (CPAP) via a tight-fitting facemask, or tracheostomy if the former is not tolerated, particularly with collapse at the carina (and in association with bronchomalacia).

Internal Stents. These have evolved significantly. Recent and bioabsorbable stents have fundamentally replaced the metal and siliconized plastic stents and avoid the inherent

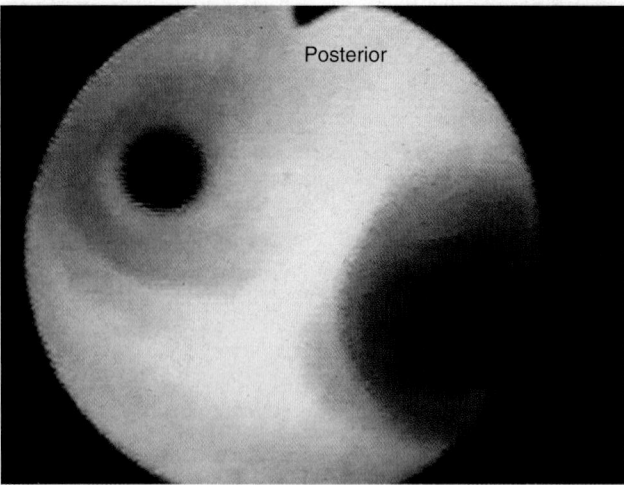

Fig. 18.22 Bronchoscopic view of a single complete cartilage ring at the origin of the right main bronchus.

dangers of both. Complications include displacement, granulation tissue, and infection.

External Stents. These represent an evolving treatment modality with conventional materials such as Gortex tubes being replaced with 3D printed bioabsorbable materials. These are still experimental, but will likely represent the future for treatment of severe intractable malacia.

CONGENITAL TRACHEAL STENOSIS (COMPLETE TRACHEAL RINGS)

In this very rare condition, there is a segment of the trachea, often distal, where the tracheal rings are truly complete. There may also be complete cartilage rings in the main bronchus (Fig. 18.22). It is often found in combination with other regional abnormalities, particularly cardiac, including pulmonary artery sling (see Fig. 18.21). In older children, large airway obstruction may be suspected from the appearances of the spirometric flow volume loop (Fig. 18.23). If the lumen of the trachea is small, this may not be compatible with life. Alternatively, the child may suffer immediate respiratory distress in the delivery room, which is not relieved by intubation or even tracheostomy. Extracorporeal oxygenation may be necessary to allow time to consider a surgical remedy.

If the child is relatively stable, it may not be necessary to consider any form of tracheal surgery, and there is potential for airway growth with the child. However, it may become necessary as the child grows if exercise tolerance is severely limited. Where the child is failing to thrive, experiencing severe respiratory distress and recurrent infections, the gold standard treatment is surgical correction via slide tracheoplasty and concurrent correction of vascular anomaly. The largest series of these from GOSH analyzing 101 patients with a follow-up of up to 235 months, shows a mean actuarial survival of 88.4% assessment with validated quality of life studies in those patients showing no significant difference from the normal healthy population.[107]

Tissue-engineered tracheal transplantation represents an exciting avenue of future research and developing surgical techniques for this condition.[108] It still remains experimental and is only for compassionate use only.

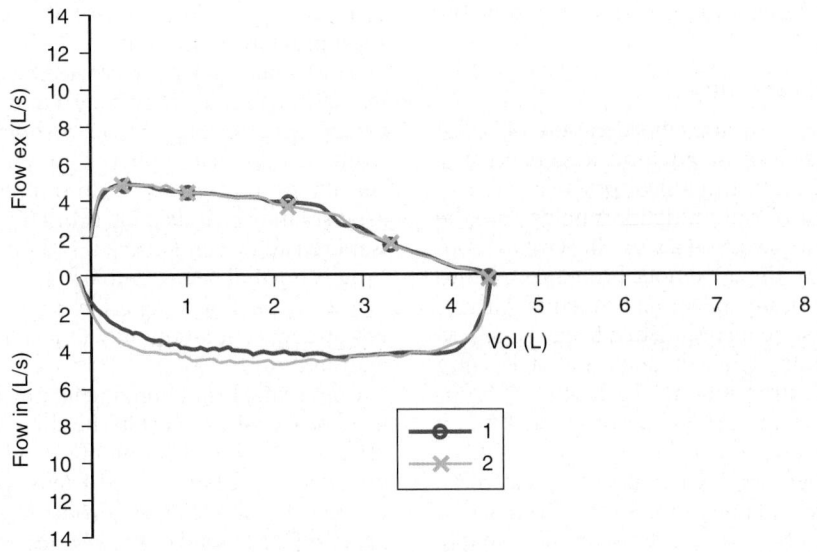

Fig. 18.23 Typical appearance of the flow volume curve in fixed upper airway obstruction. There is marked abrupt attenuation of inspiratory and expiratory flow, persisting until late near complete emptying, and then near complete filling of the lungs.

Specific Problems: Congenital Bronchial Abnormalities

CONGENITAL BRONCHIAL STENOSIS AND ATRESIA

Congenital stricture of the bronchus occurs predominantly in a main stem or middle lobe bronchus and can produce acute and/or chronic pulmonary infection. Inflammatory scarring of the congenitally stenosed bronchus provides an ideal environment for distal suppuration, atelectasis, and bronchiectasis. Atresia is usually asymptomatic and detected incidentally on radiography, but may present with recurrent infection. The airway may be blocked by a simple membrane, or there may be a discontinuity. It often results in cystic degeneration of the lobe distal to the obstruction before birth, since fetal lung liquid continues to be secreted and cannot drain into the amniotic cavity. The distal airspace is often cystic and filled with mucus, and is typically in continuity with an area of distal hyperinflation caused by collateral ventilation. Bronchial atresia may be very difficult to distinguish from a CTM until the lesion is excised. Infection and scarring may ensue, with symptomatic presentation. Failure to identify the congenital nature of the problem may lead to a misdiagnosis of mucus plugging. Unlike the situation with absent bronchus, there is no focal opacity in CLHL (congenital lobar emphysema). The continuity of the cyst with the distal airways and the hyperinflation of the distal lung distinguish absent bronchus from bronchogenic cyst (the nomenclature of which is discussed later), but the two conditions are occasionally associated.

ABNORMAL BRONCHIAL ORIGIN AND BRONCHIAL BRANCHING

Bronchi can arise from the gastrointestinal tract. Bronchial diverticula also possibly represent abnormal bronchial branching. The right upper lobe bronchus can arise from the trachea,

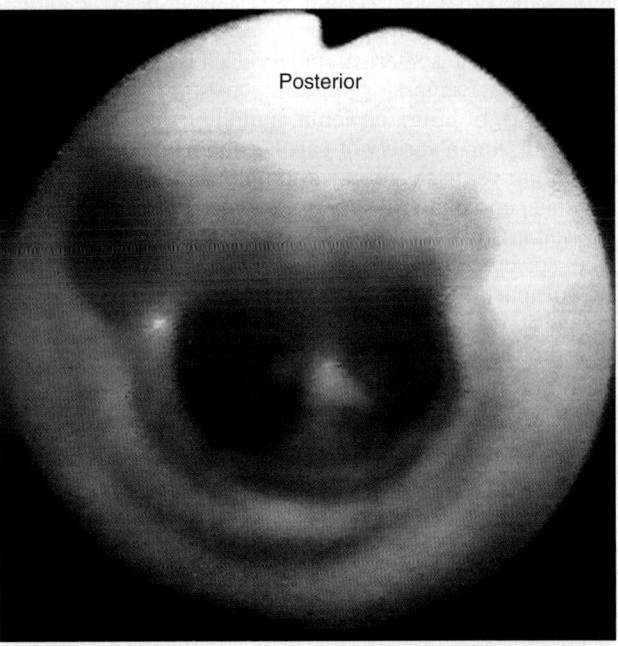

Fig. 18.24 Bronchoscopic view of the right upper lobe bronchus taking off from the trachea (pig bronchus). This abnormality is usually not of any clinical significance.

particularly in association with the tetralogy of Fallot. An accessory cardiac lobe bronchus may arise from the intermediate bronchus. A tracheal origin of one or more of the right upper lobe bronchi ("pig bronchus," Fig. 18.24) is usually of no clinical significance, but may be a cause of recurrent right upper lobe collapse in an intubated patient if the endotracheal tube (ETT) is low. The right lower lobe bronchus may also arise from the left bronchial tree, a "bridging bronchus." Lung segments may also cross over, with bronchial and arterial connections from the opposite side, usually from right to left. The crossover may simply be of vessels and bronchi, or include a tongue of parenchymal tissue, the "horseshoe" lung, where there is fusion of the lungs behind the heart.[109]

Disorders of Bronchial Laterality

Abnormal arrangements require consideration of what makes, for example, a right lung a right lung. It is not because it is in the right hemithorax. In clinical practice, the two most useful determinants of right lung morphology are the presence of three lobes, not two, and a very short main bronchus before the take-off of the upper lobe bronchus. A third criterion is the presence of an eparterial bronchus. Mirror-image arrangement must be distinguished from the superficially similar congenitally small (hypoplastic) right lung with right-sided heart (dextroposition) by determining bronchial morphology. This is important, because each has a different implication and requires different investigation. Mirror-image arrangement and other laterality disorders may be a feature of primary ciliary dyskinesia (discussed in Chapter 71), whereas a CSL must have its vascular supply delineated (see later).

The term "isomerism" is so entrenched that it is probably not feasible to replace it with, for example, bilateral right lung, which would be more logical. Nearly 80% of children with right isomerism (bilateral right lung) lack a spleen, leading to a risk of overwhelming pneumococcal sepsis. A similar proportion with left isomerism (bilateral left lung) have multiple small spleens. Ivemark's syndrome consists of right isomerism (bilateral right lung), asplenia, a midline liver, malrotation of the gut, and a variety of cardiac abnormalities including a common ventricle, totally anomalous pulmonary venous drainage, and bilateral superior caval veins and right atria. Left isomerism (bilateral left lung) is associated with multiple small spleens (polysplenia), a midline liver, malrotation of the gut, partially anomalous pulmonary venous drainage, and cardiac septal defects. Although nonfamilial, Ivemark syndrome is confined to males, whereas the other isomerism syndromes can affect either sex. A syndrome of left bronchial isomerism, normal atrial arrangement, and severe tracheobronchomalacia has been described,[110] extending the spectrum of left isomerism (bilateral left lung). Recently, the spectrum of primary ciliary dyskinesia has been broadened to include isomerism sequences (see Chapter 71).[111] Occasionally, a CSL may be so abnormal that its morphology can only be described as indeterminate. However, the contralateral lung morphology is usually obvious. Quite commonly, minor deviations from the normal bronchial branching pattern may be seen, which one study suggested may be associated with spontaneous pneumothorax.[112]

Disorders of the Bronchial Wall

Abnormalities in bronchial wall caliber may result in all or part of the bronchial tree being too large or too small. These may present with recurrent infections, steroid-unresponsive wheeze, or stridor. Congenital tracheobronchomegaly (Mounier-Kuhn's syndrome) is characterized by tracheomalacia and bronchiectasis, with greatly dilated major airways.[113] There are saccular bulges between the cartilages. Bronchial clearance is impaired, resulting in recurrent respiratory infection. This syndrome, which may be autosomal recessive, generally presents between the ages of 30 and 50 years, and is more common in males. It is occasionally associated with Ehlers-Danlos syndrome, cutis laxa, or Kenny-Caffey

syndrome.[114,115] True congenital bronchiectasis is much rarer than previously thought.

The lumen may be narrowed by complete cartilage rings (see Fig. 18.22). There may be an associated pulmonary artery sling (see Fig. 18.21). A short segment, situated relatively distally in the airway, may require no treatment. If ventilation is critically compromised, surgical excision or a Z-plasty may be indicated. Bronchoscopic balloon dilatation is increasingly being used. It is wise to ensure that the distal lung is normal before embarking on treatment; if the small airway is part of a generally maldeveloped segment, then enhancing ventilation may, in fact, only increase dead space ventilation.

Congenital bronchomalacia may be isolated, often with a good prognosis, at least in the short term, or associated with other congenital abnormalities including connective tissue disorders, and Larsen and Fryns syndrome. Williams and Campbell described a syndrome of diffuse bronchomalacia affecting the second to the seventh generations of bronchi.[116] Its occurrence in siblings, and the very early onset of symptoms, suggests a congenital etiology. Bronchomalacia also may be secondary to other congenital abnormalities, such as vascular rings. A rare cause of congenital tracheobronchomalacia is the presence of esophageal remnants in the wall of the trachea, which is generally associated with esophageal atresia and tracheoesophageal fistula. Fixed bronchial narrowing may be due to defects in the wall (e.g., complete cartilage rings) or extrinsic compression by an abnormal vessel or cyst.

PRESENTATIONS OF CONGENITAL LUNG DISEASE IN CHILDHOOD AND ADULT LIFE

Congenital lung disease may present later in childhood, or even in adult life. Respiratory distress as the sole presenting feature of congenital lung disease is rare after infancy. Many CTMs can present as an asymptomatic radiologic abnormality, including a focal solid or cystic mass, or hyperlucency. Unilateral CSL may also be a chance finding, and, if right-sided, may mimic mirror image arrangement. A cystic CTM enters the differential diagnosis of recurrent pneumonia in the same location, with failure of radiologic clearing between bouts or atelectasis due to large airway compression. More rarely, a cystic CTM may present as a lung abscess, atypical *Mycobacterial* infection,[117] focal bronchiectasis, pneumothorax, air embolism,[118] hemoptysis, or hemothorax, or even with malignant transformation, although it must be stressed that the latter is very rare; it is described in more detail below. Air embolism complicating air travel in a patient with a cystic CTM is rare, but may be fatal[119]; it is difficult to know what the best advice is for patients. The occurrence of any of this formidable but rare list of complications is extremely unusual in the first 2 years of life. Other conditions presenting with hemoptysis are any abnormalities characterized by abnormal systemic arterial supply and PAVM. The latter may also present with progressive cyanosis in a well person, which may lead to polycythemia, or with systemic abscess or embolism, including cerebral, due to bypass of the pulmonary vascular filter.

Another important presentation of congenital lung disease is as "steroid-resistant asthma." Large airway narrowing, such as tracheomalacia, vascular ring, or pulmonary artery

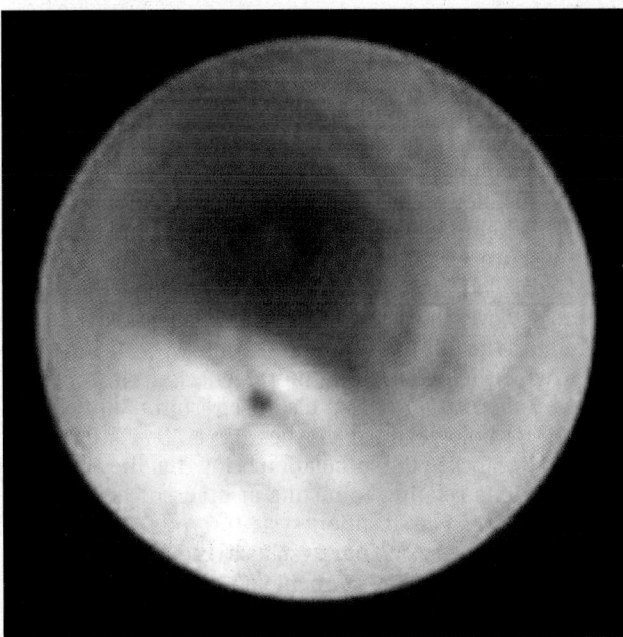

Fig. 18.25 Bronchoscopic view of an H-type fistula *(arrow)* in a 6-year-old girl with recurrent respiratory infections from birth. This was missed by a tube esophagram.

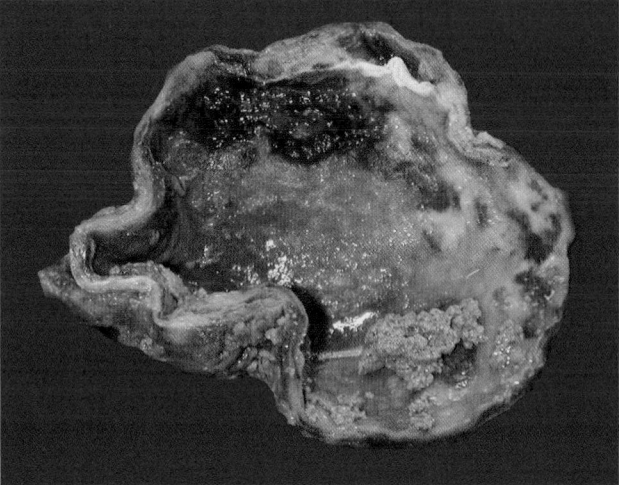

Fig. 18.26 Mediastinal bronchogenic cyst. The inner surface of this unilocular cyst is partly hemorrhagic and partly covered by purulent debris, which is indicative of recurrent infection.

sling, or complete cartilage rings enter the differential diagnosis; important physiologic clues come from the inspiratory and/or expiratory amputation of the flow volume curve, and the presence of a normal residual volume in the face of a greatly reduced FEV_1/FVC ratio (ratio of forced expiratory volume in one second to forced vital capacity).

Tracheoesophageal fistula and diaphragmatic hernia are considered the archetypal conditions presenting in the newborn period. However, both can present late. H-type tracheoesophageal fistula may present with recurrent bouts of coughing after drinking, or hemoptysis. Symptoms may have been present for more than 15 years.[120] Diagnosis is with a tube esophagram or bronchoscopy (Fig. 18.25). Diaphragmatic hernia usually presents with gastrointestinal symptoms later on, although abrupt presentation with respiratory distress has been described.[121] Whether some of these late-presenting hernias are truly congenital has been disputed.

It can be seen from the foregoing that congenital lung disease is not necessarily rare and esoteric, and important only up to the stage of early infancy, but that in many clinical scenarios it is worth asking, "Could there be a congenital thoracic disease present?" when considering the differential diagnosis. The next sections detail specific entities and their management.

Specific Problems: Parenchymal Lesions

Numerous pathologic conditions present with cystic changes in the lung, with acquired lesions outnumbering those that are developmental in origin. It is usually only after surgical excision that accurate pathologic diagnoses can be made.

FOREGUT (BRONCHOGENIC) CYSTS (CLINICALLY, CYSTIC CONGENITAL THORACIC MALFORMATIONS)

Foregut cysts can be defined as closed epithelium-lined sacs developing abnormally in the thorax from the primitive developing upper gut and respiratory tract. When these structures differentiate toward airway and contain cartilage in the wall, they are termed bronchogenic cysts, while those developing toward the gut are termed enterogenous (or enteric) cysts, although they are most likely of common origin from abnormal division of the embryonic foregut.[122] Bronchogenic cysts are the most common cysts in infancy, although many do not present until old age. About 50% are situated in the mediastinum close to the carina, and less frequently adjacent to the esophagus and alongside the tracheobronchial tree. They may present as a palpable mass in the neck; more rarely, they are found within the lung parenchyma and exceptionally in sites, such as below the diaphragm, pericardium, presternal tissues, and skin.[123] Mediastinal cysts are more common in adults than in children. Foregut cysts are usually single, unilocular, and more common on the right. They may have a systemic blood supply. Symptoms often relate to compression of the airways or complications, such as hemorrhage or infection, which may be reflected in the macroscopic appearance when the wall is thickened by fibrous scarring and shows brown discoloration due to chronic bleeding (Fig. 18.26). Diagnosis is usually after surgical excision; in adults, endobronchial ultrasound and fine needle aspiration has been deployed, but iatrogenic infection may result.[124] Microscopic examination shows a cyst lined by respiratory-type epithelium, although there may be squamous metaplasia and even ulceration with a foreign body-type granulomatous reaction depending on secondary phenomena. The wall is often fibrous and inflamed, and it may contain seromucous glands and cartilage plates (Fig. 18.27). Adenocarcinoma and mucoepidermoid carcinoma arising in bronchogenic cysts have rarely been described.[125,126] In the absence of cartilage, such a cyst should be termed a simple foregut cyst.

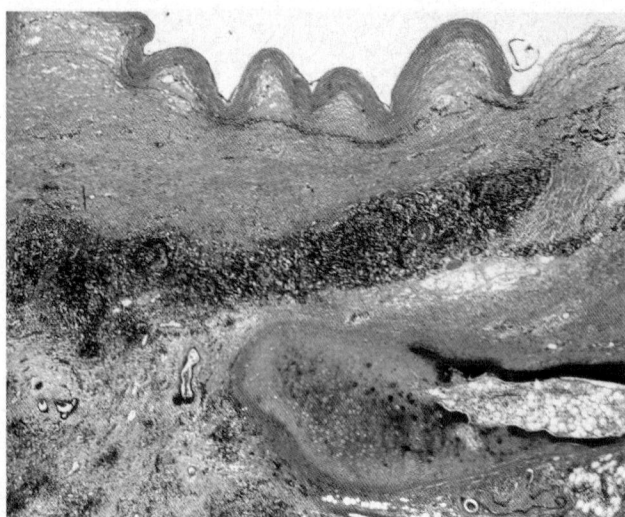

Fig. 18.27 Mediastinal bronchogenic cyst. The lining of the cyst is mainly denuded, while the wall is chronically inflamed. Note the cartilage plate that indicates bronchogenic origin.

Enterogenous cysts are subdivided into esophageal and gastroenteric (duplication) cysts, the former being more common. Esophageal cysts are intramural and do not involve the mucosa. They are lined by either squamous or respiratory-type epithelium. Gastroenteric cysts, in contrast, are typically unconnected to the esophagus, but may be in close association with the thoracic vertebrae, often in the region of the sixth to the eighth. Symptoms are typically due to pressure, infection, or hemorrhage, and there may be symptoms in association with the vertebral anomalies. In infants, they are a common cause of a posterior mediastinal mass and are typically paravertebral in location. They may extend across the diaphragm. The cysts are often saccular and are lined by gastric or intestinal mucosa with a muscle layer akin to the muscularis propria. Gastric mucosa may cause symptoms due to ulceration. Malignant transformation is exceptionally rare but is reported in gastroenteric cysts.

CONGENITAL PULMONARY AIRWAY MALFORMATION

The term CPAM (clinically, cystic CTM) encompasses a spectrum of variably sized cysts with differing histology. The etiology of CTMs (whether CPAM, sequestration, or others) is little known. Rare familial cases have been described[127] and genetic studies have implicated Hoxb-5,[40] an epidermal growth factor receptor,[128] brain type fatty acid binding protein-7,[129] *fibroblast growth factor (FGF) 7, 9, and 10*,[130,131] alpha-2 integrin, and E-cadherin.[132] *FGF10* is a mesenchymal growth factor involved in branching morphogenesis in the embryonic lung. In a rat model, focal *FGF10* overexpression led to CTMs closely recapitulating those found in humans, the nature of which depended on the site (proximal vs. distal airway) and timing (pseudoglandular vs. canalicular phase) of overexpression.[131] This work suggests that the same gene mutation may cause different types of CTM depending on developmental factors, and it underscores the need to move to molecular-based classification of mutations. Indeed, it has been suggested that strong *FGF10*, *FGFR2b*, and *sonic hedgehog* signaling may differentiate CPAM from pleuropulmonary

blastoma (PPB).[133] Other genes implicated in normal lung development, which, when knocked down or overexpressed in animal models, lead to congenital lung malformations are *FGF7*, *TGF-β1*, *TGF-β3* and *BMP4*.[134–137] Possible molecular mechanisms have recently been reviewed.[138,139]

CPAM encompasses a spectrum of variably sized cysts with differing histology. The relationship between different types and with other malformations is contentious, and their etiology is obscure. Originally classified as CCAM, the term *congenital pulmonary airway malformation* has become the favored terminology over the past decade as they are viewed as defects that relate to insults to the pulmonary airways during maturation, with the overarching more generic term *congenital thoracic malformation (CTM)* also used from a clinical perspective. Pathologically, five types (types 0–4) have been proposed by Stocker, the speculation being that they represent malformations relating to insults at different levels of the airways. In this classification system, type 0 (a condition formerly described as acinar dysplasia) is described as bronchial, type 1 as bronchial/bronchiolar, type 2 as bronchiolar, type 3 as bronchiolar/alveolar duct, and type 4 as peripheral.[2] Although lesions are not obviously distributed along the bronchial pathway, there is a high incidence of associated abnormalities of the bronchial tree on detailed analysis, and furthermore, vascularity and cellular composition in CPAMs corresponds to that seen in airways during gestation. This histologic classification is useful, because it permits identification of certain histologic patterns that rarely undergo malignant transformation in association with certain subtypes. However, this system has not been universally accepted, as discussed below, and many pathologists limit classification of CPAMs to types 1 and 2.[8]

Type 0 Congenital Pulmonary Airway Malformation

Type 0 CPAM is also termed *acinar dysplasia*. The condition is rare,[140] is nearly always incompatible with life, and is typically associated with other abnormalities. The lungs are small and firm, and histology shows bronchial-type airways with cartilage, smooth muscle, and glands that are separated only by abundant mesenchymal tissue. Associations with genetic abnormalities, such as the T-box transcription factor *TBX4* gene,[141] the *fibroblast growth factor receptor 2 (FGR2)*,[142] and cases in siblings, have been reported.[143,144] A rare variant with some lung sparing and prolonged survival has been described,[144] although arguably this may not be a true type 0 CPAM.

Type 1 Congenital Pulmonary Airway Malformation

Type 1 is the most common type of CPAM and has the best prognosis. This is because these malformations are usually localized and affect only part of one lobe.[145] Most present in the perinatal period or *in utero*, but rare cases can present later. CPAMs are usually multiloculated and range considerably in size, although the cysts in type 1 CPAMs are larger than 2 cm in diameter by definition (Fig. 18.28). There is no relationship between age and cyst size. Microscopically there is a sharp boundary between the lesion and the adjacent normal lung, but there is no capsule. The larger cystic spaces

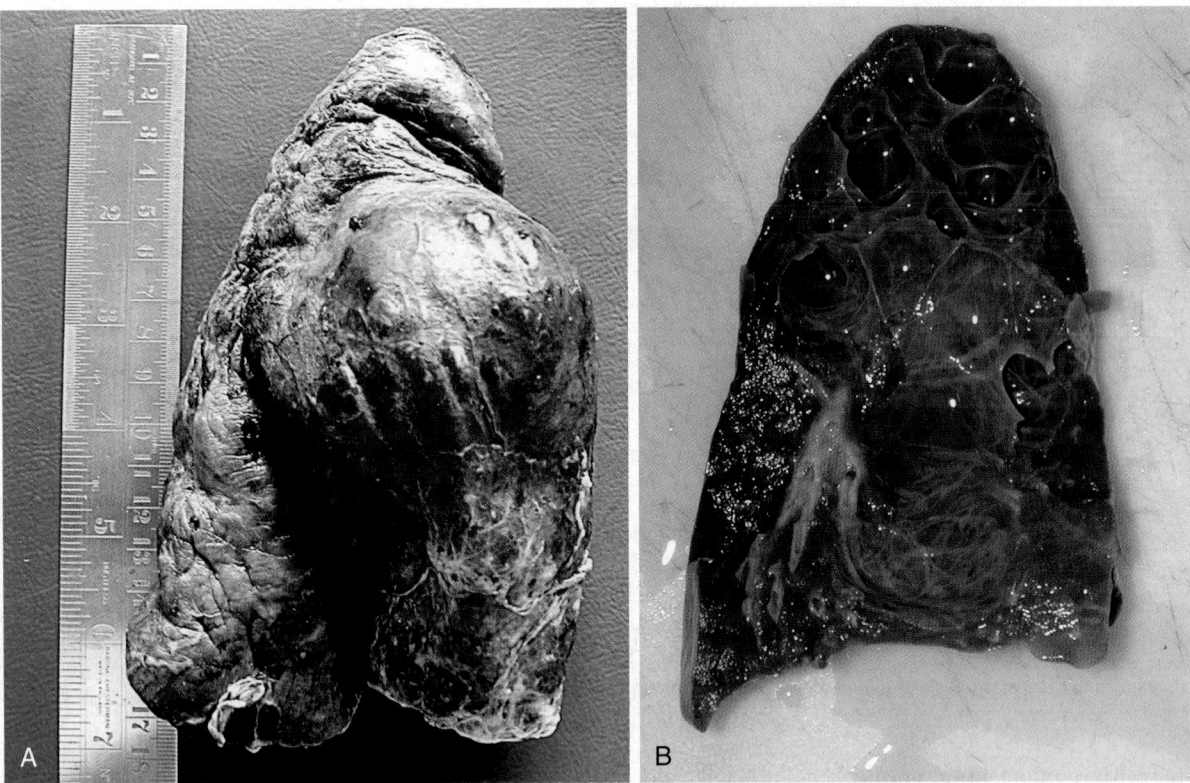

Fig. 18.28 Type 1 congenital cystic adenomatoid malformation. (A) A cystic lesion bulges to fill most of the lower lobe. (B) The cut surface shows a multiloculated cyst replacing most of the parenchyma.

are lined by pseudostratified ciliated columnar epithelium, and the lung between the cysts may show bronchiolar overgrowth and underdeveloped alveolar parenchyma like type 2 CPAMs. Historically, mucous cell hyperplasia was described in 35%–50% of cases (Fig. 18.29) Arbitrarily, hyperplasia was defined as mucous cell proliferation confined to the cyst, while extensions of this process into the alveolar parenchyma with a lepidic growth pattern were classified as bronchioloalveolar carcinoma.[146] However, there is now greater understanding of the genetics of these lesions with K-RAS mutations being identified in the mucinous cells independent of location[147,148]; therefore, they are viewed as neoplastic. With changes in the classification of adenocarcinoma,[149] any areas of mucinous proliferation within a CPAM should be classified as a mucinous adenocarcinoma. If small (5 mm or less) and localized, this should be classified as a mucinous adenocarcinoma in situ. Nearly all cases are lepidic predominant; although they are rare, more invasive patterns and nonmucinous morphology have been described, with metastases.[150] Malignant transformation is rare in CPAMs,[151] although nonresolving areas of consolidation on imaging should raise concerns. There is a very good prognosis following complete resection, although recurrent disease has been described if incompletely resected, sometimes decades after the original resection of the cyst. CPAMs may also show evidence of superimposed infection when resected, including aspergilloma.

Type 2 Congenital Pulmonary Airway Malformation

This is the second most frequent type. They generally cause respiratory distress in the first month of life and may be

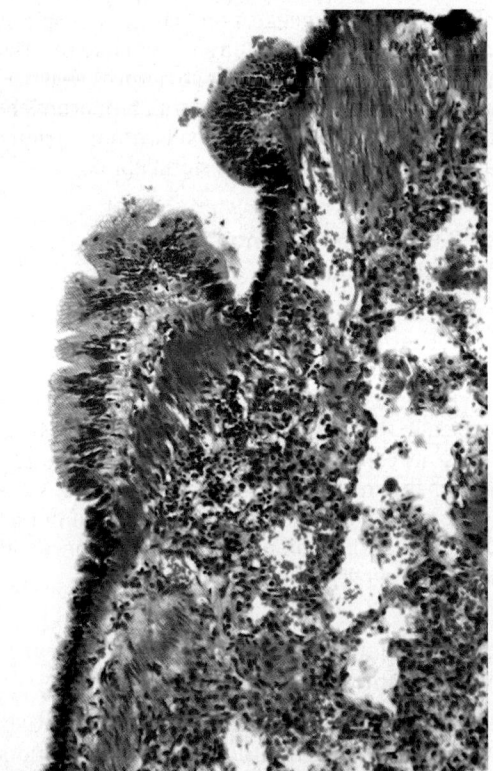

Fig. 18.29 Type 1 congenital cystic adenomatoid malformation. The cyst lining is mainly of respiratory-type, although mucous cell hyperplasia is not infrequently seen.

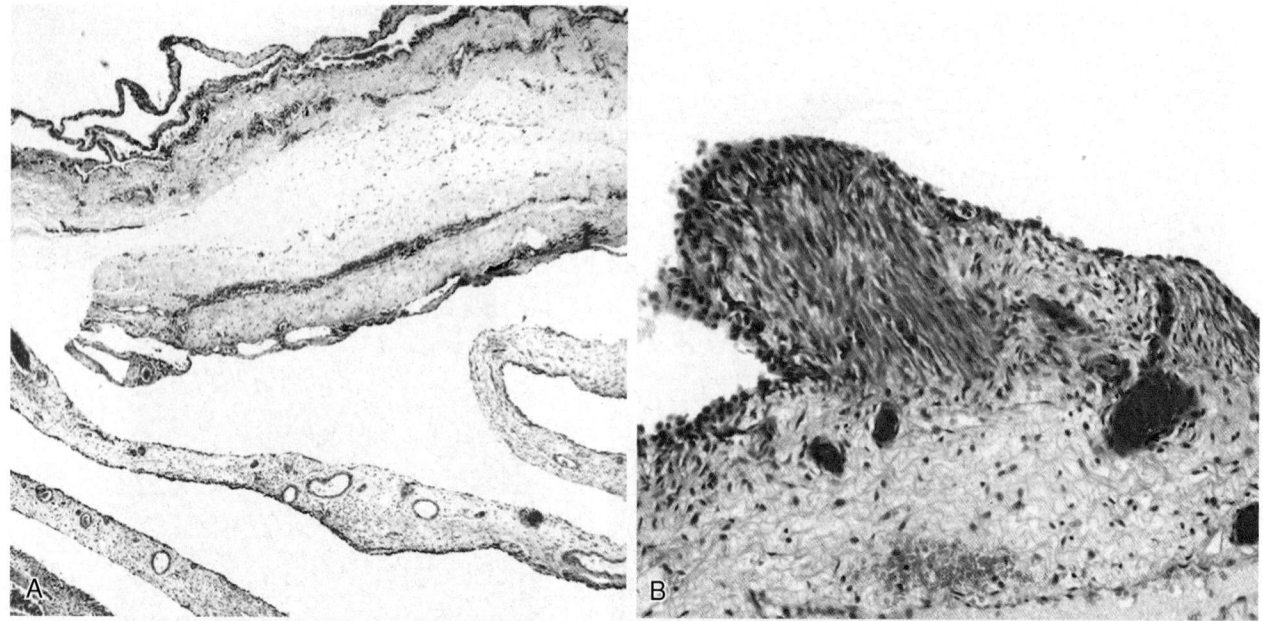

Fig. 18.30 Type 4 congenital cystic adenomatoid malformation. (A) These cysts are typically lined by pneumocytes with loose and myxoid fibrous stroma comprising the walls of variably sized thin-walled cysts. (B) Care needs to be taken to ensure that no blastematous elements are present, which would then indicate a diagnosis of pleuropulmonary blastoma.

associated with renal agenesis, cardiovascular defects, diaphragmatic hernia, and syringomyelia, which often have an additional adverse effect on the prognosis. Occasional cases present later in childhood with infection. Macroscopically, the lesions are spongelike, comprising multiple small cysts. Microscopically, the cystic airspaces relate to a relative overgrowth of dilated bronchiolar structures that are separated by alveolar tissue, which appears comparatively underdeveloped. Occasional examples contain striated muscle, although this has no clinical significance.

Type 3 Congenital Pulmonary Airway Malformation

These are uncommon and occur almost exclusively in male infants. They typically involve and expand a whole lobe with the others being compressed. Therefore, these lesions may cause hypoplasia in the remaining pulmonary tissue. Macroscopically, they appear solid and not cystic. Microscopically, there is an excess of bronchiolar structures separated by airspaces that resemble late fetal lung. There is also a virtual absence of small, medium, and large pulmonary arteries within the lesion. Some regard this lesion as identical to pulmonary hyperplasia.[8]

Type 4 Congenital Pulmonary Airway Malformation

These are also very rare and comprise peripheral thin-walled cysts that are often multiloculated. The cystic spaces are typically lined by alveolar type I or type II cells, with the intervening stroma being thin and comprising loose mesenchymal tissue (Fig. 18.30). Their etiology is obscure, and there is likely a spectrum of disease between these lesions and type 1 PPBs. Certainly, if the stroma of a suspected type 4 CPAM is even focally hypercellular, classification and management as type 1 PPB is recommended, and it has been proposed that such lesions lacking a blastematous component are better classified as regressed PPBs rather than Type 4 CPAM.[140,152,153]

A Rare Congenital Pulmonary Airway Malformation Variant: Cartilage and the Lung

Cartilage may be a feature of a number of cystic lesions; large cartilage islands have been described in giant cystic pulmonary chondroid hamartoma[154–156] and chondroid cystic malformation,[157] which may be considered a variant of CPAM.[158–160] Recently, five patients with diffuse cartilage islands scattered throughout the lung parenchyma were described.[161] Presentation was with neonatal respiratory distress in four children and a chance finding in the fifth. The initial diagnosis was of an interstitial lung disease. CT scanning showed diffuse abnormalities, including patchy ground glass change, linear opacities, and localized hyperinflation. Lung biopsy showed scattered mature cartilage islands within the lung. The prognosis was good, despite the widespread abnormalities.

POSTNATAL TREATMENT DECISIONS IN CONGENITAL CYSTIC LUNG DISEASE

Decisions about the treatment of a CTM that is symptomatic, either because of its size, compression of nearby structures, or because it has developed a complication, such as infection, are straightforward. For many abnormalities, surgery is the best and definitive treatment. For all but the smallest, sickest infants, lobectomy is a safe and well-tolerated procedure, with most surgeons reporting few, if any, significant sequelae. Segmentectomy may even be able to be done in some cases, with the preservation of normal lung tissue.[162] In one retrospective review, 14/60 patients suffered complications of surgery, including one each of tension pneumothorax, near-exsanguination, and chest wall fibromatosis close to the resection.[163] There were no deaths, and no reports of malignancy at follow-up. Increasingly, thoracoscopic surgery is used with results comparable to thoracotomy.[164] Chest tube drainage time and length of stay may be shorter with thoracoscopic procedures.[165,166] Long-term postoperative morbidity is not uncommon, and careful follow-up of patients submitted to surgery is recommended.[167] Pneumonectomy certainly carries a significant morbidity and mortality in infancy, but can be lifesaving.[168] However, it has considerable long-term morbidity, in particular scoliosis, which may worsen dramatically during the pubertal growth spurt.

It should be remembered that children with complex malformations (e.g., unilateral CSL with abnormal vasculature) may be asymptomatic for long periods despite a formidable list of abnormalities. A conservative approach, perhaps occluding any aortopulmonary collaterals, may be adequate.

Once a previously asymptomatic cystic lesion has become infected, it is probably safe to assume that recurrent infections are inevitable, and the lesion should be excised (Fig. 18.31). If medical management has failed, then surgical removal is indicated, conserving as much normal lung as possible. If the lesion is discovered as a chance finding on a chest radiograph, it is likely to be excised to establish the diagnosis and exclude a malignancy.

No area is more controversial than that of the asymptomatic CTM discovered on antenatal ultrasound. A chest radiograph should be obtained postnatally in the asymptomatic child. However, this is only around 60% sensitive, so further imaging, usually HRCT, is advised to delineate the abnormality. If infant pulmonary function tests are performed, respiratory rates are found to be elevated and tidal volumes reduced, and lung compliance reduced,[169] but how this changes after surgery and whether they are useful in selecting babies who should be operated on is unclear. The question then arises, what to do next? Even surgeons, who almost by definition are interventionists, cannot agree,[170] and there are not enough natural history data to give sound advice to the parents. Trivial lesions will probably be left alone, but some would resect even tiny malformations, to try to reduce the risk of malignancy. However, there is no evidence that this policy works (below). A worrying recent study of 69 resection specimens of asymptomatic CTMs of various sorts revealed 18 (26%) had microscopic disease; $n = 16$ infection (7 microabscesses, 9 with inflammatory cell infiltration), and $n = 2$ PPB.[171] Reasons for operation on an asymptomatic CTM would include preventing nonmalignant complications; allowing optimal lung growth; and preventing malignant transformation. Unfortunately, there are important evidence gaps in all three areas.

Even if surgery has been decided upon, the optimal timing of surgery is unclear. The longer the lesion is left, the greater the risk of complications. A small, nonrandomized follow-up study assessing lung function using radionuclide imaging suggested results were optimal with surgery at less than a year of age,[172] but another study showed no difference in spirometry at follow-up whether lobectomy was performed before or after 2 years of age.[173] Clearly more data are needed.

PREVENTION OF (NONMALIGNANT) COMPLICATIONS

The main risk is probably infection. If the CTM is cystic, then it is likely (but unproven) that infection will eventually occur. The best information is from a large meta-analysis.[174] There were 41 series published between 1996 and 2008 describing 1070 patients, nearly 80% of whom had an antenatal diagnosis of CTM. A total of 505 reached infancy without surgery with only 16 (2.3%) becoming symptomatic. Complications were significantly less likely after elective surgery. Furthermore, previous pneumonia is a risk factor for the need to convert video-assisted thoracoscopic surgery to open thoracotomy.[175] The authors recommended surgery before 10 months of age, although the numbers who actually became symptomatic were too small to be dogmatic. Conversely, in a study from a center favoring conservative management, 72/74 fetuses with an antenatal diagnosis of CTM were liveborn; one required emergency lobectomy, and three others were electively operated on at parental request. For a median of 5 years, 65/68 infants remained asymptomatic.[176]

A more recent meta-analysis of studies comparing elective resection with expectant management identified only one prospective and eight retrospective studies. A total of 70 of 168 (42%) patients underwent elective surgery when asymptomatic, with a 10% surgical complication rate; 63 of 98 (64%) patients managed conservatively developed symptoms with a 32% complication rate.[177]

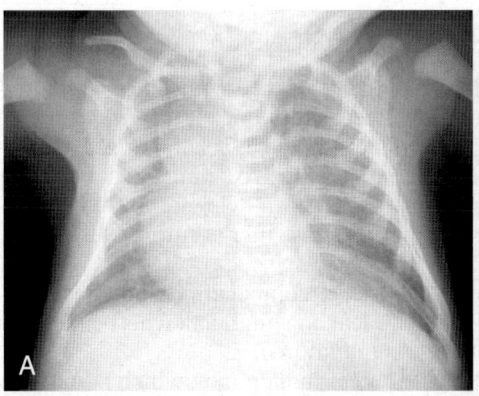
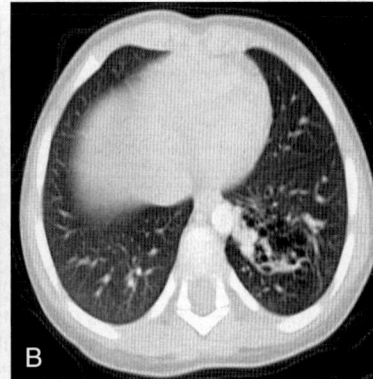
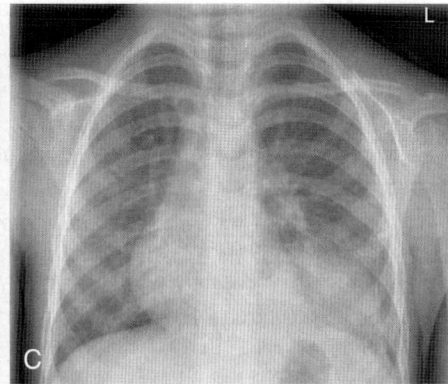

Fig. 18.31 Infection in a congenital thoracic malformation. (A) Chest radiograph and (B) high-resolution computed tomography prior to the mass becoming infected. There is a multicystic mass with arterial supply from the aorta. (C) Chest radiograph when the child was febrile with respiratory distress. The mass has become infected, and was subsequently surgically removed.

Clearly surgery will prevent nonmalignant complications of CTM, but if all CTMs were operated on, many unnecessary operations would be performed.

A final consideration is that removal of a CTM may reveal it was not as "asymptomatic" as was thought preoperatively. A single paper suggested that histiocytic inflammation may be a feature of some CTMs,[178] although no data about symptoms were given, and there was no evidence of chronic infection. However, anecdotally, the occasional infant who undergoes resection of an apparently asymptomatic malformation becomes much more alert and lively, and the family realizes that, in fact, all was not quite as well as was thought prior to resection of the CTM.

OPTIMIZING LUNG GROWTH

It seems likely that operative removal of a large mass would allow the residual lung to expand. However, evidence in support of this is scant. Indeed, CLHL (congenital lobar emphysema) may cause considerable mediastinal shift in asymptomatic infants, but as the child gets older, the shift regresses and there is no evidence of interference with lung growth or function. Indeed, CLHL may be a chance finding in a completely asymptomatic adult.[179] Such information as is available on infant lung function tests in CTMs suggests that they are associated with an mildly decreased tidal volumes, an increased respiratory rate, and decreased lung compliance,[169] but follow-up studies are lacking. Hence we do not believe that optimizing lung growth is a credible indication for removal of an asymptomatic CTM.

PREVENTION OF MALIGNANT TRANSFORMATION

This is a vexed and difficult issue.[180] A few definite background statements can be made:

- Primary intrathoracic malignancy in childhood is very rare indeed, and for most (but not all) types of CTM, there is no evidence of an increased risk, and cytogenetic studies are reassuring.[181]
- There are several case reports and case series documenting the coexistence of a CTM and primary intrathoracic malignancy, mainly invasive mucinous adenocarcinomas associated with type 1 CPAMs.[174,182,183]
- Tumor markers are found in CTMs, and these may be associated with malignancy; these include Echinoderm microtubule-associated proteinlike 4 (EML4)-anaplastic lymphoma kinase (ALK) fusion-type oncoprotein,[184] MUC5AC, CK20, erythroblastic leukemia viral oncogene homologue 2 (HER2), and K-Ras.[185–187]
- Even complete removal of a CTM does not prevent development of a malignancy.[188,189]

The most informative study came from Canada, over the period from 1998 to 2008, in a population of around 5 million with 1,187,484 live births during the study period.[190] A total of 129 children were diagnosed with a CTM (CPAM)—the incidence being one in 12,000—and 74 underwent a resection. The reasons for resection were generally poorly documented. A total of 5 PPBs were diagnosed during this time period, giving an incidence of 1 in 250,000 live births. Three were initially diagnosed as a CPAM. Thus the incidence

of PPB among apparently benign CTMs is 4%, and, worryingly, there was no clinical or radiological feature that distinguished benign from malignant. One of the two patients (both of whom were late-presenting) who had a PPB without a preexisting lung lesion, died.

Placing CPAM patients into high- and low-risk categories may be feasible with an algorithm incorporating radiological features and DICER1 mutation analysis.[191] Radiological features suggestive of uncomplicated CPAM include antenatal detection and the presence of a systemic feeding vessel and hyperinflated lung. Features suggestive of PPB included bilateral or multisegment involvement. Although this is a large study (more than 100 patients in each group) this algorithm should be used with caution until prospectively validated in another cohort. CT features overlap between CPAM/sequestration and PPB.[192,193]

It has been suggested that some CTMs may be associated with the development of sarcomas, but these are most likely PPBs with a cystic component as part of the tumor. Indeed, it has been proposed that a type 4 CPAM is better classified as a regressed PPB.[153,194] Registry data suggest that those with bilateral CTMs, a family history of PPB, lung cysts or renal anomalies, or a close relative with a childhood malignancy—especially Wilms or medulloblastoma—are at particular risk.[153,181,195,196] Recently, attention has focused on DICER1, a cytoplasmic endoribonuclease that cleaves precursor molecules into microRNAs that modulate mRNA expression. DICER1 is very important developmentally, null mutations being embryo lethal in animals.[197] Registry data show a rate of 68%[195] in PPB. At least 40 heterozygous germline mutations in DICER1 have been described, and have been shown to be important in PPB,[198] as well as a spectrum of malignancies, including cystic nephroma and Wilms tumor, ovarian sex-cord-stromal tumors, multinodular goiter, embryonal rhabdomyosarcoma of the uterine cervix, pleomorphic sarcoma of the thigh, primitive neuroectodermal tumor, pulmonary sequestration, and juvenile intestinal polyps. However, even if the clinical picture and/or the presence of DICER1 mutations puts the child in a high-risk group and leads to excision of the CTM, there is no established protocol for postoperative follow-up and imaging. Although screening for DICER1 mutations should be considered in the families of a child with PPB before this is undertaken, skilled genetic counselling is advisable to determine what should be offered to those who screen positive.[199]

SUMMARY AND CONCLUSIONS

The uncertainties as to what best to do must be shared honestly with the family. There is no one right answer in the asymptomatic child, and this should be acknowledged. Follow-up to obtain natural history data is recommended, whatever therapeutic decisions are made. Our own view is that asymptomatic congenital cystic disease merits surgery:

- There is about a 3% risk of complications, such as infection, bleeding, and air leak in childhood; whether the risk increases with age is not known.
- There is about a 4% risk of malignancy, which admittedly can be reduced but not eliminated by surgery.
- There is a very small and unquantifiable risk of complications of air travel, but these can be devastating.

- Taken together, the above risks outweigh those of elective surgery in skilled hands.

However, many would disagree, and until we have better means of assessing the risk of complications, the present unsatisfactory state of affairs will likely continue.

PULMONARY SEQUESTRATION

The etiology of these lesions is not clear, and specifically, genetic studies have tended to lump sequestrations and CPAMs together (probably logically!). Given the difficulty of distinguishing sequestration from CPAM, other than by pathological examination, and with overlapping findings even then, many of the difficulties in planning treatment are common to both. The classical definition of sequestration is pulmonary tissue that is isolated from normal functioning lung and is nourished by systemic arteries, although the separation may be purely vascular. The intrapulmonary variant is contained within otherwise normal lung parenchyma. The less common extralobar sequestration is divorced from and accessory to the lung. Sequestrations may also connect to the esophagus or stomach, or contain pancreatic tissue; they may also show histologic features of adenomatoid malformations. These complicated lesions are perhaps best classified pathologically as complex "bronchopulmonary-foregut malformation," if the simpler term CTM is not to be used.

Their etiology is far from understood, with various proposed theories. Some workers have suggested that intralobar sequestration is acquired when a focus of infection or scarring acquires its blood supply from a systemic collateral, basing this on the relative sparsity of other malformations associated with this type of sequestration and its rarity in perinatal autopsies; in such cases, intact bronchial ventilation would be expected. Those who believe sequestration to be congenital generally propose that accessory lung buds are fundamental to both forms of pulmonary sequestration and liken them to intestinal duplications, with subsequent acquisition of a blood supply from the nearest and most convenient source, which happens to be systemic.

Intralobar sequestrations are usually found in the posterior basal segment of the left lower lobe and extralobar sequestrations beneath the left lower lobe. About 15% of extralobar sequestrations are abdominal. The intralobar sequestration is encircled by visceral pleura and has no pleural separation from the rest of the lobe. The remainder of the affected lobe and lung is normal, unless secondary changes, such as infection, have supervened. More than half the cases of intralobar sequestration are diagnosed after adolescence, and symptoms in neonates and infants are uncommon. Extralobar sequestration is generally detected in infancy because of associated malformations and it affects males four times more frequently than females. Though much rarer, intralobar sequestrations also may be associated with other malformations.

The largest series of sequestrations is a retrospective review of 2625 cases from China, over the period 1998–2008[200]; it appeared that all were diagnosed postnatally, and antenatal screening was uncommonly performed, if at all. They were more common in males (gender ratio 1.58:1), 13% were asymptomatic, and the rest presented with nonspecific symptoms, such as cough, fever, and chest pain. Intralobar sequestration was more common than extralobar (84% vs.

16%). Presentation with acute chest pain due to torsion of a sequestration has been described very rarely.[201] Extralobar sequestrations tended to be asymptomatic and diagnosed later. CT appearances were variable, and included a solid mass (49%), a cystic appearance (28.6%), a cavitating mass (11.6%), and appearances suggestive of pneumonia (8%), similar to other series.[202] Only three patients had bilateral lesions. The left lower lobe was the most common site, especially left (66.4%) and right (20.1%) posterior basal segments. Arterial blood supply was most commonly from the thoracic (76.6%) or abdominal (18.5%) aorta, more than 20% had at least two arteries supplying the abnormality. A celiac, splenic, or coronary artery source of arterial supply has been described. More than 90% were drained by the pulmonary venous system; some may drain into the hemiazygous system or inferior caval vein. In nearly 60% of cases, the preoperative diagnosis was wrong. Calcification is rare in sequestrations, but may be seen in the arterial supply if there is premature atherosclerosis. In another series,[203] the mean age at presentation of 72 patients was 36.6 years. Presenting symptoms were nonspecific and more than 60% of all lesions were undiagnosed preoperatively, despite CT imaging. *Aspergillus fumigatus* and *Pseudomonas aeruginosa* were the most common organisms cultured from the resected specimens. *Mycobacterium tuberculosis* and *Nocardia* infection have been described in other series.[204–206] Changes typically associated with pulmonary hypertension (medial hypertrophy, intimal proliferation, plexogenic lesions) may be seen in many of these lesions.[207]

Treatment of sequestration may be by surgical excision (open or thoracoscopic) or embolization,[208] and both are very safe in experienced hands. Before surgery, as with all CTMs, the vascular supply should be carefully delineated by preoperative investigations (see later) and embolization of aortopulmonary collaterals at least considered. There is an increasing number of series of definitive treatment by embolization, in some cases very early in life.[209,210] The results are better for solid lesions; cystic components do not respond so well. Embolization has also been used to control massive hemoptysis.[211] Surgery is clearly the preferred option if the mass is infected or, particularly in an adult, malignancy is suspected. Embolization will abolish shunting and the risk of high-output cardiac failure, but will likely leave residual tissue. Whether this matters depends on the assessment of the (currently unquantifiable) risk of malignancy in a sequestration. There are case reports of sequestration being associated with elevated serum and intralesional tumor markers[212] and frank malignancy (adenocarcinoma[213] and primary sarcoma[214]). A benign carcinoid arising in a sequestration as a chance finding has also been described.[215]

Both types of sequestration have certain similar pathologic characteristics as well as clear-cut differences. In both types, the pulmonary tissue is largely cystic and contains disorganized, airless alveoli, bronchi, cartilage, respiratory epithelium, and a systemic artery. It is often secondarily infected, bronchiectatic, or atelectatic, and may show histology of a CPAM, particularly type 2 CPAM in extralobar variants.[216,217] The aberrant arteries may arise from the thoracic or abdominal aorta and, in the latter instance, may pierce the diaphragm and run through the pulmonary ligament before reaching the sequestration. The elastic vessel walls may become atherosclerotic, and the lumen varies considerably in size. In intralobar sequestrations, the systemic arteries are likely to be large, and the veins drain into the pulmonary system; while in extralobar variants, the systemic arteries are small and the venous drainage is likewise systemic through the azygos system. The pulmonary vessels may show features of hypertension, although this does not appear to be of clinical significance.[217]

LONG-TERM FOLLOW-UP OF CYSTIC CONGENITAL THORACIC MALFORMATIONS

There are several issues to be considered, including the effects of previous treatment (usually lung resection) and the needs of the child with a malformation that is being managed conservatively.

In general, lobectomy is well tolerated. The effects of lung resection have been reviewed[218]; issues include the total amount of resection and the age at operation (and thus the possibility of new lung tissue formation). Human and animal data are difficult to interpret, but in general it is the extent, not the age of the patient at resection that is important. Whether, when, and what imaging should be performed is controversial. The risks of radiation, especially in young children, should be taken seriously. Hopefully, in the next few years, MRI will be practicable in unsedated children, which should allow better follow-up.

Specific Problems: Overexpansion, Aplasia and Ectopia

OVEREXPANSION: CONGENITAL LARGE HYPERLUCENT LOBE (CONGENITAL LOBAR EMPHYSEMA)

A rare condition, CLHL presents in 50% of cases in the neonatal period, otherwise it is in early infancy. Some cases are caused by easily identifiable partial obstruction, such as mucosal flaps or twisting of the lobe on its pedicle. However, in many cases, a deficiency of bronchial cartilage is thought to be the cause, leading to inappropriate collapse of the airway and the trapping of air. Histologically, the majority of cases show normal radial alveolar counts, but with no apparent maturation with age when compared to age-matched controls, suggesting a postpartum arrest of acinar development within affected lung tissue. A minority of cases, however, show true alveolar hyperplasia with increased radial alveolar counts, which is sometimes referred to as a polyalveolar lobe.[219] The condition affects the left upper (42%), right middle (35%), right upper (21%), and lower lobes (2%). The affected lobe cannot deflate, but overdistends and displaces adjacent lobes, and subsequently the mediastinal structures. The emphysematous lobe may herniate into the contralateral hemithorax, usually through the anterior mediastinum. The condition may be diagnosed antenatally (see earlier), may present as respiratory distress (often with consequent failure to thrive in infancy), or may be a chance finding on a chest radiograph taken later in life.

Presentation in Infancy

Clinical features of infantile lobar emphysema are those suggestive of a tension pneumothorax: hyperresonance of the affected hemithorax associated with diminished breath sounds and deviation of mediastinal structures to the contralateral side. Usually, the chest radiograph will demonstrate a hyperlucent lobe with features of compression and collapse of adjacent lung and depression of the ipsilateral diaphragm (Fig. 18.32). The mediastinum is deviated, and the contralateral lung may be collapsed. Occasionally, initial chest radiographs may demonstrate an opaque lung field. This then clears and the affected lung becomes overinflated and hyperlucent on the radiograph. Ventilation-perfusion (V/Q) scanning may demonstrate delayed uptake and clearance of isotope and reduced blood flow in the affected lobe. This investigation is particularly useful if it is unclear whether

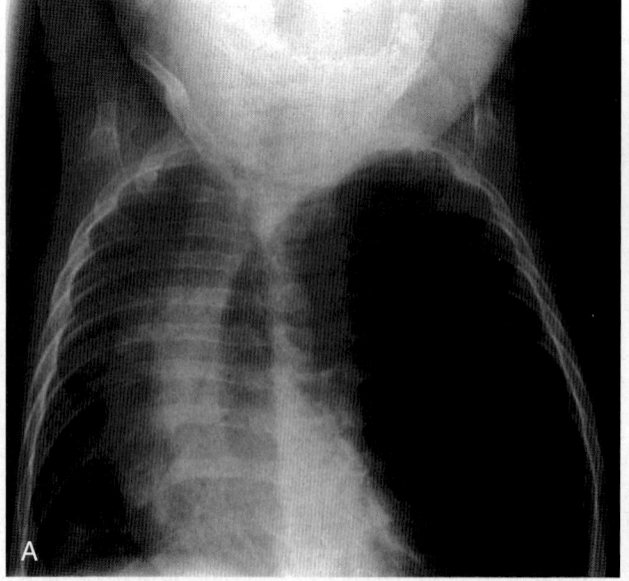
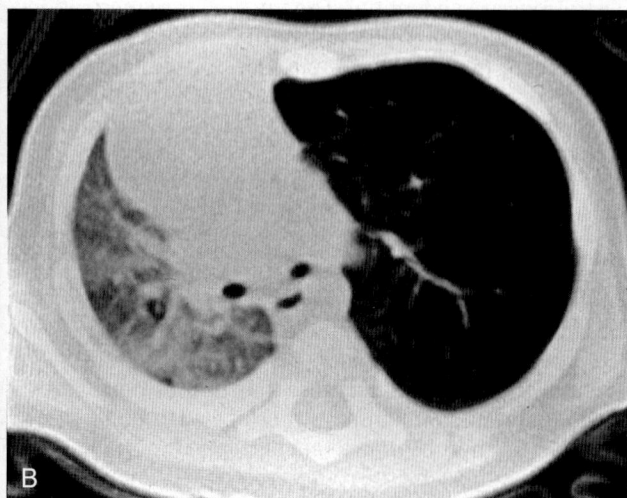

Fig. 18.32 (A) Chest x-ray and (B) computed tomography scan of a congenital large hyperlucent lobe (congenital lobar emphysema).

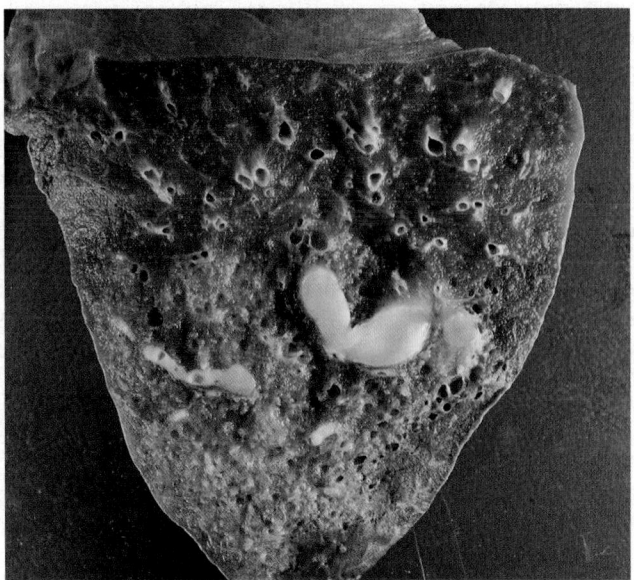

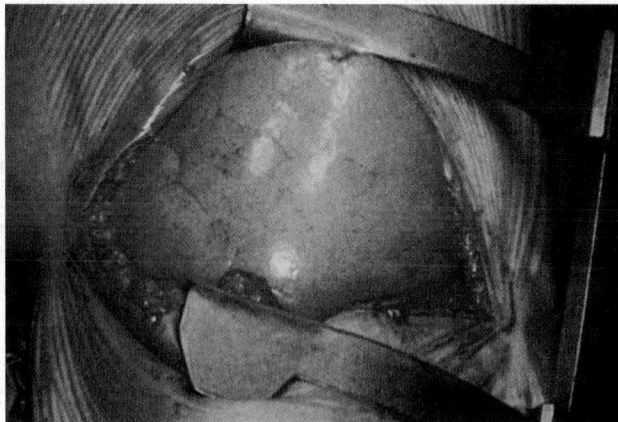

Fig. 18.34 Surgery for congenital large hyperlucent lobe (congenital lobar emphysema). The hyperexpanded lobe protrudes out of the thoracotomy incision.

Fig. 18.33 Bronchial atresia. The cut surface of the lung shows dilated airways plugged with mucus with surrounding microcystic changes. Dissection showed atresia at the origin of the apical segmental bronchus.

the problem is a pathologically distended lobe on one side or a congenitally small contralateral lung, with secondary physiologic overexpansion. Bronchoscopy may reveal causes of intrinsic obstruction and permit the removal of a foreign body or inspissated secretions. An echocardiogram is valuable in evaluating the heart and great vessels, while a contrast CT scan is useful in evaluating the anatomy of the emphysematous lobe (its size and relations), and whether it has herniated into the contralateral hemithorax.[220] It is useful in demonstrating the nature of adjacent lobes of the lung. This investigation is also useful in excluding contralateral pulmonary hypoplasia.

Differential Diagnosis

There are two broad groups of differential diagnoses. The first is any intrinsic or extrinsic cause of failure of airspace emptying. Intrinsic partial obstruction may result from inspissated mucus or aspirated material. Endobronchial granulomas due to ET suction may also result in obstruction of the airway.[221] Intrinsic obstruction due to bronchial atresia of the affected lobe is well recognized (Fig. 18.33). The affected parenchyma is ventilated collaterally, through the pores of Kohn, from adjacent normal lung. Extrinsic compression of bronchi due to congenital heart disease or anomalies of the great vessels usually presents as emphysematous changes of more gradual onset, often after the neonatal period. Less common causes of extrinsic compression include bronchogenic cysts. The other major differential diagnosis group is any cause of loss of lung volume on the contralateral side. These causes include absent lung, and lobar or lung collapse due to bronchial obstruction. Mediastinal shift with an opaque large lung, an occasional early finding in CLHL, should be distinguished from other causes of unilateral opacification and contralateral mediastinal shift in the neonate, such as chylothorax, CDH, or airless congenital CTM.

Treatment

Those children who do not suffer respiratory compromise can be managed conservatively. Their outcome is comparable those children managed by resection of an emphysematous lobe (Fig. 18.34); the distended emphysematous lobe does not compromise the growth and development of the adjacent lung.[222] Lobectomy is indicated in the event of respiratory distress, which rarely, if ever, develops de novo beyond the newborn period. The actual surgical technique is as for any other lobectomy. Ventilation in this circumstance may be difficult. Low pressure, high-frequency oscillation has been advocated to prevent barotrauma to the affected lobe and further respiratory compromise to the adjacent lung.

PULMONARY AGENESIS, APLASIA (ABSENT LUNG), AND HYPOPLASIA (SMALL LUNG)

Bilateral pulmonary agenesis is a rare malformation that may occur in anencephaly. Unilateral pulmonary agenesis is slightly more common, with the absence of the carina, and with the trachea running directly into a single bronchus. Pulmonary agenesis may be divided into three types (Box 18.4).

Pathologically, the sole lung is larger than normal in pulmonary agenesis, and this enlargement is true hypertrophy and not emphysema. Prevalence has been estimated at 0.34 per 100,000 live births.[223] Associated ipsilateral and other congenital abnormalities (cardiac, gastrointestinal, skeletal, vascular, genitourinary, and craniofacial are common.[224,225] Velocardiofacial syndromes, di George and Goldenhar syndromes, and VACTERL association have all been described in this setting. Associated pulmonary abnormalities are contralateral hypoplasia, complete tracheal rings, and tracheomalacia. There may be an association with duplications of chromosome 2.[226] The mortality of right-sided agenesis is twice that of left-sided agenesis; this is probably a result of more severe mediastinal and cardiac displacement. However, prolonged survival has been reported.[227] Pulmonary aplasia, the most common variant, consists of a carina and main-stem bronchial stump with unilateral absence of the distal lung. In this situation, secretions can pool in the stump, become infected, and possibly spill over to infect the sole lung. Lobar agenesis and aplasia are rarer than complete absence of one lung and usually affect the right upper and middle lobes together. Pulmonary hypoplasia (CSLs) consists of incompletely developed lung parenchyma connected to bronchi that may also be underdeveloped depending on when the presumed causal insult took effect in embryogenesis. There are a large number of causes of CSLs (Tables 18.9 and 18.10). The alveoli are reduced in number or size (numbers are assessed by counting alveolar wall intercepts on a line from the terminal bronchiole to the interlobular septum). However, hypoplasia is perhaps best considered to be present in term babies when the lung-to-body weight ratio is less than 0.012. There is a high incidence (around 50%) of associated diaphragmatic, cardiac, gastrointestinal, genitourinary, and skeletal malformations, as well as frequent variations in the bronchopulmonary vasculature. Correction of any underlying abnormality, if feasible, either postnatally or antenatally, may permit the growth of alveoli. However, airway branching is complete by 16 weeks, so airways will not branch after a causal abnormality has been corrected; since the airway pattern is abnormal, alveolar numbers are never likely to be normal.

Table 18.9 Causes of Bilateral Congenital Small Lungs

System Fault	Example
Lack of space	Abnormal thoracic, abdominal, or amniotic cavity contents
Abnormal vascular supply	Pulmonary valve or artery stenosis Tetralogy of Fallot
Neuromuscular disease	CNS, anterior horn cell, peripheral nerve or muscle disease (particularly severe spinal muscular atrophy and myotonic dystrophy inherited from mother) reducing fetal breathing movements

CNS, Central nervous system.

Table 18.10 Congenital Small Lungs Due to Extrapulmonary Mechanical Factors

Abnormal thoracic contents	Diaphragmatic hernia Pleural effusion Large CTM
Thoracic compression from below	Abdominal tumors Ascites
Thoracic compression from the sides	Amniotic bands Oligohydramnios (any cause) Asphyxiating dystrophy/scoliosis or other chest wall deformity

CTM, Congenital thoracic malformation.

ECTOPIA

Ectopia is growth of normal tissue in the incorrect anatomic position and, in relation to the lung, comprises either nonpulmonary tissues being present in the lung or lung tissue outside the thoracic cavity.[228,229] In relation to extrapulmonary tissues, ectopic glial tissue is well recognized within the lung, with nodules of glial tissue being implanted in anencephalics or due to embolization in relation to intrauterine trauma. Adrenocortical tissue, thyroid, liver, and skeletal muscle have also been described in the lung, and pancreatic tissue has been found in intralobar sequestrations. Ectopic lung tissue may be found in the neck, chest wall, and even in the abdomen, although some ectopias represent extralobar sequestrations. Alternative terms for this occurrence include congenital pneumatocele and congenital pulmonary hernia, although they are best regarded as true ectopias. Entire kidneys may also be intrathoracic in location.

Specific Problems: Abnormal Connections Between the Bronchial Tree and Other Structures

TRACHEOESOPHAGEAL FISTULA AND ESOPHAGEAL ATRESIA

Etiology

The environmental, chromosomal, and genetic abnormalities implicated in these conditions have recently been reviewed.[230–233] Deletions in the glutathione S-transferase gene have been implicated in isolated esophageal atresia.[234] Genetic factors implicated in esophageal atresia as part of a syndrome include *CHD7* in familial CHARGE syndrome,[235] *FOXF1* and the 16q24.1 FOX transcription factor gene cluster,[236] and polyalanine expansion in the *ZIC3* gene[237] (both VACTERL), and a 5.9 Mb microdeletion in chromosome band 17q22-q23.2 associated with TEF and conductive hearing loss.[238]

Pathology. If there is incomplete mesodermal separation of the primitive foregut, then a fistula may develop between the esophagus and the trachea (see Fig. 18.25). Most commonly, they are associated with esophageal atresia, with about 85% of such cases being associated with a fistula. Typically, the proximal part of the esophagus ends in a blind sac, and the distal part takes origin from the lower part of the trachea. The upper blind pouch is large and substantial, and usually ends about 8 cm from the superior alveolar ridge in the region of the azygos vein. Conversely, the lower esophageal segment is small and originates from the region of the distal posterior membranous trachea, carina, or right main stem bronchus.

Instances of communication between the trachea and the esophagus with an otherwise normal esophagus occur in about 3% of tracheoesophageal fistulas (Fig. 18.35). Although symptoms from this congenital abnormality are fairly severe, the diagnosis is often delayed, with considerable respiratory morbidity due to aspiration and infection. The

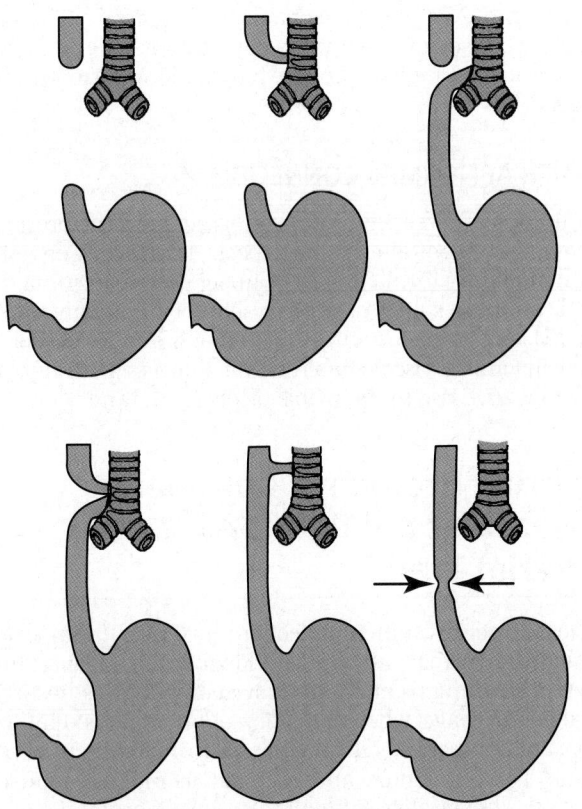

Fig. 18.35 Types of tracheo-esophageal fistulae.

Table 18.11 Waterson Classification of Esophageal Atresia, With Survival Figures

Group	Classification	Survival
A	Birthweight >2500 g, otherwise well	100%
B	Birthweight 2000–2500 g, otherwise well	85%
	Birthweight >2500 g, moderate anomalies	
	Noncardiac anomalies including patent ductus arteriosus	
	Ventricular septal defect and atrial septal defect	
C	Birthweight <2000 g, severe cardiac anomalies	65%

Table 18.12 Spitz Classification of Esophageal Atresia, With Survival Figures

Group	Classification	Survival
I	Birthweight >1500 g without congenital heart disease	97%
II	Birthweight <1500 g or major congenital heart disease	59%
III	Birthweight <1500 g and major congenital heart disease	22%

tracheoesophageal connection is almost always small, and the majority are found in the neck, from below the larynx to the thoracic inlet. Occasionally, a bronchus may communicate with the esophagus.

Associations

Tracheoesophageal fistula is more common in first and twin pregnancies of mothers of increasing age. About two-thirds have an associated abnormality.[239] Of the live births, 20% have birth weights below the fifth centile. More than 50% of infants with esophageal atresia have associated anomalies. These are most common in pure esophageal atresia without fistula and least common in H-type fistula. The acronym VATER initially described vertebral, anal, tracheoesophageal, radial, and renal anomalies. This was then modified to VACTERL to include cardiac and limb problems. Infants with this association have a high mortality rate. Almost 80% have cardiac anomalies, these being the principal cause of death. Esophageal disease is also part of the CHARGE syndrome (coloboma, heart disease, choanal atresia, retarded growth, genital hypoplasia, and ear [deafness] abnormalities), which carries a high mortality. Chromosomal abnormalities are reported in 6% of cases, in trisomy 13, 18, and 21 in particular.[240] Other associations include Potter syndrome (bilateral renal agenesis), Pierre Robin, polysplenia, and DiGeorge sequences. The incidence of cardiac anomalies has been reported to be between 30% and 50% in various series. There is also a significant incidence (47%) of tracheobronchial anomalies[241] ranging from tracheomalacia, abnormal nonciliated epithelium, lung agenesis, and hypoplasia or ectopic bronchi, to glossoptosis and airway obstruction. Pharyngeal function and aspiration on deglutition is common. The incidence of vertebral and skeletal anomalies, ranging from sacral agenesis, hemivertebrae, and rib and radial anomalies is 20%–50% overall. Cases with associated cleft lip[242] and duodenal atresia are higher risk.

Presentation

Maternal polyhydramnios has been reported in 85% of cases with pure esophageal atresia and 32% of those associated with tracheoesophageal fistula. Diagnosis by antenatal ultrasound is unreliable, with up to 50% false positives.[243] At birth, the baby is commonly frothing, choking, and suffering cyanotic episodes despite oral suction. If the condition is suspected, the initial examination should be carefully performed to identify any associated anomalies. The effect of birth weight and associated anomalies on survival is shown (Tables 18.11 and 18.12). An attempt should be made to pass an orogastric tube. Acid fluid may be aspirated from the tube if gastric contents reflux into the upper pouch across the fistula. A plain radiograph will demonstrate the tube coiled in the upper pouch and may identify pulmonary abnormalities, such as consolidation of the right upper lobe due to aspiration, plethoric lung fields due to cardiac anomalies, and vertebral and rib anomalies. The radiograph will reveal the presence or absence of gas in the stomach, indicating the presence or absence of a tracheoesophageal fistula. The intestinal gas pattern should be carefully examined on the abdominal radiograph to try to exclude distal intestinal atresia. An echocardiogram is useful to identify intracardiac structural anomalies and the possibility of a right-sided aortic arch.

Preoperative Care

The preoperative care for this condition should start from the moment it is suspected. Continuous suction of the oropharynx is important to reduce the risk of aspiration and thus protect the airway. A sump sucker, such as a Replogle tube, is useful, since it permits continuous suction and protects the esophageal mucosa from direct suction-related trauma.[243] Cyanotic episodes have been reported with the use of this form of suction of the upper pouch, and this is thought to be due to excessive negative pressure causing ineffective inspiration. The infant should be nursed prone. If pulmonary consolidation is identified, then physiotherapy and postural drainage should be employed.

Surgery

The outcomes of either thoracoscopy or open thoracotomy have a similar complication rate.[244] A right thoractomy[245] with an extrapleural approach and end-to-end single-layer anastomosis and division of fistula remains the most common technique for the majority of children presenting with esophageal atresia and tracheoesophageal fistula. Routinely, the infant is fed by a transanastomotic tube. The use of intercostal drains and postoperative contrast studies varies between institutions and cases.[245] A variety of approaches have been proposed for those cases of esophageal atresia with a large distal fistula presenting with respiratory compromise due to gastric distention: ET intubation beyond the fistula orifice, Fogarty balloon occlusion of the fistula, and formation of gastrostomy. More recently, urgent thoracotomy and fistula ligation with primary or subsequent repair of the atresia has gained wider acceptance. Several preoperative and perioperative techniques have been proposed for cases wherein the distance between the proximal and distal segments is wide. The absolute length of the gap is not as relevant as its relation to the size and strength of the wall of the esophageal segments. Per pouch bougienage either preoperatively or perioperatively to shorten the gap has been widely described and more recently modified.[246] Perioperative techniques to facilitate primary anastomosis include the use of circular, transverse, or spiral myotomies of the upper pouch. More recently, alternative techniques have been proposed to repair long-gap esophageal atresia.[247] One alternative approach, described by Scharli,[248] is to mobilize the gastric cardia into the chest by thoracoabdominal approach, permitting division of the left gastric artery; favorable long-term results have been reported.[249] The primary thoracoscopic repair of esophageal atresia and tracheoesophageal fistula is well described. The possible advantages of this approach are being assessed.[250–252] Failing these techniques, the only option may be esophageal replacement by colonic, ileocolic, or gastric interposition. Each technique is associated with vagotomy, and requires a gastric drainage procedure. Proponents of each approach have described good results. More recently, gastric transposition has become a well-established substitute for esophageal replacement.[253] What is clear is that the advantages or otherwise of this plethora of surgical techniques will only be determined if careful follow-up studies are undertaken.

Postoperative Course

Even after completely successful surgery, tracheomalacia is common, and the well-known brassy "tracheoesophageal fistula cough" (TEF cough) is a feature. Recurrent aspiration leading to bronchitis and bronchopneumonia is frequent. A missed diagnosis of laryngeal cleft should always be considered (see earlier). Occasionally, tracheomalacia may be so severe as to be life threatening, but generally the cough sounds more impressive than the consequences. Up to 17% of patients may require fundoplication for postoperative gastroesophageal reflux, and 25% have dysphagia at 2 years.[239] The early mortality associated with this condition is often related to the associated malformations, but the long-term outcome is good.[254,255]

OTHER ABNORMAL CONNECTIONS

Rare cases of direct communication between the bronchial tree and congenital cysts have been described. Congenital bronchobiliary fistula as part of upper gastrointestinal tract duplication is a source of bile in respiratory secretions. Rarely, a CTM may connect with the stomach and be associated with abdominal visceral malrotation. Conversely, the esophagus may give rise to the whole or part of a lung.[256]

Specific Problems: Congenital Disease of the Pulmonary Arterial Tree

When surgery is contemplated for any CTM, it is important that any abnormal vasculature is identified in advance. Inadvertent severing of anomalous systemic arteries has led to fatal hemorrhage, whereas ligation of anomalous veins from adjacent nonsequestered lung has led to infarction of normal tissue. The pulmonary and systemic arterial trees must be considered separately. Systemic arterial abnormalities of the great vessels of the mediastinum can be separated into those of the bronchial circulation (normally 1%–2% of the left ventricular output) and other pathologic collaterals. The pulmonary capillary bed may be bypassed, leading to direct arteriovenous communication, or absent, resulting in minimal pulmonary arteriovenous connections.

DISORDERS OF PULMONARY ARTERY ARRANGEMENT

Pulmonary arterial and venous arrangement generally mirrors bronchial arrangement. Exceptions to this rule include congenital origin of the left pulmonary artery from the right (pulmonary artery sling) (Fig. 18.36). Presentation is the same as with any vascular ring (see earlier). In this condition, the left pulmonary artery has to traverse the mediastinum from right to left, compressing the trachea as it does so. There also may be a crossover arterial segment, with the right upper lobe supplied by a branch from the left pulmonary artery, so preoperative pulmonary angiography is essential. Surgical repair of a sling with a crossover may result in infarction of the right upper lobe if the abnormal vessel has not been discovered. Another association is complete cartilage rings (above), and the infant should be evaluated for this anomaly, probably before undergoing surgery. Isolated crossover pulmonary artery branches in the absence of bronchial crossover are occasionally seen. They cross the mediastinum to supply lung segments, which often are abnormal in other ways.

Absent or Small Pulmonary Artery

Either lung may be affected by unilateral absence of a pulmonary artery (Video 18.3), and the defect may be isolated or associated with other cardiovascular anomalies, typically tetralogy of Fallot with an absent left pulmonary artery, and

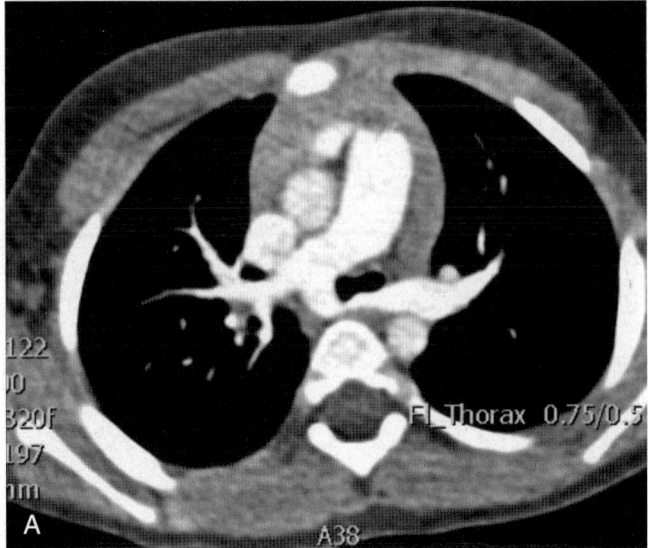

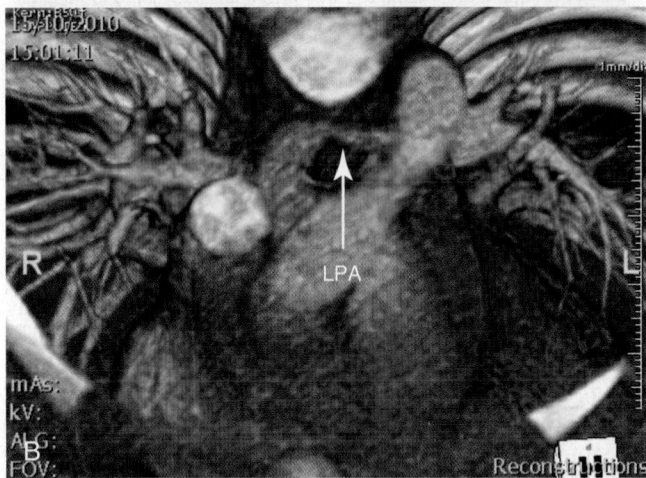

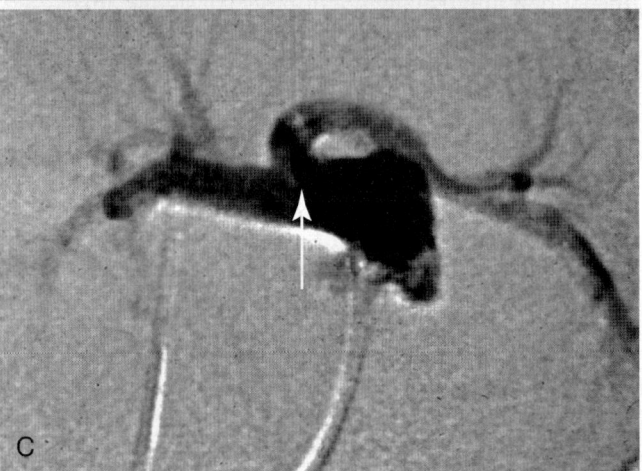

Fig. 18.36 Pulmonary artery sling. (A) Contrast CT scan showing the course of the left pulmonary artery as it takes origin from the right pulmonary artery. (B) Reconstruction demonstrating narrowing of the left pulmonary artery as it crosses the mediastinum. (C) Digital subtraction angiogram of a pulmonary artery sling. The left pulmonary artery (LPA) takes origin from the right pulmonary artery *(arrow)*.

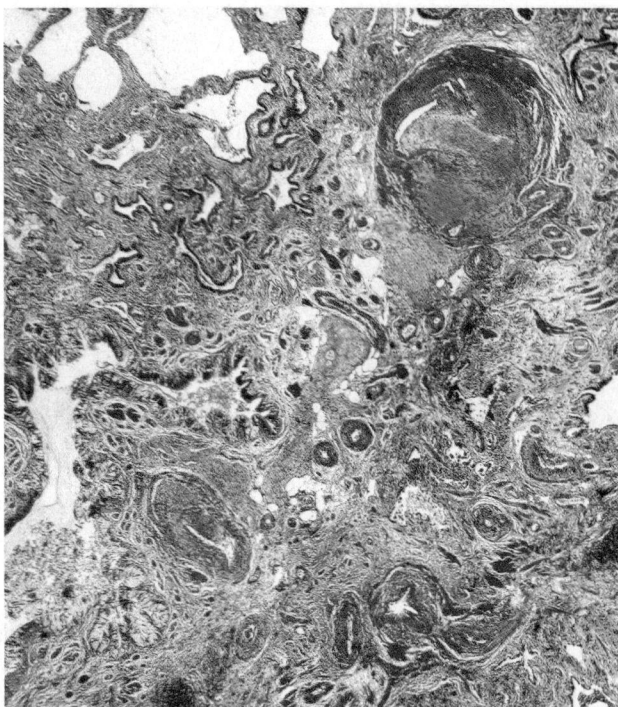

Fig. 18.37 Absence of the pulmonary artery. The parenchyma lacks pulmonary arteries, but shows very prominent bronchial arteries instead.

patent ductus arteriosus with an absent right pulmonary artery. There is an association with absent pulmonary valve syndrome. Symptoms may not arise until adult life, when they are generally due to pulmonary infection or hemorrhage. When there is only a short section absent, patients may be amenable to surgical correction, but usually the pulmonary vasculature is absent in much of the lung; histologic examination reveals hypertrophied bronchial arteries and often areas of dense fibrous scarring (Fig. 18.37). Normal pulmonary blood flow *in utero* and in the early postnatal period is needed for normal lung development. Before birth, less than 5% of the cardiac output reaches distal to the arterial duct, so it may seem surprising that interference with this small flow leads to underdevelopment of the alveolar bed and its vasculature, but there is considerable experimental evidence and clinical observation to confirm that this is so. Congenitally small unilateral pulmonary artery is usually seen in association with an ipsilateral small lung. However, it is unclear whether the primary abnormality is related to blood flow or whether both the small lung and the abnormal blood supply are due to an unknown primary event.

Pulmonary stenosis may affect lobar and segmental vessels as well as the main pulmonary arteries, and the narrowings may be multiple. Unilateral absence of a pulmonary artery leads to the lung on that side receiving only a systemic blood supply, either through anomalous systemic arteries or enlarged bronchial arteries. People with isolated unilateral absence may lead a normal life, or symptoms may not arise until adult life; one-third remain completely asymptomatic. Symptoms include pulmonary infection or bleeding from bronchopulmonary anastomoses. Ipsilateral lung tumor and pulmonary hypertension have been reported.[257] Clinically, the condition may be difficult to distinguish from embolic occlusion and obliterative bronchiolitis. The presence of other

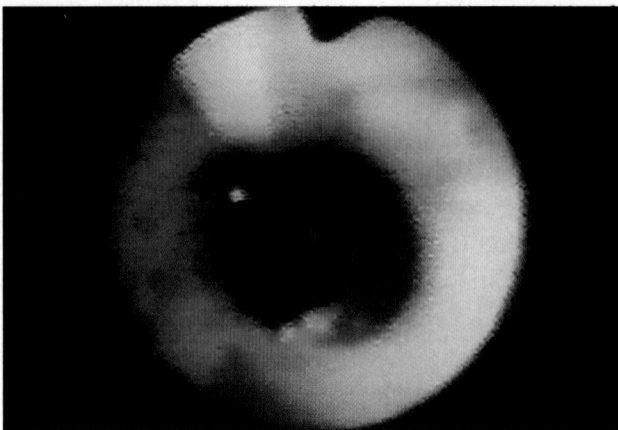

Fig. 18.38 Iatrogenic complete infarction of the trachea, which is black and necrotic. The child had undergone a unifocalization procedure, in which the bronchial arteries had been stripped from the airways and anastomosed to create a pulmonary trunk. The child is intubated; the blue line marks the endotracheal tube.

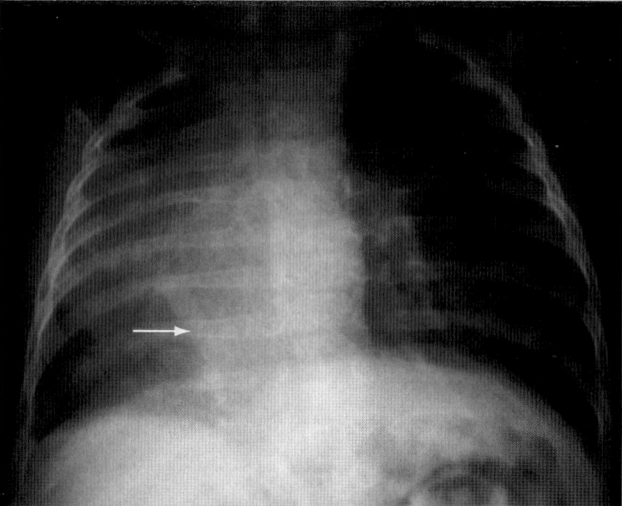

Fig. 18.39 Scimitar syndrome (congenital small right lung, venous drainage to the inferior caval vein). The abnormal right-sided venous drainage is *arrowed*.

congenital defects would militate against these, and the absence of mosaic attenuation on CT scan would point away from obliterative bronchiolitis.

It is worth noting an iatrogenic complication related to an abnormal pulmonary blood supply in children with pulmonary valve atresia and supply of the lungs solely by systemic arterial blood. In the surgical procedure of unifocalization, the collateral circulation is used to create an artificial trunk supplying the whole of the lung, which can then be anastomosed to the right ventricle via a conduit. We have reported on children with severe postoperative bronchial ischemia and even total infarction, as a result of excessively vigorous stripping of the bronchial circulation from the airways (Fig. 18.38).[258]

One or both pulmonary arteries may originate from the aorta.[259] Bilateral origin from the aorta is part of the spectrum of the common arterial trunk and usually will present to the pediatric or fetal cardiologist. Unilateral origin of a pulmonary artery from the aorta may be an isolated abnormality, sometimes presenting with persistent tachypnea.

Specific Problems: Congenital Disease of the Pulmonary Venous Tree

ABNORMAL PULMONARY VENOUS DRAINAGE

Anomalous pulmonary veins result in blood from the lungs returning to the right side of the heart rather than entering the left atrium. The anomalous veins may join the inferior caval vein or hepatic, portal, or splenic veins below the diaphragm, or above the diaphragm they may drain into the superior caval vein or its tributaries, the coronary sinus, or the right atrium. Anomalous pulmonary venous drainage may be obstructed or unobstructed. The anomaly may be total or partial, unilateral or bilateral, and isolated or associated with other cardiopulmonary developmental defects. These include bronchial isomerism, mirror-image arrangement, asplenia, pulmonary stenosis, patent arterial duct, and a small interatrial communication. The type of isomerism gives

a good indication as to whether the anomaly is total or partial; right-sided isomerism suggests totally anomalous veins and left-sided isomerism suggests a partial anomaly. Occasionally, the anomalous vein runs much of its course buried within the lung substance. Anomalous pulmonary venous connections are often narrow, and this may cause relatively mild pulmonary hypertension. Unilateral anomalous venous drainage may be part of complex lung malformations; it may also be seen in association with what appears to be a simple lung cyst. This underscores the need for accurate delineation of all abnormalities even in straightforward-appearing cases. Minor abnormalities of venous connection, such as a segment draining directly into the azygos system, are not uncommon and usually not of practical significance.

The scimitar syndrome is a particular clinical problem characterized by a small right lung, resulting in the heart moving to the right (cardiac dextroposition), and an abnormal band shadow representing the abnormal venous drainage to the systemic veins (Fig. 18.39 and Video 18.4), fancifully compared to a scimitar (a sign that is in fact often absent). Infants with this condition presenting in heart failure have a worse prognosis, often because of associated abnormalities, among which may be malformations in the left side of the heart. Aortopulmonary collaterals should be sought and occluded (Videos 18.5 and 18.6). More invasive treatment options include reimplantation of the vein or pneumonectomy. Severe pulmonary hypertension is an adverse prognostic feature. An association with horseshoe lung has been described; this usually causes early death, but occasional long-term survival has been reported.[260,261]

CONGENITAL ABSENCE OF THE PULMONARY VEINS

Absence of the pulmonary veins or narrowing of their ostia into the left atrium results in pulmonary venous obstruction. It also may be associated with partial anomalous pulmonary venous drainage. The atresia may be unilateral (Fig. 18.40) or bilateral, but in either case severe hypertensive changes develop in both lungs. Congenital pulmonary vein atresia

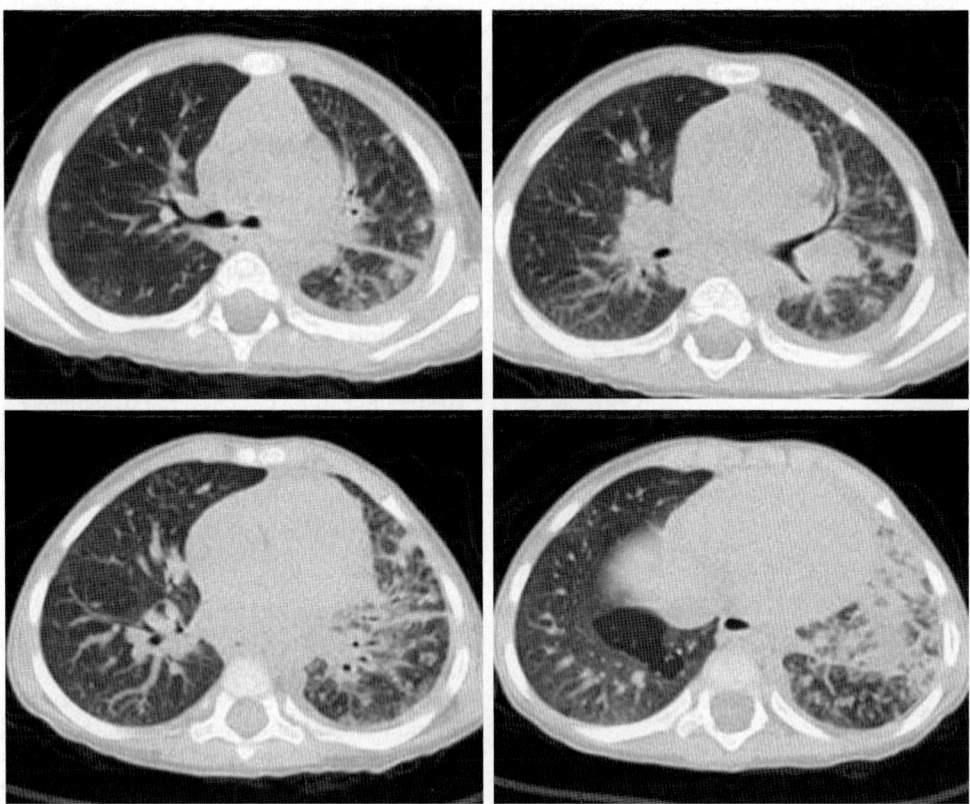

Fig. 18.40 Computed tomography scan showing changes associated with absent left pulmonary veins. The left lung is engorged, with dilated lymphatics, and a left sided pleural effusion.

carries a very poor prognosis; few children with the condition survive longer than 1 year. Stenting open the ostia via cardiac catheterization has been reported.

Specific Problems: Abnormalities of the Connections Between the Pulmonary Arterial and Venous Trees

CONGENITAL ALVEOLAR CAPILLARY DYSPLASIA

This disorder represents a misalignment of lung vessels due to a failure of capillaries to grow in appropriate number and location within the alveolar tissue of the lung. It was often thought to be associated with abnormally sited pulmonary veins within bronchovascular bundles, but in fact these are dilated bronchial veins with anastomotic connections to the pulmonary veins, which are obliterated beyond these connections.[262] It is an unusual cause of congenital pulmonary hypertension, persistent fetal circulation, and respiratory distress in the newborn. It is discussed in detail in Chapter 56, and will not be further considered in this chapter.

PULMONARY ARTERIOVENOUS MALFORMATIONS

These have been reviewed in detail recently,[263–265] and include more detailed management protocols than there is space for in this chapter.

Prevalence

The likely prevalence of significant PAVMs is around 1 in 2630 (95% confidence intervals 1 in 1315–5555).[266] The prevalence of hereditary hemorrhagic telangiectasia (HHT; Osler-Weber-Rendu disease) is 1 in 5000–8000.

Etiology

Many cases of pulmonary arteriovenous fistulae are associated with HHT, which is a genetic vascular disorder characterized by epistaxis, telangiectasia, and visceral manifestations including PAVMs. The two known disease types, HHT1 and HHT2, are caused by mutations in the endoglin (*ENG*, 9q34) and ACVRL1 (*ALK-1*, 12q13) genes, respectively.[267,268] A third locus has been described on chromosome 5[269] but the exact gene is not yet known. Recently, *SMAD4* (18q21) mutations have been described in HHT with juvenile polyposis syndrome (HHT-juvenile polyposis),[270] and the extending spectrum of these associations reviewed.[271] The unifying feature of these three genes is that they all relate to the TGF-β superfamily signaling pathway.[272] A family with diffuse PAVMs and a mutation in the nuclear prelamin A recognition factorlike (*NARFL*, 21q21.3) has recently been described.[273]

Clinical Features

PAVMs constitute an important group of abnormalities that potentially involves systemic and pulmonary arterial and venous trees (Fig. 18.41). They represent a direct intrapulmonary connection between the pulmonary artery and vein without an intervening capillary bed. This cavernous arteriovenous aneurysm is an uncommon cause of

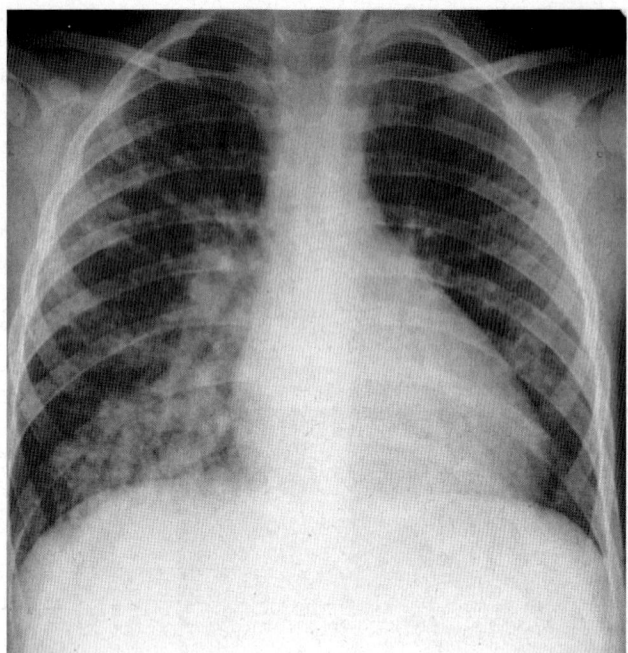

Fig. 18.41 Chest x-ray showing multiple pulmonary arteriovenous fistulae, in particular in the right lower lobe.

symptoms in the pediatric age group and is often diagnosed in adults. Presentation is with cyanosis, hemoptysis, chest pain, or neurologic complications (see later). Presentation with breathlessness is rare, and indeed these patients can exercise at a high level, which is related to compensatory secondary polycythemia restoring the blood oxygen carrying capacity.[274] Orthodeoxia and orthostatic tachycardia, if present, are useful pointers to the presence of PAVMs,[275] but relying on this as a screening test will lead to many cases being missed.[276] The chest radiograph may be normal, but more usually well-defined single or multiple opacities are seen, with vessels connecting them to the hila, which are strongly suggestive of the diagnosis. Fistulas occur in the lower lobes in about 60% of cases; they are single in 60% and unilateral in 75%. Macroscopically, lesions can be peripheral or central and may simulate a saccular, cavernous, hemangioma because of aneurysmal swelling. The fistula is fed by at least one afferent artery, usually pulmonary and less often bronchial, and may be drained by several veins, almost always pulmonary. In 80%, there is a single feeding pulmonary artery and a single draining pulmonary vein. There are numerous communications between artery and vein in this tortuous, dilated, wormlike vessel mass. On microscopic examination, the arteriovenous fistula is lined with vascular endothelium.

Diagnosis

Diagnosis is confirmed by documenting an abnormal right-to-left shunt at the pulmonary vascular level, either by contrast echocardiography (the contrast being a peripheral injection of microbubbles), a technetium Tc 99m macroaggregate lung perfusion scan, with shunt quantification by counting over the kidneys and brain, or increasingly using CT angiography. Echocardiography has excellent positive and negative predictive value, and should be the first-line investigation, since

it is estimated this approach can substantially reduce the numbers of children requiring CT,[277] and indeed the radiation burden should be a significant factor in the investigation of these patients. The large malformations may have both a systemic and a pulmonary arterial supply (see earlier). The differential diagnosis includes vascular and nonvascular mimics. The former include true and false pulmonary artery aneurysms, and pulmonary varix[263,278]; the latter include any cause of a mass, including a bronchocele and vascular tumors.

Screening

There are guidelines for screening patients with known HHT,[279] but these are often not well followed.[280] HHT patients who did not have a right to left shunt at diagnosis did not develop one during 5 years' follow-up.[281] A total of 18% of patients with a shunt at baseline increased their shunt in the next 5 years.

Treatment

When planning therapy, it is important to know if there is a systemic component, since this may cause high-output cardiac failure. Furthermore, embolization of an abnormal pulmonary arteriovenous connection via the feeding pulmonary artery may be curative, whereas more extensive procedures may be needed to deal with systemic arterial components. Embolization of PAVMs is the preferred treatment option with a feeding artery ≥3 mm,[282] even if they are extensive. Various devices, including the Amplatzer, have been used.[283–286] Although lung transplantation has been reported for this condition, the results are clearly inferior. Multiple procedures may be necessary. In one series, one-third of patients obtained normal oxygen saturation and 15% an improved exercise tolerance; generally, embolization, even of major, multiple PAVMs is preferable to transplantation.[287] Regrowth or de novo PAVMs are not rare,[288,289] so repeated echocardiographic screening is wise.[290] Diffuse microscopic disease is more difficult to treat, but there is some evidence that embolization may reduce the prevalence of neurologic complications. The molecular pathology has recently been reviewed.[291]

Associated Disorders

HHT is associated with AVMs in the brain and elsewhere. A recent meta-analysis[292] reported a prevalence of cerebral lesions around 10% with no gender difference, greater in HHT-1 (13.4%) than HHT-2 (2.4%); more than half were symptomatic. Conversely, PHT and PAVMs with liver disease were more common in HHT-2.[293] Complications include PAVMs, pulmonary hypertension secondary to high output cardiac failure with systemic AVMs, and primary pulmonary hypertension.[294] The extent to which screening should be performed for cerebral AVMS is controversial[295,296]; but this issue and other aspects of the multisystem management of the condition are beyond the scope of this chapter. PAVMs have been described in association with telomere biology disorder and dyskeratosis, some with germline *TINF2* mutations.[297,298] An association with Birt-Hogg-Dube syndrome has also been described.[299] PAVM may be the first diagnosis, before manifestations of dyskeratosis. The associations with liver disease syndrome[300,301] and after Fontan surgery[302,303] are well described.

Complications

Complications of PAVMs are related to the bypassing of the filtration function of the pulmonary circulation, and hyperviscosity due to the polycythemia secondary to systemic arterial hypoxemia. Pulmonary hypertension does not usually develop with isolated PAVMs, because there is no alveolar hypoxemia. The patient may develop systemic, in particular cerebral, abscess, or thrombosis. Cerebral complications are especially seen with larger malformations.[304,305] Particular care is needed during prolonged periods of immobility in the patient with hyperviscosity. If the child is treated before puberty, further embolizations may be needed for recurrence of PAVMs after the pubertal growth spurt. In one study, iron deficiency was found to be a risk factor for ischemic stroke,[306] possibly via an effect on platelet aggregation. Whether correction of iron deficiency reduces the risk has not been determined, but it would seem sensible to prescribe iron supplementation in iron-deficient PAVM patients

CAPILLARY MALFORMATIONS

These are only recently acknowledged as a clinical entity. They may be isolated, or part of syndromes, such as Sturge-Weber, Klippel-Trenaunay, and Parkes-Weber. They are also associated with macrocephaly and with diffuse overgrowth, and are, in effect, capillary level AVMs.[307–311]

Specific Problems: Congenital Disease of the Lymphatic Tree

This tree is the hardest to delineate, and in most malformations it will not be relevant. Lymphatic tree disorders usually require histologic confirmation. Lymphatic hypoplasia of varied distribution underlies the yellow nail syndrome in which lymphedema is accompanied by discoloration of the nails and pleural effusions.[312] Though inherited, it may not manifest until adult life. The Klippel-Trenaunay syndrome, usually characterized by varicosities of systemic veins, cutaneous hemangiomas, and soft tissue hypertrophy, is another congenital disorder in which pleuropulmonary abnormalities are described, including pulmonary lymphatic hyperplasia, pleural effusions, pulmonary thromboembolism, and pulmonary vein varicosities. Congenital chylothorax is described in Chapter 69.

Congenital pulmonary lymphangiectasia may be either secondary to obstruction to pulmonary lymphatic or venous drainage, or a primary disorder—the latter either limited to the lung or part of the generalized lymphangiectasia. There is a high association of primary pulmonary lymphangiectasia with other congenital abnormalities, particularly asplenia and cardiac anomalies. It is a rare cause of fetal hydrops,[313] and some cases are related to *PIEZO1*[314] and *FOXC2* mutations.[315] It usually causes severe respiratory distress and has been generally thought to be fatal in the neonatal period, but milder cases with prolonged survival have been described, and indeed presentation may be delayed until adult life.[316,317] The radiological features are also variable, depending on the age of presentation.[318] The lungs are heavy, with widened interlobular septa, and on the visceral pleural surface there is a pronounced reticular pattern of small cysts that accentuates the lobular architecture of the lungs. The cysts measure up to 5 mm in diameter and are situated in the interlobular septa and about the bronchovascular bundles. Near the hila of the lungs, the cysts are elongated. Microscopy confirms that the cysts are located in connective tissue under the pleura, in the interlobular septa, and about the bronchioles and arteries. Serial sections show that they are part of an intricate network of intercommunicating channels that vary greatly in width and are devoid of valves. The cysts are lined by an attenuated simple endothelium. The absence of multinucleate foreign body giant cell reaction distinguishes this condition from interstitial emphysema. The clinical history is also usually quite different; interstitial emphysema is usually (but not invariably, above) a complication of positive pressure ventilation in a very preterm infant. There is increasing interest in treating pulmonary lymphatic disease by techniques of lymphatic embolization.[319] The whole topic is reviewed in detail elsewhere.[320]

Specific Problems: Congenital Disorders of the Chest Wall

CONGENITAL DISORDERS OF THE CHEST WALL

Disorders of the bony rib cage and scoliosis are described in Chapter 72. Here we concentrate on diaphragmatic disorders. Disorders of fetal breathing movements are beyond the scope of this chapter, but these are essential for normal lung development. The abdomen is part of the chest wall, and any disorder that increases abdominal contents before birth, such as fetal ascites or a large tumor, will impede lung development and cause bilateral CSL.

Chest wall disease, such as diaphragmatic hernia and asphyxiating thoracic dystrophy, present as respiratory distress with difficulty in establishing ventilation. By contrast, neuromuscular disease, such as severe spinal muscular atrophy or myotonic dystrophy with maternal inheritance, is characterized by inadequate or absent respiratory effort, but ease of establishing ventilation, unless there are associated unilateral or bilateral CSLs. This last group of conditions is covered in Chapter 72.

CONGENITAL DIAPHRAGMATIC HERNIA

This subject has been comprehensively reviewed recently.[321]

Etiology

This is obscure, and a full review is beyond the scope of this chapter. Genetic studies have recently been reviewed.[322,323] More recent candidate genes include *HLX* gene at chromosome 1q41-1q42,[324] dispatched 1 (DISP1),[325] FGF receptor-like 1 (FGFRL1),[326,327] t-complex-associated-testis-expressed 3 (TCTE3),[328] which is interestingly also found in ciliary outer dynein arms. Animal models suggest that nitrofen-induced reduced cellular proliferation in the developing diaphragm may be important,[329] although it is possible that the primary abnormality may be maldevelopment of the ipsilateral lung.[330] There is a wide variety of abnormalities associated with CDH, including aneuploidy, in particular trisomies 18 and 13, genetic syndromes, and structural abnormalities.[331,332] Many of these will result in a stillbirth or the pregnancy being

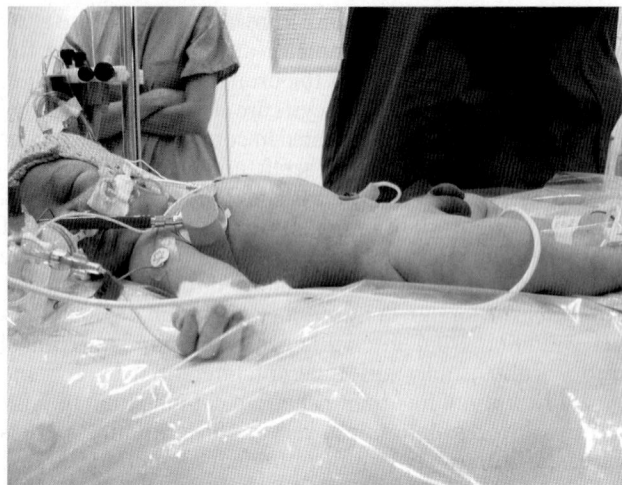

Fig. 18.42 Scaphoid abdomen in congenital diaphragmatic hernia.

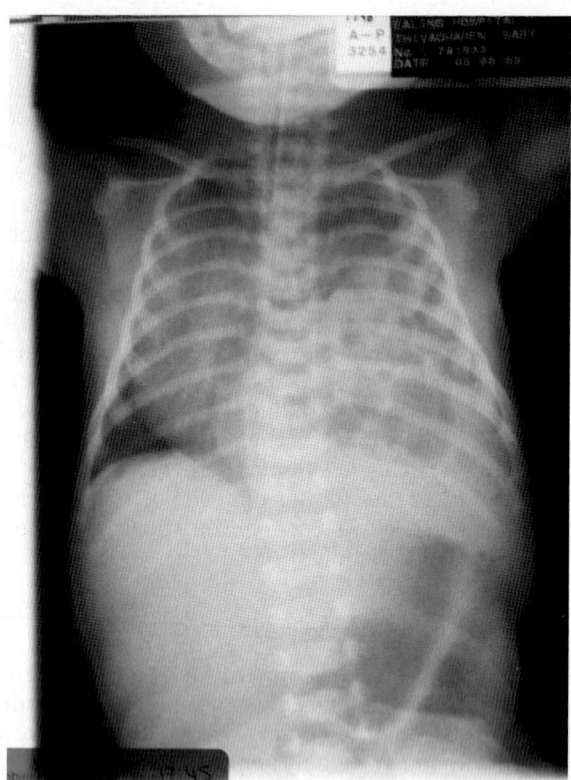

Fig. 18.43 Plain x-ray demonstrating left-sided congenital diaphragmatic hernia. There are obvious gas-filled loops of bowel in the chest.

terminated, so isolated CDH is much more common in neonates. Anomalies associated with CDH include neural tube defects (e.g., myelomeningocele), cardiac defects, and midline anomalies, such as cleft lip and palate. Genetic syndromes, such as Fryns syndrome, can account for up to 10% of cases in some series.[331]

Pathologic Anatomy

A total of 80% of CDHs are left-sided, through the left pleuroperitoneal canal. Bilateral CDHs are rare. The defect is within the diaphragm itself; there is usually no associated membranous sac. The diaphragm itself may be well developed or significantly deficient, especially at its origin from the 12th rib. Intestine, stomach, liver, and spleen may all herniate into the chest. A nonmuscular membranous sac is present in 10%–15% of cases, signifying the early occurrence of this lesion before closure of the pleuroperitoneal canal.

Postnatal Presentation

The diagnosis of CDH is usually made antenatally. From birth, infants may present with a variety of symptoms and signs. The herniation of abdominal contents into the chest inhibits normal lung development, resulting in pulmonary hypoplasia,[332] which, in isolated lesions, is the main cause of death. Typically, the abdomen is scaphoid (Fig. 18.42), the chest funnel-shaped, the trachea and mediastinum deviated to the contralateral side. The infant may be entirely well or suffer from several problems ranging from choking episodes to apnea to acute respiratory failure. Rare late presentation may be associated with chronic gastrointestinal symptoms.[333] The diagnosis of CDH is confirmed by a plain radiograph of the chest and abdomen (Fig. 18.43), after the passage of a nasogastric tube. The plain film is a poor indication of the degree of pulmonary hypoplasia.[334] If doubt persists, then an ultrasound scan of the chest demonstrating intrathoracic intestinal peristalsis is helpful. An echocardiogram should be performed to exclude intracardiac anomalies; however, fetal echocardiography should have been part of the antenatal diagnostic work-up. The postnatal differential diagnosis of CDH is similar to the prenatal one and includes extensive congenital cystic disease of the lung, Morgagni anterior diaphragmatic hernia, paraesophageal hiatus hernia, and eventration of the diaphragm.

Surgery

The management of CDH is no longer regarded as a surgical emergency. The initial management is to stabilize the baby and optimize respiratory function. Delayed surgical repair has become generally more accepted, with lower mortality rates than have been seen with immediate repair. The exact timing of surgery remains controversial. Many studies have reported varying periods of delay before surgery. One of the principal advantages of this strategy has been related to pulmonary artery pressures falling toward more normal values.[335] The operative repair may be by thoracotomy, or by subcostal or transverse abdominal approaches. The advantage of an abdominal approach is that it permits identification and correction of an associated intestinal malrotation. The laparoscopic repair of CDH has been described.[336] The principle of repair is the same as with any other hernia: reduction of herniated viscera, identification and excision of any hernia sac, and repair of the defect. Usually, primary repair can be achieved following adequate mobilization of the defect's margins. Occasionally, this is not possible because the size of the defect prevents primary suture repair. In these circumstances, a prosthetic patch may be required. An autologous muscle flap is preferred by many surgeons.[336] If extracorporeal membrane oxygenation (ECMO) therapy is anticipated, then some surgeons would prefer to minimize any dissection to reduce the risk of postoperative bleeding secondary to anticoagulation for ECMO. In these circumstances, the mobilization of the defect margins is less and the use of prosthetic patches is greater. For the same reason, malrotation will not be corrected. An intercostal chest drain is placed in the ipsilateral hemithorax by some surgeons to drain any subsequent pneumothorax or chylothorax. However, the negative pressure associated with such a device has been reported to increase barotrauma to the hypoplastic lung,[337] so some surgeons will leave the drain *in situ,* only to have negative pressure applied in the event of an accumulation that requires drainage. A thoracoscopic approach to the repair of CDH has been described. Individual centers describe the only relative contraindication to this approach as being the use of ECMO.[338] Longer operation times and higher recurrent hernia rates have been described, leading the authors to advocate for the routine use of larger wider prosthetic patches rather than primary repair of CDH. These findings have been confirmed in the most recent and wide-ranging literature review of this surgical option,[339] leading the authors to advocate a registry and review of this technique for further assessment. The need for registries and long-term follow up is a recurring theme in this field.

Chylothorax complicating repair of CDH is well recognized. It may be a persistent complication associated with significant morbidity. Octreotide has been advocated in the management of this complication.[340] In this and other causes of chylothorax, placing a thoracoabdominal shunt might be considered.[341]

Outcome

Survival of neonates reportedly varies between 39% and 95% after repair of CDH. The large variation in mortality reflects the varying severity of the pulmonary hypoplasia and abnormal pulmonary vascularity, as well as variations in the period and technique of preoperative stabilization, perioperative and postoperative mechanical ventilation, and the use of ECMO. If ECMO has to be used, the outlook is not good. Only about one-third of patients thus treated survive to 1 year of life, and substantial comorbidity (respiratory, gastrointestinal, neurodevelopmental) is common.[342] Stege and colleagues have demonstrated that the survival of this condition within one well-circumscribed geographic locus has remained unchanged over 11 years, despite the advent of new therapies. The mortality increased with the presence of other malformations.[343] A variety of neurologic abnormalities, including motor and cognitive anomalies, as well as gastroesophageal reflux, foregut dysmotility and skeletal anomalies, have been reported in infants surviving

management of this condition.[344] Significant respiratory and nutritional problems associated with gastroesophageal reflux can occur but often tend to improve with time. Respiratory findings reported in survivors include a range of abnormalities on imaging, from a completely normal examination to ipsilateral lucency on the chest radiograph. Lung function may be normal, or there may be obstructive or restrictive disease. V/Q scans are invariably abnormal. Bronchial hyperreactivity is also described, but the pattern of challenge testing suggests distal airway dysfunction rather than airway inflammation. It is suggested that most of these functional abnormalities relate to the intensity of ventilation in the perioperative period, rather than the degree of pulmonary hypoplasia at birth. However, pulmonary hypoplasia is obviously a critical determinant of survival. The incidence of gastroesophageal reflux has been reported as higher in those diaphragmatic hernias that were repaired directly.[345] Postoperative failure to thrive due to gastroesophageal reflux and oral dysfunction is common. The overall outcome of the condition is known to be worse when it is found to occur within certain syndromes, such as Fryns.

ANTERIOR DIAPHRAGMATIC HERNIA

Anterior diaphragmatic hernias occur through the foramen of Morgagni (Fig. 18.44)—a potential space that transmits the internal mammary artery, lying between the sternal and costal attachments of the diaphragm. They are much rarer than Bochdalek hernia and tend not to present in the neonatal period. If unilateral, they occur more often on the right than the left, and are almost always associated with a hernial sac. Often, these hernias are bilateral, and the hernial sacs may communicate with each other or with the pericardium.[346] Anterior diaphragmatic hernias may occur as an isolated morphologic malformation, but are often associated with cardiac anomalies and are the diaphragmatic defect associated with the pentalogy of Cantrell. The principles of repair are similar to those for Bochdalek hernia. Since the diaphragmatic defect is smaller and more easily repaired, prosthetic patches or autologous grafts are required far less frequently than with Bochdalek's hernia. Abdominal and thoracic approaches have been described for open repair.[347] Laparoscopic repair is also well established.[348] The long term outcome following repair is excellent, and is principally determined by the nature of any associated anomalies. There may be

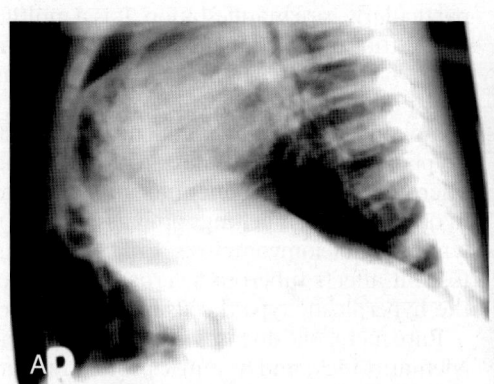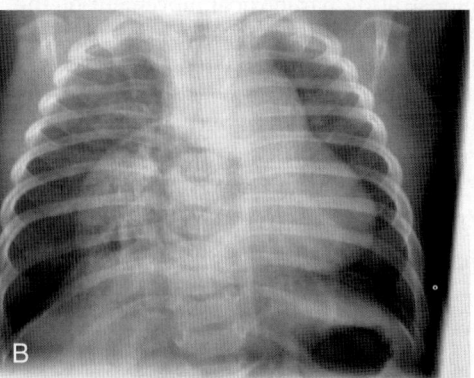

Fig. 18.44 (A) Lateral and (B) posterioranterior chest radiograph showing a Morgagni hernia.

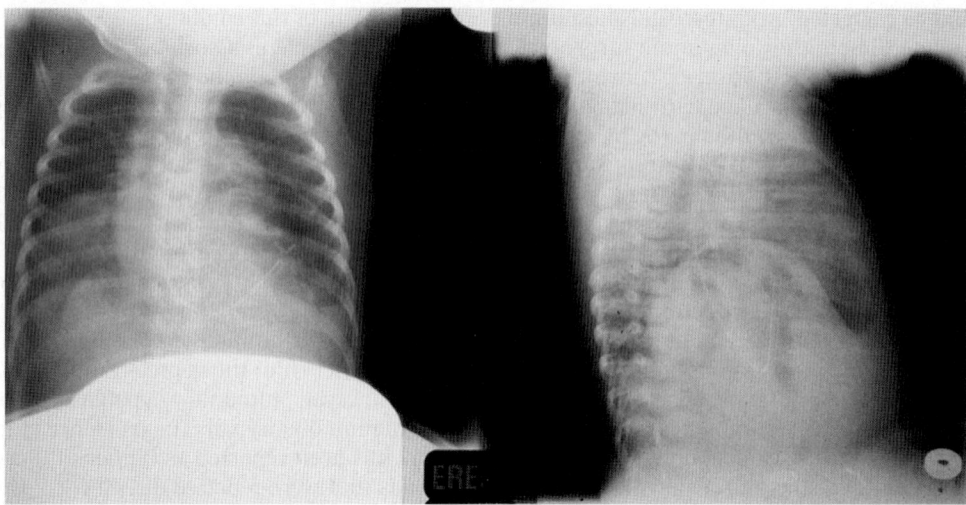

Fig. 18.45 Bilateral eventration of the diaphragm.

mild airflow obstruction and bronchial hyperreactivity to methacholine, possibly related to distal airway dysfunction. Chest asymmetry and scoliosis are not uncommon.

DIAPHRAGMATIC EVENTRATION

Eventration of the diaphragm may be congenital or acquired (Fig. 18.45). The congenital lesion is far rarer than the acquired one, which is most often either an injury to the phrenic nerve acquired during difficult instrumental delivery, insertion of a chest drain for a pneumothorax, or cardiac surgery. Should the lesion result from difficult, often breech delivery, then it may be associated with Erb palsy. The congenital lesion results from an incomplete development of the muscular portion of the diaphragm or its innervation. This has been described in neonatal cases of fetal rubella and cytomegalovirus infection. The defect is more common on the left than the right side and usually presents as a moderate to complete thinning of the diaphragmatic muscle fibers. In extreme cases, it may be very difficult pathologically to differentiate the lesion from a CDH. Bilateral lesions are rare. Several associated anomalies have been described with the congenital form of diaphragmatic eventration: rib and cardiac anomalies, renal ectopia, and exomphalos. Presentation is usually a chance finding on a chest radiograph taken for other purposes. The diagnosis is confirmed by ultrasound examination demonstrating paradoxical movement of the diaphragm. Usually, no treatment is needed, and the radiologic appearance improves with time. Bilateral large eventrations may need repair, and the best approach is through the chest, followed by radial incision and plication of the diaphragm using nonabsorbable sutures.

Specific Problems: Congenital Cardiac Disorders

Cardiac malformations may be coincidental to or a fundamental part of a pulmonary malformation. They are sufficiently common that echocardiography should be a routine part of the work-up of most suspected congenital lung abnormalities. Coincidental malformations are seen with, for example, CLHL. Around 10% have an atrial or ventricular septal defect. Lung abnormalities in which heart disease is fundamental include those with the pulmonary atresia spectrum (see earlier). By definition, lung blood supply is abnormal. However, these cases usually present to the pediatric cardiologists and are beyond the scope of this chapter. It should be noted that vascular compression of the airways in the setting of congenital heart disease is not uncommon and may be referred to the pediatric pulmonologist. The pulmonary complications of congenital heart disease are reviewed in Chapter 39.

Specific Problems: Multisystem Congenital Disorders That Affect the Lung

Most congenital lung abnormalities are isolated, but a few are part of a more generalized disorder. Tuberous sclerosis may affect the lung as well as the kidneys, heart, and brain. Complex abnormalities of lung development may be associated with chromosomal abnormalities. Micronodular type II pneumocyte hyperplasia is largely—though not exclusively—confined to patients with tuberous sclerosis, of which it is a particularly rare manifestation. It is a multifocal microscopic lesion that usually has no clinical significance, but in rare cases the lesions are of an appreciable size and so numerous that pulmonary function is compromised and the patient complains of breathlessness. The hyperplastic cells show no atypia and appear to be devoid of any malignant potential. Micronodular type II pneumocyte hyperplasia may be seen in otherwise normal lungs or in association with pulmonary lymphangioleiomyomatosis. Unlike lymphangioleiomyomatosis, it affects tuberous sclerosis patients of both sex, and the hyperplastic type II cells fail to stain for HMB-45.

Rare metabolic diseases may affect the lung. These include Niemann-Pick, and lysinuric protein intolerance. They also enter the differential diagnosis of pediatric interstitial lung disease (see Section 6).

Role of Specific Investigations

This section discusses possible investigations and their role, and does not imply that all should be performed on every child. A selective approach is essential.

CHEST RADIOGRAPHY

All infants in whom any suggestion of a lung malformation has been made antenatally will require a chest radiograph before discharge. In many it will be normal, but subsequent, more detailed imaging, may reveal even quite large malformations. Specific points in the chest radiograph in the context of congenital lung disease include the determination of bronchial (and where the gastric bubble is visible, abdominal) situs and the side of the aortic arch (Fig. 18.46); a right-sided arch may be a normal variant of no concern, but may give a clue to the presence of a vascular ring.[349] A normal chest radiograph does not exclude a significant CTM (above).

VENTILATION: PERFUSION SCANNING

Although this technique gives useful functional information, in general its use in investigating congenital lung disease is declining as CT and MRI increasingly give better anatomical and functional images. Unilateral absent perfusion and ventilation is seen in the complete absence of one lung. Unilateral absence of perfusion, which may be combined with secondary abnormalities in ventilation, is seen in the unilateral absence of the pulmonary artery, the unilateral origin of the pulmonary artery from the aorta, and the unilateral absence of the pulmonary veins. Bilateral absent or greatly reduced perfusion is seen in common arterial trunk ("truncus arteriosus"); the pattern of ventilation is normal. Focal defects are seen with large CTMs. Increased uptake of radiolabeled microspheres given by peripheral vein injection is seen in the brain and kidneys as a feature of PAVMs (as well as in congenital heart disease with right-to-left shunt) and has been used to quantitate shunt. Split lung function may be useful in determining whether operation on a unilateral bronchial or pulmonary artery stenosis is advisable. In cases of doubt, V/Q scanning can differentiate CLHL from hyperinflation of a normal lobe secondary to contralateral CSL or lobar atelectasis; in this case, the lucent area is functional, whereas congenital lobar emphysema causes a filling defect.

ULTRASOUND SCANNING (INCLUDING ECHOCARDIOGRAPHY)

Cardiac abnormality is so important when considering congenital lung malformations that it is wise to include an echocardiogram as part of the investigation of many if not most infants with suspected congenital lung disease. Indeed, fetal ultrasound will have already detected many cardiac abnormalities. Echocardiography detects relevant abnormalities of the systemic arteries in the mediastinum, such as the double aortic arch and the aberrant origin of subclavian artery. The pulmonary arteries and veins should be imaged, and unilateral abnormal (hemianomalous) venous drainage excluded. Injecting saline into a peripheral vein allows detection of a right-to-left shunt; in such cases, bubbles appear

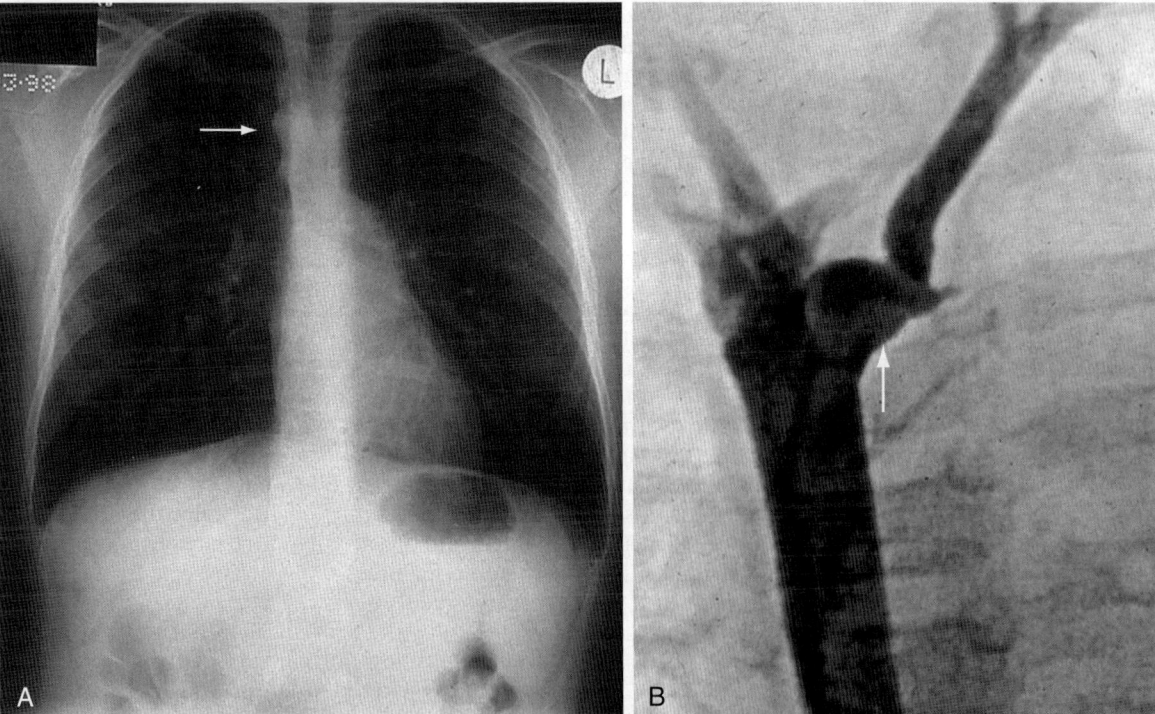

Fig. 18.46 Vascular ring. (A) Right-sided aortic arch *(arrowed)*. Note the tracheal compression by the associated vascular ring. (B) Digital subtraction angiogram showing a right-sided aortic arch, with aberrant origin of left subclavian artery from a diverticulum of Kommerel *(arrow)*. A left-sided ligamentum arteriosum completed the vascular ring.

in the left atrium. Pulmonary artery pressure may be estimated from the Bernoulli equation if there is physiologic tricuspid or pulmonary regurgitation. It may be possible to image abnormal collateral arteries arising from the abdominal aorta. Parenchymal ultrasound imaging is generally less helpful. Defects in the diaphragm may be identified and pleural disease confirmed. Ultrasound is useful in differentiating thymic abnormalities from mediastinal cysts.

A further use for this technique is endobronchial ultrasound, performed by skilled pediatric interventional radiologists, to determine if there are any complete cartilage rings in the major airways.

COMPUTED TOMOGRAPHY

CT gives the best images of parenchymal abnormalities and is currently probably the first investigation of choice in an adult with suspected CTM. A cystic CTM large enough to have the potential to be infected may be invisible on chest radiographs, so CT is recommended for all infants in whom an antenatal diagnosis of a lung malformation has been made, even if the chest radiograph after birth appears normal. Scanning after contrast injection, especially using modern reconstruction techniques, may delineate abnormal aortopulmonary collaterals, obviating the need for angiography (Fig. 18.47). This is the investigation of choice for imaging a vascular ring (see Chapter 39).

MAGNETIC RESONANCE IMAGING

As discussed above, fetal MRI is often used to delineate congenital thoracic abnormalities, but there is currently insufficient evidence to recommend that this technique be widely adopted clinically. At present, postnatal MRI requires general anesthesia in small children, but the lack of radiation exposure and ability to reconstruct vascular anatomy make this an attractive technique. MRI is the best way of detecting extension of a neurogenic tumor into the spinal canal. It can also be used to image any airway compression and its cause, and also to delineate systemic and pulmonary vasculature.

BARIUM SWALLOW

A barium swallow investigation may be used in this context to diagnose a vascular ring (Fig. 18.48), but increasingly its use is superseded by CT or MRI angiography. However, esophageal compression and hold-up of contrast may be used to confirm that the abnormality is causing dysphagia (*dysphagia lusorum*), which may be particularly useful if the vascular anatomy is of uncertain significance (anomalous subclavian artery, which may be a variant of no consequence). It is also worth considering a bronchoscopy to assess any airway compression in this anomaly. A barium swallow cannot rule out an H-type tracheoesophageal fistula.

ESOPHAGEAL TUBE INJECTION

Abnormal connections between the esophagus and the trachea or a CTM are best delineated by a tube esophagram. The pressure injection of barium will reveal a connection that a simple barium swallow will miss. This investigation

is only needed in selected cases of CTM, in which either the malformation is close to the bronchial tree, or severe infection (particularly anaerobic) is a feature. Bronchoscopy may also delineate a fistula.

ANGIOGRAPHY

In complex cases, angiography may be necessary before surgery. However, the increasing use of CT and MRI to delineate vascular anatomy means that invasive investigation is now needed much less often, and really only as part of therapeutic embolization. The operator must completely delineate the anatomy of the pulmonary and systemic trees, including establishing whether there are any arterial collaterals (see earlier). It should be remembered that a CTM may be supplied from the coronary, internal mammary, intercostals, or subclavian arteries. At the same time, any embolization that might be indicated can be performed, including occlusion of PAVMs and systemic arterial collaterals (Fig. 18.49 and Videos 18.5 and 18.6). This may be the only treatment required, or the occlusion of large aortopulmonary collaterals to a CTM may make subsequent surgery safer. It should be stated that the role of embolization in congenital disorders of the lung, other than for pulmonary arteriovenous fistula, is controversial.

BRONCHOSCOPY

The anecdotal experience with fetal bronchoscopy has been described above. Bronchoscopy may be performed with either or both a flexible or rigid instrument. Rigid bronchoscopy (MLB) was discussed in detail earlier, and it should be noted that laryngeal clefts may be missed by flexible bronchoscopy. The most clear-cut use of fiberoptic bronchoscopy is in the investigation of stridor. In all but typical cases of laryngomalacia, this investigation should be performed at an early stage. Multiple causes of stridor are not uncommon, and all of the accessible respiratory tract should be examined. Bronchoscopy should not be delayed by performing a series of nondiagnostic imaging studies. In other contexts, bronchoscopy is probably best combined with other procedures requiring a general anesthetic, such as angiography (see earlier). Other than for the investigation of stridor or other upper airway disease, an anesthetic can rarely be justified solely for bronchoscopy in the context of congenital lung disease. Ideally, the flexible bronchoscopy should be performed under general anesthesia via a facemask, so the whole of the airway can be inspected, including the larynx, under conditions of quiet respiration. First, bronchial arrangement can be verified. Second, abnormalities of the bronchial wall, such as complete cartilage rings or compression by a vascular ring, can be ascertained. Finally, the presence of blind-ending bronchial stumps can be determined; these may act as a sump for infection. Another role for bronchoscopy is the assessment of airway narrowing in the case of aberrant origin of the left subclavian artery (see earlier). This may be a harmless normal variant or may cause significant airway narrowing, if a left arterial ligament completes a vascular ring. In doubtful cases, bronchoscopic inspection of the airway is indicated. Finally, H-type fistula may be missed on esophageal tube injection, and only detected by bronchoscopy

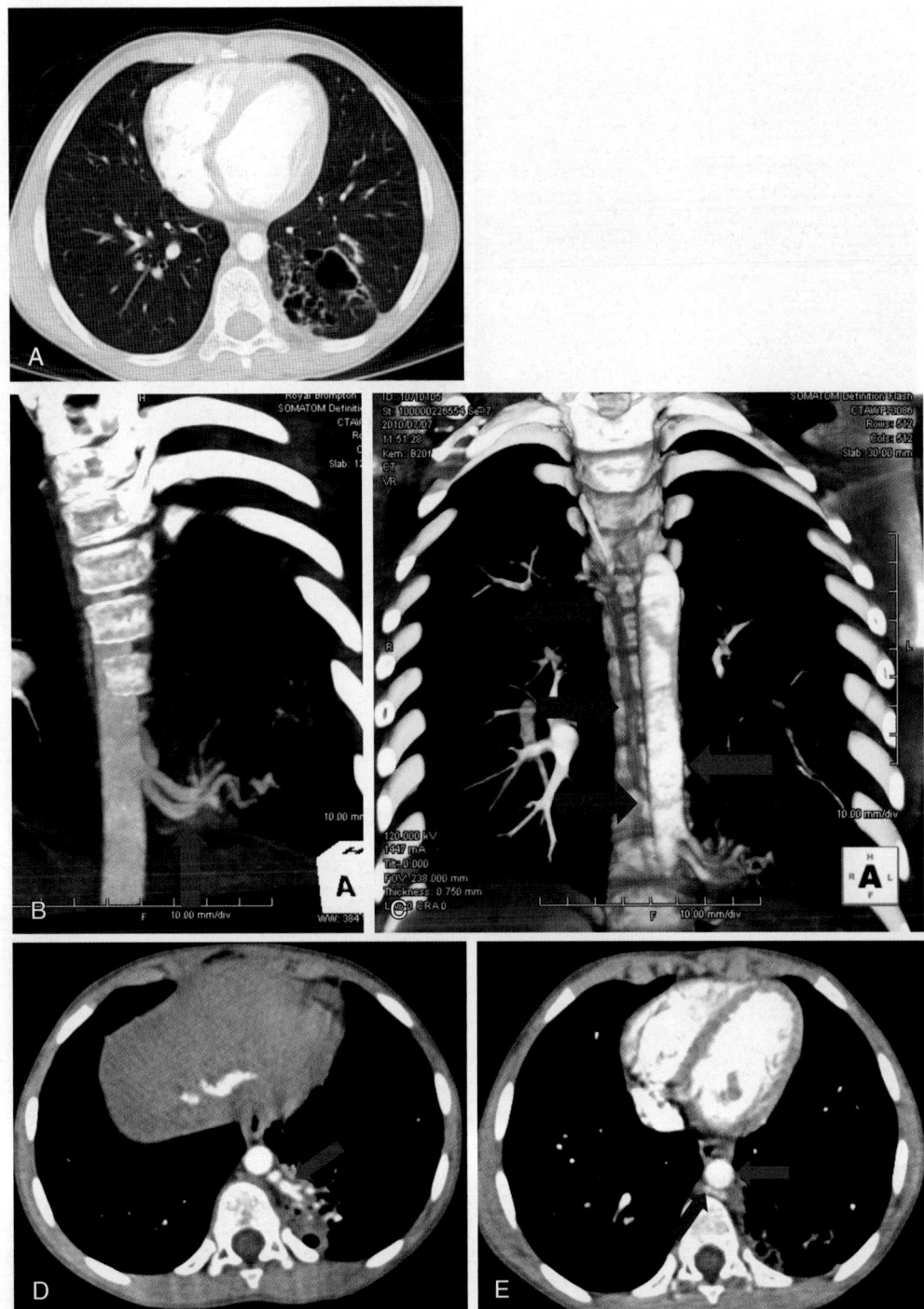

Fig. 18.47 Computed tomography with contrast injection investigation of a left-sided congenital thoracic malformation (CTM). (A) There is a large, multicystic CTM in the left lower lobe. (B) The reconstruction shows that there are large aortopulmonary collaterals to the mass *(red arrow).* (C) The venous drainage *(blue arrows)* passes behind the aorta *(red arrow)* and cranially to drain into the azygous system. (D) The CTM is supplied by collaterals arising from the aorta below the diaphragm. (E) Note the venous drainage *(blue arrow)* lying behind the aorta *(red arrow).*

Low Contrast Volume Bronchography

Airway malacia can be visualized directly and further documented by performing a limited bronchogram with a soluble contrast medium (see Video 18.2).[350] Unlike the bronchograms carried out before the advent of CT scanning, the purpose is to delineate the major airways, not to achieve alveolar filling, and only very small volumes of water-soluble contrast are required. This technique is better than flexible bronchoscopy, which may mask the severity of the condition by the inevitable application of positive end-expiratory pressure due to partial airway blockage by the bronchoscope. Low contrast volume bronchography can be used to titrate the CPAP pressures needed to overcome malacic segments.

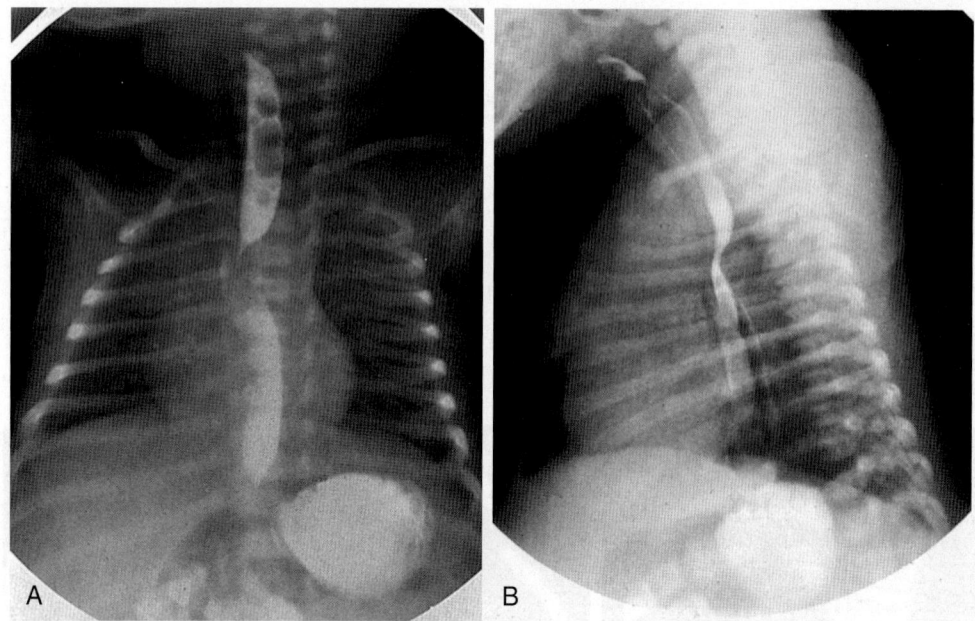

Fig. 18.48 Barium swallow showing the indentation of a vascular ring (double aortic arch). (A) Posterioranterior view. (B) Lateral view.

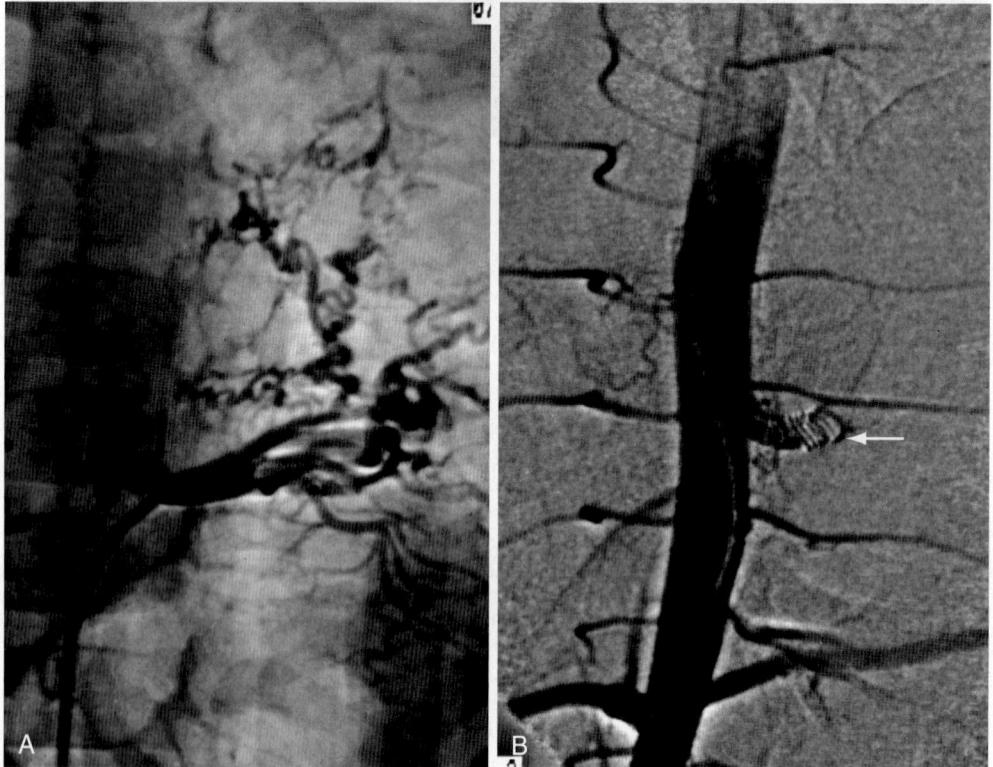

Fig. 18.49 Digital subtraction angiogram before (A) and after (B) coil embolization of a large aortopulmonary collateral, supplying a cystic congenital thoracic malformation in the left lower lobe. The *arrow* (B) points to the site of the coil occlusion.

Summary and Conclusions

Congenital lung disease can present at any time from 14 weeks of gestation to old age and should at least be considered as part of the differential diagnosis in many clinical situations. The lesions may regress to virtually nothing, require relatively straightforward surgery, or be among the most complex therapeutic challenges encountered. The chief need is for information about the long-term consequences of many of the lesions diagnosed antenatally, so that more precise counseling can be provided. Children with congenital lung disease should be enrolled in registries and followed up in a systematic manner. Another need is for refinement of MRI scanning so it can be performed without the need for general anesthesia and to give more precise information about parenchymal abnormalities to obviate the need for radiation exposure. Finally, we need to progress from a crude descriptive approach to understanding the molecular pathways underlying CTMs. This will require the formation of consortia of interested multidisciplinary teams and basic scientists to move the field forward. Only then will we have an understanding of how normal embryology deviates to produce these malformations, and it is to be hoped that gene signatures will allow us to select high-risk lesions for surgery from those that can be safely left unoperated.

References

Access the reference list online at ExpertConsult.com.

Suggested Reading

Adams S, Jobson M, Sangnawakij P, et al. Does thoracoscopy have advantages over open surgery for asymptomatic congenital lung malformations? An analysis of 1626 resections. *J Pediatr Surg.* 2017;52:247–251.

Alamo L, Gudinchet F, Meuli R. Imaging findings in fetal diaphragmatic abnormalities. *Pediatr Radiol.* 2015;45:1887–1900.

Alamo L, Vial Y, Gengler C, et al. Imaging findings of bronchial atresia in fetuses, neonates and infants. *Pediatr Radiol.* 2016;46:383–390.

Boucherat O, Jeannotte L, Hadchouel A, et al. Pathomechanisms of congenital cystic lung diseases: focus on congenital cysticadenomatoid malformation and pleuropulmonary blastoma. *Paediatr Respir Rev.* 2016;19:62–68.

Casagrande A, Pederiva F. Association between congenital lung malformations and lung tumors in children and adults: a systematic review. *J Thorac Oncol.* 2016;11:1837–1845.

Donn SM, Sinha SK. Pulmonary diagnostics. *Semin Fetal Neonatal Med.* 2017;22:200–205.

Grivell RM, Andersen C, Dodd JM. Prenatal interventions for congenital diaphragmatic hernia for improving outcomes. *Cochrane Database Syst Rev.* 2015;(11):CD008925.

Kitagawa H, Pringle KC. Fetal surgery: a critical review. *Pediatr Surg Int.* 2017;33:421–433.

Kotecha S, Barbato A, Bush A, et al. Antenatal and postnatal management of congenital cystic adenomatoid malformation. *Paediatr Respir Rev.* 2012;13:162–170.

Kotecha S, Barbato A, Bush A, et al. Congenital diaphragmatic hernia. *Eur Respir J.* 2012;39:820–829.

Laje P, Tharakan SJ, Hedrick HL. Immediate operative management of the fetus with airway anomalies resulting from congenital malformations. *Semin Fetal Neonatal Med.* 2016;21:240–245.

Oluyomi-Obi T, Kuret V, Puligandla P, et al. Antenatal predictors of outcome in prenatally diagnosed congenital diaphragmatic hernia (CDH). *J Pediatr Surg.* 2017;52:881–888.

Russo FM, Eastwood MP, Keijzer R, et al. Lung size and liver herniation predict need for extracorporeal membrane oxygenation but not pulmonary hypertension in isolated congenital diaphragmatic hernia: systematic review and meta-analysis. *Ultrasound Obstet Gynecol.* 2017;49:704–713.

Seear M, Townsend J, Hoepker A, et al. A review of congenital lung malformations with a simplified classification system for clinical and research use. *Pediatr Surg Int.* 2017;33:657–664.

Tonni G, Granese R, Martins Santana EF, et al. Prenatally diagnosed fetal tumors of the head and neck: a systematic review with antenatal and postnatal outcomes over the past 20 years. *J Perinat Med.* 2017;45:149–165.

19 Respiratory Disorders in the Newborn

NOAH H. HILLMAN, MD, and HUGH SIMON LAM, MBBChir, MD

Respiratory disorders are the most common reason for admission to a neonatal intensive care unit (NICU) and are a major source of neonatal mortality and morbidity. This chapter describes the etiology, presentation, management, and outcome of neonatal respiratory disorders, as well as the initiation of respiration at birth and resuscitation.

Initiation of Respiration at Birth

One of the most important and well-coordinated physiologic events in a person's life is the transition from the fetal state to the newborn infant. Within the first minute of life, the newborn must clear the fetal lung fluid from the airways and establish gas exchange. Although most infants complete this transition without problems, inadequate initiation of respiration at birth can be catastrophic to both the respiratory and cardiovascular system.[1]

The human fetus is breathing long before the infant is born, and fetal breathing is necessary for normal lung development. Fetal breathing is detected as early as 12–14 weeks gestational age (GA), and the frequency and duration correspond to the GA and sleep state of the fetus.[2] Fetal breathing and swallowing occur during active sleep, with limited amounts during quiet sleep.[2] During *active* sleep, the fetus has an irregular breathing pattern (20–30 bpm) characterized by long inspiratory and expiratory times with movement of fetal lung fluid into and out of the lung. Central chemoreceptors in the fetus respond to fetal hypoxia with decreased breathing (opposite of newborn physiology) and to hypercarbia by increased breathing and initiation of *active* sleep.[2] Fetal breathing is probably controlled by prostaglandin secretion. Fetal sheep given prostaglandin E2 infusions stop breathing, and treatment with prostaglandin synthetase inhibitors, such as indomethacin, cause continuous fetal breathing.[3] At birth, the rapid onset of regular breathing is likely due to a combination of removal of prostaglandin production from placenta, tactile and cold stimuli from the skin, activation of Hering-Breuer reflexes, and changes in arterial blood oxygenation levels (PaO_2).[2,4] Most of term infants (85%) will begin spontaneous breathing by 10–30 seconds of life, with another 10% requiring only drying and stimulation to begin a regular breathing pattern.[5] Most preterm infants <28 weeks and <1000 g (69%) have an audible cry and start breathing immediately after birth.[6]

Fetal Lung Fluid

The airspaces of the fetal lung are filled with fluid created by the airway epithelial cells. Production and maintenance of the normal volume of fetal lung fluid is essential for normal lung growth. Fetal lung fluid is secreted by the airway epithelium as a filtrate of the interstitial fluid of the lung by the active transport of chloride.[7] The fetal lung fluid is high in chloride but very low in protein and bicarbonate. Although the secretion rate has not been precisely measured in the human fetus, the fetal sheep during the middle of gestation has a secretion rate of about 4–5 mL/kg per hour.[8] Fetal lung fluid flows intermittently up the trachea with fetal breathing because the pressure in the trachea exceeds the amniotic fluid pressure by approximately 1 cm H_2O. Intermittent glottis closure *in utero* causes increased fetal lung fluid volume and pressure, and assists with lung development.[9] Abnormal flow and pressure in the lungs during development lead to either lung hypoplasia (e.g., in oligohydramnios) or large dysplastic lungs (e.g., in chronic upper airway obstruction). The fetal lung is fully expanded near term with a fluid volume of about 40 mL/kg, which is approximately twice the functional residual capacity (FRC) of the air breathing newborn.[8] As the pregnancy gets closer to term gestation, the rate of liquid formation and the volume of liquid within the fetal lung decreases.[10]

CLEARANCE OF LUNG FLUID FROM AIRWAYS AT BIRTH

The fetal lung fluid is cleared through (1) active transport of sodium by epithelial sodium channels (ENaCs) during labor, (2) mechanical forces during birthing process, and (3) newborn breathing after birth. Although the fetal lung fluid is generated throughout gestation by active secretion of chloride through apical epithelial cells into the airways, in late gestation the number and activity of ENaCs increase and generate a Na^+ gradient in the lung's interstitial space. Water follows the sodium out of the airspace through diffusion or through specific water channels (aquaporins). Aquaporins also increase throughout gestation and can be upregulated by antenatal steroids. Increases in fetal cortisol, thyroid hormones, and catecholamines near term gestation contribute to the reversal of fluid movement in the lungs.[11] In preterm fetal sheep, infusion of cortisol and T_3 will activate the sodium pump, which normally occurs at term.[12] Exposure to postnatal oxygen tension also increases sodium transport across the pulmonary epithelium. Blockage of or genetic mutations of the alpha-subunit of these amiloride-sensitive ENaCs leads to respiratory failure and death due to inability to clear fetal lung fluid.[13] The critical role of ENaCs at birth has been questioned by the lack of respiratory distress at birth in mice missing the other two subunits of the ENaC.[14] Cyclic nucleotide-gated channels on the type I pneumocytes also assist in Na transport out of cells.[15] Overall, activation of the ENaC assists in fluid clearance from the lungs at birth and throughout life.

338

Although there is some evidence for a small amount of lung fluid to be cleared during the progression through the vaginal vault, most lung fluid excreted through the nose and mouth, when the infants head is exposed, is due to fetal repositioning and spinal flexion caused by uterine contractions.[10] It is difficult to quantify the percent of lung fluid excreted by these physical mechanisms, but the combined relative contribution to fluid clearance is likely as high as 33% of lung fluid.[16] Elective cesarean sections (C-sections), without labor or rupture of membranes, will not have this physical clearance of lung fluid or activation of ENaCs prior to initiation of breathing.

Even with the reduction of fetal lung fluid volume during late gestation and labor and the expulsion of fluid by spinal flexion, there is greater than 15 mL/kg of fluid in the airways at the time of birth.[1] This fluid is cleared from the airways and driven into the interstitial space surrounding the airway within the first few seconds of life by a few large, negative pressure breaths.[17,18] An FRC is formed following the first breath in normal term infants. Using phase-contrast x-rays, Hooper and coworkers demonstrate that fluid leaves airways during inspiration with some reflooding during expiration (Video 19.1).[1,17] Positive end-expiratory pressure (PEEP) can decrease the backflow of interstitial fluid into airways, improve the uniformity of lung recruitment, and decrease the injury from mechanical ventilation.[1,19] The components of fetal lung fluid then are cleared directly into the vasculature or via lymphatics from the lung interstitium over multiple hours.[20]

Respiratory Depression at Birth

Although most infants initiate respirations at birth, failure can occur because of fetal hypoxia (birth asphyxia), maternal medications leading to suppression of breathing, congenital malformations, or failure of the central nervous system chemoreceptors. The combination of immature lungs and reduced respiratory drive makes preterm infants more likely to need assistance with breathing at birth.[5] Primary apnea occurs in newborns after birth and often responds to tactile stimulation. *In utero* the fetus responds to hypoxia with decreased fetal respiration thereby decreasing metabolic requirements; thus a severely hypoxic infants will not breath at birth.[21] Many of these infants will respond to stimulation and continuous positive airway pressure (CPAP). Room air (21%) has been shown to be preferable to 100% oxygen and is recommended for the initial resuscitation of the term infant.[5] If the infant in primary apnea is not assisted and hypoxia continues, the infant progresses into secondary apnea, where the heart rate (HR) decreases and responds only to positive-pressure ventilation (PPV). Continued deterioration of blood pressure will follow and metabolic acidosis will develop if respiration is not initiated. PPV through either a face mask or endotracheal (ET) tube should restore cardiopulmonary function in the majority of infants, as less than 1% of infants should need epinephrine in the delivery room.[22] Pulse oximetry is now recommended for any infant suspected of needing resuscitation.[5] Apgar scores, named after Virginia Apgar, are assigned to the infant at 1 minute, 5 minute, and 10 minutes for HR, breathing, color, reflex, and tone.[23] Although a useful guide for how a newborn

resuscitation is progressing, there is a high degree of variability in the Apgar scores assigned to infants and color has recently been removed from the algorithm for neonatal resuscitation.[5] Persistently low Apgar scores, especially <5 at 10 minutes, have been associated with higher infant mortality, cognitive delays, increased risk of cerebral palsy and increased educational needs throughout childhood.[24,25] Infants with severe birth asphyxia, metabolic acidosis, and neurologic signs of encephalopathy should receive therapeutic hypothermia.[5] Birth asphyxia can affect all the organ systems and management will be individualized based on laboratory findings.[26]

Delivery Room Resuscitation

Approximately 10% of infants require some form of assistance at birth; approximately 2% require intubation and PPV, and less than 0.5% require chest compressions and epinephrine.[5,22] The percent of infants requiring resuscitation increases with decreasing GA. Every 5 years, the International Liaison Committee on Resuscitation (ILCOR) reviews all studies on newborn resuscitation and provides treatment guidelines for infants who fail to breathe adequately at birth; the following comments reflect their most recent recommendations from 2015 (Fig. 19.1).[5] The new guidelines stress the importance of the first "golden" minute of life, when breathing should have spontaneously begun or respirations are being assisted. All newborn infants, including nonvigorous ones exposed to meconium, should receive stimulation and drying at birth.[5] Routine oropharyngeal suction should not be done unless the oral pharynx appears occluded. If the infant is not breathing, is gasping, or HR is less than 100 at 30 seconds of life, the infant should receive PPV with PEEP via a T-piece or resuscitation bag. Resuscitation with room air is recommended for term infants, whereas most preterm infants can be resuscitated with 0.21–0.30 fraction of inspired oxygen (FiO_2).[5,27] Pulse oximetry should be applied and the oxygen titrated to maintain infants within the normal ranges during the first minutes of life.[28] It should be noted that the fetal PaO_2 is low and normal transitional oxygen saturations are not greater than 85% for almost 5 minutes. If after 30 seconds of PPV ventilation, with an initial pressure of 20–25 cm H_2O, the HR is not greater than 100, the resuscitator should progress through a series of ventilation corrective steps (i.e., MR.SOPA—**M**ask adjustments/**R**eposition airway/**S**uction and **O**pen mouth and nose/increase **P**ressure/consider **A**lternative airway) and consider intubation of the infant. Intubation should be confirmed by chest rise, condensate in ET tube, improved HR, and carbon dioxide detector (PediCap). If HR remains less than 60 bpm after intubation, chest compressions should be started using a two-handed encircling chest approach.[5] The sternum is compressed approximately a third the diameter of the chest (approximately 2 cm) at a ratio of 3:1 for 120 events (90 compressions and 30 breaths) in a minute. Pulse oximetry and a three-lead electrocardiography (ECG or EKG) can be used to help assess the HR. If adequate ventilation and compressions do not return HR greater than 60, then the infant should receive intravenous (IV) epinephrine (0.01–0.03 mg/kg) through an umbilical venous catheter (UVC) or IV catheter. ET epinephrine (0.05–0.1 mg/kg) can be tried until IV access is obtained but has a decreased

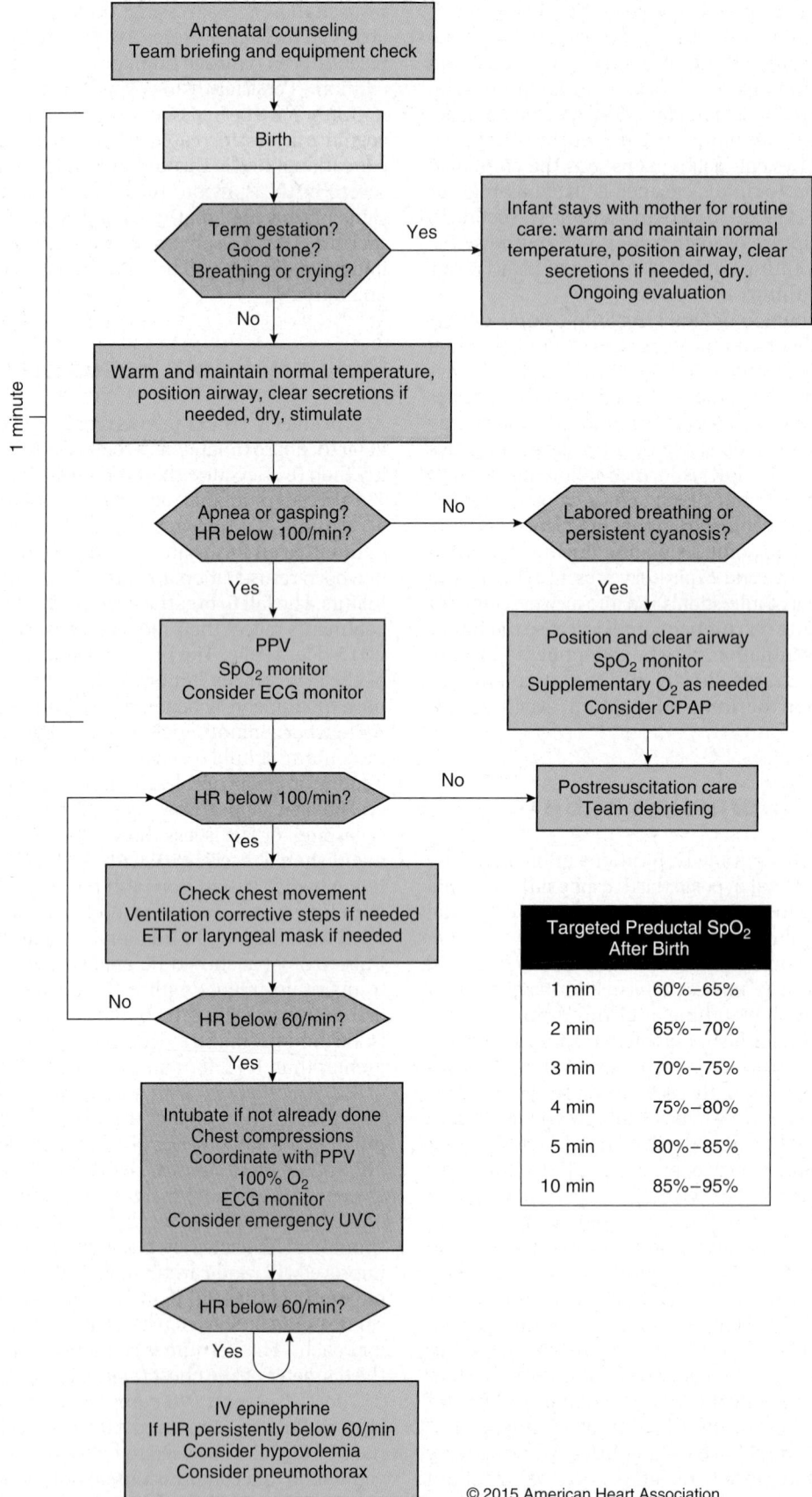

Fig. 19.1 Newborn Resuscitation Algorithm: 2015 International Liaison Committee on Resuscitation guidelines for initial management of infants in need for assistance during the transition at birth. *CPAP,* Continuous positive airway pressure; *ECG,* electrocardiography; *ETT,* endotracheal tube; *HR,* heart rate; *IV,* intravenous; *PPV,* positive-pressure ventilation; *UVC,* umbilical venous catheter. (Reprinted from American Heart Association, Wyckoff et al. Pediatrics. 2015.)

response rate compared with IV epinephrine.[29] The use of sodium bicarbonate and naloxone are no longer recommended during the newborn resuscitation. Normal saline or group O Rh-negative blood (10 mL/kg body weight) should be given over 5–10 minutes if the infant is hypotensive due to blood loss. If there is no HR and Apgar score is 0 after 10 minutes of adequate resuscitation, it is appropriate to discontinue further resuscitation due to the poor neurologic outcome.[5,29] Because most infants will respond to appropriate ventilation, resuscitators should consider other underlying conditions that might impede ventilation, such as pneumothorax, hypoplastic lungs from oligohydramnios, congenital diaphragmatic hernia (CDH), or other congenital anomalies.

RESUSCITATION OF THE PRETERM INFANT

The GA of the preterm infant will determine many of the steps taken during resuscitation. The care of late preterm infants (34–37 weeks) often follows the resuscitation guidelines for term infants, but they should be monitored closely after birth due to increased newborn morbidities (jaundice, temperature control, transient tachypnea of the newborn [TTN], feeding). Infants less than 32 weeks have immaturity of most organ systems, with the lungs and brain being the most vulnerable to injury and most likely to affect resuscitation. Antenatal steroids prior to preterm delivery stimulate maturation of many of the organs. Fortunately, more than 90% of preterm infant less than 34 weeks GA will receive some portion of a steroid course prior to delivery and this improves response to resuscitation. The extremely immature brain may have decreased respiratory drive requiring PPV ventilation. Thermoregulation is extremely important for the very preterm infant, due to brain immaturity and lack of brown fat sources, and they ought to be placed in a plastic bag or thermal wrap immediately after delivery.[29]

Lung immaturity has the largest influence on the resuscitation of the preterm infant, and many preterm infants require assistance in the transition from fetal life.[5,29] Lung development, maturation, and the surfactant system are covered extensively in other chapters in this book. Although the lack of labor may lead to increased fetal lung fluid at birth (see earlier), antenatal steroids or the maternal conditions that led to preterm birth may have primed the preterm lung for gas exchange. Although increased surfactant levels are probably not present until closer to 48 hours after antenatal steroids, preterm sheep lungs have decreased thickness of the lung parenchyma by 15 hours (likely due to decreased interstitial fluid) and decreased injury from mechanical ventilation by 24 hours after steroids.[30,31] Surfactant-deficient preterm babies may lack the muscle strength to generate sufficient negative pressure to overcome their compliant chest wall and high airway surface tension.[11] The amount of surfactant stored in type II cells is low in preterm infants not exposed to antenatal steroids, so less is available for secretion in response to birth.[32] Without the assistance of surfactant in reducing surface tension, it is difficult for very small infants to develop an FRC. Since the approval of exogenous surfactant replacement therapy in the early 1990s, there has been a trend towards intubation and treatment of the smallest infants with surfactant.[33] It should be noted that all the surfactant studies were performed prior to the American College of

Obstetricians and Gynecologists (ACOG) recommendation for antenatal corticosteroids in 1994, so it is unclear what the results would be in the current era. Multiple studies comparing CPAP and surfactant treatment have been conducted in the past 10 years, and each has shown a trend towards improved respiratory outcomes in the infants receiving CPAP.[34,35] Meta-analysis of all the trials demonstrated approximately a 10% reduction in bronchopulmonary dysplasia (BPD) with early CPAP.[36] Recently it has been recommended to attempt to support preterm infants with CPAP if they are breathing in the delivery room.[5] Remarkably, almost 50% of infants born less than 750 g will be successful on CPAP alone.[37] This is possible because an endogenous surfactant pool size of only approximately 5 mg/kg (5% of term levels) is necessary for preterm lambs to respond to CPAP and lambs with approximately 10% the endogenous pool size have reduced injury from mechanical ventilation.[38] If given the opportunity, the majority of very preterm infants will successfully initiate breathing without extensive resuscitation.[6] Extremely preterm infants that require extensive resuscitation in the delivery room have significant morbidities and increased mortality.[39]

Although there are clear benefits to resuscitation of term infants with room air, the consensus is less clear on the starting oxygen levels for preterm infants. The 2015 guidelines recommend starting preterm infants at a FiO_2 between 0.21 and 0.30 and then titrating oxygen based on pulse oximetry.[5] Preterm infants resuscitated with room air often require an increase in FiO_2 to maintain saturations.[40] Studies comparing 30%–90% oxygen for preterm infants demonstrated that most infants in the lower oxygen group had an increased oxygen requirement to 40%, whereas the higher group had decreases in oxygen requirements. Eventual oxygen requirements ended up at approximately 30% oxygen in both groups.[41,42]

To overcome the resistance created by the air-fluid interfaces in small airways of preterm infants, physicians have used prolonged inspiratory times, commonly called sustained inflation (SI), to recruit FRC.[17,43–45] In preterm lambs, SI augmented the cardiorespiratory transition at birth and improved the HR response to resuscitation after asphyxiation.[43,46] In a few small human studies, SI at birth decreased the need for mechanical ventilation at 72 hours and may lead to a decrease in BPD.[44,47] In preterm infants, SI generates an average FRC volume recruitment of only 8 mL/kg and lung volume recruitment occurs only in spontaneously breathing infants.[45,48] Adduction of the glottis, a normal fetal occurrence, blocks airflow in the nonbreathing infants.[1,48] Multiple clinical trials are currently underway to determine if clearing airway fluid with an SI to achieve FRC will benefit preterm infants. ILCOR removed the recommendation for three brief SIs (added in 2010) from the 2015 guidelines until results are known.[5]

Ventilatory Control

Complex networks of respiratory neurons within the medulla and pons generate and regulate the involuntary component of respiratory rhythm.[49] Specifically, studies suggest that this spontaneous inspiratory rhythm originates from pacemaker neurons within the pre-Bötzinger complex, one of the networks of neurons that make up the ventral respiratory group in the ventral medulla.[50,51] The phasic transition from inspiration to expiration is modulated by signals from the stretch receptors in the lungs and airways via the vagus nerves and neurons in the pneumotaxic and apneustic centers of the pons.[51] The rhythm is transmitted to the cervical and thoracic spinal motor neurons that innervate the diaphragm and intercostal muscles. These descending pathways activate the inspiratory muscles while inhibiting the expiratory muscles. Breathing pattern is further influenced by afferents from the forebrain, hypothalamus, central and peripheral chemoreceptors, muscles, joints, and pain receptors. Most areas contain multiple neuromodulators that are partly released from the same neurons, implying that neuromodulation is integrated at many levels.[52]

Several neurotransmitters play important roles in respiratory regulation. Glutamate is an excitatory neurotransmitter that activates receptors involved in generating and transmitting respiratory rhythms to spinal and cranial respiratory neurons. Serotonergic neurons in the medulla oblongata are part of a critical system that modulates autonomic and respiratory effector neurons.[53] The most consistent effect of serotonin (5HT) is to restore a normal breathing pattern after hypoxic or ischemic insult. Opioids (endorphins and exogenous drugs) suppress respiration by peripheral and central actions; the latter are due to suppression of recurrent excitation by glutaminergic input within the primary respiratory network. Both γ-aminobutyric acid (GABA) and glycine are essential for generating respiratory rhythm; they are released by late and postinspiratory neurons and inhibit inspiratory neurons, thus facilitating the transition from inspiration to expiration. Deficiency of glycinergic inhibition in knockout mice results in a slower frequency of breathing.

Central and peripheral chemoreceptors are core components of the chemical regulation of breathing patterns. These chemoreceptors modify respiratory activity in response to changes in oxygen, carbon dioxide, and acid-base balance.[54] The central chemoreceptors are situated near the ventral surface of the medulla, whereas the peripheral chemoreceptors are situated at the bifurcation of the common carotid arteries (carotid bodies) and above and below the aortic arch (aortic bodies). In the fetus the arterial chemoreceptors are active but have reduced sensitivity.[55] The peripheral chemoreceptors are not essential for the initiation of respiration and are virtually silenced when the arterial oxygen level rises at birth. Resetting of the carotid chemoreceptors to hypoxia occurs within 24–48 hours of birth[56]; this may result from changes in dopamine levels. The fetus responds to hypoxia with a suppression of ventilation. The lateral part of the lower pons mediates the hypoxic suppression of ventilation. In response to hypoxia, there is a redistribution of the circulation to favor the heart, brain, and adrenals. This minimizes oxygen consumption and conserves oxygen supplies for vital organs. The newborn has a biphasic response to hypoxia, a transient increase in minute ventilation followed by a decrease to or below baseline levels. The initial increase in ventilation may be due to activation of peripheral chemoreceptors and reconfiguration within the pre-Bötzinger complex leading to a change from eupneic rhythm to a gasping pattern.[57] The subsequent reduction in ventilation may result from a fall in carbon dioxide tension following the initial hyperventilation or the suppressant effect of hypoxia, which occurs in the fetal state and persists into the neonatal period.

Very immature infants respond to hypoxia by becoming apneic, which is like the fetal response. The biphasic response to hypoxia disappears by 12–14 days, and the adult pattern is subsequently observed (i.e., stimulation of breathing without depression). However, an animal model suggests that the acute hypoxic ventilatory response of an individual could be attenuated by exposure to sustained hypoxia followed by chronic intermittent hypoxia during the neonatal period.[58] In contrast, exposure to hyperoxia causes a temporary suppression of breathing due to withdrawal of peripheral chemoreceptor drive. After a few minutes of hyperoxia, ventilation increases to greater than control levels probably because of hyperoxic cerebral vasoconstriction resulting in increased brain tissue carbon dioxide. Immaturity and prolonged exposure to supplementary oxygen reduce the response to hyperoxia. The fetus and newborn respond to increased carbon dioxide levels with an increase in breathing activity. The slope of ventilatory response to carbon dioxide is less in term infants during active than quiet sleep, but it increases with postnatal growth. Other chemoreceptors include subepithelial chemoreceptors in the trachea, bronchi, and bronchioles that respond by changing the frequency and depth of respiration after exposure to toxic gases such as nitrogen dioxide and sulfur dioxide. This response is decreased during active sleep and in the premature infant.[59]

Respiratory activity is also regulated by nonchemical means, such as stimulation by the many respiratory reflexes.[51] Hering and Breuer described three respiratory reflexes: inflation, expiratory, and deflation. The Hering-Breuer inflation reflex is stimulated by lung inflation and results in cessation of respiratory activity. In the newborn the reflex produces a pattern of rapid, shallow tidal breathing and operates within the tidal volume range. In older subjects the reflex prevents excessive tidal volumes and can only be stimulated if the inflating volume is increased greater than a critical threshold.[60] The Hering-Breuer expiratory reflex is stimulated if inflation is prolonged; the active expiration seen in infants ventilated at slow rates and long inflation times, and which may result in pneumothoraces, may be a manifestation of this reflex.[61] In animal models the Hering-Breuer deflation reflex is evidenced by a prolonged inspiration generated in response to deflating the lung rapidly or following an unusually vigorous expiratory effort that takes the lung below its end-expiratory level.[62] In the newborn, this reflex may have a role in maintaining the FRC. Head's paradoxical reflex, also called the inspiratory augmenting reflex or provoked augmented inspiration, is the underlying mechanism of the first breath and sighing. A rapid inflation stimulates a stronger diaphragmatic contraction. The reflex improves compliance and reopens partially collapsed airways[63]; it has an important role in promoting lung expansion during resuscitation. Rapid chest wall distortion via the intercostal phrenic inhibitory reflex results in a shortening of inspiratory efforts. This reflex response is inhibited by an increase in FRC or applying CPAP. The mechanism may improve chest wall stability.[64] The airway is protected from bronchospasm induced by cold exposure by upper airway reflexes that can increase upper airway resistance and decrease inspiratory air flow. The laryngeal afferents defend the lower airway from inadvertent inhalation of foreign bodies, with maturation of the laryngeal reflex being characterized by an increase in coughing and a decrease in swallowing and apnea.[65] For a discussion of ventilatory control in sleep-disordered breathing, please refer to Chapter 81.

APNEA

Apnea is defined as cessation of breathing for at least 20 seconds or at least 10 seconds if associated with oxygen desaturation or bradycardia.[54] Apneas are classified as central, obstructive, or mixed.[66] Most apneas are central in nature (46%–69%), with the rest being either purely obstructive (6%–12%) or a combination of central and obstructive (i.e., mixed) (20%–44%).[67] Central apnea is characterized by cessation of inspiratory efforts in the absence of upper airway obstruction. In contrast, in obstructive apnea, despite the presence of central signals for breathing and the corresponding respiratory muscle activities, there is an absence of airflow through the airways due to upper airway obstruction. Bradycardia may occur within a few seconds of onset of apnea with accompanying disturbances in blood pressure and cerebral blood flow velocity. In infants without adequate cerebrovascular autoregulation, cerebral perfusion may decrease to very low levels during prolonged apnea and potentially exacerbate hypoxic-ischemic brain injury. The incidence of apnea of prematurity is inversely associated with GA and usually resolves by approximately 37–40 weeks postconceptional age.

Frequent episodes of apnea that respond to gentle stimulation may be considered normal for preterm infants. However, additional investigations and treatment are required if the apneas become frequent and/or associated with prolonged desaturation, because there are several potentially treatable associated factors that may be present (e.g., infection, intracranial abnormality or hemorrhage, anemia, metabolic disorders [e.g., hypoglycemia], temperature instability, and gastroesophageal reflux [GER] [see later in the chapter]). In addition, several pharmacologic agents (e.g., benzodiazepines and opioid analgesics) can also cause apnea. After excluding other treatable conditions, neonatal apnea may be treated with methylxanthines (e.g., theophylline) and caffeine, which have all been shown to reduce apnea in preterm infants, possibly by increasing the chemoreceptor sensitivity to carbon dioxide.[68] Caffeine is the preferred agent in view of its relatively long half-life, which allows once-daily dosing, and its higher therapeutic index compared with theophylline. Side effects of theophylline include hyperactivity, tachycardia, cardiac dysrhythmias, feeding intolerance, and seizures. Caffeine treatment in infants with, or at risk for, apnea of prematurity has also been shown to reduce BPD[69] and improve survival without neurodevelopmental delay.[70] In addition, prophylactic caffeine reduces apnea/bradycardia and episodes of oxygen desaturation in preterm infants following postoperative anesthesia.[71] Doxapram, a respiratory stimulant that is thought to act via the peripheral chemoreceptors, has been used to treat apnea in newborns but has been associated with many side effects (e.g., elevated blood pressure, abdominal distension, irritability, increased gastric residuals, and emesis). Furthermore, the long-term effects of this drug have not been adequately investigated.[68] Relatively novel treatments include olfactory stimulation,[72] inhalation of low-dose carbon dioxide,[73] and limb proprioception stimulation.[74] However, although some of these treatments show initial promise, whether they can be replicated in a wide variety of clinical situations and show any long-term advantages remain to be seen. Noninvasive ventilatory support (e.g., CPAP, noninvasive positive-pressure ventilation [NIPPV], and high-/low-flow nasal cannulas) may be considered for infants with frequent or prolonged apnea despite treatment with caffeine. The frequency of apnea has been shown to be decreased by increasing the FRC, stabilizing oxygenation, or by splinting the upper airway. Positive pressure support of the airway may be particularly effective in infants whose episodes are precipitated or prolonged by relative upper airway obstruction as both the pharynx and laryngeal aperture could be distended to reduce the risk of mixed and obstructive apneas. However, a neural component to the effects of positive pressure/flow has been suggested as even delivery of low-flow air has been shown to be effective, suggesting the possibility of the stabilization of the mechanoreceptors in the upper airway by the airflow.[68] Infants with severe and refractory apnea unresponsive to the relatively noninvasive modalities of treatment would need to be intubated and supported by mechanical ventilation.

PERIODIC BREATHING

Periodic breathing is a common breathing pattern that, unlike apnea of prematurity, can occur in infants of all GA.[75,76] In contrast to apnea of prematurity, periodic breathing does not usually occur within the first 48 hours of life[75] and can last for 6 months or longer.[76,77] The literature suggests that among healthy term babies, 78% exhibit periodic breathing within the first 2 weeks of life, decreasing to 29% by 1 year of age.[76] The definition of periodic breathing can be arbitrarily defined as three episodes of apnea of more than 3-second duration each that are interrupted by periods of breathing that are 20 seconds or less.[78] The etiology of periodic breathing is thought to be increased sensitivity of chemoreceptors involved in ventilatory control, leading to overregulation of the breathing pattern in response to small changes in PaO_2 or $PaCO_2$ levels.[79] This overcompensation leads to periodic overshooting of the target to be compensated for and the oscillation between apnea and normal breathing that is observed in this condition. Periodic breathing has previously been thought to be a benign condition. However, with improvements in computing power, detailed longitudinal analyses of neonatal breathing patterns have been made, and showed that preterm infants often exhibit increased percentage of time spent in periodic breathing before a diagnosis of necrotizing enterocolitis (NEC) or septicemia is made.[79] Furthermore, in another longitudinal study of preterm infants, it has been found that periodic breathing can be associated with significant desaturations and reduction in cerebral oxygenation, especially during sleep.[80] Although the use of CPAP or caffeine may be associated with less periodic breathing,[79] because the long-term clinical implications of these events are unknown, further follow-up studies are warranted before evidence-based diagnostic or treatment recommendations can be made.

Respiratory Distress Syndrome

Respiratory distress syndrome (RDS), also referred to as hyaline membrane disease, is a respiratory condition that occurs in many preterm infants at birth and is defined by clinical and radiographic descriptions. Infants with RDS develop oxygen requirements within 6 hours of life, typically require respiratory support at 24 hours of life, and a have a chest x-ray with findings consistent with RDS.[81] The severity of RDS has decreased with the introduction of surfactant and antenatal steroids, so the classic hyaline membranes, seen at autopsy, rarely occur in our current premature infants.[82] Because many infants are ventilated in the delivery room and given surfactant, the radiologic evidence of air bronchograms may not be present. And some infants will be maintained on mechanical ventilation due to immature respiratory drive, yet have mature lungs with plenty of surfactant. Because it is difficult to define RDS in the era of surfactant therapy and antenatal steroids, there will be variations in the number of preterm infants with RDS across studies.[82] Some may argue the alternative name for RDS may have changed from "hyaline membrane disease" to "respiratory instability of prematurity," a phrase created by Bancalari and Jobs to describe the extremely preterm infants born in recent years.[82]

EPIDEMIOLOGY

It is difficult to determine the exact incidence of RDS because multiple definitions exist. The incidence of RDS decreases as the GA increases. Prior to the introduction of antenatal steroids (1983–86), the incidence of RDS was: >95% at 25 weeks GA (average weight 800 g); 75% at 28 weeks (average weight 1000 g); 50% at 30 weeks GA (average weight 1400 g); and still approximately 20% at 34 weeks GA.[83] Antenatal steroids have been shown to reduce RDS by an average of 40% in randomized trials.[84] In the 1990s, when the more routine use of antenatal steroids was beginning (ACOG recommended steroid use in 1994), the incidence of RDS was approximately 70% between 500 and 1500 g.[85] Of note, in the Vermont Oxford network, the antenatal steroid rate increased from 23% in 1991 to 72% in 1999, but there was no difference in the rate of RDS.[85] Between 1997 and 2003, in the era of moderately high antenatal steroid use, approximately 63% of infants between 500 and 1000 g have RDS.[86] Although antenatal corticosteroids have traditionally been given to mothers at risk of preterm birth prior to 34 weeks GA, a randomized trial demonstrated a benefit of corticosteroids in late preterm infants.[87] The rates of RDS vary between races and sex. Female infants have a lower incidence of RDS than do male infants at all GAs,[88] which is consistent across most mammalian species. Late preterm males have an odds ratio (OR) of 1.68 of having RDS compared with their female counterparts.[89] Race plays an important role in the development of RDS, with African-American infants having a lower rate than do white infants.[90] In one study, only 40% of African infants less than 32 weeks GA developed RDS compared with 75% of the white infants.[91] Genetic variability as a risk factor for RDS has been confirmed in twin studies, in which monozygotic twins were more likely than dizygotic twins to both have RDS.[92,93] The largest influences on development of RDS are GA, gender, race, and antenatal steroids. Genetic polymorphisms of surfactant proteins have been found to be strongly associated with risk of RDS in preterm infants (see Chapter 57).[94]

PATHOPHYSIOLOGY

RDS is due to structural immaturity of the preterm lung and a deficiency in surfactant pool size. Increased lung fluid, inadequate respiratory efforts, and underdevelopment of the chest wall and respiratory muscles also contribute to the infant's inability to maintain expansion of the distal airspaces. Surfactant production and maturation are covered in detail in Chapter 5, so only a summary will follow. Surfactant is produced in alveolar type II cells, which are cuboidal cells covering approximately 2% of the alveolar surface that become more prominent between 22 and 24 weeks GA. Surfactant is a complex mixture of phospholipids, neutral lipids, and proteins (surfactant proteins A, B, C, and D). Lipids make up more than 90% of surfactant, with 80% being phospholipids (phosphatidylcholine [PC] and phosphatidylglycerol [PG] make up largest portion) and 10% neutral lipids (cholesterol, triacylglycerol, and free fatty acids).[95] Sphingomyelin, which is used in the lecithin to sphingomyelin (L:S) ratio, represents less than 2% of surfactant lipid. Surfactant is synthesized in the endoplasmic reticulum, collected in the lamellar bodies then released into airspace as active tubular myelin. The tubular myelin mixes with a combination of saturated and unsaturated phospholipids to make a surface film that decreases surface tension. The surface film is recycled over time by the type II cells or degraded by the macrophages. More than 90% of the PC on the alveolar surface is reprocessed, the turnover time being approximately 10 hours. The phospholipid monolayer structure allows the surfactant to change shape throughout respiration, with the most distended form allowing decreased surface tension and the most compressed form in exhalation providing stability to the alveoli. In RDS the immature lung has a lower level of PG and PC, the spreading agents for surfactant in the lung, thus the monolayer formed is unstable and does not decrease surface tension or maintain alveolar patency as well. The immature surfactant system in preterm infants with RDS leads to difficulty in generating an FRC and increased work of breathing. The addition of PEEP or treatment with exogenous surfactant allows for formation of an FRC and decreased injury from ventilation.[19,96] In RDS the resultant alveolar hypoventilation results in ventilation perfusion imbalance and hypoxia. The increased alveolar surface tension from the surfactant deficiency promotes the flow of protein-rich fluid from the intravascular space to the alveolar spaces. The leak of protein is increased by mechanical ventilation and from continued hypoxic damage to the alveolar-capillary membrane. These plasma proteins further inhibit surfactant function and make up a major component of the hyaline membrane found in infants who do not survive RDS.

The four surfactant-associated proteins, SP-A, SP-B, SP-C, and SP-D, compose approximately 10% of surfactant and play a role in the structure of tubular myelin (SP-A), the stabilization of the phospholipid monolayer (SP-B, SP-C), and in host-defense (SP-A, SP-D). ABCA3 is a protein that assists in transport of lipids with type II cells and is required for proper lamellar body formation. Genetic mutations in the surfactant proteins or ABCA3 lead to respiratory disease in the newborn that ranges from mild (SP-A) to lethal (SP-B).[97] Some of the clinical manifestations of these conditions do not appear until childhood or adulthood. The role of gene mutations in human lung diseases and surfactant production are covered in depth in Chapters 5 and 57. Term or late preterm infants with severe RDS at birth that does not have a persistent response to surfactant therapy may need to be evaluated for these mutations.

Many factors influence lung maturation and surfactant production and thus the development of RDS. Both fetal cortisol and thyroxine can stimulate lung maturation. Conversely, insulin delays the maturation of alveolar type II cells, decreasing the proportion of saturated PC, and inhibits the production of SP-A and SP-B.[98] Infants of diabetic mothers also have delayed appearance of PG, and the infant's L:S ratio is less predictive of lung maturation.[99] The increased incidence of RDS in males (1.7 : 1) may be due to the increased levels of fetal androgens. Fetal androgens delay lung maturation and PG production (by approximately a week) through direct action on lung fibroblasts.[100] Any factors that affect the integrity of the alveolar capillary membrane (asphyxia, hypothermia, or hypoxia) will lead to increased airspace protein and deactivation of surfactant function. Although often necessary in the resuscitation of preterm infants, PPV can release proteins and cause inflammation that worsens RDS.[101,102] Increased intrauterine inflammation from chorioamnionitis matures the lung and decreases the risk of RDS but may increase the risk of BPD.[103,104]

CLINICAL PRESENTATION

Infants with RDS typically present within 4 hours of birth with tachypnea (respiratory rate > 60 breaths/min), intercostal and subcostal retraction, nasal flaring, and abdominal breathing. Although severe cases of RDS present with cyanosis, milder cases of RDS are discovered by routine use of pulse oximetry in infants unable to maintain their saturations greater than 90 on RA. The high surface tension in the alveoli created by the surfactant deficiency and the weaker chest wall muscles of the preterm infant may make it difficult for the infant to develop the normal FRC of 25–30 mL/kg, and thus the infant's lungs remain in a partially deflated state. The infant may attempt to increase their FRC through an expiratory grunt, created when the infant simultaneously contracts the diaphragm and the constrictor muscles of the larynx to close the upper airway. The resultant exhalation of air is exaggerated and creates the grunting sound found in RDS. The diffuse collapse of the alveoli and smaller airways creates the classic chest radiograph findings of ground-glass appearance with air bronchograms. In infants who are not treated with exogenous surfactant, the symptoms worsen over the first 24–36 hours due to collapse of alveoli recruited by the initial breaths at birth and the deactivation of the small amounts of surfactant present in an infant with RDS. The ongoing lung injury from atelectasis and poor ventilation leads to further leak of inhibitory plasma proteins into the airspace, a cycle that can be prevented by the treatment with exogenous surfactant or CPAP.[105] Without antenatal steroids, endogenous levels of surfactant begin to increase in the airspaces by 24 hours after birth.[106] Between 36 and 48 hours of age, the endogenous production of surfactant is sufficient to maintain alveolar patency and clinical symptoms improve. Often this process is associated with a spontaneous diuresis. With eventual development of surfactant production, recovery from RDS with decreasing oxygen requirements normally occurs by approximately 1 week of age. Extremely preterm infants often require ongoing ventilator support due to chest wall weakness and central respiratory drive issues. The introduction of exogenous surfactant treatment and antenatal steroids has altered the traditional clinical progression over a course of days because most larger infants with significant respiratory distress will receive surfactant and this will be recycled by their type II cells multiple times prior to their own endogenous production.

DIAGNOSIS AND DIFFERENTIAL DIAGNOSIS

The diagnosis of RDS is made on clinical history (described previously) and chest radiographic appearance. The chest radiograph shows fine granular opacification in both lung fields due to diffuse atelectasis and air bronchograms, where the air-filled bronchi stand out against the atelectatic lungs (Fig. 19.2). In severe cases the lungs are collapsed to the extent that the cardiac silhouette is indistinguishable from the lungs. If the radiograph is taken during the first 4 hours, the retention of fetal lung fluid can make interpretation difficult. As the fluid clears, the chest radiograph appearance may show marked improvement. It should be noted that an infant on mechanical ventilation with adequate tidal volume ventilation and PEEP will have a moderately clear x-ray, even in the setting of significant surfactant deficiency. This difference can be determined clinically because the infants with surfactant deficiency will require higher pressures to maintain tidal volumes. Preterm infants with low lung compliance (i.e., requiring peak inspiratory pressure [PIP] greater than approximately 20 cm H_2O to generate a tidal volume of 5 mL/kg) would benefit from exogenous surfactant therapy. Although measurement of surfactant in a tracheal aspirate can be performed, this is currently not clinically available.[107] Tracheal secretions or gastric contents can be aspirated and a bubble shake test can be performed to give a

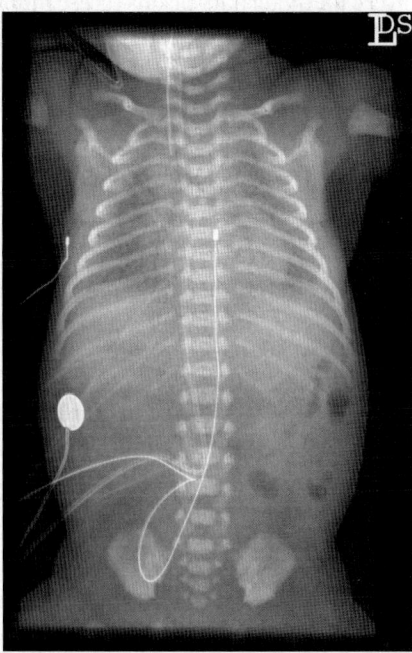

Fig. 19.2 Respiratory distress syndrome: chest x-ray demonstrates ground-glass appearance and air bronchograms due to atelectasis because of surfactant deficiency from prematurity.

basic assessment of surfactant levels, but this is rarely done in the NICU.[108]

Fetal lung fluid normally moves up the trachea and is swallowed by the fetus, but some of the fluid mixes with the amniotic fluid, allowing surfactant to be measured. As the lung matures, the amount of dipalmitoylphosphatidylcholine (DPPC) in the amniotic fluid increases, but the amount of sphingomyelin remains unchanged throughout gestation; thus lung maturity can be assessed from the L:S ratio.[109] The lower the L:S ratio, the more likely that the infant will develop RDS: 80% of infants with a L:S ratio < 1.5 have RDS, compared with 21% of infants with a ratio of 1.5–2.0, and approximately 5% if L:S ratio > 2.0 (usually is associated with lung maturity).[109] Because of the abnormalities in PG formation (not measured in L:S ratio) in infants of diabetic mothers and infants with severe hemolytic disease, these infants may have a mature L:S ratio but have significant RDS.[99] L:S ratios can be altered by the presence of blood, meconium, or vaginal secretions in the sample. Lung maturity can also be assessed by the lamellar body count in the amniotic fluid.[109,110] Lamellar body counts are more sensitive than L:S ratio and >37,000 correlates well with lung maturity, even in diabetic patients (30,000 in nondiabetic women).[109,111] Lamellar body counts can be easily obtained by running amniotic fluid through an automated hematology analyzer because they are the same size as platelets. Some investigators suggest that examining lamellar body counts in gastric aspirates of preterm infants may be helpful to guide the early use of surfactant.[112]

It is nearly impossible to differentiate severe early-onset sepsis or pneumonia from RDS, either clinically or radiographically. Because these conditions can also coexist, infants experiencing respiratory distress at birth should have an appropriate workup performed for bacterial infections (blood cultures, complete blood count [CBC], and C-reactive protein at >4 hours) and should then be started on antibiotics.[113] Clinicians may consider holding antibiotics in the setting of preterm delivery for maternal reasons (preeclampsia, Hemolysis, Elevated Liver enzymes, and Low Platelet count [HELLP] syndrome). Antibiotics should be stopped after blood cultures and other lab results are negative. Ampicillin and gentamicin act synergistically against group B streptococcus (GBS) and are also effective against many organisms that cause early-onset septicemia and pneumonia. It is important to know the local antibiotic resistance patterns as gentamicin resistant gram-negative bacteria have become more prevalent. Infants with high oxygen requirements, but a clear chest x-ray or low lung compliance, may be suffering from pulmonary hypertension. This can often be diagnosed with preductal and postductal pulse-oximetry or echocardiography and can be treated with sedation and inhaled nitric oxide (iNO). TTN (discussed later) can present with similar findings to RDS but typically improves more quickly as the excessive water in the lungs is absorbed and the function of the (already present) surfactant improves. Respiratory distress that presents after 4–6 hours of age is usually due to pneumonia; the differential diagnosis includes air leak, heart failure secondary to congenital heart disease, and aspiration.

MANAGEMENT

The appropriate management of preterm infants with RDS has been studied extensively over the past decade, yet there is not a clear consensus among neonatologists about the best approach to take in the delivery room. Everyone would probably agree that RDS is due to a combination of chest wall immaturity and surfactant deficiency and that all treatment methods are merely approaches to bridge the time until the infant begins to develop sufficient endogenous surfactant (typically over 48 hours) and grows stronger to maintain adequate respiration (days to weeks). The three typical management styles for RDS (described in detail later) all derive from these principles: (1) use of CPAP to maintain alveolar distention during spontaneous breathing,[34,35] (2) giving exogenous surfactant while the infant is spontaneously breathing (minimally invasive surfactant therapy [MIST] or less invasive surfactant therapy [LIST]),[114,115] or (3) mechanical ventilation and administration of surfactant therapy, with rapid extubation as part of INSURE (Intubation, Surfactant, Rapid Extubation) protocols.[33,116] Other forms of noninvasive respiratory support (high-flow nasal cannula and NIPPV) have also been tried for RDS.

Since its introduction in the early 1990s, exogenous surfactant therapy has had a dramatic effect on the survival and long-term morbidity from RDS. The first description of surfactant deficiency was published by Avery in 1959,[117] but it took nearly 30 years to get an animal-extracted surfactant approved for clinical use in premature infants. Surfactant therapy, when given as "rescue therapy" in infants with established RDS, decreased the rates of pneumothorax, mortality, and the combined outcome of mortality and BPD.[118] Surfactant therapy has also been shown to be more effective if given as "prophylactic therapy" to infants born less than 28 weeks gestation versus given as rescue therapy, with decreased risk of pneumothorax, pulmonary interstitial emphysema (PIE), and mortality or BPD.[33] It should be noted that the majority of the surfactant therapeutic trials were conducted prior to the ACOG recommendation for antenatal steroid use in 1994 and the infants included in the studies may be slightly less mature than extremely preterm infants who have received steroids.[119] The benefit of prophylactic surfactant in the setting of antenatal steroids has been addressed by multiple trials of surfactant versus CPAP (discussed later).[120] Most intubated extremely preterm infants, even in the setting of intubation for respiratory drive or apnea, would benefit from surfactant therapy because mechanical ventilation alone may release proteins that inhibit the endogenous surfactant.[107] Benefits are shown after a single dose of 100 mg/kg surfactant, but most studies demonstrate that better results are obtained with more than one dose.[121] The results of additional surfactant begin to diminish after the second dose of natural surfactants. There may be differences between bovine surfactant (beractant) and porcine surfactant (poractant alfa), with further benefits on BPD, mortality, and patent ductus arteriosus (PDA) seen with poractant. These differences between surfactants may be due to the higher dosing concentrations given with poractant (200 mg/kg) versus the beractant (100 mg/kg).[122] Natural (animal-derived) surfactants when compared with synthetic surfactant (protein free) are associated with a significant reduction in mortality and pneumothorax but may be associated with an increased risk of NEC.[123] The most well-studied protein-free surfactant, colfosceril palmitate (Exosurf), is no longer being produced. Synthetic surfactants are now available that contain synthetic polypeptide proteins designed to mimic surfactant proteins B or C. The most studied polypeptide is KL4, designed to mimic the C-terminal end of surfactant protein B,[124] which when mixed with DPPC, POPG phospholipids, and palmitic acid is called lucinactant (Surfaxin). KL4 appears to be more resistant to the inhibitory effects of proteins than natural surfactants.[125] Transient hypoxemia and bradycardia may be present during surfactant treatment via ET tube. A transient perturbation in cerebral hemodynamics is also present but is not associated with increased risk of cerebral hemorrhage. Pulmonary hemorrhage has been noted following surfactant administration. Surfactant, once instilled into the trachea or bronchus, will quickly spread throughout the lungs with each breath. Although surfactant dosing is approved for four quadrants, most clinicians instill surfactant with only two positions. In some surfactant-deficient preterm infants, the ET tube serves mainly as a conduit for administering surfactant, but intubation may expose the infant to injurious ventilation and cardiovascular changes. To avoid continued ventilation after surfactant treatment, the INSURE technique has been adopted by many neonatologists, especially for more mature infants (>28 weeks GA) in need of surfactant treatment.[126] To avoid intubation in spontaneously breathing infants on CPAP with higher oxygen needs, surfactant can be given through a thin catheter into the trachea of extremely preterm infants.[114,115] MIST or LIST involve direct visualization of the vocal cords by direct laryngoscopy and insertion of a feeding tube into the upper trachea (www.youtube.com/watch?v=OUvgJ57FQR8). Surfactant is then quickly instilled through the feeding tube. MIST therapy has been shown to be effective and may avoid unnecessary mechanical ventilation in preterm infants.[127] Surfactant can also be given through a laryngeal mask airway (LMA), but LMAs small enough for extremely preterm infants are still in development. Nebulization of surfactant in spontaneously breathing infants on CPAP is being studied in clinical trials. It is known that some extremely preterm infants are surfactant deficient and need surfactant treatment, but the best way to deliver it is still being determined.

Not all infants with clinical signs of RDS are surfactant deficient, especially in the setting of greater than 48 hours of antenatal steroids, and many of these infants require only CPAP to support the weak respiratory muscles and to stimulate breathing.[35,128] The mildest forms of RDS can sometimes be managed with supplemental oxygen, but most babies need some form of distending pressure to prevent atelectasis and improve oxygenation. Many centers are trialing all infants on CPAP in the delivery room, and approximately 50% of infants born less than 750 g can be maintained on only CPAP, with much higher rates in more mature infants.[36,37,129] The ability to be maintained on CPAP is likely due to the small amount of endogenous surfactant (>5% of term surfactant pool size needed in preterm sheep) necessary to maintain alveolar expansion.[38] Over the past decade, during an era of greater than 80% antenatal steroid rates, five major trials (Continuous Positive Airway Pressure or Intubation at Birth trial [COIN]; Surfactant, Positive Pressure, and Oxygenation Randomized Trial [SUPPORT]; Vermont-Oxford Network [VON] delivery room study; an international randomized controlled trial to evaluate the efficacy of combining prophylactic surfactant and early nasal continuous positive airway pressure in very preterm infants [CUPAP]; and Neocosur Network) have been conducted to compare

CPAP versus intubation and surfactant in extremely preterm infants less than 29 weeks. Even with the use of early CPAP in the delivery room, the decrease in the incidence of BPD is modest at approximately 10%.[36,129] The increased rate of pneumothorax found in the COIN trial was not found in any of the other clinical trials, with an overall pneumothorax rate in all trials of CPAP 6.3% versus surfactant 5.8%. Based on these studies, the 2015 ILCOR resuscitation guidelines recommend treating spontaneously breathing preterm infants (<30 weeks) with CPAP instead of intubation.[5] Preterm infants started on CPAP may initially do well (FiO_2 less than 30%), and then having increasing oxygen requirements and hypercapnia as alveoli begin to collapse. Although $PcCO_2 > 60$ mm Hg and a $FiO_2 > 0.6$ is used by some centers as criteria for CPAP failure (including some centers with very low BPD rates), 84% of preterm infants on CPAP with a FiO_2 of >0.4 will reach >0.6.[130] Earlier rescue surfactant, given when $FiO_2 < 0.45$, has been shown to be beneficial for air leaks,[126] and it is our practice to intubate these infants and give them surfactant if they require $FiO_2 > 0.4$ on high levels of CPAP. Increasing the level of CPAP increases the lung volume and hence improves oxygenation, but it is possible to cause overdistension, carbon dioxide retention, and air leaks. CPAP can be generated by a mechanical ventilator, a T-piece resuscitator, or an underwater seal (bubble) device (bubble continuous positive airway pressure [BCPAP]). BCPAP is attractive, especially for low-resource countries, because the CPAP is regulated by submerging the expiratory limb of the gas circuit a set distance under water (actual cm H_2O). It should be noted that the distending pressure generated by BCPAP is flow dependent and intraprong pressures may be higher (up to 1.3 cm H_2O) than expected for the depth of submersion in water.[131] Unlike ventilator-derived CPAP, BCPAP generates a variable distending pressure, often referred to as the "noise" of BCPAP.[132] In intubated sheep, BCPAP had improved gas exchange, oxygenation, and pH compared with ventilator-derived CPAP,[132] and similar benefit was seen on oxygenation in preterm infants on BCPAP.[133] When the pressure fluctuations are further increased (high-amplitude BCPAP), the oscillatory pressure wave can achieve similar blood gas values in paralyzed, saline-lavaged rabbits to conventional mechanical ventilation.[134] The transmission of the oscillatory bubbles and the CPAP pressure may differ based on the nasal interface used, with the RAM cannula losing more CPAP pressure than other nasal-prong interfaces. Heated humidified high-flow nasal cannula (HHHFNC) is used by some units to treat RDS and has been shown not to be "inferior" to CPAP in clinical trials.[135] The variability of pressures generated in preterm infants on HHHFNC, often caused by leaks through the mouth, makes it a less predictable form of distending pressure.

Preterm infants may need PPV due to poor respiratory drive (apnea of prematurity), inability to maintain chest expansion on CPAP (surfactant deficiency, respiratory muscle weakness), or ineffective gas exchange (hypoxia or hypercarbia). PPV can be given via an ET tube (traditional mechanical ventilation) or through nasal prongs (NIPPV). In meta-analysis of studies comparing NIPPV with CPAP following extubation, NIPPV reduced the incidence of extubation failure but had no effect on BPD or mortality.[136] Although earlier studies demonstrated a benefit of synchronized NIPPV on BPD, more recent, larger studies, which used unsynchronized NIPPV with lower average PIPs, found no difference.[137] In unsynchronized NIPPV, only 25% of breaths were coordinated with infant's breaths and only these breaths led to an increase tidal volume. The ability to synchronize breaths can now be done with neurally adjusted ventilatory assist (NAVA), which uses an esophageal catheter to measure diaphragmatic electrical activity to both synchronize breaths and adjust ventilator pressures. NAVA has been shown to decrease BPD in some small studies[138] but needs to be studied in a randomized trial for prevention of BPD. Conventional mechanical ventilators deliver intermittent positive-pressure inflations and PEEP at a preset rate and inspiratory time. The ventilator inflations are often not synchronized with the infant's breaths, and this can contribute to air leak syndromes. Many neonatologists now use higher rates and lower tidal volumes to improve asynchrony and decrease possible lung injury from alveolar overdistention. Volutrauma, from high tidal volumes, and atelectrauma, from inadequate stenting of the airways with PEEP at the end of expiration, are likely more dangerous to the developing lung than the pressures used to generate these volumes. The development of infant mechanical ventilators with accurate flow sensors at the end of the ET tube has allowed for the more reliable use of volume ventilation in the NICU. Studies comparing volume to pressure ventilation in preterm infants demonstrate a benefit for volume ventilation of reduced death or BPD, duration of ventilation, pneumothoraces, periventricular leukomalacia, and severe intraventricular hemorrhage.[139] Volume ventilation also allows for rapid changes in inspiratory pressures in response to changes in lung compliance, especially in the setting of exogenous surfactant administration or use of postnatal corticosteroids. An alternative approach to conventional mechanical ventilation, which generates a tidal volume of 4–6 mL/kg through either pressure or volume control, is to use extremely small volumes but very high rates. During high-frequency jet ventilation (HFJV), high-velocity bursts of gas are fired at rates of 200–600 per minute to generate gas flow down the ET tube. There are few randomized trials comparing HFJV with conventional ventilation, but the largest included approximately 130 infants and demonstrated a slight decrease in BPD rates and need for home oxygen.[140] High-frequency oscillatory ventilation (HFOV) uses a piston to generate a gas gradient within the dead space of the trachea, with gas exchange reliant on oxygen moving down the gradient into the lungs and carbon dioxide diffusing along its gradient out of the lung. Because HFOV relies on forming oxygen and carbon dioxide gradients, extremely active infants or those breathing against the ventilator may affect the gas exchange ability of the ventilator. Randomized trials comparing HFOV to conventional ventilation have variable results, but a meta-analysis demonstrated that HFOV is associated with a modest reduction in BPD, with no excess of intraventricular hemorrhage (IVH) or periventricular leukomalacia (PVL).[141] Surprisingly, especially because many clinicians use HFOV in setting of PIE, HFOV was also associated with a mild increase in air leaks.[141] Use of open lung strategies with HFOV, where mean airway pressure (MAP) is increased until there is no longer an improvement in oxygenation and then decreased by 2 cm H_2O, may lead to improved pulmonary responses in preterm infants. Infants with RDS whose hypoxia is more severe than would be anticipated from the chest radiograph, and who have low lung compliance, should be evaluated for pulmonary hypertension.

PREVENTATIVE STRATEGIES

Antenatal steroids (dexamethasone or betamethasone) can cross the placenta to mature the fetal lung and brain.[142] In the lung, antenatal steroids can decrease the fetal lung fluid through activation of ENaCs, induce the production of surfactant proteins and lipid synthesis, and alter preterm responses to oxidative stress.[142,143] Randomized trials have demonstrated that administration of antenatal corticosteroids significantly reduces the incidences of RDS, neonatal death, cerebral hemorrhage, and NEC.[84] Guidelines recommend the routine use of antenatal steroids for mothers at risk for preterm delivery from 24 weeks to 34 weeks GA.[144] Betamethasone (two doses 24 hours apart), rather than dexamethasone (four doses 12 hours apart), is preferred. Antenatal steroids can be considered at 23 weeks GA but are not currently recommended at 22 weeks GA.[144] Studies have also demonstrated decreased respiratory complications in late preterm infants (34–36 weeks) randomized to antenatal corticosteroids, and revisions to ACOG guidelines are underway.[87,142] Studies of antenatal steroids prior to elective C-section also demonstrate some benefit on respiratory symptoms at birth.[145] The benefit of steroids is maximal in infants delivered between 24 and 168 hours after maternal therapy, but benefits on the lungs are seen in less than 24 hours.[119] The use of repetitive courses of antenatal steroids showed some benefits for respiratory outcomes, but more than five weekly courses caused decreased fetal growth and head circumference.[142] Infants who received repetitive dosing did not show differences in adverse neurologic outcomes at 18-month follow-up. Some obstetricians will give an additional dose of steroids to a mother with persistent threat of preterm delivery 1–2 weeks after initial course. Antenatal steroids do not increase the risk of infection in pregnancies complicated by preterm prelabor rupture of the membranes. There is not a consensus opinion about the use of antenatal steroids for infants of mothers with possible chorioamnionitis.

Thyroid hormones induce surfactant synthesis in animal models. Randomized trials of antenatal administration of thyrotropin-releasing hormone (the only component of the pathway that crosses the placenta) did not reduce the risk of neonatal respiratory distress or BPD, and unfortunately increased the risk of lower 5-minute Apgar scores and caused transient suppression of the pituitary system.[146] Other drugs such as aminophylline, ambroxol, and terbutaline have also been tried, with variable success.

MORTALITY AND MORBIDITY

Overall the mortality from RDS is 5%–10%; the mortality rate is inversely proportional to GA. The use of antenatal steroids and exogenous surfactant therapy has decreased the mortality from RDS, but significant morbidities still exist in the extremely preterm infants that survive. The acute complications of RDS include air leaks, PDA, and pulmonary hemorrhage (discussed separately later). BPD, defined as either oxygen dependency 28 days after birth or at 36 weeks corrected GA, develops in more than 40% of infants born prior to 29 weeks of gestation. BPD is discussed at length in

Chapter 20. Some of these infants require tracheostomy and prolonged mechanical ventilation (see Chapter 21). Changes in antenatal steroid use, modes of respiratory support, and endogenous surfactant have fortunately created a very different form of RDS than was first described by Northway in 1967.

Transient Tachypnea of the Newborn

EPIDEMIOLOGY

Although the exact numbers are unclear, TTN occurs in less than 1% of term vaginal deliveries but is more frequent in late preterm infants.[87] Each week of GA after 35 weeks reduces the risk of respiratory symptoms, particularly if primary C-section is performed.[147] Other risk factors for TTN include C-section birth, with or without labor (threefold higher risk), male sex, macrosomia, maternal diabetes, and maternal history of asthma. Infants of asthmatic mothers may have a genetic predisposition to decreased responsiveness of β-adrenergic stimulation of ENaCs, increasing the risk of TTN and RDS.[148] Antenatal corticosteroids given to women at risk for preterm labor at 34–36 weeks decreased the risk of respiratory support and oxygen need.[87]

PATHOPHYSIOLOGY

This syndrome is thought to result directly from ineffective clearance of fetal lung fluid at the time of birth (see previous description of lung clearance). The lack of uterine contractions causing spinal flexion, and catecholamine surge from labor, lead to increased fetal lung fluid at birth and an increased risk of TTN with elective C-section.[1] The excessive fluid in the lung interacts with the surfactant, which is often at adequate levels to maintain alveolar expansion, and leads to relative inactivation of the surfactant until the fluid is absorbed. A subpopulation of term infants with TTN, often ones who have prolonged hypoxia and tachypnea, have a degree of surfactant deficiency that contributes to the respiratory distress.[149] Inadequate Na$^+$ transport out of the airways, either because of decreased numbers of ENaCs or lack of activation of these channels, contributes to the excess fluid.[14,150] The number of water channels (aquaporins) may also differ in infants with TTN.[15] Preterm infants also have decreased Na$^+$ transport, and late preterm infants with TTN have low amounts of surfactant.[151] The increased fluid accumulates in the interstitial space generating increased pressure and increased refilling of the airways with fluid during expiration, which can be overcome by CPAP in many infants.[1]

CLINICAL PRESENTATION

Infants with TTN are tachypneic with respiratory rates that can be greater than 80 breaths/min. The clinical presentation can resemble mild RDS, although the infants have grunting less often.[152] The chest may be barrel shaped because of hyperinflation. The chest radiograph shows hyperinflation, prominent perihilar vascular markings due to engorgement of the periarterial lymphatics, edema of the interlobar septae,

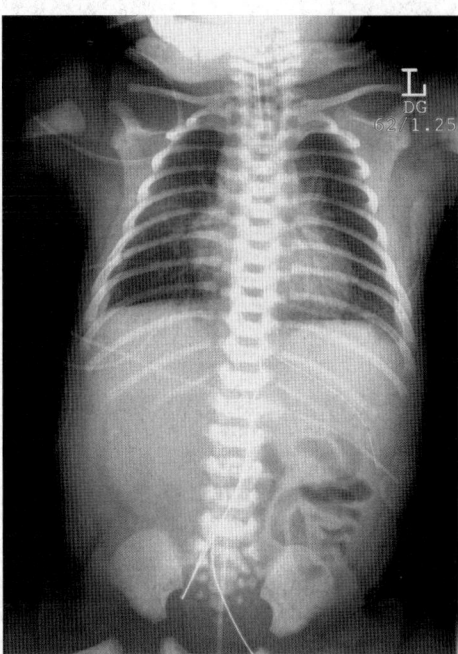

Fig. 19.3 Transient tachypnea of the newborn: excess lung fluid causes transient deactivation of surfactant and similar appearance to mild respiratory distress syndrome. Increased fluid is visible in fissures, with increased vascular markings in the lungs.

and fluid in the fissures (Fig. 19.3). Some infants with TTN will develop pulmonary hypertension, and this should be suspected in infants requiring high concentrations of oxygen.

MANAGEMENT

Most infants with TTN can be managed with supplemental oxygen or CPAP. CPAP will help to drive the excessive fluid out of airways and into the interstitial spaces, where it is absorbed over a few hours. Except in the setting of elective C-section or C-section for maternal reasons not related to infection, IV antimicrobials should be considered because sepsis and pneumonia in the term infant can mimic TTN clinically. TTN is usually self-limiting, and affected infants usually have significant clinical improvement within the first 24 hours and complete recovery within a few days of birth. Complications are rare, but air leaks may occur. Many infants with TTN have respiratory rates too high for safe oral feeding, so intravenous fluids or gavage feeds may be necessary until the tachypnea improves. Trials of furosemide or racemic epinephrine to increase fluid clearance have not shown clear benefits. More recently, it has been suggested that affected infants may derive clinical benefit from inhaled β-adrenergic agonist therapy[153,154]; however, larger trials are required.

Meconium Aspiration Syndrome

EPIDEMIOLOGY

Meconium-stained amniotic fluid (MSAF) complicates approximately 13% of live births,[155,156] affecting term more than preterm infants. MSAF occurs in less than 5% of preterm pregnancies, and when it does occur it suggests infection.

Five percent of babies born through MSAF will develop meconium aspiration syndrome (MAS). In a large study of perinatal registry data in a developed setting, it was found that the overall incidence of MAS was 0.43/1000 live births. The incidence has been decreasing with time; it is associated with factors including advanced GA, low Apgar scores, and C-section delivery.[157] MAS is therefore a condition that predominantly affects term and postterm babies.

PATHOPHYSIOLOGY

MASF occurs when there is antenatal passage of meconium. This phenomenon has been associated with fetal distress and hypoxic-ischemic insult. MAS is an inflammatory lung condition caused by aspiration of MSAF by the infant into the airways during the peripartum period.

It has been found that antenatal passage of meconium is associated with higher levels of motilin in the baby.[158] Motilin is produced mainly by endocrine M cells of the duodenojejunal mucosa and stimulates peristalsis.[159] Levels are very low in preterm infants and nonasphyxiated term infants but are raised in asphyxiated term babies who pass meconium during the peripartum period. Prolonged severe fetal hypoxia can stimulate fetal gasping *in utero* leading to inhalation of MSAF. It is also thought that inhalation can occur perinatally with the first breaths of the baby who is delivered through MSAF. Although meconium is mainly made up of water (approximately 80%), it is chemically complex, containing components of various substances, including digestive juices, lipids, intestinal epithelial cells, lanugo hair, bile, and amniotic fluid.[160,161] It is of variable consistency and, when inhaled, can create a ball-valve mechanism within the airways. This obstructive pathology predisposes the lungs to air trapping and hyperinflation. In addition, meconium irritates the lungs, activating numerous inflammatory mediators, toll-like receptors, and the complement system.[161] An inflammatory pneumonitis and systemic inflammatory response can ensue, with an associated release of vasoactive substances that can cause vasoconstriction and raised pulmonary arterial pressure. In addition, meconium impairs surfactant function, increasing the possibility of atelectasis. Meconium harbors microbiota that are associated with amniotic fluid and placental microbiota.[162] In addition, meconium is thought to enhance bacterial growth by serving as a growth factor and inhibiting bacteriostatic properties of amniotic fluid,[163] facilitating the growth of pathogens such as *Escherichia coli*. Meconium has been suggested to significantly impair mechanisms of intracellular microbial killing, inhibiting phagocytosis and the neutrophil oxidative burst.

CLINICAL FEATURES

Infants with MAS generally present with signs of respiratory distress such as tachypnea and use of accessory muscles of respiration. The obstructive pathology can lead to increased anteroposterior diameter of the chest, whereas the ventilation-perfusion mismatch and pulmonary hypertension can lead to cyanosis. Initial chest radiographs may show hyperinflated lung fields and widespread patchy infiltrates (Fig. 19.4). Small pleural effusions occur in approximately 20% of patients. With development of pneumonitis and interstitial edema the radiographic appearance can progress to diffuse, homogeneous opacification of both lung fields. Air leaks, such as

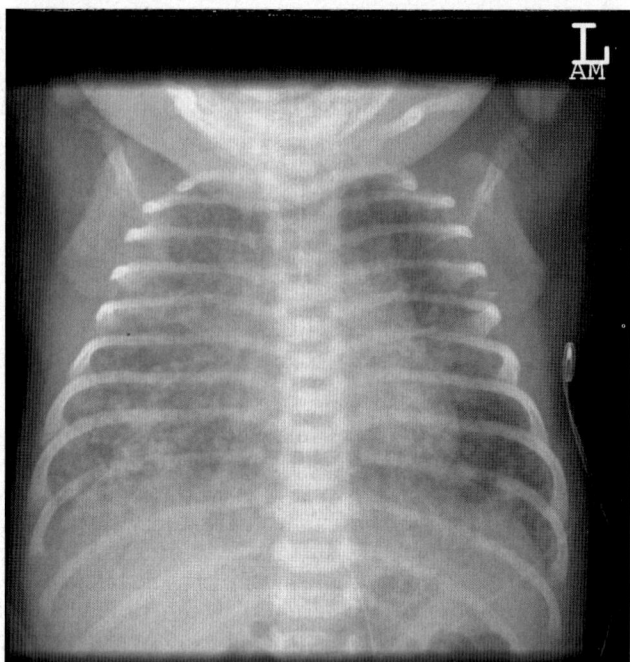

Fig. 19.4 Meconium aspiration syndrome: chest x-ray with hyperinflation and patchy infiltrates throughout both lung fields.

pneumothorax and pneumomediastinum, are very common, occurring in approximately 20% of infants. In those with pulmonary hypertension, right-to-left shunting at ductal and atrial levels may be seen by echocardiography. Differential diagnoses include pneumonia, surfactant deficiency, persistent pulmonary hypertension of the newborn (PPHN), congenital cardiac disease, and aspiration of blood.[164]

MANAGEMENT

Although infants mildly affected by MAS may require no specific treatment, a substantial proportion of infants will require intensive care management of the many complications that can arise. The risk of pulmonary hypertension is high in infants with MAS, and hypoxemia should be avoided. Supplemental oxygen should be administered to keep oxygen saturations greater than 94%. One should also consider using PaO_2 to guide oxygen use. With increasing evidence that high oxygen concentrations can cause harm, ventilatory support measures such as CPAP or mechanical ventilation should be considered if the FiO_2 requirement is persistently high. Traditionally MAS has been conceptualized as a primarily obstructive condition; however, it is now increasingly recognized that areas of hyperinflation may coexist with atelectasis in a setting of ventilation-perfusion mismatch.[164] It is therefore essential that ventilatory support should be initiated with close monitoring of the progress of the infant. Use of CPAP or mechanical ventilation may improve oxygenation but may also increase the risk of air leak. The thresholds at which ventilatory support should be initiated are therefore not evidence based and may need to be adjusted depending on the condition of the individual baby. In general, mechanical ventilation would be considered in infants with $PaCO_2 > 8$ kPa (>60 mm Hg) and $PaO_2 < 6$ kPa (<50 mm Hg) despite initial oxygen supplementation, especially in infants with evidence of PPHN. Conventionally, the ventilator strategy should be based on a relatively low PEEP and long expiratory time, but in practice, the appropriateness of this strategy will depend on the relative balance between atelectasis and hyperinflation. In infants with severe disease, and particularly if associated with pulmonary hypertension, HFOV and adjunctive use of inhaled NO should be considered.[165,166] In a meta-analysis that included four randomized trials, it was suggested that surfactant administration could reduce the severity of respiratory illness and decrease the number of infants with progressive respiratory failure requiring support with extracorporeal membrane oxygenation (ECMO),[167] especially if administered as a bolus. Surfactant administration both as lung lavage and as a bolus reduced duration of mechanical ventilation and length of hospital stay but did not reduce mortality.[168] The use of antibiotics has not been shown to benefit infants with MAS in terms of duration of ventilation, hospital stay, or mortality.[168,169] However, despite this, it is widespread practice to commence broad-spectrum antibiotics empirically in view of the difficulty in differentiating between MAS and pneumonia. Results of a randomized trial suggested that ECMO improved survival in infants with an oxygenation index (OI) of >40.[170] However, with improving intensive care strategies, the need for ECMO has been reduced.[165] There has been interest in the protective effects of hypothermia for lung conditions such as MAS, and some centers have started to incorporate it into the management of these infants.[171]

PREVENTION

There is an inverse association between amniotic fluid volume and fetal HR decelerations, possibly due to either cord or head compression. Amnioinfusion has been thought to dilute meconium, especially in cases of thick MSAF, and correct oligohydramnios, thereby relieving umbilical cord compression.[172] However, results of a meta-analysis suggested that amnioinfusion did not improve perinatal outcomes in settings of standard peripartum surveillance and was only beneficial in settings with limited facilities to monitor the baby during labor.[172] Furthermore, amnioinfusion carries increased risk of several adverse outcomes, including cord prolapse, infection, and requirement for instrumental delivery. There has been much debate in the value of meticulous clearing of the airway during and after delivery in an infant delivered through MSAF,[173] with recommendations being based more on biologic plausibility and expert opinion than a strong body of evidence. Avoidance of postterm delivery is the key factor in reducing the incidence of MSAF and thus MAS. With increasing numbers of studies and meta-analyses, there has been a failure to obtain evidence that routine efforts to clear the airway of meconium by ET or oropharyngeal suctioning can prevent MAS or lead to improved outcomes of affected infants.[174] It has been argued that MAS incidence in these studies was low. However, even in a setting with a high incidence of MAS, intrapartum suctioning was not shown to be of benefit.[175] In another recent study in a developing setting, ET suctioning was not shown to be superior to routine resuscitation even for nonvigorous babies delivered through MSAF.[162] Because of the accumulating evidence of lack of benefit of routine suctioning to prevent MAS, ILCOR no longer recommends routine ET suctioning of nonvigorous babies delivered through MSAF.[176] Clinical judgement regarding the presence of significant airway obstruction should be exercised when deciding whether to initiate ET suctioning, taking care not to delay PPV and other important resuscitation measures in the process.

PROGNOSIS

The mortality of MAS in a developed setting has been reported to be 2.5%.[157] In contrast, mortality can be as high as 32% in developing regions of the world.[177] Most deaths are from respiratory failure, pulmonary hypertension, or air leaks. Fifty percent of babies who require mechanical ventilation because of MAS suffer an air leak. Neurodevelopmental delays have been observed even in infants who respond well to conventional ventilation.[178] Children with a history of MAS have been found to exhibit long-term lung function abnormalities, increased bronchial hyperreactivity, and higher reported rates of recurrent cough and wheeze.[179]

Acute Respiratory Distress Syndrome

PATHOPHYSIOLOGY

Acute respiratory distress syndrome (ARDS) in the newborn occurs when a systemic injury leads to lung inflammation and injury in previously healthy lungs and is often associated with multiorgan failure.[180] Like adults, ARDS can occur following asphyxia, shock (cardiogenic or hypovolemic), or sepsis. Myocardial dysfunction from birth asphyxia or from severe metabolic acidosis can lead to pulmonary edema and need for ventilator support. The direct injury from the hypoxia on the lung tissue or the injury sustained from mechanical ventilation leads to release of proteins into the air spaces, thus worsening the lung disease by inactivation of surfactant.[105] Sepsis will lead to increased capillary leak of fluid and protein into the lungs. Preterm infants may be predisposed to lung inflammation from chorioamnionitis, and severe chorioamnionitis may have systemic responses—fetal inflammatory response syndrome (FIRS).[181]

CLINICAL PRESENTATION

ARDS presents with worsening tachypnea and oxygen requirements after a systemic event. Clinically it may look very like primary lung diseases such as pneumonia or MAS (discussed in other sections of this chapter). Some infants who have the clinical appearance of RDS, but who are not premature and do not have a good response to exogenous surfactant therapy, may have underlying lung disease more consistent with ARDS. The tachypnea may result initially from stimulation by metabolic acidosis or damage to the central nervous system, but the hypoxia will progressively worsen as the lung tissue becomes edematous and inflammation develops. The chest radiograph demonstrates diffuse pulmonary infiltrates, with some severe cases having complete opacification of the lungs. Blood cultures and tracheal aspirates may guide the antibiotic management of these infants.

MANAGEMENT

Treatment of the underlying cause of the ARDS (sepsis, birth asphyxia, cardiogenic shock) is essential for the lungs to recover. The newborn lung is moderately resistant to chronic injury and should be able to recover if the infant can survive the initial insult. Surfactant administration can improve oxygenation in ARDS, similar to MAS, but may require larger doses than used in RDS.[180] Efforts to increase the mean airway pressure, through either higher PEEP or longer inspiratory time, will help to increase FRC and improve oxygenation. HFOV, especially when using a series of recruitment steps to reach an open lung, may have benefits for improving oxygenation in ARDS though its superiority over conventional ventilation has not been demonstrated.[182] In recent studies in adults with ARDS, HFOV did not decrease mortality over conventional mechanical ventilation.[183] Fluid management is important in treating ARDS as the clinician tries to decrease flooding of the lung with fluid restriction, while still maintaining proper perfusion of other organs. Broad-spectrum antimicrobials (usually ampicillin plus an aminoglycoside if in the first few days after birth but with broader coverage, especially for staphylococcus, when systemic infection is suspected after 3 days) should be administered. Aminoglycoside levels must be carefully monitored because these infants are at high risk of renal dysfunction. Air leaks and infection are commonly seen in infants with ARDS. Pulmonary hypertension can occur in ARDS and infants may benefit from sedation or inhaled NO therapy. Severe ARDS that does not respond to HFOV may require ECMO, often arteriovenous due to cardiac dysfunction, until the lungs recover. The mortality and morbidity of ARDS are high, and this is due to a combination of the hypoxia from the lung disease and the effects of the systemic disease that caused the ARDS.

Early-Onset Pneumonia

Early-onset pneumonia presents clinically within the first 48 hours to 1 week after birth.[184] Because early-onset or congenital pneumonias are often present at birth, it is sometimes difficult to distinguish pneumonia from RDS, TTN, or MAS. Radiographically diagnosed pneumonia was found in 1.5% of infants born at 34 weeks versus 0.2% of infants born at term.[185] Pneumonias can be acquired either transplacentally from mother, during labor with prolonged rupture of membranes or chorioamnionitis, or during delivery. The timing of clinical presentation will depend on the mode of transmission. The term newborn lung is immature with respect to ciliary clearance of microbes, lung macrophage function, and humoral immune responses (immunoglobulin A, surfactant protein A and D); and this predisposes the newborn lung to pneumonias. Although originally thought to be sterile, the normal lung is now known to be colonized with its own microbiome and the interactions between normal and pathologic bacteria may play a role in the development of pneumonia or other respiratory diseases.[186] The mode of delivery affects the respiratory microbiome, with infants delivered vaginally having bacteria closer to the mother's vaginal secretions, whereas C-section infants have a lung biome closer to maternal skin.[186] Transplacentally acquired organisms associated with pneumonia include *Listeria monocytogenes* (often found in unpasteurized cheeses), *Mycobacterium tuberculosis*, *Treponema pallidum*, rubella virus, cytomegalovirus (CMV), herpes simplex virus (HSV), adenovirus, and influenza type A virus. A high percentage (more than 20%) of stillborn infants or infants that die soon after birth are found to have pneumonia at autopsy.[184] Most cases caused by ascending infection are due to *Streptococcus agalactiae* (GBS), and antenatal testing for GBS is recommended for all pregnant women. The use of antenatal GBS prophylaxis has decreased the rates of early onset GBS sepsis and pneumonia but has not changed the rates of late-onset disease. There are 10 identifiable subtypes of GBS based on capsular polysaccharide antigens; most neonatal infections are caused by types Ia, II, III, and V, but the pathogenic subtypes differ between countries.[187] The incidence of early-onset GBS sepsis is 0.67 per 1000 live births in the Americas and 0.53 per 1000 in Europe. Countries reporting no use of intrapartum antibiotics have had a 2.2-fold increase in early-onset disease.[187] *E. coli* is the second most common cause of early-onset neonatal sepsis and pneumonia.[188,189] A large percentage of *E. coli* strains that cause early-onset sepsis possess the capsule type K1, which confers antiphagocytic properties and resistance to complement mediated killing; antibiotic resistance to both ampicillin and gentamicin have been increasingly reported in *E. coli*. Other organisms that cause ascending infection include *Haemophilus influenzae*, *Streptococcus pneumoniae*, *L. monocytogenes*, *Klebsiella pneumoniae*, *Candida albicans*, and viruses such as adenovirus, CMV, HSV, and echovirus.

Risk factors for early-onset pneumonia include prolonged rupture of the membranes, premature labor, and colonization of the vagina with GBS or other pathogens. Chorioamnionitis increases the risk of early-onset pneumonia and may predispose the infant to an altered immune/inflammatory response to microorganisms acquired during labor.[189] In developed countries, approximately 20%–30% of women are colonized with GBS in the vaginal vault and 50% of infants born vaginally will become colonized. Fortunately, only 1% of these infants will develop invasive GBS disease.[187] Although not routinely tested clinically, the highest transmission rate is in GBS colonized women who have low levels of circulating anti-GBS immunoglobulin. Women infected with HIV are considerably more susceptible to many perinatal infections, especially *L. monocytogenes*. HSV is usually transmitted during delivery through an infected maternal genital tract.

CLINICAL PRESENTATION

The timing of presentation depends on whether the infection was acquired transplacentally, usually present at birth, or during labor, when it may take up to 48 hours to develop. GBS is a fast-growing microorganism, and most of these infections will present in the first 12 hours, and rapid deterioration can occur without prompt treatment. In the setting of chorioamnionitis, sepsis may present within 6 hours of birth.[189] Many infants with pneumonia or sepsis have normal Apgar values at birth but develop progressive tachypnea, respiratory distress, hypoxia, and other signs of sepsis. Some infants will have more subtle findings, such as poor feeding, irritability, hypothermia, or fever.[152] Infants who are overtly septic with poor peripheral perfusion, cyanosis, and inadequate respiration have a poor prognosis.[189] Infants with severe congenital pneumonia may require high PIPs to open the inflamed lungs. Infants with congenitally acquired Listeria infection are often extremely ill at birth, with severe pneumonia and hepatomegaly, and at autopsy have small pinkish-gray granulomas throughout the lung, liver, skin,

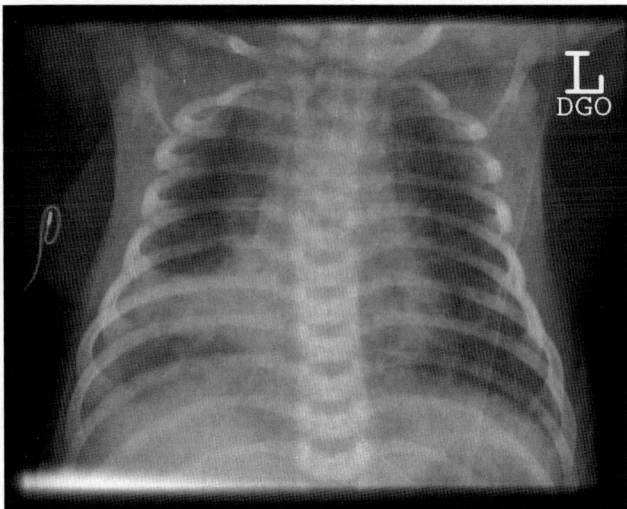

Fig. 19.5 Lobar pneumonia: right lower lobe is consolidated on chest x-ray and streaky infiltrates can be seen in other portions of the lungs.

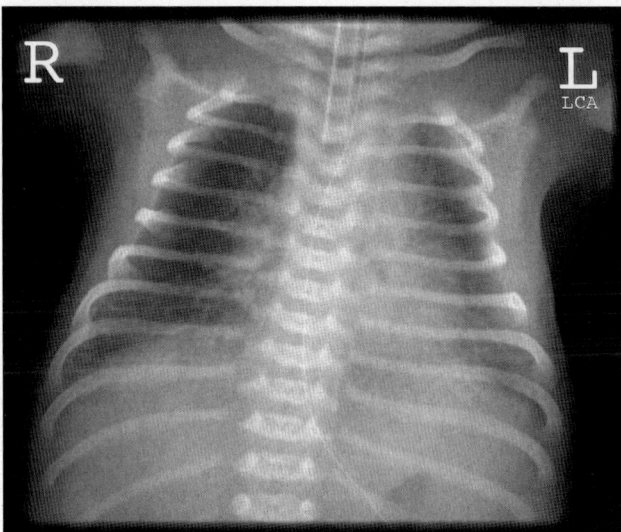

Fig. 19.6 Newborn pneumonia. Diffuse opacifications are visible throughout lungs. Clinical correlation will often determine pneumonia verses transient tachypnea of the newborn or respiratory distress syndrome.

and other organ systems. Viruses such as CMV and HSV can present with pneumonia or more generalized pneumonitis.

The chest radiograph appearance is variable and can range from an entire lobe (Fig. 19.5) to segmental consolidation, atelectasis, or diffuse opacification (Fig. 19.6). Many pediatric radiologists will not distinguish between neonatal pneumonia, TTN, or RDS, and often a follow-up image is needed (TTN should have resolved on repeat x-ray). Pleural effusions can be present and sometimes abscesses or pneumatoceles. For intubated infants, a tracheal aspirate from a new ET tube can sometimes be useful and should be evaluated by microscopy for white blood cell, and culture. Blood cultures are important because many of the infections are hematogenously spread or have secondary bacterial release into the bloodstream. Systemic markers of infection and inflammation, such as a CBC or C-reactive protein, may help to guide the clinician regarding antibiotic use. In the setting of suspected chorioamnionitis, histologic evaluation and culture of the placenta

may provide additional information on the organism. If herpes infection is likely, viral cultures from the maternal lesions and the infant should be obtained.

MANAGEMENT

Because it is difficult to determine whether respiratory distress is caused by pneumonia or TTN, many clinicians will treat any respiratory distress requiring additional monitoring with antibiotics. All infants who were well appearing at birth and then develop respiratory distress require a work-up for sepsis, pneumonia, and congenital heart disease. Initial treatment for early-onset pneumonia should be a combination of ampicillin or benzylpenicillin and an aminoglycoside, most often gentamicin. The initial management regiment should be modified once culture results are available, or if certain resistance patterns are present within the local community. Cefotaxime can be substituted for gentamicin in infants with birth asphyxia or concerns about renal failure. Certain bacteria, such as *H. influenza*, may require cefotaxime due to development of antibiotic resistance. *E. coli* is often resistant to ampicillin, and bacterial strains resistant to both ampicillin and gentamicin have been reported. For Listeria, the most effective antimicrobial therapy is the combination of ampicillin plus gentamicin because Listeria is resistant to all cephalosporins. The length of treatment depends on the severity of the disease, the presence of systemic response, and the organism isolated. Most early-onset cases of pneumonia will respond to antibiotic therapy of 7–10 days, with no clear evidence for one treatment length or the other. Lung abscesses and empyemas should be drained, and with these complications IV antimicrobials should be administered for at least 2 weeks. Infections due to HSV require long-term therapy with high-dose acyclovir.

Late-Onset Pneumonia

Late-onset pneumonia typically occurs in infants after approximately 1 week to 3 weeks of life and can be caused by a variety of bacteria and respiratory viruses. The most common causes are gram positive cocci (coagulase-negative Staphylococci, *Staphylococcus aureus*, streptococci) and gram-negative bacilli (including *Klebsiella, E. coli, Serratia marcescens*, and *Pseudomonas*). These infections often occur in infants with prolonged mechanical ventilation, and hospitals have developed respiratory hygiene protocols to attempt to decrease ventilator-associated pneumonias.[190] Increasing respiratory support while on mechanical ventilation should be investigated for development of pneumonia. *Chlamydia trachomatis* is a well-recognized cause of late-onset pneumonia, often presenting at 1–3 months of age, and may develop in 7% of infants born to mothers infected with Chlamydia.[184] Two weeks of oral erythromycin is recommended for chlamydial pneumonia. *Ureaplasma urealyticum* is a common cause of chorioamnionitis and pneumonia in infants, but the bacterium does not grow well on typical culture media and is often not identified. In areas of the world where tuberculosis is prevalent, tuberculosis pneumonia should be considered because the symptoms are nonspecific, and tuberculosis can be acquired by transplacental spread, aspiration, ingestion of infected amniotic fluid, or airborne inoculation from close contacts.[184] Respiratory viruses have an increasing role in late-onset pneumonia, with adenovirus, rhinovirus, respiratory syncytial virus, influenza, and human metapneumovirus being the most common. With the use of respiratory virus polymerase chain reaction (PCR) panels, many previously undiagnosed infections can be found and proper isolation of the infant can be instituted. Viral pneumonias are often nosocomial and usually occur when there are high levels of infection in the community. Fungal pneumonias, often due to candida species, can be found in very low birth weight (VLBW) infants, especially after prolonged exposure to third-generation cephalosporins, but are typically caused by hematogenous spread. CMV pneumonia is rare in the term infant but can be a cause of persistent CMV pneumonitis in immunocompromised or very preterm infants. CMV can be acquired from CMV-infected amniotic fluid or through feeding with thawed frozen breast milk from HCMV-Ig–positive mothers.[191] Although many of the bacteria that cause late-onset pneumonia are covered by the combination of ampicillin and gentamicin, initial treatment with a third-generation cephalosporin and vancomycin may be warranted. If the infant is worsening on current antimicrobials, the regime should broadened to cover nosocomial organisms such as *Pseudomonas* and *Serratia*.[184]

Aspiration Pneumonia

Aspiration pneumonia occurs in newborns either through aspiration of GER into airways or from inappropriate closure of the airways during feedings. The aspirated fluid can cause inflammation of the airways or cause physical obstruction of the airways.[192] The airway obstruction can lead to lung collapse or increased propensity for bacterial infection (Fig. 19.7), with the right upper lobe being the most affected region. The low pH of gastric secretions may lead to worsening chemical irritation of the airways and lung parenchyma. Infants with chronic microaspirations may develop hypoxia and respiratory distress.[193] Severe aspiration pneumonia often requires mechanical ventilation until inflammation has resolved. Broad-spectrum antimicrobial cover should be prescribed for aspiration pneumonia with consolidation but may not

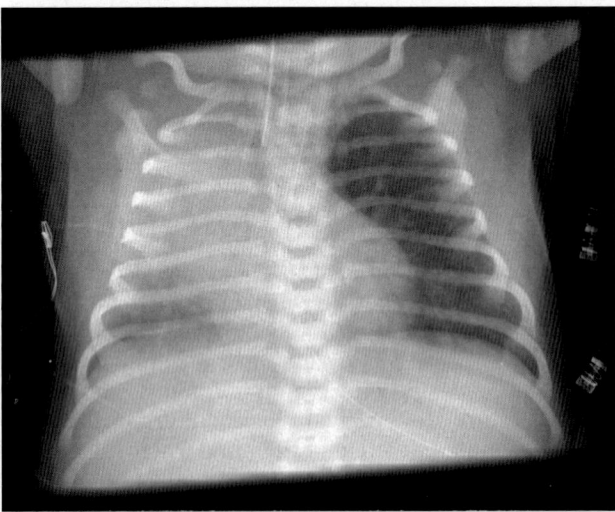

Fig. 19.7 Aspiration pneumonia: aspiration often causes lobar pneumonitis or pneumonia. The right upper lobe is most often involved.

be necessary for microaspiration. Infants with consolidation of the right upper lobe may benefit from positioning this side up to allow increased aeration and drainage of the lung segment. Aspiration pneumonia is more common in infants with neurologic disease or injury, and surgical intervention with Nissen procedure or gastrostomy tube may be necessary to prevent recurrent events.[194] Preterm infants with BPD and a developmentally normal neurologic examination can be fed while on CPAP without increased risk of aspiration pneumonia.

Interstitial Lung Disease

Childhood interstitial lung disease (chILD) should be in the differential of term newborns with severe respiratory distress, or preterm infants with prolonged ventilator support that do not have normal responses to surfactant therapies. These conditions include problems with the surfactant system (e.g., surfactant protein deficiency and ABCA3 deficiency—reviewed in Chapters 5 and 57), pulmonary interstitial glycogenosis (PIG), neuroendocrine cell hyperplasia of infancy (NEHI—previously called persistent tachypnea of infancy), or alveolar capillary dysplasia (ACD). Interstitial lung disease is diagnosed through high-resolution computed tomography (CT) scan or lung biopsy. Corticosteroids are commonly used in many chILD and may decrease lung inflammation and interstitial thickening. Interstitial lung disease is covered in detail in Chapters 54–57.

Persistent Pulmonary Hypertension of the Newborn

PPHN is caused by failure of the pulmonary vascular resistance (PVR) to rapidly decrease at birth, leading to right-to-left shunts at the level of the ductus arteriosus and the foramen ovale and difficulty with oxygenation. Although PPHN is sometimes referred to as persistent fetal circulation, the removal of the low-resistance, high-volume placental circuit creates additional work for the cardiopulmonary system. Understanding the alterations in the normal physiologic transition at birth helps clinicians to develop therapeutic interventions for these critically ill infants.

CHANGES IN THE CIRCULATION AT BIRTH

During fetal circulation, the PVR is high and only 10%–20% of the cardiac output goes through the pulmonary vasculature. The low resistance, high volume of the placenta enhances shunting of the blood away from the lungs through the foramen ovale or the ductus arteriosus. Pulmonary blood flow and PVR changes throughout the pregnancy in a U-shaped curve. The PVR is high at 20 weeks GA, with 13% cardiac output going to lungs, then PVR drops around 30 weeks gestation to increase blood flow to lungs to 25%–30% of cardiac output, before an increase in PVR near term causes a drop in pulmonary blood flow to around 20%.[195] The combination of increased arterial oxygen content, removal of the low resistance of the placenta, and removal of placental derived prostaglandins lead to rapid transitions from fetal to newborn circulations. Removal of the placenta decreases venous return to the right atrium, decreases right atrial (RA) pressure, and increases systemic vascular resistance (SVR) leading to increased left atrial pressure, which leads to closure of the foramen ovale. The flow through the ductus arteriosus decreases such that it passively closes within 3–7 days after birth. In normal newborns, PVR falls rapidly in the first minutes after birth, with recruitment of FRC and then more gradually over the next days. Aeration of the lungs, through stimulation of stretch receptors, vasodilates the pulmonary vascular bed and increases the pulmonary blood flow.[196,197] Opening of the alveoli also leads to decrease perivascular fluid and improved gas exchange (see clearance of airway fluid). *In utero* the PVR remains high due to low levels of pulmonary vasodilators (oxygen, prostacyclin [PGI_2] and NO), and high levels of vasoconstrictors (endothelin-1 [ET-1]).[198] PGI_2 is produced by the vascular endothelial cells, pulmonary stretch increases its release, and causes relaxation of smooth muscle surrounding the arterioles. Blockade of prostaglandins *in utero* does not affect resting PVR, whereas exogenous PGI_2 causes vasodilation after birth.[199] NO is also produced by the vascular endothelial cells through the cleavage of L-arginine by NO synthase. NO diffuses into the smooth muscles cells to stimulate vessel relaxation through production of guanosine monophosphate. Because oxygen tension helps to regulate NO production, fetal NO levels are low in the relative hypoxic environment. Endogenous NO production responds to the increased PaO_2 associated with initiation of ventilation at birth. PGI_2 activity may be modulated by NO because NO synthase inhibitors decrease the effectiveness of exogenous PGI_2. Along with increasing vasodilators, endogenous vasoconstrictors (thromboxane and ET-1) decrease at birth to allow relaxation of the vasculature. In newborns with significant hypoxia or sepsis, levels of ET-1 and thromboxane A2, along with leukotrienes, are increased and can cause severe pulmonary hypertension. Prostaglandin E_2, which helps to maintain ductal patency *in utero*, is produced by the placenta and PGE_2 metabolism within the lungs is enhanced by ventilation, thus decreasing levels of PGE_2 help to facilitate ductal closure. Although there is some variation, most infants complete this cardiovascular transition by 8 hours of age and the ductus arteriosus typically closes by 24 hours of age. Pulmonary vascular pressure decreases to 50% of systemic vascular pressure by 24 hours of life, and adult levels of PVR are typically reached by 6 weeks of age.[198]

PATHOPHYSIOLOGY

PPHN can be secondary to systemic conditions (birth asphyxia, sepsis, metabolic disorders, maternal exposure to selective serotonin reuptake inhibitor, BPD) or due to congenital conditions (CDH, congenital heart disease, ACD, pulmonary hypoplasia). There is an increased incidence of pulmonary hypertension in some genetic disorders (trisomy 21, Noonan syndrome, DiGeorge) and with rare familial mutations.[200] The newborn pulmonary vasculature responds quickly to changes in pH, PaO_2, and $PaCO_2$. Acidosis (either respiratory or metabolic) leads to pulmonary vasoconstriction, whereas alkalosis can temporarily improve PVR and oxygenation. Caution should be used with induction of chronic respiratory alkalosis, because overventilation and hypocapnia can injure the lung and may potentiate cerebral vasoconstriction.[200] Hypoxia also

causes pulmonary vasoconstriction, with PaO_2 levels less than 60 mm Hg causing exponential increases in PVR.[201,202] Intrauterine growth restriction infants with chronic hypoxia and placental insufficiency also have increased muscularization of the pulmonary arterioles and extension of muscle layer into smaller arteries. Hypoxia leads to increase in vasoconstrictor and smooth muscle mitogens (ET-1, platelet-derived growth factor B, vascular endothelial growth factor) and decreases in endothelial NO synthase.[203] In the setting of meconium aspiration, where the release of meconium is a response to *in utero* stress and chronic hypoxia over a period of days, there may be changes to the vascular walls that contribute to pulmonary hypertension. Higher hematocrits (Hcts) have also been associated with increased pulmonary hypertension, but this may be due to changes from fetal hypoxia that also stimulate red cell production. ACD (discussed in Chapter 56) cause disruption of the alignment of the pulmonary vasculature with the distal airspaces, creating pulmonary hypertension and failure to oxygenate. Infants with pulmonary hypoplasia, due to either physical obstruction in CDH or from loss of distending pressure in severe oligohydramnios, have decreased arteriole numbers and increased musculature. These infants often have both a fixed anatomic component and a reactive component (responds to treatments listed later) to their pulmonary hypertension creating a mixed response to treatment. Infants with PPHN typically have a normal number and muscularization of the arteries, but the arterioles fail to respond to normal transitional cues of increased oxygen tension and expansion of the lung at birth. PPHN is more common in infants with African-American or Asian mothers, and who are male.[204] With current therapies, the PVR of most infants will eventually decrease over the first week. Prolonged need for treatment warrants further evaluation for rare conditions such as ACD or surfactant deficiency.

CLINICAL PRESENTATION

Infants with PPHN usually present within 6 hours of birth with cyanosis and mild respiratory distress. Because the lungs are often fully expanded in PPHN, grunting and nasal flaring are uncommon with these infants. On cardiac examination, the second heart sound may be louder due to the increased pulmonary pressures and there may be a soft systolic murmur from tricuspid regurgitation (TR). Infants with pulmonary hypertension from structural changes to the lung parenchyma (CDH, pulmonary hypoplasia) will present with increased respiratory symptoms and other physical examination findings associated with these conditions. Pulmonary hypertension can occur in severe GBS infection and birth asphyxia, and these infants may have systemic signs of shock or neurologic changes.

DIAGNOSIS AND DIFFERENTIAL DIAGNOSIS

Pulmonary hypertension should be suspected when the severity of hypoxemia does not correspond to the severity of radiologic or clinical symptoms. Infants with pulmonary hypertension secondary to other systemic diseases may have radiographic changes consistent with the original disease process. Evidence of right-to-left shunting across the ductus arteriosus can be determined by pulse oximetry readings between the right wrist (preductal) and the lower extremity (postductal). PaO$_2$ levels can be compared between a radial artery and the umbilical artery, but this is normally not necessary due to the reliability of saturation differences on pulse oximetry. Response to oxygen therapy is more common in pulmonary hypertension than congenital heart disease, although some infants with severe PPHN will have PaO$_2$ < 100 mm Hg on 100% oxygen. Infants with congenital heart disease may have a similar presentation, so echocardiogram is necessary to rule out structural heart disease. Although cardiac catheterization is the only way to directly measure pulmonary arterial pressures, echocardiogram is primarily used clinically to diagnosis pulmonary hypertension.[200] The TR jet velocity is the most accurate echocardiographic predictor of pulmonary hypertension in children.[200] Because many infants do not have a measurable TR, other echocardiographic findings in PPHN include RA enlargement, right ventricular (RV) dilation, pulmonary artery dilation, septal flattening, and directional shunting at PFO or PDA.[200] Infants with fixed pulmonary hypertension from congenital changes to the lung (CDH, lung hypoplasia) may not respond to oxygen therapy. ACD should be suspected in infants with severe pulmonary hypertension that is persistent and unresponsive to conventional therapies, but it requires a lung biopsy to establish the diagnosis. The severity of the pulmonary hypertension can be measured by either oxygen index or alveolar-arterial oxygen difference, and these parameters can be used to determine response to therapies and need to escalate care towards ECMO.

MANAGEMENT

Overstimulation can worsen pulmonary hypertension and oxygenation in infants with PPHN. Minimal handling by staff and family and reduction in nursing interventions such as routine ET suctioning can improve oxygenation. The infant should be maintained in a normothermic environment, unless undergoing therapeutic hypothermia for birth asphyxia, because extremes of temperature can alter PVR. Because sepsis and neonatal pneumonia are often causes of pulmonary hypertension in the newborn, broad-spectrum antibiotics should be considered in the initial days of treatment. The infant's Hct should be maintained in a normal range (40%–50%) to optimize oxygen delivery without causing the increased viscosity and PVR seen with polycythemia.[203] In situations of extreme polycythemia (Hct > 70%), a partial exchange transfusion should be considered. Many infants with moderate to severe pulmonary hypertension will require continuous sedation and pain control to improve oxygenation. In some situations, pharmacologic paralysis can be used to reduce PVR and prevent ECMO use; up to 73% of infants received paralysis prior to routine NO use.[205]

Two of the most basic therapies for PPHN, available in low-resource environments, are optimizing lung expansion and oxygen therapy. Many infants with mild PPHN can be treated with nasal cannula oxygen to decrease PVR. Maintaining lung expansion and avoiding atelectasis is important for improving ventilation-perfusion mismatch in PPHN and can often be achieved with CPAP. Infants with moderate to severe PPHN normally require intubation and mechanical ventilation. The addition of surfactant to infants receiving mechanical ventilation, especially in the setting of meconium aspiration, should be considered.[200,206] Surfactant therapy has been shown to reduce the need for ECMO in MAS, but

not in PPHN. Current European guidelines for management of acute PPHN recommend maintaining partial pressure of carbon dioxide (pCO$_2$) between 45 and 60 mm Hg and pH > 7.25.[206] Lower pH levels increase the reactivity of the pulmonary vasculature to hypoxia. Alkalosis, either by mechanical ventilation to induce hypocapnia or through metabolic alkalosis with sodium bicarbonate, can transiently increase oxygenation. Hyperventilation, once a main therapy in PPHN, is not routinely recommended because prolonged alkalosis can worsen lung disease and can cause changes in cerebral blood flow and neurodevelopmental outcome.[200,205] Lung overdistention from high inflating pressure and PEEP can also cause barotrauma and worsening of pulmonary hypertension. Some centers use high-frequency oscillation or jet ventilation to maintain higher mean airway pressures to keep the lungs inflated. ECMO is used as a rescue therapy for infants unresponsive to additional therapies listed later. Oxygen is the other main therapy for PPHN available in most parts of the world. Oxygen is a potent vasodilator of the pulmonary vasculature, and this drug should be titrated in infants with PPHN to both avoid hypoxia and hyperoxia. Hypoxia causes vasoconstriction in animals at PaO$_2$ < 50 mm Hg with exponential increases in PVR as hypoxia worsens.[202] Increasing PaO$_2$ to greater than 60 mm Hg does not decrease the PVR further. High oxygen tension can lead to free radical formation and worsening of the pulmonary hypertension. NO is directly inactivated by superoxide forming peroxynitrite which is toxic, and hyperoxia enhances phosphodiesterase-5 (PDE-5) activity, leading to increased break down of NO. Hyperoxia can also cause vasoconstriction through activation of xanthine oxidase.[207] To avoid hypoxia and hyperoxia, infants with PPHN are recommended to be maintained at an oxygen saturation by pulse oximetry (SpO$_2$) level between 90% and 95% with avoidance of SpO$_2$ levels less than 85 or greater than 97%.[200,206,207] These saturation levels correspond to a PaO$_2$ of 60–80 mm Hg. Although many infants with mild to moderate PPHN can have oxygenation maintained through oxygen, CPAP, and sedation, an increasing OI should signal a need for a higher level of NICU care and initiation of therapies listed later.

iNO is the only US Food and Drug Administration (FDA)-approved gas for treatment of pulmonary hypertension in term and late preterm infants. iNO is typically bled into a ventilator circuit, although it can be given via nasal cannulae (NC) or CPAP in noninvasive ventilation. iNO diffuses across the capillary membrane into the vascular smooth muscle to relax the arterioles. iNO then binds to hemoglobin and is quickly converted to an inactive form leaving methemoglobin (metHg) and nitrite. This conversion limits the systemic effects of NO, making it a selective pulmonary vasodilator. MetHg is normally reduced by metHg reductase in erythrocytes, but this enzyme can be low in premature infants and some ethnic groups (Native Americans, Siberians, Turkish). Because MetHg poorly binds oxygen, metHg levels need to be followed on infants on NO. iNO has also been associated with an increased bleeding time and possible effects on surfactant function. For the treatment of PPHN, iNO is usually started at 10–20 parts per million (ppm) and has vasoactive properties as low as 5 ppm. Studies have compared 20 ppm and 80 ppm in term infants with PPHN and found no difference in the efficacy but an increased risk of metHg.[208] Guidelines recommend the use of iNO in infants with an OI > 25 or a PaO_2 < 100 mm Hg on 100% FiO_2.[200,206] iNO improves oxygenation and decreases the need for ECMO when started on infants with OI > 25 but has no effect on mortality or neurologic outcome.[200,206,207] Approximately 30% of infants do not have a sustained response to NO.[209] There are conflicting data on whether starting iNO when OI is >15 but <25 is beneficial.[200,207] The combination of surfactant and NO may lower OI. The use of HFOV has been advocated by some research groups because the open lung ventilation styles may decrease the ventilation-perfusion mismatch and improve iNO delivery.[200] Once the infants PVR improves, iNO should be weaned to avoid risks of metHg. iNO can be weaned quickly to 5 ppm but then should be slowly weaned to 1 ppm over a period of hours.[200] Abrupt discontinuation of iNO will lead to rebound pulmonary hypertension due to a decrease in endogenous NO production caused by the therapy. The use of iNO in premature infants is controversial. The NIH released a consensus statement in 2011 that discouraged the use of iNO is preterm infants, except in the infant with prolonged rupture of membranes or oligohydramnios, because of lack of efficacy.[210] Multiple large studies of preterm infants have been conducted to test if iNO could decrease BPD, but none have shown a benefit for lung disease or neurologic outcomes.[211]

Because more than 30% of infants do not have a sustained improvement in oxygenation with iNO, other medications have been used to decrease pulmonary hypertension in the newborn. Like iNO, these medications are designed to modulate the pathways discussed earlier (PGI_2, ET-1, PDE5) and have been used in adults with pulmonary hypertension (see Chapter 35). These medications can be given either intravenously or by nebulization with the mechanical ventilator. PGI_2 modulates vascular muscle contraction by increasing cyclic-adenosine monophosphate to cause relaxation. In adults, PGI_2 analogs (epoprostenol, treprostinil, iloprost, beraprost) play a vital role in treatment of pulmonary hypertension but are often given intravenously and can lead to systemic hypotension. To avoid systemic hypotension, epoprostenol and iloprost (the only FDA-approved PGI_2 analog for inhalation) can be nebulized through the ventilator and have shown good results in PPHN refractory to iNO.[199] Bosentan, an ET-1 antagonist, is used for chronic therapy in adults with pulmonary hypertension but is normally only available in an oral solution. In the setting of iNO, the addition of bosentan to infants with PPHN did not show additional effects.[199] One of the most common adjuvant therapies to iNO in PPHN is sildenafil.[200,206] Sildenafil, a PGE5 inhibitor, inhibits the breakdown of cyclic guanosine monophosphate (cGMP) (the secondary messenger of NO pathway) to inactive GMP in the vascular smooth muscles. Sildenafil, which is available in IV and oral forms, can be given in combination with iNO for PPHN or for helping wean infants from iNO.[199,200,206] Guidelines recommend that sildenafil should be considered as first-line therapy for PPHN in settings where iNO is not available.[200,206] Sildenafil is often used in infants with BPD and pulmonary hypertension, and adjustments have been made to FDA warnings about its use in pediatric patients.[199] Tolazoline hydrochloride and magnesium sulfate have been used with moderate success in PPHN, but their systemic effects and the availability of iNO have limited their use in recent years.

Maintaining adequate systemic blood pressure is crucial to the management of PPHN. The right-to-left shunt across the PDA and PFO is dependent on the ratio of the PVR to the SVR. Increasing the systemic blood pressure will decrease this ratio and divert blood into the pulmonary vasculature.[212] Management of systemic perfusion involves both the RV dysfunction due to increased afterload with pulmonary hypertension and left ventricular dysfunction from preload reduction due to decreased pulmonary return. Increasing SVR without increasing pulmonary resistance may be more difficult in some cases of pulmonary hypertension where increased muscularity of the arterioles, due to chronic in utero hypoxia, may create similar increases in PVR. Dopamine and epinephrine may have the highest risk of similar increases in both PVR and SVR but are often used to maintain systemic blood pressure in the setting of PPHN. Norepinephrine may have less effect on PVR than SVR and has been shown to improve oxygenation in PPHN.[212] Dobutamine improves cardiac contractility and at lower doses (2–5 micrograms/kg per minute) increases PVR. Milrinone, a selective phosphodiesterase-3 (PDE3) inhibitor, can improve cardiac output by increasing contractility and decreasing left ventricular afterload, and improve PVR through interactions with NO and PGI_2. In the setting of 100% O2, iNO upregulates PDE3, thus milrinone may have additional benefits in PPHN refractory to iNO.[199,200,212] Milrinone can cause systemic hypotension, which may limit its use in neonates; thus it is often used in combination with other vasoactive medications.

When medical therapies fail to improve oxygenation and OI remains higher than 40 (protocols differ between centers), ECMO can be used to treat PPHN.[200,203,206] ECMO is not advisable for PPHN in infants with chromosomal anomalies, lethal congenital malformations, uncorrectable heart defects, and major intracranial bleeds. Due to size limitations and increased risk of IVH, ECMO is not recommended for severe PPHN in preterm infants less than 34 weeks GA or less than 2000 g.[206] ECMO can be done via either venovenous or venoarterial methods, depending on the size and cardiac function of the infant, and many centers have protocols for duration of use of ECMO.[203] The chance of an intracranial bleed is 10%–15%, and adverse neurologic outcome may be due to the underlying hypoxia or the vascular compromise from ligation and cannulation. With the introduction of iNO, the use of ECMO for PPHN has dramatically decreased.

MORTALITY AND MORBIDITY

Before the use of ECMO and iNO, the mortality from PPHN was nearly 50%.[200,205] Even with advanced therapies, the mortality rate for PPHN remains between 8% and 10%.[200] The mortality rate varies according to the underlying condition. The mortality rate for PPHN, or pulmonary hypertension due to RDS or MAS, is lower than that of infants with septic shock (e.g., GBS). ACD is a uniformly fatal condition without lung transplantation. Infants with severe PPHN have increased risk for neurodevelopmental delays and audiologic impairment.

Pulmonary Hypertension in Bronchopulmonary Dysplasia

BPD in the modern era, discussed in Chapter 20, is due to both alveolar and capillary simplification. Infants with

BPD have increased risk of pulmonary hypertension (25%–37% of infants) and may progress to right heart failure.[213] Screening echocardiograms should be done on infants with established BPD.[200] In infants with BPD and increased PVR, oxygen saturations of 92%–95% may be appropriate.[200] iNO and sildenafil can be used to treat pulmonary hypertension with BPD.

Pneumothorax

Spontaneous pneumothoraces likely occur in 1%–2% of newborn deliveries, but only 10% of them are symptomatic.[214,215] Elective C-section increases the risk of pneumothorax compared with spontaneous vaginal delivery, probably due to the increased fetal lung fluid present at birth.[215] PPV and ET intubation increase the incidence to almost 6%.[214] High transpulmonary pressure, generated by the first spontaneous breaths to clear the fetal lung fluid from the airways, can cause local overdistention of the alveoli and air leaks. Prematurity and congenital lung malformations increase the risk of pneumothoraces. Rarely, pneumothoraces are caused by direct trauma to the airways by suction catheters or ET tubes, but these injuries more often lead to pneumomediastinum.

Small asymptomatic pneumothoraces are often found on chest films taken for other reasons. Most small pneumothoraces can be monitored clinically without intervention. Larger pneumothoraces will present with respiratory symptoms, including tachypnea, retractions, and an oxygen requirement. Pneumothoraces large enough to cause a shift of the central structures of the chest (tension pneumothorax) will presents with severe desaturations and signs of shock. Breath sounds may be decreased with a pneumothorax, and transillumination with a fiberoptic light can be used to evaluate for pneumothorax (area with pneumothorax will appear brighter). If the infant is clinically stable, a chest radiograph should be obtained to determine the diagnosis. A moderately large pneumothorax will demonstrate absent lung markings and a collapsed lung on the ipsilateral side. Tension pneumothorax will have eversion of the diaphragm and displacement of the central structures to the contralateral side (Fig. 19.8). Congenital lung malformations, such as pulmonary lobar emphysema or congenital pulmonary airway anomalies, can appear like pneumothoraces (see Chapter 18) and should be included in the differential diagnosis of atypically appearing air within the chest.

Asymptomatic pneumothoraces do not require treatment and will reabsorb over time. Although many institutions use 100% oxygen for 6 hours to wash out the nitrogen in the pneumothorax, this practice has not been shown to decrease the time of resolution of pneumothoraces and may increase length of stay in the special care baby unit (SCBU).[216] In a cohort of infants >36 week GA with symptomatic spontaneous pneumothorax, approximately 71% could be managed with oxygen therapy, whereas 29% required thoracentesis or a thoracotomy tube.[217] Infants with significant respiratory distress or a tension pneumothorax require manual drainage of the pneumothorax. Immediate evacuation of the pneumothorax can be accomplished with an 18–22-gauge butterfly needle attached to a three-way stopcock and syringe. After cleaning with alcohol, the needle can be inserted into the

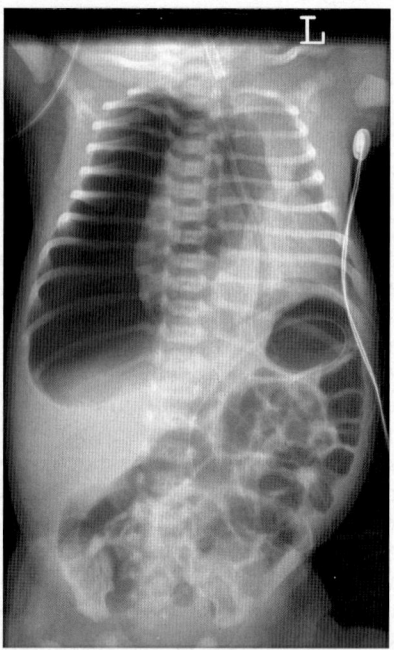

Fig. 19.8 Tension pneumothorax: right-sided tension pneumothorax with collapse of the right lung, midline shift of the cardiac and trachea to the left.

second intercostal space above the rib at the midclavicular line and air aspirated. This can also be done through the mid-axillary region between the fourth and sixth ribs. In some larger infants, removal of the initial air by needle thoracentesis will be enough to resolve the pneumothorax. With larger pneumothoraces or reaccumulation of air after needle thoracentesis, a thoracotomy tube can be placed through the mid-axillary region and aimed in the direction of the pocket of air. Using sterile techniques and local anesthesia, either a standard chest tube (French gauge 10–14) or a pigtail angiocath can be inserted into the pleural space and positioned in the anterior chest (Fig. 19.9). The chest tube should be connected to an underwater seal drain with suction of 5–10 cm H_2O. Often the chest tube is removed from suction and placed to water seal for approximately 24 hours prior to removal of the chest tube.

Pneumomediastinum

Pneumomediastinum occurs in up to 2% of births, with similar risk factors to pneumothorax.[214] Most pneumomediastinums are asymptomatic and do not require treatment. On the chest radiograph, a pneumomediastinum is often seen near the borders of the heart or in the mediastinal region behind the sternum. The thymus can be elevated away from the central structures to form a spinnaker sail sign (Fig. 19.10) or the heart can be elevated off the diaphragm to create the appearance of a continuous diaphragm. Drainage of a pneumomediastinum is difficult because the gas is collected in multiple independent lobules. Because multiple vital vascular structures occupy the mediastinum, drainage should only be done in situations of severe respiratory distress.

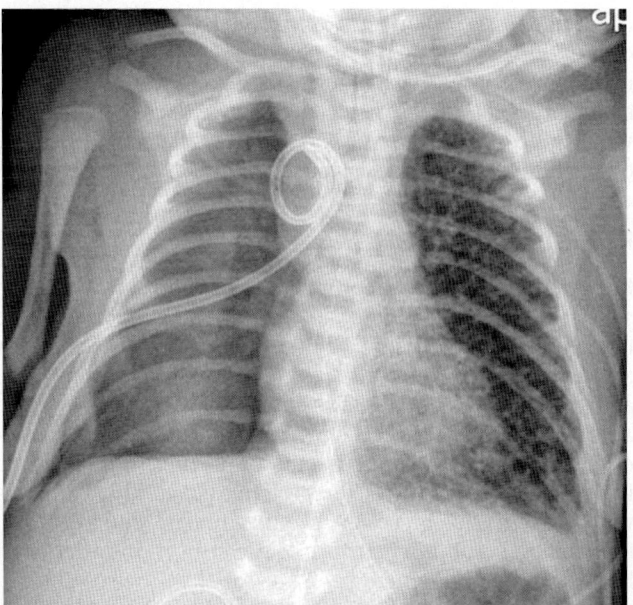

Fig. 19.9 Pigtail catheter placement: chest tube catheter placed in right chest through axillary approach has resolved majority of pneumothorax. Small residual air is present on right chest and significant pulmonary interstitial emphysema is present on the left.

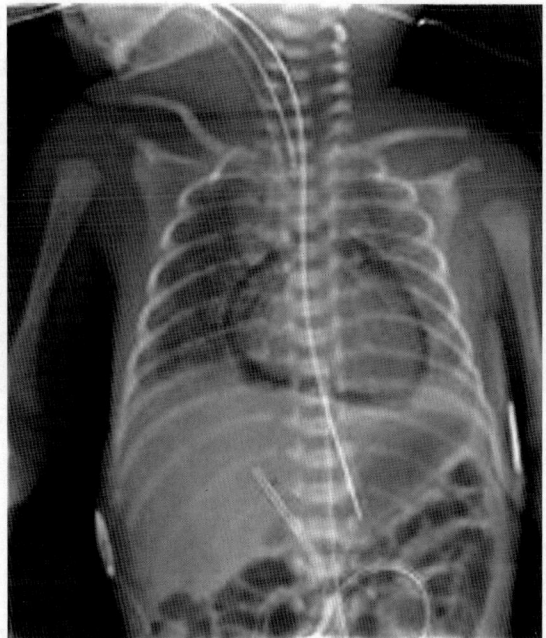

Fig. 19.11 Pneumopericardium: often a medical emergency due to cardiac tamponade, the chest x-ray demonstrates air within the pericardium.

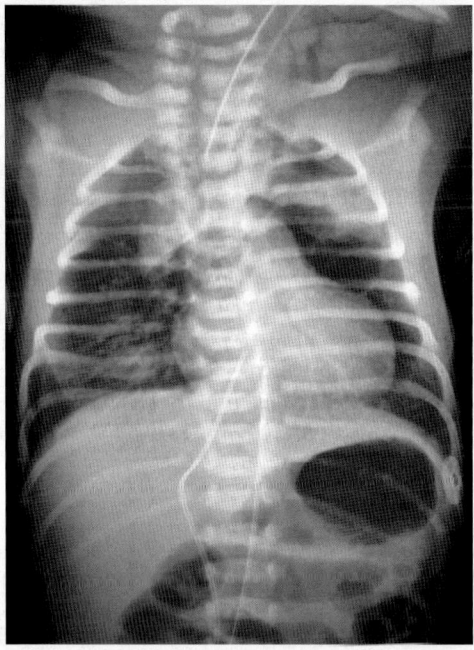

Fig. 19.10 Pneumomediastinum: chest x-ray demonstrates air within the mediastinum causing upward displacement of the thymus (spinnaker sign).

Pneumopericardium

Pneumopericardiums are rare and usually associated with other air leak syndromes. The gas, initially released into the space around the lungs, may dissect through a hole in the pericardial sac. It is more common in ventilated preterm infants and may be a consequence of severe PIE. Clinically, pneumopericardium presents with sudden hypotension and bradycardia due to cardiac tamponade. On chest radiograph,

gas surrounds the heart and outlines the great arteries (Fig. 19.11). Infants with symptomatic pneumopericardium require immediate drainage due to impaired cardiac output. An angiocath or pigtail catheter can be inserted into the pericardial space using a subxyphoid approach. Blood pressure changes and bradycardia may suggest reaccumulation of the air within the pericardial sac. The mortality and long-term morbidity from pneumopericardium is high.

Pulmonary Interstitial Emphysema

PIE is collection of air that escapes the alveoli and tracks along the sheaths of the small blood vessels of the lung. It rarely occurs spontaneously and is associated with PPV, especially with high pressures in small preterm infants. PIE occurs when the extraalveolar air remains within the lung parenchyma and does not escape into other regions of the chest (pneumothorax, pneumomediastinum, pneumopericardium, and rarely pneumoperitoneum). PIE commonly involves both lungs, but it may be lobar in distribution. The trapped gas can compress the vasculature and decreases pulmonary perfusion. The lung parenchyma is expanded leading to airway obstruction, increased lung compliance, and areas of hyperinflation. As a result, infants with severe PIE can be profoundly hypoxemic and hypercarbic on presentation. PIE is usually diagnosed by chest radiograph which demonstrates hyperinflation and diffuse, multiple, or small nonconfluent cystic radiolucencies (Fig. 19.12). Bilateral, diffuse PIE may have a narrow cardiac silhouette due to mediastinal compression. As the amount of air collects within the lung parenchyma, large bullae or pneumatoceles may form and are visible as circular air collections on the chest radiograph. Lobar emphysema and congenital pulmonary

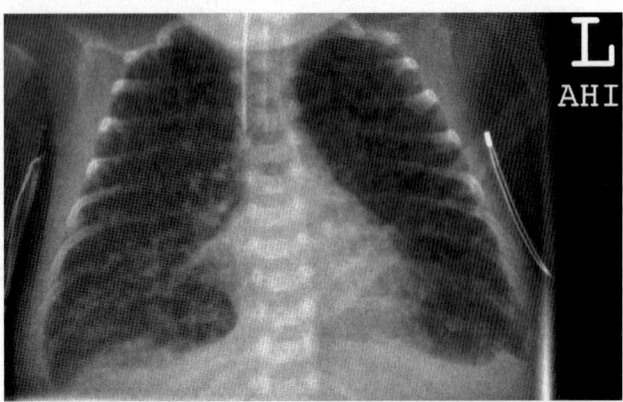

Fig. 19.12 Pulmonary interstitial emphysema: small cystic changes throughout both lungs represent air dissection into the parenchyma.

airway malformations are in the differential for these large cystic formations but are typically seen on earlier chest radiographs.

If PIE is localized to one lobe of the lung, then placing the infant with this side down will cause partial collapse of the lung and may improve the PIE. This is not possible in severely ill preterm infants. Selective intubation of the opposite side from the PIE has been studied, but left mainstem intubation is often not possible in small infants. If the infant has diffuse PIE, the PEEP and peak inflating pressures should be reduced to the minimum compatible with acceptable oxygenation and ventilation. Pneumatoceles also respond to decreased ventilator pressures. HFJV and HFOV are often used clinically in PIE to decrease the pressure fluctuations within the injured lungs, but studies have not shown a conclusive benefit over conventional ventilation. One study supports the use of low-frequency settings (5–6 Hz) on HFOV to decrease severe PIE.[218] Overall, PIE is associated with severe lung disease in the preterm infant and is thus associated with high overall morbidity.

Secondary Pulmonary Hypoplasia

See also Chapter 18.

EPIDEMIOLOGY

The incidence of pulmonary hypoplasia is estimated to range from 9 to 11 per 10,000 live births.[219] Most cases are secondary in nature, with primary cases reported to be rare.[220] It is possible that mildly affected infants may not exhibit any clinical features, and thus the true incidence may be higher than reported.

ETIOLOGY

The causes of secondary pulmonary hypoplasia may be divided into four main categories: (1) space-occupying lesions within the thoracic cavity (e.g., CDH, pulmonary sequestration, congenital pulmonary airways malformation [CPAM], and pleural effusions); (2) chest wall deformities leading to reduced intrathoracic space (e.g., asphyxiating thoracic dystrophy); (3) causes of severe oligohydramnios (e.g., bilateral

renal agenesis, prolonged rupture of the membranes); (4) disorders impacting on normal lung development (e.g., neuromuscular disorders with reduced fetal breathing movements, congenital heart disease associated with abnormal pulmonary vasculature, large anterior abdominal wall defects affecting diaphragmatic, and chest wall development).[219,221–223]

PATHOGENESIS

Lung development is a complicated process that has been shown to occur in stages.[219,224] The pseudoglandular stage takes place between approximately 6 and 17 weeks of GA and is the period when the conducting airways and initial acinar framework develop. The canalicular stage follows from approximately 17–26 weeks GA, during which further development of the lung parenchyma occurs. There is an increase in canaliculi, widening of the peripheral respiratory tubules with concurrent increase in pulmonary capillarization, forming the respiratory surface of the lung.[224] Disorders that impact lung development before 17 weeks GA also substantially impact lung growth, bronchiolar branching, cartilage development, acinar complexity, and capillarization. Disorders affecting lung growth during the canalicular stage (i.e., after 17 weeks GA) mainly affect acinar complexity.[219] Risk of pulmonary hypoplasia is much decreased by late canalicular stage, with higher risk of pulmonary hypoplasia associated with earlier insults. A review of 28 studies suggested that GA of preterm prelabor rupture of membranes was better associated with pulmonary hypoplasia than either degree of oligohydramnios or latency period.[225] A lack of intrathoracic space within which to grow and develop in the presence of space-occupying lesions or chest wall deformities is thought to physically limit the growth of the lungs. Further limitations in space can also impact fetal breathing movements and the usual movements of amniotic fluid in and out of the airways. This limitation in fetal breathing movements is also seen in infants with neuromuscular conditions, such as type 1 spinal muscular atrophy. Lack of adequate amniotic fluid can occur with all causes of severe oligohydramnios (e.g., bilateral renal agenesis) and prolonged and premature leakage of amniotic fluid, which has been shown to be associated with abnormal lung growth.[226,227]

CLINICAL FEATURES

A proportion of infants may be diagnosed antenatally. Pulmonary hypoplasia may be suspected if commonly associated conditions (e.g., oligohydramnios, CDH, or pleural effusion) are present. Once suspected, there are numerous antenatal features that have been reported to be useful to determine severity of pulmonary hypoplasia.[219,225] Of importance is the need to be able to distinguish between lethal and nonlethal forms. For example, investigators have suggested that persistent severe oligohydramnios after preterm prelabor rupture of membranes with onset <25 weeks GA was associated with greater than 90% mortality from pulmonary hypoplasia.[219] Other antenatal parameters include ultrasonic detection of absence of fetal breathing movements and biometric indices, such as thoracic circumference to abdominal circumference ratio, thoracic circumference to head circumference ratio, thoracic area minus heart area and thoracic area to heart area ratio. More recently, other imaging

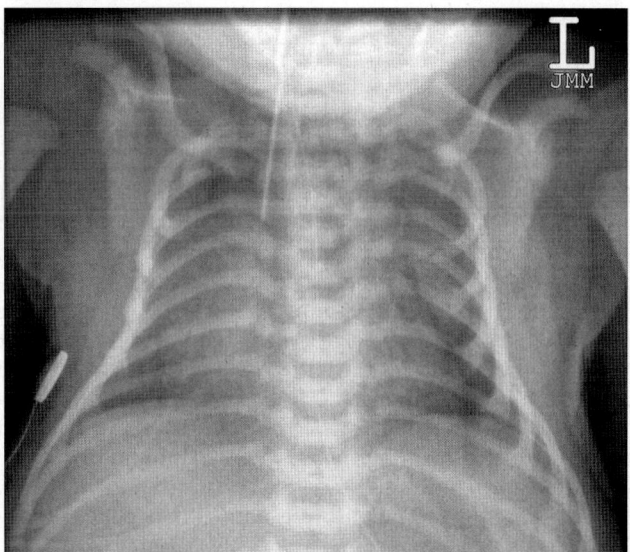

Fig. 19.13 Pulmonary hypoplasia: chest x-ray demonstrates bell-shaped chest with low lung volumes. Severe lung hypoplasia due to prolonged oligohydramnios may be incompatible with successful gas exchange.

modalities, such as magnetic resonance imaging (MRI), have been explored.[228]

After birth, infants with secondary pulmonary hypoplasia can present with the clinical features of the condition to which the hypoplastic lung is secondary. For infants where the pulmonary hypoplasia is not associated with an intrathoracic space-occupying lesion, the chest wall may appear disproportionally small compared with the overall size of the infant. For those with underlying conditions not immediately apparent, the hypoplasia may be clinically undetectable, but, in those who present, the signs may range from tachypnea and mild respiratory distress to severe hypoxemic respiratory failure requiring ventilatory support with high ventilatory pressures. Chest radiography may reveal crowded ribs and low thoracic-to-abdominal ratio and a bell-shaped chest (Fig. 19.13). Imaging may also reveal features of the underlying condition or commonly associated complications. Pulmonary hypoplasia is not uncommonly complicated by air leaks, such as pneumothorax. The pathologic criteria for the diagnosis of pulmonary hypoplasia are relatively well established and usually include an assessment of lung weight to body weight ratio and radial alveolar count.[219] Ratios greater than 0.018 suggest that pulmonary hypoplasia is unlikely, whereas a ratio of <0.012 suggests likely or probable pulmonary hypoplasia and need for further confirmation of the diagnosis. In cases with low lung weight to body weight ratio, the diagnosis is confirmed if the radial alveolar count is <75% of the mean normal value for GA.

MANAGEMENT

Severely affected infants have small lungs with poor compliance, oxygenation failure, and high ventilatory requirements. There is a substantial risk of air leaks, and thus some experts suggest low-pressure fast-rate ventilation or HFOV.[229] In cases with pulmonary hypertension, pulmonary vasodilators such as iNO should be considered.[230] Some infants may need home oxygen therapy for several months after discharge, and, in

view of the considerable risk of respiratory exacerbations, annual influenza vaccine, pneumococcal vaccine, RSV prophylaxis, and stringent infection control should be recommended. Lung development and growth should be facilitated by careful attention to nutrition.

PREVENTION

Prevention of pulmonary hypoplasia is theoretically possible if the underlying cause has been detected sufficiently early during the antenatal period and if the condition is amenable to intervention. Examples of conditions that have been treated *in utero* include pleural effusions, congenital lung lesions, fetal urinary obstruction, and CDH.[231-234] *In utero* thoracoamniotic shunting can drain fetal pleural effusions and cystic lung lesions and have been associated with resolution of hydropic features, in infants presenting with hydrops fetalis, and improved survival.[231] There is currently insufficient evidence to support *in utero* surgical repair of CDH.[233] More recently, efforts have been made to investigate the potential of early fetal endoscopic tracheal occlusion by balloon with subsequent deflation and removal at 34 weeks GA.[234,235] This approach has seen some improvements in infant survival for those predicted to have severe CDH (lung to head ratio < 0.7).[236]

PROGNOSIS

The prognosis of infants with pulmonary hypoplasia can be very poor depending on severity, with estimated mortality of >90% in those associated with severe persistent oligohydramnios due to preterm prelabor rupture of membranes with onset <25 weeks GA.[219] Mortality improves when the underlying condition impacting on lung development occurs later during pregnancy (>25 weeks) and is of relatively short duration (<6 days) and if there are no other associated conditions, such as PPHN.[219,237,238] Long-term morbidity includes limb abnormalities (incidence 27%–80%) due to the compression if associated with oligohydramnios,[239] BPD and recurrent wheezy episodes,[240] and neurodevelopmental deficits (incidence 28% if associated with rupture of membranes before 26 weeks GA).[241]

Patent Ductus Arteriosus

EPIDEMIOLOGY

The incidence of PDA is inversely related to GA, with estimated incidences of <0.1% and 42% for term infants and extremely low-birth-weight infants, respectively.[242,243]

ETIOLOGY

PDA is caused by a failure of the ductus arteriosus to close during the transition of the infant from a fetal to extrauterine circulation after birth.

PATHOGENESIS

Gas exchange in the fetus occurs at the placenta rather than the lungs. Blood is therefore shunted from the right ventricle and pulmonary artery away from the lungs and directly to the aorta via the ductus arteriosus. After birth, functional closure of the ductus arteriosus occurs. In term infants the process is complete in 20% of cases by 24 hours, 82% by 48 hours, and 100% by 96 hours. In preterm infants >30 weeks GA, 8% close by 24 hours, 60% by 48 hours, and almost 100% by 96 hours.[244] In preterm infants, especially <30 weeks GA, there is decreased ductal sensitivity to oxygen, poor intrinsic tone of the ductal wall, and the balance of vasodilators to vasoconstrictors favor ductal patency. Ductal closure is therefore often delayed. Anatomic closure relies on changes that occur after functional closure is complete; ductal patency therefore prevents this process from taking place. Other factors that are associated with delayed ductal closure include thrombocytopenia, respiratory distress, and persistently low PaO_2.[244,245]

CLINICAL FEATURES

Clinical features of PDA typically arise because of hemodynamically significant left-to-right shunting of blood from the aorta to the pulmonary artery. In view of the relatively high pulmonary pressure of newborn infants, the chance of clinical features developing before normal functional closure of the ductus is very low. As the PVR decreases, left-to-right shunting through the PDA increases and signs of left heart failure may develop. Clinically the infant may exhibit a harsh systolic murmur best heard at the upper left sternal border, hyperdynamic precordial impulse, and bounding peripheral pulses with widened pulse pressure. As the left-to-right pressure gradient increases, the murmur may become continuous. With worsening of the heart failure, the infant will develop increasing tachycardia, tachypnea, cardiomegaly, and hepatomegaly. The chest radiograph illustrates cardiomegaly, pulmonary plethora, and a wide angle between the left and right main bronchi due to left atrial dilation (Fig. 19.14). Particularly in preterm infants, the

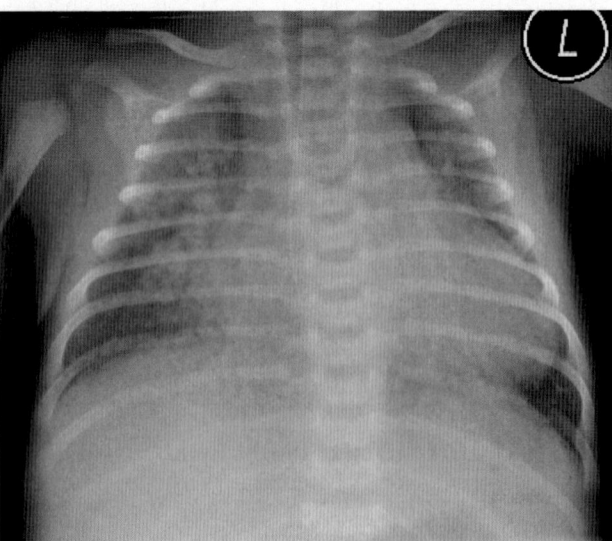

Fig. 19.14 Patent ductus arteriosus: left-to-right shunting through the patent ductus arteriosus can lead to signs of congestive heart failure, including chest x-ray findings of cardiomegaly, pulmonary vessel congestion, and diffuse haziness.

increased pulmonary blood flow could lead to pulmonary congestion and decreased pulmonary compliance. These infants may exhibit increasing oxygen and ventilatory requirements. Echocardiography is the gold standard for diagnosing PDA. In general, the PDA can be visualized by echocardiography in the parasternal short-axis view as a third branch of the main pulmonary artery alongside the left and right branch pulmonary arteries. Color Doppler could help to determine whether the flow through the PDA is left to right, right to left, or bidirectional. Additional features of a moderate to large left-to-right ductal shunt are bowing of the interatrial septum to the right with enlargement of the left atrium and ventricle. Left atrial enlargement with a left atrial to aortic root (LA:Ao) ratio > 1.4:1[245] is considered hemodynamically significant. The PDA size can be determined from the ductal size on color Doppler examination. If the shunt is large, flow reversal will be throughout diastole. Echocardiography is helpful to exclude other possible congenital cardiac abnormalities.

PREVENTION

In a meta-analysis,[246] PDA prophylaxis with ibuprofen showed reduced PDA incidence and need for rescue therapy/surgical closure but no improvement in any other short-term outcomes. In a randomized study, use of ibuprofen as PDA prevention showed a trend towards decreased PVL but did not affect any other clinical outcome.[247] In summary, despite the availability of several ductal closure strategies, whether the intervention is medical[246,248] or surgical,[249] no long-term benefits in terms of outcomes such as BPD, neurodevelopment or mortality have been demonstrated. Nevertheless, avoiding factors that may increase risk of PDA, such as excessive fluids,[250] hypoxia, and sepsis, would be prudent.

MANAGEMENT

Ductal closure occurs naturally, and the clinical impact of PDA on individual patients can vary greatly. As with PDA prevention, there is very little evidence of long-term benefit of treatment of PDA.[251] It has therefore been controversial when, whom, and even whether to treat.[251,252] PDA spontaneously closes in a small proportion of extremely preterm infants (approximately 24%) and is more likely to be refractory to treatment.[253] Initial management of PDA in a preterm infant includes fluid restriction and diuretics. Cyclo-oxygenase inhibitors are the most commonly used drugs for ductal closure in preterm infants. Nonsteroidal antiinflammatory drugs (NSAIDs) such as indomethacin and ibuprofen are nonselective cyclo-oxygenase inhibitors which reduce the synthesis of prostaglandin E and thus shift the balance toward ductal closure. Indomethacin was previously the drug of choice; however, in recent studies, ibuprofen has been shown to be as effective in terms of ductal closure but associated with fewer side effects, such as transient renal impairment and NEC.[254] Ibuprofen is usually given as a 3-day course at 10 mg/kg on the first day, 5 mg/kg on the second day, and 5 mg/kg on the third day; however, there are small studies that report that higher doses may be more effective with no increase in side effects.[255] Side effects are increased with concomitant use of other drugs such as diuretics and corticosteroids. Use of diuretics in conjunction with indomethacin for the treatment of PDA did not improve urine output but increased serum creatinine and hyponatremia.[256] It has also been shown that concurrent use of NSAIDs and corticosteroids increases the risk of gastrointestinal perforation 10-fold.[257] Increasingly, paracetamol (acetaminophen) has been used as an alternative therapeutic option for treatment of PDA.[258] Meta-analyses suggest that paracetamol is as effective as ibuprofen for ductal closure.[259] However, maternal use of paracetamol during pregnancy has been associated with neurodevelopmental disorders in children,[260] and before more definitely long-term outcome data are available, use of paracetamol for ductal closure cannot be considered first-line therapy. Medical treatment by administration of the drugs via the oral route has been suggested to be feasible,[261,262] especially for countries with limited access to IV forms of ibuprofen, indomethacin, and paracetamol. Treatment failure is more common in infants with sepsis and extremely preterm infants.[263] Even for those infants with hemodynamically significant PDA, there is currently insufficient evidence to conclude whether surgical ligation or medical ductal closure is preferable as first-line treatment. Although surgery offers decreased closure failure rate, there is an increased risk of pneumothorax and retinopathy of prematurity.[264] Furthermore, despite surgical closure, infants may still go on to develop BPD.[265] Many neonatal units reserve surgical closure for infants with hemodynamically significant PDA refractory to treatment or when medical therapy is contraindicated. However, there is evidence that even in these infants, a nonintervention approach despite failure of medical closure may be associated with decreased incidence of BPD without increase in risk of NEC or IVH.[266] The question of management ultimately rests on clinical judgment on whether the PDA is hemodynamically significant with a trend towards conservative management in those who remain "asymptomatic."

PROGNOSIS

Complications associated with hemodynamically significant PDA include heart failure, BPD, neurodevelopmental impairment, NEC, and increased mortality.[267] The complications associated with both medical and surgical therapeutic options are substantial, and optimizing outcomes for an affected infant involves a balance of the risks of treatment versus the potential risks of the PDA. Objective, validated assessment tools to determine the hemodynamic significance of a PDA to an individual infant could potentially help to solve the difficult clinical problem of whether to intervene.

Pulmonary Edema

EPIDEMIOLOGY

Although there are very little data on the epidemiology of neonatal pulmonary edema, it is a well-known association of several common neonatal conditions.

ETIOLOGY

Pulmonary edema is associated with several cardiopulmonary conditions, including TTN, perinatal asphyxia, left ventricular failure, RDS, hemodynamically significant PDA, and inflammatory pulmonary conditions.[268,269]

PATHOGENESIS

Pulmonary edema occurs because of abnormal leakage of fluid from pulmonary capillaries into the lung parenchyma and alveolar spaces. This occurs when the pulmonary capillary pressure exceeds the plasma oncotic pressure or when there is disruption of the respiratory membrane. Pulmonary capillary pressure is increased in conditions with pulmonary congestion secondary to left ventricular dysfunction or fluid overload. Abnormalities of the pulmonary lymphatics can also lead to accumulation of fluid in the lungs. Plasma oncotic pressure can be decreased in hypoproteinemia, which is common in preterm infants and when inappropriately large volumes of crystalloids have been infused into the infant. The integrity of the respiratory membrane can be disrupted in many conditions, especially those associated with inflammatory or hypoxic insults. High ventilator settings can also cause excessive stretching of the alveoli and subsequent epithelial protein leaks.[268] In addition, epithelial ion transport plays an important role in lung lumen fluid clearance (see earlier section on pulmonary lung fluid clearance) and may offer new strategies for managing this condition.[270]

CLINICAL FEATURES

Newborn infants with pulmonary edema present with signs of respiratory distress and may exhibit tachycardia, tachypnea, and other signs related to the underlying condition. Chest radiograph features of pulmonary edema include increased vascular markings, perihilar shadowing (Fig. 19.15), linear septal opacities (Kerley B lines) in the lower lung fields, linear opacities along the horizontal and oblique fissures, cardiomegaly, and hazy lung fields. Investigations to determine the underlying cause should also be considered, such as echocardiography for cardiac causes. Lung ultrasonography may be helpful for detecting pulmonary edema, especially in cases in which the chest radiograph is

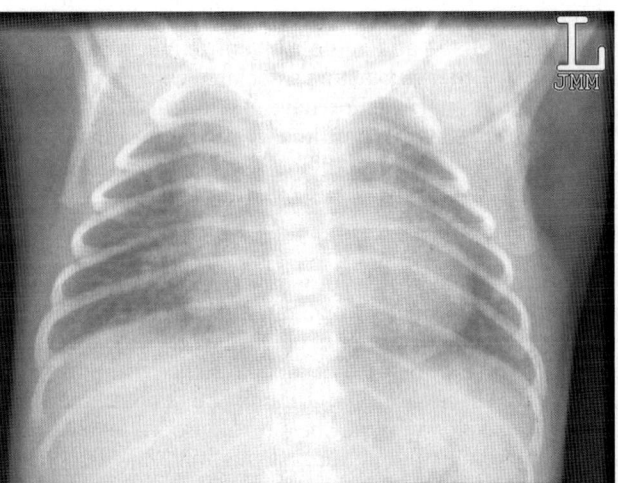

Fig. 19.15 Pulmonary edema: increased vascular markings and linear septal opacities (Kerley B lines).

indeterminate.[269] Important differential diagnoses that may also coexist with pulmonary edema include pneumonia, RDS, and MAS.

MANAGEMENT

Fluid restriction, administration of diuretics, appropriate ventilatory support, and treatment of the underlying condition are the cornerstones of the management of pulmonary edema. Some investigators have shown that corticosteroids can upregulate epithelial ion transporters, which explains why antenatal and postnatal corticosteroids have been found to be helpful in conditions that are associated with pulmonary edema.[270]

PREVENTION

The risk of neonatal pulmonary edema can be decreased by management strategies that decrease pulmonary congestion, increase plasma oncotic pressure, and minimize lung injury. Avoidance of excessive fluid administration and reduction of ventilator pressures may be helpful.

PROGNOSIS

Outcomes of pulmonary edema usually depend on the severity of the underlying condition, with excellent prognosis for self-limiting conditions such as TTN.

Pulmonary Hemorrhage

EPIDEMIOLOGY

Pulmonary hemorrhage has increased from 0.1% to 1.2% in the presurfactant era[271] up to 5.9%, according to a meta-analysis of surfactant trials.[272] However, its incidence may be underestimated because it has been reported to be the cause of death of 9% of newborns who underwent autopsy.[273]

ETIOLOGY

Pulmonary hemorrhage has been shown to be associated with the presence of a hemodynamically significant PDA in preterm infants[274] and acute left ventricular failure due to asphyxia.[273] Other risk factors associated with increased risk of severe pulmonary hemorrhage include surfactant administration (especially if synthetic),[275] hypothermia, Rhesus hemolytic disease, and small for GA.[276]

PATHOGENESIS

Analysis of hemorrhagic lung fluid from infants diagnosed with pulmonary hemorrhage revealed a relatively low Hct of only 10% and the presence of plasma proteins, suggesting that the fluid is composed of blood diluted with plasma filtrate.[273] It is believed that, although the hemorrhagic fluid appears to be bloody, it may be more appropriate to describe it as hemorrhagic pulmonary edema fluid. The association with acute left ventricular dysfunction suggests that pathogenesis of pulmonary hemorrhage is related to left-to-right shunting, pulmonary congestion, and pulmonary edema.

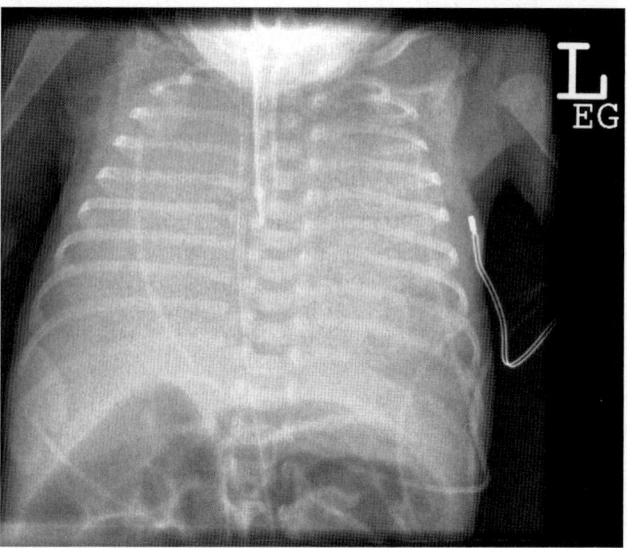

Fig. 19.16 Pulmonary hemorrhage: diffuse bilateral opacification of the lungs, usually associated with blood in endotracheal secretions and clinical deterioration in oxygenation.

Presence of clotting abnormalities[273] or hypoxic damage to the pulmonary capillaries also appears to play important roles in the pathogenesis.[271]

CLINICAL FEATURES

Infants who develop severe pulmonary hemorrhage often deteriorate suddenly on the first few days of life, with an earlier onset associated with more mature infants.[271] There is no standard definition of pulmonary hemorrhage but is usually recognized as the appearance of frank blood originating from the airway (usually seen in the ET tube) which is accompanied by acute clinical deterioration (e.g., increasing ventilator requirements and hemodynamic instability).[271,274] Pulmonary hemorrhage is usually associated with chest radiograph changes such as whiteout lung fields and air bronchograms (Fig. 19.16). Differential diagnoses include severe RDS, pneumonia, sepsis with disseminated intravascular coagulopathy, and airway injury.

MANAGEMENT

Conventional management of infants with severe pulmonary hemorrhage includes mechanical ventilation with high PEEP.[271,277] Heavy sedation and even paralysis is frequently used. Despite the association between surfactant use and pulmonary hemorrhage, it has been shown that a single dose of surfactant after the pulmonary hemorrhage has occurred may improve oxygenation.[278] In view of the clinical deterioration, broad-spectrum empirical antibiotics are usually commenced if not already in use. Anemia and coagulopathy should be corrected, with some authors suggesting the use of activated recombinant factor VII.[277] Management of associated heart failure should be considered. Some authors suggest that use of 4% cocaine (0.1 mL/kg, i.e., 4 mg/kg) or 1:10,000 epinephrine (0.1 mL/kg, i.e., 0.01 mg/kg or 0.5 mL, i.e., 0.05 mg) via the ET route may be helpful for short-term outcomes.[271,279]

PREVENTION

Prophylactic indomethacin reduces the rate of early serious pulmonary hemorrhage, possibly because of its action on the PDA, but it is less effective in preventing severe pulmonary hemorrhage that occurs after the first week of life.[280] Judicious fluid management and prevention of heart failure may possibly decrease the risk of pulmonary hemorrhage.

PROGNOSIS

Mortality of severe pulmonary hemorrhage is high. Risk factors for higher mortality include early GA, lower birth weight, and small for GA.[271,280] The high ventilator settings and oxygenation failure often lead to long-term morbidity in survivors, including BPD and neurosensory impairment.

Upper Airway Obstruction

EPIDEMIOLOGY

Neonatal upper airway obstruction can occur at any level and reflect many different underlying conditions. The overall incidence of neonatal upper airway obstruction is unknown because the exact incidence of even laryngomalacia, one of the most common causes, remains unknown in the general population. It has been reported that the prevalence can range from 8% to 50% in infants with neuromuscular disease.[281] Rarer causes include choanal atresia, where the incidence is 1–2 per 10,000 live births.[282]

ETIOLOGY AND PATHOGENESIS

Causes associated with neonatal upper airway obstruction vary with the level of obstruction encountered. Examples include: choanal atresia, basal encephalocele (nasal); Pierre-Robin syndrome, Down syndrome, Crouzon syndrome (pharyngeal); laryngomalacia and vocal cord palsy (laryngeal).[283] The most common congenital cause of nasal obstruction is choanal atresia, which can occur in isolation or as part of a syndrome such as CHARGE (Coloboma of the iris and retina, Heart disease, Atresia choanae, Retarded growth, Genital hypoplasia, Ear defects) syndrome.[282] Obstruction at the pharyngeal level can occur from craniofacial anomalies. For example, if the tongue is too large (macroglossia) or the mandible is small (retrognathia/micrognathia), the base of the tongue can fall backwards, especially when the infant is in a supine position and it can obstruct the airway in the hypopharynx.[281] At the laryngeal level, causes of obstruction include structural lesions (e.g., laryngeal polyps/cysts) and functional causes (e.g., vocal cord palsy and laryngomalacia). Approximately 20% of vocal cord palsy is associated with injury to the recurrent laryngeal nerve caused by traction to the neck during delivery. Where vocal cord palsy is bilateral, neurologic causes should be sought. Other causes include surgical complications during ductal ligation or repair of tracheoesophageal fistula. In the neonate the epiglottis and the aryepiglottic folds can collapse upon the airway in laryngomalacia. In these cases, structural causes should also be sought because an associated airway lesion is seen in 18.9%

and an associated cardiac lesion is present in as many as 31% of cases.[281]

CLINICAL FEATURES

Partial obstruction can vary in severity, and presenting features range from mild tachypnea or stridor to complete obstruction. Infants born with complete upper airway obstruction present immediately after birth with persistent cyanosis and ineffective respirations; they will remain refractory to conventional airway management measures[284] and can rapidly deteriorate with fatal consequences if not promptly treated.[285]

Infants with unilateral choanal atresia may not exhibit any clinical signs unless the unaffected side is blocked, at which point they may develop respiratory distress. The classical presentation of bilateral choanal atresia is respiratory distress at rest, which is absent when crying or mouth breathing. Differential diagnoses include choanal stenosis, nasal injury, and abnormal structures, (e.g., encephalocele or meningocele). Imaging by CT or MRI may be necessary to differentiate these causes.

Infants at risk of pharyngeal obstruction often present with dysmorphic features (e.g., retrognathia/micrognathia in Pierre-Robin syndrome, craniosynostosis and dysmorphic features in Crouzon syndrome, and characteristic facies in Down syndrome). Pharyngeal obstruction may produce stertor which is usually worse when the baby is nursed in a supine position. In cases in which it is unclear whether apneas are central or obstructive, infant polysomnography may be helpful to identify obstructive events.

Infants with laryngeal obstruction may present with stridor. One of the most common conditions causing laryngeal obstruction is laryngomalacia, which may present during the first 10 days of life. The stridor is usually worse with crying and feeding but improves when the infant is at rest. The severity of obstruction cannot be judged from the severity of the stridor, but rather from the presence of failure to thrive, respiratory distress, obstructive sleep apnea, and feeding difficulties.[281] Another commonly encountered example of airway obstruction is subglottic stenosis. This can be due to congenital structural abnormality but is more usually acquired secondary to intubation. Infants present with stridor or hoarseness after extubation with subsequent difficulty in intubation with the original sized tube. Vocal cord palsy can also present with stridor and hoarseness, and affected infants may also develop signs of aspiration pneumonia in view of the increased risk of aspiration. It may be life-threatening if both vocal cords are affected. Most causes of laryngeal obstruction can be diagnosed endoscopically, so a newborn presenting with stridor should undergo laryngoscopy and/or bronchoscopy to identify dynamic lesions. For extrinsic structural lesions, imaging by CT or MRI should be considered.

MANAGEMENT

Nasal causes of obstruction can be relieved by an appropriately sized oropharyngeal airway. Choanal atresia requires surgical intervention to correct the occlusion. For cases with pharyngeal obstruction, some may respond to prone positioning. In the prone position, the base of the tongue can fall forwards and relieve obstruction of the pharyngeal airway. Oropharyngeal or nasopharyngeal airways may be helpful, but ET intubation or tracheostomy may be required in more severe cases.

In the absence of associated structural obstructive lesions, many of the common causes of laryngeal obstruction may resolve with expectant management. For example, laryngomalacia usually resolves by the age of 18–24 months,[281] whereas unilateral vocal cord palsy may resolve within weeks after resolution of the underlying cause.[286] If there are no signs of severe disease, conservative management is recommended. For those with substantial risk of life-threatening airway obstruction (e.g., bilateral vocal cord palsy), the infant may require ET intubation or tracheostomy. For infants with subglottic stenosis secondary to ET intubation, preextubation corticosteroids may be useful. Surgical intervention may be indicated in cases with severe disease (e.g., failure to thrive) and respiratory compromise.

PREVENTION

The occurrence of acquired subglottic stenosis is associated with ET intubation. Minimizing the use of intubation and invasive ventilation by increasing the use of noninvasive ventilation may help to prevent subglottic stenosis. There are no effective means to prevent the other causes of upper airway obstruction.

PROGNOSIS

Mortality of upper airway obstruction can be high if complete or critical airway obstruction is present. However, this is relatively uncommon. The more common forms of obstruction, such as laryngomalacia and unilateral vocal cord palsy, are often mild and resolve without specific intervention.

Gastroesophageal Reflux

GER is common in preterm infants, but its correlation with respiratory issues and apnea are small. Reflux of fluid up the esophagus will cause a reflexive closure of the vocal cords to protect the airway and may cause obstructive apnea until the infant is able to swallow the fluid. Inability to successfully close the larynx during GER can lead to recurrent aspiration pneumonia (discussed earlier in the chapter). Apnea may also trigger GER because the lower esophageal sphincter pressure decreases when hypoxia occurs.[287] Using a combination of esophageal impedance probes, pH probes, and respiratory monitors, it was demonstrated that approximately 3% of respiratory events/apneas followed a GER, whereas GER occurred in 9% of infants after an apnea event.[288] The GER events are associated with the clinical symptoms of apnea/bradycardia approximately 10% of time in term and preterm infants.[289] Aspiration of gastric secretions should be suspected in neonates with recurrent respiratory problems, especially if there is right upper lobe collapse or consolidation on the chest radiograph. Significant levels of fat-laden macrophages or pepsin have been shown in the tracheobronchial secretions of infants who are fed and have clinical

features of aspiration; however, the diagnostic utilities are not high enough for these methods to diagnose aspiration as a standalone test.[290,291] The extent of reflux can be assessed using contrast and fluoroscopy in an upper gastrointestinal study, through pH or impedance monitoring, or through visualization of edema and irritation at the vocal cords. Even when GER is documented, there are still questions about the benefits of treatment.

MANAGEMENT

Up to 25% of extremely preterm infant are discharged home on medications for GER, usually due to a belief that it helps with apnea.[287,292] According to recent surveys, more than 70% of these infants were started on medications for GER and apnea without any investigations.[287] Most neonatologists stop the medications when the infants are apnea free and greater than 36 weeks GA. Gastric acid suppressors, H2 blockers and proton pump inhibitors, are more commonly used than motility promoting agents (erythromycin, cisapride, metoclopramide). Randomized trials of proton pump inhibitors have not shown a benefit for GER and apnea but have shown increased adverse events. There is an association of acid-blocking agents with increased risk of NEC and sepsis, especially with gram-negative bacteria.[293] Routine use of medications to treat GER should be avoided in preterm infants. Promotility agents have had limited success in treating GER in preterm and term infants.[294] Erythromycin has had the most success; however, the risk of hypertrophic pyloric stenosis should be balanced against the potential benefits, especially during the first 2 weeks of life.[295] Thickening agents have not been shown to decrease symptoms of GER, and one was removed from the market because of an increased risk of NEC. Continuous feeds or transpyloric feedings have also not been shown to decrease apnea or GER.[294] Nissen fundoplication may be necessary in some infants with severe GER, as documented by upper gastrointestinal (GI) tract contrast studies, and signs of aspiration pneumonia.

References

Access the reference list online at ExpertConsult.com.

Suggested Reading

Abman SH, Hansmann G, Archer SL, et al. Pediatric pulmonary hypertension: guidelines from the American Heart Association and American Thoracic Society. *Circulation.* 2015;132(21):2037–2099.

Bancalari EH, Jobe AH. The respiratory course of extremely preterm infants: a dilemma for diagnosis and terminology. *J Pediatr.* 2012;161(4):585–588.

Laudy JA, Wladimiroff JW. The fetal lung. 2: pulmonary hypoplasia. *Ultrasound Obstet Gynecol.* 2000;16(5):482–494.

Lindenskov PH, Castellheim A, Saugstad OD, et al. Meconium aspiration syndrome: possible pathophysiological mechanisms and future potential therapies. *Neonatology.* 2015;107(3):225–230.

Oei JL, Vento M, Rabi Y, et al. Higher or lower oxygen for delivery room resuscitation of preterm infants below 28 completed weeks gestation: a meta-analysis. *Arch Dis Child Fetal Neonatal Ed.* 2017;102(1):F24–F30.

Perlman JM, Wyllie J, Kattwinkel J, et al. Part 7: neonatal resuscitation: 2015 International Consensus on Cardiopulmonary Resuscitation and Emergency Cardiovascular Care Science With Treatment Recommendations. *Circulation.* 2015;132(16 suppl 1):S204–S241.

Schmolzer GM, Kumar M, Pichler G, et al. Non-invasive versus invasive respiratory support in preterm infants at birth: systematic review and meta-analysis. *BMJ.* 2013;347:f5980.

20 *Bronchopulmonary Dysplasia*

LAURIE SHERLOCK, MD, and STEVEN H. ABMAN, MD

Introduction

Improved survival of very immature infants has contributed to an increase in the number of infants who develop bronchopulmonary dysplasia (BPD). BPD is a chronic lung disease that occurs in roughly 10,000–15,000 infants per year in the United States alone. This has important implications for the utilization of health resources, as follow-up studies have demonstrated that BPD infants require frequent readmission to the hospital in the first 2 years after birth for respiratory infections, asthma, and related problems; they also have persistent lung function abnormalities as adolescents and young adults. BPD most commonly occurs in prematurely born infants who have required mechanical ventilation (MV) and oxygen therapy for acute respiratory distress,[1-3] but it also can occur in immature infants who have had minimal initial lung disease.[4-6] Although BPD is most commonly associated with premature birth, it can occur in term or near-term infants due to severe acute lung injury, as reflected by a need for high mechanical ventilator support or extracorporeal membrane oxygenation (ECMO) therapy.

Over the past 40 years, the introduction of prenatal steroid use, surfactant therapy, new ventilator strategies, aggressive use of early continuous positive airway pressure (CPAP), changes in approach to managing patent ductus arteriosus (PDA), improved nutrition and other treatments have resulted in dramatic changes in the clinical course and outcomes of premature newborns with respiratory distress syndrome (RDS). Whereas the overall incidence of BPD has not declined over the past decade,[6] its severity has been clearly modulated by changes in clinical practice. There is now growing recognition that infants with chronic lung disease after premature birth have a different clinical course and pathology than had been traditionally observed in infants who were dying with BPD during the presurfactant era (Fig. 20.1).[4-8] The classic progressive stages with prominent fibroproliferation that first characterized BPD are often absent, and the disease has changed to being predominantly defined by a disruption of distal lung growth; this has been termed "the new BPD."[4] In contrast to classic BPD, the new BPD develops in preterm newborns who may have required minimal or even no ventilatory support and relatively low inspired oxygen concentrations during the early postnatal days (Fig. 20.2).[5,6] At autopsy, the lung histology of infants who die with the new BPD displays more uniform and milder regions of injury, but impaired alveolar and vascular growth remain prominent (Table 20.1). The implications of how these changes in BPD alter long-term pulmonary outcomes remain unknown. The new BPD is likely the result of disrupted antenatal and postnatal lung growth that leads to persistent abnormalities of lung architecture. It is unclear whether such infants subsequently experience sufficient catch-up lung growth to achieve and sustain improved lung function over time. To date, there

are limited safe and effective preventative therapies for BPD, but there are promising new therapies directed either at reducing lung injury or improving lung growth.

Overall, BPD may perhaps be best considered as a "syndrome" rather than a single disease because etiologies, clinical course and respiratory outcomes are diverse and modulated by therapeutic interventions. The changing nature of BPD suggests that a standard binomial definition will not adequately predict long-term pulmonary outcomes. Importantly, there is growing recognition that prematurity itself, even in the absence of BPD and even in late preterm infants, is associated with significant late respiratory morbidity.[9-12] Additionally, there is a growing appreciation that interventions designed to prevent BPD should focus on late pulmonary and neurodevelopmental outcomes that have the most impact on the health and welfare of prematurely born children and their families rather than short-term outcomes (e.g., supplemental oxygen requirement at 36 weeks corrected age). Such a change in thinking about BPD requires the development of multidisciplinary teams of health care professionals and clinician-scientists, an appreciation of the magnitude, nature and chronic manifestations of prematurity and BPD and novel programs that provide continuity of long-term care. This chapter reviews the epidemiology, pathophysiology, and long-term outcomes of infants with BPD.

Definition

Despite extensive studies of premature infants with chronic lung disease, the definition of BPD remains problematic. Northway's initial diagnosis incorporated a clinical assessment, radiologic findings, and histopathology. Today current definitions of BPD diagnose the disease based on the treatment: oxygen requirement at 28 days or 36 weeks corrected gestational age. Ideally a diagnosis of BPD would act as an accurate surrogate to predict long term pulmonary morbidity, would be a meaningful outcome measure for evaluating prevention and therapeutic interventions and would be consistently defined between units so it could be used to compare performance and identify best practices, identifying quality improvement measures and targeting future investigation. Unfortunately the current definition falls short on all counts. Owing to inconsistencies in how different institutes were defining BPD, a National Institutes of Health–sponsored conference developed a new definition of BPD that incorporates several components of previous definitions and adds a BPD severity categorization according to the level of respiratory support required at 36 weeks corrected gestational age or at the time of discgharge (Table 20.2).[13] The potential advantage of this approach is that BPD is defined as a spectrum of disease with early markers that may be predictive of long-term pulmonary morbidity. However, even with the improved current definition, sensitivity and specificity are

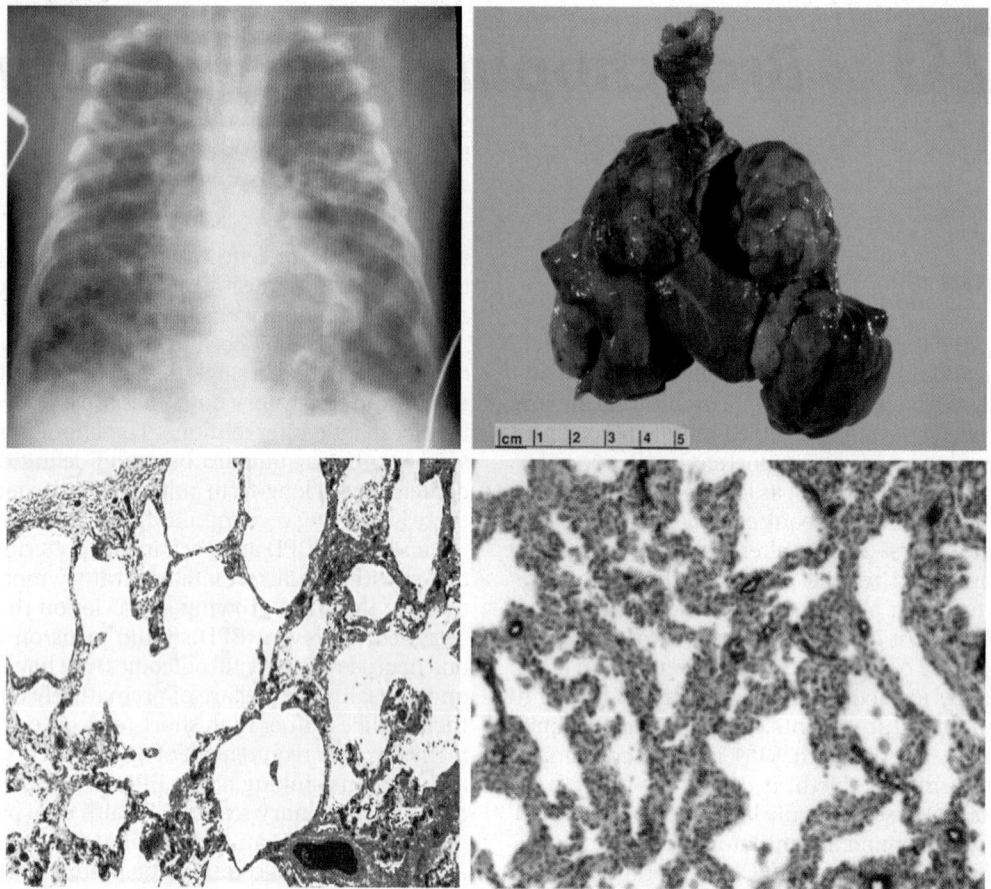

Fig. 20.1 Radiographic, anatomic, and histologic features of severe bronchopulmonary dysplasia (BPD). Upper left panel shows a chest radiograph with hyperinflation, diffuse but patchy parenchymal infiltrate and cor pulmonale. Upper right panel shows gross appearance of severe fibroproliferative BPD. Note the cobblestone pattern with pseudofissures. Lower left panel shows marked alveolar simplification in an older child who died from a nonrespiratory cause. Lower right panel shows immunostaining for factor VIII to highlight a dysmorphic and simplified vascular bed.

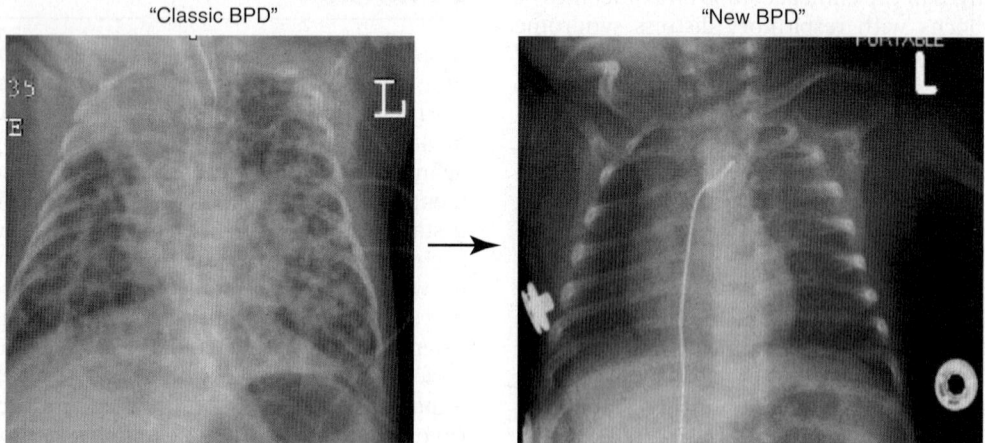

Fig. 20.2 Chest radiographs illustrating the transition from severe bronchopulmonary dysplasia (BPD; Northway stage IV) in the presurfactant era (classic BPD) compared with a typical x-ray pattern from the new BPD.

lacking in predicting long-term pulmonary adverse outcomes. In one study evaluating pulmonary outcomes with different definitions of BPD, even with the improved definition, 20%–27% of very low birth weight (VLBW) neonates without a diagnosis of BPD still had long-term pulmonary morbidity requiring respiratory medications or rehospitalization for respiratory etiology.[14] For the VLWB neonates with a

diagnosis of severe BPD, up to 50% did not have any long-term pulmonary morbidities (Fig. 20.3).[14]

An additional problem in defining BPD is the wide center-to-center variability in diagnosing the need for supplemental oxygen. A survey from the Vermont Oxford Network revealed striking variations in thresholds for instituting supplementary oxygen based on pulse oximetry, ranging from less than 84%

Table 20.1   Changing Pathologic Features of Bronchopulmonary Dysplasia

PRESURFACTANT ERA ("OLD BPD")	POSTSURFACTANT ERA ("NEW BPD")
Alternating atelectasis with hyperinflation	Less regional heterogeneity
Severe airway epithelial lesions (e.g., hyperplasia, squamous metaplasia)	Rare airway epithelial lesions
Marked airway smooth muscle hyperplasia	Mild airway smooth muscle thickening
Extensive, diffuse fibroproliferation	Rare fibroproliferative changes
Hypertensive remodeling of pulmonary arteries	Fewer arteries but "dysmorphic"
Decreased alveolarization and surface area	Fewer, larger and simplified alveoli

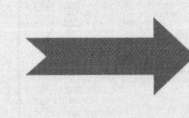

BPD, Bronchopulmonary dysplasia.

Table 20.2   National Institute of Health Consensus Conference: Diagnostic Criteria for Establishing Bronchopulmonary Dysplasia

Gestational Age	<32 Weeks	>32 Weeks
Time point of assessment	36 weeks PMA or discharge, whichever comes first	>28 days but <56 days postnatal age or discharge, whichever comes first
	Treatment with oxygen >21% for at least 28 days	
Mild BPD	Breathing room air at 36 weeks PMA or discharge, whichever comes first	Breathing room air by 56 days postnatal or discharge, whichever comes first
Moderate BPD	Need for <30% O_2 at 36 weeks PMA or discharge, whichever comes first	Need for <30% O_2 to 56 days postnatal age or discharge, whichever comes first
Severe BPD	Need for >30% $O_2 \pm$ PPV or CPAP at 36 weeks PMA or discharge, whichever comes first	Need for >30% $O_2 \pm$ PPV or CPAP at 56 days postnatal age or discharge, whichever comes first

BPD, Bronchopulmonary dysplasia, *CPAP,* continuous positive airway pressure; *PMA,* Postmenstrual age; *PPV,* positive pressure ventilation.

Definition	Oxygen at 36 weeks		Mild	Moderate	Severe
	No	Yes			
% meeting criteria	56.3%	43.7%	30.8%	29.7%	16.7 %
Pulmonary medications (%)	28.5%	43.3%	29.7%	40.8%	46.6%
Pulmonary rehospitalization	25.6%	36.1%	26.7%	33.5%	39.4%

No BPD:	Severe BPD:
Almost 1/3rd still had pulmonary morbidity	Over half did not have pulmonary morbidity

Fig. 20.3 Current definitions of bronchopulmonary dysplasia (BPD) lack sensitivity and specificity to predict long-term pulmonary morbidities. (Modified from Ehrenkranz RA, Walsh MC, Vohr BR, et al. Validation of the National Institutes of Health consensus definition of bronchopulmonary dysplasia. *Pediatrics.* 2005;116(6):1353-1360.)

Health and Human Development (NICHD) definition.[18] Further work is needed to identify early physiologic, structural, and genetic or biochemical markers of BPD that are predictive of critical long-term endpoints, such as the presence of late respiratory disease evidenced by recurrent hospitalizations, reactive airways disease, the need for prolonged oxygen, the need for respiratory medications or exercise intolerance during childhood.[19]

Epidemiology

Pulmonary immaturity is the primary risk factor for BPD owing to incomplete structural and biochemical development, including inadequate surfactant, antioxidant, and antiprotease activities.[20] In the early 1960s, oxygen and MV were selectively used for premature infants with acute respiratory failure due to apnea and hyaline membrane disease. As these therapies were applied more widely, there was a growing recognition of premature infants who survived but developed chronic pulmonary disease with hypoxemia and chest radiographic abnormalities. In 1964, Shepard and colleagues reported that 50% of premature neonates who received oxygen and MV developed chronic lung disease.[21] In 1967, Northway and coworkers provided a comprehensive characterization of the clinical, radiologic and pathologic features of chronic lung disease in infants who had received high concentrations of oxygen and MV from birth.[1] On average, these premature infants were born at 34 weeks' gestation and weighed 2200 g, yet their mortality was 67%, and the surviving infants had persistent respiratory distress and abnormal chest radiographs beyond the first 4 weeks after birth. In the latter study, the term *bronchopulmonary*

to less than 96%, with only 41% of the respondents using the same criterion (<90%).[15] This alone has a marked impact on the reported incidence of BPD. For a given study population, the incidence of BPD decreased from 37% to 24% if the need for supplemental oxygen was defined by accepting oxygen saturations above 92% or 88% while breathing room air, respectively.[16] Use of an oxygen reduction test may better help to diagnose ongoing supplemental oxygen requirements.[16,17] Despite efforts to improve the diagnosis of BPD, the emerging practice trend of using of noninvasive positive pressure through heated high flow leaves up to 2.1% of infants unclassifiable with the current National Institute of Child

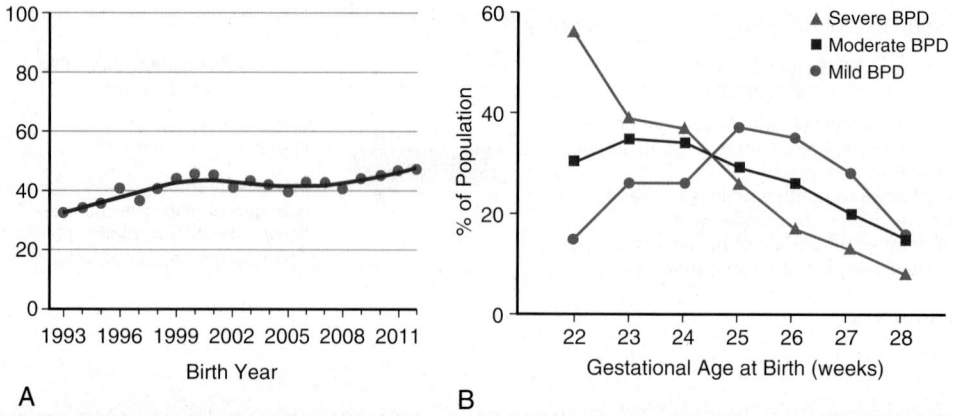

Fig. 20.4 (A) The incidence of bronchopulmonary dysplasia (BPD) may be increasing. (B) Early gestational age is associated with increased BPD severity. (A, Modified from Stoll BJ, Hansen HI, Bell EF, et al. Trends in Care Practices, Morbidity, and Mortality of Extremely Preterm Neonates, 1993-2012. *JAMA.* 2015;314(10):1039-1051. B, Modified from Stoll BJ, Hansen NI, Bell EF, et al. Neonatal outcomes of extremely preterm infants from the NICHD Neonatal Research Network. *Pediatrics.* 2010;126(3):443-456.)

dysplasia was first applied, referring to the striking disruption of airway structure. This seminal study identified the interactive roles of three key pathogenic factors: lung immaturity, acute lung injury, and inadequate repair of the initial lung injury. This basic concept still provides an important paradigm for our current understanding of BPD.

Currently most infants who develop BPD are born with extreme prematurity, and 97% have birth weights below 1250 g.[22] The risk of BPD increases with decreasing gestational age, with an incidence of 85% for infants born at 22 weeks and 23% for those born at 28 weeks (Fig. 20.4).[7] It is also inversely associated with birth weight. The incidence has been reported to be as high as 85% in neonates between 500 and 699 g, but only 5% in infants with birth weights over 1500 g. Although the overall incidence of BPD is reported at about 20% of ventilated newborns, marked variability exists between centers.[23–26] This likely reflects regional differences in the clinical definitions of BPD, the number of infants born at the hospital versus born at outside facilities and transferred in, the proportion of newborns with extreme prematurity, and specific patient management. In the most immature infants, even minimal exposure to oxygen and MV may be sufficient to contribute to BPD. Two-thirds of infants who develop BPD have only mild respiratory distress at birth (Fig. 20.5).[6] Other observers have recognized this change in patterns of respiratory diseases[6,7] and have emphasized the importance of enhancing our understanding of the mechanisms of progressive respiratory deterioration and the lack of clinical improvement during the first week of life.

Despite advances in neonatal care, the incidence of BPD has not decreased; some reports suggest that it is actually increasing.[7] Whether this increase in incidence is a result of improved survival of the most immature and vulnerable infants is unclear. Whatever the case may be, it is a strong impetus to identify improved strategies for prevention and treatment.

Etiology

Implications regarding the impact of extremely premature birth on lung growth and structure are best appreciated in

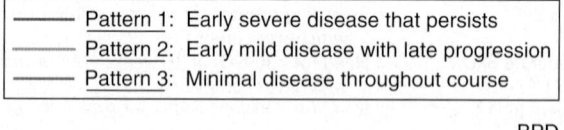

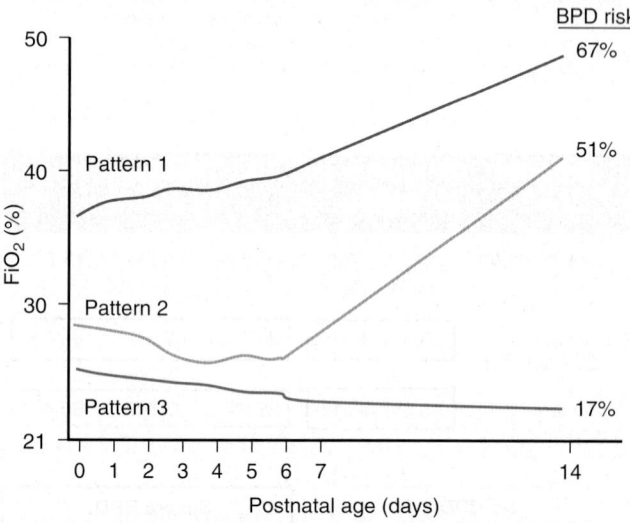

Fig. 20.5 Changing patterns of respiratory disease with risk for bronchopulmonary dysplasia (BPD). (Modified from Laughon M, Alfred EN, Bose C, et al. Patterns of respiratory distress during the first 2 postnatal weeks in extremely premature infants. *Pediatrics.* 2010;123:1124-1131.)

the context of the stages of lung development (Fig. 20.6). The fetal lung at 24 weeks' gestation is generally at the late canalicular or early saccular stage of growth, which is characterized by immature airway structure, undifferentiated epithelial cells, a paucity of capillaries, and reduced surface area. Thus premature birth and injury at this early stage of development have profound implications for the risk of BPD, which provides additional challenges beyond those of premature birth at later stages of lung development.

Epidemiologic studies of BPD have identified many factors that modify the risk. Endogenous factors linked with BPD include gestational immaturity, lower birth weight, male sex, white or nonblack race, family history of asthma, and being small for gestational age.[27] Epidemiologic studies of

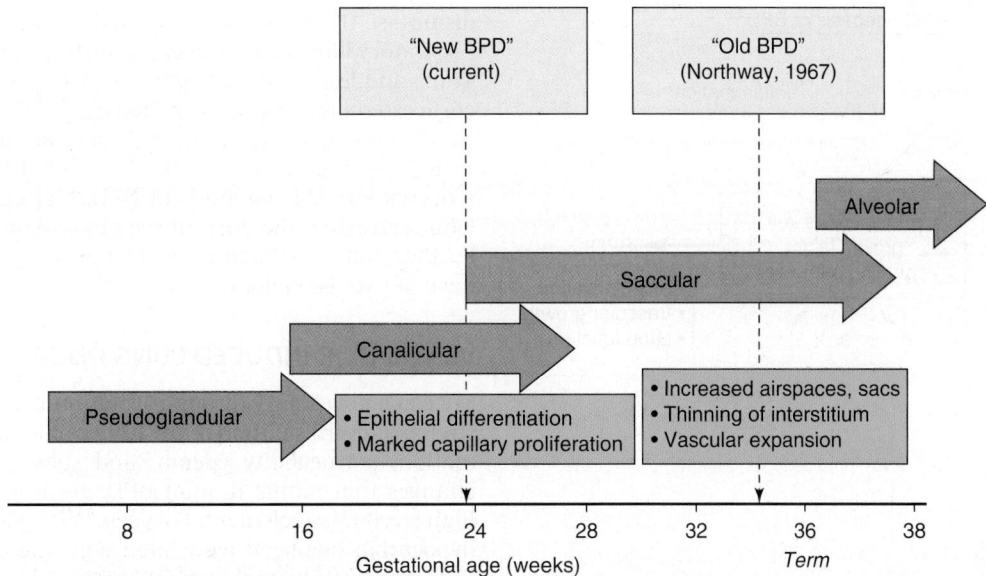

Fig. 20.6 Relationship between the stages of lung development, gestation and average birth of infants with classic bronchopulmonary dysplasia (BPD) versus the more extreme premature newborn that typifies the new BPD. (Modified from Laughon M, Alfred EN, Bose C, et al. Patterns of respiratory distress during the first 2 postnatal weeks in extremely premature infants. *Pediatrics.* 2010;123:1124-1131.)

BPD have yielded a number of predictive models.[28] Although none is routinely applied in caring for infants at risk of BPD, such models might serve as valuable tools for providing risk adjustment for clinical trials and other clinical research studies.

GENETIC SUSCEPTIBILITY

The risk for developing BPD is now recognized as being markedly influenced by complex interactions between genetic and environmental risk factors.[29] Variability in the incidence and severity of BPD among premature infants with similar environmental risk factors suggests that genetic susceptibility plays a critical role in the pathogenesis of BPD. Parker and colleagues first reported that genetic factors increase the risk for BPD in preterm twin pairs independent of birth weight, gestational age, gender, RDS severity, PDA, infection, antenatal steroids and other factors.[30] Lavoie and colleagues found that genetic effects accounted for about 80% of the observed variance in BPD susceptibility.[31] Initial genomewide association studies implicated SPOCK2 (SPARC/osteonectin, cwcv and kazal-like domains proteoglycan 2 gene) as significant in the development of BPD[32]; however, two subsequent genome wide association studies (GWAS) did not confirm this or find other genes to be significant.[33] Exome sequencing from newborn blood spot samples has identified numerous mutated genes in infants with BPD and could provide further insight into genetic risk moving forward.[34] Numerous genes are required for normal lung growth and development, and they are likely to contain sequence variations that modulate the risk for BPD. Published studies have identified several potential candidate genes, especially regarding surfactant proteins and cytokines.[35–38] However, many studies report small sample sizes, and the findings from most of the studies have not been replicated in subsequent cohorts. The current challenge is to specifically identify the candidate genes that

contribute to the development of BPD and their interaction with the specific environmental stimuli that adversely affect lung injury, repair, and structure after preterm birth.

PRENATAL FACTORS

Recent studies have strongly implicated prenatal factors, including maternal smoking, preeclampsia, placental abnormalities, chorioamnionitis, and intrauterine growth restriction as key factors in the risk for BPD after preterm birth.[39–50] The interactions of prenatal and postnatal factors, such exposure to hyperoxia in growth-restricted infants or after exposure to endotoxin, may be critical factors as well. The question of how these epidemiologic observations are mechanistically linked with premature birth and poor respiratory outcomes is currently under intense laboratory and clinical investigation. Additional perinatal risk factors for BPD include absence of maternal glucocorticoid treatment and perinatal asphyxia.

POSTNATAL FACTORS

BPD risk has also been linked with early neonatal influences, including lower Apgar scores, RDS, PDA,[51] higher weight-adjusted fluid intake,[52] earlier use of parenteral lipid, light-exposed parenteral nutrition, and duration of oxygen therapy. Among at-risk infants, the duration and approach to MV (including the use of high inspired oxygen, high peak inspiratory pressure, lower positive end-expiratory pressure, and higher ventilation rate) are also associated with BPD—relationships that could be causal or simply reflect the underlying severity of acute respiratory disease.[53–56] Increased BPD risk has been associated with hypocarbia (indicated by highest PCO_2 <40 at 48 or 96 hours), suggesting that aggressive ventilation can contribute to lung injury and BPD.[57] Colonization or infection with *Ureaplasma urealyticum*, postnatal

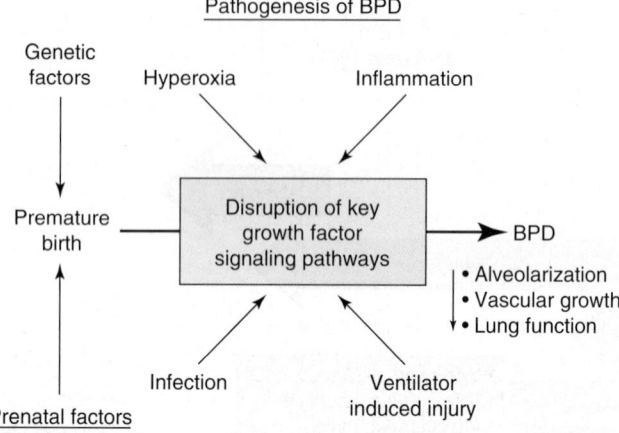

Fig. 20.7 Pathogenesis of bronchopulmonary dysplasia (BPD): multi-factorial mechanisms. *IUGR,* In utero growth restriction.

cytomegalovirus infection and postnatal sepsis also appear to predispose to BPD.[58–60]

Pathogenesis

Preterm infants are especially susceptible to injury caused by mechanical forces, oxidative stress, and inflammation due to the extreme structural and biochemical immaturity of the preterm lung. As Northway first observed, BPD has diverse, multifactorial etiologies, including hyperoxia, ventilator-induced lung injury (VILI), inflammation, and infection (Fig. 20.7).[1] Animal studies suggest that lung injury due to each of these adverse stimuli is at least partly mediated through increased oxidative stress, which further augments inflammation, promotes lung injury, and impairs growth factor–signaling pathways.

OXYGEN TOXICITY

Oxygen toxicity due to high levels of supplemental oxygen markedly increases the production of reactive oxygen species (ROS), which overwhelm host antioxidant defense mechanisms in the immature lung and thus cause adverse molecular, biochemical, histologic, and anatomic effects.[1,61,62] Prematurely born infants are especially vulnerable to oxidative stress because their lungs are relatively deficient in antioxidant enzyme systems (e.g., superoxide dismutase, catalase and others) at birth. Early animal studies clearly demonstrated that high levels of supplemental oxygen promote lung inflammation, impair alveolar and vascular growth, and increase lung fibroproliferation. Experimentally, even relatively mild levels of hyperoxia may be sufficient to induce oxidative stress and impair growth of the immature lung.

A potential method for preventing the development of BPD appears to be prophylactic supplementation of human recombinant antioxidant enzymes.[63] In a multicenter randomized controlled trial (RCT), intratracheal treatment of premature infants at birth with recombinant human CuZn superoxide

dismutase (rhSOD) was associated with fewer episodes of respiratory illness (i.e., wheezing, asthma, pulmonary infections) and less need for treatment with bronchodilators or corticosteroids at 1 year corrected age.[63,64] This suggests that rhSOD may prevent long-term pulmonary injury from ROS in high-risk premature infants. This trial failed to demonstrate a decrease in the diagnosis of BPD, highlighting the challenges posed by the current way in which BPD is defined. Further studies evaluating recombinant antioxidants enzymes have not yet been done.

VENTILATOR-INDUCED LUNG INJURY

MV can induce injury through "volutrauma," in which phasic stretch or overdistention of the lung can induce lung inflammation, permeability edema, and subsequent structural changes that mimic human BPD, even in the absence of high levels of supplemental oxygen.[65,66] Aggressive MV with hypocarbia has been associated with the development of BPD, as reports have shown an inverse relationship between low $PaCO_2$ levels and BPD development.[57] High tidal volumes should be avoided during MV and even during resuscitation in the delivery room.[67] In an experimental study demonstrating a relationship between the size of manual inflations and lung damage in lambs, adverse effects were demonstrated even with inflations of 8 mL/kg.[67–69] Although small tidal volumes may reduce the risk for VILI in preterm infants, failure to recruit and maintain adequate functional residual capacity (FRC), even with low tidal volumes, is injurious in experimental models.[69]

INFLAMMATION

Experimental and clinical studies have shown that inflammation clearly plays a central role in the pathobiology of BPD.[70–72] Oxygen toxicity, volutrauma, and infection can induce early and sustained inflammatory responses that promote the recruitment and activation of neutrophils, which persist in infants who develop BPD.[73] Levels of multiple proinflammatory cytokines (e.g., interleukins [ILs] such as IL-1β, IL-6 and soluble intracellular adhesion molecule 1 [ICAM-1]) and growth factors (e.g., transforming growth factor-β [TGR-β], vascular endothelial growth factor, and others) are present and altered in lung lavage and blood samples from premature infants who subsequently develop BPD versus controls.[71–73] IL-1β induces the release of inflammatory mediators, activating inflammatory cells and upregulating adhesion molecules on endothelial cells. ICAM-1 is a glycoprotein that promotes cell-to-cell contact. Direct contact between activated cells leads to further production of proinflammatory cytokines, such as IL-8, which induces neutrophil chemotaxis, inhibits surfactant synthesis and stimulates elastase release.[73] The levels of collagenase and phospholipase A2 are also increased, and oxidative modification results in the inactivation of alpha-1-antiprotease, which further tips the protease-antiprotease imbalance to favor injury. Lung inflammation is associated with loss of endothelial basement membrane and interstitial sulfated glycosaminoglycans,[74] which are important in inhibiting fibrosis. Tumor necrosis factor alpha (TNF-α) and IL-6 induce fibroblast and collagen production.[70,75,76] Increased TGF-β and impaired vascular endothelial growth factor (VEGF) signaling have been strongly linked with the risk for BPD.[77–80] Leukotrienes are present at high levels in the lungs of infants developing BPD and remain elevated even at 6 months of age.[81,82]

Evidence that a systemic inflammatory response contributes to the pathogenesis of BPD led investigators to explore the contributions of antenatal, perinatal, and postnatal inflammation to lung injury.[83] Observational studies have suggested an association between amniotic fluid markers and placental and umbilical cord pathology of chorioamnionitis with BPD.[84,85] The combined effects of antenatal infection or inflammation and clinical factors might contribute to the occurrence of BPD via a number of mechanisms: direct injury of pulmonary parenchyma, disruption of the developmental milieu, impaired angiogenesis,[86,87] or activation (priming) of immune cells in the lung, thus provoking an exaggerated inflammatory injury in response to a variety of prenatal, perinatal, and postnatal insults.[83] BPD may be increased in infants whose mothers had chorioamnionitis.[49] This is because intraamniotic endotoxin exposure can disrupt alveolar and vascular development and thus lead to a decreased alveolar number and pulmonary hypertension (PH).[88] In a case-control study of 386 infants born at or below 1500 g (after adjusting for other BPD risk factors), chorioamnionitis alone appeared to be associated with reduced risk of BPD; however, chorioamnionitis followed by 7 days of MV or postnatal sepsis had a synergistic effect that substantially increased the risk of BPD.[89] These data suggest that chorioamnionitis might make the lung more susceptible to postnatal injury from a "second hit" of hyperoxia or ventilator-induced injury. Alternatively, these findings also suggest variable effects of chorioamnionitis on lung maturation versus arrested development, in which greater prenatal injury is reflected by an increased need for more ventilator and oxygen support.[88]

Pathophysiology

RESPIRATORY FUNCTION

Nonuniform damage to the airways and distal lungs results in variable time constants for different areas of the lungs. Inspired gas may be distributed to relatively poorly perfused lung, thereby worsening ventilation-perfusion matching. Decreased lung compliance appears to correlate strongly with morphologic and radiographic changes in the lung. Dynamic lung compliance is markedly reduced in infants with established BPD, even in those who no longer require oxygen therapy.[90] The reduction in compliance is due to small airway narrowing, interstitial fibrosis, edema, and atelectasis. Established BPD is primarily characterized by reduced surface area and heterogeneous lung units in which regional variations in airway resistance and tissue compliance lead to highly variable time constants throughout the lung. As a result, MV of severe BPD, especially beyond the first few months of life, requires strikingly different ventilator strategies than commonly used earlier in the disease course (Fig. 20.8). Such strategies generally favor longer inspiratory times, larger tidal volumes, higher positive end-expiratory pressure (PEEP), and lower rates to allow more effective gas exchange and respiratory function.[91]

Although the new BPD has been characterized as an arrest of distal lung and vascular growth, most of these observations

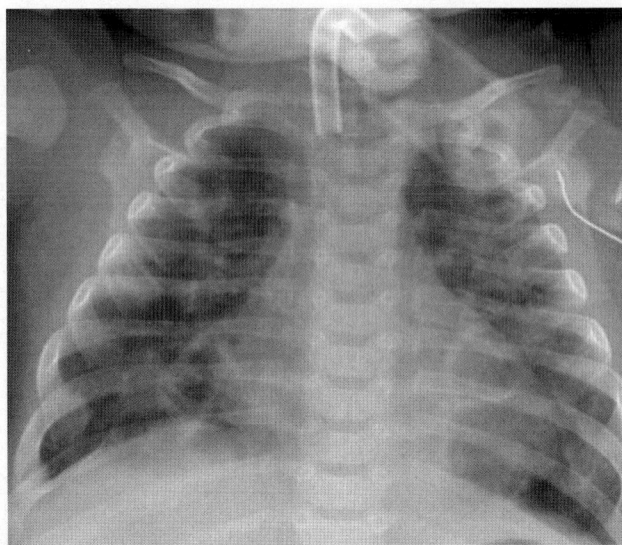

Fig. 20.8 Chest radiograph of bronchopulmonary dysplasia in an infant with tracheostomy and chronic ventilation.

were based on lung histology; evidence that provided direct physiologic data to support this finding was lacking. Tepper and colleagues have demonstrated the important finding of reduced lung surface area in infants with BPD by utilizing novel methods of assessing diffusion capacity.[92] Their recent work provides in vivo evidence for impaired diffusion capacity secondary to both decreased alveolar surface area and decreased pulmonary capillary bed.[93]

PULMONARY CIRCULATION

Acute lung injury also impairs growth, structure, and function of the developing pulmonary circulation after premature birth.[94,95] Endothelial cells are particularly susceptible to oxidant injury due to hyperoxia or inflammation. The media of small pulmonary arteries may also undergo striking changes, including smooth muscle cell proliferation, precocious maturation of immature pericytes into mature smooth muscle cells, and incorporation of fibroblasts into the vessel wall and surrounding adventitia.[96] Structural changes in the lung vasculature contribute to high pulmonary vascular resistance (PVR) due to narrowing of the vessel diameter and decreased vascular compliance. Decreased angiogenesis may limit vascular surface area, causing further elevations of PVR, especially in response to high cardiac output with exercise or stress. The pulmonary circulation in BPD patients is further characterized by abnormal vasoreactivity, which also increases PVR (Fig. 20.9).[97] Abnormal pulmonary vasoreactivity is evidenced by a marked vasoconstrictor response to acute hypoxia.[98] Cardiac catheterization studies have shown that even mild hypoxia causes marked elevations in pulmonary arterial pressure, even in infants with modest basal levels of PH. Maintaining oxygen saturation levels above 92%–94% effectively lowers pulmonary arterial pressure.[97,98] Strategies to lower pulmonary arterial pressure or limit lung injury to the pulmonary vasculature may limit the subsequent development of PH in BPD.

Early injury to the lung circulation leads to the rapid development of PH, which contributes significantly to the morbidity

LUNG PATHOPHYSIOLOGY OF BPD

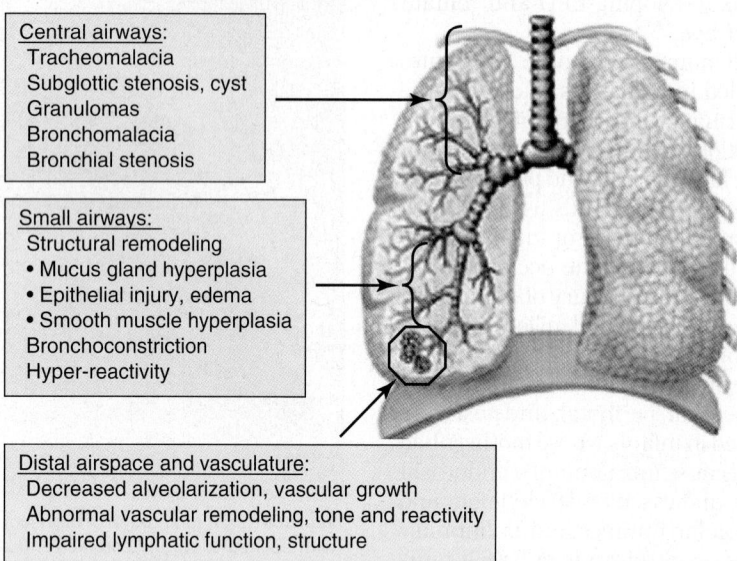

Central airways:
 Tracheomalacia
 Subglottic stenosis, cyst
 Granulomas
 Bronchomalacia
 Bronchial stenosis

Small airways:
 Structural remodeling
 • Mucus gland hyperplasia
 • Epithelial injury, edema
 • Smooth muscle hyperplasia
 Bronchoconstriction
 Hyper-reactivity

Distal airspace and vasculature:
 Decreased alveolarization, vascular growth
 Abnormal vascular remodeling, tone and reactivity
 Impaired lymphatic function, structure

Fig. 20.9 Lung pathophysiology of bronchopulmonary dysplasia.

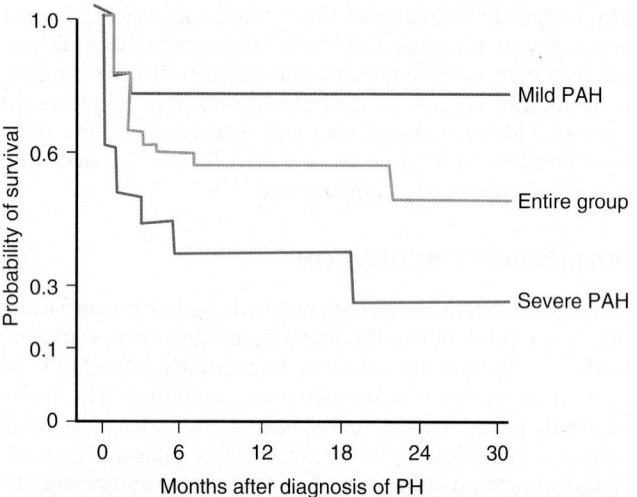

Fig. 20.10 High mortality associated with late pulmonary arterial hypertension (PAH) in bronchopulmonary dysplasia. (Modified from Khemani E, McElhinney DB, Rhein L, et al. Pulmonary artery hypertension in formerly premature infants with bronchopulmonary dysplasia: clinical features and outcomes in the surfactant era. *Pediatrics.* 2007;120:1260-1269.)

and mortality of severe BPD.[99] Persistent echocardiographic evidence of PH beyond the first few months has been associated with up to 40% mortality in infants with BPD.[100] High mortality rates have been reported in infants with BPD and severe PH, especially in those who require prolonged ventilator support (Fig. 20.10).[101] Although PH is a marker of more advanced BPD, elevated PVR also causes poor right ventricular function, impaired cardiac output, limited oxygen delivery, increased pulmonary edema, and perhaps a higher risk for sudden death.

In addition to the adverse effects of PH on the clinical course of infants with BPD, the lung circulation is further characterized by persistence of abnormal or "dysmorphic" growth, including a relative paucity of small pulmonary

arteries with an altered pattern of distribution within the interstitium of the distal lung.[86,102] In infants with severe BPD, decreased vascular growth occurs in conjunction with marked reductions in the formation of alveoli, suggesting that the new BPD is primarily characterized by growth arrest of the developing lung. This reduction of alveolar-capillary surface area impairs gas exchange, thereby increasing the need for prolonged supplemental oxygen and ventilator therapy. This causes marked hypoxemia with acute respiratory infections and late exercise intolerance and further increases the risk for developing severe PH. Experimental studies have further shown that early injury to the developing lung can impair angiogenesis, which contributes to decreased alveolarization and simplification of distal lung airspace (the "vascular hypothesis").[86] Thus, abnormalities of the lung circulation in BPD are related not only to the presence or absence of PH but also, more broadly, to *pulmonary vascular disease* after premature birth. This becomes manifest by decreased vascular growth and structure, thus also contributing to the pathogenesis and abnormal cardiopulmonary physiology of BPD.

Clinical studies have shown that the metabolic function of the pulmonary circulation is also impaired, as reflected by the lung's reduced clearance of circulating norepinephrine (NE).[103] Normally, 20%–40% of circulating NE is cleared during a single passage through the lung, but infants with severe BPD have an increase, suggesting a net production of NE across the pulmonary circulation. It is unknown whether impaired metabolic function of the lung contributes to the pathophysiology of BPD or is simply a marker of severe pulmonary vascular disease. It has been speculated that high catecholamine levels may lead to left ventricular hypertrophy (LVH) or systemic hypertension, known complications of BPD.

In addition to pulmonary vascular disease and right ventricular hypertrophy, other cardiovascular abnormalities associated with BPD include LVH, systemic hypertension, and the development of prominent systemic-to-pulmonary collateral vessels.[104,105] Infants with severe BPD can develop

LVH in the absence of right ventricular hypertrophy. Left ventricular diastolic dysfunction can contribute to lung edema, diuretic dependency, and PH in some infants with BPD.[106]

Prominent bronchial or other systemic-to-pulmonary collateral vessels were noted in early morphometric studies of infants with BPD and can readily be identified in many infants during cardiac catheterization.[107,108] Although these collateral vessels are generally small, large collaterals may contribute to significant shunting of blood flow to the lung, resulting in edema and the need for higher levels of supplemental oxygen. Collateral vessels have been associated with high mortality in some patients with both severe BPD and PH. Some infants have improved after embolization of large collateral vessels, as reflected by a reduced need for supplemental oxygen, ventilator support, and diuretics. The contribution of collateral vessels to the pathophysiology of BPD, however, is poorly understood.

Clinical Findings

PHYSICAL FINDINGS

Multiple abnormalities of lung structure and function contribute to late respiratory disease in BPD (see Fig. 20.5). Depending on the severity of BPD, findings on physical examination are variable and some infants may not have any abnormal findings. Chronic respiratory signs in children with BPD include tachypnea with shallow breathing, retractions, head bobbing, and a paradoxical breathing pattern. Auscultation may reveal coarse rhonchi, crackles, and wheezes. Some infants may demonstrate systemic hypertension during the first year of life. This systemic hypertension in BPD may be mild, transient, or striking. It usually responds to medication.[104,105] The etiology remains obscure, but further evaluation of some affected infants reveals significant renovascular or urinary tract disease.

IMAGING

Chest radiography is easily and frequently obtained in infants with BPD; however, its utility in diagnosis is limited owing to variable findings and the fact that many infants may have minimal radiologic abnormalities. Some patients may show lung fields with diffuse haziness. Patients with severe disease may demonstrate areas of hyperinflation and air trapping alternating with areas of fibrosis and atelectasis. Pulmonary edema may be present, especially during acute exacerbations.

Computed tomography (CT) of the chest has been used to identify structural abnormalities in patients with BPD, demonstrating increased airspace area reflecting alveolar simplification, hyperexpansion, emphysema, fibrosis and interstitial abnormalities, and mosaic attenuation.[109] Several different scoring systems have been developed correlating with the severity of BPD.[110] Longitudinal assessment by chest CT is not routinely used owing to concerns of exposing patients to large doses of ionizing radiation. New low-dose high-resolution CT protocols decrease this exposure, with dosing equivalent to 10–15 chest x-rays.[111] Nevertheless, the risk of serial radiation exposure limits the utility of this imaging modality.

Magnetic resonance imaging (MRI) of the lung is an alternative imaging modality without the risk of ionizing radiation; however, this is complicated, in that lungs have low proton density and alveolar spaces contribute to rapid signal decay, making imaging technically challenging. MRI with a hyperpolarized noble gas such as helium or xenon can improve sensitivity in identifying airway abnormalities. A proof-of-concept study demonstrated the safe performance of a nonsedated hyperpolarized-gas MRI in a healthy infant,[112] and this technique may facilitate longitudinal assessment of patients with BPD in the future.[113]

PULMONARY FUNCTION TESTS

Increased airway resistance can be demonstrated even during the first week after birth in preterm neonates at risk for BPD.[114] Infants with BPD at 28 days of age have an increased total respiratory and expiratory resistance with severe flow limitation, especially at low lung volumes.[115] The presence of tracheomalacia may also result in airflow limitation, which is worsened by bronchodilator therapy. In the early stages of BPD, the functional lung volume is often reduced due to atelectasis, but during later stages there is gas trapping with hyperinflation. The use of pulmonary function testing to follow the progression of BPD and the response to therapeutic interventions has increased but is still not commonly applied in the clinical setting.

LABORATORY FINDINGS

There is no specific laboratory test for the diagnosis of BPD. Patients with BPD may demonstrate hypercarbia and elevated bicarbonate levels in compensation for respiratory acidosis. Although not routinely used in clinical practice, changes in cytokine profiles have been associated with the development of BPD.[72,73] Increased concentrations of IL-1β, IL-6, IL-8, IL-10, and interferon-γ and decreased concentrations of IL-17, RANTES (regulated on activation, normal T cell expressed and secreted), and TNF-β have been observed. A recent study identified markers of urinary inflammation and oxidative stress that are associated with an increased risk of developing BPD.[116] Increased 8-hydroxydeoxyguanosine levels, a marker of oxidative stress–derived DNA damage, were associated with increased BPD. Greenough and colleagues have shown increased exhaled nitric oxide on day of life (DOL) 28 is associated with increased risk of BPD.[117] Research continues to seek improved markers to predict or identify infants at risk for long-term pulmonary morbidities.

ECHOCARDIOGRAPHIC FINDINGS

Routine echocardiograph monitoring is recommended at 36 weeks' corrected gestational age to assess for evidence of PH. Cardiac catheterization remains the gold standard for diagnosing PH. However, owing to its invasive nature, it is typically performed only in patients with severe disease. Tricuspid regurgitant jet velocity (TRJV) is used to estimate right ventricular systemic pressure (RVSP); however, other findings used to diagnose PH include right ventricular hypertrophy, right atrial enlargement, and interventricular septal flattening.[99]

Prevention

As described earlier, diverse mechanisms contribute to the pathogenesis of BPD, which perhaps makes it less surprising that there is no single therapy or prevention strategy except for the prevention of premature birth. The use of antenatal steroids in mothers at high risk of delivering a premature infant has reduced the incidence of neonatal death and RDS by 50%[118] but failed to decrease the incidence of BPD, even in combination with postnatal surfactant. Thus far, there has been no clear advantage to one antenatal steroid dosing regimen.[119] Similarly, antenatal thyrotrophin-releasing hormone therapy did not reduce BPD in randomized trials.[120]

Postnatally prevention of BPD begins in the delivery room. Emerging evidence suggests that avoiding or limiting MV leads to a decreased incidence of BPD.[6,121-123] Rapid establishment of FRC has become an early goal for all VLBW infants in attempts to avoid MV. Use of a T-piece resuscitator as opposed to a self-inflating bag has been shown to decrease intubation rates.[124] Sustained lung inflation immediately after birth is being investigated as a strategy to establish FRC and avoid lung injury. One RCT demonstrated a decreased need for MV at 72 hours; yet there was no difference in BPD at 36 weeks and an increase in pneumothorax.[125] Results of a larger RCT are pending.[126]

There has been a practice trend supporting early and aggressive use of noninvasive ventilation to avoid MV in hopes of decreasing BPD.[127] Several RCTs have compared the use of early nasal continuous positive airway pressure (nCPAP) with intubation.[128-130] A meta-analysis of these results reveals a small but significant decrease in the incidence of BPD or death.[123] Additionally, early nCPAP reduced the need for subsequent intubation and was associated with a reduced rate of steroid prescription and shorter duration of ventilation.

Despite efforts to avoid intubation, 85% of infants born between 22 and 28 weeks are exposed to MV[15] and CPAP failure rates remains high, between 40% and 60%.[128-130] Although no optimal ventilation mode has emerged, it is clear from physiologic studies that tidal volumes and inspired oxygen concentrations should be reduced as low as possible to avoid hypocarbia, volutrauma, and oxygen toxicity and that lung recruitment strategies should be employed. The association of volutrauma with the development of BPD has led to the use of strategies such as permissive hypercapnia to minimize lung injury.[131] Despite the physiologic plausibility of permissive hypercapnia as a prevention strategy for BPD, the recent permissive hypercapnia in extremely low birthweight infants (PHELBI) trial did not show a difference in BPD or death between groups targeting high compared to low carbon dioxide, suggesting that more research is needed to better understand optimal early ventilator strategies.[132] Meta-analysis of randomized trials has demonstrated that patient-triggered ventilation does not reduce BPD; if started in the recovery phase of RDS, however, it significantly shortens weaning from MV.[133] The results of randomized trials of high-frequency oscillatory ventilation (HFOV) or high-frequency jet ventilation (HFJV) have been inconsistent.[134] Two large studies that incorporated prenatal steroid and surfactant replacement therapy yielded different results. In one study (which restricted entry to VLBW infants with moderate to severe hypoxemic respiratory failure following surfactant administration), there was a significant benefit from HFOV of higher survival without BPD.[135] No substantial benefit or adverse effects of HFOV were found in the other study, however, which randomized premature infants (younger than 29 weeks) within 1 hour of birth regardless of the degree of lung disease.[136] An explanation for those conflicting results may be that in the current era, in which modified conventional ventilation strategies are used, pulmonary benefit from HFOV may be demonstrable only in infants with moderate to severe disease. Clearly the strategy applied for either conventional or HFOV is more important than the device itself. HFOV is frequently used as "rescue" therapy in premature newborns with severe respiratory failure despite treatment with exogenous surfactant. Whether such an approach reduces BPD or improves long-term outcomes requires appropriate testing.

Exogenous surfactant therapy to treat RDS has changed the face of neonatology in the last century. Surfactant reduces the combined outcome of death and BPD but not BPD alone.[137] Arguably, this may be due to the increased survival of very immature infants at high risk of BPD. The "intubate, surfactant, extubate" (INSURE) technique was originally described in 1994, combining early surfactant administration with rapid extubation to minimize duration of MV.[138] This technique has been evaluated as both an early and a prophylactic intervention (within the first hour of life or in the delivery room) as well as a rescue technique once infants develop symptoms of RDS. A meta-analysis of early INSURE showed improved outcomes including decreased oxygen requirement at 28 days and less exposure to MV; however, there was no decrease in BPD or mortality.[137] Studies of late or rescue INSURE have had a small number of participants and more studies are needed to determine if this technique should be used broadly. Several groups are currently investigating techniques to deliver surfactant to spontaneously breathing infants while avoiding intubation altogether.[139-141] Ongoing multicenter RCTs are currently recruiting and hopefully will provide greater insight in the coming years.[142]

The use of late surfactant for preterm infants on prolonged MV and thus at high risk for BPD has been evaluated in two recent RCTs. Hascoet et al. showed that late surfactant administration did not decrease the incidence of BPD; however, it did decrease long-term pulmonary morbidities including rehospitalization for respiratory illnesses and need for chest physiotherapy.[143] Ballard et al. and the TOLSURF (Trail Of Late SURFactant) study group recently published initial data showing no difference in BPD between infants treated with late surfactant or placebo; however, long-term pulmonary data are still being collected.[144]

Several nutritional and fluid balance strategies have been considered to decrease BPD. Although fluid restriction in the first week after birth does not reduce BPD,[145] it is important to avoid fluid overload, administration of colloid and sodium supplementation. A retrospective evaluation of 400- to 1000-g infants demonstrated that a higher fluid intake and less weight loss in the first week of life was associated with a higher incidence of BPD.[146] Aggressive treatment of symptomatic PDA may reduce the severity of BPD, but this remains controversial.

Appropriate nutrition, both in utero as well as postnatally, is critical in helping to promote normal lung growth, maturation, and repair. Infants born with in utero growth restriction (IUGR) have an increased risk of developing BPD.[147,148] Rapid weight gain and crossing of centiles, however, may be undesirable, particularly in infants that are small for gestational age.[149] Long-chain polyunsaturated fatty acids (LCPUFAs) are important for cell membrane function as well as for their antiinflammatory role, and animal data support that docosahexaenoic acid (DHA) in particular is critical for alveolarization. Cohort studies suggest that low levels of DHA are associated with increased BPD, and maternal DHA supplementation while breastfeeding is associated with decreased BPD.[150,151] Additionally, a small clinical trial comparing soy-based versus fish oil–based lipid suggests that soy-based lipids are associated with an increased risk of BPD.[152] Meta-analysis of seven randomized trials has demonstrated that systemic supplementation with vitamin A in sufficient quantities to establish normal serum retinol concentrations reduces oxygen dependence at 36 weeks postmenstrual age (PMA).[153] However, follow-up studies showed no improvement in long-term respiratory outcomes in vitamin A–treated infants. Additionally, after a national vitamin A shortage, units reported no difference in BPD during the period when they were unable to provide this treatment.[154–155]

One of the only pharmacologic approaches or supplements shown to reduce the risk for BPD is caffeine. A large-scale clinical trial (the Caffeine for Apnea of Prematurity, or CAP, trial) was initially developed to examine the effects of early and prolonged use of caffeine on late neurocognitive outcomes. Analysis of other endpoints related to this study suggests that caffeine significantly reduced the risk of BPD.[156] This effect is more striking than the benefit previously observed with vitamin A treatment.[153] Although mechanisms whereby caffeine reduced BPD risk are uncertain, treated infants also had a decreased need for surgical PDA closure, and respiratory support was discontinued earlier. A subgroup analysis of the CAP trial suggested that early initiation of caffeine (before DOL 2) provided greater reduction in BPD incidence than late initiation (DOL 3–10).[157] This finding was replicated in three retrospective cohort studies.[158–160] An ongoing RCT will compare early (DOL1) caffeine administration with late (DOL 2 or beyond).

Corticosteroid therapy, primarily directed at reducing lung inflammation, remains one of the most controversial areas of BPD care. Acute treatment with steroids improves lung mechanics and gas exchange and reduces inflammatory cells and mediators in tracheal samples of patients with BPD.[161,162] Meta-analysis of randomized trials suggests that corticosteroids reduce chronic oxygen dependency at 28 days and 36 weeks PMA, both when given early (before 8 days) and late.[163,164] However, there are significant concerns regarding increased mortality and adverse effects on head growth, neurodevelopmental outcomes, and lung structure, particularly with the use of dexamethasone.[165,166] Other side effects include systemic hypertension, hyperglycemia, cardiac hypertrophy, intestinal perforation, poor somatic growth, sepsis, intestinal bleeding, and myocardial hypertrophy. Currently the routine use of early high-dose steroids in premature newborns is strongly discouraged, as reflected in editorial statements from the American Academy of Pediatrics.[166] The adverse findings, however, are generally based on data from older studies that have used high doses of dexamethasone

for prolonged periods of time, and many questions persist regarding the risk-benefit relationship with the use of other steroids for shorter study periods. The DART trial (Dexamethasone: A Randomized Trial) was designed to investigate if lower dose courses of dexamethasone would be safe; however, it was unable to recruit the target number of patients. The investigators showed improved extubation rates in the short term and no significant difference in long-term adverse outcomes; however, these results should be interpreted with caution given insufficient power to determine long-term safety.[167,168] Doyle et al. published a meta-analysis of postnatal corticosteroid therapy and long-term outcomes, showing that the risk of death or neurodevelopment delay is inversely related to the risk of BPD.[169] As a result, some centers advocate the use of steroids at lower doses and shorter durations (5–7 days) in ventilator-dependent infants with severe, persistent lung disease after 1–2 weeks of age.[170] A recent study on prophylactic low-dose hydrocortisone therapy demonstrated a decreased incidence of BPD; however, it also showed a nonsignificant trend toward culture-proven sepsis.[171] Interestingly, this study demonstrated sex-specific differences, with hydrocortisone showing greater benefit in female infants than males.

To avoid the adverse effects associated with systemic administration, steroids have also been given by inhalation. Although meta-analysis has shown no significant benefits using this route, a recent trial of early inhaled budesonide demonstrated significantly decreased rates of BPD.[172,173] However, infants treated with budesonide showed a nonsignificant trend toward increased mortality and culture-proven sepsis, leaving uncertainty regarding the risk/benefit profile of inhaled steroids.

Owing to the association of *U. urealyticum* infection with the subsequent development of BPD, several studies have tried to determine whether treatment with macrolides would decrease the incidence of BPD. Although none of the individual studies demonstrated benefit, a meta-analysis showed a small decrease in the incidence of BPD in infants treated with azithromycin, with a number needed to treat (NNT) of 9.6 infants.[174] Owing to the small sample size, heterogeneity of patients and unclear blinding in some of the trials, this has not yet become widespread in clinical practice and larger RCTs are needed. A subgroup analysis of one of the trials revealed a benefit in infants who were colonized with *Ureaplasma*.[175]

In clinical studies, inhaled nitric oxide (iNO) therapy acutely lowered PVR and improved oxygenation in patients with PH in various settings, including premature infants with severe RDS and established BPD.[176–178] Experimental data have demonstrated that iNO therapy may be lung-protective in several animal models of experimental BPD and, importantly, may be associated with increased alveolar and vascular growth.[179] The potential role of iNO in the prevention of BPD has received considerable attention over the past decades, but the results of randomized trials for the prevention of BPD have yielded conflicting results. A large multicenter trial showed a 50% reduction in BPD and death in preterm infants who weighed more than 1000 g at birth.[180] Another large multicenter study suggested that prolonged iNO therapy at higher doses reduces BPD when started before the second week of life and improves some respiratory outcomes during infancy.[181] However, a third large-scale study showed no effects when administered to preterm infants with minimal respiratory disease.[182]

Overall, these findings suggest that iNO therapy may lower the risk for BPD in some preterm infants. However, because of the differences between studies (including gestational age, onset and duration of therapy, dose, and related questions), recommendations for its routine use for the prevention of BPD were not supported at a recent NICHD-sponsored Consensus Conference.[183]

Treatment

OXYGEN

Supplemental oxygen remains a mainstay of therapy for infants with BPD, yet the most appropriate target for oxygen saturation levels remains controversial. Growing concerns regarding the adverse effects of even moderate levels of oxygen therapy have led many neonatologists to accept oxygen saturations below 85%–90% early after birth of preterm newborns. Studies have shown that levels of equal to or less than 92% compared with equal to or greater than 95% are associated with a shorter duration of supplemental oxygen requirement[184] and perhaps fewer respiratory exacerbations.[185] Results from the NeOProM (Neonatal Oxygenation Prospective Meta-analysis) large multicenter collaborative trials found that targeting oxygen saturations between 85% and 89% was associated with higher mortality in comparison with infants treated with oxygen saturations targeted between 91% and 95%.[186,187] There were no differences in rates of BPD, retinopathy of prematurity, or neurodevelopment adverse outcomes. These results must interpreted with caution, as there was significant overlap in the oxygen saturation range that infants realistically spent time in as well as a problematic algorithm in pulse oximeters, potentially skewing results.[186,187] Currently most pulmonologists recommend maintaining infants with established BPD at oxygen saturations of 92%, with slightly higher levels for BPD infants with growth failure, recurrent respiratory exacerbations, or PH. Concerns persist that targeting higher levels (>95%) may be associated with ongoing lung injury due to oxidative stress. Prolonged monitoring of oxygenation while the infant is awake, asleep, and during feeds is important to ensure the avoidance of hypoxia while adjusting oxygen therapy.

In most neonatal intensive care units (NICUs), nCPAP, high-flow nasal cannulas, and noninvasive positive pressure ventilation (NIPPV) are used to maintain adequate oxygenation and ventilation while avoiding the need for prolonged ventilation or reintubation. Recent data from the Prematurity and Respiratory Outcomes Program (PROP) show a probability of 230- to 286-week infants being on different forms of respiratory support based on postnatal age (Fig. 20.11).[18] These prospectively collected data from multiple centers reflect current practice trends in respiratory support and include infants treated with heated high flow (HHF). HHF is being increasingly used, with benefits including improved perceived comfort, less nasal trauma, and easier positioning for feeding and holding infants.[188] Drawbacks are the imprecision and uncertainty in generated pressure delivered as well as lack of robust safety data. Studies that have compared HHF to

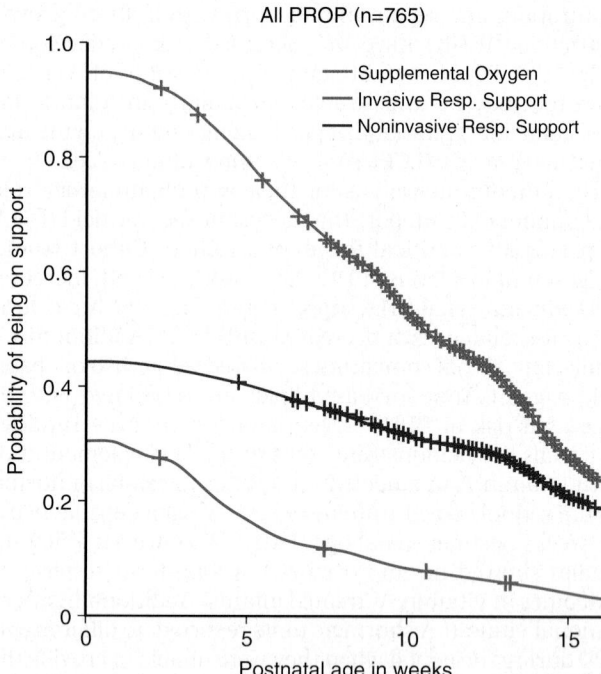

Fig. 20.11 Respiratory support for infants of very low birth weight over the initial postnatal course. *PROP,* Prematurity and Respiratory Outcomes Program. (From Poindexter BB, Feng R, Schmidt B, et al. Comparisons and limitations of current definitions of bronchopulmonary dysplasia for the prematurity and respiratory outcomes program. *Ann Am Thorac Soc.* 2015;12:1822-1830.)

nCPAP as the either the primary mode of respiratory support or for preventing extubation failure have evaluated older gestational-aged infants, excluding those at highest risk for BPD.[188] The HIPSTER (nasal high-flow therapy for primary respiratory support in preterm infants) trial, a large ongoing multicenter noninferiority trial comparing HHF to CPAP for infants born between 28 and 36 weeks, was stopped early as interim analysis showed that HHF was inferior to CPAP for respiratory support in VLBW infants.[189] Additionally, a recent retrospective evaluation suggested that use of HHF in infants weighing 1000 g or less was associated with an increased number of ventilator days, increased need for postnatal steroids and prolonged length of hospitalization, again raising concerns that HHF may not provide adequate support for the most at-risk infants.[190]

Whereas several studies have examined the role of early nCPAP in lieu of endotracheal intubation during the first week after birth, there are no studies regarding benefits of the prolonged use of nCPAP in established BPD with chronic respiratory failure. There have been conflicting results concerning whether NIPPV is equal to or superior to nCPAP for supporting infants with evolving BPD. The largest RCT showed no difference in death or incidence of BPD when comparing infants extubated to NIPPV versus nCPAP[191]; however, a meta-analysis suggests that NIPPV may be superior in preventing extubation failure.[192] This will be an ongoing area for investigation. One additional ventilatory strategy, neurally adjusted ventilatory assist, or NAVA, is being used to improve synchronization with the infant. Noninvasive NAVA has been used in infants as young as 24 weeks, but minimal literature currently exists in terms of feasibility and safety for this technology in infants at risk for BPD.[193]

In some infants with BPD, signs of severe respiratory distress persist despite nCPAP or high-flow nasal cannula therapy, including marked dyspnea, head bobbing, retractions, tachypnea, intermittent cyanosis, and CO_2 retention. If subsequent attempts at weaning are not successful, these infants may benefit from reintubation and the consideration of tracheostomy for chronic ventilator support. The timing and patient selection for tracheostomy and the commitment to more prolonged ventilator support are highly variable between centers. Tracheostomy and chronic ventilator support may provide a stable airway to allow for more effective ventilation and less respiratory distress, with enhanced cardiopulmonary function as reflected by lower oxygen requirements and less PH. Greater respiratory stability often improves tolerance of respiratory treatments, physical therapies and handling by staff and family members, thereby improving maternal-infant interaction and neurodevelopmental outcome. Detailed care of ventilator-dependent BPD infants is beyond the scope of this chapter, but successful management requires well-organized, multidisciplinary teams to address the complexity of issues.

DRUG THERAPIES

Multiple pharmacologic therapies have been used in the management of BPD, including diuretics, bronchodilators, and steroids. Despite observations that suggest acute improvement with many of these interventions, data are limited regarding the long-term safety and efficacy of many drugs used in infants with BPD.

DIURETICS

Diuretics improve pulmonary compliance and airway resistance by reducing lung edema. Two Cochrane Systematic Reviews assessed the effects of loop diuretics (furosemide) and those acting on the distal renal tubule (thiazides and spironolactone) for preventing or treating BPD in preterm infants.[194,195] Chronic furosemide therapy can improve oxygenation and lung compliance in infants with BPD.[196] A small study suggested that furosemide (1 mg/kg q12h intravenously or 2 mg/kg q12h orally) can improve weaning from the ventilator when compared with placebo.[197] Thiazides and spironolactone can improve lung function, but this finding has not been consistent.[198,199] Although diuretics generally cause short-term improvements in lung compliance, there is little evidence of sustained reduction in ventilator support, length of hospital stay, or other long-term benefits.

BRONCHODILATORS

Infants with BPD have airway smooth muscle hypertrophy and often have signs of bronchial hyperreactivity that acutely improve with bronchodilator therapy, but response rates are variable.[200,201] Data showing long-term benefit of bronchodilators (including beta agonists and anticholinergic agents) for the prevention or treatment of BPD are lacking. In addition to their roles in apnea, aminophylline and caffeine can reduce airway resistance in infants with BPD and may have an additive effect with diuretics. Methylxanthines can improve

weaning of infants from MV,[202] but side effects such as jitteriness, seizures, and gastroesophageal reflux are recognized. As described earlier, caffeine use has been shown to reduce BPD, PDA, and cerebral palsy.

STEROIDS

Steroids are generally used to reduce lung inflammation in BPD. The use of corticosteroids to prevent BPD has already been discussed. Late systemic glucocorticoids can be used to improve lung mechanics and gas exchange, facilitating earlier extubation. Although commonly used in infants with asthma, inhaled steroids have not consistently showed improvement in lung function in BPD. As discussed earlier regarding BPD prevention, the side effects of poor head growth and neurocognitive outcomes with early and prolonged high-dose strategies are unacceptable risks for preterm infants at risk for BPD. However, steroid bursts (high doses for 3–5 days) may be helpful in the management of BPD infants with acute deterioration of lung function.

ANTIVIRAL IMMUNIZATION

Infants with BPD are at increased risk of recurrent respiratory tract infections, especially those due to respiratory syncytial virus (RSV). Treatment with RSV immunoglobulin or RSV monoclonal antibodies is effective in preventing hospital readmissions. A large multicenter study of palivizumab, a humanized monoclonal antibody against RSV, found that monthly injections of 15 mg/kg for 5 months reduced hospitalization rates for RSV infection by 5% in infants with BPD.[203,204] The American Academy of Pediatrics recommendations include the use of palivizumab or RSV intravenous immunoglobulin prophylaxis for infants and children with BPD during the first year of life during RSV season. Older infants with more severe BPD, with continued oxygen requirement, diuretic requirement, or steroid requirement during the 6 months prior to RSV season, may benefit from prophylaxis for two RSV seasons.[204]

PULMONARY HYPERTENSION

The initial clinical strategy for the management of PH in infants with BPD begins with treating the underlying lung disease. This includes extensive evaluation for chronic reflux and aspiration, structural airway abnormalities (e.g., tonsillar and adenoidal hypertrophy, vocal cord paralysis, subglottic stenosis, and tracheomalacia), assessments of bronchial reactivity, improving lung edema and airway function, and other pulmonary considerations. Periods of acute hypoxia, whether intermittent or prolonged, can often contribute to late PH in BPD. A sleep study may be necessary to determine the presence of noteworthy episodes of hypoxia and whether hypoxemia has predominantly obstructive, central, or mixed causes.

Additional studies that may be required include flexible bronchoscopy for the diagnosis of anatomic and dynamic airway lesions (e.g., tracheomalacia) that may contribute to hypoxemia and poor clinical responses to oxygen therapy. An upper gastrointestinal series, pH or impedance probe, and swallow study may be indicated to evaluate for gastroesophageal reflux and aspiration that can contribute to ongoing lung injury. If the findings are positive or even if clinical suspicion remains high in the face of negative findings and in the setting of lung disease that fails to improve, consideration should be given to gastrostomy tube placement and fundoplication. For patients with BPD and severe PH who fail to maintain near-normal ventilation or require high levels of FiO_2 despite conservative treatment, consideration should be given to chronic MV support.

Despite the growing use of pulmonary vasodilator therapy for the treatment of PH in BPD, data demonstrating efficacy are extremely limited; the use of these agents should only follow thorough diagnostic evaluations and aggressive management of the underlying lung disease. We strongly encourage cardiac catheterization prior to the initiation of chronic therapy. Current therapies used for PH therapy in infants with BPD generally include inhaled NO, sildenafil, endothelin-receptor antagonists (ETRAs), and calcium channel blockers. Calcium channel blockers (e.g., nifedipine) benefit some patients with PH, and short-term benefits of these blockers in infants with BPD have been reported.[205] In comparison with an acute study of iNO reactivity in infants with BPD, the acute response to calcium channel blockers was poor, and some infants developed systemic hypotension. We generally use sildenafil or bosentan (an ETRA) for chronic therapy of PH in infants with BPD. Sildenafil, a highly selective type 5 phosphodiesterase (PDE-5) inhibitor, augments cyclic GMP content in vascular smooth muscle. It has been shown to benefit adults with PH as monotherapy and in combination with standard treatment regimens.[206] In a study of 25 infants with chronic lung disease and PH (18 with BPD), prolonged sildenafil therapy as part of an aggressive program to treat PH was associated with improvement in PH by echocardiogram in most (88%) patients without significant rates of adverse events.[207] Although the time to improvement was variable, many patients were able to wean off mechanical ventilator support and other PH therapies, especially iNO, during the course of sildenafil treatment without worsening of PH.

The recommended starting dose for sildenafil is 0.5 mg/kg per dose every 8 hours. If there is no evidence of systemic hypotension, this dose can gradually be increased over 2 weeks to achieve the desired pulmonary hemodynamic effect or a maximum of 2 mg/kg per dose every 6–8 hours. Data are largely lacking on other agents (e.g., ETRAs and prostacyclin analogues) in BPD infants who fail to respond to other approaches.

Prognosis

Most follow-up data have been obtained from patients from the presurfactant era. Approximately 50% of infants with BPD will require hospital readmission during early childhood for respiratory distress, particularly if they develop respiratory syncytial virus (RSV) infection.[208] Importantly, late readmissions are not exclusively a problem of preterm infants with BPD; increased rehospitalizations, including the need for intensive care, are also observed in late preterm infants without BPD.[209] This high rate of hospitalization generally declines during the second and third years of life,[210] but lung function studies often show limited reserve even in patients with minimal overt respiratory signs.[211] This observation

likely explains the severity of presentation in some infants with BPD after acquiring RSV or other infections.

Infants with severe BPD often develop chronic obstructive pulmonary disease (COPD), but impaired flows may reflect disproportionate or abnormal growth patterns between airways and the distal lung. In the majority of BPD infants, lung growth and remodeling during infancy results in progressive improvement of gas exchange, lung function, and level of oxygen therapy; few BPD patients remain oxygen-dependent beyond 2 years of age. Lung function is usually in the low-normal range by 2–3 years of age, but air flow abnormalities may remain. Infants with BPD have reduced absolute and size-corrected flow rates in comparison with age- and size-matched control patients, suggesting poor airway growth with age. Filipone and colleagues have reported a strong correlation between V_{max} FRC at 2 years of age with FEV_1 at school age, suggesting persistent air flow limitation in selected patients with BPD.[211]

Although pulmonary function in most survivors with BPD improves over time and permits normal activity, abnormalities detected by pulmonary function testing often persist through adolescence, including increased airway resistance and reactivity.[212] Unfortunately, comprehensive longitudinal studies of the pulmonary course and lung function of adult patients with a previous history of premature birth are lacking. More studies are needed to determine the long-term respiratory course of premature neonates, with or without severe BPD, and their relative contribution to the growing adult population with COPD.

Summary

Nearly 40 years after its original description, BPD has changed. However, it remains a significant complication of premature birth and is a persistent challenge for the future. BPD has evolved from the classical stages described initially to a disease characterized largely by inhibition of lung development. Future strategies that improve long-term outcomes will depend on successful integration of basic research on the fundamental mechanisms of lung development and response to injury, will incorporate precision medicine to apply targeted therapies given the heterogeneity of etiologies contributing to BPD, and will test novel interventions to lower the occurrence and severity of the cardiopulmonary sequelae of BPD.

References

Access the reference list online at ExpertConsult.com.

Suggested Reading

Abman SH, Collaco JM, Keszler M, et al; for the BPD Collaborative. Interdisciplinary Care of Children with Severe Bronchopulmonary Dysplasia. *J Pediatr.* 2017;181:12–28.e1.

Isayama T, Chair-Adisaksopha C, McDonald SD. Noninvasive ventilation with vs without early surfactant to prevent chronic lung disease in preterm infants: a systemic review and meta-analysis. *JAMA Pediatr.* 2015; 169(8):731–739.

Islam JY, Keller RL, Aschner JL, et al. Understanding the short- and long-term respiratory outcomes of prematurity and bronchopulmonary dysplasia. *Am J Respir Crit Care Med.* 2015;192(2):134–156.

Lal CV, Ambalavanan N. Genetic predisposition to bronchopulmonary dysplasia. *Semin Perinatol.* 2015;39(8):584–591.

Maitre NL, Ballard RA, Ellenberg JH, et al. Respiratory consequences of prematurity: evolution of a diagnosis and development of a comprehensive approach. *J Perinatol.* 2015;35:313–321.

Manja V, Lakshminrushimha S, Cook DJ. Oxygen saturation target range for extremely preterm infants: a systemic review and meta-analysis. *JAMA Pediatr.* 2015;169(4):332–340.

Manley BJ, Owen LS. High-flow nasal cannula: mechanisms, evidence and recommendations. *Semin Fetal Neonatal Med.* 2016;21:139–145.

Poindexter BB, Feng R, Schmidt B, et al. Comparisons and limitations of current definitions of bronchopulmonary dysplasia for the prematurity and respiratory outcomes program. *Ann Am Thorac Soc.* 2015;12:1822–1830.

Stoll BJ, Hansen HI, Bell EF, et al. Trends in care practices, morbidity, and mortality of extremely preterm neonates, 1993-2012. *JAMA.* 2015;314(10):1039–1051.

21 *Children Dependent on Respiratory Technology*

HOWARD B. PANITCH, MD

Introduction

Children who require technology for chronic respiratory insufficiency or failure constitute a small but varied group. The US Congress's Office of Technology Assessment (OTA) defines a technology-dependent child as "one who needs both a medical device to compensate for the loss of a vital body function and substantial and ongoing nursing care to avert death or further disability."[1] This definition does not take into account either site of care (hospital, home, or skilled facility) or credentials of the caregiver (professional nurse or trained layperson). Further, the OTA identifies four separate groups of children that would be considered technology-dependent. Two of these include children dependent on mechanical ventilation for at least part of the day and children dependent on other device-based respiratory support such as tracheostomy tubes, airway suctioning, and the use of supplemental oxygen. This chapter discusses only those children requiring technology for the treatment of chronic respiratory failure, a condition for which mechanical ventilatory support is required for at least 4 hours/day for a month or longer.[2,3]

Epidemiology

The large-scale need for chronic respiratory support of children began with the polio epidemics of the 1930s, 1940s, and 1950s. The development of subspecialties in neonatology and pediatric critical care in the 1960s resulted in advances in medical therapies that allowed children with previously fatal conditions to survive, albeit occasionally with chronic conditions such as respiratory failure.[4] A focus on pediatric chronic respiratory failure did not occur in the United States until the early 1980s. In 1981, President Ronald Reagan waived the eligibility rules for Supplemental Security Income to allow Katie Beckett, a ventilator-dependent child, to be cared for at home without losing Medicaid benefits, thus bringing the population of children with chronic respiratory failure into the national spotlight.[5] In 1982, the surgeon general then convened the Workshop on Children with Handicaps and Their Families, where he noted that advances in medical interventions created a new type of disability: infants chronically dependent on ventilatory support as a result of other medical interventions, which he referred to as "a creature of our new technology."[6]

The causes of chronic dependency on mechanical ventilation or supplemental oxygen can be categorized as (1) those that affect the respiratory pump (respiratory muscles, rib cage, ventral abdominal wall); (2) those that affect respiratory drive; (3) extrathoracic and central airway lesions; and (4) pulmonary parenchymal and vascular abnormalities (Table 21.1). Individual patients can have more than one cause for chronic ventilator dependency (i.e., neuromuscular weakness and severe kyphoscoliosis, or anoxic encephalopathy with abnormal respiratory drive, recurrent aspiration, and obstructive sleep apnea).

In the United States, there is no national registry that tracks the population of ventilator-assisted individuals. Center-specific surveys of children cared for in acute pediatric hospitals in the 1980s demonstrated that bronchopulmonary dysplasia (BPD) and noncardiac congenital anomalies were the most common diagnoses of infants and toddlers who required prolonged mechanical ventilation,[7–9] whereas spinal cord injury and underlying neuromuscular diseases were more common among those cared for in rehabilitation facilities.[10] In Massachusetts, surveys of children receiving chronic mechanical ventilatory support outside of acute care hospitals showed that the chief cause of chronic respiratory failure (CRF) was sequelae of prematurity or congenital malformations in the 1980s[11] and early 1990s.[12] However, over the next 15 years the major causes of CRF became neuromuscular disease and central nervous system injury or malformations.[13] In addition, the number of children receiving such care outside a hospital had nearly tripled from 1990 to 2005.[13] National surveys from Canada, Europe, and Japan have similarly demonstrated that neuromuscular disease and central nervous system injuries are the most common indications for chronic ventilation in children.[14–22] This probably reflects a philosophical change toward providing chronic respiratory support to patients with progressive neuromuscular disorders,[23,24] an increasing role of noninvasive ventilation for these patients,[25] and a reflection of the types of patients most commonly requiring prolonged care in pediatric intensive care units.[26]

The prevalence of children requiring chronic mechanical ventilation has grown over the last three decades. In 1987, the OTA estimated that there were between 600 and 2000 ventilator-dependent children in the United States.[1] Ten years later, extrapolations of a survey from Minnesota estimated that there were 17,824 ventilator-assisted individuals in the United States, of whom 5534 would be below 21 years of age.[25] It was also shown that subjects below 20 years of age represented about one-third of all ventilator-assisted individuals in the state, with those below age 11 years being the largest group and those between 11 and 20 years accounting for the greatest increase since the prior survey of 1992. This survey included only patients in whom a backup ventilator rate was used; thus the number was likely an underestimate. In the 1990s, the prevalence of children requiring chronic mechanical ventilation was estimated to be 0.5 per 100,000 in the United Kingdom,[16] 0.68 per 100,000 in Japan[18] and 1.2–1.5 per 100,000 in the United States.[9,27] Extrapolating

Table 21.1 Conditions Leading to Technology Dependence

Respiratory pump	■ Neuromuscular diseases ■ Chest wall deformity/ kyphoscoliosis ■ Spinal cord injury ■ Prune-belly syndrome
Respiratory drive	■ Congenital central hypoventilation syndrome ■ Brain/brainstem injury ■ Central nervous system tumors ■ Metabolic disorders
Airway	■ Craniofacial malformations ■ Obstructive sleep apnea ■ Tracheomalacia ■ Bronchomalacia
Pulmonary parenchymal and vascular problems	■ Chronic lung disease of infancy (bronchopulmonary dysplasia) ■ Lung hypoplasia ■ Recurrent aspiration syndromes ■ Cystic fibrosis ■ Congenital heart disease

data from Massachusetts[13] and Pennsylvania.[28] King estimated the prevalence of ventilator-assisted children cared for at home in the United States in 2010 to be 4.7–6.4 per 100,000.[29] Recent international prevalence rates of home mechanical ventilation in children below 18 years of age are similar, ranging from 4.2 to 6.7 per 100,000.[30,31] The method of mechanical ventilation has changed over time as well, with most recent surveys demonstrating a marked rise in the percentage of children supported by noninvasive ventilation and far fewer receiving ventilation via tracheostomy.[17,32–34] The overall increase in prevalence of ventilator-dependent children cared for at home is likely multifactorial, reflecting advances in the medical care of critically ill children, improved technology in home equipment and pediatric noninvasive interfaces, increased use of polysomnography in children to detect nocturnal hypoventilation and philosophical changes in the willingness of physicians to apply these technologies to children with progressive diseases.

Goals of Therapy

The objectives of technology dependence support are largely independent of the cause of respiratory failure. They include reversing or ameliorating the cause of respiratory compromise, extending life, improving physiologic function, and reducing morbidity.[35] In infants and young children, respiratory failure can also be associated with slow growth and developmental delay; therefore chronic ventilatory support is sometimes used to avoid these consequences. Occasionally, ventilatory support is augmented during periods of physical activity to promote the child's potential for rehabilitation, or it may be increased if the child fails to maintain adequate growth velocity. Thus in formulating the daily prescription for mechanical ventilation, the desire to reduce support must be balanced with a more global view of the child's needs.

Psychosocial development and quality of life can be enhanced when chronic ventilatory support is safely accomplished outside the intensive care unit.[36] The home setting

has long been considered the best place for technology dependent children in terms of their psychological and somatic development,[7,37,38] but excellent medical, psychosocial, and developmental support, including weaning from mechanical ventilation when appropriate, can be safely accomplished in inpatient rehabilitation facilities (within or outside the acute care hospital).[39–42] The setting for postacute care will depend on the degree of medical stability of the patient, the willingness and ability of family caregivers to provide care in the home, and community resources. Although the number of ventilator-dependent children has increased over the years and home care of this population has become more common, it should never be assumed de facto that home care is the best setting for an individual child or family. This can be concluded only once a full assessment of the child, family, resources, home care setting, and available alternative settings has been made. Additionally, the best location might change throughout a child's course—for instance, as the child's medical condition improves or worsens, or if caregiver availability changes.

PATHOPHYSIOLOGY OF RESPIRATORY FAILURE

Respiratory failure can result from an imbalance between the output of the respiratory pump and the load against which it has to work, development of respiratory muscle fatigue, inadequate respiratory drive, pulmonary parenchymal disease or pulmonary vascular disease.[43] The disparity between the abilities of the respiratory pump and its load refer to either inadequate pump output for the imposed load, as in the case of a child with respiratory muscle weakness, or an increased load for the output. This could be the result of a reduction in lung compliance, an increase in pulmonary resistance, or stiffening of the chest wall itself. In theory, "pump failure" results in hypercapnia, whereas parenchymal disease causes hypoxemia. In practice, however, the two often coexist, and hypoventilation from pump failure will result in hypoxemia. An understanding of the causes of respiratory failure often provides a rationale for the type of assisted ventilation that will provide the best support for the individual. It is critical to recognize that although chronic mechanical ventilation will not alter the ultimate prognosis for chronic progressive disorders like Duchenne muscular dystrophy, spinal muscular atrophy (SMA), or cystic fibrosis, its use can still prolong survival, relieve dyspnea, and improve daytime function and quality of life for children with such disorders.

INADEQUATE PUMP OUTPUT (E.G., NEUROMUSCULAR DISEASE, SPINAL CORD INJURY)

There is a typical progression of respiratory morbidity in patients with neuromuscular disease (NMD).[44] Once weakness of respiratory muscles is present, airway clearance becomes compromised, predisposing patients to recurrent episodes of lower respiratory tract infections and atelectasis. This results in a decrease in lung compliance and therefore an increase in the load against which the respiratory pump must work. Infants and young children with NMD are more likely to experience complications from mucus plugging because their airways are smaller and peripheral airways contribute a greater proportion of intrathoracic resistance in children under 5 years.[45] Early in childhood, the chest wall of children with NMD is abnormally compliant[46]; as a result, the effect of chest wall recoil on lung volume and airway caliber is reduced, and this contributes to intrathoracic airway narrowing.

There are also ventilatory consequences of this alteration of chest wall compliance. In the young child with neuromuscular weakness and a highly compliant chest wall, much of the work of the respiratory muscles can be wasted as chest wall retractions reduce the contribution of the thoracic compartment to ventilation. Contraction of intercostal muscles can help to maintain tidal volume, but at the cost of increased respiratory energy expenditure; thus adequate ventilation can be maintained, but growth failure might ensue. In very young children, the imbalance between the highly compliant chest wall and relatively stiff lungs can result in an acquired pectus excavatum deformity.[47–49] Acquired chest wall deformity like this has led to the theoretical concern that when chronic low-volume breathing is present in infants, it can also impair lung growth and development,[50] although this has never been demonstrated. Nevertheless, noninvasive ventilation has been used to correct or prevent the development of pectus excavatum in young children with NMD.[47–49]

Over time, the chest wall of subjects with neuromuscular weakness becomes stiffer than normal because of prolonged periods of low-tidal-volume breathing without deep sigh breaths. This leads to the development of ankylosis around costovertebral joints, with stiffening of ligaments and tendons. When present, the progression of kyphoscoliosis will contribute to a mechanical disadvantage around the costovertebral joint, making the respiratory muscles less efficient. The sum of these imbalances results in a restrictive pattern of lung function, with reduced vital capacity and total lung capacity. If subjects have significant expiratory muscle weakness, however, the residual volume and functional residual capacity can be normal or even slightly elevated, because the rib cage cannot be reduced below its normal resting volume.

As weakness progresses, patients experience episodes of hypoventilation during sleep, especially during rapid-eye-movement (REM) sleep. Obstructive apnea can also occur because of weakness of the bulbar musculature or physical features of certain neuromuscular diseases such as macroglossia, retrognathia or flattening of the malar eminences.[51] When respiratory muscle weakness becomes sufficiently severe to cause hypoventilation during sleep, the patient will compensate with an arousal response. This protective mechanism causes sleep disruption and fragmentation, poor sleep quality, and reduced sleep time.[44] These phenomena, in turn, can cause daytime somnolence and fatigue as well as poor school performance.[52] Initially, patients will demonstrate hypercapnia during sleep, but they will be able to maintain normocapnia while awake. As the severity of sleep-disordered breathing increases, either because of prolonged periods of nocturnal hypoventilation, mechanical alterations of the respiratory system or both, central drive becomes blunted and the patient does not respond in an appropriate way to the challenge of elevated $PaCO_2$. At this point, diurnal hypercapnia will occur, but the daytime hypercapnia can be corrected if nocturnal mechanical support of breathing is instituted.[53] Further progression of weakness, however, will result in ineffective ventilation during the day and diurnal hypercapnia, even when nocturnal ventilation has been instituted.[54]

Timing of the progression of respiratory failure varies with different NMDs. In the absence of ventilatory support, infants with SMA who are unable to sit typically die by 2 years of age.[55] Boys with Duchenne muscular dystrophy, in contrast, do not exhibit respiratory compromise until their second decade of life. Respiratory muscle weakness in congenital myopathies is often static, but as children grow, their status may deteriorate because the respiratory muscles cannot compensate for the increase in body mass. Respiratory failure often ensues during the pubertal growth spurt. Some disorders, like myotonic dystrophy or myelomeningocele with Chiari malformation, are associated with primary disorders of ventilatory control.[56,57]

Paralysis of the diaphragm results from cervical injury above C-3 or from phrenic nerve injury, often in the setting of birth trauma, cardiac surgery or other thoracic surgery. Infants can occasionally compensate for unilateral paralysis, but bilateral diaphragmatic paralysis requires ventilatory support. When unilateral diaphragmatic paralysis causes respiratory failure, plication of the affected diaphragm often improves ventilation sufficiently that mechanical support is not required. If the paralysis is the result of trauma, plication does not prohibit recovery of function of the diaphragm.

ABNORMAL RESPIRATORY PUMP (E.G., EARLY-ONSET SCOLIOSIS, ASPHYXIATING THORACIC DYSTROPHY, SEVERE KYPHOSIS)

The respiratory pump itself can present a load too great to be overcome by the muscles of respiration. Distortion of the thoracic cage from early-onset scoliosis results in a restrictive pattern of lung function.[58,59] A reduction in chest wall compliance can occur when ribs are congenitally fused, the intercostal muscles are replaced by fibroconnective tissue after years of disuse or when costovertebral joints become ankylosed from chronic low-tidal-volume breathing without sigh breaths. Alternatively, distortion of the thoracic cage can place the inspiratory muscles at sufficient mechanical disadvantage that their force-generating ability is compromised. Then the thoracic compartment is noncompliant, and the majority of the volume change that occurs with ventilation is in the abdominal compartment. *Thoracic insufficiency syndrome* is a term used to describe conditions where the thorax cannot support normal ventilation or lung growth.[60] Since the volume of the thorax is small in these patients, tidal volume targets during mechanical ventilation are smaller as well.

ABNORMAL RESPIRATORY DRIVE (E.G., CONGENITAL CENTRAL HYPOVENTILATION SYNDROME, CHIARI MALFORMATION, BRAIN STEM LESIONS, LEIGH DISEASE)

Several rare disorders result in an abnormal response to hypercapnia and hypoxemia. Congenital central hypoventilation syndrome (CCHS) represents a failure of autonomic control of breathing; it is caused by a defect in the paired homeobox 2B *(PHOX2B)* gene, which produces a transcription factor essential to migration of neural crest cells and development of the autonomic nervous system.[61–63] There is a range of ventilatory abnormalities in children with CCHS, so that some children present in the neonatal period with chronic alveolar hypoventilation, requiring around-the-clock ventilatory support, while others may not present until adulthood.[63] Often, as infants grow older, they are able to breathe adequately without support while awake but require ventilatory assistance during sleep and with acute illnesses. Because patients with CCHS do not respond appropriately to hypoxemia or hypercarbia, their mechanical ventilation strategy requires a mandatory rate to assure adequate ventilation. Since the underlying lung parenchyma and chest wall are normal, the delivered tidal volume should be normal as well.

Prader Willi syndrome and rapid onset obesity with hypothalamic dysfunction, hypoventilation, and autonomic dysregulation (ROHHAD) represent two other disorders associated with potentially severe hypoventilation.[61,62] The majority of children with Prader-Willi syndrome have a deletion of the long arm of chromosome 15, whereas the genetic abnormality leading to ROHHAD is currently unknown. Both conditions are associated with hyperphagia and the rapid onset of obesity, but children with ROHHAD also have problems with salt and water balance. The presence of obesity in both conditions can also cause obstructive sleep apnea and contribute to sleep-related hypoventilation. Obesity hypoventilation syndrome—defined as a body mass index (BMI) greater than 30 kg/m^2, daytime hypercapnia and hypoxemia, and sleep-disordered breathing—is another cause of respiratory failure in children,[64] although its pathophysiology is not well understood.

Children with Chiari malformation demonstrate a blunted response to hypercapnia, suggesting a central chemoreceptor problem.[62] They may also have both central and obstructive apnea during sleep. Thus assuring adequate minute ventilation and providing necessary distending pressure to overcome upper airway obstruction are both important strategies in supporting these patients. If the Chiari malformation is accompanied by myelomeningocele and kyphoscoliosis, adjustment of the tidal volume will be necessary.

PARENCHYMAL LUNG OR INTRATHORACIC AIRWAY DISEASE (BRONCHOPULMONARY DYSPLASIA, CYSTIC FIBROSIS, TRACHEOMALACIA, BRONCHIECTASIS)

The majority of children in this category of respiratory failure are those with chronic sequelae of neonatal lung disease. Approximately 1.5% of all newborns develop bronchopulmonary dysplasia (BPD) (chronic lung disease of infancy),[65] making it the most common cause of chronic obstructive lung disease among infants. A recent point prevalence study showed that 36.5% of infants hospitalized in eight tertiary referral neonatal intensive care units fulfilled criteria for severe BPD, defined as those born after less than 32 weeks' gestation and receiving ≥30% or more supplemental oxygen and/or positive pressure ventilation at 36 weeks postmenstrual age (PMA).[66] Among the infants with severe BPD, 41% were still supported by positive pressure ventilation at 36 weeks PMA, suggesting that they are at greater risk to

require prolonged mechanical ventilation.[67] BPD is associated with lung hypoplasia resulting from the arrest of alveolar development, but there is also evidence of parenchymal scarring, air trapping and distortion of lung architecture. The central airways can become deformed from cyclic positive pressure distension, leading to acquired tracheomalacia or bronchomalacia. These abnormalities lead to a decrease in lung compliance and conductance, increasing the respiratory pump load. Severe air trapping can impair diaphragm contractility by altering its length-tension relationships. These can all result in an unfavorable balance between respiratory pump output and load, leading to chronic respiratory failure and a need for prolonged mechanical ventilation. The energetics of breathing may comprise as much as 25% of the infant's caloric needs. Thus, if weaning from mechanical ventilation is too aggressive, some infants with BPD can maintain adequate gas exchange, but only at the expense of growth and development. The need for supplemental oxygen will depend on the extent of parenchymal damage, hypoplasia, or ventilation/perfusion mismatch. Most infants with BPD who require chronic mechanical ventilation develop respiratory failure while in the neonatal intensive care unit and do not recover before the time when they are otherwise considered ready for discharge. Occasionally, however, chronic respiratory failure ensues after discharge in the setting of an acute viral lower respiratory illness. Prolonged mechanical ventilation is appropriate in both settings, as lung function is expected to improve with growth and postnatal lung development.

In recent years chronic mechanical ventilation of patients with cystic fibrosis (CF) has been performed, first as a bridge to lung transplant and subsequently as a palliative measure. Like other patients whose respiratory pump becomes inadequate for the load, patients with CF and severe airway obstruction develop a rapid, shallow breathing pattern that is inefficient.[68,69] When challenged with an increased load or imposed hypercapnia, the mechanics of the respiratory system limit the patient's response.[68–70] As obstruction worsens, dynamic compliance of the lung falls as well, contributing to an increased respiratory load.[69] At the same time, downward displacement of the diaphragm from hyperinflation places it in a less favorable mechanical position, contributing to inefficiency of the respiratory pump.

General Considerations for Home Care

Often, the need for chronic mechanical ventilatory support is determined following an acute illness, when the child is unable to wean from mechanical ventilation. In other children, the requirement for chronic mechanical ventilation is recognized following an abnormal polysomnogram or identification of other nonacute indicators such as poor growth or chronic dyspnea. No matter the presentation, once it has been decided that chronic mechanical ventilation is necessary for the support of a child, the eventual site of long-term care must be determined. This requires assessment not only of the medical stability and suitability of the child but also of the family as potential medical caregivers. Other decisions regarding the approach to the child's care (e.g., the performance

Table 21.2 Criteria for Medical Stability

Home	General Hospital Ward/ Transitional Care Facility
CLINICAL	
Positive trend on growth curve	No need for 1:1 nursing care
Stamina for periods of play	No invasive monitoring
No frequent fevers or infections	No need for intravenous vasopressors or vasodilators
PHYSIOLOGIC	
Stable airway	Mature tracheostomy ≥ 1 week postoperatively
PaO_2 ≥60 torr in FiO_2 ≤0.4	SpO_2 >92% in FiO_2 ≤0.40
$PaCO_2$ <50 torr (parenchymal disease) or <45 torr (chest wall or neuromuscular disease)	Stable blood gases within normal range for the diagnosis
No need for frequent ventilator setting changes	Stable ventilator settings ≥1 week

Modified from Make BJ, Hill NS, Goldberg AI, et al. Mechanical ventilation beyond the intensive care unit. Report of a consensus conference of the American College of Chest Physicians. *Chest* 1998;113:289S-344S and Ambrosio IU, Woo MS, Jansen MT, Keens TG. Safety of hospitalized ventilator-dependent children outside of the intensive care unit. *Pediatrics* 1998;101:257-259.

of a tracheostomy) require careful consideration as to how the choice of the child's site of care will be affected.

A child's medical stability must be evaluated within the context of the site of care. The required level of stability at the time of transfer from a pediatric intensive care unit (PICU) will differ between home and a care site within a hospital or a subacute care facility (Table 21.2).[35,39] In any setting, the child must have a stable airway (natural or tracheostomy), have blood gas values that are appropriate for the underlying diagnosis, and not have care demands that exceed the resources of the site of care. When a child goes home supported by mechanical ventilation for the first time, there should be no changes in the medical plan for at least 1 week before discharge to assure that the child is adequately supported on the proposed regimen. In addition, any change to the medical regimen within 1 week of the initial hospital discharge has been associated with unanticipated readmission within 1 month of the child's going home.[71]

When a technology-dependent child is being discharged to home, two adults must be willing and able to learn and assume all aspects of the child's daily care, including dosages and indications for all medications being used, feedings, respiratory assessment, ventilator assessment and troubleshooting, and equipment care.[72] For children with weak or ineffective cough, caregivers must learn various techniques of airway clearance to avoid atelectasis or treat acute illnesses. If the child will receive mechanical ventilation through a tracheostomy, the family caregivers must also learn how to suction the artificial airway and perform routine and emergency tracheostomy tube changes. In addition, there must be adequate financial support from third-party payers to provide the equipment and supplies necessary to care for the child at home. The residence in which the child will be cared for must have adequate space for the child, equipment, and visiting health care providers. The home must have running water, heat, electricity and a working telephone. Entrances must be accessible for a patient confined to a wheelchair.

The amount of skilled nursing care the family will require must also be included in the discharge plan. All families of children who cannot correct an airway or ventilator problem, or call for help, should be offered skilled nursing care for at least a portion of the day to allow caregivers to sleep with the reassurance that the child's welfare is not at risk. Funding for those services, which are the most expensive component of the home care of technology-dependent children,[2] should be guaranteed by third-party payers with periodic reassessments established to determine ongoing needs. In some health care systems outside of the United States, personal care attendants rather than nurses are funded to perform some of these services and to facilitate the patient's full participation in society at a lower cost.[73,74] Although there are no uniform criteria for establishing the number of nursing hours provided, this should be determined by the medical needs of the child, the capabilities of the family, and other demands on family providers (work, other children in the home, etc.). Funded respite care, to allow caregivers time off from continuous medical care and monitoring of the child, should also be built into the discharge plan, as this has repeatedly been identified as an essential component to help relieve stress and caregiver burnout.[75-80]

Treatment of Chronic Respiratory Failure

NONINVASIVE VENTILATION

Noninvasive ventilation (NIV) refers to correction of alveolar hypoventilation or upper airway obstruction without the use of artificial airways (endotracheal or tracheostomy tubes). It is usually used at night, rather than continuously, but if a child has a progressive disorder or experiences an acute decompensation, NIV can be used 24 hours/day.[81] For patients with NMD or chest wall restriction who develop symptomatic hypercapnic respiratory failure, 4 hours or more of nocturnal NIV per day can cause a sustained decrease in daytime $PaCO_2$ and resolution of symptoms related to sleep-disordered breathing.[82] For instance, nocturnal NIV corrected diurnal hypercapnia and severe nocturnal hypoventilation and maintained normal daytime $PaCO_2$ for an extended period in a group of 23 young men with Duchenne muscular dystrophy.[83] In this series, nocturnal NIV was associated not only with improved survival (85% at 1 year, and 73% from 2 through 5 years) but also with sustained improvement in daytime gas exchange throughout the 5-year duration of the study.

The proposed mechanisms by which nocturnal NIV improves overall function in patients with restrictive disorders include resting of the respiratory muscles to reverse fatigue,[84] improving lung and chest wall mechanics by reversing areas of microatelectasis, increasing chest wall excursion[82,85-88] and resetting central chemoreceptor sensitivity to CO_2.[82,85] These mechanisms are not necessarily mutually exclusive, but evidence that NIV improves lung or chest wall mechanics in a sustained way is lacking. Several series involving subjects with a variety of neuromuscular diseases failed to demonstrate an increase in vital capacity after the institution of NIV,[82,85-87] and the institution of NIV in young men with Duchenne muscular dystrophy before the onset of respiratory failure failed to slow the expected decline in vital capacity.[88] It may be that episodic chest inflations closer to total lung capacity, or "lung volume recruitment maneuvers," are required to alter the decline in vital capacity.[89,90] Furthermore, direct measurements of lung and chest wall compliance after 3 months of NIV did not change in a series of 20 patients with neuromuscular disease and restrictive defects.[82] By contrast, the investigators demonstrated enhanced responsiveness to CO_2 in these subjects after 3 months of NIV, suggesting a resetting of central chemoreceptors and enhancement of respiratory drive. Another study showed that nocturnal NIV can restore CO_2 responsiveness by an alternate method: reduction of respiratory muscle fatigue and improvement in respiratory muscle endurance.[54] Investigators calculated the tension time index of the respiratory muscles, a noninvasive measurement of the likelihood of muscle fatigue, in 50 subjects with Duchenne muscular dystrophy just after they ended a night of NIV support (8 a.m.) and again just before they resumed nocturnal NIV (8 p.m.). To assess respiratory muscle endurance, the authors also measured the time to fatigue (T_{lim}) after pressure threshold loading under the same conditions. There was a progressive increase in the tension time index and a decrease in T_{lim} that correlated with the progression of symptoms. In the most affected subjects, however, the tension time index decreased and T_{lim} increased significantly following a night of NIV support. Thus these data suggest that nocturnal NIV can unload weakened respiratory muscles, thereby improving their daytime capacity and reducing their fatigability.

Although noninvasive ventilation is usually confined to those who require support for 16 hours/day or less, it has been used successfully in patients who require continuous support.[81,91] This can be achieved either by a nasal interface or by mouthpiece.[81,91,92] Contraindications include poor glottic function, inability to achieve adequate ventilation noninvasively, patient preference, and lack of caregiver expertise.[81] However, sometimes NIV has been used successfully in infants with SMA and children with static encephalopathy who have impaired glottic function.[93] The use of NIV has been recommended by some over ventilation via tracheostomy for palliation of dyspnea in severely affected infants with SMA type I.[55]

Complications of positive-pressure NIV are related to either the interface itself or misdirection of the applied pressure. Choices of nasal or oronasal interfaces for infants and small children are limited, so adaptation of adult interfaces is often necessary.[94] Poorly fitting interfaces lead to leaks that not only interfere with adequacy of ventilation but also can cause eye irritation. In response, straps are often tightened to reduce the leak. This can cause facial erythema and skin ulceration.[95,96] Use of a custom-molded mask[95,97] or an alternate interface with different pressure points can reduce this complication, but attention to skin integrity is an integral component of care of the child receiving positive-pressure NIV. Skin ulceration can preclude the ability to provide effective NIV and force a decision to advance to tracheostomy. Prolonged application of pressure by nasal interfaces on the growing face has been associated with midface flattening.[95,98,99] Although special devices have been created to correct this,[99] use of more than one interface with different pressure points or a custom-molded mask[100] should be considered.

High flows related to NIV can cause nasal congestion and mouth dryness[101]; these deleterious side effects can be ameliorated by humidifying the circuit. The positive pressure applied during NIV has been associated with ear and sinus pain in adults[102] and retrograde lacrimal duct flow in children,[103] and higher positive pressures can cause aerophagia. Gastric distension, in turn, can impair the effectiveness of NIV by creating abdominal competition for lung expansion.

VENTILATION VIA TRACHEOSTOMY

Invasive ventilation via tracheostomy is typically used in infants and children with parenchymal lung or congenital heart disease. In addition it is used in young children who require continuous mechanical ventilation, those with severe craniofacial malformations (or other causes of upper airway or central airway obstruction that cannot be corrected by NIV) and those with severe developmental delay.[3,8,104] Whenever possible, relatively small tracheostomy tubes are used to allow for a leak[35,105]: this facilitates speech and avoids damage to the tracheal wall. When leak around the tracheostomy tube is large, however, effective mechanical ventilation can be compromised. This is especially true if the child is being ventilated in a volume-control mode, since the large leak will prevent adequate development of intrathoracic pressure to expand the chest because the ventilator breath escapes through the mouth and nose. The leak may be variable, so that even when mechanical ventilation is adequate during awake hours, significant hypoventilation can occur during sleep.[106] This is remedied either by changing to a pressure-control mode of ventilation or by using a cuffed tracheostomy tube.

The presence of a tracheostomy increases the complexity of care for most patients requiring ventilatory assistance. Caregivers must be taught how to suction, clean and change the tracheostomy tube and how to assess for displacement and obstruction.[105] The presence of a tracheostomy tube interferes with the child's speech and swallowing, increases risk for infection and aspiration and is associated with airway complications such as infection at the stoma site, granuloma formation, tracheal stenosis and traumatic tracheoinnominate or tracheoesophageal fistula formation.[107–109] Although the presence of a tracheostomy alone can increase caregiver stress,[110] in some situations (such as the need for continuous ventilatory assistance and difficulty with secretion management in a young child) it can ease the burden of care. Thus the decision to advance from noninvasive to invasive ventilation must be individualized, considering the impact on both the child and the child's caregivers.

OPTIONS FOR VENTILATORY SUPPORT

Body Ventilators

Initially, negative-pressure body ventilators were used to augment the ventilatory efforts of patients with restrictive lung disease.[102] Devices like the iron lung (tank ventilator), chest shell, poncho and cuirass ventilators can all successfully reverse respiratory failure in children.[102,111,112] Negative-pressure body ventilators, however, are cumbersome and can cause upper airway obstruction.[102,112,113] This may result from phasic collapse of the epiglottis or a lack of preinspiratory upper airway muscle activation before the ventilator supplies a negative-pressure breath.[114,115] Negative-pressure ventilators are difficult to get into and out of; thus they are not well suited for subjects who require frequent access for care. They are not portable, so the user cannot readily travel or sleep at other people's homes. Nevertheless, a negative-pressure ventilator can be an excellent alternative for the patient who cannot tolerate placement of a nasal device or the sensation of nasal positive pressure. Positive-pressure body ventilators, like the pneumobelt, are used to only a limited degree in children. The pneumobelt must be used while the patient is in a seated position so it is not suitable for the treatment of nocturnal hypoventilation.

Positive-Pressure Devices

The most common way for children to receive ventilatory assistance noninvasively is by positive pressure delivered via nasal, oronasal or mouthpiece interfaces. Application of positive pressure can relieve upper airway obstruction as well as improve minute ventilation and unload inspiratory muscles. The source of positive pressure can be a portable volume- or pressure-preset ventilator, bilevel positive-airway-pressure (B$_i$PAP) device, or continuous positive-airway pressure (CPAP) device. B$_i$PAP and CPAP devices use a blower to generate flow adequate to achieve the desired pressure set by the practitioner. Portable ventilators use pistons or turbines to generate the selected volume or pressure and can do so at lower flow rates. Newer positive-pressure ventilators can also provide continuous flow, which allows for spontaneous breathing without imposing additional work and dead space. In general, B$_i$PAP units are smaller than portable ventilators, but newer portable ventilators generally weigh less than 15 pounds. B$_i$PAP devices operate more quietly, compensate for leaks better and are also less costly than portable ventilators.[116] On the other hand, B$_i$PAP devices cannot generate such high peak pressures and have higher rates of energy consumption than portable ventilators.[117] Unlike portable ventilators, most B$_i$PAP devices do not contain an internal battery. Because they use a single-limb circuit for inspiration and exhalation, they are also more likely to promote rebreathing than systems with a double-limb circuit.

Newer portable ventilators blur some of these distinctions and combine features of standard ventilators with those of B$_i$PAP devices. They can compensate for leaks well and are suitable for noninvasive use. They can also be adapted from "open system" single-limb circuits with passive exhalation valves and leak compensation to "closed-circuit" systems with a mechanical exhalation valve. These machines have an internal battery, the ability to control several ventilation variables and more extensive monitoring capabilities than B$_i$PAP devices.[118]

Some consider that CPAP is not a form of noninvasive ventilation, since the patient receives neither mandatory breaths nor assistance during spontaneous efforts. CPAP can, however, unload respiratory muscles and enhance minute ventilation by relieving upper airway obstruction, offsetting intrinsic PEEP or improving lung compliance. B$_i$PAP devices provide pressure-support ventilation, in which the patient's spontaneous effort is supported to a preset pressure. The supported breath is initiated by the patient, and the support is cycled off when inspiratory flow falls to a preset percent of

peak flow. Many B$_i$PAP devices have, in addition to a spontaneous mode, timed or combined spontaneous/timed modes in which mandatory breaths can be delivered in the event that the patient's drive or ability to trigger the machine is inadequate. The sensitivity of trigger and cycle variables differs according to the manufacturer,[119,120] making some machines a poor choice to use in infants or patients who are very weak.[121] In such circumstances, the practitioner can set a mandatory rate higher than the child's spontaneous rate to overcome the mechanical shortcomings of the system.[93] When supplemental oxygen is required, the amount bled into the system can mask the patient's inspiratory efforts by contributing additional flow that must be overcome to trigger the device. The final FiO$_2$ delivered to the patient will vary depending not only on the flow rate of oxygen bled into the system but also on where in the circuit the oxygen is introduced and the inspiratory pressure measured.[122] It is unusual to be able to deliver an FiO$_2$ above 0.5–0.7 noninvasively.[122,123]

Older first-generation portable ventilators, which are still in use, are able to provide only volume-preset breaths in which a desired tidal volume is set by the practitioner. The breaths can be delivered in a synchronized intermittent mandatory ventilation (SIMV) mode, where the patient breathes spontaneously but unsupported through the ventilator circuit in between mandatory positive pressure breaths delivered according to a set rate, or in Assist/Control (A/C) mode. Here the practitioner sets a rate at which mandatory breaths are delivered, but if the patient wishes to breathe above that rate, each effort results in a fully supported positive-pressure breath. Such machines also require the use of an external PEEP valve if end-distending pressure is required. When large leaks are present in children with tracheostomies who use this type of ventilator, it is usually not possible to maintain the set PEEP.

Newer second- and third-generation portable ventilators can provide either pressure preset or volume preset breaths, pressure support breaths, and continuous flow. Thus they are more versatile, allowing for more modes of ventilatory support that can enhance ventilator-patient synchrony and hence patient comfort. The PEEP valve is integrated into the machine. These machines can be used to provide CPAP with or without pressure support, SIMV with or without pressure support and A/C ventilation. Both trigger and cycle variables can be adjusted on most models. All have internal batteries that differ widely among models in duration,[124] whereas external lightweight lithium batteries allow for their use away from an electrical power source for several hours.

No single type of positive-pressure device is ideal for all patients. Patient characteristics, as well as machine characteristics like trigger and cycle sensitivities, and sensitivity to leaks, can influence the degree of patient-ventilator dyssynchrony and adequacy of ventilatory assistance.[119–121] Patients who breathe spontaneously will benefit from features like continuous flow and pressure support. Patients with no spontaneous respiratory effort (e.g., children with cervical spinal cord injury) do not require such accessories, and their presence can occasionally be detrimental. When there is a large leak around the child's tracheostomy or interface, the leak will be interpreted by the ventilator as a patient-initiated breath and will result in unintended excessive ventilation or ventilator auto triggering. If trigger or cycle sensitivities are not adequate, the child will make inspiratory efforts that are not supported, or have to exhale while the device continues to provide a positive pressure breath.[125] In the best of circumstances the needs of the patient are matched to the capabilities of the device, and interactions between device and child are assessed critically before the child is given that machine for long-term use.[121]

Ancillary Equipment

In addition to the actual ventilator, other equipment needs of children requiring chronic mechanical ventilation will vary. This will depend on the interface being used (noninvasive versus tracheostomy), whether or not the child requires assistance with airway clearance and coughing, how many hours the child can tolerate being without ventilator support and whether or not the child spends most waking hours in a wheelchair. In addition, how far the child lives from the medical center or durable medical equipment company and how frequently power outages occur in the child's community are important considerations.

Those children who use nasal or oronasal interfaces should have a second, different style interface available to interchange with the primary one. In this way, different areas of the face are exposed to pressure from the mask, and discomfort or skin injury can be minimized or avoided. Small children, those who perspire excessively and those who have difficulty controlling secretions should have backup headgear available for noninvasive interfaces. Fixation devices for noninvasive interfaces come in a variety of materials and, often because nasal interfaces are used that were designed for adults, straps must be altered or extra hook and loop (Velcro) straps added to fit a child's head and keep the interface in place. Whenever the mask or tubing touches the child's skin, adequate padding must be provided and frequent assessments performed to avoid skin injury. Children with tracheostomies should have a second tracheostomy tube available for emergencies and another tube one size smaller in case there is difficulty reinserting the tube during an unplanned tube change. Children who drool excessively may require extra tracheostomy tube holders to allow for frequent changes so that skin breakdown under the ties can be avoided. Twill tape, Velcro, neoprene and beaded chain tracheostomy holders all are available and are chosen based on patient/family preference and the experience of the health care team. Standards for tracheostomy care in children have been published that detail the equipment required.[105]

Children with neuromuscular weakness develop a stereotypical progression of respiratory involvement that begins with difficulty clearing the central airways of secretions, even before they develop ventilatory insufficiency.[44] Cough is the mechanism primarily responsible for clearing the central airways of secretions and particulate matter, while mucociliary clearance is the chief mechanism by which debris is removed from the peripheral airways.[126] Weakness of inspiratory, bulbar or expiratory muscles can impair effectiveness of coughing and predispose toward chronic atelectasis or recurrent pneumonia.[127]

To address this, several methods have been developed for subjects whose cough is inadequate to clear the central

airways. These include techniques such as manual or mechanical insufflation to raise precough lung volume, manually assisted cough, and mechanical exsufflation with negative pressure.[128] Mechanical insufflation/exsufflation (MI-E) combines mechanical insufflation and exsufflation with negative pressure; it has been utilized in patients with inadequate cough since the polio epidemics of the 1940s and 1950s.[129] MI-E has gained increasing popularity in children over the last two decades, and has been used safely across the spectrum of pediatric ages.[130] The device can be used with a face mask, a mouthpiece, or attached directly to a tracheostomy tube. Among 62 patients ranging in age from 3 months to 28.6 years, no correlation existed between the pressures used with MI-E and the age of the patient or the type of underlying neuromuscular disease.[130] Generation of cough peak flows high enough to achieve airway clearance requires a pressure span ($P_{insufflation} - P_{exsufflation}$) of at least 30 cm H_2O.[131] But during acute illness when increased airway resistance or decreased lung compliance might occur, higher pressures are probably required to achieve adequate precough volumes and cough peak flows.[132] In addition, increasing insufflation time can result in higher exsufflation flows, whereas increasing exsufflation time does not significantly increase expiratory flows.[131,133]

Most studies that evaluate the effectiveness of MI-E in patients with neuromuscular weakness report the short-term results of a single MI-E treatment; there are no randomized controlled trials that evaluate long-term effects like survival, quality of life, duration and number of hospitalizations, or serious side effects of MI-E use.[134] There have, however, been smaller studies that report a reduction in the number of hospital days in the 6 and 12 months following MI-E use compared with a similar period before its use. In addition, improved quality of life for the child and parents was reported resulting from their enhanced ability to manage illnesses or acute episodes of airway obstruction at home, thereby avoiding emergency rooms and hospital visits.[135,136] Serious side effects of MI-E use are only rarely reported in children and include cardiac dysrhythmias, aggravation of gastroesophageal reflux, gastric distention and dynamic central airway collapse.[130,137] Complications related to barotrauma, like pneumothorax, have only rarely been reported in adults[138] and never in children. The author has, however, cared for a 16-year-old boy with Duchenne muscular dystrophy who experienced recurrent pneumothoraces while being treated with both MI-E and positive-pressure ventilation via tracheostomy.

Home mechanical ventilators are generally reliable pieces of equipment, but the addition of microprocessor technology and increased complexity of the machines increases the risk for ventilator malfunction. In a survey of 150 ventilator users followed over 1 year, of whom 44 were 18 years of age or younger, defective equipment or failure of mostly first-generation ventilators occurred on average of only once per 1.25 years of continuous ventilator use.[139] Of the 189 incidents of suspected ventilator failure, actual equipment malfunction or failure was responsible for the report in only 73 (39%). Two patients required rehospitalization, and in both cases, the problem was due to a change in the patient's condition that mimicked equipment failure rather than a true ventilator malfunction. King accessed the FDA Manufacturer and User Facility Device Experience (MAUDE) database, which reported more than 150 home mechanical ventilation failures or malfunctions in the United States in 2010.[29] In a recent European review of ventilator problems among both pediatric and adult home ventilator users, the likelihood of ventilator malfunction was fairly small (involving 28% of more than 3000 calls received over a 6-month period).[140] The risk of ventilator malfunction was greater if the machine was more than 8 years old, if it was a model newly introduced to the market or if it was used 16 hours/day or more.[140] Given these considerations, if a child cannot tolerate absence of ventilatory support for more than 4 hours of the day[35] or if the child lives more than 1 hour from the tertiary care center or home equipment company,[139] the child should have a second ventilator and complete circuit setup in the home in case of emergency. If the child spends most of the day in a wheelchair, two setups are usually made available: one left on the chair for daytime use and a second kept at the bedside. To assure proper functioning, mechanical ventilators and other equipment should undergo a routine check at least monthly and receive preventive maintenance as needed.[35] These checks should include not only assessment of various ventilator functions (i.e., inspiratory and expiratory pressures, trigger sensitivity, oxygen delivery, alarms, etc.) but also of whether the actual settings match the patient's prescription.[141]

Most of the newer ventilators designed for home use have an internal battery that can be used during transfers or a brief power outage. In some models, the internal battery lasts only about 1 hour, depending on the amount and mode of support required by the child.[124,142] External batteries are necessary when the child is expected to spend longer away from an electrical power source. These periods can last up to 12 hours, again depending on the child's ventilator requirements.[142] Some systems also permit the ventilator to use power from the battery of an electric wheelchair to reduce the bulk of equipment that must be transported. Batteries enhance the child's portability and can be used in emergencies when electrical power is not available. If the child lives in an area where electrical power outages are frequent, a backup generator may be required to keep the child safely at home during outages and to run other equipment such as suction machines and monitors.

Infants and children who are supported by mechanical ventilation via tracheostomy require humidification of the ventilator circuit, since bypassing the natural upper airway results in delivery of cool, dry air to the central airways. This can result in ineffective secretion clearance and plugging of the artificial airway. Inspired gas should be humidified to 28–35 mg/L, and heated to 29–35°C.[105,143] This can be achieved with heated humidifiers or heat-moisture exchangers. The effectiveness of heat-moisture exchangers varies by manufacturer,[144] and their efficiency decreases with increasing tidal volume, inspiratory flow, and minute ventilation.[143] Heat-moisture exchangers are not as efficient as heated humidifiers when used in infants and small children and should be confined to use during travel or waking hours, with a heated humidifier used during sleep. The addition of heating devices to the ventilator circuit can increase ventilatory demands: heated humidifiers increase ventilator circuit compliance, and heat-moisture exchangers add dead space to the circuit. In both cases, the set tidal volume may have to be increased to accommodate these changes. Children

who use noninvasive ventilation do not necessarily require humidification of the circuit. Patients who complain about nasal congestion or dryness, however, can benefit from humidification and they are often more comfortable when the delivered air is humidified.

Patients ventilated via tracheostomy and those with neuromuscular or neurologic conditions using noninvasive ventilation require suction equipment. Both stationary and portable devices should be available to facilitate patient mobility.[78] Portable suction machines are capable of developing pressures in excess of the 60–150 torr recommended for airway suctioning.[145] All patients with tracheostomies and those who use noninvasive ventilation to treat alveolar hypoventilation require a manual ventilation system (e.g., self-inflating resuscitation bag) for use with suctioning or during emergencies. The self-inflating bag can also be used for lung volume recruitment in patients with neuromuscular weakness.[89,90] Patients with impaired cough also can use a self-inflating bag to provide insufflation before manually assisted cough, or use specialized equipment (e.g., a mechanical in-exsufflator) to aid with airway clearance.[78]

Home positive-pressure mechanical ventilators have internal alarms, as do many newer B$_i$PAP machines. These include alarms for low pressure or patient disconnect, power failure, low battery, high pressure, apnea, low minute volume, and low tidal volume. These alarms provide early warning in the case of machine failure, ventilator disconnection, inadvertent decannulation, tracheostomy tube obstruction or excessive leak of a noninvasive circuit. The low-pressure alarm present on ventilators delivering positive pressure via tracheostomy is typically set 5 cm below the desired peak pressure to be delivered.[35] However, the low-pressure alarm might not sound in the setting of an inadvertent decannulation when used with children who require small tracheostomy tubes (<4.5-mm inside diameter) because of the high resistance of the tube.[146] For this reason, additional monitoring with external devices is used for the early detection of emergencies.

The use of external monitors remains driven by practice, not data. No author advocates recreating an ICU environment at home, but considerable differences of opinion exist regarding the roles of home cardiorespiratory impedance monitoring, pulse oximetry, and capnometry.[3,4,35,78,147,148] Monitoring practice also varies depending on the method of ventilatory assistance between tracheostomy-delivered, noninvasive positive pressure, and negative-pressure ventilation.[13] Impedance monitors are advocated generally by some[4,148] or recommended for use in certain circumstances, such as in the child who requires a tracheostomy tube smaller than 4.5 mm.[35] Others feel that such monitoring is both redundant and unnecessary.[147] Importantly, the cardiorespiratory monitor will not alarm in the event of a tube obstruction, inadvertent decannulation or ventilator disconnection until the child has become sufficiently hypoxemic to experience bradycardia. Pulse oximetry monitoring is not universally advocated,[147,148] but a recent clinical practice guideline on pediatric home mechanical ventilation from the American Thoracic Society recommends the use of pulse oximetry instead of a cardiorespiratory monitoring device for children who are invasively ventilated, especially when asleep or unobserved.[72] A decrease in the number of deaths and cases of severe hypoxic encephalopathy related to airway accidents has been attributed to this approach,[9] as oximetry will detect hypoxemia associated with ventilator failure, tube obstruction, or accidental disconnection sooner than these events can be discovered by cardiorespiratory monitoring. Pulse oximetry is also used to assist in weaning supplemental oxygen or ventilator support and as an early warning of lower respiratory tract complications (such as bronchospasm or infection) that might require an increase in ventilatory support. Pulse oximetry monitoring is an integral component for monitoring patients with neuromuscular disease, where hypoxemia heralds the need for increased airway clearance, or delay in airway extubation to noninvasive ventilatory support after an acute illness.[93] Importantly, absence of nocturnal hypoxemia by pulse oximetry monitoring does not preclude significant episodes of hypercapnia in children who require nocturnal ventilation for treatment of alveolar hypoventilation.[149] Capnometry or capnography is not advocated by all,[147] but its intermittent use can be helpful in assessing a child's ability to sustain adequate ventilation during weaning trials. Continuous capnography or capnometry is not indicated for home monitoring. Recently a transcutaneous oximeter/capnometer was shown to be accurate and effective in assessing gas exchange in children with chronic respiratory failure using noninvasive ventilation at home.[149]

In general the recommendation for external monitoring must be individualized. Although such monitoring can be lifesaving, the monitors themselves can also increase caregiver stress and anxiety.[110] False alarms can disrupt parents' sleep, contributing to caregiver sleep deprivation.[76,150] No monitoring system can fully replace direct patient observation,[151] and none of the external monitors should be considered as a surrogate for appropriate ventilator alarms.

Patient Follow-Up

The course of children with chronic respiratory failure is either one of gradual improvement with ability to be liberated from mechanical ventilation or a trajectory of worsening, depending largely on the natural history of the underlying disease. The frequency with which children need to be seen will vary according to where they are in their disease process and the comfort of the health care team and family to perform interventions at home. For instance, an adolescent with type 2 SMA might require only semiannual visits, once growth has stopped, if the progression of the underlying disease is slow. An infant with type 1 SMA is likely to require visits every 2–3 months to reassess the adequacy of ventilation and airway clearance.

Growth and stamina for play or developmental activities are key determinants of adequacy of ventilatory support for children with chronic respiratory failure. Yet nutritional assessments in this population often do not take into account the metabolic state of the patient, resulting in undernutrition or overnutrition.[152] A recent study of 20 children ventilated at home via tracheostomy showed that 35% had mild to moderate undernutrition while 13 of 19 were either overfed or underfed.[153] Furthermore, 11 of 19 received less than the daily recommended protein intake. In addition, 45% were hypermetabolic, while 30% were hypometabolic. These findings highlight the need for expert nutritional input and

assessment to evaluate the needs of ventilator-dependent children who often have complex conditions and who are at risk for malnutrition.

Children with chronic respiratory failure can be weaned partially or completely from mechanical ventilation in post-acute rehabilitation facilities[41,42] or in the home.[154,155] In our practice, once a child has demonstrated tolerance for reduction in ventilator support during an office visit, the family is given guidelines for reduction in support and clinical indicators for tolerance of reduction of support. Through weekly telephone interviews, changes in vital signs, weight gain, tolerance for physical activity, and overall mood are assessed, and if the child tolerates the reduction in support, orders are given for a continued slow reduction of ventilator assistance. Often, several days of reduction of mechanical ventilation are required before intolerance becomes apparent, either through an alteration in mood, reduction of activity, or failure to continue to gain weight. Thus reductions occur only weekly or at most twice weekly. A 20% increase in heart rate or respiratory rate from the resting condition or failure to maintain adequate gas exchange as determined by oximetry and capnometry are indicators to curtail further weaning immediately. There is no single best way to liberate a child from mechanical ventilation. Some programs use polysomnography to guide nocturnal weaning of mechanical ventilation[155] whereas others do not.[154] Some practitioners gradually reduce the level of pressure support or number of mandatory breaths delivered to the patient. Our practice usually is to begin weaning trials either to CPAP or complete nonsupport for short periods once or twice a day, returning the child to the usual level of support for the duration of the day. The weaning trials are gradually lengthened as tolerated while the child is awake until the child is breathing independently for all waking hours. Further reduction of support then occurs during naps and finally during sleeping hours overnight. The ability to liberate a child from daytime mechanical ventilation, even if nocturnal support is still required, minimizes the need for community health services and promotes school attendance.[156]

If a child had undergone tracheostomy placement to facilitate chronic mechanical ventilation and has weaned from ventilator support, decannulation of the trachea should be considered. There is no single best approach to tracheal decannulation. Most authors recommend bronchoscopy before attempted decannulation to assess for airway obstruction from granulation tissue, suprastomal collapse, tracheomalacia, enlarged tonsils or adenoids or vocal cord paralysis.[154,157–159] Once airway patency is assured, the tube is often downsized and capped for a period of time,[158–160] whereas other authors simply remove the tube.[161] Other programs remove the tracheostomy tube only in the sleep laboratory with overnight polysomnography to assure adequate nocturnal ventilation.[162] In all cases, however, the child is hospitalized for 24–48 hours to be certain that airway compromise does not develop after tube removal. Polysomnography with the tube downsized and capped can be used as an adjunct when concern about patency of the airway during sleep affects the decision to decannulate the airway.[160] In each case, the approach to tracheal decannulation should be tailored to the individual's condition.[158]

Children with tracheostomies require routine tube changes. Recommendations, based on practice rather than evidence, range from daily to monthly with most experts suggesting a weekly timetable.[105] However, a panel of experts in otolaryngology failed to reach consensus on the proper interval for tracheostomy tube changes.[163] More frequent changes may be required in the setting of an acute infection, when thick secretions can obstruct the tube. Bacterial colonization of the airway is almost ubiquitous in patients with tracheostomies,[164] but most experts do not advocate the routine use of oral or inhaled antibiotics for prophylaxis against pneumonia.[165] Although *Pseudomonas aeruginosa* and *Staphylococcus aureus* are the two most commonly isolated organisms from patients on long-term mechanical ventilation, anaerobes may also play an important role and should be considered when antibiotic treatment is contemplated.[166] Routine bronchoscopic evaluation to assess for airway lesions or narrowing and appropriate sizing of the tube is recommended every 6–12 months or more frequently in a child experiencing rapid changes in growth or medical condition.[105] However, in the absence of bleeding or difficulty with tracheostomy tube changes, some otolaryngologists do not perform routine bronchoscopic evaluation.

Infants and toddlers with BPD experience exacerbations of respiratory failure most commonly because of acute wheezing illnesses and nonbacterial respiratory infections. During such episodes, ventilatory support may have to be increased. The first intervention for respiratory distress in a child with a tracheostomy is to perform a tracheostomy tube change so as to ensure that there is not partial obstruction of the tube causing the distress. Occasionally, antibiotics are administered when tracheal secretions remain purulent, increased neutrophils are identified on sputum Gram stain, and a predominant bacterial organism is recovered from the sputum culture.[165] Thereafter, if minor changes in ventilator support do not correct gas-exchange abnormalities or if the family or skilled caregivers are not comfortable with continuing care at home, the child should be hospitalized.

Patients with neuromuscular weakness can experience acute deterioration in respiratory function when impaired mucus clearance leads to atelectasis or respiratory infections cause increased mucus production with airway obstruction. The first intervention is to increase airway clearance to resolve the obstruction or to keep pace with increased mucus production. Experts also recommend judicious use of antibiotics for respiratory infections,[55] even when the illness begins as a viral infection, because stasis of mucus predisposes to secondary bacterial infections. Patients supported by NIV may require longer (up to continuous) periods of ventilatory support during the acute illness, or an increase in applied positive pressure. Distending pressure (expiratory positive airway pressure [EPAP]) is often increased to overcome atelectasis, while inspiratory positive airway pressure (IPAP) may have to be increased to offset increases in airways resistance or a decrease in lung compliance. If the child requires airway intubation for an acute illness, some experts advocate waiting until the child has weaned from supplemental oxygen before attempting extubation to noninvasive support.[93] Progression of the underlying neuromuscular disease can lead to inadequate support, so symptoms of sleep-related hypoventilation should be sought at each office encounter and reassessment of ventilatory requirements during sleep should occur at least annually.[167]

Outcomes

WEANING FROM VENTILATOR SUPPORT

The underlying cause of respiratory failure is the principal determinant of whether a child will eventually be liberated from ventilator support.[3,4,41,156,168–171] Several studies suggest that those children receiving long-term mechanical ventilation for parenchymal lung disease such as bronchopulmonary dysplasia or central airway lesions like tracheomalacia are more likely to be able to be weaned from mechanical ventilation than are those with neuromuscular weakness or multiple congenital anomalies.[3,41,156,168,169,171] This finding probably reflects the propensity for improvement in a child's lung mechanics or respiratory pump function over time in the former group and deterioration in lung and respiratory pump function in the latter. In a series of 102 patients with BPD supported by home mechanical ventilation via tracheostomy, 69 (83% of survivors) were liberated from mechanical ventilation, and 97% of those children were liberated by 5 years of age[172]; 58 of 60 children who could be decannulated accomplished that before 6 years of age. In contrast, among 449 children supported with long-term NIV, only 42 (9%) were liberated over 18 years[173]; 60% of the population had neuromuscular or chest wall disease. One of these reviews, in which 20% of the 228-patient cohort carried a diagnosis of central hypoventilation syndrome, included transitioning from chronic mechanical ventilation to diaphragm pacing as a reflection of successful weaning.[169] Severity of underlying disease also may influence weaning outcome: of 35 children requiring chronic mechanical ventilation via tracheostomy in association with congenital heart disease, only those patients with less severe underlying disease, as reflected by a Risk Adjustment for Congenital Heart Surgery (RACHS-1) score ≤3, were able to wean from mechanical ventilation.[170]

SURVIVAL

There is no question that chronic ventilatory support, even when confined to nocturnal use alone, improves survival among patients with neuromuscular and other restrictive chest wall diseases. In the absence of ventilatory support, mean duration of survival for patients with Duchenne muscular dystrophy and diurnal hypercapnia was 9.7 months.[174] In contrast, among 23 young men with Duchenne muscular dystrophy and diurnal hypercapnia who began NIV, survival was 85% at one year and 73% at 5 years.[83] Because of the increased longevity of patients with diseases such as Duchenne muscular dystrophy resulting from improved respiratory care and other technologies, new complications and medical issues are being described that will require greater recognition and surveillance.[173,175,176] In addition, the success of home ventilation in prolonging survival of ventilator-dependent children with little likelihood of weaning from support highlights the need to create adult-care transition programs for these patients as they reach the age of majority.[32,173,177,178]

Among all children with chronic respiratory failure cared for at home, mortality is generally low; the greatest predictor of long-term survival is the prognosis of the underlying condition.[179] Teague abstracted the average 5-year cumulative survival from published reports of 265 pediatric patients and reported approximately 85% survival in children treated with home mechanical ventilation between 1983 and 1998.[179] Of the 137 patients with neuromuscular diseases who were receiving home mechanical ventilation, the 5-year cumulative survival estimate was 75%. A single-center experience from Canada involving 379 children followed between 1991 and 2011 described an annual mortality rate of only 0.73%.[32] Once again, severity of the underlying disease has been suggested as a predictor of survival in some diseases: the cumulative 5 year survival of children with chronic respiratory failure associated with congenital heart disease was 68%, but it was 90% when considering only those with a RACHS-1 score of ≤3 and 12% for those with a score ≥4.[170]

Most studies suggest that the primary cause of death of ventilator-dependent children cared for outside hospital relates to progression of the underlying disease.[8,171,179,180] A recent single-center review, however, noted that death among tracheostomy and ventilator-dependent children was often unexpected and may have been related to comorbidities as well.[169] Similarly, comorbidities contributed to mortality in children supported with long-term NIV.[173] Although it is unlikely for ventilator malfunction to be the cause of death,[181] one series in which 17 patients died over a 20-year period described 3 deaths resulting from unwitnessed ventilator disconnections and 1 from an overnight power failure of a negative-pressure body ventilator. This led the author to speculate that at least 3 and perhaps as many as 7 deaths could have been prevented if the patients had been monitored visually or electronically.[10]

The presence of a tracheostomy increases the risk of death as well as other negative outcomes. Edwards et al. calculated that tracheostomy-related deaths accounted for 8% of all reported deaths among published accounts.[169] In their cohort, tracheostomy-related deaths were responsible for 19% of all deaths, with complications that included obstruction of the tube, bleeding from tracheal granulomas and misplacement of the tracheostomy tube into a false track. Downes and Pilmer compared the incidence of life-threatening tracheostomy-related accidents between those ventilator-dependent children cared for in the home and those in the hospital in the early 1980s.[9] Although the rate was low, they found it to be 9 times greater among those cared for at home (2.3 of 10,000 patient days) versus the pediatric ICU (0.3 of 10,000 patient days). The authors speculate that the recent use of home pulse oximetry helped to reduce the disparity. Tracheostomy-related deaths have also been reported after children had already been weaned from chronic mechanical ventilation. Of 30 deaths among 101 infants with chronic respiratory failure over an 18-year period, 10 occurred after ventilation had been discontinued.[8] Six of the deaths were considered airway-related accidents, and all but one occurred following hospital discharge.

QUALITY OF LIFE

When surveyed, ventilator-dependent children generally view the use of the ventilator as positive, because it helps them breathe more easily, giving them more energy and an overall sense of better health.[182,183] Mechanical ventilatory support is associated with a reduction in hospital admission frequency, improved sleep quality, and better daytime functioning in children with nocturnal hypoventilation from neuromuscular and chest wall disorders.[184–186] Subjects who have diurnal hypercapnia or who complain of dyspnea by the end of the day experience relief of dyspnea by using daytime mechanical ventilator support for as little as 2 hours in the afternoon.[54] When patients were surveyed, quality of life of those with neuromuscular disease was independent of the need for mechanical ventilation.[187] Ventilator users have a generally positive outlook and are interested in making plans.[186,188–190] Ventilator-dependent children attend school, including college and graduate school, and vacation with their families.[186,189] They are generally happy with how they spend their time, although adolescents with chronic respiratory failure may be less satisfied with their daily activities than younger children.[189] Children dependent on mechanical ventilation view their equipment as adaptive technology, in much the same way that a wheelchair helps with mobility.[182] Nevertheless, children who are ventilator users feel ostracized by people outside of immediate circle of friends and family because of their need for breathing support,[75,182,183] and they express a concern for being excluded from society and everyday relationships with others.[191] Both they and their families express feelings of isolation because of the disability,[75] and siblings feel that they have to shoulder more adult responsibilities.[191]

In fact, there is disparity between the perceived good quality of life of ventilator-dependent children and that of their families. Home care of a ventilator-dependent child is stressful, and the degree of stress increases with duration of care.[75,190,192,193] Parents focus more on the possibility of their child's death and dying than do the ventilator users themselves.[75,182] One single-center study found that whereas parents of ventilator-dependent children rated their children's quality of life higher than did parents of children dependent on gastrostomy tubes, parents of both groups rated their children's health quality of life lower than that of healthy children and children with other complex conditions like cystic fibrosis.[194] Additionally, home care of ventilator-dependent children adversely affects the health of caregivers, resulting in sleep disruption and inadequate amounts of sleep, feelings of depression and being overwhelmed, as well as limited time for the caregiver to pursue health-promoting activities.[76,192,195,196] Nevertheless, parents typically express a desire to have their child at home and satisfaction with their choice to do so.[75,77] Regardless of these stresses, parents and ventilator users themselves typically rate the child's quality of life higher than do health professionals,[24,197] and recognition of this by parents adds to their sense of frustration and isolation.[75,182]

Summary

The number of children requiring prolonged mechanical ventilatory support continues to grow because of improved care of critically ill neonates, infants, and children; advances in medical technology and changing practices regarding children with neuromuscular diseases. Whereas negative-pressure body ventilators gave way to positive-pressure ventilation via tracheostomy in the 1970s and 1980s, recent trends have been toward noninvasive positive pressure ventilation. Significant improvement in equipment, monitoring and understanding of the pathophysiology of respiratory failure has led to a wider array of therapeutic options that benefit patient tolerance. Significant challenges remain, especially concerning the design of interfaces and equipment for very young patients, supporting patients and their families to avoid caregiver fatigue and improving general societal access. This includes access to public transportation, housing choices (e.g., group homes for ventilator-assisted individuals), and employment opportunities. Older children who remain ventilator-dependent will require programs designed to transition their care to adult care providers.

References

Access the reference list online at ExpertConsult.com.

Suggested Reading

Caring for the Ventilator Dependent Child. A Clinical Guide. New York: Springer; 2016.

Make BJ, Hill NS, Goldberg AI, et al. Mechanical ventilation beyond the intensive care unit. Report of a consensus conference of the American College of Chest Physicians. *Chest.* 1998;113:289S–344S.

Mehta S, Hill NS. Noninvasive ventilation. *Am J Respir Crit Care Med.* 2001;163:540–577.

Sterni LM, Collaco JM, Baker CD, et al. An official american thoracic society clinical practice guideline: ediatric chronic home invasive ventilation. *Am J Respir Crit Care Med.* 2016;193:e16–e35.

Teague WG. Long-term mechanical ventilation in infants and children. In: Hill NS, ed. *Long-Term Mechanical Ventilation.* Vol. 152. New York: Marcel Dekker, Inc.; 2001:177–213.

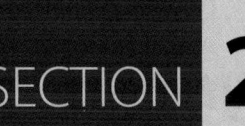

Infections of the Lung

22 Microbiological Diagnosis of Respiratory Illness: Recent Advances

DAVID R. MURDOCH, MD, MSc, DTM&H, FRACP, FRCPA, FFSc(RCPA),
ANJA M. WERNO, MD, PhD, FRCPA, and LANCE C. JENNINGS,
MSc, PhD, MRCPath, FFSc(RCPA)

Infections of the respiratory tract are among the most common health problems in children worldwide, and are associated with substantial morbidity and mortality.[1] A wide variety of microorganisms are potential respiratory pathogens; knowledge about the likely etiologic agents of respiratory infections can help direct management and can also play an important role in disease surveillance. Beyond the identification of specific pathogens, the clinical microbiology laboratory can also provide valuable information on antimicrobial susceptibility and strain typing. Continued liaison between clinicians and laboratory staff is vital to facilitate the most cost-effective use of laboratory diagnostics.

Presently, we are still reliant on many traditional diagnostic tools that have been used for decades to determine the microbial etiology of respiratory infections.[2,3] However, these tools have been increasingly supplemented by newer methods, particular molecular diagnostic techniques, which have enabled the more rapid detection of many pathogens that were previously difficult to detect.[4] These advances have particularly led to improvements in the ability to detect respiratory viruses and other microorganisms that do not normally colonize the respiratory tract. Moreover, recent discussions about the existence of a lung microbiome have challenged traditional paradigms about the pathogenesis of respiratory infections.[5,6] The concept that the healthy lung may not be a sterile organ is reshaping our interpretation of laboratory diagnostics.

This chapter focuses on the use of the clinical microbiology laboratory to determine the microbial causes of respiratory infections in children. Diagnostic aspects of some specific respiratory infections, such as tuberculosis and pertussis, are also covered in other chapters.

Respiratory Pathogens and Syndromes

Tables 22.1–22.17 show the etiologic agents associated with respiratory infections broken down by respiratory syndrome. These lists represent our current understanding and have changed little over recent decades; there have been only a relatively small number of newly discovered pathogens. The latter include human bocavirus, human metapneumovirus, and a variety of coronaviruses (SARS-CoV, CoV-NL63,

CoV-HKU1 and MERS-CoV).[7] Pathogen discovery efforts using unbiased next-generation sequencing methods have shown considerable promise but have not yet identified major new respiratory pathogens.[8,9]

In general, upper respiratory infections tend to be monomicrobial and are predominantly caused by viruses, with a few notable exceptions caused by specific bacteria (e.g., acute pharyngitis caused by *Streptococcus pyogenes*). Lower respiratory infections are caused by a wide variety of viral and bacterial pathogens. For pneumonia at least, sequential or concurrent polymicrobial infection may be relatively common, and the exact roles of individual microorganisms and how they interact in this context are still poorly understood.[10,11] The incidence of many respiratory infections follows a cyclical pattern aligned with the typical seasonal transmission of specific pathogens. Secular trends have also been noted for some vaccine-preventable infections, such as those caused by *Streptococcus pneumoniae* and *Haemophilus influenzae* type b, with decreasing burden following the successful implementation of vaccine programs.

Use of the Clinical Microbiology Laboratory

Before ordering a diagnostic test, it is important to be clear about the key clinical questions and expectations of diagnostic testing. Is knowledge about the cause of a particular respiratory infection important for patient treatment, outbreak management, epidemiological surveillance, or to reassure the clinician or caregiver of the child? It is also important to have an understanding about which specimens to collect, what tests are available, test limitations, and how to interpret results to appropriately integrate the findings into their clinical management.

The most useful specimens for diagnostic testing are those collected directly from the site of infection. Unfortunately, it is not always possible to collect these specimens, and this particularly applies to the lower respiratory tract, which is difficult to access safely in a manner that avoids contamination with colonizing organisms.

When bacteria are isolated from specific body sites, such as a throat swab, nasopharyngeal swab, or sputum, it is important to know which bacteria can be found as commensals or colonizers in the upper respiratory tract and which

Table 22.1 Etiologic Agents Associated With Pharyngitis

Viral	Bacterial	Fungal
Adenoviruses	*Streptococcus pyogenes*	*Candida* species
Coronaviruses	Other β-hemolytic streptococci	
Parainfluenza viruses	*Corynebacterium diphtheriae*	
Respiratory syncytial virus	*Corynebacterium ulcerans*	
Human metapneumovirus	*Arcanobacterium haemolyticum*	
Rhinoviruses	*Neisseria gonorrheae*	
Influenza viruses	Mixed anaerobes	
Epstein-Barr virus	*Treponema pallidum*	
Enteroviruses	*Chlamydophila pneumoniae*	
Herpes simplex viruses	*Mycoplasma pneumoniae*	
Measles	*Streptobacillus moniliformis*	
Rubella		
Cytomegalovirus		
HIV		

HIV, Human immunodeficiency virus.

Table 22.2 Etiologic Agents Associated With Croup

Viral	Bacterial
Parainfluenza viruses	*Mycoplasma pneumoniae*
Influenza viruses	
Respiratory syncytial virus	
Human metapneumovirus	
Coronaviruses	
Human bocavirus	
Adenoviruses	
Measles	
Rhinoviruses	
Enteroviruses	
Herpes simplex viruses	

Table 22.3 Etiologic Agents Associated With Sinusitis

Viral	Bacterial	Fungal
Rhinoviruses	*Haemophilus influenzae*	*Aspergillus* species
Influenza viruses	*Streptococcus pneumoniae*	*Alternaria* species
Parainfluenza viruses	Anaerobes	*Penicillium* species
Adenoviruses	*Moraxella catarrhalis*	Zygomycetes
	Staphylococcus aureus	
	Streptococcus pyogenes	
	Mycoplasma pneumoniae	

Table 22.4 Etiologic Agents Associated With Acute Bronchitis

Viral	Bacterial
Adenoviruses	*Mycoplasma pneumoniae*
Influenza viruses	*Bordetella pertussis*
Parainfluenza viruses	*Bordetella parapertussis*
Respiratory syncytial virus	*Chlamydophila pneumoniae*
Rhinoviruses	*Haemophilus influenzae*
Coronaviruses	*Streptococcus pneumoniae*
Human metapneumovirus	*Moraxella catarrhalis*
Herpes simplex viruses	*Streptococcus pyogenes*
Enteroviruses	
Measles	
Mumps	
Human bocavirus	

Table 22.5 Etiologic Agents Associated With Bronchiolitis

Viral	Bacterial
Respiratory syncytial virus	*Mycoplasma pneumoniae*
Parainfluenza viruses	
Adenoviruses	
Influenza viruses	
Human metapneumovirus	
Rhinoviruses	
Enteroviruses	
Mumps	
Herpes simplex viruses	

Table 22.6 Etiologic Agents Associated With Pneumonia

Viral	Bacterial	Fungal
Respiratory syncytial virus	*Streptococcus pneumoniae*	*Pneumocystis jiroveci*
Parainfluenza viruses	*Haemophilus influenzae*	*Aspergillus* species
Influenza viruses	*Staphylococcus aureus*	Zygomycetes
Coronaviruses	*Mycoplasma pneumoniae*	*Coccidioides immitis*
Adenoviruses	*Bordetella pertussis*	*Cryptococcus neoformans*
Human metapneumovirus	*Legionella* species	*Histoplasma capsulatum*
Rhinoviruses	Enterobacteriaceae	
Epstein-Barr virus	*Pseudomonas aeruginosa*	
Enteroviruses	*Acinetobacter* species	
Human bocavirus	Mixed anaerobes	
Herpes simplex viruses	*Streptococcus agalactiae*	
Varicella zoster virus	*Chlamydophila pneumoniae*	
Measles	*Chlamydia psittaci*	
Rubella	*Chlamydia trachomatis*	
Cytomegalovirus	*Burkholderia pseudomallei*	
HIV	*Streptococcus pyogenes*	
	Neisseria meningitidis	
	Coxiella burnetii	
	Mycobacterium species	

HIV, Human immunodeficiency virus.

when found would indicate definitive infection. Table 22.15 outlines microorganisms that are regarded as part of the normal respiratory flora.[12–15] Importantly, given the right conditions, some bacteria that can harmlessly colonize the respiratory tract may also be respiratory pathogens. As will be discussed further in this chapter, several microbiological diagnostic tests employed in the diagnosis of childhood respiratory disease have limited ability to differentiate between colonization and disease and are therefore of limited value when considered in isolation.

Table 22.7 Etiologic Agents Associated With the Common Cold

VIRAL	
Rhinoviruses	Human metapneumovirus
Coronaviruses	Adenoviruses
Parainfluenza viruses	Influenza viruses
Respiratory syncytial virus	Enteroviruses
	Human bocavirus

Table 22.8 Etiologic Agents Associated With Epiglottitis

BACTERIAL	
Haemophilus influenzae type b	*Staphylococcus aureus*
Streptococcus pneumoniae	*Haemophilus parainfluenzae*
	Other streptococci

Table 22.9 Etiologic Agents Associated With Pleural Effusion and Empyema

BACTERIAL	
Streptococcus pneumoniae	Gram-negative bacilli
Staphylococcus aureus	*Mycoplasma pneumoniae*
Haemophilus influenzae	*Mycobacterium* species

Table 22.10 Etiologic Agents Associated With Lung Abscess

Bacterial	**Parasitic**
Staphylococcus aureus	*Entamoeba histolytica*
Anaerobes	
Streptococcus pneumoniae	
Other gram-negative bacilli	
α-Hemolytic streptococci	

Table 22.11 Etiologic Agents Associated With Cystic Fibrosis

BACTERIAL	
Staphylococcus aureus	*Burkholderia cepacia*
Haemophilus influenzae	*Stenotrophomonas maltophilia*
Pseudomonas aeruginosa	*Mycobacterium* species

Table 22.12 Respiratory Specimens and Diagnostic Testing

Specimen Type	Microbiological Investigations	Comment
Sputum/induced sputum	Microscopy; culture; susceptibilities; DFA; PCR	Provided it is a good-quality specimen, it can be a highly informative specimen; can be difficult to obtain in children
Nasopharyngeal aspirate/swab	Microscopy; culture; susceptibilities; DFA; PCR	Most useful in viral infections; requires a skilled operator to obtain specimen; in some ways, it is easier to obtain than a throat swab, because the nares are always accessible
Nasal swab	Microscopy; culture; susceptibilities; DFA; PCR	Limited usefulness as it only recovers organisms present in the nasal cavity and not beyond
Throat swab	Microscopy; culture; susceptibilities; DFA; PCR	Probably the most representative specimen for disease of the upper respiratory tract; many bacterial pathogens are also common colonizers at various stages of childhood; can be difficult to obtain without child and parent cooperation; may represent organisms present in the nose as well as the oropharynx
Endotracheal aspirate	Microscopy; culture; susceptibilities; DFA; PCR	Invasive specimen, but is likely to represent pathogens from the lower respiratory tract; can be contaminated by organisms present in the oropharynx that can make result interpretation difficult
Bronchoalveolar lavage fluid	Microscopy; culture; susceptibilities; DFA; PCR	Invasive specimen but is likely to represent pathogens from the lower respiratory tract; can be contaminated by organisms present in the oropharynx, which can make result interpretation difficult
Transthoracic needle aspiration	Microscopy; culture; susceptibilities; DFA; PCR	Highly invasive specimen; risk of complications; microbiologically of high value provided the correct area has been biopsied
Lung tissue	Microscopy; culture; susceptibilities; DFA; PCR	Highly invasive specimen; risk of complications; microbiologically of high value provided the correct area has been biopsied
Pleural fluid	Microscopy; culture; susceptibilities; DFA; PCR	Invasive specimen but is the specimen of choice in a child with empyema
Blood cultures	Microscopy; culture; susceptibilities;	Very helpful if positive, but the positivity rate in pneumonia is relatively low
Serum/whole blood	Immunoassays; DFA; PCR	Serology per se is of limited value, since a diagnosis is dependent on paired sera that then makes it a retrospective tool; a single high titer can occasionally be obtained in acute disease; PCR on whole blood may be helpful in severe disease to detect viremia, but viremia is generally short lived
Urine	Antigen detection tests; microscopy; culture	Antigen detection tests are of limited value in children; pathogen is rarely cultured from urine

DFA, Direct fluorescent antibody; *PCR,* polymerase chain reaction.

Table 22.13 Gram Stain Appearance of Bacterial Respiratory Pathogens

Pathogen	Typical Gram Stain Appearance	Likely to Be Significant
Streptococcus pneumoniae	Gram-positive lancet-shaped diplococci	Predominant pathogen in Gram stain with abundant neutrophils
Staphylococcus aureus	Gram-positive cocci in clumps	
Haemophilus influenzae	Small pleomorphic gram negative coccobacilli	
Streptococcus pyogenes	Gram-positive cocci in chains	
Arcanobacterium haemolyticum	Gram-positive diphtheroid-shaped bacilli	
Corynebacterium diphtheriae	Pleomorphic diphtheroid gram-positive bacilli; special stain (Loeffler's methylene blue stain) demonstrates typical club-shaped ends	
Mycoplasma pneumoniae	Absence of organisms as they lack a cell wall and cannot be visualized on Gram stain	

Table 22.14   Screening of Respiratory Specimen Quality

Specimen	Acceptable for Culture
Sputum	<10 SEC/average 10× field
Endotracheal aspirate	<10 SEC/average 10× field and bacteria seen in at least 1 of 20 oil immersion fields
Bronchoalveolar lavage fluid	<1% of cells present are SEC

This table has been modified from Jorgensen JH, Pfaller MA, Carroll KC, et al. *Manual of Clinical Microbiology*, 11th ed. Washington, DC: American Society of Microbiology; 2015.
SEC, Squamous epithelial cells.

Table 22.15   Normal Respiratory Flora

Streptococcus species
  ▪ including *Streptococcus pneumoniae*
Staphylococcus species
  ▪ including *Staphylococcus aureus*
Corynebacterium species
Moraxella species
  ▪ including *Moraxella catarrhalis*
Neisseria species
  ▪ including *Neisseria meningitidis*
Haemophilus species
  ▪ including *Haemophilus influenzae*
Cardiobacterium species
Kingella species
Eikenella corrodens

Table 22.16   Molecular Assays Commonly in Use for the Diagnosis of Respiratory Diseases

Molecular Assay	Principle	Main Use	Comment
Singleplex PCR	Single DNA or RNA target that is amplified	Can be designed for the detection of any known DNA or RNA sequence	Generally higher sensitivity than multiplex PCR as the targets are not competing
Multiplex PCR	Simultaneous amplification of several DNA or RNA targets	Respiratory pathogens; immunocompromised protocols; detection of various pathogens in blood cultures	Wide coverage of pathogens in a single test informs clinical management in a timely manner
16S rRNA sequencing	Amplification of 16S ribosomal RNA followed by sequencing of the product	Used to detect bacterial species in a clinical specimen that has failed to detect pathogens in culture.	Covers a wide range of pathogens listed in accessible sequence databases
Next-generation sequencing	Sequencing of a whole bacterial or viral genome or simultaneous sequencing of multiple bacterial or viral genes	Resistance testing and outbreak investigations	Can offer multiple gene sequences simultaneously or whole genome sequencing as well as de novo sequencing; currently, high cost prohibits routine use

PCR, Polymerase chain reaction.

Table 22.17   Molecular Terms Commonly Used in Diagnostics

Molecular Term	Explanation
PCR	An in vitro chemical reaction that leads to the synthesis of large quantities of a target nucleic acid sequence.
Reverse transcriptase PCR	RNA targets are converted into cDNA that is then amplified. This is needed for the amplification of RNA viruses (most common respiratory viruses).
RT PCR	The target amplification and the detection step occur simultaneously in the same tube. These assays require special thermal cyclers.
SNPs	Useful markers of genetic differences between strains, e.g., in outbreak investigations.
Target amplification techniques	Copies of a specific target nucleic acid are synthesized, and the products of amplification are detected by specifically designed oligonucleotide primers that bind to the complementary sequence on opposite strands of the double-stranded targets.
Signal amplification techniques	The target itself is not amplified; instead, the concentration of labeled molecules attached to the target nucleic acid is increased and measured

PCR, Polymerase chain reaction; *RT,* real-time; *SNPs,* single-nucleotide polymorphisms.

CLINICAL SPECIMENS FOR RESPIRATORY PATHOGEN DIAGNOSIS

Detection of respiratory pathogens is dependent on the type and quality of specimen collected, the timing of collection after the onset of clinical symptoms, the age of the patient, and transportation and storage of the sample before being tested in the laboratory. Ensuring high-quality collection of the right specimens is essential for making an accurate and interpretable laboratory diagnosis.

A range of specimens can be used for identifying the microbial etiology of respiratory infections in children and are shown in Table 22.12. Not all specimens are easily obtainable, and the diagnostic utility varies with each specimen type. The inability to obtain good-quality specimens from the lower respiratory tract is a fundamental problem with pneumonia diagnostics, and obtaining representative and uncontaminated specimens from the lungs is a challenge. Specimens collected by sputum induction or bronchoscopy may be contaminated by normal respiratory flora. Transthoracic needle aspiration is the best technique to obtain specimens from the site of infection in pneumonia, but it is performed in few centers despite a good safety profile.[16]

Specimens should be collected as early as possible in the acute stage of an infection, preferably prior to administration of antimicrobial or antiviral drugs. During this period, higher pathogen concentrations are likely to be present; however, the duration of pathogen shedding depends on the microorganism involved and the severity of the infection and other factors. With uncomplicated influenza virus infections, virus shedding is usually 3 to 5 days following symptom onset; however, this may be extended in severe respiratory disease to 5 to 10 days.[17] Children may also shed for up to 10 days and many weeks in immunocompromised individuals.

Throat and Nasopharyngeal Specimens

The majority of respiratory tract specimens received in the diagnostic laboratory from children are aspirates or swabs obtained from the upper respiratory tract. Nasopharyngeal aspirates are generally superior to swabs for the detection of respiratory viruses, since large numbers of respiratory epithelial cells are aspirated during the collection process.[18] However, aspirates are more difficult to obtain, especially outside the hospital setting, as they require a specific suction device. A range of commercial swabs are available, which include rayon tipped swabs and polyurethane sponges with wooden, plastic, or wire shafts. The availability of flocked nylon swabs, designed for the collection of respiratory samples, allows for the improved collection and release of respiratory epithelial cells and secretions from both children and adults.[19] Their use for obtaining nasopharyngeal specimens has been shown to have a similar performance to nasopharyngeal aspirates for the detection of common respiratory viruses in children, and the technique is relatively noninvasive.[20]

Nasal or oropharyngeal samples are generally not recommended for routine diagnostic use. The combining of nasal and throat swabs has been trialed in children in hospital and community settings and shown to have a reduced sensitivity.[21] In general, viral loads are higher in the nasopharynx than in the oropharynx, but with some respiratory virus infections, avian influenza H5N1, for example, titers may be highest in the lower respiratory tract. There may also be a higher yield from throat swabs compared to other samples for the detection of *Mycoplasma pneumoniae*.[22]

Induced Sputum

Culture of sputum specimens is commonly used as part of the evaluation of pneumonia in adults. Despite difficulties with interpretation of results,[3] carefully collected and processed sputum specimens have been shown to be useful in some contexts.[23] Nonetheless, there is still ongoing controversy about the value of routinely examining sputum.[24–28] Furthermore, sputum microscopy and culture are not routinely performed in children due to difficulties in obtaining specimens in this age group who are typically unable to expectorate.[29]

To overcome specimen collection problems, methods such as hypertonic saline nebulization have been used to induce sputum production. Induced sputum is now widely used to investigate lower respiratory infections in immunocompromised adults, especially for diagnosing *Pneumocystis jirovecii* infection,[30] and has also been used to diagnose pneumonia in children from settings with a high prevalence of tuberculosis.[31] However, few studies have collected induced sputum routinely from children with pneumonia. Recent studies of children hospitalized with community-acquired pneumonia from Finland, Kenya, and New Caledonia showed that collection of induced sputum was well tolerated, with

a diagnostic yield from culture ranging from 12% to 65% using different interpretative criteria.[32–34]

The most rigorous evaluation of induced sputum for the diagnosis of pneumonia in children was performed as part of the Pneumonia Etiology Research for Child Health (PERCH) study. In this large study, there was no clear evidence that isolation of specific potential pathogens by culture or detection by polymerase chain reaction (PCR) was associated with pneumonia case status.[35,36] In addition, for PCR, there was no evidence that induced sputum provided additional evidence over and above testing a nasopharyngeal specimen.[36] In contrast, a recent longitudinal study from South Africa found that testing of induced sputum in addition to nasopharyngeal swabs provided incremental yield for detection of *Bordetella pertussis* and several respiratory viruses.[37]

Bronchoscopy Specimens

Although obtaining a lower respiratory sample via bronchoscopy is more invasive than sputum collection and is only available in certain facilities, there are potential advantages in being confident that the sample actually comes from the lower respiratory tract and in the avoidance of upper airway contamination. However, despite best efforts to avoid contamination with normal upper airways flora (including with use of protected specimen brushes), this is often difficult to achieve and must be considered when interpreting routine bacterial culture findings.[38] In practice, the use of bronchoscopy to obtain specimens in the context of childhood respiratory infections is largely restricted to immunocompromised individuals and those with problematic cystic fibrosis or with persistent focally abnormal chest radiographic changes.[39] Bronchoscopy can also have an important role in the diagnosis and management of pediatric pulmonary tuberculosis.[40]

Endotracheal Aspirates

Despite widespread use, the value of endotracheal aspirates to diagnose the cause of ventilator-associated pneumonia is debatable. Even though quantitative culture methods have been recommended, tracheal aspirate microscopy and culture do not appear to distinguish between infection and colonization.[41] There is also evidence that specimens should be rejected from further processing if no organisms are seen on Gram stain.[42]

Transthoracic Lung Aspiration

Needle aspiration of an area of suspected pneumonia is theoretically most likely to obtain the ideal clinical specimen for determining microbial etiology of pneumonia. Experience with large numbers of procedures at some locations has demonstrated the good safety profile of this technique. In The Gambia, which has the greatest experience with transthoracic lung aspiration in children, a review of over 500 lung aspirates over 25 years reported complications in six patients (all transient) and no deaths from the procedure.[16] Diagnostic yield with both culture and nucleic acid detection methods is appreciable,[16,43] with about a two-fold increase in yield with nucleic acid detection over culture alone.[43] However, the interpretation of results from highly sensitive molecular diagnostic techniques needs to consider new concepts of the lung microbiome that question whether the lungs are normally sterile. Transthoracic needle aspiration is not indicated for all children with pneumonia and is only appropriate for peripheral lesions confirmed on chest radiography.

Lung Tissue

The use of lung tissue to determine the microbial etiology of pneumonia is largely restricted to postmortem studies.[44] These are rarely performed on children but may provide valuable information on the causes of fatal cases of pneumonia and can confirm antemortem microbiological diagnoses.

Blood Specimens

Blood can be collected for culture, serological testing and, occasionally, nucleic acid tests. The yield from blood cultures is enhanced by obtaining adequate specimen volume, collecting the specimen prior to antimicrobial therapy, and avoidance of skin contamination through good phlebotomy technique.[45,46] Although there is good evidence that yield increases with increasing blood volume, the optimal collection volume in children is unclear. One current guideline recommends the collection of 3% to 4% of total patient blood volume in patients weighing less than 12.7 kg and 1.8% to 2.7% in patients weighing greater than 12.8 kg.[47] Anaerobic blood culture is usually unnecessary in children.

Urine

The main reason to collect urine specimens as part of the workup of respiratory infections in children is to test for specific antigens. For this purpose, the timing of specimen collection in relation to antimicrobial therapy is less important than for urine culture for suspected urinary tract infection. Collection of acute phase urine specimens can be challenging in young children, and a variety of techniques have been deployed to enhance collection in a clinically relevant time frame.

Testing of urine for antimicrobial activity by simple bioassay methods has been a valuable tool for detecting prior antimicrobial administration in epidemiological studies, although the timely collection of urine samples in young children can be challenging.[48]

MICROBIOLOGICAL TOOLS

Microscopy

As part of the investigation of respiratory infections, specimens obtained from the lower respiratory tract, pleural space, or abscesses that are sent for bacterial culture are usually examined first by Gram stain microscopy. Microscopy provides information on specimen quality and can provide early clues about the cause of infection. For example, the presence of large numbers of polymorphonuclear leukocytes indicates an inflammatory response, while the presence of bacteria with characteristic morphology may provide an early indication of the culture result and give guidance about treatment. When performed by experienced microscopists, some findings can be very specific. For example, the detection of Gram-positive cocci in clusters in a pleural fluid sample is highly suggestive of *Staphylococcus aureus*. The presence of a predominance of small gram-negative pleomorphic coccobacilli in a good-quality sputum sample is suggestive of infection with *H. influenzae*. Table 22.13 lists the typical Gram stain picture of three commonly found pathogens.

Microscopy is also an important tool to assess the quality of lower respiratory samples, which itself has a large impact on the interpretation of culture results.[49] Specimens from the lower respiratory tract can be contaminated by upper respiratory secretions during collection. Also, a poorly collected "lower respiratory" specimen may be predominantly composed of upper respiratory secretions. Either situation can lead to incorrect interpretations of culture results. To overcome this issue, it is standard practice for diagnostic laboratories to assess the quality of lower respiratory samples before they are cultured. This typically involves assessing the number of squamous epithelial cells (SECs) and polymorphonuclear cells (PMNs) in a Gram-stained smear of the specimen.[50,51] The presence of low numbers of SECs and high numbers of PMNs per low-power field are regarded as being indicative of a high-quality specimen.[52] Conversely, specimens with relatively low numbers of PMNs and high numbers of SECs are likely to represent oropharyngeal contamination and are rejected for routine culture. Detection of a potential pathogen in such a specimen that is contaminated with oropharyngeal flora may represent nothing more than the patient's oropharyngeal microbiota.

Table 22.14 summarizes some commonly used criteria for assessment of lower respiratory specimens. Other rejection criteria have been described that also include the presence of PMNs,[51] and it is the responsibility of the laboratory to have a standard operating procedure that specifies rejection criteria. Although there is a paucity of data from children, quantity of SECs alone was demonstrated to be a useful quality measure for induced sputum from young children with pneumonia.[53] Notable exceptions to sputum rejection criteria are specimens for detection of *Legionella* spp.[54] and *Mycobacterium tuberculosis*; any specimen submitted for investigation of legionellosis or tuberculosis should be processed by the laboratory regardless of the specimen quality.

Culture

Traditional bacterial culture techniques continue to be a fundamental diagnostic tool in diagnostic laboratories. In contrast, viral culture is now infrequently performed as a routine test, as it is time-consuming, requires a specialist laboratory area and has been largely superseded by molecular diagnostic techniques.

Although most important bacterial pathogens grow on standard laboratory media, such as sheep blood agar, special media environmental conditions are required to optimize the growth of some bacteria. For example, chocolate agar is the usual medium used to isolate *H. influenzae*, an atmosphere of 5% CO_2 is required to isolate *S. pneumoniae*, and special media are required for culturing *Legionella* species and *B. pertussis*. As a rule of thumb, it takes most bacterial pathogens 24 to 48 hours to grow in culture, and a further 24 to 48 hours are required to perform antimicrobial susceptibility testing.

The recent availability of matrix-assisted laser desorption ionization time-of-flight mass spectrometry (MALDI-TOF MS) has revolutionized the workflow in diagnostic laboratories.[55-57] MALDI-TOF MS allows the rapid identification of cultured microorganisms at a relatively low cost. The identification is based on the generation of mass spectra from whole cell extracts that are then compared to a library of well-characterized protein profiles. Although this method still

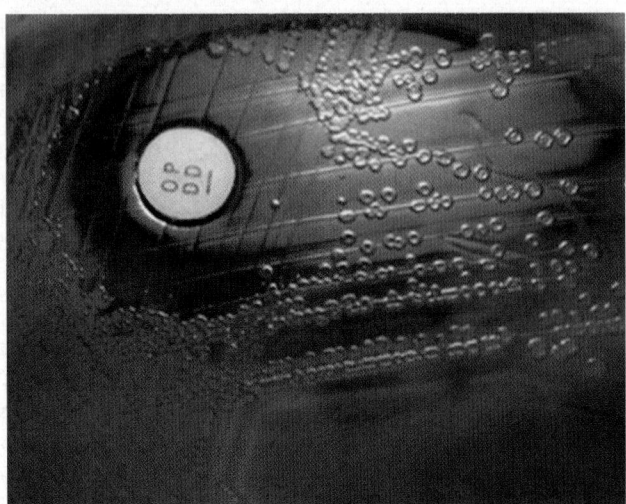

Fig. 22.1 Typical "draughtsman" phenomenon (ringed colonies with raised edges and depressed centers) and optochin-susceptibility of *Streptococcus pneumoniae*.

relies on traditional culture methods to obtain a pure isolate, MALDI-TOF MS provides full identification within minutes, including for all major bacterial respiratory pathogens.[58]

When reporting respiratory tract culture results, which are typically mixed cultures, laboratory scientists will focus on predominant organisms and those known to be important pathogens, such as *S. pyogenes* in throat swabs and *S. pneumoniae* in sputum samples (Fig. 22.1). Background oropharyngeal flora will normally not be worked up or reported in any detail, as this information will not contribute to patient care and, indeed, may give the false impression that they need to be treated.

The isolation of a bacterial organism from blood conclusively provides evidence of the cause of severe respiratory disease in children. The drawback is that recovery of bacterial pathogens from blood cultures in the context of respiratory infections is very low in children.[59,60] The typical blood culture yield in children admitted to hospital with community-acquired pneumonia is under 10%.[49,61] As discussed previously, the yield is greater when larger volumes of blood are collected, careful measures are taken to avoid skin contamination, and when samples are collected before antibiotics are commenced.[46]

Antigen Detection Assays

A variety of antigen detection assays for respiratory pathogens have been introduced into routine use by diagnostic laboratories. Direct fluorescent antibody (DFA) assays have been used for many years as rapid tests for respiratory viruses, although they have now been largely replaced by molecular methods or rapid antigen detection tests (RADTs). DFA looks for characteristic fluorescent staining patterns in cellular material from clinical specimens. Currently available assays detect respiratory syncytial virus (RSV), influenza A and B, parainfluenza viruses 1, 2, and 3, human metapneumovirus and adenovirus with sensitivities of about 80% to 90% and very high specificity.[62] DFA requires particular technical expertise but has the advantages that sample quality can be directly evaluated, and test results can be available within 60 minutes.

Among the most common antigen detection assays for respiratory infections are the RADTs for respiratory viruses, particularly influenza viruses and respiratory syncytial virus. The usefulness of RADTs is limited by variable and often suboptimal sensitivity, typically 50% to 98% for RSV and 10% to 85% for influenza viruses, although specificities are generally high (80% to 100%).[63,64] The clinical usefulness of these tests is affected by disease prevalence, being poor when there are few cases in the community (positive predictive value is low and false-positive cases are more likely). During peak virus circulation, although the positive predictive value approaches 100%, the negative predictive value is lower and false-negative results are more likely.[65,66] Due to concerns about poor sensitivity, most authorities recommend that RADTs for influenza are only used with caution outside the influenza season and only when a result will influence patient management; they emphasize that negative RADT results do not exclude influenza in patients with typical signs and symptoms.[67,68]

Other commonly used antigen detection assays for respiratory infections are those that detect *S. pneumoniae* and *Legionella pneumophila* serogroup 1 antigens in urine. These assays, typically in immunochromatographic test format, provide results within a short time frame, but are almost exclusively used on adults with suspected pneumonia. The specificity of currently used pneumococcal urinary antigen tests in children is poor, with frequent false positives due to nasopharyngeal carriage of *S. pneumoniae*.[69–71] This has limited the clinical utility of this test in children, but there may be some value as a diagnostic adjunct in cases with radiologically confirmed pneumonia. There is considerable interest in the development of serotype-specific pneumococcal urinary antigen tests.[72–74] Early assessments in children indicate that these next-generation assays may have some diagnostic value, at least in epidemiological studies, but assay cutoffs need to differ from adults to distinguish between carriage and disease.[75] Pneumococcal antigen detection assays have also been successfully applied to pleural fluid samples in children with pleural effusion or empyema.[76,77] A positive test result has high specificity in this context.

RADTs are also available for the diagnosis of *S. pyogenes* in throat swab specimens. These tests have high specificity for detection of *S. pyogenes*, but have relatively low sensitivity (70% to 90%), which is even lower in those with less severe disease.[78] As a consequence of suboptimal sensitivity, it is commonly recommended to perform bacterial culture on any samples that test negative by RADTs.[79,80]

Serology

Serological testing for respiratory pathogens was commonly performed in the past, relying either on the detection of immunoglobulin M (IgM) in the acute phase of the disease or the demonstration of seroconversion. More recently, the use of serological testing has largely been replaced by molecular-based assays that provide a rapid diagnosis with greater sensitivity and specificity.

Serological assays still have a limited place in the diagnosis of childhood respiratory disease. Detection of IgM antibodies is still a routine diagnostic tool for *M. pneumoniae* infection. However, older children may not mount an IgM response because of reinfection rather than primary infection, and IgM antibodies may persist for months after the acute infection.[81,82] For detection of *B. pertussis* infection, IgG antibody responses to pertussis toxin may be an indicator of infection, although these assays cannot differentiate between an immune response induced by infection and that due to vaccination. Serological diagnosis of pertussis has largely been replaced by molecular-based assays.[83,84] The serological diagnosis of *Chlamydophila pneumoniae* infection is complicated by the lack of species-specific tests and the resultant potential of cross-reactions in the assay. A single positive IgM response in any disease investigation may represent possible cross-reactivity or nonspecific interference in the assay and needs to be interpreted with caution and in the context of the clinical presentation.

Although detection of antistreptolysin O (ASO) and deoxyribonuclease (DNase) antibodies can be used when investigating the potential complications of *S. pyogenes* infections, such as glomerulonephritis and rheumatic fever, they are not useful for the diagnosis of acute *S. pyogenes* pharyngitis.[85]

Molecular Methods

The development and implementation of molecular methods is the single biggest recent advance in the diagnostics of respiratory infections.[4] While nucleic acid detection tests (NATs), such as PCR, have been used to detect respiratory pathogens for over two decades, the widespread adoption of these tests by diagnostic laboratories has occurred only recently, largely due to the increased availability of commercial assays. Table 22.16 discusses some of the more commonly used molecular assays, and Table 22.17 gives explanation of commonly used terms in molecular diagnostics.

NATs have several advantages over other diagnostic tools, including rapid turnaround time, the ability to detect low levels of all known pathogens, the lack of dependence on the viability of the target microorganism, little influence of antimicrobial therapy on diagnostic sensitivity, and the ability to be automated.[4] NATs may also provide additional information, such as antimicrobial susceptibility data and strain typing.

For the diagnosis of respiratory infections, the most widely used NATs are those that detect respiratory viruses and noncolonizing bacteria (e.g., *M. pneumoniae*, *Legionella* species, *B. pertussis*). For these microorganisms, detection in a respiratory sample from a child with a compatible clinical syndrome is regarded as sufficient evidence to assign causation. In contrast, NATs for other bacteria that may also be found in normal respiratory flora, including some of the most important pneumonia pathogens (e.g., *S. pneumoniae*, *H. influenzae*, and *S. aureus*), have struggled for a role outside research laboratories. As with culture-based methods, the problem with detection of these targets by NAT is the inability to distinguish colonization and carriage from disease.

NATs have particularly revolutionized the diagnosis of viral respiratory tract infections,[86,87] and are now the testing method of choice. Respiratory viruses are now commonly detected by large multiplex panels that typically include influenza A and B viruses, respiratory syncytial virus, parainfluenza viruses, human metapneumovirus, human rhinoviruses, enteroviruses, parechovirus, adenoviruses, human bocavirus, and several coronaviruses (OC43, 229E, NL63, HKU1). There are now many commercial multiplex assays available in a variety of formats, and the landscape is continually changing. In the right clinical context, the detection

of a respiratory virus in a respiratory sample is generally regarded as being sufficient to assign causation.[88] However, this assumption is not always reliable as there is uncertainty about the pathogenic role of some viruses,[89] leading some to question the wisdom of using large multiplex NAT panels as first-line tests for respiratory pathogens, given potential problems with interpretation of positive results.[90] Furthermore, respiratory viruses are often detected in a similar proportion of both subjects with and without pneumonia in childhood pneumonia etiology studies,[32,91] although this observation typically does not apply to influenza A and B viruses, respiratory syncytial virus, and human metapneumovirus, which are disproportionately associated with case status.

NATs have also been used to detect *S. pyogenes* in throat swab samples, although these methods have not been used widely.[92–94] This situation is likely to change with the recent increased availability of commercial methods[92,94] and the motivation to improve turnaround times to better guide antimicrobial therapy.

Detection of microbial load by quantitative molecular methods has been explored in the effort to help distinguish infection from contamination or colonization. Microorganisms detected in greater quantities may be more likely to be clinically significant. Quantitative multiplex PCR has been used to determine the etiology of community-acquired pneumonia in adults using cutoffs developed for interpretation of culture results from lower respiratory tract specimens.[95,96] Greater confidence in the diagnostic cutoffs will be needed before this approach can be introduced into routine diagnostic use. Quantitative approaches using NATs have also been applied to nasopharyngeal specimens. Among human immunodeficiency virus (HIV)-infected adults in South Africa, quantitative PCR testing of nasopharyngeal samples distinguished between pneumococcal pneumonia and asymptomatic pneumococcal colonization with reasonable diagnostic accuracy.[97,98] Nasopharyngeal pneumococcal load also distinguished colonization from microbiologically confirmed pneumococcal pneumonia in a large pediatric study, although the diagnostic accuracy was inadequate for clinical use.[99]

NATs have also been applied, with limited success, to nonrespiratory specimens for determining the microbial etiology of respiratory infections in children. There has been particular interest in the testing of blood for *S. pneumoniae* by PCR. Among Italian children, blood PCR detected invasive pneumococcal disease with high specificity.[100–104] However, in other populations positive results have been reported in control participants who do not have suspected pneumococcal disease,[105] with false-positive results being relatively common in children from developing countries where there is a high prevalence of pneumococcal carriage.[106]

The potential application of whole genome sequencing in the diagnostic laboratory is still being realized. This method is already being increasingly used for strain characterization of bacterial isolates as part of epidemiological investigations.[107] However, its precise role in determining the etiology of respiratory infections is uncertain.

Antimicrobial Susceptibility Testing

Most antimicrobial susceptibility testing methods are performed on pure live bacterial cultures using a variety of standard methods.[108] Several guidelines have been established for interpretation of findings; the most commonly used guidelines are produced by the European Committee on Antimicrobial Susceptibility Testing (EUCAST)[109] and the Clinical and Laboratory Standards Institute (CLSI).[110] These guidelines are comparable, and it is essential that each diagnostic laboratory chooses an approved guideline for interpretation of their antimicrobial susceptibility test results. Increasingly, molecular methods with rapid turnaround times are being used to detect specific antimicrobial resistance mechanisms.[111] This trend is likely to continue given the constant demands for rapid identification of resistant pathogens.

Antiviral susceptibility testing against respiratory pathogens is rarely indicated and has mainly focused on influenza viruses.[112]

DIAGNOSTIC APPROACH BY SYNDROME

Common Cold

Manifestations of the common cold are so typical that diagnostic testing is usually unnecessary. If there is a reason to determine the specific virus involved, testing a nasopharyngeal specimen for respiratory viruses by NAT is the current test of choice.

Pharyngitis

The main reasons to diagnose the cause of acute pharyngitis are to detect cases caused by *S. pyogenes* and to identify the occasional case due to less common causes, such as *Arcanobacterium haemolyticum* and *Corynebacterium diphtheriae*. Throat swab culture is still the mainstay although antigen detection assays are available. In future, molecular point of care tests are likely to become available to clinicians in primary care.

Croup

The diagnosis of croup is usually based on the characteristic clinical picture (fever, hoarseness, barking cough, inspiratory stridor, and varying degrees of respiratory distress) and epidemiology. Identification of specific microbial causes can be accomplished by testing a nasopharyngeal specimen for respiratory viruses by NAT.

Sinusitis

Diagnostic testing is not usually performed on cases of acute sinusitis as the microbial etiology is well described. However, sinus puncture should be performed to obtain specimens for bacterial culture in patients with severe sinusitis, in those who have not responded to empiric antibiotics, and in patients with severe immunosuppression.

Epiglottitis

H. influenzae type b is isolated in cultures of blood and/or epiglottis in most children with epiglottitis. Direct visualization of the epiglottis should be performed in a setting where immediate securing of the airway is possible.

Bronchiolitis

A specific diagnosis of the causative agent of bronchiolitis can be made by testing a nasopharyngeal specimen for respiratory viruses by NAT.

Pneumonia

Determining the microbial etiology of pneumonia in children remains challenging, largely due to difficulties obtaining a sample from lungs.[2] Current guidelines for the management of community-acquired pneumonia in children generally recommend that diagnostic tests should mainly be used on patients with severe disease, with a focus on blood cultures and detection of respiratory viruses.[61,113] The development of improved urinary antigen tests and quantitative molecular assays holds hope for the future.

Pleural Effusion and Empyema

Gram stain and culture of fluid aspirated from the pleural cavity is indicated in patients for whom a diagnosis of infection is considered. The sample can also be tested for pneumococcal antigen by a RADT and nucleic acid detection methods. Testing of pleural fluid increased the yield of *S. pneumoniae* detection by 31% in South African children with empyema.[114]

Lung Abscess

Needle aspiration provides the best opportunity to identify the microbial cause of an abscess. Abscess fluid may also be recovered by bronchoscopy if it has ruptured. Blood cultures should also be performed in children with suspected lung abscess.

Infections Associated With Cystic Fibrosis

There is often a close working relationship between clinicians caring for patients with cystic fibrosis and laboratory scientists. Special attention is given by the laboratory to lower respiratory specimens from patients with cystic fibrosis with a particular focus on classic pathogens associated with this disease, such as *Pseudomonas aeruginosa*, *Burkholderia cepacia* complex, and *S. aureus*.[115] The use of synergy testing to assess antimicrobial combinations is often used in cystic fibrosis patients with multiresistant organisms, although the value of this practice has been questioned.[116]

Microbiome

Recognition of the possible existence of the lung microbiome has been a major recent revelation in respiratory medicine.[6] Until recently, the lungs in health were regarded as sterile, but the use of modern culture-independent techniques has consistently found evidence of bacteria in the lower airways.[6] Most of these studies have been performed on bronchoscopic specimens, which may be susceptible to contamination, but there is certainly mounting evidence supporting the non-sterility of the lung.

The existence of the lung microbiome has challenged our traditional paradigm of pneumonia pathogenesis, as the traditional view is that pneumonia is caused by a single invasive pathogen in a normally sterile site. There is increasing recognition that bacteria and viruses frequently interact in the causative pathway to pneumonia,[117,118] and the common finding of polymicrobial infection[10] adds further complexity to our understanding of how pneumonia develops. The traditional bacterial versus viral pneumonia concept may be too simplistic. Consequently, we are likely to need more sophisticated approaches to pneumonia diagnosis and interpretation of laboratory results than simply using assays that target single specific putative pathogens.

We have a lot to learn about the lung microbiome and are only just beginning to understand changes in the lung ecosystem during acute infections.[6,119–121] Analysis of the lung microbiome may provide insights into pneumonia etiology and reveal novel markers for pneumonia prognosis and treatment guidance.[122] The following are some examples of recent findings about the respiratory microbiome that may have clinical implications, and they give an indication of the applications that may be available in the future.

Using 16S ribosomal RNA sequencing, a recent study showed that certain taxa in the respiratory microbiota were associated with the clinical course of pediatric pneumonia.[123] In children aged 6 months to 5 years, high relative abundance in sputum of *Actinomyces, Veillonella, Rothia*, and Lactobacillales was associated with decreased odds of length of stay ≥4 days, and high relative abundance of *Haemophilus* and Pasteurellaceae was associated with increased odds of intensive care unit admission. In children aged 5 to 18 years, high relative abundance in sputum of Porphyromonadaceae, Bacteriodales, Lactobacillales, and *Prevotella* was associated with increased odds of length of stay ≥4 days.

In another recent study, the composition of the nasopharyngeal bacterial community of children was related to the prior history of acute sinusitis.[124] History of acute sinusitis was associated with significant depletion in relative abundance of taxa including *Faecalibacterium prausnitzii* and *Akkermansia* spp. and enrichment of *Moraxella nonliquefaciens*. Children who experienced more frequent upper respiratory infections had significantly diminished nasopharyngeal microbiota diversity.

Other recent data indicate that interactions between RSV and nasopharyngeal microbiota might modulate the host immune response, potentially affecting clinical disease severity,[125] that the nasopharyngeal microbiome at the time of upper respiratory viral infections during infancy may contribute to the ensuing risk for development of asthma,[126] and that the microbiome of children with cystic fibrosis is susceptible to environmental influences, suggesting that interventions to preserve the community structure found in young patients and slow disease progression might be possible.[127]

We can expect to see an exponential increase in publications on the role of the respiratory microbiome in health and disease over the next few years. The extent to which these findings can be readily translated into clinical applications is uncertain.

Future Prospects

The trend towards increased use of molecular diagnostic tools will probably continue with increased availability of point of care testing. It is also likely that measurement of bacterial and viral pathogen load will be part of those developments, both for distinguishing between colonization and disease and for monitoring response to treatment. Any future developments in diagnostics for respiratory infections must incorporate new knowledge about the lung microbiome. For lower respiratory infections, there is likely to be a move away from the detection of specific known pathogens to measurement of markers of change in the lung microbial ecology during disease. The development of new and better urinary antigen tests would be welcome, as these can be readily adapted to point of care testing.

References
Access the reference list online at ExpertConsult.com.

23 Acute Infections That Produce Upper Airway Obstruction

IAN MICHAEL BALFOUR-LYNN, BSC, MBBS, MD, FRCP, FRCPCH, FRCS(Ed), and
MARIE WRIGHT, MBChB, MRCPCH

Upper airway obstruction due to acute infection is not uncommon in children, and many parents have experienced an anxious night with a "croupy" child. Although infants and young children are most commonly affected because they have relatively narrow upper airways, older children and adults can also have significant symptoms. Fortunately, these are mostly due to self-limiting viral laryngotracheobronchitis (LTB), but there is also a group of bacterial infections (e.g., epiglottitis, bacterial tracheitis, diphtheria, retropharyngeal abscess, and peritonsillar abscess) that can occasionally cause significant obstruction. It is the job of the emergency physician, pediatrician, pediatric pulmonologist, or otorhinolaryngologist to diagnose more serious infections promptly so that treatment can be instituted early and disastrous obstruction avoided. It is also important to recognize when a simple viral LTB is causing significant problems, so that appropriate treatment can be given immediately. This chapter is clinically oriented and outlines the principal infective causes of upper airway obstruction, with an emphasis on diagnosis and treatment. Confusion exists regarding the nomenclature for these disorders, with some using the term *croup* to refer to any inflammatory disorder of the upper airway, whereas others restrict its use to subglottic disease (i.e., LTB, which is usually of viral origin). Therefore, for the sake of clarity, the term *croup* will be largely avoided in this chapter.

The consequence of these upper airway infections is usually stridor, which is a clinical sign and should not be considered a definitive diagnosis. This section briefly outlines the principles behind what causes stridor, which should clarify why this condition mostly affects infants and young children. The appendix in Holinger and colleagues' *Pediatric Laryngology and Bronchoesophagology* discusses the physics of air flow and fluid dynamics.[1] The laws of fluid dynamics are based on flow through fixed tubes and may not always apply to dynamic airways in vivo. Normally, air flow through the upper airways is laminar, and the moving column of air produces slight negative pressure on the airway walls.[2] Inflammation resulting from infection causes a degree of airway narrowing, which increases the flow rate through the narrowed segment (the Venturi effect). This, in turn, causes a reduction in the pressure exerted on the airway wall. This is the Bernoulli principle. In other words, negative intraluminal pressure increases. This enhances the tendency of the airway to collapse inward, further narrowing the airway and causing turbulent air flow. The respiratory phase (inspiration or expiration) has a differential effect on air flow, depending on whether the obstruction is intrathoracic or extrathoracic (Fig. 23.1). Stridor is the sound made by rapid, turbulent flow of air through a narrowed segment of a large airway. It is most often loud, with medium or low pitch, and inspiratory. It usually originates from the larynx, upper trachea,

or hypopharynx.[3] Progression of the disease process may make stridor softer, higher-pitched, and biphasic (inspiratory and expiratory). With the onset of complete obstruction, stridor may become barely audible as minimal air moves through the critically narrowed airway.[4]

The laryngeal anatomy of children makes them particularly susceptible to narrowing of the upper airways. The larynx of a neonate is situated high in the neck, and the epiglottis is narrow, omega-shaped (ω), and vertically positioned.[5] The narrowest segment of the pediatric airway is the subglottic region (in adults, it is at the glottic level), which is encircled by the rigid cricoid cartilage ring. There is nonfibrous, loosely attached mucosa in this region that is easily obstructed in the presence of subglottic edema. In addition, the cartilaginous support of the infant airway is soft and compliant, easily allowing dynamic collapse of the airways during inspiration. Young children have proportionally large heads and relatively lax neck support; this combination increases the likelihood of airway obstruction when supine.[6] Also, their tongues are relatively large for the size of the oropharynx. Simple mathematics shows why a small amount of edema has such a profound effect on the cross-sectional area and hence air flow. The diameter of the subglottis in a normal newborn is approximately 5 mm, and 0.5-mm edema in this region reduces the cross-sectional area to 64% of normal (area = $\pi \infty$ radius^2). Air flow is directly proportional to the airway radius to the fourth power (Poiseuille's law), so a small reduction in caliber has a major effect on flow rate. The same 5-mm airway with 0.5 mm edema will have a flow rate of only 41% of baseline, assuming that pressure remains unchanged—a situation that is not necessarily the case if the Bernoulli principle is in play. Because the caliber of the airway is almost inevitably reduced further in accord with the Bernoulli principle, and Poiseuille flow is not established, the flow rate is much further reduced, and the work of breathing is greatly increased to maintain ventilation.

Viral Laryngotracheobronchitis

EPIDEMIOLOGY

Viral LTB is the most common cause of infective upper airway obstruction in the pediatric age group. Affected children are usually of preschool age, with a peak incidence between 18 and 24 months of age.[7] Although viral LTB episodes become uncommon beyond 6 years of age, cases have been reported during later childhood and adolescence, and rarely described in adults. Reported annual incidence rates in preschool children vary from 1.5% to 6%, but less than 5% of these require

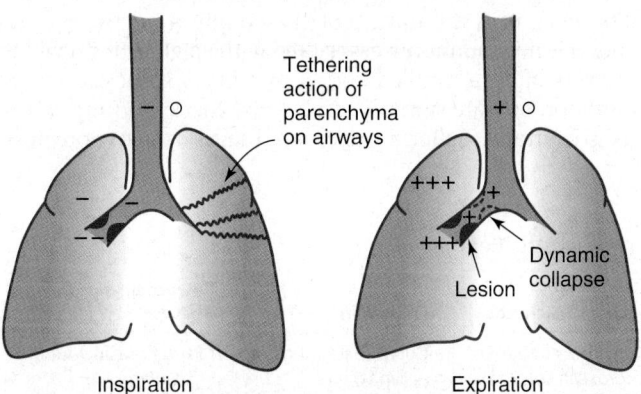

EXTRATHORACIC OBSTRUCTION

Lesion →

Pressure drop across obstruction

Dynamic collapse →

Inspiration

Expiration

INTRATHORACIC OBSTRUCTION

Tethering action of parenchyma on airways

Dynamic collapse

Lesion

Inspiration

Expiration

Fig. 23.1 The effect of the respiratory phase on extrathoracic and intrathoracic obstruction is shown. During inspiration, negative intratracheal pressure (relative to atmospheric pressure) leads to dynamic collapse of the extrathoracic airway, thus worsening the effects of an extrathoracic obstructive lesion. In contrast, intrathoracic obstruction improves during inspiration because the elastic recoil of the lung parenchyma opens the intrathoracic airways. During expiration, intratracheal pressure is positive relative to atmospheric pressure, opening the extrathoracic trachea and lessening the obstructive effect of lesions. In contrast, intrathoracic obstruction worsens because of lower pressure in the airways relative to the surrounding parenchyma, collapsing the airways. (From Loughlin GM, Taussig LM. Upper airway obstruction. *Semin Respir Med.* 1979;1:131-146.)

hospital admission, and only 1% to 2% of those admitted require endotracheal intubation and intensive care.[8] This proportion has fallen dramatically since the use of corticosteroids has become routine. Mortality is low, reported by one 10-year follow-up study as less than 0.5% of intubated patients.[9] There is a male preponderance in children younger than 6 years of age (1.4:1), although both sexes appear to be affected equally at an older age.

Children with a specific CD14 genetic polymorphism (C/C variant of CD14 C-159T) have recently been described as having a reduced prevalence of croup. It has been hypothesized that this relates to the role of the CD14 gene as a pattern recognition receptor in the mediation of the innate immune system response to LTB-causing viruses.[10]

Cases may occur in epidemics, with those caused by parainfluenza virus (PIV) type 1 typically presenting in fall and winter months. Infections caused by other common organisms, including other PIV subtypes, occur more commonly as isolated infections. Infection is via droplet spread or direct inoculation from the hands. Viruses can survive for long periods on dry surfaces, such as clothes and toys, emphasizing the importance of infection-control practices.

ETIOLOGY

The most common etiologic agents are the PIVs, of which PIV 1 is found most frequently and leads to epidemics. PIV 2 may account for many sporadic cases, and PIV 3 is a less common cause of viral LTB, usually targeting the epithelium of the smaller airways and leading to bronchiolitic illness. Less is known about the clinical presentation of PIV 4, but it is reported to result in milder clinical illness and is infrequently associated with croup symptoms.[11] The PIVs belong to the *Paramyxoviridae* family, along with respiratory syncytial virus, measles, mumps, and the recently identified human metapneumovirus.[12] Together the PIVs account for more than 75% of viral LTB cases, although other respiratory viruses (e.g., respiratory syncytial virus, rhinovirus, adenovirus, coronavirus, human bocavirus, and enteroviruses) can produce a similar clinical syndrome. Herpes viruses and influenza viruses tend to cause a more severe and protracted form of the disease.[13] LTB can also occur with some systemic infections, such as measles and, less commonly, mycoplasma. In general, however, it is not usually possible to identify the cause of infection from the child's symptoms because severity does not correlate with any particular etiologic agent.

PATHOLOGY

Infection affects the larynx, trachea, and bronchi, although swelling and inflammation in the subglottic area leads to the characteristic clinical features of viral LTB. In addition to relative differences in airway size (discussed earlier in the chapter), it is suggested that poor cell-mediated immunity in younger age groups also accounts for differences observed between adults and children.[14] The epithelium of the subglottis possesses abundant mucous glands, secretions from which can further narrow the airway lumen in response to infection. The PIVs are trophic for the respiratory epithelium, binding in particular to ciliated cells via an interaction between the viral hemagglutinin-neuraminidase protein and its receptor, sialic acid. Other viral proteins (the F protein in particular) are important in membrane fusion and the passage of viral particles between cells. Many strains of PIV are cytopathic, with infection leading to the formation of giant cells and cell death. As with many infective processes, the ensuing inflammatory response is involved in the evolution of symptoms. Both polymorphonuclear and monocytic leukocytes infiltrate the subepithelium, which leads to vascular congestion and airway wall edema. In addition, the symptoms of viral LTB are believed to be caused by the release of spasmogenic mediators, leading to decreased airway diameter. This may result from a type I hypersensitivity response to PIV, and some authors have postulated a role for anti-PIV-specific immunoglobulin E (IgE) in the development of airway narrowing.[15] These factors may play a relatively greater role in patients with recurrent (spasmodic) croup, and these patients may have hyperreactivity of the extrathoracic and intrathoracic airways.[16]

The etiology of recurrent, spasmodic croup remains unclear, with authors expressing differing views on whether it is usually virus-related[17] or is a separate disease entity; suggested triggers include gastroesophageal reflux, eosinophilic esophagitis,[18] and anatomical abnormalities, in addition to an allergic predisposition.[19]

CLINICAL FEATURES

Mild

Most children are affected mildly by viruses that cause LTB.[7] The exact incidence remains unknown, because many of them do not receive medical attention, but are managed by parents at home. Children have a barking cough and a hoarse cry or voice; these symptoms are worse in the evening and at night. They may also have inspiratory stridor on exertion, but stridor at rest is usually absent, as are other signs of respiratory distress. There is most commonly a coryzal prodrome accompanied by a low-grade fever, but children are not particularly unwell or toxic. They remain interested in their surroundings, are playful, and still eat and drink.

Moderate

Features of moderate viral LTB include those discussed earlier, but with inspiratory stridor present at rest, as well as a degree of respiratory distress manifest by chest wall recession, tachypnea, and the use of accessory muscles of respiration. There is usually accompanying tachycardia, but children remain interactive and are able to take at least liquids orally.

Severe

Progression from moderate to severe infection can occur rapidly and may be precipitated by the distress caused by clinical examination. Worrisome signs include those of increasing respiratory distress, with the child appearing anxious or preoccupied and tired. Drooling may occur (but not as commonly as in epiglottitis), and the child will often refuse liquids or be unable to coordinate swallowing and breathing. However, the child with viral LTB will not appear toxic, with high fever and flushed face, as do those with the classic signs of bacterial epiglottitis (Table 23.1). Another difference is in the nature of the cough; a harsh, barking cough is not commonly associated with epiglottitis (in which there is often a muffled cough and cry). Restlessness and agitation are late signs of airway obstruction of any cause, as is cyanosis, pallor, or decreased level of consciousness.

Table 23.1 Differentiation of Principal Infective Causes of Upper Airway Obstruction

	Viral Laryngotracheobronchitis	Epiglottitis	Bacterial Tracheitis	Diphtheria	Retropharyngeal Abscess
Principal organisms	Parainfluenza 1–3 Adenovirus respiratory syncytial virus	*Haemophilus influenzae,* Streptococcus	*Staphylococcus aureus, Moraxella catarrhalis, H. influenzae*	Corynebacterium diphtheria	Mixed flora, including *S. aureus, Streptococcus, H. influenzae,* anaerobes
Age range	6 months–4 years (peak, 1–2 years)	2–7 years	6 months–8 years	All ages	<6 years
Incidence	Common	Rare	Rare	Rare if vaccinated	Uncommon
Onset	Insidious usually follows upper respiratory tract infection	Rapid	Slow, with sudden deterioration	Insidious	Gradual
Site	Below the vocal cords	Supraglottis	Trachea	Tonsils, pharynx, larynx, nose, skin	Retropharyngeal space
Clinical manifestations	Low-grade fever Nontoxic barking (seallike) cough Stridor hoarseness Restlessness	High fever Severe sore throat Minimal nonbarking cough Toxic stridor Drooling Dysphagia Muffled voice Tripod position	High fever Toxic, brassy cough Stridor Hoarse voice Neck pain Choking	Fever Toxic stridor Sore throat Fetor oris Cervical lymphadenopathy Bull neck	Fever Sore throat Neck pain and stiffness (especially on extension) Dysphagia Stridor (less common) Drooling Retropharyngeal bulge
Endoscopic findings	Deep red mucosa Subglottic edema	Cherry-red or pale and edematous epiglottis Edematous aryepiglottic folds	Deep red mucosa Ulcerations Copious, thick tracheal secretions Subglottic edema, with normal epiglottis and arytenoids	Gray, adherent membrane on the pharynx	N/A
Intubation	Occasional	Usual	Usual	Occasional	Unusual
Therapy	Corticosteroids Nebulized epinephrine	Intubation (1–3 days) IV antibiotics	Intubation (3–7 days) IV antibiotics Tracheal suction	Diphtheria antitoxin IV antibiotics Immunization during convalescence	IV antibiotics ± surgery

IV, Intravenous.

Pulse oximetry should be performed, but limitations must be recognized. Oxygen saturation may be well preserved until the late stages of severe viral LTB, and it can lead to significant underestimation of respiratory compromise in a patient who is receiving supplementary oxygen. Conversely, desaturation may be seen in children with relatively mild airway obstruction (presumably reflecting lower airway involvement and ventilation-perfusion mismatch).[20] Pulsus paradoxus is present in the group with severe disease, but in clinical practice, it is difficult to assess, and attempts to do so could worsen symptoms by causing distress.

Diagnosis and Differential Diagnosis

The diagnosis of croup is made clinically, based on the features described earlier; there is no role for laboratory tests or radiography in the assessment of acute airways obstruction. In skilled hands, plain lateral neck radiographs may demonstrate sites of obstruction, but this rarely influences management; it also wastes time and can be dangerous. The neck extension that is required could precipitate sudden worsening of airway obstruction, which can be fatal in severe cases. Investigations during the acute illness should be reserved for children with an atypical presentation or who fail to respond to conventional treatment. In such cases, alternative infective (e.g., epiglottitis) and noninfective (e.g., inhaled foreign body) causes of acute airway obstruction require careful exclusion (see Box 23.1 and Table 23.1). Advice from a senior clinician is vital when croup is severe.

RECURRENT OR SPASMODIC CROUP

Symptoms are similar to those of the more typical forms of viral LTB, but children are often older, do not have the same coryzal prodrome, and may be afebrile during the episode. There may be links with atopy, often with a positive family history. Episodes are often similar to acute asthma except the child has stridor rather than wheeze. Attacks often occur suddenly, at night, and may resolve equally quickly. Treatment must be guided by the degree of severity, and is similar to that for viral LTB. Some practitioners prescribe oral or inhaled corticosteroids (via a nebulizer) to be kept at home and administered by the parents in case of an episode, although there is a paucity of evidence for or against this practice in spasmodic croup.

Box 23.1 Infectious and Noninfectious Causes of Acute Upper Airway Obstruction

Infectious	Noninfectious
Viral laryngotracheobronchitis	Foreign body
Epiglottitis	Trauma
Bacterial tracheitis	Caustic burns
Diphtheria	Spasmodic croup
Retropharyngeal abscess	Angioneurotic edema
Peritonsillar abscess	Hypocalcemia (e.g.,
Infectious mononucleosis	hypoparathyroidism)

NONINFECTIVE CAUSES OF ACUTE AIRWAY OBSTRUCTION

There are a number of noninfective causes of upper airway obstruction, and these must be considered in the differential diagnosis of infective causes (see Box 23.1). Foreign body inhalation is the most common noninfective cause in children. Symptoms may partly mimic those of viral LTB and will depend on the location of the foreign body, the degree of resultant airway obstruction, and (to a lesser extent) the nature of the foreign body. Onset of symptoms may be either acute or insidious; a large foreign body may cause severe obstruction, whereas a smaller one may simply lead to laryngeal and tracheal irritation and airway edema. In cases of severe airway obstruction, the voice may be lost and breath sounds quiet. This condition is an emergency, and requires immediate visualization of the larynx and trachea and removal of the foreign body by a physician or surgeon experienced in this procedure. Occasionally an unrecognized inhaled foreign body leads to chronic stridor. Acute upper airway obstruction may also result from the ingestion of caustic substances, with resulting pharyngeal burns, edema, and inflammation of the epiglottis, aryepiglottic folds, larynx, and trachea. This diagnosis is usually clear from the history. Rarely, angioneurotic edema may cause acute laryngeal swelling and airway obstruction. Patients appear nontoxic and may exhibit other signs of allergic disease, such as urticaria and abdominal pain. In hereditary angioneurotic edema due to C1 esterase inhibitor deficiency, the family history may be positive, although the first presentation is more common in adults than in children. Hypocalcemia, for example, due to hypoparathyroidism, can lead to laryngospasm (a form of tetany), which can cause stridor with significant airway obstruction.[21]

There are numerous causes of chronic airway obstruction that are discussed elsewhere in this book. Confusion may arise when an upper respiratory tract infection unmasks a previously asymptomatic congenital abnormality. For example, mild subglottic stenosis may cause symptoms only with the additional burden of airway edema due to a simple viral upper respiratory infection. It is important to ensure that there is no history of intubation (which may have been brief, as in resuscitation of a newborn in the maternity unit) or of any coexisting signs (e.g., a cutaneous hemangioma) that may increase the index of suspicion for a congenital airway abnormality. One catch with subglottic hemangiomata is that they may initially respond to systemic steroids, and thus their diagnosis may be masked with the assumption that stridor was due to viral croup.[22]

MANAGEMENT OF VIRAL LARYNGOTRACHEOBRONCHITIS

Management of viral LTB must be based on clinical assessment of severity. Several scoring systems have been devised,[23] and the most commonly applied system (the 17-point Westley scale, which assesses degree of stridor, chest retractions, air entry, cyanosis, and level of consciousness) has been well validated. However, these are mainly used in the context of clinical trials and are not a substitute for experienced clinical assessment.

Supportive Care

Children with mild croup can be managed at home. They should be treated with plenty of fluids and antipyretics as required. Because the vast majority of cases are of viral etiology, there is no role for the routine use of antibiotics in the absence of other features suggestive of bacterial infection. Parents should be warned that symptoms are usually worse at night and may recur after apparently disappearing during the day.

Humidification

Both at home and in the hospital setting, humidified air (either steam or cool mist) has been used for more than a century to produce symptomatic relief from croup. Despite this, there is very little supportive evidence; most early studies, some of which may have been underpowered, generally suggested no benefit.[24–26] A larger study of 140 moderately affected children showed no differences in signs or requirement for additional treatments with optimally delivered 100% humidity,[27] and the most recent Cochrane Systematic Review has also concluded there is no evidence of benefit.[28] Case reports have described severe burns caused by spilling of boiling water and facial scalds from the use of steam, so this type of treatment is not without the potential for harm.[29]

Corticosteroids

The use of corticosteroids has received much attention for more than a decade, and their therapeutic role is well established. Their mechanism of action, however, remains unclear, although is believed to relate to rapid-onset antiinflammatory properties. The cumulative evidence strongly supports their use in children with moderate to severe symptoms, although there are still outstanding questions, including the optimal route of administration, the most appropriate dosing regimen, and the best oral agent.

The role of corticosteroids in the management of croup in children has been the subject of several Cochrane reviews, with the most recent update in January 2011.[30] In this review, the authors identified 38 studies that fulfilled their criteria for inclusion—namely, randomized controlled trials in children measuring the effectiveness of corticosteroids (any route of administration) against either a placebo or another treatment. A total of 4299 children were included, the majority from double-blind, placebo-controlled trials. Outcome measures included the croup score (most commonly the Westley scale), the requirement for admission or return visit, the length of stay, the requirement for additional therapeutic interventions, and overall assessment of "improvement" (indicated by a minimum incremental improvement in croup score or subjective relief of symptoms). Overall, treatment led to an improvement in the croup score at 6 and 12 hours, with a number needed to treat (NNT) of 5 calculated in order to achieve clinical improvement in one child at both those time points. The improvement was no longer apparent at 24 hours, but this was thought to be a reflection of reduced statistical power due to the small number of participants evaluated at 24 hours. The length of time spent in either the emergency department or the hospital was also significantly decreased, as was the requirement for nebulized epinephrine. Importantly, and in contrast to the first version

of this Cochrane review, the authors concluded with funnel plots and other statistical methods that these results were not influenced by publication bias. In conclusion, there is convincing evidence that corticosteroids provide effective and sustained treatment of croup symptoms, leading to clinical improvement within 6 hours of administration. In severe disease, rates of intubation are significantly decreased and the duration of intubation is reduced, and in moderate disease admission, the need for additional treatment and return visits are reduced.[8] More recent studies have focused attention on the optimal formulation, dose, and treatment regimen.

Optimal Route of Administration, Formulation, and Dosing Regimen

Studies included in the Cochrane review (discussed earlier in the chapter) and others conducted since then have used the intramuscular, oral, or nebulized route to administer different corticosteroid preparations. This area has been well reviewed recently.[8] From the studies that have attempted to address the route of administration, nebulized, oral, and intramuscular routes appear, in general, to be roughly equivalent. Nebulization could potentially increase distress of the child and worsen upper airway obstruction, although it may be preferable in a child who is vomiting or having difficulty swallowing.

Similarly, studies using oral agents have used either dexamethasone or prednisolone, and both in varying doses. Many primary care physicians who visit homes do not routinely carry dexamethasone but do carry oral prednisolone. There is no strong evidence in support of one preparation over the other, although one recent study favored dexamethasone, which led to a reduced frequency of re-presentation.[31] In contrast, a recent Australian trial compared 1 mg/kg prednisolone with a single dose of oral dexamethasone using two different dosing regimens (0.15 and 0.6 mg/kg) and found no difference in croup score, requirement for further treatment, or re-presentation.[32] Similarly, a community-based double-blind trial comparing a single dose of dexamethasone 0.6 mg/kg with three doses of 2 mg/kg prednisolone on consecutive days found no difference in additional health care attendances, duration of symptoms, parental stress, or sleep disturbance.[33] With regard to dexamethasone, 0.6 mg/kg has been the dose most widely used, but several studies have demonstrated that this dose may be higher than required and that 0.15 mg/kg is just as effective.[32,34–36] A practical approach might be to use dexamethasone, if available, at a dose of 0.15 mg/kg. If this preparation were not available at a home visit, prednisolone (at an equivalent dose of 1 mg/kg) could provide a useful substitute. Due to the short duration of symptoms in a typically episode of croup, one dose of steroid is usually sufficient treatment. However, a second dose should be considered if residual symptoms are still present the following day, and can be given to the parents to administer at their discretion.

Nebulized Epinephrine (Adrenaline). The most recent update of the Cochrane Review of nebulized epinephrine use in croup was published in 2013.[37] It included eight randomized controlled studies, with a total of 225 subjects comparing the efficacy of nebulized epinephrine to placebo (six studies), or comparing different epinephrine formulations and delivery methods (two studies).

All studies involved the management of moderate to severe croup in either an emergency department or hospital setting. Outcome measures used were croup score, intubation rates, side effect profile, and total health care utilization. Nebulized epinephrine was associated with improved clinical severity score 30 minutes posttreatment, but this effect was not sustained at 2 or 6 hours posttreatment. Magnitude of benefit was consistent between studies, and similar, irrespective of whether epinephrine was administered in an inpatient or outpatient setting.

Duration of hospitalization was also significantly reduced with epinephrine (mean difference of 32 hours), although this outcome was only assessed in one study. No studies provided a comparison of intubation rate or side effect profile. In summary, nebulized epinephrine has been shown to improve clinical severity in the short term and reduce hospital admission in cases of moderate to severe croup. It should be used in any child who has severe signs and symptoms, and it should be considered for those with moderate signs and symptoms, depending on the signs of respiratory distress and possible response to corticosteroid administration. It can be administered in the home setting while awaiting an ambulance, but clearly any child requiring this treatment at home must be transferred promptly to the hospital for monitoring. Multiple doses may be administered, although the requirement for this must lead to consideration of the need for intensive care management. Although rebound worsening of symptoms after administration of nebulized epinephrine is often alluded to, in practice, this phenomenon does not appear to be a real risk. Traditionally, children treated with epinephrine have been admitted to the hospital, but recent studies have confirmed that discharge home is safe after 3 to 4 hours of observation if the child has made significant improvement.[38]

Most clinical trials have used the racemic form of this drug,[39] although there is evidence that the L-isomer used alone (which is the only available formulation in some units) may be equally effective and has a longer duration of action.[40] The mechanisms of action are believed to be a combination of rapid reduction in airway wall edema and bronchodilation. The recommended dose is 0.4 to 0.5 mL/kg (to a maximum of 5 mL) of the 1:1000 preparation that is put undiluted into the nebulizer cup. Intramuscular epinephrine is not used in severe stridor, so it is important to ensure the stridor is not due to acute anaphylaxis, in which case it should be given.

Other Treatments for Severe Cases. Oxygen should be administered to any child with severe airway obstruction, even in the absence of severe hypoxia, because it will aid respiratory muscle function. As mentioned earlier, a child with severe respiratory distress and obstruction may have normal pulse oximetry readings when breathing oxygen, which can be dangerous if misinterpreted by staff who are unaware of this limitation. Heliox (70% to 80% helium with 20% to 30% oxygen) has been used in both upper airway obstruction[41] and severe asthma, and it is the focus of a recent Cochrane review.[42]

Three randomized controlled trials were identified totaling 91 participants with croup of varying severity. Heliox was compared with either 30% humidified oxygen, 100% oxygen plus epinephrine, or against no treatment. No pooled analysis was possible, as each study used a different comparator. Collectively, these studies provided evidence of a short-term benefit of Heliox inhalation, with improved croup scores at 60 to 90 minutes following administration. However, this clinical improvement was not sustained over subsequent hours. The authors summarized that no additional benefit appeared to have been provided by Heliox beyond that delivered by administration of 30% oxygen in cases of mild croup, or 100% oxygen plus nebulized epinephrine in moderate to severe croup. Adequately powered studies are required to further evaluate the role of Heliox in the management of moderate to severe croup.

Endotracheal Intubation

Some children with severe croup either do not respond to the usual therapies or are too severely compromised at presentation to permit their use. These children require urgent endotracheal intubation and mechanical ventilation to avoid potentially catastrophic complete airway obstruction and the serious sequelae of hypoxia and hypercapnia (e.g., hypoxic ischemic encephalopathy). Intubation should be performed by the most experienced person available, and it should be attempted with an uncuffed endotracheal tube one size smaller than the usual size for the child.[43] Facilities for immediate tracheostomy must be available at the time of intubation. Children may have coexisting lower airway and parenchymal involvement that impairs gas exchange and may lead to slower than expected clinical improvement after intubation. Rarely, pulmonary edema may develop after relief of airway obstruction, particularly if the disease course has been prolonged. Most children without severe parenchymal involvement require respiratory support for 3 to 5 days.[43] This is one context in which multiple rather than single doses of corticosteroids are often administered. The timing of extubation will depend on the development of an air leak around the endotracheal tube, indicating resolution of airway narrowing.[43] Reintubation rates of approximately 10% have been reported.[44]

PREVENTION

Because of the substantial health care costs associated with management of PIV infections (estimated annual costs of $43, $58, and $158 million for hospitalizations in the United States for PIV-associated bronchiolitis, croup, and pneumonia, respectively), there is much interest in development of an effective PIV vaccine.[45] The most promising candidate vaccine developed to date is an intranasally administered cold-adapted PIV 3 vaccine that appears to be well-tolerated and immunogenic in infants as young as 1 month of age.[46] Also under evaluation is a PIV 3-vectored RSV vaccine that would confer protection against both of these common respiratory viruses. Results from efficacy studies into each of these promising vaccine candidates are awaited.

PROGNOSIS AND FURTHER EVALUATION

Most children with viral LTB were previously well, have short, self-limiting symptoms, and make a full recovery. The lack of complete immunity and the variety of agents that can cause viral LTB mean that more than one episode is not uncommon, particularly in separate seasons.

Recurrent (≥3) episodes have been reported in more than 60% of affected children, with family history of croup identified as the most significant risk factor for recurrence in one case-control study.[47] Although further evaluation is not necessary in every case of recurrent croup, it should be considered in cases that are particularly severe or frequent, if symptoms are particularly slow to resolve, or if symptoms occur between or in the absence of obvious infections. Evaluation of patients in this group is aimed at identifying an underlying airway abnormality that would predispose the child to more severe airway narrowing with viral infections, or that could cause problems independently of such infection. Investigation is usually centered on airway endoscopy. This must be performed in a unit and by an operator who is experienced in the technique because there is a risk of exacerbating the airway obstruction. Spontaneous breathing is necessary to identify vocal cord problems or airway malacia, and anesthetic techniques must be carefully considered. If an inhaled foreign body is considered likely, rigid bronchoscopy is the study of choice. Additional studies that might be considered once the acute episode has resolved include plain lateral neck and chest radiographs, computed tomography or magnetic resonance imaging, contrast assessment of the upper airway (e.g., videofluoroscopy, barium swallow), and a pH probe study. Polysomnography may help determine the severity of chronic symptoms. Rarer causes of recurrent stridor (e.g., hypocalcaemia or angioneurotic edema) are diagnosed by blood testing.

Epiglottitis

EPIDEMIOLOGY

Haemophilus influenzae type B (HiB) vaccines were first licensed in the United States in 1988, with widespread immunization programs in place by the early 1990s. Since then, reported cases of invasive HiB disease (including epiglottitis) in children younger than 5 years of age have declined by 99%.[48]

By 2008, the overall incidence in the United States had fallen to 1.55 per 100,000, having been 4.39 per 100,000 in 1989.[49] The same pattern has been repeated in Europe, with significant reductions in the United Kingdom.[50,51] Immunization was introduced in the United Kingdom in 1992, and with immunization coverage exceeding 90%, the decline in incidence was more than 95%.[51] In 1998, the incidence in those younger than 5 years of age was 0.6 per 100,000, compared with 31 to 36 per 100,000 in England and Wales before the introduction of the vaccine.[51] However, in 2003 there was a resurgence of HiB infections in the United Kingdom, which led to the launch of a booster program. By 2012, in England and Wales, the incidence had fallen further to 0.06 per 100,000 aged less than 5 years (0.02 per 100,000 for all ages).[49] Ethnicity plays a part in vaccine efficacy. Data from 1996 to 1997 in the United States show that the average annual incidence of HiB invasive disease per 100,000 children younger than 5 years of age was 0.5 among non-Hispanic whites, 0.6 among Asians and Pacific Islanders, 0.7 among non-Hispanic blacks, 0.7 among

Hispanic Americans, and 12.4 among Native Americans and Alaskan natives.[48] Nevertheless, cases of epiglottitis due to HiB continue to be reported,[52] as do cases due to other organisms.[53]

Cases of invasive HiB occur principally in nonimmunized children, but also rarely in some true vaccine failures. Clinical risk factors for vaccine failure include prematurity, Down syndrome, malignancy, developmental delay, and congenital or acquired immunodeficiency, principally with reduced immunoglobulin concentrations (IgG_2 subclass, IgA, IgM) or neutropenia.[54] However, these factors explain fewer than 50% of cases of vaccine failures.[54] An HiB IgG antibody titer of ≥0.15 µg/mL confers protection from disease, but given the natural waning in antibody levels, it is estimated that a titer of ≥1.0 µg/mL should provide long-term protection.[52] However, sometimes there are qualitative functional problems with antibody responses that are not yet fully elucidated.

Among the pediatric cohort, epiglottitis tends to occur in children 2 to 7 years of age, but cases have been reported in those younger than 1 year of age.[2] Since the introduction of HiB vaccine, the peak age distribution has increased slightly.[55] A review of a national US dataset from 1998 to 2006 has shown that the mean age of a patient admitted with epiglottitis is 45 years, and the national mortality rate is 0.89%; there is a decrease in admissions for those under 18 years of age (with greatest risk at <1 year) and an increase in the 46- to 64-year-old group.[56] This is similar in England and Wales, where 68% of culture-positive cases of epiglottitis occurred in patients aged 45 or over.[49] Most cases occur in the fall and winter.

ETIOLOGY

Historically, HiB was responsible for almost all (approximately 99%) cases of epiglottitis in otherwise healthy children. Since the introduction of HiB immunization, other organisms have been implicated, including groups A, B, C, and G β-hemolytic *Streptococcus*. Other responsible organisms include *H. parainfluenzae*, *Staphylococcus aureus*, *Moraxella catarrhalis*, *Streptococcus pneumoniae*, *Klebsiella*, *Pseudomonas*, Candida, and viruses (e.g., herpes simplex, varicella, PIV, influenza, and Epstein-Barr virus).[2,53,57]

PATHOLOGY

Although HiB has a low point-prevalence of nasopharyngeal carriage (1% to 5%), most young children become colonized with HiB in the first 2 to 5 years.[58] The relationship between asymptomatic carriage, immunity, and the development of invasive disease is not clearly understood. Viral coinfection may have a role in the transition from colonization to invasion.[59] Colonies of HiB organisms reside in the nasal mucosal epithelium and submucosa. Invasive disease occurs when organisms disseminate from the mucosa of the upper respiratory tract via the bloodstream; bacteremia increases over a period of hours, and metastatic seeding can occur.[58] Thus, although situated in close proximity to the nose, the supraglottic area is likely to be affected via the bloodstream; direct spread along mucosal surfaces may also play a part. This may account for the relatively high yield of positive blood cultures in epiglottitis and the relatively low incidence of epiglottitis among carriers of HiB.

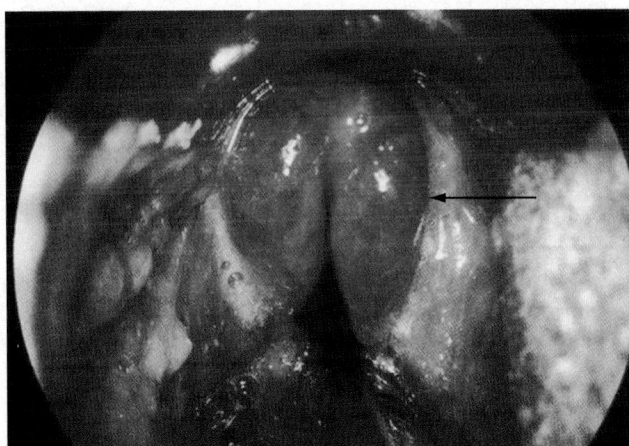

Fig. 23.2 Swollen epiglottis *(arrow)* caused by acute epiglottitis in an intubated child. (From Benjamin B, Bingham B, Hawke M, et al. *A Colour Atlas of Otorhinolaryngology*. London: Taylor & Francis; 1995:292, with permission.)

Epiglottitis is more correctly called *supraglottitis*. It is a bacterial cellulitis of the supraglottic structures, particularly the lingual surface of the epiglottis and the aryepiglottic folds.[2] Destruction of the infected epithelial tissue results in mucosal ulcerations, which may appear on the epiglottis, larynx, and trachea. The submucosal glands are involved as well, with the formation of epiglottic abscesses. Infection of the epiglottis itself causes a local inflammatory response that results in a cherry-red edematous epiglottis when caused by HiB (Fig. 23.2), although it tends to be pale and edematous and accompanied by edematous aryepiglottic folds when caused by *Streptococcus*.[48,53] As supraglottic edema worsens, the epiglottis is displaced posteriorly, and it may obstruct the airway.

CLINICAL FEATURES

Classic epiglottitis caused by HiB is a fulminant disease in an otherwise healthy child, who can be near death in a few hours. It is a medical emergency that can be alarming for the medical staff and devastating for the family. Epiglottitis clearly has not been eliminated, but due to its rarity there are concerns about a potential lack of familiarity with its management among emergency physicians, pediatricians, anesthesiologists, and otolaryngologists.[60] Up to 20% of infants with epiglottitis are misdiagnosed initially, usually with viral LTB.[4] Typically there is a short history of fever, severe throat pain, stridor, and respiratory distress, but the symptoms progress rapidly. Children become toxic and tend to sit anxiously in the classic tripod position (sitting upright, with the chin up, mouth open, bracing themselves on their hands) as air hunger develops (Fig. 23.3). They often drool because they cannot swallow their secretions, and the voice is muffled due to pain and soft tissue swelling. Stridor may progress, and when marked (or if it disappears completely), signals almost complete obstruction of the airways. Complete, fatal airway obstruction may occur suddenly and without warning. The most serious complication of this disease process (and any infective upper airway obstruction) is hypoxic ischemic encephalopathy resulting from respiratory arrest. This tragic complication is almost always preventable with clinical suspicion, prompt diagnosis, and correct management.

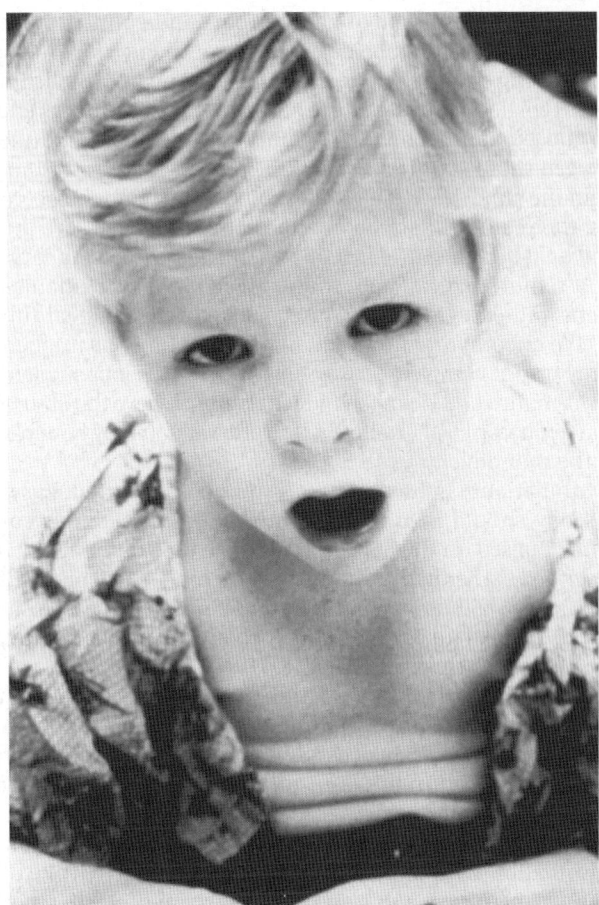

Fig. 23.3 Characteristic posture in a patient with epiglottitis. The child is leaning forward and drooling, with a hyperextended neck. (Courtesy of Dr. Robert Berg.)

However, a 13-year case series demonstrated that cardiac arrest occurred in 3 of 40 cases (7.5%), although there were no long-term sequelae.[52] Secondary sites of HiB infection may be present in approximately half of cases, and include meningitis, otitis media, pneumonia, and cellulitis; descending necrotizing mediastinitis has been reported. Therefore repeated physical examination during the admission is critical.[2] The pneumonia may contribute to poor gas exchange.

In general, distinction from standard viral LTB is based on the older age of the child, the lack of history of upper respiratory tract infection, the speed of progression, the degree of toxicity, the extent of drooling, the use of the tripod position, and minimal cough (see Table 23.1). However, it is important to remember that most of these symptoms can be present in acute severe upper airway obstruction from other causes.

The presentation and clinical course of epiglottitis caused by the various types of β-hemolytic streptococcal pathogens are similar to each other, but they differ from those associated with HiB.[53] The onset of disease is more gradual, but the resolution of tissue damage and the time to recovery are longer, with a mean intubation time of 6 days.[53,61]

MANAGEMENT

The first priority and key response to the diagnosis must be to secure the airway in a controlled environment. Physical examination (especially of the throat) and cannulation or venipuncture should be deferred, because emotional upset and crying may precipitate complete airway obstruction. When epiglottitis is suspected clinically, the child (and parents) should be approached in a calm and reassuring manner. Oxygen should be given, even if the mask is held at a distance from the child's face. The child should be taken to the operating room, anesthetic room, or pediatric intensive care unit, and held by a parent. The child should also be accompanied by a senior medical team that is skilled in airway management and carrying a laryngoscope, an endotracheal tube, needle cricothyroidotomy kit, and a percutaneous tracheostomy tray. If complete airway obstruction develops suddenly, performance of a Heimlich maneuver may relieve the obstruction temporarily; alternatively, forward traction may be applied to the mandible.

Inhalational induction of anesthesia is preferred. Laryngoscopy should then be performed and the diagnosis confirmed, based on the appearance of the epiglottic region, as described earlier in the chapter (erythema and edema of the supraglottis). Endotracheal intubation is then achieved using an orotracheal tube, which is later changed to a nasotracheal tube, because this is less likely to be displaced leading to a potentially disastrous extubation. Intubation may be done using the Seldinger technique over a bronchoscope. Although tracheostomy is rarely necessary, a surgical team should be prepared to perform this immediately if intubation is unsuccessful. Once the airway is secured, the emergency is over, and the remaining studies can be performed. Intravenous cannulation and blood sampling can be done. The white cell count is increased, and blood culture findings are often positive (70% in one series).[52] Airway secretions and swabs from the epiglottic region should be sent for bacterial culture and viral detection. Urinary antigen testing may be useful for those already receiving antibiotics.[59]

Some authors have advocated the use of a lateral neck radiograph if the child is stable before intubation, claiming it to be the "single most useful study."[2,6] We strongly disagree, and this is not our recommendation, because it can precipitate respiratory arrest as a result of complete obstruction. We take the same view as Goodman and McHugh, who state that "plain radiographs have no role to play in the assessment of the critically ill child with acute stridor."[62]

Once the airway is secured, intravenous antibiotics are started which must cover HiB and *Streptococcus;* the response is usually rapid.[2] A third-generation cephalosporin (e.g., ceftriaxone or cefotaxime) is usually given and may be changed once antibiotic sensitivities are available. Antibiotics have traditionally been given for 7 to 10 days; however, a randomized controlled trial showed that a two-dose course of intravenous ceftriaxone was as efficacious as 5 days of intravenous chloramphenicol.[59] Contacts of patients with HiB should be given appropriate prophylaxis, usually rifampicin (patients must be warned about orange secretions [e.g., tears, urine], and also that oral contraceptives can be inactivated, and the fact that this warning has been given should be recorded). There is some empiric evidence that corticosteroids may improve the course of epiglottitis, but racemic epinephrine has not been shown to be of benefit. The duration of intubation for epiglottitis due to HiB averages 1 to 3 days,[6,52] but it is longer when caused by *Streptococcus*[3]; as always, there is great individual variation. A decision to extubate

may be made when an air leak develops around the endotracheal tube, but repeat endoscopy may be useful to aid this decision. Again, facilities for emergency tracheostomy must be available. Some give dexamethasone before extubation to reduce post extubation stridor.[4]

Bacterial Tracheitis

Bacterial tracheitis has also been known as bacterial, or membranous LTB; nondiphtheritic laryngitis with marked exudate; and pseudomembranous croup.

EPIDEMIOLOGY

Bacterial tracheitis is a rare disease, with a large case series (from 1998) describing only 46 cases.[63] The estimated annual incidence is 0.1 case per 100,000 children.[63] The peak incidence is during fall and winter (consistent with its postviral etiology), and it predominantly affects children 6 months to 8 years of age (mean 5 years of age). Most affected children were previously well, but it has been reported as a complication of elective tonsillectomy and adenoidectomy.[64] A large case series of life-threatening upper airway infections from Vermont in the United States between 1997 and 2006 showed that bacterial tracheitis has now superseded viral croup and epiglottitis, and was three times more likely as a cause of respiratory failure than the other two diagnoses combined.[65]

ETIOLOGY

The most common pathogen is *S. aureus,* although other organisms implicated include HiB, α-hemolytic *Streptococcus, Pneumococcus,* and *M. catarrhalis.*[6] Occasionally, gram-negative enteric organisms and *Pseudomonas aeruginosa* are isolated (the latter is associated with a more severe clinical course).[66] In one case series, *M. catarrhalis* (27%) was more common than *S. aureus* (22%), although this represents data from a single center over the course of 14 months.[67] One series of 94 cases over 10 years found that *M. catarrhalis* was associated with a greater rate of intubation: 83% versus 49% with other organisms, although they were a younger group.[68] In addition, PIV and influenza viruses are commonly isolated from tracheal secretions; measles and enteroviruses have also been detected. Although it may be a primary bacterial infection, bacterial tracheitis is considered secondary to primary viral LTB. Presumably, viral injury to the tracheal mucosa and impairment of local immunity predisposes to bacterial superinfection.

PATHOLOGY

Bacterial tracheitis is characterized by marked subglottic edema, with ulceration; erythema; pseudomembranous formation on the tracheal surface; and thick, mucopurulent tracheal secretions. The thick exudate and sloughed mucosa frequently obstruct the lumen of the trachea and the main-stem bronchi.[2] The epiglottis and arytenoids are usually normal in appearance, although epiglottitis and bacterial tracheitis may coexist. Tracheal stenosis can be a complication, especially after prolonged intubation.[66]

CLINICAL FEATURES

The clinical picture is initially similar to that of viral LTB, with mild fever, cough, and stridor for several days. However, the patient's condition deteriorates rapidly, with a high fever and often a toxic appearance, with respiratory distress and airway obstruction. Other symptoms include choking episodes, orthopnea, dysphagia, and neck pain.[67] The clinical picture differs from that of epiglottitis in that its onset tends to be more insidious. Patients have a substantial brassy cough, are more able to lie flat, and tend not to drool (see Table 23.1).[6] Children are more ill than with simple viral LTB and do not respond to expected therapies (e.g., corticosteroids or nebulized epinephrine). There may be other coinfections, particularly pneumonia. Other reported complications include cardiopulmonary arrest, with subsequent hypoxic encephalopathy and seizures, pneumothorax, subglottic stenosis, septicemia, toxic shock syndrome, pulmonary edema, and adult respiratory distress syndrome.[69]

The white blood cell count shows polymorphonuclear leukocytosis, often with a left shift. A lateral neck radiograph may show a hazy tracheal air column, with multiple luminal soft tissue irregularities due to pseudomembrane detachment from the soft tissue, but radiographs should be taken only after the patient is stabilized and safe. There are, however, no clinical or radiographic features capable of confirming the diagnosis.[2] This must be confirmed by upper airway endoscopy and a positive bacterial culture.

MANAGEMENT

Diagnostic rigid endoscopy, which should be done under general anesthesia, is also therapeutic because it enables removal of secretions and sloughed tissue from the airway lumen; sometimes the procedure must be repeated. Many patients (especially younger ones) require endotracheal intubation and mechanical ventilation to overcome airway obstruction (reports of 50% to 100% intubation rates),[70] usually for 3 to 7 days. Frequent tracheal suction is necessary. In a 1998 case series, 57% of patients required intubation, which is lower than the rate previously reported.[67] The decision to extubate is based on clinical improvement, with reduction of fever, decreased airway secretions, and development of an air leak around the endotracheal tube. Corticosteroids may be given before extubation. Tracheostomy is required less often than in the past. There has been a case reported that was successfully managed with extracorporeal membrane oxygenation (ECMO) required for bilateral pneumothoraxes and pneumomediastinum.[71] Initially, intravenous broad-spectrum antibiotics are given, and these can be refined once cultures and antibiotic sensitivities are known, usually for 10 to 14 days. Mortality is now uncommon, estimated at 3%.[63]

Diphtheria

EPIDEMIOLOGY

Diphtheritic laryngitis was once the most common infectious cause of acute upper airway obstruction in children. In the 1920s, in the United States, there were up to 200,000 cases

and nearly 15,000 deaths per year due to diphtheria.[72] Although it became uncommon due to widespread immunization programs started in the 1940s, it remains a serious disease in parts of the world. Large outbreaks occurred in the 1990s throughout Russia and the independent countries of the former Soviet Union (nearly 50,000 cases were reported). In 2005, 36 countries reported almost 13,000 cases to the World Health Organization, and 80% were from India.[73] However, in the United States, there were only five cases reported between 2000 and 2015.[72] The last childhood deaths reported in the United Kingdom were 1 in 1994 and 1 in 2008.[74] In 2013, in a refugee camp in Afghanistan, there were 50 cases and 3 deaths. Most life-threatening cases occurred in unvaccinated or inadequately vaccinated persons, and it is important for children traveling to these countries, particularly for extended periods, to be vaccinated. A list of endemic countries is available on the Centers for Disease Control website, last updated July 2015.[75] It is also important to take into account a history of recent travel in potential cases. Global coverage of a three-dose course of diphtheria-tetanus-pertussis vaccination is estimated to be 86% in 2014.[76] Adults are particularly at risk because protective levels of diphtheria antibodies decrease progressively with time from immunization, so reimmunization is recommended before travel. The Third National Health and Nutrition Examination Survey of US residents (1988–1994) indicated that fully protective levels ($\geq$0.1 IU/mL) were found in 91% of children 6 to 11 years of age, but only in 30% of adults 60 to 69 years of age.[77]

ETIOLOGY

Diphtheria is caused by toxigenic strains of the bacterium *Corynebacterium diphtheriae* and, less frequently, *C. ulcerans*. The organism may be isolated on bacterial culture of nasal and pharyngeal swabs, and serologic studies may detect antibodies to diphtheria toxin. Polymerase chain reaction can confirm *C. diphtheriae tox* genes.[72] There has been a case reported where nontoxigenic *Corynebacterium diphtheria* caused necrotizing epiglottitis in an immunocompromised child.[78]

PATHOLOGY

Diphtheria is an acute disease, primarily involving the tonsils, pharynx, larynx, nose, skin, and occasionally other mucous membranes. In the milder, catarrhal form, there is no membrane formation, but in the more severe, membranous form, there is a characteristic lesion of one or more patches of an adherent grayish-white membrane, surrounded by inflammation. The toxin causes local tissue destruction at the site of membrane formation, which promotes multiplication and transmission of the bacteria.[79]

CLINICAL FEATURES

The incubation period is 1 to 6 days. Classic respiratory diphtheria is characterized by an insidious onset, and patients typically present with a 3- to 4-day history of upper respiratory infection. They have a fever, membranous pharyngitis with a sore throat, characteristic fetor oris, cervical lymphadenopathy, and sometimes edema of the surrounding soft

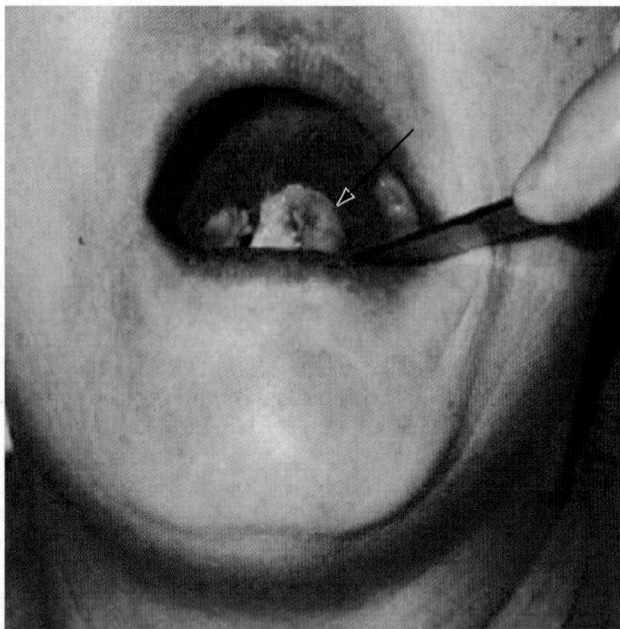

Fig. 23.4 Diphtheritic membrane *(arrow)* extending from the uvula to the pharyngeal wall in an adult. (From Kadirova R, Kartoglu HÜ, Strebel PM. Clinical characteristics and management of 676 hospitalized diphtheria cases. Kyrgyz Republic 1995. *J Infect Dis.* 2000;181[suppl 1]:S110-S115. Photograph by P. Strebel.)

tissues (bull-neck appearance). They may have a serosanguineous nasal discharge. Although not always present, the membrane is typically gray, thick, fibrinous, and firmly adherent, so it may bleed on attempted removal (Fig. 23.4). Laryngeal diphtheria most commonly occurs as an extension of pharyngeal involvement in children, leading to increasing hoarseness and stridor. The patient appears toxic, with symptoms of LTB, and signs of severe airway obstruction may develop quickly if the pharyngeal membrane dislodges and obstructs the airway. Complications include secondary pneumonia and toxin-mediated disease including myocarditis or cardiomyopathy, neuritis or paralysis, and adrenal failure with hypotension.[74] Cardiomyopathy can be predicted from a combination of a pseudomembrane score greater than 2 (range is up to 4) and a bull-neck appearance.[80] Case fatality rates vary and can reach 20%, but the mortality rate was only 3% in a series of 676 patients (30% younger than 15 years of age) reported from the 1995 Kyrgyz Republic outbreak.[81] Deaths are usually a result of airway obstruction, myocarditis/cardiomyopathy, or sepsis (disseminated intravascular coagulation and renal failure).

MANAGEMENT

Because diphtheria is now rare, a high index of suspicion is important to make the diagnosis and institute prompt treatment. Patients should be strictly isolated. Diphtheria antitoxin, which is a hyperimmune equine antiserum (available from the Centers for Disease Control and Prevention), should be administered without waiting for laboratory confirmation because it neutralizes circulating toxin, but not toxin bound to tissues. Antibiotics are not a substitute for antitoxin, but they are given to eradicate the organism, stop toxin production, and reduce the likelihood of transmission.[79] Intravenous

penicillin or erythromycin is used, and once the child can swallow comfortably, treatment can be given orally, for a total of 14 days.[79] Mechanical ventilation and tracheostomy may be required. Intravenous dexamethasone has been given to children with laryngeal diphtheria and airway obstruction, and a small case series suggested that it was beneficial.[82] Because the disease may not confer immunity, patients should be given a diphtheria toxoid-containing vaccine during convalescence. Antibiotic prophylaxis (penicillin or erythromycin) is recommended for close contacts after nasal and pharyngeal specimens are taken, and immunization should be given to those who have not been vaccinated in the preceding 5 years.[79]

Retropharyngeal Abscess

EPIDEMIOLOGY

The majority of cases occur in children younger than 6 years of age, probably due to the fact that retropharyngeal lymph nodes are so abundant at this age (they tend to atrophy later in life). Analysis of the US-based Kid's Inpatient Database (KID) for 2003 covering 36 states revealed 1321 admissions with a mean age of 5.1 years, and 63% were boys; there were no deaths reported.[83] Another large series reported a median age of 3 years, with 75% of those affected younger than 5 years of age and 16% younger than 1 year of age.[84] In a large series from 1995 to 2006, there was a linear increase in incidence through the period.[85] The KID database has extended this and found a significant increase in incidence of retropharyngeal abscesses from 0.10 per 10,000 in 2000 to 0.22 in 2009, although the overall incidence of pediatric deep space neck infections has not changed.[86] The reason for this increase in the United States is unknown, but it has been thought that perhaps it is due to a change in bacterial flora (especially community-acquired methicillin-resistant *Staphylococcus aureus* [MRSA]),[87] and perhaps artifactual due to the increased use of diagnostic computed tomography (CT) scanning. Additionally, in England it has been suggested that the 39% rise in retropharyngeal and parapharyngeal abscess admission rate (children and adults) between 1996 and 2011 may be correlated with the National Health Service drive to reduce tonsillectomies in that same period, which resulted in a 41% fall in overall tonsillectomy rate.[88]

ETIOLOGY

Retropharyngeal abscesses generally result from lymphatic spread of infection, although direct spread from adjacent areas, penetrating pharyngeal trauma (e.g., a fall with a pencil in the mouth), or foreign bodies can also play a role.[6] It has also been reported as a complication of adenoidectomy and adenotonsillectomy.[89,90] Infection is usually due to mixed flora, including *S. aureus* (methicillin-sensitive and resistant), various streptococcal species (in particular group A betahemolytic *Streptococcus*), HiB, and anaerobes.[84] A case has been reported due to tuberculosis (cervical Pott's disease).[91]

PATHOLOGY

The retropharyngeal space (between the posterior pharyngeal wall and the prevertebral layer of deep cervical fascia) contains loose connective tissue and lymph nodes that drain the nasopharynx, paranasal sinuses, middle ear, teeth, and adjacent bones. The space extends from the base of the skull down to vertebra C7 or T1. Acute bacterial infection in this region may start as retropharyngeal cellulitis with localized edema of the tissues, which can progress to purulent inflammation of the tissues and retropharyngeal adenitis. However, when this process is caused by lymphatic spread, it starts as adenitis. If liquefaction of one of the nodes occurs, an abscess can form and is usually contained within the inflammatory rind of the infected node.

CLINICAL FEATURES

Presentation is often nonspecific, and there may be overlap with the presentation of croup, epiglottitis, tracheitis, and peritonsillar abscess (see Table 23.1).[6] Children with acute epiglottitis tend to appear more toxic and progress to respiratory distress more rapidly.[92] Excluding causes secondary to foreign bodies or trauma, patients usually have a history of a viral upper respiratory infection that lasts several days and then worsens. Children then have high fever, sore throat, dysphagia, poor feeding, neck pain, and stiffness. Limitation of neck extension and torticollis are more common than limited neck flexion.[84] Although the occurrence of neck signs with fever may suggest meningitis, affected children tend not to be as toxic as those with meningitis. Further deterioration may lead to extrathoracic airway compromise, with drooling, stridor, and respiratory distress. The classical picture of stridor and airway obstruction seems to be less common now, and in a series of cases reported by pediatricians from 1993 to 1998, only 3% of 64 children in Salt Lake City had stridor or wheezing.[84] However in a series of cases from 2002 to 2007 from the same center, but published by the otolaryngologists, 14/130 (11%) presented with airway obstruction, and 50% required intubation, with an average age of 1.4 years.[93] Older series have reported a higher incidence of stridor. Reported rates include 71% in patients younger than 1 year of age, 43% in patients older than 1 year of age, and no stridor in those older than 3 years of age in a series of 31 children in Sydney, Australia[94]; a rate of 56% in 17 patients in Denver[95]; and a rate of 23% in 65 children in Los Angeles.[96] It is possible that the spectrum of disease is changing, but it is more likely that the diagnosis is being made earlier, before the airways are compromised.[84] Sometimes a retropharyngeal mass is visible in the mouth, seen as an asymmetrical bulge of the posterior pharyngeal wall (Fig. 23.5), or a neck mass (marked lymphadenopathy or parapharyngeal abscess) is visible and palpable. Complications include rupture of the abscess with aspiration, asphyxiation or pneumonia, extension to a mediastinal abscess with or without mediastinitis, and Lemierre syndrome with vascular complications (e.g., anaerobic septic thrombophlebitis of the internal jugular vein with multiple septic pulmonary emboli, and potential erosion through the carotid artery sheath).[89,92]

Once the child is stable and safe, a lateral neck radiograph with the neck in full extension may confirm the diagnosis. Widened prevertebral soft-tissue shadow and air-fluid levels in the retropharyngeal space are all indicators.[6] The radiograph must be taken in the correct position (true lateral orientation, with the neck in extension, and if possible, during full inspiration) to ensure that the retropharyngeal space is

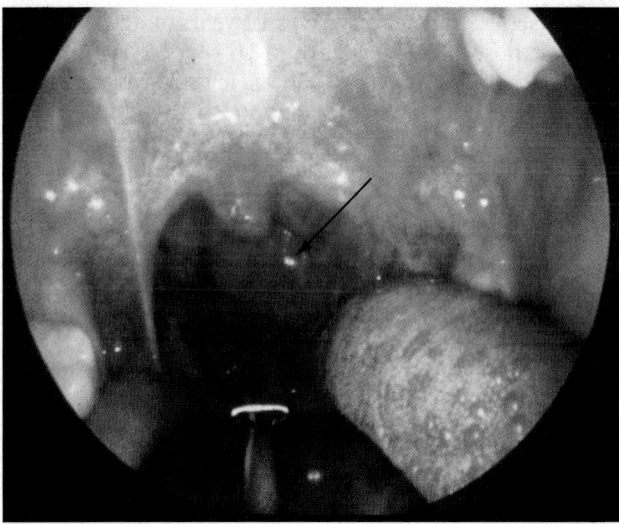

Fig. 23.5 Retropharyngeal abscess behind and to the left of the uvula *(arrow)* is shown. The tongue is pressed down and to the left with a **tongue depressor.** (Photograph courtesy of the Otolaryngology Teaching Set, Department of Ear, Nose & Throat, Great Ormond Street Hospital for Children NHS Trust, London.)

not falsely thickened.[84] A contrast-enhanced computed tomography scan is useful because it differentiates a fully developed abscess from cellulitis and delineates the full extent of the abscess. Blood cultures findings are usually negative, but the white blood cell count will be increased.

MANAGEMENT

Traditionally, management involves surgical drainage of the abscess (plus antibiotics). However, more cases are being managed by intravenous antibiotics alone, although surgery must be considered early if there is a compromised airway. Percutaneous CT-guided aspiration has also been described.[97] In one older series, 25% of patients required no surgery,[95] but in the Salt Lake City series that covered 1993–1998, 58% of 64 patients had antibiotics alone, with no treatment failures.[84] Data from KID 2003 (discussed earlier in the chapter) showed that 43% of cases admitted required surgical drainage.[83] Update of the KID database shows that surgical management has continued to fall to 38% in 2009.[86] Many children start treatment with antibiotics before the diagnosis is made, and certainly retropharyngeal cellulitis can be treated with antibiotics alone. When necessary, surgical drainage is performed through the intraoral route. Care must be taken to avoid aspiration of the infected material. Occasionally, if there is extension lateral to the great vessels, external drainage through the neck is necessary. Mortality is rare now, with no deaths in recent reports.

Peritonsillar Abscess (Quinsy)

EPIDEMIOLOGY

Peritonsillar abscess is the most common deep-space head and neck infection in both adults and children. However, it is more common in young adults than in children. It tends to affect older children and adolescents, and in one large,

10-year series, the mean age was 12 years of age, with two-thirds of those affected older than 10 years of age.[98] In this series, 62% of cases occurred on the left side versus 38% on the right (with no obvious explanation).[98] There is no seasonal predilection. The reduction of antibiotic prescribing to children by general practitioners in the United Kingdom from 1993 to 2003 has not been accompanied by an increase in hospital admissions for peritonsillar abscess.[99] The KID database in the United States found no significant change in incidence of peritonsillar abscess between 2000 and 2009 (0.82 to 0.94 per 10,000 children).[86] In England, there was a 31% rise in peritonsillar abscess admission rate for children and adults between 1991 and 2011, that was thought to be associated with the 41% fall in overall tonsillectomy rate in that same period.[88]

ETIOLOGY

A peritonsillar abscess is usually a complication of acute tonsillitis, but it may follow pharyngitis or a previous peritonsillar abscess. The infection usually involves mixed bacterial flora, with *Streptococcus pyogenes* as the predominant organism. In a small series of children younger than 5 years of age, *Streptococcus viridans* was the most common organism detected.[100] In a large series of 457 children and adults in Israel, while *S. pyogenes* was the most common organism isolated, there was a sharp rise in anaerobes cultured, particularly *Prevotella* and *Peptostreptococcus*.[101]

PATHOLOGY

Peritonsillar abscess is believed to arise from the spread of infection from the tonsil or the mucous glands of Weber, located in the superior tonsillar pole.[98] There is a spectrum of peritonsillar cellulitis that may then result in a collection of pus located between the tonsillar capsule (pharyngobasilar fascia), the superior constrictor, and the palatopharyngeus muscle.[98] There is a risk of spread through the muscle into the parapharyngeal space or other deep neck spaces. The abscess pushes the adjacent tonsil downward and medially, and the uvula may be so edematous, as to resemble a white grape.

CLINICAL FEATURES

The child who is already affected by acute tonsillitis becomes more ill with a high fever and has a severe sore throat or neck pain, as well as marked dysphagia with referred earache. Absent or decreased oral intake can lead to dehydration, particularly in younger children.

Cervical lymphadenopathy is almost always present. The uvula is edematous and deviated to one side, and there is fetor oris. A striking feature may be trismus, with limited mouth opening. Examination may be difficult in a young, uncooperative child who refuses to open the mouth. The white blood cell count will be elevated.

The relevance of this condition to pediatric pulmonologists is that acute enlargement of the tonsils can cause airway compromise, and a ruptured abscess can lead to aspiration of infected material and subsequent pneumonia. In one large series of 169 children under 18 years of age, 8% presented with airway compromise.[102]

MANAGEMENT

Children may need intravenous fluids. Antibiotics are necessary, and intravenous penicillin is as effective as broad-spectrum antibiotics, although additional anaerobic coverage should be considered.[103] Analgesia is important. Corticosteroids are not uncommonly used but are of no obvious benefit (or harm).[102] Treatment often involves needle aspiration or incision and drainage; a meta-analysis of 10 studies with 496 patients revealed an average 94% success rate with simple needle aspiration.[104] The KID database revealed that about a third of cases required incision and drainage in 2009, with an increase over the decade (26% to 34%).[105] Nevertheless, an initial period of medical treatment is appropriate in the absence of airway compromise and systemic toxicity, especially in younger children.[106] One case series of 88 children from Korea suggested that younger age (<7.5 years), fewer episodes of acute tonsillitis, and smaller abscess size predicted successful nonsurgical treatment.[107] There is some debate among otolaryngologists about the role and timing of tonsillectomy, and peritonsillar abscess is no longer considered an absolute indication for tonsillectomy, although a history of recurrent tonsillitis prior to developing the peritonsillar abscess leads to a higher recurrence rate.[108] In the United States, the KID database found a significant reduction in tonsillectomy carried out between 2000 and 2009 (13% to 8% cases).[105] In a large nationwide study from Taiwan of almost 29,000 cases of peritonsillar abscess, the recurrence rate was 5% and was associated with the incidence of prior episodes of tonsillitis in all ages, and management by needle aspiration (vs. incision and drainage) in children.[109]

Infectious Mononucleosis

Infectious mononucleosis is caused by Epstein-Barr virus (EBV) and is common in adolescents and young adults. The clinical syndrome is characterized by fever, fatigue, malaise, lymphadenopathy, and sore throat. Diagnosis is confirmed by positive EBV serology, and positive heterophile antibodies (Monospot), although the latter are only positive in 50% of children and 90% of adults. The illness is usually self-limiting, but malaise and exhaustion can persist.

Some degree of airway obstruction is not uncommon (reported in 25% to 60% cases),[74] but significant airway compromise is rare, occurring in an estimated 1% to 3.5% cases.[110] Nevertheless, given the high frequency of EBV infection, this small proportion still represents many patients. Acute upper airway obstruction may occur, but the cardinal signs of acute obstruction (stridor and respiratory distress with recession and tachypnea) can be absent until late in the process.[111] Obstruction arises from a combination of inflammation and hypertrophy of the palatal and nasopharyngeal tonsils, edema of the pharynx and epiglottis, and pseudomembrane formation in the large airways.[112] Acute onset of obstructive sleep apnea has also been described in a child who required continuous positive airway pressure when asleep, until recovery after 3 days.[113] Peritonsillar abscess formation is a rare complication that can further compromise the airway, and it is now believed that this is not significantly associated with the use of corticosteroids, which contradicts earlier reports.[114]

Management is with systemic corticosteroids (in the presence of obstruction) and supportive care, which may include ventilation. A tracheostomy is sometimes necessary, as the severity of the inflammation in the oropharynx can make intubation difficult. If corticosteroids do not help, the role of acute tonsillectomy has been advocated,[115] but it is controversial due to the high risk of perioperative bleeding.[112]

References

Access the reference list online at ExpertConsult.com.

Suggested Reading

Bjornson CL, Johnson DW. Croup. *Lancet.* 2008;371:329–339.
Jenkins IA, Saunders M. Infections of the airway. *Pediatr Anesthesia.* 2009;19(suppl 1):118–130.
Johnson D. Croup. *Clin Evid.* 2004;12:401–426.
Loftis L. Acute infectious upper airway obstructions in children. *Semin Pediatr Infect Dis.* 2006;17:5–10.

24 Bronchiolitis

STEVE CUNNINGHAM, MBChB, PhD

Epidemiology

Bronchiolitis is the most common lower respiratory tract infection in children. The condition forms part of the spectrum of viral lower respiratory tract infection that includes bronchiolitis, viral pneumonia, and viral-induced wheeze. In polar hemispheres (north and south), bronchiolitis is a seasonal disease, dominating winter months, with a peak over 6 to 8 weeks around the winter solstice. In tropical climates, the disease is associated with rainy months and is seasonally more dispersed.[1] Climate and environment appear to influence both season and severity.[2,3]

Bronchiolitis is diagnosed clinically by integrating characteristic but variable signs and symptoms across a broad age range, though the majority of cases occur in children under 1 year of age. The condition can be caused by any respiratory virus and has a wide spectrum of disease severity.[4]

A "classic" case would be an infant aged 3 to 5 months of age[5] who develops coryza and over the subsequent 3 to 4 days has increased difficulty with breathing, and consequent inability to maintain adequate oral feeding. Wheeze or crackles can be heard on auscultation. Improvement occurs by days 5 to 7, though a characteristic harsh cough may persist for 21 days or more.[6,7]

While the diagnosis often appears straightforward, the wide range of disease severity across a skewed but broad age range and the need for clinical diagnosis (with associated inconsistency) creates difficulty in establishing precise data.[8] In addition, while bronchiolitis is a clinical diagnosis applied to any infecting agent, the majority of data available relate to bronchiolitis caused by respiratory syncytial virus (RSV) infection; and within RSV bronchiolitis is a focus on those at high risk, in particular, those born prematurely. Reference to these groups synonymously with bronchiolitis can make interpretation of epidemiological data difficult and may reduce the understanding of bronchiolitis caused by non-RSV and in lower risk patients (particularly children born at term).

POPULATION RISK FOR BRONCHIOLITIS ASSOCIATED WITH ALL RESPIRATORY VIRUSES

There are only limited estimates of population risk for bronchiolitis associated with all respiratory virus infections, but approximately 40% of infants are affected by bronchiolitis in the first year of life.[9] In the United Kingdom, using primary care databases, the 1 year incidence of children given a specific diagnosis of bronchiolitis is 58 to 65 per 1000 children,[8,10] rising to 204 per 1000 when a broader definition of bronchiolitis was used to capture potential cases.[8] This study highlights that in children with typical lower respiratory tract signs and symptoms, clinicians may not ascribe the discrete diagnosis of bronchiolitis; a finding also found

in other countries such as Spain[11] and across health care systems,[12] with evidence that a diagnosis of bronchiolitis is more likely to be made in secondary than primary care. The hospital admission rate for bronchiolitis in children without high-risk conditions is 1.9% in the United States using coded hospital data,[13] showing a decline from 2.7% in the period 2000–2009. In contrast, UK data suggest that admission rates are continuing to increase over time (to 4.0% in 2011).[14] Of those admitted to hospital, 85% are born at term and 15% are born preterm.[15] Additional factors also place children at higher risk of admission including, age (<3 months), male sex, being bottle-fed, multiple birth, and family smoking. Rates of admission for infants with a diagnosis of bronchiolitis can vary up to threefold across hospitals in the same country.[14] Duration of admission is also highly variable within countries and internationally.[16]

Mortality for bronchiolitis is low[17]; United States 0.03% overall, with an adjusted odds ratio (OR) of 0.25 for mortality in children less than 1 year of age without previous health condition and primary diagnosis of bronchiolitis.[13] Admissions to intensive care have remained constant over time[14] although related costs are increasing.[13]

POPULATION RISK FOR RESPIRATORY SYNCYTIAL VIRUS BRONCHIOLITIS

RSV infects 69% to 98% of infants in the first year of life.[18,19] The rapid development of vaccines and treatment therapies for RSV has added impetus to the need to better define the burden of RSV disease. Globally there are an estimated 33.8 million cases of RSV lower respiratory tract infection each year in children under 5 years of age, resulting in 3.4 million admissions to the hospital and 66 to 199 thousand deaths (with the majority in low- and middle-income countries).[20]

In the United States an estimated 20% of children will attend primary care each year with RSV bronchiolitis, and up to 7% attend an Emergency Department (ED).[21] Admission to hospital with RSV bronchiolitis is typically around 2.4% of all infants,[15,22] though in previously healthy term infants, the admission rate to hospital with RSV bronchiolitis can be as low as 0.7%.[23]

HIGH-RISK POPULATION FOR BRONCHIOLITIS ASSOCIATED WITH ALL RESPIRATORY VIRUSES

In infants who are born preterm at 32 to 35 weeks' gestation, 48% will develop bronchiolitis and 6% require admission to the hospital.[24] The risk of bronchiolitis is increased in a range of conditions compared with term infants, including preterm birth (respiratory rate [RR] 1.89), cystic fibrosis (RR 2.45), congenital heart disease (RR 3.35), chronic lung disease (RR 1.61), immunodeficiency (RR 1.73), Down syndrome (RR 2.53), and cerebral palsy (RR 2.43).[25,26]

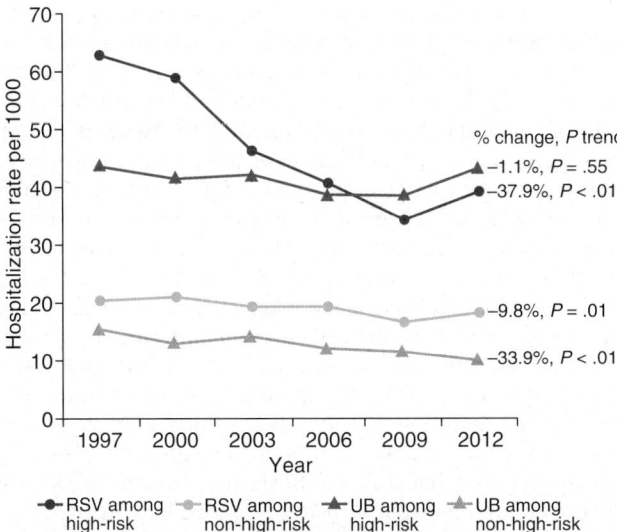

Fig. 24.1 Rate of hospitalizations due to respiratory syncytial virus (RSV) or unspecified bronchiolitis (UB) according to high-risk status in the United States Kids Inpatient Database, 1997–2012. (Doucette A, Jiang X, Fryzek J, et al. Trends in respiratory syncytial virus and bronchiolitis hospitalization rates in high-risk infants in a United States Nationally Representative Database, 1997–2012. *PLoS One.* 2016;11(4):e0152208.)

HIGH-RISK POPULATION FOR RESPIRATORY SYNCYTIAL VIRUS BRONCHIOLITIS

For infants born ≤ 32 weeks gestation, 75% of infants will have a lower respiratory tract infection in the first year of life, with 35% RSV positive and 40% RSV negative; of these infants, 41% of RSV positive will be admitted to the hospital versus 18% of RSV negative.[27] Recent studies suggest that hospitalization rates for high-risk infants due to RSV are reducing over time and are now similar to those for RSV negative, possibly as a result of improvements in neonatal care or immunoprophylaxis in high-risk groups (Fig. 24.1).[28,29] Risk of death is much higher amongst high-risk groups who are RSV positive, including preterm (1.2%), congenital heart disease (5.2%), and bronchopulmonary dysplasia (7.0%).[17]

Etiology

Bronchiolitis has a viral etiology, with RSV the most common cause, reported in 43% to 75%[30,31] of cases. Other viruses associated with bronchiolitis are human rhinovirus (18%), influenza, coronavirus, human metapneumovirus, adenovirus, parainfluenza virus and human Boca virus[30,31]; that is, "any respiratory virus."

RSV has two strains, A and B, with RSV A associated with more severe disease.[32,33] Reinfection in the same season with the same or different strain is possible.[34] As a sole infecting agent, RSV is associated with more severe bronchiolitis than other single respiratory virus infections.[5] Coinfection of RSV with rhinovirus can produce even more severe disease.[35] RSV is the most common infectious agent in children admitted to the hospital with radiological features consistent with pneumonia (occurring in 28% of children—most commonly those under 5 years of age).[36] In young children who are well immunized, RSV represents the most common cause of lower respiratory tract infection.[37]

Pathology/Pathogenesis

What commences as an upper respiratory tract infection becomes a lower respiratory tract infection over the course of 2 to 5 days. Infants are particularly susceptible as they have small bronchi that are more likely to become blocked by secretions and edema, and a less well-developed ability to respond to and clear viral infection.[38]

Histopathology is naturally limited to the most severe cases who have died, where the bronchioles are edematous and blocked by necrotic epithelium and neutrophils, with some mucus binding this debris together.[39] Airway obstruction is intensified by poor airway clearance associated with loss of cilia function occurring within 24 hours and persisting for up to 3 months after the illness.[40] Destruction of cilia is considered to be caused by virus replication and not mediated by inflammation.[38] RSV is associated with more severe airway pathology than that found in children dying from other respiratory viruses, even in those not mechanically ventilated.[39]

Viral shedding is higher and more prolonged in younger infants and those with more severe disease.[41] Increased disease severity, longer hospital stay and use of intensive care is associated with higher viral load for RSV in nasopharyngeal secretions.[42,43] Severity of disease is associated with both infant risk factors (including lack of adaptive T cell response),[26,44] but also RSV virus specific factors (viral antigen load and direct cytotoxic effects).[45] Determining the relative contribution of both of these to disease severity will be important; if the latter is dominant, antiviral agents provided early in the course of the disease may reduce severity, whereas dominance of the former might need additional immunomodulators.[4]

Biomarkers are now sought to better characterize those at risk of greater disease severity and to indicate recovery. Infants hospitalized with RSV bronchiolitis have increased interleukin (IL)-33 and IL-13 in secretions.[46] Polymorphisms of surfactant protein A are associated with increased risk of intensive care admission.[47] Cysteinyl leukotrienes are increased in infants with RSV bronchiolitis and are still increased 1 month following infection.[48] More severe disease is also associated with increased serum cathelicidin,[49] lactate dehydrogenase, caspase[50] and IL-15.[51] There is some evidence that more severe disease may be associated with an insufficient inflammatory response.[52] The interrelationship of the microbiome in bronchiolitis is also being actively explored.[53]

Clinical Features

Bronchiolitis is diagnosed clinically. Variance in the clinical interpretation of symptoms and physical findings lead to inconsistency in diagnosis, particularly in milder cases and children over 1 year of age.

SYMPTOMS

Typical symptoms are rhinorrhea, proceeding over 2 to 4 days to a characteristic harsh moist cough with pyrexia that is typically below 39°C, although fever above 38.5°C is seen in 50% of infants.[54] Ability to achieve adequate oral feeding declines as nasal obstruction with secretions develops and work of breathing increases. The time to peak symptoms of 4 days is associated with the peak in viral load,[42,55] varying from infant to infant.

In younger children (particularly <6 weeks of age), apnea may be a presenting sign, sometimes in the absence of other features of bronchiolitis. Apnea may be temporarily improved by nasal suctioning, but it is most likely a direct viral effect in young infants.[56] Apnea is a "red flag" sign in bronchiolitis that warrants a period of review in a supervised clinical setting to ensure that it has resolved.

Patients more likely to require intensive care include preterm infants and those with apnea, low birth weight, or a respiratory rate greater than 70/min.[57,58] Children tend not to relapse during the improving phase of the illness, which should give confidence to clinicians when considering discharge from ED or hospital.[58,59]

PHYSICAL FINDINGS

Physical findings include an increased respiratory rate, chest recession, use of accessory muscles, hyperinflation, wheezing, crackles, and reduced arterial oxygen saturations.[60] Physical findings vary depending on sleep state (and associated changes in tidal volume). Respiratory rate is a key marker of disease severity, with ≥60/min considered severe and ≥70/min critical.[26,61] Oxygen saturation may be improved (at least temporarily) by removal of nasal secretions.[62]

CLINICAL SCORES

Bronchiolitis is a highly variable disease that requires assessment of disease severity by clinicians for decision making, some of which is subjective. Clinical scoring systems have been developed in an attempt to standardize care and minimize variance. Many early scores derived from asthma scores. The most commonly applied scores for bronchiolitis are outlined in Table 24.1. Within this table, the most widely quoted is the Respiratory Distress Assessment Instrument (RDAI)[63] (and the resulting Respiratory Assessment Change Score, RACS). More recent scores were developed to have more detailed validation (Liverpool Infant Bronchiolitis Severity Score–Proxy Reported Outcome Measure [LIBSS PRO][64] and Genetics, Vaccines and Infectious Diseases Paediatrics Research Group [GENVIP][65]) and to improve the ability to identify those at risk of deterioration. The ability of clinical scores to retain precision and reliability, when scoring is performed by larger numbers of health care professionals in the context of multicenter Phase III trials, is of current interest.

DISEASE SEVERITY

Symptoms in bronchiolitis vary across a wide but skewed continuum from mildly increased work of breathing with cough to respiratory failure and death. Often divided into mild, moderate, and severe disease, the perspective on these gradations varies across health care systems. A World Health Organization (WHO) workshop has provided candidate definitions differentiating a diagnosis of RSV lower respiratory tract infection (SpO_2 <95%) from severe (<93%) and very severe RSV disease (SpO_2 <90%, inability to feed orally, or reduced level of consciousness).[66] Infants can display variance in SpO_2 within this range (90% to 95%) over short periods of observation without significant change in clinical status,[58,62,67] which may limit the discriminatory reliability of these definitions. From a secondary care perspective, moderate severity is often considered a need for admission to hospital and severe by need for critical care (positive pressure support). Clinical scores are often designed to identify transition points in the level of care required.[64] The currently available evidence concerning transition points in level of care is poor. Treatment guidance, particularly benefit from use of interventions at the ED/Ward (i.e., SpO_2)[68] and ward/critical care floor interface (i.e., high-flow nasal cannula [HFNC] oxygen and continuous positive airway pressure [CPAP]) is much needed. Guidelines have provided signs and symptoms that should alert clinicians to a child at risk of deterioration and suggested criteria for admission to the hospital.[26] In hospitals, those most likely to deteriorate to the extent of being provided with critical care support are of lower birth weight (<5 lbs, 2.25 kg) and/or have a respiratory rate ≥70/min on day 1 of admission.[57]

IMAGING, LABORATORY FINDINGS

Chest radiography is not required to confirm a diagnosis of bronchiolitis. A chest radiograph often leads to increased diagnostic uncertainty as the features may be similar to those of pneumonia (atelectasis, mucous plugging, and loss of volume) and consequently lead to greater inappropriate use of antibiotics.[69] Chest radiography should be reserved for a child who is atypical, for example, showing persistently focal crackles, a temperature remaining above 39°C despite antipyretics, or respiratory failure requiring critical care support.[26,70]

Laboratory tests do not aid in the clinical diagnosis of bronchiolitis. Serious bacterial infection is unusual and complete blood counts and blood cultures are unhelpful (though recent evidence suggests that although still uncommon, it may be more frequent than previously considered).[65] Dehydration is usually mild and best assessed clinically without electrolyte measurement. Approximately 6% of infants with bronchiolitis can have concurrent urinary tract infection, so urine culture may be of value in persistently febrile infants, particularly those under 3 months of age.[71]

Measurement of arterial/capillary carbon dioxide is commonly performed, but can be restricted to those children with increased respiratory rate and work of breathing despite oxygen supplementation.[72]

Diagnosis and Differential Diagnosis

The clinical interpretation of signs and symptoms is difficult in a condition where age boundaries are loose (and skew to older ages in those with comorbidity) and symptoms vary from patient to patient and time to time. This naturally leads to variation in diagnosis and differential diagnosis. There is a common understanding that a clearer diagnosis is possible in those under 1 year of age and most guidelines reflect this. However, constraining a diagnosis of bronchiolitis to those less than 1 year of age may reduce the ability to identify the whole population of children with bronchiolitis who could benefit from potential interventions. In general, a broader

Table 24.1 Clinical Scores for Bronchiolitis

Score	Tal[a]	Lowell[b]	Wang[c]	Wilson[d]	Jacobs[e]	Liu[f]	Walsh[g]	Marlais[h]	Van Miert[i]	Cebey-Lopez[j]
Name	Tal and later Modified Tal (SpO₂, not cyanosis)	Respiratory Distress Assessment Instrument (RDAI)	No names	Comprehensive Severity Index (pediatric component)	Canadian Acute Respiratory Infection and Flu Scale (CARIFS)	No name	Bronchiolitis Assessment Severity Tool	Bronchiolitis Risk of Admission Scoring System	LIBSS-PRO	GENVIP
General respiratory or bronchiolitis specific	General	General	General	General	General	General	Bronchiolitis	Bronchiolitis	Bronchiolitis	General
Date published	1983	1987	1992	2000	2000	2004	2006	2011	2015	2016
Number of items	4	7 (in 3 domains)	4	27 (in 7 domains)	18 (in 3 domains)	4 (age specific ranges)	4	5	10	7
Subjective/objective	2/2	2/1	3/1	11/14	18/0	3/1	2/2	0/5	3/7	3/4
Scoring	0–3 per item	0 to max 4 per item. Total max = 17	0–3 per item	1–4	0–3 per item	0–3 per item	0 to max 3 + age	0–1	0 to max 8 per item	0–3 (max 20)
Score	Mean score	Sum	Sum	Sum	Sum	Sum	Sum of weighted scores	Sum	Sum	Sum
Interpretation	Relative change	Change in score >4 = improvement, <4 no improvement	Relative change	Relative change	Relative change	Relative change	≤0.654 mild disease, >1.866 severe	≥3 predicted admission	Cut of scores for mild, moderate, and severe	Relative change
For completion by	Health care	Health care	Health care	Health care	Parents	Health care	Health care	Health care	Health care	Health care
Interrater reliability Correlation				Length of stay $r^2 = 0.23$				PPV 67% NPV 83%		
Kappa	0.7[k]	Not provided for total score	0.48		0.36–0.52	0.52–0.65	0.68		0.83	0.74

[a]Tal A, Bavilski C, Yohai D, Bearman JE, Gorodischer R, Moses SW. Dexamethasone and salbutamol in the treatment of acute wheezing in infants. *Pediatrics.* 1983;71(1):13-18.

[b]Lowell DI, Lister G, Von Koss H, McCarthy P. Wheezing in infants: the response to epinephrine. *Pediatrics.* 1987;79(6):939-945.

[c]Wang EE, Milner RA, Navas L, Maj H. Observer agreement for respiratory signs and oximetry in infants hospitalized with lower respiratory infections. *Am Rev Respir Dis.* 1992;145(1):106-109.

[d]Wilson DF, Horn SD, Smouth R, Gassaway J, Torres A. Severity assessment in children hospitalized with bronchiolitis using the pediatric component of the comprehensive severity index. *Pediatr Crit Care Med.* 2000;1(2):127-132.

[e]Jacobs B, Young NL, Dick PT, et al. Canadian Acute Respiratory Illness and Flu Scale (CARIFS): development of a valid measure for childhood respiratory infections. *J Clin Epidemiol.* 2000;53(8):793-799.

[f]Liu LL, Gallaher MM, Davis RL, Rutter CM, Lewis TC, Marcuse EK. Use of a respiratory clinical score among different providers. *Pediatr Pulmonol.* 2004;37(3):243-248.

[g]Walsh P, Gonzales A, Satar A, Rothenberg SJ. The interrater reliability of a validated bronchiolitis severity assessment tool. *Pediatr Emerg Care.* 2006;22(5):316-320.

[h]Marlais M, Evans J, Abrahamson E. Clinical predictors of admission in infants with acute bronchiolitis. *Arch Dis Child.* 2011;96(7):648-652.

[i]van Miert C, Abbott J, Verheoff F, Lane S, Carter B, McNamara P. Development and validation of the Liverpool infant bronchiolitis severity score: a research protocol. *J Adv Nurs.* 2014;70(10):2353-2362.

[j]Cebey-Lopez M, Pardo-Seco J, Gomez-Carballa A, et al. Bacteremia in children hospitalized with respiratory syncytial virus infection. *PLoS One.* 2016;11(2):e0146599.

[k]McCallum GB, Morris PS, Wilson CC, et al. Severity scoring systems: are they internally valid, reliable and predictive of oxygen use in children with acute bronchiolitis? *Pediatr Pulmonol.* 2013;48(8):797-803.

LIBSS PRO, Liverpool Infant Bronchiolitis Severity Score–Proxy Reported Outcome Measure.

definition of bronchiolitis is used in North America and Asia that captures a higher percentage of older children with wheezing, where rhinovirus is the dominant infecting agent.[73] Such children may be given a diagnosis of viral induced wheeze in other countries. There is most likely a continuum of viral lower respiratory tract infection across age ranges that moves from current diagnoses of viral bronchiolitis to viral pneumonia and viral-induced wheeze/wheezy bronchitis.[74,75]

The clinical features consistent with a diagnosis of bronchiolitis across different guidelines are presented in Table 24.2. Diagnosis has a typical onset of a viral respiratory tract prodrome proceeding to lower respiratory symptoms over 3 to 4 days. The South African guideline (2010) considers hyperinflation the most reliable clinical sign in bronchiolitis.[76] The UK guideline (2015) provides a more proscriptive definition.[26]

Testing of nasal secretions for virus may help consolidate the clinical diagnosis of bronchiolitis and inform health care logistics. Most commonly used, and with highest precision, are polymerase chain reaction (PCR) diagnostics for a range of respiratory viruses, but point of care (PoC) testing for a more limited range of viruses (most often RSV) is increasingly precise and cost effective.[77] Testing for RSV (as the most common infecting agent in bronchiolitis) is often performed to aid cohorting of patients within hospitals. The increasing recognition that multiple viruses may be identified in those with acute bronchiolitis has called into question the benefit of cohorting based on RSV status.[78] PCR diagnostics may sometimes be considered oversensitive to the detection of virus fragments postinfection, and multiplex PCR results should be interpreted with this understanding.

Differential diagnosis includes bacterial pneumonia or an alternative cause of crackles, wheeze, and increased work of breathing in a young child. Persisting crackles (crepitations) in one lung zone, fixed focal wheeze, persistent pyrexia (>39°C) or persistently increased work of breathing in a child who appears otherwise recovered warrant further evaluation.

Prescient in the mind of most clinicians is that a bacterial pneumonia may be missed. Chest radiographs have similar appearances and are poor discriminators. We can assume that bacterial coinfection risk is low, as the use of antibiotics in bronchiolitis is not associated with faster recovery.[79] Further investigation could be limited to those with the persisting clinical features noted above. In children with more severe disease, there may be a role for antibiotics as bacteria are isolated in 33% to 44% of lavage samples in children with severe bronchiolitis who are intubated and ventilated.[80–82]

Table 24.2   Guideline Recommendations in Bronchiolitis

	Spain (2010)	South Africa (2010)	Canada (2014)	United States (2014)	United Kingdom (2015)	Finland (2016)	Recent Evidence That May Influence Future Recommendations[a]
Age	<24 months	Children	≤2 years	1–23 months	Children (mostly under 1 year)	Children (mostly under 6 months)	
Clinical definition	Not stated	Viral URTI, with poor feeding, low-grade fever, hyperinflation of the chest, wheezing, tachypnea, lower chest wall retractions	Viral URTI, cough or rhinitis followed by some of tachypnea, costal retractions, apnea, wheezing or crackles, nasal flaring, hypoxemia	Rhinitis and cough, followed by tachypnea, wheezing, rales, use of accessory muscles and/or nasal flaring	Coryza followed by persistent cough and tachypnea or chest recession (or both) and wheezing or crackles (or both). Apnea may be presenting symptom in absence of above.	Not stated. Fine crackles on auscultation considered characteristic.	
THERAPIES							
Oxygen supplementation threshold	<92%	<92% (<90% above 1800 m)	<90%	<90%	<92%	"Low"—not defined	Cunningham
Bronchodilator	No	Trial in hypoxic infant	No	No	No	No	
Hypertonic saline	No	Trial in hypoxic infant	?Equivocal	Trial in hospitalized child	No	No	Everard Florin Teunissen Jacobs Wu Silver
Corticosteroids	No	No	No	No	No	No	
Epinephrine	No	No	?Equivocal	No	No	No	
Antibiotics	No	Consider if severe	No	No	No	No	

[a]See "Suggested Reading" section.
URTI, Urinary tract infection.

There are no trials of outcome for antibiotic use in children with bronchiolitis receiving intensive care.

Though uncommon, congenital lesions may masquerade as bronchiolitis, and this should be borne in mind for children with atypical clinical features or those slow to recover. Congenital heart disease may present as bronchiolitis when pulmonary vascular resistance falls increasing left to right shunt. More difficult to differentiate are children with congenital (or less commonly acquired) pulmonary malformations. Fixed focal wheeze may be a sign of tracheomalacia or bronchomalacia, stenosis, or compression from lobar emphysema or a bronchogenic cyst and would warrant a chest radiograph. A slow recovering course with persistent chest signs could be an infected congenital pulmonary malformation (such as a congenital cystic adenomatoid malformation [CCAM] or sequestration). Children with persistent fine crackles, tachypnea, and low (often borderline) oxygen saturation may have an interstitial lung disease, particularly neuroendocrine cell hyperplasia (NEHI) presenting as recurrent "bronchiolitis." Young children with persistent, sometimes focal, crackles postadenovirus (though may also be other respiratory viruses and mycoplasma pneumonia) should be evaluated for postinfectious bronchiolitis obliterans (PIBO); see section 6 of the book.

Management and Treatment

Management of bronchiolitis is supportive, assisting hydration and hypoxemia until improvement. With increased respiratory rate and nasal secretions, oral feeding is challenged, and those with severe disease require assistance with feeding by enteral or parenteral means. The threshold for supporting hydration is typically when an infant's intake is reduced to 50% to 75% of usual volume. The chosen percentage of intake depends on the child's status: an expreterm 10-week-old infant on day 3 of illness may be supported at 75% understanding that they most likely will deteriorate, whereas a robust 8-month-old term infant may be able to tolerate 50% feed volume for a couple of days until disease resolution. Nasogastric feeding is easier to administer than intravenous fluids but has no advantage in recovery from acute disease.[83]

Oxygen may be used to treat hypoxemia. The threshold oxygen saturation at which to use supplemental oxygen varies across guidelines and is typically set between 90% and 94% at sea level. In children admitted to hospital with bronchiolitis, management at a threshold of 90% SpO$_2$ is safe and as clinically effective as a 94% target.[84] The threshold oxygen saturation for admission to hospital is often 92%, as some data suggest that infants have a higher risk of desaturating further at this oxygen saturation.[85] Oxygen desaturation may however have a disproportionate influence on decisions to admit children to the hospital,[68] and much like hydration status (previously mentioned), the context of the measurement should be considered. Many infants discharged home from ED with bronchiolitis experience desaturation events subsequently that are not associated with clinical deterioration.[67] In hospitals, the use of intermittent oxygen saturation monitoring is much discussed, and though the benefit below 90% SpO$_2$ is not established, once stable above 90% SpO$_2$, oxygen saturation monitoring should be stopped.[86] Use of

therapies in addition to supplemental oxygen and hydration are poorly supported by current evidence. There is some evidence that infants handled less get better quicker,[87] and the use of additional therapies should be considered with that in mind.

There is widespread variation across hospitals and countries in the management and treatment of bronchiolitis reflecting local custom and individual clinician practice.[88] Reducing variation and associated health care costs is a key aim of bronchiolitis management presented through guidelines. Guidelines for the care of infants with bronchiolitis based on systematic review and published in English are available from the United Kingdom (2015),[89] United States (2014),[90] Canada (2014),[61] Spain (2010),[91] Finland (2016),[92] and South Africa (2010),[76] which has been updated as a critical review 2016.[93] No therapies receive support across all guidelines for use with the exception of supplemental oxygen. Chest physiotherapy does not speed recovery. Antibiotics, though still widely used, are of no benefit in bronchiolitis.[79] In addition, bronchodilators are less likely to be recommended in more recent guidelines, and the theory that they may be of greater benefit in infants more likely to develop asthma has been refuted.[94] Nebulized hypertonic saline has been of benefit in cystic fibrosis and in early trials in bronchiolitis,[95] but larger well-designed trials have not demonstrated a persuasive benefit.[96–100]

Recent years have seen the increasing use of HFNC oxygen in acute bronchiolitis.[101] Though clinical trials have not yet demonstrated important clinical or physiological benefits,[102] large well-designed trials are in progress and are beginning to report.[102a,103] CPAP has some benefit in bronchiolitis, and may prevent deterioration when used early.[104] As with all management in bronchiolitis, the use of HFNC oxygen, CPAP, and intubation varies across sites irrespective of disease severity,[105] and better understanding of the risks and benefits of these interventions is required.[106]

There are no current effective pharmacological treatments for RSV. While ribavirin was previously used as an antiviral treatment for RSV, it is now considered ineffective.[107] Novel treatments for acute infection are in development: antivirals and nebulized immunoglobulin. In this rapidly moving field, it seems probable that a treatment for RSV will become available in the next 5 years.[108] Reduction in viral load has been demonstrated in adult challenge models of RSV treated with the antivirals ALS-8176[109] and GS-5806[110]

Prevention

Prevention of spread of RSV depends on good hygiene, in particular, hand washing, as RSV may survive for up to 6 hours on surfaces contaminated by droplets.[111] Similar precautions are appropriate for other respiratory virus infections associated with bronchiolitis. Many hospitals use PoC testing for RSV to determine cohorting of infants as inpatients.[107] While this is still common, the practice is called into question by the range of coinfection with other respiratory viruses revealed by PCR panel testing; up to 62% of children with viral respiratory tract infection have more than one virus detected.[112]

Prevention of RSV (as the most common cause of bronchiolitis) has been a long-term goal. Early formalin inactivated vaccines were associated with more severe enhanced RSV disease and deaths, possibly resulting from inadequate T cell priming.[113] Subsequent vaccine development has been cautious in view of this experience.

In the 1990s, RSV intravenous immunoglobulin was developed[114,115] but was rapidly superseded by palivizumab, a monoclonal antibody delivered by monthly intramuscular injection. When administered over the RSV season, it reduces hospital admission in high-risk infants.[116] Palivizumab's monthly injections and limited efficacy have prompted the development of extended life monoclonal antibodies that are undergoing licensing trials in preterm infants.[117] They will hopefully be evaluated in the future for high-risk infants born at term.

RSV vaccine development has gained significant impetus over the last 15 years with a wide range of candidate vaccines in development both for pediatric and maternal use; maternal immunization could provide passive transplacental protection to infants in the first 3 to 6 months of life (http://www.path.org). A Phase III trial of maternal immunization by Novovax is expected to conclude in 2020.

Prognosis

For most children, bronchiolitis is a self-limiting disease, with cough as the most persistent symptom resolving at a median of 12 to 15 days.[84,118] Many children, however, develop recurrent respiratory symptoms. In the first few months following illness, this is considered in part to result from loss of cilia from the airway epithelial surfaces during the acute illness.[40] For those who experience chronic symptoms, the debate continues on whether children with more severe bronchiolitis and recurrent postinfectious wheezing have premorbid susceptibility, with some evidence suggesting poorer preexisting lung function.[119] Recurrent wheeze in the year following

bronchiolitis occurs in 62% of those who are RSV positive and 32% of those who are RSV negative.[120] Recurrent postinfectious wheeze is not reduced by montelukast[121] or inhaled corticosteroids,[122,123] but there is good evidence of benefit from Palivizumab,[124] and potentially azithromycin,[125] though the latter requires further study.

In the longer term, there is good evidence that children who have had an admission to the hospital for RSV bronchiolitis are 3 times more likely to have a diagnosis of asthma and lower lung function at age 6 years[23] and a higher incidence of asthma at age 13[126] and 18[127] years. The question remains whether such children are predisposed to bronchiolitis because of premorbid anatomy[119] and the consequent interrelationship between host and virus specific effects on the development of asthma.

References

Access the reference list online at ExpertConsult.com.

Suggested Reading

Cunningham S, Rodriguez A, Adams T, et al. Oxygen saturation targets in infants with bronchiolitis (BIDS): a double-blind, randomised, equivalence trial. *Lancet.* 2015;386(9998):1041–1048.

Everard ML, Hind D, Ugonna K, et al. SABRE: a multicentre randomised control trial of nebulised hypertonic saline in infants hospitalised with acute bronchiolitis. *Thorax.* 2014;69(12):1105–1112.

Florin TA, Shaw KN, Kittick M, et al. Nebulized hypertonic saline for bronchiolitis in the emergency department: a randomized clinical trial. *JAMA Pediatr.* 2014;168(7):664–670.

Jacobs JD, Foster M, Wan J, et al. 7% Hypertonic saline in acute bronchiolitis: a randomized controlled trial. *Pediatrics.* 2014;133(1):e8–e13.

Silver AH, Esteban-Cruciani N, Azzarone G, et al. 3% hypertonic saline versus normal saline in inpatient bronchiolitis: a randomized controlled trial. *Pediatrics.* 2015;136(6):1036–1043.

Teunissen J, Hochs AH, Vaessen-Verberne A, et al. The effect of 3% and 6% hypertonic saline in viral bronchiolitis: a randomised controlled trial. *Eur Respir J.* 2014;44(4):913–921.

Wu S, Baker C, Lang ME, et al. Nebulized hypertonic saline for bronchiolitis: a randomized clinical trial. *JAMA Pediatr.* 2014;168(7):657–663.

25 Pneumonia in Children

MARCELO C. SCOTTA, MD, PAULO J.C. MAROSTICA, MD, and RENATO T. STEIN, MD

Pneumonia is broadly defined as inflammation in the lung caused by an infectious agent that stimulates a response resulting in damage to lung tissue. Different definitions for pneumonia vary from "detection of pulmonary pathogens in lung specimens" to the "presence of pulmonary infiltrates on chest radiographs," or even clinically based criteria, such as age-specific tachypnea or lower chest retractions.[1,2]

Epidemiology and Etiology

Community-acquired pneumonia (CAP) is one of the most important health problems affecting children worldwide, and is the leading single cause of mortality in children younger than 5 years of age, especially in low- and middle-income countries. Annually, there are 4–5 million deaths reported in children younger than 5 years of age, and pneumonia is estimated to account for approximately 1 million of these.[3]

The estimated median global incidence of pneumonia in 2010 in children younger than 5 years of age was 0.22 episodes per child-year, 11.5% of which are sufficiently severe to require hospitalization; this was at least 25% lower than previous estimates a decade earlier. The estimated incidence for high-income countries is 0.015 episodes per child-year.[4]

The proportion of pneumonia cases obtained from efficacy estimates of vaccine trials was used to demonstrate the burden of pneumonia caused by *Streptococcus pneumoniae* and *Haemophilus influenzae* type b (Hib). Over 13 million new cases of pneumococcal pneumonia were estimated, with a global yearly incidence of 2228 cases per 100,000 children younger than 5 years of age, ranging from 462/100,000 cases in Europe to 3397/100,000 cases in Africa.[5] The case fatality rate ranged from 2% in the Western Pacific to 11% in Africa. The estimated global incidence of Hib pneumonia in the absence of vaccination was 1304 per 100,000 children younger than 5 years of age.[6]

A recent prospective study, including more than 2300 children in the United States, reported an overall incidence of radiologically confirmed CAP requiring hospitalization of 15.7 cases per 10,000 children and 62.2 cases per 10,000 among children younger than 2 years.[7] In South Africa, a birth cohort study following 697 infants during the first year of life has shown that the incidence of clinically defined pneumonia was 0.27 episodes per child-year, with 23% of those classified as severe pneumonia.[8]

Pneumonia can be caused by several different microorganisms, with viruses and bacteria being the most frequent agents. Viruses are, by far, the most prevalent cause of pneumonia throughout childhood, with the highest burden observed among infants. However, pathogens are epidemiologically interconnected, and coinfections, both with two or more viruses, or with viruses and bacteria, are very common. Coinfection rates up to 75% are commonly reported in infants.[7,8]

There are substantial age-related differences in the etiology of CAP during childhood (Table 25.1).[7] From birth to 28 days of life, most CAP is caused by group B streptococci, or Gram-negative enteric bacteria, although respiratory syncytial virus (RSV) also has a prominent role in this age group.[9] Beyond the neonatal period, RSV, influenza, and human metapneumovirus are among the most common viruses associated with a diagnosis of pneumonia.[7,9] *Chlamydia pneumoniae* and particularly *Mycoplasma pneumoniae* infections occur more often in school-age children and during adolescence, although there are many reports of these agents causing CAP in younger children as well.[7,10] In the first 6 months of life, *Chlamydia trachomatis*, a variety of respiratory viruses, *Bordetella pertussis* (see Chapter 32), or even *Ureaplasma urealyticum* may have a role (data are inconsistent).[11]

The frequency rates for *S. pneumoniae*, the most prevalent bacteria causing CAP, are less affected by age. *S. pneumoniae* is a common pathogen throughout both infancy and childhood[7]; however, the incidence, severity, and complications from pneumococcal pneumonia have substantially reduced since the introduction of pneumococcal conjugate vaccine (PCV).[12–14]

Various pneumococcal serotypes have been associated with CAP, with specific and distinct prevalence rates in different parts of the world. The majority of the most important serotypes are included in PCV, especially the 13 valent pneumococcal vaccine (PCV13).[15,16]

Hib was a more frequent cause of CAP, before the widespread use of Hib immunization. It is still an important cause of CAP in countries where these vaccines are not universally available. Hib is more frequently observed in children younger than 5 years of age.[4] Nontypable *H. influenzae* may be more frequently associated with pneumonia than *S. pneumoniae* in immunocompetent and immunized children, as shown in studies from low- and middle-income countries.[17,18] Recently, several studies have reported on the impact of new conjugate vaccines (Hib and PCV) on pneumonia incidence, severity, and complications (see section "Prevention" of this chapter).[19,20]

As for other pathogens, pneumonia secondary to *Streptococcus pyogenes* is an infrequent cause of CAP nowadays; bacteremia or scarlet fever are more frequently diagnosed, especially among small children. Chickenpox (*Varicella zoster* virus) pneumonia may be associated with group A streptococcus since it seems to transiently affect host defenses and predispose to infection from commensal bacteria.[21,22]

Staphylococcus aureus pneumonia usually occurs secondary to inhalation of the pathogen. In rare cases, it can be the result of bacteremic spread, usually when there is a predisposing factor (e.g., a catheter, or use of intravenous [IV] drugs). *S. aureus* pneumonia tends to present as an acute, severe illness, especially because many first-line antibiotics commonly used to treat CAP do not provide appropriate coverage. Radiologic findings include bronchopneumonia

Table 25.1   Most Common Agents Causing Community-Acquired Pneumonia According to Age Group

		AGE		
Newborns	**1–6 Months**	**6–12 Months**	**1–5 Years**	**Older Than 5 Years**
Group B Streptococcus	Viruses	Viruses	Viruses	Viruses
Enteric Gram-negative	*Streptococcus pneumoniae*	*Streptococcus pneumoniae*	*M. pneumoniae*	*M. pneumoniae*
RSV	*Haemophilus influenzae*	*Haemophilus influenza*	*S. pneumoniae*	*S. pneumoniae*
	Staphylococcus aureus	*S. aureus*	*C. pneumoniae*	*C. pneumoniae*
	Moraxella catarrhalis	*Moraxella catarrhalis*		
	Chlamydia trachomatis			
	Ureaplasma urealyticum			
	Bordetella pertussis			

with alveolar infiltrates, mostly unilateral. These infiltrates may coalesce and evolve to large areas of consolidation and cavitation. Destruction of bronchial walls may lead to air trapping and pneumatocele formation in at least 30% of cases. Pleural effusion and empyema are found in as many as 60% of the cases, and pneumothorax or pyopneumothorax are common complications. In the case of hematogenous spread of *S. aureus*, the radiologic picture is one of multiple bilateral pulmonary infiltrates that may cavitate. An increase in white blood cell counts is usual, but is not sufficiently sensitive or specific to suggest the etiologic diagnosis. Although the appearance of staphylococcal pneumatoceles may be dramatic, usually once the infection is controlled, the pneumatoceles resolve completely in the following few months.[23,24]

In recent years, community-associated methicillin-resistant *S. aureus* (CA-MRSA) has been increasingly recognized in otherwise healthy adults and children. CA-MRSA usually affects younger patients compared to hospital-acquired MRSA, and it is often susceptible to clindamycin, trimethoprim-sulfamethoxazole, and tetracyclines. Many strains of CA-MRSA carry the gene for Panton-Valentine leukocidin, an exotoxin that is lethal to leukocytes, which causes tissue necrosis, skin lesions, necrotizing pneumonia, and necrotizing fasciitis.[25–27]

Mycobacterium tuberculosis should also be considered in the differential diagnosis of acute pneumonia, especially in high endemic areas (see Chapter 29). A recent systematic review reported 7.5% positive cultures in children with acute pneumonia, especially in endemic areas with a tuberculosis yearly incidence higher than 50 cases per 100,000 people.[28]

Pathogenesis

The upper airways are commensally colonized by a variety of organisms, differently from the lower respiratory tract, which, until recently, was considered to be sterile. However, evolving knowledge of the human microbiome, using high-throughput sequencing-based studies, has shown that the lower airways are transiently or even chronically colonized.[29] Upper respiratory infections usually precede lower respiratory tract invasion by microorganisms, such as bacteria and viruses. Viruses usually reach the lower airways through contiguous spread and replication, and a similar mechanism of invasion is believed to occur with atypical bacteria. Microaspiration from the upper respiratory tract is the most common mechanism for most bacterial pneumonia.

Macroaspiration, which is associated with an overwhelming inoculum, and hematogenous spread may also occur, with this latter mechanism more common in pneumonia caused by *S. aureus*.[30–32] In children, significant aspiration may occur due to swallowing dysfunction, gastroesophageal reflux, or congenital malformations.[33]

In the lower airways, the infectious process begins with an immune response leading to leukocyte infiltration, edema, and consequent small airway obstruction; this is followed by loss of tissue compliance, increase in airway resistance, atelectasis, abnormalities in ventilation-perfusion ratios, and necrosis. Virulence factors also facilitate the evasion of immune defenses, causing lung invasion and tissue destruction, such as occurs with the protein NS1 from some influenza strains, and with surface proteins of *S. pneumoniae*.[34–36] Impairment of the epiglottic and cough reflexes, interruption of mucociliary clearance by virus-induced changes in ciliary structure and function, and virus-induced enhancement of bacterial adherence are some of the mechanisms believed to contribute to this chain of events, which eventually leads to pneumonia. Evidence suggests that tumor necrosis factor-alpha (TNF-α) and specific interleukins play a role in the exaggerated immune response observed in severe pneumonias.[37,38] Both humoral and cellular immune responses are crucial to protect children against pneumonia.[34,35,39]

Clinical Features

SYMPTOMS

Children with pneumonia usually present with an acute illness, and some have no specific respiratory signs or symptoms. Common clinical findings include fever, chills, tachypnea, productive cough, lower chest indrawing, abdominal pain, and chest pain, all of which suggest—but do not prove—pneumonia. For Hib, the clinical picture is similar to other typical bacteria, although a more insidious onset is the rule.[40] A more gradual clinical onset associated with a combination of symptoms, such as headache, malaise, nonproductive cough, and low-grade fever/no fever, is generally associated with infection by atypical pathogens such as *M. pneumoniae*.[7,41]

Children can have fever and pneumonia without overt manifestations of respiratory disease. In a Canadian series of 570 pediatric patients with signs and symptoms suggestive of lower respiratory tract infection (LRTI), fever was the most sensitive sign, while grunting and retractions were the most specific, associated with alveolar infiltrates found on a chest radiograph.[42] A retrospective study from the United States showed that 5.3% of children with fever and no signs of LRTI, respiratory distress, or hypoxia may have a confirmed diagnosis of pneumonia by chest radiograph. The presence of a cough, as well as a longer duration of both a fever and a cough, was more likely associated with occult pneumonia. When a cough was absent, only 0.28% of the children had pneumonia.[43] The clinical presentation of pneumonia in the first months of life is generally different from that in older children. Infants in the first 3 months of life may present with a cough and respiratory distress associated with low-grade or no fever.[11]

PHYSICAL FINDINGS

The presence of age-specific tachypnea or lower chest indrawing is the main clinical sign used by the World Health Organization (WHO) for the diagnosis of pneumonia. According to the updated WHO guidelines, children with tachypnea or lower chest indrawing are classified as having pneumonia. Formerly, pneumonia in children with chest indrawing was classified as severe. However, evidence suggests that this last group is successfully treated with oral antibiotics. Children with danger signs (inability to drink, persistent vomiting, convulsions, lethargy, impaired level of consciousness, stridor, and severe malnutrition) are classified as having severe or very severe pneumonia.[2] The best way to assess the respiratory rate is over a 60-second period with the child alert and calm. Other respiratory signs may also indicate pneumonia, but no sign by itself can be used to diagnose or to rule out pneumonia. The respiratory rate seems to provide better interobserver agreement than auscultation of the chest, especially when examining infants.[44] Usually, the cut-off points are a respiratory rate of 60 breaths per minute in infants younger than 2 months of age, 50 breaths per minute for infants from 2 to 12 months of age, and 40 breaths per minute for children 1–5 years of age. Tachypnea is usually more sensitive and specific than crackles on auscultation, after the exclusion of a diagnosis of bronchiolitis or asthma. Tachypnea is highly sensitive for pneumonia, but is nonspecific; therefore it is widely used to diagnose CAP in low- and middle-income countries, where pneumonia is highly prevalent. By contrast, in affluent countries, most children (especially infants) who present acutely with an increased respiratory rate have either viral bronchiolitis or asthma associated with a viral infection. Systemic toxicity is less common in viral compared to bacterial infection because respiratory viruses rarely cause viremia.[45]

Wheezing is most frequently associated with infection by viral agents, and bacterial pneumonia, except for *Mycoplasma* or *Chlamydia*, is an unlikely cause.[46] In a case series of pneumonia from Wubbel and colleagues, pneumococcal infection was the most frequent diagnosis among patients without wheezing. On the other hand, viruses were the most frequent pathogens among those who wheezed.[46]

LABORATORY TESTS

Higher white blood cell counts and concentrations of C-reactive protein, as well as procalcitonin, have been associated with bacterial pneumonia, but there is great overlap

with pneumonia of viral etiology; therefore these tests are of little clinical utility for an individual subject.[47] Although consistent studies in children are scarce, evidence from adults suggest that inflammatory markers are useful for follow-up, especially to detect a possible treatment failure.[48]

RADIOLOGIC FINDINGS

In general, chest radiographs are standard practice in hospitalized children for whom a diagnosis of pneumonia is being considered. In the early clinical stages of disease, patients with bacterial pneumonia may have normal chest radiographs. There is also significant variation in the interpretation of these radiographs in children, with considerable intraobserver and interobserver disagreement. Specificity ranges from 42% to 100% in different studies because of the varying definitions of pneumonia.[49,50] Whether accuracy is improved by adding lateral chest radiographs is controversial, as studies have shown conflicting results.[51–53] WHO criteria for the standardization of chest radiograph interpretation defined primary end-point pneumonia as consolidation ("a dense opacity that may be a fluffy consolidation of a portion or whole of a lobe or of the entire lung, often containing air bronchograms") or pleural effusion, and such an approach is reported to improve agreement. When comparing the presence of any infiltrate (end-point or other infiltrates not matching this definition), agreement was lower.[1]

A considerable proportion of children younger than 5 years of age with fever and leukocytosis, and without a well-defined source of infection, may have radiographic abnormalities consistent with pneumonia. In a study by Bachur and colleagues, 26% of the patients younger than 5 years of age who presented to the emergency department with fever, leukocytosis greater than 20,000 cells/mm^3, and no clinical findings suggestive of pneumonia, had a confirmed diagnosis of pneumonia on radiograph.[54] Therefore a plain chest radiograph is part of the investigation of nonspecific clinical signs of infection in this age group.

Because chest radiographs do not change the outcome of LRTIs, guidelines do not recommend them for children older than 2 months of age who are cared for in an outpatient setting.[42,45,55]

Although alveolar or lobar pneumonia (Fig. 25.1) is more frequently observed in infection from typical bacteria, when compared with interstitial pneumonia (which occurs more frequently in viral pneumonia or with *Mycoplasma* or *Chlamydia* infection), it is usually impossible to make an etiologic diagnosis based on a chest radiograph.[44] No follow-up radiographs are needed to evaluate a CAP with good clinical response, except for cases of round pneumonias, lobar collapse, or whenever clinical deterioration may occur.[45]

Recent reports have shown that bedside lung ultrasound (US) may be an option for the diagnosis of pneumonia in children.[56] The accuracy is similar or higher than chest radiographs, with the possibility of bedside use and avoidance of radiation exposure.[57] However, this technique requires specialized training, and further studies are needed.[58]

Computed tomography (CT) scans should not be used routinely unless another underlying diagnosis is suspected (e.g., a tumor or abscess) because of radiation concerns, and because less invasive imaging techniques usually suffice for

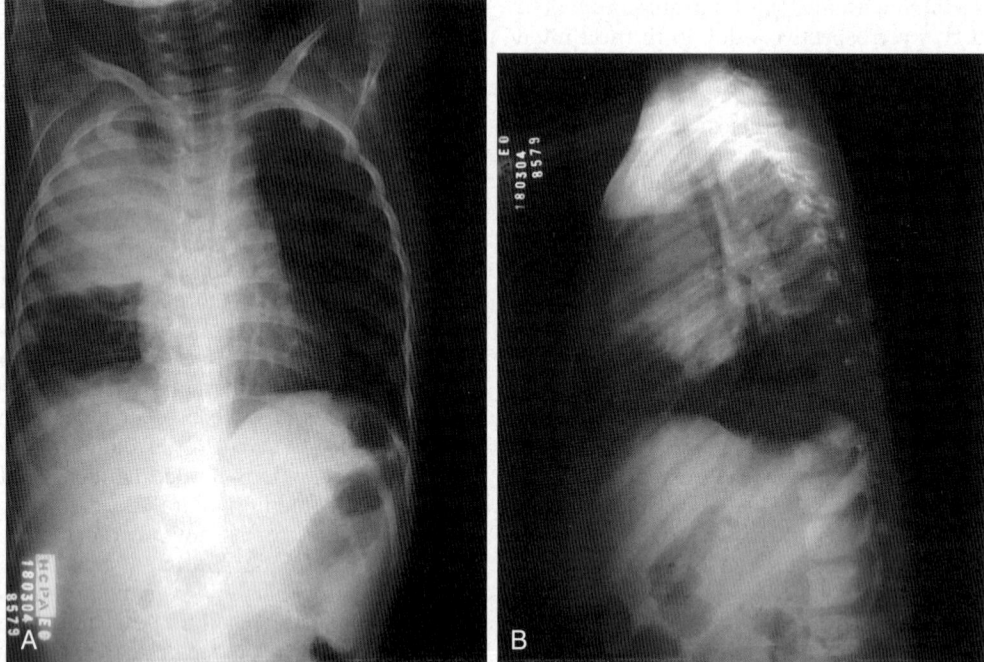

Fig. 25.1 Pneumococcal pneumonia. Positive blood cultures for *Streptococcus pneumoniae*. Dense consolidation of right upper and middle lobes with air bronchogram. (A) Anteroposterior view. (B) Lateral view.

diagnosis and management.[59] A possible exception would be in cases where a surgical approach is being considered.[60]

Some studies have also compared lung magnetic resonance imaging (MRI) to conventional chest radiography. High agreement was reported, with greater sensitivity of MRI for complications, such as lung abscess and necrosis, with the advantage of it being a radiation-free procedure. However, the role of MRI is yet to be determined, since accuracy is not clearly superior, and it is not readily available in most settings; also, it requires sedation or a cooperative patient, and is more expensive than traditional methods.[61,62]

Etiologic Diagnosis

Confirmation of pneumonia etiology may be difficult. Various approaches have been used to try to address this issue. Diagnostic methods for etiologic identification can be divided into microbiologic, immunologic, and molecular methods of detection (see Chapter 22). The gold standard for etiologic diagnosis in CAP is either by collecting direct lung specimens or by performing a bronchoalveolar lavage (BAL), but these methods are unacceptable for routine clinical purposes. BAL in children is helpful in nonresponding patients with severe infections, and for nosocomial or life-threatening infections. Blood cultures are positive in less than 10% of the samples and should be considered only in hospitalized children or those with complicated pneumonia. Repeating blood cultures to document resolution of bacteremia is not recommended for patients who are clinically improving, except for those with *S. aureus* pneumonia.[27,45]

A sputum examination is a viable alternative for respiratory sampling. It is practical for adolescents and school-aged children and can be induced in young children, but it should be interpreted with caution because upper airway commensals, which can be pathogenic in the lower airways, are usually contaminants. Bacterial cultures of the throat or nasopharynx do not correlate well with lung parenchyma and are more likely to confound than to help, with the known exception of the high correlation between upper and lower airway cultures in sick patients with cystic fibrosis.[27]

Pleural fluid cultures may grow potential pathogens, but the usual practice of empiric antibiotic use in the early phases of pneumonia decreases the sensitivity of this method. However, pleural fluid should be cultured whenever technically accessible, unless the effusion is too small or when clinical recovery is uneventful.[27]

ANTIGEN AND SEROLOGIC TESTS

Detection of bacterial antigens in urine or plasma has been used, but results are conflicting, and sensitivity and specificity are low. In children, pneumococcal urinary antigen has a high sensitivity, but a positive test is frequently due to nasal carriage.[27,45]

For respiratory viruses, tests based on antigen detection are more often available and, in general, have greater specificity than sensitivity. Rapid immunoassay tests for influenza and RSV have a sensitivity of 66% and 80% and a specificity of 98% and 97%, respectively.[63,64] Despite specificity values greater than 94% for viruses overall, direct immunofluorescence assays do not reach sensitivity levels above 75% for most viruses, with the exception of RSV, which is around 90%.[65,66]

Serology is useful for some agents such as *M. pneumoniae*, *C. pneumoniae*, and *S. pneumoniae*; paired acute and convalescent titers are the gold standard, with the caveat of the diagnosis having only retrospective value in most situations.[67] For *M. pneumoniae*, detection of immunoglobulin (Ig)M antibodies in acute disease is usually less than 80%.[68,69]

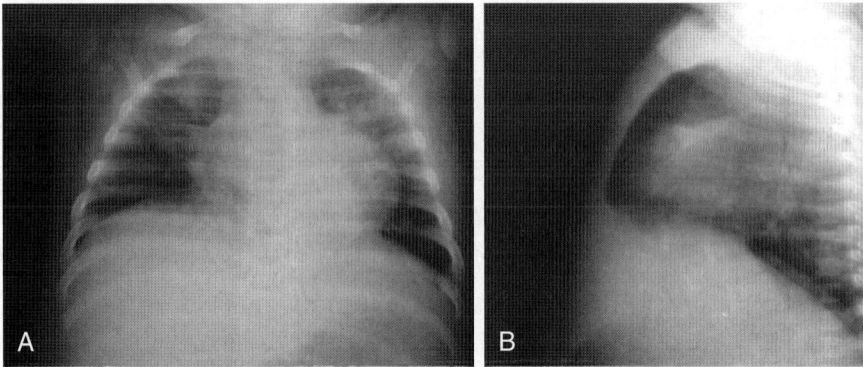

Fig. 25.2 Viral pneumonia in a 6-month-old infant with respiratory-syncytial-virus–positive nasopharyngeal aspirate. (A) Anteroposterior radiograph with bilateral interstitial infiltrates and patchy atelectasis. (B) Lateral radiograph with hyperinflated lungs; increased anteroposterior diameter, flattening of the diaphragm, and mediastinal air cushion.

POLYMERASE CHAIN REACTION

Respiratory secretions, pleural effusion, lung aspirate samples, or blood, are sources for specimen testing. Molecular biology techniques have uniformly high sensitivity and specificity in diagnosing viral infections, apart from agents whose pathogenicity is still not well established, such as human bocavirus (which remains polymerase chain reaction [PCR] positive for months after acute infection).[45,70] PCR is a good diagnostic tool in research and can be used by clinicians in special situations, but it does not differentiate carrier state from disease. Quantitative PCR may solve these problems if cut-off levels for disease and carrier state can be adequately defined.

Diagnosis and Differential Diagnosis

Pneumonia should be suspected in children with fever, cough, tachypnea, lower chest indrawing, or crackles on chest auscultation. However, no single clinical feature has sufficient accuracy to diagnose pneumonia. Abdominal pain or nausea, when associated with fever, can present as the sole clinical finding in pneumonia affecting the lower pulmonary lobes.[45,71]

The differential diagnosis of CAP includes viral bronchiolitis, asthma, cardiogenic causes of tachypnea, interstitial lung diseases, and chemical pneumonitis, especially those secondary to aspiration syndromes. Infants and small children presenting with fever and respiratory signs are frequently sent for a chest radiograph and often receive antimicrobial treatment for a presumptive diagnosis of bacterial pneumonia. Importantly, a chest x-ray cannot reliably differentiate between viral and bacterial etiologies, which may coexist.[72] Radiologic signs of bilateral interstitial lung infiltrates or atelectasis, signs of bronchitis (true wheeze on auscultation), and generalized hyperinflation, though not definitive markers, are very likely to indicate viral pneumonia (Fig. 25.2).

Although "atypical" pneumonia is often described with several different presentations, in clinical practice neither signs nor symptoms alone, or with radiologic findings have sufficient accuracy to differentiate *M. pneumoniae* infections from other agents.[68,73] Tuberculosis should always be considered as a possible diagnosis, especially among children living in, or in families that have recently moved from, endemic

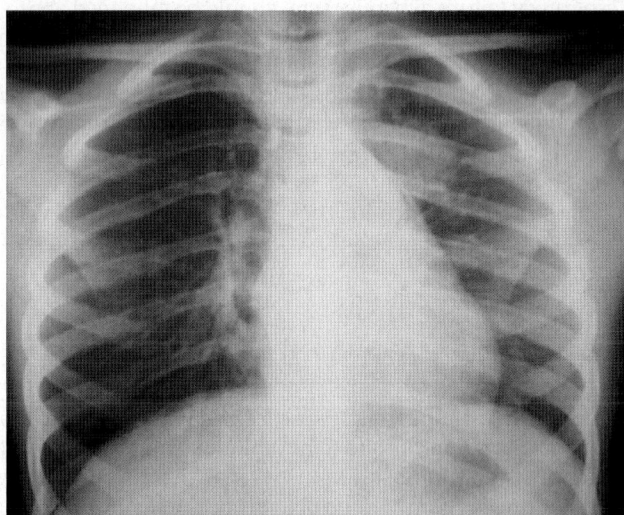

Fig. 25.3 Round pneumonia. Opacity in the left upper segment, partially concealed by the mediastinal shadow.

areas. Nonresolving pneumonia with persistence or recurrent radiologic findings should alert the physician to possible noninfectious primary causes or infection with bacterial agents, such as *M. tuberculosis*.[74] Another important differential diagnosis is that of round pneumonia, since these and infected congenital malformations or thoracic masses may have similar radiologic presentations (Fig. 25.3).

General Management

Infants and children with CAP without danger signs can be safely cared for at home. In this situation, the child usually should be reexamined within 48 hours after beginning treatment. According to the most current guidelines, for infants aged less than 2 months, SaO_2 of 90%–92% or less, cyanosis, a respiratory rate greater than 70 breaths per minute, difficulty breathing, intermittent apnea, grunting, an inability to feed, failure after oral therapy, severe malnutrition, or a family incapable of providing appropriate care, are all indications for hospital admission.[2,27,45,75,76] In older children, the indicators are a SaO_2 of 92% or less, cyanosis, respiratory rate greater than 50 breaths per minute, grunting, difficulty breathing, signs of dehydration, or a family incapable of providing appropriate observation or supervision.[45]

General management for hospitalized children includes oxygen delivery through a mask or nasal cannula to keep oxygen saturation above 92%, antipyretics, and IV fluids if the child is unable to drink. Fluid intake should be carefully monitored because pneumonia can be complicated by hyponatremia secondary to the syndrome of inappropriate antidiuretic hormone secretion. The benefit of nasogastric tube feeding should be weighed against its potential for respiratory distress due to the obstruction of a nostril, or by inducing gastroesophageal reflux.

Supplemental oxygen should be given when oxygen saturation is 92% or lower.[45,76] In most mild cases, this can easily be administered via a nasal cannula, a head box, or a facemask.

No randomized, controlled trials have addressed the use of noninvasive ventilation for children with pneumonia. Respiratory failure, when present, should be managed appropriately and noninvasive ventilation may be used to avoid tracheal intubation. Children should be admitted to an intensive care facility with continuous cardiorespiratory monitoring capabilities when invasive ventilation is required, or pulse oximetry measurements are below 92% with the child on inspired oxygen concentrations of 50% or more.[27,45]

There is no evidence for the usefulness of chest physiotherapy in the management of CAP; therefore it is not currently indicated.[45,77]

Treatment With Antimicrobials

Since viruses are the main cause for many cases of CAP in childhood, it is appropriate to be cautious and not overtreat these rather common situations with antibiotics. However, therapeutic decisions can be difficult because most tests do not adequately differentiate viral from bacterial infection in an individual child. An additional issue is the fact that many patients harbor mixed viral and bacterial agents.[46]

The problem of bacterial resistance to antibiotics has increased steadily in the last few years, so antibiotics should be used judiciously and narrow-spectrum agents used whenever appropriate. Prior antibiotic therapy, daycare attendance, travel, and coexisting morbidities are risk factors for resistance. It is also important to keep in mind that, in an era of effective vaccines against Hib and *S. pneumoniae*, previous antibiotic regimens may have to be reevaluated.[78]

Antibiotics should be started whenever bacterial pneumonia is the most probable diagnosis.[79] Since a definitive etiologic diagnosis is more the exception than the rule, usually antibiotics are started on an empirical basis. The local prevalence of CAP-causing agents should be considered.

Several randomized studies assessing different antibiotics for pneumonia have shown that children under 5 years with tachypnea or indrawing of the lower chest without danger signs can be safely treated with oral amoxicillin.[79,80] Cotrimoxazole is no longer recommended, since it is less effective than amoxicillin. Furthermore, higher doses of amoxicillin, that is, 80–90 mg/kg per day in two doses, are more effective than a lower dose and are now recommended.[2,79]

Some studies have recently reviewed the issue of treatment duration. A multicenter study from Pakistan, which enrolled 2188 children between the ages of 2 and 59 months, showed the equivalence of a 3-day or 5-day course of amoxicillin in the treatment of nonsevere pneumonia, as diagnosed by the WHO criteria. Of note were a low prevalence of positive radiographic findings (14%) and a relatively high rate (20%) of treatment failure, which suggests that there may have been a high proportion of viral pneumonia.[81]

For severe pneumonia or very severe pneumonia, according to the WHO classification, there is no evidence supporting a shortened course, and patients should be treated with IV antibiotics.[2,82] Interestingly, although not yet universally adopted as the standard of care, there is growing evidence from both adult and pediatric studies that the use of procalcitonin as a biomarker for bacterial infection allows for the reduction of antibiotic duration, without any increase in adverse outcomes in bacterial pneumonia.[83,84]

CHOICE OF ANTIBIOTICS

The choice of antibiotics is based on clinical features, prevalence data for different organisms in different age groups, and regional variations in pathogens. All current guidelines recommend oral amoxicillin as the first choice, and penicillin or ampicillin if IV treatment is required.[2,27,45,75,76]

Penicillins (either intramuscular [IM], IV, or orally) can be used for most pneumococcal pneumonias, unless highly resistant strains are identified. The prevalence of penicillin resistance also varies widely throughout different countries and continents.[85,86] The degree of penicillin resistance does not appear to cause adverse outcomes for hospitalized patients with a diagnosis of pneumococcal CAP, since high parenteral penicillin serum concentrations are obtained with usual dosage regimens, which are much higher than the observed levels of resistance for these bacteria.[87] Hospitalized patients with pneumococcal pneumonia caused by strains with minimum inhibitory concentration (MIC) up to 2 µg/mL respond well to adequate doses of β-lactam antibiotics (e.g., 200,000–250,000 U/kg per day of penicillin). Susceptibility breakpoints have been revised due to the cumulative evidence of clinical improvement even with conventional doses of penicillin for strains that were previously considered intermediately resistant. Consequently, current breakpoints of resistant *S. pneumoniae* for parenteral penicillin in the case of nonmeningeal infections are ≤2 µg/mL (susceptible), 4 µg/mL (intermediate), and ≥8 µg/mL (resistant). However, for oral penicillin, the previous breakpoints are still valid, due to lower serum levels achieved with enteral presentations.[27,87] High doses of oral penicillin, ampicillin, and amoxicillin have been recommended whenever intermediately susceptible pneumococcus strains are considered. As mentioned above, the WHO recommends oral amoxicillin in higher doses twice daily as the first-line treatment for pneumonia.

Vancomycin or teicoplanin should be reserved for severely ill patients, when coverage for highly resistant pneumococcus is desired, because overuse may lead to increased resistance from other pathogens. Antibiotic resistance is usually associated with changes in the penicillin-binding sites of the transpeptidases of the bacteria, and it may be associated with cross-resistance to other β-lactams and carbapenems. Worldwide, most resistant pneumococcus strains were from serogroups 23F, 6A, 6B, 9V, 19A, 19F, and 14; five of these

Table 25.2   Choice of Antibiotic Treatment for Community-Acquired Pneumonia When Typical Bacteria Are Identified

Pathogen	First Choice	Other
Streptococcus pneumoniae, penicillin susceptible or intermediate	Penicillin, ampicillin, or high-dose amoxicillin	Cefuroxime, ceftriaxone, azithromycin
S. pneumoniae, penicillin resistant (MIC ≥ 4 µg/mL)	Second- or third-generation cephalosporins for sensitive strains; vancomycin	
Staphylococcus aureus	Methicillin/oxacillin	Vancomycin or teicoplanin (for MRSA)
Haemophilus influenzae	Amoxicillin	Amoxicillin/clavulanate, cefuroxime, ceftriaxone, other second- and third-generation cephalosporins
Moraxella catarrhalis	Amoxicillin/clavulanate	Cefuroxime

MIC, Minimum inhibitory concentration; *MRSA,* methicillin-resistant *S. aureus.*

are covered by the heptavalent PCV7, and all are included in the PCV13.[88]

Resistance to macrolides is associated with the alteration of the 50S ribosomal binding site, preventing the drug from inhibiting protein synthesis, or the presence of efflux pumps to macrolides. Overall macrolide resistance is around 30%.[89]

When a causative agent is known, narrow-spectrum antibiotics are preferred. Table 25.2 shows appropriate antibiotic choices, based on bacteriologic tests and MICs.

In real-life situations, causative agents are rarely identified, and the choice of antibiotics is based on models that include both the age of the child and the clinical presentation.

Neonates with CAP can be treated with a combination, such as IV ampicillin and gentamicin. Methicillin/oxacillin may be the best choice if the clinical picture is suggestive of *S. aureus* infection. For symptomatic children between 3 weeks and 3 months of age with interstitial infiltrates visible on chest radiograph, if a viral etiology is not the most likely diagnosis, a macrolide should be used to cover for agents such as *C. trachomatis, B. pertussis,* and *U. urealyticum.* Children between 4 months and 5 years of age with CAP are most likely infected by pneumococcus, viral agents, or both, and amoxicillin, penicillin, or ampicillin are the drugs of choice (see Tables 25.1 and 25.2). Some experts suggest macrolides (e.g., azithromycin, clarithromycin, or erythromycin) as optional choices because they cover both typical and atypical bacteria. Of note, azithromycin has a distinct pharmacokinetic profile and it does not reach high serum levels, which is a potential disadvantage in the treatment of bacterial pneumonia.[90] Pneumococci have become increasingly macrolide resistant, indicating that macrolides should be reserved as second-line treatment or for situations in which atypical infections are either probable or confirmed by laboratory tests.[89]

Infants and young children with CAP can receive ampicillin, amoxicillin, penicillin, or even a third-generation cephalosporin orally, unless there is vomiting, or when the patient is so sick that hospitalization and parenteral antibiotics are needed. In a recent Cochrane review, three controlled trials comparing oral with parenteral antibiotics in severe pneumonia, according to the WHO criteria, were evaluated and there were no differences in outcomes between oral and parenteral antibiotics.[91] Since children with serious signs and symptoms (e.g., inability to drink, cyanosis, and convulsions) were not included, no definitive conclusions can be drawn from the review for this specific group of patients.[91] In regions of the world where Hib immunization is not available, clinicians should consider amoxicillin/clavulanate, cefprozil, cefdinir, cefpodoxime proxetil, cefuroxime, or ceftriaxone as drugs

of choice. The addition of a β-lactamase inhibitor does not confer additional coverage for pneumococcus because this is not its resistance-associated mechanism.

Whenever there is a positive culture or a clinical picture suggestive of *S. aureus,* specific antibiotic coverage against this pathogen should be added (e.g., methicillin, oxacillin, clindamycin, or vancomycin in the case of MRSA strains).

The diagnosis of CA-MRSA should be considered in cases presenting with necrotizing pneumonia. Atypical bacteria causing CAP are not common in infancy and early childhood, and should be considered only in deteriorating cases. Recent data on the use of ceftaroline (a fifth-generation cephalosporin with anti-MRSA activity) in children suggest that it is effective against CA-MRSA pneumonia. Nonetheless, specific epidemiologic or treatment data on MRSA pneumonia in children are still very scarce.[92] If the clinical and radiologic findings suggest the possibility of an atypical agent, then a macrolide is the first choice, and a β-lactam should be added in cases of poor response.[27]

Both cefuroxime and cefixime should be considered as good options whenever cost is not a main issue. If atypical pneumonia is suspected, a macrolide or azalide (e.g., azithromycin) should be used for 5–7 days. The role of azithromycin, clarithromycin, and erythromycin is limited to extending the antimicrobial spectrum to atypical organisms, because these agents are relatively inactive against *H. influenzae,* and there is increasing resistance among *S. pneumoniae.* Thus, such choices should be tailored to treat organisms that do not respond to first-line therapy.[93] Pneumonia in HIV-infected children may present with a broader spectrum of pathogens, requiring a specific pattern of antibiotic cover (see Chapter 66).

Table 25.3 and Box 25.1 summarize these recommendations, including suggested drug regimens.

Slowly Resolving Pneumonia

This term refers to the persistence of either clinical or radiologic findings of pneumonia beyond the normal time course during which one would expect the infection to resolve (i.e., between 48 and 96 hours after empiric "adequate" antimicrobial treatment). However, radiologic resolution may take several weeks. Radiologic abnormalities are found 3–7 weeks after initial episode in a substantial proportion of patients.[94] One example of slowly resolving pneumonia is when patients fail to respond to conventional treatment, and another is when clinical symptoms or radiologic signs persist, even in the presence of clinical improvement. During this period, it

Box 25.1 Suggested Antibiotic Dosages for the Treatment of Community-Acquired Pneumonia

Penicillin 200,000 U/kg per day IV q4h or q6h (if resistant strains are to be covered, up to 400,000 U/kg per day, for 7–10 days)

Ampicillin 50 mg/kg per day PO q6h, for 7–10 days and 100–200 mg/kg per day IV q6h for 7–10 days

Amoxicillin 80–90 mg/kg per day PO q12h, for 5 days (if resistant strains are to be covered, dose can be increased up to 100 mg/kg per day)

Amoxicillin/clavulanate 40 mg/kg per day PO of amoxicillin for 5 days

Oxacillin/nafcillin 150 mg/kg per day IV q6h, maximum 12 g/day, for 14–21 days

Cefuroxime 30 mg/kg per day PO q12h, for 5–7 days and 150 mg/kg per day IV q8h, for 7–10 days

Ceftriaxone 50–75 mg/kg per day IM/IV qd, for 7–10 days

Cefotaxime 200 mg/kg per day IV q8h, for 7–10 days

Cefprozil 15–30 mg/kg per day PO q12h, maximum 1 g/day, for 7–10 days

Cefdinir 14 mg/kg per day PO q12h, for 7–10 days

Cefpodoxime proxetil 10 mg/kg per day PO q12h, maximum 400 mg/day, for 7–10 days

Azithromycin 10 mg/kg per day PO qd, for 3–5 days

Clarithromycin 15 mg/kg per day PO q12h, maximum 1 g/day, for 5–7 days

Erythromycin 40 mg/kg per day PO q6h, for 5–7 days

Vancomycin 40–60 mg/kg per day IV q6h, for 7–10 days (14–21 days for *Staphylococcus aureus*)

Gentamicin 7.5 mg/kg per day IM/IV q8h, for 7–10 days

is not recommended that antimicrobials be changed unless there is clear evidence that other microorganisms, not covered by the initial empiric choice of therapy, are involved (e.g., *S. aureus* with developing pleural effusion or in the presence of pneumatoceles, when initial therapy was amoxicillin). The presence of empyema or an underlying lung abscess should be considered whenever there is persistence of fever with or without pleuritic pain (basal segment pneumonias may mimic acute abdominal pain). These situations often require additional interventions, rather than a change in antibiotic regimen (Fig. 25.4).

Factors such as an inappropriate choice of drugs, unexpectedly resistant microorganisms, inadequate dosage, complications, or poor compliance of oral therapy can result in slowly resolving CAP and should always be considered. Antibiotic failure may be the case in either slow or unresponsive pneumonia. The inappropriate choice of antibiotics may be an issue; for example, when there is inadequate coverage for atypical organisms. In endemic areas, tuberculosis should always be considered because its radiologic appearance may mimic bacterial pneumonia.

Inadequate host defenses or other coexisting diseases (e.g., ciliary dyskinesia, cystic fibrosis, HIV, or noninfectious causes) may also be associated with slowly responding or nonresponsive pneumonia. Several differential diagnostic tests for such possible comorbidities may be considered, including bronchoscopy with BAL, chest CT scan, or lung biopsy. Blood, pleural, and sputum cultures, as well as PCR, should be considered for the diagnosis of possible atypical microorganisms.

Table 25.3 Choice of Antibiotic Treatment for Community-Acquired Pneumonia According to Age and Clinical Picture

Age/Clinical Picture	Inpatient	Outpatient
Newborn	Ampicillin + gentamicin	—
1 month to 5 years	Penicillin or ampicillin[a]	Amoxicillin[a]
5 years and older: alveolar infiltrate, pleural effusion, toxic appearance	Penicillin or ampicillin; add macrolide if not responding	—
5 years and older: interstitial infiltrate	Macrolides; consider adding a β-lactam if not responding	Macrolide
Necrotizing pneumonia	Oxacillin/nafcillin; vancomycin. Consider adding third-generation cephalosporin	

[a]Macrolides if atypical pneumonia suspected.

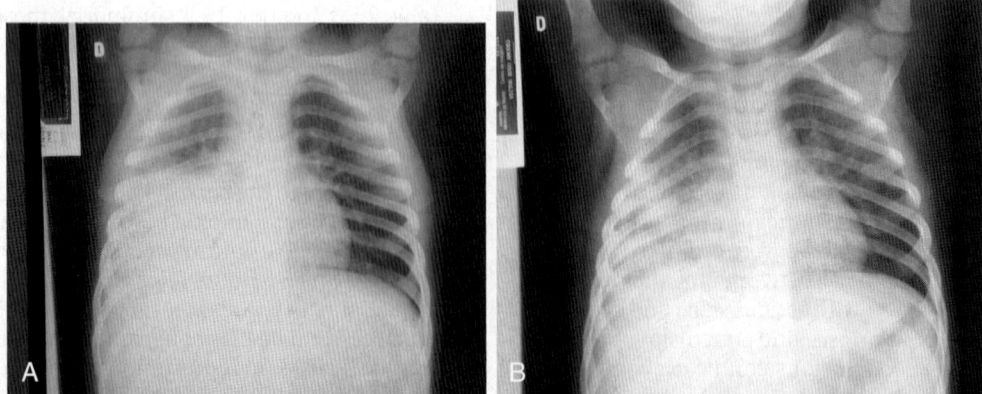

Fig. 25.4 Slowly resolving pneumonia. (A) A 3-year-old child with presumptive diagnosis of pneumococcal pneumonia. Lower and middle lobe consolidation is shown; treatment started with intravenous benzyl penicillin. This evolved into a pleural effusion, which later necessitated a thoracotomy. (B) The same child 3 weeks after the first diagnosis; the child was in a good clinical condition on discharge. Aeration of previously consolidated areas.

Other conditions, such as persistent alveolar collapse or atelectasis, may be secondary to obstruction of the bronchial lumen, from either foreign body aspiration or lymph node enlargement. Congenital malformations, such as pulmonary sequestration, bronchogenic cysts, or other mediastinal masses, also may be causes for delayed radiologic improvement, especially if the appearance resembles round pneumonia. It is important to ensure adequate follow-up of all children with CAP who do not have a typical course with full resolution of their symptoms and signs.[27,45,95]

Major Clinical Complications

NECROTIZING PNEUMONIA

Necrotizing pneumonia is characterized by necrosis and liquefaction of consolidated lung tissue, which may be complicated by solitary, multiple, or multiloculated radiolucent foci, bronchopleural fistulas, and intrapulmonary abscesses. Most cases are confined to a single lobe, but sometimes there is multilobar involvement. Pneumatoceles are commonly associated with and develop after localized bronchiolar and alveolar necrosis, which allows for the one-way passage of air into the peripheral airways and alveoli. Necrotizing pneumonia is usually secondary to pneumococcus, S. aureus, or, less commonly, Pseudomonas aeruginosa infections. CA-MRSA is often associated with this clinical presentation, since there is production of Panton-Valentine leukocidin, an exotoxin that causes tissue necrosis. In Europe, methicillin-sensitive S. aureus (MSSA), producing this same exotoxin, has been associated with necrotizing pneumonia.[25,96,97]

PLEURAL EFFUSION AND EMPYEMA

Pleural effusion occurs when an inflammatory response to pneumonia causes an increase in permeability of the pleura with an accumulation of fluid in the pleural space. There is increased capillary permeability after parenchymal lung injury, favoring the migration of inflammatory cells (neutrophils, lymphocytes, and eosinophils) into the pleural space. When bacteria enter the pleural space, pus appears, characterizing empyema. Empyema may also be secondary to bronchiectasis and lung abscess.[98,99]

Either the child presents with typical, but usually more severe, signs of pneumonia or, after a few days of usual pneumonia symptoms, children deteriorate clinically, with persistent fever or respiratory distress. Pleuritic pain is common. In cases where infection is in the lower lobes, abdominal pain is often present. On physical examination, there is reduced air entry and dullness to percussion over the affected area.[98] Radiographic findings may progress to complete hemithorax opacification with mediastinal contralateral deviation (Fig. 25.5). Unlike adults, where mortality rates around 40% are expected, the typical clinical outcome of children is good with full recovery. Bronchopleural fistula, lung abscess, and perforation through the chest wall (empyema necessitatis) are uncommon complications in children.[60]

After the introduction of PCV7, a rise in empyema incidence was reported in some settings.[100–103] However, a reduction after PCV13 introduction was detected, probably due

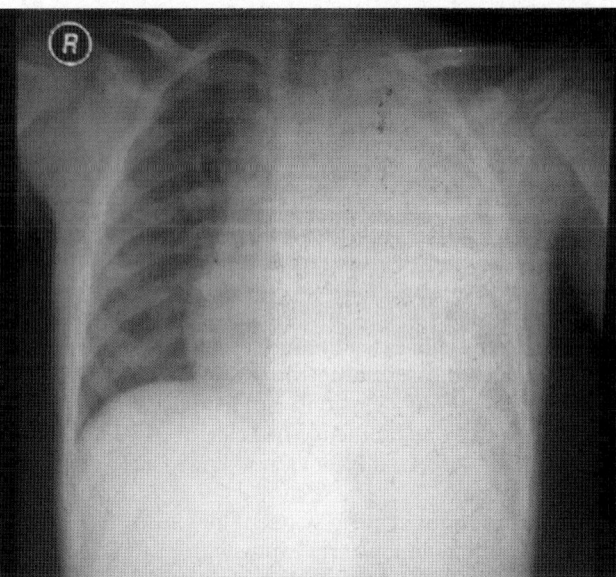

Fig. 25.5 Empyema with complete hemithorax opacity and mediastinal deviation to the contralateral side.

to better coverage of serotypes related to complications, such as serotype 1.[14,104,105]

Blood culture is recommended to identify the causative organism, but positive cultures in patients with empyema occur only in 10%–22% in most series. Acute phase reactants are not helpful in detecting parapneumonic effusions or differentiating them from empyema. Other biochemical tests from the pleural fluid are usually inadequate to identify the causal agent or to differentiate empyema from an uncomplicated parapneumonic effusion.[60,98]

Chest radiographs should always be obtained when there are signs indicating an inadequate clinical course. Obliteration of the costophrenic angle and a rim of fluid may be seen ascending the lateral chest wall (meniscus sign) on posterior-anterior or anterior-posterior radiographs. If the film is taken when a child is supine, the appearance can be of a homogeneous increase in opacity over the whole lung field. A complete whiteout of a hemithorax may be seen with a large pleural effusion. Another radiographic finding of empyema is that of scoliosis, concave to the side of the collection, reflecting that the child may be choosing a protective position to avoid pain.

Loculation, defined as fluid not moving freely due to pleural fibrinous adhesions, can be diagnosed by evaluating the chest dynamically (i.e., in different positions) by means of plain radiographic films or by US. Statically, loculation can probably be inferred when a collection adopts a lenticular shape with internal convexity, while a freely moving collection should form an internally concave meniscus paralleling the chest wall.[99] Although chest radiographs are helpful in diagnosing pleural effusions, they are not useful for clinical follow-up because full radiologic recovery may be slow, and findings may not be clinically significant. Chest radiographs will normalize in two-thirds of the children 3 months after the acute event; 90% should have normal radiographs by 6 months, and all should be normal by 18 months.[106]

US is very useful to differentiate between solid and liquid content in the chest, and to mark the best spot for tube insertion in the case of empyema. It is particularly valuable in the case of whiteout of a lung, where atelectasis, consolidation, and effusion should be differentiated. Either US or CT scans are advocated to identify fibrin deposition, but fibrinous septations are better visualized using US. US can estimate the size of the effusion, can differentiate free from loculated pleural fluid, and can determine the echogenicity of the fluid. It can be used to guide chest drain insertion or thoracentesis with the radiologist or radiographer marking the optimum site for drainage on the skin. In most cases, plain radiographs or US can distinguish an abscess from a septated pleural effusion, although sometimes a CT is needed. US is considered essential in the management of children with parapneumonic effusions. Guidelines from the British Thoracic Society recommend the referral of such patients if the health care facility does not have these diagnostic options available.[60]

Pleural fluid should always be sent for Gram stain, microbiological testing, and, wherever possible, for PCR diagnosis. Culture and PCR (Xpert) for *M. tuberculosis* should also be done in tuberculosis (TB) endemic areas. A cell count should be considered, and when lymphocytosis is prominent, tuberculosis or malignancies are more likely. In parapneumonic effusions, one should expect a predominance of neutrophils. Low glucose, low pH, and high lactate dehydrogenase (LDH) in adults have long been used to predict empyema development, but in children their role to guide management remains undetermined. Although it is probable that biochemical characteristics from parapneumonic effusions in children are not that different from those in adults, such tests do not change the management nor the outcome.[27,60]

All children with parapneumonic effusion and empyema should be admitted to a hospital. Children who need drainage of the effusion should preferably be managed at a tertiary center under the supervision of a specialist. Different outcomes have been used to compare the efficacy of different treatment strategies (e.g., length of hospitalization, radiologic resolution, or pulmonary function tests) because mortality rates are very low. Smaller effusions less than 10 mm thick can usually be managed with antibiotics alone, and these should especially cover *S. pneumoniae*; *S. aureus* should be considered when pneumatoceles are present and the child is toxic. Although not based on specific randomized trials, a panel of experts from the British Thoracic Society recommends one of the following: cefuroxime, co-amixiclav, penicillin plus flucloxacillin, amoxicillin plus flucloxacillin or clidamycin when effusion follows CAP. Broader coverage should be the choice in cases of hospital-acquired pneumonia and following surgery, trauma, or aspiration. The same panel recommends continuation of antibiotics for 1–4 weeks after discharge or even longer when there is residual disease.[60]

Antibiotics alone should not be the main strategy for managing effusions that are enlarging, or those that are big enough to cause respiratory distress. Therapeutic options besides antibiotics are thoracentesis, chest drain insertion with or without the instillation of fibrinolytic agents, and surgical techniques, such as video-assisted thoracoscopic surgery (VATS), minithoracotomy, and standard thoracotomy with decortication. Few studies have compared repeated thoracentesis versus catheter drainage. In prospective, uncontrolled studies, where chest drain alone (i.e., without further surgical intervention) was used, the length of hospital stays varied between 14 and 24 days, and all children fully recovered.[107]

After chest tube placement, a chest radiograph should be obtained to check the tube position and to ensure there is no pneumothorax. Even though drainage with tube thoracotomy and antibiotics may be all that is needed for the exudative stage, the presence of loculation and fibrinous adhesions may limit the success of this therapy. The objectives of treatment of stage 2 empyema (fibrinopurulent), apart from antibiotics, are fluid removal and debridement of the fibrinous layer of the pleura to allow the lung to expand. In these situations, fibrinolytic drugs are used to lyse the fibrinous strands in loculated empyemas, thereby clearing lymphatic pores, which restores pleural fluid circulation. Different fibrinolytics (e.g., streptokinase, urokinase, and alteplase) have been studied in randomized, clinical trials comparing them to saline or to VATS, and the results were variable. The success rate of fibrinolytics is 80%–90% in case series, with pain being the major side effect. Bleeding diathesis and pneumothorax are contraindications to fibrinolytics. Other possible side effects are fever and, less commonly, bleeding and allergic reactions.[60,107]

The American Pediatric Surgical Association recommends fibrinolytics as the first choice of treatment for empyema that requires drainage, particularly when it is associated with loculations, since fibrinolytic therapy can shorten the duration of treatment and length of hospital stay. On the other hand, systematic reviews have not shown outcome differences when comparing fibrinolytics to VATS. There was no evidence of a clinically significant difference in the length of stay between VATS and chest drain with fibrinolytics, except in one of the trials; insertion of a small-bore chest drain used with fibrinolytics was associated with lower hospital costs.[108–112] It should be emphasized that children virtually always recover irrespective of the treatment they receive, and that the long-term outcome is not affected.[98,107]

While sequelae occur in many adults, full recovery is the rule in children, although a temporary restrictive pattern can be seen in pulmonary function tests soon after hospital discharge.[27,60]

LUNG ABSCESS

Another possible complication of pneumonia is a lung abscess. A pulmonary abscess is a thick-walled cavity that contains purulent liquid. The pathogenesis of a lung abscess begins with inflammation of the parenchyma, which progresses to necrosis, cavitation, and abscess formation. The abscess may be secondary to predisposing conditions (e.g., pulmonary aspiration), especially in children with neurodevelopmental delay, congenital malformations, immunodeficiency, or endocarditis. In the case of pulmonary aspiration, this may be associated with either large or frequently aspirated small volumes. Usually, the most dependent segments of the lung, especially the upper lobes and the apical segments of the lower lobes, are affected. Primary abscesses are associated with a pulmonary infection, especially due to gram-positive cocci (*S. pneumoniae, S. aureus, S. pyogenes*) and gram-negative bacteria (*P. aeruginosa* and *Klebsiella*). *S. pneumoniae, S. aureus, P. aeruginosa*, anaerobic bacteria, and fungi also cause secondary abscesses.[113]

The initial clinical presentation of a lung abscess is like that of uncomplicated CAP, with fever and cough as the key features. Other common signs are dyspnea, chest pain, anorexia, nausea, vomiting, malaise, and lethargy. A main difference from usual CAP is that it progresses indolently. A typical patient may show tachypnea, dullness to percussion, locally reduced air entry, and localized inspiratory crackles. Plain chest radiography usually confirms the diagnosis. A cavity with thick walls and an air-fluid level is the characteristic finding, although the initial presentation may not be significantly different from a simple consolidation. US is very useful in defining a lung abscess and to differentiate an abscess from a loculated empyema. A contrast-enhanced CT scan is usually considered the investigation of choice, being able to better define a thick wall cavity filled with fluid. It helps to differentiate an abscess from empyema, necrotizing pneumonia, sequestration, pneumatocele, and underlying congenital abnormalities, such as a bronchogenic cyst. It is the usual preferred test to guide an invasive drainage procedure.[113]

The mainstay of treatment is the use of a parenteral antibiotic. There is no controlled trial addressing the duration of antimicrobial therapy, which is usually recommended for 4–6 weeks. Ampicillin-sulbactam or a cephalosporin with clindamycin (if CA-MRSA is suspected) are the usual choices to cover the most prevalent pathogens. If an MRSA strain resistant to clindamycin is a possibility, vancomycin should be used.[27,114] In most cases, this will be the only treatment, but interventional radiology-driven drainage or surgery can be considered. The routine use of CT-guided aspiration for abscesses, and the more recent use of CT-guided pigtail drainage catheters at the time of presentation, has been associated with a decrease in the length of hospital stay. Surgery is the last resource after medical therapy has failed.

In a secondary abscess, the outcomes are more closely related to the predisposing factors. In the case of a primary abscess, the prognosis is usually good, no matter the choice of treatment. Complications of lung abscess are empyema, pyothorax, pneumothorax, and, occasionally, bronchopleural fistula.[113,115]

Prevention

As mentioned earlier, viruses are the most common etiology of childhood pneumonia in populations with high PCV and Hib vaccination coverage.[7] Since respiratory viruses are ubiquitous, complete prevention is difficult. Hygiene measures, such as hand washing and respiratory etiquette, are universally helpful. In health care settings, cohorting and contact isolation, together with droplet precautions, are additional measures that help reduce transmission.[116]

For influenza prevention, annual vaccination with inactivated vaccine is recommended in all children older than 6 months, especially in high-risk groups. Children at an elevated risk of influenza complications include those aged younger than 2 years, those on long-term aspirin therapy, and those with comorbidities (pulmonary, cardiovascular, hematologic, metabolic, neuromuscular, and immunosuppression). Children younger than 8 years should receive two doses at the first year of immunization and one dose per year thereafter. Children aged 9 years or older are considered immunized with a single dose even if receiving influenza vaccination

for the first time. An inactivated influenza vaccine has been shown to be more effective than live attenuated vaccines. Antivirals also may be used as chemoprophylaxis under specific situations.[117] For RSV, prophylaxis with a specific monoclonal antibody (palivizumab, IM) is effective in infants at high risk of RSV disease.[118] Several potential vaccines against RSV are under development, although none is approved for clinical use.[119] Live attenuated measles-mumps-rubella and varicella vaccines are recommended to prevent complications, including pneumonitis, especially associated with measles and varicella.[120,121]

S. pneumoniae and Hib conjugate vaccines have recently become widely available; however, many children are still not vaccinated globally, especially in low- and middle-income countries. Several studies evaluated the impact of Hib immunization in the prevention of childhood pneumonia, showing reductions of up to 44% in radiology-confirmed cases and up to 100% of bacteremic cases.[20]

Many studies have also reported reductions in clinical and radiological pneumonia, hospitalizations, and mortality due to pneumococcal disease in low- and middle-income and affluent countries following the introduction of PCV, mostly 10- and 13-valent vaccines.[19,122–129] In settings where immunization with the PCV7 was first implemented and switched to the PCV13, further declines in incidence and hospitalization, as well as decreases in complications with empyema, have been observed.[12,13,130–132] The incidence of penicillin-resistant strains of *S. pneumoniae* due to the 19A subtype also decreased after the introduction of PCV13. Nonetheless, replacement with a disease caused by non-PCV serotypes is still a concern.[133,134] Although rare, infection due to PCV-included serotypes can also occur and seems more common in children with comorbidities.[135]

The incidence of pertussis was reduced dramatically after the introduction of immunization. However, its reemergence in recent years has become a public health concern due to waning immunity or the lack of immunization (see Chapter 32).[136] Moreover, prevention strategies for pneumonia in low- and middle-income countries must address a series of important variables that play a role in mortality and morbidity, such as malnutrition, low birth weight, HIV infection, exposure to unprocessed solid fuel, tobacco exposure in the home, poor breastfeeding regimens, and crowding. Reductions in these risk factors may substantially reduce the incidence of pneumonia in the 21st century.[4,137,138]

Prognosis

The overall prognosis of pneumonia in most children, especially those who were previously healthy, is complete recovery. A younger age is associated with an increased risk of admission and readmission.[139,140] In high-income countries, death occurs in less than 1 per 1000 patients per year.[7] In low- and middle-income countries, overall mortality can be as high as 65 per 1000 patients per year.[141] Bacterial pneumonia, although less common than viral pneumonia, accounts for a high proportion of deaths.[4] Chronic underlying disease, as well as severe malnutrition and lack of vaccination, are associated with an increased risk of death for both viral and bacterial infections.[141–145] Viral coinfection has a prevalence around 25%–30% of hospitalized children, but it has not been associated with an increased risk of severity, including death.[146] The prognostic significance of viral-bacterial coinfection is unclear, and difficulties in detecting bacteria from the lower respiratory tract remain a challenge.[147]

A systematic review assessing the long-term outcomes of childhood pneumonia with a median follow up of 11 years described a risk of major sequela of 5.5% and 13.6% for outpatients and hospitalized children, respectively.[148] Adenovirus disease was related to an important increase in chronic morbidity (54.8%), and restrictive lung disease was the most common complication. However, a high loss of follow-up in many of the included studies may limit the applicability of these findings.[148] Recently, pneumonia, or LRTI, in the first year of life have been associated with a reduction in lung function at 1 year of age; the effect was compounded by episodes of recurrent pneumonia.[149] Further, an increased risk of wheezing in childhood following pneumonia or LRTI, especially in association with human rhinovirus C and RSV, has been described.[150–153]

References

Access the reference list online at ExpertConsult.com.

Suggested Reading

Bradley JS, Byington CL, Shah SS, et al. The management of community-acquired pneumonia in infants and children older than 3 months of age: clinical practice guidelines by the Pediatric Infectious Diseases Society and the Infectious Diseases Society of America. *Clin Infect Dis.* 2011;53(7):e25–e76.

Cannavino CR, Nemeth A, Korczowski B, et al. A randomized, prospective study of pediatric patients with community-acquired pneumonia treated with ceftaroline versus ceftriaxone. *Pediatr Infect Dis J.* 2016;35(7):752–759.

Harris M, Clark J, Coote N, et al. British Thoracic Society guidelines for the management of community acquired pneumonia in children: update 2011. *Thorax.* 2011;66(suppl 2):ii1–ii23.

Jain S, Williams DJ, Arnold SR, et al. Community-acquired pneumonia requiring hospitalization among U.S. children. *N Engl J Med.* 2015;372(9):835–845.

le Roux DM, Myer L, Nicol MP, et al. Incidence and severity of childhood pneumonia in the first year of life in a South African birth cohort: the Drakenstein Child Health Study. *Lancet Glob Health.* 2015;3(2):e95–e103.

26 *Bronchiectasis and Chronic Suppurative Lung Disease*

ANNE B. CHANG, MBBS, FRACP, MPHTM, PhD, FAAHMS, and
GREGORY J. REDDING, MD

Introduction

Worldwide, there are more people with bronchiectasis unrelated to cystic fibrosis (CF) than with CF and although regarded in affluent countries as an "orphan disease," bronchiectasis remains a major contributor to chronic respiratory morbidity in affluent[1,2] and less affluent countries.[3,4] With the increasing appreciation of bronchiectasis in adults,[5–7] the renewed interest in bronchiectasis has resulted in greater research depth, albeit[7–9] there is still proportionately little research in children. Indeed, bronchiectasis is regarded by the European Respiratory Society[10] as "one of the most neglected diseases in respiratory medicine." This chapter addresses childhood bronchiectasis, chronic suppurative lung disease (CSLD), and protracted bacterial bronchitis (PBB) unrelated to CF. Other underlying pulmonary host defense deficiencies such as ciliary dyskinesia syndromes and immunodeficiencies are covered elsewhere in this textbook.

Definitions

BRONCHIECTASIS, CHRONIC SUPPURATIVE LUNG DISEASE, PROTRACTED BACTERIAL BRONCHITIS

Bronchiectasis, CSLD, and PBB share common features but are different diagnostic entities with overlaps (Fig. 26.1).[11] Bronchiectasis is a pathologic state of the conducting airways manifested by radiographic evidence of bronchial dilation and clinically by chronic productive cough. Bronchiectasis can be focal with recurrent wet or productive cough and infectious exacerbations, or it can be diffuse, resulting in generalized airway obstruction and destruction with eventual respiratory failure. The diagnostic criteria for bronchiectasis are based on radiographic features of chest high-resolution computerized tomography (c-HRCT), although the sensitivity of adult-defined radiographic criteria has been questioned when applied to children.[12,13] Bronchiectasis may also occur in patients with interstitial lung diseases, because traction on the airways causes secondary bronchial dilation. Traction bronchiectasis in the absence of wet or productive cough will not be considered further.

CSLD describes a clinical syndrome where symptoms of chronic endobronchial suppuration exist without c-HRCT evidence of bronchiectasis. The presenting symptoms are identical to bronchiectasis, including a prolonged moist or productive cough responsive to antibiotics with or without exertional dyspnea, increased airway reactivity, and recurrent chest infections. The absence of physical signs and symptoms other than wet or productive cough do not reliably exclude either bronchiectasis or CSLD. Lung abscess and empyema (previously included as CSLD) have distinct radiological characteristics and will not be discussed further. Whether bronchiectasis and CSLD are different clinical entities or simply reflect a spectrum of airway disease remains undetermined.[12] Both are chronic suppurative airway diseases and respond to similar treatment regimens.

The sole reliance of radiographic features to distinguish between bronchiectasis and CSLD is in question for several reasons:

1. It is unknown when radiological changes consistent with bronchiectasis occur in the context of a patient with symptoms of CSLD/bronchiectasis. Adult studies have shown that bronchography (the old gold standard for diagnosis of bronchiectasis) is superior to c-HRCT scans in mild disease.[14,15] In the last decade, studies have shown that contiguous 1-mm slices of c-HRCT images identify more bronchiectasis than conventional techniques (1 mm slice every 10 to 15 mm).[16,17] Hill et al. reported that the contiguous 1-mm slices protocol demonstrated 40 extra lobes with bronchiectasis not identified on conventional HRCT in 53 adults.[16] False negative results are more likely to occur when the disease is mild and localized.[14] Thus, in the current era, tertiary centers generally use multidetector CT (MDCT) scans with HRCT reconstructions used to define airway lesions. It is likely that c-HRCT protocols (without MDCT scans) have insufficient sensitivity to detect early signs of bronchiectasis in some children with symptoms of bronchiectasis.

2. A significant number of children have clinical characteristics of bronchiectasis, but their c-HRCT do not meet the criteria for the adult-based radiological bronchiectasis criteria. c-HRCT findings of bronchiectasis were derived from adult studies,[13] but scans in adults are not necessarily equivalent to those in children. Airway and morphologic changes in the lung occur with maturation and aging.[18] One of the key signs of bronchiectasis is increased bronchoarterial ratio (diameter of the bronchial lumen divided by the diameter of its accompanying artery) of greater than 1 to 1.5. This ratio is influenced by age.[19] Thus, a lower bronchoarterial ratio should be used in children to diagnose bronchiectasis. In young children (aged <5 years), the normal bronchoarterial ratio is around 0.5[20]; and in older children (<18 years), the upper limit is less than 0.8.[13]

3. To fulfill the criteria of "irreversible dilatation," at least two scans are required. Performing more than one c-HRCT scan purely for diagnostic reasons may be impractical

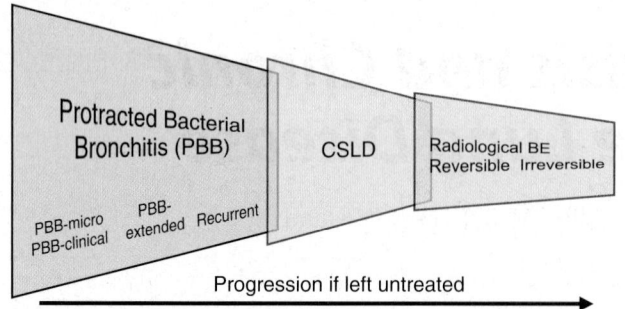

Fig. 26.1 Schema of the interrelationship between protracted bacterial bronchitis (PBB), chronic suppurative lung disease (CSLD), and bronchiectasis (BE). "Using the pathobiologic model, PBB, CSLD and radiographic-confirmed bronchiectasis likely represents different ends of a spectrum with similar underlying mechanisms of airway neutrophilia, endobronchial bacterial infection and impaired mucociliary clearance. Untreated it is likely some (but not all) children with PBB will progress to develop CSLD and some will ultimately develop bronchiectasis, initially reversible and subsequently irreversible if left to progress. There is a degree of overlap between each of the entities." (Chang AB, Upham JW, Masters IB, et al. State of the art. Protracted bacterial bronchitis: the last decade and the road ahead. *Pediatr Pulmonol*. 2016;51:225-242; Reproduced with permission from John Wiley and Sons Pediatr Pulmonol 2015; epub ahead doi: 10.1002/ppul.23351.)

and poses safety concerns regarding cancer risks from radiation in children, adolescents, and young adults.[21]

4. The timing of c-HRCT scans to diagnose bronchiectasis is important. Scans performed in different clinical states, such as during an acute pulmonary exacerbation, immediately following treatment, or when clinically stable, may yield different results. C-HRCT scans are ideally performed in a "non-acute state," but this state may differ from a posttreatment state. Bronchial dilatation resolved completely in 6 of 21 children with radiologically defined bronchiectasis when c-HRCT scans were repeated immediately following intensive medical therapy.[22]

Thus, we recommend that HRCT scans are best performed in a nonacute state and bronchiectasis be diagnosed if symptoms of CSLD are present when HRCT findings meet the pediatric[13] rather than adult radiological criteria.

PBB is a condition that is likely a prebronchiectasis state. It was first described as a diagnostic entity in 2006 with clear clinical criteria supported by laboratory studies,[23] although astute clinicians had long recognized PBB-like conditions.[11] PBB is discussed later in the chapter as a separate entity.

Bronchiectasis and Chronic Suppurative Lung Disease

EPIDEMIOLOGY, PREVALENCE, AND BURDEN OF DISEASE

Prevalence Across Time and Countries

In most affluent countries, the prevalence of childhood bronchiectasis has substantially declined since the 1940s. Field reported on 160 children with bronchiectasis over a 20-year period noting a decline in the incidence from 48 to 10 cases

per 10,000 people from the 1940s to the 1960s.[24] By 1994, an English study found that only 1% of 4000 children referred to a respiratory specialty service had bronchiectasis.[25] The reduced incidence over time has been ascribed to reduced crowding, improved immunization programs, better hygiene and nutrition, and early access to medical care. However, bronchiectasis is now increasingly recognized worldwide as an important contributor to chronic respiratory morbidity in less affluent countries[4] and both indigenous[26] and non-indigenous populations in affluent countries.[27] Indeed bronchiectasis is not rare in affluent countries,[1,5,27] but is more common among certain groups for example, the Alaskan Yupik children in the United States, Aboriginals in Australia, and Maori and Pacific Islanders in New Zealand.[26,28] Among these populations, the prevalence of childhood bronchiectasis is 147 to 200 per 10,000 children.[26] A Canadian study conservatively estimated that the prevalence of bronchiectasis among Inuit children living in Nunavut was 20 per 10,000.[29] The only available national incidence data on children is that from New Zealand with a rate of 3.7 per 100,000 under 15 year old children per year,[30] which is almost twice that of CF. In the Northern Territory (Australia with a high proportion of Indigenous people) the incidence in the first year of life is 12 per 10,000.[31]

In adults, the estimated prevalence rate has been increasing (annual change of 8.8% from 2000 to 2007) based on a 5% sample of outpatient Medicare claims in the United States.[32] In the United Kingdom (UK), the prevalence of bronchiectasis in people aged 18 to 29 years increased from 29.3 (95% confidence interval [CI] 20.4 to 41.9) per 100,000 in 2004 to 43.4 (32.3 to 58.4) per 100,000 in 2013.[2] These estimates far exceed the prevalence of CF. Given the need for a CT scan to diagnose bronchiectasis, prevalence or incidence data would be an underestimation. Furthermore, recognition of bronchiectasis is physician dependent and it is not surprising that many cases in children and adults are misdiagnosed as "difficult asthma"[33,34] or chronic obstructive pulmonary disease (COPD). A proportion of adults with COPD (29% of 110) have underlying bronchiectasis.[35] Importantly, the majority of bronchiectasis in adulthood has its roots in childhood.[36,37] One study of adults with bronchiectasis found that 80% of patients had chronic respiratory symptoms from childhood.[38]

Hospitalization rates for adults with non-CF bronchiectasis in the United States have also increased in the last two decades; from 1993 to 2006, the age-adjusted rate increased significantly with an average annual percent increase of 2.4% among men and 3.0% among women.[39] German hospital statistics for 2005–2011 have also increased over that period with an annual age-adjusted rate for bronchiectasis of 9.4 hospitalizations per 100,000 population.[40] Likewise, an Australian state (Queensland) documented an increase in hospitalization from 65 to 83 per 100,000 population between 2005 and 2009.[41]

Data from less affluent countries suggest that bronchiectasis is still associated with poor outcomes, for example, 22% with respiratory failure in a 6.6-year Tunisian follow-up study.[42] Mortality from pediatric bronchiectasis is rarely reported. Arguably, no child without a serious comorbidity should die from bronchiectasis. However, an England and Wales study reported 12 deaths in the 0 to 14 years age group between 2001 and 2007,[43] and 6 (7%) of 91 children died while attending a single New Zealand center between 1991 and 2006.[44] The premature mortality from bronchiectasis may carry over into young adulthood particularly in circumstances with nonoptimal management. This is depicted by a retrospective cohort study of 120 Central Australian Indigenous adults with bronchiectasis (50 diagnosed as children) hospitalized between 2000 and 2006 that reported 34% died during the period at a median age of 42.5 years.[45] In the UK, a recent study described that the crude mortality for men aged 18 to 49 years with bronchiectasis was 13.1 (95% CI 3.4 to 22.8) per 1000 population and 6.4 (0.8 to 12.0) for women compared to the general population, which are rates of 1.3 (1.3 to 1.4) and 0.8 (0.7 to 0.8), respectively.[2] These represent excess mortality rates of 8 to 10 times the general population.

Economic Cost

There is little data on the economic cost of bronchiectasis and none specific to children. In an United States-based case-control study involving 9146 children and adults (6.7% were aged <18 years), the direct medical cost increased by US$2319 per patient per year relative to the matched control from the preceding year.[46] The cost specifically for children was not described. An earlier study found that in the United States, adults with bronchiectasis averaged 2.0 (95% CI 1.7 to 2.3) additional days in hospital and that the average total annual medical-care expenditures (in 2001) were US$5681 ($4862 to $6593) higher for bronchiectasis patients than age, gender matched controls with other chronic diseases such as diabetes, COPD, and congestive heart failure.[47]

Other Burden of Disease

In recent years, four pediatric studies in three different continents evaluated the impact of bronchiectasis on the child's and/or parents' health-related quality of life (QoL).[3,48–50] Using the Parent Cough-Specific Quality of Life (PC-QoL)[51] and the Depression, Anxiety and Stress (DASS-21) questionnaires, a Malaysian[3] study described that children with CF had better parental mental health compared to children with non-CF CSLD. Overall, 77% of parents had abnormal DASS-21 scores (54% stressed and 51% depressed).[3] An Australian study[49] examined PC-QoL and DASS-21 scores during the stable-state and exacerbations in 69 children (median age 7 years) and their parents. In the stable state, the median PC-QoL was 6.5 (interquartile range [IQR] 5.3 to 6.9) and DASS-21 was 6 (0 to 20). Both scores were significantly worse during exacerbations (PC-QoL = 4.6 [3.8 to 5.4], $P \leq .001$ and DASS = 22 [9 to 42], $P < .001$).[49] DASS score showed that 38% had elevated anxiety and that 54% had abnormal depression/stress scores during the exacerbation. In the stable state, poorer QoL was significantly recorded with younger children, but QoL did not relate to the radiological extent, lung function, or underlying etiology.[49] In contrast, a Turkish study[48] described that the severity and frequency of symptoms were inversely related to the pulmonary function and the QoL scores (nonpediatric scales were used) in 42 children aged 9 to 18 years. Another Turkish study[50] involving 76 Caucasian children with bronchiectasis and 65 controls used self-reported questionnaires to evaluate the psychological status (using the Child Depression Inventory, State-Trait Anxiety Inventories for Children, and Pediatric Quality of Life Inventories). In this older cohort of children (mean age

11.7, SD 2.6 years), depression and trait anxiety scores were not elevated in those with bronchiectasis, but the child-rated physical health QoL scores were significantly lower in those with bronchiectasis compared to controls.[50] The determinants of QoL were related to age, forced expiratory volume in one second (FEV_1)/forced vital capacity (FVC) % predicted, and dyspnea severity.[50]

The differences between the Australian[49] and Turkish[48,50] studies likely relate to the different QoL scales used and severity of disease. It is likely that QoL scores correlate to disease severity only in more severe disease, similar to the relationship between spirometry and radiological extent of bronchiectasis; spirometry is often normal in mild or localized disease,[52] and significant correlations between spirometry indices and radiology scores are seen only in more severe disease.[53] Nevertheless, all studies showed the negative impact of bronchiectasis on the children and/or their parents QoL and mental health. Poor sleep quality has also been reported.[54]

Etiologic Risk Factors

Bronchiectasis is the result of a variety of airway insults and predisposing conditions that ultimately injure the airways and lead to recurrent or persistent airway infection and destruction. Examples of these conditions are listed in Table 26.1. Bronchiectasis develops in some individuals when structural airway abnormalities, such as bronchomalacia, endobronchial tuberculosis, central airway compression, or retained aspirated foreign bodies impair mucus and bacterial clearance. However, there is currently no evidence of airway malacia causing bronchiectasis in human studies. *Persistent* airway injury and narrowing associated with bronchiolitis obliterans (BO; due to viral injury or following lung transplantation) can lead to bronchiectasis. *Recurrent* airway injury, such as occurs with aspiration syndromes, can also result in bronchiectasis. Selected pediatric cohorts from various settings and countries that describe the frequencies of these associated conditions are summarized in Table 26.2.

Impaired upper airway defenses may also predispose to bronchiectasis based on the common association between rhinosinusitis and bronchitis/bronchiectasis. Indeed, the sinuses and Eustachian tubes have been considered a "sanctuary site" for bacterial pathogens and cytokines that may predispose to recurrent lower airway infection. Finally, there are variations in host inflammatory responses, for example, cytokine and metalloproteinase levels, and counterbalancing antiinflammatory mechanisms, for example, antioxidants and antiproteases, which may explain why some children develop bronchiectasis, while others do not despite similar exposures and living conditions.[26]

Previous Acute Lower Respiratory Infections

It is well documented that acute lower respiratory tract infections (ALRIs) in children can lead to subsequent respiratory morbidity and lung function abnormalities.[60,61] Classic epidemiological studies have linked acute ALRIs from adenovirus and other infections with chronic bronchitis and productive cough later in childhood.[62,63] Recent large epidemiological studies have also shown that those with ALRIs in early childhood are at risk of lower lung function in adulthood.[64,65] Although low lung function at birth may be the underlying

Table 26.1   Causes of Bronchiectasis

Primary Pathophysiology	Diseases	Major Associations
Impaired immune function[a]	Severe combined immunodeficiency	Gastrointestinal bacterial infections
	Common variable immunodeficiency	
	Natural killer cell deficiency	EBV infection
	Bare lymphocyte syndrome	
	X-linked lymphoproliferative disease	
	Ectodermal dysplasia	Abnormalities of teeth, hair, eccrine sweat glands
	Ataxia-telangiectasia	Cerebellar ataxia, telangiectases
	Bloom syndrome	Telangiectasia, altered pigmented skin
	DNA ligase I defect	Sun sensitivity
	T-cell deficiency	Thymus aplasia
	HIV	
	Cartilage-hair hypoplasia	Short-limb dwarfism
Ciliary dyskinesia	Primary	Sinusitis
	Functional	
Abnormal mucous	Cystic fibrosis	Pancreatic insufficiency
Clinical syndromes	Young's syndrome	Azoospermia
	Yellow nail lymphedema syndrome	Nail discoloration
	Marfan syndrome	Phenotypic appearance
	Usher syndrome	Retinitis pigmentosa
	Autosomal Dominant Polycystic kidney disease	Kidney disease
Congenital tracheobronchomegaly	Mounier-Kuhn syndrome, Williams-Campbell syndrome	
	Ehlers-Danlos syndrome	Phenotype appearance
Aspiration syndromes	Recurrent small volume aspiration	Neurodevelopmental problems
	Primary aspiration	
	Tracheoesophageal fistula	
	Gastroesophageal reflux disease	
Obstructive bronchiectasis	Foreign body, tumors, lymph nodes	
Other pulmonary disease associations	Interstitial lung disease	Systemic disease, dyspnea
	Bronchiolitis obliterans	Past severe ALRI
	Allergic bronchopulmonary aspergillosis	Wheeze
	Bronchopulmonary dysplasia	Extreme prematurity
	Tracheobronchomalacia	Brassy cough
Others	Alpha-1 trypsin or protease inhibitor deficiency	Liver disease
	Posttransplant	
	IgG4 related disease	Pancreatitis, skin lesions
	Autoimmune diseases	
	Post toxic fumes	
	Eosinophilic lung disease	
	Prolidase deficiency	Leg ulcers, pulmonary cysts

[a]List is incomplete for immune deficiency.
ALRI, Acute lower respiratory tract infection; *EBV*, Epstein-Barr Virus; *HIV*, human immunodeficiency virus; *IgG4*, immunoglobulin G_4.

factor of the significant association found, single severe ALRIs and multiple ALRIs in early childhood can undoubtedly lead to CSLD and bronchiectasis.[1,66] These single ALRIs associated with bronchiectasis have been described with tuberculosis, pertussis, adenovirus, measles, and severe viral pneumonia. Although these infections do not frequently cause bronchiectasis, they remain common ALRIs in less affluent countries[4] and are still considered important antecedents to childhood bronchiectasis.

In cohort studies, the most common associated cause or ascribed etiology for the bronchiectasis is past pneumonic events with lobar or diffuse alveolar infiltrates (see Table 26.2). In the sole case-control study of childhood pneumonia and radiographically proven bronchiectasis, a strong association between hospitalized pneumonia and bronchiectasis was found.[67] Children who had been previously hospitalized due to pneumonia were 15 times more likely to develop bronchiectasis.[67] A dose effect was also shown; recurrent (>1) hospitalization for pneumonia and more severe pneumonia (episodes with longer hospital stay or oxygen requirement) increased the risk of bronchiectasis later in childhood.[67] Bronchiectasis was 3 times more likely in children with four

or five episodes of pneumonia and 21 times more likely if they had 6 or more pneumonias. The overall number of pneumonias rather than the site of pneumonia were associated with bronchiectasis.[67] In an Alaskan cohort, there was no association between lobe affected by first ALRI and the eventually bronchiectatic lobe, but there was an association between lobe most severely affected by ALRI and the lobes later affected by bronchiectasis.[56] Specific infectious etiologies were not described in these studies. A review on the long-term effects of pneumonia in young children[66] described a mixture of obstructive and restrictive lung deficits when followed up long term. However, the majority of studies in the review[66] were limited with case ascertainment and follow-up issues.

Some authors have suggested that bronchiolitis is an important precursor of bronchiectasis. An Alaskan 5-year case-control follow-up of children hospitalized in infancy specifically with severe RSV infections described that they were not more likely to have been diagnosed with bronchiectasis.[68] In contrast, a study of Indigenous children hospitalized with bronchiolitis in Australia found that on CT scans performed at a median 13 months (range 3 to 23)

Table 26.2 Selected Studies on Etiologies of Childhood Bronchiectasis Published in Last 20 Years From Various Regions and Settings

Study	Nikolaizik et al.[25] N = 41	Edwards et al.[55] N = 60	Singleton et al.[56] N = 46	Chang et al.[52] N = 65	Santamaria et al.[57] N = 105	Kapur et al.[58] 2012 N = 113	Brower et al.[59] 2014 N = 989[a]
Setting n (%)	City, England	City, New Zealand	Remote, Indigenous, Alaska	Remote, Indigenous, Australia	City, Italy	City, Australia	Mixed locations
Postinfectious (severe pneumonia)	12 (29)	15 (15)	42 (92)	58 (90)	7 (6.7)	14 (12)	174 (19)
Tuberculosis	0	0	2 (4)	1 (1)	0	0	Not described
Inherited immune deficiency	8 (20)	7 (12)	0	2 (3)	11 (10.5)	13 (12)	158 (17)
Primary ciliary dyskinesia	7 (17)	0	0	0	25 (23.8)	2 (2)	66 (7)
Congenital malformations	6 (15)	1 (1)	0	1 (1)	0	0	34 (4)
Secondary immune defects	3 (7)	0	0	0	0	5 (4)	29 (3)
Aspiration of exogenous toxicants or foreign body	2 (5)	1 (2)	1 (2)	0	0	2 (2)	Combined with below
Aspiration or GERD	0	6 (10)	1 (2)	3 (5)	4 (3.8)	12 (11)	91 (10)
Unknown	2 (5)	30 (50)	0	0	58 (55.2)	62 (55)	308 (34%)
CF-like or CF	1 (2)	0	0	0	0	0	0
Interstitial lung disease including bronchiolitis obliterans	0	0	0	0	0	3 (3)	12 (1)
"Asthma"	0	0	0	0	0	0	Not described
Others	0	0	0	0	0	0	18 (2)

[a]Although this study was called systematic review, the review was incomplete with several studies omitted.
CF, Cystic fibrosis; *GERD,* gastroesophageal reflux disease.

posthospitalization, infants with persistent cough at 3 week (n = 31) after hospitalization were significantly more likely to have bronchiectasis compared to those without a cough (n = 126), OR 3.0, 95% CI 1 to 7, P = .03.[69] We surmise that bronchiectasis is not a consequence of specific viruses that produce bronchiolitis.

Upper Airway Infection and Aspiration

Mechanisms by which upper respiratory infections predispose to lower airway inflammation and injury are reviewed elsewhere.[70] Bacterial pathogens colonizing the nose and mouth are shed into saliva and contaminate the lower airways. Proinflammatory cytokines from the oropharynx may also be aspirated and augment neutrophilic responses in the lower airways. Hydrolytic enzymes in infected upper airway secretions impair protective secretory molecules such as mucins in the lower airways, and thereby predispose the lower airways to infection. *In vitro* studies have shown that some bacteria produce factors that cause ciliary slowing, dyskinesia, and stasis, setting the stage for chronic bacterial colonization of the lower airways.[71] Whether the concentration or persistence of these pathogens in upper airways represents a significant risk factor for development or progression of bronchiectasis is unknown. In indigenous Australian children with bronchiectasis, a study relating nasopharyngeal to bronchoalveolar lavage (BAL) bacteria found a high density and diversity of respiratory bacteria along with strain concordance between upper and lower airways.[72] The study suggests a possible pathogenic role of recurrent aspiration of nasopharyngeal secretions.[72]

Bronchiectasis and other forms of suppurative lung disease have been described among individuals with neurologic and neuromuscular conditions that reduce the frequency and effectiveness of cough and also increase the risk of aspirating oropharyngeal contents. Brook reported on 10 children with

such conditions who developed anaerobic pulmonary infections; six had poor oral hygiene.[73]

Public Health Issues

In 1949, Field wrote "Irreversible bronchiectasis is not commonly seen in the better social and economic classes. Good nutrition and home conditions probably give the child a better chance of more complete recovery from lung damaging disease."[74] Poor public health conditions, including malnutrition, crowding, lack of running water, and environmental pollution, increase the risk of ALRIs and bronchitis.[75,76] These issues are particularly important in developing countries. In affluent countries, those communities with higher prevalence of bronchiectasis are also those where poverty and low standards of housing are common.[26] In a qualitative study, community members and health care providers believed that potential contributing factors to acute and chronic lung diseases were smoke, dust, feeding practices, socioeconomic conditions, and mold.[77]

Macro and selected micro malnutrition increases infection risks, as it creates an immune deficiency state and leads to the malnutrition-infection-malnutrition cycle.[78] However, data on malnutrition specifically preceding bronchiectasis are limited and inconsistent. In Central Australia, Indigenous children with bronchiectasis are 3 times more likely to have had malnutrition in early childhood prior to the diagnosis of bronchiectasis,[67] but this is not seen in Alaska or New Zealand.[26] Breast-feeding is a known protective factor against development of bronchiectasis.[67] Bronchiectasis may itself predispose to malnutrition as a result of chronic pulmonary infection, diminished appetite, and reduced caloric intake. The caloric needs and daily oxygen consumption of children with non-CF-related bronchiectasis have not been reported. One series described that children with bronchiectasis and low (<80%) baseline FEV$_1$ % predicted values, and those with immunodeficiency had significantly lower body mass index at diagnosis, and they significantly improved after appropriate therapy was instituted.[79] Also, in a double-blind randomized controlled trial on the effect of long-term azithromycin, Indigenous children randomized to the azithromycin group (c.f. placebo) had a significant improvement in weight z-score, concurrent with a reduction in exacerbations (incidence rate ratio = 0.5, 95% CI 0.35 to 0.71).[80] This suggests that effective management of children with bronchiectasis improves nutrition.

Another predisposing factor to bronchiectasis is the presence of inhaled irritants, including indoor and outdoor pollutants, particularly in the presence of impaired airway clearance. The effects of environmental tobacco smoke (ETS) on children's respiratory system are well known from both *in utero* and *ex utero* exposure and include reduced airway caliber, increased lower respiratory tract infections, and middle ear disease. Reviews of ETS and its effects on the developing lung and accelerated lung decline are available elsewhere.[81] Exposure to indoor biomass combustion increases coughing illness associated with ALRIs with an exposure-response effect.[82] Exposures to other indoor pollutants (nitrogen dioxide, gas cooking) and traffic are also associated with increased cough in children in both cross-sectional and longitudinal studies.[75] There is no direct evidence of pollutants causing bronchiectasis, and the pathogenic role is likely indirect through an increased frequency of ALRIs and increased airway mucus production. In Chile, increased arsenic exposure has been associated with a variety of chronic disorders including bronchiectasis.[83]

Genetics

The interplay between genotype, epigenetics, and environment is increasingly recognized as the key in phenotypic expression of respiratory diseases. An increased frequency of cystic fibrosis transmembrane conductance regulator (CFTR) genotypes associated with CF, presenting as heterozygotes, has been described in several case series of adults with diffuse bronchiectasis.[84] While heterozygotes for alpha-1 antitrypsin have also been described more frequently in those individuals with diffuse bronchiectasis, a causal relationship remains controversial. Older guidelines suggest optional screening for alpha-1 antitrypsin deficiency for patients with idiopathic diffuse bronchiectasis,[85] but newer guidelines described a lack of evidence and do not suggest alpha-1 antitrypsin deficiency testing for people with bronchiectasis.[86] A Turkish study (where consanguinity of parents is common) described transporter associated with antigen presentation (TAP) gene polymorphisms in their cohort of children with bronchiectasis.[87] It is interesting to note the high rate of consanguinity in several series of children with bronchiectasis from different countries.[88,89] As with other diseases, an increasing number of gene aberrations have been associated with syndromes where bronchiectasis may occur. Examples include primary ciliary dyskinesia, autosomal dominant polycystic kidney disease (PKD1 on chromosome 16p13.3 and PKD2 on chromosome 4p21),[90] and prolidase deficiency[91] (PEPD gene).

Aside from variations in specific gene frequencies, overexpression of innate pulmonary immune mechanisms, such as proinflammatory cytokine and adhesion molecule production, and receptor expression, may contribute to the development of bronchiectasis in certain children. An increased or exaggerated neutrophilic response in Australian Indigenous children as a group has been described.[92] Similarly, metalloproteinases, for example, MMP-2 and 9, have been isolated from the sputum and BAL of bronchiectatic subjects, suggesting a role in airway destruction by gelatinases and collagenases.[93,94] Whether proinflammatory cytokine and collagenase overexpression are associated with early onset disease or, particularly, progressive disease in childhood remains unknown.

PATHOLOGY AND PATHOPHYSIOLOGY

The histopathology of bronchiectasis was first described by Laënnec[95] in 1819. It includes alterations in subsegmental bronchial structure accompanied by neutrophilic inflammation, intraluminal secretion accumulation, and obliteration of distal airways. There are accompanying changes of peribronchial inflammation and fibrosis, distal lung collapse, bronchial and pulmonary vascular changes, and pleural adhesions. The macroscopic and microscopic features of bronchiectasis change as the disease progresses. Classical papers on bronchiectasis divided morphological types of bronchiectasis into tubular or cylindrical, early fusiform, late fusiform, fuso-saccular, and saccular types as different stages in the progression of disease.[36] The most commonly used classification is that of Reid's subtypes: cylindrical, varicose and cystic,[96] which were based on bronchographic findings. The latter findings are illustrated in Figs. 26.2 and 26.3 and they reflect progression of increasing severity. More recent HRCT scoring systems describe cylindrical and saccular changes as markers of disease severity.[97] Saccular and cystic changes tend to reflect clinically more advanced, severe, and irreversible disease.

Macroscopically, the airways are tortuous and dilated, at times extending to the pleural surface. Early histologic changes include bronchial wall thickening, edema, presence of inflammatory cells, development of lymphoid nodules and follicles, and mucus gland hyperplasia. Intraluminal secretions are purulent or mucopurulent (Video 26.1). Microscopic changes include loss of ciliated epithelial cells and epithelial ulcerations. With time, chronic inflammation leads to squamous cell metaplasia and fibrotic obliteration of distal conducting

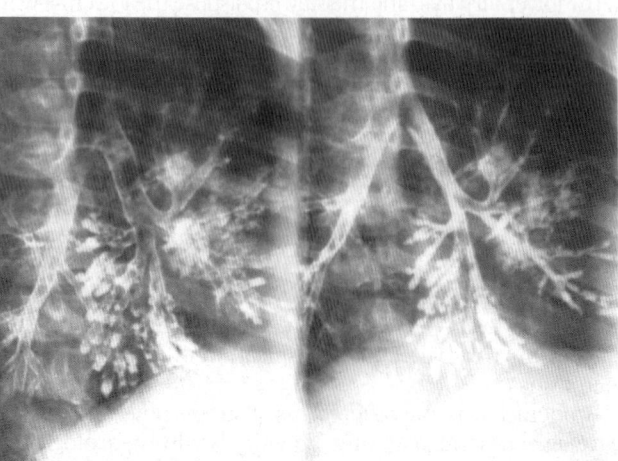

Fig. 26.2 Varicose and cystic changes characteristic of severe bronchiectasis by bronchogram.

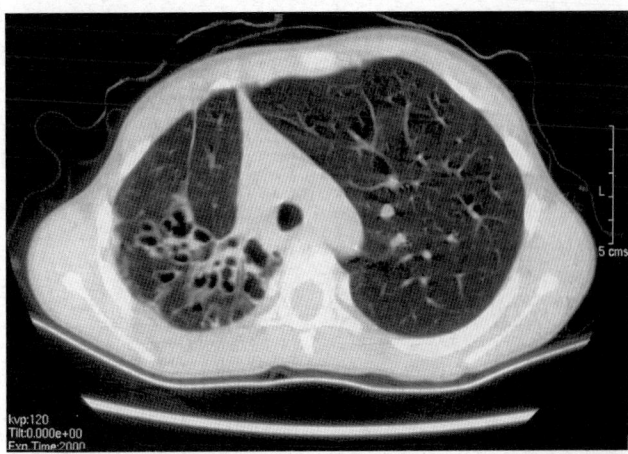

Fig. 26.3 CT scan findings of saccular bronchiectasis in the right upper lobe of a 9-year-old boy.

airways and peribronchial tissue. As bronchiectasis becomes more severe, the airway walls become thin and saccular with destruction of the airway's muscular, elastic, and cartilaginous elements.[96,98] The saccular airway walls are composed of fibrous and granulation tissue with only remnants of normal tissue. In advanced disease, mucus-filled saccular airway changes can be severe enough to appear as cystic microabscesses.

Vascular changes accompany bronchial structural changes in bronchiectasis. Large bronchopulmonary anastomosis can develop, and total bronchial arterial blood flow is increased. Extensive precapillary anastomoses between the two arterial systems can serve as a shunt between the pulmonary and systemic systems, increasing cardiac work.[98] Bronchopulmonary vascular anastomoses most often occur near distal subsegmental bronchi that have undergone saccular changes. Abnormal bronchopulmonary anastomoses and enlargement of aberrant bronchial arteries are thought to be associated with the metabolic demands of hypertrophied muscle, lymphoid tissue, and peribronchial granulation tissue during the course of the organizing pneumonitis that precedes the development of bronchiectasis.[99] The presence of significant hemoptysis is likely related to these abnormalities. Additional vascular remodeling of the pulmonary arteries and arterioles occurs in association with chronic airway obstruction and alveolar hypoxia, predisposing patients to pulmonary hypertension and cor pulmonale in severe cases.

The initial trigger for the bronchiectasis process is unknown, and there is little doubt that both host and pathogen factors play a role (Fig. 26.4). Animal models of bronchiectasis suggest that inadequate mucus clearance and persistent infection are necessary prerequisites.[101] Mucus clearance in bronchiectasis is reduced by a combination of factors including airflow limitation,[102,103] abnormal quantity and quality of mucus produced,[104] and factors produced by bacteria that cause ciliary slowing, dyskinesia, and mucus stasis.[71] Mucociliary clearance is enhanced by cough, exercise, and hyperventilation,[103,105,106] and is decreased in situations where airway caliber is diminished.[102,103] Decreased mucociliary clearance in turn leads to increased bacterial colonization and infection, setting up a vicious cycle. This concept is schematically presented in Fig. 26.4. Importantly, reduced mucociliary clearance is localized to the affected regions when

bronchiectasis is produced by local injury rather than underlying deficiencies in pulmonary host defenses.[107] The role of bacteria in the pathogenesis of chronic lung infection and bronchiectasis is reviewed elsewhere.[8,108,109]

Airway and Systemic Markers

The majority of studies on airway inflammation have been performed in adults where, unlike children, assessment by using sputum is easy. Airway secretions are usually excessive in those with more severe bronchiectasis. The sputa from Alaskan native children with stable idiopathic bronchiectasis are less viscous (by one-third), less elastic (by one-fifth), less adhesive (by half), and more transportable (by 50%) compared to sputum from children with CF.[110]

Neutrophilia is the dominant type of airway inflammation,[58] although eosinophilia has also been described in some populations[111] and when treated, airway inflammation may be absent.[58] Increased percentages of neutrophils, neutrophil elastase, myeloperoxidase, mellatoproteinases, tumor necrosis factor-α (TNF-α), interleukin (IL-8), and IL-6 have been described in lower airway secretions.[112] These generally reflect neutrophilic inflammation and are not specific to bronchiectasis. The intensity of the airway and systemic inflammation is ameliorated by treatment.[112,113] An adult cohort involving 385 patients described a direct relationship between airway bacterial load and markers of airway inflammation (myeloperoxidase, neutrophil elastase, TNF-α, IL-8, and IL-1β) with a dose response such that higher inflammation correlated with higher bacterial loads.[112] High bacterial loads were associated with higher serum intercellular adhesion molecule-1 (ICAM-1), E-selectin, and vascular cell adhesion molecule-1 (VCAM-1), reflective of systemic inflammation. Using both short (14 days)- and long (12 months)-term antibiotic treatments, the study demonstrated a significant reduction in the airway bacterial load and inflammation (both airway and systemic) compared to those who did not receive antibiotic therapies.[112] However, there is a poor correlation between systemic and bronchial inflammatory mediators, suggesting that the inflammatory process is mostly compartmentalized to the airways.[114] There is paucity of data on BAL or sputum markers in children. A small study in children described increased median values of systemic markers (white cells, C-reactive protein [CRP], and fibrinogen) in children whose airways were colonized (n = 14) compared to those without identified bacteria in their sputum (white cell count: 8.2 [IQR 6.4 to 9.5] vs. 6.4 [5.8 to 7.7] × 10³/mm³; CRP: 0.91 [0.45 to 1.29] vs. 0.42 [0.30 to 0.77] mg/dL; fibrinogen: 433.5 [390.3 to 490.3] vs. 392.0 [327.0 to 416.0] mg/dL, $P < .05$ for all).[115] While the authors concluded that systemic inflammation was absent in children with bronchiectasis compared to controls, it is highly likely that a type-1 error was present in the study. In an in-depth study, the blood of children with bronchiectasis had a significant increase in the percentage of CD8+ T cells and T and natural killer T-cells (NKT)-like subsets expressing perforin/granzyme, interferon gamma (IFNγ), and TNFα compared with controls.[116] The proinflammatory cytotoxic T cells were more marked in Indigenous children compared to non-Indigenous children.[116]

Exaggerated or persistent pulmonary inflammation present in bronchiectasis leads to increased lung destruction by many mechanisms.[8] The balance between proteases and

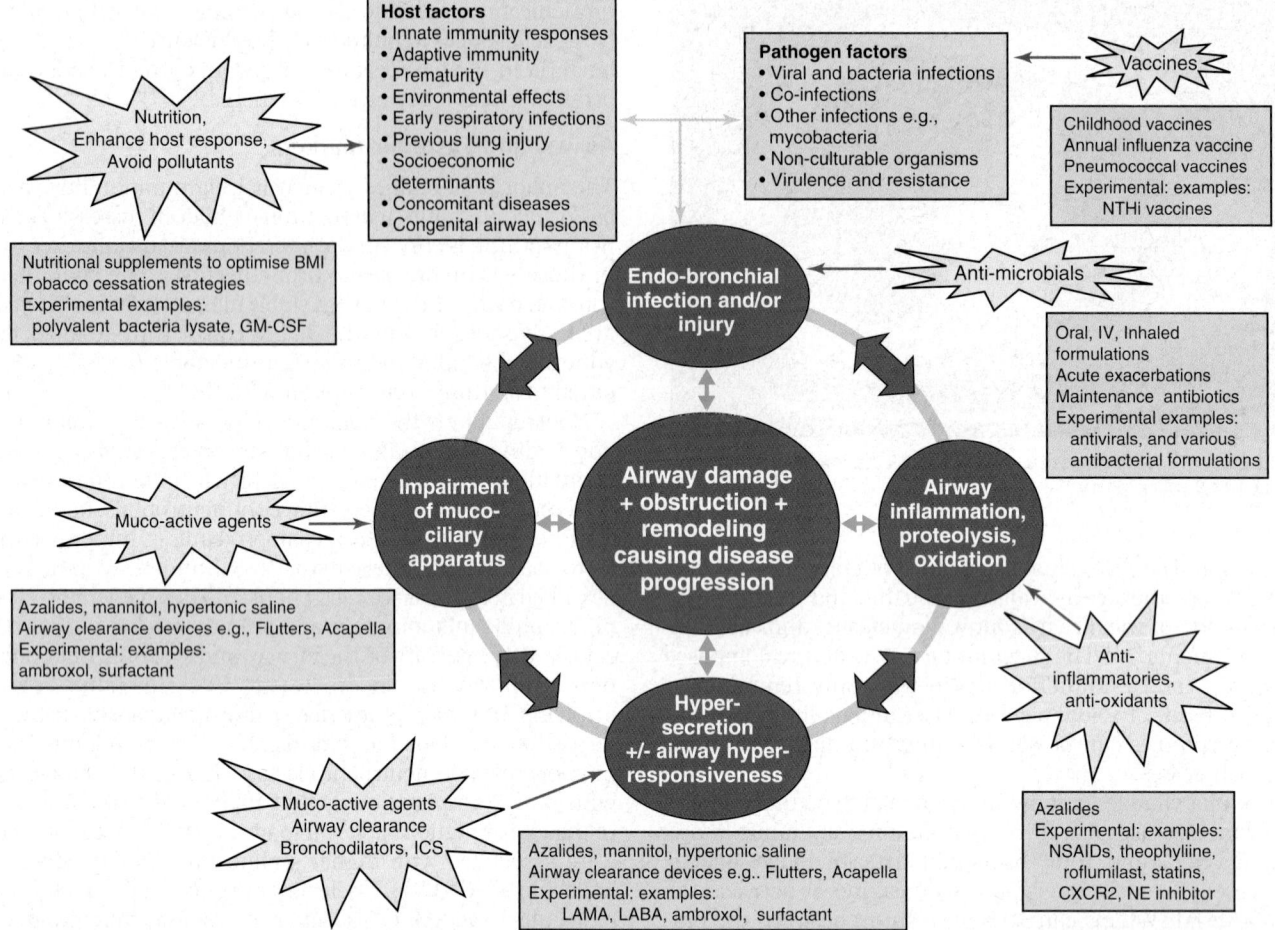

Fig. 26.4 A simplified schematic diagram of the factors contributing to the development of bronchiectasis. The initial trigger causing persistence of endobronchial infection and injury is dependent on host, environmental, and pathogen factors. This infection leads to inflammation, proteolysis, oxidation and subsequent mucous hypersecretion and/or airway hyperresponsiveness, with impairment of the mucociliary apparatus. Each factor influences each other (as in Cole's vicious cycle postulate)[100] and may lead to development, or increasing severity, of bronchiectasis (central circle) if left untreated. Possible therapeutics affecting each factor are presented in the jagged shapes. *BMI,* Body mass index; *CXCR2,* CXC chemokine receptor 2 antagonist; *GM-CSF,* granulocyte-macrophage colony-stimulating factor; *ICS,* inhaled corticosteroids; *IV,* intravenous; *LABA,* long acting beta$_2$-adrenoceptor agonist; *LAMA,* long acting muscarinic antagonists; *NE,* neutrophil elastase; *NTHi,* nontypeable *Haemophilus influenzae.*

antiproteases is increasingly recognized as important to the protection of airways against hostile agents and destruction of lung tissue. Upregulation of circulating adhesion molecules (E-selectin, ICAM-1, and vascular adhesion molecule VCAM-1) have also been suggested as playing a role in the pathogenesis of bronchiectasis.[117] Collagenase activity present in the BAL of adults with moderately severe bronchiectasis originates from neutrophils and bacteria. These collagenolytic proteases are likely contributors to tissue destruction.[118] As described above, the airways of people with bronchiectasis contains collagenolytic proteinases of bacterial origin.[118] and neutrophilic-associated cytokines that, unabated, lead to increased tissue damage (e.g., metalloproteinases [MMP-2,8, and 9]).[117] MMP-9 (but not tissue inhibitors of metalloproteinase-1) measured in exhaled breath condensate of children with non-CF bronchiectasis (42.8 ± 18.1 ng/mL) were similar to those with CF (48.9 ± 26.8) and significantly higher than controls (30 ± 3.7).[119] Endobronchial biopsies in adults with bronchiectasis demonstrated an overexpression of neutrophil matrix metalloproteinases (MMPs).[117] Using sputum from adults with bronchiectasis, Shum et al. showed that serine proteases derived from neutrophils were responsible

for degradation of proteoglycans in a matrix model and that the protease secretion was stimulated by TNF-α in the presence of factors found in the sputum sol.[120]

There are additional pathogenic processes associated with bronchiectasis that contribute to the persistence of airway inflammation and obstruction. Increased airway permeability has also been described with bronchiectasis when purulent sputum and significant colonization of the respiratory tract by bacterial pathogens are present.[121] Also, resolution of inflammation is normally associated with the orderly removal of apoptotic inflammatory cells, and impaired removal of apoptotic inflammatory cells has been described in children[122] and adults[123] with bronchiectasis. The pediatric study[122] also examined specifically for phagocytic activity for nontypeable *Haemophilus influenzae* (NTHi), whereas the adult study[123] investigated apoptosis in relation to inflammation. The adult study[123] reported that impaired apoptosis occurred in a dose-response fashion with increasing neutrophil elastase, a marker of neutrophilic inflammation. In children with bronchiectasis, the macrophage phagocytic capacity of BAL cells to apoptotic cells (efferocytosis) and to NTHi was significantly lower than in controls (efferocytosis: 14.1%, IQR 10 to 16 vs. 18.1%,

IQR 16 to 21 respectively, $P < .001$ and NTHi: 13.7%, IQR 11 to 16 vs. 19.0%, IQR 13 to 21 respectively, $P = .004$).[122] Mannose receptor expression in BAL was also found to be significantly reduced in the bronchiectasis group compared to controls ($P = .019$).[122]

Other Immune Markers and Response

Innate defense mechanisms also play a role in the pathogenesis and upregulated response to infection in people with bronchiectasis.[8] However, there is little data specific to children.[27] In a study involving 26 children with human immunodeficiency virus (HIV)-related bronchiectasis,[124] the soluble triggering receptor expressed on myeloid cells-1 (sTREM-1), an innate immune marker, was upregulated and more highly expressed than in children with CF. sTREM-1 also correlated with IL-8 and neutrophil elastase derived from BAL.[124]

The increased expression of innate immune receptors (e.g., receptors TLR2, TLR4, and CD14) and cytokine responses (e.g., IL-8 and IL-1β) seen in adults with bronchiectasis are also found in those with neutrophilic asthma and children with PBB,[125,126] a likely forerunner of bronchiectasis.[11] This raises the possibility that some people with neutrophilic asthma have unrecognized CSLD. Indeed, many of children with PBB were previously misdiagnosed with asthma[11,34] and in some settings has been classified as "difficult or severe asthma."

There is an emerging body of evidence that impaired cell-mediated immune responses and dysregulated airway inflammation are linked and could contribute to the pathobiology of CSLD. A study on systemic immunity found that children with CSLD or bronchiectasis produced significantly less IFN-γ in response to NTHi than healthy control children, whereas mitogen-induced IFN-γ production was similar in both groups.[127] The production of systemic NTHi-specific IFN-γ was significantly negatively associated with the BAL IL-6 ($P = .001$) and IL-1β ($P = .001$).[128] The presence of bacterial or viral infection and severity of bronchiectasis using modified CT Bhalla score did not influence systemic NTHi-specific IFN-γ response.[128]

CLINICAL FEATURES

Presenting Clinical Features: Symptoms and Signs

The clinical case definition of bronchiectasis is imprecise, but the diagnosis should be considered when children have a chronic "wet" sounding or productive cough with or without exertional dyspnea, recurrent wheezing and chest infections, hemoptysis, growth failure, clubbing, or hyperinflation. The most common symptom is persistent or recurrent wet/productive cough with purulent or mucopurulent sputum. Sputum color reflects neutrophilic airway inflammation.[129,130] The frequency of chest wall deformity (hyperinflation) and digital clubbing vary among case series (5% to 60%).[24,52,131] Digital clubbing can disappear after medical or surgical treatment in association with the disappearance of purulent sputum.[24,131] Although hemoptysis is much less common among children than in adults with bronchiectasis, a presenting finding of hemoptysis should raise the possibility of airway bleeding due to bronchiectasis. Chest auscultation may be entirely normal or reveal coarse inspiratory crackles over the affected regions. Reduced oxygen saturations and abnormal cardiac sounds associated with pulmonary hypertension are very late signs in bronchiectasis. Similar to any other serious chronic respiratory illness, children with bronchiectasis may have growth failure[52] that is associated with delayed diagnosis of bronchiectasis.

The median age of diagnosis of bronchiectasis unrelated to CF in affluent countries is 4 to 5 years.[52,56] A New Zealand cohort[55] was older at 9 to 10 years old at diagnosis but also experienced more advanced disease. Idiopathic bronchiectasis is rare in infancy, but when present, it is likely to reflect congenital pulmonary malformations, such as cystic lung disease or tracheobronchomegaly, or alternatively, primary ciliary dyskinesia. Only 50% of those with ciliary dyskinesia have the Kartagener triad of situs inversus, bronchiectasis, and sinusitis.[132]

Radiological risk factors for development of bronchiectasis are the presence of atelectasis[67,133] and persistent lobar abnormalities.[134] In Alaska, children were more likely to develop bronchiectasis if chest radiographs obtained in children less than 2 years of age showed lung parenchymal densities, persistent parenchymal densities greater than 6 months duration, or repeated parenchymal densities.[134] Among Aboriginal Australian children hospitalized with lobar changes on admission chest radiographs, children with alveolar abnormalities were more likely to have bronchiectasis on follow-up.[133] In a prospective radiographic study of alveolar changes (179 lobes in 112 hospitalized children), the two most common involved lobes were the right upper lobe and left lower lobes.[133] Both lobes had similar rates of radiological clearance on follow-up (22% and 27% respectively).

Comorbid Conditions

Children with postinfectious bronchiolitis obliterans and CSLD share some common clinical features (airway obstruction, chronic cough, recurrent ALRIs) in addition to the same etiological insult.[60,135] In an Australian study, 6 of 19 children with postinfectious BO developed bronchiectasis.[60] A South American cohort follow-up study (mean period of 12 years, SD 3.5) described that mean FVC increased by 11%/year (95% CI 9.3 to 12.6), FEV_1 by 9%/year (95% CI 7.7 to 10.2), and FEV_1/FVC ratio decreased by 1.9%/year (95% CI 1 to 2.8).[136] Seventy-eight percent of the 46 children in that cohort had bronchiectasis.[136]

Phenotypes of childhood wheeze have been recognized and airway hyperreactivity occurs in some individuals with bronchiectasis.[135] The presence of features of asthma has been described as a bad prognostic factor in both children[24,131] and adults[137] with bronchiectasis. The frequency of airway hyperreactivity in children with bronchiectasis varies from 26% to 74%.[52,56] As a corollary, clinicians must recognize that wheeze and cough may not be related to asthma but to increased airway secretions and airway collapse as features of bronchiectasis.

Gastroesophageal reflux disease (GERD) may coexist with any chronic respiratory illness and should be appropriately treated. However, data in adults indicate that GERD may resolve or significantly improve once the underlying respiratory disorder has been treated.[138] There is, however, no evidence-based approach to the management of GERD associated with bronchiectasis. Caution is necessary with regard to overdiagnosis, and unnecessary treatment of GERD is given the increasing evidence of increased risk of respiratory infections in children and adults receiving proton pump inhibitors in community and hospital cohorts.[139,140] Readers are referred to the pediatric guidelines on diagnosis and treatment of GERD.[141]

Hypertrophic osteoarthropathy (clubbing, periostosis of the tubular bones, and arthritis-like signs and symptoms) may occur in children with bronchiectasis.[142] Systemic amyloidosis has also been reported as a complication or comorbidity.[143] Cardiac dysfunction, although rare, has also been reported and may not be accompanied by pulmonary hypertension. A study of 21 children with bronchiectasis showed that the ventricular systolic function was normal but some patients had changes in left ventricular diastolic function.[144] The authors also found that isovolumetric relaxation time had a significant negative correlation with the clinical severity score. Other reported comorbid conditions associated with bronchiectasis are osteopenia,[145] scoliosis, chronic suppurative ear disease, social problems, past urinary tract infections, and developmental delay.[52,56]

In adults, vitamin D deficiency has been reported to be associated with increased severity of bronchiectasis and chronic bacterial colonization of the airways.[146] However, as serum vitamin D is a negative acute phase reactant (i.e., values fall with increased inflammation), deciphering cause and effect is problematic.[147]

DIAGNOSTIC EVALUATIONS

The goals of evaluating children with suspected bronchiectasis are: (1) to confirm the diagnosis, (2) to define the distribution and severity of airway involvement, (3) to characterize extrapulmonary organ involvement associated with bronchiectasis (such as cor pulmonale), and (4) to identify familial and treatable underlying causes of bronchiectasis and contributors to its progression.

Diagnostic Criteria

Chest HRCT is the gold standard for diagnosis,[27] because plain chest radiographs are insensitive. It has been long recognized that chest x-rays can be normal in people with bronchiectasis.[148] With modern CT scanners, the images are best acquired using an MDCT scan with HRCT reconstruction which provides the best sensitivity.[27] The scan protocol must be child-appropriate to minimize radiation risk. Radiology centers inexperienced in dealing with children often utilize adult protocols that subject children to higher doses of radiation. Radiological features of bronchiectasis can also occur in association with pulmonary fibrosis, congenital lesions such as Mounier-Kuhn, and Williams-Campbell syndrome,[97] and as a result of traction in nonsuppurative lung disease.[149]

The characteristic radiographic finding on HRCT in bronchiectasis is the presence of a "signet ring" where a dilated bronchus is greater than the diameter of the accompanying blood vessel in cross section (Fig. 26.5).[97,150] However, the cutoff (>1 to 1.5) whereby the ratio is considered abnormal should be reduced to 0.8 in children when CSLD symptoms are present.[13] While this is generally appreciated by pulmonologists, radiologists may still use the adult criteria. The presence of bronchial dilatation relative to the accompanying vessel does not always equate to the presence of bronchiectasis,

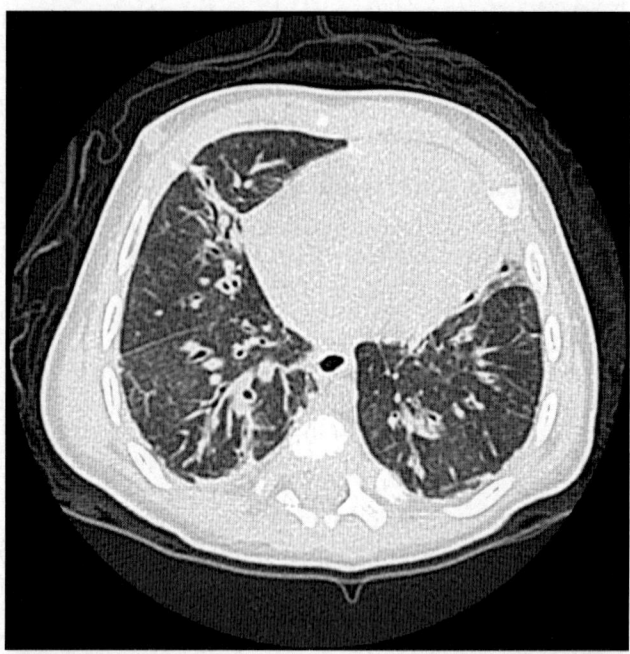

Fig. 26.5 High resolution CT finding in bronchiectasis. Image illustrates the "signet ring" appearance of a dilated airway adjacent to smaller associated pulmonary vessels. In adults, abnormal dilatation is considered present when the bronchoarterial ratio (inner diameter of bronchus: external diameter of adjacent artery) is greater than 1. In children, a cutoff of 0.8 is considered abnormal when clinical features of bronchiectasis are present.

Box 26.1   Features of Bronchiectasis on Chest High Resolution Computed Tomography Scans

1. Signet ring sign: internal diameter of bronchi is larger than accompanying vessel (diameters of both should be short axis)
2. Enlarged internal bronchial diameter
3. Failure of airway to taper normally while progressing to lung periphery
4. Presence of peripheral airways at CT periphery
5. Presence of associated abnormalities
   - Bronchial wall thickening
   - Mucoid plugging or impaction (seen as branching or rounded/nodular opacities in cross sections, tubular or Y-shaped structures or tree in bud appearance)
6. Mosaic perfusion
7. Air trapping on expiration
8. Air-fluid levels in distended bronchi

Compiled from references 97, 151-153.

---

as this finding can also be present in other conditions (Box 26.2). Other c-HRCT signs of bronchiectasis include abnormalities in the surrounding lung may include parenchyma loss, emphysema, scars and nodular foci,[150] a linear array or cluster of cysts, dilated bronchi in the periphery of the lung, and bronchial wall thickening (Box 26.1).[154] Image quality and hence detection of bronchiectasis is dependent on the radiological technique used (tube setting, radiation dose, collimation distance, and image intervals).[155] False positive and false negative situations that may occur are listed in Box 26.2. HRCT does not differentiate the etiologies of bronchiectasis.[156]

Etiologic Evaluation

As most patients are usually diagnosed with bronchiectasis after many years of symptoms, it may be difficult to define the etiology. Differentiating idiopathic from postinfectious bronchiectasis is particularly problematic. A common feature of many patients is impaired local or systemic host defenses to infection.[127,157] Often, no cause is found even with extensive investigation, and many retain the label of idiopathic or presumed postinfectious bronchiectasis (see Table 26.2). Difficulties with ascribing an etiology to CSLD/bronchiectasis arise due to unavailability of certain tests, for example, functional tests for ciliary motility and extended immune testing, lack of a standardized approach to diagnosis, the population studied, and the CT definitions used.

Identifying etiology and assessing disease severity can influence surveillance frequency, treatment intensity, and prognosis.[157,158] Investigations for specific causes of CSLD/bronchiectasis are recommended, even though many patients will lack an identifiable etiology.[79] Current best practices for investigating possible etiology are outlined in Table 26.3. The diagnosis of ciliary dyskinesia[159] is addressed in another chapter (see Chapter 71).

Bronchoscopic Findings

Bronchoscopy is indicated to identify obstructive bronchiectasis, which can be intraluminal (tumors and foreign body), in the wall (tracheobronchomalacia [TBM]), or extramural from external airway compression. Bronchiectasis is a complication of inhaled foreign bodies and occurs among 25% of patients whose diagnosis of aspiration was delayed by greater than 30 days.[160] In a prospective study involving 56 children with bronchiectasis undergoing flexible bronchoscopy, there were 25 occasions in 23 children where bronchoscopic results altered empiric treatment.[111] BAL microbiology results led to antibiotic changes in five (9%) children, and an unsuspected foreign body was found in one (2%).[111]

Bronchoscopic findings of major airways related to bronchiectasis have been described as five types: type I: mucosal

---

Box 26.2   Pitfalls in Diagnosis of Bronchiectasis on Chest High-Resolution Computed Tomography Scans

False Positives

1. Physiologic constriction of pulmonary artery (creates relative bronchial enlargement)
2. Artefacts from cardiac pulsation and respiratory motion (creates pseudocystic pattern)
3. Pseudobronchiectasis or transient bronchial atresia (related to acute pneumonia or atelectasis)
4. Increased bronchoarterial ratio in normals, asthmatics or at high attitude

False Negatives

1. Inappropriate HRCT protocol (wrong electronic windows or collimation)
2. Poor image due to movement artefacts
3. Nonuse of high-resolution techniques

HRCT, High-resolution computed tomography.
Compiled from references 97, 151-153.

Table 26.3   Evaluation for Underlying Etiologies

Investigation Type	Details	Evaluation for:
ROUTINE		
Baseline immune function	IgG, A, M, IgG subclasses, IgE, hemagglutinins, antibodies to vaccinations	Immune deficiency states
Full blood count	White cell count	Neutropenia
HIV status	HIV antibody, HIV PCR assay	HIV infection
Sweat test and consider genotype	Sweat chloride and CF genotype	Cystic fibrosis
Radiology	Chest HRCT scan Chest radiograph	Diagnosis, congenital malformation and disease severity
Aspergillosis serology	Aspergillus specific IgE Skin test, total IgE	Allergic bronchopulmonary aspergillosis
Cilial biopsy and consider genetic testing	Electron microscopy and ciliary beat function	Ciliary dyskinesia
Sputum	Microscopy, sensitivity and culture	Number of polymorphs, microbiology
ADDITIONAL TESTS DEPENDING ON CLINICAL CHARACTERISTICS		
Bronchoscopy	Airway abnormalities BAL	Obstructive bronchiectasis Congenital airway abnormalities Microbiological assessment when sputum cannot be obtained Cellular differential count
Investigations for GERD	Esophageal pH studies, manometry and/or upper endoscopy	GERD with or without aspiration syndromes
Barium meal		Tracheoesophageal fistula, esophageal abnormalities causing secondary aspiration such as achalasia
Mantoux	PPD tuberculin and atypical	Mycobacterium TB and atypical mycobacteria
Further immune tests	Neutrophil function, CH50, etc.	Immune function
Video fluoroscopy	Oro-palatal function and assessment of laryngeal protection	Primary aspiration lung disease
Genetic tests		

BAL, Bronchoalveolar lavage; *GERD,* gastroesophageal reflux disease; *HRCT,* high-resolution computed tomography; *PPD,* purified protein derivative skin test; *TB,* tuberculosis.

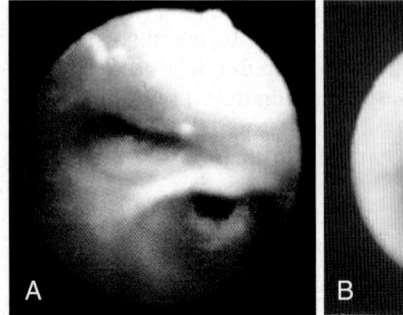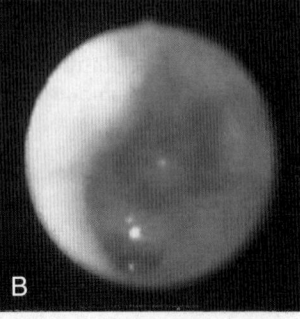

Fig. 26.6 Major airway bronchoscopic findings in bronchiectasis. (A) Bronchomalacia (airway type II) of the right middle lobe. (B) Obliterative-like lesion (airway type III) seen in the segmental bronchi (middle of picture) while the adjacent bronchi are widely patent and more inflamed. (Reproduced with permission from the BMJ Publishing Group—Chang AB, Boyce NC, Masters IB, et al. Bronchoscopic findings in children with non-cystic fibrosis chronic suppurative lung disease. *Thorax* 2002;57:935-938.)

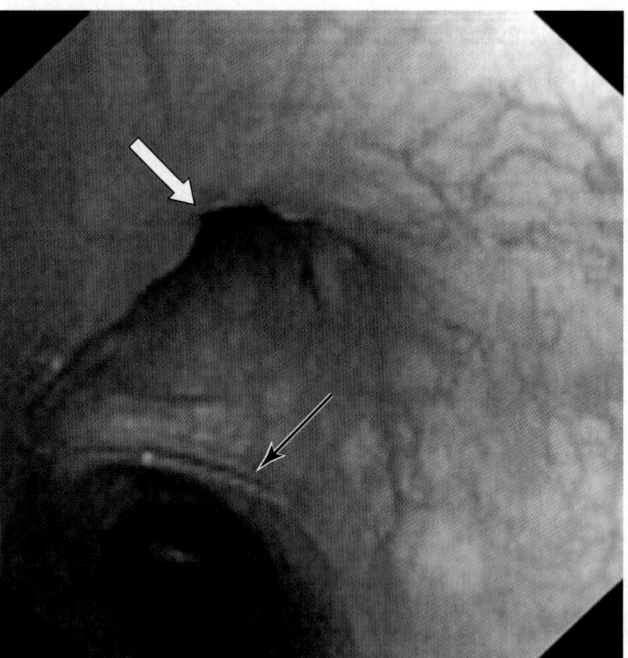

Fig. 26.7 Bronchoscopic picture from a child with bronchiectasis. Airway mucosal abnormality in child with bronchiectasis depicting mucosa erythema and irregularity, muscularis ridging *(black arrow)*, and bronchomalacia *(white arrow*, right middle lobe).

abnormality/inflammation only; type II: bronchomalacia (Fig. 26.6A); type III: obliterative-like (Fig. 26.6B); type IV: malacia/obliterative-like combination; and type V: no abnormality.[161] The frequencies of these findings among 28 children with non-CF bronchiectasis were 58%, 17%, 17%, 4%, and 2% for types I through V respectively.[161] In the 33 children with postinfectious bronchiectasis and CSLD, structural airway lesions were present in 40%.[161] A retrospective study involving 93 Greek children (0.6 to 16.4 years) described that type III (OR 5.4, 95% CI 1.9 to 15.4) and type IV (OR 8.9, 95% CI 2.5 to 15.4) bronchoscopic lesions significantly correlated to worse radiological scores, reflecting severity, and correlated with the percentage of BAL neutrophils (r = 0.23, P = .036).[162]

Bronchomalacia associated with bronchiectasis can be related to chronic inflammation,[163] although it is unknown if bronchomalacia predates recurrent respiratory infections. Airway mucosal changes typical of chronic bronchitis are usually present in bronchiectatic airways at bronchoscopy. Bronchoscopic findings include atrophic mucosa, increased secretions, and airway friability. Airway flaccidity, hypertrophy of elements in wall, longitudinal corrugations, mucosal reddening, increased vascularity, dilated ducts, and displacement due to lobar collapse have also been described in the proximal conducting airways (Fig. 26.7).[163]

Assessment of Severity

Pulmonary Function. In children, spirometry is insensitive in detecting early structural lung damage in children with bronchiectasis, both in CF[164] and non-CF.[52] Spirometric values may be normal, but when a spirometric abnormality is present[52,165]; it is usually obstructive in the earlier stages and becomes a mixed obstructive and restrictive process when bronchiectasis is more severe. Although FEV_1 correlates with chest HRCT abnormalities in some populations, it is not a sensitive measure, especially if bronchiectasis is localized.[52,165] FEV_1 can also be normal, as in CF, in the early stages of disease even when radiological bronchiectasis was present.[164] However, when bronchiectasis is diffuse, spirometric abnormalities, although insensitive to disease activity, reflect disease severity.[164] Other pulmonary function test abnormalities described are a high residual volume, lower aerobic capacity, and lower maximal ventilation at maximal exercise.[166] Effort

limitation during cardiopulmonary exercise testing does not relate to HRCT scores.[167]

There are limited data on how bronchiectasis alters respiratory system resistance or reactance measured by forced oscillatory techniques (FOT). In children, indices obtained from impulse oscillometry during exacerbations were not significantly different from the stable state.[168] In the stable state, resistance at 5 Hz was poorly sensitive to lung disease.[168] In children with CF, indices from FOT are not only insensitive at baseline but also cannot detect lung progression over 12 months.[169]

Another tool to assess severity of bronchiectasis is lung clearance index (LCI). The LCI reflects ventilation inhomogeneity in peripheral airways. Data in children with CF suggest that LCI changes occur early and before other physiological measurements when evaluating lung damage.[170] Among adults with stable non-CF bronchiectasis, the LCI negatively correlated with FEV_1 % predicted and was abnormal more often than FEV1.[171] However, a study involving 25 paired measurements of adults with non-CF bronchiectasis found that LCI was less sensitive than FEV_1 when evaluating improvement after treatment with intravenous antibiotics and physiotherapy for respiratory exacerbations.[170] While FEV_1 and vital capacity significantly improved, there was no significant change in LCI after intravenous antibiotics and physiotherapy.[170] The same study also undertook paired measurements in 25 adults with stable bronchiectasis and described that LCI indices were reproducible and, compared to controls, LCI was significantly higher.[170] There are no studies in children with non-CF bronchiectasis to know its sensitivity to early disease.

Radiology. There are at least eight radiographic scoring systems to assess severity of bronchiectasis using plain films. However, given the insensitivity of chest radiographs in detecting bronchiectasis, these scoring systems have been superseded by chest HRCT scoring systems described by Webb et al.,[97] Bhalla et al.,[172] and Reiff et al.[156] These chest HRCT scoring systems are based on composite scores of multiple radiological findings. Some systems utilize expiratory scans,[173] while others do not.[97] The Webb composite score[97] is a summation score of severity, extent, and features of emphysema and consolidation/atelectasis. The Bhalla score[172] comprises the sum of scores assigned to each of nine categories: severity of bronchiectasis, peribronchial thickening, extent of bronchiectasis, extent of mucus plugging, sacculations, generations of bronchi involved, number of bullae, emphysema, and collapse/consolidation. One study compared these three scoring systems in a group of 59 children with non-CF bronchiectasis.[52] The correlation between the scores ranged from 0.61 to 0.8 but none related to FEV_1 values. Magnetic resonance imaging (MRI) is an emerging technique for assessing bronchiectasis, but it is currently poorer than CT in evaluating airway diseases.[174,175]

Other Markers. A UK group developed the bronchiectasis severity index for adults[6] as a stratification tool for morbidity and mortality. The index includes features that are rare in children (e.g., FEV_1 of <30% predicted) and is thus not used in children.

The world of "omics" is blooming, but there currently are no studies relevant to clinical care in bronchiectasis. In children with CF, metabolomics using mass spectrometry have described possible biomarkers of BAL neutrophilic inflammation.[176] Techniques such as expired breath analysis and breath condensate measurements described almost two decades ago have not advanced in bronchiectasis.

Assessment of Disease Progression

To date, there is little research on the most sensitive and appropriate method of assessing progression of bronchiectasis in children. Clinicians rely on frequency of respiratory exacerbations and on daily clinical symptoms, which may be perceived differently by children and their parents. There is no bronchiectasis severity score for children. QoL scores that are not specific for cough have been used in children with bronchiectasis, but to date, there is no pediatric bronchiectasis-specific QoL score.

The most sensitive objective assessment of early disease progression is based on HRCT changes, as these precede most pulmonary function changes.[52,165] However, repeated HRCT scans are not recommended purely for assessment of disease progression given the known risks of radiation in young children.[177] Other assessments of disease progression include chest radiographs which are insensitive, lung function, markers of neutrophilic airway inflammation, and possibly assessments of airway proteases. One small cross-sectional study showed significant correlations between HRCT severity scores and symptoms, FEV_1, sputum IL-8, and TNF-α levels (r values of 0.64, −0.68, 0.41 and 0.41, respectively).[53] However, there are no data relating these airway markers to imaging assessments longitudinally and disease progression.

Assessment of Infection

Sputum sampling is the easiest method of obtaining an endobronchial microbiologic profile, but young children often do not expectorate sputum even when they have substantial lower airway secretions. Hence, in young children, assessment of lower airway microbiology requires bronchoscopy to obtain BAL and lower airway samples. BAL remains the gold standard, although the criteria for defining infection remains controversial.[11,178] Studies have generally used a threshold of bacterial growth of $\geq 10^4$ colony forming unit (cfu)/mL BAL to indicate infection.[11,179]

Other methods for identifying airway pathogens from children with bronchiectasis are oropharyngeal or nasopharyngeal swabs and induced sputum. In adults with bronchiectasis, sputum culture is generally reflective of lower airway organisms obtained by bronchoscopic catheter protected brushings.[180] One study on children with bronchiectasis described that the sensitivity and negative predictive value of nasopharyngeal cultures for individual respiratory bacterial pathogens, causing lower airway infection using BAL for comparison, ranged from 75% to 100%, and the specificity and positive predictive value were lower (32% to 72%).[72]

Common respiratory pathogens in children with bronchiectasis are *Streptococcus pneumoniae* and *H. influenzae* nontype b. Other organisms include *Moraxella catarhallis* and *Pseudomonas aeruginosa*. In pediatric bronchiectasis, the pathogen isolation rate from sputum or BAL is 53% to 67%.[58,109] Pseudomonas is commonly found in adults with severe bronchiectasis, but it is uncommon in children until adolescence or when bronchiectasis is severe.[58] In adults, a systematic review[181] found that persistent pseudomonas endobronchial infection was associated with increased disease severity measured radiographically, with spirometry, with death (threefold), and with more hospitalizations and poorer QoL; there are no such data in children. While nontuberculous mycobacteria and Aspergillus are commonly found in adults with bronchiectasis, they are rarely present in children with bronchiectasis.[58,72]

A number of children with bronchiectasis are persistently colonized with potential pathogenic microorganisms.[180] The largest study to report on microbiology in children with bronchiectasis was undertaken when they were clinically stable.[58] *H. influenzae* was identified in 32%, *S. pneumoniae* in 14%, *M. catarrhalis* in 8%, and *S. aureus* in 5% of BAL cultures.[58] *P. aeruginosa* was present in seven (6%) children of whom six had bronchiectasis involving multiple lobes, and five had other comorbidities.[58] The study also reported that respiratory viruses (principally respiratory syncytial virus and adenovirus) were present in 14 (12%) children; codetection of respiratory pathogens was found in more than half of those with positive microbiology results.[58] When the adenovirus was genotyped, almost all were type C, and the presence of adenovirus was significantly associated with bacterial coinfection with *H. influenzae, M. catarrhalis,* or *S. pneumoniae* (OR 3.27; 95% CI 1.38 to 7.75) and negatively associated with *S. aureus* infection (P = .03) in the BAL.[182] Studies on the microbiota (using bacterial 16S rRNA gene pyrosequencing) in children[9] and adults[183] with bronchiectasis have been reported. However, their impact on clinical management is yet to be defined. Nevertheless, one study that compared the microbiota of children and adults with bronchiectasis reported that the respiratory microbiota significantly differed from each other.[9]

Pulmonary exacerbations among children with non-CF bronchiectasis are often triggered by viruses and an increased density of known bacterial pathogens in sputum. The single prospective study in children that evaluated the point prevalence of viruses associated with exacerbations reported that respiratory viruses were detected during 37 of 77 (48%) exacerbations.[184] As the viruses reported included those commonly found in well children (rhinovirus [n = 20], enterovirus [n = 4] bocavirus [n = 4] coronavirus [n = 1]), it is possible that the percentage of true virus-associated triggers is lower. Classical respiratory viruses (adenoviruses, metapneumovirus, influenza, respiratory syncytial virus, parainfluenza [n = 3 each]) were found in only 15 (20%) exacerbations.[184]

Assessment and Importance of Exacerbations

There is one published study that developed a standardized definition of exacerbation in children.[168] In 69 children over 900 child months, the study described validated major and minor criteria that can be used in the hospital or primary care setting. The major criteria were the presence of a wet cough and a cough severity score of ≥2 over 72 hours (area under the curve [AUC] of 0.85 [95% CI 0.79 to 0.92] and 0.84 [95% CI 0.77 to 0.91] respectively).[168] The minor criteria were change in sputum color, chest pain, dyspnea, hemoptysis and new chest signs on physical examination. The inclusion of investigations (investigatory criteria: elevated serum C-reactive protein, amyloid-A, or IL6) to the definition improved its specificity and positive predictive value.[168] Other infrequent features of importance are reduced exercise tolerance and energy.[185] Fever and hemoptysis are uncommon in exacerbations of bronchiectasis in the pediatric age group.[168,185]

Determinants of accelerated lung function decline in adults with bronchiectasis are frequency of hospitalized exacerbations, increased systemic inflammatory markers, and colonization with *P. aeruginosa*.[186] In one study of 52 children over a 3-year interval, the only significant predictor of FEV$_1$ decline was frequency of hospitalized exacerbations[79]; with each exacerbation, the FEV$_1$ % predicted decreased by 1.95% adjusted for time.[79] It is likely that interventions that can reduce exacerbations prevent further lung dysfunction.[187] Also, exacerbations, particularly when recurrent, are one of the strongest predictors of poor QoL among adults with bronchiectasis.[188,189] A prospective study involving 93 Indigenous children in Alaska and Australia showed that factors associated with recurrent (≥2) exacerbations included age less than 3 years, respiratory-related hospitalization in the first year of life, and pneumonia or hospitalization for exacerbations in the year preceding enrollment.[1] The study also reported that with clinical care and time exacerbations occurred less frequently.[1]

Exacerbations should be treated such that at the end of treatment, there are improvements in cough character, general well-being, QoL indicators, and inflammatory markers with reduced sputum volume and purulence, decreased sputum bacterial load or pathogen clearance, and a return toward the patient's stable baseline state.[109,190]

MANAGEMENT AND TREATMENT PRINCIPLES

As early as 1933, Roles and Todd emphasized the importance of early diagnosis and treatment in reducing mortality associated with bronchiectasis.[36] Over the ensuing years, other authors such as Field[74] emphasized the importance of treatment "Even with simple medical treatment, the progress of most cases can be arrested...."[74] In bronchiectasis secondary to CF and primary ciliary dyskinesia, aggressive management of infections with antimicrobials, regular use of airway clearance methods, attention to nutrition, coupled with vigilant monitoring of long-term clinical trends, and proactive care led to improved survival and preservation of lung function.[191] CF produces a specific type of progressive bronchiectasis that differs from other forms of bronchiectasis with respect to mucus rheology, airway surface abnormalities, salt content, airway microbial pathogens, and extrapulmonary organ involvement. Although blind extrapolation of management used in CF to non-CF bronchiectasis can be harmful,[192] management of children with bronchiectasis should be arguably as intensive in children with idiopathic bronchiectasis to minimize acute exacerbations, daily symptoms, and functional limitations; thus improving the prognosis. Indeed, more recent data have provided evidence that intensive treatment of children who either have bronchiectasis or who are at risk of developing severe bronchiectasis prevents poor lung function in adulthood.[79,193] Even among children with serious underlying conditions, such as congenital immunodeficiencies and bronchiectasis, comprehensive regular care and surveillance programs have delayed decline in lung function over a period of a year.[194]

The aims of regular review include optimal postnatal lung growth, prevention of premature respiratory decline, maximal QoL, and prevention of complications due to bronchiectasis. Issues that require regular monitoring are listed in Box 26.3. Ideally, a team approach with incorporation of allied health expertise (nursing, physiotherapy, nutritionist, social work) should be used, as this model has been shown to improve health outcomes for several chronic diseases.[195] Evidence-based guidelines of management of bronchiectasis in children have been published since 2002 and subsequently updated,[190] and adults have been included.[196] An umbrella Cochrane review on the interventions for bronchiectasis has been published.[197]

Box 26.3 Management Issues for Regular Review

1. Accurate diagnoses of underlying etiology and conditions that aggravate bronchiectasis
2. Philosophy of antibiotics use (maintenance, intermittent, regular hospitalizations)
3. Airway pathogens and drug-sensitivity profiles
4. Effectiveness of mucociliary clearance techniques
5. Nutritional state and support
6. Psychosocial support and adherence issues
7. Pattern and frequency of acute respiratory exacerbations
8. Presence of comorbid conditions
9. Education and promotion of self-management
10. Preventive measures (environment assessment, vaccines)
11. Indications for surgical resection of bronchiectatic regions
12. Complications related to bronchiectasis (e.g., hemoptysis, lung abscess, pulmonary hypertension, sleep disorders, reactive airway disease)
13. Review of new therapies and therapeutic strategies as they emerge, for example, macrolide use for antiinflammatory, antisecretagogue effects.

Antimicrobials

Antimicrobial treatment is a key intervention in the management of patients with bronchiectasis.[109] In stable adult patients, there was a direct relationship between bacterial load and the risk of both subsequent and severe exacerbations (ORs of 1.2, 95% CI 1.1 to 1.3 and 1.1, 95% CI 1.0 to 1.2; respectively).[112] However, there are few published randomized controlled treatment trials on childhood bronchiectasis and none that focus on acute exacerbations.[198] Brief antimicrobial interventions significantly improve the inflammatory profile in the airways,[199,200] and blood,[199,200] sputum production, cough frequency, and QoL measures.[200,201] Use of antimicrobials for bronchiectasis was recently summarized.[109]

In general, the type of antimicrobial should target known pathogens and the route dependent on the severity of the illness and response to previous treatments.[109,190] Ideally, a sputum culture should be obtained prior to initiating antibiotics. Oral antibiotics are usually prescribed initially, but more severe episodes, or failure to improve with oral agents, require intravenous antibiotics combined with more intensive airway clearance techniques. Although robust evidence is lacking, a course of antibiotics for 14 days has been recommended by respiratory specialists.[112,190]

Comprehensive care programs for bronchiectasis have used both intermittent antibiotics to treat exacerbations and chronic or maintenance antibiotic treatment strategies. The use of maintenance antimicrobials may be suitable in selected situations where frequent exacerbations are likely to occur. Old studies in adults demonstrated that regular use of macrolides and trimethoprim reduced pulmonary inflammation, infective exacerbations and improved lung function.[202,203] A pediatric randomized controlled trial (RCT) involving 25 children (12 weeks of roxithromycin 4 mg/kg twice a day or placebo) also described a significant improvement in sputum markers and of airway responsiveness in the roxithromycin group, but improvements in FEV_1 were not observed in either group.[204] More recent studies in adults and children have confirmed these findings.[205] However, many questions remain, such as when should maintenance antibiotics be started and in whom, what is the optimal duration (studies suggest effects are evident only after 3 months), whether macrolides are the best choice of maintenance treatment, and which macrolides to use. Other questions are the optimal type and dosing regimen (daily-to-weekly) and whether associated increases in S. aureus and other macrolide-resistant bacteria are harmful at individual or community levels.[206] The latest Cochrane review (children and adults included) consisted of 18 studies whereby the meta-analysis showed that in patients with at least one exacerbation, the use of maintenance antibiotics (for >4 weeks) significantly reduced exacerbations compared to placebo or usual care with a reduction of 275 exacerbations per 1000.[205] Hospitalization was also reduced (50 fewer hospitalizations per 1000 people treated).[205] There was a threefold higher likelihood of antibiotic resistance in the group using maintenance antibiotics.[205] However, in the sole RCT that reported on use of antibiotics for conditions other than respiratory exacerbations, those in the antibiotic arm required 50% less other antibiotics (Incidence Rate Ratio = 0.5, 95% CI 0.31 to 0.81).[80] The factors affecting the risk of development of resistance to long-term macrolide therapy are adherence (adherence ≥70% reduces risk OR 0.34, 95% CI 0.14 to 0.81 compared to <70%) and baseline macrolide resistance rate.[207] The majority of the long-term studies used macrolides that have antiinflammatory and antisecretagogue effects.[208]

Antiinflammatory and Antioxidant Agents

In 18 children with CF and 15 children with idiopathic bronchiectasis, 6 months of beta-carotene supplementation reduced plasma levels of TNF-α and malondialdehyde, a marker of lipid peroxidation,[209] but did not change clinical status. In adults with bronchiectasis, nonsteroidal antiinflammatory agents have a major effect on peripheral neutrophil function, significantly reducing neutrophil chemotaxis and fibronectin degradation by resting and stimulated neutrophils, but they had no effect on bacterial colonization of the airways or superoxide anion generation by neutrophils.[210] There are no studies on oral nonsteroidal antiinflammatory drugs (NSAIDs), but a Cochrane review on inhaled NSAIDs found a single trial in CSLD.[211] In adults with bronchiectasis, Tamaoki et al. reported a significant reduction in sputum production over 14 days in the treatment group (4 days of inhaled indomethacin) compared to placebo and significant improvement in a dyspnea score.[212] There was no significant difference between groups in lung function or blood indices. Emerging drugs in development have been recently reviewed.[213]

Antisecretagogues and Mucoactive Agents

Mucoactive agents enhance mucus clearance from the respiratory tract in conditions where mucus clearance is impaired.[104] Mucolytics reduce mucus crosslinking and viscosity by disruption of polymer networks in the secretions through severing disulfide bonds, depolymerizing mucopolysaccharides, liquefying proteins, and degrading DNA filaments and actin.[104] In adults, high doses of bromhexine (not available in some countries) used with antibiotics eased difficulty in expectoration and reduced sputum production.[197] Recombinant deoxyribonuclease (rhDNAse) is efficacious in CF but is contraindicated in non-CF bronchiectasis. In a double-blind, RCT, multicenter study for 24-weeks in 349 adults with bronchiectasis, those given rhDNAse had higher exacerbation and hospitalization rates and more rapid pulmonary decline (decrease in FEV_1 3.6% in rhDNase group; 1.6% in placebo group).[192] Inhaled osmotic agents, such as 7% hypertonic saline and mannitol, improve airway clearance and lung function and reduce exacerbation frequency in people with CF but studies in adults with non-CF bronchiectasis show a benefit only in time to first exacerbation and QoL and not in exacerbation rates.[214] There are no studies in children and clinically selected children can be commenced on hypertonic saline. When used, pretreatment with a short-acting bronchodilator is recommended to avoid bronchospasm, which occurs in up to 30% of patients.

Antisecretagogues reduce airway mucus production and secretion. These agents include anticholinergic agents, macrolide antibiotics, and bromhexine. Fourteen-member-ring macrolides are antibiotics with antiinflammatory activities and their use is discussed in the antimicrobials section. There are no RCTs on anticholinergics in the treatment of acute or stable bronchiectasis. Some anticholinergic agents such as atropine and glycopyrrolate slow mucociliary transport and predispose to further mucus stasis. An uncontrolled trial of tiotroprium in adults with hypersecretory states, including bronchiectasis that was resistant to macrolides, reduced daily symptoms and improved QoL with short-term use,[215] but it is not currently recommended in children.

Airway Clearance Methods

Although it is lacking a robust evidence-base,[216] airway clearance techniques (encompassing various types of chest physiotherapy) are recommended in children and adults.[190,196] Available studies suggest that airway clearance techniques are beneficial with improved QoL and exercise capacity and reduced cough and sputum volumes.[216] Thus daily chest physiotherapy is recommended in a form that maximizes potential benefit and minimizes burden of care. In the past, postural drainage was standard therapy for children with CSLD/bronchiectasis. However, this treatment may increase gastroesophageal reflux and possible aspiration.[217] Given the availability of multiple techniques for airway clearance and the lack of clear superiority of any one technique, specific choices should be individualized and pediatric-specific physiotherapist expertise sought. In addition, children with bronchiectasis should be encouraged to participate in exercise activities.

Asthma Therapy

Asthma in children with bronchiectasis should be treated on its own merits. Inhaled corticosteroids (ICS), at best, have a modest benefit in those with severe CSLD/bronchiectasis and those with *P. aeruginosa*.[218] The Cochrane review (six studies in adults, no pediatric studies) found that in the short term (ICS for <6 months duration), adults on very high doses of ICS (2 g per day of budesonide equivalent) had significantly improved FEV_1, FVC, QoL, and sputum volume but no improvement in peak flow, exacerbations, cough, or wheeze when compared to adults in the control arm (no ICS). When only placebo-controlled studies were included in the review, there were no significant differences between groups in any of the outcomes examined (spirometry, clinical outcomes of exacerbation or sputum volume). A single study on medium-term (>6 months) outcomes showed no significant effect of inhaled steroids on any of the outcomes.[218] There is no published RCT on the use of ICS for children with CSLD/bronchiectasis.[218] One study reported that 12-week withdrawal of ICS resulted in a significant increase in bronchial hyperreactivity and decrease in neutrophil apoptosis but no change in the children's clinical parameters or sputum inflammatory markers.[219] This suggests that ICS have little role in the management of CSLD/bronchiectasis in children when asthma does not coexist.

Short- and long-acting β-2 agonists also have an indeterminate role in the management of bronchiectasis,[197] and their use must be individualized. Although the presence of asthma is associated with advanced bronchiectasis and a worse prognosis, treatment of asthma to alter long-term outcomes has not been studied. It may be that the asthmatic features associated with diffuse bronchiectasis reflect the disease itself rather than a concurrent condition. Whether published guidelines for asthma care pertain to patients with wheeze and airway hyperactivity is unclear. Increased cough in children with bronchiectasis should be initially treated as an exacerbation of bronchiectasis.

Environmental Modification

In utero tobacco smoke exposure alters respiratory control and pulmonary development and physiology.[81,220] Tobacco smoke also skews the early immune function,[81] but its role in permanently altering local and systemic pulmonary immunity is unknown. Exposure to ETS increases susceptibility to respiratory infections, causes adverse respiratory health outcomes, and increases coughing illnesses.[81] Cessation of parental smoking reduces children's cough.[221] Behavioral counseling and motivational interviewing for smoking mothers reduces young children's ETS exposure in both reported and objective measures of ETS.[222]

Indoor wood smoke also increases acute respiratory infections, demonstrating an exposure-response effect.[223] Thus efforts to reduce smoke and biomass exposure including *in utero* exposure and children's exposure in the home must be maximized. There is low to moderate quality evidence that repairing houses decreases respiratory tract infections.[224]

Prevention: Vaccines

Vaccination as per national schedules is recommended. Many of the diseases described as causing bronchiectasis (e.g., pertussis and measles) are now controlled in developed countries. Vaccinations for prevention of influenza are recommended despite the lack of evidence specific for bronchiectasis.[225,226] While there is no specific evidence for influenza vaccine in those with CSLD/bronchiectasis,[225] indirect evidence suggests that annual influenza vaccinations reduce morbidity, mortality, and health care cost in "at risk" groups.[227] For pneumococcal vaccination, limited evidence supports the use of the 23-valent pneumococcal vaccine in reducing acute infective exacerbations.[226] 23-valent pneumococcal vaccine is recommended for high-risk children, including those with bronchiectasis.[228,229] Current evidence support revaccination, although the frequency of revaccination is controversial.[228] A recent study found that vaccination with the pneumococcal 10-serotype with *H. influenzae* protein D conjugate vaccine was associated with improvements in NTHi-specific cell-mediated and humoral immune responses in children with CSLD.[230] While this is promising, further confirmatory data are required.

Surgical Considerations

Surgery is considered most often when bronchiectasis is focal and medical therapy has failed. Surgery is very rarely undertaken now in affluent countries but is still a common intervention in less affluent countries.[231] Perioperative mortality for lobectomy and pneumonectomy has fallen dramatically. In a retrospective series of 109 children (mean age 7.6 years, range 1 to 15.5), 36% had minor postoperative complications (transient atelectasis in 26%, air leak 6%) and one child died within the 30-day postoperative period. Of the 83 children with an average follow-up period of 667 days, 76% showed improvement of clinical symptoms. This is similar to several reviews of surgical therapy for bronchiectasis; the compiled group of adult and pediatric patients experienced 1% mortality (6/597) and an operative complication rate of 8.5% (51/597).[232,233] Complications included empyema, bronchopulmonary fistula, hypotension, and bleeding, but surgical treatment of bronchiectasis was more effective in patients with localized disease.[233] Appearance of new

Box 26.4   Indications and Contraindications for Lobectomy

Indications

1. Poor control of symptoms (purulent sputum, frequent exacerbations) despite optimal medical therapy
2. Poor growth despite optimal medical therapy
3. Severe and recurrent hemoptysis uncontrolled by bronchial artery embolization

Relative Indications

1. Localized disease with moderate persistent symptoms

Contraindications

1. Widespread bronchiectasis
2. Young child (<6 years)
3. Minimally symptomatic disease

bronchiectasis following surgical management has been described.[52,234] Indications for surgical intervention are controversial, and data from the 1940 to 1950's cannot be applied given the major advances in antibiotics, airway clearance techniques, and nutrition supplementation, and socioeconomic standards among underserved populations. Our suggested indications for surgical intervention are outlined in Box 26.4. Although lung transplantation has been reported widely for patients with CF, this option has only been used for adults with end-stage non-CF bronchiectasis,[235] and outcomes following lung transplantation in children without CF have not been reported.

Social Determinants and Health Care

Finally, health cannot be isolated from social, economic, environmental, and educational issues. Health and health behaviors are closely linked to socioeconomic factors,[236,237] and increased poverty, with its associated consequences such as poor housing and poor water supply, is an independent risk factor for increased respiratory infections and associated mortality.[237] To effectively reduce the morbidity and mortality from CSLD and bronchiectasis in children, a multifaceted approach encompassing good clinical care and public health concerns bears consideration. Although it is beyond the scope of this article to address this important issue, future work must focus on the public health issues predisposing to childhood bronchiectasis if the disparity between developed and developing countries is to be reduced.

Delivery of chronic disease programs requires comprehensive and highly skilled culturally competent primary health care. Education of primary health providers should ideally focus on identifying children for appropriate referral and high quality local management. Initial assessment requires specialist expertise, and specialist evaluation is recommended to confirm diagnosis, investigate etiology, assess baseline severity, and develop a management plan. Similar to other chronic illnesses, individualized and multidisciplinary case management operating within an interprofessional framework is optimal. Similarly, deterioration should prompt early referral for specialist care. In addition, those with moderate or severe disease are best managed by a multidisciplinary team approach.

PROGNOSIS

Given the heterogeneity of etiological factors and host responses, regional severity, and distribution of bronchiectasis, it is not surprising that the prognosis is varied, ranging from mild respiratory morbidity to death from airway obstruction, pulmonary infection, and respiratory failure with hypercapnia. There are cases where bronchiectasis resolves radiographically with treatment.[22] However, these children remain at risk of developing bronchiectasis and should be monitored regularly for reemergence of symptoms and obstructive lung disease. More often, bronchiectasis persists on HRCT but becomes less severe clinically with fewer infectious exacerbations and less cough evident later in childhood. In a series of 46 children with HRCT–documented bronchiectasis, a third improved, a third remained symptomatic but stable, and a third worsened while receiving medical therapy[56] Both Field[131] and Landau et al.[238] reported reductions in exacerbations during the second and third decade of life despite persistence of bronchiectasis radiographically. What happens in the following decades is inferred from case series of adults with bronchiectasis, many of whom had onset of respiratory problems, if not bronchiectasis in childhood. However, these series do not depict the era of minimal symptoms that occur at adolescence and anecdotally reappear at age 35 to 40 years old.

There are three published studies (all retrospective) on longitudinal FEV_1 changes in children with non-CF bronchiectasis studied over variable intervals with varying results.[79,239,240] A British study (n = 59 over 2 years, n = 31 over 4 years) found that lung function improves with intensive treatment but does not necessary normalize.[239] Likewise, an Australian study (n = 52 over 3 years, n = 25 over 5 years)[79] found that lung function and anthropometric parameters remain stable over a 3- to 5-year follow-up period once appropriate therapy is instituted, and those with low function at diagnosis (FEV_1 % predicted <80%) improved with time.[79] In contrast, a New Zealand (NZ) study of 44 children over 4.5 years found that FEV_1 declined at 1.9% per annum.[240] The explanations for this contrast are speculative but likely include the different age groups, children from different ethnicities, and health care differences. Also, the NZ cohort had more extensive radiological disease with 89% bilateral disease (median of four diseased lobes, 95% with multilobar involvement). The Brisbane study found that the only significant predictor of FEV_1 decline (over 3 years) was frequency of exacerbations requiring hospitalization[79] The other two cohorts[239,240] did not examine for determinants of lung function decline.

Published data also suggest that delayed diagnosis is associated with poorer outcomes.[27,79] A large study of adults newly diagnosed with bronchiectasis showed that the decline in FEV_1 correlates with the duration of chronic wet cough,[37] the most common symptom of bronchiectasis.[241] For each additional year of productive cough, FEV_1% predicted declined by 0.51% in nonsmokers.[37] Adults with bronchiectasis who were symptomatic from childhood have much poorer lung function and worse chest CT scan scores than those with adult-onset symptoms.[37] In the Brisbane longitudinal study, children diagnosed earlier and hence managed earlier were significantly younger and had better long-term spirometry and growth parameters.[79] FEV_1% predicted decreased by

1.64% points for each year increase in age at diagnosis, but this was statistically nonsignificant.[79]

When bronchiectasis worsens, it may become increasingly saccular within a local lung region (see Figs. 26.2 and 26.3). Alternatively, bronchiectasis can extend to additional airways, either due to endobronchial spread of infection or evolution of disease at multiple airway sites. The frequency with which bronchiectasis extends to new lung regions varies with different series, from 2% to 35%.[242,243] Local progression of disease rather than extension to new areas is likely more common.

The most severe cases of bronchiectasis have diffuse airway involvement and are accompanied by airflow limitation, with or without concomitant airway hyperreactivity. The diagnosis of asthma in the context of an underlying lung disease may be difficult. Wheeze and asthma symptoms are common in people with CSLD/bronchiectasis, although reported prevalence varies from 11% to 46%.[57,244] While some studies describe asthma as a cause of bronchiectasis, it is more likely that wheezing illness is a secondary or coexistent condition or that asthma was initially misdiagnosed. Asthmalike symptoms in adults with bronchiectasis may be associated with an accelerated decline in lung function.[137] King reported that increased use of bronchodilators led to a trend of a greater FEV_1 decline over time in adults.[245] The NZ cohort found that while the presence of asthma was associated with lower FEV_1 at diagnosis, asthmatics had a slower rate of decline over the 5-year follow-up.[240]

Unfavorable prognostic factors for patients with bronchiectasis include presence of asthma, bilateral lung involvement,[131,246] saccular bronchiectasis,[246] frequency of exacerbations, and presence of *P. aeruginosa* in the airways.[181] The advent of better antibiotics, inhaled antibiotics, long-term oxygen therapy, and improved nutrition has improved prognosis. Cor pulmonale and right heart failure are now uncommon complications of advanced bronchiectasis in children. In one series, echocardiography in 50 children with bronchiectasis found only one child with pulmonary hypertension.[52] In addition, chronic lung infection and inflammation are independent risk factors for developing cardiovascular disease in adults.[247]

Protracted Bacterial Bronchitis

EPIDEMIOLOGY AND DISEASE BURDEN

Prior to a diagnosis of PBB, most children with a chronic wet cough received multiple medications and consulted several health physicians.[34,248] An Australian multicenter study found 70% of 138 children with PBB had received asthma medications, and 76% had seen greater than five doctors previously because of persistent cough.[249] However, these findings were also similar to children with a chronic cough from other causes.[249] QoL scores of children with PBB were similar to children with cough due to asthma or bronchiectasis presenting to pediatric pulmonologists.[249,250] Importantly, QoL scores normalized once the cough resolved.[251] While the prevalence of PBB cases in the community clinics is unknown, studies from specialist clinics (pediatrics and/or pediatric pulmonology) from Australia[23,34] and Turkey[252,253] found PBB to be among the top three diagnoses in children

with chronic cough, with the prevalence ranging from 6% to 42%.[11]

PATHOLOGY AND PATHOGENESIS

Microbiology

In the first description of PBB,[23] BAL cultures grew the common respiratory bacterial pathogens, *S. pneumoniae*, *H. influenza*, and *M. catarrhalis* (Fig. 26.8). Subsequent studies confirmed this finding, although one retrospective study also identified *S. aureus* (11 of 50 children),[254] but quantitative bacteriology was not performed, making interpretation difficult. One study examined the presence of respiratory viruses in children with PBB.[255] This study reported rates of 39% for viruses detected by polymerase chain reaction (PCR) in the BAL fluid from 104 PBB cases compared to 9% of 49 other chronic respiratory disease controls (OR = 6.3, 95% CI 2.1 to 19.1). The most common virus identified was adenovirus (AdV),[255] which upon genotyping, belonged predominantly to AdV species C.[182]

The presence and role of biofilms in the BAL of children with PBB have not been studied, but their presence has been speculated.[11] The microbiota of the lungs of children with PBB has been examined in a single cross-sectional study.[9] One-way analysis of variance showed the Shannon-Weiner index (a measure of species diversity) of the lower airway microbiota in children with PBB, and bronchiectasis were similar and statistically higher (i.e., richer) than in CF. The lung microbiota in children were significantly different from those observed in adults with CF and bronchiectasis, suggesting that chronic airway infections begin similarly with

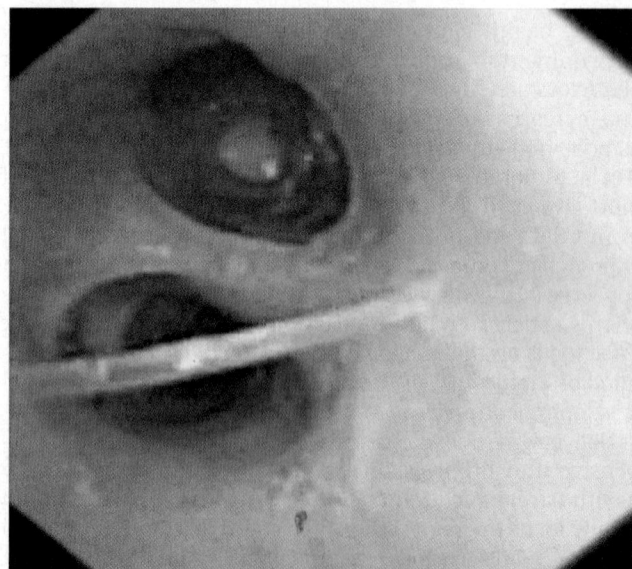

Fig. 26.8 Bronchoscopic picture from a child with protracted bacterial bronchitis. The picture shows a strand of mucus just proximal to the left lower lobe bronchus and prominent secretions in the left lingula bronchus. The bronchoscopic appearances in children with protracted bacterial bronchitis are similar to those seen in mild bronchiectasis. The bronchoalveolar lavage from this child cultured *Haemophilus influenzae* and *Streptococcus pneumoniae*, both at a density of greater than 10^5 cfu/mL. Polymerase chain reaction for respiratory viruses (influenza A and B, RSV, parainfluenza 1-2, adenovirus, human metapneumovirus), *Mycoplasma* and *Chlamydia* were negative.

defective airway clearance of otherwise normal airway microbiota. Over time with antibiotic treatment and perhaps the effects of the underlying disease, the microbiota in these disease groups progressively diverge.[11,182]

Immunity and Inflammation. Studies on immunity in children with PBB[11] reported the following features: (1) absence of an overt systemic immunodeficiency (normal serum IgA, IgM, IgG, and IgE levels), (2) robust responses to protein (tetanus) and conjugated protein-polysaccharide (*H. influenzae type b*) vaccines,[255] and (3) upregulated innate immunity (e.g., elevated TLR-2, TLR-4, human β-defensin 2 [hBD2], and mannose-binding lectin [MBL][125]). A small BAL-based study described significantly decreased ability of alveolar macrophages to phagocytose apoptotic bronchial cells and NTHi in children with PBB (n = 13) compared to controls (n = 13).[122] For both types of impaired phagocytosis, the values in children with PBB were intermediate to those with bronchiectasis and controls (median phagocytosis of NTHi: bronchiectasis = 13.7% [IQR 11% to 16%], PBB = 16% [11 to 16], controls = 19.0% [13 to 21]; and median efferocytosis values were 14.1% [10 to 16], 16.2% [14 to 17] and 18.1 [16 to 21], respectively).[122]

BAL from children with PBB typically shows intense airway neutrophilia (median 40% to 44%).Whether this is a pathologically disproportionate response to infection is unknown.[11] There are also marked proinflammatory mediator responses (increased IL-8, MMP-9, and IL-1β) that correlate with BAL neutrophil percentages.[256,257] Median BAL levels of IL-8 and MMP-9 in children with PBB were 5- to 19-fold higher than controls and children whose cough resolved without treatment.[256] Children with PBB had significantly higher BAL fluid levels of IL-1β, α-defensin, IL-1 pathway members and CXCR2 gene and protein expression than non-PBB disease controls.[257] IL-1β levels correlated with duration and severity of cough,[257] and with elevated expression of α-defensins 1 to 3 in PBB cases. In those with recurrent PBB (>3 in the next 12 months), gene expression of the IL-1β signaling molecules pellino-1 and IL-1 receptor associated kinase (IRAK)-2 (in BAL at initial bronchoscopy) were significantly higher than those without recurrent PBB, suggesting this pathway's involvement in recurrence.[257] Thus, "PBB is characterized by increased IL-1β pathway activation. IL-1β and related mediators were associated with BAL neutrophils, cough symptoms, and disease recurrence, providing insight into PBB pathogenesis."[257]

Large Airway Lesions. While some clinicians believe TBM causes chronic ineffective cough, it is as likely that the airway malacia predisposes individuals to prolonged, inefficient airway clearance and hence increases risk of infection. Since the cough resolves once the underlying infection is treated, this suggests malacia has a limited causative role.[23] Nevertheless, TBM is found commonly in children with PBB.[23,258] This association may be primary (airway malacia predisposes to PBB through reduced efficiency in airway clearance) or secondary (malacia developing because of intense airway inflammation and infection).[161,259] One retrospective study reported TBM was present in 52/74 (74%) children with PBB.[258] However, a prospective study involving 104 children with PBB found that these airway abnormalities were no more common in children with PBB than in those undergoing bronchoscopy for other respiratory indications at a tertiary pediatric hospital (68% vs. 53%, respectively).[255] However, it has been shown in a prospective study that, children with TBM (c.f. controls) have a higher frequency of respiratory infections and symptoms.[260,261]

CLINICAL FEATURES

Symptoms and Signs

Children with PBB have a chronic wet cough but otherwise typically appear well with an absence of recurrent nasal or ear disease. They have normal growth and development, and lack signs of underlying CSLD. The prevalence of atopic features (eczema, systemic and airway eosinophilia, elevated IgE, or positive radioallergosorbent test) is similar to children without PBB.[255] While many parents report previous "ever wheeze" (41% to 81%),[255,262] wheeze on auscultation confirmed by doctors is unusual. Occasionally, a "rattly chest" can be palpated and crackles are heard.

Imaging and Pulmonary Function Tests

The chest radiograph is normal or near-normal, showing only peribronchial changes.[12,249,263] When performed, both spirometry[249] and respiratory system reactance and resistance measured by FOT are normal.[11] Laboratory findings, when undertaken, show absence of serum neutrophilia or systemic inflammation (CRP and erythrocyte sedimentation rate [ESR] normal).

DIAGNOSIS AND DIFFERENTIAL DIAGNOSIS

Defining Protracted Bacterial Bronchitis

When PBB was first described in 2006,[23] its existence as a distinct diagnostic entity was controversial. However, it is becoming recognized increasingly and is now incorporated into all national pediatric chronic cough guidelines.[11] It is also forms part of the European pediatric respiratory training curriculum.[264] PBB was first defined *a priori* and was based on clinical experience before being applied to a subgroup of children in a prospective study evaluating the etiology of chronic cough.[23] The diagnostic criteria were (1) history of chronic wet cough, (2) positive BAL cultures for respiratory bacterial pathogens at densities ≥10⁴ cfu/mL without serologic or PCR assay evidence of infection by either *Bordatella pertussis* or *Mycoplasma pneumoniae*, and (3) cough resolution after a 2-week course of oral antibiotics (amoxicillin-clavulanate).[23] The consideration of feasibility in day-to-day clinical practice and further research has resulted in definitions (Box 26.5) based on recurrence and clinical setting.[11] Each criteria has been validated.[11] However, uncertainties remain and include (1) diagnosis can only be determined after a trial of therapy, (2) lack of research data on an optimal length of antibiotics, and (3) uncertainty of the diagnostic threshold for determining lower airway infection.[11]

Differentiation between acute bronchitis and PBB is because acute bronchitis cough usually resolves within 2 to 4 weeks. Difficulties arise when recurrent and acute bronchitis episodes overlap, especially during the "respiratory virus" season.[11] Furthermore, PBB can coexist with other illnesses, including asthma, and recurrent episodes need to be differentiated from bronchiectasis when chronic wet cough does not respond to greater than 4 weeks of oral antibiotics.[268] Among 105 children with persistent cough despite at least 4 weeks of antibiotics, 88 (83.8%) had bronchiectasis; of the 24 children whose cough resolved after antibiotics, only six (25.0%)

received this diagnosis (adjusted OR 20.9; 95% CI 5.4 to 81.8).[268]

Differential Diagnosis

There are many causes of chronic wet cough in children, and further investigation to elucidate the cause is necessary when the child does not respond to antibiotics and/or has other clinical features, for example, coughing with feeds.[11,179] These are addressed elsewhere in this textbook.

Bronchitis is a component of many airway diseases. In the literal translation of the word, bronchitis refers to inflammation of the bronchus or bronchi. However, bronchitis has different major overlapping constructs based on duration (acute, subacute, chronic), inflammation type (neutrophilic, eosinophilic, lymphocytic, neurogenic), phenotype, or clinical syndromes (e.g., acute bronchitis, larygnotracheobronchitis, PBB, aspiration bronchitis). A diagnostic entity may have varying types of airway inflammation (Table 26.4). For example, acute viral bronchitis is associated with both lymphocytic and neutrophilic inflammation. Although the types of airway inflammation do not distinguish etiology of the bronchitis in children, it provides support for the diagnosis. Cough usually occurs when bronchitis is present.

Chronic (>4 weeks) wet cough in children signifies the persistence of increased airway secretion production or decreased airway clearance in the large airways.[283] The greater the amount of secretions seen at bronchoscopy, the higher the likelihood of bacterial infection and intense neutrophilia in the airways.[284] Clinicians need to be cognizant that recognition of wet cough is dependent on the clinical setting, and it is also likely age dependent. It is easier to detect a wet cough in young children, while older children may have a productive cough but may have a dry cough when asked to cough. Parents and clinicians have varying ability to recognize cough quality. In Australia, Brisbane-based parents were more accurate in determining the type of cough (compared to pulmonologists [kappa = 0.75, 95% CI 0.58

Box 26.5 Diagnostic Criteria for Protracted Bacterial Bronchitis

1. Original microbiologic-based case definition[23] (also termed PBB-micro)
   a. Presence of chronic wet cough (>4 weeks)
   b. Lower airway infection (recognized respiratory bacterial pathogens growing in sputum or BAL at density of a single bacterial specifies ≥10^4 colony-forming units/mL)
   c. Cough resolved following a 2-week course of an appropriate oral antibiotic (usually amoxicillin-clavulanate)
2. Modified clinical-based case definition[265] (also termed PBB-clinical)
   a. Presence of chronic wet cough (>4 weeks)
   b. Absence of symptoms or signs of other causes of wet or productive cough[a]
   c. Cough resolved following a 2-week course of an appropriate oral antibiotic (usually amoxicillin-clavulanate)
3. PBB-extended = PBB-clinical or PBB-micro, but cough resolves only after 4 weeks of antibiotics.
4. Recurrent PBB = recurrent episodes (>3 per year) of PBB.

[a]Specific cough pointers[265–267] are: chest pain, history suggestive of inhaled foreign body, dyspnea, exertional dyspnea, hemoptysis, failure to thrive, feeding difficulties (including choking/vomiting), cardiac or neurodevelopmental abnormalities, recurrent sinopulmonary infections, immunodeficiency, epidemiological risk factors for exposure to tuberculosis, signs of respiratory distress, digital clubbing, chest wall deformity, auscultatory crackles, chest radiographic changes (other than perihilar changes), lung function abnormalities.

BAL, Bronchoalveolar lavage; *PBB*, protracted bacterial bronchitis.

Chang AB, Upham JW, Masters IB, et al. State of the art. Protracted bacterial bronchitis: the last decade and the road ahead. Pediatr Pulmonol. 2016;51:225-242.

Table 26.4 Dominant Type of Airway Cellularity in Selected Childhood Diseases With Bronchitis

Inflammation Type	Examples of Disease	Other Key Airway Makers
Neutrophilic	Acute viral infection[269]	Soluble intercellular adhesion molecule-1
	Bronchiectasis[116,128]	Elevated IL-8, neutrophil elastase, TNF-α, IL-1β
	Cystic fibrosis[270]	Elevated IL-8, neutrophil elastase, proteases
	Protracted bacterial bronchitis[11,257]	Elevated IL-8, MMP-9, IL-1β and related mediators that reflect IL-1β pathway activation
	Chronic lung disease of prematurity[271]	Proinflammatory cytokines and chemokines
	Severe bronchiolitis[272,273]	Myeloperoxidase, CD11b
		RSV proteins and mRNA transcripts in severe RSV bronchiolitis
	Bronchiolitis obliterans[274]	Elevated IL-6, IL-8, TNF-α, IL-1β
	Aspiration lung disease[275]	Index of lipid-laden macrophages (nonspecific marker), amylase, pepsin (still needs validation)
Eosinophilic	Atopic asthma[276]	Elevated nitric oxide in steroid naive
	Helminth infections[111] e.g., toxocara and strongyloides	
	Allergic bronchopulmonary aspergillosis[277]	Neutrophilic inflammation may also be present with elevated IL-8 and MMP-9
	Hypersensitivity, eosinophilic pneumonia[278]	
Lymphocytic	Acute viral infection[269]	Soluble intercellular adhesion molecule-1
	Bronchiolitis obliterans[279,274]	CD8+T lymphocytes
	Autoimmune disease*[280]	
Neurogenic	Post RSV infection[281]	substance P, nerve growth factor
	Cough with gastroesophageal reflux[282]	Calcitonin G-related peptide

to 0.93] and flexible bronchoscopy findings),[283] whereas Indigenous caregivers were less accurate.[285]

MANAGEMENT AND TREATMENT

There is high-quality evidence that in children with greater than 4 weeks' duration of wet or productive cough, the use of appropriate antibiotics improves cough resolution.[179] In PBB, the child's cough resolves only after a 2-week course of appropriate antibiotics, in contrast to shorter durations of treatment.[23,286] Meta-analyses of three RCTs that used 10 to 14 days of antibiotics for chronic wet cough found that the number needed to treat (for benefit by end of study) was 3 (95% CI 2.0 to 4.3) Although the British Thoracic Society (BTS) cough guidelines[287] suggest all children with PBB should receive 4 to 6 weeks of antibiotics, there is no prospectively derived evidence for this. While some children with PBB may need longer antibiotic treatment, we advocate the shorter 2-week course initially.[11]

PROGNOSIS

The rate and risk factors of PBB recurrence are likely dependent on the sampling frame and definition. Factors in those severe enough to need to bronchoscopy and BAL sampling are probably different from those enrolled from the community. The sole prospective study to date was undertaken in 106 children with PBB followed for a median of 25 months (IQR 24 to 28).[288] Their median age at bronchoscopy was 23 months (IQR 14 to 53). At the 24-month follow-up, children with PBB were more likely to be coughing compared with controls (44% vs. 12% of respective cohort, $P = .005$) and to have had parent-reported wheeze in the preceding 12 months (58% vs. 16%, $P = .001$). By the end of the study, 66 (62%) of those with PBB had experienced recurrent episodes (>3 per year) and 13 (12%) had bronchiectasis diagnosed by chest CT scans.[288] The major independent risk factors for bronchiectasis were *H. influenzae* (mainly NTHi) lower airway infection and having ≥2 siblings. *H. influenzae* infection conferred greater than six times higher risk of bronchiectasis than a *H. influenzae* negative state (hazard ratio = 6.8, 95% CI 1.5 to 30.8).[288]

ACKNOWLEDGMENT

We are grateful to Dr. Rosalyn Singleton for her expert comments and critique on the chapter published in the 7th edition of this textbook.

References

Access the reference list online at ExpertConsult.com.

Suggested Reading

Chang AB, Oppenheimer JJ, Weinberger M, et al. Children with chronic wet or productive cough: treatment and investigations: a systematic review. *Chest.* 2016;149(1):120–142.
Chang AB, Upham JW, Masters IB, et al. State of the Art: protracted bacterial bronchitis: the last decade and the road ahead. *Pediatr Pulmonol.* 2016;51(3):225–242.
Goyal V, Grimwood K, Marchant JM, et al. State of the Art: bronchiectasis in children: no longer an orphan disease. *Pediatr Pulmonol.* 2016; 51(5):450–469.

27 Influenza

SUCHITRA RAO, MBBS, ANN-CHRISTINE NYQUIST, MD, MSPH, and PAUL C. STILLWELL, MD

Introduction

Influenza viruses are enveloped ribonucleic acid (RNA) viruses and belong to the family Orthomyxoviridae. There are three virus types within this family: influenza A, B, and C. Influenza A and B viruses are the types that predominantly infect humans, and A viruses are responsible for pandemic outbreaks of influenza and annual epidemics.[1]

The virus contains three important envelope glycoproteins: hemagglutinin (HA), neuraminidase (NA), and matrix proteins (M1 and M2). HA is the viral attachment protein responsible for entry of the virus into cells; it is an important surface antigen to which virus-neutralizing antibodies are directed. NA is an enzyme whose main function is to facilitate the cell-to-cell spread of virus; it is the target for the antiviral drugs zanamivir and oseltamivir. Antibody against HA is very protective against infection and illness, and antibody against NA can reduce illness severity. The matrix protein 2 (M2) is a structural protein linking the viral envelope with the virus core and is integral to the infectivity of the influenza virion. Influenza viruses have a segmented genome, containing eight strands of RNA. This property enables gene reassortment to occur among different subtypes of influenza, allowing new subtypes to form. Variation in the structure of HA and NA between influenza virions is the basis of the subtype H and N classification nomenclature (e.g. influenza A H1N1) (Fig. 27.1).

Influenza viruses have developed ways to evade the body's immune response using an antigenic variation known as antigenic *shift* and *drift*. Antigenic shift is seen only with influenza A viruses and results from the replacement of HA (or occasionally NA) with novel subtypes from other nonhuman influenza viruses. Introduction of a new HA into human viruses results in a pandemic, or worldwide epidemic, with the potential to cause millions of influenza-related deaths.[2]

Antigenic drift results from the accumulation of mutations within the antibody-binding sites in HA, NA, or both. These mutations prevent antibodies against previous strains from being effective against the current strain, enabling spread throughout a partially immune population. Antigenic drift occurs in both influenza A and B viruses.[3] Antigenic shift and drift must be taken into account when strains are being considered for inclusion in annual influenza vaccines.

Epidemiology

Human-to-human transmission of influenza occurs through small-particle aerosols or droplets, which enter the environment from an infected individual. The virus then binds to epithelial cells of the upper and lower respiratory tract. The incubation period from exposure to illness averages 2–3 days but can be as rapid as 18 hours or as long as 5 or more days. Healthy adults will shed influenza virus for 3–7 days, and young children may shed for 10 days or longer with generally higher viral titers.

Influenza occurs each year in winter through early spring and is associated with significant morbidity and mortality in certain high-risk populations (Table 27.1). In the United States up to 36,000 deaths per year are attributable to influenza, with people above 65 years of age accounting for more than 90% of deaths. Influenza is responsible for 5%–15% of upper respiratory tract infections in children.[4–6]

Healthy children aged 6–23 months are at substantially increased risk of influenza-related hospitalizations, and children aged 24–59 months remain at increased risk of influenza-related clinic and emergency department visits and hospitalizations but less so than younger children.

Pathology/Pathogenesis

Influenza virus infection begins with the attachment of viral HA to terminal sialic acids on the surface of target host cells. In the lungs, the target cells of the influenza virus are typically ciliated columnar epithelial or alveolar epithelial cells (AECs), with each HA subtype displaying a unique tropism. Attachment of the influenza virus triggers receptor-mediated endocytosis by host cells and thus entry into the cell. To effectively release influenza RNA into the cytosol, viral M2 forms ion channels in the viral envelope. Liberated viral RNA then travels to the nucleus of the infected cell, where messenger RNA (mRNA) and viral RNA are synthesized. Assembly and budding of daughter virions occurs at the cell surface, where NA facilitates virion release by cleavage of sialic acid attachments to viral HA. Without this cleavage, influenza virions aggregate at the cell surface and are not released, which is the mechanism by which NA inhibitors are effective.

Ultimately, viral infection leads to apoptosis of the infected epithelial cells, which denudes the airways, resulting in acute tracheobronchitis.[7–10] When type I AECs are damaged, the tight junctions of the alveolar capillary membrane allow a transudate of fluid and proteins to enter the alveolar spaces, producing acute alveolar damage with the potential of progressing to acute respiratory distress syndrome (ARDS).[11,12] Viral HA and M2 also inhibit the resorption of alveolar fluid by the epithelial sodium channel, further promoting alveolar edema. Influenza infection and resultant cytokine induction can also activate the endothelial pole of the alveolar capillary barrier, facilitating neutrophil influx and further disruption of barrier function.[11]

The host immune response to influenza infection is complex and redundant, incorporating both innate and adaptive processes (see Chapter 8 for details of innate and adaptive

AN INFLUENZA VIRUS

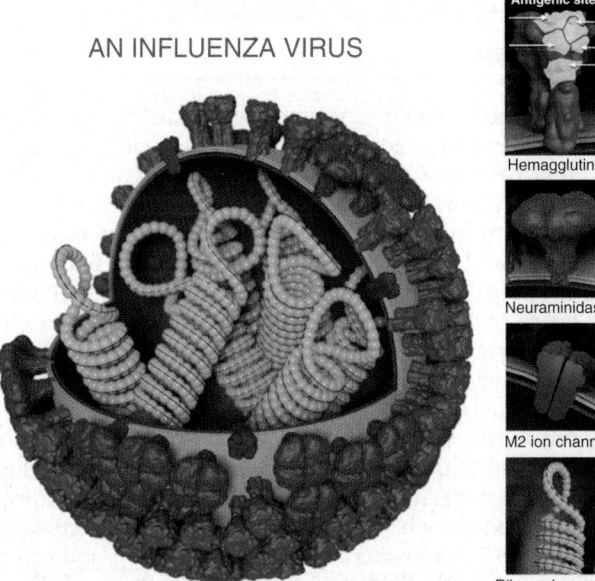

Antigenic sites

Hemagglutinin

Neuraminidase

M2 ion channel

Ribonucleoprotein

Fig. 27.1 Graphic representation of an influenza virion showing its structure and important components. *RNP,* Ribonucleoprotein. (From http://www.cdc.gov/flu/images.htm.)

Table 27.1 Individuals at High Risk for Influenza Complications

Hospitalized
Severe, complicated, or progressive illness
Children aged <2 years[a]
Individuals <19 years receiving long-term aspirin therapy
Adults aged ≥65 years
People of all ages with:
chronic pulmonary (including asthma), cardiovascular, renal, hepatic, metabolic (including diabetes), hematologic, neurologic (including seizure disorders) conditions; intellectual disability (mental retardation), moderate to severe developmental delay, and neurodevelopmental conditions
People with immunosuppression
Pregnant or recently postpartum women
American Indians/Alaska Natives
People who are morbidly obese (body mass index ≥40)
Residents of nursing homes or chronic care facilities

[a]Although all children below 5 years of age are considered at higher risk for complications from influenza, the highest risk is for those younger than 2 years, with the highest hospitalization and death rates among infants younger than 6 months.

immune responses).[8–10,13] In response to infections, activated macrophages and neutrophils work to eliminate viral particles and damaged or apoptotic epithelial cells. Although this is a key element in viral elimination and the recovery of epithelial integrity, the inflammatory by-products—such as myeloperoxidase, neutrophil elastases, and increased nitric oxide synthase—may cause further injury to the airway.[8,9] Increased risk of secondary bacterial infection may be due to delayed epithelial healing after influenza infection, excessive interferon gamma production, and type I interferons.[8,9]

The majority of systemic symptoms observed in acute influenza infection are attributable to the cytokines produced and released during the host immune response. Viremia is uncommon in an immunocompetent host. Similarly, dysfunction in nonrespiratory organs—such as myocarditis, encephalopathy, encephalitis, and rhabdomyolysis—is not usually associated with viral infection in those tissues.[9]

Viral infections can also stimulate the Th2 arm of the immune system by producing thymic stromal lymphopoietin (TSLP), IL-25, and IL-33. TSLP stimulates dendritic cells to induce Th2 cells and predisposes the host to allergic airway inflammation and asthma. IL-25 and IL-33 stimulate type 2 cytokine–producing innate lymphoid cells (ILC-2) to synthesize IL-5 and IL-13, which are promoters of eosinophilic inflammation, excessive mucus secretion, and bronchial hyperresponsiveness. This may explain, in part, how acute influenza infection exacerbates asthma and potentiates a subsequent asthma phenotype.[14,15]

Clinical Features

SYMPTOMS

There is great overlap in the symptomatology of influenza and other respiratory pathogens. The influenza syndrome usually has a sudden onset, associated with fever, headache, cough, sore throat, myalgia, nasal congestion, weakness, and loss of appetite.[16,17] In a retrospective study of adolescents and young adults with influenza-like illness, the best predictors of influenza infections were cough and fever, with a positive predictive value of 79%.[18] Young children, however, have a less classic presentation compared with adults and tend to have higher fevers, less prominent respiratory symptoms, and more gastrointestinal symptoms such as abdominal pain, vomiting, diarrhea, and decreased appetite.[16,19,20] Influenza infection is also an important cause of febrile seizures.[21]

Lower respiratory tract manifestations in young children are virtually indistinguishable from those due to other viral infections. Influenza, similar to other respiratory viruses, may cause bronchiolitis, interstitial pneumonia, laryngotracheitis (croup), bronchitis, exacerbations of asthma, wheezing, and pneumonia.[22] Extrapulmonary manifestations include myocarditis, hepatitis, encephalitis, myositis, renal insufficiency, Guillain-Barré syndrome, rhabdomyolysis, and multiorgan system failure.[23–28]

PHYSICAL FINDINGS

Findings on examination include tachypnea, conjunctival erythema, nasal injection, edema, nasal discharge, and cervical adenopathy. Rash is an uncommon manifestation of influenza, but when it occurs it is usually a generalized maculopapular rash sparing the palms and soles. Other rashes associated with influenza infection have been characterized as petechial, macular, papular, reticular, or purpuric; they can be localized and pruritic or nonpruritic.[29–34]

RADIOGRAPHIC FINDINGS

The chest radiographic features of influenza pneumonia are indistinguishable from those of pneumonia caused by other organisms.[35,36] The most common radiographic findings are

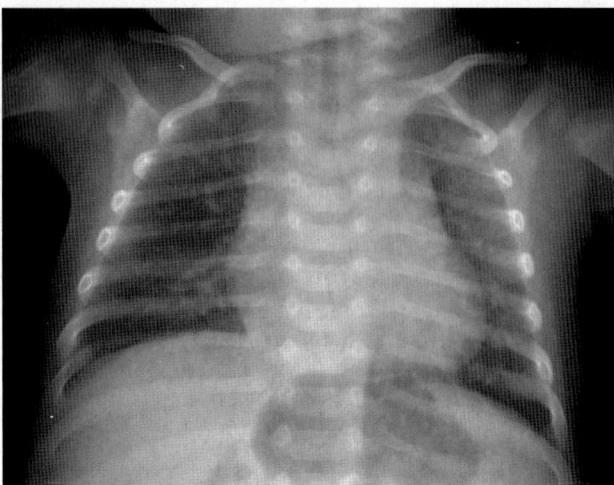

Fig. 27.2 Characteristic chest radiographic appearance of influenza pneumonia in a 13-month-old with influenza A (H3). (Courtesy Dr. Jason Weinman, University of Colorado School of Medicine Anschutz Medical Campus and Children's Hospital Colorado.)

bilateral, symmetric, perihilar, and peribronchial opacities, but focal opacities and asymmetric disease may also occur (Fig. 27.2).[36] Lymph node enlargement can occur, but pleural effusions are rare. The nonspecific findings make it challenging to differentiate viral from bacterial pneumonia based on the radiographic appearance alone. Younger children with influenza pneumonia may have bilateral patchy opacities that probably reflect the retention of mucus.[35] Progression of the pneumonia can lead to diffuse airspace disease with an ARDS picture and acute respiratory failure. Complete resolution to a normal chest radiograph should be expected following mild disease.

COMPLICATIONS

Children with chronic lung disease, asthma, airway disease, cardiovascular disease, neuromuscular disease, and immuno-compromised states are at highest risk of complicated influenza infection (see Table 27.1).[37] Severe influenza infection can present with bilateral pulmonary infiltrates and hypoxemia, leading to ARDS and death.[11,38-40] In particular, the 2009 H1N1 pandemic influenza virus was associated with higher rates of life-threatening lower respiratory tract illness, including ARDS, which was thought to be due to an increased predilection to infection of ciliated epithelial cells of the lower respiratory tract.[41-43] Pneumonia and secondary bacterial infection is a common cause of hospitalization from influenza.[44] Although *Streptococcus pneumoniae* is the most common pathogen identified, *Staphylococcus aureus* is a commonly associated copathogen. Methicillin-resistant *S. aureus* (MRSA) coinfections with influenza are increasingly being identified and are a risk factor for mortality in previously healthy children and adolescents.[45] Clinical features that support a bacterial superinfection among children with influenza include secondary fever after a period of defervescence, focal findings on pulmonary auscultation, lobar consolidation on chest imaging, and new onset of respiratory compromise occurring several days after initial symptoms.[46]

Diagnosis and Differential Diagnosis

Testing for influenza is recommended if positive or negative results will influence clinical management or clinical practice for other patients. Testing should be considered, regardless of immunization status, during the influenza season among children with fever and acute onset of respiratory signs and symptoms, and those with acute exacerbations of underlying chronic lung disease. Infants and young children with fever and no other signs and symptoms, hospitalized children with acute respiratory symptoms who develop an acute febrile respiratory illness, and severely ill children with fever or hypothermia should also be tested. Testing should occur at any time of the year for children who are epidemiologically linked to an influenza outbreak (e.g., household and close contacts of people with suspected influenza, returned travelers from countries where influenza viruses may be circulating, participants in international mass gatherings, and cruise ship passengers).[47] Testing 5 days or more beyond illness onset may result in false-negative test results because of decreased viral shedding; this occurs in particular among older children.

Testing modalities available include influenza-specific reverse transcription polymerase chain reaction (RT-PCR), multiplex respiratory pathogen PCR, direct fluorescent antibody (DFA) tests, and rapid influenza antigen tests. RT-PCR is the most accurate testing modality for influenza; it is useful for differentiating between influenza types and subtypes and is significantly more sensitive than rapid influenza antigen detection tests (>95% vs. 10%–70%, respectively). Rapid antigen tests have less sensitivity and specificity than RT-PCR tests. A meta-analysis of children demonstrated sensitivity of 64.6% for influenza A and 52.2% for influenza B.[48] These and other studies indicate that rapid antigen tests are not reliable during periods of low influenza activity. Immunofluorescent antibody testing can distinguish between influenza A or B and other respiratory viruses. However, the test performance is dependent on the quality of the respiratory specimen and expertise of the laboratory.

Viral culture is usually unhelpful in the clinical setting because results are not available until 48–72 hours later. However, it is helpful for the confirmation of screening results, surveillance, and research. Serologic testing is also not helpful in the clinical setting because acute and convalescent (obtained 10 days later) sera are required for diagnosis. Testing platforms include hemagglutination-inhibition, enzyme-linked immunosorbent assays (ELISA) and complement fixation assays. A fourfold rise or greater in antibody titers between acute and convalescent specimens confirms the diagnosis of influenza.

The differential diagnosis of influenza infection is listed in Table 27.2.[22]

Management and Treatment

TREATMENT

Clinical trials and observational data show that early antiviral treatment can shorten the duration of fever, influenza symptoms, and hospitalization; it may also reduce the risk of complications from influenza (e.g., otitis media in young children, pneumonia, respiratory failure, and death).[49-54] Clinical benefit is greatest when antiviral treatment is administered early, especially within 48 hours of influenza illness onset.[49,55,56] Treatment should not wait for laboratory confirmation of influenza but should be started as soon as possible when clinically indicated.

Antiviral treatment is recommended regardless of the day of illness for any patient with confirmed or suspected influenza who is hospitalized; has severe, complicated, or progressive illness; or is an outpatient who is at higher risk for influenza complications based on age or underlying medical conditions. Clinical judgment—based on the patient's disease severity and progression, age, underlying medical conditions, likelihood of influenza, and time since onset of symptoms—is important in making decisions regarding antiviral treatment for high-risk outpatients. Antiviral treatment may be considered for any outpatient with confirmed or suspected influenza who is otherwise healthy if treatment can be initiated within 48 hours of illness onset.

Neuraminidase inhibitors (NAIs) oseltamivir and zanamivir are the antiviral medications still recommended for the treatment and chemoprophylaxis of influenza A and influenza B virus infections owing to near universal susceptibility. They inhibit the viral NA enzyme that helps progeny escape from infected cells. NAIs may also have efficacy against the novel influenza viruses. Oseltamivir is given orally for 5 days with dose adjustments required for renal impairment and weight (Table 27.3). The most common side effects of oseltamivir are nausea and/or vomiting. Transient neuropsychiatric events (self-injury or delirium) have been reported, mainly among Japanese adolescents and adults.[57] Zanamivir is a dry powder administered via oral inhalation. It is not FDA-approved for the treatment of children under 7 years of age. The dose is two breath-activated inhalations twice daily for 5 days. The prophylactic dose is two inhalations once daily for children 5 years of age and older. It is not recommended for children with underlying airway disease including asthma owing to lack of safety and efficacy data in these individuals. Serious adverse events include bronchospasm and decline in lung function, most commonly seen in patients with underlying airway disease. (If zanamivir is used in patients with underlying airway disease, they should be instructed to have a short-acting bronchodilator available.) Allergic reactions including rashes and oropharyngeal or facial edema have been reported. Side effects include diarrhea, nausea, sinusitis, rhinitis, nasal congestion, bronchitis, cough, headache, dizziness, and ear/nose/throat complaints. Peramivir is an intravenous NAI indicated for the treatment of acute, uncomplicated influenza in patients 18 years of age and older who have been symptomatic for no more than 2 days; it is given as a single 600-mg administration.

Matrix protein inhibitors amantadine and rimantadine target the M2 protein and are potentially effective against only influenza A owing to the lack of a M1/M2 protein channel in influenza B viruses. These antiviral medications are not currently recommended for treatment or chemoprophylaxis since most circulating influenza A strains have developed resistance to them.[58-60]

Steroids have been proposed as an adjunctive therapy for influenza pneumonia; however, several studies failed to demonstrate clinical benefit in the treatment of patients

Table 27.2 Differential Diagnosis of Influenza Infection

Upper Respiratory Infection	Lower Respiratory Tract Infection	Exacerbations of Wheezing/Asthma
Rhinovirus	hMPV	RSV
hMPV	Adenovirus	hMPV
Adenovirus	RSV	Rhinovirus
RSV	PIV	Adenovirus
PIV	Coronaviruses	PIV
Coronaviruses	Chlamydophila pneumoniae	Coronaviruses
Enteroviruses	Mycoplasma pneumoniae	Chlamydophila pneumoniae
	Bocavirus	Mycoplasma pneumoniae
	Streptococcus pneumoniae	Bocavirus
	Staphylococcus aureus	
	Haemophilus influenzae	
	Streptococcus pyogenes	

hMPV, Human metapneumovirus; *PIV*, parainfluenza virus; *RSV*, respiratory syncytial virus.

Table 27.3 Treatment and Prophylactic Dosing of Oseltamivir

Age	Treatment Dose	Prophylactic Dose
2 weeks–3 months[a]	3 mg/kg per dose twice a day	Not recommended unless situation judged critical
Children 3–11 months[b]	3 mg/kg per dose twice a day	3 mg/kg per dose once daily
Children 1–12 years old and weighing		
≤15 kg	30 mg/dose twice a day	30 mg once daily
>15–23 kg	45 mg/dose twice a day	45 mg once daily
>23–40 kg	60 mg/dose twice a day	60 mg once daily
>40 kg	75 mg/dose twice a day	75 mg once daily
Children ≥13 years of age and adults	75 mg/dose twice a day	75 mg once daily

[a]Although not part of the US Food and Drug Administration (FDA)-approved indications, use of oral oseltamivir for treatment of influenza in infants less than 14 days old and for chemoprophylaxis in infants 3 months to 1 year of age is recommended by the Centers for Disease Control and Prevention (CDC) and the American Academy of Pediatrics.
[b]The American Academy of Pediatrics recommended an oseltamivir treatment dose of 3.5 mg/kg orally twice daily for infants aged 9–11 months for the 2013–14 season on the basis of data indicating that a higher dose of 3.5 mg/kg was needed to achieve the protocol-defined targeted exposure for this cohort as defined in the Capability Acquisition and Sustainment (CASG) 114 study (Kimberlin, 2013).[68] It is unknown whether this higher dose will improve efficacy or prevent the development of antiviral resistance. However, there is no evidence that the 3.5-mg/kg dose is harmful or causes more adverse events to infants in this age group.

with severe influenza infection. Furthermore, studies indicate an increase in overall mortality, increased incidence of hospital-acquired pneumonia, and longer duration of mechanical ventilation and ICU stay in patients treated with steroids.[61,62]

Prevention

Routine annual influenza vaccination is recommended for all children 6 months of age and older. Ideally, vaccination should occur before the onset of influenza in the community and should be administered as soon as a vaccine supply is available. Vaccination should be continued as long as influenza viruses are circulating. Multiple different vaccine formulations are available, and some are licensed for specific age groups or are more appropriate for particular patient populations. Recommendations regarding influenza and vaccine dosing are updated by the CDC each year and are available via the Centers for Disease Control and Prevention (CDC) influenza website (http://www.cdc.gov/flu/); they are also published in the *Morbidity and Mortality Weekly Report* by the CDC.[63,64] Two formulations of vaccine are approved for children: inactivated influenza vaccine (IIV) and live-attenuated influenza vaccine (LAIV). LAIV is an intranasal vaccine and is offered solely in quadrivalent form. IIV is available in trivalent or quadrivalent formulations. The Centers for Disease Control and Prevention (CDC) has recommended that LAIV should not be used until further notice due to low vaccine effectiveness against influenza A during the 2013–2014 and 2015–2016 seasons. Recombinant influenza vaccine (RIV) is available for adults with egg allergy.

Children 6 months through 8 years of age receiving vaccine for the first time require two doses of vaccine at least a month apart. Influenza vaccine contraindications are provided in Table 27.4. Data demonstrate that IIV and LAIV[65] given in a single, age-appropriate dose is well tolerated by virtually all recipients who have egg allergy. Children with anaphylaxis to eggs may receive influenza vaccine by a health care provider who is familiar with the potential manifestations of egg allergy in a setting where anaphylaxis can be recognized and treated. Such children should be observed for at least 30 minutes for signs of a reaction after administration of each vaccine dose.

CHEMOPROPHYLAXIS

NAIs are 70%–90% effective in preventing influenza. Yet the CDC does not recommend widespread or routine use of chemoprophylaxis owing to the possibility that resistant viruses could emerge, thus limiting the usefulness of these medications for high-risk or severely ill people. Oseltamivir can be used for chemoprophylaxis of influenza among infants below 1 year of age when indicated, although, owing to limited data in this age group, children less than 3 months of age should not receive prophylaxis unless the situation is judged to be critical.

Chemoprophylaxis is not usually recommended if more than 48 hours have elapsed since the last exposure to an infected person. For effective prophylaxis, an antiviral medication must be taken each day for the duration of potential exposure to a person with influenza and continued for 7 days after the last known exposure. Postexposure prophylaxis should be considered for family members and close contacts of infected patients if they are at high risk of complications from influenza.

Prognosis/Outcome

With or without antiviral treatment, most children have a full and uneventful recovery after an acute, uncomplicated influenza infection. Unfortunately, some will have a fatal outcome. Death from influenza is more frequent in children with comorbidities such as asthma or severe neurologic impairment and in those who develop ARDS.[66] A small proportion of children may develop asthma after experiencing an acute influenza infection, although asthma subsequent to infection seems

Table 27.4 Influenza Vaccine Contraindications and Precautions

Vaccine	Contraindications	Precautions
Inactivated influenza vaccine (II₃ or II₄) Cell culture–based IIV₃ High-dose IIV₃	Severe allergic reaction to any component of the vaccine, including egg protein, or after previous dose of any influenza vaccine.	Moderate to severe illness with or without fever; history of Guillain-Barré syndrome within 6 weeks of receipt of influenza vaccine.
Recombinant influenza Vaccine (RIV₃)	Severe allergic reaction to any component of the vaccine.	Moderate to severe illness with or without fever; history of Guillain-Barré syndrome within 6 weeks of receipt of influenza vaccine.
Live-attenuated influenza vaccine (LAIV₄)ᵃ	Severe allergic reaction to any component of the vaccine, including egg protein, or after previous dose of any influenza vaccine. Concomitant use of aspirin or aspirin-containing medications in children and adolescents. In addition, Advisory Committee on Immunization Practices recommends LAIV₄ not be used for pregnant women, immunosuppressed people, people with egg allergy, and children aged 2–4 years who have asthma or who have had a wheezing episode noted in the medical record within the past 12 months, or for whom parents report that a health care provider stated that they had wheezing or asthma within the last 12 months.	Moderate to severe illness with or without fever. History of Guillain-Barré syndrome within 6 weeks of receipt of influenza vaccine. Asthma in people 5 years of age and older. Medical conditions that might predispose to higher risk for complications attributable to influenza.

ᵃLAIV should not be used until further notice due to low vaccine effectiveness against influenza A during the 2013–2014 and 2015–2016 seasons.

to be more common with other viral lower respiratory tract infections such as RSV or human rhinovirus.[67]

References

Access the reference list online at ExpertConsult.com.

Suggested Reading

Barr CE, Schulman K, Iacuzio D, et al. Effect of oseltamivir on the risk of pneumonia and use of health care services in children with clinically diagnosed influenza. *Curr Med Res Opin.* 2007;23(3):523–531.

Harper SA, Bradley JS, Englund JA, et al. Seasonal influenza in adults and children—diagnosis, treatment, chemoprophylaxis, and institutional outbreak management: clinical practice guidelines of the Infectious Diseases Society of America. *Clin Infect Dis.* 2009;48(8):1003–1032.

Treanor J. Influenza vaccine—outmaneuvering antigenic shift and drift. *N Engl J Med.* 2004;350(3):218–220.

Wright PF, Kirkland KB, Modlin JF. When to consider the use of antibiotics in the treatment of 2009 H1N1 influenza-associated pneumonia. *N Engl J Med.* 2009;361(24):e112.

New and Emerging Infections of the Lung

PAUL TAMBYAH, MD, MAS SUHAILA ISA, MBBS, MRCPCH (UK), and
CHRISTELLE XIAN-TING TAN, MBBS (S'pore), MRCPCH (UK), MMed (Paeds)

Introduction

In this era of rapid globalization and frequent travel, emerging viral infections have gained an immense potential to spread at an unprecedented speed and scale compared with the past. This poses a significant challenge to coordinated international efforts in global surveillance and infection control.

Significantly, respiratory viral infections, spread mostly via droplet transmission, are extremely contagious and have caused significant morbidity and mortality during outbreaks in the last decade. Molecular diagnostics via reverse transcriptase polymerase chain reaction (RT-PCR) have been key in the rapid diagnosis of most of these viral infections. However, a high index of suspicion and early institution of appropriate isolation measures remain as the mainstay in the control and containment of the spread of these viral infections. Although treatment for most of the viral infections remains supportive, efficacious antiviral agents against influenza infections exist.

The infections discussed in this chapter include those first described in the 2000s: Middle East respiratory syndrome coronavirus (MERS-CoV) and metapneumovirus and rhinovirus C as well as those that have been described in the past but have reemerged in the last decade in outbreaks resulting in significant morbidity and mortality, including adenovirus, influenza virus, and enterovirus D68 (EV-D68).

EPIDEMIOLOGY

EV-D68 was first isolated in 1962 in California and had been rare with occasional reports of clusters. Since the late 2000s, EV-D68 has been increasingly reported in various parts of the world. In August 2014, the US Centers for Disease Control and Prevention (CDC) reported cases beginning in the Midwest, with more than 1000 cases reported in 49 states in 2014.[1]

ETIOLOGY

EV-D68 is a single-stranded, nonenveloped RNA virus. It belongs to the genus *Enteroviruses* and family Picornaviridae. It is one of the five EV-D serotypes identified so far. It has virologic characteristics including the ability to bind to α-2, 6-linked sialic acids that are present in the upper respiratory tract, which facilitate respiratory infections (Table 28.1).[2]

PATHOLOGY/PATHOGENESIS

The pathogenesis of EV-D68 has been studied in animal models. Schieble and colleagues noted that the Rhyne strain demonstrated a neurotropic virulence with paralysis of mice. However, despite the predominant respiratory symptoms seen in humans, no effective animal models have been established. Humans are at the moment the only known natural reservoirs of the disease.

CLINICAL FEATURES

The incubation period for EV-D68 is between 1–5 days, similar to many other viral respiratory infections, and the infectious period lasts from a day prior to symptom onset to about 5 days after onset. Spread of infection occurs by droplet transmission and through the fecal-oral route or indirect contact with contaminated surfaces, as with other enteroviruses.

SYMPTOMS

EV-D68 primarily causes acute respiratory symptoms, unlike other enteroviruses. Presenting symptoms range from mild upper respiratory symptoms such as rhinorrhea, sore throat, fever, and rash to severe pneumonia. Most reported cases were associated with difficulty breathing and wheezing, but this may affected by reporting bias.[3]

Patients can also present with aseptic meningitis or encephalitis. EV-D68 infection has been reported to have a predilection for patients with a personal or family history of atopy.[1] The respiratory symptoms have also been reported to be more severe in those with underlying respiratory illnesses such as asthma, often requiring intensive care treatment. Prior to virological diagnosis, many of these cases were often discharged with a diagnosis of asthma exacerbation.

During the outbreak in California and Colorado, a significant group of children was reported to have presented with acute flaccid myelitis, symptoms of sudden asymmetric limb weakness, facial weakness, ophthalmoplegia, or bulbar signs; they were found to be positive for EV-D68 in their nasopharyngeal swabs. However, the spectrum of neurologic disease associated with EV-D68 has not been fully characterized.

PHYSICAL FINDINGS

The physical findings for infected patients are similar to those associated with most respiratory viral infections and

Table 28.1 Summary Table of Characteristics of Emerging Viral Respiratory Infections

Virus	Mode of Transmission	Incubation Period	Clinical Features	Diagnosis[3]	Management and Treatment	Prophylaxis
Enterovirus D68 (EV-D68)	▪ Droplet ▪ Fecal-oral ▪ Fomites	1–5 days	▪ Respiratory ▪ Rarely flaccid myelitis ▪ Predilection to atopic individuals	▪ PCR ▪ Viral cultures ▪ (including serum)	Supportive	
MERS-CoV	▪ Droplet	2–14 days, median of 5 days	▪ ARDS ▪ Myalgia ▪ Gastrointestinal ▪ Asymptomatic	▪ RT-PCR (including stool specimens)	Supportive	
Human metapneumovirus	▪ Droplet ▪ Fomites	4–6 days Shedding can last 1–2 weeks	▪ Respiratory ▪ Gastrointestinal ▪ Predisposes to severe bacterial infections	▪ RT-PCR ▪ Immunofluorescence assay (IFA)	Supportive Intravenous immunoglobulin Ribavirin Investigational therapies	
Rhinovirus C	▪ Aerosol or droplet ▪ Fomites	0.5–3 days	▪ Respiratory ▪ Coinfection with bacterial infections common	▪ RT-PCR	Supportive	
Adenovirus	▪ Aerosol or droplet ▪ Fomites ▪ Fecal-oral	2–14 days Shedding up to 2 years in stool	▪ Pharyngoconjunctival fever ▪ Respiratory ▪ Gastrointestinal ▪ Renal-hematuria	▪ DFA ▪ PCR (throat, sputum and rectal swabs; blood and stool in immunocompromised) ▪ Serologic rise in antibody titers	Supportive Cidofovir for severe infections[b]	Oral vaccine (types 4 and 7)

ARDS, Acute respiratory distress syndrome; *ARF,* acute renal failure; *DFA,* direct fluorescent assay; *MERS-CoV,* Middle East respiratory syndrome coronavirus; *RT-PCR,* reverse transcriptase polymerase chain reaction.
[a]Unless otherwise stated, samples were obtained from the nasopharynx or oropharynx.
[b]Off-label use.

are not specific to the disease. However, a significant number of EV-D68 patients have been reported with wheezing as the main clinical feature. Patients with more severe EV-D68 respiratory infections present with tachypnea and retractions.[3] As already mentioned, neurologic symptoms including flaccid myelitis have also been associated with EV-D68 infections.

IMAGING, PULMONARY FUNCTION TESTS, LABORATORY FINDINGS

Chest radiographs often demonstrate peribronchial thickening and infiltrates, often with areas of atelectasis.[4,5]

DIAGNOSIS AND DIFFERENTIAL DIAGNOSIS

EV-D68 can be identified using molecular methods, polymerase chain reaction (PCR), or viral cultures of fluid samples from the nasopharynx, oropharynx, and serum. Most commercially available respiratory multiplex PCR assays may not be able to distinguish enteroviruses from rhinoviruses, so specific assays for EV-D68 may be needed to identify infections with EV-D68 if the clinical suspicion is high.

MANAGEMENT AND TREATMENT

Supportive care remains the mainstay of treatment. No specific treatment is currently available.[4] Pleconaril has not been shown to be effective for EV-D68 to date.

PREVENTION

There are currently no available vaccines. Good hand hygiene and prompt diagnosis with subsequent isolation of

cases is the main approach to containing the spread of these infections.

PROGNOSIS

Initial studies had suggested that patients with EV-D68 infection, compared with other pulmonary pathogens such as rhinoviruses or non EV-D68 enteroviruses, were more likely to have severe respiratory symptoms and to require hospitalization.[1] However, in a more recent retrospective analysis of the outbreak at the St. Louis Children's Hospital,[3] the cases analyzed have shown no significant difference in severity of illness in EV-D68 patients compared with those with other viral etiologies. This may have been due to ascertainment bias, as more severely affected children were tested and thus the case fatality rate appeared to be much higher than it probably really was. This has happened with a number of respiratory viruses, including influenza A H1N1 in 2009, when it was first recognized.

In most cases of EV-D68 infection, with supportive care recovery is expected over a few days. Fatalities have been associated with neurologic complications or occasionally cardiac events.[6,7]

Middle East Respiratory Syndrome Coronavirus

EPIDEMIOLOGY

First reported in April 2012 in Jordan,[8] MERS-CoV spread rapidly to the Middle East, including the Kingdom of Saudi Arabia (KSA), the United Arab Emirates (UAE), and Qatar.

Subsequent imported cases were then reported in European countries including France, the United Kingdom, Italy, and Germany and in North Africa (Tunisia). After the 2012 outbreak, there were only sporadic cases and nosocomial outbreaks reported from the Middle East until 2015, when a large outbreak occurred in Korea and Guangdong (China) involving 184 cases and 33 deaths.[9] Since 2012, according to statistics from the World Health Organization (WHO), there have been 1365 laboratory-confirmed cases of MERS-CoV infection, including 487 related deaths.

ETIOLOGY

MERS-CoV is an enveloped single-stranded RNA virus belonging to the family Coronaviridae. As with most coronaviruses, the reservoir of infection is thought to originate from animals. MERS-CoV is postulated to have originated from the dromedary camels within the Arabian Peninsula. Molecular isolation of several alphacoronaviruses and betacoronaviruses from bats in Saudi Arabia and other parts of the world has suggested the involvement of bats in human infection as well. The actual route of zoonotic transmission has not been clearly defined despite the publication of a large case-control study.[10]

PATHOLOGY/PATHOGENESIS

The exact pathogenesis of MERS-CoV is being elucidated. Studies looking at ex vivo infected hepatoma cells demonstrate severe cytopathic effects.[11] Hocke and colleagues[12] have demonstrated, through spectral microscopy, significant MERS-CoV antigen expression in type I and II alveolar cells, ciliated bronchial epithelium, and unciliated cuboidal cells of terminal bronchioles as well as pulmonary vessel endothelial cells. Evidence of alveolar epithelial damage with detachment of type II alveolar epithelial cells and associated disruption of tight junctions, chromatin condensation, nuclear fragmentation, and membrane blebbing were seen on electron microscopy.[12] The receptor for MERS-CoV has been identified as dipeptidyl peptidase 4 (DPP4) (CD26), an exopeptidase, which has been demonstrated in cells on spectral microscopy.[11]

MERS-CoV infection causes significant host immune dysregulation with downregulation of genes involved in the antigen-presenting pathway, leading to subsequent impaired adaptive immune responses, possibly explaining the rapid progression of the illness and the high mortality rate.

CLINICAL FEATURES

Most of the MERS-CoV infections were spread via travel to or residence in countries near the Arabian Peninsula. Infection occurs via droplet transmission from patients to close contacts. The risk of person-to-person transmission is generally low, but superspreading events have been identified similar to the severe acute respiratory syndrome (SARS) coronavirus, in which single individuals have been associated with transmission to large numbers of others. The median incubation period for secondary cases of human-to-human transmission is about 5 days (range 2–14 days).[13]

SYMPTOMS

In adults, infection results in fever as well as upper and lower respiratory tract symptoms including cough and breathlessness, which can rapidly deteriorate to severe acute respiratory distress syndrome. Other symptoms of myalgia and gastrointestinal symptoms of diarrhea, vomiting, and abdominal pain were commonly present.[14] However, two case series from the Middle East[15,16] have reported that MERS-CoV infection ran a milder course in children, with the majority being asymptomatic carriers who were contacts of symptomatic adult cases. Severe respiratory symptoms occurred more commonly in those with existing comorbidities.

The reported patients' age range has been from below 1 year to 99 years of age, although children have formed a minority of cases. This may be due to limited exposure to animals or health care settings where most infections have occurred.

The respiratory symptoms in symptomatic cases are rapidly progressive, with the median time from onset of symptoms to hospitalization being about 4 days and from onset to intensive care admission for severe cases approximately 5 days. Complications include acute respiratory failure, acute respiratory distress syndrome, refractory hypoxemia, and extrapulmonary complications (ischemic hepatitis, septic shock, hypotension, acute renal failure). The median time from onset to death was about 12 days.[13]

PHYSICAL FINDINGS

Patients presenting with symptomatic MERS-CoV infection have mainly lower respiratory findings, including tachypnea, rhonchi, and retractions, although upper respiratory symptoms have been reported.

IMAGING, PULMONARY FUNCTION TESTS, LABORATORY FINDINGS

Reported chest x-ray findings have included unilateral or bilateral patchy opacities, consolidation, interstitial infiltrates, and pleural effusions.[13]

DIAGNOSIS AND DIFFERENTIAL DIAGNOSIS

Laboratory confirmation of active MERS-coV infection is based on real-time reverse transcription PCR (RT-PCR) detection of at least two specific genomic targets or a single positive target with sequencing of a second target.[17] Confirmation with nucleic acid sequencing may be required for epidemiologic investigation of the origin and spread of the disease. Specimen collection sites for RT-PCR include lower respiratory samples (bronchoalveolar lavage, tracheal, or sputum aspirates) and upper respiratory samples (nasopharyngeal and oropharyngeal swabs) as well as serum and stool specimens, although the highest yield has been from respiratory samples.[17]

Serologic testing by enzyme-linked immunosorbent assay (ELISA), immunofluorescence assay (IFA) or microneutralization assay is available for the detection of previous infection and is used mainly for surveillance purposes; it should not be used as a diagnostic tool as there is a risk of cross-reactivity with other coronaviruses.

A single negative result on a recommended specimen sent is sufficient to demonstrate no active MERS-CoV infection according to the definition of the US CDC. However, if the clinical suspicion remains, more samples should be sent, as false-negatives do occur.

Patients who have been diagnosed with MERS-CoV are considered clear of active infection and can be deisolated when two consecutive specimen tests are negative on RT-PCR.

Other infectious etiologies presenting similarly with acute, rapidly progressive respiratory distress syndrome include SARS and influenza virus (H5N1). Noninfective causes of acute respiratory distress syndrome (ARDS) should be considered as well. The epidemiologic history and a high index of clinical suspicion are critical.

MANAGEMENT AND TREATMENT

No specific antivirals have developed at this point, and the mainstay of treatment remains supportive care.

PREVENTION

Currently no vaccine is available against MERS-CoV. Strict infection control measures, including standard, contact, and droplet precautions, with airborne precautions for aerosol-generating procedures, must be taken when care is being provided for suspected or confirmed cases. These have been shown to be effective in controlling nosocomial outbreaks in both the KSA and South Korea. Continued vigilant epidemiologic surveillance, good hand hygiene, and cough etiquette remain the mainstays of prevention for areas not affected by outbreaks.

PROGNOSIS

The prognosis is guarded in symptomatic cases, especially in adults, with 3–4 of every 10 patients reported to have died. The number of children infected has been small, so it remains to be seen if the disease runs a more benign course in the pediatric age group. In the adult population, patients admitted to the intensive care unit had a 58% mortality rate at 90 days post admission.[18]

Human Metapneumovirus

EPIDEMIOLOGY

Human metapneumovirus (HMPV) was first isolated in pediatric patients with acute respiratory infections in the Netherlands in 2001.[19] Subsequent retrospective serologic studies demonstrated the presence of antibodies to HMPV in humans more than 50 years prior,[20] and the virus has since been found worldwide. HMPV accounts for up to 10% of viral respiratory tract infections, occurring commonly during the months of January through April in the United States.[21] However, a recent 7-year surveillance study in the United States reported that the HMPV season occurred after the respiratory syncytial virus (RSV) and influenza seasons.[22] Serologic studies have demonstrated that most children in Europe and North America have acquired a HMPV infection at

least once by the age of 5 years.[20] Although this is a common childhood respiratory infection, immunity is believed to be transient, and HMPV infection is reported to contribute to acute respiratory illnesses in the elderly (above age 65) who have comorbid respiratory conditions such as asthma or chronic obstructive pulmonary disease or conditions resulting in an immunocompromised status. The overall rate of detection of HMPV was 6% among hospitalized children with respiratory studies.[21] Although there have been questions as to whether HMPV is truly a pathogen, asymptomatic carriage among children is estimated to be only 1%.[21]

ETIOLOGY

HMPV is an enveloped single-stranded RNA virus and is a member of the Paramyxoviridae family, belonging to the subfamily Pneumovirinae under the genus *Metapneumovirus*. Two genotypes of HMPV exist, A and B; subgroups are based on the fusion (F) and attachment (G) surface glycoproteins.[20]

PATHOLOGY/PATHOGENESIS

The pathogenesis of HMPV infection has been extensively studied in multiple animal models. Studies on young adult cotton rats inoculated with the virus demonstrate inflammation within and surrounding the bronchi and bronchioles with significant leukocytosis. The HMPV was found mostly on the apical surface of the columnar cells. In the same animal model, upregulation of mRNAs related to interferon gamma (IFN)-α, CCL5, CCL2, CCL3 and interleukin (IL)-2 was demonstrated. Previous infection conferred partial protection in these rats, with lower viral loads within the respiratory tract and a neutralizing antibody response on subsequent infection.[23] However, long-term immunity seems unlikely given the incidence of disease in older adults.

CLINICAL FEATURES

HMPV infection is transmitted via close or direct contact with contaminated secretions; the incubation period of HMPV is estimated to be 4–6 days.[20] The duration of symptoms varies according to severity, but it is commonly less than a week. However, shedding of the virus in infected cases can last from 1 to 2 weeks after the acute illness, with viral RNA found in stools 5 days to 2 weeks after symptom initiation.[20] A large prospective surveillance study done by the US CDC on HMPV infection in children[21] found that infected children were mostly without comorbidities and most were younger than 5 years of age, with many infants less than 6 months of age. The annual rate of hospitalization associated with HPMV infection was similar to that of influenza virus (1 per 1000) but lower than that for RSV (3 per 1000).[19]

SYMPTOMS

Clinical infection with HMPV results in initial upper respiratory tract symptoms such as cough, rhinorrhea, and fever and can progress to lower respiratory tract symptoms of shortness of breath and wheezing. Sore throat, conjunctivitis, poor appetite, rash, and other gastrointestinal symptoms such as vomiting and diarrhea have been reported.[23–25] The diagnosis is often not made clinically. In a 2-year population-based prospective surveillance study, outpatient cases subsequently found to be positive for HMPV were discharged mostly with the diagnosis of viral illness and bronchiolitis, while inpatient cases were mostly discharged with a diagnosis of bronchiolitis, asthma, or pneumonia.[25] Although infections are usually mild and self-limiting, some studies suggest that HMPV infections can predispose to severe bacterial infections, which complicate the course of the disease.[20]

PHYSICAL FINDINGS

Clinical findings in infected cases are like those seen in other respiratory viral infections, although fever was less common in children with HMPV infections than those with influenza in one study.[25] However, findings of respiratory distress, tachypnea, and wheezing were more common in patients with HMPV infections than in those with influenza in the same study.

IMAGING, PULMONARY FUNCTION TESTS, LABORATORY FINDINGS

Initial laboratory findings may reveal lymphopenia, neutropenia, and transaminitis,[26] or they may be completely normal. Chest x-ray findings for lower respiratory tract involvement in severe disease, especially in the immunocompromised, have demonstrated ground-glass opacities with parenchymal airspace consolidation, ill-defined nodular-like centrilobular opacities and bronchial wall thickening (Fig. 28.1).[26] Compared with RSV pneumonia, in one series HMPV pneumonia showed more asymmetrical findings.[26]

DIAGNOSIS AND DIFFERENTIAL DIAGNOSIS

Diagnostic tests for HMPV infection include various techniques of culture, the nucleic acid amplification test (NAAR), antigen detection and serologic testing. As culturing the virus is technically challenging owing to its slow growth and

cytopathic effects in vitro, the most commonly used detection technique is via RT-PCR from nasopharyngeal or oropharyngeal samples. Direct IFA testing can be done in outbreak settings because of the shorter turnaround time, but IFA has a lower sensitivity.[20] Serologic testing has been used mainly for epidemiologic purposes.

Differential diagnoses for similar upper respiratory tract presentations would include other viral etiologies including RSV, influenza, parainfluenza, and adenovirus. In the immunocompromised host with lower respiratory tract signs, fungal etiologies would have to be considered as well.

MANAGEMENT AND TREATMENT

Treatment of HMPV infections, like that of other viral infections, is mainly supportive; however, there is much interest in developing therapeutic options. Ribavirin, a nucleoside inhibitor licensed for the treatment of RSV and hepatitis C infections, has demonstrated good in vitro and in vivo activity against HMPV in animal models. Antiviral fusion inhibitors are also currently being investigated.

Other promising treatment options include therapeutic antibodies. Following the successful introduction of monoclonal antibodies such as palivizumab for RSV infections, development of specific monoclonal antibodies against HMPV is ongoing. An example is MAb338, an antibody targeting the HMPV fusion protein, which has shown therapeutic potential in mouse models. Another example is the intranasally administered Human Fab DS7.[27] Standard intravenous immunoglobulin preparations have also been shown to inhibit replication of HMPV in vitro.[28]

RNA interference is a new approach to treating RNA viral infections by regulating gene expression through the silencing of specific mRNAs.[20] Two extremely efficient small interfering RNAs against HMPV have been identified by Deffrasnes and colleagues,[29] These are still in the investigation phase. Finally, Wyde and colleagues have investigated the antiviral properties of sulfated sialyl lipid and heparin and have found activity against HMPV in vitro.[30]

Although there has yet to be a randomized controlled trial on therapeutics in HMPV infections, in severe case, in uncontrolled studies a combination of oral and aerosolized ribavirin with polyclonal intravenous immunoglobulin had some effect.[20]

PREVENTION

An effective vaccine against HMPV remains to be developed. Strategic targeting of the F and G surface proteins for both live attenuated and inactivated vaccine development is in progress. Particularly challenging is the fact that natural infection confers only transient immunity and reinfections are common into adulthood. This raises questions about the protective effect of any future vaccine.

Infection control remains the mainstay of prevention, especially within the hospital. Droplet isolation of infected cases with lower respiratory tract symptoms should be implemented until symptom recovery.

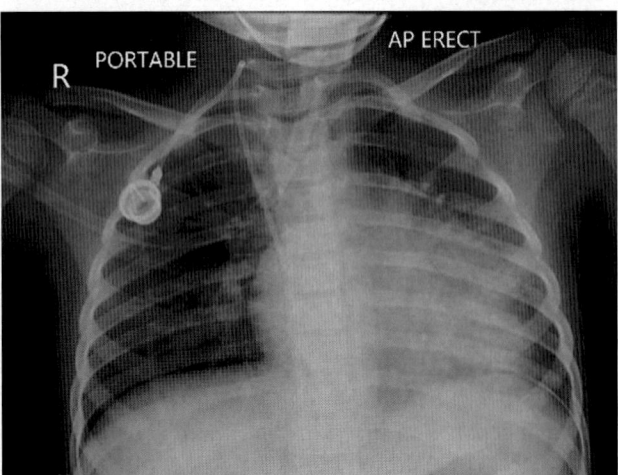

Fig. 28.1 Chest x-ray in a 4-year-old patient with underlying acute lymphoblastic leukemia demonstrating left mid- to lower-zone consolidation consistent with a left-sided pneumonia. The bronchoalveolar lavage fluid was positive for human metapneumovirus on reverse transcriptase polymerase chain reaction testing.

PROGNOSIS

Although children infected with HMPV had a higher likelihood of supplemental oxygen use and were noted to have a longer intensive care unit (ICU) stay compared to respiratory infections from other causes, the rates of ICU admission and intubation remained similar to other respiratory infections. The lengths of stay in hospital were not significantly different[21] and fatal HMPV infections are rare.

Rhinovirus C

EPIDEMIOLOGY

Human Rhinovirus C (HRV-C) is the newest member of the HRV family, having been discovered only in 2006 after retrospective VP4 sequence analysis, done with respiratory samples from patients in Queensland and New York City, showed distinct clustering from known HRV-A and HRV-B species.[31] Shortly after being described, these rhinoviruses were quickly reported worldwide in countries including Africa, Asia, Australia, America, and Europe and are now estimated to contribute to greater than 5% of tested specimens, highlighting their importance as a cause of respiratory tract infections.[31] In Asia and the United States, HRV-C and HRV-A are the most prevalent of the three species. There appears to be a seasonality in HRV-C infections, with a peak incidence in the fall and winter, as well as the rainy season in tropical countries, but also occurring throughout the year.[31] HRV-C infection has a predilection for the young, with most infections occurring in children less than 5 years of age, especially those below the age of 36 months.[32] Part of the apparent rise in rhinovirus C infection may be due to improved virus detection methods that have led to an increase in its recognition as a cause of severe pneumonia in the elderly and the immunocompromised, specifically in pediatric oncology and patients who have undergone hematopoietic stem cell transplantation.

ETIOLOGY

HRV-C is a positive-sense, single-stranded nonenveloped RNA virus from the Picornaviridae family. It is one of the three species of HRV based on phylogenetic sequence analysis and is distinctly distinguished from other previously described species (HRV-A and HRV-B) on the basis of genomic features.[33]

PATHOLOGY/PATHOGENESIS

In healthy individuals, HRV-C infection mostly causes rhinosinusitis through a neutrophilic inflammatory response resulting in increased vascular permeability and mucus hypersecretion in the upper respiratory tract. Cough, though less common, is thought to be due to direct infection of the bronchi or irritation from the posterior pharyngeal drainage of secretions.[34] In patients with asthma or underlying lung disease, lower respiratory symptoms are more common. Despite the fact that rhinoviruses grow optimally at 33°C, which favors the upper respiratory tract, it is postulated that the warmer temperature in the lower respiratory tract is not an absolute barrier to replication. In many children with pneumonia, rhinoviruses have been isolated together with bacterial pathogens suggesting that HRV infection may lead to a predisposition to other respiratory pathogens.[34] This has been supported by studies demonstrating that human tracheal epithelial cells had increased adherence to *Streptococcus pneumoniae* when coinfected by HRV.[35] Other studies have also demonstrated that HRV-exposed macrophages had suboptimal responses to bacterial toll-like receptor agonists,[36] which may predispose to secondary bacterial infections in humans.

The true prevalence and pathogenic role of HRVs in the community has not been investigated in detail, and HRV has been found in lower airway fluids and cells of healthy volunteers.[37,38] Cohort studies, though, have shown high rates of HRV-C detection (up to 75%) in hospitalized children with lower respiratory illnesses.[39-41]

There are also increasing data linking wheezing secondary to HRV in early infancy with a higher risk of subsequent development of asthma compared with wheezing caused by other viruses. The Childhood Origins of Asthma (COAST) study showed that HRV-related wheezing in the first year of life led to a threefold risk of having asthma at 6 years. HRV wheezing in year 2 was associated with a more pronounced increase in asthma risk (odds ratio [OR] ~7), while HRV-related wheezing during year 3 of life was associated with an even dramatic (OR ~32) increase in asthma at school age.[42] A similar birth cohort study in Australia reported that HRV-related wheezing in infancy was associated with an increased asthma risk at 5 years.[43] The exact mechanisms by which HRV triggers or contributes to the inflammatory changes often seen in asthma is unclear, but it is suggested that it evolves from a combination of host susceptibility, other aeroallergen sensitization and the ability of HRV to activate proinflammatory and airway remodeling pathways.[44]

CLINICAL FEATURES

Symptoms of HRV-C infection typically occur after an incubation period of 12–72 hours. The disease is spread through aerosol or droplet transmission or direct person-to-person contact with contaminated secretions. Symptoms generally last 7–11 days.

SYMPTOMS

Symptoms of HRV-C infection in children include fever greater than 38°C, and both upper and lower respiratory symptoms of cough, wheezing and shortness of breath.[45] Infections commonly associated with HRV-C include acute upper respiratory tract infection, acute laryngitis, suppurative tonsillitis, otitis media, bronchitis, bronchiolitis, and bronchopneumonia. Although the clinical course is generally mild, HRV-C has been found to be more virulent than HRV-A[32] and can run a more severe course in immunocompromised hosts—for example, children with hematologic malignancies, hematopoietic stem cell transplant recipients, and those on long-term steroid use.

PHYSICAL FINDINGS

Common findings in HRV-C infection include upper respiratory tract signs of nasal congestion, cough, facial tenderness with sinus involvement, and inflammation of the tympanic membrane with otitis media. With lower respiratory tract involvement, symptoms such wheezing, cough, and dyspnea are common.

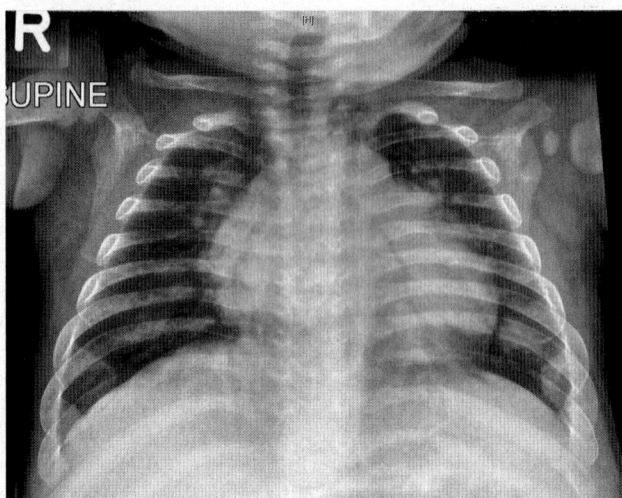

Fig. 28.2 Chest x-ray of an 11-month-old infant with underlying decompensated liver disease and rhinovirus bronchiolitis. Bilateral perihilar infiltrates are demonstrated on this film.

IMAGING, PULMONARY FUNCTION TESTS, LABORATORY FINDINGS

Chest x-ray findings include increased haziness in the perihilar or lower zone regions (Fig. 28.2). Consolidative changes and pleural effusions were less commonly noted in children and more commonly found in adult patients.[31]

DIAGNOSIS AND DIFFERENTIAL DIAGNOSIS

Conventional methods of viral testing such as immunofluorescence have often missed the presence of HRV-C; hence the recommended gold standard for the diagnosis of HRV-C infection is molecular testing with RT-PCR from nasopharyngeal or oropharyngeal secretions. Coinfection with bacterial infections is common, and the degree of rhinovirus identification in asymptomatic individuals in the community is not known. Hence isolation of rhinovirus C in a single sample with lack of clinical improvement over time may require analysis for the presence of a concomitant bacterial pathogen.

MANAGEMENT AND TREATMENT

Similar to the other common viral upper respiratory tract pathogens already mentioned, treatment remains supportive and symptomatic. Pleconaril, an antiviral agent known to be effective against enterovirus and rhinovirus infections, seems to be an option for severe HRV-C infections. However, owing to the distinct genomic differences of HRV-C compared with the earlier discovered HRV-A, it is likely that HRV-C may be resistant to this drug.[46]

PREVENTION

Despite the significant global burden of rhinovirus infection, no vaccine exists at this point because of antigenic heterogeneity between the greater than 150 rhinovirus strains.[47] Strict hand hygiene and droplet precautions for patients with upper respiratory tract symptoms remain the mainstays of prevention.

PROGNOSIS

Despite the initial reports of high mortality from rhinovirus C infections,[48–50] most cases are associated with a good prognosis. A recent study of hematology and oncology patients did not detect any deaths associated with HRV-C infection.[48] In a study from the Philippines, although rhinoviruses were the most common pathogens identified in children hospitalized with pneumonia, there were no fatalities associated with HRV infections, unlike influenza A.[51]

Adenovirus

EPIDEMIOLOGY

Adenovirus has been recognized as a pathogen since its discovery in 1953. However, recent interest in this virus as an emerging or (more accurately) reemerging respiratory pathogen arose from continued small outbreaks worldwide in both the United States and Asia. These have affected infants and young children, with 90% of them below the age of 60 months.[52] Significantly, in Taiwan, there was a noted surge in cases in 2010–2011, triggering the establishment of a national surveillance system that found an acute rise of adenovirus-positive respiratory tract specimens from a baseline of 5.75% to a peak of 37.3% of all respiratory viruses isolated.[53] Outbreaks across Asia appear to be linked by molecular epidemiology, although the mode of international spread is not clear.[54]

ETIOLOGY

Adenoviruses are icosahedral, nonenveloped, medium-sized, double-stranded DNA viruses with more than 50 immunologically distinct serotypes; they belong to the family Adenoviridae. The serotypes linked to epidemic keratoconjunctivitis include types 8, 19, 37, 53, and 54. Those that typically cause acute respiratory disease are types 3, 4, and 7, while the enteric adenoviruses in children are mainly types 40 and 41.[55]

Adenoviruses are known to be resistant to common disinfectants and can remain on surfaces and in the water of pools and lakes for long periods of time.[56]

TRANSMISSION AND INFECTION

Adenovirus is spread by droplet transmission of respiratory secretions or direct contact with infected secretions (respiratory, urine, stool, or ocular). The virus can also spread through water and via the fecal-oral route. Shedding of the virus in stools has been documented for up to 2 years after an infection, and shedding can occur in the urine as well. The virus can cause latent infection in lymphoid tissue such as the adenoidal and tonsillar tissues of the throat,[57] but the clinical significance of this is unclear.

CLINICAL FEATURES

The incubation period of adenoviral infections ranges from 2 to 14 days. Infection has been known to cause pharyngitis, adenoiditis, tonsillitis, otitis media, and keratoconjunctivitis, commonly known as pharyngoconjunctival fever. Lower respiratory tract involvement with pneumonia and bronchitis has also been seen. Adenoviral infections are also known to cause extrapulmonary manifestations, which are commonly seen as acute gastroenteritis and acute hemorrhagic cystitis, with some cases of hepatitis and rarely meningoencephalitis. Infection is particularly severe and prolonged in the immunocompromised, especially those who have undergone hematologic stem cell transplantation.

Certain serotypes, particularly 3, 7, and 21, have been reported to result in epidemics or fulminant events associated with long-term respiratory complications of bronchiolitis obliterans, bronchiectasis, and Swyer–James syndrome.[58,59] Bacterial coinfection in patients with adenoviral infections is noted to be rare, with a minimal role in the course of the disease in severe adenoviral infections.[53]

SYMPTOMS

The main symptoms of adenoviral infection include fever, cough, rhinorrhea, sore throat, and bilateral conjunctivitis, which can last from 3 to 5 days. Occasionally adenoviral infections cause prolonged fevers. Lower respiratory tract involvement is much less common. Extrapulmonary manifestations include diarrhea, abdominal pain, vomiting, and hematuria.

PHYSICAL FINDINGS

Pharyngoconjunctival fever typically manifests with bilateral conjunctivitis, an injected pharynx and tonsils with significant bilateral cervical lymphadenopathy. In adenoviral pneumonia, findings include significant hypoxia, wheezing, and features of pulmonary consolidation.

IMAGING, PULMONARY FUNCTION TESTS, LABORATORY FINDINGS

Adenoviral infections can easily be confused with bacterial infections, as they are known to cause leukocytosis and neutrophilia on peripheral blood counts as well as elevated inflammatory markers.[59] Transaminitis is also often noted with adenoviral infections. Because of high fevers, which can be more prolonged than with other viral causes, children with adenoviral infections are often presumptively treated for bacterial infections, with blood and urine cultures, and antibiotics before the diagnosis is made.

For patients with lower respiratory tract involvement, chest x-ray findings typically show interstitial pulmonary infiltrates; less commonly, lobar consolidation is seen (Fig. 28.3).[59]

DIAGNOSIS AND DIFFERENTIAL DIAGNOSIS

Pharyngoconjunctival fever in adenoviral infections can mimic other viral infections and is a common differential of the inflammatory condition Kawasaki disease due to conjunctival involvement as well as significant cervical lymphadenopathy. Gastroenteritis caused by adenoviral infections is similar to that caused by other viruses, such as astrovirus or norovirus. In immunocompromised patients, cytomegalovirus and Epstein-Barr virus are differentials for adenoviral enterocolitis.

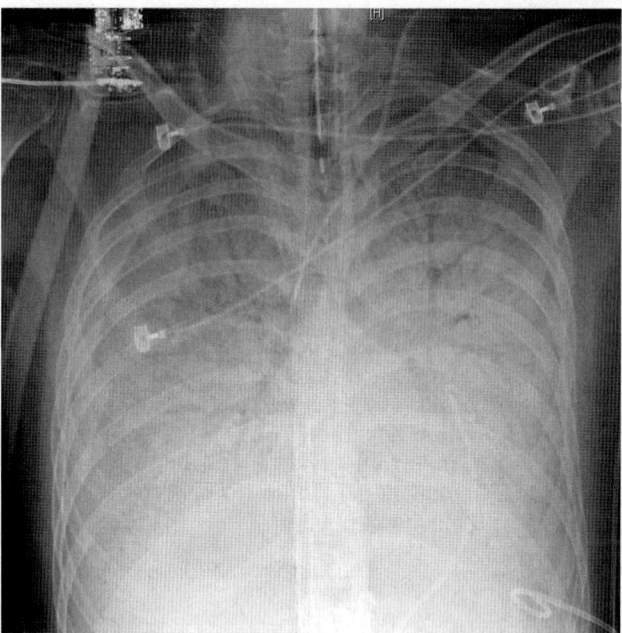

Fig. 28.3 Chest x-ray of an adolescent boy admitted for severe adenoviral pneumonitis with acute respiratory distress syndrome requiring support with extracorporeal membrane oxygenation. The figure demonstrates extensive bilateral pulmonary infiltrates consistent with severe pneumonitis.

Detection of the virus can be performed via antigen detection, PCR, virus isolation, or serology. Antigen testing by direct fluorescent assay of respiratory secretions (nasopharyngeal) has been shown to have a sensitivity of about 62.5% and a specificity of up to 100%.[52] PCR testing for adenovirus can be done on throat swabs, sputum, and rectal swabs with a reported sensitivity of 91%, 88%, and 86%, respectively. However, pleural effusion fluid has low pickup rates of adenovirus, estimated to be only 39%.[53] Adenoviral PCR on blood and stool samples is most useful for immunocompromised patients in cases with severe manifestations.

Blood serologic testing demonstrating a fourfold rise in the antibody titers between the acute and convalescent phases is the gold-standard diagnosis but is less commonly done owing to the development of more rapid diagnostic methods. Serotyping is not routinely performed and is used mainly for epidemiologic surveillance purposes.

MANAGEMENT AND TREATMENT

No specific treatment exists for adenoviral infections in immunocompetent individuals, and most infections are self-limited. In immunocompromised hosts, the antiviral agent cidofovir has been used to treat severe infections, and several novel therapies have been explored.[60]

The treatment of postadenoviral bronchiolitis obliterans remains largely supportive, with oxygen supplementation and bronchodilators. Corticosteroids would be an ideal theoretical treatment, since bronchiolitis obliterans is largely an immune-mediated inflammatory response, but there have been mixed results. In a study of 31 children, the use of systemic steroids in adenoviral pneumonia did not alter the progression to bronchiolitis obliterans.[61] Case series showing possible clinical benefit with intravenous methylprednisolone to treat bronchiolitis obliterans have been limited by small sample sizes and other confounders such as bronchodilator therapy. There have been no large clinical trials of the effectiveness of inhaled corticosteroids in the treatment of bronchiolitis obliterans.[62] There is evidence suggesting that latent adenoviral infection causes eosinophilic airway inflammation, leading to the ineffectiveness of steroid treatment.[63]

PREVENTION

Military recruits in the United States from 1971 to 1999 were routinely vaccinated against adenovirus due to the occurrence of outbreaks. After the cessation of vaccination, more cases became apparent. A new oral live attenuated adenoviral vaccine against types 4 and 7 was approved in 2011 for use in military personnel. However, no vaccine has been used in the general public.[56]

PROGNOSIS

Most immunocompetent individuals recover from the infection with no sequelae. However, severe cases of adenoviral pneumonia have been reported to result in bronchiectasis or bronchiolitis obliterans, and there have been deaths from severe adenoviral lung disease, mostly in patients with major underlying illnesses. Immunocompromised hematology and transplant patients have had fatal outcomes from disseminated adenoviral infections with liver failure, respiratory disease, and disseminated infection. Fatal cases have been associated particularly with serotype 7, but other serotypes have also been reported to be associated with fatalities.[53]

References

Access the reference list online at ExpertConsult.com.

29 *Tuberculosis*

HEATHER YOUNG HIGHSMITH, MSc, MD, JEFFREY R. STARKE, MD, and
ANNA MARIA MANDALAKAS, MD, PhD

Despite advances in diagnostic tests, availability of inexpensive curative treatment, and the nearly universal use of the bacillus Calmette-Guérin (BCG) vaccines, tuberculosis (TB) was the leading infectious cause of mortality in the world in 2015. The World Health Organization (WHO) estimates that TB leads to 1.8 million deaths and 10.4 million new cases annually. One million of these cases and 210,000 deaths occur in children.[1] As long as contagious TB persists in adults, children will be affected. However, many aspects of the epidemiology, pathophysiology, and natural history of childhood TB are fundamentally different from the features of the disease in adults.

In all populations, TB, caused by the organism *Mycobacterium tuberculosis*, has several stages. *TB exposure* is the first stage, which occurs when an individual has been in close proximity to a person with contagious TB disease. The second stage is *TB infection*, which occurs when an individual has inhaled the causative organism but has no overt physical symptoms or findings on radiographic examination. *TB disease* exists when an individual manifests symptoms, signs, or radiographic manifestations consistent with *M. tuberculosis* pathology. Because the organism can develop resistance to the drugs used to treat it, the proliferation of resistant strains has become a growing public health threat. It is also important to differentiate between drug-susceptible *M. tuberculosis*—susceptible to all first-line medications used to treat it, and drug-resistant *M. tuberculosis*. A thorough understanding of TB in all its stages and resistance patterns is essential to treating individual children and designing effective interventions to control it.

Epidemiology

TRANSMISSION

Transmission of *M. tuberculosis* is generally from person to person and occurs via inhalation of mucous droplets that become airborne when an individual with pulmonary or laryngeal TB coughs, sneezes, speaks, laughs, or sings. After drying, the droplet nuclei can remain suspended in the air for hours. Only small droplets (<10 μm in diameter) can reach alveoli. A video from the Centers for Disease Control and Prevention illustrates the transmission process as well as the pathogenesis of the disease, and is available at https://youtu.be/9112brXCOVc. Droplet nuclei can also be produced by aerosol treatments, sputum induction, aerosolization during bronchoscopy, and through the manipulation of lesions or processing of tissue or secretions in the hospital or laboratory. Transmission occurs rarely by direct contact with infected body fluids or fomites.

Many factors are associated with the risk for acquiring *M. tuberculosis* infection, including the extent of contact with a contagious person, the burden of organisms in the person's sputum and the frequency of a person's cough. Adults with pulmonary TB and bacilli present on acid-fast staining of sputum are more likely to transmit infection. Recent evidence from adult patients suggests that the magnitude of the inhaled dose of *M. tuberculosis* as measured by cough aerosols can predict an individual's risk of TB progression following exposure.[2] In addition, the risk for transmission correlates directly with the closeness of contact and amount of time spent with a contagious case.[3] Most transmission to children occurs in the home. Markers of close contact such as urban living and overcrowding correlate with acquisition of infection.[4] An increased risk for infection has been demonstrated in several institutional settings, including nursing homes, schools, correctional institutions, and homeless shelters. A growing problem concerns TB transmission in refugee and orphanage settings.[5–7] There is some evidence that the risk for acquiring infection increases with age from infancy to early adulthood, likely because of increasing likelihood of contact with infectious persons.[8]

It has been noted for decades that children with TB rarely infect other children or adults.[9] In the typical case of childhood pulmonary TB, tubercle bacilli in endobronchial secretions are sparse, and when young children with TB cough, they lack the tussive force of adults. Sputum production is rare in children, and collected specimens usually do not show acid-fast bacilli (AFB) upon staining, indicating a low concentration of organisms. However, specimens from young infants with extensive TB infiltrates, children and adolescents with cavitary lesions, or intubated children with TB are potentially infectious. The few documented cases of transmission from children have been in individuals with typical findings of adult-type TB, with lung cavities and sputum production, or infants with congenital TB who have a large burden of organisms in the lungs.[10–12] When transmission of *M. tuberculosis* has been documented in schools, orphanages or children's hospitals, it has almost invariably been from an adult or adolescent with undiagnosed pulmonary TB.[7,13,14] In fact, when a child is suspected clinically of having TB disease, the adults who accompany the child should undergo urgent testing for TB (usually by chest radiograph or AFB) sputum smear to be sure they do not spread infection in the facility.[14]

A few classic studies have investigated the factors that influence whether or not an infected person will develop TB disease. It is clear that the risk for disease is highest shortly after initial infection and declines thereafter. From infancy to age 10 years, age is inversely associated with the risk for developing disease. Children under the age of 2 are at high risk of progressing from infection to disease (25%–30%, and this risk is even higher for children under 1 year of age, 40%–50%). Furthermore, children less than 1 year of age are more likely to develop severe forms of disease, such as miliary or meningeal TB.[15] For unknown reasons, there is a second peak in the risk for developing disease during late adolescence and early adult life. Most young children who develop TB disease do so within the first year after infection, with most cases occurring within 6 months of transmission of the organism. There is also increasing evidence that certain strains of *M. tuberculosis* create an increased risk of progression to disease and an increased risk of severe disease.[16,17]

INCIDENCE AND PREVALENCE

The WHO estimates that 2 billion people are infected with *M. tuberculosis*.[18] This reservoir of TB infection leads to approximately 10.4 million new TB cases and 1.8 million deaths annually.[1] Estimates of childhood TB disease did not exist prior to 2012. Several reasons contributed to the lack of reporting: (1) children not coming to health services, (2) the difficulties in diagnosis of TB disease in resource-poor settings, (3) the lack of age-disaggregated data for many countries and (4) underreporting of clinically diagnosed childhood cases. Once the WHO first started reporting global childhood TB estimates in 2012, the efforts were plagued by methodologic limitations.[19]

Mathematical modeling has since provided figures that are probably more accurate. Within the 22 countries that carry 80% of the world's burden of TB disease, it is estimated that 7.6 million children acquire TB infection each year, while 53 million children harbor the infection at any given time; of these, at least 650,000 develop TB each year.[20] Systematic review with modeling to adjust for underreporting has led to an estimate of 850,000, or 1 million children with incident TB disease annually.[21,22] In 2015, with increasing numbers of countries reporting age-disaggregated data and using similar methodology to the aforementioned studies, the WHO estimated that 1 million children develop incident TB disease annually, and 210,000 children die from TB.[1] Despite the improvement in methodology and reporting, the true number of cases remains unknown. The majority of childhood cases occur in resource-limited areas where diagnostic tests include only acid-fast staining of sputum, which is positive in up to 70% of adults but in less than 10% of children with pulmonary TB. As a result, when microbiologic confirmation is required, only one-third of the estimated number of childhood cases are ever reported to national TB programs.[1] In regions where improved case finding has been initiated, children may represent up to 39% of all cases, with a skew toward more serious and complicated cases.[1]

M. tuberculosis can develop resistance to therapeutic drugs if individuals are improperly treated, as discussed later in the chapter. Once an isolate has developed resistance to isoniazid (INH) and rifampin (RIF), it is considered a multidrug-resistant (MDR) organism, and when individuals develop disease from a MDR organism, it is referred to as MDR-TB. The WHO estimates that 3.3% of new TB cases in 2015 were MDR-TB cases.[1] India, China and the Russian Federation have the majority of cases of MDR-TB, but the areas with the highest rates of MDR-TB cases are clustered in eastern Europe and Central Asia, where more than 18% of new TB cases were estimated to be MDR.[1]

Children usually develop MDR-TB after inhaling already resistant organisms from an older individual with contagious TB who has been treated improperly (secondary resistance) instead of developing MDR-TB during his or her own treatment (primary resistance). Because it is difficult to isolate the organism, especially from children, on which to perform drug susceptibility testing (DST), it is difficult to estimate the number of children with MDR-TB. Two mathematical modeling studies have estimated that, globally, between 25,000 and 32,000 children develop MDR-TB annually.[21,22]

In high-resource settings, such as the United States, Canada, Australia, the United Kingdom, and many western European countries, TB incidence declined upon the advent of effective therapy and prevention. In such settings, foreign-born individuals and racial and ethnic minorities bear a disproportionate amount of TB infection and disease. Screening of immigrants and high-risk populations with connection to appropriate evaluation and treatment are key to TB control in these settings.

THE EPIDEMIOLOGY OF TUBERCULOSIS IN INDIVIDUALS INFECTED WITH HUMAN IMMUNODEFICIENCY VIRUS

The United Nations Program on Human Immunodeficiency Virus (HIV)/Acquired Immunodeficiency Syndrome (AIDS) estimates that there are 3.2 million children living with HIV. More than 91% of these children live in sub-Saharan Africa in high-burden TB settings.[23] Despite dramatic gains in the fight against HIV owing to successful prevention of mother-to-child transmission and the robust rollout of antiretroviral therapy, TB is the leading cause of death in people living with HIV. In 2014, HIV-associated TB deaths among adults accounted for 25% of all TB deaths (among HIV-uninfected and HIV-infected people and one-third of the estimated 1.2 million deaths from HIV/AIDS).[24] In high-burden settings, HIV-infected children are at increased risk of acquiring TB infection.[25] TB is a major cause of mortality in HIV-infected children, who have a high risk of progression to TB disease and death following TB infection.[26] HIV-infected infants and young children are at least 24 times more likely to develop culture-confirmed TB than are HIV-uninfected infants and young children.[27] Other populations to consider are HIV-uninfected and HIV-exposed but uninfected children living in a household with HIV-infected individuals. As adult caregivers with HIV infection are at risk for TB disease, all children living in HIV-affected households are more likely to be exposed and to consequently develop TB disease. Maritz has shown that HIV-infected and HIV-exposed children in a high-burden setting have similar rates of TB exposure, with TB disease being found in 19% of the HIV-infected children and 8% of the HIV-exposed children.[28] Although Madhi and colleagues have shown a high incidence of TB disease in HIV-exposed but uninfected children (41 cases per 1000 child-years), TB incidence was threefold greater in HIV-infected children (121 per 1000 child-years in the same high-burden setting).[29]

Immune-compromised HIV-infected children are prone to developing disease manifestations indicative of poor organism containment, such as cavitation of the Ghon focus and disseminated (miliary) disease.[30–32] This presentation is notably similar to that of very young non–HIV-infected children, suggesting that the immune system of both populations has difficulty controlling *M. tuberculosis*.[30,33,34] HIV-infected individuals are also at risk for other HIV-related lung pathology, such as lymphocytic interstitial pneumonia (LIP), which can present with similar symptoms and radiographic findings (see Chapter 66). The nonspecific clinical and radiographic presentations of TB disease in HIV-infected children make this a challenging diagnosis.

Mycobacteriology

The genus *Mycobacterium* consists of a diverse group of obligate aerobes that grow most successfully in tissues with high oxygen content, such as the lungs. These nonmotile, nonspore-forming, pleomorphic rods range in length from 1 to 10 μm and in width from 0.2 to 0.6 μm. Their cell wall has a complex structure that includes a large variety of proteins, carbohydrates, and lipids. The mycolic acids are the most distinctive lipids. The lipid-rich cell wall makes them impermeable to many stains unless the dyes are combined with phenol. Once stained, the cells resist decolorization with acidified organic solvents, resulting in their hallmark trait of being "acid-fast." This property is demonstrated with basic fuchsin stain techniques, such as the Ziehl–Neelsen and Kinyoun methods, or the more sensitive fluorochrome method using auramine and rhodamine stains. It is not possible to distinguish one species of *Mycobacterium* from the others using only acid-fast staining.

Of the more than 60 species of *Mycobacterium* that have been described, about half are pathogenic in humans.[35] The *M. tuberculosis* complex consists of five main closely related species: *M. tuberculosis, M. bovis, M. microti, M. canetti,* and *M. africanum.* These organisms are commonly grown on solid media that contain an egg-and-potato base, such as Lowenstein–Jensen media or on synthetic media, such as Middlebrook agars 7H9 and 7H10. Visible growth on solid media can take 3–6 weeks. *M. tuberculosis* complex grows in only 7–10 days in liquid media; a broth formulation of Middlebrook agars is most commonly used.[36]

DST for *M. tuberculosis* can be performed on either solid or liquid media that contain standard concentrations of antimicrobial agents; the growth is compared to a control inoculation.[37] The results can take several weeks to return, as these tests depend on growth of the organism. Other newer methods of identification and DST are available and are discussed in more detail in the section titled "Diagnosis of Disease."

Immunology

Humans display a wide spectrum of immunologic responses to *M. tuberculosis.* The varied immunologic response is reflected in the diverse clinical manifestations, ranging from asymptomatic infection with a positive tuberculin skin test (TST) or the interferon-γ release assay (IGRA) to hematogenous dissemination with severe or fatal disease.[38–40] Immunologically competent cells of the human host recognize *M. tuberculosis* by its antigens; an extraordinarily large number of these antigens have been described. In a few individuals, the innate immune system represented by macrophages, natural killer cells, and neutrophils control infection as part of the initial response to *M. tuberculosis.*[41] In the majority of infected persons, the acquired immune response is responsible for control of *M. tuberculosis* and the subsequent pathophysiologic events.

T cells, as antigen-recognition units, have critical regulatory and effector roles in the immune response to *M. tuberculosis.* In the traditional model, macrophages present antigens from phagocytosed bacilli to T cells. Antigen-activated T cells secrete cytokines, which in turn stimulate macrophages, making them more effective at controlling mycobacterial growth. Recent advances in studies of the human immune response to mycobacteria have expanded on this simple model.[42] First, a large variety of circulating and tissue-bound T-lymphocyte subsets (CD4[+], CD8[+] and γδT cells) have antigen receptors with high affinity for mycobacterial antigens.[39] Second, T cells also serve as cytotoxic effector cells against *M. tuberculosis*–infected macrophages. Third, macrophages sensitized to nontuberculous mycobacteria (NTM) or BCG vaccine produce a large number of cytokines in response to a repeat exposure to mycobacterial antigens. Of note, B lymphocyte–mediated humoral responses to mycobacterial antigens occur in patients, but they have no clearly demonstrated role in the pathogenesis of disease.

The course of infection is influenced largely by the host immune response to *M. tuberculosis.*[38–40] Most children infected with *M. tuberculosis* develop infection characterized by a positive TST or IGRA but no symptoms or radiographic abnormalities.[39] These children have an effective macrophage- and lymphocyte-activated response with a rapid expansion of T cells and production of protective cytokines and mediators. In children who develop disease, the most common manifestation is pulmonary disease, including a Ghon focus, enlarged lymph nodes or bronchial disease. However, the immune system in these children often contains the disease, which may resolve without chemotherapy.[15] A few children experience severe forms of disease, including progressive pulmonary TB, miliary or disseminated TB or TB meningitis. These forms of disease result from an immune response that fails to contain the growth of the bacilli. The risk for disease development in childhood following initial infection is inversely related to age, suggesting an inadequate or immature immune response in young children.[15,43]

Although children classically have been thought to progress from exposure to TB infection to TB disease in a linear, unidirectional fashion, a growing body of evidence suggests that a more complex, dynamic bidirectional continuum of responses exists, leading to a spectrum of TB infection and disease states (Fig. 29.1).[44] Several lines of evidence suggest that the specific acquired host defenses against mycobacteria are genetically determined. Twin studies indicate that there is a higher concordance of TB among monozygotic compared with dizygotic twins,[45,46] and segregation analysis of TB in families indicates an oligogenic pattern of inheritance.[47]

Pathophysiology

After inhaling *M. tuberculosis,* most children do not develop disease but rather develop TB infection. These children have a positive TST or IGRA result and no clinical or radiographic evidence of TB disease. It is presumed that these children are infected with a low number of viable tubercle bacilli that do not immediately cause clinical disease. Once the organisms are inhaled, they are ingested by alveolar macrophages, which form caseating granulomas to contain the bacilli. Macrophages transport some bacilli to the regional lymph nodes. Before an adequate immune response is mounted, the bacilli can transit from the regional lymph nodes via the lymphatic duct or directly into the systemic circulation. This occult lymphohematogenous spread disseminates bacilli to various organs, where they may survive for decades.[48] Disseminated TB disease results if the dissemination is not controlled by the developing acquired immune response. The occult dissemination also provides the seed organisms for extrapulmonary TB, which accounts for 20%–30% of childhood TB cases.

In some children, tubercle bacilli reach a terminal airway and induce a localized pneumonic parenchymal inflammatory process referred to as the primary (Ghon) focus. Approximately 70% of the primary foci are subpleural. All lobes are equally affected, and 25% of children have multiple parenchymal foci. Bacilli originating from this focus drain via local lymphatics to the regional lymph nodes. The triad of the

primary focus, local tuberculous lymphangitis, and enlarged regional lymph nodes is referred to as the primary complex.

EVOLUTION OF CLINICAL DISEASE IN CHILDREN

A review of information available from the prechemotherapy era provides a rich understanding of the natural evolution of clinical disease in children.[15,49] Following infection, all children progress through an asymptomatic incubation period generally lasting 3–8 weeks. The subsequent development of clinical disease is determined by the interaction of the host and the organism and is highly age-dependent (Table 29.1).[49]

The various manifestations of TB tend to occur according to a predictable timetable.[48] Disseminated TB and TB meningitis tend to be early manifestations, often presenting 2–6 months after initial infection has occurred. The primary complex and its complications become apparent most often 3–6 months after infection. It is common for untreated primary complex TB to result in calcification of the lung parenchyma and/or regional lymph nodes, a process that occurs at least 6 months after infection (Fig. 29.2). Although pleural and lymph node TB often develop within 3–9 months after infection, other extrapulmonary forms of TB, especially skeletal and renal disease, may not develop for several years.

Children younger than 2 years of age are at greatest risk for both the development of disease and severe manifestations of disease. Children between 2 and 5 years of age have the next highest risk. Children between 5 and 10 years of age are at the lowest risk of progressing from infection to disease; this time span is often called the "favored age." The risk increases again in adolescence, when children are more likely to manifest adult-type disease, including cavitary disease.

Clinical Features

INTRATHORACIC TUBERCULOSIS

Following inhalation of *M. tuberculosis* and the formation of the primary complex (see Fig. 29.2), a child can develop

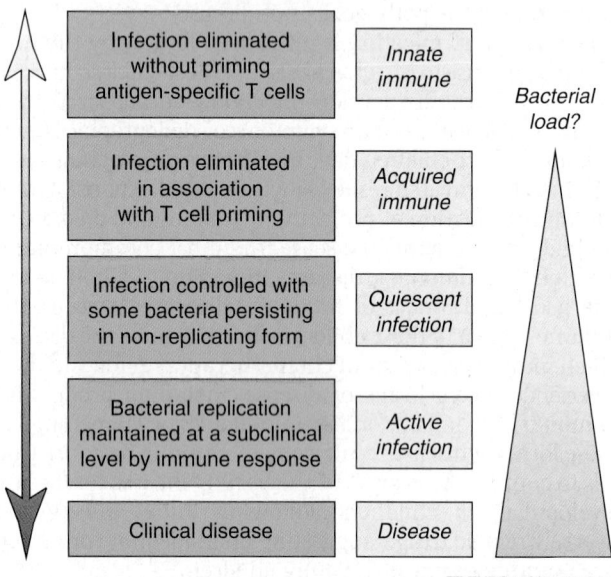

TRENDS in Microbiology

Fig. 29.1 A spectrum of responses to tuberculosis infection.

Table 29.1   Average Age-Specific Risk for Disease Development Following Primary Infection

Age at Primary Infection	Immune-Competent Children (Dominant Disease Entity Indicated in Parentheses)	Risk of Disease Following Primary Infection
<1 year	No disease	50%
	Pulmonary disease (Ghon focus, lymph node or bronchial)	30%–40%
	TBM or disseminated disease	10%–20%
1–2 years	No disease	70%–80%
	Pulmonary disease (Ghon focus, lymph node or bronchial)	10%–20%
	TBM or disseminated disease	2%–5%
2–5 years	No disease	95%
	Pulmonary disease (lymph node or bronchial)	5%
	TBM or disseminated disease	0.5%
5–10 years	No disease	98%
	Pulmonary disease (lymph node, bronchial effusion or adult type)	2%
	TBM or disseminated disease	<0.5%
>10 years	No disease	80%–90%
	Pulmonary disease (effusion or adult type)	10%–20%
	TBM or disseminated disease	<0.5%

TBM, Tuberculous meningitis.

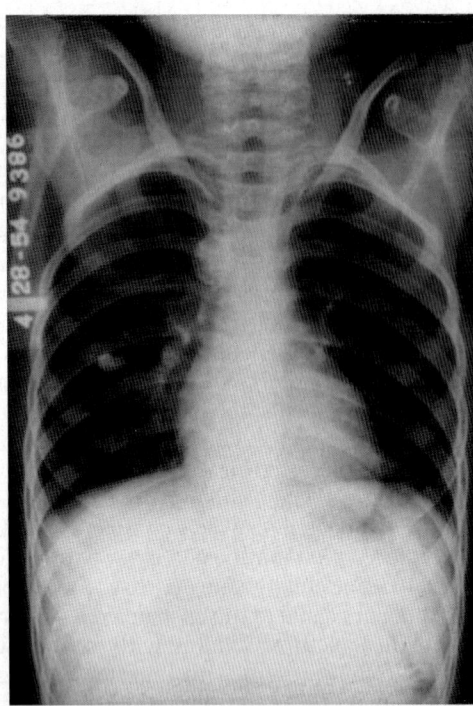

Fig. 29.2 A calcified parenchymal lesion and lymph node in a child with tuberculosis infection. These lesions contain a small number of viable *Mycobacterium tuberculosis* organisms.

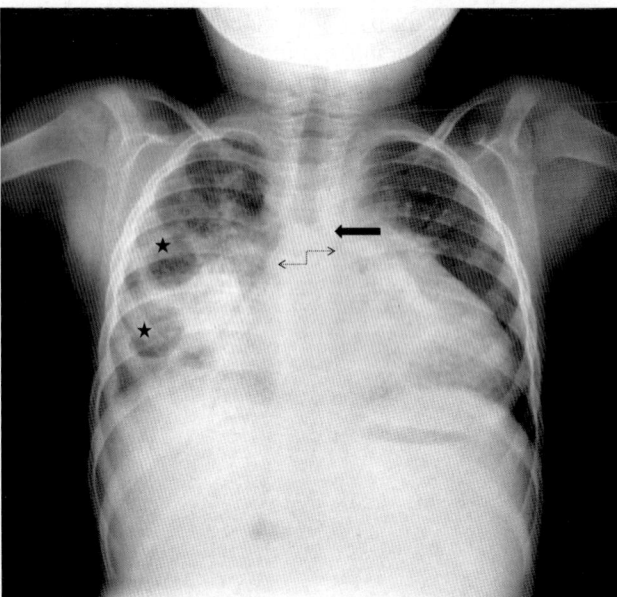

Fig. 29.3 A young child with pulmonary tuberculosis who has developed cavitation of the lung parenchyma *(asterisk)*. The *solid arrow* shows narrowing of left mainstem bronchus, while *dotted arrows* show splaying of the main bronchi.

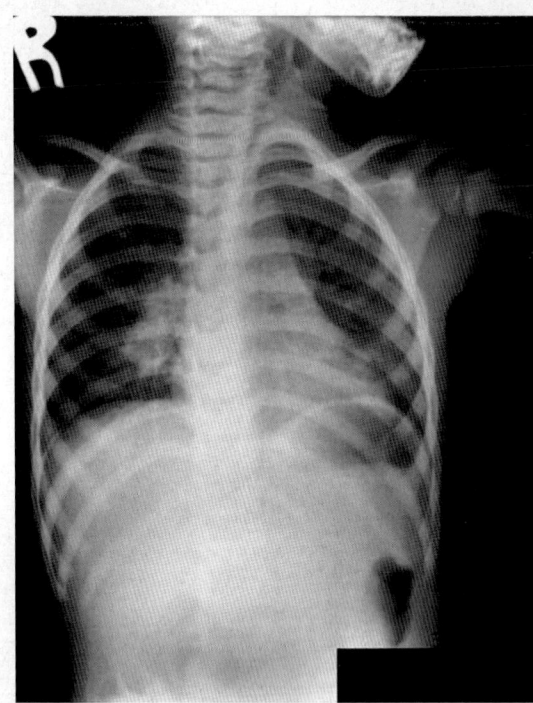

Fig. 29.4 Hilar adenopathy in a child with early pulmonary tuberculosis. Most children with this radiographic appearance have few or no symptoms.

intrathoracic TB, which is the most common manifestation of TB disease. Intrathoracic TB consists of a spectrum ranging from subclinical to severe manifestations, which are described in the following sections.

ISOLATED LYMPHADENOPATHY

The hallmark of childhood pulmonary TB is enlargement of the regional hilar, mediastinal, or subcarinal lymph nodes on chest x-ray (Fig. 29.3).[50,51] When thoracic adenopathy is isolated without other findings, it usually causes few or no clinical signs or symptoms. This manifestation is most common soon after exposure, usually as part of active case finding.

PROGRESSIVE PRIMARY INFECTION

A primary focus, without or occasionally with cavitation, may be seen in symptomatic children who have weight loss, fatigue, fever, and chronic cough.[52] If the host is unable to contain the tubercle bacilli, progressive caseation occurs in the lung parenchyma surrounding the primary focus. The area of caseation may discharge into a bronchus, resulting in the formation of a primary cavity with possible endobronchial spread (Fig. 29.4; see also Fig. 29.3). The tubercle bacilli disseminate further to other parts of the lobe and can involve an entire lung. On rare occasions an enlarging primary focus ruptures into the pleural cavity, creating a pneumothorax, bronchopleural fistula, or caseous pyopneumothorax. Profound fever, cough, and weight loss accompany a severe progressive lesion. Before the advent of chemotherapy, 25%–65% of children with progressive

primary disease died. However, with appropriate therapy, the prognosis is excellent.

BRONCHIAL DISEASE

In some children, particularly infants who have smaller-caliber airways, infected lymph nodes continue to enlarge, resulting in lymphobronchial involvement, where the affected bronchus may become partially or totally obstructed because of nodal compression, inflammatory edema, polyps, granulomatous tissue, or caseous material extruded from ulcerated lymph nodes (Fig. 29.5). Although chest radiography rarely delineates the specific pathologic process causing the abnormalities, it is often apparent if bronchoscopy or a computed tomography (CT) scan of the chest is performed. The most frequently affected lobes are the right upper, right middle, and left upper lobe. Symptoms vary according to the degree of airway irritation and obstruction but frequently include

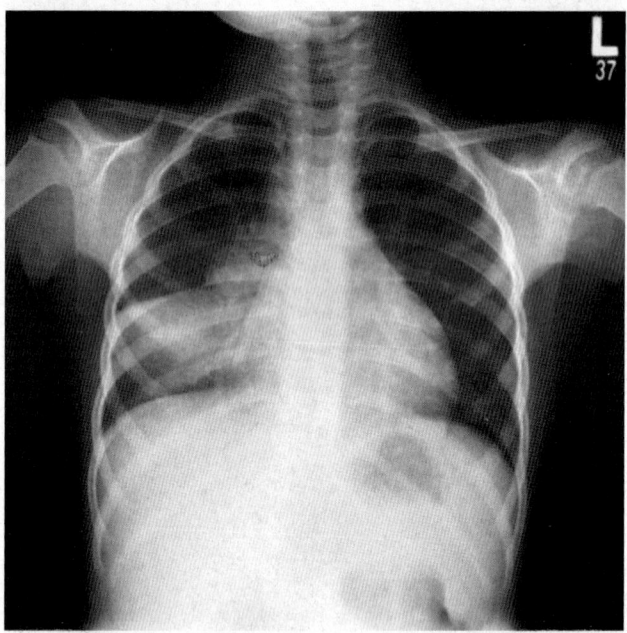

Fig. 29.5 A classic collapse-consolidation lesion with hilar adenopathy in a child with pulmonary tuberculosis.

localized wheezing or persistent coughing, which may mimic pertussis. A common radiographic sequence is adenopathy followed by localized hyperinflation and then atelectasis of contiguous parenchyma, referred to as collapse-consolidation or segmental lesions (Fig. 29.6A, B). However, collapse-consolidation lesions rarely produce symptoms unless the area affected is quite substantial.[53] The radiographic and clinical picture mimics foreign-body inhalation and other obstructive disorders.

Additional pathology that may accompany bronchial disease includes airway allergic consolidation, caseating consolidation, and bronchopneumonia. Children with allergic consolidation typically experience high fevers, acute respiratory symptoms, and signs of consolidation on chest radiography. Children with caseating consolidation are very ill, with high undulating fevers, chronic cough, and occasional hemoptysis (Fig. 29.7). These children are likely to have positive cultures. The affected airway is completely obstructed, and surgical intervention may be necessary to provide symptomatic relief. In some children, an acute secondary bacterial infection that occurs distal to the obstructed bronchus plays a role in the clinical picture. Children with secondary bacterial pneumonia often present with high fever, cough, and crackles. The clinical signs and symptoms often respond to antibiotics, but the chest radiographic findings do not clear because of the underlying TB.

COMPLICATED LYMPH NODE DISEASE

Although segmental lesions and hyperaeration are the most common findings produced by enlarging thoracic lymph nodes, other problems may occur. Enlarged paratracheal nodes may cause stridor and respiratory distress. Subcarinal nodes may impinge on the esophagus and cause difficulty in swallowing, followed occasionally by the formation of an esophageal diverticulum, or the nodes may rupture directly

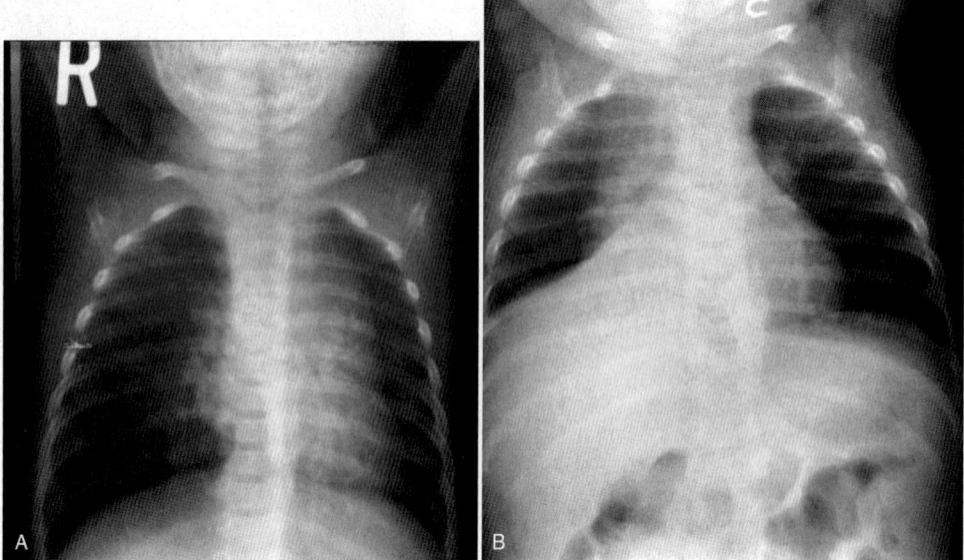

Fig. 29.6 (A) Hyperinflation of the right lower lobe in an infant with pulmonary tuberculosis and airway obstruction. At this point the child had respiratory distress. (B) A chest radiograph from the same child several hours later shows complete collapse of the right lower lobe. At this point the respiratory distress had ceased.

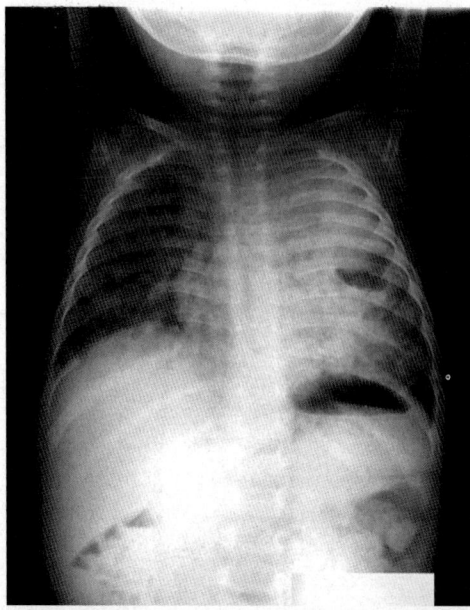

Fig. 29.7 Pronounced caseating consolidation in a young child with pulmonary tuberculosis.

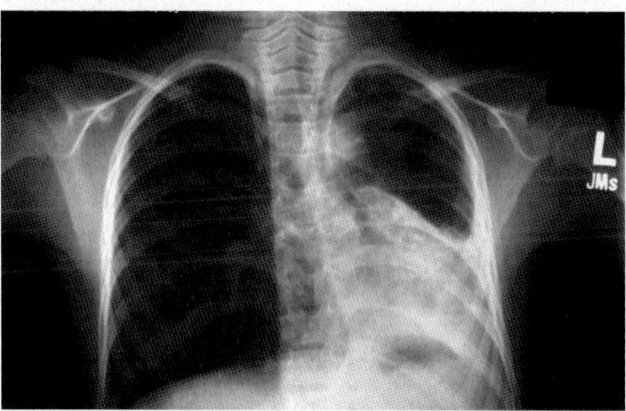

Fig. 29.8 Bronchiectasis of the left lower lobe in a child with tuberculosis who was nonadherent to appropriate treatment.

into the esophagus and produce a bronchoesophageal fistula. Enlarged lymph nodes may compress the subclavian vein and produce edema of the hand and arm, or they may erode major blood vessels, including the aorta. They also may rupture into the mediastinum and point in the left, or more often the right, supraclavicular fossa. Compression of the left recurrent laryngeal nerve has been reported. Rupture into the pericardial sac causes tuberculous pericarditis. The late results of bronchial obstruction include the following possibilities: (1) complete reexpansion of the lung and resolution of the radiographic findings; (2) disappearance of the segmental lesion, with residual calcification of the primary focus or the regional lymph nodes; or (3) scarring and progressive contraction of the lobe or segment usually associated with bronchiectasis (Fig. 29.8). Permanent anatomic sequelae result from segmental lesions in approximately 60% of all cases, even though the abnormality is usually not apparent on plain radiographs. Cylindric (rarely saccular) bronchiectasis, stenoses, and elongation or shortening can be demonstrated

on bronchography. Fortunately most of these abnormalities are asymptomatic in the upper lobes. However, secondary infection may occur in the middle and lower lobes and cause the middle-lobe syndrome.

In adults, symptomatic endobronchial TB has been treated with various interventional bronchoscopic techniques including endobronchial stenting, balloon dilation, and argon plasma coagulation.[54] There are no data supporting these interventions in children. When children are symptomatic from endobronchial disease, corticosteroids are a useful adjunct to antitubercular therapy in order to decrease the amount of airway inflammation.

Acute Pneumonia

TB can also produce an acute infection that is clinically and radiographically indistinguishable from acute pneumonia. A systematic review assessing the contribution of TB to pneumonia in children in high-burden areas found many studies reporting that children with TB had a cough duration of less than 1 week. This is in contrast to many case management guidelines calling for evaluation for TB in the presence of a chronic cough. Inpatient case-fatality rates for pneumonia associated with TB ranged from 4% to 21% in the four clinical studies that reported pathogen-related outcomes.[55] A seminal study from Zambia found that among hospitalized children who died of acute respiratory disease, 20% had TB on necropsy.[56] Many children in this study were also found to have simultaneous pyogenic pneumonia with TB (12 of 80 patients with dual diagnoses). In another study in Uganda, 18.9% of children presenting with acute pneumonia had pulmonary TB, which was associated with being less than 5 years of age and having a TB contact.[57] Providers in high-burden settings should be aware that TB can present as an acute pneumonia or with simultaneous pyogenic infection, especially in younger children and those with a history of a TB contact.

Adult-Type Disease

Chronic pulmonary TB, often called the adult type, or reactivation TB, occurs when pulmonary tissue has been previously sensitized to *M. tuberculosis* at primary infection and an isolated focus of organisms begins proliferating in that tissue. Chronic pulmonary TB rarely develops in children who acquired infection with *M. tuberculosis* before 10 years of age and is especially rare among children less than 2 years of age. It occurs more common when TB infection is acquired close to the onset of puberty. The preponderance of evidence supports the concept that most cases of reactivation TB result from endogenous reinfection with the dormant bacilli. However, reinfection with a different strain of *M. tuberculosis* leading to typical adult-type TB has been documented.

Reactivation pulmonary TB arises from the small round foci of organisms in the apices of the lungs (often called Assmann or Simon foci) resulting from the lymphohematogenous spread at the time of the initial infection.[58] Fibronodular infiltrates in one or both upper lobe apices are most common, but more extensive pulmonary involvement leads to diffuse consolidation or cavitation (Fig. 29.9). Involvement of thoracic lymph nodes is usually absent. Cough, remitting fevers, night sweats, chest pain, sputum production, and hemoptysis are the most common clinical manifestations.

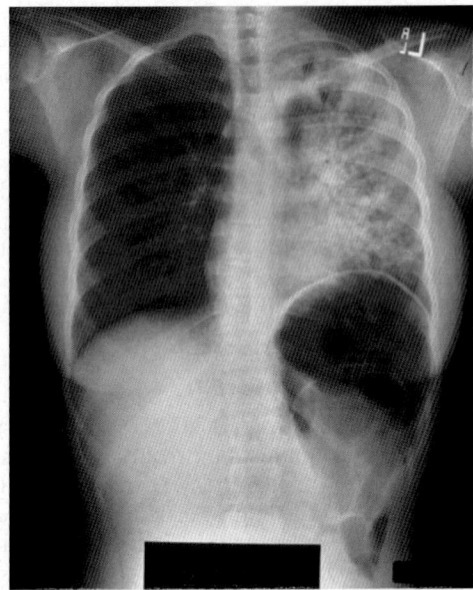

Fig. 29.9 A chest radiograph of an adolescent girl with chronic pulmonary tuberculosis.

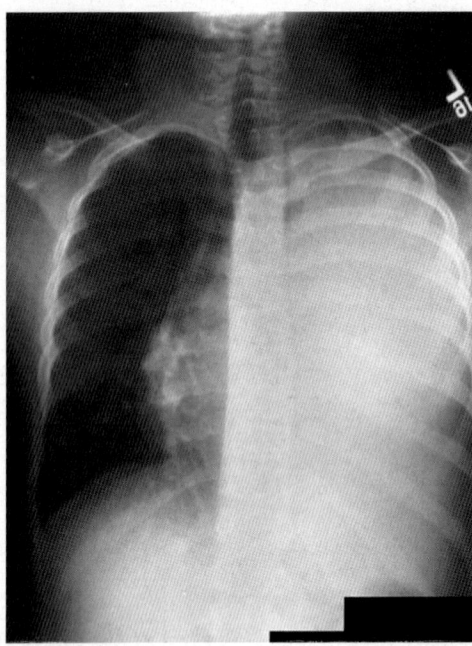

Fig. 29.10 A large tuberculous pleural effusion in an 11-year-old girl.

Pleural Disease

Pleural TB results from the direct spread of caseous material from a subpleural parenchymal or lymph node focus or from hematogenous spread.[58–60] Pleural TB is uncommon in children younger than 6 years of age and rare in those younger than 2 years of age. The presence of caseous material in the pleural space may trigger a hypersensitivity reaction, with the accumulation of serous straw-colored fluid containing few tubercle bacilli. This exudate has a high protein concentration and lymphocyte predominance; the number of polymorphonuclear cells depends on the acuteness of onset. Although direct microscopy is usually negative, culture yields may be as high as 40%–70%. However, molecular tests such as GeneXpert are not recommended for pleural fluid owing to their low sensitivity.[61] Pleural biopsy often demonstrates caseating granulomas and increases the culture yield if ample tissue is collected. The clinical course associated with pleural involvement characteristically begins with acute chest pain, accompanied by high fever in the absence of acute illness, an ill-defined loss of vigor, and a dry cough. Active caseation in the pleural space may cause thick loculated pus containing many tubercle bacilli (Fig. 29.10). The prognosis for children with tuberculous pleural effusion has always been good compared with other overt forms of TB, even before chemotherapy was available.

Extrapulmonary Disease

Tubercle bacilli from the lymphadenitis of the primary complex are disseminated during the incubation period in all cases of TB infection. The clinical picture produced by lymphohematogenous spread is probably determined by host susceptibility at the time of spread and by the quantity of tubercle bacilli released. Three clinical forms of dissemination are recognized:

1. The lymphohematogenous spread may be occult, in which case it usually remains so, or it may be occult initially with metastatic extrapulmonary lesions appearing months or years later (e.g., renal TB).
2. So-called protracted hematogenous TB, rarely seen today, is characterized by high spiking fever, marked leukocytosis, hepatosplenomegaly, and general glandular enlargement, sometimes with repeated evidence of metastatic seeding in the choroid plexus, kidney, and skin. Calcifications may appear subsequently, often in large numbers, in the pulmonary apices (Simon foci) and in the spleen, thus attesting to the earlier dissemination of tubercle bacilli via blood. The TST is usually strongly positive. Bone marrow biopsy may confirm the clinical impression, but treatment must often be started on a presumptive basis. Although this type of TB often ended tragically in TB meningitis in past years, today it is completely treatable if diagnosed in time.
3. The third form of lymphohematogenous spread, analogous to sepsis with pyogenic bacteria, is miliary TB. It usually arises from discharge of a caseous focus, often a lymph node, into a blood vessel such as a pulmonary vein. It may be self-propagating, with repeated discharge arising at various sites. Most common during the first 2–6 months after infection in infancy, it can arise even in adults who have apparently well-healed calcified lesions.

The clinical picture of miliary TB varies greatly, probably depending on the number of bacilli in the bloodstream.[34,62] Sometimes the patient is afebrile and appears to be well, and the condition is diagnosed by chance during contact investigation of another individual with infectious TB. The onset can be insidious, often occurring after the patient has had another precipitating infection. In rare cases, the onset is abrupt. Drowsiness, loss of weight and appetite, persistent fever, weakness, rapid breathing with a rustling sound on auscultation of the lungs, occasionally cyanosis and almost always a palpable spleen are the clinical manifestations that lead the clinician to obtain a chest radiograph.

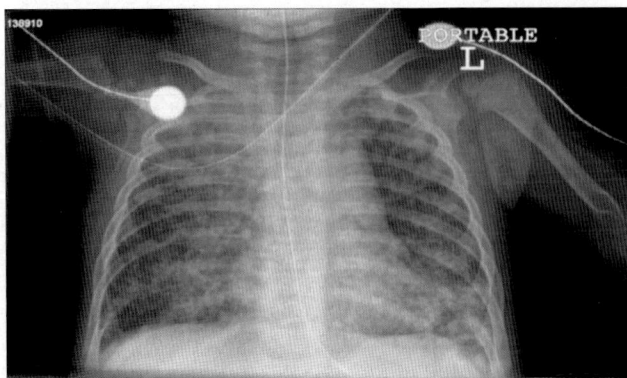

Fig. 29.11 The appearance of miliary tuberculosis in the chest radiograph of an infant.

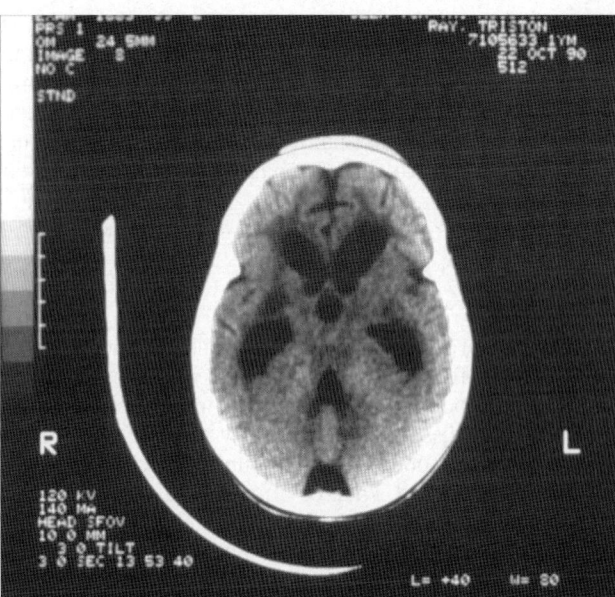

Fig. 29.12 A computed tomography scan of the head demonstrating the communicating hydrocephalus that is typical of tuberculosis meningitis.

Usually, within no more than 3 weeks after the onset of symptoms, tubercles, sometimes tiny and at times large, can be seen evenly distributed throughout both lung fields (Fig. 29.11). In the initial stages, they are often detected best on a lateral view of the retrocardiac space. Recurrent pneumothorax, subcutaneous emphysema, pneumomediastinum, and pleural effusion are less serious but well-recognized complications of miliary TB. Cutaneous lesions—including painful nodules, papulonecrotic tuberculids and purpuric lesions—may appear in crops. In addition, choroid tubercules can be noted on ophthalmologic exam and are specific for the diagnosis of miliary TB. The diagnosis of disseminated TB is usually established by means of the clinical picture and a chest radiograph; sometimes by a liver or skin biopsy; by culturing *M. tuberculosis* from the gastric aspirate, sputum, urine, or bone marrow; or by fiberoptic bronchoscopy. Treatment is usually very successful.

EXTRATHORACIC TUBERCULOSIS

A complete description of extrathoracic TB is beyond the scope of this chapter. However, pulmonologists may encounter this possibility in evaluating children with pulmonary involvement and other manifestations. The most common forms of extrathoracic disease in children include TB of the superficial lymph nodes (scrofula) and the central nervous system. Other rare forms of extrathoracic disease in children are osteoarticular, abdominal, gastrointestinal, genitourinary, cutaneous, and congenital disease.

TB of the superficial lymph nodes (scrofula) is the most common form of extrathoracic disease.[63,64] Although this disease is also associated with *M. bovis* acquired by drinking unpasteurized cow's milk or cheese, most current cases occur after primary pulmonary infection with *M. tuberculosis* within 6–9 months of initial infection. Children between the ages of 5 and 10 years, followed by children over the age of 10 years, are most likely to have this presentation, but scrofula can occur in any age group. Scrofula occurs when primary lesions of the upper lung fields or abdomen extend to involve the supraclavicular, anterior cervical, tonsillar and submandibular nodes. In children, TB of the skin or skeletal system rarely leads to involvement of the inguinal, epitrochlear, or axillary lymph nodes. Early during infection, lymph nodes are discrete, firm, and nontender. The lymph nodes become fixed to surrounding tissues and feel matted as the infection

progresses. Low-grade fever may be the only systemic symptom. Although usually present, a primary pulmonary complex is visible radiologically only 30%–70% of the time. TST or IGRA results are usually reactive. Although spontaneous resolution is possible, untreated lymphadenitis frequently progresses to caseating necrosis, capsular rupture and spread to adjacent nodes and overlying skin. Rupture through the skin results in a draining sinus tract that may require surgical removal. Excisional biopsy and culture of lymph nodes are often required to differentiate between TB and NTM disease.

Central nervous system disease is the most serious complication of TB in children and complicates approximately 0.5% of untreated primary infections. It is most common in children 6 months to 4 years of age and generally occurs within 2–6 months of primary infection.[65] Central nervous system disease arises from the formation of a caseous lesion in the cerebral cortex or meninges that results from early occult lymphohematogenous spread.[66] Lesions enlarge and discharge bacilli into the subarachnoid space, leading to an exudate that infiltrates the cortical and meningeal blood vessels. This results in inflammation, obstruction, and subsequent infarction of the cerebral cortex. The clinical onset of TB meningitis can be rapid or gradual. Infants and children are more likely to experience a rapid progression to hydrocephalus, seizure, and cerebral edema over several days (Fig. 29.12). In most children, signs and symptoms progress over several weeks, beginning nonspecifically with fever, headache, irritability, and drowsiness. Disease often advances abruptly with symptoms of lethargy, vomiting, nuchal rigidity, seizures, hypertonia, and focal neurologic signs. The final stage of disease is marked by coma, hypertension, decerebrate and decorticate posturing, and eventual death. Rapid confirmation of TB meningitis can be extremely difficult, with wide variability in cerebrospinal fluid characteristics and nonreactive TSTs in 40% of cases. Although some older studies reported normal chest radiographs in 50% of cases, more recent reports indicate that 80% of young children with TB meningitis have significant abnormalities on chest radiography. Since improved outcomes are associated with prompt treatment, empiric antituberculosis therapy should be instituted for any child with basilar meningitis and hydrocephalus or cranial nerve involvement that has no other apparent cause.

TUBERCULOSIS AND HUMAN IMMUNODEFICIENCY VIRUS

Immune-compromised HIV-infected children have a higher risk of developing extrapulmonary disease manifestations indicative of poor organism containment, such as tuberculomas and disseminated (miliary disease).[30–32] Their presentations are notably similar to those of very young non–HIV-infected children. Lack of an age-related difference in disease presentation suggests that immune maturation is less relevant in HIV-infected children.[30] Because of the common presence of other HIV-related lung pathology on chest x-ray, such as LIP, it is often challenging to diagnose TB accurately, particularly disseminated (miliary) disease. These tremendous diagnostic difficulties result in a tendency to overdiagnose TB in this vulnerable group of children. When pulmonary TB develops in an HIV-infected child, the response to standard short-course TB therapy has lower cure rates and higher mortality, but HIV-infected children can still recover with appropriate therapy.[32,67] However, these children can develop sequelae such as bronchiectasis if TB therapy and antiretroviral therapy (ART) are delayed.[68] TB may further hasten the progression of HIV disease by increasing viral replication and depleting CD4+ T lymphocytes.[69] The confirmation of TB disease in HIV-infected children is complicated by the low yield of culture and chronic HIV-related comorbidities.[31]

Diagnosis

DIAGNOSTIC IMAGING

Various imaging modalities can be used to evaluate for intrathoracic TB. Ultrasonography is increasingly used as a point-of-care test in many settings to detect mediastinal lymphadenopathy and pleural fluid because of it has the advantages of lack of radiation, ease of interpretation, potential for portability and rapid results. However, this requires significant performer training. CT is another option that is available in some settings. It provides high definition of the lung parenchyma and mediastinal structures, which is useful if the chest x-ray findings require further delineation, such as determining if a density is due to prominent vasculature or lymphadenopathy. However, CT uses a significant amount of radiation, requires intravenous contrast and is costly. These issues limit CT use in low-resource settings.

CHEST RADIOGRAPHY

Chest radiography was the first diagnostic test outside of stain and culture that assisted in the diagnosis of TB. Radiography services are available in high-burden low-resource settings but are more likely to be located at referral centers than at decentralized providers. Many of the pathognomonic

findings of TB can be seen on plain chest radiographs. Posteroanterior and lateral images have the most utility. Parenchymal disease, such as that found early in progressive primary infection or in acute pneumonia, appears to be identical to other airspace diseases as a nonspecific infiltrate. These areas can calcify and subsequently appear as hyperlucencies on imaging. If parenchymal disease is untreated, the area can develop a cavity, which manifests itself as a hyperlucent ring devoid of airspace markings on the interior (see Fig. 29.3).

The hallmark of pediatric TB is intrathoracic lymphadenopathy, which can manifest in a multitude of ways on radiography. Lymph nodes appear as a soft tissue density on radiography. Because these nodes commonly occur in the hilum and mediastinum, it is often difficult to differentiate these densities from the other soft tissues, such as the thymus and major blood vessels. It is often easier to see the consequence of lymphadenopathy rather than the lymph node itself. Once the lymph nodes become enlarged, they can affect nearby structures in several ways. Large lymph nodes can exert mass effect on the airways. For example, enlarged subcarinal nodes can push on the mainstem bronchi and cause the bronchi to appear splayed (see Fig. 29.3). Lymph nodes can also impinge on the airway, causing a narrowing of the airway that is notable on imaging (Fig. 29.13), with distal hyperinflation from a ball-valve effect (see Fig. 29.6A), or they may cause secondary collapse of the distal segment, manifesting as a fan-shaped consolidation (see Fig. 29.6B). When not exerting a mass effect, hilar lymph nodes can also be noted on posteroanterior images as enlargement of the mediastinal silhouette (Fig. 29.14A). On lateral images, lymphadenopathy densities can produce what is known as the "donut sign" in the posterior mediastinum, comprising the great vessels of the heart superiorly and the hilar lymphadenopathy inferiorly (Fig. 29.14B).

Interpretations of chest radiography findings can vary between clinicians. Du Toit compared three experienced pediatric radiologists' interobserver and intraobserver interpretations of chest radiographs and found that the radiologists

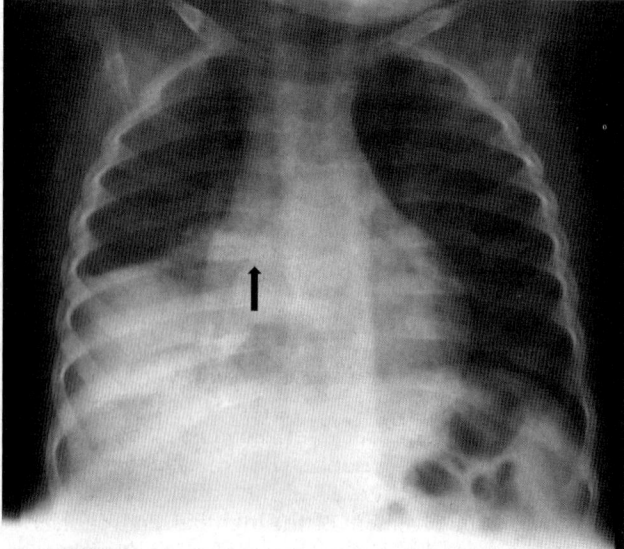

Fig. 29.13 Posteroanterior view of a child with right-lower-lobe infiltrate and narrowing of the right mainstem bronchus (*solid arrow*).

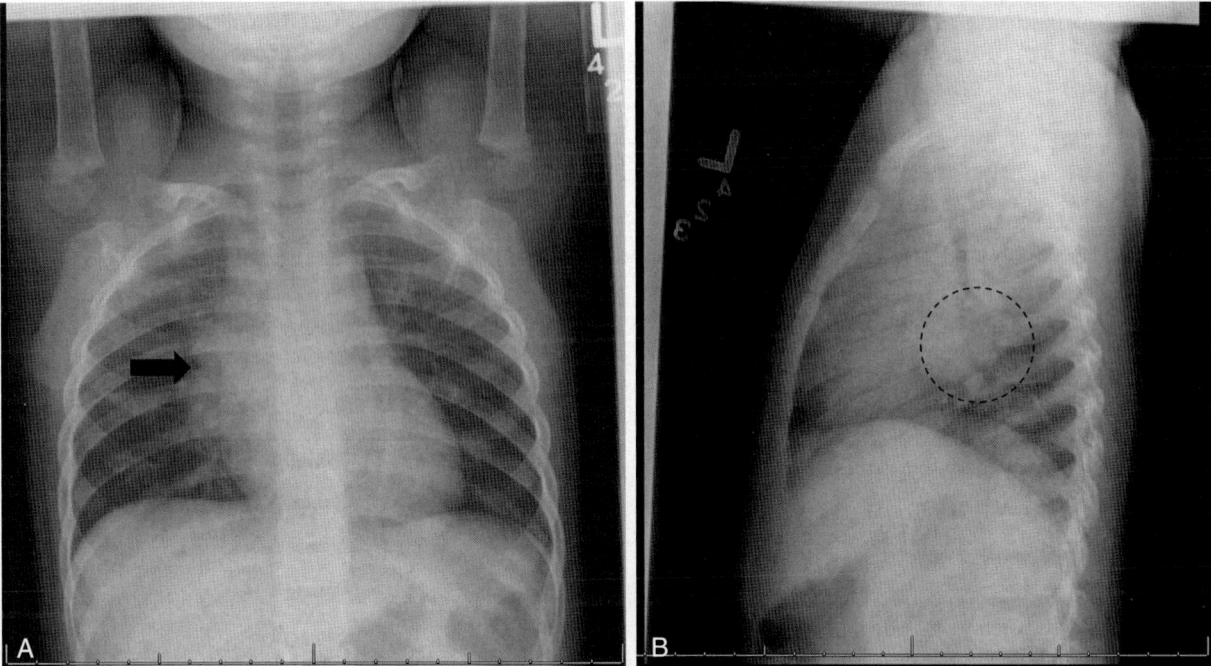

Fig. 29.14 (A) Posteroanterior view of a child with right hilar lymphadenopathy *(solid black arrow)*. (B) Lateral view of same child with a "donut sign" within the dotted circle comprising the great vessels superiorly and subcarinal lymph nodes inferiorly.

agreed on the presence of lymphadenopathy with a kappa of 0.40, which indicates only moderate agreement. Agreement between a radiologist's first read of an image and a second read after weeks of delay was higher but still offered only moderate agreement (a kappa of 0.55).[70] This illustrates the difficulties in assessing intrathoracic lymphadenopathy, and consequently TB, in pediatric films. Several standardized approaches have been recommended for radiologic interpretation of childhood TB, but these are not always utilized.[49,71–73]

Tests of Infection

TUBERCULIN SKIN TEST

The TST remains the most widely employed test for the diagnosis of TB disease and infection in children. The sensitivity and specificity of the TST are significantly affected by several factors; these are reviewed in this section.

Infection with *M. tuberculosis* produces a delayed-type hypersensitivity reaction to specific antigenic components of the bacilli that are contained in extracts of culture filtrates called *tuberculins*. A batch of purified protein derivative (PPD), called PPD-S, produced by Siebert and Glenn in 1939, serves as the standard reference material worldwide. In response to the antigen, previously sensitized T cells release lymphokines that induce local vasodilation, edema, fibrin deposition and recruitment of other inflammatory cells.[74] The reaction begins 5–6 hours after injection and reaches maximal induration at 48–72 hours, the time when the test should be interpreted. Variability of the results of the TST may be reduced by careful attention to details of administration and reading, which should be done by trained professionals. The diameter of induration should be measured transversely to the long axis of the forearm and recorded in millimeters.

Use of the ballpoint pen method developed by Sokal minimizes interobserver variability. In some individuals, the reaction may peak after 72 hours, and the largest reaction size at any time after 48 hours is considered the result. Vesiculation and necrosis occur rarely. In these cases, the result is always considered positive and repeat tuberculin testing should be avoided. A video from the Grey Bruce Health Unit in Ontario demonstrates TST administration and is available at https://www.youtube.com/watch?v=bR86G-itrTQ.

The size of the area of induration should be interpreted within the view of the child's risk of having acquired TB infection and the risk of progressing to TB disease. TST interpretation is dependent on the clinical setting. In the United States and Canada, 5 mm is used as the smallest area of induration that can be positive for the highest-risk groups, such as children with HIV infection, signs of TB disease, or recent exposure to a known TB case. An area of induration 15 mm or greater is positive even for an individual with no risk factors for disease. Guidelines for TST interpretation in the United States are available in Box 29.1. The United Kingdom now uses a universal size of 5 mm as positive.[75] The WHO recommends use of a cutoff of 10 mm for most children and a cutoff of 5 mm in immunosuppressed children.[76] WHO guidelines are followed in most countries.[77] A nonreactive TST does not exclude TB infection or disease. Several factors can diminish tuberculin reactivity resulting in a false-negative reaction (Box 29.2). The administration of live-attenuated vaccines results in immune system suppression that appears more than 48 hours after vaccination. Tuberculin skin testing may be performed on either the same day as vaccination with live virus or 4–6 weeks later. Studies have demonstrated that up to 10% of immunocompetent children with reactive anergy tests and culture-confirmed pulmonary TB have false-negative reactions to tuberculin testing.[78]

Box 29.1 Definitions of a Positive Tuberculin Skin Test Result in Infants, Children, and Adolescents

Induration ≥5 mm

- Children in close contact with known or suspected contagious case of tuberculosis disease
- Children suspected to have tuberculosis disease: Findings on chest radiograph consistent with active or previously active tuberculosis
- Clinical evidence of tuberculosis disease
  Children receiving immunosuppressive therapy or with immunosuppressive conditions, including human immunodeficiency virus (HIV) infection

Induration ≥10 mm

- Children at increased risk for disseminated disease: those younger than 4 years of age
- Those with other medical conditions, including Hodgkin disease, lymphoma, diabetes mellitus, chronic renal failure or malnutrition
  Children with increased exposure to tuberculosis disease:
- Those born or whose parents were born in high-prevalence regions of the world
- Those frequently exposed to adults who are infected with HIV, homeless, users of illicit drugs, residents of nursing homes, incarcerated or institutionalized or migrant farm workers
- Those who travel to high-prevalence regions of the world

Induration ≥≥15 mm

Children 4 years of age or older without any risk factors

Box 29.2 Factors Causing False-Negative Tuberculin Skin Test Results

Factors Related to the Person Being Tested

Infections
Viral (measles, mumps, chickenpox, human immunodeficiency virus)
Bacterial (typhoid fever, brucellosis, typhus, leprosy, pertussis, overwhelming tuberculosis, tuberculosis pleurisy)
Fungal (blastomycosis)
Live virus vaccinations (measles, mumps, polio, varicella)
Metabolic derangements (chronic renal failure)
Low protein states (severe protein depletion, afibrinogenemia)
Diseases affecting lymphoid organs (Hodgkin disease, lymphoma, chronic leukemia, sarcoidosis)
Drugs (corticosteroids and other immunosuppressive agents)
Age (newborns, elderly patients with "waned" sensitivity)
Stress (surgery, burns, mental illness, graft-versus-host reactions)

Factors Related to the Tuberculin Used

Improper storage (exposure to light and heat)
Improper dilutions
Chemical denaturation
Contamination
Adsorption (partially controlled by adding Tween 80)

Factors Related to the Method of Administration

Injection of too little antigen
Subcutaneous injection
Delayed administration after drawing into syringe
Injection too close to other skin tests

Factors Related to Reading the Test and Recording Results

Inexperienced reader
Conscious or unconscious bias
Error in recording

In many of these children, TST conversion occurs after several months of treatment, suggesting that the infection was recently acquired or resulted in suppression of the immune response. Skin testing results were available in nearly all (95.4%) children reported to have newly diagnosed TB in the United States between 1993 and 2001. Of these children, 11% had negative skin test results as defined by CDC guidelines.[79] Of note, children who were diagnosed with disseminated or meningeal TB were less likely to have a positive TST result (57.6% and 54.6%, respectively) than those with pulmonary TB (90.6%).

A number of factors have been associated with false-positive tuberculin reactions and decreased tuberculin test specificity. Because some antigens in PPD are shared with other mycobacteria, false-positive reactions can occur in children who have been infected with other mycobacteria or who have been vaccinated with BCG. Exposure to NTM varies geographically and generally results in smaller, transient indurations than those caused by *M. tuberculosis*. The degree of BCG cross-reactivity is dependent on a number of factors, including strain of BCG employed, repeated BCG vaccination, age and nutritional status at vaccination, frequency of skin testing, and years since vaccination.[80–83] In most studies of children who received a BCG vaccine during the newborn period, only 50% reacted to tuberculin testing at 12 months, and 80%–90% lose reactivity within 2–3 years. Although BCG vaccination of older children or adults results in greater initial and more persistent cross-reactivity, most of these individuals lose cross-reactivity within 10 years of vaccination. Most guidelines currently suggest that the TST should

be interpreted in the same way for patients who have and have not received a BCG vaccination; however, this will lead to some children with false-positive TST results being treated. A growing body of evidence now demonstrates that the impact of infant BCG vaccination on TST responses in children exposed to TB wanes with age, but in young BCG-vaccinated children, a TST cutoff of 5 mm is associated with poor specificity.[83–86] Nevertheless, as young children have the greatest risk of progression from infection to disease and are also the most susceptible to severe disseminated forms of TB disease, test sensitivity remains more important than specificity in evaluating children in this age group.

INTERFERON-GAMMA RELEASE ASSAYS

The identification of genes in the *M. tuberculosis* genome that are absent from *M. bovis* BCG[87] and most NTM[88] has supported the development of more specific tests for the detection of *M. tuberculosis*.[89] *M. bovis* BCG has 16-gene deletions, including the region of difference 1 (RD-1) that encodes for early secretory antigen target-6 (ESAT-6) and culture filtrate protein 10 (CFP-10).[88,90] ESAT-6 and CFP-10 are strong targets of the cellular immune response in patients with *M. tuberculosis* infection and disease.[91,92] In people with TB infection or disease, sensitized memory/effector T cells produce IFN-γ in response to *M. tuberculosis* antigens, forming the biologic basis for both the TST and IGRAs. Research over the past two decades[89,93] has resulted in the development of two commercial brands of IGRAs that are approved for use in Europe and the United States. In brief, the Quantiferon assays (QFTs; Cellestis Limited, Australia)[94] are enzyme-linked immunosorbent assay (ELISA)–based whole blood assays measuring the amount of IFN-γ produced in response to *M. tuberculosis*–specific antigens. In contrast, the enzyme-linked immunospot (ELISPOT)–based test (T.SPOT.TB; T.Spot; Oxford Immunotec, Abingdon, Oxfordshire, United Kingdom)[95] uses peripheral mononuclear cells to detect the number of INF-γ– producing T cells. Of note, both commercial IGRAs also measure a response to a negative control and a nonspecific positive control stimulant, such as phytohemagglutinin (PHA). Results are then interpreted on the basis of a comparison of the magnitude of the response to the *M. tuberculosis*–specific stimulus compared with the negative controls. A lack of response to the positive control is interpreted as an indeterminate (Quantiferon) or invalid (T-SPOT.TB) result. Similarly, a robust response to the negative stimuli is considered an invalid or indeterminate result.

In the absence of a gold standard for infection, studies have assessed the performance of IGRAs in children with bacteriologically confirmed and clinically diagnosed TB disease. A systematic review of these pediatric studies estimated the specificity of commercially approved IGRAs for detecting *M. tuberculosis* infection at 91% for the ELISA-based tests and 94% for the ELISPOT-based test, compared with 88% for the TST (positive defined as 10 mm).[96] Estimates of test sensitivity were similar for the three tests: 83% (QFT assays), 84% (T.SPOT) and 84% (TST), respectively. Similarly, a second pediatric systematic review found the performance of the TST and QFT assays to be no different but noted that a qualitative review of four pediatric studies suggested that the QFT assays were more specific for the detection of TB infection in children compared with the TST.[97] Like the TST, IGRAs cannot differentiate between TB infection and TB disease.

The lack of a gold standard for the detection of TB infection complicates studies of diagnostic accuracy,[98] many of which have employed surrogate measures of infection to serve as the reference standard for TB infection.[96] The association between IGRA positivity and the presence of TB exposure is well described in low-burden countries.[99-101] Results from high-burden countries examining IGRA positivity and the presence of TB exposure are conflicting and demonstrate both advantages of the T.SPOT[102] and no difference in T.SPOT performance compared with TST and QFT.[103] A few key studies have illustrated that exposure may be quantified to support direct comparison of tests of TB infection.[100,102-105] The largest of these studies, including over 1300 children, demonstrated that IGRAs were more strongly associated with quantified TB exposure than the TST.[105] Pooled analysis of studies employing a measure of TB exposure also demonstrates that positive IGRA results are more strongly correlated with quantified TB exposure than the TST results.[96]

There is limited and conflicting evidence regarding IGRA use in young or impoverished children. Studies have demonstrated variable association between indeterminate IGRA results and young age, with some studies showing an association[106-111] and others showing no association.[103,105,112,113] A seminal study of European immigrant children found that indeterminate IGRA results were more frequent among young children but occurred at clinically insignificant rates of 1.8% and 1.6 % for the QFT and T.SPOT, respectively.[111] Most studies have reported indeterminate rates less than 10%.[96] Emerging evidence further demonstrates that a number of factors related to poverty (malnourishment,[105,113,114] micronutrient deficiency[115] and helminth infection)[116,117] may lead to diminished IGRA sensitivity.

Limited data are available regarding IGRA performance in immune-compromised HIV-infected children, in whom the performance of the TST is impaired.[118-120] Two studies suggest that test failures described as indeterminate or invalid results are common among pediatric oncology patients.[121,122] Two studies have shown a noncommercial IFN-γ ELISPOT assay to have higher sensitivity for detecting TB infection compared with the TST in HIV-infected children.[118,123] A comparison of the QFT–gold assay and the TST for the detection of TB infection in 36 young HIV-infected children with culture-confirmed TB disease found comparable sensitivity in children with CD4+ cell counts below 200/mL; unfortunately indeterminate QFT-gold results were reported in 25% of children tested.[124] In a head-to-head comparison among 130 HIV-infected and 120 HIV-uninfected children, the TST and IGRAs performed similarly for the detection of TB infection in well-nourished HIV-uninfected children, but test performance was differentially affected by chronic malnutrition, HIV infection and age.[113] In a study of over 1300 children, indeterminate QFT results were more frequent in HIV-infected (4.7%) than HIV-uninfected children (1.9%), while T.SPOT invalid results were rare (0.2%) and were not affected by HIV infection.[105] Conversion, reversion and operational measures were not associated with HIV status. Among HIV-infected children, test sensitivities declined as malnutrition worsened. As a conclusion from the available evidence, clinicians should take age, nutritional status, and HIV status into consideration in interpreting IGRAs.

Both the TST and IGRAs have limitations, but use of the tests in targeted populations with increased risk of TB infection or TB disease maximizes the impact of testing. IGRAs are commonly used in children living in upper-income, low-burden countries and have influenced clinical decision making.[123] National guidelines continue to change and vary dramatically among countries in light of rapidly emerging evidence. Pragmatic approaches to the use of IGRAs and TST have emerged through clinical practice and are emerging in formal guidelines.[125]

The purpose of the TST and IGRAs is to determine whether the person is infected with *M. tuberculosis*, which can serve as a useful tool in the diagnosis of TB, and guide subsequent care for infection or disease. Attributes of the child and the purpose of the testing should inform the choice of which diagnostic test to use (Fig. 29.15). Per the American Academy of Pediatrics (AAP), "Only children who have risk of TB exposure, underlying health conditions that require immune suppression, or suspected TB disease should be tested for TB infection in TB low-burden settings."[125] In low-risk, BCG-vaccinated or NTM-exposed children in whom the TST will result in a considerable number of false-positive results, high specificity is desired, making the IGRAs preferable. In young or immune-compromised children with significant risk of TB progression following TB infection, testing strategies should optimize sensitivity. Although it may compromise specificity of the testing strategy, both an IGRA and a TST should be

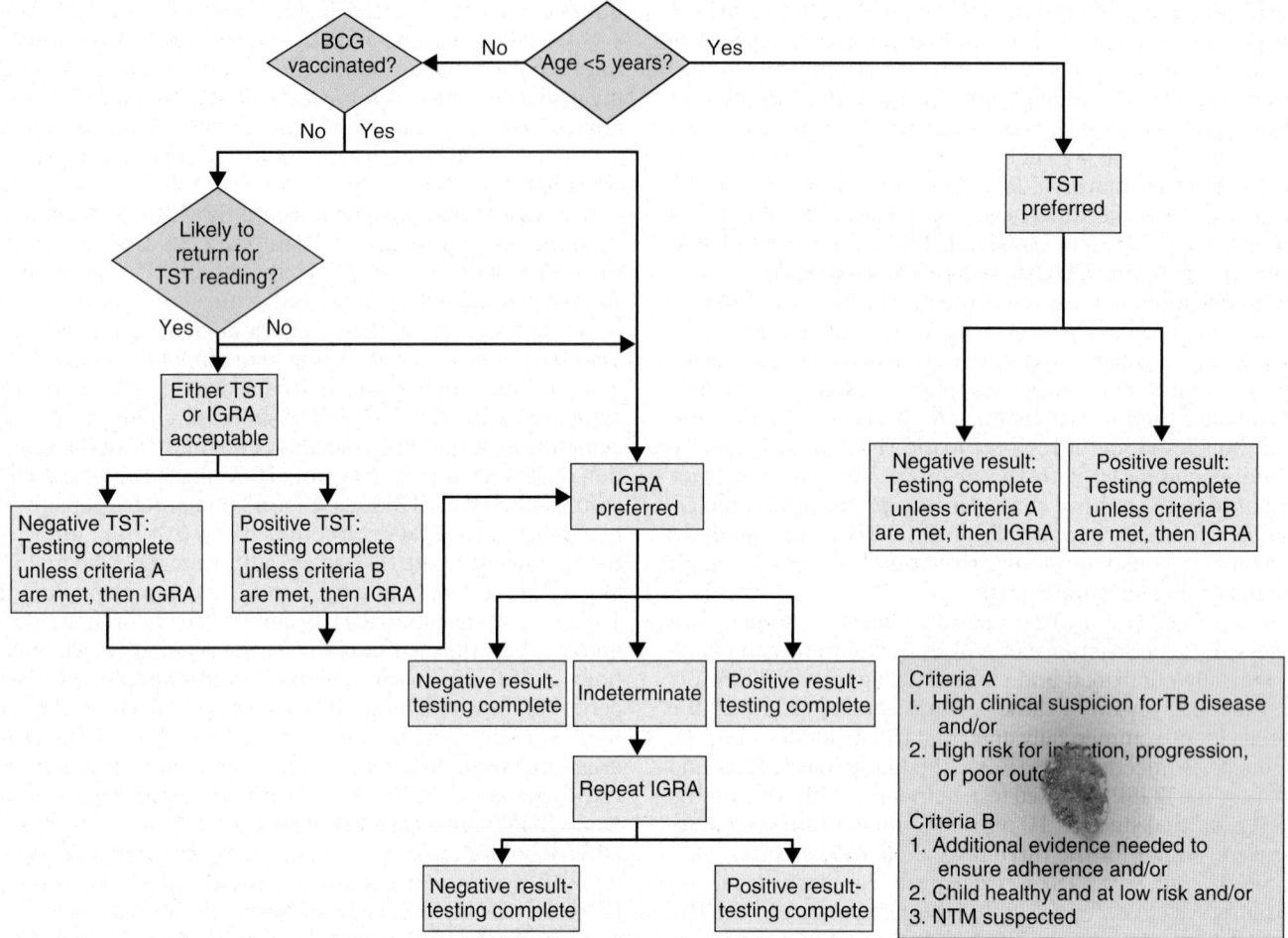

Fig. 29.15 An algorithm for the use of tuberculin skin test (TST) and interferon-γ release assays (IGRAs) in children with risk of tuberculosis (TB) infection in low-burden settings. *BCG,* Bacillus Calmette-Guérin; *NTM,* nontuberculous mycobacteria. (Reproduced with permission from the American Academy of Pediatrics. *Pediatrics.* 2014;134(6):e1770.)

performed in a child with a high suspicion of TB disease or a high risk of progression to TB disease. In these instances, a positive result with either the TST or IGRA should be considered evidence of TB infection. Although this approach may result in overtreatment, the benefits of avoiding disease progression generally outweigh the risk of overtreatment, particularly since children tolerate treatment of TB infection with few side effects.

IGRAs offer several pragmatic advantages compared with the TST (Table 29.2). Use of *M. tuberculosis*–specific antigens improves specificity and decreases the chance of false-positive responses, particularly in young BCG-vaccinated children. Use of internal positive controls assesses anergy, which can be useful in immune-compromised and young children. Because IGRAs do not require a second visit to measure the response, they afford an advantage in testing patients who may have difficulty returning, such as emergency department patients, migrants, and homeless individuals. Although the direct cost of IGRAs is greater than that of the TST, evidence from studies of adults suggests that IGRAs are cost-effective in certain populations and in high-income settings by decreasing the number of false-positive results and reducing the subsequent evaluation and treatment of patients.[126–129] However, the WHO has recommended against the use of

IGRAs in low- and middle-income countries for several reasons, including but not limited to a lack of evidence of on their performance in high-burden, low-income countries and the increased cost and technical skill required as compared to the TST.[130]

Laboratory Diagnosis

Careful attention to the details of specimen collection and handling can optimize the isolation and identification of *M. tuberculosis*. A variety of specimens can be collected, including sputum, induced sputum, gastric aspirates, bronchial washings, bronchoalveolar lavage, transbronchial biopsy, urine, blood, tissue, cerebrospinal fluid and other body fluids.[131,132] Because children cannot easily produce sputum, gastric aspirates are frequently obtained. Optimal collection of gastric aspirates usually entails hospitalization to acquire about 50 mL of early-morning gastric contents after the child has fasted for at least 8–10 hours and preferably while he or she is still in bed.[133] Alternatively, trained public health nurses may perform this procedure in the home or clinic. *M. tuberculosis* may be recovered from gastric aspirates in roughly 40% of children with radiographic evidence of significant pulmonary disease.[134] Because many specimens contain an abundance of bacteria other than mycobacteria, specimens should be collected in a sterile fashion and held under conditions that minimize the growth of contaminating organisms.

In addition to gastric aspiration, sputum induction is a means of sample collection. In this process, a child is treated first with an inhaled beta agonist followed by hypertonic saline. As the child begins coughing, the practitioner suctions the child's mouth and throat to obtain the specimen. Sputum induction offers advantages as it can easily be performed in outpatient settings and only requires 3 hours of

fasting as opposed to overnight fasting, which is considered optimal for gastric aspiration. In studies from Cape Town, sputum induction has yielded more positive cultures than gastric aspiration—51 of 250 (20%) versus 38 of 250 (15%)—with yield improving with the sampling of multiple specimens.[135]

The yield of any diagnostic test is increased if adequate specimens are obtained. In addition, yield increases for both gastric aspirates and induced sputum if multiple specimens are obtained. However, obtaining multiple specimens can be a difficult endeavor in outpatient settings, where children and their caregivers may have to travel far to access care. Both procedures require frequent training of health care workers and availability of necessary supplies to promote their use, which is often an obstacle in high-burden settings. Despite ongoing academic debate regarding the preferred sputum collection technique, providers should be supported to perform the procedure that they are most comfortable with, as this will likely lead to the greatest number of specimens being collected and ultimately improve diagnostic yield. Videos are available from the Francis Curry TB Center and Medecins Sans Frontieres South Africa to demonstrate how both gastric aspirates (https://www.youtube.com/watch?v=21Rjk2E-Lsc) and induced sputum (https://www.youtube.com/watch?v=sbGITrNP8j8) are obtained.

Diagnostic tests for TB disease either detect the presence of *M. tuberculosis* in a clinical sample or demonstrate a host response to the organism. Methods for diagnosis of TB are summarized in Table 29.3. Tests of infection, either IGRA or TST, can help clinicians who are considering a diagnosis of TB disease. If either test of infection is positive, it increases the likelihood that a child's symptoms are caused by *M. tuberculosis*, but as tests of infection can be negative during disease, a clinical index of suspicion should have more weight than a negative test of disease.

STAINING AND MICROSCOPIC EXAMINATION

Acid-fast staining and microscopic examination are the easiest, quickest, and least expensive diagnostic procedures.

Table 29.2 Comparison of the Tuberculin Skin Test and Interferon-Gamma Release Assay

Consideration	TST	IGRA
Sampling	Intradermal injection	Blood draw
Patient visits required	Two	One
BCG cross-reactivity	Yes	No
NTM cross-reactivity	Yes	Infrequent[a]
Boosting associated with repeat testing	Yes	No
Population specific interpretation	Yes	No
Internal controls for anergy	No	Yes
Subject to human variability	Yes	No
Subject to laboratory error	No	Yes
Requires trained clinical staff	Yes	No
Requires trained laboratory staff	No	Yes
Relies on host immune function	Yes	Yes
Distinguishes TB infection from disease	No	No
Predicts progression from TB infection to disease	No	No
Distinguishes remote versus recent infection	No	No
Monitors treatment efficacy	No	No

[a]IGRA positivity results from infection with the following organisms thereby decreasing test specificity: *Mycobacterium marinum, M. kansasii, M. szulgai* and *M. flavescans*.

BCG, Bacillus Calmette-Guérin; *IGRA*, interferon-gamma release assay; *NTM*, nontuberculous mycobacteria; *TB*, tuberculosis; *TST*, tuberculin skin test.

Table 29.3 Summary of Laboratory Methods for the Diagnosis of Tuberculosis

Identification Method	Test System	Use
Culture	Conventional media (Lowenstein Jensen, Middlebrook agars) Colony morphology (3–5 weeks) Biochemical tests	Preliminary identification Species identification
Microscopic-observation drug-susceptibility (MODS)	Positive growth (1–2 weeks)	Identification and drug susceptibility Easy, inexpensive, highly sensitive
Radiometric methods	Positive growth index (5–14 days)	Differentiates *Mycobacterium tuberculosis* from nontuberculosis mycobacterial species
Chromatography	HPLC mycolic acid profile Gas chromatography–fatty acid profile	Speciates all common mycobacteria
DNA probes	Gen-Probe ACCUPROBE Syngene SNAP probes	Identifies *M. tuberculosis* complex, *M. avium, M. intracellulare-avium* complex, *M. kansasii, M. gordonae* Identifies *M. tuberculosis* complex, *M. avium* complex
Rapid direct tests Direct smear	Acid-fast or fluorochrome stains	Easy, inexpensive, moderately sensitive
Nucleic acid detection	PCR amplification Line probe assays	Moderately sensitive, highly specific, technically complex
Cartridge-based nucleic acid detection	GeneXpert	Highly specific, moderately sensitive, easy performance but high initial cost

DNA, Deoxyribonucleic acid; *EIA*, enzyme immunoassay; *HPLC*, high-performance liquid chromatography; *PCR*, polymerase chain reaction.

Yield of microscopy is dependent on stain selection because the auramine-rhodamine fluorescent stain is more sensitive than the traditional Kinyoun or Ziehl–Neelsen stains. However, these methods can provide physicians with only preliminary confirmation of the diagnosis because of the inability to differentiate between *M. tuberculosis* and NTM. Additionally, there must be 5000–10,000 bacilli present per milliliter of specimen to allow detection of the bacteria in stained smears, resulting in low sensitivity in children. Acid-fast staining of gastric aspirates and sputum is positive in fewer than 10% of children with pulmonary TB.

CULTURE

Culture is the most important laboratory test for the diagnosis and management of TB. A positive culture may result from as few as 10 organisms per milliliter of specimen. Growth of bacilli is necessary for precise speciation and DST. Genotyping of the organism may be useful to identify epidemiologic links. Unfortunately bacteriologic confirmation of TB in children is generally poor. For example, in the United States from 1997 to 2007, over 70% of adult pulmonary TB cases had a positive culture, compared with 45% in children.[136] In three studies evaluating the role of bronchoscopy, only 13%–62% of cultures in children with pulmonary TB were positive.[134,137,138] The yield from gastric aspirates was higher in these studies. Bronchoscopy can be useful to define anatomy or clarify the diagnosis, but it cannot be recommended solely to collect culture specimens in children.

Reliance on detection of *M. tuberculosis* using available methods will lead to misdiagnosis of the majority of cases of childhood pulmonary TB. Even in developed countries, the gold standard for diagnosis of childhood TB is a triad of (1) an abnormal chest radiograph and/or clinical findings consistent with TB, (2) a positive TST or IGRA result and (3) a history of contact with an infectious TB case within the past year. If the results of DST on the organism isolated from the contact case are available, obtaining a culture from the child adds little sensitivity or specificity to the diagnosis if the triad is present.[51,58]

As noted in the section on mycobacteriology, specimens can be isolated on either solid or liquid media, taking 7–10 days for growth in liquid media and 3–6 weeks for growth on solid media. Standard concentrations of antitubercular drugs can be added to the media to provide DST. A certain amount of growth in media containing antitubercular therapy versus controls indicates phenotypic resistance.

The microscopic-observation drug-susceptibility (MODS) assay is a variation of traditional DST, where the organism is inoculated into several wells containing concentrations of antitubercular drugs in addition to a control well. The wells are examined daily by inverted light microscopy to visualize cord formation, which indicates *M. tuberculosis* growth. The growth in wells with antitubercular drugs indicates resistance. This assay has been shown to perform better than traditional culture methods in two settings. In Peru, two cohorts showed that MODS detected more TB cases (87%–91%) versus traditional culture methods (55%–59%).[139] In Vietnam, MODS performed better than smear (46% vs. 8.8%) and culture (46% vs. 38.9%), even on nonsputum samples.[140] MODS is endorsed by the WHO for use at reference laboratories.[141]

DNA METHODOLOGIES

DNA probe methods use nucleic acid hybridization with specifically labeled sequences to rapidly detect complementary sequences in the test sample. Various systems are commercially available. Although the *M. tuberculosis* complex probe tests have been 99%–100% specific, the dependence of these methods on large numbers of bacilli means that they can be used only in the laboratory on cultured organisms.[142]

Direct detection of the DNA of *M. tuberculosis* in clinical samples has been performed using nucleic acid amplification, most often utilizing the polymerase chain reaction (PCR). Most techniques have used the mycobacterial insertion element IS6110 as the DNA marker for *M. tuberculosis* complex organisms.[143] Evaluation of traditional PCR for childhood TB has been limited. As compared with the clinical diagnosis of pulmonary TB in children, the sensitivity of PCR on sputum or gastric aspirates has varied from 25% to 83%, and the specificity has varied from 80% to 100%.[144-146] A negative PCR never eliminates TB as a diagnostic possibility, and a positive result does not completely confirm it.

However, in 2010, the WHO endorsed the use of a newer PCR method, the GeneXpert MTB/RIF assay (Xpert) (Cepheid, Sunnyvale, California). The WHO commissioned its use in resource-limited settings for both adult and pediatric specimens as well as pulmonary and extrapulmonary specimens.[147] Xpert is a cartridge-based PCR platform that detects the presence of *M. tuberculosis* DNA as well as the presence of mutations in *rpoB* gene, which confer resistance to RIF. A systematic review and meta-analysis of 15 pediatric studies that were performed across a wide range of settings showed no difference in the performance of Xpert between induced sputum, expectorated sputum, or gastric lavage. The sensitivity of Xpert ranged widely in all the studies, but the pooled sensitivity was 66%, versus the 28% sensitivity of smear microscopy. In contrast, the specificity of Xpert had little variation between the studies and yielded a pooled specificity of 98%.[148] Xpert's limit of detection is 131 CFU/mL, as compared with smear's 5000–10,000 CFU/mL and culture's 10 CFU/mL.[149-151] Given the paucibacillary nature of childhood TB and the limited specimen volumes children can produce, Xpert's limits of detection are not able to capture all cases of childhood TB, and it does not replace the use of culture or clinical diagnosis.

Xpert also provides information regarding potential RIF resistance. In studies in Cape Town, Xpert has been shown to have good correlation with DST, with one study showing the sensitivity and specificity for RIF resistance to be 83.3% and 99.1%, respectively.[152-154] However, the presence or absence of the *rpoB* gene mutation does not equal phenotypic resistance or susceptibility, as not all RIF resistance is related to this specific gene mutation.[155] Therefore Xpert's RIF resistance results should be used only to evaluate potential drug resistance in a timely manner and should always be confirmed with phenotypic testing. Other diagnostic measures should be used to evaluate the full drug susceptibility profile of the organism.

In addition to its specificity and improved sensitivity versus microscopy, Xpert has further advantages over other nucleic acid detection techniques. The methodology is user-friendly and does not require extensive training, which allows it to be potentially used in decentralized clinics. Furthermore, the processing time for a specimen is only 2 hours once the specimen has reached the laboratory, thus decreasing wait times for patient results substantially. Unfortunately, in many TB high-burden settings, the health systems do not have the capacity to relay Xpert results to the clinician immediately, which negates the advantages that Xpert was designed to provide.

LINE PROBE ASSAYS

Newer molecular assays, termed line probe assays (LPAs), are also available in some settings; these are PCR tests that detect mutations in the genes that confer resistance. The DNA is amplified and hybridized to probes that bind to colorimetric strips. The operator then interprets the resistance profile from the pattern of colorization. LPAs are endorsed by the WHO and are used increasingly around the world, but limitations are noted on their sensitivities, specifically among the injectable agents used as second-line drugs used to treat resistant TB.[156] Furthermore, because they indicate the presence of genetic mutations, they do not indicate the phenotypic expression of these mutations.

Treatment

Each of the distinct clinical stages of disease caused by *M. tuberculosis* has a distinct treatment regimen, as further described in the following sections and illustrated in Table 29.4.

TREATMENT OF TUBERCULOSIS EXPOSURE

If a child has been exposed to an individual with potentially contagious TB, there is the possibility that child could have become infected with the organism. Children take up to 3 months to develop an immune response sufficient to produce a positive TST or IGRA result,[157] and children younger than

5 years of age may develop severe disease before these tests become positive.[158] Because of this risk, in low-burden settings with active contact tracing, children under the age of 5 with a known or suspected exposure to an adult with potentially contagious TB, should have an initial test of infection performed at the time of presentation. If the initial test of infection is negative, then the child should receive treatment with INH, as he or she may have already acquired infection but not yet developed an immune response to a test of infection. Children younger than 5 are at increased risk of developing potentially severe disease in the meantime; thus INH offers critical protection for this at-risk population. A test of infection should then be repeated 8–10 weeks after the child is no longer exposed to TB. If the result of the second test of infection is negative, therapy may be discontinued. If the result of the second test of infection is positive, a full course of treatment for TB infection should be given, as detailed in a later section.

Isoniazid Preventative Therapy

In areas where tests of infection are not readily available, the WHO recommends initiation of Isoniazid Preventative Therapy (IPT) in HIV-uninfected children under the age of 5 who have been in contact with an individual with contagious TB. These children must first be evaluated for disease with at minimum a symptom screen assessing for fever, cough and weight loss. If they lack any signs or symptoms of TB disease, they are given daily INH for 6 months. Given the low rate of side effects in this age group and the resource constraints of the setting, tests of infection are not used but rather infection is presumed, given the proximity of the child to the individual with contagious TB. Treatment is typically with INH for 6 months in high-burden settings.

Another form of IPT is specific for HIV-infected individuals regardless of age. In high-burden settings where presumably an HIV-infected individual is continually exposed to TB, the WHO has recommended that HIV-infected individuals be screened regularly for TB symptoms—including fever, cough,

Table 29.4 Preventive Regimens for Tuberculosis Infection in Children

Resistance Pattern of Source Case	Antimycobacterial Agent Dosage and Duration	Comments
INH-susceptible or unknown	1 INH, 10–20 mg/kg as single daily dose × 9 months (maximum 300 mg per dose) 2 INH, 20–40 mg/kg/dose twice weekly × 9 months (maximum, 900 mg per dose) 3 INH + rifamycin (3HP): INH 15 mg/kg (max dose 900 mg) Rifapentine 10.0–14.0 kg: 300 mg 14.1–25.0 kg: 450 mg 25.1–32.0 kg: 600 mg 32.1–49.9 kg: 750 mg >50 kg: 900 mg once weekly × 12 weeks 4 INH 10 mg/kg + RIF 10 mg/kg as single daily dose × 3 months (maximum, 900 mg INH + 600 mg RIF)	Optimal duration for children is debated CDC and AAP recommend 9-month intermittent schedule should be given only by DOT
INH-resistant or INH not tolerated	RIF, 10–20 mg/kg/dose as single daily dose × 4 months (maximum, 600 mg per dose)	
MDR-TB (resistant to INH and RIF)	Guided by susceptibility testing on a child or source case isolate	Should be provided in consultation with an expert DOT strongly recommended

AAP, American Academy of Pediatrics; *CDC,* Centers for Disease Control and Prevention; *DOT,* directly observed therapy; *INH,* isoniazid; *MDR-TB,* multidrug-resistant tuberculosis; *RIF,* rifampin.

weight loss/poor weight gain, and night sweats—and individuals who have a negative TB screen be given 36 months of INH to treat potential TB infection and prevent future TB disease and transmission.[159]

Despite international and national guidelines, recommending IPT in children, delivery and monitoring of IPT to children remains poor. Existing data demonstrate that poor IPT delivery is due to missed opportunities for IPT,[27,160,161] poor uptake and adherence,[162,163] and limited administrative systems to support IPT delivery.[164] In order to improve IPT delivery in TB high-burden settings, IPT must become a core intervention of both TB and HIV control programs that is supported by regionally appropriate tools, implementation, monitoring, and evaluation systems.

TREATMENT OF TUBERCULOSIS INFECTION

Asymptomatic TB infection is the most common presentation of children exposed to TB. These children have a reactive TST or IGRA, normal chest radiograph, no clinical evidence of TB disease, and presumed infection with small numbers of viable tubercle bacilli. Children with TB infection should receive treatment for the following reasons: (1) infants and children less than 5 years of age have been infected recently and are immunologically immature, so risk for progression to disease is high; (2) risk for severe disease, including meningitis and disseminated disease, is inversely related to age; (3) children with TB infection have more years at risk for the development of disease later in life; (4) children with TB infection become adults who may transmit organisms if they develop disease; and (5) the risk of developing disease is higher than the risk of developing significant adverse reactions from treatment for TB infection.[125]

Several large clinical trials have demonstrated the efficacy of INH to reduce the risk for TB in children with TB infection. In 1958, the US Public Health Service (USPHS) conducted a randomized trial to prevent TB in boarding schools in Alaska.[165] Two dosing regimens of INH were studied, 1.25 mg/kg per day versus 5 mg/kg per day given for 6 months to 1701 attendees 5–20 years of age for either 5 days per week or daily. In 10 years of follow-up, participants who received the higher dose of INH had significantly less progression to disease (1.9%), 10 of 513, than participants receiving the lower dose (5.8%), 31 of 536. The study also demonstrated that an intermittent therapy course (5 days per week) was efficacious. Additional randomized controlled trials completed by the USPHS in the 1950s and 1960s found the protective efficacy of INH treatment of TB infection to be approximately 90% when analysis was restricted to adherent participants.[166] Secondary analysis of two USPHS household contact studies has suggested that the efficacy of INH treatment of TB infection plateaus at 9–10 months of therapy.[167] Similarly, in a study among the Inuit in Alaska, a second year of INH treatment did not result in additional benefit beyond that conferred by the first year of treatment.[168,169] Although the International Union against Tuberculosis and Lung Disease (IUATLD) evaluated the efficacy of various durations of INH therapy in adults with TB infection, similar studies have not been conducted in children. There have also been no comparison studies between 6 and 9 months of INH. In the IUATLD trial, individuals who completed 12 months of INH therapy with good adherence had a reduced TB incidence by 93%, compared with a 69% reduction if a 6-month INH course was completed with good adherence.[170] Comparing the overall benefit regardless of adherence showed a more equivocal comparison between 6 and 12 months of therapy.[132] In addition, cost-effectiveness studies have suggested no increased benefit between 6 and 12 months of therapy.[171] Difficulties with adherence as well as the cost/benefit ratio have led the WHO to recommend 6 months of INH therapy for TB infection. However, the current AAP recommendation for treatment of TB infection in children is 9 months of INH given either daily (10–15 mg/kg, maximum 300 mg usually under self-supervised administration) or twice weekly (20–30 mg/kg, maximum 900 mg) under directly observed therapy (DOT).

RIF has been used for the treatment of TB infection in children and adolescents when INH was not tolerated or the child was exposed to an individual with an INH-resistant, RIF-susceptible isolate. A daily 4-month-long course is considered an alternative treatment to INH in the United States.[172] In addition, a new regimen consisting of INH and a long-acting rifamycin called rifapentine is available in some areas. This regimen is given once weekly for 12 weeks. It has been shown to be as effective as and safer than 9 months of daily self-administered INH. This regimen is well tolerated in teens and older children. Its use is limited in younger children owing to the lack of a liquid formulation and pharmacokinetic data for children under the age of 2 years.[173]

In some areas, a 3-month regimen of daily INH and RIF in combination is used to treat TB infection. This regimen has been shown in several studies to be as effective and as safe as other regimens, although randomized controlled studies in children are lacking.[174] The majority of a data supporting this regimen come from British observational studies, which show a reduced incidence of childhood TB disease on daily INH and RIF.[175,176]

Treatment of TB infection should be tailored according to host immune factors, drug susceptibility, tolerance, and compliance (see Table 29.4). Any treatment can be used in HIV-infected children with documented evidence of TB infection, although care should be taken to avoid drug interactions between RIF/rifamycin and the protease inhibitors used in highly active retroviral therapy (HAART). Treatment of infection with an organism must be individualized and should be delivered via DOT, if resources are available. In instances where the MDR isolate is susceptible to fluoroquinolones, such as levofloxacin or moxifloxacin, these agents can be used to treat infection. This can be given alone or in combination with another agent to which the organism is susceptible, often ethionamide or ethambutol. However, the combination of pyrazinamide and a fluoroquinolone should be avoided owing to an increased risk of adverse events. There are no studies indicating the exact duration of treatment, but daily administration for 6 months is recommended. Any child exposed to MDR-TB should be followed closely for 18 months, whether treated or not, in order to identify disease quickly and initiate appropriate therapy in order to avoid poor outcomes.[177]

Providers should follow otherwise healthy children on treatment for TB infection with periodic physical exams. Laboratory investigations are required only if children experience side effects of the medications. Both INH and RIF can cause elevated transaminases, usually associated with abdominal pain and vomiting. The fluoroquinolones tend to be well tolerated in children but have been associated with transient arthralgias.

TUBERCULOSIS DISEASE

Principles of Treatment

Treatment of TB disease is designed to prevent the complications of disease in the host and the development of drug resistance in the organism. Antitubercular agents should be bactericidal and effective against intracellular and extracellular organisms. Three or more drugs are used empirically for initial therapy and adjusted when DST is available. Initial use of a single agent will select for emergence of a dominantly resistant population of bacilli in individuals with TB disease. Therapy should be provided for extended periods via DOT to ensure compliance. Length of therapy is dependent on the site of infection.

Pulmonary Tuberculosis

The first-line drugs used to treat TB disease in children are shown in Table 29.5. Many therapeutic trials have been reported in children with pulmonary TB. A 6-month regimen consisting of INH and RIF was effective in some patients with isolated hilar adenopathy and without drug-resistant organisms.[178] Limited data are available to support a 6-month, INH-RIF regimen for the treatment of drug-susceptible pulmonary TB.[179] At least a dozen studies have examined the efficacy of 6-month regimens consisting of three or more drugs in children with pulmonary TB. The most common regimen studied consisted of INH and RIF, supplemented with pyrazinamide during the first 2 months. Most trials used daily therapy for the first 2 months, followed by daily or twice-weekly therapy to complete 6 months. In these trials, the overall success rate was greater than 95% for cure and 99% for significant improvement during a 2-year follow-up.

Although current guidelines recommend that all patients be started on a four-drug regimen,[180] a three-drug regimen may be used in children exposed to a source case with pansusceptible TB. Hence, in children with suspected INH-susceptible pulmonary TB, the recommended treatment is a 6-month regimen consisting of INH and RIF, supplemented during the first 2 months with pyrazinamide. The first 2 months of multidrug therapy are frequently referred to as the *intensive phase*. Daily administration of the regimen during the first 2 weeks to 2 months may be followed by at minimum twice-weekly therapy to complete 6 months, a period referred to as the *continuation phase*. All treatment for TB disease should be administered by DOT unless there is a compelling reason to avoid it.

In children or adolescents with adult-type pulmonary TB or epidemiologic circumstances suggesting an increased risk for infection with an organism that is resistant to INH, the American Thoracic Society (ATS) recommends an initial 2-month treatment phase consisting of daily administration of four drugs: INH, RIF, pyrazinamide, and ethambutol. This initial treatment is followed by 4 months of INH and RIF twice-weekly therapy administered under DOT if the organism is susceptible to both drugs.[180] Although there have been concerns about the use of ethambutol because it can cause optic neuritis, which is difficult to detect in children, this adverse effect is extraordinarily rare in children and should not preclude the use of ethambutol.

The optimal treatment of pulmonary TB in children and adolescents with HIV infection is unknown. In HIV-infected children with TB disease who received three to four drugs in the initiation phase followed by INH and RIF in the continuation phase for 6 months, a recurrence risk of 13% has been reported despite good adherence.[181] The AAP and ATS recommend initial therapy that should consist of four drugs for the first 2 months with a total duration of therapy that can go up to 9 months for HIV-infected children not on antiretroviral therapy.[180] The WHO recommends that TB in HIV-infected children should be treated with a 6-month regimen similar to the treatment of HIV-uninfected children, but treatment should not be delivered using intermittent schedules.[182,183] In HIV-infected adults with TB disease, prolonged TB treatment duration[184–186] and use of HAART.[186–189] reduce the risk of TB recurrence. In children, reduced TB incidence rates in those on HAART compared with the rates of those not on HAART are seen in retrospective and observational cohort studies.[190,191] The optimal timing for initiating HAART in HIV-infected children with TB disease is not known, but the WHO recommends initiation of HAART within 2–6 weeks of starting TB therapy.[182] Newer recommendations from the ATS, Centers for Disease Control and Prevention, and Infectious Disease Society of America recommend initiating HAART at the same time as TB therapy, as there is evidence of improved outcomes. In treating HIV-infected children with TB disease, a number of special issues must be considered, including drug-drug interactions, immune reconstitution

Table 29.5 Commonly Used Drugs for the Treatment of Tuberculosis in Children

Drug	Dosage Forms	Daily Dose (mg/kg)	Twice-Weekly Dose (mg/kg Per Day)	Maximum Dose
Ethambutol	Tablets: 100 mg, 400 mg	20	50	Daily: 1 g Twice weekly: 2.5 g
Isoniazid[a,b]	Scored tablets: 100 mg, 300 mg Syrup: 10 mg/mL	10–15	20–30	Daily: 300 mg Twice weekly: 900 mg
Pyrazinamide	Scored tablets: 500 mg	20–40	50	2 g
Rifampin[a]	Capsules: 150 mg, 300 mg Formulated in syrup from capsules	10–20	10–20	Daily: 600 mg Twice weekly: 900 mg

[a]Rifamate is a capsule containing 150 mg of isoniazid and 300 mg of rifampin. Two capsules provide the usual adult (>50 kg body weight daily doses of each drug).
[b]Most experts advise against the use of isoniazid syrup because of its instability and a high rate of gastrointestinal adverse reactions (diarrhea, cramps).
IM, Intramuscular.

inflammatory syndrome (IRIS), and drug-resistant TB.[192] See Chapter 66 for a full discussion of ART regimens options to be used in childhood TB.

Extrapulmonary Tuberculosis

Controlled therapy trials have not been reported for children with extrapulmonary TB. In general, recommended treatment for extrapulmonary TB is the same as for pulmonary TB. Osteotuberculosis and TB meningitis are exceptions. Recommended treatment of drug-susceptible osteotuberculosis includes 9–12 months of INH and RIF or 6 months of INH and RIF supplemented by two other drugs during the first 2 months of therapy. There are inadequate data to support any 6-month treatment regimen for TB meningitis.[193] Recommended regimens consist of the standard intensive phase regimen during the initial 2 months followed by 7–10 months of therapy with INH and RIF.

Drug-Resistant Tuberculosis

The incidence of drug-resistant TB is increasing in the United States and the world because of poor patient adherence, the availability of some antituberculosis drugs in noncontrolled over-the-counter formulations, migration of at-risk people and poor medical management. In the United States, approximately 10% of M. tuberculosis isolates are resistant to at least one drug. Of the 480,000 cases of MDR-TB estimated by WHO to have occurred in the world in 2014, only about a quarter of these—123,000—were detected and reported. Of note, mathematical modeling predicts that 25,000–32,000 children fall ill to MDR-TB each year, suggesting an even greater reporting gap than that estimated by WHO.[21,22] Certain epidemiologic factors—recent immigration, homelessness in some communities, and history of previous antituberculosis therapy—correlate with drug resistance in adult patients. Drug-resistant cases are classified in categories based on DST of clinical isolates confirmed to be M. tuberculosis:

- **Monoresistance:** resistance to one first-line anti-TB drug only.
- **Polydrug resistance:** resistance to more than one first-line anti-TB drug (other than both INH and rifampicin).
- **MDR:** resistance to at least both INH and rifampicin.
- **Extensive drug resistance (XDR):** resistance to any fluoroquinolone and to at least one of three second-line injectable drugs (capreomycin, kanamycin, and amikacin, in addition to MDR).
- **Rifampicin resistance:** resistance to rifampicin detected using phenotypic or genotypic methods, with or without resistance to other anti-TB drugs. It includes any resistance to rifampicin, whether monoresistance, multidrug resistance, polydrug resistance, or XDR.

Patterns of drug resistance in children tend to mirror those found in adult patients in the population.[194] Outbreaks of drug-resistant TB in children occurring at schools have been reported. Individual cases also have been recognized. Since it is difficult to isolate M. tuberculosis from children because of the paucibacillary nature of childhood TB, the determination of drug resistance in childhood TB is often inferred from the contact with contagious TB. Hence it is critically important to identify the adult source case that infected the child, as the drug susceptibility patterns of the culprit organism are required to determine an effective therapy regimen.

Therapy for drug-resistant TB is successful only when four to five drugs to which the strain of M. tuberculosis is susceptible, at least two of which are bactericidal, are given. If only one effective drug is given, secondary resistance will develop. The drugs used to treat MDR-TB are listed in Table 29.6. Treatment typically requires a backbone of (1) a fluoroquinolone [group A], (2) an injectable agent [group B], (3) at least two other second-line drugs with evidence of activity against the isolate [group C] and (4) whichever first-line drugs to which the isolate remains susceptible [group D1].[195] This should result in a regimen consisting of at least five agents. If this cannot be achieved because of the isolate's susceptibility profile, agents from D3 can be used until five agents compose the regimen.[195]

The D2 agents, bedaquiline and delamanid, are the first new TB medications in 40 years. Bedaquiline, a dairylquinoline that inhibits mycobacterial adenosine triphosphate (ATP) synthase, was approved by the US Food and Drug Administration (FDA) and the European Medicines Association (EMA) in 2012. Delamanid, a nitroimidazole that inhibits synthesis of the mycobacterial cell wall, was approved by the EMA and the Japanese Regulatory Authority in 2014. Owing to limited to nonexistent pediatric data, the medications are not approved for use in children but may be used on a compassionate release basis when other options are unavailable.

Traditionally, MDR-TB in children has been treated for 18–24 months of therapy. In children with widespread disease or cavitary lung lesions, the treatment is an 18-month regimen with the injectable agents used for the first 4–6 months.[196] However, given newer evidence, the WHO has issued new MDR-TB guidelines stating that children with uncomplicated disease can complete a shorter 9-month treatment course composed of the "Bangladesh regimen," named for the country where the shorter regimen was first investigated. It consists of an intensive phase of 4 months with gatifloxacin or moxifloxacin as well as kanamycin, prothionamide, clofazimine, ethambutol and high-dose INH. If an individual who is smear-positive is started on the regimen and fails to convert the smears before the end of the intensive phase, the guidelines recommend continuing the intensive phase until smear conversion occurs. After the intensive phase, the regimen consists of a 5-month-long continuation phase with the following medicines: gatifloxacin or moxifloxacin, clofazimine, ethambutol and pyrazinamide. Individuals should be excluded from this shorter-course regimen if they have had prior treatment with second-line TB drugs for the past month or have documented resistance to any medicines in the regimen.

The second-line TB drugs are associated with more side effects than the first-line therapy agents (see Table 29.6). In addition, few of these agents come in pediatric formulations, so children are frequently required to take halved and quartered tablets in order to obtain the correct dose. Potentially inaccurate dosing combined with a lack of pharmacokinetic studies of these drugs in children place children at risk for adverse events on treatment. Thus health care providers should closely monitor for adverse events, suggest mitigating factors, and make appropriate changes to therapy when able. In fact, the adverse events profile of the injectable agents, which includes nephrotoxicity and permanent hearing loss, has given rise to the newer WHO guidelines, which suggest that the harms associated with injectable agents may

Table 29.6 Drugs Used to Treat Multidrug-Resistant *Mycobacterium Tuberculosis*

Drug Group	Agents Within Group		Side Effects	Side-Effect Monitoring
Group A: Fluoroquinolones	Levofloxacin Moxifloxacin Gatifloxacin		Arthralgias/arthritis, GI disturbance, sleep disturbance,	Signs and symptoms
Group B: Second-line injectable agents	Amikacin Kanamycin Capreomycin Streptomycin[a]		Pain at injection site, nephrotoxicity, ototoxicity	Monthly creatinine and potassium, monthly audiology
Group C: Other core second-line agents	Ethionamide/prothionamide		Hypothyroidism GI upset	Monitor TSH, T4 at baseline and every 3 months
	Cycloserine/terizidone		Neurologic and/or psychologic side effects	Monitor for signs and symptoms
	Linezolid		Bone marrow suppression, optic neuritis, lactic acidosis	Blood counts at baseline, then monthly for the first 2 months, then then every 2 months × 2 then every 3 months
	Clofazimine		Skin discoloration, dry skin, abdominal pain	Monitor for signs and symptoms
Group D: Add-on agents	D1	Pyrazinamide	Hepatitis, arthritis	HIV-uninfected: no LFTs unless symptomatic HIV-infected: LFTs at baseline, 6 months, and 15 months
		Ethambutol	Optic neuritis	Color vision testing every month for first 6 months, followed by every 3 months thereafter
		High-dose isoniazid	Hepatitis, peripheral neuropathy	HIV-uninfected: no LFTs unless symptomatic HIV-infected: LFTs at baseline, 6 months, and 15 months
	D2	Bedaquiline/delamanid	QT prolongation	ECG at baseline, months 1 and 2, 4 and 6; every 3 months thereafter
	D3	p-aminosalycilic acid	Diarrhea	Monitor for signs and symptoms
		Imipenem-cilastin[b] Meropenem[b]	Seizures	Monitor for signs and symptoms
		Amoxicillin-clavulanate[b]	Diarrhea	Monitor for signs and symptoms
		Thioacetazone[c]	Stevens–Johnson syndrome in HIV-infected individuals	Monitor for signs and symptoms

[a]Only to be used when other injectables cannot be used and the organism is susceptible to streptomycin.
[b]Must use amoxicillin-clavulanate with either imipenem-cilastin or meropenem.
[c]Thioacetazone can only be used in individuals who are not infected with HIV.
ECG, Electrocardiogram; *GI,* gastrointestinal; *HIV,* human immunodeficiency virus; *LFTs,* liver function tests; *TSH,* thyroid stimulating hormone.
Modified from the WHO 2016 Guidelines for Drug Resistant Tuberculosis.

outweigh the potential benefits and that these agents may be excluded in children with mild disease.

The management of childhood MDR-TB is a complicated affair, and treatment guidelines change often as new evidence becomes available. The International Union against TB and Lung Disease provides a free interactive online module that covers the diagnosis and management of these patients at https://childhoodtb.theunion.org/courses/CTB2/en/intro. However, given the complexity of treatment and the rapidly changing knowledge base, a childhood TB expert should always be involved in the care of a child with MDR-TB.

ADJUNCTIVE THERAPY

Because INH competitively inhibits pyridoxine metabolism, resulting in a peripheral neuritis, pyridoxine (25–50 mg/day) is recommended for infants, children, and adolescents treated with INH who have nutritional deficiencies, symptomatic HIV infection, or diets low in milk or meat products and in breastfed infants. Corticosteroid administration is beneficial in the management of children when the host inflammatory reaction contributes significantly to tissue damage or impaired function. Administration of corticosteroids decreases mortality and morbidity in patients with TB meningitis by reducing vasculitis, inflammation, and intracranial pressure.

Corticosteroid administration may significantly reduce compression of the tracheobronchial tree caused by hilar lymphadenopathy, reduce the alveolar-capillary block associated with miliary disease, to improve symptoms from pleural effusions, and to reduce symptoms and mortality from pericardial effusion.[180] Prednisone (1–2 mg/kg per day for 4–6 weeks) is most commonly employed.

FOLLOW-UP DURING ANTITUBERCULOSIS THERAPY

The major goals of following children during treatment include promoting adherence, monitoring for toxicity and adverse effects of therapy and assessing clinical response. Patients should be evaluated monthly and receive only enough medication for the intervals between follow-up appointments. During all phases of treatment, clinicians should assess potential nonadherence with treatment. Children with missed appointments and questionable adherence should be referred to the responsible public health agency, which likely has programs incorporating incentives or behavioral modification.

Rates of adverse reactions caused by first-line antituberculosis medications are low in children. INH and RIF are associated with elevated serum alanine aminotransferase in less than 2% of children and rarely cause overt hepatitis.

Elevated alanine aminotransferase levels are generally less than three times normal values, do not predict hepatotoxicity and are not an indication for discontinuing treatment. Routine biochemical monitoring is indicated only if the child has existing liver disease or is taking other potentially hepatotoxic drugs. It is preferable to educate caregivers relative to potential adverse events and clinical symptoms (abdominal pain, vomiting, jaundice necessitating medical evaluation) and immediate discontinuation of medication. Monitoring of adverse reactions in second-line drugs is shown in Table 29.6.

Frequent radiographic monitoring is not indicated. Because improvement of intrathoracic TB in children occurs slowly, chest radiographs are generally obtained at diagnosis. Some providers with available resources prefer to repeat a radiograph at completion of therapy to establish a new baseline for the patient. Radiographic resolution of hilar lymphadenopathy and associated pulmonary lesions may not occur for 2–3 years following treatment; a normal chest radiograph appearance is not necessary for completion of therapy. If resolution of radiographic abnormalities has not occurred by completion of therapy, radiographs may be obtained at 3- to 6-month intervals to assess continued improvement. Radiographs should also be repeated if the patient is not clinically improving.

Control and Prevention

BACILLUS CALMETTE-GUÉRIN VACCINATION

BCG vaccines have been administered to nearly 4 billion people and have been routinely administered to newborns in most countries except the United States and the Netherlands. Nevertheless, the immune response to BCG and its mechanism of action are not well understood. Large clinical trials have shown the efficacy of BCG vaccination to range from 0% to 80%. A number of factors contribute to the heterogeneity of results from these trials, including eligibility criteria, strain of vaccine employed, vaccine administration, diagnostic criteria, disease surveillance, and environmental factors.[197] Although BCG does not prevent primary pulmonary TB, studies have demonstrated that BCG vaccination decreases the risk for developing severe forms of disease in very young children, including meningitis and miliary TB.[198,199] The clinical presentation of TB disease in older individuals who have received a BCG vaccination tends to be similar to that in nonimmunized persons.

BCG-induced immune responses in HIV-infected children are significantly lower compared with those in uninfected children.[200] Nevertheless, in the absence of antiretroviral therapy, HIV-infected infants have a significant risk of developing disseminated BCG disease, which is associated with a case fatality rate exceeding 75%.[201,202] Following initiation of antiretroviral therapy, 5%–10% of HIV-infected infants experience BCG IRIS.[203] The risk of serious BCG-related adverse events can be reduced by delaying BCG vaccination in HIV-exposed infants until their HIV status has been definitely established and in HIV-infected infants by rapid initiation of antiretroviral therapy.[204] Based on the high risk of disseminated BCG disease in HIV-infected infants, the WHO has recommended that infants with known HIV-infection should not receive BCG vaccination.[204] The practical feasibility of this recommendation has been questioned by TB experts in countries with high burdens of HIV and TB, where the feasibility of selectively deferred vaccination and potential disruption of general vaccination coverage is a concern.[205]

PUBLIC HEALTH INVOLVEMENT

Childhood TB is a direct reflection of the incidence of adult TB within a community. Childhood TB usually represents recent transmission from an infectious adult or adolescent and is considered a sentinel event in public health. TB control programs should respond to a case of childhood TB by seeking to identify the source of infection and additional cases. Two distinct types of public health investigations exist. Contact investigations evaluate all contacts of an infectious adult or adolescent for TB disease or infection. Contact investigations have the highest yield for finding infected persons and are considered the cornerstone of reducing the incidence of TB disease. The WHO recommends contact investigation and treatment of exposed children, but this is often not performed in resource-limited settings. Some public health experts recommend that public health authorities develop estimates of numbers of children living in households with active TB cases. These estimates can then provide targets for the children investigated, which can help public health authorities plan financial and logistical resources that would allow for robust investigation and treatment.[206]

Source case investigations evaluate all contacts of a child with TB to identify an infectious adult or adolescent and other infected persons. Source case investigations are less successful because the child may have moved into the jurisdiction of the public health authorities and away from the source case. It is the public health authority's responsibility to ensure that all persons with suspected TB are identified and evaluated promptly and that appropriate treatment is prescribed and successfully completed. These responsibilities are accomplished through several activities, including epidemiologic surveillance and investigations, direct provision of diagnostic services and treatment and monitoring of treatment decisions and outcomes. The approach should be tailored for each patient to account for individual needs and ensure completion of therapy. DOT is the preferred, core management strategy to ensure adherence and involves providing the antituberculous drugs directly to the patient and watching that he or she swallows them.

References

Access the reference list online at ExpertConsult.com.

Suggested Reading

Chiang SS, Swanson DS, Starke JR. New diagnostics for childhood tuberculosis. *Infect Dis Clin North Am.* 2015;29(3):477–502.

Colditz GA, Brewer TF, Berkey CS, et al. Efficacy of BCG vaccine in the prevention of tuberculosis. Meta-analysis of the published literature. *JAMA.* 1994;271:698–702.

Cruz AT, Ahmed A, Mandalakas AM, et al. Treatment of latent tuberculosis infection in children. *J Pediatr Infect Dis Soc.* 2013;2(3):248–258.

Cruz AT, Ong LT, Starke JR. Mycobacterial infections in Texas children: a 5-year case series. *Pediatr Infect Dis J.* 2010;29:772–774.

Horsburgh CR, Barry CE, Lange C. Treatment of tuberculosis. *N Engl J Med.* 2015;373(22):2149.

Mandalakas AM, Kirchner HL, Lombard C, et al. Well-quantified tuberculosis exposure is a reliable surrogate measure of tuberculosis infection. *Int J Tuberc Lung Dis.* 2012;16(8):1033–1039.

Marais BJ, Gie RP, Schaaf HS, et al. The natural history of childhood intra-thoracic tuberculosis: a critical review of literature from the pre-chemotherapy era. *Int J Tuberc Lung Dis.* 2004;8:392–402.

Nahid P, Dorman SE, Alipanah N, et al. Official American Thoracic Society/Centers for Disease Control and Prevention/Infectious Diseases Society of America Clinical Practice Guidelines: treatment of drug-susceptible tuberculosis. *Clin Infect Dis.* 2016;63(7):e147–e195.

Starke JR. Transmission of *Mycobacterium tuberculosis* to and from children and adolescents. *Semin Pediatr Infect Dis.* 2001;12:115–123.

WHO. *Global Tuberculosis Report 2015.* Geneva: World Health Organization. Available online at: http://apps.who.int/iris/bitstream/10665/191102/1/9789241565059_eng.pdf.

WHO. *WHO Treatment Guidelines for Drug Resistant Tuberculosis.* Geneva: World Health Organization. Available online at: http://www.who.int/tb/MDRTBguidelines2016.pdf.

30 Nontuberculosis Mycobacterial Disease

STACEY L. MARTINIANO, MD, JERRY A. NICK, MD, and CHARLES L. DALEY, MD

There is widespread agreement that detection of nontuberculous mycobacteria (NTM) is increasing worldwide within surveys of the general population[1–9] and among specific vulnerable disease groups.[10–12] The true incidence of disease caused by NTM is difficult to accurately track. Available data almost certainly underestimate the burden of infection due to the low clinical suspicion, the low sensitivity of available diagnostic techniques, and the lack of mandatory public health reporting of NTM infections. The most common presentation of NTM disease in children is cervical lymphadenitis, and skin and soft tissue infection. Pulmonary NTM disease in children occurs in the setting of preexisting lung disease, and is most often associated with cystic fibrosis (CF).[13] Disseminated disease may occur in the setting of immune compromise, often due to HIV/AIDS[13] or a variety of rare conditions.[14] The accurate diagnosis of pulmonary NTM disease can be challenging because of the limitations of available diagnostic tests and the common occurrence of transient or indolent infections in the absence of new or worsening symptoms.[15]

Microbiology

The genus *Mycobacterium* consists of a diverse group of obligate aerobes that grow most successfully in tissues with high oxygen content, such as the lungs. These nonmotile, nonspore-forming, pleomorphic rods feature a cell wall rich in mycolic acids. The lipid-rich cell wall makes them impermeable to many stains unless the dyes are combined with phenol. Once stained, the cells resist decolorization with acidified organic solvents, resulting in their hallmark trait of "acid-fastness." This property is demonstrated with basic fuchsine stain techniques, such as the Ziehl-Neelsen and Kinyoun methods, or the more sensitive fluorochrome method using auramine and rhodamine stains.

More than 170 species of *Mycobacterium* have been described, with new species being identified each year.[16] Many NTM are nonpathogenic in humans, and others have been described to cause disease very rarely in case reports or small cases series of immunocompromised individuals.[17] NTM species are often categorized using the Runyon classification system based on rate of growth and pigmentation. The most commonly encountered NTM are among the "slow growers" and classified together as the *Mycobacterium avium* complex (MAC), which includes the species *M. avium*, *M. intracellulare*, *M. chimaera* among several other species and subspecies.[18] MAC is genetically close to the *Mycobacterium tuberculosis* complex, and is susceptible to several of the antibiotics effective in the treatment of tuberculosis. Another disease-causing slow growing NTM is *Mycobacterium kansasii*. Also of clinical significance is the *Mycobacterium abscessus* species complex (MABSC), which includes three subspecies, *M. abscessus*, *M. massiliense*, and *M. bolletii*. MABSC are classified as "rapid growers," and are genetically quite distinct from MAC.

Advances in diagnosis and treatment of NTM infection have lagged, in part, due to challenges relating to the culture, detection, and identification of the organisms. Methods developed for the isolation of *Mycobacterium tuberculosis* from clinical samples have been adapted for the isolation of NTM. Current recommendations are that both liquid and solid media are used for NTM culture with incubation for at least 6 weeks.[19] Isolation on solid media of slow-growing NTM takes 2–6 weeks; only the rapid growers reliably form visible colonies in less than 10 days. However, automated systems using liquid media allow detection of most species of mycobacteria more rapidly. Sensitivity is increased and the time for isolation is decreased by a larger specimen size and a higher bacterial burden. In the setting of CF, adequate sample decontamination to remove overgrowth of *Pseudomonas aeruginosa* and other coinfections is essential to permit culture-based detection of NTM.[20] Importantly, decontamination protocols can reduce NTM viability in samples, resulting in false negative results.[21] Current best practice for CF isolates consists of a two-step approach of (N-acetyl-L-cysteine–2% sodium hydroxide (NALC-NaOH) decontamination prior to mycobacterial culture with the addition of a second decontamination using 5% oxalic acid or 1% chlorhexidine to permit the recovery of NTM from persistently contaminated samples, albeit with reduced sensitivity.[20,22]

Traditional identification of NTM relies on statistical probabilities of a characteristic reaction pattern in a battery of biochemical tests. Molecular methods have now surpassed biochemical tests for NTM identification in many laboratories. These tests include line probe assays,[23] polymerase chain reaction (PCR) product restriction analysis,[24] and partial gene sequencing.[25] For subspeciation of MABSC, a multilocus sequence typing approach has recently been validated.[26] Each of these methods has significant strengths as well as disadvantages, and there is no consensus regarding the gold standard for NTM identification. However, recently published guidelines sponsored by the CF Foundation (CFF) and the European CF Society (ECFS) recommend that all NTM isolates from individuals with CF should undergo molecular identification.[20] All MABSC isolates from individuals with CF should be identified to the subspecies level, and other NTM identified to the species level, except for *M. avium*, *M. intracellulare*, and *M. chimaera*, where identification can be limited to MAC.[20]

Epidemiology

PREVALENCE

General Population

Several problems compound the epidemiologic description of NTM infections in children.[19] NTM infection is rarely a cause of death, with an overall mortality rate of 2.3 deaths per 1,000,000 person-years attributed to NTM in the United States.[27] In individuals age 24 years and younger, age-adjusted mortality rates range from 0.04 to 0.12 per 1,000,000 in the absence of an HIV diagnosis, and are even lower in the presence of an HIV diagnosis.[27] Smaller laboratories that isolate NTM often do not refer isolates to reference laboratories for identification and drug-susceptibility testing, so statistics from reference laboratories grossly underestimate the incidence of NTM disease. Finally, as opportunistic environmental bacteria with relatively low pathogenic potential, isolation of an NTM from a clinical specimen is rarely sufficient for the diagnosis of disease. Distinguishing among environmental contaminants, transient recovery of the bacteria, colonizers, and truly pathogenic organisms requires clinical correlation that is not available based simply on laboratory reports. A recent study of NTM disease prevalence in the United States estimated 27.9 cases per 100,000 population,[28] based primarily on Medicare beneficiary data. These authors estimated 31% of cases were less than 65 years old, but the actual number of pediatric cases is unknown.[28] Substantial differences in susceptibility to NTM pulmonary disease appear linked to race and ethnicity.[1] Within the Hawaiian Islands, which has a rate of NTM pulmonary disease four times greater than the national average in the United States,[2] prevalence was highest among Japanese, Chinese, and Vietnamese patients (>300/100,000 persons) and lowest among Native Hawaiians and Other Pacific Islanders (50/100,000).[1]

Cystic Fibrosis

The best estimates for the prevalence of positive NTM cultures comes from CF populations, where the rate of infection has been studied in prospective and retrospective clinical trials, as well as in extensive longitudinal data collection through national registries. In the largest studies, the overall prevalence is 6%–13%.[29-35] Since 2010, the US CF Patient Care Registry has tracked the presence of positive NTM culture, and over a 4-year span (2011–2015), 19% of patients who were cultured had one or more species isolated.[10] There is widespread agreement that the prevalence of NTM is increasing in the CF population[10-12]; however, it is often difficult to compare reports from single centers or even national surveys because of widely differing methods of ascertainment, regional environmental differences, culture methods, and the definitions of colonization, infection, and disease. CF features underlying progressive pulmonary disease and chronic airway infections with highly pathogenic bacteria such *P. aeruginosa* and *Staphylococcus aureus*.[36] In this setting, it is challenging to assess the role of an NTM infection in an individual patient. While the isolation of an NTM from a CF patient's sputum may be associated with a worsening clinical and radiographic course, in the majority of patients a positive NTM culture may be a transient occurrence or not associated with measurable acceleration of disease.[15]

In CF patients in whom NTM disease is diagnosed, there are apparent differences between those infected with MABSC and MAC. Patients infected with MABSC are often younger, and may include children, with relatively more severe lung disease.[12,37] Those infected with MAC are often older and more frequently heterozygous for residual function cystic fibrosis transmembrane conductance regulator (CFTR) mutations, resulting in a less severe phenotype, which may not be diagnosed until adulthood.[30,37,38] There are, of course, many exceptions to this general observation, and children with CF can develop NTM disease from either MAC or MABSC. Disease from MABSC is the more feared infection due to a more difficult course of treatment, a poorer response to antibiotic therapy, an often more severe clinical course, and frequent exclusion from lung transplant in the setting of failure to eradicate the bacteria.[12,20,39]

Human Immunodeficiency Virus Infection/Acquired Immune Deficiency Syndrome

Clinical disease due to NTM is common in adults and children with AIDS. MAC accounts for most cases, followed in incidence by *M. kansasii*.[40] The predominant risk factor appears to be a CD4 cell number below 50 cells/mm^3, and can occur as either disseminated or localized disease.[41] Other NTM that have been described as disease-causing in HIV/AIDS include *Mycobacterium xenopi*,[42] *Mycobacterium haemophilum*,[17] *Mycobacterium fortuitum* or *Mycobacterium chelonae*,[43] *Mycobacterium genavense*,[44] *Mycobacterium simiae*,[45] and *Mycobacterium szulgai*.[46] A high clinical suspicion is needed for either unexplained lymphadenitis, cutaneous or systemic presentations in patients with CD4 cell < 50 cells/mm^3.

Mendelian Susceptibility to Mycobacterial Disease and Other Immunocompromised Conditions

Mendelian susceptibility to mycobacterial diseases (MSMD, MIM #209950) is caused by genetic defects in the mononuclear phagocyte/T helper cell type 1 (Th1) arm of host defense.[14] Patients with MSMD have increased susceptibility to systemic NTM infections, even including the Bacillus Calmette-Guérin vaccine strain. All the MSMD conditions feature defects in the interferon gamma (IFN-gamma)-interleukin-12 pathway and/or supporting accessory pathways (Table 30.1). In about half of patients with MSMD, the genetic etiology has yet to be identified.[47]

Disseminated disease with pulmonary involvement caused by NTM has been described in patients with a variety of other rare immunodeficiency states, as well as malignancies including leukemia and lymphoma. Inherited and acquired defects in the host immune response include auto-antibodies to IFN-gamma, CD4 lymphopenia due to HIV or other causes, and use of tumor necrosis factor-alpha inhibitors, particularly infliximab and adalimumab. A wide variety of biologic and synthetic small molecules target aspects of host defense against NTM, and carry high theoretical risks for the infection.[48] NTM disease also has been reported in adults and children after organ transplantation.

ENVIRONMENTAL RISK FACTORS AND SPATIAL CLUSTERS

Distribution of NTM in the general population and in vulnerable populations varies dramatically by regions,[2,30,31] reflecting,

Table 30.1 Diseases Associated With Nontuberculous Mycobacteria Infection

Mendelian susceptibility to mycobacterial diseases (MSMD)	Autosomal recessive complete interferon-gamma receptor deficiencies[140]
	Autosomal dominant partial interferon-gamma receptor deficiencies[140,141]
	IFN-gamma-R1 (IFNGR1)[141] or IFN-gamma-R2 (IFNGR2)[142]
	Autosomal recessive partial IFN-gamma receptor deficiencies[143,144]
	IL-12 receptor beta1 (IL12RB1) deficiency[14,145,146]
	IL-12 p40 (IL12B) deficiency[147]
	Autosomal recessive signal transducer and activator of transcription 1 (STAT1) deficiency[14,148,149]
	Autosomal dominant STAT1 (STAT1) deficiency[150]
	Tyrosine kinase 2 (TYK2) deficiency[151]
	Autosomal recessive IFN regulatory factor 8 (IRF8) deficiency[152–154]
	Autosomal dominant IFN regulatory factor 8 (IRF8) deficiency[152–154]
	GATA2 (GATA2) deficiency (monoMAC syndrome)[155,156]
	Autosomal recessive IFN-stimulated gene 15 (ISG15) deficiency[84]
	RAR-related Orphan Receptor C (RORC) dysfunction[157]
X-linked MSMD	Nuclear factor-κB essential modulator (IKBKG) (NEMO) deficiency[158]
	X-linked chronic granulomatous disease due to mutations in gp91(phox) subunit (CYBB) of NADPH oxidase[159]
Other immune disorders	Anti-IFNγ autoantibody formation[160,161]
	Natural-resistance-associated macrophage protein 1 (NRAMP1) gene polymorphisms[162]
T-cell disorders	Severe combined immune deficiency[163]
	Isolated CD4+ T cell deficiency[164]
	HIV/AIDS[165]
Phagocyte defects	Chronic granulomatous disease[166]
Iatrogenic immunosuppression	Recipients of solid organ transplants[167]
	Recipients of hematopoietic or stem cell transplants[76,168]
	Anti-TNFα treatment[169]
	Inhaled or systemic corticosteroids[170–172]
	Other immunosuppressive medications[171]
Structural lung disease[48]	Cystic fibrosis (CF)[36]
	Alpha-1 antitrypsin deficiency[173]
	Non-CF bronchiectasis[174]
	Pneumoconiosis[175]
	Pulmonary alveolar proteinosis[176]
	Chronic obstructive pulmonary disease[177]

IFN, Interferon; *IL*, interleukin; *TNFα*, tumor necrosis factor alpha.

in part, the environmental origin of the bacteria.[50] In the United States, the greatest number of estimated cases per 100,000 populations was 164.6 in Hawaii, followed by Florida (53.6), Mississippi (52), and Arizona (48.9). The states with the lowest rates were largely clustered in the upper Midwest, including Montana (5.4), South Dakota (6.5), North Dakota (7.4), and Minnesota (9.3).[28] These differences likely reflect a combination of host and environmental risk factors within these regions. A greater understanding of environmental risk factors and spatial clusters of NTM infection has come from the analysis of Medicare and Medicaid data, combined with population and socioeconomic data from the US Census Bureau, and environmental and climatic data from the US

Census Bureau, US Forest Service, and the US Geological Survey.[51] Counties in high-risk areas were significantly larger, had greater population densities, and higher education and income levels than low-risk counties. High-risk counties also had higher mean daily potential evapotranspiration levels and percentages covered by surface water, and were more likely to have greater copper and sodium levels in the soil, with lower manganese levels.[51] Similar conclusions have been found from combining CF Patient Registry data with climatic databases, where higher saturated vapor pressure increased the risk for NTM (odds ratio = 1.06; 95% confidence interval = 1.02–1.10).[52]

The species of NTM causing infection also demonstrates significant regional differences. Nearly all surveys from European countries have established that MABSC is the most frequent NTM isolated from CF patients in those regions.[12,30,53] In contrast, reports from the United States have consistently shown MAC to be the predominant NTM infection.[15,31,52] In somewhat isolated regions, other NTM may be highly represented. For example, *M. simiae* is reported as the most frequent cause of NTM pulmonary disease in CF patients on the Island of Gran Canaria[54] and is also common in Israel.[11] Even within the US CF population, dramatic state-by-state differences in prevalence of various NTM species have been reported. When CF Patient Registry data were analyzed, 60% of positive cultures nationwide were identified as MAC, ranging by state from 29% in Louisiana to 100% in Nebraska and Delaware.[52]

Acquisition and Potential for Transmission

Nearly all acquisition of NTM by children occurs from environmental sources, including soil, water, dust, and aerosols.[50] MAC species are found frequently in animals, particularly birds and swine, which may be important natural reservoirs for the organisms. However, there is little evidence to suggest that animal-to-human transmission is a major factor in human infection.

The number of reported clusters of health-care-associated disease caused by various species of NTM is growing. Most common are outbreaks by the rapid growers. Both clusters and sporadic NTM infections have been associated with a variety of surgical procedures, including sternal wound infections after open heart surgery, augmentation mammoplasty, corneal surgery, implantation of pressure equalizing tubes in the tympanic membranes, and insertion of central venous catheters.[55–63] A number of outbreaks or pseudo-outbreaks of respiratory tract colonization caused by various NTM species have been associated with contaminated ice machines, showers, potable water supplies, laboratory supplies, topical anesthetics, and tap water in hospitals.[64–66] Contamination of endoscopes, bronchoscopes or bronchoscopy supplies has been implicated in some of these outbreaks.[61,67]

There is also growing concern over the potential for human-to-human transmission. Until recently, this was believed to never occur,[19] but with improved surveillance and increased availability of whole genome sequencing, several outbreaks have been reported. Well-described clusters of highly similar strains of *M. massiliense* have been reported in CF centers in Seattle, Washington, and Papworth, United Kingdom, in patients who were seen within the same clinic or hospital ward over a relatively short interval of time.[68,69] Mechanisms of NTM transmission are not well understood, but in well-defined localized outbreaks, it seems that shared exposure of a contaminated clinical space is a more plausible mechanism of pathogen spread than direct patient-to-patient transmission.[68] Strict infection control procedures following the Seattle outbreak have been associated with a cessation of any additional cases.[70] More recently, a much larger study found highly similar clusters of both *M. massiliense* and *M. abscessus* represented in collections of clinical isolates from United States, European, and Australian CF centers, indicating transcontinental dissemination of these clades.[71] Unlike the previous outbreaks in Seattle or Papworth, there was no clear epidemiologic link between patients or physicians traveling between these different centers worldwide. In many cases, shared strains have been associated with increased virulence, antibiotic resistance and/or worse outcomes.[68,69,71] There is ongoing debate about whether these findings represent global transmission of strains of MABSC between CF centers through yet-to-be-defined mechanisms, or dominant environmental strains that are present worldwide with extremely low genetic diversity, or a combination of both.[72]

Apparent Increase in Nontuberculous Mycobacteria Vulnerable Populations and in the Modern Environment

The incidence of detecting various NTM organisms in surveys of the general population, as well as individuals with CF appears to be increasing.[1–12] The underlying cause of this apparent increase is almost certainly multifactorial and interconnected. Within the CF population, impressive gains in projected lifespan puts greater numbers of patients at risk for NTM. Infection with MAC, in particular, is clearly age-related[37] and associated with long-term survivors with a milder phenotype.[37,38] Certainly, improved culture techniques and greater awareness among providers to consider NTM infection has contributed to the increase in positive NTM cultures.[20,22] There is also considerable debate as to whether various medications and CF treatment strategies directly place patients at increased risk. Some reports have implicated systemic steroids, high-dose ibuprofen, the higher use of antipseudomonal antibiotics, and chronic azithromycin therapy as being associated with higher prevalence of NTM-positive cultures and/or disease. However, for each of these medications, the opposite findings have also been reported.[36,73]

To a certain extent, these same considerations may apply to individuals within the general population with less well-defined risks for NTM. Certainly, humanity has never before included as many individuals with various forms of immunosuppression, ranging from HIV/AIDS to malignancies, and to the use of steroid and immunomodulatory drugs.[74] Presumably, physicians caring for these individuals are increasingly aware of the potential risks for NTM infection, and are practicing appropriate culture surveillance. Certainly, nosocomial risks for acquisition of NTM are well described, particularly

in the setting of surgery or other invasive procedures,[56–67,75,76] and this may extend to patient-to-patient transmission in some settings, as discussed above. Finally, there is growing evidence that many features of the modern environment may favor NTM survival and a higher potential burden of exposure. These factors may include high density urban populations,[30,51] plumbing and water supply systems,[77,78] the use of showers,[79] and lower temperatures of hot water heaters in homes and hospitals.[60,77] Climate change has also been implicated in the apparent increase in NTM, as higher temperatures are linked to increased evaporation of water, and the increase in natural disasters, which have been correlated with local outbreaks of NTM.[9] While risks related to nosocomial acquisition can be addressed, most of the other factors identified as relating to increased prevalence of NTM in the modern environment, and in vulnerable patient populations, are expected to increase for the foreseeable future, and to result in a continued increase of infections by NTM.

Clinical Manifestations of Nontuberculous Mycobacteria Pulmonary Disease

Clinical and radiographic manifestations of NTM pulmonary disease are described in Table 30.2. Children can present with any combination of clinical signs and symptoms, though most patients experience chronic cough and sputum production that do not improve with the antibiotic treatment that is used for more typical lung pathogens, or with the use of corticosteroids.[19,80] Radiographic signs include presence of single or multiple pulmonary nodules, tree-in-bud opacities, large areas of consolidation, or bronchiectasis (Fig. 30.1).[81] Additionally, cavitation is an important finding representing more significant tissue destruction. Importantly, in patients with CF, there is significant overlap of both clinical and

Table 30.2 Clinical and Radiographic Manifestations of Nontuberculous Mycobacteria Pulmonary Disease

Symptoms	■ Constitutional ▪ Fever ▪ Night sweats ▪ Fatigue ▪ Weight loss ■ Respiratory ▪ Chronic cough ▪ Sputum production ▪ Chest pain ▪ Dyspnea on exertion ▪ Hemoptysis
Physical Exam	■ Pulmonary crackles ■ Clubbing
Imaging	■ Chest x-ray ▪ Consolidation ▪ Bronchiectasis ▪ Nodules ▪ Cavities ■ High resolution chest computed tomography ▪ Nodules ▪ Tree-in-bud opacities ▪ Cavities ▪ Bronchiectasis ▪ Consolidation

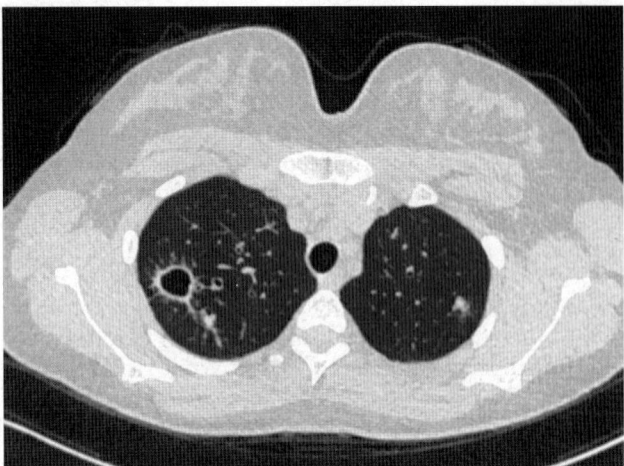

Fig. 30.1 Radiographic findings of nontuberculous mycobacteria pulmonary disease in a patient with cystic fibrosis (CF). The patient is a 16-year-old with CF with multiple positive cultures for *Mycobacterium abscessus*, a decline in pulmonary function, and the presence of clinical syndrome symptoms that persisted despite several courses of prolonged intravenous, oral, and inhaled antibiotics. This computed tomography image shows bilateral bronchiectasis and airway wall thickening, bilateral pulmonary nodules, and the presence of a new 2.1 cm cavitary lesion in the right upper lobe in the region of a previously identified small pulmonary nodule.

radiographic NTM manifestations with underlying pulmonary disease and chronic airway infection due to more common CF pathogens such as *P. aeruginosa* or *S. aureus*, as well as symptoms related to CF comorbidities, including CF-related diabetes and allergic bronchopulmonary aspergillosis (ABPA). In patients with CF, one should suspect NTM infection in those with constitutional or respiratory symptoms above baseline, unexplained increased decline in lung function, and progressive radiographic disease that are not responsive to typical CF therapies and antibiotics.[15,20,82,83]

Diagnosis of Nontuberculous Mycobacteria Pulmonary Disease

CLINICAL CRITERIA

To make the diagnosis of NTM pulmonary disease in a child, a patient must meet both microbiologic and clinical criteria with appropriate exclusion of other diagnoses (Box 30.1).[19] Clinical and radiographic findings are described above. In patients with CF, it is essential to first treat underlying typical CF pathogens, maximize airway clearance, and adequately assess for and treat CF-related comorbidities to ensure the clinical syndrome is not a consequence of underlying CF alone, prior to diagnosing NTM pulmonary disease.[20]

MICROBIOLOGIC CRITERIA

In contrast to *M. tuberculosis*, a single positive culture for NTM does not necessarily constitute a disease that requires treatment in patients both with and without CF. Individuals should have two or more positive sputum cultures for the same NTM species. An exception is that a positive culture from a single bronchial wash or lavage, or from transbronchial or

other lung tissue biopsy, can be sufficient if NTM is highly suspected. Expert consultation should be obtained when NTM that are either infrequently encountered or that usually represent environmental contamination are recovered from culture.[19] Patients who are suspected of having NTM lung disease, but who do not meet the diagnostic criteria, should be followed closely with increased surveillance of sputum acid-fast bacilli (AFB) smears and cultures until the diagnosis is firmly established or excluded. Importantly, making the diagnosis of NTM pulmonary disease does not necessarily require initiation of treatment. Due to the burden of treatment, risk of emergence of resistance with partial treatment, and potential treatment-related side effects, the risks and benefits of therapy for the individual patient must be considered and discussed prior to initiating therapy.[19,80]

EXTRAPULMONARY NONTUBERCULOUS MYCOBACTERIA DISEASE

Extrapulmonary NTM disease in children most commonly occurs as lymphadenitis, typically in the cervical lymph nodes.[84] Localized disease can happen in both immunocompetent and immunocompromised children and presents with fever, leukocytosis, and focal inflammation in a lymph node (cervical, intraabdominal, or mediastinal). The diagnosis is confirmed by AFB culture from an aspirate of the node.[85] Less common are skin and soft-tissue infections due to NTM. A high level of suspicion when evaluating a nonhealing wound should prompt collection of AFB cultures. Disseminated NTM disease is uncommon in children, most typically occurring in an immunocompromised child. Disseminated MAC presents as fever, night sweats, abdominal pain, diarrhea, and weight loss, with the diagnosis confirmed through isolation of MAC from blood cultures. *M. kansasii* can present similarly with features that resemble *M. tuberculosis*.[86] Notably, in extrapulmonary or disseminated disease, a single culture from a wound or blood is sufficient for diagnosis, and treatment should be initiated.

Management and Treatment

Treatment of NTM disease depends on the location and extent of disease, the species causing infection, and the drug resistance pattern of the organism.[19] Precise speciation is critical for directing antimicrobial therapy as treatment outcomes vary depending on the causative species. Unfortunately, drug susceptibility test results do not correlate well with treatment outcomes, except for the macrolides and amikacin in pulmonary MAC,[19,87] rifampin in pulmonary *M. kansasii*,[19] and macrolides in MABSC.[88,89]

The drugs most commonly used to treat NTM infections are listed in Table 30.3. Multiple-drug therapy is used for all mycobacterial infections because of the propensity of these organisms to develop resistance.[19] The treatment regimens for children with NTM disease are based on either limited clinical trials in adults or anecdotal evidence from small series or case reports. Standard treatment regimens typically include at least three drugs directed against the specific NTM pathogen, in the oral, inhaled, and/or intravenous forms.[19] Empirical therapy is not advised in most settings as treatment varies significantly between species. However, in settings where tuberculosis is endemic or clinically suspected, empirical therapy for tuberculosis is recommended pending the results of diagnostic studies.

NONTUBERCULOUS MYCOBACTERIA PULMONARY DISEASE

There have been no clinical trials evaluating antibiotic treatment regimens for NTM lung disease in children, including those with CF. Treatment of NTM pulmonary disease should be based on American Thoracic Society and Infectious Disease Society of America (ATS/IDSA) guidelines[19] that were developed for the general population and CFF/ECFS guidelines developed specifically for treatment in the setting of CF.[20] While there is general agreement on which drug regimens should be used for the initial treatment of NTM infections, it is unclear what the optimal length of therapy is for children with NTM disease. The ATS/IDSA and CFF/ECFS recommend that patients be treated for 12 months beyond culture conversion, which is defined as three consecutive negative cultures with the time of conversion being the date of the first negative culture, and assuming there are no additional positive cultures during the 12 months.[19,20]

TREATMENT OF *MYCOBACTERIUM AVIUM* COMPLEX PULMONARY DISEASE

Recommended regimens for the treatment of MAC lung disease in children are based entirely on the results of clinical trials in adults. Although there is only anecdotal information

available for treatment of MAC pulmonary infections in children, the regimens used in adults seem to be effective in children. The most important determinants of treatment are the presence of macrolide resistance and cavitation. In macrolide-susceptible MAC disease, the initial treatment for noncavitary NTM lung disease due to MAC utilizes a three-drug regimen that includes a macrolide, rifamycin, and ethambutol.[19] Azithromycin is the macrolide usually chosen due to once daily dosing and reduced interactions with rifampin and the CYP3A enzyme system compared to clarithromycin.[19] Also, chronic azithromycin therapy has been shown to have benefits in people with CF due to immunomodulatory properties of the drug, in particular those patients with chronic *P. aeruginosa* infection.[90–92] Although azithromycin has recently been shown to reduce macrophage autophagy of *M. abscessus* in CF, suggesting that it has the potential to impair host defense independent of its antibiotic properties,[93] this potential detriment has not been identified in patients with NTM disease.

For patients without CF, with noncavitary disease, intermittent (i.e., three times weekly) oral therapy is recommended.[19] However, intermittent therapy is not recommended in patients with CF due to concerns about abnormal absorption of antimycobacterials and altered pharmacokinetics.[20] Instead, daily administration of the same mediations is preferred. In CF patients with MAC which is macrolide-resistant, or who are systemically ill or AFB smear positive, or who have evidence of a cavitary lesion on chest imaging, a 1- to 3-month course of intravenous daily amikacin may be added at the beginning of the treatment course along with the standard three oral antibiotics.[20]

Macrolide resistance is associated with a very poor prognosis. Risk factors for the development of macrolide-resistant MAC are macrolide monotherapy and prior macrolide therapy with inadequate companion drugs.[87] In non-CF patients, macrolide resistant MAC lung disease has been associated with sputum culture conversion rates as low as 5%–15%.[87,94] Patients with macrolide-resistant MAC should generally be managed in collaboration with an expert in the treatment of NTM disease.

TREATMENT OF *MYCOBACTERIUM KANSASII* PULMONARY DISEASE

Because *M. kansasii* is rarely a contaminant, most patients with *M. kansasii* isolated from respiratory specimens should be considered to have the disease and should be treated accordingly.[19] While there have been no randomized, controlled trials of treatment for *M. kansasii*, treatment outcomes are usually good with rare treatment failures or relapses.[19] The current recommendation for treatment of pulmonary disease caused by *M. kansasii* is a regimen of isoniazid, rifampin, and ethambutol given daily for at least 12 months after the sputum culture has become negative.[19] Because the concentrations of drugs used in susceptibility testing were chosen for their usefulness with *M. tuberculosis* and not *M. kansasii*, some *M. kansasii* isolates may be reported to be resistant to isoniazid. However, these isolates are susceptible to slightly higher drug concentrations, and laboratory reports showing resistance to the lower concentrations have no clinical or therapeutic significance if a rifampin-containing regimen is being used.

Table 30.3 Commonly Used Drugs for Nontuberculous Mycobacterial Infections With Adverse Reactions and Suggested Monitoring

Drug	Route of Administration	Pediatric Dosage	Adverse Reactions	Suggested Monitoring
Amikacin	Intravenous	Children: 15–30 mg/kg per dose once daily Adolescents:10–15 mg/kg per dose once daily (maximum dose 1500 mg daily)	Nephrotoxicity, auditory-vestibular toxicity	Creatinine Serum amikacin levels Hearing exams Clinical symptoms
Amikacin	Nebulized	250–500 mg/dose once or twice daily	Auditory-vestibular toxicity	Hearing exams Clinical symptoms
Azithromycin	Oral	Children: 10–12 mg/kg per dose once daily (maximum dose 500 mg daily) Adolescents: 250–500 mg daily	Nausea, vomiting, diarrhea, auditory-vestibular toxicity, prolonged QT	Clinical symptoms Hearing exams EKG
Cefoxitin	Intravenous	50 mg/kg per dose three times daily (maximum dose 12 g/day)	Fever, rash, cytopenias, eosinophilia	Complete blood count Clinical symptoms
Clarithromycin	Oral	7.5 mg/kg per dose twice daily (maximum dose 500 mg daily)	Hepatitis, taste disturbance, inhibits metabolism of rifabutin	Clinical symptoms
Clofazimine	Oral	1–2 mg/kg per dose once daily (maximum dose 100 mg daily)	Discoloration of skin, enteropathy, nausea, vomiting, prolonged QT	Liver function tests[120] Clinical symptoms EKG[120]
Ethambutol	Oral	15 mg/kg per dose once daily	Optic neuritis, peripheral neuropathy	Liver function tests Eye exams Clinical symptoms
Imipenem	Intravenous	15–20 mg/kg per dose twice daily (maximum 1000 mg per dose)	Nausea, vomiting, diarrhea, hepatitis, fever, rash	Liver function tests Complete blood count Clinical symptoms
Isoniazid	Oral	5 mg/kg per dose once daily	Hepatitis, peripheral neuropathy	Liver function tests Clinical symptoms
Linezolid	Oral, intravenous	<12 years: 10 mg/kg per dose three times daily ≥12 years: 10 mg/kg per dose once or twice daily (maximum 600 mg per dose)	Cytopenias, peripheral neuropathy, optic neuritis	Complete blood count Eye exams Clinical symptoms
Minocycline	Oral	2 mg/kg per dose once daily (maximum dose 200 mg)	Photosensitivity, nausea, vomiting, diarrhea, vertigo, tooth discoloration	Clinical symptoms
Moxifloxacin	Oral	7.5–10 mg/kg per dose once daily (maximum dose 400 mg)	Nausea, vomiting, diarrhea, insomnia, agitation, anxiety, tendonitis, photosensitivity, prolonged QT	Clinical symptoms EKG
Rifabutin	Oral	5–10 mg/kg per dose once daily (maximum dose 300 mg)	Cytopenias, orange discoloration of fluids, hepatitis, nausea, vomiting, diarrhea, hypersensitivity/flulike syndrome, increased metabolism of many drugs, uveitis	Liver function tests Complete blood count Clinical symptoms
Rifampin	Oral	10–20 mg/kg per dose once daily (maximum dose 600 mg)	Cytopenias, orange discoloration of fluids, hepatitis, nausea, vomiting, diarrhea, fever, chills, increased metabolism of many drugs, renal failure	Liver function tests Complete blood count Clinical symptoms
Tigecycline	Intravenous	8–11 years: 1.2 mg/kg per dose twice daily (maximum 50 mg per dose) ≥12 years: 50 mg once or twice daily	Nausea, vomiting, diarrhea, pancreatitis, hypoproteinemia, hepatitis	Liver function tests Complete blood count Clinical symptoms
Trimethoprim-sulfamethoxazole	Oral	10–20 mg/kg per dose twice daily	Nausea, vomiting, diarrhea, cytopenias, fever, rash	Complete blood count Clinical symptoms

EKG, Electrocardiogram.

Adapted with permission from Griffith DE, Aksamit T, Brown-Elliott BA, et al. An official ATS/IDSA statement: diagnosis, treatment, and prevention of nontuberculous mycobacterial diseases. *Am J Respir Crit Care Med.* 2007;175(4):367-416; and Floto RA, Olivier KN, Saiman L, et al. US Cystic Fibrosis Foundation and European Cystic Fibrosis Society consensus recommendations for the management of non-tuberculous mycobacteria in individuals with cystic fibrosis. *Thorax.* 2016;71(suppl 1):i1-i22.

Macrolides have excellent in vitro activity against *M. kansasii* and, in a murine model, clarithromycin was the most active single agent followed by rifampin and gatifloxacin.[95] Moreover, at least two clinical studies have reported excellent treatment outcomes when a macrolide is substituted for isoniazid.[96,97] Surgical resection is seldom required.

TREATMENT OF *MYCOBACTERIUM ABSCESSUS* SPECIES COMPLEX PULMONARY DISEASE

Treatment of pulmonary disease due to MABSC is complicated because of significant levels of in vitro resistance, the need for intravenous antibiotics, common adverse reactions, and generally poor treatment outcomes. As described previously, MABSC can be divided into three subspecies: *M. abscessus*, *M. massiliense*, and *M. bolletii*. Studies in CF[98] and non-CF[99–101] patients have clearly demonstrated that culture conversion is much more likely to occur in patients infected with *M. massiliense* compared with *M. abscessus*.[98] These differences are presumably related to the presence of a functional erm[41] gene in *M. abscessus* that results in inducible macrolide resistance, whereas in *M. massiliense* the gene is nonfunctional.[99]

The typical treatment regimen for MABSC involves an intensive phase followed by a continuation phase. The intensive phase should include 3–12 weeks of intravenous amikacin, plus one or more of the following agents: intravenous tigecycline, imipenem, or cefoxitin.[19,20] This regimen should also include oral drugs for which some degree of in vitro activity has been demonstrated. Whether a macrolide should be included in the regimen for *M. abscessus* or *M. bolletii* is debatable given the presence of an erm[41] gene in most strains. However, if this cannot be determined, or there is a potential benefit from the immunomodulatory activity of the macrolide, then the drug should be given. As noted previously, azithromycin is preferred over clarithromycin and there is some evidence to suggest it is associated with better treatment outcomes in non-CF adults.[101] The duration of the intensive phase will be determined by the severity of disease, the response to therapy, and the tolerability of the regimen.

After intravenous therapy, patients typically continue a combination of oral and inhaled treatments with adjustments of therapy based on culture conversion as well as clinical and radiographic response. The continuation phase should include inhaled amikacin in conjunction with 2–3 of the following daily oral antibiotics: minocycline, moxifloxacin, linezolid, and clofazimine.[19,20] If macrolides are used, they should be continued throughout the continuation phase. Changes to the drug regime are common, due to drug intolerance, side-effects, and lack of efficacy. In some cases, patients must be treated with intermittent courses of intravenous antibiotics to control spread of the infection. These patients should generally be managed in collaboration with an expert in the treatment of NTM disease.

SURGICAL TREATMENT OPTIONS

Resection lung surgery (pneumonectomy, lobectomy, or segmentectomy) is sometimes performed in adults with NTM lung disease to improve treatment outcomes, particularly infections caused by *M. abscessus*. An initial period of chemotherapy to contain the infection followed by resection surgery and a more prolonged course of chemotherapy leads to high rates of sputum culture conversion. In primarily non-CF patients with NTM lung disease, culture conversion rates after surgical resection have been reported to be 80%–100% with relapse rates of 0%–16%.[102–107] Among cohorts of non-CF patients with MABSC lung disease, surgical resection increased culture conversion rates by 25%–30%.[89,108] In patients with CF, the disease is generally more diffuse and it is difficult to identify, with certainty, a focus of NTM infection in the setting of coinfection with typical CF pathogens, such as *P. aeruginosa* and *S. aureus*. Furthermore, CF patients with a history of NTM are at a very high risk of acquiring a second NTM in their lifetime.[15] For these reasons, surgical resection is rarely recommended.[20] As this surgery is difficult to perform, it is important that the thoracic surgeon has experience in performing the procedures.

NONPHARMACOLOGIC TREATMENT OPTIONS

For patients with underlying bronchiectasis, nonpharmacologic therapies that target the clearance of airway mucus are essential. This is particularly important in patients with CF where the NTM treatment regimen should be part of a comprehensive CF care plan that includes effective airway clearance, nutrition management, and treatment of CF comorbidities, such as sinus disease and CF-related diabetes.[36] This care is most effectively delivered at a CF care center, which utilizes a multidisciplinary approach, providing access to a respiratory therapist, a dietitian, and a social worker, in addition to nurses and physicians experienced in CF care.

EXTRAPULMONARY NONTUBERCULOUS MYCOBACTERIA DISEASE

In general, treatment of extrapulmonary and disseminated NTM disease follows the same principles used in pulmonary disease with the exception that surgical debridement/excision plays a more critical role in the treatment of lymphadenitis, skin, and soft tissue infections. Cervical lymphadenitis is the most common clinical presentation of NTM in children.[109–111] Treatment is generally divided into observation without intervention, surgical excision, and antimicrobial therapy (with or without surgery). Without intervention, most children who develop cervical adenitis will eventually resolve the infection; however, the time to resolution may be prolonged (6–12 months) and result in significant scarring.[110,111] Surgical excision can involve total excision, partial excision, or curettage. Factors in favor of complete surgical excision include a greater chance of isolating the organism, higher cure rates, faster healing times, less need for repeat surgery, and improved esthetic outcomes.[110–114] Antimicrobial agents may be indicated in some patients alone or in combination with surgery. In a randomized, controlled trial comparing surgical excision with antimicrobial therapy alone (clarithromycin and rifabutin), cure was reported in 90% versus 66%, respectively.[113] Temporary facial palsy occurred in 14% of those undergoing surgery but was permanent in only one patient.

Skin and soft tissue infections are the next most common form of extrapulmonary disease in children, and are often due to rapidly growing mycobacteria.[109] Treatment usually involves surgical debridement, abscess drainage, and foreign-body removal. Treatment is based on susceptibility testing of the specific isolate because susceptibility patterns vary greatly even within a species.[114] Successful treatment of disease due to *M. fortuitum* can be accomplished sometimes with chemotherapy alone, although this is seldom the case with *M. abscessus*.

MONITORING OF DRUG TOXICITY AND CLINICAL RESPONSE

Routine monitoring of drug toxicity is required, and a plan for monitoring should be set in place at the initiation of treatment. Patients should be evaluated for evidence of hearing loss, visual loss, renal impairment, and liver function abnormalities.[19,20] Monitoring is particularly important for patients on intravenous aminoglycosides. Patients with CF are commonly treated with aminoglycosides for other lung pathogens; therefore, they are prone to auditory-vestibular toxicity and renal injury, making baseline and regular audiology evaluations and monitoring of renal function essential.[36] Even with oral agents, the potential for drug-related side effects and toxicity is considerable, including bone marrow suppression and hepatitis. Patients receiving ethambutol, rifabutin, or linezolid should have their vision monitored routinely and the drug should be discontinued immediately at the first sign of vision disturbance. Suggested monitoring guidelines are depicted in Table 30.3.

ALTERNATIVE DRUGS

Several additional drugs have been used to treat NTM infections, including fluoroquinolones, clofazimine, inhaled amikacin, linezolid, and bedaquiline. The fluoroquinolones are widely available and have variable in vitro and in vivo activity against MAC and typically poor activity against *M. abscessus*.[115–119] However, in refractory disease, there may be an indication for their use.[119] Clofazimine has historically been used with success as an alternative agent for patients with MAC, and more recently for those with MABSC.[120,121] Clofazimine is generally well tolerated with 6%–14% of patients having to stop due to drug-related intolerance. Inhaled amikacin has been used for many years in patients intolerant to parenteral aminoglycosides, or as an adjuvant to oral therapy, but adverse effects may limit its use.[122–124] Linezolid is an oxalidinone with broad antimycobacterial activity that has been used to treat multidrug-resistant tuberculosis as well as NTM. However, efficacy remains unknown, and use of the drug has been limited by high rates of adverse reactions, including peripheral neuropathy, optic neuritis, and cytopenias.[125,126] Bedaquiline is a diarylquinoline approved for the treatment of multidrug-resistant tuberculosis in adults with broad in vitro antimycobacterial activity for MAC.[127] Based on early data, there may be future potential for using bedaquiline in the treatment of refractory MAC or MABSC.[128]

Outcomes

Outcomes associated with NTM in children are not well reported in the literature,[129] though there is increasing evidence that NTM has the ability to affect clinical status and to accelerate the progression of lung disease, which causes an increased rate of decline in pulmonary function.[15,83]

Additionally, older adults with NTM respiratory isolates have higher mortality compared to those without; however, there is lack of evidence of causality.[130,131] Importantly, there are also reports that have shown no clinical impact,[132] and other reported cohorts of patients with positive NTM cultures that are either transient or not associated with evidence of pulmonary disease.[15,32,81,133–135]

With various treatment regimens among patients with and without CF, clearance of sputum in patients with MAC pulmonary disease is reported to range from 45% to 75%, while MABSC culture conversion rates are lower, and are typically reported in the 40%–50% range.[15,108,136,137] *M. massiliense* subspecies clearance rates are higher than *M. abscessus*, and are thought to be secondary to a lack of inducible macrolide resistance,[99] and *M. kansasii* treatment is successful in about 90% of patients.[19] Relapse following treatment occurs in up to 35% for MAC[138] and 23% for MABSC.[108,137] Additionally, in patients with CF previously infected with NTM, the presence of a future, second NTM species is common, and is reported in up to 26% of patients at 5 years and 36% at 10 years following the first NTM species cultured.[15] With treatment, stabilization or improvement in clinical symptoms of NTM pulmonary disease, including cough, sputum production, and fatigue, as well as radiographic measures have been shown.[89,108,139] Longitudinal follow-up of cases of CF patients with NTM have also shown evidence of stabilization of pulmonary function.[15,136]

PREVENTION

Little is known about the prevention of NTM infection in any group of individuals. Because these organisms are ubiquitous in nature, it is impossible to prevent exposure to them except under the most extreme circumstances. There has been no recommendation about the use of chemotherapy to prevent NTM infection in patients with or without CF. Until the risk factors for acquisition are better delineated, chemoprophylaxis will not be a part of the management of this disease.

References

Access the reference list online at ExpertConsult.com.

Suggested Reading

Floto RA, Olivier KN, Saiman L, et al. US Cystic Fibrosis Foundation and European Cystic Fibrosis Society consensus recommendations for the management of non-tuberculous mycobacteria in individuals with cystic fibrosis. *Thorax.* 2016;71(suppl 1):i1–i22.

Griffith DE, Aksamit T, Brown-Elliott BA, et al. An official ATS/IDSA statement: diagnosis, treatment, and prevention of nontuberculous mycobacterial diseases. *Am J Respir Crit Care Med.* 2007;175(4):367–416.

31 The Pulmonary Mycoses

AARON SAMUEL MILLER, MD, MSPH, and
ROBERT WILLIAM WILMOTT, BSc, MB, BS, MD, FRCP (UK)

Introduction

There is a wide range of pathogens that causes pneumonia in children. Fungal pathogens account for only a small percentage of community-acquired and nosocomially acquired pneumonias. When fungal infections of the lungs do occur, they can be caused by either endemic or opportunistic fungi. The endemic mycoses are a diverse group of fungal organisms that share several characteristics, including the ability to show temperature dimorphism (i.e., mold in the environment, yeasts/spherules at body temperature), ability to cause disease in otherwise healthy humans, and the tendency to occupy specific geographical regions. Fungi that cause opportunistic infections are typically seen in children with compromised immune systems, altered microbiota, or those with disrupted integumentary barriers. In some cases, however, the fungi that cause opportunistic infections can occur in normal hosts.

Pulmonary mycoses in humans can occur after inhalation of fungal spores, reactivation of a latent infection, or via hematogenous dissemination. Immunocompromised children, as well as those from geographic regions where endemic fungal infections occur, are at highest risk. The diagnosis of pulmonary fungal infection can be difficult, as the signs and symptoms of disease can be nonspecific and noninvasive diagnostic tests often have a low sensitivity. For these reasons, the diagnosis of pulmonary mycoses is often made presumptively based on a combination of factors including the clinical setting, chest imaging, and negative bacterial or viral studies. The prognosis of pulmonary fungal infections depends on the clinical scenario, as most children with endemic fungal infections recover from their illness, while the prognosis for immunocompromised patients is more guarded. The highest morbidity and mortality is seen in patients with prolonged or irreversible immunosuppression.

Antifungal Drugs

Antifungal drugs for systemic fungal infections have evolved significantly over the past 25 years. Amphotericin B deoxycholate was initially developed in the early 1950s and is part of the polyene class.[1] For many decades this was the primary antifungal used for invasive fungal infections. This class of antifungals binds to ergosterol in the fungal cell membrane, which results in cell death. Amphotericin B has activity against a wide range of fungal pathogens and is still considered the treatment of choice for various pathogens and clinical scenarios in children. It is absorbed poorly by the gastrointestinal tract and is solubilized with sodium deoxycholate for intravenous (IV) administration. Amphotericin B has dose-dependent renal toxicity and hypokalemia. In the mid-1990s, various lipid formulations were released, including amphotericin B lipid complex (ABLC; Abelcet) and a small, unilamellar vesicle formulation (L-AmB; Ambisome). These drug preparations have decreased toxicity compared with the deoxycholate formulation. In regard to the pulmonary mycoses mentioned in this chapter, most experts believe that a lipid formulation should be used over the deoxycholate formulation when available.[2] One exception may be in neonates, where limited retrospective data suggest that the deoxycholate formulation has improved efficacy.[3] Another possible exception involves the use of the deoxycholate formulation for fungal infections of the kidneys, as a study of a murine candidiasis model showed that the lipid preparations did not penetrate well into the renal parenchyma.[4] Efforts are being made to develop an effective oral formulation of amphotericin B by using polymeric nanoparticles to facilitate absorption across the gastrointestinal epithelium.[5]

The azole class of antifungal drugs acts by inhibiting the synthesis of ergosterol, which is the major sterol in fungal cell membranes. This drug class can be divided into the imidazoles (e.g., clotrimazole, miconazole, ketoconazole), and the triazoles (e.g., fluconazole, itraconazole, voriconazole, posaconazole). The imidazoles are primarily limited to topical use, given their hepatic toxicity and antiandrogen effects. The azole class is fungistatic against yeasts and fungicidal against molds. The development of the triazole fluconazole in 1981 was a major advance in the treatment of systemic antifungal infections, as it has excellent activity against *Cryptococcus neoformans* and many *Candida* spp. while also having good cerebral spinal fluid (CSF) penetration. Some of the disadvantages of fluconazole are that it has no activity against molds and has variable activity against certain *Candida* spp. (i.e., *Candida glabrata* and *Candida krusei*). Fluconazole was followed by the introduction of other important azoles, such as itraconazole in 1992 (activity against *Aspergillus* spp. and *Histoplasma capsulatum*), voriconazole in 2002 (expanded activity against fluconazole-resistant *Candida* spp. and *Aspergillus* spp.), and posaconazole in 2006. Posaconazole is notable for being the first available azole with activity against the agents that cause mucormycosis. In 2015, the US Food and Drug Administration (FDA) approved isavuconazole for adults with invasive aspergillosis (IA) or mucormycosis. Although no pharmacokinetic studies have been performed in children, this drug is promising for those patients with IA or mucormycosis who are not able to tolerate amphotericin B or posaconazole therapy.[6,7] Transaminase elevation and peripheral neuropathy are notable adverse reactions to the azole class. Voriconazole is known for its visual side effects

AREAS ENDEMIC FOR HISTOPLASMOSIS

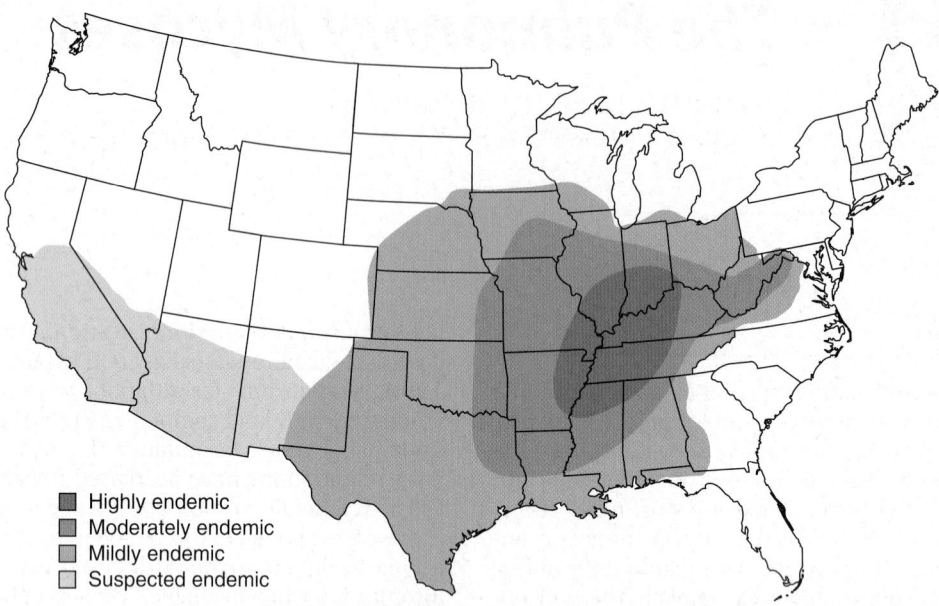

- ■ Highly endemic
- ■ Moderately endemic
- ■ Mildly endemic
- □ Suspected endemic

Fig. 31.1 Areas endemic for histoplasmosis (CDC reference map).

(e.g., photophobia, altered color discrimination) and central neurologic toxicity, which can manifest as hallucinations. These adverse reactions are typically reversible upon discontinuation of the drug.

The echinocandins are the newest class of antifungal agents that work by inhibiting beta-1,3-D-glucan synthase, resulting in the destruction of the fungal cell wall. This enzyme is not present in mammalian cells, resulting in a drug class with a low side-effect profile. In contrast to the azole class of antifungals, the echinocandin class is fungicidal against yeasts and fungistatic against molds. These drugs include caspofungin (approved in 2001), micafungin (approved in 2004), and anidulafungin (approved in 2006). The echinocandins are poorly absorbed through the digestive tract and are therefore available only in IV formulations. The echinocandins are not ideal for fungal infections of the central nervous system (CNS), eye, or urinary tract owing to poor tissue penetration. The echinocandins can occasionally cause elevation of the aminotransferases.

Flucytosine (also known as 5-fluorocytosine, or 5-FC) is a fluorinated pyrimidine analogue. It has activity against *Candida* spp. and *C. neoformans.* Given that resistance develops quickly when used as monotherapy, flucytosine is typically used in combination with amphotericin B or an azole. Bone marrow suppression and gastrointestinal upset are the most notable adverse reactions to this drug.

As of 2017, there are 14 individual antifungal agents approved by the FDA, some of which have several formulations.[2] Up-to-date pediatric-specific dosing recommendations of the previously mentioned antifungal drugs can be found in many sources.[2,8] It should be noted that some of the newer antifungal agents have not been adequately tested in neonates in regard to efficacy, safety, and pharmacokinetics/pharmacodynamics. For these reasons, until new data are available, the drugs of choice for neonates with invasive fungal infections are amphotericin B deoxycholate, fluconazole, and micafungin.[9]

Endemic Mycoses

HISTOPLASMOSIS

Epidemiology

Histoplasmosis is caused by the organism *Histoplasma capsulatum.* It is typically found in soil throughout the world and is endemic in the central United States (Ohio and Mississippi River valleys) (Fig. 31.1). This organism thrives in areas with a high concentration of bird or bat excrement in the soil. As a mold, *H. capsulatum* forms microconidia that can be aerosolized and inhaled by humans. The infection risk is highest when people are exposed to disturbed soil in endemic areas (e.g., construction, farming). Caves and abandoned buildings can also put people at risk of inhalation. Person-to-person transmission is not thought to occur. Skin test reactivity is common in hyperendemic areas, with as many of 80% of the population having a positive skin test by 18 years of age.[10]

Etiology

H. capsulatum is a thermally dimorphic fungus that exists as a mold in the environment and as a yeast at human body temperature. At 25°C–30°C, the mold grows as a fluffy colony with spore-bearing aerial mycelia containing small oval microconidia and larger macroconidia. These infectious particles become airborne when soil is disrupted. At 37°C, the spores develop into a budding yeast form over a period of 7 days.

Pathology/Pathogenesis

After inhalation, the microconidia germinate within the alveoli and distal bronchioles and transition to a yeastlike form. The yeast phase can enter and proliferate within macrophages.[11] Similar to tuberculosis, there is early transport to regional lymph nodes with formation of a primary complex.

The normal host develops specific T-lymphocyte immunity with proinflammatory cytokine stimulation of the macrophages to kill the fungus. This results in an acute inflammatory reaction in the lungs. The histopathologic features of this process include granulomas and caseous necrosis. As these lesions heal, fibrosis and calcification can develop. Although uncommon in children, an exuberant fibrous response can cause destruction and obstruction of the lung parenchyma and other mediastinal structures.[12]

Symptoms and Physical Findings

The majority of people exposed to *H. capsulatum* do not develop symptoms. Symptomatic infection occurs in fewer than 5% of infected individuals.[13] The risk of developing disease after exposure depends on inoculum size, degree of immunosuppression, strain-specific virulence factors, and preexisting immunity. The incubation period for the disease is typically 1–3 weeks after exposure. The clinical manifestations of histoplasmosis are classified according to physical location (pulmonary or disseminated), course of disease (acute, subacute or chronic), and whether the disease is a primary infection or due to reactivation of previous infection.[14]

Pulmonary Histoplasmosis. The most common symptomatic manifestation of histoplasmosis is acute pulmonary histoplasmosis. This begins as an acute inflammatory pneumonitis characterized by fever, nonproductive cough, and malaise. It is often a self-limited illness. For patients who develop more significant disease, the presenting signs and symptoms include persistent cough, nonpleuritic chest pain, wheezing, headache, fever, fatigue, myalgias, and arthralgias. These symptoms can last for 2–3 days or, in the subacute form, as long as 2–3 weeks. The acute form can also be accompanied by erythema nodosum, pericardial effusion, hypercalcemia, pleural effusion, or chylothorax. Unilateral wheezing is a classic pulmonary sign in patients with acute pulmonary histoplasmosis and is associated with bronchial compression. In the most severe cases of acute pulmonary histoplasmosis (typically due to a high inoculum), patients develop significant hypoxemia, diffuse reticulonodular infiltrates and acute respiratory distress syndrome (ARDS). Although acute disease is rare in children, adults with acute disease can go on to develop chronic cavitary pulmonary histoplasmosis. This process is associated with the "marching cavity," in which continuing necrosis leads to a progressively larger cavity that can consume the entire lobe.[11]

Acute pulmonary histoplasmosis can result in hilar or mediastinal lymphadenitis. In routine cases, a limited number of lymph nodes enlarge until the host's immune response is able to control the infection. In these cases, the lymph nodes eventually recede and calcify. In a smaller subset of patients, there is more significant enlargement of multiple hilar lymph nodes that become matted together and progress to granulomatous inflammation (mediastinal granuloma). This process can result in compression or obstruction of contiguous structures within the thorax, such as bronchi, trachea, pericardium, and pulmonary vasculature. Such compression can result in distal pneumonitis, pleural effusions, pulmonary infarction, pericarditis, and tracheoesophageal fistula formation. It is thought that the pericarditis and pleural effusions associated with acute pulmonary histoplasmosis are secondary to the inflammation of adjacent lymph nodes rather than direct fungal invasion.[14] The term *fibrosing mediastinitis* applies to excessive proliferation of invasive fibrous tissue within the mediastinum. It is thought to represent an abnormal immunologic host response rather than an active fungal infection. This leads to invasion of normal mediastinal structures such as the pulmonary vasculature, the superior vena cava, or the airways. Fibrosing mediastinitis occurs only rarely in children.[15]

Disseminated Histoplasmosis. Disseminated histoplasmosis can occur early in infection and is usually self-limited in the immunocompetent host. The term *progressive disseminated histoplasmosis* (PDH) applies to infections where there is overwhelming reticuloendothelial involvement; this is typically fatal if untreated. PDH can develop after acute infection or with recrudescence of previous histoplasmosis.[11] PDH is rare in children but can be seen in a variety of clinical situations. One form of PDH occurs in children with immunocompromising conditions such as hematologic malignancy, acquired immunodeficiency syndrome (AIDS), or those who have undergone a solid organ transplant (SOT). There is also an increased risk in those children who receive tumor necrosis factor (TNF) antagonists such as infliximab, adalimumab, and golimumab.[16,17] In these cases, the presenting symptom can be fever alone or respiratory distress.

Another rare but notable subset of patients with histoplasmosis is those with PDH of infancy. This form of PDH is subacute and has been described in otherwise healthy children less than 2 years of age. These infants typically present with fever, failure to thrive, hepatosplenomegaly, pancytopenia, pneumonitis, meningitis and disseminated intravascular coagulation. This clinical picture can initially be mistaken for leukemia. The expected cure rate is greater than 85% if the infection is recognized and treated promptly.[18]

Imaging, Pulmonary Function Testing, Laboratory Findings

Patients with no known history of histoplasmosis can have incidental findings on their chest radiographs showing single or multiple calcified nodules in the lungs as well as mediastinal and hilar lymphadenopathy. Imaging of the chest of those with acute infection is variable and ranges from normal, to focal pneumonitis with mediastinal adenopathy, to extensive interstitial or reticulonodular infiltrates (Fig. 31.2A). Chest computed tomography (CT) can be used to better define pericardial involvement, along with bronchial or vascular compression (see Fig. 31.2B). Calcification of the liver or spleen can also be seen. Chronic pulmonary histoplasmosis with cavitary lesions is rarely seen in children and is more commonly seen in adults with preexisting obstructive pulmonary disease.[19]

Diagnosis

The diagnosis of histoplasmosis can be challenging. Techniques used in this regard include histopathology, fungal culture, antigen detection, and serologic testing for *Histoplasma*-specific antibodies. Historically, an intradermal skin test was used, but this has fallen out of favor owing to

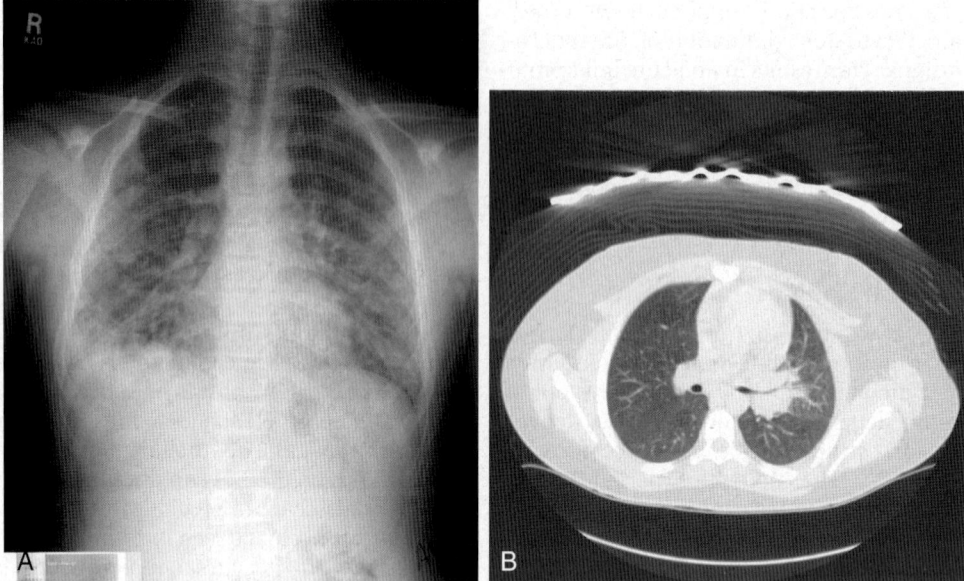

Fig. 31.2 (A) Chest x-ray in acute histoplasmosis showing a diffuse interstitial process. (B) Cross-sectional computed tomography with narrowing of the right main stem bronchus attributable to hilar adenopathy in histoplasmosis.

a high rate of false-positive results in adults from endemic areas.[20]

H. capsulatum can be cultured from sputum, tissue specimens, and bone marrow on standard fungal culture media. Unfortunately the sensitivity is low in acute disease. Growth is seen in 1–6 weeks.[21] Histopathologic examination of biopsy specimens can allow for a rapid diagnosis. Specimens from lung, bronchoalveolar lavage (BAL) fluid, lymph nodes or bone marrow can show intracellular yeast forms using Gomori methenamine silver stains (Fig. 31.3E and F).[15,22]

Detection of *H. capsulatum* antigen from serum, urine, or BAL fluid can be done with a commercially available enzyme immunoassay (EIA). This test is most sensitive for severe pulmonary infections or progressive disseminated disease in adults but has a low sensitivity in primary disseminated disease in childhood or in the setting of immunosuppression. When positive, the antigen test can also be helpful in monitoring response to treatment and determining length of treatment. False-positive results are occasionally seen with other endemic fungal infections.[23]

The serologic diagnosis of histoplasmosis also has limitations. Acute pulmonary disease may be missed with this test, as serology does not become positive until 2–6 weeks after infection. Two different types of assays are available: an immunodiffusion test using antibodies to the M and H antigens of *H. capsulatum* and a complement fixation test that uses antigens from the yeast and mycelial forms. The complement fixation test is slightly more sensitive, while the immunodiffusion test has been found to be more specific. Complement fixation titers equal to or greater than 1 : 32 are highly suggestive of acute or recent infection. In the immunodiffusion test, results are reported as M or H bands. The H band is detectable in less than 20% of cases and is typically found to be positive in cases of disseminated infection or severe acute pulmonary histoplasmosis. Serologic tests are often negative in immunocompromised patients.[15]

Differential Diagnosis

Pulmonary histoplasmosis with mediastinal lymph node involvement can mimic tuberculosis or lymphoma. Disseminated histoplasmosis of infancy can mimic leukemia or sepsis.

Management and Treatment

Histoplasmosis in the normal host is usually a self-limited disease, and antifungal therapy is not required for mild to moderate disease in the immunocompetent host. Children who have persistent symptoms lasting longer than 4 weeks should receive a 6- to 12-week course of oral itraconazole. For severe or disseminated disease, the lipid formulation of amphotericin B is recommended for 1–2 weeks, followed by oral itraconazole for an additional 12 weeks (longer courses may be required for immunocompromised patients). Children being treated for PDH should not be transitioned to oral itraconazole until they have demonstrated clinical improvement and a decline in their serum *Histoplasma* antigen level. When using oral itraconazole, serum trough concentrations should be checked after 2 weeks of therapy to ensure that levels are greater than 1 μg/mL. Methylprednisolone should also be considered during the first 1–2 weeks of therapy in cases of severe respiratory disease. All children with chronic pulmonary histoplasmosis should be treated with a prolonged course of itraconazole (typically 1–2 years), and severe cases may require an initial course of amphotericin B.[15]

Children with the inflammatory mediastinal manifestations of histoplasmosis (e.g., mediastinal adenitis, pericarditis) may not require antifungal therapy. Mild to moderate cases of pericarditis or rheumatologic syndromes can be treated with nonsteroidal antiinflammatory drugs. In severe cases of mediastinal disease (e.g., adenitis leading to obstruction, severe pericarditis), corticosteroids can be used. In cases where corticosteroids are used, itraconazole should be used concurrently and continued for 6–12 weeks thereafter. General recommendations for the treatment of histoplasmosis

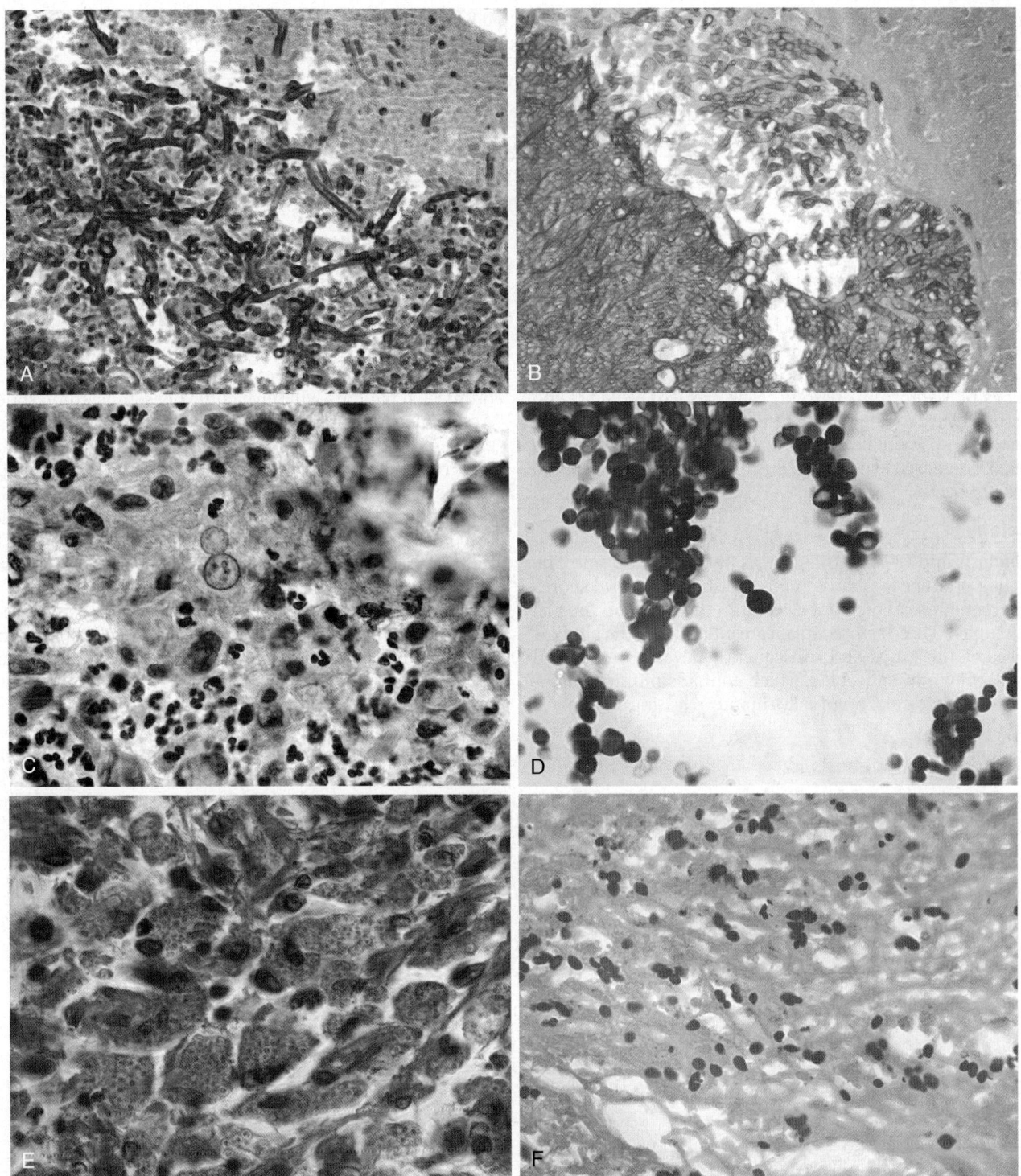

Fig. 31.3 Panels showing the typical morphology of invasive aspergillosis (A and B), blastomycosis (C and D), and histoplasmosis (E and F). (A, C, and E) Hematoxylin and eosin. (B, D, and F) Gomori's methenamine silver stain.

in children and adults have been published by the Infectious Disease Society of America (IDSA).[15]

Prevention

Children with impaired cellular immunity should be counseled about the risks of histoplasmosis if they are living in or visiting endemic areas. These patients should avoid activities that increase the risk of exposure, including cleaning household areas with significant dirt or dust (e.g., garages, basements, and barns), cutting firewood, gardening, or exposure to soil contaminated by bird or bat guano. If such activities are unavoidable, an appropriate mask should be worn.

Prognosis

The prognosis of children with histoplasmosis varies greatly based on the clinical scenario. In most children, the disease is unrecognized or self-limited. The cure rate for immunocompetent children with acute disease is high. PDH of infancy was considered uniformly fatal before effective antifungal agents were available, but survival rates are high with modern therapies.[18] Immunocompromised children with disseminated histoplasmosis have a more guarded prognosis.

COCCIDIOIDOMYCOSIS

Epidemiology

Coccidioidomycosis, also known as San Joaquin Valley fever, is a systemic fungal infection caused by *Coccidioides immitis* and *Coccidioides posadasii*. Both organisms are found in geographic regions with low rainfall, high summer heat, and alkaline soil. Such geographic locations include the central valleys of California, Arizona, New Mexico, Nevada, and northern Mexico (Fig. 31.4). Children are at greatest risk of disease acquisition during the dry seasons of the year when there is increased exposure to dust. Person-to-person spread does not occur.

Etiology

C. immitis and *C. posadasii* grow as mycelia in the soil. The mycelia produce hyphae composed of barrel-shaped spores (arthroconidia), which are swept into the air when the soil is disrupted. These arthroconidia are inhaled into the alveolar spaces of the lungs and subsequently develop into round forms known as spherules, which contains multiple endospores. The spherules eventually rupture, releasing endospores into the adjacent tissues.[24]

Pathology/Pathogenesis

The arthroconidia and spherules induce an immune response by neutrophils and macrophages, but phagocytosis is made difficult by the size of the fungal elements. Macrophages and dendritic cells exposed to the coccidioidal antigens stimulate the production of interferon gamma and other cytokines. This leads to further activation of phagosome-lysosome fusion and killing, followed by granulomatous inflammation of the affected area of the lung. Natural infection leads to lifelong immunity.[25]

Clinical Features

Approximately 60% of humans infected with coccidioidomycosis have a subclinical infection. The remainder of infected individuals have symptomatic disease ranging from a self-limited influenza-like illness to more severe disease.[26] After inhalation of arthroconidia, there is an incubation period of 1–4 weeks. This is followed by cough, chest pain, fever, night sweats, arthralgias, and extreme fatigue. About one-third of infected patients will have clinically significant dyspnea. Acute infection can also be accompanied by a papular rash, erythema nodosum, or an erythema multiforme-like eruption. The combination of erythema nodosum, fever, and arthralgia has been described as "desert rheumatism." Other extrapulmonary manifestations are rare in children and include osteomyelitis and pustules that can ulcerate over time. The most severe manifestation of coccidioidomycosis is meningeal disease, which is seen in less than 1% of patients.[24]

Chronic forms of pulmonary coccidioidomycosis are seen but are uncommon in children. Patients with chronic disease may have had a mild primary infection that was not initially recognized as coccidioidomycosis. Chronic infection can result in cavitary lesions. Hemoptysis may often be the only symptom of a pulmonary cavity infected by *Coccidioides* spp. Risk factors for chronic pulmonary coccidioidomycosis include diabetes mellitus or an immunocompromising condition.

In one study of 41 children's hospitals in the United States from 2002 to 2007, Fisher et al. identified 199

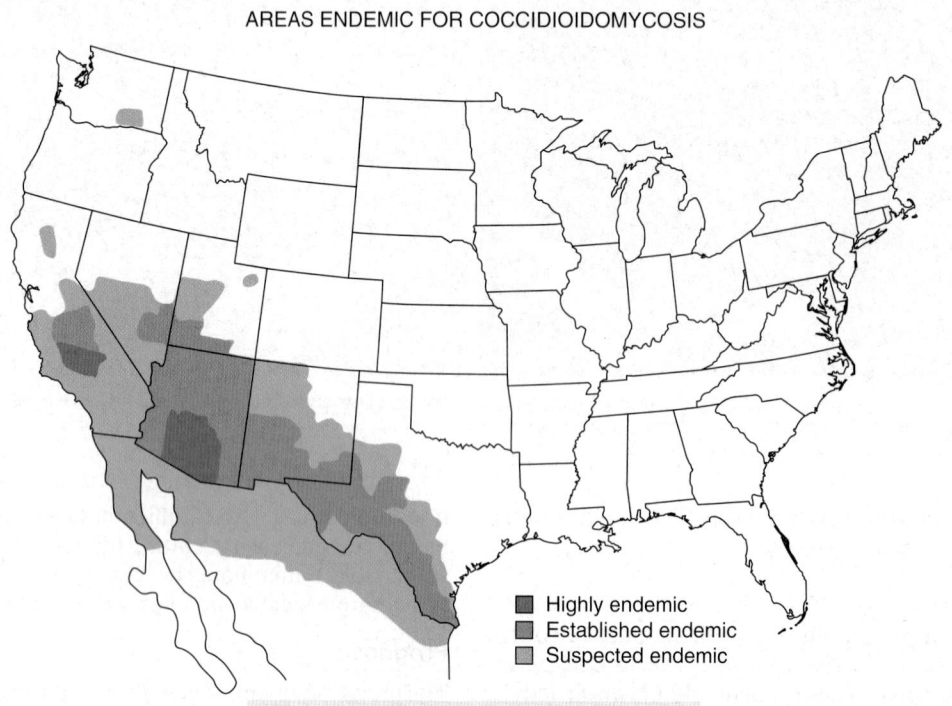

AREAS ENDEMIC FOR COCCIDIOIDOMYCOSIS

- Highly endemic
- Established endemic
- Suspected endemic

Fig. 31.4 Areas endemic for coccidioidomycosis.

children who required hospital admission for coccidioidomycosis. The authors found that 34% of the children had an underlying comorbid condition and 22% required at least one readmission for their disease during the study period.[27]

Imaging, Pulmonary Function Testing, Laboratory Findings

Radiographic findings in pulmonary coccidioidomycosis are variable. Pulmonary nodules and thin-walled cavities can be seen on chest imaging, and some nodules will show calcification over time. Lobar, nodular, and patchy pulmonary infiltrates are all seen in acute disease, with or without hilar lymphadenopathy and pleural effusion. Cavitary lesions and bronchiectasis are all late features of pulmonary *Coccidioides* infection. In rare cases, rupture of a cavity may lead to severe disease with pyopneumothorax.[14]

Diagnosis

Coccidioidomycosis may not be clinically recognized outside of endemic areas. Children with community-acquired pneumonia, especially with the dermatologic and rheumatologic symptoms already mentioned, should be considered for testing. The diagnosis of coccidioidomycosis is most often made with specific serologic tests utilizing EIA, immunodiffusion, or complement fixation–based tests. Antibody detection of IgG and IgM by EIA is the most sensitive assay and multiple commercially tests are available. Assays that utilize immunodiffusion or complement fixation are more specific. In general, approximately 50% of patients have IgM detected by 1 week of illness, and 90% have IgM detected by 3 weeks of illness. Unlike the case with other infections, IgG returns to normal levels after the infection resolves rather than remaining positive for life. Persistent high titers equal to or greater than 1 : 16 are seen with severe disease or disseminated infection.[28]

A second approach to the diagnosis of coccidioidomycosis is use of an EIA to detect *Coccidioides* antigens in urine, blood, or BAL fluid. This may prove useful in diagnosing coccidioidomycosis in patients who may not produce *Coccidioides*-specific antibodies. A small retrospective study of mostly immunocompromised patients found that *Coccidioides* antigenuria occurred in approximately 70% of patients with culture-proven infection, most of whom had severe disease. The assay proved to have a high negative predictive value except in patients who had infections with another endemic fungal infection.[29] Finally, coccidioidomycosis can be diagnosed by direct identification of the organism in its spherule form in biopsy tissue or BAL fluid. Isolation of *Coccidioides* from fungal culture is diagnostic. The organism grows rapidly on appropriate artificial media, with visible colonies of mold forming in 5–7 days. There is risk of infection to laboratory workers and the microbiology laboratory should be alerted prior to sending a sample if the disease is suspected.[24]

Differential Diagnosis

Primary pulmonary coccidioidomycosis can resemble viral pneumonia, atypical pneumonia, bacterial pneumonia, tuberculosis, or other endemic fungal infections of the lungs.

Management and Treatment

Treatment is not indicated for all patients. Asymptomatic patients who are found to have a pulmonary nodule from coccidioidomycosis and are otherwise healthy do not require treatment.[28] The benefit of treatment in immunocompetent patients with mild to moderate acute symptomatic infection is controversial. Some experts believe that antifungal therapy may decrease the length of illness or decrease the likelihood of severe infection. Suggested criteria to indicate severe disease include the need for hospitalization, weight loss of greater than 10%, persistent night sweats for greater than 3 weeks, pulmonary infiltrates involving both lungs or greater than half of one lung, prominent hilar lymphadenopathy, symptoms persisting over 2 months, inability to work or attend school, or a complement fixation titer of at least 1 : 16. Treatment should be strongly considered for those of African or Filipino descent, given higher rates of disseminated infection as compared with Caucasians. Although meningitis is uncommon in children with this infection, clinicians should have a low threshold for evaluating for the presence of CNS disease.

When treatment for coccidioidomycosis is indicated, an oral azole such is fluconazole is recommended for 3–6 months, depending on the clinical response. Regardless of whether antifungal therapy is started, patients with coccidioidomycosis should be followed every 1–3 months to document resolution of disease on chest x-ray (CXR) and monitored for new pulmonary or extrapulmonary complications.

Patients with active pulmonary coccidioidomycosis who are at increased risk for severe or disseminated infection should be treated with antifungal therapy. This includes patients with a history of human immunodeficiency virus (HIV) infection, hematopoietic stem cell transplant (HSCT), solid organ transplantation, prolonged exposure to corticosteroids or TNF inhibitors, or those who are pregnant. Treatment in these populations involves fluconazole or amphotericin B, depending on the extent of disease. Patients started on amphotericin B can be switched to oral fluconazole after clinical improvement. General recommendations for treatment of coccidioidomycosis in adults have been published by the IDSA and were last updated in 2016.[24]

Prevention

Patients with impaired cellular immunity who live in or are visiting endemic areas should be counseled about the risks of coccidioidomycosis. This includes children with HIV, those on high-dose corticosteroids, those on anti-TNF therapies, those on antirejection medications after organ transplant, and women in their third trimester of pregnancy. Such patients should avoid activities that increase the risk of exposure, including environments where they would be exposed to large amount of dust from disrupted soil. If such activities are unavoidable, an appropriate mask should be worn. Preemptive therapy for coccidioidomycosis in special at-risk populations is recommended and is described in the IDSA guidelines.[24]

Prognosis

The prognosis of children with coccidioidomycosis varies greatly based on the clinical scenario. The majority of patients have a self-limited disease process with complete recovery

AREAS ENDEMIC FOR BLASTOMYCOSIS IN THE UNITED STATES

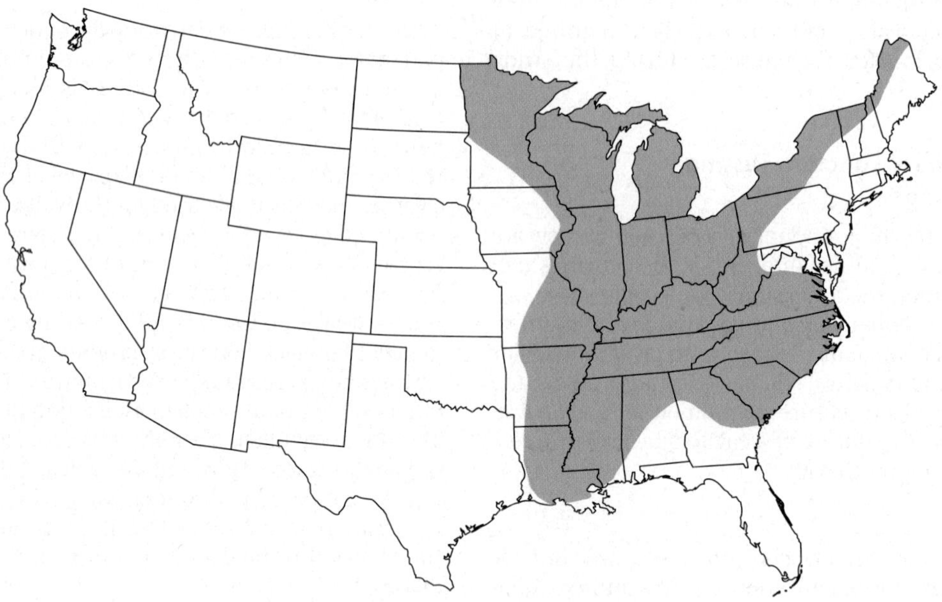

Fig. 31.5 Areas endemic for blastomycosis.

in 1–3 weeks. Mortality is low, even in children hospitalized for coccidioidomycosis. In the previously mentioned study by Fisher et al., the authors found that the overall in-house mortality for children admitted with coccidioidomycosis was 3 of 199 patients (1.5%).[27]

BLASTOMYCOSIS

Epidemiology

Blastomycosis is another endemic fungal infection that has a geographic localization similar to that of histoplasmosis. This fungus grows best in warm, moist soil, and is endemic in the Ohio and Mississippi River valleys, in addition to the borders of the Great Lakes and the St. Lawrence River (Fig. 31.5). Blastomycosis is uncommon in children, with an estimated 3%–10% of all cases occurring in the pediatric population.[30]

Etiology

Blastomyces dermatitidis is a thermally dimorphic fungus that exists in nature in a mycelial form and converts to a yeast at body temperature. The mycelial form is primarily found in the soil and consists of hyphae that produce conidia. These conidia are released into the air from the soil when it is disrupted and can subsequently be inhaled by humans.[31]

Pathology/Pathogenesis

Blastomycosis can occur in immunocompetent and immunocompromised hosts. Population studies show that the infection is asymptomatic in 50% of children.[32] After *B. dermatitidis* conidia are inhaled by humans, the organism converts to pathogenic yeast. Alveolar macrophages and neutrophils are capable of phagocytizing and destroying conidia. The adaptive immune response is coordinated by T lymphocytes and is critical in activating a TNF-α response, which further enhances fungicidal activity. Conidia that evade this immune

response can convert to the pathogenic yeast form in the lung and may subsequently disseminate.[30]

Clinical Features (Symptoms/Physical Findings)

Blastomycosis is primarily a disease of the lungs. Children typically present with a prolonged illness consisting of fever, fatigue, cough, myalgias, and chest pain. In rare cases, a more severe ARDS presentation is seen. Between 38% and 50% of children with blastomycosis develop disseminated disease,[33,34] which can manifest as skin lesions (pustular, nodular, or ulcerative lesions), osteomyelitis, septic arthritis, or involvement of the genitourinary tract (prostatitis or epididymitis). Pulmonary blastomycosis can occasionally persist in the chronic form as chronic pulmonary blastomycosis. Symptoms may include productive cough, hemoptysis, and weight loss.[31]

Imaging, Pulmonary Function Testing, Laboratory Findings

Chest imaging can show patchy pneumonitis, nodular lesions or lobar consolidation, which can occur with or without cavitation. Hilar and mediastinal lymphadenopathy is uncommon and should suggest an alternative diagnosis such as tuberculosis or histoplasmosis.[30]

Diagnosis

The diagnosis of blastomycosis is based on visualization of the thick-walled, budding yeast cells on smears from sputum, tracheal aspirates, urine or tissue specimens (see Fig. 31.3C and D). In cases where the organism cannot be identified by examining sputum, BAL fluid can be cultured on brain/heart infusion or Sabouraud dextrose agar. Serologic testing by immunodiffusion or complement fixation assays lacks sensitivity.[32] A *Blastomyces* urine antigen test is commercially available, but a high degree of cross-reactivity is seen with other endemic mycoses. Real-time polymerase chain reaction (PCR) assays have been developed that can identify *B. dermatitidis* in various clinical specimens (e.g., pleural fluid, BAL fluid, sputum) with high sensitivity and specificity.[35]

Differential Diagnosis

Acute pulmonary blastomycosis can mimic bacterial pneumonia, tuberculosis, sarcoidosis, or a malignant neoplasm. Chronic pulmonary blastomycosis can be mistaken for malignancy or tuberculosis. The skin lesions can be misdiagnosed as pyoderma gangrenosum.[30]

Management and Treatment

Unlike acute pulmonary histoplasmosis or coccidioidomycosis, for which treatment is unnecessary in milder forms of disease, treatment of all forms of acute pulmonary blastomycosis is generally recommended.[31] The high rate of disseminated disease in children underscores this recommendation. For mild to moderate acute pulmonary disease, oral itraconazole is recommended for 6–12 months. For patients with moderate to severe pulmonary disease or those with disseminated extrapulmonary disease, amphotericin B (lipid or deoxycholate) should be given for 1–2 weeks or until improvement is noted. This should be followed by oral itraconazole for 6–12 months for pulmonary disease and at least 12 months for disseminated disease. Serum levels of itraconazole should be determined after the patient has received this agent for at least 2 weeks, to ensure adequate drug levels. It is recommended that serum itraconazole levels be greater than 1.0 mg/mL. General recommendations for the treatment of blastomycoses were last published in 2008 by the IDSA.[31]

Prognosis

Overall mortality in adults with blastomycosis is reported to be 4%–6%, with an 18% mortality rate in those with CNS disease. Limited data are available in children, but mortality is thought to be lower in children than in adults due to the presence of less comorbidity.[30]

Pulmonary Mycoses Primarily Seen in Hosts With Impaired Immunity

INTRODUCTION

Children with altered immunity constitute a growing proportion of pediatric patients and the lungs are a frequent site of opportunistic fungal infections in this population.[36] Susceptibility to opportunistic fungi is increased in patients who undergo HSCT and receive cytotoxic chemotherapy, as these interventions result in decreased function and number of lymphocytes and phagocytes. Patients who receive such treatment often require indwelling catheters and invasive procedures, which further disrupt the normal barriers to immunity. Other risk factors for opportunistic fungal infections in children include those with AIDS, primary immunodeficiency syndromes, neonates with extreme prematurity and those with exposure to broad-spectrum antibiotics.

Diagnosis of pulmonary fungal infections in the immunocompromised child can be difficult, as the clinical presentation is often nonspecific. Likewise, radiographic patterns of disease in this population lack etiologic specificity, and microbiologic diagnosis is difficult without the use of invasive procedures to obtain specimens. For these reasons, clinicians must maintain a high index of suspicion for fungal infections in the immunocompromised child. Procedures such as bronchoscopy and lung biopsy must be carefully timed because the risks associated with an invasive procedure may become too high as the underlying disease progresses.

ASPERGILLOSIS

The term *aspergillosis* can refer to disease related to allergy, airway or pulmonary invasion, cutaneous disease or extrapulmonary dissemination. This section focuses on the invasive forms of aspergillosis. The inflammatory syndrome of allergic bronchopulmonary aspergillosis (ABPA) and allergic sinusitis is covered in the chapter titled "Hypersensitivity Pneumonitis and Eosinophilic Lung Diseases" (Chapter 65).

Epidemiology

Aspergillus species are an important cause of life-threatening infection in immunocompromised children. Humans with normal pulmonary host defenses rarely develop IA, despite routine exposure to airborne conidia. It has been estimated that the average person inhales several hundred *Aspergillus* conidia spores per day.[37] Hospital construction and renovation have been linked to nosocomial infection in immunocompromised patients.[38] Specific groups of children are at risk of IA. This includes those with leukemia and other malignancies, neutropenia secondary to cytotoxic chemotherapy, HSCT, SOT, inherited or acquired immunodeficiencies, corticosteroid use, as well as low-birth-weight infants. In a retrospective study of pediatric patients with probable or proven IA, 63% had a hematologic malignancy, 38% had a history of a hematopoietic transplant, 11.5% had an inherited immunodeficiency, 6.5% had a history of a SOT and 0.7% had HIV infection.[39]

Of the primary immunodeficiencies, chronic granulomatous disease (CGD) has the best-characterized association with IA. There is a 33% lifetime risk of IA in CGD.[40] Severe combined immune deficiency (SCID) is the other primary immunodeficiency for which the risk of IA is known to be significant. Approximately 4% of children with SCID develop IA, resulting in a high mortality rate.[41]

Of the commonly used immunosuppressive medications, corticosteroids have been identified as an important risk factor for IA. Although the mechanisms are still incompletely understood, corticosteroids have been shown to impair the anticonidial activity of macrophages and suppress neutrophils, both in recruitment and antifungal activity.[42] Newer immunomodulating drugs that inhibit TNF have also been shown to increase the risk of pulmonary and IA.[17,43,44] There have also been reports of pulmonary aspergillosis in adults with critical illness secondary to influenza A H1N1.[45]

Aspergillosis has occasionally been described in premature neonates. In this population, risk factors for *Aspergillus* infection include skin maceration from adhesive tape or venous arm boards, percutaneous catheter insertion sites and necrotizing enterocolitis, all of which reflect mucocutaneous portals of entry.[46]

Etiology

Species within the genus *Aspergillus* are ubiquitous worldwide; they are found in soil, water, air, and decaying vegetation. The classification of the genus *Aspergillus* is complex, as there are more than 200 different species that are divided amongst multiple subgenera.[47] Given that some species can be distinguished only by molecular typing, it has been proposed that isolates are referred to as a "species complex." *Aspergillus fumigatus* is a species complex that causes the majority of invasive disease in humans, and most of what is known about *Aspergillus* virulence factors and host immune response comes from research on this organism. *Aspergillus flavus* is the principal species found in sinusitis and accounts for up to 10% of all invasive isolates. *Aspergillus niger, Aspergillus terreus,* and *Aspergillus nidulans* are less common causes of invasive disease. *Aspergillus terreus* is a notable species given that it is resistant to amphotericin B, and infection from this organism is associated with a high mortality rate. *Aspergillus nidulans* has been found to occur at an unusually high frequency in children with CGD.[48] The varying pathogenicity of these different species is thought to be related to variables such as the ability to grow at 37°C, conidial size, growth rate, and the production of various virulence factors.

The infective components of the organism are conidia, which are readily aerosolized from the end of hyphal stalks. Inhalation and subsequent germination of conidia leads to the formation of hyphae in the distal airways. These hyphal forms of *Aspergillus* subsequently invade pulmonary blood vessels and parenchyma, resulting in thrombosis and ischemic necrosis of the affected lung. The time required for this sequence of events to occur is variable; the incubation period of IA is estimated to be as short as 2 days and as long as 3 months. After invasion of pulmonary tissue, spread to contiguous thoracic structures or hematogenous dissemination may occur.[49]

Pathology/Pathogenesis

Anatomic barriers play an important role in the host defense against inhaled *Aspergillus* conidia. An intact respiratory mucosa, bronchial mucus, surfactant, and ciliated respiratory epithelium eliminate inhaled conidia and prevent germination. Innate immunity is clearly another important part of the host defense. Alveolar macrophages are responsible for the ingestion of conidia. Neutrophil recruitment and activation of cellular immunity also play key roles in the control of invasive hyphae. Once the *Aspergillus* conidia have germinated into invasive hyphal forms, vascular invasion is seen. One of the histopathologic hallmarks of IA is tissue infarction and necrosis.[41]

Clinical Features (Symptoms/Physical Findings)

IA can be classified into four main clinical presentations: pulmonary aspergillosis, tracheobronchitis, rhinosinusitis, and disseminated disease. Of all these clinical presentations, invasive pulmonary aspergillosis (IPA) is the most common. In a study of aspergillosis in children with cancer, 70% of the 66 children with culture-proven disease had lung involvement.[50] In children with either CGD or HIV/AIDS, pulmonary disease is also the most common manifestation.[40,51] The classic triad of presenting symptoms for IPA is fever, pleuritic chest pain and hemoptysis, although this triad is seen in only a minority. More often, the presenting symptoms of IPA in children are nonspecific, with the most common complaints being fever, cough, and dyspnea.[50]

Aspergillus tracheobronchitis has been described in lung transplant recipients and those with other immunocompromising conditions. These patients present with cough, dyspnea, and wheezing. Three different patterns of *Aspergillus* tracheobronchitis have been described: obstructive, ulcerative, and pseudomembranous. Patients with obstructive tracheobronchitis have thick mucus plugs obstructing the airways, which consist of *Aspergillus* hyphae. These patients often present with expectoration of mucous plugs. Ulcerative tracheobronchitis represents the focal invasion of the mucosa and/or cartilage with *Aspergillus* hyphae. A final pattern is pseudomembranous tracheobronchitis, which is characterized by diffuse inflammation and invasion of the airway mucosa. This inflammatory process results in a pseudomembrane composed of necrotic debris from *Aspergillus* hyphae.[52]

Invasive rhinosinusitis due to aspergillosis can cause disease similar to mucormycosis. This can present acutely with fever, facial pain, epistaxis, and visual changes. Extension into the orbits and CNS can be seen. Early nasal endoscopic evaluation by an otolaryngologist is important in the immunocompromised patient, where necrotic lesions are seen from fungal invasion of the mucosal tissues. Disseminated aspergillosis can spread from the respiratory tract to multiple different organs including the skin, CNS, eyes, liver, and kidneys. *Aspergillus* spp. can also cause endocarditis, particularly in those with prosthetic heart valves.[49]

Imaging, Pulmonary Function Testing, Laboratory Findings

The radiographic appearance of IPA is variable. Overall, the most common findings on plain radiographs of the chest are peripherally distributed lung nodules or masses.[53] Chest radiographs can also be normal early in diagnosis, or they may show a variety of nonspecific findings such as segmental or multilobar consolidation, perihilar infiltrates, pleural effusions or nodular lesions.[54] Chest CT is the imaging modality of choice for early diagnosis and has allowed for earlier preemptive therapy for patients at high risk for IA. Classic CT findings of the "halo sign" (a distinct nodular lesion with surrounding areas of decreased attenuation) and the "air crescent sign" (a late finding of nodular cavitation, usually occurring after recovery of neutrophil counts) are less common in children with IPA than in adults.[36,39] In a large retrospective study of children with IA, only 11% demonstrated the halo sign and 2.2% showed the air crescent sign.[39]

Diagnosis

The diagnosis of IA involves multiple testing modalities including fungal culture of various clinical specimens, histopathologic examination of tissue, imaging studies and serum biomarkers such as the galactomannan assay.[55] The definitive diagnosis of IA requires the growth of *Aspergillus* spp. on culture in addition to the visualization of tissue-invasive hyphal forms from biopsy tissue obtained from the same organ (e.g., lung tissue and culture of airway secretions; see Fig. 31.3A and B). Given that humans are exposed to *Aspergillus* conidia on a daily basis, a positive culture of *Aspergillus* spp. from the airways does not necessarily indicate infection. Although lung biopsy is a valuable tool in the diagnosis of IPA, the risks involved in obtaining a biopsy makes this technique unfeasible in some children. For patients at risk of IPA who also have clinical and radiographic findings consistent with the diagnosis, the detection of *Aspergillus* spp. from respiratory tract secretions has been used as a surrogate method of diagnosis.[49]

When respiratory specimens are obtained from sputum or bronchoalveolar lavage fluid, both direct examination for hyphal elements (via staining with calcofluor or methenamine silver) and fungal culture should be performed. Growth of *Aspergillus* in the laboratory typically requires 1–3 days of incubation. Once growth is seen, identification of the species requires sporulation so that the spore-bearing structures can be seen on microscopy. If growth of *Aspergillus* spp. is present in culture and patients are suspected to have an azole-resistant isolate or are unresponsive to initial antifungal agents, susceptibility testing can be performed.[49]

Although a negative culture from sputum or BAL fluid cannot rule out the diagnosis, a positive culture in a neutropenic or bone marrow transplant (BMT) patient with new pulmonary infiltrates is putative evidence of IPA. However, in solid-organ transplant patients, nonneutropenic patients with chronic lung disease, and HIV-infected patients, the positive predictive value of respiratory tract cultures is much lower. There is evidence that the overall culture isolation rate of *Aspergillus* spp. from BAL or bronchial washing specimens is higher than that from biopsy tissue specimens (8.1% vs. 1.5%).[56]

When lung biopsy is performed, tissue from both the peripheral and central areas of the affected lung should be sampled. Thoracoscopic lung biopsy for diagnosis of IPA has not been systematically studied in children but has been used in this population. Given that biopsy is often not possible, due to comorbidities such as thrombocytopenia, alternative methods of diagnosis are needed in patients at risk of aspergillosis. Despite the angioinvasive nature of *Aspergillus* spp., positive blood cultures for the mold are rarely reported in IA.[56]

Various biomarker assays have been developed to help in the diagnosis of IA, including the galactomannan assay, PCR-based assays, and tests to detect the (1-3)-β-D-glucan found in the fungal cell wall. The galactomannan antigen assay uses a double-sandwich EIA to detect galactomannan, a polysaccharide cell wall antigen of *Aspergillus* spp. The assay recognizes circulating galactomannan in patients with IA and was approved in 2003 for use in the United States on serum and BAL specimens.[49] The galactomannan assay is best validated for neutropenic patients with hematologic malignancy and HSCT. In some of the early studies, the galactomannan antigen assay was reported to have a sensitivity as high as 81% and a specificity as high as 89%.[57] Subsequent studies in more diverse populations have shown significantly more variability in test sensitivity, with rates ranging from 30% to 100%.[58] Data on the galactomannan assay in children are limited. In a retrospective study of children receiving chemotherapy or those with a history of HSCT, the galactomannan antigen assay showed poor sensitivity (32%) and positive predictive value (70%), but good specificity (98%) and negative predictive value (92%).[59] Variables such as cutoff values for positivity, specimen treatment, preceding antifungal treatment, pretest probability of IA

based on risk factors, and false-positive results in patients receiving piperacillin/tazobactam are thought to contribute to the variability of the results.[58,60]

Detection of *Aspergillus* spp. in BAL fluid has been studied using the galactomannan assay and PCR technology, but the precise role of these techniques in diagnosis remains to be seen. In a study of 85 children (59 of whom were immunocompromised), the use of the galactomannan assay on BAL fluid showed a sensitivity of 78% and specificity of 100% for pulmonary aspergillosis.[61] In a study of adult patients with hematologic malignancies, the authors found that the galactomannan assay of BAL fluid had a sensitivity of 92% and specificity 98%.[62] In the same study, PCR of BAL fluid for *Aspergillus* spp. was compared to the galactomannan assay. The authors found that PCR showed a decreased sensitivity compared with the galactomannan assay but had a similar specificity. *Aspergillus* PCR from blood specimens of immunocompromised patients has also been studied. In a meta-analysis of 18 primary studies (4 of which included pediatric patients), the authors found that the *Aspergillus* blood PCR had a mean sensitivity and specificity of 80.5% and 78.5% when tested in patients at high risk of IA. The authors also found a high negative predictive value of 96%.[63]

Several assays (e.g., Fungitel, Fungitec, and Endosafe-PTS) have been developed to detect another component of the fungal cell wall, (1-3)-β-D-glucan (BDG). As a nonspecific marker of invasive fungal infections, BDG assays have varying predictive values in studies of adult patients. However, the assay does not distinguish *Aspergillus* from the other fungi that contain BDG (various other molds, *Candida* spp., *Pneumocystis*). Furthermore, the performance of the BDG assays in pediatric patients is largely unknown.[36]

Differential Diagnosis

IA can mimic multiple other disease processes depending on the clinical and radiographic features. Pulmonary aspergillosis can be difficult to distinguish from tuberculosis or other invasive fungal infections (e.g., mucormycosis, *Fusarium* spp.). Rhinosinusitis due to *Aspergillus* spp. can be clinically and radiographically similar to invasive mucormycosis.[49]

Management and Treatment

Effective treatment of IA involves a combination of antifungal therapy, reversal of immunosuppressing drugs or interventions and in some cases surgery. For over 40 years, amphotericin B was recommended as primary therapy for IA.[65] Monotherapy with amphotericin B has historically had only modest success in the treatment of IA. Mortality with amphotericin B as sole therapy for IA was 65% in one large retrospective review.[49] The toxicity of amphotericin B deoxycholate is well known, with nephrotoxicity being the most common dose-limiting side effect. The newer lipid formulations of amphotericin B offer reduced toxicity, but these compounds have not shown an increase in efficacy relative to the deoxycholate formulation.

In a seminal randomized trial published in 2002, primary therapy with voriconazole was shown to be superior to amphotericin B.[66] Subsequent studies have supported this conclusion, with an estimated 15% improved survival at 12 weeks in patients who received voriconazole compared with other antifungal therapies.[49] The IDSA guideline on the management of aspergillosis published in 2016 recommends that voriconazole be used as the primary treatment of IA in adults and children. The intravenous form should be used for patients with severe illness. When the oral form is used, trough levels should be greater than 1–1.5 µg/mL for efficacy but less than 5–6 µg/mL. Treatment should continue for a minimum of 6–12 weeks, depending on the duration of immunosuppression and evidence of disease improvement. Isavuconazole has shown promise as a treatment option for IA, as it is associated with a lower rate of hepatobiliary and visual disturbances as compared with voriconazole. In a randomized double-blind trial comparing voriconazole with isavuconazole in 527 adults with invasive mold infections (primarily with *Aspergillus* spp.), isavuconazole was found to be noninferior to voriconazole.[67] Based on these data, isavuconazole was approved by the FDA as an alternative primary therapy for IPA. Amphotericin B should still be used for situations in which hepatic toxicities or drug interactions warrant an alternative to azoles or when voriconazole-resistant molds (e.g., mucormycosis) are still in the differential diagnosis.[49]

Primary therapy with an echinocandin is not recommended for aspergillosis unless the patient is intolerant to both the azoles and amphotericin B or has failed alternative therapy (i.e., salvage therapy).[49] The combination of either voriconazole or amphotericin B with an echinocandin shows some evidence of benefit based on in vitro studies and small nonrandomized clinical trials.[68,69] The authors of the IDSA guideline recommend that combination antifungal therapy be reserved for severe disease, especially in patients with profound and persistent neutropenia.[49]

Treatment of IA should involve the reduction or elimination of immunosuppressive agents when possible. Adjunctive therapies such as interferon gamma (INF-γ), colony-stimulating factor, and infusions of granulocytes harvested from donors pretreated with granulocyte colony-stimulating factor (GCSF) have a role in the treatment of aspergillosis in certain patients. Although these modalities have not yet been well studied, experience with certain patient populations has led to recommendations for their use. GCSF or granulocyte macrophage colony-stimulating factor (GM-CSF) should be considered in severely neutropenic patients who do not respond to standard therapy. Granulocyte transfusions can be considered for patients with prolonged neutropenia and disease that is refractory to standard therapy. In patients with CGD, recombinant INF-γ is recommended as prophylaxis against IA and other infections.[49]

Therapeutic surgical excision of IPA also has a role in the treatment of certain patients. Surgical resection can provide a definitive diagnosis and can completely eradicate a localized infection of the lung. Patients with IPA that has invaded the great vessels, pericardium, or pleural space may also benefit from surgical intervention. In a retrospective review of 43 pediatric patients with IPA, most of whom were significantly immunosuppressed, the authors found a significantly higher survival rate in the 18 patients who underwent surgical intervention compared with those who received only medical therapy.[70] The retrospective nature of the study, high overall mortality rate in the series (91%) and limitations of medical therapy available at the time of the study (i.e., before the approval of voriconazole) make it difficult to know if such findings can be generalized to current care. In the absence of chest wall extension or uncontrolled bleeding, there is no consensus regarding the benefit of surgical resection prior to HSCT or intensive chemotherapy. General recommendations for the treatment of aspergillosis were published in 2016 by the IDSA.[49]

Prevention

Children with prolonged neutropenia who are at risk of IA should receive prophylaxis with posaconazole or voriconazole. For children previously treated for IA who will require subsequent immunosuppression, antifungal therapy should be restarted to prevent recurrent infection. Children who have had a lung transplant should receive antifungal prophylaxis for 3–4 months after lung transplant with either an azole such as voriconazole or itraconazole or inhaled amphotericin B. Hospitalized allogeneic HSCT recipients should be roomed in a protected environment to reduce exposure to mold. Routine environmental sampling of fungal spores in the hospital is not recommended in the absence of a known outbreak.[49]

Prognosis

In a retrospective analysis of 139 children with IA, the overall mortality rate was found to be 52.5%. The highest mortality rate was seen in patients with allogeneic HSCT, where 78% of the patients had died by 12 weeks or at the end of therapy.[39]

CANDIDIASIS

Epidemiology

Invasive infections due to *Candida* species can cause significant morbidity and mortality in certain populations of children. *Candida* spp. are the third most common cause of nosocomial bloodstream infections in children.[71] Risk factors include the use of broad-spectrum antibiotics, invasive devices such as central venous catheters, organ transplant, immunosuppressive chemotherapy regimens, and neonates born with very low birth weights. Infections occur primarily via tissue invasion from endogenously acquired strains rather than by person-to-person spread.

Etiology

Candida spp. are yeasts that reproduce by budding. Most members of the genus can produce only pseudohyphae, which are chains of elongated yeast that result from incomplete budding. An exception to this is seen with *Candida albicans* and *Candida dubliniensis*, which can produce true hyphae under conditions found in the human host.

Candida spp. commonly colonize the human gastrointestinal tract, genital mucosa and skin. Of the approximately 150 known species of *Candida*, only 15 species are known to cause human disease.[72] *C. albicans* is by far the most common species to cause disease and represents about 50% of pediatric invasive candidiasis.[73] Other important *Candida* species include *Candida krusei*, *glabrata*, *parapsilosis*, *tropicalis*, *lusitaniae* and *dubliniensis*.

Pathology/Pathogenesis

Most studies related to the pathogenicity of *Candida* spp. have utilized *C. albicans*. This microorganism has several notable virulence factors including adhesion to host mucosal cells, morphologic switching between the yeast and hyphal forms and the ability to form biofilms. The formation of biofilms plays a significant role in infections of medical devices including central venous catheters and cardiovascular devices. The immune response to *Candida* is complex and involves the innate and adaptive arms. Neutrophils, macrophages, and monocytes play a particularly important role in preventing disseminated candidiasis, as evidenced by the high risk of disseminated disease in neutropenic patients.[74]

Clinical Features (Symptoms/Physical Findings)

Candida spp. are well known for their ability to cause mucocutaneous infections in normal hosts, including oralpharyngeal (thrush) infection, diaper rash and paronychia. Immunocompromised patients can develop laryngeal or esophageal candidiasis. Disseminated or invasive candidiasis can occur in almost any organ system or anatomic site. In children with disseminated candidemia, the lungs were found to be involved in 45%–58% of cases. Less common sites of dissemination include the liver, kidney, brain, heart, spleen, and eyes.[74,75]

When pulmonary candidiasis does occur, three different patterns of disease have been described: primary pneumonia due to tracheobronchial colonization and aspiration, secondary pneumonia in the setting of candidemia with disseminated disease, and secondary pneumonia in the setting of septic emboli.[76] In all of these cases, the clinical manifestations are nonspecific, with fever, cough, and a sepsis-like picture being the most common presentation. Primary candidal pneumonia (i.e., with no evidence of candidemia or other sites of disseminated disease) is rare and is thought to be limited to neutropenic patients and low-birth-weight infants. In patients with disseminated disease, bilateral lung involvement is typical, and microscopic examination of the lung shows pseudohyphae in the pulmonary capillaries. In embolic disease, the lungs (and other organs) are seeded with infected emboli from an endovascular source, resulting in hemorrhagic infarcts at the periphery of the lungs. Invasive candidiasis in neonates differs from disease in older children in that neonates are more likely to present with nonspecific or subtle signs and symptoms of infection.[73]

Imaging, Pulmonary Function Testing, Laboratory Findings

Patterns on chest radiographs have been described most often as patchy consolidations, with larger areas of consolidation limited to severe disease. Nodular lesions with central necrosis can be seen in disseminated disease and are best detected by CT of the lungs. Cavitation and pleural effusions are rare findings.[53]

Diagnosis

Candida grows well on routine agar and does not require specialized fungal media. Culture of *Candida* spp. from a sterile body site (e.g., blood or CSF) or the demonstration of organisms from tissue biopsy are still the "gold standard" for diagnosis. Growth is typically seen after 2–3 days of incubation, but occasionally >7 days. Automated blood culture systems can allow for earlier detection, but overall sensitivity of candidemia by blood culture is still less than 50%.[77] There are multiple nonculture diagnostics for invasive candidiasis (BDG,

antigen/antibody detection assays, PCR), but none are currently recommended by the IDSA guideline for routine use in children.

In immunocompetent children, growth of *Candida* spp. from the sputum or tracheostomy cultures usually indicates colonization and not infection. In a study of nonneutropenic patients, nearly 90% of bronchoalveolar lavage cultures positive for *Candida* spp. were judged to be probably or definitely contaminated, despite the fact that the majority of the cultures had been done on protected brush specimens.[78] Candidal pneumonia after aspiration is rare in immunocompetent children.

In immunocompromised patients, growth of *Candida* from a respiratory tract culture should prompt clinicians to investigate for invasive candidiasis, although it can be difficult to distinguish oropharyngeal or tracheobronchial colonization from invasive pulmonary disease. In a large study of adult cancer patients, the positive predictive value of various cultures for pulmonary candidiasis was determined using histopathology from autopsy specimens as the gold standard. The authors found that the positive predictive value of a sputum culture for pulmonary candidiasis was 42%; from BAL fluid culture it was 29%.[79]

In intubated patients, histologic evidence of candidal invasion of the lung tissue is the only widely accepted definition of pulmonary candidiasis.[76] In patients with candidemia and new respiratory symptoms or radiographic abnormalities, the diagnosis of invasive pulmonary candidiasis should be strongly suspected.

Differential Diagnosis

Invasive candidiasis, depending on the organ system involved or the clinical situation, can mimic multiple disease processes. Candidemia can mimic septic shock. Pulmonary candidiasis can be confused for bacterial or viral pneumonia or other pulmonary mycoses such as aspergillosis or cryptococcosis.

Management and Treatment

The approach to the treatment of invasive candidiasis depends on a variety of factors including the status of the host immune system, source of infection (e.g., medical device–associated, endovascular), identified *Candida* spp. susceptibility profile, and age of the patient. For neonates with invasive candidiasis, treatment recommendations differ from those for nonneonates given the distinct epidemiology and pathogenesis of the disease in this population as well as the distinct pharmacokinetic and pharmacodynamics of antifungal drugs.

Multiple antifungal drug classes play a role in the treatment of invasive candidiasis, each with strengths and weaknesses based on the clinical scenario. These drug classes include the polyenes (amphotericin B), the azoles, the echinocandins, and flucytosine. Amphotericin B is effective against most *Candida* species with notable exceptions being resistance in *C. lusitaniae* and decreased susceptibly in *C. krusei and C. glabrata.* As mentioned in the section on antifungal drugs at the beginning of this chapter, the lipid preparations of amphotericin B are generally recommended over the deoxycholate form. In the azole family of antifungals, fluconazole should not be used prior to identification of the *Candida* species, as *C. krusei* is resistant to fluconazole and increasing rates of resistance have been seen with *C. glabrata* (~50%) and *C. tropicalis.* Other drugs in the azole family have broader anticandidal activity than fluconazole, but resistance is still seen in some cases (e.g., voriconazole is often ineffective against *C. glabrata*). The echinocandins (caspofungin, micafungin, and anidulafungin) have good activity against almost all *Candida* species, have a good safety profile, and are approved as first-line agents for severely ill or neutropenic patients. Of note, there is an overall trend of increasing resistance of *Candida* species to the triazoles and echinocandins.[80] The use of flucyctosine is generally limited to children with candidal infections of the CNS. Therapeutic drug monitoring may be needed in patients on itraconazole, voriconazole, posaconazole, and flucytosine. Standards for susceptibility to the triazole and echinocandin antifungals have been established for *Candida* spp., and testing is available commercially.

Outside the neonatal population, nonneutropenic children with invasive candidiasis can be treated with fluconazole or an echinocandin. In neutropenic patients or those with critical illness, an echinocandin or liposomal amphotericin B should be used. Voriconazole can be used in children in situations where additional mold coverage is needed. In both of these situations, fluconazole can be used as step-down therapy for patients who have susceptible isolates and documented blood culture clearance.

In patients with a vascular or peritoneal catheter, removal of the catheter is recommended, in addition to antifungal therapy. Full details of management of patients with candidal infection of central venous catheters can be found in guidelines published by the IDSA.[81] In patients with persistent disease despite adequate treatment, a search for a disseminated infection should be conducted. This diagnostic evaluation may need to include evaluation of the liver, spleen, lung, heart, and genitourinary tract. The length of treatment for patients without metastatic complications is generally 2 weeks after clearance of the bloodstream and resolution of symptoms. In disseminated candidiasis, other sites of infection may dictate the type and length of treatment (e.g., endocarditis, meningitis, endophthalmitis). All patients with candidemia should have a dilated fundoscopic evaluation. A lumbar puncture is recommended for all neonates with candidemia.[82]

In neonates with invasive candidemia, amphotericin B deoxycholate is the drug of choice with disseminated disease, including meningitis. The lipid formulations of amphotericin B should be used with caution in neonates, especially if urinary tract involvement is suspected. Oral or IV fluconazole is an alternative to amphotericin B deoxycholate in patients who have not been on fluconazole prophylaxis. The echinocandins should be used with caution in neonates because there are limited data in this population. The IDSA guidelines recommend that this class of antifungals should be limited to salvage therapy or to situations in which resistance or toxicity preclude the use of amphotericin B or fluconazole.[73]

Full details of the treatment of neonatal and nonneonatal candidemia can be found in the guidelines published by the IDSA. These guidelines were last published in 2016 and were endorsed by the American Academy of Pediatrics (AAP) and the Pediatric Infectious Diseases Society (PIDS).[73]

Prevention

Fluconazole prophylaxis is recommended for infants of extremely low birth weights who are admitted to a neonatal intensive care unit with at least moderate rates (≥5%) of invasive candidiasis. Prophylactic fluconazole is also sometimes used in patients with advanced HIV disease, allogenic HSCT, and severe neutropenia.[82]

Prognosis

The mortality rate of invasive *Candida* infection in neonates is high. In a multicenter study of infants weighing less than 1000 g at birth, the mortality rate was 34% in those with invasive candidiasis, compared to 14% in those without invasive candidiasis.[83] Outside the neonatal period, children with candidemia were also found to have a significant mortality rate. In studies of candidemia in children of all ages, mortality rates range from 10% to 28%.[71,84,85]

CRYPTOCOCCOSIS

Epidemiology

C. neoformans and *Cryptococcus gattii* are two species of *Cryptococcus* known to be human pathogens. *Cryptococcus* is an encapsulated yeast that is found worldwide. Exposure to soil that has been contaminated with bird excrement has been found to be associated with infection. In the pre-AIDS era, symptomatic cryptococcal disease (cryptococcosis) was thought to be an uncommon condition, primarily associated in those with hematologic malignancies or recipients of organ transplants. In the HIV era, rates of cryptococcal disease increased significantly. Currently cryptococcosis is most associated with HIV infection, with an estimated 1 million new cases a year worldwide.[86]

Cryptococcosis is an AIDS-defining illness and is seen most often in HIV-infected patients with CD4+ lymphocyte counts fewer than 100/μL. In adults with AIDS, cryptococcosis occurs in approximately 5% of patients annually. In children with AIDS, this rate is significantly lower, with reported rates of approximately 1% annually.[87] Reasons for the lower incidence in children with AIDS are not known, but potential reasons include a decreased number of lifetime exposures, differences in infecting strains, and inadequate time to reactivate a prior infection.[88] *C. neoformans* infection in children is also associated with leukemia, lymphoma, prolonged courses of corticosteroids, and SOT as well as in those with congenital immunodeficiencies such as hyperimmunoglobulin M (IgM) and hyperimmunoglobulin (IgE) syndromes.

Cryptococcosis has also been found to occur in immunocompetent children. In a study utilizing a national database of 42 children's hospitals from the United States, the authors identified 63 children who were hospitalized with cryptococcal disease between 2003 and 2008. Of these children, 64% had an immunocompromising medical condition, 21% were immunocompetent, and 16% had HIV.[89] In another study from Colombia, the authors identified 41 children with the diagnosis of cryptococcosis from 1993 to 2010. Of this cohort, 24.4% had AIDS and 46.3% had no known risk factors.[90]

The incubation period for *C. neoformans* has not been determined, as infection with this organism often represents reactivation of latent disease. The incubation period for *C. gattii* is 2–13 months.[82]

Etiology

Cryptococcus is a polyphyletic genus of encapsulated yeasts that compromises more than 70 species. Two of these species,

C. neoformans and *C. gattii,* are known to be pathogenic in humans. *C. neoformans* primarily causes disease in immunocompromised patients and represents 90% of infections worldwide. *C. gattii* also causes disease in immunocompromised patients but is more likely than *C. neoformans* to cause illness in immunocompetent hosts. This phenomenon recently gained attention when *C. gattii* was found to be the cause of disease in otherwise healthy hosts in the Pacific Northwest of the United States and adjacent parts of Canada.[91]

Cryptococcus has been isolated from soil, trees, and fruit. Dried pigeon droppings have been found to be a particularly effective culture medium for *Cryptococcus* spp. *C. neoformans* grows as yeast and replicates by budding. The organism's sexual state creates basidiospores at the end of the hyphae. The basidiospores are aerosolized and can be inhaled by humans. After inhalation, the organism initially grows in the alveoli without a significant inflammatory response, which is thought to be due in part to the antiphagocytic effect of the polysaccharide capsule. Once within the lung, *Cryptococcus* may either be contained in a dormant state or disseminate to other organs prior to an adequate host immune response. The CNS is a common site of dissemination for *C. neoformans*, although the reason for this CNS tropism is not known.[92]

Pathology/Pathogenesis

Both innate and adaptive immune responses are necessary to control infection due to *C. neoformans*. T cells activate alveolar macrophages via cytokines and promote ingestion of the encapsulated yeast. Humoral immunity plays a role in opsonization, activation of natural killer cells, and clearing of capsular polysaccharide. Conditions associated with defective cellular immunity are at increased risk of symptomatic cryptococcal infections.[92]

Clinical Features (Symptoms/Physical Findings)

Although the most common route of acquisition of cryptococcosis is via inhalation, the pulmonary manifestations of the disease are often mild or asymptomatic.[93] It is estimated that less than 10% of patients with disseminated cryptococcosis have pulmonary symptoms at the time of diagnosis.[92] In individuals with symptomatic pulmonary disease, the typical presentation includes fever, cough, pleuritic chest pain, and weight loss. In cases of disseminated cryptococcosis, virtually any organ system can be involved. The most important sites of extrapulmonary infection include the CNS, skin, prostate and eyes. Cryptococcal meningitis often presents in an indolent manner with progressive symptoms of fever, headache, visual changes, and altered mental status. Isolated cryptococcal fungemia without concurrent organ involvement can occur in adults with HIV but is rare in children.[82]

Imaging, Pulmonary Function Testing, Laboratory Findings

For patients with pulmonary cryptococcal infection, imaging of the chest by plain radiographs and CT is usually nonspecific. An isolated pulmonary nodule, with or without hilar adenopathy, may be the only manifestation of pulmonary cryptococcal infection in immunocompetent individuals. In patients with more severe manifestations of pulmonary cryptococcosis, a variety of imaging findings have been well described, including multiple lung nodules, lobar consolidation with a predilection for the lower lobes, cavitary lesions, pleural effusion, diffuse interstitial infiltrates, and an ARDS-like appearance.[92,94] If signs of increased intracranial pressure or CNS infection are present, magnetic resonance imaging (MRI) or CT of the head to rule out hydrocephalus and cryptococcomas is indicated. In patients with CNS disease, common CSF indices such as cell count, protein and glucose values can be normal.

Diagnosis

The sensitivity of diagnostic tests for cryptococcal disease are different depending on whether there is isolated pulmonary disease or disseminated disease. For disease isolated to the lungs, noninvasive diagnostic tests have a relatively low sensitivity. Serum cryptococcal antigen testing is usually negative in isolated pulmonary disease. Likewise, sputum culture has a low sensitivity. Bronchoscopy with fungal culture and antigen testing of the lavage fluid can be helpful, although the sensitivity of this approach is variable for patients with isolated pulmonary cryptococcosis.[93] Antibodies to *C. neoformans* can develop in response to either colonization or infection and are not useful in diagnosis.[92]

Given the limitations of noninvasive methods for isolated pulmonary cryptococcal disease, more invasive procedures such as transthoracic or transbronchial fine-needle aspiration or open lung biopsy may be required to confirm the diagnosis. Direct histopathologic identification of *C. neoformans* from tissue biopsy specimens is both sensitive and specific for the diagnosis of isolated pulmonary disease. Several different stains can be used to identify the yeast in tissue, including silver stains or stains that target the polysaccharide capsule (e.g., mucicarmine stain).[92] Caution should be used in interpreting the significance of growth of *Cryptococcus* from sputum culture, as this may represent colonization.[95]

Cryptococcus can be grown on standard automated blood culturing systems, although growth is best seen with Sabouraud dextrose agar. This media can be used to culture the organism from tissue, sputum, blood, BAL fluid, or CSF. Growth can be slow, sometimes taking up to a week for cultures to become positive. When pleural effusions are present, cultures of thoracentesis fluid are positive in about 40% of AIDS patients.[95] Selective media are available to differentiate *C. neoformans* and *C. gattii.* Susceptibility testing for cryptococcal organisms is available, although resistance to antifungals is uncommon.

In contrast to patients with cryptococcal pulmonary disease, the diagnosis of cryptococcal meningitis is less difficult. The latex agglutination test and EIA can be used to provide a rapid diagnosis for those with suspected meningitis. All of these tests detect cryptococcal capsular polysaccharide antigen and are approved for use on serum or cerebrospinal fluid. The sensitivity of these antigen assays in patients with cryptococcal meningitis is greater than 90%. Visualization of encapsulated yeast cells in CSF using India ink has sensitivity ranging from 50% to 80%. Given the frequency of concomitant meningitis, it is generally recommended that a lumbar puncture be performed on patients with pulmonary disease even in the absence of overt signs of CNS infection.[92]

Patients who are severely immunocompromised with cryptococcal disease have been found to have significant incidence of coinfection with other pathogens such as *Mycobacterium tuberculosis,* nontuberculous mycobacteria, cytomegalovirus, *Nocardia* spp., and *P. jirovecii.* For this reason, patients with cryptococcal disease should be tested for additional pathogens as appropriate to the clinical situation.

Differential Diagnosis

The differential diagnosis of a patient with suspected cryptococcal pulmonary disease depends on the clinical scenario and radiographic findings. Patients with an ARDS-like clinical picture and immunodeficiency may present like cases of *P. jirovecii* infection. Patients with an indolent course of fever, cough, and multiple pulmonary nodules on chest radiograph may be suspected to have a lung malignancy. Children with fever, cough, sputum production, and lobar consolidation are often treated for bacterial pneumonia prior to the diagnosis of pulmonary cryptococcosis.[96]

Management and Treatment

There are no prospective trials in children for the treatment of cryptococcosis. The IDSA guideline on cryptococcosis makes treatment recommendations for both adults and children.[92] For otherwise healthy children with mild-to-moderate pulmonary cryptococcosis, fluconazole is recommended for 6–12 months. If fluconazole cannot be used, itraconazole, voriconazole, and posaconazole are effective alternatives. Echinocandins should not be used as they do not have activity against *Cryptococcus* spp. Children with severe pulmonary cryptococcosis should be treated similarly to those with CNS disease, regardless of immune status.

All immunocompromised patients and those with CNS cryptococcal infection should be treated aggressively. Corticosteroid treatment may be considered if ARDS is present. Immunocompromised patients with isolated pulmonary cryptococcosis that is mild to moderate in severity (i.e., absence of diffuse pulmonary infiltrates) can be treated with fluconazole orally for 6–12 months. For patients with cryptococcal meningitis, the preferred regimen for induction and consolidation therapy is amphotericin B deoxycholate plus oral or intravenous flucytosine for 2 weeks (or until CSF cultures are negative). This should be followed by oral fluconazole for a minimum of 8 weeks. Lipid formulations of amphotericin B can be substituted for deoxycholate formulations in children with abnormal renal function. After induction and consolidation therapy, maintenance (suppressive) or prophylactic therapy may be indicated depending on the immunosuppressing condition. The IDSA guidelines provided detailed recommendations regarding the length of maintenance and prophylactic therapy for children with HIV and other immunosuppressive conditions.[92]

Prognosis

The prognosis for patients with isolated pulmonary cryptococcosis has not been studied thoroughly, but in the absence of dissemination outcomes appear to be favorable.[95] Prognosis in patients with cryptococcal meningitis is predicted by various CSF parameters, such as organism load, opening CSF pressure, CSF glucose and leukocyte count, and titers of cryptococcal antigen in CSF or blood.[96]

MUCORMYCOSIS (FORMALLY ZYGOMYCOSIS)

Epidemiology

Mucormycosis is caused by environmental molds found primarily in soil and organic matter. The organism has a near worldwide distribution. The main route of transmission is inhalation of spores from an environmental source. Outbreaks of disease have been linked to construction, excavation, and contaminated air-conditioning filters. Nosocomial clusters of cutaneous infections have been traced to contaminated wooden tongue depressors and various adhesive bandages used in the hospital.[97] Ingestion of spores can also result in gastrointestinal disease. Invasive mucormycosis is typically limited to those with an impaired immune system. Diabetic patients, particularly during ketoacidosis, are known to be at risk for developing rhinocerebral mucormycosis.[98] In nonneutropenic HSCT recipients, mucormycosis can be seen as a late (1–6 months) or very late (>6 months) infection.[99]

Etiology

As with many fungal pathogens, the taxonomy of these organisms has changed. The phylum name Zygomycota has been reorganized based on new molecular phylogenic analyses, and the species that cause human disease are no longer limited to this phylum. For this reason, the term *zygomycosis* is no longer considered valid. Given that the clinically significant causative agents of mucormycosis belong to the order *Mucorales,* the term mucormycosis has been proposed as the most valid mycologic reference.[98] Within the family of *Mucorales,* the most clinically significant genera are *Rhizopus* and *Mucor. Mucorales* are filamentous fungi that produce sporangiospores (asexual spores) contained within a saclike structure called a sporangium. When this structure ruptures, the sporangiospores are released and can be inhaled by the human host. Therefore sinus and pulmonary infections are the most common manifestation of this disease.

Pathology/Pathogenesis

Both macrophages and neutrophils are responsible for controlling infection due to mucormycosis. Alveolar macrophages control the germination of inhaled spores through phagocytosis. Neutrophils and mononuclear cells also prevent germination via generation of oxidative metabolites. Dysfunction of macrophage phagocytosis, neutrophil chemotaxis, and oxidative killing by neutrophils have been demonstrated in diabetic ketoacidosis.[100] Other important risk factors include use of corticosteroids, broad-spectrum antibiotics, and hematologic and organ transplantation. One other established at-risk patient group are those receiving iron chelation therapy with deferoxamine. It is thought that this drug acts as a siderophore where it can deliver iron to the fungus, thus promoting growth.[101]

Clinical Features (Symptoms/Physical Findings)

Mucormycosis can be classified into the following forms: rhinocerebral, pulmonary, cutaneous, gastrointestinal, and disseminated disease. Pulmonary disease is the most common clinical manifestation and is found to account for 30% of mucormycosis in a recent series from Europe.[102] The clinical symptoms of pulmonary mucormycosis can initially be subtle or nonspecific in immunocompromised patients. When symptoms are seen, children with pulmonary mucormycosis develop persistent fever, cough, chest pain, and dyspnea. The disease is sometimes found in at-risk patients with pulmonary infiltrates that persist despite treatment for presumed bacterial pneumonia. In advanced disease, hemoptysis can occur because of angioinvasion and hemorrhagic infarction, which characterize this group of infections. Clinicians should be especially alert to the possibility of mucormycosis in children who are receiving antifungal prophylaxis with agents that have activity against *Aspergillus* but not the *Mucorales* (e.g., voriconazole or the echinocandins).[99]

Imaging, Pulmonary Function Testing, Laboratory Findings

The radiographic findings of mucormycosis are quite variable. Isolated nodules, lobar consolidation, cavitary lesions, wedge-shaped areas of infarction, and disseminated pulmonary involvement have all been described.[103]

Diagnosis

The diagnosis of invasive mucormycosis is difficult, as the sensitivity of fungal cultures from blood and respiratory tract specimens is low. Testing modalities such as serology and antigen detection are not clinically useful for mucormycosis. PCR assays to detect *Mucorales* from tissue specimens have shown promise but have not yet become a standardized adjunctive diagnostic test.[104] A tissue-based approach is essential to the diagnosis assuming that the patient can tolerate the necessary procedure.[105] As with *Aspergillus* spp., histopathology performed on tissue specimens from patients with mucormycosis often shows angioinvasion, with resulting vessel thrombosis and tissue thrombosis.[99] Given these diagnostic limitations, a high index of suspicion is needed in at-risk patients to identify mucormycosis as early as possible. Unfortunately the diagnosis is often made after severe disease or at autopsy.

Differential Diagnosis

Pulmonary mucormycosis can be difficult to distinguish from IPA. In patients with hematologic malignancies, factors that favor the diagnosis of mucormycosis are the presence of concomitant sinusitis, the presence of more than 10 pulmonary nodules, and multiple negative serum *Aspergillus* galactomannan antigen assays. The diagnosis of mucormycosis is favored if the patient was receiving prophylactic antifungal agents with activity against *Aspergillus*, such as voriconazole or echinocandins.[106]

Management and Treatment

Treatment of mucormycosis involves a combination of antifungal therapy, aggressive debridement of necrotic lesions, and, when possible, reversal of the predisposing condition that originally led to the infection. Amphotericin B (lipid formulation if available) is the recommended antifungal in patients with mucormycosis. In a study of 70 patients (primarily adults) with hematologic malignancy who had mucormycosis, the authors found that a delay of 6 or more days of an amphotericin B–based therapy resulted in a twofold increase in mortality rate compared with early treatment (82.9% vs. 48.6%).[107]

Most azoles and echinocandins lack significant activity against the organisms that cause mucormycosis, although a few notable exceptions have been found. Both posaconazole and isavuconazole have in vitro activity against the *Mucorales*.[108,109] There are multiple published reports of success with posaconazole as part of combination therapy or salvage therapy for mucormycosis.[110–113] Another exception has been found with caspofungin. Although caspofungin has no activity against the fungi that cause mucormycosis in standard in vitro susceptibility tests, there is some evidence in animal and human studies that caspofungin is synergistic with amphotericin B. In a study of diabetic ketoacidotic mice with disseminated mucormycosis, caspofungin combined with amphotericin B resulted in better outcomes than amphotericin B alone.[114] This combination of caspofungin combined with amphotericin B was also associated with improved outcomes in a retrospective study of primarily diabetic patients with rhino-orbital-cerebral mucormycosis.[115] Isavuconazole has been studied as primary or salvage treatment in adults with mucormycosis. In an open-label trial, the authors found that isavuconazole showed similar efficacy to historical controls who were treated with amphotericin B.[116]

The optimal length of treatment with antifungals has not been studied in patients with pulmonary mucormycosis. Most successfully treated patients require at least 4–6 weeks of therapy, although longer courses may be needed based on clinical response and ability to reverse the underlying immunocompromised state.

Mucormycosis is associated with tissue infarction; therefore antifungal therapy alone may not allow for clinical cure without debridement of devitalized tissue.[117] In a retrospective review of 255 cases of pulmonary mucormycosis, mortality of patients treated with debridement and antifungal therapy was significantly lower than those who received antifungal therapy alone.[118]

Prognosis

Mucormycosis is associated with high mortality, with reported rates of 100% for disseminated disease, 76% for pulmonary disease, and 46% for rhinocerebral disease.[106]

SPOROTRICHOSIS

Epidemiology

Sporotrichosis is caused by the fungus *Sporothrix schenckii* and is seen most commonly in Central America, South America, and the Midwest of the United States. Cutaneous sporotrichosis is the most common form of the disease in both adults and children. Pulmonary sporotrichosis is typically seen in adult males with alcoholism or other chronic medical illnesses such as diabetes mellitus. Disseminated sporotrichosis is rare in children and is typically seen in those who are exposed to immunosuppressive therapy, prolonged treatment with corticosteroids, or in those with AIDS.[119]

Etiology

S. schenckii is a dimorphic fungus with a worldwide distribution in soil and plant products such as straw, wood, and sphagnum moss. Direct inoculation of exposed skin is the most common form of exposure, especially among those working with thorny plants (e.g., florists or rose gardeners).

Household transmission has also been attributed to domestic cats.[120] Pulmonary sporotrichosis is thought to be secondary to the inhalation of spores rather than part of disseminated infection. In immunocompromised children, dissemination can occur after cutaneous inoculation or from primary pulmonary infection.[119]

Pathology/Pathogenesis

The immunological mechanisms involved in host control of *S. schenckii* infections are not well understood. It is thought that both humoral and cellular responses are involved in response to fungal surface and secreted antigens. The factors that influence localized versus disseminated disease include inoculum load, immune status of the host, virulence of the inoculated strain, and depth of traumatic inoculation.[120]

Clinical Features

Sporotrichosis is most commonly a cutaneous or lymphocutaneous infection that manifests as a chronic, papulonodular lesion with or without central ulceration. It is often associated with regional lymphadenopathy. In addition to cutaneous disease, sporotrichosis can occasionally occur as pulmonary, osteoarticular or meningeal infection. The primary pulmonary form of sporotrichosis results in a granulomatous pneumonitis that often cavitates. Signs and symptoms of pulmonary disease include productive cough, fever, weight loss, and hemoptysis. The presentation can be subacute or chronic. Patients with multifocal sporotrichosis are much more likely to be immunocompromised.[121]

Imaging, Pulmonary Function Testing, Laboratory Findings

Radiographs often reveal unilateral or bilateral cavitary lesions with associated parenchymal infiltrate. Hilar lymphadenopathy or pleural effusions are occasionally seen.

Diagnosis

The diagnosis of children with the classic lymphocutaneous form of sporotrichosis is relatively straightforward, given its characteristic pattern of presentation. The diagnosis of pulmonary or disseminated disease can be more difficult given that pulmonary or osteoarticular presentation can mimic other disease processes. The gold standard of diagnosis of sporotrichosis is fungal culture. Tissue biopsy, sputum, or BAL fluid can be inoculated onto Sabouraud's dextrose agar and incubated at room temperature. Growth typically occurs within 5 days. Fungal staining can be performed on tissue or respiratory specimens, but the small number of fungal organisms may limit visualization. Serology is not used routinely in the diagnosis of sporotrichosis, as the available assays lack adequate sensitivity and specificity. PCR assays have been developed for identifying *S. schenckii* in tissue specimens, but they are not widely available.[119]

Differential Diagnosis

The skin lesions of sporotrichosis can resemble *Nocardia brasiliensis*, cutaneous leishmaniasis, or mycobacterial infection. The differential diagnosis of disseminated disease depends on the clinical scenario and location of disease. Pulmonary sporotrichosis can mimic mycobacterial infections, histoplasmosis, or coccidioidomycosis.

Management and Treatment

Treatment of sporotrichosis involves a combination of antifungal therapy and, in some cases, surgical excision. Amphotericin B is the preferred antifungal treatment for life-threatening or extensive pulmonary sporotrichosis. After the patient has shown a favorable response to amphotericin B, therapy can be switched to itraconazole to complete a total course of therapy of at least 12 months. Localized pulmonary disease, particularly cavitary lesions, should be treated with a combination of surgical excision and amphotericin B.[121] In children with less severe pulmonary disease, itraconazole administered for at least 12 months is recommended. Lifelong suppressive therapy with itraconazole may be required for patients with AIDS and other causes of immunosuppression. Serum levels of itraconazole should be measured after the patient has received this medication for at least 2 weeks so as to ensure adequate drug levels. It is recommended that serum itraconazole levels be greater than 1.0 mg/mL.[119]

Prognosis

Cutaneous sporotrichosis responds well to antifungal therapy. Disseminated disease in immunocompromised children can be difficult to treat and is associated with significant morbidity and mortality.

TRICHOSPORONOSIS

Epidemiology

Trichosporon infections are caused by a group of related fungi that can occasionally cause invasive infections in humans. *Trichosporon* spp. have been found to colonize the gastrointestinal tract, respiratory tract, skin and vagina. Opportunistic invasive infections are thought to result from preexisting *Trichosporon* spp. that colonizes these locations. Invasive trichosporonosis can occur in patients with hematologic malignancies and other immunosuppressive states. This pathogen has also been proposed as a cause of severe exacerbations in patients with cystic fibrosis.[122] Immunocompetent patients typically have disease that is limited to the skin, nails or mucosal surfaces.[123]

Etiology

Trichosporon species (*asahii*, *mucoides*, *mycotoxinivorans* and others) and the closely related *Blastoschizomyces capitatus* are related fungi that can occasionally cause disease in humans. For the purposes of this chapter, we will refer to these fungi collectively as *Trichosporon* species. These fungal organisms are commonly found in soil but can colonize the skin, hair shafts, sputum, and mucosal surfaces.

Pathology/Pathogenesis

Invasive infection from *Trichosporon* spp. is thought to begin with cutaneous and mucosal endogenous flora. Alteration of integrity of these surfaces by an intravascular catheter or chemotherapy-induced mucosal injury may lead to bloodstream infection. Some *Trichosporon* spp. can form biofilms on implanted devices.[124]

Clinical Features (Symptoms/Physical Findings)

Disease in immunocompetent patients is usually limited to the superficial infections of the skin and hair shafts, particularly in tropical climates. Invasive infections are limited to immunocompromised patients, particularly in those with prolonged neutropenia. The resulting fungemia can lead to subsequent dissemination of the lungs. It is not known how often the lungs are the primary site of disseminated *Trichosporon* infection, as pulmonary disease is not consistently seen in these cases. In one study of immunocompromised adults with disseminated trichosporonosis, 26.9% were found to have pulmonary involvement.[125] The typical clinical presentation in these cases included fever, dyspnea, cough, and hemoptysis. Renal involvement is also common and may initially manifest as microscopic hematuria or proteinuria. Disseminated *Trichosporon* infection is also associated with erythematous papules that can progress to bullae and necrotic lesions. Life-threatening disease can occasionally progress rapidly with hypotension, respiratory distress, and renal failure.[126]

Imaging, Pulmonary Function Testing, Laboratory Findings

Chest radiographs in patients with pulmonary trichosporonosis infection typically show diffuse infiltrates with an alveolar pattern, although cavitary lesions and lobar consolidation have been described.

Diagnosis

Trichosporon species grow well on standard fungal media, although differentiating *Trichosporon* spp. from *Candida* spp. can be difficult. The importance of distinguishing these two organisms is highlighted by the observation that *Trichosporon* spp. has shown decreased susceptibility to amphotericin B. Distinguishing between the various *Trichosporon* species is typically not performed in most clinical laboratories. Disseminated infection can be diagnosed when *Trichosporon* species is isolated from a sterile site such as blood, CSF or lung tissue. Skin biopsies can be helpful when skin lesions are associated with disseminated infection. Diagnosis can also be made by fungal culture from BAL fluid. Given that *Trichosporon* species can colonize mucosal surfaces, isolation from sputum and tracheal cultures should be interpreted based on the clinical context. Pseudoinfections due to inadequately sterilized bronchoscopes has also been reported.[127] Given that the genus *Trichosporon* is closely related to Cryptococcus, the *C. neoformans* polysaccharide antigen assay may be positive in patients with disseminated *Trichosporon* infection.[126]

Management and Treatment

Patients with disseminated *Trichosporon* infection are typically severely immunocompromised. The degree of immunosuppression should be reduced if possible (e.g., GCSF administration, reducing glucocorticoids or other immunosuppressive medications). The azole class of antifungal drugs (particularly voriconazole) has good activity against *Trichosporon* spp., while significant resistance has been seen with amphotericin B based on in vitro susceptibility studies. The echinocandins are not active against *Trichosporon* spp.[128]

Prognosis

Pulmonary infections due to disseminated trichosporonosis are associated with a high mortality rate. Patients who recover from their neutropenia have the best prognosis.[125]

HYALOHYPHOMYCOSIS (*FUSARIUM* SPP., *TALAROMYCES* [PENICILLIUM] *MARNEFFEI, PSEUDALLESCHERIA BOYDII, CHRYSOSPORIUM* SPP.)

Epidemiology and Etiology

Hyalohyphomycosis is caused by a heterogeneous group of filamentous molds that produce hyaline (translucent) hyphae on microscopic examination of clinical tissue specimens. These organisms are ubiquitous molds that are found in the soil and can occasionally cause disease in immunocompromised hosts.

Fusarium spp. (*F. solani, F. oxysporum*, and *F. moniliforme*) are a group of filamentous fungi that have long been known to cause infections of the nails, skin, and cornea of humans. These organisms have more recently been recognized as an infrequent but important cause of sinusitis, pulmonary disease, and disseminated infection in patients undergoing chemotherapy and HSCT. Corticosteroid therapy has also been found to be an important predisposing factor in developing fusariosis. The respiratory tract is the primary portal of entry for disseminated infection, although access through vascular catheters has also been reported.[129]

Talaromyces (formerly *Penicillium*) *marneffei* is a dimorphic fungus that has been identified as an important opportunistic infection in HIV-infected patients who live in or have traveled to eastern Asia. The lungs are the likely portal of entry, as conidia from the environment convert to the yeast form prior to dissemination. Pulmonary alveolar macrophages are thought to be the primary pulmonary host defense[123] and impaired cell-mediated and alveolar phagocytic function are the main predisposing risk factors in AIDS patients. In more recent years, *T. marneffei* has been associated with non-HIV immunosuppressive conditions, including various autoimmune diseases, SOTs, HSCT, T lymphocyte–depleting immunosuppressive drugs, and anti-CD20 monoclonal antibodies.[130]

Pseudallescheria boydii and its asexual form, *Scedosporium apiospermum*, are fungi found in soil as well as polluted and stagnant water. In immunocompetent hosts, these organisms are an important cause of eumycetoma, a chronic granulomatous fungal disease of the subcutaneous tissues. Eumycetoma is rare in children and is typically seen in parts of Southeast Asia, Africa, and Central America. In immunocompromised hosts, disseminated disease can occur, with spread to the lungs or brain.

Pathology/Pathogenesis

The pathogenesis of hyalohyphomycosis has not been well defined, as these organisms are minimally pathogenic in normal hosts.

Clinical and Laboratory Features (Symptoms/Physical Findings)

The clinical features of hyalohyphomycosis are similar to those of IA, with sinus, pulmonary, cutaneous, and disseminated disease being seen. *Fusarium* spp. are best known as causes of sinusitis, pulmonary infections and fungemia. Chest imaging shows nonspecific alveolar or interstitial infiltrates, nodules, and cavities. Papular skin lesions with necrotic centers are common.[129]

Disseminated *T. marneffei* infection can present with the clinical syndrome of fever, lymphadenopathy, hepatosplenomegaly, pulmonary infiltrates, weight loss, and anemia. Patients with disseminated infection can also develop a papular rash with central necrosis that can initially be mistaken for molluscum contagiosum.[130] *T. marneffei* can mimic other infections such as tuberculosis, *Pneumocystis jirovecii* pneumonia, and cryptococcosis.

P. boydii (and its asexual form *S. apiospermum*) are causes of pulmonary disease in immunocompromised patients and are associated with a high mortality rate. Children with CGD are known to be at increased risk of pulmonary infection with *S. apiospermum*.[131] *P. boydii* has been reported to be an important cause of pneumonia in children with near-drowning events.[132]

Diagnosis

Fusarium spp. is unusual in that it is the only mold that is commonly associated with fungemia. Fungal blood cultures are positive in 60%–82% of disseminated cases. Diagnosis can be made by isolation of the organism from culture of infected tissues.[56,133] The diagnosis of *T. marneffei* and *P. boydii* is typically made by histopathology or fungal culture of bone, bone marrow, or biopsy tissue from skin or lungs.[130]

The diagnosis of *P. boydii* (and *S. apiospermum*) is also made by culture and histopathologic examination of tissue. The septate hyphae of *P. boydii* can be indistinguishable from those of *Aspergillus* hyphae.

Management and Treatment

Treatment for fusariosis includes amphotericin B or voriconazole. Combination antifungal therapy with amphotericin B or voriconazole showed no benefit when compared to those treated with monotherapy. Mortality from disseminated fusariosis has historically been greater than 50% despite antifungal therapy. Amphotericin B is the favored acute treatment of *T. marneffei* infection. After induction therapy, the patient can be transitioned to itraconazole as maintenance/suppressive therapy.[134] *P. boydii* and *S. apiospermum* can be resistant to amphotericin B but are typically susceptible to voriconazole, posaconazole and itraconazole.[133]

PHAEOHYPHOMYCOSIS (*BIPOLARIS* SPP., *ALTERNARIA* SPP., *EXOPHIALA* SPP., *CURVULARIA* SPP., AND *SCEDOSPORIUM PROLIFICANS*)

Epidemiology and Etiology

Phaeohyphomycosis refers to infections caused by a heterogeneous group of fungi (also known as the dematiaceous molds) that can occasionally cause invasive disease in immunocompromised hosts. More than 150 species have been identified as human pathogens, with the most important species causing invasive disease being *S. prolificans*, *Bipolaris* spp., *Alternaria* spp., *Exophiala* spp., and *Curvularia* spp.[135] The agents of phaeohyphomycosis are ubiquitous filamentous molds that are found in the soil and characterized by their darkly pigmented cell walls, which include melanin (the prefix *phaeo* is derived from Greek meaning "dark"). As with many molds that are responsible for invasive human disease, the respiratory tract is the usual portal of entry for these fungi. Extrapulmonary dissemination is known to occur in immunocompromised patients. This group of organisms is also known to contribute to allergy in humans, including asthma and allergic fungal sinusitis.[136] Various agents of phaeohyphomycosis (e.g., *S. prolificans*, *Exophiala* spp.) have been found to colonize the lungs of patients with cystic fibrosis, although it is unclear if these organisms play a role in the progression of this disease.[137]

Clinical and Laboratory Features

Invasive infections are generally limited to immunocompromised hosts and localize to the sinuses, lungs, blood, CNS, skin and eyes. *Bipolaris* spp., *Exophiala* spp., *Curvularia* spp., and *S. prolificans* have been found to cause the majority of the cases of pneumonia and disseminated disease. The pulmonary manifestations of phaeohyphomycosis include lobar consolidation, asymptomatic solitary pulmonary nodules, and endobronchial lesions. *Bipolaris* spp. and *Curvularia* spp. are both known to cause fungal sinusitis.[136]

Diagnosis

The primary method of diagnosis for all agents of phaeohyphomycosis is fungal culture and histopathologic examination of tissue. Microscopic examination is aided using Fontana-Masson stain, which will strongly stain the melanin within the conidia, spores, or hyphae. Even with proper staining, histopathologic interpretation can be difficult and may require referral to a mycology reference laboratory. No commercially available serologic, antigen or PCR assays are available for these organisms.[136]

Management and Treatment

Therapy for invasive phaeohyphomycosis involves antifungal therapy and possible surgical resection of fungal lesions. In addition to diagnosis, isolation of the fungal pathogen allows for susceptibility testing to various antifungal agents. Amphotericin B has activity against many of the fungal organisms responsible for phaeohyphomycosis, although *S. prolificans* is usually resistant. Other antifungal agents with activity against certain organisms that cause phaeohyphomycosis include voriconazole, itraconazole, and posaconazole. Regardless of antifungal regimen, the mortality of disseminated invasive phaeohyphomycosis is greater than 70%.[136]

Acknowledgments

The authors thank the following collaborators for their roles in obtaining radiographs and pathologic specimens used for the figures in this chapter: Richard M. Heller, Sharon M. Stein, and James D. Chappell. We also would like to thank Dennis O'Connor for his careful review of the manuscript.

References

Access the reference list online at ExpertConsult.com.

Suggested Reading

The clinical guidelines produced by the Infectious Diseases Society of America are excellent resources for diagnosis and treatment of systemic fungal diseases. These include guidelines on: Aspergillosis, Blastomycosis, Coccidioidomycosis, Cryptococcal Disease, Candidiasis, Histoplasmosis, and Sporotrichosis. Full text is published free at their website: https://www.idsociety.org/Organism.

Ankrah AO, Sathekge MM, Dierckx RA, et al. Imaging fungal infections in children. *Clin Transl Imaging.* 2016;4:57–72.

Bradley JS, Nelson JD. Chosing among anti-fungal agents: polyenes, azoles and echinocandins and Prefered Therapy for Specific Fungal Pathogens. In: Cantey JB, Kimberlin DW, eds. *2016 Nelson's Pediatric Antimicrobial Therapy.* 22nd ed. Elk Grove Village, IL: American Academy of Pediatrics.; 2016.

Dornbusch HJ, Manzoni P, Roilides E, et al. Invasive fungal infections in children. *Pediatr Infect Dis J.* 2009;28(8):734–737.

Montenegro BL, Arnold JC. North American dimorphic fungal infections in children. *Pediatr Rev.* 2010;31(6):e40–e48.

Ramos-Martín V, O'Connor O, Hope W. Clinical pharmacology of antifungal agents in pediatrics: children are not small adults. *Curr Opin Pharmacol.* 2015;24:128–134.

Steinbach WJ. Invasive aspergillosis in pediatric patients. *Curr Med Res Opin.* 2010;26(7):1779–1787.

32 Pertussis and Other Bordetella *Infections of the Respiratory Tract*

ULRICH HEININGER, MD

Pertussis ("whooping cough") is an acute bacterial infection of the respiratory tract. The illness occurs worldwide and affects all age groups, but it is most serious in young, unprotected infants. It is caused by *Bordetella pertussis* (first described in 1906) and, less frequently, by *Bordetella parapertussis* (1937).[1–3] The term *pertussis* was coined in 1670 and means "violent cough." The clinical picture was described for the first time in 1640 by Guillaume de Baillou, based on a 1578 epidemic in Paris.[3]

Epidemiology

Pertussis occurs worldwide, and humans are the only host of *B. pertussis*. Transmission occurs effectively by droplets, with secondary attack rates close to 100% in exposed susceptible individuals.[3] The incubation period is usually 7–10 days but may vary substantially. In a household contact study, secondary cases were noted to have their onset up to 6 weeks after the onset of illness in the primary case, especially when antibiotics were used.[4] Several studies have shown that females and males are equally affected by pertussis in childhood, whereas a female preponderance (55%–69%) is noted in adolescents and adults.[5–7] Most likely, this is due to more frequent contact of females with young children, from whom they acquire infection. The seasonal pattern of pertussis varies between different geographic locations.[6,7]

The epidemiology of pertussis caused by *B. pertussis* infection is incompletely understood. Reasons for this are the lack of a uniform case definition, inconsistent use of diagnostic laboratory tests, variable surveillance systems, and incomplete case ascertainment due to underconsulting, underrecognition, underdiagnosis, and underreporting.[8] Furthermore, epidemiology is greatly influenced by pertussis immunization programs that, with high coverage rates, confer not only individual protection but also herd protection to some extent. In contrast to *B. pertussis*, *B. parapertussis* infections appear to occur independent of immunization activities, and their relative frequency varies considerably by geography and time.[9,10]

Although in most countries pertussis still mainly affects infants and young children, it is increasingly diagnosed in adolescents and adults, who are also important sources of infection in young, unprotected infants in their families and households (Table 32.1).[11] In recent years, a shift from mothers to siblings as the predominant source of *B. pertussis* transmission to infants has been noted in the United States.[12]

Among 1306 cases of pertussis in infants, the source of infection was identified in 569: overall, 35.5% were siblings, 20.6% were mothers, and 10.0% were fathers.

A resurgence of cases and a gradual shift toward an increase of pertussis in adolescents and adults has been noted in North America and elsewhere.[5] Whether this increase is caused by waning vaccine immunity and a decreased chance for natural boosters, a consequence of increased awareness and diagnostic tools or both is an ongoing debate. Of note, pertussis in adolescents and adults is frequently atypical, and true numbers of cases are certainly higher than reported.[5,13] Furthermore, in support of a true change in epidemiology, a rise in fatalities due to pertussis has been observed in infants in the United States during the last decades. Whereas 1.67 deaths per million infants per year were reported in the 1980s, the rate increased to an average of 2.40 in the 1990s. This increased incidence almost exclusively affected infants under 4 months of age.[14]

The crucial role that mass immunization plays in controlling pertussis has been clearly demonstrated in countries such as Japan, England, and Sweden, where infant pertussis vaccination was either discontinued or markedly curtailed as a result of unsubstantiated concerns about vaccine-related adverse events.[3]

Etiology

Bordetella organisms are small, aerobic, gram-negative coccobacilli. Today, the genus comprises 10 different species, of which 9 have been shown to cause respiratory tract illness in humans; these species include *B. pertussis* and *B. parapertussis*, the causative agents of whooping cough; *B. bronchiseptica* and *B. holmesii*, which can cause variable respiratory symptoms; *B. trematum*, which has been found in ear and wound infections, and *B. petrii*, isolated from respiratory tract secretions in patients with cystic fibrosis and from a patient with mastoiditis.[1–3] However, the overwhelming majority of *Bordetella* infections are caused by *B. pertussis* and *B. parapertussis*.

Pathology/Pathogenesis

The organism is transmitted by aerosol droplets from infected to susceptible humans. After transmission, adhesion of the bacteria to ciliated cells of the upper and lower respiratory tract establishes colonization, followed by multiplication and

Table 32.1   Household Members as the Source of Pertussis in Infants

Country	Investigator (Year)	Study Population	Observation[a]
United Kingdom	Crowcroft (2003)[64]	25 infants <5 months of age admitted to ICU because of proven pertussis	Primary case: Parent: $N = 11$ (44%) Sibling: $N = 6$ (24%)
United States	Bisgard (2004)[65]	616 infants with proven pertussis	Source discovered in 264 (43%) cases: Parent: $N = 123$ (47%; 20% of total) Grandparent: $N = 22$ (8%; 4% of total) Sibling: $N = 52$ (20%; 8% of total)
France	Bonmarin (2007)[66]	1668 hospitalized infants <6 months of age with proven pertussis	Source discovered in 892 (53%) cases: Parent: $N = 491$ (55%; 29% of total) Sibling: $N = 223$ (25%; 13% of total)
Multinational	Kowalzik (2007)[67]	99 infants admitted to ICU because of proven pertussis	≥1 source ($N = 30$) discovered in 24 (24%) cases: Parent: $N = 18$ (60%; 18% of total) Other adult: $N = 6$ (20%; 6 % of total) Sibling: $N = 5$ (17%; 5% of total)
Multinational	Wendelboe (2007)[68]	95 infants <6 months of age admitted to hospital because of proven pertussis	≥1 source discovered in 44 (46%) cases: Parent: $N = 27$ (55%; ≈25% of total) Grandparent: $N = 3$ (6%; ≈3% of total) Sibling: $N = 8$ (16 %; ≈5% of total)
The Netherlands	de Greef (2010)[69]	201 infants <6 months of age admitted to hospital because of proven pertussis	≥1 source discovered in 96 (48%) cases: Parent: $N = 53$ (55%; ≈25% of total) Sibling: $N = 39$ (41%; ≈19% of total)
United States	Skoff et al. (2015)[12]	Cases of pertussis in infants, identified through "enhanced pertussis surveillance" in seven US states	Source identified in 569 (44%) cases: siblings (35.5%), mothers (20.6%), fathers (10.0%), grandparents (7.6%), aunts/uncles (6.5%), and other source, not specified (6.3%)

[a]Restricted to household contacts; other sources, if any, were nonhousehold contacts.
ICU, Intensive care unit.

spread on the epithelium, local mucosal damage, and finally, induction of respiratory symptoms. Invasiveness is extremely rare.[15] Asymptomatic, transient colonization frequently occurs during reinfection in immune individuals.[16] Animal studies suggest that a variety of virulence factors is involved in the various steps of infection of the respiratory tract (Table 32.2). Expression of these factors is regulated in response to environmental changes by BvgAS, a two-component signal transduction system.[17] The precise mechanisms during *B. pertussis* and *B. parapertussis* infection in the human host are unknown. Laboratory studies suggest that several factors working in concert allow adherence of the organisms to the epithelium, and filamentous hemagglutinin (FHA) inhibits phagocytosis. Later on, effects caused by adenylate cyclase toxin and pertactin expression allow effective phagocytosis and killing of the bacteria by the host. The popular belief that pertussis is a single-toxin illness caused by pertussis toxin (PT), exclusively produced by *B. pertussis*, is refutable by the observation that a similar illness results from infection with *B. parapertussis*, which does not express PT.[10] Further insight into the pathogenesis of *Bordetella* infection will be gained now that several members of the genus have been sequenced.[18]

The pathology of pertussis has been characterized by studies of *B. pertussis* infection. It causes inflammation, congestion, and infiltration of the respiratory mucosa with lymphocytes and granulocytes and leads to accumulation of viscous secretions in the lumens of the bronchi, bronchiolar obstruction, and occasional atelectasis.[3] Later in the infection, necrosis of the midzonal and basilar parts of the bronchial epithelium result in necrotizing bronchitis (Fig. 32.1). Subsequently, bronchopneumonia may develop, either caused by *B. pertussis* itself or by secondary infections with other pathogenic bacteria.

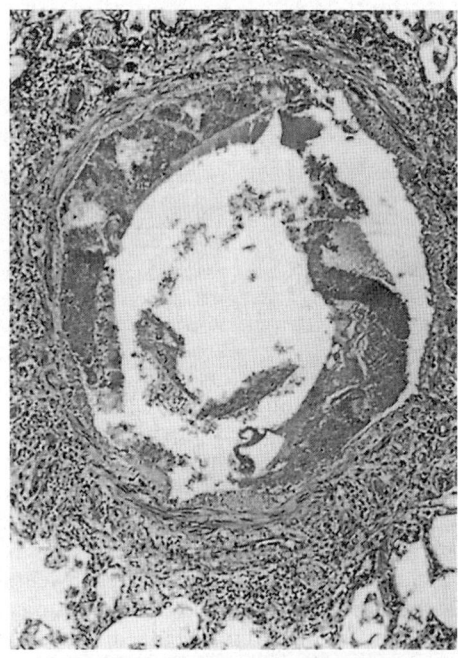

Fig. 32.1 Necrotizing bronchitis (×100).

Infection with *B. pertussis* of a previously naive host results in the production of serum and salivary antibodies against a number of antigens such as PT, FHA, pertactin, and adenylate cyclase toxin.[19–21] Enzyme-linked immunosorbent assay techniques allow discrimination of class-specific antibodies, with Immunoglobuline G (IgG) being more reliably detectable than Immunoglobulines A, E, and M. In individuals who have been "primed" by *B. pertussis* infection or immunization, reinfection will elicit a secondary immune response

Table 32.2   Virulence Factors of *Bordetella Pertussis* and Their Specific Characteristics

Factor (Gene)	BVG Regulation	Molecule	Major Role	Other Functions	Comments
Pertussis toxin (PTX)	Yes	"A" protomer and "B" subunits	Toxin and first-line adhesion factor	Causes leukocytosis by lymphocytosis	Precise role in disease unknown
Filamentous hemagglutinin (FHA)	Yes	Large, filamentous protein (220 kDa)	Major adhesion; predominantly in trachea	Not known	Need for inclusion in vaccine questionable
Fimbriae 2 and 3 (fim2, fim3, fimX)	Yes	Small, filamentous proteins (23 kDa)	Adhesion factor; predominantly in trachea	Agglutinogens; sustain infection	Important stimulator of host's immune response
Pertactin (prn1, prn2, prn3)	Yes	69-kDa outer membrane protein	Adhesion factor, induces type-specific antibody	Major protective antigen (mouse model)	Important vaccine antigen, used for genotyping
Adenylate cyclase (cyaA)	Yes	Protein toxin	Toxin; inhibits phagocytosis by ↑ cAMP	Inhibits chemotaxis and induces apoptosis of macrophages	Candidate for future vaccines!
Tracheal cytotoxin (TCT)	No	Peptidoglycan derivative	Toxin; paralyzes mucociliary clearance system	Inhibits DNA synthesis and cell death	Nonimmunogenic → not suitable for vaccine
Dermonecrotic toxin (DNT)	Yes	Heat-labile toxin (140 kDa)	Toxin; dermal necrosis and vasoconstriction	Effect only after injection in skin	Role in human disease unknown
Tracheal colonization (tcfA)	Yes	Proline-rich protein	Adhesion factor; predominantly in trachea	Not known	C-terminal homology to prn, factor brkA, and vag-8
Bordetella resistance to killing factor (brkA)	Yes	Outer membrane protein (32 kDa)	Adhesion factor	Provides resistance to complement	C-terminal homology to prn, tcfA, and vag-8
Virulence-activated gene 8 (vag-8)	Yes	Outer membrane protein (95 kDa)	Adhesion factor (?)	Not known	C-terminal homology to prn, tcfA, and brkA
Lipooligosaccharide (wlb)	Yes	Lipid A and trisaccharide	Presumably required for nasal colonization	Not known	Substantially species-specific structure within *Bordetella*
BVG intermediate-phase (bipA)	Yes	Outer membrane protein (137 KDa)	Transmission (?) and adhesion factor	Not known	First of a new class of *Bordetella* protein A antigens ("intermediate phase")
Type III secretion system (bsc)	Yes	Several, not yet specified proteins	Secretes effector proteins into host cells	Downregulation of the host immune system	Appears to be functional only in *B. bronchiseptica* (and some *B. parapertussis* strains)
bteA (bteA)	Yes	Linked to type III secretion system (72 kDa)	Induction of cytotoxicity	Persistent infection (animal model)	Potential vaccine antigen

BVG, Bordetella virulence gene; CAMP, cyclic adenosine monophosphate; wlb, Bordetella pertussis lipopolysaccharide biosynthesis locus (formerly Bpl).
Modified and updated from Heininger U. Recent progress in clinical and basic pertussis research. *Eur J Pediatr.* 2001;160:203-213.

with or without concomitant symptoms.[16] Of note, infection with *B. pertussis* does not provide lifelong immunity, and apparently no cross protection exists between different species of *Bordetella*.[11,22] After natural infection, sustained IgG and IgA serum antibody levels against FHA, pertactin, and—though less—PT have been observed before returning close to baseline values after approximately 5 years.[23,24] Yet the precise role of serum antibodies in immunity against pertussis is a matter of ongoing debate, and various studies show conflicting results.[25,26]

Cell-mediated immune responses to *B. pertussis* have been shown to play an important role in protection against pertussis. In mice, challenge with *B. pertussis* resulted in a predominant T helper 1 (Th1) cell–mediated immune response followed by complete bacterial clearance.[27] Specific protection could be conferred by adoptive transfer of immune spleen cells into immunosuppressed mice, further underlining the role of Th1 cells. Interestingly, persistent vaccine efficacy has been documented in young children several years after immunization despite significant antibody decline, and it was also preferentially mediated by Th1 cells.[28]

Clinical Features

SYMPTOMS

Typical pertussis is a three-stage illness, comprising catarrhal, paroxysmal, and convalescent phases.[3] The catarrhal stage lasts for about 1–2 weeks and is characterized by flulike symptoms such as coryza, sneezing, lacrimation, conjunctival injection, malaise, and nonspecific cough. It is followed by the paroxysmal stage, which in classical cases is marked by an increase of frequency and severity of coughing, with paroxysms as the most typical feature; characteristically, repetitive series of 5–10 or more hacking spells of cough occur during a single expiration. At the end of a paroxysm, a typical whoop, which is caused by the sudden rush of inspired air through a narrowed glottis, is noted. Paroxysms may occur up to several times per hour, during both day and night, triggered by various stimuli such as eating and drinking and physical or emotional stress. The paroxysmal stage may last from a few days to several weeks, until the convalescent stage is reached; this phase is marked by a decrease in the frequency and severity of coughing spells. However, over a period of several months, similar coughing episodes may again occur, often associated with other respiratory tract infections. Notably, *B. pertussis* infections present with considerable variability, which primarily depends on age, previous immunization, or infection. Other variables—including the presence of passively acquired antibody (in young infants), degree of exposure to the source of infection, specific bacterial inoculum, host genetic and acquired factors, and genotype of the organism—may contribute to attenuation of symptoms.

The variability of symptoms is exemplified by results from a study of 1860 culture-positive cases in unvaccinated children and adolescents in Germany. In that study, 38% of patients had a total coughing illness duration of 4 weeks or less, 18% had nonparoxysmal cough, 21% did not whoop, and 47% did not have posttussive vomiting.[7] On rare occasions, *B. pertussis* infection has been found to cause otitis media and to be associated with unilateral hyperlucent lung (MacLeod or Swyer-James syndrome) and the hemolytic uremic syndrome.[29–31]

Overall symptoms with *B. parapertussis* infection are similar to those caused by *B. pertussis*, but illness is usually less severe and of shorter duration.[10] Dual infections of *B. pertussis* and *B. parapertussis* have been observed.[32] Occasionally *B. bronchiseptica* and *B. holmesii* have been isolated from children with pertussis-like illness.[33,34] The clinical role of *Bordetella* species isolated from sputum specimens in patients with cystic fibrosis is currently unknown.[35]

PHYSICAL FINDINGS

Cyanosis, neck vein distention, bulging eyes, tongue protrusion, salivation, lacrimation, sweating, and posttussive vomiting of food or viscous mucus may occur with pertussis. Fever is usually minimal or absent. There is a wide spectrum of complications of pertussis, most of which predominantly occur in young infants (Table 32.3). Respiratory complications include bronchopneumonia with or without atelectasis, pulmonary hypertension, and otitis media mainly secondary to other respiratory tract pathogens. Pertussis has also been associated with activation of latent tuberculosis. Additional complications that have been observed as a consequence of

pertussis include ulcer of the frenulum of the tongue, epistaxis, melena, subconjunctival hemorrhages, meningoencephalitis, encephalopathy with cerebral seizures, tetanic seizures caused by severe alkalosis as a result of loss of gastric contents due to persistent vomiting, subdural hematomas, spinal epidural hematoma, rupture of the diaphragm, rib fracture, umbilical hernia, inguinal hernia, rectal prolapse, dehydration, syndrome of inappropriate antidiuretic hormone secretion, apnea, and nutritional disturbances.[3] Death secondary to pneumonia, pulmonary hypertension, or sudden death, probably due to severe hypoxemia, occurs mainly in infants, for whom the mortality rate is 0.6%.[6,36]

Imaging, Pulmonary Function Testing, Laboratory Findings

Uncomplicated pertussis does not require any imaging studies. The role of radiographic imaging in pertussis is limited. The most frequent abnormalities are consolidation, atelectasis, and hilar lymphadenopathy. In a case series of 238 hospitalized patients with pertussis, radiographic abnormalities were detected in 63 patients (26%). Pulmonary consolidation was seen in 50 patients (21%), atelectasis in 9 (4%), and lymphadenopathy in 22 (9%). Most consolidations were peribronchial (72%). For unknown reasons, both atelectasis and consolidation were more common on the right and predominantly involved the lower and middle lobes of the lung. Radiographic abnormalities were more common beyond infancy. Follow-up radiographs after 1 month demonstrated no significant radiographic sequelae.[37] One can conclude that chest radiographs should be limited to severe cases and when pulmonary complications are suspected on the basis of clinical findings.

Most cases of pertussis caused by primary *B. pertussis* infection in unvaccinated individuals will demonstrate leukocytosis due to lymphocytosis. This is caused by the effects of PT, which appears to reduce L-selectin expression by the T cells and thus prevents their homing to the lymphoid tissues.[38] Hyperleukocytosis ($>30,000/mm^3$) correlates with severity of pertussis in young infants. In a case series of 31 infants 3 months of age or less with pertussis severe enough

Table 32.3 Complications in 1640 Unvaccinated Patients With *Bordetella Pertussis* Infections by Age Group as Reported in Follow-Up Questionnaires

Complication	<6 Months (N = 63) N (%)	6–12 Months (N = 59) N (%)	1–4 Years (N = 610) N (%)	4–9 Years (N = 846) N (%)	>9 Years (N = 62) N (%)	Total (N = 1640) N (%)
Pneumonia	2 (3.2)	—	8 (1.3)	18 (2.1)	—	28 (1.7)
Apnea/cyanosis	10 (15.9)	1 (1.7)	—	1 (0.1)	—	12 (0.7)
Otitis media	—	—	6 (0.9)	4 (0.5)	—	10 (0.6)
Poor feeding/severe vomiting	2 (3.2)	—	2 (0.3)	2 (0.2)	1 (1.6)	7 (0.4)
Cardiopulmonary failure	1 (1.7)	—	—	—	—	1 (0.1)
Death	—	1 (1.6)	—	—	—	1 (0.1)
Others[a]	—	2 (3.4)	5 (0.8)	15 (1.8)	—	22 (1.3)
Unspecified	1 (1.6)	—	8 (1.3)	5 (0.6)	2 (3.2)	16 (1.0)
Any	15 (23.8)	3 (5.1)	29 (4.8)	45 (5.3)	3 (4.8)	95 (5.8)

[a]Includes cases of epistaxis, inguinal hernia, frequent paroxysms, and bronchitis.

From Heininger U, Klich K, Stehr K, Cherry JD. Clinical findings in Bordetella pertussis infections. Results of a prospective multicenter surveillance study. *Pediatrics*. 1997;100:e10.

to require intensive care, those with pulmonary hypertension or who died had higher leukocyte counts (>30,000/mm^3) and were more likely to have tachycardia, tachypnea, and pneumonia than those who did not have pulmonary hypertension or survived.[39]

In contrast, secondary infections and breakthrough cases of pertussis in vaccinated patients (with preexisting IgG antibodies to PT) usually lack leukocytosis, as do patients infected with *B. parapertussis* (which does not express PT).[10]

Diagnosis and Differential Diagnosis

In typical cases, a diagnosis of pertussis can be established on the basis of characteristic symptoms. Isolation of *B. pertussis* or *B. parapertussis* from a person with a cough illness provides certainty of the diagnosis. Nasopharyngeal specimens (NPSs), obtained by aspiration, calcium alginate or Dacron swabs, and specific media (Regan-Lowe or Bordet-Gengou agar and modified Stainer-Scholte broth) are necessary to recover *Bordetella* species. Direct fluorescent antibody staining is no longer recommended due to lack of sensitivity and specificity. Sensitivity of culture is optimal (≈95%) in unvaccinated, untreated individuals early in the course of the illness, when clinical suspicion of pertussis is usually low. During the paroxysmal phase, sensitivity of culture rapidly declines to 50% or lower. Over the last two decades, the polymerase chain reaction (PCR) technique applied to NPSs has markedly improved the diagnosis of pertussis. Recently a combination of induced sputum and NPS has been shown to increase the diagnostic yield of *B. pertussis* by PCR considerably (i.e., from 17 [NPS only] to 32 [NPS plus induced sputum] positive results in 460 South African children hospitalized for lower respiratory tract infections).[40] PCR is particularly useful in oligosymptomatic cases, in patients who have been started on antibiotics (where PCR may remain positive for prolonged periods of time) and in patients with progressed illness.[41] In addition, the sensitivity of PCR in general is higher than that of bacterial culture; PCR is therefore the preferred diagnostic tool. Advanced technology today allows discrimination between different species of the *Bordetella* genus, and recent developments such as real-time detection of the amplification products and LightCycler PCR now provide results within a few hours.[42,43]

Serologic tests are the most sensitive technique for the diagnosis of *Bordetella* infections. Enzyme immunoassays have been most widely applied, and although whole-cell preparations of *B. pertussis* can be used as antigens, purified proteins such as PT, FHA, and pertactin are preferable for their better specificity. IgG antibody assays provide sufficient sensitivity, but the addition of IgA assays may be helpful. Although paired acute- and convalescent-phase serum samples are optimal, analysis of a single serum specimen is more appropriate for routine purposes. Unfortunately, however, serology tests are not standardized and interpretation of results is difficult in the presence of vaccine-induced preexisting antibodies.[44] Therefore test results have to be interpreted cautiously, and cutoff values derived from age-matched control groups are required. IgA antibodies have traditionally been considered to be reliable indicators of recent or acute infection. A recent study, however, has shown persistently high IgA antibodies against both FHA and pertactin and, though less pronounced, also against PT for as long as 30 months after infection.[24] This observation further complicates the serologic diagnosis of *B. pertussis* infection in single-serum analyses.

Several microorganisms other than *B. pertussis* or *B. parapertussis* can cause cough illnesses that can occasionally be confused with pertussis. In one study from Germany, the frequency of serologic evidence for an infection with microorganisms other than *B. pertussis* was assessed in children with pertussis-like illnesses.[45] Of 149 such children, a diagnosis of adenovirus (*n* = 33); parainfluenza viruses 1, 2, and 3 (*n* = 18); *Mycoplasma pneumoniae* infection (*n* = 15); and respiratory syncytial virus infection (*n* = 14) was made. In studies of concurrent outbreaks of *Mycoplasma* and *B. pertussis* infections, it has been shown that clinical symptoms alone lacked adequate specificity to distinguish pertussis from mycoplasma infection.[46] Moreover, in populations with high immunization rates, atypical presentations of *B. pertussis* may be more frequent than classical illness, and a high index of clinical suspicion is imperative in the diagnosis of pertussis.[7] These observations underscore the need for appropriate laboratory tests if there is any doubt about the diagnosis.

Management and Treatment

Several antibiotics have proven in vitro activity against *B. pertussis* and *B. parapertussis*.[1] Sufficient minimal inhibitory concentrations have been demonstrated for macrolides and for fluoroquinolones. In contrast, minimal inhibitory concentrations of oral beta-lactam antibiotics, including cephalosporins, are unacceptable and render them unsuitable for the treatment of pertussis. Oral erythromycin (succinate formulation at 50 mg/kg body weight per day given every 6–8 hours or estolate formulation at doses of 40 mg/kg per day at 12-hour intervals for 14 days) is still the preferred treatment in neonates and young infants. When given in the catarrhal or early paroxysmal stage of the illness, this will ameliorate the symptoms, eradicate the bacteria from the nasopharynx within a few days, and terminate contagiousness of the patient. Of the different formulations, erythromycin is favored by most experts. Erythromycin remains the first-line drug, although resistance has been observed in single isolates and ongoing surveillance of antibiotic susceptibility is a challenge in the era of PCR diagnostics.[47] The mechanism underlying resistance is currently unknown. Seven days of treatment with erythromycin estolate was shown to be as effective as 14 days of treatment in a large Canadian study.[48] It should be noted, however, that this investigation was carried out in a highly vaccinated community, and results may have been different in unvaccinated children.

Macrolide antibiotics with improved gastrointestinal tolerability, such as clarithromycin or azithromycin, demonstrate efficiency comparable to that of erythromycin and are preferred in older children and adolescents.[49] In Canada, the microbiologic and clinical efficacy and the clinical safety of a 7-day course of clarithromycin (15 mg/kg per day in two doses for 7 days) was compared with a 14-day course of erythromycin (40 mg/kg per day in three doses for 14 days) in a prospective, randomized, single-blind (investigator) trial in children from 1 month to 16 years of age with culture-proven pertussis.[50] Nasopharyngeal cultures for *B. pertussis* were performed at enrollment and the end of treatment. Microbiologic eradication and clinical cure rates were equal: 100% (31/31) for clarithromycin and 96% (22/23) for erythromycin. Patients on clarithromycin had significantly fewer adverse events (45%) than those on erythromycin (62%).

In an open, uncontrolled study in the United States, 34 subjects (most of them children) with culture or PCR-proven *B. pertussis* infection received a 5-day course of azithromycin (10 mg/kg in a single dose on the first day and 5 mg/kg per day as single doses on the following 4 days). *B. pertussis* was eradicated from the nasopharynx in 33 (97%) of 34 patients after 72 hours, and all were negative on follow-up after 2–3 weeks.[51] Azithromycin is also the preferred antibiotic in neonates.[3] It is noteworthy that when azithromycin or erythromycin is used in young infants (<6 weeks, particularly <2 weeks of age), the increased risk for hypertrophic pyloric stenosis should be borne in mind, and parents need to be educated about the symptoms of this disease.[52]

Young infants, who are threatened by hyperleukocytosis and hypoxemia associated with apneic spells, should be hospitalized and their blood oxygen saturation closely monitored. Careful removal of respiratory secretions and oxygen supplementation may be necessary. Uncontrolled observations indicate that corticosteroids and/or β-adrenergic drugs adjunctive to antibiotics may ameliorate respiratory distress associated with pertussis, but evidence of efficacy is lacking.[3] Pneumonia, frequent apneic spells, and significant respiratory distress may require assisted ventilation, especially in neonates and young infants.[3] In young infants, extreme leukocytosis (>50,000/μL) and pulmonary hypertension carry a high risk for respiratory and cardiovascular failure. In spite of intensive treatment efforts—such as pulmonary artery vasodilators, exchange transfusion to reduce leukocytosis, and extracorporeal membrane oxygenation—the outcome of these complicated courses is frequently fatal.[53,54]

General supportive medical treatment is important for patients with pertussis. Physical and emotional stress, which may trigger paroxysms, should be avoided. Furthermore, if posttussive vomiting is present, careful attention should be paid to adequate fluid and food intake. Respiratory isolation precautions should be implemented until 5 days of effective antibiotic treatment have been received. There is no role for intravenous antipertussis immunoglobulin treatment and no such products are commercially available.

Prevention

Prevention of pertussis is possible by avoidance of exposure, postexposure antibiotic treatment, and immunization. Avoidance of exposure is usually impossible in clinical practice, given that contagiousness is highest during the early stage of illness in the primary case where commonly a diagnosis of pertussis has not yet been made. Prophylactic use of erythromycin (or clarithromycin or azithromycin) has been shown to protect from *B. pertussis* infection when given to close contacts and is most useful when administered before the occurrence of the first secondary case.[55] Recommended antibiotic dosage and duration is the same as for treatment and should be given to all close contacts regardless of age

and immunization status according to recommendations by the American Academy of Pediatrics.[56] Postexposure active immunization should also be considered in unimmunized or incompletely immunized individuals by use of a dose of age-appropriate pertussis vaccine.

Active immunization is the most effective way to prevent pertussis. Over the last decades, acellular pertussis vaccines (containing various numbers and quantities of *B. pertussis* antigens) have been developed and studied for safety, immunogenicity, and efficacy; these have been implemented in most countries worldwide.[1] Virtually all countries recommend a primary series of two or three vaccine doses in infancy and usually also a reinforcing dose in the second year of life. Timely initiation of the immunization series, usually at 6 weeks to 2 months of age, is crucial, because the risk of severe pertussis in immunized infants decreases from dose to dose as compared with the risk in unimmunized infants.[57] The optimal timing and number of further booster immunizations is a matter of ongoing debate.[8] Because vaccine-induced efficacy is sustained despite declining antibody values, observational studies are needed to answer these questions. Investigations conducted so far indicate ongoing efficacy for several years after three or four doses of acellular pertussis vaccine.[1] Today most countries recommend booster doses at preschool age and/or in adolescents. Furthermore, several countries—including the United States, Canada, France, and Germany—have introduced a universal pertussis booster dose in adults regardless of age.[58]

Overall, when compared with conventional whole-cell pertussis vaccines, acellular component vaccines have been shown to cause lower rates of local and systemic reactions such as fever.[3] Also, severe reactions such as febrile seizures and hypotonic-hyporesponsive episodes declined significantly (79% and 60%, respectively) with the broad dissemination of acellular pertussis vaccines.[59] Of some concern is that local reactions after pertussis immunization increase from dose to dose, and whole-limb swelling at the site of injection may occur. Yet these side effects are only temporary, usually do not interfere with the child's well-being, and are without known sequelae. Furthermore, they are considered to be less severe than those seen after five consecutive doses of whole-cell vaccine.[60] Providing timely and complete immunizations against pertussis for all infants and young children, followed by regular booster doses as needed throughout life, will be crucial to better control of pertussis in the future.

A new concept that holds promise in protecting young infants from death by pertussis is that of immunizing women during pregnancy, ideally around 28–32 weeks of gestation.[61,62] Hence maternal IgG antibodies against PT will be boosted and transferred to the fetus via the placenta, so that they will persist at comparatively high levels throughout the first weeks of life. When a young infant is then infected with *B. pertussis*, this passive immunity is then thought to reduce the risk for hyperleukocytosis, the major risk factor for fatal disease. This mechanism is assumed to be the basis for the protective effect provided to infants by maternal immunization.

Prognosis

There is no evidence for long-term sequelae such as allergic sensitization after pertussis.[63]

References

Access the reference list online at ExpertConsult.com.

Suggested Reading

Cherry JD, Heininger U. Pertussis and other bordetella infections. In: Feigin RD, Cherry JD, Harrison GJ, et al, eds. *Textbook of Pediatric Infectious Diseases*. 7th ed. Philadelphia: WB Saunders; 2014:1616–1639.

Dabrera G, Amirthalingam G, Andrews N, et al. A case-control study to estimate the effectiveness of maternal pertussis vaccination in protecting newborn infants in England and Wales, 2012–2013. *Clin Infect Dis*. 2015;60:333–337.

Kilgore PE, Salim AM, Zervos MJ, et al. Pertussis: Microbiology, disease, treatment, and prevention. *Clin Microbiol Rev*. 2016;29:449–486.

Mortimer EA. Pertussis and its prevention. A family affair. *J Infect Dis*. 1990;161:473–479.

Winter K, Zipprich J, Harriman K, et al. Risk factors associated with infant deaths from pertussis: a case-control study. *Clin Infect Dis*. 2015; 61:1099–1106.

33 Toxocariasis, Hydatid Disease of the Lung, Strongyloidiasis, and Pulmonary Paragonimiasis

AYESHA MIRZA, MD, FAAP, and
MOBEEN RATHORE, MD, CPE, FAAP, FPIDS, FIDSA, FSHEA, FACPE

Toxocariasis

Toxocariasis is a soil-transmitted zoonotic roundworm infection transmitted to humans by contact with canine and feline feces. It causes two main diseases in humans: visceral toxocariasis (VT), formerly known as visceral larva migrans, and ocular toxocariasis (OT), formerly known as ocular larva migrans.[1] VT results from an inflammatory response to the migration of immature, second-stage larvae through the viscera of a host that is not suitable for completion of the parasite's life cycle. The lung parenchyma is commonly involved in this form of the disease.

EPIDEMIOLOGY

Toxocara species are found worldwide in domesticated and wild dogs and cats. Infection with *Toxocara* spp. is more prevalent than realized, because many individuals do not express the complete VT syndrome. Current seroprevalence data place toxocariasis among the most common zoonotic infections worldwide.[2] The global prevalence of *Toxocara* spp. in humans varies widely and is dependent upon factors such as population density, sanitation, poverty, education, and enforcement of laws regarding proper disposal of animal excreta.[1,2]

Toxocariasis is also endemic throughout the United States.[3] In one seroprevalence study conducted more than 20 years ago by the Centers for Disease Control and Prevention (CDC), using a nationally represented set of banked sera from the First National Health and Nutrition Examination Survey (NHANES 1971–1973), the seroprevalence of *Toxocara* antibodies, as measured by enzyme-linked immunosorbent assay (ELISA), varied from 4.6% to 7.3%.[4] However, rates approaching 30% were seen among black children of lower socioeconomic status.[4] A second seroprevalence study, also conducted by the CDC (NHANES 1988–1994), found an overall prevalence of 13.9%.[3] As in the prior survey, rates varied between different geographic regions and were influenced by socioeconomic conditions.[5] Similarly, seroprevalence rates also vary in other industrialized countries, particularly those that are resource rich versus resource poor, with higher rates seen in rural or underserved areas with high rates of poverty, overcrowding, and poor hygiene.[2,6,7]

Infection in the definitive host may be through multiple routes including vertical, transplacental (not in cats), and transmammary, as well as horizontal. The ability to survive and develop to sexual maturity in the intestinal tract of several vertebrate species has contributed to the worldwide propagation of the species. Puppies are especially dangerous, because transplacental infection results in 77%–100% of puppies becoming infected, and many pups are born with congenital canine toxocariasis.[6,8] They can then shed millions of eggs into the environment depending on the immune status of the host as well as the intensity of the *Toxocara canis* infection. By the time the animals are 3 weeks old, mature egg-laying worms can be present. Adult female worms can produce and shed more than 200,000 ova per day, which are then passed unembryonated onto the soil in the feces of the infected animal. Under suitable soil conditions (temperature 10–30°C, availability of light, suitable pH and humidity), the ova become embryonated and infectious after a minimum of 2–3 weeks. Because of the thick shell, the embryonated ova can survive in moist soil for months or even a few years. Most infections in children affect those with a history of pica or individuals who have accidentally ingested contaminated soil. Children also become infected commonly while playing in backyards, parks, playgrounds, and sandboxes where it is easy to come in contact with infectious ova.[2,9]

ETIOLOGY

Two species of the genus *Toxocara* are primarily responsible for most cases of VT: dogs, wolves, coyotes, and foxes are the definitive hosts for *T. canis*, whereas domestic cats are the host for *T. cati*. Other *Toxocara* spp. have been implicated in human infection, including *T. vulpis (canine whipworm) and T. vitulorum (found in cattle)*. The role of *T. lyncus* (wild cats) and *T. malaysiensis* (domestic cats) in causing human infection is not clear. In addition, *Baylisascaris procyonis (raccoon roundworm), Capillaria hepatica (rodent nematode), Ascaris suum (pig roundworm)*, and rarely *Ascaris lumbricoides*, hookworm larvae, as well as *Strongyloides stercoralis* can cause a VT-like syndrome.[2,10]

PATHOLOGY/PATHOGENESIS

In the natural host, infectious ova are ingested and hatch in the upper alimentary tract. The second-stage larvae then migrate through the intestinal walls into the bloodstream and then into the liver and lungs of the infected animal. From the lungs, the larvae mature by migrating through the tracheobronchial tree and passing into the upper alimentary tract. There, the mature worm can begin laying eggs, which pass out in the feces to begin the cycle anew.

In aberrant hosts, such as humans, the initial stages of infection are identical: infectious second-stage larvae hatch in the small intestine and then begin migrating through blood and lymphatics to the liver, lung, brain, and other organs such as the eye. Before the larvae can complete their transtracheal passage and maturation to adult worms, however, host defenses block further migration of the larvae by encasing them within a granulomatous reaction, which is generally eosinophilic in nature. The pathogenesis of VT is the direct result of the immunologic response of the body to the dead and dying larvae. Multiple eosinophilic abscesses may develop in the infected tissues. The larvae remain alive and infective for an indefinite period of time, often as long as 7 years. The inflammation appears as an eosinophilic granuloma, and an open biopsy of a granulomatous lesion will often show the *Toxocara* larva. Host antibodies are generated against the *Toxocara* excretory-secretory (TES) antigens of the larvae. These glycoprotein antigens contain protease, acetylcholinesterase, and eosinophil-stimulating activity. They also elicit Th 2 immune responses and high levels of interleukins 4 and 5.[11]

CLINICAL FEATURES

Symptoms

It is the immediate hypersensitivity response to the larvae that manifests as symptoms of VT. The specific signs and symptoms depend on the organ affected. *Toxocara* is mainly an infection of young children, since they have a greater opportunity to ingest the infectious ova. The classic case occurs in a male child, younger than 6 years, with a history of pica and exposure to dogs. A child with fever of unknown etiology and eosinophilia with the appropriate epidemiological history should be assumed to have *Toxocara* infection until proven otherwise. The extent of signs and symptoms depends on the number and location of granulomatous lesions and the host's immune response.

Pulmonary toxocariasis is generally asymptomatic or may present with symptoms such as mild cough and dyspnea.[12] The initial symptoms may include a prodrome of anorexia, fever, and malaise. The so-called "covert toxocariasis" has been implicated as responsible for many subtle clinical manifestations. In a study of children in Ireland, a plethora of clinical manifestations were seen including fever, headache, anorexia, abdominal pain, nausea, vomiting, lethargy, sleep and behavior disorders, pharyngitis, pneumonia, cough, history of wheezing, limb pain, cervical lymphadenitis, and hepatomegaly.[13,14] Another case-control study in French adults led to the term "common toxocariasis," a syndrome comprising chronic dyspnea and weakness; cutaneous rash; pruritus and abdominal pain, often with eosinophilia; elevated levels of immunoglobulin E (IgE); and high titers of *Toxocara*-specific antibodies.[15] Both "covert" and "common" toxocariasis probably represent variations in the clinical spectrum of mild *Toxocara* childhood and adult disease.

The time course for VT may be quite prolonged. The initial stage of the illness lasts several weeks, beginning with low-grade fevers and nonspecific symptoms and progressing to eosinophilia and hepatomegaly. Episodes of bronchitis, asthma, or pneumonia may occur. Over the next month, intermittent high fevers occur along with the major manifestations of the disease. Recovery may take as long as 1–2 years, during which time the eosinophilia resolves along with the hepatomegaly. Resolution of pulmonary infiltrates occurs more rapidly.

With more severe involvement, various combinations of abdominal pain, arthralgias, myalgias, weight loss, high intermittent fevers, and neurologic disturbance may be seen. Acute respiratory failure has been reported from *Toxocara* infection.[16]

Other symptoms can include idiopathic seizure disorder, functional intestinal disorders, skin diseases (prurigo and chronic urticaria), eosinophilic and reactive arthritis, and angioedema.

Physical Findings

These depend on the extent of the infection, the organ system involved, and whether the disease is systemic or limited to a specific organ. The lung is one of the most common organs affected in children with toxocariasis. Cough, if present, is generally nonproductive. Wheezing is the most frequent finding on chest examination, although rhonchi and crackles also have been described.[17] Because of the wheezing, some patients are diagnosed initially as suffering from asthma. Multiple studies have looked at the relationship between the seroprevalence of *Toxocara* infection and asthma and found that there is a significant positive correlation. In fact, toxocariasis is a well-recognized environmental risk factor for asthma in endemic regions.[18] Apart from pulmonary involvement as noted previously, other symptoms in VT depend on organ involved; hepatomegaly of varying degrees is almost always present.

Imaging, Pulmonary Function Tests (PFTs), Laboratory Findings

There is no typical chest radiographic finding. Multiple pulmonary infiltrates or nodules may be seen; however, these are not pathognomonic.[19,20] A recent study reported that all nodules seen in children with *Toxocara* infection on computed tomography (CT) scan, whether they were single or multiple, were in the peripheral area of the lungs. Less commonly pleural effusion has also been reported in association with the infection.[21] Descriptions of imaging studies range from patchy airspace disease with pseudonodular infiltrates on CT scan to diffuse interstitial pneumonitis to an asymptomatic pulmonary mass. The latter may at times raise the suspicion for malignancy on initial evaluation.[22,23] As with other eosinophilic pneumonias, pulmonary involvement in toxocariasis may present as patchy ground-glass opacities on initial CT scan findings. A recent study reported the presence of focal linear opacities on CT scan.[24] A pattern similar to miliary tuberculosis (TB) has also been reported in severe cases. The varied radiologic patterns may reflect whether direct larval invasion of lung tissue or a hypersensitivity reaction to larval antigens is the primary pathologic process present in that particular patient.

Pulmonary function testing may reveal diminished lung function with decreased forced expiratory volumes in one second (FEV1).[25] Bronchiectasis may result from chronic lung infection.[26]

Neutrophilia occurs during the first few days but rapidly gives way to the eosinophilia classically seen in the disease. Eosinophilia can range up to 50%–90% of the total white blood cell count. Leukocytosis is generally present, with extreme values of over 100,000 cells/mm^3 occasionally reported.[27]

Other laboratory findings also may be helpful in supporting a diagnosis of VT. Serum IgE levels are above 900 UI/mL in 60% of patients tested. Hypergammaglobulinemia is frequently reported and characterized by elevations of any one or all of the immunoglobulin classes.[28,29] Because of cross-reactivity between larval and blood group antigens, many patients will develop high anti-A and anti-B isohemagglutinin titers that persist for months after the initial infection.[29] Bronchoalveolar lavage fluid also may exhibit a relative eosinophilia.

DIAGNOSIS AND DIFFERENTIAL DIAGNOSIS

ELISA and Western blot (WB) using the larval TES antigens to detect the host's antibodies are the most widely available and accepted tests for confirmation.[30] If a titer above 1 : 32 is considered, the diagnostic sensitivity is approximately 78% with a specificity of over 92%.[31] Because antibodies against *Toxocara* are present for years, an antigen-capture ELISA has been developed to separate acute from dormant infection.[32] Most recently, polymerase chain reaction (PCR) tests and recombinant antigen based assays on the Luminex platform, have also been developed.[33] The latter perform similarly to the existing TES-antigen WB and better than the TES-antigen ELISA method. However, they may not be widely available in underresourced countries where there is a high burden of disease.

Examination of the stool for ova and parasites is not helpful because the larvae rarely mature in humans. Before the ELISA against TES antibodies was developed, tissue biopsy to demonstrate the larvae in eosinophilic granulomas was the definitive test for diagnosis. Skin tests, other serologic testing, and fluorescent antibody techniques were troubled by low sensitivities and unacceptably high cross-reactivity with other parasitic infections.

Differential diagnosis should include the visceral lesions that may be produced by other nematode worms, as well as immature stages of certain nematodes and filarial worms. Invasion of the liver by *Fasciola hepatica*, a nematode worm, or *Capillaria hepatica*, a trematode, might be included. Also

to be considered in this diagnosis are trichinosis, hepatitis, leukemia, other causes of intense eosinophilia, TB, asthma, lead poisoning, and the leukemoid reaction occurring in severe bacterial pneumonia.

MANAGEMENT AND TREATMENT

Treatment depends on the severity and location of the infection. Albendazole or mebendazole are the treatments of choice for *Toxocara* infections, although albendazole is not approved by the Food and Drug Administration (FDA), for this particular indication, and mebendazole is no longer available in the United States (Table 33.1). Thiabendazole and ivermectin have also been used. Most patients recover without any specific anthelmintic therapy. Corticosteroids along with antihelminthic treatment have been useful in patients with severe pulmonary and ocular involvement, possibly by also treating the hypersensitivity component of the disease as well.[34] Surgery may be indicated in some cases with ocular disease. Otherwise, treatment is symptomatic.

PROGNOSIS

Prognosis depends on the extent of the disease. The few deaths described with VT have resulted from myocardial, neurologic, or overwhelming systemic involvement. Neurologic disturbances have been described in severe cases because of invasion of the central nervous system (CNS) by larvae.[35] Seizures, encephalopathy, meningoencephalitis, and transverse myelitis have all been reported. Manifestations of peripheral nervous system involvement include radiculitis and cranial nerve palsy. Renal, pancreatic, and cardiac invasion rarely occur. Cardiac involvement, while rare, can be a potentially life-threatening complication of the disease.[36] *T. canis* also may produce the Pulmonary Infiltrates and Eosinophilia (PIE) syndrome.[37] Finally, various dermatologic manifestations have been reported with toxocariasis.[38] These include chronic urticaria, eczema, and pruritis.

Measures that decrease the ingestion of contaminated soil reduce the incidence of the disease. Anticipatory guidance

Table 33.1 Recommended Treatment Options: Toxocariasis, Echinococcosis, Strongylodiasis, Paragonimiasis[e]

Disease	Drug	Dose and Duration
Toxocariasis	Albendazole	400 mg by mouth twice a day for 5 days (adult & child)
	Mebendazole	100–200 mg by mouth twice a day for 5 days (adult & child)
Echinococcosis	Albendazole	Adults: 400 mg by mouth twice a day for 1–6 months
		Children: 10–15 mg/kg/day (max 800 mg) by mouth twice a day for 1–6 months
	Mebendazole	50–60 mg/kg/day in three divided doses for 3–6 months up to 1 year[a]
Strongyloides	Ivermectin[b]	200 μg/kg given as a single dose for 1–2 days
	Albendazole	400 mg by mouth 2 times daily for 7 days
Paragonimus	Praziquantel	25 mg/kg given orally three times a day for 2 days[c]
	Triclabendazole[d]	10 mg/kg once or twice

[a]100–200 mg/kg/day for 3 months has also been used successfully in children without any serious complications reported.
[b]Oral Ivermectin is available for human use in the United States. Relative contraindications for the use of ivermectin include: pregnant women, confirmed or suspected *Loa loa* infection, and those weighing less than 15 kg. For Strongyloides associated hyperinfection syndrome, Ivermectin should be given until stool and sputum exams are negative for the parasite for 2 weeks.
[c]Safety of praziquantel not established in children less than 4 years old. In endemic areas, risks and benefits of treatment should be considered.
[d]Not available in the United States, not FDA approved.
[e]Contents of table adapted from the CDC and more information is available at the following websites:
http://www.cdc.gov/parasites/toxocariasis/health_professionals/index.html
http://www.cdc.gov/parasites/echinococcosis/health_professionals/index.html#tx
http://www.cdc.gov/parasites/strongyloides/health_professionals/index.html#tx
http://www.cdc.gov/parasites/paragonimus/health_professionals/index.html#tx.

should focus on the risks of pica and elimination of the behavior. Regular deworming of puppies and lactating or pregnant female dogs should be performed, and the risks of indiscriminate disposal of dog feces, especially in children's play areas, should be emphasized.

Recently, the CDC announced an initiative to prioritize five neglected parasitic infections in the United States, including toxocariasis.[39] Among the major priorities outlined are efforts to better define risk factors and further research to elucidate the natural history of toxocariasis and its complications. There is also a need to develop improved and easily available diagnostic tests for detecting active infection and studies to optimize current treatment regimens using anthelminthic drugs.[29]

Echinococcosis (Hydatid Disease)

EPIDEMIOLOGY

Tapeworms of the genus *Echinococcus* are the causative agents of Echinococcosis, which has been recognized as one of the 17 neglected tropical diseases by the World Health Organization (WHO).[40] The disease has a worldwide distribution. It is endemic in most parts of the world where sheep rearing is common including South America, the Mediterranean region, Central Asia, Western China, and East Africa.

There are three major forms of echinococcosis that affect humans: cystic echinococcosis, alveolar echinococcosis, and polycystic echinococcosis. Of these, cystic echinococcosis predominantly affects the lungs, whereas the latter two affect the liver and will not be discussed in detail. Polycystic echinococcosis is the least common form seen and is restricted to South and Central America.[41,42]

Echinococcosis is known to affect all age groups and any body cavity, organ, or site, although it most frequently affects the liver and the lungs, with the lung more commonly affected in children.[41–47] Infection occurs mostly during childhood, although years may elapse before manifestations are seen. While overall there is no gender preference, more cases are reported in males, and this slight difference in gender incidence is probably related to activity or occupation.

ETIOLOGY

Currently, nine species of *Echinococcus* have been identified with the two major species of medical importance being *E. granulosus sensu lato* (formerly recognized as a single species *E. granulosus*) and *E. multilocularis*.[48] Phylogenetic sequencing now shows that there are several different genotypes of *E granulosus sensu lato*, some of which are considered different species.[49] Of these *E. granulosus sensu stricto*, *E. equinus*, *E. ortleppi* and *E. Canadensis* all cause cystic echinococcosis. *Enterococcus multilocularis* is the causative agent of alveolar echinococcosis, while *E. vogeli* and *E. oligarthrus* cause polycystic echinococcosis.[48] In addition, another species *E. shiquicus* has been recently described in the Qinghai-Tibet highlands, and while no human disease has been described thus far, further studies are needed.[50] *Echinococcus granulosus sensu stricto* is responsible for the majority (up to 88%) of human cases globally.[48,49]

The parasites are maintained in nature by canines (primarily dogs, coyotes, dingoes, and wolves), which act as the definitive host. Herbivores (sheep, goats, or other livestock) are the intermediate hosts and harbor the larval stage. The life cycles of *E. granulosus*, *E. multilocularis*, and *E. vogeli* are similar, with the major difference being that the fox is the major definitive host for *E. multilocularis* and rodents are the intermediate hosts for both *E. locularis* and *E. vogeli*. For this review, we will be focusing primarily on *E. granulosus (sensu lato)*.

PATHOLOGY/PATHOGENESIS

The first developmental stage is the tapeworm, which reaches sexual maturity only in the intestinal tract of its definitive mammalian host: dogs or other canines. Adult *Echinococcus* worms typically produce thousands of eggs each day that are extremely resistant to climatic conditions and survive for at least 2 years in northern regions. Infectious ova are released during defecation, contaminating fields, irrigated lands, and wells. Once the eggs are swallowed by humans, the outer shell is digested and the embryos penetrate the intestine and are hematogenously disseminated to various parts of the body, mostly to the liver and lung. In the lung, the embryos form fluid-filled cysts (hydatid cysts) (Fig. 33.1).

Under ideal conditions, tapeworm heads, or protoscoleces, develop within the cysts. The minimum time for protoscoleces to develop has been estimated to be 10 months or longer after infection. Humans are accidental hosts and are highly unlikely to be involved in disease transmission. They can become infected from contaminated water and food or through close contact with infected dogs, sheep, or other livestock. Human-to-human transmission does not occur.

Lung cysts develop when embryos pass through the liver, through lymphatic ducts bypassing the liver, by contiguous extension from the liver, or through the bronchi. The cyst slowly enlarges, and its rate of growth is dependent on the distensibility of the tissue and the age of the host. It has also been suggested that different biological attributes such as the rate of attaining fertility as well as the size of a hydatid cyst can be related to the genotype.[40] Pulmonary cysts grow faster in children. At a size of 1 cm, three layers can be identified within the cyst: (1) an inner layer of germinal epithelium or endocyst that is responsible for formation of daughter cysts by endogenous vesiculation; (2) a middle noncellular,

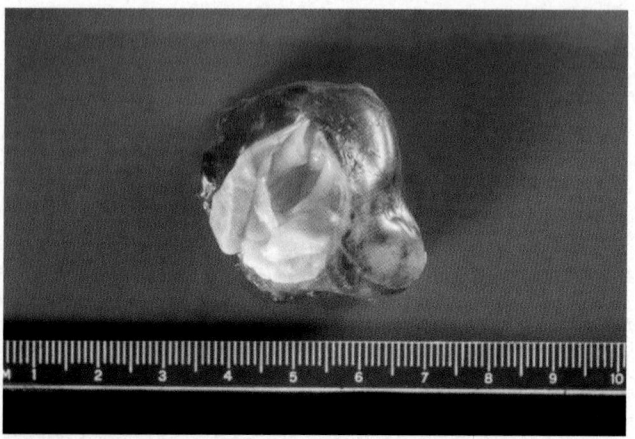

Fig. 33.1 Gross pathology of membrane and hydatid daughter cysts from human lung.

laminated layer or ectocyst; and (3) an adventitia or pericyst, an outer capsule of fibrous tissue, vasculature, giant cells, and eosinophils resulting from a weak host reaction. With time, blood capsules and daughter cysts may develop and disintegrate, liberating free floating hooklets or "hydatid sand."[40]

Involvement of the diaphragm and transdiaphragmatic extension into the lung has been described in patients with primary hydatid cysts of the liver. Virtually any organ including the brain, eye, heart, mediastinum, blood vessels, pleura, diaphragm, pancreas, spleen, endocrine glands, bone, and genitourinary tract may be affected.[47] The CNS is affected more often in children than in adults.

CLINICAL FEATURES

Symptoms

Cyst size, location, and the potential for impairment of vital structures determine the clinical manifestations.[51] The more common symptoms of pulmonary cysts are cough, chest pain, hemoptysis, fever, and malaise. Other manifestations include sputum production, chest discomfort, loss of appetite, dyspnea, vomiting of cyst elements, dysphagia, and hepatic pain.[52–54] Bronchospasm has been reported with relief of "bronchial asthma" after removal of the cyst.[55] Growth retardation patterns have been observed in many children.

A large proportion of pulmonary cases may be discovered incidentally on a routine chest radiograph. The intact cyst is most commonly asymptomatic and may account for a third of all cases. This is usually seen in children where the cyst may be an incidental finding. Most individuals harboring small lung cysts often remain asymptomatic 5–20 years after infection until the cyst enlarges sufficiently to cause symptoms.[56] Awareness of symptoms is due to pressure from the enlarging cyst, secondary infection, and cyst rupture. Up to 30% of lung cysts may be complicated by rupture into the pleural space or bronchus, precipitated by coughing, sneezing, trauma, or increased abdominal pressure. Chills, fever, increased cough, mild hemoptysis, and change in appearance on radiographs suggest rupture.

Physical Findings

Physical examination is rarely definitive. Occasionally, a hydatid thrill (fluid wave) can be felt while percussing a large cyst. Demonstration of scoleces and hooklets of the parasite in vomitus, stool, urine, or sputum is pathognomonic but is rarely observed and may be seen only during surgery.

Children with echinococcosis may present to the emergency room because of complications of the disease. These complications may be mechanical, with hydatid growth affecting the bronchial tree or pleura; they also may result from hematogenous spread, infection, or allergic reaction. Cyst rupture, pneumothorax, atelectasis, bronchopleural fistula, empyema, saprophytic mycosis have been reported.[55,57,58] A rare complication is rupture into the cardiovascular system with dissemination or sudden death.

Secondary hydatidosis in the pleura, acute asphyxia by bronchial obstruction, and allergic reactions, including anaphylaxis, may follow cyst rupture and leakage.[57] Bronchobiliary fistula occurs in 2% of cases and is commonly, but not always, preceded by suppuration. The right side and posterior basal segment of the lung are most frequently affected. Pyrexia and weight loss may mimic malignancy, but bile expectoration is pathognomonic.

Imaging, PFT, Laboratory Findings

Lung cysts are readily detected on plain radiographical films, and the possibility of a hydatid cyst should always be considered in an endemic area.[59] An intact cyst is seen as a round or oval homogeneous lesion with a sharply defined smooth border surrounded by normal lung or a zone of atelectasis. It may be located in the periphery, center, or hilum; be single or multiple; and unilateral or bilateral (Fig. 33.2). The final form depends on the location and neighboring structures. With an increase in size, bronchial displacement occurs without obstruction, as has been demonstrated by CT or bronchography. On fluoroscopy, good elasticity of the cyst wall is demonstrable, and there is no interference with movement of the diaphragm.

As the cyst grows, air passages and surrounding vessels are eroded, producing bronchial air leaks into the cyst adventitia. The bronchial connection is actually nonpatent before rupture because of pressure of the endocyst against bronchial passages, and it may be recognized only during surgery. With varying stages of air dissection into the cyst, different classical radiologic signs may be seen.[59,60] Pericystic emphysema is seen before rupture. A "meniscus sign" or "crescent sign" is a crescentic radiolucency above the homogeneous cyst shadow on deep inspiration that is seen when air penetrates between the adventitia and ectocyst. As air dissection continues, the parasite's membrane is torn, and some hydatid fluid flows out. An air-fluid level is seen within the cyst lumen as well as an air cup between ectocyst and adventitia, known as "double air-layer appearance" or the Cumbo sign. This is also referred to as the onion peel or double arch sign and is pathognomonic for a ruptured pulmonary hydatid cyst.[61] With free connection to a bronchus, the cyst wall is detached from the adventitia, crumbles, collapses, and floats on remaining cyst fluid. This result is seen on the radiograph as air between the collapsed floating cyst wall and the adventitia, known as the "water lily sign" or Camellote sign.[62] The adventitial wall does not collapse at once, so the obliteration of the cyst cavity is not an immediate outcome.

Ultrasonography helps distinguish cystic lesions from solid tumors and has become the diagnostic study of choice for cystic and alveolar echinococcosis due to its low cost and high specificity and sensitivity.[63–66] Pathognomonic signs on ultrasonography are multiple daughter cysts within a cyst, separation of the laminated membrane from the wall of the cyst, and collapsed cysts (Fig. 33.3). A simple cyst with a thick wall in patients from an endemic area is suggestive. Abdominal ultrasonography is also recommended for liver cyst detection. Specific features identified on sonogram are similar to those seen on plain radiographs and include the double-walled cyst, water lily sign, honeycomb appearance, ball of wool sign, and cyst wall calcification with pseudosolid content.[67] The honeycomb sign is caused by multivesiculated cysts in which the walls of adjacent cysts give the impression of "septa." The ball of wool sign is caused by multiple degenerating hypoechoic cyst membranes folded inside the pseudosolid cyst content.

Cystic hydatidosis of the lung occurs most often as a single unilocular cyst. Only about 7%–38% occur as multiple

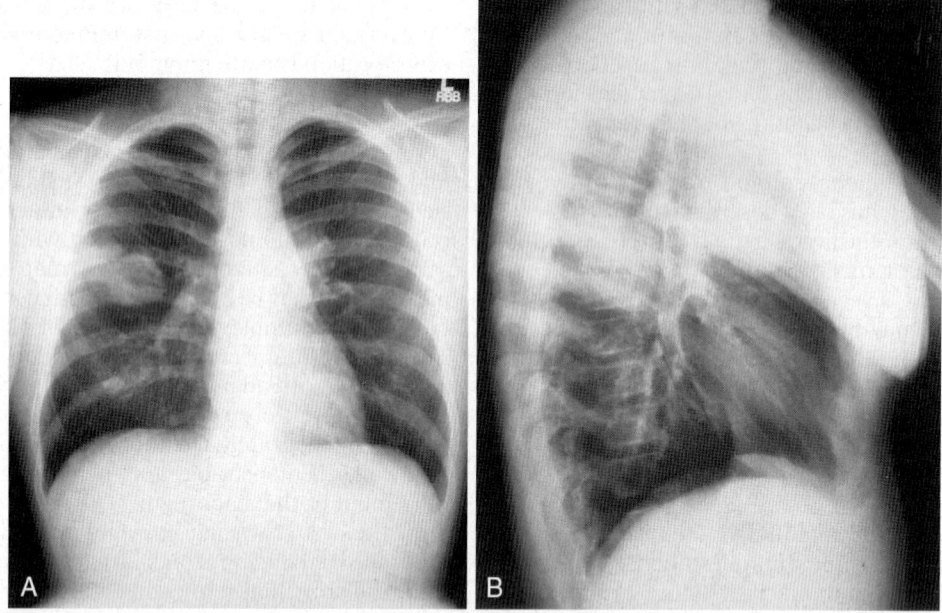

Fig. 33.2 The posteroanterior (A) and lateral (B) chest radiographs from a 15-year-old boy with cough of several months' duration show bilateral circumscribed densities in the anterolateral right upper lobe and the superior left lower lobe. Histopathology after excision confirmed the diagnosis of hydatid cysts.

WHO-IWGE Classification of Ultrasound Images of Cystic
Echinococcosis Cysts

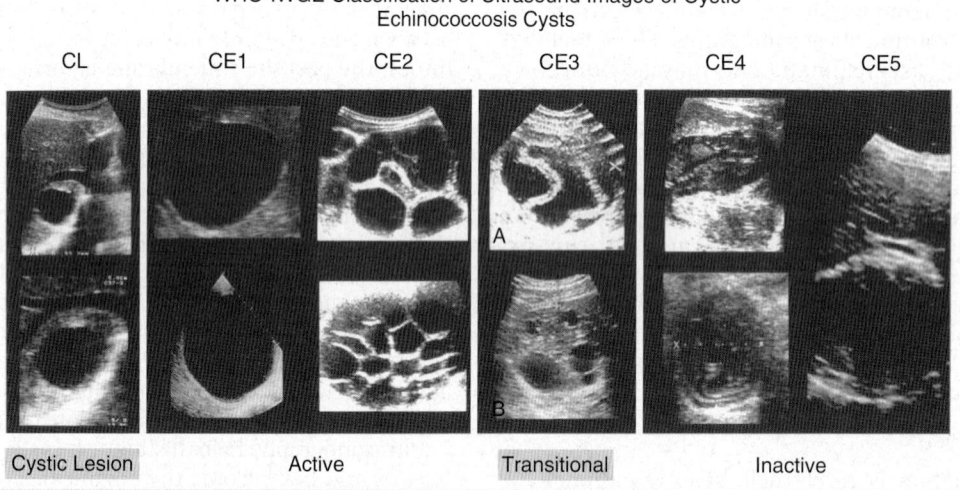

Fig. 33.3 WHO Informal Working Group on Echinococcosis (IWGE) classification of echinococcal cysts on ultrasound.

unilocular cysts. The inferior lobes are most commonly affected. In children, the ratio of intact to ruptured cysts is 3 : 1, which is the inverse of that in adults. Unlike spleen and liver hydatid cysts, calcification of lung cysts is rare. A high right hemidiaphragm and right basal bronchiectasis suggest bronchobiliary fistula. A tract on sinogram or bronchogram is diagnostic. CT and magnetic resonance imaging (MRI) can also be used and may help with better documentation and definition of the vascular and biliary anatomy in complicated cases (Fig. 33.4).[68,69]

Hepatic function may be abnormal in one-half of patients with liver cysts. An increased specific serum IgE may be observed, but eosinophilia is more often absent than present and is completely unreliable in areas endemic for other parasites.

DIAGNOSIS AND DIFFERENTIAL DIAGNOSIS

The coughing up of hydatid cyst elements, described as "coughing up grape skins," is diagnostic (see Fig. 33.1). Awareness of the disease is most important. Lung involvement is very likely if a cyst is present elsewhere in the body. Cystic hydatid disease is suspected based on a history of current or previous residence in an endemic area, clinical observations, and radiographic evidence. In 10% of cases, a diagnosis is suspected on routine radiographic study alone.[54] A history of contact with possibly infected dogs may be obtained in only half the cases.

The Casoni skin test involves injection of hydatid fluid in the dermis, which produces an erythematous papule in 50%–80% of patients in less than 60 minutes (Fig. 33.5).[70]

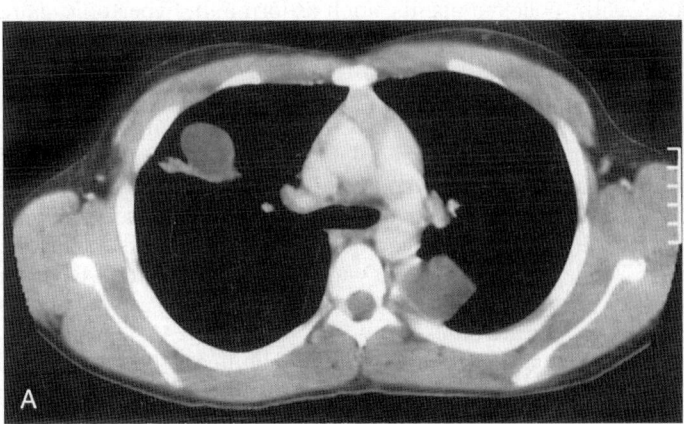
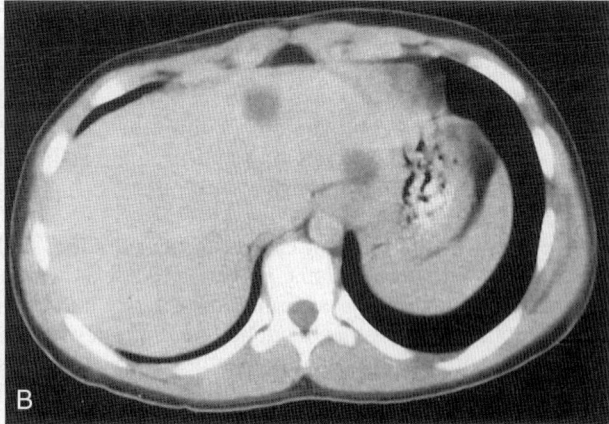

Fig. 33.4 Computed tomography (CT) of the chest (A) confirms the location of fluid-filled cysts in the anterior right upper lobe and the superior left lower lobe (same patient as in Fig. 33.1), and liver involvement is seen on abdominal CT (B).

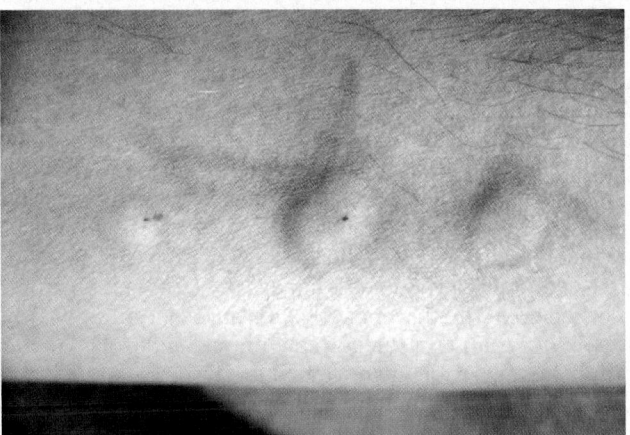

Fig. 33.5 Casoni reaction.

False-negative results, sometimes due to infected cysts, and false-positive results occur in 30% of those tested. With the development of improved serologic tests, the Casoni skin test is less commonly used.

Serologic tests include latex agglutination, indirect hemagglutination, complement fixation, agar gel diffusion, enzyme immunoassay, and immunoblot.[71,72] Cross-reactivity between echinococcosis and cysticercosis (*Taenia solium* infection) is a problem with any test that employs whole-cyst antigens. Serum antibody testing by indirect hemagglutination is 91% sensitive and 83% specific at a titer greater than or equal to 1:128. Immunoblot is 86% sensitive and 99% specific. It has been suggested that the Casoni test and indirect haemagglutination tests be used together in the diagnosis of hydatid disease to establish the diagnosis particularly in endemic areas where this remains a problem.[73] Most recently, rapid diagnostic tests have been developed that may be useful and may complement ultrasound findings in uncertain cases.[74]

After surgical removal of the cyst, there is generally a rapid decline in antibodies within 3 months although they may persist for years. Failure to observe the decline suggests incomplete cyst removal. Serum antibody tests can be referred to the CDC. False-negative results are more common in children and with pulmonary cysts. Up to 50% of patients with hydatid cysts in the lung or calcified cysts are seronegative.

Laboratory tests may be more sensitive in complicated cysts, but at present, no single test is infallible, and there is still no serologic test that can effectively rule out the disease. Thus, disease awareness is most important.

Differential diagnosis of hydatid disease includes abscess, hamartoma, pulmonary arteriovenous fistula, benign granuloma, malignant tumor, metastases, and cysts of different origin. When present, the Cumbo sign is pathognomonic.

MANAGEMENT AND TREATMENT

The treatment options for cystic echinococcosis include surgery, ultrasound-guided aspiration, and chemotherapy. Each method has limitations depending on the specific case. Spontaneous cure is possible after coughing out the cyst and its contents, but more commonly, infection and toxemia follow from the residual cyst. Up to two-thirds of symptomatic patients may die without intervention. Surgery used to be the treatment of choice along with antihelminthic treatment prior to the introduction of ultrasound guided percutaneous drainage, which is now used widely.[75] Endoscopic retrograde cholangiopancreatography should be performed prior to the procedure to ensure that no connections exist with the biliary tree. The acronym PAIR has been used to describe the process that is puncture, aspiration, injection, and then reaspiration.[76] This process has shown a percent reduction in cyst size of 73%–99%.

Once the diagnosis has been confirmed by serology, followed by imaging, the patient should be pretreated with albendazole for a few days prior to percutaneous removal of the cyst.[60] Preoperative treatment has been reported to reduce intracystic pressure and simplify removal. However, it has also been reported that use of albendazole prior to surgery may itself contribute to rupture of the cyst.[77] This is much more likely to occur with large cysts (>6 cm in diameter) due to degenerative changes that occur in the cyst wall. Presurgical use of albendazole or mebendazole can reduce the recurrence of cystic echinococcosis.

Use of albendazole following removal is also controversial.[78] One group suggested treatment should continue for up to 1 month and less if the cyst is smaller (i.e., <6 cm in diameter). In another study, the authors reported that they only used albendazole if there was cyst spillage after surgery, partial cyst removal, or biliary rupture.[79] Most would agree, however, that there is a risk of recurrence if not treated with albendazole as high as 11% in one older report.[80]

Percutaneous removal of hydatid cysts has been reported, but has its limitations and generally cannot be used in the case of multiple cysts or cysts that appear solid, although successful percutaneous drainage of multiple cysts has been reported.

More recently, minimally invasive surgical techniques such as video assisted thoracoscopic surgery (VATS) as well as laparoscopic removal of cysts has also shown to be successful for uncomplicated cysts.[81,82] In addition, techniques such as staged thoracotomy and pneumonostomy have been used for the treatment of multiple lung cysts as well as residual cavities in large complicated cysts.[83,84]

When percutaneous drainage is not possible, surgery is recommended, although conservative management with benzimidazoles may be equally effective in asymptomatic patients.[85] The success of surgery is dependent on the size and location of the cyst and on the skill of the surgeon. If surgery is indicated, it is important to perform surgery immediately after diagnosis, because a weak adventitial reaction and bronchial communications may lead to rupture with intrapulmonary dissemination. Only in the benign Alaskan-Canadian variant is conservative treatment recommended.

The aims of surgery are total eradication of the parasite with evacuation of the cyst and removal of the endocyst, prevention of cyst rupture and consequent dissemination during the operation, along with extirpation of the residual cavity. The lung parenchyma should be preserved and resection should be avoided in children if possible, because the damaged lung parenchyma has great capacity for recovery. Lung resection may be done in cases with bronchiectasis, severe inflammation, and large or multiple cysts that have destroyed lung parenchyma. The posterolateral approach is favored.[60] Surgical techniques to eradicate the parasite may include puncture and aspiration of cysts *in situ*, excision of the entire cyst by enucleation, wedge resection, segmentectomy, lobectomy, or pneumonectomy. Surgical procedures such as enucleation with or without obliteration of the residual cavity by sutures (capitonnage) and cystectomy are mainly used for uncomplicated cysts.[60] Lobectomy or segmental resection is reserved for lungs destroyed by large cysts or bronchobiliary and biliary-pleural fistulas.

The following YouTube video links show removal of hydatid lung cysts both using VATS and open surgical procedures:

https://www.youtube.com/watch?v=1a5DCaSgsuQ
https://www.youtube.com/watch?v=CT-cf-BNazc
https://www.youtube.com/watch?v=SP6qgL8dMZE

Rupture and spillage may occur during surgery and lead to dissemination and anaphylaxis, which can be fatal. This complication, although uncommon even with spillage during surgery, is greatly feared. Anaphylaxis remains a concern, although an extensive literature search showed that lethal anaphylaxis has been a relatively rare event.[86] The differences in surgical techniques therefore reflect the desire to prevent spillage of viable cyst contents. Commonly, the operative field is protected with saline-moistened gauzes, and the cysts are gently manipulated.

After extirpation of the parasite, bronchial fistulas are closed. To prevent recurrence, the residual cavity is injected with scolicidal agents, such as formalin, hypertonic saline, povidone-iodine, or absolute alcohol and albendazole.[87] Because of extremely grave complications with the use of formalin and hypertonic solutions, some have used hydrogen peroxide with good results. The residual cavity is then either obliterated by sutures or left open to communicate with the pleural space. Alternatively, the pericystic membrane is resected with repair of bronchial leakage. Bronchobiliary fistulas may rarely occur following liver hydatid cyst disease. While the management was traditionally thought to be surgical, conservative management has been used with success in less severe cases.[88]

Medical treatment alone has limited success, although results may vary according to the individual case. Between 30% and 50% of cases show some improvement after medical treatment based on imaging findings. Chemotherapy alone is indicated when percutaneous drainage and/or surgery is impractical or impossible, when patients have multiple cysts in two or more organs, when peritoneal cysts are present, and for recurrent disease.[89]

According to the WHO guidelines, benzimidazoles (e.g., mebendazole or albendazole) are the chemotherapeutic agents of choice.[66] Albendazole is the preferred treatment option in the United States, since mebendazole is no longer available in the United States. Albendazole differs from mebendazole in two respects: it is absorbed at a higher rate and it undergoes almost total first-pass metabolism to its effective protoscolicide metabolite, albendazole sulfoxide.[85] Its plasma concentration in hydatid-infested patients is about 10–40 times higher than that achieved with mebendazole. Cyst fluid concentrations also are higher than those achieved with mebendazole. Further enhancement of drug concentration in target tissues may be possible with the concurrent use of cimetidine or administration with a fat-rich meal. Albendazole is usually well tolerated. Liver function may be abnormal in 10%–20% of patients during treatment, but side effects are rarely severe. Use of albendazole has been shown to be a safe and effective alternative to surgery for treating uncomplicated liver cystic *Echinococcosis* and requires a shorter hospital stay. Albendazole should not be used during the first trimester of pregnancy because it has teratogenic effects in animals, although these have not been observed in humans.

Mebendazole interferes with uptake of glucose by cestodes and disrupts their microtubule system, but it is poorly absorbed and produces low blood concentrations.[85] Absorption is enhanced with meals. Repeated courses may be necessary. Cure of hydatid disease has been achieved in 35%–75% of patients, and recurrence rates have been low. Adverse reactions to mebendazole may occur within the first month and include fever and allergic reactions, alopecia, glomerulonephritis, and reversible leukopenia. With hepatobiliary disease, high blood levels and toxicity have been observed. Monitoring of clinical status, liver function, renal function, and complete blood count should be done weekly for the first month and biweekly thereafter.

Patients with chronic liver disease or bone marrow suppression should not undergo benzimidazole treatment. Another benzimidazole compound oxfendazole is available for use in veterinary practice only.

In addition to benzimidazoles, praziquantel may be added especially after surgery, when the risk of spillage is high.[90] Praziquantel when given alone is not effective, but it does act synergistically with albendazole. Although limited data are available, the dose recommended is 40 mg/kg per week.

PROGNOSIS

The more common surgical complications in children include atelectasis, hydropneumothorax, wound infection, pleural reaction, and hemothorax. Other reported complications from surgery are chest infection, abscess, empyema, septic shock, bronchial rupture, pneumothorax, bronchobiliary and/or biliary-pleural fistula, hemorrhage, massive aspiration, prolonged drainage, bronchiectasis, and allergic reactions, including anaphylactic shock and death with rupture.

The cysts' unusual location is the cause of the following reported rarer complications: arterial emboli, portal hypertension, systemic venous obstruction, paraplegia, pleural effusion, phrenic nerve paralysis, transitory paralysis of cervical sympathetic chain, lower extremity thrombophlebitis, and stress ulcer.[91–93]

Hydatid lung disease is preventable. The use of veterinary taeniacides for dogs; proper disposal of carcasses and entrails of animals to prevent dogs from gaining access; and the proper practice of hand, food, and drink hygiene to prevent contamination from dog excrement are appropriate preventive measures. Follow-up abdominal ultrasonography should be done annually for 5 years or more after successful treatment of hydatid disease. A cyst cavity may remain, and serologic findings may be positive for several years.

SYLVATIC ALASKAN-CANADIAN VARIANT

The Alaskan-Canadian *Echinococcal* species is clinically and morphologically distinct and has been named *E. granulosus* var. *Canadensis*.[94] It is seen in the tundra and northern coniferous forests of North America, south to the Great Lakes, mainly among the native population, including the Eskimo, Aleut, and Native American Indians, 75% of whom live in areas where *E. granulosus* occurs. The wolf is the definitive host, and sometimes the dog, which ingests the tapeworm by eating the viscera of infected deer. Elk, reindeer, moose, and caribou also are intermediate hosts. Pig, sheep, and cattle resist the infection. In contrast, humans are not very suitable hosts.

The Alaskan-Canadian sylvatic infection is more benign; the cysts are smaller and more delicate, do not grow as rapidly, and produce fewer symptoms than the classic or pastoral *E. granulosus*. The risk of anaphylaxis with rupture is less, and the prospect for spontaneous cure without significant complications is excellent.

Most commonly affected organs are the liver and the lung, with lung involvement in 61% of the cases. Most cysts are simple, intact, and uninfected. For pulmonary cysts, the mean age is 22 years (5–77 years), and for liver cysts, it is 65.3 years (24–96 years). In patients with lung cysts, 71% are younger than 20 years. Only 6%–8% of cases are symptomatic, mostly because of cyst rupture, which occurs in some 26% of patients. Cough, purulent expectoration, and hemoptysis are usual complaints. Serious complications are rare, and no cases of anaphylaxis or seeding have been seen in the Alaskan or Canadian experience.

Diagnosis is based on a history of residence in an endemic area, exposure to dogs, and characteristic findings on routine radiographic study. Typically, a round or oval homogeneous waterlike density with clear-cut borders and no surrounding reaction is seen. Classic signs such as the water lily and crescent sign are rare. Laboratory tests are of little value. Eosinophilia is positive in only 29% of cases, hemagglutination in 10%, and the Casoni test in 56% of cases. With cyst leak or rupture, test results are usually but not always positive.

The surgical risk is minimal. Extrusion of the intact vesicle is not appropriate, and an open wedge resection of adventitia with intact cyst is favored. Gentleness is very important. The bronchial stump should be closed, and the defect in the lung obliterated. Alternatively, cystectomy may be performed.

Quite commonly, the cyst evacuates into the bronchi, and the symptoms disappear. Thus, surgery is not recommended for asymptomatic patients who are managed by observation. No serious morbidity and mortality have been reported with this approach.

Strongyloidiasis

EPIDEMIOLOGY

Strongyloidiasis is caused by the nematode *Strongyloides stercoralis*. It is considered one of the most neglected among the neglected tropical diseases.[95] Information on the prevalence of the infection is lacking from many countries; however, it is considered endemic in the tropical and subtropical as well as temperate regions of the world including countries where hygiene and sanitation are lacking; this includes parts of the southeastern United States.[96] Humans are the primary hosts, but primates, cats, and dogs also are frequently infested. Prevalence in the United States has been shown to be 0%–6.1% in selected populations. The numbers among immigrant populations as would be expected are higher, ranging from 0% to 46.1%.[97,98] Infections have also been reported among solid organ transplant recipients.[99,100] A strong association exists between *Strongyloidosis* and immunosuppression such as that seen in patients with malignancies and those on high-dose corticosteroid therapy.[101,102] While once believed to be an acquired immunodeficiency syndrome (AIDS) defining illness in individuals with human immunodeficiency virus (HIV) infection, it is now known that these individuals are not at particular risk for *Strongyloides* infection unless they are immunocompromised due to other concomitant conditions as opposed to HIV infection alone.[103]

ETIOLOGY

The etiologic agent is *Strongyloides stercoralis*. Other species that are known to cause disease in humans include *S. fuelleborni*, while *S. myopotami* and *S. procyonis* are reported to infect animal hosts.[104]

PATHOLOGY/PATHOGENESIS

The life cycle of *S. stercoralis* is more complex than other nematodes because of its alteration between free-living and parasitic cycles and its potential for autoinfection and multiplication within the human host. The female worm is infectious and lays its embryonated eggs in the intestine; the rhabditiform larvae hatch in the mucosa and then bore through the epithelium and migrate into the intestinal lumen and are excreted in stool. The rhabditiform larvae in the soil, under suitable warm and moist conditions, develop into filariform larvae (direct developmental cycle). However, the rhabditiform larvae can also develop into free-living (non-parasitic) adult male and female helminthes who can mate and lay eggs in the soil (indirect developmental cycle). These eggs then hatch into rhabditiform larvae that can develop into infectious filariform larvae. Similar to the hookworm, these infectious larvae can penetrate human skin, enter the bloodstream, and reach the heart and lungs. In the lung, they molt, climb up the bronchi and trachea, and are swallowed. Once in the intestinal mucosa and crypts, they complete their life cycle. Internal autoinfection can occur, when rhabditiform larvae in the lower bowel develop directly into filariform larvae that in turn penetrate the intestinal mucosa and gain access into lymphatic and hematogenous systems and reach the lung and bowel to complete their life cycle. Massive autoinfection can induce hyperinfection syndrome (HS).[105] Another phenomenon referred to as external autoinfection occurs when the filariform larvae penetrate the perianal skin. The larvae are sensitive to dryness and extreme temperatures.

CLINICAL FEATURES

Symptoms

Strongyloides stercoralis infection encompasses five clinical syndromes: (1) acute infection with Loeffler syndrome, (2) chronic intestinal infection, (3) asymptomatic autoinfection, (4) symptomatic autoinfection, and (5) HS with dissemination.[106] The latter is of particular concern in immunocompromised and transplant patients. The pathogenesis of HS may involve disruption in Th 2 cell-mediated, humoral, or mucosal immunity, which triggers conversion of the rhabditiform larvae into filariform larvae, which then migrate from the small intestines to other organs. The mortality of HS is 15% increasing to 87% when there is dissemination.[105,107] Because of the autoinfection phenomenon, patients may have symptoms for years.

Symptoms fall into three broad categories: cutaneous, intestinal, and pulmonary and can occur during acute or chronic disease and during HS. The acute disease is often recognized by its cutaneous manifestations followed by pulmonary and intestinal symptomatology.[108–112] The hallmark of cutaneous symptoms is pruritus at the site of larval entry, usually at the foot or ankle but sometimes also the perianal area. The site of entry has erythema and edema with a petechial or urticarial localized skin rash. Within a week or so, the migration of larvae into the trachea-bronchopulmonary tree causes itching of the throat, dry cough, and Lofflerlike pneumonia with eosinophilia. This is followed by intestinal manifestations that include colicky abdominal pain (often epigastric), diarrhea, flatulence, and malaise.

Symptoms may be recurrent or continuous as the patient enters the chronic stage of the disease. This stage, if not treated, can last decades. With chronic infection, the cutaneous features include stationary urticaria and larva currens (similar to larva migrans).[108] Gastrointestinal symptoms are similar to those in the acute disease and can range from mild to severe. Burning or colicky abdominal pain can accompany diarrhea that can contain blood and mucus and alternate with constipation. In addition, patients may complain of anorexia, nausea, vomiting, flatulence, and perianal pruritus. There also may be epigastric tenderness.

Chronic pulmonary manifestations include dry cough and wheezing. Patients may present with asthma.[113,114] It has been suggested that patients with asthmalike symptoms from endemic areas should be screened for *Strongyloides* infection.[113] With worsening infection, patients may complain of fever, malaise, dyspnea, weakness, and weight loss. One-half of affected patients with chronic strongyloidiasis may be asymptomatic.

HS occurs because of disseminated strongyloidiasis from massive autoinfection, resulting in an overwhelming larval burden and increased dissemination of the larvae to the lungs and other organ systems. This results in severe pulmonary and extrapulmonary systemic symptoms. Although this syndrome can occur without a predisposing cause, it is usually associated with depressed cellular immunity caused by malnutrition, hematologic malignancies, or immunosuppressive therapy (e.g., steroids or anti-tumor necrosis factor [TNF]-α).[101,102]

Pulmonary manifestations in patients with HS include increasing cough and dyspnea along with mucopurulent or blood-tinged sputum. Severe hypoxemia may also occur. Occasionally, hemoptysis or pulmonary hemorrhage may be seen.[110] Pneumonia, bronchitis, and pleural effusion have all been associated with *Strongyloides* infection. Rarely, miliary abscesses may form.[115,116]

Physical Findings

These depend mainly on the extent of the disease. Wheezing, rhonchi, and crackles on lung exam may all be noted. Tenderness on abdominal examination and skin rashes may be present.

Imaging, PFT, Laboratory Findings

The chest radiograph is normal in most infected patients.[108] During pulmonary larval migration, there may be irregular and transient patches of pneumonitis or fine nodularity.[117] Hyperinfection is accompanied by chest radiographic changes that range from focal to diffuse pulmonary infiltrates, to cavitation and abscess formation.

As with many parasitic infections, peripheral blood eosinophilia is seen, although this is usually absent in HS, since use of corticosteroids reduces the levels of circulating eosinophils by inhibiting their proliferation and increasing apoptosis.[118]

DIAGNOSIS AND DIFFERENTIAL DIAGNOSIS

Similar to the other helminthic infections, the diagnosis of strongyloidiasis is best made by visual identification. For *S. stercoralis*, identifying the characteristic rhabditiform larvae in stool, sputum, or duodenal fluid is diagnostic. However, a single stool specimen has a sensitivity of only 15%–30%.[108,117] Stool concentration techniques may be required. Sensitivity increases to nearly 100% if seven consecutive daily stool specimens are examined in an expert laboratory, although this may not always be very practical. Serologic tests (gel diffusion and ELISA) are sensitive but often cross-react with other filarial parasites, thus limiting their usefulness, particularly in endemic settings. PCR of stool has been developed but may not be widely available, particularly in resource-poor countries.[118–121] CDC can provide confirmation of serologic tests that are equivocal or difficult to interpret.[122]

The combination of cutaneous, intestinal, and pulmonary symptoms, with eosinophilia on peripheral smear, and potential exposure in an endemic area provide essential clues for making the diagnosis. Pulmonary symptoms should be differentiated from pneumonitis caused by TB, mycoses, paragonimiasis, ascariasis, tropical pulmonary eosinophilia, and Löffler syndrome due to other causes.

The treatment is medical, and the goal is elimination of all the worms; therefore, repeated treatment is sometimes needed. Ivermectin is the drug of first choice followed by albendazole (see Table 33.1).[123,124] Thiabendazole in a dose of 25 mg/kg twice daily for 2–3 days (or 2–3 weeks for HS) has also been used and appears to have equal efficacy to Ivermectin with fewer side effects. Thiabendazole is only available for veterinary use in the United States; however, it is still used in other countries.[124] A recent report described the use of the veterinary preparation of Ivermectin in two patients with severe HS with successful outcomes.[125] After completion of initial treatment, patients must be followed for years to ensure complete eradication of all worms.

Screening strategies should be considered in patients who may be particularly vulnerable to *Strongyloides* infections.[126–128] These include patients who are on or about to start corticosteroid or other immunosuppressant therapy, those known to have human T-lymphotropic virus (HTLV)-1 infection, individuals with hematologic malignances, those about to undergo organ transplantation, those with persistent and unexplained eosinophilia, and individuals with recent or remote travel histories to endemic areas. As with any of the other parasitic infections, the best method of prevention includes proper disposal and treatment of sewage material.

Pulmonary Paragonimiasis (Lung Fluke Disease)

EPIDEMIOLOGY

Paragonimiasis, also known as lung fluke disease, Japanese lung fluke, oriental lung fluke, and pulmonary distomiasis, is caused by the genus *Paragonimus* and causes a zoonotic infection of carnivorous animals, including those in the canine and feline families (which also serve as reservoir hosts). Most human disease is caused by *Paragonimus westermani* and occurs following consumption of raw, undercooked, or alcohol pickled crustaceans (namely shellfish). Occasionally ingestion of raw meat from a mammalian host may also cause the disease.[129] The disease is endemic in parts of Southeast (SE) Asia (including China, Philippines, Thailand, Vietnam, and Japan) but is also seen in North America and Africa. More than 30 species have been reported worldwide with at least 10 that can infect humans. Paragonimiasis is rare in children, because they are less likely to indulge in consumption of exotic food and because this helminth is not transmitted by fecal-oral transmission, by person-to-person contact, or from consumption of infested water.

ETIOLOGY

Apart from *P. westermani*, other species that can cause human disease include *P. heterotremus*, *P. skrjabini*, and *P. miyazakii*, which are all found predominantly in Southeast Asia; *P. africanus* and *P. uterobilateralis* in Africa; and *P. caliensis* and *P. mexicanis* in South and Central America. *P. kellicotti* is the only species that is endemic in North America.[130–132]

PATHOLOGY/PATHOGENESIS

P. westermani adult lung cysts have two adult flukes in them that lay eggs that reach the bronchi of the mammalian host either by penetrating the intact cyst wall or through rupture of the cyst wall. From the bronchi, the eggs reach the mouth and are either spit out or swallowed and then excreted in stool. In the water, these eggs embryonate and hatch in approximately 3 weeks. The hatched miracidium invades the first intermediate host (one of several families of snails), and after a protracted asexual cycle, they form sporocytes that turn into cercariae. These then enter the second intermediate host (crustaceans); here they encyst and form the infectious metacercariae that reach the definitive mammalian host. Once eaten by the definitive host, the metacercariae encyst in the duodenum, penetrate the intestinal wall to reach the liver, and change into flukes. These flukes migrate through the diaphragm into the lung. In the lung, over a period of 5–6 weeks, they mature into adult flukes and are encysted as a result of host immune response. Adult flukes begin to lay eggs 8–10 weeks after the infection. Human infection occurs by eating crustaceans that contain the parasite metacercariae.

As the life cycle of the fluke suggests, it can cause both pulmonary and extrapulmonary disease involving the brain, liver, skin and rarely eyes as well as other parts of the body.[129,133–136] The lesions are a result of direct mechanical damage by the flukes or their eggs or by the toxins released by the flukes. The host response also adds to the damage in the lungs when the host immune response takes the form of eosinophilic infiltration and the subsequent development of a cyst of host granulation tissue around the flukes. Besides the adult flukes, the cyst also contains eggs and Charcot-Leyden crystals.[137] The cysts are in the parenchyma of the lungs close to the bronchioles. The release of cyst contents can cause bronchopneumonia, and the cyst wall may fibrose and become calcified. In extrapulmonary infections, the flukes may form cysts, abscesses, or granulomata.

CLINICAL FEATURES

Symptoms

The symptoms depend on the site infected and the infectious burden. Some individuals may remain asymptomatic because of low inoculum burden. Pulmonary paragonimiasis has acute and chronic stages with different clinical manifestations. The main clinical manifestations of paragonimiasis are respiratory symptoms and eosinophilia. Once the flukes reach the lungs, the patient can have cough, dyspnea, and chest tightness or even pain; systemic symptoms of fever, malaise, and night sweats may also be present. The patient may recall being sick days or weeks before their current illness with fever, diarrhea, and abdominal pain. Chills and urticarial rash may occur, leading to the diagnosis of a viral syndrome. A peripheral smear at this time shows eosinophilia. The diagnosis of paragonimiasis is frequently not made in the acute stage of the disease. The chronic stage usually follows 2–4 months later. Most patients look well, and the disease may resemble chronic bronchitis or bronchiectasis with a worsening cough that starts out dry and becomes productive and profuse. The sputum is gelatinous and blood streaked or rusty brown in color. Hemoptysis can be frequent and life threatening.[138] Low-grade fever along with vague pleuritic chest pain may be present. Patients also may have weight loss and complain of muscular weakness. Given the similarity of the clinical complaints, patients are frequently misdiagnosed and treated for pulmonary TB.[139–142]

Physical Findings

In uncomplicated pulmonary paragonimiasis, the chest examination may be remarkably normal. Children rarely have digital clubbing. Other physical findings would depend on disease manifestations. Pulmonary paragonimiasis can be complicated by lung abscess, pneumothorax, pleural adhesions, empyema, and interstitial pneumonia. As noted previously, pulmonary disease may be associated with abdominal (hepatic or peritoneal) and cerebral disease.

Imaging, PFT, Laboratory Findings

Chest radiography may be normal in acute pulmonary paragonimiasis, or it may show peribronchitis and hilar lymphadenopathy. However, in chronic paragonimiasis, chest radiography may show various abnormalities, including patchy nodular or linear infiltration, well-defined homogeneous densities, pleural thickening, effusion, and calcification.[143,144] The pathognomonic radiographic picture shows a ring shadow with a crescent-shaped opacity along one side of the border.[145] CT scan may define the cavities much better.[146] In addition, the detection of a migration track may also help narrow the differential and point to the diagnosis.[147] Similar findings may be seen on MRI.[148] On routine laboratory investigation, eosinophilia may be seen although leukocytosis is not common. Pleural fluid findings may include eosinophilia and increased lactic dehydrogenase levels, as well as low glucose[139]

DIAGNOSIS AND DIFFERENTIAL DIAGNOSIS

History is important in the diagnosis. In the United States, the most likely patient is a refugee, a recent immigrant, or someone with a recent history of travel. Similar to other protozoal infections, the definitive diagnosis can be made by identifying the characteristic golden brown, ellipsoidal operculated protozoal eggs. The characteristic operculated eggs can be identified in sputum or stool specimens, although the sensitivity of the tests is low. Repeat examination may increase the sensitivity of these tests. Bronchoalveolar lavage also has been successful in identifying the eggs and making the diagnosis. In complicated pulmonary paragonimiasis, the eggs can be identified in pleural fluid or lung abscess material. Rarely, adult flukes can be identified in the sputum. Serologic tests using various techniques (immunoblot,

counterimmunoelectrophoresis, complement fixation, and ELISA) are sensitive (96%) and specific (99%).[149] They are more useful in diagnosing extrapulmonary paragonimiasis. Skin testing cannot be used to make a diagnosis.

Pulmonary TB is the major differential diagnosis because the same endemic areas also have a high prevalence of TB. Other conditions to consider include bronchial asthma, chronic bronchitis, pulmonary neoplasm, and other parasitic infections endemic for the region.

MANAGEMENT AND TREATMENT

Treatment is with praziquantel 25 mg/kg 3 times daily after meals for 2 days (see Table 33.1). Cure rates greater than 95% have been reported.[150] Another drug used more recently with promising results is triclabendazole.[150]

PROGNOSIS

Prevention efforts should be aimed at educating the public against the use of untreated fresh water for drinking or cooking and avoiding improperly prepared or raw crustaceans.

References

Access the reference list online at ExpertConsult.com.

Suggested Reading

American Academy of Pediatrics. Toxocariasis. In: Kimberlin DW, Brady MT, Jackson MA, et al, eds. *Red Book. 2015 Report of the Committee on Infectious Diseases*. 30th ed. Elk Grove Village, IL: American Academy of Pediatrics; 2015:786–787.

Budke CM, Carabin H, Ndimubanzi PC, et al. A systemic review of the literature on cystic echinococcosis frequency worldwide and its associated clinical manifestations. *Am J Trop Med Hyg*. 2013;88:1011–1027.

Chai JY. Praziquantel treatment in trematode and cestode infections: an update. *Infect Chemother*. 2013;45:32–43.

Craig JM, Scott AL. Helminths in the lungs. *Parasite Immunol*. 2014; 36:463–474.

Fürst T, Duthaler U, Sripa B, et al. Trematode infections: liver and lung flukes. *Infect Dis Clin North Am*. 2012;26:399–419.

Giovannini-Chami L, Blanc S, Hadchouel A, et al. Eosinophilic pneumonias in children: a review of the epidemiology, diagnosis, and treatment. *Pediatr Pulmonol*. 2016;51:203–216.

Lal C, Huggins JT, Sahn SA. Parasitic diseases of the pleura. *Am J Med Sci*. 2013;345:385–389.

Mazur-Melewska K, Jończyk-Potoczna K, Kemnitz P, et al. Pulmonary presentation of *Toxocara sp.* Infection in children. *Pneumonol Alerol Pol*. 2015;83:250–255.

Parise ME, Hotez PJ, Slutsker L. Neglected parasitic infections in the United States: needs and opportunities. *Am J Trop Med Hyg*. 2014;90:783–785.

Rubinsky-Elefant G, Hirata CE, Yamamoto JH, et al. Human toxocariasis: diagnosis, worldwide seroprevalences and clinical expression of the systemic and ocular forms. *Ann Trop Med Parasitol*. 2010;104:3–23.

Vijayan VK. Parasitic lung infections. *Curr Opin Pulm Med*. 2009;15:274–282.

Weatherhead JE, Hotez PJ. Worm infections in children. *Pediatr Rev*. 2015;36(8):341–352, quiz 353-354.

WHO-Preventive chemotherapy in human helminthiasis. http://apps.who.int/iris/bitstream/10665/43545/1/9241547103_eng.pdf. Accessed March 15, 2016.

Woodhall DM, Eberhard ML, Parise ME. Neglected parasitic infections in the United States: toxoxcariasis. *Am J Trop Med Hyg*. 2014;90:810–813.

Woodhall DM, Fiore AE. Toxocariasis: a review for pediatricians. *J Pediatric Infect Dis Soc*. 2014;3:154–159.

SECTION 3

Pulmonary Disease in the Intensive Care Unit

34 Principles of Mechanical Ventilation

BHUSHAN KATIRA, MB, BS, DNB, TAKESHI YOSHIDA, MD, PhD, and
BRIAN P. KAVANAGH, MB, FRCPC

History

Historical descriptions of artificial respiration include 18th-century devices for intubation, bag and mask ventilation, and application of negative extrathoracic pressure.[1] The widespread use of mechanical ventilation (MV) did not occur until the polio outbreaks of the 1950s when iron lungs (negative pressure chambers) were deployed. Bjorg Ibsen, a Danish anesthesiologist, was the first to deploy positive pressure ventilation for the care of these patients as the iron lung did not prevent aspiration and was inefficient in the presence of significant atelectasis.[2] Approximately 200 medical students manually ventilated patients via tracheostomies, and the overall mortality was 25%, compared with an anticipated rate of 90%. This laid the foundation for modern critical care medicine. Since then, devices for MV have become more sophisticated facilitating synchrony between the patient and the ventilator, the use of graphics, added measurements, and user friendliness.

Indications for Mechanical Ventilation

In most situations, the indications for MV are evident. The principal indications for MV in the critically ill are inadequate respiratory effort, or to recruit lung units and improve oxygenation. Causes of inadequate respiratory effort include a sustained increase in respiratory and metabolic demand (e.g., pneumonia, asthma, lung injury, sepsis, or metabolic acidosis), or underlying neuromuscular failure, such as acute or chronic paresis or fatigue.

MV is used during general anesthesia if respiration is inhibited or blocked by deep sedation, opioids, or neuromuscular blockade. Indications for intubation also include "protection" of the airway, when the patency of the airway is diminished from proximal airway obstruction due to edema or tumor, or is at risk from the aspiration of gastric contents or hemorrhage; in such situations, MV is usually added.

In addition to providing a "pumping" action that facilitates tidal gas exchange, MV is also used to provide elevated airway pressure, which recruits collapsed lung units (or maintains local recruitment), thereby improving oxygenation.

Finally, ventilation may be used in an emergency to provide hyperventilation when hypocapnia is temporarily sought in the management of acute intracranial hypertension.

Composition of a Mechanical Ventilator

The ventilator consists of a gas delivery system, in addition to several subsystems (Fig. 34.1). The delivery system in turn consists of a breath controller, a mode controller, and a demand sensor. The breath controller generates the flow (i.e., the tidal volume [V_T]), which may be entirely derived from the ventilator, or in part, from the patient's effort.

There are three elements at play in the delivery of a V_T. First, the breath is triggered (by ventilator timing, or is initiated by the detection of patient inspiratory effort). Second, the flow of gas is controlled either by attaining a certain pressure, or volume, during inspiration. If "pressure" is targeted, then the inspiratory gas flow will vary depending on the difference between the pressure in the airway at the trachea (measured) and that in the alveoli (not measured), and will decrease as the inspiration progresses. If the "volume" is targeted, then the volume is delivered equally during each fraction of the inspiratory time (i.e., at a constant flow rate). Third, the ventilator "cycles off," to end inspiration and permit (passive) exhalation; as with initiating inspiration, cycling off can be initiated by ventilator timing or by detecting the patient's expiratory effort.[3]

Where initiation or termination of inspiration is governed by the patient, effort sensors are key. These detect changes in pressure (or flow), and the sensitivity (how sensitive is the ventilator to change in airway pressure or flow) and responsiveness (speed of response by the ventilator to such a change) of "effort sensors" are major determinants of satisfactory patient-ventilator interaction.[4]

Important additional components include gas blenders that mix air (21% O_2) and oxygen (100% O_2) to achieve the required F_IO_2. An "expiratory pressure generator" is required to maintain a certain pressure in the airway during expiration (termed: positive end-expiratory pressure, PEEP), to recruit atelectatic lung units, or to prevent their collapse.

Effective humidification and temperature control of the inspired gas is achieved by the use of special humidifiers, and the gas delivery circuit connects the ventilator to the interface (usually an endotracheal tube [ET], noninvasive ventilation mask, or ventilation hood).

Modes of Ventilation

Modes of MV can be described in terms of the type of "control" (pressure vs. volume) and the initiation of the breath (Fig. 34.2).[5]

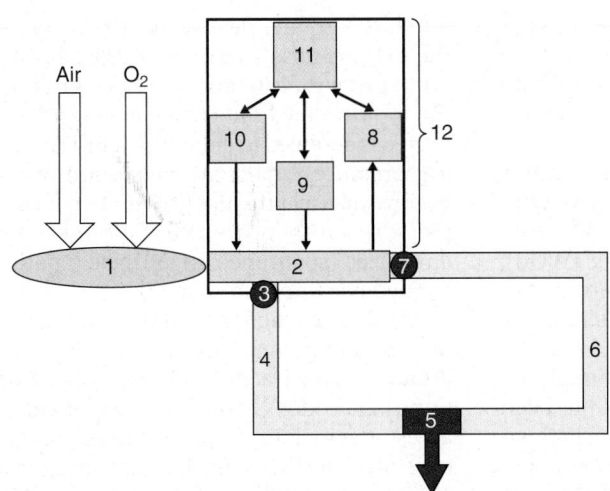

1. Gas Blender
2. Valving Systems
3. Inspiratory Flow/Pressure Controller
4. Inspiratory Limb of Ventilator Circuit
5. To Patient
6. Expiratory Limb of Ventilator Circuit
7. Expiratory Flow/Pressure Controller
8. Demand Sensors
9. Continuous Flow/Pressure Generator
10. Positive Pressure Breath Generator
11. Mode Controller
12. Gas Delivery System

Fig. 34.1 Basic ventilator design principle. The schematic illustrates the essential components of a mechanical ventilator: gas delivery system, gas blender, and patient circuit.

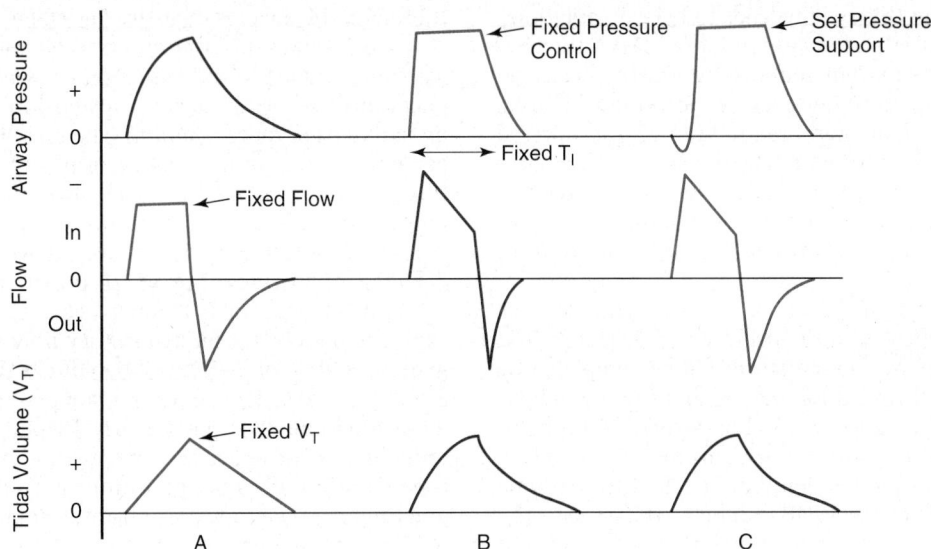

Fig. 34.2 Basic ventilation modes. The graph depicts changes in pressure, flow, and volume during a respiratory cycle for three commonly used modes: volume control (A), pressure control (B), and pressure support (C) ventilation. In volume control ventilation (A), tidal volume (V_T) is determined by the clinician, and so the inspiratory flow (volume per minute) is therefore also fixed. The pressure required to achieve the tidal volume depends on the lung compliance and resistance (which may change from breath to breath). During pressure control ventilation (B), the pressure, as well as the start time, duration, and finishing time of the inspiration are decided by the clinician. The resulting V_T depends on the lung compliance and resistance. Pressure support ventilation (C) is a spontaneous mode during which the breath is triggered by the patient (negative airway pressure deflection). The level of support (i.e., inspiratory airway pressure; pressure support) is chosen by the clinician. Inspiration ends and expiration begins when the inspiratory flow rate decreases to a predetermined level (usually 20%–30% of peak inspiratory flow). In contrast to pressure control ventilation, where inspiration is started and stopped by the ventilator timing, inspiration in pressure support ventilation is controlled by the patient. V_T, Tidal volume; T_I, inspiratory time.

The control reflects either volume or pressure. Volume control ventilation indicates that the V_T is predetermined. Because the inspiratory time is fixed, the volume is delivered through inspiration at a constant flow ("square wave" pattern); thus, inspiratory pressure reflects any changes in lung mechanics. The V_T is controlled at the set value by the ventilator, and is delivered independent of the chosen level of PEEP.

In pressure control ventilation the inspiratory pressure is constant; therefore, the pressure-time waveform is a "square wave" pattern. The flow (therefore the volume) of gas, which

depends on the pressure difference between the ventilator (gas source) and the alveoli (gas destination), diminishes over time (as the lungs fill). In addition, any changes in compliance, resistance or patient effort will alter the flow (but not the pressure). The initiation and termination of a pressure control breath depend on timing, that is the rate (breaths per minute), and the duration of inspiration (T_I), which are set on the ventilator.

In pressure support ventilation, the profile of pressure and principles of flow are the same as in pressure control. However, the initiation of a breath needs to be triggered by an inspiratory effort by the patient; in contrast, termination of inspiration occurs when the inspiratory flow rate falls to 20%–30% (chosen by the clinician) of the peak (initial) inspiratory flow rate, which occurs when a patient attempts to exhale.

The "type" of breath is the second main factor, and this describes the interaction between the patient and the ventilator. Continuous mandatory ventilation (CMV) indicates that the ventilator provides all the work of breathing (WOB); indeed, there is no ability for the patient to breath as the ventilation is set by the clinician and cannot be altered by the patient.

Assist control (AC) indicates that the patient can initiate (trigger) the breath, but as soon as the inspiration has been initiated, the ventilator completes the breath. The clinician sets the "minimum" (or back-up) number of breaths per minute, which is the number of breaths that will occur if the patient makes no effort. However, each breath initiated by the patient will be completed by the ventilator (regardless of the rate). Weaning is difficult with this mode, because every breath results in a full V_T—even if the AC rate is set to a low value—and this readily leads to hyperventilation.

With intermittent mandatory ventilation (IMV), the ventilator provides intermittent mandatory breaths based on the set minute ventilation; however, between these breaths, patients can make their own breaths that are not altered (assisted, completed, or inhibited) by the ventilator. In contrast to AC, patient breaths are not assisted by the ventilator; therefore, weaning the IMV rate means that the patient can make intermittent breaths of variable size without resultant hyperventilation.

Modern IMV is "synchronized" so that the ventilator sets windows of time each minute during which if a sufficient V_T is not completed by the patient it will be completed by the ventilator; synchronization means that these windows are reset every time an adequate V_T has occurred. This helps achieve better patient–ventilator synchrony.[6]

Continuous spontaneous ventilation refers to a simple mode wherein most of the WOB is done by the patient; the ventilator provides constant pressurization of the circuit (continuous positive airway pressure, CPAP), on which pressure support (see above) can be superimposed.

Although important for understanding the classification of ventilators, pure forms of CMV or IMV are almost never used in contemporary practice.

Noninvasive Ventilation

Noninvasive ventilation (NIV) describes the delivery of mechanical support through an interface (e.g., nasal prongs or mask, face mask, or helmet) and without the need for an ET. NIV offers the ability to reduce patient WOB and improve respiratory gas exchange while avoiding the risks and complications related to the placement of an ET, including sedation and neuromuscular blockade. In addition, it can easily be initiated during transport or in settings where intubation in not commonly performed.[7]

Conventional NIV is delivered using nasal cannula, nasal mask, full face mask, and helmet. A full-face mask or helmet more reliably provides positive airway pressure, but it may cause agitation, especially in infants and younger children,

and has a greater dead-space (requiring high flows to clear the CO_2). A nasal cannula or mask is often better tolerated but a pressure leak due to a poor interface seal or through the mouth may limit effectiveness.

NIV is designed to either deliver CPAP: Continuous distending pressure for the whole respiratory system) or bilevel positive airway pressure (BiPAP: two levels of positive airway pressure—inspiratory and expiratory). BiPAP is either synchronized (spontaneous) with each patient effort or with a defined back up rate (Timed).

NIV is particularly used in bronchiolitis, asthma, pneumonia, pulmonary edema, cystic fibrosis, acute chest syndrome, laryngotracheomalacia, and acute hypoxemic failure. Contraindications to the use of NIV include cardiopulmonary arrest, the inability to protect upper airway, poor neurological status, shock (requiring escalating vasopressors), upper gastrointestinal bleed, facial injuries, and untreated pneumothorax. The appropriate selection of interface and mode of NIV are key to optimizing support for children. It is clinically titrated to WOB, heart rate, subjective comfort, and oxygenation. Frequently BiPAP is used for ventilation failure; therefore, the effect is measured as efficacy of CO_2 removal.

Air leak syndrome, aspiration, and hemodynamic instability from cardiac preload reduction are serious but rare complications, whereas gastric distension and facial skin breakdown are more common. The inability to humidify the gas may lead to nasal/oral mucosal damage. Eye irritation, trauma, and inflammation can also result from improper mask fit and continuous exposure to high gas flow.

Heated high flow O_2 is a newer delivery system used to deliver gas flow rates of up to 8 L/min in an infant (or about 60 L/min in large child). It allows delivery of flow rates higher than the patient's peak inspiratory flow with fixed FiO_2. It generates PEEP of 2–5 cm H_2O, reduces WOB, improves tolerance of the oxygen delivery system, and reduces the need for intubation. It is particularly helpful in children with bronchiolitis and airspace disease without ventilation failure.[8] Importantly, it does not guarantee a fixed airway pressure, and thus may generate lower transpulmonary pressure than NIV, when a patient adds a significant inspiratory effort to the external ventilator support.

High-Frequency Ventilation

High-frequency ventilation (HFV) applies continuous distending pressure to maintain lung expansion, and superimposes small V_Ts at a rapid rate; the main type of HFV used is high-frequency oscillatory ventilation (HFOV). The small V_Ts result from oscillating air movements produced by the ventilator diaphragm or piston at frequencies of 600–900 breaths per minute (10–15 Hz), which result in both positive (inspiratory) and negative (expiratory) pressure fluctuations.

Two major concepts differentiate HFOV and so-called conventional ventilation (although HFOV has been in use for over 40 years). First, CO_2 is cleared despite using a V_T that is less than physiological dead-space, a phenomenon that is not possible using standard "bulk flow" kinetics. However, with HFOV, multiple mechanisms contribute to CO_2 removal. Second, CO_2 removal (which is increased by greater V_T, but not in a linear relationship), is increased by decreasing the frequency; this counterintuitive finding is because with a lower rate, the time to develop a V_T is increased, and this increases CO_2 clearance.

In most circumstances, the major use for HFOV is lung recruitment, and this is primarily a function of the mean airway pressure employed, and is assessed in terms of oxygenation response. The other key adjustments are the amplitude and frequency of the pressure wave, to achieve CO_2 clearance, as well as the inspired O_2 concentration (FiO_2).

HFOV has a long history in pediatric critical care. One subset of potential priority is ventilated children with neonatal pulmonary hypertension (e.g., congenital diaphragmatic hernia), where the major rationale is enhanced CO_2 clearance (below).

Neurally Adjusted Ventilator Assistance

Conventional MV tracks changes in airway pressure (and flow), and the assumption is that these parameters account for changes in the patient's respiratory "need" (i.e., respiratory drive). However, increased respiratory drive may not translate into increased diaphragmatic contraction, perhaps due to partial paralysis or muscle weakness. Further, increased diaphragm contractility may not translate into an adequately negative deflection of the pressure–time curve during expiration, due to lung injury and poor pressure transmission from the pleural space to the airway. Because the conventional ventilator only senses changes in airway pressure (or flow), there may be a significant discrepancy between the patient "need" (i.e., phrenic nerve output to the diaphragm) and the level of support supplied by the ventilator.[9]

Neurally adjusted ventilator assistance (NAVA) senses the electric activity of the diaphragm (EA_{di}), which is independent of ventilator, circuit, and respiratory mechanics, using a catheter embedded in a gastric tube. When electrical activity is greater than a set threshold ($0.5\ \mu V$) a mechanical breath is delivered; the size of the breath (of level of pressure) is based on the amplitude of EA_{di} and the level of assistance determined by the clinician. This results in breath-to-breath variation of V_T, and adjustment is made to the assist level such that a satisfactory V_T is delivered and a diminished EA_{di} signal is detected that reflects lessened patient demand. This approach should improve patient comfort and prevent over or under ventilation, relative to neutrally determined need.

Hemodynamic Effects of Mechanical Ventilation

The most important hemodynamic effects of MV are the impact on ventricular preload and afterload (Fig. 34.3). Positive ventilator pressure increases alveolar pressure and lung volume, and compressed the heart and the great veins in the thorax. Therefore, the compressed veins and right atrium can accommodate lower blood volume (than with spontaneous ventilation, i.e., "negative pressure"), and thus the venous return and preload (i.e., end-diastolic volume) are decreased. The lower preload results in a lower stroke volume, and therefore a lower cardiac output, which if severe, will result in hypotension. Patients particularly susceptible to the impact on preload are those with hypovolemia, tamponade, air

trapping (e.g., status asthmaticus), or those in incipient shock from any cause. The optimization of intravascular volume may mitigate this problem.

The effects of positive pressure ventilation on "compressing" the heart may be beneficial if the ventricle is less sensitive to reduced preload, but more sensitive to increased afterload. The afterload against which the ventricle contracts is the ventricular wall stress (i.e., the "transmural" pressure divided by the wall thickness):

Ventricular afterload
= [pressure inside – pressure outside]/(wall thickness)

Thus, positive pressure, by increasing the "outside" (i.e., pericardial = pleural, pressure) decreases wall stress, and this effect is proportionally greater if the ventricular performance is impaired (i.e., generates lower values of intraventricular pressure). In this situation, positive airway pressure assists the ventricle to eject, and provided the preload is adequate, this increases the cardiac output. In situations where the afterload is limiting the ventricular output (e.g., impaired contractility, mitral valve regurgitation), positive pressure ventilation increases cardiac output.

Finally, the effects of MV are especially useful in cardiogenic pulmonary edema where the rate of formation of edema is slowed, due to lower venous return to the thorax; and, the cardiac output is increased, which augments forward flow of blood out of the lungs.

Mechanical Ventilation in Specific Conditions

NORMAL LUNGS

General anesthesia is certainly the commonest indication for MV and most of these children have normal lungs. Here, evolving clinical evidence (from adult studies) raises the possibility that high V_T should be avoided in patients with normal lungs during general anesthesia. Children are commonly intubated (and ventilated) in the setting of encephalopathy, brain injury, or neuromuscular weakness (e.g., Guillain-Barré syndrome, myopathy, etc.), because of either impaired airway protection (e.g., inadequate airway reflexes or cough strength) or hypoventilation.

The main complications include atelectasis of dependent lung, or rarely, ventilator-associated pneumonia. The use of PEEP, endotracheal toilet, and the prevention of airway contamination offset most of these issues. Depending on the primary illness, recovery of strength and level of consciousness may be delayed, and tracheostomy may be indicated to maximize comfort, and to facilitate nursing care as well as weaning from MV.

ACUTE RESPIRATORY DISTRESS SYNDROME

Acute respiratory distress syndrome (ARDS) is an acute pathological condition characterized by inflamed, atelectatic lungs, resulting from an underlying condition (most commonly sepsis). While pathologically it is represented by characteristic histology termed "diffuse alveolar damage," it is

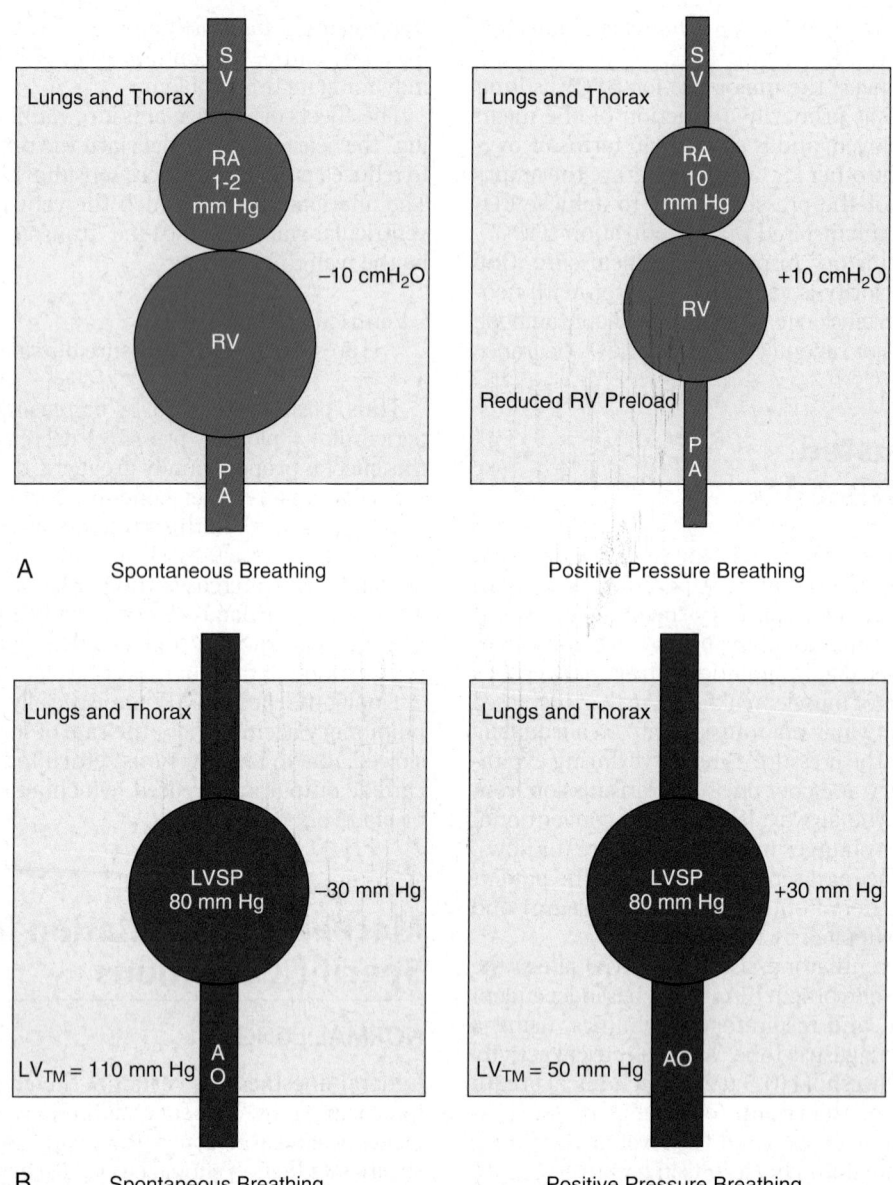

Fig. 34.3 Effect of positive pressure on hemodynamics. The schematic illustrates key effects of mechanical ventilation on preload (A) and afterload (B). During spontaneous breathing, the intrathoracic pressure is negative and the RA pressure is low; this draws blood into the thorax. During positive pressure, the intrathoracic pressure is positive and the major veins, RA and RV are compressed. This reduces venous return and, hence, the preload to the right (and left) heart. During spontaneous ventilation, due to negative intrathoracic pressure, the transmural LV pressure (i.e., pressure inside—pressure outside) is higher, whereas during positive pressure ventilation the transmural LV pressure is lower, but the inside pressure remains unchanged. Thus, positive pressure ventilation reduces LV wall stress and increases cardiac output. *AO*, Aorta; *LVSP*, left ventricular systolic pressure; *PA*, pulmonary artery; *RA*, right atrium; *RV*, right ventricle; *SV*, systemic veins.

suspected clinically in the setting of an acute respiratory deterioration accompanied by pulmonary infiltrates and impaired oxygenation. MV in these patients serves to reduce the WOB, and provide increased airway pressure to recruit atelectatic lung.

Perhaps the most important issue, having secured adequate oxygenation, is to minimize ventilator-associated lung injury (VALI). The mainstay of this approach is avoidance of high V_T although the optimum V_T[10] for children with ARDS, or for any child in particular, is not known.

A key principle in ventilator management is to keep the lung "open," and this likely represents sound practice in cases where it is possible. The use of recruitment maneuvers, and

the maintenance of the recruited lung (if recruitable) with elevated PEEP, is a standard approach. Where higher levels of PEEP are being contemplated (especially where the chest wall is noncompliant, e.g., obesity), an esophageal manometer might be used to determine the (real) transpulmonary distending pressure and thereby permit use of higher levels of PEEP. Alternative approaches to recruitment include prone positioning or the use of HFOV.

STATUS ASTHMATICUS

In status asthmaticus, ventilation failure due to exhaustion from prolonged or profound airway obstruction, is the major indication for assisted ventilation. Such failure is usually manifest as the inability to speak more than one or two words, or as a diminished level of consciousness.

In many cases, noninvasive ventilation with CPAP (or bi-level ventilation, BiPAP) can be effective via a facemask, while aggressive bronchodilator therapy and steroids are administered. The impact of positive airway pressure may be two-fold. First, there may be a simple reduction in the WOB due to the ventilator assistance with inspiration. Second, in rare cases, the positive airway pressure may maintain patency of the distal airways that are closed because of raised pleural pressure from intense expiratory effort; in this situation, the positive pressure "stents" open the airways and facilitate exhalation. Endotracheal intubation is reserved for cases in which NIV is ineffective; this is fraught because laryngeal and tracheal stimulation can worsen bronchospasm, and should involve expert airway management whenever possible.

BRONCHIOLITIS

Bronchiolitis due to childhood respiratory viruses is often complicated by airway inflammation, obstruction, mucus plugging, and atelectasis. This culminates in increased work of breathing (WOB) and impaired gas exchange. NIV or High Flow O_2 can reduce WOB by distending the airway and preventing its collapse, but progressive increases in WOB or worsening hypoxemia may be indications for invasive ventilation. Dynamic hyperinflation also can be a problem due to widespread bronchial inflammation, although mucus plugging is more common. Thus, balancing PEEP to reduce hyperinflation, and opening areas of atelectasis, is important. In this situation, V_T is targeted to 6–8 mL/kg, and the respiratory rate is titrated to allow better expiration.

THE NEONATE

Premature newborns may need respiratory support at birth for resuscitation, respiratory distress syndrome (RDS), persistent pulmonary hypertension (PPHN), sepsis, or simply to facilitate growth and development.[11]

During neonatal resuscitation, intubation is often elective and the duration of MV variable; however, in neonatal RDS, MV is specifically used to reduce WOB. In addition, MV facilitates the delivery of surfactant, and the prevention of elevated pressure after surfactant delivery is key to avoiding the pulmonary air leak syndrome.

PPHN is an entity unique to neonates, where oxygenation failure occurs in the absence of acute lung disease or congenital heart disease; here, there is a prepost ductal oxygenation gradient reflecting profound pulmonary hypertension (which can be identified and quantified using an echocardiogram). The goal of MV in this disease is to provide O_2, recruit lung (if recruitable), and to assist in clearing CO_2 to minimized respiratory acidosis and to alleviate pulmonary hypertension. The use of HFOV in this setting (as in congenital diaphragmatic hernia) should exploit the technique's unique ability to effectively clear CO_2 in neonates, and should not be used to recruit (nonrecruitable) lung; the mechanism of improved oxygenation is usually through the relief of pulmonary hypertension, and thereby reduced right to left shunting. The judicious use of high FiO_2 (a pulmonary vasodilator), longer T_{Ins}, lowering $PaCO_2$, and the use of inhaled nitric oxide arc important elements in the management of PPHN.

CONGENITAL HEART DISEASE

In patients with elevated pulmonary blood flow (e.g., caused by a large left-to-right shunt or single ventricle physiology), the use of lower FiO_2, adequate PEEP to maintain functional residual capacity, and hypercapnia to increase pulmonary vascular resistance, may each help limit pulmonary blood flow.

Where the pulmonary blood flow is primarily low (e.g., teratology of Fallot), adjusting the level of PEEP and V_T volume may allow increased lung blood flow. With a Glenn circulation, (bidirectional cavo-pulmonary shunt), the presence of hypercapnia increases cerebral blood flow, and thereby increases pulmonary perfusion. In addition, early extubation (and resumption of spontaneous ventilation) may be beneficial in right heart failure, and the Glenn and Fontan circulation. In contrast, for left heart failure or mitral regurgitation, positive pressure ventilation augments cardiac output.

Management During Mechanical Ventilation

MONITORING

Monitoring assists in the ongoing management of all patients. The key monitoring of the ventilated child is for comfortable ventilation, including oxygenation and WOB. Deterioration in WOB mandates immediate attention to consider the status of the underlying condition and the possible development of a complication, such as a poor mask fit, obstructed or dislodged ET, or ventilator equipment failure. In the sedated and paralyzed patient pulse oximetry, end-tidal carbon dioxide and blood gas analysis are especially important. Chest roentgenography may help to determine the ET position, the evidence of air leak, and the development of new infiltrates, in addition to monitoring the baseline condition for which MV was instituted.

COMFORT

The presence of an ET, as well as pain from operative incisions or following trauma, coupled with anxiety associated with being in the intensive care unit, warrant judicious use of sedation and analgesia. This will assist in optimizing patient-ventilator synchrony.

SUCTIONING

Normal airway ciliary action, and coughing, moves respiratory secretions towards the mouth but the presence of the ET tube impedes this process, and an impaired cough, due to sedation (and perhaps paralysis), compounds the problem. Secretion volume and tenacity are increased with pulmonary infection or inflammation, and thus secretion clearance is a problem. Therefore, the presence of pneumonia, ARDS, bronchiolitis, or especially pulmonary hemorrhage, mandates careful and thorough suction, often with irrigation, to prevent airway occlusion from inspissated secretions.

SYNCHRONIZATION

Patient-ventilator dyssynchrony manifests as respiratory distress while receiving MV, and this is often observed as "fighting" the ventilator. This requires a careful review, first of the patient, to ensure that deterioration in the underlying condition or a treatable complication (e.g., blocked or displaced ET tube, pneumothorax) have not developed. The nature of the dyssynchrony then needs to be carefully examined to determine if the level of support (pressure, V_T, respiratory rate, FiO_2) is sufficient for the patient's demands, and, thereafter, if the patient is able to trigger the ventilator.[6] In many cases, the first step is to disconnect the ventilator circuit from the ET to facilitate independent assessment of the patient. Discomfort may cause asynchrony (and certainly asynchrony can be uncomfortable); determining the cause, and optimizing sedation and analgesia, is important.

GAS HUMIDIFICATION

The gas in the ventilator circuit is dry and can cause airway erosion. When ventilating children, humidification of the air-oxygen mixture is achieved by a chamber in the inspiratory limb of the ventilator circuit that contains water at 2–3°C above body temperature. In larger children, passive humidification can be accomplished by inserting a heat-moisture exchanger between the circuit and the ET.

FLUID MANAGEMENT

Aside from during active resuscitation, fluid restriction is preferred in most mechanically ventilated patients, because the insensible losses due exhaled humidified air are minimal. In addition, positive pressure ventilation can cause fluid retention (reduced renal perfusion, increased secretion of antidiuretic hormone). Obviously, the assessment of ongoing fluid losses will dictate the approach.

WEANING AND EXTUBATION

Weaning is the process of transferring all WOB from the ventilator to the patient. While a major problem in debilitated adults, this appears to be less of an issue in pediatric critical care medicine. The major concerns in preparing for extubation are adequacy of respiratory drive, muscle strength for coughing and ventilation, airway integrity, oxygenation, adequacy of analgesia (in burns or postoperative cases) and fluid status.[6] A brief trial of spontaneous breathing (T-piece, flow inflating bag) will make clear the child's respiratory drive and the neuromuscular status; it is usually not necessary to slowly reduce ventilator settings, and most children who are awake and pain-free can simply be extubated. Finally, planning should always address the likely cause of respiratory failure (should it occur) in a child before extubation, as well as the approach to airway management, if required.

NEUROMUSCULAR BLOCKADE

Neuromuscular blockade is commonly used in ventilated patients. It may be an important component of care in specific settings such as intracranial hypertension, or more recently,

in patients with ARDS (likely to minimize the additive lung injury from strong spontaneous effort superimposed on mechanical breaths). A major concern is use of paralysis when a patient is distressed: care must be taken that the airway is secure and that ET malposition is not the cause of agitation. In addition, sedation must be sufficient to prevent awareness during paralysis.

Complications of Mechanical Ventilation

Positive pressure ventilation can injure lungs directly, and this is called VALI; it primarily results from use of high V_Ts. This problem likely compounds any underlying lung injury (e.g., from pneumonia), and worsens the outcome. Pressure-induced damage (barotrauma) causes pulmonary air leak syndromes, which can vary from pulmonary interstitial emphysema to pneumothorax or bronchopleural fistula. Excessive recruitment maneuvers, extreme levels of PEEP, or high inspiratory pressure, lead to this kind of injury. Although 6 mL/kg is a widely recommended V_T for adults with ARDS, the optimal V_T in children is unknown.

Ventilator induced diaphragmatic dysfunction is being increasingly recognized and results from disuse (or overuse) of the diaphragm during MV. Steroids and paralysis can aggravate this problem.

Ventilation associated pneumonia (VAP) is defined as onset of new lung infection within 48 hours of intubation and ventilation. It is thought to result from aspiration of oropharyngeal secretions. However, VAP is poorly understood and most centers now look to alternative quality measures to manage the issue.

Subglottic stenosis secondary to intubation occurs in 1%–2% of intubated children in the intensive care unit. The incidence increases with the length of intubation, traumatic intubation, and preexisting airway inflammation. Steroids can reduce airway inflammation and may reduce the chances of subglottic stenosis. A subset of children may eventually need laryngoplasty to treat this condition.

Conclusion

MV is a life-saving supportive therapy in critically ill children, and is deployed for a variety of indications. Choosing the optimal mode, defining the goals, optimizing mechanics and gas exchange, enhancing patient–ventilator synchrony, and preventing ventilator-associated complications, are important principles of practice. Finally, ongoing monitoring and expert care are the keys to success.

References

Access the reference list online at ExpertConsult.com.

Suggested Reading

Amaddeo A, Frapin A, Fauroux B. Long-term non-invasive ventilation in children. *Lancet Respir Med.* 2016;4(12):999–1008.

Brower RG, Matthay MA, Morris A, et al. Ventilation with lower tidal volumes as compared with traditional tidal volumes for acute lung injury and the acute respiratory distress syndrome. *N Engl J Med.* 2000;342(18):1301–1308.

Chatburn RL, El-Khatib M, Mireles-Cabodevila E. A taxonomy for mechanical ventilation: 10 fundamental maxims. *Respir Care*. 2014;59(11):1747–1763.

Ibsen B. The anaesthetist's viewpoint on the treatment of respiratory complications in poliomyelitis during the epidemic in Copenhagen, 1952. *Proc R Soc Med*. 1954;47(1):72–74. No abstract available.

Levy SD, Alladina JW, Hibbert KA, et al. High-flow oxygen therapy and other inhaled therapies in intensive care units. *Lancet*. 2016;387(10030):1867–1878.

Owen LS, Manley BJ, Davis PG, et al. The evolution of modern respiratory care for preterm infants. *Lancet*. 2017;389(10079):1649–1659.

Sinderby C, Navalesi P, Beck J, et al. Neural control of mechanical ventilation in respiratory failure. *Nat Med*. 1999;5(12):1433–1436.

Tobin MJ. Advances in mechanical ventilation. *N Engl J Med*. 2001;344(26):1986–1996.

Tobin MJ. Conventional methods of ventiatory support. In: Tobin MJ, ed. *Principle and Practice of Mechanical Ventilation*. 3rd ed. New York: McGraw Hill; 2013.

Tobin MJ. Mechanical ventilation. *N Engl J Med*. 1994;330(15):1056–1061.

35 Childhood Pulmonary Arterial Hypertension

USHA KRISHNAN, MD, DM, and ERIKA BERMAN-ROSENZWEIG, MD

Introduction

Pulmonary arterial hypertension (PAH) is a serious progressive condition with a poor prognosis if not identified and treated early. Until recently, the diagnosis of idiopathic pulmonary arterial hypertension (IPAH, formerly termed primary pulmonary hypertension [PPH]) was virtually a death sentence, particularly for children, with a median survival of less than 1 year.[1–4] The data in the Primary Pulmonary Hypertension-National Institutes of Health (PPH NIH) Registry illustrated the worse prognosis for children than adults.[1] In this registry, the median survival for all of the 194 patients was 2.8 years, whereas it was only 0.8 years for children. Fortunately, there has been promising progress in the field of PAH over the past several decades, with significant advances in treatment that can improve quality of life, exercise capacity, hemodynamics, and survival.[5–7] Nevertheless, extrapolation from adults to children is not straightforward. This chapter will review childhood PAH, with an emphasis on the latest therapeutic advances.

Definition and Classification

In children, per the pediatric American Heart Association/American Thoracic Society (AHA/ATS) guidelines, PAH is defined as having a mean pulmonary artery pressure (PAPm) ≥ 25 mm Hg at rest, beyond 3 months of age at sea level with a normal pulmonary artery wedge pressure (<15 mm Hg), and an elevated pulmonary vascular resistance (PVR > 3 Wood Units $\times$ m^2). PH is defined as mPAP >25 mm Hg in children >3 months of age at sea level. PAH occurs in the "precapillary" pulmonary vascular bed and therefore excludes causes of pulmonary venous hypertension (e.g., mitral stenosis). Although exercise hemodynamic abnormalities are no longer included in the updated definition of PAH, they may still be an important measure in some children, because children with PAH often have an exaggerated response of the pulmonary vascular bed to exercise.[8,9] The exclusion of exercise-induced PAH was based on the difficulty in reliably obtaining complete exercise hemodynamics and the concern that some subjects could be misdiagnosed as having exercise-induced PAH. Children also have a greater vasoreactive response to hypoventilation than adults. Not uncommonly, children with a history of recurrent exertional or nocturnal syncope have a resting PAPm that markedly increases with exercise and with modest systemic arterial oxygen desaturation during sleep.

EVOLUTION OF THE CLASSIFICATION OF PULMONARY HYPERTENSION

The first WHO World Symposium in 1973 classified PH into primary and secondary PH. In 1998, at the second World Symposium in Evian, clinical investigators from around the world proposed a new diagnostic classification; this classification categorized pulmonary vascular disease by similar clinical features, histopathology, hemodynamics, and management. PH was classified into five basic groups: PAH (group 1), left heart disease (group 2), lung disease (group 3), chronic thromboembolic PH (CTEPH; group 4), and multifactorial PH (group 5). At the 2003 Venice meeting, the term "PPH" was changed to "IPAH," reflecting the fact that this is a diagnosis of exclusion with exact cause(s) yet unknown.[10–12] Thus, in addition to IPAH (both sporadic and familial), PAH associated with congenital heart disease (CHD); connective tissue disease (CTD); portal hypertension; HIV infection; drugs and toxins (including anorexigens); and persistent pulmonary hypertension of the newborn (PPHN) were classified along with IPAH as group I PAH. In 2008 at Dana Point, the diagnostic classification system was updated further, and the term "familial pulmonary arterial hypertension" (FPAH) was abandoned in favor of heritable PAH (HPAH), defined to include all subjects with FPAH, plus any patients with an identified genetic mutation, regardless of whether there was a family history of PAH. Pulmonary veno-occlusive disease and pulmonary capillary hemangiomatosis, which share many similarities with group I PAH but have subtle variations, was separated out to group I'. Finally, in 2013, at the fifth World Symposium held in Nice, France, although the basic framework was maintained, it was decided in conjunction with the pediatric PH task force to add elements related to pediatric PH and have a comprehensive classification common for all age groups, reflecting the understanding that many children with PH will grow up to become adults with PH (Box 35.1).[11]

Although the classification helps our understanding of the pathophysiology of PAH patients, it also has implications for the natural history. Despite the different physiologic classifications of group 1 PH, the histopathologic changes are virtually identical, so similar treatment strategies have evolved. As insight is advanced into the mechanisms responsible for the development of PAH, the introduction of novel therapeutic modalities will hopefully increase the overall efficacy of therapeutic interventions for PAH. In 2011, the members of the pediatric task force of the pediatric pulmonary vascular research institute (PVRI) proposed a functional classification of PH in children that describes assessment of functional capacity in children of different age groups, as well as a 10-category scheme of further categorizing pulmonary hypertensive vascular disease in children (Boxes 35.2 and 35.3).[13,14] They divided the functional classes to class I, II,

Box 35.1   Updated Clinical Classification of Pulmonary Hypertension

1. Pulmonary arterial hypertension
   - 1.1 Idiopathic PAH
   - 1.2 Heritable PAH
     - 1.2.1 BMPR2
     - 1.2.2 ALK 1, ENG, **SMAD9, CAV1, KCNK3**
     - 1.2.3 Unknown
   - 1.3 Drug and toxin induced
   - 1.4 Associated with:
     - 1.4.1 Connective tissue disease
     - 1.4.2 HIV infection
     - 1.4.3 Portal hypertension
     - 1.4.4 Congenital heart diseases
     - 1.4.5 Schistosomiasis
   - **1′ Pulmonary veno-occlusive disease and/or Pulmonary capillary hemangiomatosis**
   - **1″ Persistent Pulmonary Hypertension of the Newborn (PPHN)**
2. Pulmonary hypertension due to left heart disease
   - 2.1 Left ventricular systolic dysfunction
   - 2.2 Left ventricular diastolic dysfunction
   - 2.3 Valvular disease
   - 2.4 **Congenital/acquired left heart inflow/outflow tract obstruction and congenital cardiomyopathies**
3. Pulmonary hypertension due to lung diseases and/or hypoxia
   - 3.1 Chronic obstructive pulmonary disease
   - 3.2 Interstitial lung disease
   - 3.3 Other pulmonary diseases with mixed restrictive and obstructive pattern
   - 3.4 Sleep-disordered breathing
   - 3.5 Alveolar hypoventilation disorders
   - 3.6 Chronic exposure to high altitude
   - 3.7 Developmental lung diseases
4. CTEPH
5. Pulmonary hypertension with unclear multifactorial mechanisms
   - 5.1 Hematologic disorders: **chronic hemolytic anemia,** myeloproliferative disorders, splenectomy
   - 5.2 Systemic disorders: sarcoidosis, pulmonary histiocytosis, lymphangioleiomyomatosis
   - 5.3 Metabolic disorders: glycogen storage disease, Gaucher disease, thyroid disorders
   - 5.4 Others: tumoral obstruction, fibrosing mediastinitis, chronic renal failure, **segmental PH**

BMPR, Bone morphogenic protein receptor type II; *CAV1,* caveolin 1; *CTEPH,* chronic thromboembolic pulmonary hypertension; *ENG,* endoglin; *PAH,* pulmonary arterial hypertension; *PH,* pulmonary hypertension.
Fifth WSPH Nice 2013. Main modifications to the previous Dana Point classification are in **bold**.
Simonneau G, Gatzoulis MA, Adatia I, et al. Updated clinical classification of pulmonary hypertension. J Am Coll Cardiol. *2013;62 (25 suppl):D34-D41.*

Box 35.2   Broad Schema of 10 Basic Categories of Pediatric Pulmonary Hypertensive Vascular Disease

CATEGORY	DESCRIPTION
1	Prenatal or developmental pulmonary hypertensive vascular disease
2	Perinatal pulmonary vascular maladaptation
3	Pediatric cardiovascular disease
4	Bronchopulmonary dysplasia
5	Isolated pediatric pulmonary hypertensive vascular disease (isolated pediatric PAH)
6	Multifactorial pulmonary hypertensive vascular disease in congenital malformation syndromes
7	Pediatric lung disease
8	Pediatric thromboembolic disease
9	Pediatric hypobaric hypoxic exposure
10	Pediatric pulmonary vascular disease associated with other system disorders

PAH, Pulmonary arterial hypertension.
Cerro MJ Del, Abman S, Diaz G, et al. A consensus approach to the classification of pediatric pulmonary hypertensive vascular disease: Report from the PVRI Pediatric Taskforce, Panama 2011. Pulm Circ. *2011;1(2):286-298.*

IIa, IIb, and IV, and also described them separately for age groups 0–0.5 years, 0.5–1 year, 1–2 years, 2–5 years, and 5–16 years. Of particular importance is the acknowledgement of single ventricle circulation, where pulmonary vascular disease may be present without a mean PAP reaching 25 mm Hg, as these patients may benefit from targeted therapy.[14,15] Thus the definition of PAH may be further expanded in single ventricle circulations to include a transpulmonary gradient of >6 mm and a PVRi >3 WU × m²[.15,16]

Epidemiology and Etiology

Because PAH remains an "orphan" disease with multiple potential etiologies, registries have been developed to better describe the populations with PAH and categorize them into various etiologies and study the disease epidemiology better.[1,18] McLaughlin et al. discussed the importance of the various registries and stressed their role in generating future prospective studies of the clinical course and management of a rare disease like PH.[19,20] The Dutch national pediatric PH registries suggested an annual incidence of 0.7 cases per million for IPAH, and a prevalence of 4.4 per million and 2.2 and 15.6 cases per million children with CHD-PAH.[21,22] Two major registries describing the adult populations are the French registry, which reported a distribution of IPAH 39.2%, FPAH 3.9%, CTD 15.3%, and CHD 11.3%, whereas the Registry to Evaluate Early And Long-term PAH Disease Management (REVEAL) registry revealed slightly different estimates of IPAH 42.7%, FPAH 2.7%, CTD 25%, and CHD 10%.[8,23,24] The pediatric pulmonary hypertension network (PPHNet) is currently establishing a registry of pediatric pulmonary hypertension in the United States and Canada, and results are pending.[25] Studies from national databases in countries with centralized care for PAH, such as France and Britain, have been very helpful in estimating the prevalence of the disease.[26,27] The UK registry reports an incidence and prevalence of 0.48 per million and 2.1 per million children for IPAH, and the French study reported a prevalence of 2.2 cases per million children. CHD-PH is more common in children as compared with adults; however, with increasing survival of CHD patients into adulthood, these statistics are rapidly changing. A report on the treatment and survival of children from the national pediatric PH service in the United

Box 35.3 Detailed Classification of Pediatric Pulmonary Hypertensive Vascular Disease

1. Prenatal or developmental pulmonary hypertensive vascular disease
   1.1. Associated with maternal or placental abnormalities
      1.1.1 Preeclampsia
      1.1.2 Chorioamnionitis
      1.1.3 Maternal drug ingestion (nonsteroidal antiinflammatory drugs)
   1.2. Associated with fetal pulmonary vascular maldevelopment
      1.2.1. Associated with fetal pulmonary hypoplasia
         1.2.1.a. Idiopathic pulmonary hypoplasia
         1.2.1.b. Familial pulmonary hypoplasia
         1.2.1.c. Congenital diaphragmatic hernia
         1.2.1.d. Hepatopulmonary fusion
         1.2.1.e. Scimitar syndrome
         1.2.1.f. Associated with fetal pulmonary compression
            oligohydramnios
            omphalocele/gastroschisis
            cystic adenomatosis
            fetal tumors or masses
         1.2.1.g. Associated with fetal skeletal malformations
      1.2.2. Associated with fetal lung growth arrest/maldevelopment
         1.2.2.a. Acinar dysplasia
         1.2.2.b. Congenital alveolar dysplasia
         1.2.2.c. Alveolar capillary dysplasia with/out misalignment of pulmonary veins
         1.2.2.d. Lymphangiectasia
         1.2.2.e. Pulmonary artery abnormalities
         1.2.2.f. Pulmonary venous abnormalities
   1.3. Associated with fetal cardiac maldevelopment
      1.3.1. Premature closure of foramen ovale or ductus arteriosus
         1.3.1.a. Idiopathic
         1.3.1.b. Drug induced
      1.3.2. Congenital heart defects associated/causing pulmonary vascular disease in the fetus
         1.3.2.a. Transposition of the great arteries (TGA) with intact ventricular septum
         1.3.2.b. Hypoplastic left heart syndrome with intact atrial septum
         1.3.2.c. Obstructed total anomalous pulmonary venous connection
         1.3.2.d. Common pulmonary vein atresia
2. Perinatal pulmonary vascular maladaptation (persistent pulmonary hypertension of the neonate, PPHN)
   2.1. Idiopathic PPHN
   2.2. PPHN associated with or triggered by
      2.2.1. Sepsis
      2.2.2. Meconium aspiration
      2.2.3. Congenital heart disease
      2.2.4. Congenital diaphragmatic hernia
      2.2.5. Trisomy[13,18,21]
      2.2.6. Drugs and toxins
         Diazoxide
3. Pediatric heart disease
   3.1 Systemic to pulmonary shunts
      3.1.1. PAH associated with systemic to pulmonary shunt with increased PVRi, no R-L shunt
         3.1.1.1. Operable
         3.1.1.2. Inoperable

   3.1.2 Classical Eisenmenger syndrome
      3.1.2.1. Eisenmenger–simple lesion (ASD, VSD, PDA)
      3.1.2.2. Eisenmenger–complex lesion (truncus, TGA/VSD, single ventricle)
   3.1.3. Small defect with elevated pulmonary arterial pressure/PVRI out of proportion to the size of the defect
      Coexistent with pulmonary hypoplasia
      Coexistent with inherited or idiopathic pulmonary hypertensive vascular disease
   3.2. Postoperative pulmonary arterial hypertension following
      3.2.1. Closure of shunt with
         3.2.1.1 Persistent increase in PVRI>3 WU $\times$ m^2
         3.2.1.2 Recurrent increase in PVRI>3 WU $\times$ m^2
      3.2.2. Arterial or atrial switch operation for TGA with intact ventricular septum
      3.2.3. Repair of left heart obstruction
      3.2.4. Repair of tetralogy of Fallot
      3.2.5. Repair of pulmonary atresia with VSD and MAPCAs
      3.2.6. Surgical aortopulmonary shunt
   3.3. Pulmonary vascular disease following staged palliation for single ventricle physiology
      3.3.1. After stage 1 (PA banding, modified Norwood, hybrid procedure, aortopulmonary or ventricular pulmonary shunt, stenting PDA)
      3.3.2. After SVC to PA anastomosis (Glenn)
      3.3.3. After total cavopulmonary anastomosis (Fontan)
   3.4. Pediatric pulmonary hypertensive vascular disease associated with congenital abnormalities of the pulmonary arteries/veins
      3.4.1. PPHVD associated with congenital abnormalities of the pulmonary arteries
         3.4.1.1. Origin of a pulmonary artery from the aorta
         3.4.1.2. Unilateral isolation/ductal origin/"absence" of a pulmonary artery
      3.4.2. PPHVD associated with congenital abnormalities of the pulmonary veins
         3.4.2.1. Scimitar complex
         3.4.2.2. Pulmonary vein stenosis
         3.4.2.3. Cantú syndrome[157]
   3.5. Pulmonary venous hypertension
      3.5.1. Pulmonary venous hypertension due to congenital left heart inflow or outflow disease: aortic stenosis, aortic incompetence, mitral stenosis, mitral regurgitation, supramitral ring, pulmonary vein obstruction, cor triatriatum, endocardial fibroelastosis, left ventricular hypoplasia/Shone complex, congenital cardiomyopathy, restrictive atrial septum in hypoplastic left heart syndrome
      3.5.2. Pulmonary venous hypertension due to acquired left heart disease
         Left-sided valvar heart disease (rheumatic/postendocarditis/rheumatoid arthritis)
         Restrictive/dilated/hypertrophic cardiomyopathy
         Constrictive pericardial disease
4. Bronchopulmonary dysplasia
   4.1 With pulmonary vascular hypoplasia
   4.2 With pulmonary vein stenosis
   4.3 With left ventricular diastolic dysfunction
   4.4 With systemic to pulmonary shunts
   4.5. With significant hypercarbia and/or hypoxia

Box 35.3   Detailed Classification of Pediatric Pulmonary Hypertensive Vascular Disease—cont'd

5. Isolated pediatric pulmonary hypertensive vascular disease (PPHVD) or isolated pulmonary arterial hypertension (PAH)
   5.1. Idiopathic PPHVD/Idiopathic PAH
   5.2. Inherited PPHVD/PAH
      5.2.1. BMPR2
      5.2.2. ALK 1, endoglin
      5.2.3. Unidentified genetic cause
   5.3. Drugs and toxins
      5.3.1. Definite association: toxic oil
      5.3.2. Likely association
         Amphetamine
      5.3.4. Possible association
         Cocaine
         Methylphenidate
         Diazoxide
         Cyclosporin
         Phenylpropanolamine
   5.4. Pulmonary veno-occlusive disease (PVOD) and/or pulmonary capillary hemangiomatosis[156]
      5.4.1 Idiopathic PVOD
      5.4.2 Inherited PVOD
6. Multifactorial pulmonary hypertensive vascular disease associated with multiple congenital malformations/syndromes
   6.1. Syndromes with congenital heart disease
   6.2. Syndromes without congenital heart disease
   Both 6.1 and 6.2 may include VACTERL, CHARGE, Poland, Adams-Oliver Syndrome, Scimitar complex, Trisomy, Di George, Noonan, von Recklinghausen disease, Dursun syndrome, Cantú syndrome
7. Pediatric lung disease
   7.1. Cystic fibrosis
   7.2. Interstitial lung diseases: surfactant protein deficiency, etc.
   7.3. Sleep-disordered breathing
   7.4. Chest wall and spinal deformities
   7.5. Restrictive lung diseases
   7.6. Chronic obstructive lung diseases
8. Pediatric thromboembolic disease causing pulmonary hypertensive vascular disease
   8.1. Chronic thromboemboli from central venous catheters
   8.2. Chronic thromboemboli from transvenous pacing wires
   8.3. Ventriculoatrial shunt for hydrocephalus
   8.4. Sickle cell disease
   8.5. Primary endocardial fibroelastosis
   8.6. Anticardiolipin/antiphospholipid syndrome
   8.7. Methylmalonic acidemia and homocystinuria
   8.8. Due to malignancy: osteosarcoma, Wilms tumor
   8.9. Post splenectomy
9. Hypobaric hypoxic exposure
   9.1. High-altitude pulmonary edema (HAPE)
   9.2. Infantile subacute mountain sickness
   9.3. Monge disease
   9.4. Hypobaric hypoxic exposure associated with PPHN
      Congenital heart disease
      Isolated PPHVD or PAH
10. Pulmonary hypertensive vascular disease associated with other system disorders
    10.1. Pediatric portal hypertension
       10.1.1. Congenital extrahepatic portocaval/portosystemic shunt (e.g., Abernethy syndrome, left atrial isomerism, trisomy,[21] portal vein atresia or thrombosis)
       10.1.2. Liver cirrhosis
    10.2. Pediatric hematological disease
       10.2.1. Hemolytic anemias: β-thalassemia, sickle cell disease
       10.2.2. Post splenectomy
    10.3. Pediatric oncologic disease
       10.3.1. Pediatric pulmonary arterial hypertension associated with malignancy
       10.3.2. Pulmonary veno-occlusive disease after bone marrow transplantation and chemotherapy[156]
    10.4. Pediatric metabolic/endocrine disease
       10.4.1. Gaucher disease
       10.4.2. Glycogen storage disease[1,111]
       10.4.3. Nonketotic hyperglycinemia
       10.4.4. Mitochondrial depletion syndrome
       10.4.5. Mucopolysaccharidosis
       10.4.6. Hypothyroidism/hyperthyroidism
    10.5. Pediatric autoimmune or autoinflammatory disease
       10.5.1. POEMS
       10.5.2. Mixed connective tissue disease
       10.5.3. Scleroderma–limited and diffuse disease
       10.5.4. Dermatomyositis
       10.5.5. Systemic lupus erythematosis (SLE)
       10.5.6. Antiphospholipid/anticardiolipin syndrome
       10.5.7. Systemic-onset juvenile arthritis
       10.5.8. Pulmonary veno-occlusive disease and SLE[156]
    10.6. Pediatric infectious disease
       10.6.1. Schistosomiasis
       10.6.2. HIV infection
       10.6.3. Pulmonary tuberculosis
    10.7. Pediatric chronic renal failure
       10.7.1 Pulmonary arterial hypertension predialysis and with hemodialysis or peritoneal dialysis
       10.7.2 Pulmonary veno-occlusive disease after renal transplantation

Cerro MJ Del, Abman S, Diaz G, et al. A consensus approach to the classification of pediatric pulmonary hypertensive vascular disease: Report from the PVRI Pediatric Taskforce, Panama 2011. Pulm Circ. 2011;1(2):286-298.

Kingdom over a 5-year period from 2001 to 2006 showed that 60/216 patients had IPAH and 156 had associated pulmonary arterial hypertension (APAH).[10,12,18] Of the APAH group, there were 49 patients with Eisenmenger syndrome (ES), 47 repaired CHD, 29 chronic lung disease, 9 CTD, and 8 complex CHD. The mean age in the UK report for IPAH was 7.4 years, and the French registry reported a mean age at inclusion of 8.9 years. The mean age at diagnosis of the 216 pediatric patients recruited from 54 centers in the United States included in the REVEAL registry was 7 years.[8,28]

GENDER

The gender distribution in adults is weighted toward more women with IPAH, whereas in pediatric patients, this distribution has been more variable, depending on the inclusion criteria, with female to male ratio varying from 1.09 : 1 in the French and Swiss registries to 1.7 : 1 reported by the UK group. Other studies have found a more even gender distribution, with the Dutch study reporting 55% of IPAH patients to be female.[22,29] When all etiologies of PAH are included, the female to male ratio gets closer to 1 : 1 because there is no significant gender predominance for CHD with PAH. The REVEAL registry reported a 2 : 1 female to male ratio in children and a 4.1 : 1 in adults with IPAH.[8]

GENETICS OF PAH

The first report of familial PPH was published as early as 1954 by Dresdale, and since then it has been increasingly evident that heritable PAH has a very strong association with germline mutations.[30–33] By the1980s it was evident that FPAH had an autosomal dominant mode of inheritance, and by 1997, two independent groups localized the defect to a region on chromosome 2 Q33. Mutations of the transforming growth factor β (TGFβ) family of receptors, particularly bone morphogenetic protein receptor (BMPR2), are found in kindreds with FPAH. More than 300 germline BMPR2 mutations have been identified in FPAH patients, with the mutations being usually similar within families. These mutations are located throughout the gene. BMPR2 mutations are seen in more than 80% of patients with HPAH, while the remaining have mutations in other genes encoding the TGFβ superfamily of receptors. In addition, mutations of ACVRL 1, activin receptor–like kinase 1 (ALK 1) located on chromosome 12, and endoglin (ENG) on chromosome 9 have been described in association with hereditary hemorrhagic telangiectasia (HHT).[34–36] A third locus, the SMAD8 gene identified on chromosome 13, ties in with the role of SMADs in BMP signaling.

The BMPR2 mutations are germ line mutations and are potentially heritable, regardless of whether they appear de novo in an index case or have been inherited. Because of reduced penetrance, only approximately 20% of people with a BMPR2 mutation develop the disease. Females have a greater incidence and prevalence of HPAH, suggesting either that the male fetuses with the disease die in utero or there are hitherto undetected risk factors increasing the predilection for developing the disease in women. The clinical expression of PAH is variable, even within families having the same mutation. Genetic anticipation has been described with HPAH (i.e., affected individuals in successive generations in a family pedigree express the disease earlier with earlier age of death); however, this has been recently been questioned.[37] BMPR2 mutations are seen in 80% of subjects with FPAH and are also seen in approximately 10%–25% of patients with no family history of PAH, suggesting that these represent de novo mutations. Individuals with BMPR2 mutation have more severe disease phenotype associated with earlier disease manifestation, worse hemodynamics, less vasoreactivity, and earlier mortality.[30] This is also seen with the ACVRL 1 mutation.[36] Male carriers of the BMPR2 mutations tend to have a worse prognosis. It has been suggested that genetic testing for BMPR2 mutations be performed in children with PAH and healthy siblings. Because of the large number of potential mutations in the gene, and the fact that mutations within a given pedigree are constant, testing should start with the proband and then the family members of the affected individual.

Whole exome sequencing (WES) techniques have shown a rare mutation in the caveolin 1 (CAV1) gene in members of a family with PAH.[34] More recently, a novel channelopathy has been described in the potassium channel (KCNK3),

which may have implications for finding a therapeutic pathway.[38]

Neonatal Pulmonary Hypertension

PERSISTENT PULMONARY HYPERTENSION OF THE NEWBORN

PPHN is a unique form of PAH, which usually resolves completely with appropriate intervention. PPHN is a syndrome characterized by increased PVR, right to left shunting (at the atrial and/or ductal level), and severe hypoxemia.[39] It is frequently associated with pulmonary parenchymal abnormalities (e.g., meconium aspiration, pneumonia, or sepsis) or may occur when there is pulmonary hypoplasia, maladaptation of the pulmonary vascular bed postnatally as a result of perinatal stress, or maladaptation of the pulmonary vascular bed in utero from unknown causes. In some instances, there is no evidence of pulmonary parenchymal disease and the cause of PAH is unknown. Although some children die during the neonatal period despite maximal cardiopulmonary therapeutic interventions, PPHN is almost always transient, with infants recovering completely without requiring long-term medical therapy. In contrast to these infants, patients with IPAH, as well as PAH related to the other conditions discussed previously, appear to require treatment indefinitely. It is possible that in some neonates the PVR does not fall normally after birth and goes unrecognized during the neonatal period; the patient is then diagnosed with PAH at a later date as the pulmonary vascular disease progresses. Pathologic studies examining the elastic pattern of the main pulmonary artery suggest that IPAH is present from birth in some patients, although it is acquired later in life in others. The histopathologic changes have illustrated increased muscularity of the peripheral pulmonary arterioles, similar to IPAH.

BRONCHOPULMONARY DYSPLASIA AND PULMONARY HYPERTENSION

Bronchopulmonary dysplasia (BPD) is a chronic lung disease of infancy that occurs in premature infants after oxygen and ventilator therapy for acute respiratory failure at birth. When first characterized nearly 50 years ago, BPD was originally described as severe chronic respiratory disease with very high morbidity and high mortality in relatively late-gestation preterm infants, because infants below 28 weeks gestation rarely survived in that era.[40,41] With improved care in very premature infants in modern neonatal units, including gentle ventilation techniques, appropriate oxygenation and acid-base balance, nutrition, and other interventions, survival of infants beyond 23 weeks has dramatically improved. However, these successes have not led to a reduction in persistence of BPD, which remains a major problem, occurring in an estimated 10,000–15,000 infants per year in the United States alone, or in 68% of infants born at less than 29 weeks gestation and weighing less than 1500 g. In the previous era, BPD was related to airway injury, inflammation, and fibrosis due to ventilator damage and oxygen toxicity. The "new BPD" in the current era is characterized by impaired angiogenesis and alveolarization, with decreased vascular branching and persistent precapillary arteriovenous anastomotic vessels.[42–44] Despite the differences in the pathology and epidemiology of BPD over time, PH continues to contribute significantly to high morbidity and mortality and is present early in the course of disease. Even the original descriptions of BPD noted striking pulmonary hypertensive vascular remodeling in severe cases and that the presence of PH beyond 3 months of age was associated with high mortality. Now in the "postsurfactant era" or the "new BPD," late PH continues to be strongly linked with poor survival, with reports suggesting mortality rates of greater than 50% for infants with severe PH.[45] Furthermore, the chronic lung disease can persist after infancy, with frequent hospitalizations due to respiratory problems in childhood and exercise limitations extending into adulthood.[46]

Associated Pulmonary Arterial Hypertension With Congenital Heart Disease

PAH is an important determinant of morbidity and mortality in patients with CHD. An updated shunt-related classification (Table 35.1) was proposed at the fifth World Symposium on Pulmonary Hypertension in Nice, France (the Nice-CHD classification).[11,47] The value of this classification in determining survival of adult patients with CHD was recently described by Manes et al. and by Zijlstra in pediatric patients.[48] By definition, Nice group 1 includes ES, with reversal of a previous large shunt; group 2—hyperkinetic PAH with large left to right (L-R) shunts; group 3—PAH with coincidental CHD, which could not be causative to the PAH, such as small ventricular septal defects or atrial septal defects of <2 cm in size; and group 4—postoperative PAH with or without residual shunts.[47] PAH related to unrepaired CHD (i.e., ES) is thought

to develop after exposure to hyperkinetic shear stress, following a period of normal PVR and increased pulmonary blood flow. Several types of congenital heart defect are associated with a greater risk for the development of pulmonary vascular disease. In patients with transposition of great arteries (TGA), truncus arteriosus, and atrioventricular canal (AVC) defects, pulmonary vascular changes are accelerated and seen in very early infancy. Repair should be performed in the neonatal period for TGA and truncus and in the first few months of life for AVC defects.[49–52] The progression of PH is also determined by coexisting genetic defects, including Down syndrome and other genetic syndromes, developmental lung disease, and metabolic and other systemic diseases. There is a whole group of patients with CHD-PAH who do not fit into the Nice-CHD classification, including segmental PH, as seen in aortopulmonary collaterals, patients with TGA after atrial switch surgery, and single ventricle physiology; the prognosis for these is variable.[22] The PVRI pediatric task force attempted to classify pediatric pulmonary hypertensive vascular disease into 10 categories, to try and include all of these issues; however, further large outcome studies are needed to validate the classification.[15] In children whose CHD is diagnosed later in life, one needs to determine whether the patient is "operable" or has "irreversible" pulmonary vascular disease. In the past, the evaluation of "operability" included anatomic criteria (Heath-Edwards classification) based on microscopic findings from lung biopsies to aid in the determination of "operability." However, lung biopsies carry a significant risk of morbidity and mortality in this population. Furthermore, because the pulmonary vascular disease can be quite heterogeneous, a biopsy from one area of the lung may not necessarily represent the vascular disease in both lungs. Cardiac catheterization with acute vasoreactivity testing (AVT) is performed in children with CHD to assess whether the PVR will decrease sufficiently for surgical repair to be undertaken in borderline cases. The vast majority of children with CHD do not require cardiac catheterization

Table 35.1 Pharmacological Therapy for Pediatric PH

Drug Class	Agent	Dosing	Adverse Effects	COR/LOE Comments
Digitalis	Digoxin	Usual age and weight dosing schedule 5 µg/kg orally twice daily up to 10 years, then 5 µg/kg once daily Maximum dose, 0.125 mg/d orally	Bradycardia is dose limiting and may limit effectiveness in PH	COR IIb LOE C Limited data and now rarely used in pediatric PH Not effective for acute deterioration Monitor renal function
Diuretics	Several agents	Loop diuretics, thiazides, and spirolactone are all dosed by weight and are not different than for other forms of heart failure	Care is needed because overdiuresis can reduce the preload of the failing RV	COR IIa LOE C
Oxygen	Oxygen	Flow rate as needed by nasal cannula to achieve target O_2 saturations	Too high a flow rate can dry the nares and cause epistaxis or rhinitis	COR IIb LOE C Oxygen is not usually prescribed for children with PH unless the daytime Saturations are low (<92%) Polysomnography is helpful in delineating the need for O_2 therapy at night May be helpful for symptomatic class IV patients

Continued

Table 35.1   Pharmacological Therapy for Pediatric PH—cont'd

Drug Class	Agent	Dosing	Adverse Effects	COR/LOE Comments
Vitamin K antagonists (anticoagulation)	Warfarin	Goal INRs in the range of 1.5–2.0 are usually chosen for this indication Higher INR may be needed for history of thrombosis or hypercoagulability	Risk of anticoagulation in pediatrics must be balanced with the hypothetical benefits Teratogenic effects	For IPAH/HPAH: COR IIa LOE C Use of warfarin in children before they are walking well or with developmental or neurological problems, including seizures or syncope, adds risk May be useful in PH with heart failure, central venous line, or right-to-left shunt Use of warfarin in patients with hypercoagulable state is reasonable For APAH: COR IIb LOE C Use of warfarin in this population is poorly studied Use of warfarin in patients with hypercoagulable state is reasonable
CCB	Nifedipine	Starting dose: 0.1–0.2 mg/kg orally 3 times daily Dose range: 2–3 mg·kg^{-1}·d^{-1} Maximum adult dose: 180 mg/d orally Always uptitrate from a lower dose If possible, use extended-release preparations	Bradycardia Decreased cardiac output Peripheral edema Rash Gum hyperplasia Constipation	COR I LOE B Duration of benefit may be limited even with initial favorable response; periodic repeat assessments for responsiveness are indicated
CCB	Diltiazem	Starting dose: 0.5 mg/kg orally 3 times daily Dose range: 3–5 mg·kg^{-1}·d^{-1} orally Maximum adult dose: 360 mg/d orally Always uptitrate from a lower dose If possible, use extended-release preparations	Bradycardia Decreased cardiac output Peripheral edema Rash Gum hyperplasia Constipation	COR I LOE B Duration of benefit may be limited even with initial favorable response; periodic repeat assessments for responsiveness are indicated May cause bradycardia more than other CCBs Suspension useful in younger children
CCB	Amlodipine	Starting dose: 0.1–0.3 mg·kg^{-1}·d^{-1} orally Dose range: 2.5–7.5 mg/d orally Maximum adult dose: 10 mg/d orally Always uptitrate from a lower dose	Bradycardia Decreased cardiac output Peripheral edema Rash Gum hyperplasia Constipation	COR I LOE B Duration of benefit may be limited even with initial favorable response
PDE5 inhibitor	Sildenafil	Age <1 year: 0.5–1 mg/kg 3 times daily orally Weight <20 kg: 10 mg 3 times daily orally Weight >20 kg: 20 mg 3 times daily orally Delay use in extremely preterm infants until retinal vascularization is established	Headache Nasal congestion Flushing Agitation Hypotension Vision and hearing loss may be concerns Priapism Avoid nitrates	COR I LOE B Avoid higher dosing in children because a greater risk of mortality was noted in the STARTS-2 study in children with IPAH treated with high-dose sildenafil monotherapy Sildenafil approved in Europe and Canada FDA warning for use in children 1–17 years of age
PDE5 inhibitor	Tadalafil	Starting dose: 0.5–1 mg·kg^{-1}·d^{-1} Maximum dose: 40 mg orally daily Evaluated only in children >3 years of age	Headache Nasal congestion Flushing Agitation Hypotension Vision and hearing loss may be concerns Priapism Nosebleeds Avoid nitrates	COR IIa LOE B Once-daily dosing Safety and efficacy data in children are limited

Table 35.1 Pharmacological Therapy for Pediatric PH—cont'd

Drug Class	Agent	Dosing	Adverse Effects	COR/LOE Comments
ERA	Bosentan (dual ET$_A$ and ET$_B$ antagonist)	Starting dose is half the maintenance dose. Maintenance dose: Weight <10 kg: 2 mg/kg twice daily orally. Weight 10–20 kg: 31.25 mg twice daily. Weight >20–40 kg: 62.5 mg twice daily. Weight >40 kg: 125 mg twice daily	Monthly LFTs required due to risk for hepatotoxicity. HCG and pregnancy test required monthly. Incidence of AST/ALT elevation is less in children compared with adults. Fluid retention. Teratogenicity. Male infertility. May decrease sildenafil level	COR I. LOE B. Data have been published on efficacy in Eisenmenger PH. 2 Forms of birth control required. Drug interaction with sildenafil
ERA	Ambrisentan (a highly selective ET$_A$ antagonist)	Dose range: 5–10 mg orally daily. Use in pediatric patients <5 years of age is unstudied	Routine LFTs recommended. HCT and pregnancy test required. Incidence of AST/ALT elevation is less in children compared with adults. Fluid retention. Teratogenicity. Male infertility	COR IIa. LOE B. Safety and efficacy data in children are limited. Avoid use in neonates or infant because glucuronidation is not mature
Prostacyclin	Epoprostenol (Flolan), Veletri (thermostable)	Continuous intravenous infusion. Drug interaction with sildenafil. Starting dose: 1–2 ng·kg^{-1}·min^{-1} IV without a known maximum. In pediatric patients, a stable dose is usually between 50 and 80 ng·kg^{-1}·min^{-1} IV. Doses >150 ng·kg^{-1}·min^{-1} IV have been used. Dose increases are required. High-output syndrome at high doses can occur	Flushing, jaw, foot and bone pain, headaches, and diarrhea. Systemic hypotension is possible. Half-life is short (2–5 min), so PH crises occur rapidly if the infusion is stopped. Icepack cooling and remixing every 24 h needed. Central line complications occur	COR I. LOE B. Standard therapy for severe PH. A temperature-stable formulation is available
Prostacyclin	Treprostinil (Remodulin)	Intravenous or subcutaneous: Starting dose: 2 ng·kg^{-1}·min^{-1} without a known maximum. In pediatric patients, a stable dose is usually between 50 and 80 ng·kg^{-1}·min^{-1} IV or SC. Dose increases are required. Inhaled: 1–9 patient-activated breaths every 6 h. Oral: dosing not fully evaluated in children	Flushing, muscle pain, headaches, and diarrhea are common side effects. Frequency and severity of side effects are less than with epoprostenol. Elimination half-life is 4.5 h. The drug is stable at room temperature. Central line complications can occur, including gram-negative infections with intravenous route. Subcutaneous injection site pain may limit this route. Inhaled drug can worsen reactive airway symptoms. GI side effects may be greater than with intravenous, subcutaneous, or inhaled	For intravenous and subcutaneous: COR I. LOE B. For inhalation: COR IIa. LOE B. The nebulizer requires patient activation and controlled inhalation limited by age and development
Prostacyclin	Iloprost (intermittent inhalation)	Pediatric dosing has not been determined but 6–9 inhalations per day are required, each lasting 10–15 min. Start with 2.5-μg dose and uptitrate to 5-μg dose as tolerated	Flushing and headaches are common side effects. Systemic hypotension is rare. Half-life is short. Inhaled drug can worsen reactive airway symptoms	COR IIa. LOE B. In pediatrics, the dosing frequency may limit usefulness

ALT, Alanine aminotransferase; *APAH,* pulmonary arterial hypertension associated with disease; *AST,* aspartate aminotransferase; *CCB,* calcium channel blocker; *COR,* class of recommendation; *ERA,* endothelin receptor antagonist; *ET,* endothelin; *FDA,* US Food and Drug Administration; *GI,* gastrointestinal; *HCG,* human chorionic gonadotropin; *HCT,* hematocrit; *HPAH,* heritable pulmonary arterial hypertension; *INR,* international normalized ratio; *IPAH,* idiopathic pulmonary arterial hypertension; *LFT,* liver function test; *LOE,* level of evidence; *PDE5,* phosphodiesterase type 5; *PH,* pulmonary hypertension; *RV,* right ventricular; *STARTS,* Sildenafil in Treatment-Naïve Children, Aged 1–17 years, With Pulmonary Arterial Hypertension.
COR and LOE grading are based on pediatric data.
From Abman SH, Hansmann G, Archer SL, et al. Pediatric Pulmonary Hypertension Guidelines from the American Heart Association and American Thoracic Society. *Circulation.* 2015;132:2037-2099. Table 3, pp 2043-2045. doi:10.1161/CIR.0000000000000329.

as a prelude to repair. It is important to determine whether the elevated PVR index (PVRi) responds favorably to acute pharmacologic vasodilatation.[52] The availability of pulmonary vasodilators for the perioperative management of pulmonary hypertension have allowed for surgical "correction" in select patients who present later in life with borderline elevated PVRi in the range 3–5 Wood units $\times$ m^2. If a patient with elevated PVR is being considered for surgery, there is an increased risk of postoperative pulmonary hypertensive crises. Thus knowing if the pulmonary circulation will respond favorably to inhaled nitric oxide (NO) can help guide the management of this potentially life-threatening postoperative complication. In general, positive AVT for borderline cases with posttricuspid shunts is defined as a decrease in PVRi to <6–8 WU $\times$ m^2 or pulmonary vascular resistance/systemic vascular resistance (PVR/SVR) ratio <0.3.[14] However, AVT is only one measure used to define operability, and the whole clinical picture, the age of the patient, and the type of lesion should be taken into consideration. For patients with borderline elevated PVRi, partial or complete surgical closure may be attempted after treatment with targeted pulmonary vasodilators for a period of time and repeated hemodynamic studies. Partial closure of shunts may sometimes improve the clinical and hemodynamic status of such patients by reducing the shear damage with continued increased pulmonary blood flow from persistent shunts.

SURVIVAL IN APAH-CHD

Barst et al. compared patients with IPAH or HPAH ($n = 1,626$) to those with CHD-associated PAH ($n = 353$) who were enrolled in the REVEAL registry.[8,53] Of patients with CHD-associated PAH, 151 had ES. They showed that there was no significant survival rate at 4 and 7 years in patients with APAH-CHD (regardless of presence of a shunt) versus IPAH. Analysis of 240 patients with APAH-CHD enrolled in the Spanish registry (REHAP) revealed that within the group, patients with ES had better survival than postoperative PAH (which had outcomes similar to IPAH). Among ES, a pretricuspid shunt predicted worse survival.[12,54] Data from the German national register revealed 1-, 5-, and 10-year survival rates of 92, 75, and 57%, respectively, in the entire cohort of ES patients, with treatment-naïve patients having survival rates of 86, 60, and 34%, respectively.[55]

IDIOPATHIC/HERITABLE PULMONARY ARTERIAL HYPERTENSION

IPAH and HPAH, subtypes of PH group 1 PAH, are characterized by progressive pulmonary arterial vascular obliteration and subsequent right heart failure if untreated. A PAH patient is subclassified as having IPAH when a patient meets the hemodynamic criteria of PAH and all other associated forms of PAH (APAH) have been ruled out. HPAH previously referred to as FPAH occurs when there is a family history of PAH or identification of one of the genetic mutations associated with PAH, regardless of whether there is a family history or not. Although HPAH may represent a different clinical phenotype, both IPAH and HPAH likely represent overlapping diagnostic subgroups of PAH and are classified with other forms of PH group 1 PAH because of similar characteristics, histopathologic changes, and treatment responses.

EPIDEMIOLOGY

The exact incidence and prevalence of IPAH/HPAH in children worldwide is unknown. Adult studies have reported an overall incidence of approximately 1–2 new IPAH cases per million in industrialized countries.[18,28,56,57] In the French and Scottish registries, the prevalence of group I PAH was reported as 15–50 PAH cases per million adults and included cases of APAH.[27] With respect to children, a national cohort study of IPAH children in the United Kingdom followed over 7 years reported a lower incidence and prevalence compared with adults.[58] The incidence of childhood IPAH was 0.48 cases per million children per year, and the prevalence was 2.1 cases per million. Of these patients, 7.8% had HPAH similar to reports in adults. The difference between the prevalence in the French registry and the UK childhood registry may be in part attributable to cases of PAH (including anorexigen related and CTD) included in the adult French registry that are not seen in children. A French pediatric registry reported a 4.4 per million prevalence of pediatric IPAH/HPAH.[24] However, this prevalence does not include APAH-CHD, a subgroup of PAH that is considered to make up at least 50% of pediatric PAH. Thus the "best" estimate for pediatric PAH prevalence is approximately 10 per million.

Although the disease is rare, with improved diagnostics and increased awareness, it appears that more patients (both children and adults) have PAH than was previously recognized. On occasion, infants who died with the presumed diagnosis of sudden infant death syndrome had IPAH diagnosed at postmortem examination. The female preponderance in adult patients with IPAH previously reported as approximately 1.7 : 1 females:males is similar to earlier reports in children with IPAH (i.e., 1.8 : 1), with no significant difference in younger children compared with older children.[59] More recent reports from the United States have reported a higher female preponderance in adults with PAH (i.e., approximately 4 : 1), with the gender ratio in the pediatric patients more similar to previous reports (i.e., approximately 2 : 1).

NATURAL HISTORY

Historically, untreated IPAH exhibited a course of progressive right heart failure and early death. In contrast, patients with unrepaired CHD with shunts often lived for at least several decades without targeted treatment. Several large survival studies of primarily adult patients with IPAH were conducted in the 1980s prior to the current treatment era. These retrospective and prospective studies yielded quite uniform results: adult patients with IPAH who did not have lung or heart/lung transplantation had actuarial survival rates at 1, 3, and 5 years of 68%–77%, 40%–56%, and 22%–38%, respectively.[1] In the era before the use of continuous intravenous epoprostenol (approved in 1995), in children who were nonresponders to acute vasodilator testing and therefore not candidates for oral calcium channel blockade, the 1-, 3-, and 5-year survival rates were 66%, 52%, and 35%, respectively[3] In more recent times, with the use of epoprostenol treatment for nonresponders, and calcium channel blockade for responders, the 10-year survival for children was reported by Yung et al. at 78%.[53,60] However, there is significant biological variability in the natural history of the disease in both adults and children, with some patients having a rapidly progressive downhill course resulting in death within several weeks after diagnosis and others surviving for at least several decades.

PATHOGENESIS AND PATHOBIOLOGY OF PEDIATRIC PULMONARY ARTERIAL HYPERTENSION

Although the exact mechanism of PAH development has not been completely elucidated, endothelial cell dysfunction with smooth muscle cell (SMC) proliferation, dysfunction, and altered apoptosis secondary to imbalance of vasoactive mediators is the most consistent common factor (Fig. 35.1).[61] A thorough understanding of the factors underlying the pathogenesis is the mainstay for developing targeted treatment modalities. As more and more factors involved in this complex process are uncovered, molecules targeting these individual pathways are concomitantly undergoing testing on animal and cellular models, giving rise to a whole new generation of medications recently added to the armamentarium available to clinicians.

Pulmonary vascular disease is a multifactorial disease with several causes that lead to a final common histopathologic vasculopathy. Recent investigations in the basic science arena have uncovered several different biochemical/mechanistic features of pulmonary vascular obstructive disease that have led to novel treatments. These include abnormalities of the prostacyclin pathway, the endothelin (ET) system, and NO production/availability. Wagenvoort and Wagenvoort

hypothesized that "PPH" (IPAH) afflicts individuals with hyperreactive pulmonary arterioles in whom various stimuli initiate vasoconstriction, with subsequent development of the characteristic vascular lesions.[62] Although the early focus for treatment of this disease stemmed from this hypothesis (i.e., finding the ideal pulmonary vasodilator), evidence over the past two decades has pointed to other vasoproliferative abnormalities. In infants, the pathobiology suggests failure of the neonatal vasculature to relax, in addition to a striking reduction in arterial number/surface area. However, with time, the changes become fixed, with a vasodilator-unresponsive component that appears temporally related to the development of thickened vascular media and adventitia with dramatic increases in the deposition of structural matrix proteins such as collagen and elastin in the pulmonary arterial wall.[63,64] In older children, intimal hyperplasia, occlusive changes, and plexiform lesions are found in the pulmonary arterioles. Despite significant advances in the understanding of the pathobiology of IPAH, the mechanisms that initiate and perpetuate this disease remain speculative. Adults with IPAH often have severe plexiform lesions and what appear to be "fixed" pulmonary vascular changes. In contrast, children with IPAH have more pulmonary vascular medial hypertrophy with less intimal fibrosis and fewer plexiform lesions. In the classic autopsy studies by Wagenvoort and Wagenvoort, medial hypertrophy was severe in patients younger than 15 years of age, and it was usually the only abnormality seen in infants. With increasing age, intimal fibrosis and plexiform lesions were seen more frequently. These postmortem studies

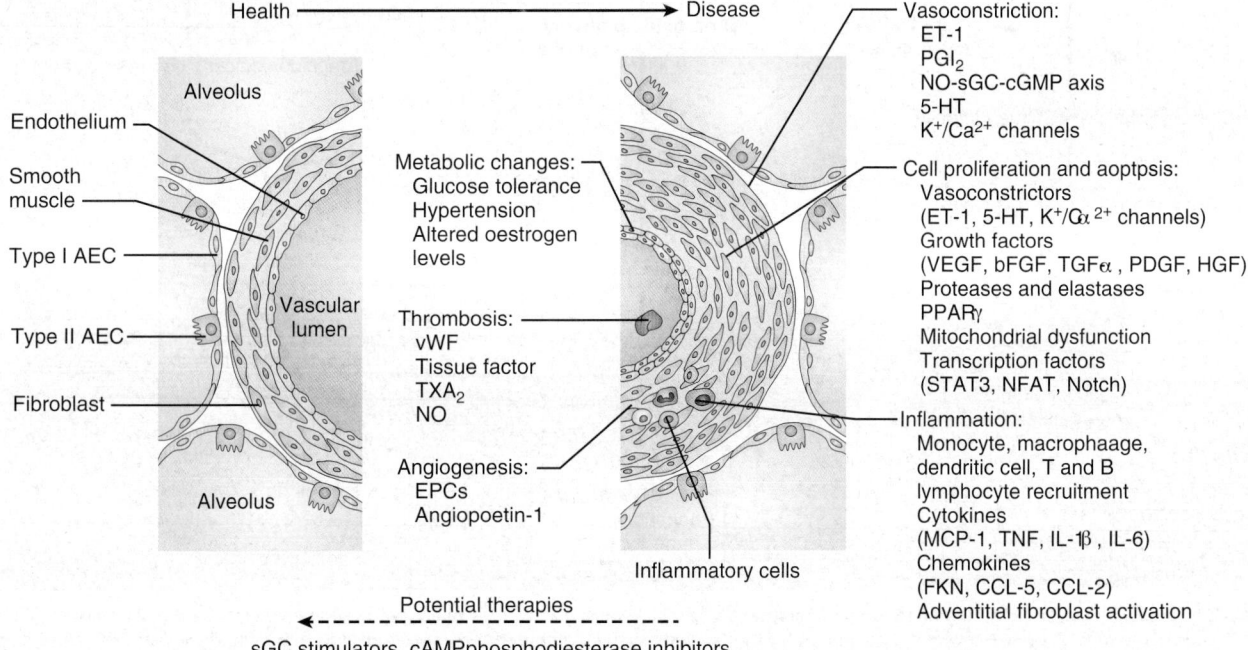

Fig. 35.1 The key pathologic mechanisms underlying vascular changes in pulmonary hypertension (PH). Potential new therapies for PH are also indicated. *5-HT*, 5-hydroxytryptamine; *AEC*, alveolar epithelial cell; *bFGF*, basic fibroblast growth factor; *cAMP*, cyclic adenosine monophosphate; *CCL*, chemokine ligand; *cGMP*, cyclic guanosine monophosphate; *EPC*, endothelial progenitor cell; *ET-1*, endothelin-1; *FKN*, fractalkine; *HGF*, hepatocyte growth factor; *IL*, interleukin; *MCP-1*, monocyte chemoattractant protein-1; *NFAT*, nuclear factor of activated T-cells; *NO*, nitric oxide; *PDGF*, platelet-derived growth factor; *PGI₂*, prostaglandin I₂; *PPAR γ*, peroxisome proliferator-activated receptor γ; *sGC*, soluble guanylate cyclase; *STAT3*, signal transducer and activator of transcription 3; *TNF*, tumor necrosis factor; *TGFα*, transforming growth factor α; *TXA₂*, thromboxane A₂; *VEGF*, vascular endothelial growth factor; *vWF*, von Willebrand factor. (From Wilkins MR. Pulmonary hypertension: The science behind the disease spectrum. *Eur Respir Rev.* 2012;21(123):19-26.)

suggested that pulmonary vasoconstriction, leading to medial hypertrophy, may occur early in the course of the disease and may precede the development of plexiform lesions and other fixed pulmonary vascular changes. The observations may offer clues to the observed differences in the natural history and factors influencing survival in children with IPAH compared with adult patients. In general, younger children appear to have a more reactive pulmonary vascular bed relative to both vasodilatation and vasoconstriction. Severe acute pulmonary hypertensive crises occur in response to pulmonary vasoconstrictor "triggers" more often in young children than in older children or adults. Based on these pathologic studies, the most widely proposed mechanism for IPAH until the late 1980s and early 1990s was pulmonary vasoconstriction.[65]

Important Pathways Thought to Be Responsible for Vasoconstriction

The three important pathways that have been well studied are the prostacyclin pathway, NO pathway, and ET pathway (Fig. 35.2).[66]

1. Prostacyclin—PGI2, generated from arachidonic acid via the cyclooxygenase pathway, causes SMC relaxation and inhibits platelet aggregation via cyclic adenosine monophosphate (cAMP) production. Thromboxane (TX) synthetase, which is derived from the same substrate as PGI2 synthetase, generates TXA_2, which is a potent vasoconstrictor and leads to platelet aggregation. In IPAH the balance between PGI2 and TXA_2 is tilted in favor of the

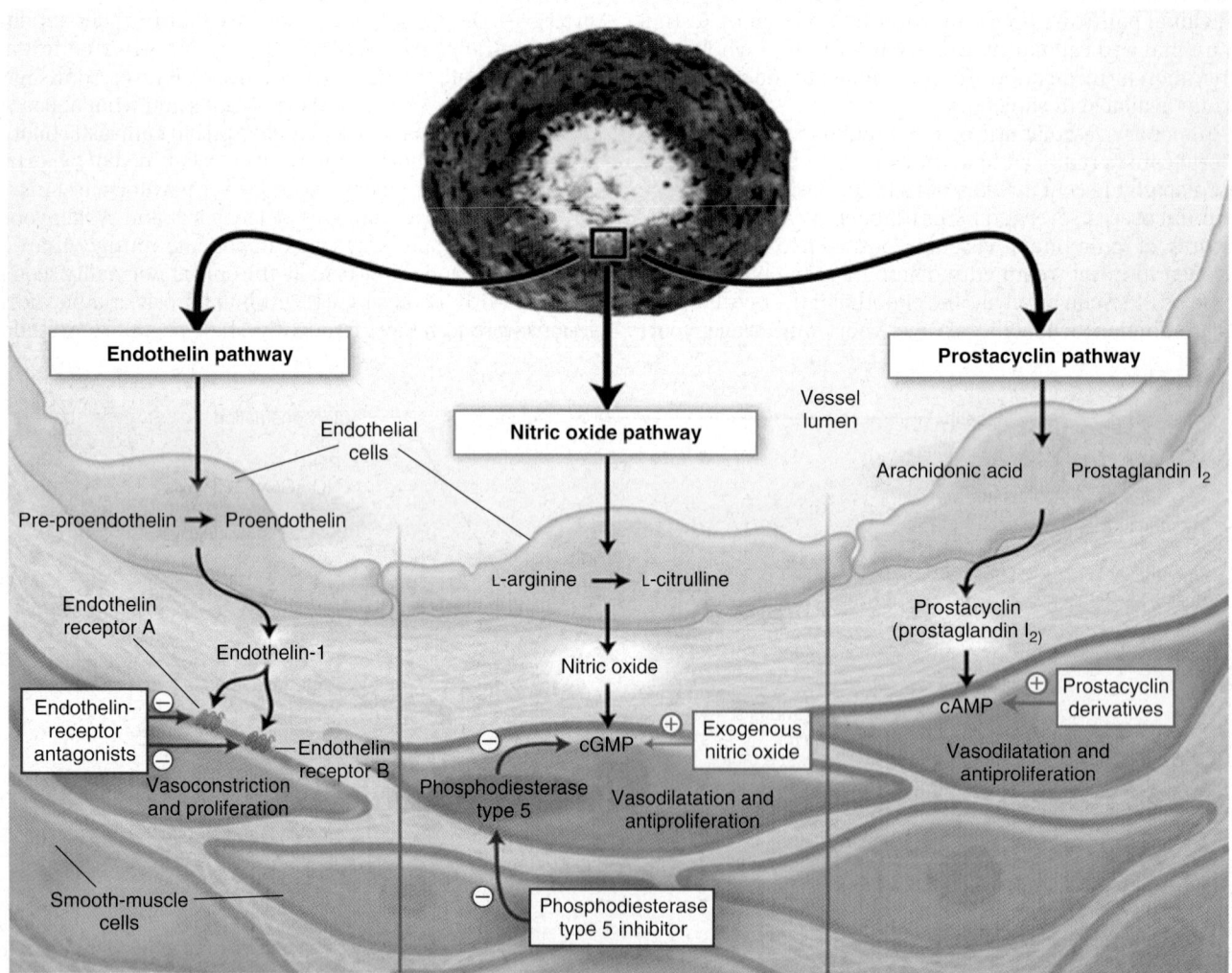

Fig. 35.2 Targets for current or emerging therapies in pulmonary arterial hypertension. Three major pathways involved in abnormal proliferation and contraction of the smooth muscle cells of the pulmonary artery in patients with pulmonary arterial hypertension are shown. These pathways correspond to important therapeutic targets in this condition and play a role in determining which of four classes of drugs—endothelin-receptor antagonists, nitric oxide, PDE5 inhibitors, and prostacyclin derivatives—will be used. At the top of the figure, a transverse section of a small pulmonary artery (<500 μm in diameter) from a patient with severe pulmonary arterial hypertension shows intimal proliferation and marked medial hypertrophy. Dysfunctional pulmonary artery endothelial cells *(blue)* have decreased production of prostacyclin and endogenous nitric oxide, with an increased production of endothelin-1—a condition promoting vasoconstriction and proliferation of smooth muscle cells in the pulmonary arteries *(red)*. Current or emerging therapies interfere with specific targets in smooth muscle cells in the pulmonary arteries. In addition to their actions on smooth muscle cells, prostacyclin derivatives and nitric oxide have several other properties, including antiplatelet effects. *Plus signs* denote an increase in the intracellular concentration; *minus signs* blockage of a receptor, inhibition of an enzyme, or a decrease in the intracellular concentration. *cAMP*, Cyclic adenosine monophosphate; *cGMP*, cyclic guanosine monophosphate; *PDE5*, phosphodiesterase 5. (From Wilkins MR. Pulmonary hypertension: The science behind the disease spectrum. *Eur Respir Rev.* 2012;21(123):19-26.)

latter. Thus use of epoprostenol (PGI2) leads to pulmonary vasodilation and improvement in long-term outcomes by correcting this imbalance.

2. NO is synthesized in the endothelium by endothelial NO synthetase (eNOS). NO stimulates guanylate cyclase to produce cyclic guanosine monophosphate (cGMP), which has vasodilatory and antiproliferative properties. Identification of this pathway has led to the use of inhaled NO (iNO) therapeutically in the treatment of PAH, as well as development of other medications that lead to release of endothelial cGMP. In various forms of PAH, there is reduced bioavailability of eNO, either because of reduced eNOS expression or secondary to oxidative free radical production, which consumes NO. Asymmetric dimethyl arginine (ADMA) is elevated in many forms of PAH, and it acts either by inhibition of eNOS or via its direct effects on gene expression. Increased expression of the phosphodiesterase 5 (PDE5) enzyme also degrades cGMP and leads to vasoconstriction. PDE5 inhibitors replenish cGMP and act as rescue agents, preventing rebound PAH when iNO is weaned off in patients, and also act as potent pulmonary vasodilators in various forms of PH.

3. The third pathway that has stirred a lot of interest in PAH research is the ET-1 pathway. ET-1 leads to vasoconstriction, fibrogenesis, and cell proliferation and acts via ET_A and ET_B receptors in the SMC. ET-1 levels are found to be increased in lung tissue and circulation in IPAH, APAH secondary to lung disease, and thromboembolism, as well as congenital diaphragmatic hernia patients. ET_B receptors on endothelial cells are involved with release of eNO and PGI2; however, there seems to be no added advantage to selective ET_A inhibition, suggesting that the relative expression of the two receptors in disease states may play a role.

Other vasoactive mediators at play are serotonin (5 hydroxytryptamine [5HT]), which is increased in patients with PAH and is a potent vasoconstrictor that causes remodeling. The roles of potassium and calcium channel function, caveolin, ADMA, and TNFα are all undergoing intense investigation.

Endothelial Dysfunction

Endothelial dysfunction appears to be a key factor in mediating the structural changes that occur in the pulmonary vasculature in PAH. The integrity of the pulmonary vascular endothelium is critical for maintaining vascular tone, homeostasis, barrier function, leukocyte trafficking, transduction of luminal signals to abluminal vascular tissues, production of growth factors, and cell signaling with autocrine and paracrine effects.[67,68] In addition, abnormalities in vasoactive mediators appear to contribute to the pathobiology of PAH. Whether these perturbations are a cause or consequence of the disease process remains to be elucidated.

The vascular endothelium is now recognized as an important source of locally active mediators that contribute to the control of vasomotor tone and structural remodeling, and appears to play a crucial role in the pathogenesis of PAH. Various studies suggest that imbalances in the production or metabolism of vasoactive mediators produced in the lungs, as well as substances involving control of pulmonary vascular growth, may be important in the pathogenesis of PAH. These may include increased TX, ET, and serotonin,

and decreased prostacyclin and NO, as well as changes in VEGF and xanthine oxidoreductase.[65,69] The endothelial cell dysfunction seen in association with PAH leads to the release of vasoproliferative substances in addition to vasoconstrictive agents that ultimately result in the progression of the pulmonary vascular remodeling and progressive vascular obstruction and obliteration. Stewart et al. and Giaid et al. reported elevated circulating levels of ET, a potent vasoconstrictor and mitogen, in patients with various forms of PAH and PH with increased local production of ET by the pulmonary arterial endothelium reported in the PAH patients.[63,70,71] Endothelial dysfunction also likely results in the release of chemotactic agents, leading to the migration of SMCs into the vascular wall, which may lead to the characteristic pulmonary arteriolar medial hypertrophy and hyperplasia. This endothelial dysfunction, coupled with the excessive release of locally active thrombogenic mediators, promotes a procoagulant state, leading to further vascular obstruction. Therefore the process is characterized by an inexorable cycle of endothelial dysfunction leading to the release of vasoconstrictive, vasoproliferative, and prothrombotic substances, ultimately progressing to vascular remodeling and progressive vascular obstruction and obliteration. Despite our lack of complete understanding of the pathogenesis of PAH, these imbalances and abnormalities have changed the focus of clinical drug development from chronic vasodilator therapy alone, to the evaluation of therapeutic agents that may reverse the vasoproliferation, and ultimately result in pulmonary vascular regression and reverse remodeling. Although various studies have demonstrated endothelial dysfunction in patients with PAH, whether the dysfunction is the primary problem or secondary to another insult remains unknown.

The theory that certain individuals are genetically susceptible has led to genetically oriented research. It is now clear that gene expression in pulmonary vascular cells responds to environmental factors, growth factors, receptors, signaling pathways, and genetic influences that can interact with each other. The molecular processes behind the complex vascular changes associated with PAH include phenotypic changes in endothelial and SMCs in hypertensive pulmonary arteries, the recognition that cell proliferation contributes to the structural changes associated with the initiation and progression of PAH, the role of matrix proteins and matrix turnover in vascular remodeling, and the importance of hemodynamic influences on the disease process. Examples of effector systems controlled by gene expression include transmembrane transporters, miRNA, ion channels, transcription factors, modulators of apoptosis, kinases, and cell-to-cell interactive factors, such as integrins, membrane receptors, growth factors, and cytokines.[32,38]

In addition, defects in the KCNK3s of pulmonary vascular SMCs may be involved in the initiation or progression of IPAH. Inhibition of the voltage regulated (Kv) KCNK3s in pulmonary artery SMCs taken from IPAH patients has been reported. Ma et al. described the association of a novel gene KCNK3 with HPAH.[38] Mutations of this gene reduced KCNK3 current, which has potential for developing a therapeutic target.

These studies suggest that IPAH is a disease of "predisposed" individuals, in whom various "stimuli" may initiate the pulmonary vascular disease process. By identifying molecular mechanisms that are linked to epidemiologic risk factors, as well as developing molecular, genetic, biochemical, and physiologic tests to monitor and diagnose IPAH, novel treatment strategies will improve therapeutic interventions for IPAH. There may be different subsets of patients in whom vasoconstriction is the predominant feature, and those in whom vascular injury or endothelial dysfunction is the primary problem. Even so, these components appear closely intertwined. Whether these physiologic processes (vasoconstriction vs. vascular injury) are a cause or a consequence of the disease remains unclear.

Cell Proliferation and Apoptosis

Many of the mediators described previously also play an important role in cell proliferation and remodeling in addition to vasoconstriction. Abnormalities in signaling pathways lead to impairment of apoptosis and increase in proliferation. Both endothelial and SMCs in patients with PAH demonstrate mitochondrial abnormalities, which lead to a shift in metabolism favoring glycolysis for ATP generation and possibly altering the apoptosis potential. Mutations in BMPR2 ALK-1 and ENG lead to vascular remodeling and are potential pathways for therapeutic intervention. When loss of BMPR2 is experimentally induced, PA endothelial cells and SMCs are more susceptible to apoptosis, migration, and proliferation in response to TGFβ1.[72]

Growth Factors

Several growth factors act as potent mitogens and chemotactic agents in PAH. Increased vascular endothelial growth factor (VEGF) and fibroblast growth factor (FGF) levels have been recorded in various forms of PAH, including neonatal PPHN. Other growth factors, including TNFα and platelet-derived growth factor (PGDF), are also implicated in PAH. Most of these growth factors act by activating tyrosine kinase receptors, which initiates major signaling cascades within the cells, resulting in an antiapoptotic and proproliferative phenotype. Human trials using tyrosine kinase inhibitors are ongoing, with promising results in selected patient groups with PAH. Peroxisome proliferator activated receptor γ (PPAR γ) expression is reduced in endothelial cells of plexiform lesions in PAH patients. This is important for BMP2-mediated inhibition of SMC proliferation and reduces ET-1 levels.

Apoptosis

The plexiform lesion forms a fascinating substrate for studying the mechanism of vascular proliferation and remodeling. Selective apoptosis of endothelial cells results in unbridled proliferation of apoptosis-resistant precursor cells driven by changes in BMPR2, mitochondrial metabolism, altered signaling factors (Notch-3), TK activation, and potassium and Ca channel derangements. This process also requires activation of prosurvival transcription factors linked to development of PAH. Abnormalities in proteases and elastases are also implicated in abnormal lung remodeling.

Inflammation and Thrombosis

Inflammation has long been implicated to play a triggering role in PAH, as evidenced by an increase in cytokines, interleukins, and chemokines, especially in PAH crisis.[73–76] Endothelial dysfunction and inflammation predispose to *in situ* thrombosis in PH. Patients with IPAH have increased von Willebrand factor levels and also have increased platelet aggregation and a hypercoagulable state. Use of anticoagulants has been shown to reduce the incidence of thrombosis both in IPAH and chronic thromboembolic pulmonary hypertension (CTEPH).

PATHOPHYSIOLOGY

Although the histopathology and pathobiology in children with IPAH is similar to that seen in adult patients, there may be differences in the pathophysiology that alter the clinical presentation, natural history, and outcome in children. For example, children appear to have differences in their hemodynamic parameters at the time of diagnosis compared with adult patients.[59] Children with IPAH most often have a normal cardiac index at the time of presentation, as opposed to adults who frequently present in clinical right heart failure with a low cardiac index. This may reflect earlier diagnosis and explain why children tend to have a greater response rate to acute vasodilator testing than adults.

A brief review of the normal physiology of the pulmonary circulation will enable a better understanding of the pathophysiology of the pulmonary vascular bed.[77,78] The normal fall in PVR occurs soon after birth and reaches normal adult levels by 4–6 weeks of life. The normal pulmonary vascular bed is a low pressure, low resistance, highly distensible system that can accommodate large increases in pulmonary blood flow with minimal elevations in pulmonary arterial pressure (PAP). In PAH, however, this capacity to accommodate increases in pulmonary blood flow is lost due to the increase in PVR, leading to increases in pulmonary artery pressure at rest and further elevations in pulmonary artery pressure with exercise. The right ventricle hypertrophies in response to this increase in afterload. If there has been a gradual exposure over time, the right ventricle has the ability to remodel and adapt to the pressure overload by recruitment of sarcomeres and hypertrophy of myocytes. The adaptation of the right ventricle to increased afterload, such as in IPAH or congenital heart defects with increased right ventricular afterload (e.g., pulmonic stenosis), is a double-edged sword. The right ventricular hypertrophy will assist the right ventricle in pumping against the increased afterload; however, this occurs at a cost to left ventricular integrity. Under normal conditions, the right ventricle is crescent shaped with the right ventricular free wall and interventricular septum concave around the left ventricle at both end diastole and end systole. During systole, the left ventricle contracts toward a central axis, while the right ventricular free wall and septum contract in parallel. With right ventricular hypertrophy, the interventricular septal orientation flattens and ultimately commits to the right ventricle in severe cases. This may lead to a vicious cycle of left ventricular diastolic dysfunction and subsequent worsening of right heart failure in severe cases.[79–81] In the early stages the right ventricle is capable of sustaining normal cardiac output at rest, but the ability to increase cardiac output with exercise is impaired. As pulmonary vascular disease progresses, the right ventricle fails and resting cardiac output decreases. As right ventricular dysfunction progresses, right ventricular diastolic pressure increases with clinical onset of right ventricular failure, the most ominous sign of pulmonary vascular disease. Dyspnea is the most frequent presenting complaint in adults and children with IPAH; it is due to impaired oxygen delivery during physical activity as a result of an inability to increase cardiac output in the presence of increased oxygen demands. Syncopal episodes, which occur more frequently with children than with adults, are often exertional or postexertional and imply a severely limited cardiac output, leading to a decrease in cerebral blood flow. Peripheral vasodilatation during physical exertion can exacerbate this condition. However, syncope may also reflect a very vasoactive circulation with rapid changes in the pulmonary vascular reactivity in response to various stimuli.

The two most frequent mechanisms of death in PAH are progressive right ventricular failure and sudden death, with the former occurring more often, especially in adults. Progressive right ventricular failure leads to dyspnea and a progressive decrease in cardiac output.[8] Complicating illnesses such as pneumonia can be fatal because alveolar hypoxia causes hypoxic pulmonary vasoconstriction, leading to an inability to maintain adequate cardiac output, which results in cardiogenic shock and death. When arterial hypoxemia and acidosis (respiratory or metabolic) occur, life-threatening arrhythmias may develop. Postulated mechanisms for sudden death include bradyarrhythmias and tachyarrhythmias, acute pulmonary emboli, acute pulmonary artery aneurysm rupture, massive pulmonary hemorrhage, and sudden right ventricular ischemia. Hemoptysis appears to be due to pulmonary infarcts from secondary arterial thromboses.

CLINICAL PRESENTATION

The clinical presentation of pediatric pulmonary hypertension is often indistinguishable from other chronic cardiorespiratory diseases. Specific neonatal conditions such as PPHN and BPD-PH or congenital diaphragmatic hernia with PH have signs and symptoms attributable to the causative condition.

Data from 216 children enrolled in the REVEAL registry showed that the median age at PAH diagnosis was 7 years, and the most frequent presenting symptoms were exertional dyspnea, seen in 53% of IPAH and 30% in CHD-PAH, and fatigue in 25% and 21% in the two groups.[3,59,82] Effort intolerance arises from the inability of the cardiac output to increase appropriately to the oxygen demands from effort in these children. In children with CHD-PAH, fatigue and exertional dyspnea may be underreported because of these patients adapting their lifestyle to a more sedentary one, because of long-standing disease. Presyncope/syncope was present in 36% of IPAH and only 4% of CHD-PAH, possibly reflecting the effect of having a shunt to pop off during PH crisis. Syncopal episodes, which occur more frequently with children than with adults, are often exertional or postexertional and imply a severely limited cardiac output, leading to diminished cerebral blood flow.[29,83] Peripheral vasodilatation during physical exertion can exacerbate this condition. In the TOPP registry, syncope was noted to be twice as common in children (25% vs. 12%) and is often the presenting symptom.[29] Syncope occurs because of the acute drop in left ventricular output with the ventricular septum bowing into the left ventricle, restricting its stroke volume and ejection fraction. In patients with shunts, PH crisis is associated with a greater right to left shunting, thereby maintaining left ventricular output at the cost of oxygen saturation. Thus, rather than syncope, these children present with increased

cyanosis and an increased oxygen requirement at the time of PH crisis. Cyanosis is commonly seen in patients with right to left shunts at baseline or shunts that reverse with exertion due to increased RV work. In IPAH, cyanosis occurs in the presence of an atrial shunt. With increasing cyanosis in ES patients comes the risk of increasing hematocrit with all the side effects of polycythemia, including headaches, coagulopathies, and microthrombosis. Hemoptysis can occur secondary to pulmonary infarcts with secondary arterial thrombosis; in patients with HHT, due to pulmonary telangiectasia; and, in some patients, because of overzealous or unsupervised anticoagulation. Chest pain was described in 16% of IPAH as compared with 3% of ES patients and is likely from right ventricular endothelial ischemia. Dilated pulmonary arteries compressing the coronary circulation have also been described to cause acute angina. A small proportion of patients, 3% and 7%, reported no symptoms in the two groups. In infants with PAH, failure to thrive is another significant symptom, in addition to those attributed to right heart failure, including irritability, feed intolerance, pedal and sacral edema, and malabsorption from intestinal edema. Patients with portopulmonary hypertension, metabolic disorders, and hematologic diseases and those with CTD associated PAH will exhibit symptoms related to the primary disease conditions.[84,85] The two most frequent mechanisms of death are progressive right ventricular failure and sudden death. Comorbidities such as pneumonia and other systemic infections result in alveolar hypoxia, leading to a downward spiral of pulmonary vasoconstriction and compromised cardiac output, resulting in cardiogenic shock and death. In addition to right ventricle hypertrophy (RVH) and right ventricle (RV) dilatation, elevated RV end diastolic pressures lead to right atrial dilatation and atrial arrhythmias, including atrial fibrillation and ventricular arrhythmias. Acidosis can make the arrhythmias worse, and the loss of atrial kick in atrial fibrillation and flutter can lead to low cardiac output and death. Possible mechanisms for sudden death include ventricular arrhythmias, acute pulmonary emboli, massive pulmonary hemorrhage, sudden right ventricular ischemia, and acute increases in RV pressure, leading to posterior septal bowing into the left ventricle and an acute drop in cardiac output.

PHYSICAL EXAMINATION FINDINGS

Failure to thrive, with reduced height and weight percentiles, is often present, and is an indicator of chronic disease. APAH with other diseases such as scleroderma or lupus will have the skin and joint manifestations of the primary disease. Genetic syndromes associated with PH, such as trisomies, CHARGE syndrome, Dursen syndrome, glycogen storage diseases, and other metabolic disorders, all have specific phenotypes.[36,86] Signs of heart failure, including tachycardia, tachypnea, edema, and hepatosplenomegaly, may be present. Hypotension is often associated with PH crises and is associated with a grave prognosis. Cardiac examination in children with IPAH may reveal a right ventricular heave, a loud pulmonary component of the second sound, a pulmonary artery systolic click, the holosystolic murmur of tricuspid regurgitation (TR), a right ventricular gallop, and a prominent early diastolic murmur of pulmonary regurgitation (PR). In CHD-PAH the cardiac findings will depend on the

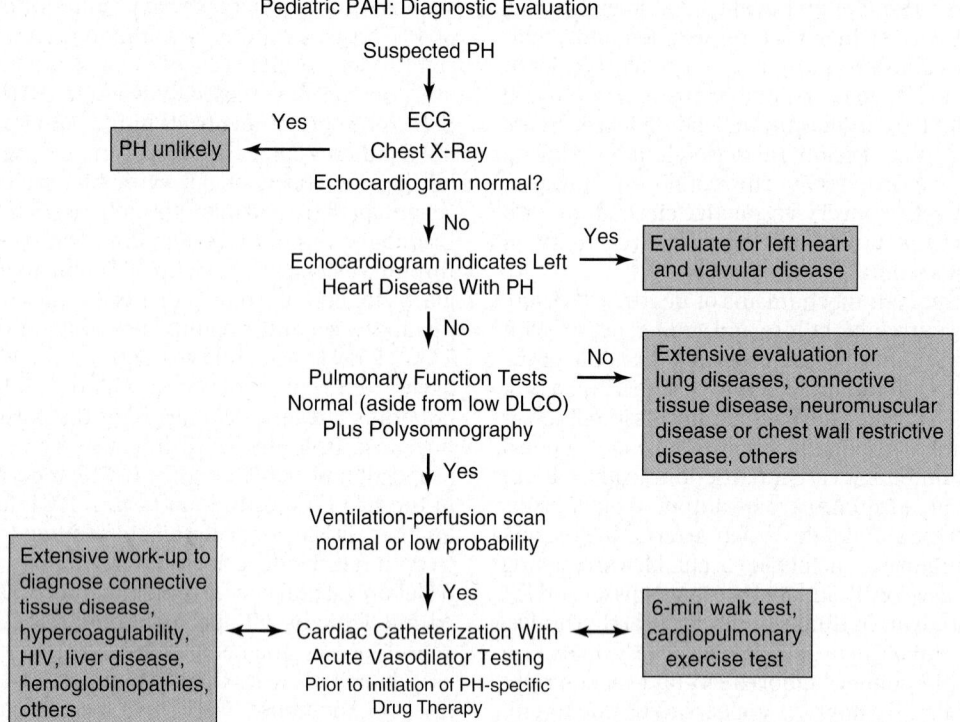

Fig. 35.3 Algorithm illustrating general diagnostic workup for pediatric pulmonary arterial hypertension. *DLCO,* Diffusing capacity of the lungs for carbon monoxide; *ECG,* electrocardiogram; *HIV,* human immunodeficiency virus; *PH,* pulmonary hypertension. (From Abman SH, Hansmann G, Archer SL, et al. Pediatric pulmonary hypertension: guidelines from the American Heart Association and American Thoracic Society. *Circulation.* 2015;132(21): 2037-2099.)

underlying heart disease. Clubbing and cyanosis are usually associated with ES. Unless there is associated lung disease or pleural effusions from heart failure, the lung exam should be normal.

DIAGNOSIS AND ASSESSMENT

It is important that the diagnosis and evaluation of children with suspected PH be done at a specialty center with expertise in the management of PH.[87] An algorithm illustrating the diagnostic workup for pediatric PAH is shown in Fig. 35.3. The diagnosis of IPAH is one of exclusion. It is critical to exclude all likely related or associated conditions that might be managed differently. A detailed history and physical examination, as well as appropriate tests, must be performed to uncover potential causative or contributing factors, as well as to assess cardiac function and functional class of the patient at baseline. A detailed family history, including a diagnosis of pulmonary hypertension, connective tissue or rheumatologic/immune disorders, CHD, other congenital anomalies, and unexplained deaths, may be contributory. If the family history suggests FPAH, careful screening of all first-degree relatives is recommended. Genetic testing should ideally be performed in all patients presenting with PH. Additional issues to address include obtaining a detailed birth/neonatal history, a medication history, exposure to high altitude or to toxic cooking oil, travel history, and any history of frequent respiratory tract infections, or venous or arterial thrombi.[88] The medication history should also include psychotropic drugs; appetite suppressants; chemotherapy, including tyrosine kinase inhibitors (dasatinib); use of glucagon

in infants; selective serotonin reuptake inhibitors (SSRIs) in pregnancy; and over-the-counter drugs. The answers to these questions may offer clues to a possible "trigger" for the development of the PAH.

The diagnostic evaluation in children suspected of having PAH is similar to that of adult patients. Follow-up evaluations are done 3–6 monthly to assess detailed functional class, both on history as well as testing, which should include a 6-minute walk test, cardiopulmonary exercise testing (CPET), imaging studies, and laboratory testing.

Echocardiography in Pediatric Pulmonary Arterial Hypertension

Echocardiography has a very important role to play in the diagnosis and follow-up of patients with PAH. It is used to screen for PH, rule out associated structural heart disease, determine heart function, and estimate the PAP by Doppler.[89,90]

The echo protocol suggested for an IPAH patient includes two-dimensional (2D) and Doppler evaluation for atrial and ventricular enlargement and hypertrophy. Pulmonary artery systolic pressure (PASP) can be determined by measuring the peak systolic pressure gradient from the right ventricle to the right atrium (calculated using the Bernoulli equation $P = 4v$ [2], where v is the maximum velocity of the TR jet measured by continuous wave Doppler) and adding the estimated right atrial pressure. The TR jet may be inadequate to estimate peak velocity in 10%–25% of patients, and simultaneous systemic blood pressure (BP) should be measured and documented in all studies. Using the TR jet velocity (TRV) as an estimate of PASP can overestimate or underestimate the PAP, and the clinician uses other features of the echo-cardiogram to support the diagnosis.[90–93] Adult studies estimate the sensitivity and specificity of TRV Doppler to be 0.79–1 and 0.68–98, respectively, but it is lower in infants with lung disease. Estimation of RV function is challenging due to the complex geometry of the RV compared with the left. Several measures have been described to estimate the degree of RV dysfunction, including the Tei index, (myocardial performance index), tissue Doppler, RV ejection fraction, RV fractional area change, and tricuspid annular plane systolic excursion (TAPSE).[94] The pulmonary artery Doppler also provides helpful clues toward indirect estimation of PVR.[92] Prolongation of the PA preejection time suggests elevated PVR. Shortened PA acceleration time and presence of systolic notching on PA Doppler suggest elevated PVR. When PR is present, the velocity profile of the pulmonary regurgitant jet can be used to estimate the pulmonary artery diastolic pressure. The peak PR and the end diastolic PR gradients correlate with mean and end diastolic PA pressures. In the presence of ventricular or great artery level shunts, the Doppler gradient across the shunts can give an estimate of RV and PA systolic pressures. Ventricular septal flattening and posterior systolic bowing occur as the right ventricular pressure increases and then exceeds the left ventricular pressure. The ratio of the left ventricle (LV) minor and major axes in the parasternal short axis view at the level of mitral valve chordae is the eccentricity index, which quantifies septal flattening and RV-LV interactions. With severe right ventricular hypertension, as the septum bows posteriorly pancaking the LV, the LV size and diastolic filling is reduced, and hence LV diastolic function gets compromised. The LV systolic function is usually preserved at this time. A redistribution of left ventricular filling from early to late diastole as demonstrated by Doppler reflects reduced compliance.[91,92,95,96] Diastolic dysfunction of the ventricles can be quantified by mitral and tricuspid diastolic inflow velocities, pulmonary and systemic venous flow patterns, and tissue Doppler imaging of the mitral and tricuspid annulus.

Hemodynamics/Cardiac Catheterization

Despite advances in noninvasive technology, cardiac catheterization remains the "gold standard" for the diagnosis of PAH. Cardiac catheterization is necessary (1) to confirm the diagnosis and assess the severity of PH; (2) to exclude other potentially treatable conditions, such as pulmonary thromboembolic disease; (3) to rule out left heart disease; (4) to assess response to vasodilators before starting therapy (and to reassess on therapy to determine need for escalation or change in treatment); (5) to determine operability in patients with APAH-CHD; and (6) to determine suitability for lung transplantation. Cardiac catheterization is performed under general anesthesia or conscious sedation. It is important that the procedure is performed at centers with multispecialty experience in management of PH, as there can be significant morbidity and mortality. In experienced hands the risk of complications is 0%–1%.[97–101] As shown in the diagnostic algorithm (see Fig. 35.3), all children should undergo a diagnostic cardiac catheterization with acute pulmonary vasodilator testing using a short-acting vasodilator to determine acute vascular responsiveness.[14] In very small premature infants with PH or in critically ill children presenting with severe PH in heart failure, treatment may be initiated with

prostanoids or other appropriate targeted therapy prior to cardiac catheterization, which is then performed when the patient is a more suitable candidate from a size and stability standpoint. The younger the child is at the time of diagnosis, the more likely that the child will respond to acute testing, but there is wide variability. The presence of a robust response to acute vasodilator testing usually predicts long-term response to high-dose oral calcium channel blockade therapy. Unfortunately there are no additional hemodynamic or demographic variables that accurately predict whether or not a child will respond to acute vasodilator testing. It appears that HPAH patients are less likely to respond to acute vasodilator testing and therefore less likely to respond to chronic calcium channel blockade treatment. Acute vasoreactivity has been defined differently by different authors. In adults, the most accepted definition is the Sitbon criteria: reduction in mean PAP by at least 10 mm Hg to <40 mm Hg, with no change or increase in the cardiac index.[102] The REVEAL registry used the modified pediatric criteria of a decrease in mPAP >20%, with an increase or no change in the cardiac index and a decrease or no change in the PVR/SVR ratio, to analyze their pediatric subgroup.[82] They found 35% of their IPAH (36/102 patients of which 5/13 were HPAH) and 15% of their APAH (9/60) were acute responders. When the Sitbon criteria were used, this proportion dropped to 19% of IPAH and 7% of APAH-CHD patients, which is similar to adult values. The REVEAL registry analyzed 5-year survival based on the pediatric criteria and found no death in the 22 acute responders who were treated with calcium channel blockers, in the 5 years following diagnostic right heart catheterization.[8] These observations underscore the marked biological variability in the time course of IPAH and emphasize the need to individualize the therapeutic approach. The currently recommended vasodilators for acute vasodilator drug testing are iNO (20–80 PPM), 100% oxygen, inhaled iloprost, intravenous epoprostenol, intravenous adenosine, and intravenous sildenafil. Patients who do not manifest a response to acute vasodilator testing are unlikely to have clinical benefit from chronic oral calcium channel blockade therapy. Furthermore, acute deterioration and decompensation may occur with empiric calcium channel blockade therapy in patients who are not acutely responsive, particularly in children with underlying lung disease. Patients with veno-occlusive disease or WHO group 2 PH may develop acute pulmonary edema during vasodilator testing and require very close monitoring if testing is done. Cardiac catheterization is also essential in patients with APAH-CHD to evaluate shunts and determine operability, as well as response to therapy. Left heart catheterization is done to assess pulmonary venous, left atrial, and left ventricular pressures and to evaluate for covert or overt diastolic dysfunction, and angiograms are performed to evaluate for aortopulmonary collaterals, pulmonary vein stenosis, and peripheral pulmonary artery stenosis or occlusion with thrombus. Cardiac catheterization is repeated in the setting of clinical worsening on therapy, after a change in therapy, or every 1–2 years during follow-up to assess continued response to therapy (AHA guidelines).

Other imaging studies include computerized tomography (CT) scans to evaluate parenchymal lung disease and vascular lesions, and CT angiograms to help in diagnosing pulmonary venous and arterial abnormalities, as well as to detect pulmonary embolism.[103–105] Ventilation-perfusion scans are performed in older children to diagnose pulmonary embolism and also to evaluate differential blood flows in children with PH after surgery for CHD.

Magnetic Resonance Imaging

Because the shape of the right ventricle limits the ability of echocardiography to accurately assess RV volume, mass, and function, magnetic resonance imaging (MRI) has become the gold standard for evaluating the RV. It is particularly useful in serial follow-up after surgery. In young children, MRI still requires sedation to ensure adequate imaging, and this may be an added risk factor in children with PAH. However, in adults with PAH, indices of ventricular size and function are useful in predicting mortality, and the use of MRI is more widespread.[98,106,107]

Assessment of Functional Capacity

The 6-Minute Walk Distance (6MWD) Test. This is used in children older than 6–8 years, who are capable of performing an adequate 6MWD, for baseline assessment and serial follow-up on therapy. It is a useful test to follow patients on therapy; however, in pediatrics, one must take into account age, height, and weight while interpreting the results, and its utility has not been well-validated in children.

Cardiopulmonary Exercise Testing. This test is performed in children older than 7–8 years, who are capable of using a bicycle ergometer. Variables measured include maximal oxygen consumption, carbon dioxide elimination, cardiac output, and anaerobic threshold. Yetman et al. reported in a series of 40 children with PAH who underwent CPET that parameters such as peak oxygen consumption (pVO_2), anaerobic threshold, end tidal carbon dioxide, and change in ventilation per amount of expired carbon dioxide (VE/VCO_2) correlated with invasive measures of disease severity, including pulmonary vascular resistance.[108–111]

Laboratory Testing. Baseline and follow-up laboratory testing performed include the following: (1) Those required to diagnose etiology of disease include hematologic tests for coagulopathy, factor V Leiden abnormalities, hemoglobinopathies, and connective tissue disorders. (2) Monitoring effects of treatment includes complete blood counts, liver function tests, and thyroid function tests. (Anemia and elevated aminotransferases may be caused by ET receptor antagonists, low platelets may be a marker for worsening PH, and thyroid dysfunction is a side effect of prostanoids.) (3) Biomarkers for ventricular function are brain natriuretic peptide (BNP) and N-terminal pro B-type natriuretic peptide (NT-proBNP), which are useful in following improvement or worsening of PH in response to therapy.[112,113] Circulating endothelial cells have been described by Levy et al. from Paris as another biomarker to assess severity of PH and response to therapy.[70,114,115] (4) Genetic tests, including BMPR2, ALK1, ENG, SMAD, KNCK3, ELF2AK4, and Cav1, should ideally be performed in all patients at the time of initial evaluation, especially in children with FPAH.

A sleep study is recommended in patients at risk for sleep-disordered breathing, including children with genetic syndromes, former preterm infants, obese children, and those who do not respond appropriately to targeted therapy.[116]

Management

Although there is no cure for PAH, nor a single therapeutic approach that is uniformly successful, therapy has dramatically improved over the past several decades, resulting in sustained clinical and hemodynamic improvement, as well as increased survival in many children with various types of PAH.[58,117] An overview of our current approach and guidelines for treatment is shown in Fig. 35.3. Noninvasive studies obtained prior to initiating therapy, as well as periodically thereafter, are useful in guiding changes in therapeutic regimens, particularly in light of advances with various novel therapeutic agents.

GENERAL MEASURES

The pediatrician plays an invaluable role in the care of children with PAH. Because children often have a more reactive pulmonary vascular bed than adult patients, any respiratory tract infection that results in ventilation/perfusion mismatching from alveolar hypoxia can result in a serious or even catastrophic acute pulmonary hypertensive crisis if not treated aggressively. Influenza and pneumococcal vaccinations are recommended unless there are contraindications. Antipyretics should be administered for temperature elevations greater than 101° F (38° C) to minimize the consequences of increased metabolic demands on an already compromised cardiorespiratory system. Children may also require aggressive therapy (e.g., iNO) for acute pulmonary hypertensive crises occurring during episodes of pneumonia or other infectious diseases. Patients may require antitussive medications during upper respiratory infections to prevent excessive coughing, which increases pulmonary artery pressures and can result in acute pulmonary hypertensive crises. Decongestants with pseudoephedrine should be avoided because they may exacerbate the pulmonary hypertension. Diet and medical therapy should be used to prevent constipation because Valsalva maneuvers transiently decrease venous return to the right side of the heart and may precipitate syncopal episodes.

ANTICOAGULATION

Consideration of chronic anticoagulation in children with PAH is based on observational studies in adults with IPAH.[118] The lung histopathology often demonstrates thrombotic lesions in small pulmonary arterioles in both adult and pediatric patients with IPAH and other forms of APAH. Some patients have an underlying coagulopathy (e.g., antiphospholipid syndrome or protein C/S deficiency). In patients with poor right ventricular function, thrombi can form within the ventricle, and postmortem examinations of patients with pulmonary vascular disease who have died suddenly often demonstrate fresh clot in the pulmonary vascular bed. Whether or not secondary thrombosis *in situ* is a significant exacerbating factor in patients with a normal resting cardiac output is unknown. In addition, even a small pulmonary embolus can be life-threatening in patients who cannot vasodilate or recruit additional pulmonary vessels. Clinical data supporting the chronic use of anticoagulation are limited.[119,120] Warfarin has been shown to be associated with improved survival in two retrospective adult observational studies, and one prospective adult observational study (in patients who were not responsive to acute vasodilator testing); all three studies were in adult patients with IPAH/HPAH or PAH associated with anorexigen exposure. The dosage of anticoagulation usually recommended is that to achieve an international normalized ratio (INR) of 1.5–2; however, certain clinical circumstances (e.g., positive lupus anticoagulant, positive anticardiolipin antibodies, factor V Leiden, factor II 20210A variant, and documented chronic thromboembolic disease) may require dose adjustment to maintain a higher INR. For patients at a higher risk of bleeding (e.g., patients with significant thrombocytopenia), the dosage should be adjusted to maintain a lower INR. Whether or not chronic anticoagulation is efficacious and safe for children with pulmonary hypertension remains to be determined. The guidelines suggest anticoagulation in older children who are hypercoagulable or in right heart failure, similar to the approach for adult patients.[14] In children who are extremely active, particularly toddlers, anticoagulation can be risky and not routinely recommended, unless there is a proven coagulation disorder. Antiplatelet therapy with aspirin or dipyridamole does not appear to be effective in areas of low flow, where thrombosis *in situ* is known to occur. However, studies have not been done to evaluate such agents in PAH. Parents should be advised to avoid administering other medications that could interact with the warfarin unless the possible interactions are known, and the dose of the warfarin is adjusted as needed. Similar to the approach with adult pulmonary hypertension patients, if anticoagulation with warfarin is contraindicated or dose adjustments are difficult, low-molecular-weight heparin at a dose of 0.75–1 mg/kg by subcutaneous administration once or twice daily may be a reasonable alternative. However, the long-term side effects of heparin, such as osteopenia and thrombocytopenia, are of concern. To date there are no studies comparing the safety and efficacy of anticoagulation with warfarin to heparin. There may be additional benefits of heparin on the pulmonary vascular bed.

CALCIUM CHANNEL BLOCKADE

Calcium channel blockers are a chemically heterogeneous group of compounds that inhibit calcium influx through the slow channel into cardiac and SMCs. Their usefulness for select patients with PAH is based on their pulmonary vasodilator effects. Acute vasodilator testing during right heart catheterization is a critical part of the initial assessment of patients with PAH to determine the appropriate initial treatment course. Chronic calcium channel blockade is efficacious for patients ("responders") who demonstrate a robust acute response to vasodilator testing, although not all acute "responders" have a sustained long-term response.[5,102,121] In contrast, patients who do not respond acutely fail to respond to long-term calcium channel blockade. In general, these "nonresponders" will respond to long-term treatment with an intravenous prostacyclin, such as epoprostenol, and may respond to other novel treatments. The term "nonresponder" is only used with respect to acute vasodilator testing and calcium channel blockade response.

For acute responders, most adult studies have used calcium channel blockers at relatively high doses (e.g., long-acting nifedipine 120–240 mg daily or amlodipine 2.5–10 mg daily), with lower doses appropriate to weight in children. Calcium channel blockers are also not recommended in infants.[14] Because of the frequent occurrence of significant adverse effects with calcium channel blockade therapy in nonresponders, including systemic hypotension, pulmonary edema, right ventricular failure, and death, treatment with calcium channel blockers is not recommended for patients in whom acute effectiveness has not been demonstrated. This supports the importance of an initial assessment by cardiac catheterization with acute vasodilator testing before prescribing a long-term pulmonary vasodilator.

Serial Reevaluations

Serial reevaluations, including repeat vasodilator testing to maintain an "optimal" chronic therapeutic regimen, are essential to the care of children with PAH. In our experience, acute "responders" who are treated with chronic oral calcium channel blockade therapy continue to do exceedingly well as long as they remain acutely reactive to vasodilator testing on repeat cardiac catheterizations. In contrast, children who are initially acute "responders" and are treated with chronic calcium channel blockade, and who then stop demonstrating active vasoreactivity on repeat testing, usually deteriorate clinically and hemodynamically despite continuation of chronic calcium channel blockade therapy. If they are then treated with continuous intravenous epoprostenol, they will probably demonstrate improvement similar to the experience with children who are "nonresponders." Other novel therapeutic agents, discussed later, may also be considered for these patients.

Targeted Pulmonary Arterial Hypertension Therapy

Prior to 1995, there were no approved therapies for PAH. However, since then, multiple randomized controlled trials with nine compounds as monotherapy have been completed in adult PAH patients. In addition, six randomized controlled trials evaluating combinations of agents (e.g., ET-receptor antagonists [ERAs] and PDE5 inhibitors, or prostacyclin analogues and ERAs or PDE5 inhibitors) have been completed. More than 5000 patients, the vast majority being adults, have participated in these studies aimed at developing effective treatments for PAH. The conclusions derived from clinical trials over the past 20 years have permitted development of an evidence-based treatment algorithm for adult patients with PAH.[14] However, despite there being multiple drugs currently approved for adults, until recently, none were approved for pediatric use. In September 2017, bosentan, an endothelin receptor antagonist, became the first drug to be FDA approved for use in children over 3 years of age diagnosed with idiopathic or congenital PAH. Based on similarities between pediatric and adult PAH, consensus recommendations for pediatric PAH have to date been extrapolated from adult data with off-label use in children. Although off-label use in pediatric patients appears to have significantly improved the overall quality of life and outcomes for many children with PAH, without adequate long-term safety studies and determination of optimal dosing, we may not be treating them optimally. Nevertheless, treatment for pediatric PAH currently uses the adult evidence-based guidelines. In 2015, the ATS/AHA pediatric pulmonary hypertension guidelines were published, outlining suggested pediatric dosages for medications used for PAH. The fifth World Symposium on Pulmonary Hypertension published a treatment algorithm based on risk stratification of PAH (Figs. 35.4 and 35.5).

Treatment of IPAH initially focused on the use of vasodilators in the hope that an increase in pulmonary vascular tone significantly contributed to the high PAPs. Although the bulk of the pulmonary vascular obstruction was clearly anatomic, vasodilators offered the prospect not only of decreasing PAPs somewhat, and therefore the hemodynamic burden on the right ventricle, but also of prompting reversibility of the anatomic lesions. Unfortunately, results from the use of vasodilators, which could affect the systemic as well as the pulmonary circulation, led to progressive disenchantment with one agent after another.

Less than 10% of adult IPAH patients and even fewer patients with PAH associated with other conditions such as CTD or CHD respond acutely to vasodilator testing and are

AHA/ATS Consensus Pediatric PAH: Disease Severity

LOWER RISK	DETERMINANTS OF RISK	HIGHER RISK
No	Clinical evidence of RV failure	Yes
I,II	WHO class	III,IV
None	Syncope	Recurrent syncope
Minimal RV enlargement/dysfunction	Echocardiography	Significant RV enlargement/dysfunction Pericardial effusion
PVRI <10 WU × m² CI >3.0 L/min/m² PVR/SVR <0.5	Hemodynamics	PVRI >20 WU × m² CI <2.0 L/min/m² PVR/SVR >1.0
Minimally elevated	BNP/NTproBNP	Significantly elevated
Longer (>500 m)	6MWD	Shorter (<300 m)
Peak VO₂ >25 mL/kg/min	CPET	Peak VO₂ <15 mL/kg/min

Fig. 35.4 Features that distinguish severity of disease in pediatric pulmonary arterial hypertension. *6MWD*, 6-minute walk distance; *BNP*, brain natriuretic peptide; *CI*, cardiac index; *CPET*, cardiopulmonary exercise testing; *PVR*, pulmonary vascular resistance; *PVRI*, pulmonary vascular resistance index; *RV*, right ventricular; *SVR*, systemic vascular resistance; *WHO*, World Health Organization; *WU*, wood units. (From Abman SH, Hansmann G, Archer SL, et al. Pediatric pulmonary hypertension: guidelines from the American Heart Association and American Thoracic Society. *Circulation*. 2015;132(21):2037-2099.)

AHA/ATS Consensus Pediatric PAH Treatment Algorithm

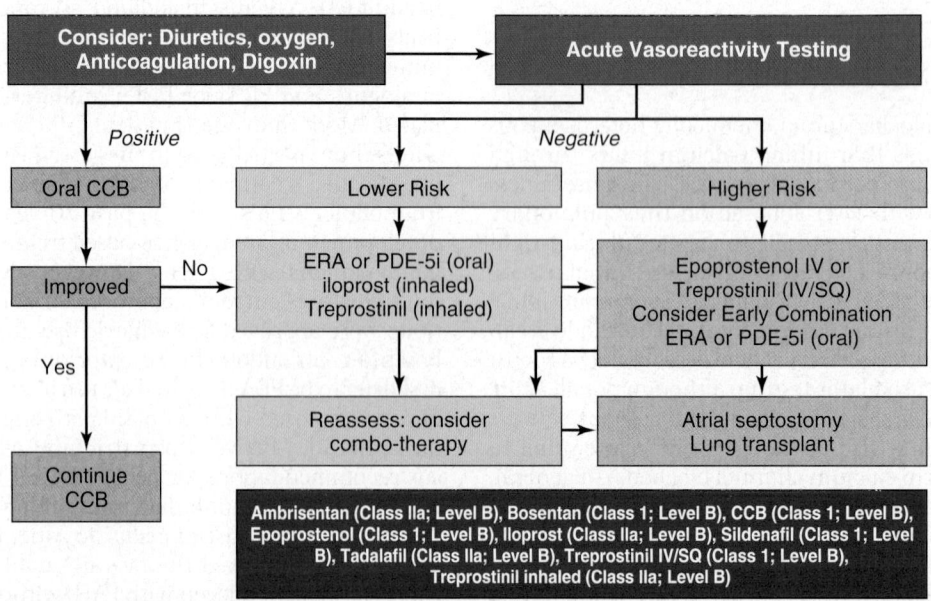

Fig. 35.5 Algorithm illustrating the pharmacological approach to pediatric pulmonary arterial hypertension. *CCB*, Calcium channel blocker; *ERA*, endothelin receptor antagonist; *PDE5i*, phosphodiesterase type 5 inhibitor. (From Abman SH, Hansmann G, Archer SL, et al. Pediatric pulmonary hypertension: guidelines from the American Heart Association and American Thoracic Society. *Circulation*. 2015;132(21):2037-2099.)

candidates for calcium channel blockade. A landmark development for patients who failed to satisfy the criteria for a good hemodynamic response to acute vasodilator testing was the demonstration that such patients respond to continuous infusions of epoprostenol. That is, patients who fail to respond acutely to intravenous epoprostenol can respond chronically. Indeed, a substantial number of such patients have been treated this way for many years or have used continuous intravenous epoprostenol as a transition to transplantation or newer drug therapies. During this evolution, heart-lung and then lung transplantation became increasingly feasible and available, although the donor supply is still a significant limiting factor. Since 2002, the development of oral medications that block the receptors for ET or that augment the effects of endogenous NO by inhibiting PDE5 (the enzyme responsible for the inactivation of cyclic guanosine monophosphate) have been shown to be effective therapies and are extensively used. Alternative forms of delivery of longer-acting prostacyclin analogues, including subcutaneous and inhaled, are approved in adults and being used in children. They may delay the need for intravenous prostacyclin therapy in many patients.

As a result of these advances, a patient with PAH has several therapeutic options. However, none of these modalities are free from complications, and one must remember that all of these drugs were evaluated primarily in adult patients and not in children. Thus safety concerns for a class of drugs may be greater or less in children, based on their metabolism being different from adults. Many affected children are still growing, with ongoing lung development, and the optimal doses are not necessarily being used (or known). ET receptor antagonists can cause hepatic injury. The continuous infusion of a prostacyclin analogue has the risks associated with a permanently placed intravenous catheter, such as bacteremia, sepsis, or thromboembolic events. Transplantation offers the substitution of immunosuppression and its attendant risk of infection as a "better" or alternative option to RV failure. Despite the limitations of each of these therapeutic modalities, together they provide a graduated therapeutic approach that has provided, at each stage, a better quality of life for many children with PAH.

PROSTACYCLIN ANALOGUES

Intravenous Prostacyclin (Epoprostenol)

Epoprostenol (prostacyclin) has been used since its approval in 1995 with great success. It improves hemodynamics, quality of life, and exercise capacity in patients with IPAH and PAH associated with other conditions such as CHD, CTD, HIV infection, and portal hypertension, and increases survival in IPAH/HPAH. By the late 1990s, epoprostenol became the "gold" standard for treatment of IPAH in patients who were not responsive to acute vasodilator testing and therefore would not benefit from chronic oral calcium channel blockade. Epoprostenol (prostacyclin, prostaglandin I_2), a metabolite of arachidonic acid, and its analogues continue to be a major focus for treatment for a variety of forms of PAH. The pulmonary endothelium naturally elaborates prostacyclin into the bloodstream, where it has a short biological half-life (2–3 minutes). In principle, prostacyclin is attractive for the treatment of PAH on several accounts. It has been shown to (1)

be a pulmonary vasodilator, (2) inhibit platelet aggregation, (3) inhibit proliferation of vascular smooth muscle, (4) improve endothelial dysfunction, and (5) possibly be a cardiac inotrope.

The use of prostacyclin or other prostacyclin analogues for the treatment of IPAH is supported by the demonstration of an imbalance in the TX to prostacyclin metabolites in patients with IPAH, as well as the demonstration of a reduction in prostacyclin synthase in the pulmonary arteries of patients with IPAH.[4,6,122] Although chronic intravenous epoprostenol improves exercise tolerance, hemodynamics, and survival in patients with IPAH, its mechanism(s) of action remains unclear. Epoprostenol lowers pulmonary artery pressure, increases cardiac output, and increases oxygen transport. These effects occur with long-term use, even if there is no acute response to vasodilator testing supporting the premise that epoprostenol has additional properties (other than as a pulmonary vasodilator), resulting in pulmonary vascular remodeling. The optimal dose of intravenous epoprostenol is unclear. The dose (ng/kg/min) is titrated incrementally, with the most rapid increases during the first several months of epoprostenol use. Although a mean dose at 1 year in adult patients is approximately 20–40 ng/kg/min, the mean dose at 1 year in children, particularly young children, is closer to 50–80 ng/kg/min, but there is significant patient variability in the "optimal" dose.[60]

Because epoprostenol is chemically unstable at neutral pH/room temperature and has a short half-life (1–2 minutes), chronic epoprostenol treatment requires a continuous intravenous delivery system with cold packs to maintain stability. A thermostable and PH stabilized molecule of epoprostenol is now available and is approved for use in adult PH. Permanent central venous access is required to administer the medication. Thus serious complications are associated with its use such as line sepsis, local site infection, and catheter dislodgment. In addition, pump malfunction may lead to a sudden bolus of epoprostenol (rare) or interruption of the medication that can cause severe rebound PAH. Therefore a search for alternate routes of drug delivery has led to the clinical development of oral, inhaled, and subcutaneous prostacyclin analogues. Treprostinil, a longer-acting prostacyclin analogue, is approved for continuous subcutaneous, continuous intravenous, or inhaled (administered four times daily) use, and can also be administered using a mini-pump that is more portable.

Inhaled Prostacyclin Analogues (Iloprost, Treprostinil)

Iloprost, an inhaled prostacyclin analogue, may be advantageous because of the potential benefits of inhaled delivery that may avoid some of the systemic side effects, including hypotension, that can accompany epoprostenol use. Iloprost is a more stable synthetic analogue of prostacyclin.[123,124] It has a similar molecular structure to prostacyclin and acts through prostacyclin receptors on vascular endothelial cells. Iloprost has both vasodilator and platelet aggregation inhibition properties similar to prostacyclin. It has a biological half-life of approximately 20–25 minutes in humans, and it has been shown to have more pronounced short-term hemodynamic effects than iNO in patients with IPAH.

Inhaled iloprost (2.5–7.5 mcg, 6–9 times a day [median adult dose 30 µg/day]) was approved in 2004 for the treatment of PAH. The noninvasive delivery method makes it appealing, but the need for 6–9 treatments a day (each lasting 5–15 minutes) can be a considerable burden for patients, particularly children. Furthermore, the currently approved inhalation devices may be challenging for routine administration in young children. Randomized trials of inhaled iloprost versus intravenous epoprostenol are warranted, although the feasibility of such trials is problematic. It also has use in the intensive care setting where it has been used even more frequently (hourly and continuously) to prevent PH crises.

The acute effects of iNO have also been compared with aerosolized iloprost for children with pulmonary hypertension and congenital heart defects and found to be equally efficacious.[124,125] Although additive effects have been suggested when the two agents are used together, in this study there were no additive or synergistic effects.

In 2009 the prostacyclin analogue treprostinil was approved in its inhalation form for PAH. Based on a longer half-life than iloprost, inhaled treprostinil is given four times a day as opposed to six to nine times a day for inhaled iloprost. A two-institution case series described the safety and tolerability of this medication in the pediatric population.[126,127] The delivery system may be easier for younger children to administer effectively compared with inhaled iloprost.

Subcutaneous/Intravenous Prostacyclin Analogue (Treprostinil)

Treprostinil sodium is a chemically stable prostacyclin analogue that shares at least some of the pharmacologic actions of epoprostenol. Acute hemodynamic effects with treprostinil are similar to those observed with intravenous epoprostenol in patients with IPAH; however, treprostinil is stable at room temperature and neutral pH and has a longer half-life, 2–3 hours, when administered subcutaneously. Similar to epoprostenol, treprostinil is infused continuously by a portable pump and can be administered either subcutaneously or intravenously. Treprostinil was approved in 2002 for subcutaneous infusion and in 2004 for intravenous infusion. The risk of central venous line infection is eliminated when treprostinil is used subcutaneously. Although no serious adverse events have been reported related to treprostinil or the delivery system when used subcutaneously, discomfort at the infusion site is common and may not be tolerated by older children.[126] There are recent literature describing use in infants and young children suggesting that the tolerability in this population is better than in older patients, indicating a difference in response to pain in infants with chronic lung disease of prematurity.[128–131]

Oral Prostacyclin Analogues

Oral Prostacyclin Analogue. Oral treprostinil was approved for use in adults with PAH in 2013 and was found in trials to improve exercise capacity in PAH. This medication is associated with gastrointestinal side effects and headaches that are often dose limiting. Doses can begin with 0.125 mg or 0.25 mg twice a day with gradual increases as tolerated. No pediatric data are available for this medication. Oral selexipag, a prostacyclin receptor agonist, has also been studied and approved in adults with group 1 PAH, but there are currently no data on its use for pediatric PAH.[132] It was studied in the Prostacyclin (PGI2) Receptor Agonist In Pulmonary Arterial HypertensiON (GRIPHON) trial, a multicenter, double-blind, randomized, parallel-group, placebo-controlled, event-driven, phase III study which showed that among patients with PAH, the risk of the primary end point of death or PAH complication was significantly lower with selexipag as compared with placebo.[132–134] The adverse effects were similar to prostanoid therapy.

ENDOTHELIN RECEPTOR ANTAGONISTS

ET-1 is a potent mitogen and vasoconstrictor that is produced in excess by the hypertensive pulmonary endothelium.[70,135] Circulating levels of ET are increased in patients with PAH, and the magnitude of elevation correlates with survival. There are at least two different receptor subtypes: ET_A receptors are localized on SMCs and mediate vasoconstriction and proliferation, whereas ET_B receptors are found predominantly on endothelial cells and are associated with (1) endothelium-dependent vasorelaxation through the release of vasodilators (i.e., prostacyclin and NO), (2) clearance of ET, and (3) vasoconstriction (on SMCs) and bronchoconstriction. The use of ERAs, both dual receptor and selective ET_A receptor antagonists, appears promising for children with PAH. For patients who do not have an acute response to vasodilator testing or have failed treatment with oral calcium channel blockade, ERAs may offer a viable treatment option. Bosentan, an orally active twice-daily dual ET_A and ET_B receptor antagonist, was approved in 2001 for adults with PAH and in September 2017 for children over 3 years of age with PAH.[50,136,137] This was a significant advance in the field of PAH in that prior to 2001 there were no oral therapies approved for PAH. This drug is generally well-tolerated; however, liver function must be monitored monthly because bosentan can produce significant hepatic dysfunction in approximately 8% of adult patients and approximately 3% of pediatric patients. In addition, because of potential teratogenicity, dual contraception is recommended, and care is advised while handling the medication by female caregivers. The FormUlation of bosenTan in pUlmonary arterial hypeRtEnsion (FUTURE)-2 study was an open-label long-term safety and tolerability phase III extension study of the FUTURE-1, which was a pharmacokinetic study of pediatric bosentan, showing that bosentan in a dose of 2 mg/kg twice a day was safe and effective.[138] A 5-year retrospective study of 101 children in the United Kingdom who received bosentan as monotherapy or combination showed that bosentan was safe and effective in slowing disease progression in pediatric PAH.[136,139]

Two selective oral ET_A receptor antagonists, sitaxsentan and ambrisentan, have also been developed.[140] The rationale for selective ET_A receptor blockade is that it may benefit patients by blocking the vasoconstrictor effects of the ET_A receptor while maintaining the vasodilator and clearance effects of the ET_B receptor. Sitaxsentan was found to be associated with fatal hepatotoxicity and was withdrawn from commercial use in 2010. Ambrisentan is a longer-acting (once a day) selective ET_A receptor blocker. The safety and tolerability of ambrisentan in the pediatric age group was described in a two institution case series, and the medication was shown to improve functional class and hemodynamics in a group of 38 pediatric patients.[141-143] Macitentan is a newer tissue-specific ERA that has been shown to reduce morbidity and mortality in patients with PAH in a multicenter, double-blind, randomized placebo controlled, event-driven phase III trial (Endothelin Receptor Antagonist in Pulmonary Arterial Hypertension to Improve Clinical Outcome [SERAPHIN] trial).[144] This trial included patients older than 12 years. There are no studies describing the use of macitentan in patients younger than 12 years.

Inhaled Nitric Oxide

NO is synthesized in endothelial cells from one of the guanidine nitrogens of L-arginine by the enzyme NO synthase. It has proved to be the endothelium-derived relaxing factor that contributes to the low initial tone of the pulmonary circulation. It has the advantage over other vasodilators of selectively relaxing pulmonary vessels without affecting systemic arterial pressure. It is currently being used as an acute test of vasoreactivity in a wide variety of pulmonary hypertensive states and is approved for PPHN.[145,146] When inhaled, the rapid combination of NO and hemoglobin inactivates any NO diffusing into the blood, preventing systemic vasodilatation. NO is therefore a potent and selective pulmonary vasodilator when administered by inhalation. NO may also have antiproliferative effects on smooth muscle and inhibit platelet adhesion. iNO has been demonstrated to be safe and efficacious in the treatment of PPHN. iNO has been useful for determining "operability" of patients with CHD. It has also been used for the treatment of IPAH exacerbations, perioperative pulmonary hypertension following cardiac surgery, and other forms of PAH. Clinical trials are in progress evaluating the safety and efficacy of chronic iNO in patients with inadequate responses to the currently approved PAH therapies.

PHOSPHODIESTERASE INHIBITORS

PDE5 inhibitors prevent the breakdown of cGMP, thereby raising cGMP levels. This effect should potentiate the pulmonary vasodilatation with NO. Sildenafil (orally active three times daily) and tadalafil (orally active once daily), both PDE5 inhibitors, enhance NO activity by inhibiting PDE5, the enzyme responsible for catabolism of cGMP. They were approved for the treatment of PAH in 2005 and 2009, respectively. PDE5 inhibitors may also be particularly beneficial in conjunction with chronic iNO, where withdrawal of NO may lead to rebound pulmonary hypertension. Intravenous, long-acting oral, or aerosolized forms of PDE5 inhibitors all have therapeutic appeal. The effects of intravenous sildenafil were compared with iNO in preoperative and postoperative patients with CHD and elevated pulmonary vascular resistance.[147-149] In this study, intravenous sildenafil was as effective as iNO in children with CHD. The Sildenafil in Treatment-Naive Children, Aged 1-17 Years, With Pulmonary Arterial Hypertension (STARTS-1) trial was a multicenter, placebo-controlled double-blind study of low-, medium-, and high-dose oral sildenafil monotherapy in treatment naïve pediatric PAH.[150,151] Improvement in VO2, functional class, and hemodynamics were seen with medium- and high-dose sildenafil. The STARTS-2 extension study, done over 3 years, showed an increased signal of mortality in the higher dose range in IPAH but not in APAH-CHD, and there was a favorable

survival for children on sildenafil across groups.[151] Based on these results, the European medicines agency approved sildenafil in children at a dose of 10 mg three times a day between 10 and 20 kg and 20 mg three times a day for >20 kg. The same data initially elicited a warning from the US Food and Drug Administration (FDA) in 2012, which was subsequently tempered down in 2014 to "judicious use by healthcare professionals when there is a favorable risk-benefit ratio for the patient" after publication of the STARTS 2 study and a review from the members of the pediatric pulmonary hypertension network.[152,153]

Tadalafil is a PDE5 inhibitor that is longer acting and suitable for once daily use. The initial experience describing its use in 33 children, either as a transition from sildenafil or initial therapy, suggested improved hemodynamics and functional class, with a similar side effect profile.[154] Larger studies are necessary to study the long-term effects of this drug in children.

The other available medication approved for adult PAH but have no reported pediatric experience is soluble guanylate cyclase stimulator riociguat, which is approved for WHO group 1 and 4 PH based on the randomized placebo-controlled phase III Pulmonary Arterial Hypertension Soluble Guanylate Cyclase–Stimulator Trial 1 (PATENT-1) and 2 (extension) and Chronic Thromboembolic Pulmonary Hypertension Soluble Guanylate Cyclase–Stimulator Trial 1 (CHEST-1) and 2 trials for PAH and inoperable CTEPH patients.[67,140,155]

Gene Therapy

With the identification of an HPAH gene, a mutation in the BMPR2 protein at chromosomal locus 2q33 that is associated with FPAH in selected families, attention has focused on gene replacement therapy. An alternative therapeutic approach has been to induce the overexpression of vasodilator genes, notably endothelial NO synthase and prostacyclin synthase, because patients with various forms of PAH have been shown to have deficiencies in both. Given the preliminary clinical observations that exogenous administration of chronic NO or epoprostenol may have salutary effects on even advanced forms of the disease, it seems worthwhile to pursue these alternative modes of "drug delivery." Advances in our understanding of the genetic predisposition associated with at least some, if not all, patients with PAH suggest that gene therapy may be possible in the future.

Oxygen

Some patients who remain fully saturated while awake demonstrate modest systemic arterial oxygen desaturation with sleep, which appears to be due to mild hypoventilation. During these episodes, children with pulmonary hypertension may experience severe dyspnea, as well as syncope, with or without hypoxic seizures. Desaturation during sleep usually occurs during the early morning hours and can be eliminated by using supplemental oxygen. We recommend that children have supplemental oxygen available at home for emergency use. Children with PAH should be treated with supplemental oxygen during any significant upper respiratory tract infections if systemic arterial oxygen desaturation occurs. Children with desaturation due to right to left shunting through a patent foramen ovale usually do not improve their oxygen saturation with supplemental oxygen, although oxygen supplementation may reduce the degree of polycythemia in these children. A small study of children with ES demonstrated improved long-term survival with supplemental oxygen. However, in a subsequent study with 23 adult patients with ES, there was no significant improvement in survival with nocturnal oxygen. Some children experience arterial oxygen desaturation with exercise as a result of increased oxygen extraction in the face of fixed oxygen delivery and may benefit from ambulatory supplemental oxygen. In addition, children with severe right ventricular failure and resting hypoxemia, resulting from a markedly increased oxygen extraction, should also be treated with chronic supplemental oxygen therapy. Supplemental oxygen is also recommended for air travel to avoid alveolar hypoxia and exacerbation of the pulmonary hypertension.

Additional Pharmacotherapy: Cardiac Glycosides, Diuretics, Antiarrhythmic Therapy, Inotropic Agents, and Nitrates

Although controversy persists regarding the value of digitalis in IPAH, children with right-sided heart failure may benefit from digitalis in addition to diuretic therapy. Diuretic therapy must be initiated cautiously because these patients are preload dependent to maintain optimal cardiac output. Despite this, relatively high doses of diuretic therapy are often needed. Although malignant arrhythmias are rare in pulmonary hypertension, treatment is appropriate for documented cases. Atrial flutter or fibrillation often precipitates an abrupt decrease in cardiac output and clinical deterioration due to loss of the atrial component. As opposed to healthy children, in whom atrial systole accounts for approximately 25% of the cardiac output, atrial systole in children with IPAH often contributes as much as 70% of the cardiac output. Therefore aggressive treatment of atrial flutter or fibrillation is advised.

Although there are no studies on the usefulness of intermittent or continuous treatment with inotropic agents, dobutamine can be used for additional inotropic support in conjunction with continuous intravenous epoprostenol in children with severe right ventricular dysfunction, as a bridge to transplantation. Children have also benefited from short-term inotropic support during acute pulmonary hypertensive crises to augment cardiac output during a period of increased metabolic demand.

Oral and sublingual nitrates have been used to treat chest pain in some children with IPAH, although the experience with these agents remains limited. Children who complain of chest tightness, or pressure, or vague discomfort that is responsive to sublingual nitroglycerin should be treated with chronic oral nitrates as well as sublingual nitroglycerin.

Atrial Septostomy

Children with recurrent syncope in severe right heart failure have a very poor prognosis.[156] Exercise-induced syncope is due to systemic vasodilation, with an inability to augment cardiac output (through a fixed pulmonary vascular bed) to maintain adequate cerebral perfusion. If right to left shunting through an interatrial or interventricular communication is present, cardiac output can be maintained or increased if necessary. In addition, right to left shunting at the atrial level alleviates signs and symptoms of right heart failure by decompression of the right atrium and right ventricle. Increased survival has been reported in patients with IPAH with a patent foramen ovale, although this remains controversial. Patency of the foramen ovale may improve survival if it allows sufficient right to left shunting to maintain cardiac output. Successful palliation of symptoms with atrial septostomy has been reported in several series.[157–159] In our experience, patients with PAH with recurrent syncope or right heart failure improve clinically, as well as hemodynamically, following atrial septostomy: patients experience no further syncope, and signs and symptoms of right-sided heart failure improve. Although systemic arterial oxygen saturation decreases, overall cardiac output and oxygen delivery improve, despite the right to left shunting at the atrial level. In our experience, atrial septostomy results in a survival benefit; the survival rates at 1 and 2 years are 87% and 76%, respectively, compared with conventional therapy (64% and 42% at 1 and 2 years, respectively).[158,159] Thus, although atrial septostomy does not alter the underlying disease process, it may improve quality of life and represent an alternative for selected patients with severe IPAH. However, this invasive procedure is not without risk; our indications for the procedure include recurrent syncope or right ventricular failure despite maximal medical therapy, and as a bridge to transplantation. Closure of the atrial septal defect can be performed at the time of transplantation.

POTTS SHUNT IN SEVERE PULMONARY ARTERIAL HYPERTENSION

Until the past decade, balloon atrial septostomy and lung transplant were the only available options for severe refractory pulmonary hypertension with heart failure. Because of better prognosis in Eisenmenger patients with great artery level shunts, the Potts shunt was proposed as an attractive alternative. The physiologic advantage is sparing the cerebral and coronary circulation of desaturated blood (as with an atrial septostomy) and also a more effective decompression of the hypertensive RV through the creation of a descending aorta-left pulmonary anastomosis. Baruteau et al. reported their experience in 24 children who underwent a Potts shunt over an 11-year period, of which five were done transcatheter. There were three early surgical deaths, but in the 21 of 24 survivors, there was dramatic improvement in functional class to 1 or 2, normalization of BNP, weaning off prostanoids, and catch up in growth. To prevent left to right shunting through the shunt and flooding of the lungs, this group also developed a unidirectional valved shunt, which would act as a pop-off only during suprasystemic right-sided pressures, without flooding the lungs.[160–163]

Lung Transplantation

Although successful heart-lung transplantation, as well as single and double lung transplantation with repair of congenital heart defect(s), has been available for more than 20 years, there are several limitations to these procedures. A limited number of centers perform the procedures in children, and the availability of suitable donors is limited. Furthermore, the high incidence of chronic allograft rejection or bronchiolitis obliterans in the transplanted organs of these patients (25%–50%) and the potential consequences of lifelong immunosuppression are of great concern. Both single and bilateral lung transplantation have been performed in pediatric patients with pulmonary vascular obstructive disease, including patients with severe right ventricular failure.[164] Currently, the overall 1-, 5-, and 10-year survival following lung transplantation for PAH patients is 64%, 44%, and 20%, respectively. There has been no significant improvement in survival in more recent years (e.g., 1998–2001 versus 1992–1998). For untreated Eisenmenger patients, the natural history is much more favorable. The 5- and 25-year survival is greater than 80% and 40%, respectively, for untreated Eisenmenger patients, as opposed to following lung transplantation with a 1- and 5-year survival of 52% and 39%, respectively. Thus transplantation is most often reserved for WHO functional class III and IV patients with PAH who have progressed despite optimal medical therapy (see Box 35.2). As progress is made in the medical management of PAH, the indications for transplantation will change. The course of the disease and the waiting time must be taken into account when referring for transplantation. Ideally, children should be listed when their probability of 2-year survival without transplantation is 50% or less. Although there are advantages and disadvantages to each operation (i.e., lung [single or double] versus heart-lung transplantation), there is currently no consensus regarding the optimal procedure. The availability of donor organs often influences the choice of procedure. It is possible that data on long-term survival will demonstrate a survival advantage of one procedure over another. Although lung and heart/lung transplantation are imperfect therapies for PAH, when offered to appropriately selected patients, transplantation may improve survival with an improved quality of life. Early referral to a center with expertise in pediatric lung and heart-lung transplantation will decrease pretransplantation mortality and allow families to have adequate time to make an informed and thoughtful choice about this therapy. Living-related donor transplantation remains controversial; although it has been successful, there is limited experience.

Conclusions

Recent therapeutic advances have significantly improved the prognosis for children with PAH. Nevertheless, PAH remains a serious condition that is extremely challenging to manage. Chronic vasodilator therapy with calcium channel blockade in "acute responders" to vasodilator testing, and continuous intravenous epoprostenol in "nonresponders" appears to be effective in children, with observational studies reporting improved survival, hemodynamics, and symptoms. In addition, prostacyclin analogues administered by inhalation, continuous subcutaneous or continuous intravenous infusion, or oral ERAs and oral PDE5 inhibitors are available for the treatment of PAH. Although not approved for PAH, iNO is frequently used in the acute setting, with chronic administration undergoing evaluation. In a carefully controlled setting, there may be a role for transitioning PAH children who have had an excellent response to long-term intravenous epoprostenol therapy to oral or inhaled agents. In the future, there will undoubtedly be more treatment options for patients with PAH. However, in the early stages of use and without controlled studies for comparison, the newer agents should be used cautiously with close monitoring for treatment failure. Based on distinct mechanism(s) of action, combination therapy may further improve the overall efficacy of treating a child's PAH. Future developments in vascular biology will improve our understanding of the etiologies of PAH and its pathobiology, as well as provide rationale for more specific medical therapies. The current treatment algorithm for pediatric patients, extrapolated from adult evidence-based guidelines, will continue to evolve as newer agents become available (see Fig. 35.5). Whether these new agents will prove to be as effective as intravenous epoprostenol in selected children remains unknown. In addition, with increasing collaborative efforts between pharmaceutical companies, regulatory agencies, and academia, the future of clinical drug development for pediatric patients looks bright. Such studies should further the advances made to date in treating children with PAH, as even when the disease is similar between children and adults, children are not merely "small adults." Optimal care for pediatric patients requires knowledge of the therapies assessed in pediatric patients in addition to study in adult patients.

We hope that by increasing our understanding of the pathobiology of PAH, novel treatment strategies will continue to evolve and one day we will be able to prevent and cure this disease.

References

Access the reference list online at ExpertConsult.com.

36 *Pulmonary Edema*

HUGH O'BRODOVICH, MD

Improvements in the intensive care and monitoring of patients with serious illnesses led to a greater appreciation of the significance of fluid movement into the lung as a complication of a variety of conditions. This, coupled with an improved understanding of the pathogenesis of pulmonary edema, has enhanced our ability to treat various illnesses in which pulmonary edema develops.

The chapter first outlines the relevant anatomy, factors that control fluid movement within the lung, mechanisms responsible for the genesis of pulmonary edema, and how this edema fluid is cleared from the lung's interstitium and airspaces. This background will enhance the reader's understanding of the pathophysiologic consequences of edema formation, including the clinical and laboratory findings. Common disorders associated with pulmonary edema are then described along with the approach to therapy, which is based on understanding the underlying pathophysiologic mechanisms.

Anatomic Considerations

Certain structural features of the lung are worth pointing out because they have a bearing on gas exchange during pulmonary edema. The capillaries are placed eccentrically within the alveolar septum (Fig. 36.1A). In some areas, the basement membranes of the capillary endothelium and the alveolar epithelium are fused with no additional space between them, even during edema formation. This situation is ideal for preserving gas exchange, at least until such time as the alveoli themselves are filled with liquid. In other areas, there is an interstitial space between the endothelial and epithelial basement membranes that contains secreted matrix. This matrix consists of structural proteins (e.g., collagens and elastin), attachment proteins for cells (e.g., laminin), and proteoglycans and glycosaminoglycans (e.g., hyaluronic acid, chondroitins, and heparan sulfate). In addition to supplying support to the capillary network, this widened portion of the alveolar-capillary membrane provides a channel for water and protein *en route* to the lymphatics and larger interstitial fluid spaces (see Fig. 36.1B). As long as fluid can be confined to these channels, gas exchange can be preserved. Morphometric studies have shown that the majority of interstitial edema accumulates within the thick, and not the thin, portion of the alveolar-capillary membrane.[1]

Pulmonary capillaries, similar to muscle capillaries, have a continuous endothelium with relatively tight intercellular junctions. The bronchial microvasculature, much like visceral capillaries, is discontinuous, with intercellular fenestrations or gaps. Whether these gaps account for the greater fluid movement across the bronchial capillaries, but not the pulmonary capillaries, remains to be determined. The role of bronchial circulation in the genesis of pulmonary edema may have been underestimated, but it is certain that bronchial circulation plays an important pathophysiologic role in inflammatory airway diseases such as asthma and inhalational lung injury.

At the ultrastructural level, the available evidence from tracer studies indicates that the alveolar epithelial membrane contains tighter intercellular junctions than does the capillary endothelial membrane. These epithelial tight junctions (zonulae occludentes) are estimated by both morphologic and physiologic studies to have an effective molecular radius of approximately 4 Å. This has two implications. First, they markedly restrict the movement of small ions, thereby making ions the most important solute in the genesis of osmotic pressure across the epithelial membrane. Second, fluid leaking from the vascular spaces is likely to be confined initially to the interstitial and lymphatic spaces; alveolar edema results only when the volume that can be handled by these spaces is overwhelmed. In contrast to the epithelium, the pores between endothelial cells have an effective molecular radius of approximately 40 Å. This 10-fold difference in interendothelial junction size allows the free movement of small ions and noncharged solutes, such as urea, but restricts the movement of larger macromolecules such as albumin and globulins. Thus, it is the protein concentration that is the most important solute in the genesis of transvascular osmotic pressure. These large macromolecules move across the microvasculature; however, the relative contributions of movement via pinocytotic vesicles (vesicular shuttle) versus across pores that can enlarge ("stretched pores"), especially when there is increased intravascular pressure or injury, is unclear.

Although the alveoli are often portrayed as spherical, a polyhedral model is closer to reality (see Chapter 6). From the perspective of fluid movement in the lung, the importance of this shape is that the walls of the alveolar septa are flat, except at the corners where the septa meet. Thus, it is only at the corners, where the alveolar air-liquid interface is curved, that the force exerted by surface tension can lower alveolar fluid and interstitial fluid pressures as predicted by the LaPlace relationship. The lower interstitial pressures at the corners favor movement of interstitial fluid that has traversed the alveolar capillary wall toward the corners of the alveolus. This is important from a lung fluid balance perspective. Alveolar type II epithelial cells are also predominately found in the corners of the alveoli.

Pulmonary blood vessels have been defined using both anatomic and physiologic criteria (see Chapter 6). Anatomically, the vessels have been classified traditionally by their morphologic characteristics as arteries, arterioles, capillaries, venules, or veins. Physiologically, these divisions are included under two broad classifications—alveolar and extraalveolar vessels—based on their behavior relative to the hydrostatic pressures of the interstitium surrounding the vessels, the interstitial fluid pressure. Alveolar vessels are in the alveolar walls and behave as if their outer walls were exposed to alveolar pressure. These vessels may collapse if airway

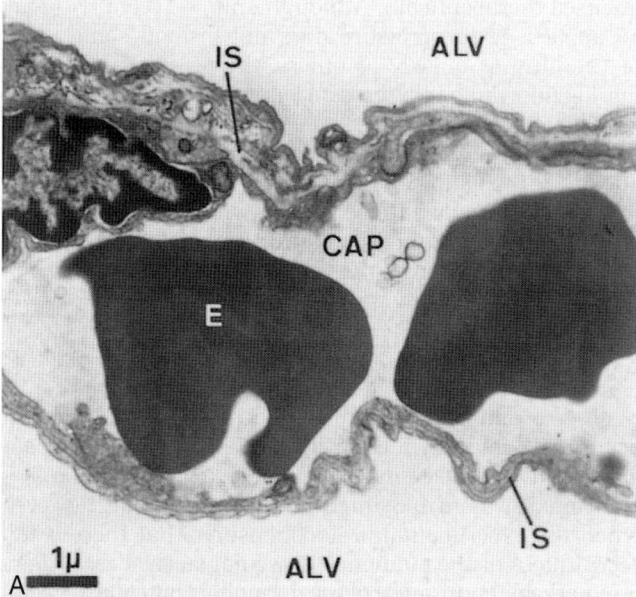

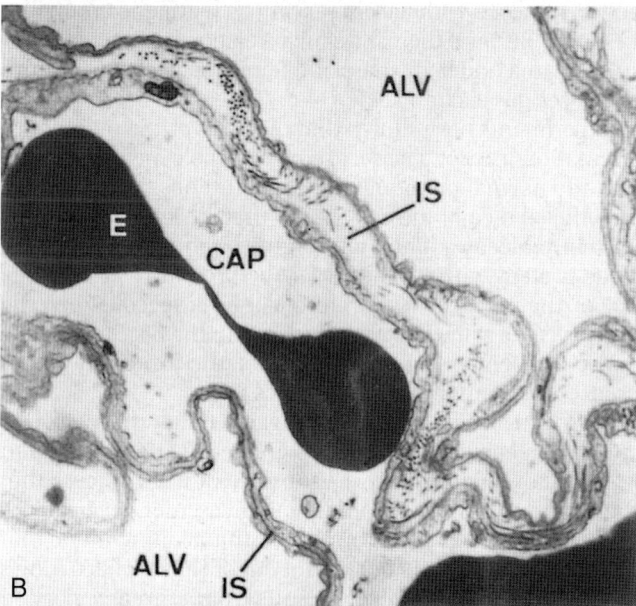

Fig. 36.1 (A) The normal alveolar septum in which the epithelial and endothelial basement membranes are fused in some areas and separated by an interstitial space of connective tissue in others. (B) The alveolar septum in pulmonary edema. The areas where the basement membranes are fused remain thin; only the areas with a connective tissue interstitial space widen. *ALV,* Alveolar lumen; *CAP,* capillary; *E,* erythrocyte; *IS,* interstitial space. (From Mellins RB, Levine OR, Skalak R, Fishman AP. Interstitial pressure of the lung. *Circ Res.* 1969;24:197.)

the bulk of fluid movement occurs at the level of the capillaries, with approximately three-fourths arising from the alveolar vessels.[2]

Anatomically, the lung has two main compartments, each possessing markedly different potential volumes, into which edema fluid can move. The interstitial spaces of the alveolar capillary septae and peribronchovascular compartment can only accommodate small amounts of fluid. When this small interstitial safety reservoir, estimated to be a few hundred milliliters in an adult lung,[3] is filled with edema fluid, subsequent accumulation must take place in the alveolar space, which at functional residual capacity (FRC) has a volume of approximately 30–40 mL/kg body weight or approximately 2000–3000 mL in the adult lung. This anatomic difference, in part, explains why interstitial edema may resolve quickly, whereas alveolar edema takes significantly longer periods of time.

Juxtacapillary (J) receptors are distributed throughout the lung's interstitium and are stimulated by the presence of edema. They induce an increase in respiratory rate and their continued activation is responsible, in large part, for the continued tachypnea seen in pulmonary edema even when hypoxemia has been corrected through the use of supplemental oxygen and positive airway pressure.

Factors Responsible for Fluid Movement

The factors responsible for fluid accumulation include intravascular and interstitial hydrostatic and colloid osmotic pressures, permeability characteristics of the fluid-exchanging membrane, and lymphatic drainage.

The equilibrium of fluid across fluid-exchanging membranes is generally expressed as the Starling equation:

$$Q_f = K_f[(Pmv - Ppmv) - \sigma(\pi mv - \pi pmv)]$$

wherein, Q_f = the net transvascular flow; K_f = the hydraulic conductivity and filtration surface area of the fluid-exchanging vessels; Pmv = microvascular hydrostatic pressure; $Ppmv$ = perimicrovascular (interstitial fluid) hydrostatic pressure; πmv = colloid osmotic pressure in the microvasculature; πpmv = colloid osmotic pressure in the perimicrovasculature, the interstitial fluid colloid osmotic pressure; and σ = the reflection coefficient, which is a measure of the resistance of the membrane to the movement of protein. Thus, σ influences the "effective" osmotic pressure of the protein. If the endothelium were completely impermeable to protein ($\sigma_{protein}$ = 1), then the 5 g/dL of plasma would yield approximately 28 mm Hg osmotic pressure (each 1 mOsm/L of solute yields 19 mm Hg pressure). The osmotic pressure resulting from proteins is also termed the "oncotic pressure."

As discussed subsequently, the absolute values for the variables within the Starling equation may change during health and disease. However, it should be emphasized that in the normal lung, Q_f is positive and there is a continuous movement of fluid from the vascular to the interstitial spaces of the lung. Experimentally derived values are approximately: Pmv = 20 cm H_2O, $Ppmv$ = −2 cm H_2O, πmv = −33 cm H_2O, πpmv = 20 cm H_2O, and 0.7 < σ < 0.95.

The term *microvasculature* is used to describe the vessels from which fluid leaks because fluid exchange is not limited

pressures exceed vascular pressures, as is the case in zone I perfusion conditions. Extraalveolar vessels lie in the larger interstitial spaces and behave as if their outer walls were exposed to a pressure that is as negative as or more negative than pleural pressure and that tends to vary with pleural pressure. In addition, there are vessels lying in the intersections of alveolar septal walls (corner vessels) that are exposed to more negative pressures than the alveolar vessels. Unfortunately, there is no clear-cut correlation between the functional and the anatomic classifications. Fluid movement occurs at the level of the arterioles, capillaries, and venules;

to the capillaries alone. In the following discussion, each of the above factors and the pathophysiologic influences on them are described in detail.

VASCULAR FORCES

The pressure in the pulmonary microvasculature (Pmv) is frequently, but not precisely, referred to as pulmonary capillary pressure. For technical reasons, this pressure is extremely difficult to measure *in vivo*. The pulmonary artery wedge pressure (Pw), also known as the pulmonary artery occlusion pressure, reflects the pressure in the first pulmonary veins where there is flow from nonobstructed vascular routes. Pmv is higher than left atrial (LA) pressure by approximately 40% of the difference between LA pressure and pulmonary arterial (PA) pressure. The relative amounts of arterial and venular resistance within the pulmonary vasculature is altered during hypoxia, the infusion of vasoactive agents (e.g., catecholamines) or during disease (e.g., endotoxinemia). An increase in either PA or LA pressure will tend to increase the hydrostatic pressure, favoring movement out of the fluid-exchanging vessels. For example, Pmv may be increased by the elevation in LA pressures in left-sided heart failure or by increases in PA pressure as seen in large left-to-right shunts. Although both PA and Pw pressures increase in a linear relation to exercise-induced increases in cardiac output, the ratio is significantly less than 1 : 1 in healthy young adult humans.[4] Because the pulmonary vascular membrane is only slightly permeable to proteins and freely permeable to ions and small uncharged solutes, the plasma proteins normally are responsible for osmotic pressure (πmv). The πmv is significantly above the pulmonary microvascular hydrostatic pressure. The plasma colloid osmotic pressure may be markedly reduced in clinical conditions in which the plasma proteins are low (e.g., malnutrition, nephrosis, and massive burns) and thus may facilitate the formation of pulmonary edema.

INTERSTITIAL FORCES

The interstitial hydrostatic pressure throughout the lung is normally negative relative to alveolar pressure,[5] and there is a positive alveolar-hilar pressure gradient[6] that facilitates the movement of interstitial fluid from alveolar to perihilar interstitial areas. The pressure surrounding the corner and extraalveolar vessels is less than pleural pressure[5] and becomes considerably more negative at high lung volumes. In disease, these negative pressures may be amplified many fold because of "mechanical interdependence" of lung units.[7] When the expansion of some units of the lung lags behind surrounding lung units because of disease, the force per unit area distending the lagging unit is increased. Amplification of transpulmonary (distending) pressures by mechanical interdependence is seen in conditions characterized by increased respiratory resistance, decreased lung compliance, and expansion of the lung from the airless state. Mechanical interdependence can act on diseased areas of the lung to produce distending pressures that are exceedingly high. When transmitted to the interstitial space around blood vessels, these pressures can enhance edema formation and can cause the rupture of vessels. These considerations become especially important, because various forms of constant distending pressures

are used therapeutically. Although only 5–10 cm H_2O may be applied, if the pressure does not distend some areas of the lung as quickly as others, the pressure surrounding lagging units may be considerably greater because of amplification.

Surfactant alters the liquid pressure within the airspace and, by extrapolation, the alveolar interstitial pressure.[8] Thus increased air-liquid surface tension, whether as a result of inadequate or dysfunctional surfactant, will promote the movement of fluid from the vessels into the lungs.

MICROVASCULAR FILTRATION COEFFICIENT AND VASCULAR PERMEABILITY

There are significant technical difficulties in obtaining an accurate estimate of the K_f within intact lungs and, dependent upon the species and experimental approach, estimates had varied by more than three orders of magnitude. However, when the experimental protocol ensures that there is full recruitment of the pulmonary vascular surface area, there is remarkable consistency of the normalized baseline K_f values between species with widely varying body weights from mice to sheep.[9] Because there is a similar relation between alveolar surface area and body mass of different species, this feature optimizes gas exchange.

Experiments have shown that the walls of the pulmonary circulation are not a perfect semipermeable membrane and that the normal pulmonary vasculature has $0 < \sigma < 1$. The endothelial membrane has "pores" that are larger than some protein molecules. Fluid filtering through a pore will drag some protein with it. The larger the protein relative to the size of the pore, the less protein will be dragged. When the protein is the same size as or larger than the pore, the reflection coefficient σ is 1. As the size of the protein becomes progressively smaller, σ approaches zero.[10]

Early experimental evidence suggested that the microvascular permeability to protein is greater in the young than in the adult animal; however, subsequent work showed that there was no difference in lung microvascular permeability to protein between late-term and postnatal animals and that the higher rate of fluid movement out of the newborn lung's microvasculature bed likely results from a greater portion of the younger smaller lung being in West's zone III perfusion status.[11]

LYMPHATIC CLEARANCE

Whether there is fluid accumulation in the lung depends on the balance between fluid filtration into the lung and lymphatic clearance. Early in the onset of interstitial edema, lymphatic drainage of fluid is an important protective mechanism to prevent alveolar flooding. Although early work had indicated that increased motion or ventilation of the lung increased the lymphatic fluid drainage, suggesting a passive milking action, it is now known that there are active contractions of the lymphatic smooth muscle that can be further augmented by vasoactive agents. Indeed, rhythmic inflation and deflation is not required for normal lymphatic function in lungs that have normal or increased vascular permeability.[12] Lung lymph flow can increase up to tenfold acutely, and when there is chronic edema, the maximal ability of the lymphatics to clear fluid may increase many fold, presumably as the result of proliferation of the lymphatic vasculature. Because the lymphatics ultimately drain into the great veins, elevation of systemic venous pressure might be expected to increase fluid accumulation, not only by raising pressure in the fluid-exchanging vessels, but also by opposing lymphatic drainage.

SURFACE TENSION

Surface tension at the air-liquid interface on the inner surface of the alveolus tends to pull fluid away from the alveolar epithelium with a force of at least 2 mm Hg. This surface tension at the alveolar air-liquid interface would be expected to expand the perivascular space and to lower perimicrovascular pressure. As pulmonary edema fluid enters the airspace, it first collects in the corners, but as fluid continues to accumulate, the filling of an alveolus with fluid is self-accelerating once there is a critical amount of fluid present.

SAFETY FACTORS THAT OPPOSE EDEMA FORMATION

A variety of clinical observations have indicated that transvascular hydrostatic pressures must be raised by 15–20 mm Hg before edema develops. Several factors provide this protection against edema formation. The interstitial fluid pressure, as previously described, is below alveolar pressure[13] and will rise when there is even minimal amounts of fluid accumulation within the lung[5,6] and thus oppose fluid movement. At the same time, the filtered fluid will dilute the interstitial plasma protein, thus lowering the interstitial colloid osmotic pressure and diminishing the movement of fluid out of the microvasculature. Lymphatic drainage of fluid and protein also contributes to this "margin of safety." The interstitial space itself, especially around the bronchi and blood vessels (bronchovascular cuffs), can sequester fluid (several hundred milliliters in the adult) and thus can provide an additional safety factor before fluid floods the alveoli.

Mechanisms That Cause Pulmonary Edema

There has been much effort to classify the different causes of pulmonary edema into cardiogenic and noncardiogenic pulmonary edema. Although this is useful to some degree, it should be remembered that in many lung diseases characterized by pulmonary edema, there are both increased transvascular pressure gradients and increased permeability to solutes. For example, 30% of patients diagnosed with acute lung injury (ALI) have a pulmonary artery wedge (occlusion) pressure greater than 18 mm Hg.[14] The various etiologies of pulmonary edema are introduced by using the Starling equation as the basis for the discussion.

INCREASED HYDROSTATIC PRESSURE IN THE PULMONARY MICROVASCULATURE

Increased hydrostatic pressure in the Pmv is the most common and perhaps most easily understood cause of pulmonary edema in the pediatric and adult population. A variety of clinical conditions are associated with increased hydrostatic pressures in the Pmv, either as the result of elevation of vascular pressures distal to the lung's parenchyma, increased blood flow, increased blood volume, or PA or venular hypertension. In each case, there would be an increase in the amount of water and solute leaving the microvasculature and entering the interstitium. Although hypoxia increases PA pressures, it does not by itself increase vascular permeability to solutes.[15]

DECREASED PLASMA COLLOID OSMOTIC PRESSURE

If a patient has no other disorders, hypoproteinemia will not, by itself, cause pulmonary edema. Large pleural effusions may develop in diseases such as the nephrotic syndrome, but there is no evidence of lung edema as assessed by gas exchange and chest radiography. However, in patients where vascular pressure or alveolar capillary membrane permeability increases, pulmonary edema is more likely to develop and be more severe when the plasma protein concentration is low. This is seen in various conditions including severe malnutrition, massive burns, protein-losing enteropathies, and nephrosis. Hypoproteinemia also can be seen in patients with a variety of other conditions when withdrawal of multiple blood samples for diagnostic purposes is coupled with the administration of large amounts of noncolloid-containing fluids.

DECREASED INTERSTITIAL HYDROSTATIC PRESSURE

As a result of mechanical interdependence of adjacent lung units, when inflation of some units lags behind that of others, large negative interstitial pressures can be generated around and within the lagging units. These negative pressures can be transmitted to the fluid-exchanging vessels (when there is airway closure), enhancing edema formation, especially in obstructive lung diseases such as asthma, bronchiolitis, and bronchopulmonary dysplasia (BPD), as well as in nonobstructive "stiff lung" disorders such as the respiratory distress syndrome (RDS).

INCREASED PULMONARY VASCULAR SURFACE AREA

The normal adult lung usually has approximately one-third of its microvascular bed perfused under resting conditions. Infants and young children have a greater percentage of their vascular bed distended with blood. Regardless of the absolute percentage, the lungs of all age groups can undergo significant recruitment and distention of the pulmonary vasculature. Although it had been suggested that various regions of the normal lung might have different permeability to solutes, most studies suggest that lung fluid movement simply increases in direct proportion to the increase in perfused pulmonary vascular surface area. Under normal conditions, the lung lymphatics can easily accommodate the threefold to fourfold increase in lung water and solute movement that is associated with full recruitment of the vasculature. However, when pulmonary vascular permeability is increased, similar amounts of recruitment can lead to marked increases in fluid movement as vessels with high permeability are recruited.[16,17]

INCREASED VASCULAR PERMEABILITY IN FLUID-EXCHANGING VESSELS

Increased alveolar-capillary membrane permeability to solutes can occur by different routes. Classic modeling of the Pmv uses the concept of various sized "pores" through which various-sized solutes move under normal physiologic conditions. Thus, permeability could increase via an increase in the total number of pores, the diameter of the pores, or a combination of the two phenomena. For example, vasoactive agents could increase the size of the interendothelial junctions. Alternatively, or in addition, direct and extensive damage to the alveolar epithelium or endothelium occurring during overventilation lung injury[18,19] or stress-induced endothelial injury[20] will open up large nonphysiologic pathways for fluid and solute movement.

A variety of clinical conditions are believed to alter the permeability of the alveolar capillary membrane, presumably by damage to epithelial and endothelial cells. The cellular mechanisms for this injury can be divided into two major categories: direct and inflammatory-mediated lung injury.

Direct lung injury can occur when a toxic substance directly causes cell injury without a preceding inflammatory response. Direct lung injury is seen during the inhalation of a variety of noxious gases, including the oxides of sulfur and nitrogen, hydrocyanic acid, and aldehydes. Similarly, the inhalation of gastric acid can directly damage lung epithelium. These produce denaturation of proteins, cellular damage, and pulmonary edema.

Inflammation-mediated lung injury, as occurs in ALI and acute respiratory distress syndrome (ARDS), most frequently arises from leukocytes and their products. The unregulated release of leukocyte-derived toxic products occurs in response to direct injury or in response to various infective and inflammatory stimuli. These toxic products include reactive oxygen species (e.g., superoxide, hydrogen peroxide, hypochlorous acid, hydroxyl radical, peroxynitrite), proteolytic enzymes (e.g., elastase, collagenase, lysozyme), products of arachidonic acid (e.g., platelet-activating factor), and cationic proteins. Leukocytes have been implicated in animal models of ALI induced by the administration of endotoxin, hyperoxia, microembolization, and mechanical ventilation. Nonleukocyte-derived vasoactive mediators also can increase vascular permeability. Examples include histamine, prostaglandins, cytokines, proteases, and reactive oxygen intermediates.

Increased permeability of the microvasculature also occurs in a variety of disorders characterized by aberrant regulation of the immune system. These include hypersensitivity pneumonitis and pulmonary vasculitis, which can occur in various disorders such as acute pulmonary systemic lupus erythematosus.

When there is increased pulmonary vascular permeability, an increase in microvascular hydrostatic pressure[16] or pulmonary blood flow[17] produces a much greater outward flow of fluid. As such, the combination of increased permeability and high LA pressures represents an especially difficult clinical challenge.

Clearance of Pulmonary Edema Fluid

Once the basic condition producing the edema is reversed, how quickly pulmonary edema resolves depends on whether the fluid is confined to the interstitium, from which it can be cleared in hours, or is also located in the alveolar space, from which it may take many hours or days to clear.

Interstitial fluid has two pathways for clearance. The lymphatics play the most important major role; however, a second site is the venular end of the microvascular bed where Pmv has decreased and the balance of Starling forces can favor reabsorption. Alveolar edema fluid, after being actively transported across the epithelium, is returned to the circulation either by direct entry into the Pmv across the thin side of alveolar capillary membrane or by the lymphatics after it has been translocated back to the interstitial space. Both of these potential pathways, however, require water and solutes to have first traversed the distal lung epithelium.

In both high-pressure and high-permeability pulmonary edema, there is a substantial amount of protein within the alveolar fluid that opposes protein osmotic reabsorption, and it has been shown that passive forces cannot explain the clearance of alveolar fluid from the intact lung.[21] Long-term studies have demonstrated that as edema fluid is reabsorbed, the protein concentration in the alveolar space actually increases to levels above those in the plasma. This suggests that an active transport of salt and water was involved in the clearance of airspace fluids. Numerous studies, as reviewed recently,[22] have demonstrated that nonprimate mammalian and human distal lung epithelium actively transports Na^+ with Cl^- and water following (Fig. 36.2). Although most research, for reasons of feasibility only, have focused on the alveolar type II epithelium's ability to actively transport salt, it is known that both the alveolar type I epithelium and Clara cells play important roles in this active epithelial Na^+ transport.[22] Studies in adult patients[23,24] have indicated that active alveolar fluid clearance rates in the human are in the range of 25% per hour.

Protein clearance from the alveolar spaces is significantly slower than salt and water, and in animals, it is in the range of 1% per hour.[21] The relative amount of protein cleared by metabolic degradation and macrophage ingestion versus active transport by the pulmonary epithelium is unknown, but active transport is involved in the clearance of at least some proteins from the airspaces of the lungs.[25] Protein clearance from the interstitial space is believed to occur primarily by lymphatic clearance, but direct penetration into the circulation either before or after metabolic degradation might also occur.

The presence of protein in the alveolar and interstitial spaces may attract inflammatory cells. In ALI syndromes, there is marked leakage of plasma protein into the alveolar space, and resultant activation of the coagulation cascade results in fibrin formation. The coagulum opposes the efficient reabsorption of fluid, and fibrin and fibrin degradation products are potent stimuli for fibrosis within the lung. Circulating monocytes and alveolar macrophages likely play a major role in the clearance of inflammatory edema protein from the lung's airspaces.

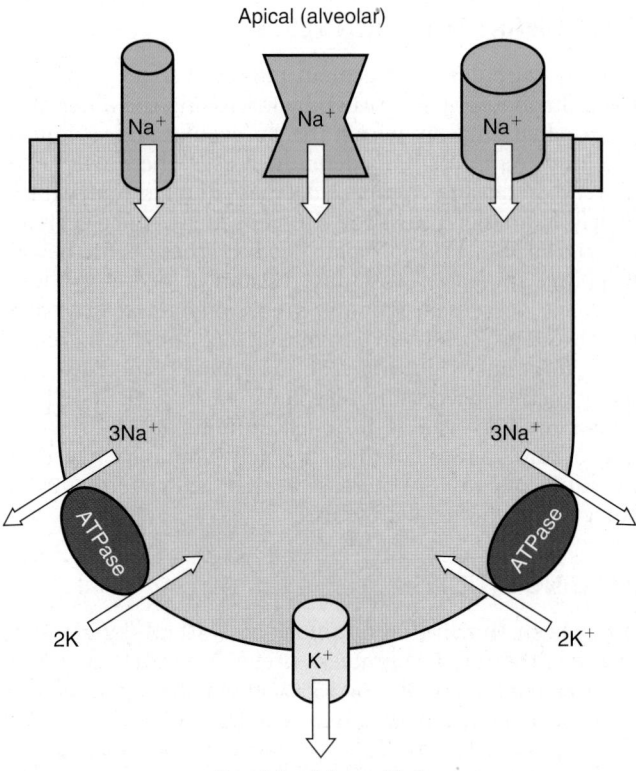

Apical (alveolar)

3Na⁺

2K

ATPase

K⁺

2K⁺

ATPase

3Na⁺

Basolateral (interstitial)

Fig. 36.2 Model for Na⁺ transport by the alveolar epithelium. The Na⁺/K⁺ ATPase located on the basolateral membrane is responsible for the creation of the marked intracellular/extracellular (10:150 mM) Na⁺ concentration gradient. This chemical gradient along with the negative intracellular electrical potential arising from the permeability of the K⁺ channels attracts Na⁺ ions into the cell through Na⁺-permeant ion channels located in the apical membrane to be extruded across the basolateral membrane. There are different types of Na⁺ channels in the apical membrane, the most important of which is the amiloride sensitive epithelial Na⁺ channel (ENaC). The activity of these Na⁺-permeant ion channels represents the rate-limiting step in Na⁺ transport. Chloride (Cl⁻) follows both via the paracellular pathway past the tight junctions and through the cell via the Cl⁻ channel encoded by the cystic fibrosis transmembrane conductance regulator (CFTR). Water follows in response to the osmotic gradient created by the active ion transport. For more details, see reference 22.

In summary, a wide variety of mechanisms and sites exist for protein and electrolyte clearance and fluid removal, including pulmonary and bronchial circulations, lymphatics, active transport of ions, macromolecular metabolism and degradation, and mononuclear cell activity.

Pathophysiologic Consequences of Edema

The pathophysiologic consequences and clinical findings in pulmonary edema are best understood by reviewing the sequence of events that lead from interstitial to airspace edema. Edema accumulates within the lung in a step-wise fashion (Fig. 36.3). Distal lung units in different regions of the lung will be at different stages of fluid accumulation because of their regional differences in pressure, alveolar-capillary membrane integrity, and gravitationally dependent factors.

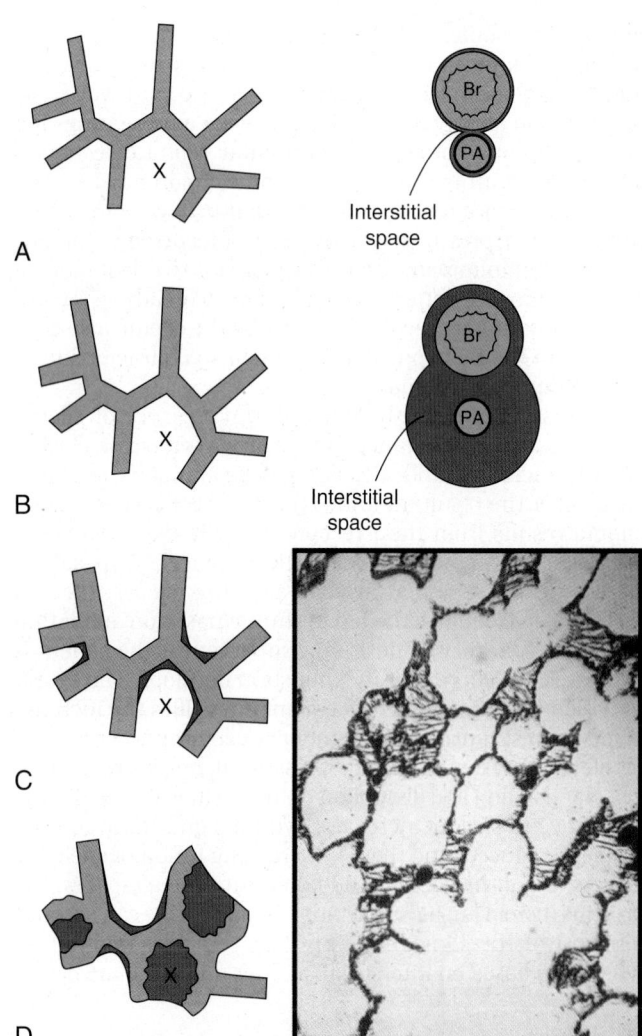

Fig. 36.3 Schematic representation of the sequence of fluid accumulation during acute pulmonary edema. (A) Normal alveolar walls and no excess fluid in perivascular connective tissue spaces. (B) Initial fluid leak. Fluid flows to the interstitial space (at subatmospheric pressure) around the conducting vessels and airways. (C) Tissue space fills, alveolar edema increases, and fluid begins to overflow into the alveoli, notably at the corners where curvature is pronounced. (D) Quantal filling. Individual alveoli reach a critical configuration at which existing inflation pressure can no longer maintain stability. Note that the fluid filled alveoli are smaller in size than their adjacent air-filled alveoli. The insert is a photomicrograph of a flash frozen lung with pulmonary edema that illustrates the above scheme of fluid filling. (From Staub NC, Nagano K, Pearce ML. Pulmonary edema in dogs, especially the sequence of fluid accumulation in lungs. *J Appl Physiol.* 1967;22:227-240.)

Increased pulmonary blood volumes, even without associated pulmonary edema, have been shown to cause a small decrease in lung compliance. Consistent with these findings, clinical studies have shown that infants with left to right congenital heart disease have low lung compliance that improves after correction of their shunt.[26]

In humans, the increase in airway resistance that occurs when there are small amounts of interstitial edema arises largely from a vagally mediated reflex.[27] Once interstitial edema worsens, the peribronchiolar cuffs of fluid would be expected to lead to increased closing volume and airway resistance, although this has been difficult to prove in morphometric studies of adult nonprimate lungs.[28] When small airways contribute a relatively greater proportion of the total airway resistance, as is the case in infants in contrast to adults, edema can lead to a greater increase in airway resistance. Small airway obstruction has been a presenting sign of a group of infants with ventricular septal defects and left-to-right shunts.[29] In addition, some children with interstitial edema as a result of LA obstruction (e.g., cor triatriatum) have also presented with a history of recurrent asthmatic attacks. To minimize the markedly increased work of moving their stiff lungs, a pattern of rapid, shallow breathing is used. The stimulation of vagal J receptors by the edema also contributes to the tachypnea and dyspnea so characteristic of early pulmonary edema.

For reasons previously outlined, the presence of edema increases airway resistance. As the airways narrow, closing volume increases and alveolar gas exchange is impaired because of the resultant low V/Q ratio. At this stage, hypocapnia results from the J receptor vagally mediated reflex hyperventilation independent of the presence of hypoxemia. As edema worsens and alveolar flooding occurs, there is further hypoxemia as the blood shunts past nonventilating alveoli. Respiratory acidosis may supervene if the patient is depressed by sedation or if exhaustion develops. The extent to which bronchial mucosal edema intensifies the increase in airway resistance when pulmonary edema is accompanied by elevated systemic venous pressure is not known. With alveolar flooding and disruption of the normal alveolar lining, resistance to airflow increases, dynamic and static compliance are reduced, and there is increasing inhomogeneity of airflow. Once the edema fluid floods into the airspaces, the proteins therein impair surfactant function.[30] One can account for most of the clinical findings (e.g., crackles and diffuse wheezing) based on interstitial, airway, and alveolar edema.

Clinical Presentation

PHYSICAL EXAMINATION

In a general way, small increases in lung fluid are too subtle to be detected by currently available clinical methods, and only when the extravascular fluid volume has increased considerably is the condition clinically obvious. The patient will be tachypneic not just when hypoxemia stimulates ventilation but also because of the stimulation of the J receptors. This latter point explains, at least in part, the continuing tachypnea even after correction of arterial hypoxemia by supplemental oxygen therapy. On auscultation, crackles occur when edema fluid is present in the terminal airways, and they are produced by the sudden opening of peripheral lung units (terminal bronchioli and alveolar ducts). When the fluid moves up to larger airways, rhonchi and wheezes are to be expected. The relative contribution of bronchial wall edema and bronchoconstriction to rhonchi and wheezes is not known. Chest wall retractions will be observed as the spontaneously breathing patient must generate more negative pleural pressures to overcome the markedly decreased total respiratory system compliance and mild increases in airway resistance. Grunting may be present in pulmonary edema and represents a useful maneuver to create a positive end expiratory pressure to prevent derecruitment of distal lung units.

PULMONARY FUNCTION TESTS

Initially, vascular engorgement may lead to an *increase* in the diffusing capacity (DLCO) by increasing the amount of perfused vasculature within the gas exchanging regions of the lung. As interstitial edema increases, there will be an increase in closing volume, a decrease in maximum expiratory flow, an increase in V/Q inhomogeneity, and a decrease in arterial PO_2. With alveolar flooding, there is further air trapping, increased vascular resistance, decreased lung volumes, decreased dynamic lung compliance, decreased DLCO, and progressive hypoxemia arising from the increased intrapulmonary right-to-left shunting and rising $PaCO_2$, the latter further decreasing alveolar PO_2. In patients with a patent foramen ovale, right-to-left shunting at the atrial level may occur as a result of the associated pulmonary hypertension and concomitant increase in right ventricular end diastolic and right atrial pressures.

IMAGING STUDIES

It has been shown that an infusion of 30 mL/kg of saline into healthy adult volunteers over 30 minutes increases extracellular fluid volume by 15% without altering the density of the lungs on computed tomography (CT) or the amount of Compton scattering; the only change on chest radiography and 1980 era CT studies was an increase in the size of the azygos vein.[31] To this author's knowledge, human studies such as these have not been repeated and modern imaging techniques would likely be more sensitive.

The Chest Radiograph

Pulmonary edema can be detected in adult humans on a chest radiograph when extravascular lung water (EVLW) is increased by approximately 35%. Although most of the radiographic signs of pulmonary edema are nonspecific, improved radiographic techniques in conjunction with improved understanding of the pathophysiology of pulmonary edema have enhanced the usefulness of the chest roentgenogram in the diagnosis of pulmonary edema.

The Kerley lines represent interlobular sheets of abnormally thickened or widened connective tissue that are tangential to the x-ray beam (Fig. 36.4). These are more properly referred to as septal lines. Thickened septal lines may occur from a variety of processes, including fibrosis, pigment deposition, and pulmonary hemosiderosis. However, when they are transient, these lines are usually caused by edema. These septal lines of edema are more clearly visible in older children and adults with chronic edema than in infants, presumably because they are wider. Perivascular and peribronchial cuffing are also radiographic signs of interstitial edema fluid. For hydrostatic reasons, perivascular edema is greatest in the gravitationally dependent regions, and the normal tethering action of the lung is therefore less in this region. Increased resistance in the lower lobe vessels promotes the redistribution of blood to the upper lobes. This sign is, of course, of limited value in infants, because they are most likely to be in the supine position, have smaller gravitational induced differences because of their size, and normally have only slightly increased PA pressures relative to children and adults.

More severe forms of pulmonary edema commonly produce a perihilar haze, presumably because the large perivascular

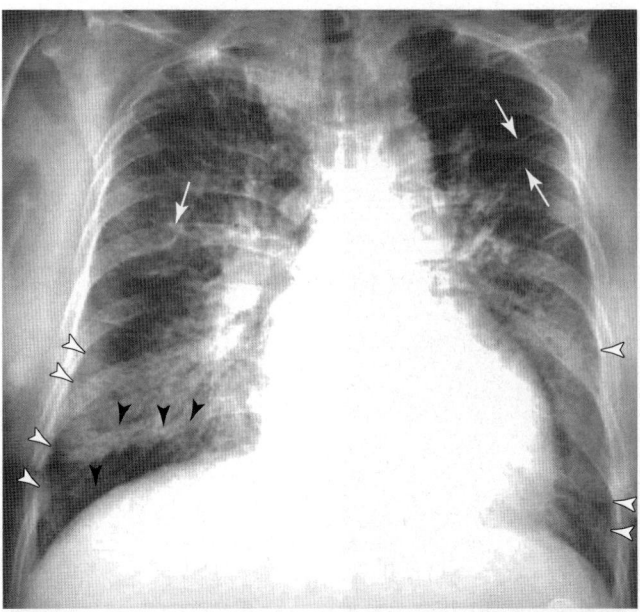

Fig. 36.4 Kerley's A lines *(arrows)* occur in the upper lung zone and point towards the hilum and are directed toward, but do not extend to, the pleural surface. Kerley's B lines *(white arrowheads)* are usually in the lung base and are at right angles to, and in contact with, the pleural surface. Kerley's C lines *(black arrowheads)* are reticular opacities representing Kerley's B lines seen *en face.* (Reproduced from Koga T, Fujimoto K. Images in clinical medicine. Kerley's A, B, and C lines. *N Engl J Med.* 2009;360[15]:1539.)

and peribronchial collections of fluid are in this location. A reticular or latticelike pattern also may be present and is more common inferiorly in an upright individual. Once the magnitude of pulmonary edema is sufficiently severe to lead to persistent airway closure or alveolar flooding, it is very difficult to separate edema, atelectasis, and inflammation on chest radiographs. Air bronchograms indicate airless distal lung units and not the underlying cause.

Because pulmonary edema can lead to airway obstruction in children from both vagal reflex[27] and bronchial froth,[32] airway closure can occur and produce air trapping.[29] Thus, low diaphragms may be a useful sign of interstitial edema, provided there are no other reasons for airway obstruction. Although studies in children are limited, a summary of findings that allows separation of cardiogenic or hemodynamic edema, renal or overhydration edema, and injury or ARDS edema has been provided in adults.[33,34] There is an inverted base-to-apex redistribution of blood flow in patients with heart failure. The progressive recruitment of connective tissue spaces by edema fluid in both cardiac and renal disease gives rise to hilar blurring, peribronchial cuffing, and a hazy pattern of increasing lung density. In ARDS, there is more likely to be a patchy peripheral distribution of edema and a paucity of such findings as septal lines and peribronchial cuffing.

Computed Tomography and Magnetic Resonance Imaging

Thin-section CT imaging of the thorax has provided new information regarding pulmonary edema (Fig. 36.5). For example, studies in ARDS have shown that the lung densities, presumably representing regional edema and microatelectasis, are very heterogeneous and shift with the position of the patient, with densities appearing in the most gravitationally dependent lung regions.[35–37] However, alterations in lung density have to be interpreted with caution. Increases in regional lung density can result from increases in EVLW (i.e., edema), a decrease in regional gas volume, or both.

To date, magnetic resonance imaging (MRI) has had limited use in the management of patients with pulmonary edema. Its major advantage is that it does not require ionizing radiation. One major limitation is that despite obtaining excellent imaging of the larger pulmonary vessels, MRI provides relatively poor resolution of the lung's parenchyma. The safe transport to and the management of the patient within the MRI suite are also pragmatic limitations to this imaging modality. However, one center with a MRI within their critical care unit has used this approach to document that there is increased lung water content in premature babies with RDS.[38] Their findings are consistent with earlier studies of gravimetric measurement of lung water content in postmortem premature infants[39] and research studies on experimental RDS in nonhuman primates (see Neonatal Respiratory Distress Syndrome).[40]

DISTINGUISHING HIGH-PRESSURE FROM LOW-PRESSURE PULMONARY EDEMA

Direct measurements of Pmv would be useful in the differentiation of high-pressure from high-permeability edema. However, the use of pulmonary artery occlusion pressures to estimate Pmv has its limitations (see Vascular Forces), and patients with pulmonary edema often have both increased permeability and elevated pulmonary artery occlusion pressures.[14] Although B-type natriuretic peptide (BNP) has been found useful in identifying congestive heart failure (CHF), it does not reliably distinguish CHF-induced from ARDS-induced pulmonary edema.[41]

When patients with pulmonary edema have undergone endotracheal intubation, one can collect airway fluid that may reflect alveolar fluid. On this basis, investigators attempted to differentiate high-pressure from increased permeability pulmonary edema[42] by comparing the concentration of the protein in the airspace fluid with the simultaneously measured plasma protein concentration. Although this ratio was statistically significantly different between the two groups, there is such significant scatter that it is of little diagnostic utility for the individual patient. The reason for this variation and lack of clinical utility is now understood: the alveolar fluid's protein concentration not only depends on the leakiness of the alveolar-capillary membrane, but also on the efficiency and amount of time available for the epithelium to actively pump salt and water out of the airspace with the resultant concentration of the protein that remains in the distal lung unit (see Clearance of Pulmonary Edema Fluid).

Endothelial cell injury has been assessed by the ability of the pulmonary circulation to remove or metabolize a variety of substances; however, these tests are neither sufficiently sensitive nor specific. Similarly, although the clearance rate of inhaled and deposited small solutes (e.g., [99m]technetium diethylenetriamine-pentaacetic acid [Tc-DTPA]) from the lungs provides an index of pulmonary epithelial integrity,[43] this approach is hampered by the inability to differentiate increased epithelial permeability from marked increases in regional lung volume.[44] Analysis of airspace fluid may be

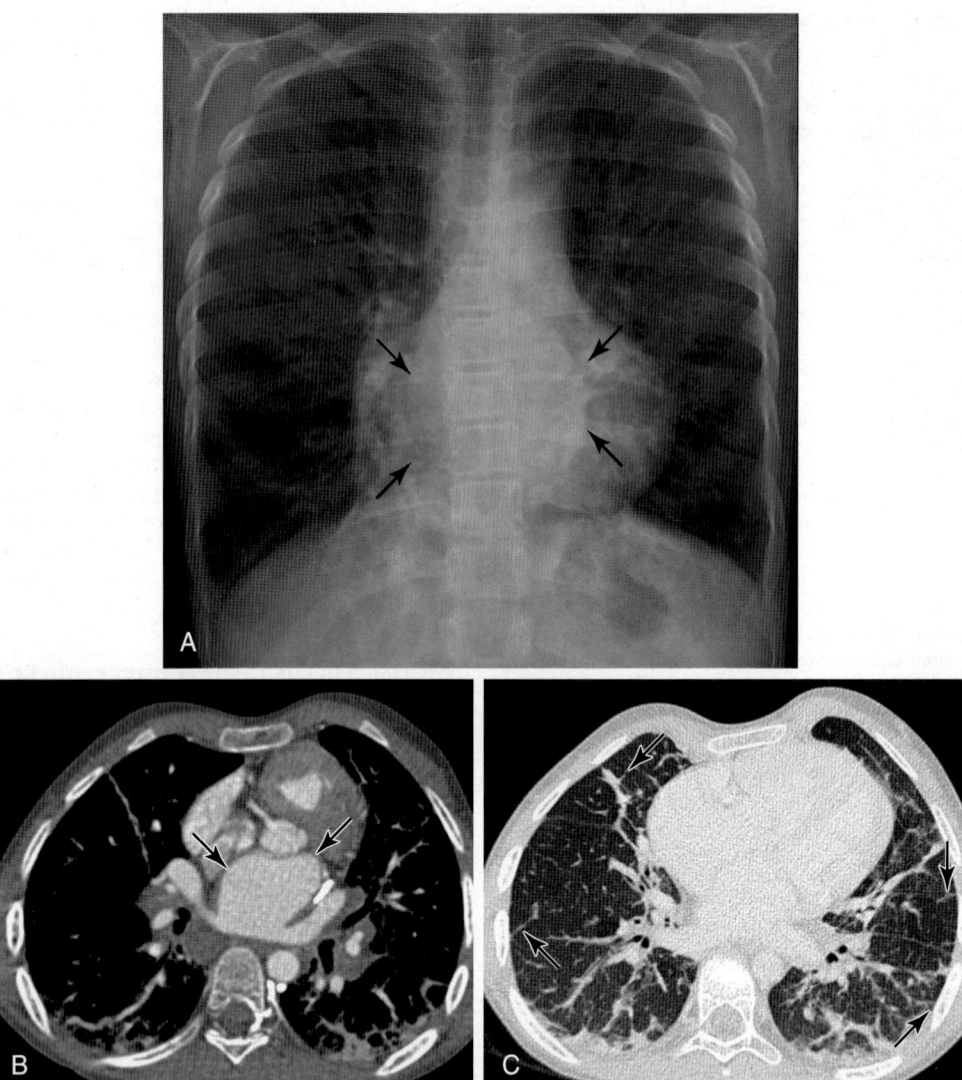

Fig. 36.5 Images of a 7-year-old patient with Shone syndrome and long-standing mitral stenosis. (A) Frontal chest radiograph reveals mild cardiomegaly with an enlarged left atrium *(arrows)*. There is vascular prominence of the upper lobes and features of the interstitial edema, including hyperinflation, perihilar prominence of vessels, and indistinct vascular margins. (B) CT (mediastinal windows) illustrates the enlarged left atrium *(arrows)* and pulmonary veins. (C) CT (lung windows) illustrates prominent vessels, areas of mosaic perfusion (darker and lighter regions) indicating small airway dysfunction and interlobular septal thickening *(arrows)*, which are the CT equivalent of Kerley B lines on plain chest radiographs. (Images courtesy of Dr. Beverley Newman, Stanford University.)

beneficial, as proteomic analysis may reveal qualitative changes in the expression of some proteins and might provide markers for lung injury.[45] Similarly, investigators have attempted to use plasma biomarkers to detect ALI.[46]

QUANTITATION OF PULMONARY EDEMA IN PATIENTS

Indicator dilution techniques have been used to measure EVLW content in humans. Traditional techniques have used a technique that depends on one tracer being confined to the vascular space and another tracer that diffuses into the perfused tissue. The difference in the sum of the two time concentration curves has been used to calculate the amount of EVLW. Measurements of EVLW are improved when results are normalized to lung volumes as predicted by height and gender rather than the previous approach of body weight,

which is affected by obesity.[47] Useful information has been obtained using this approach. For example, EVLW correlates with mortality in critically ill adults (Fig. 36.6).[47,48] The major assumption, and limitation, of these techniques is that it can only measure that portion of the lung that is perfused; therefore, it may underestimate the total lung water or measurements may assess differing amounts of the lungs at different time points.[49]

Clinical Disorders Causing Pulmonary Edema

HIGH-PRESSURE PULMONARY EDEMA

This diagnostic label refers to conditions where there is a demonstrable increase in the forces promoting fluid movement

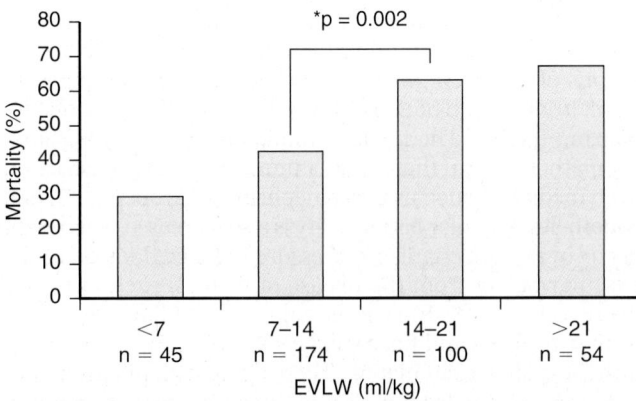

Fig. 36.6 Mortality as a function of extravascular lung water (EVLW). Patients were classified into four groups according to their highest EVLW value. The asterisk indicates statistical significance to the next higher EVLW group (chi-squared). (Reproduced from Sakka SG, Klein M, Reinhart K, Meier-Hellmann A. Prognostic value of extravascular lung water in critically ill patients. *Chest.* 2002;122[6]:2080-2086.)

out of the microvasculature. By far the most common cause is left-sided heart disease, which results in marked elevations of pulmonary venous and hence microvasculature hydrostatic pressure.

Obstructive lesions such as cor triatriatum, mitral stenosis, congenital obstruction of pulmonary venous drainage, and pulmonary venoocclusive disease directly cause pulmonary venous hypertension. In contrast, other obstructive lesions such as coarctation of the aorta and severe aortic stenosis only cause pulmonary edema once left ventricular failure has occurred.

Myocardial failure with subsequent pulmonary venous hypertension may arise from either congenital or acquired heart disease. Examples of the former include hypoplastic left heart syndrome, and the latter includes intrinsic myocardial disease (e.g., cardiac glycogen storage diseases, endocardial fibroelastosis, viral and rheumatic myocarditis) and myocardial ischemia (e.g., anomalous left coronary artery or Kawasaki disease).

Markedly increased pulmonary blood flow occurs in patients with congenital arteriovenous fistulas or congenital heart defects that promote left-to-right shunting of blood (e.g., ventricular septal defect, patent ductus arteriosus). This leads to pulmonary vascular engorgement, especially in the case of anatomic left-to-right shunting. In either case, there is a marked increase in left ventricular output. When the burden on the left ventricle becomes too great and left-sided heart failure supervenes, pulmonary microvascular pressures are increased by both high flow and increased LA pressures.

Significant increases in blood volume can result in pulmonary vascular engorgement and edema. Fluid retention rapidly occurs in acute renal disease as a result of the expanded extracellular fluid volume. Nephrosis and chronic renal disease also may predispose an individual to pulmonary edema by the associated hypoproteinemia. Perhaps the most common cause of increased pulmonary blood volume is the overzealous administration of fluids. This will intensify the development of pulmonary edema by raising hydrostatic pressures and diluting plasma proteins. Finally, to what extent the inappropriate secretion of antidiuretic hormone, which occurs in disorders such as pneumonia, asthma, and BPD,

complicates and intensifies the development of pulmonary edema in these diseases is incompletely understood.

AIRWAY OBSTRUCTION

Severe obstruction of the extrathoracic airways predisposes the patient to pulmonary edema (see Interstitial Forces). For example, croup and epiglottitis are associated with pulmonary edema.[50,51]

Diffuse small airway obstruction, as occurs in status asthmaticus, also promotes the development of pulmonary edema as a result of a lag in the expansion of the lung in spite of the development of very negative intrathoracic pressures.[52] Although airway inflammation is recognized as an important part of the pathogenesis of asthma, it is not clear to what extent edema of the airways, per se, plays in the airway obstruction. Certainly, any inflammation-induced increase in permeability would dramatically increase the amount of fluid moving across the vascular bed in response to a more negative interstitial pressure. Clinically, significant short-term improvements in gas exchange may be seen in some patients with asthma and bronchiolitis with the use of diuretics. Because these diuretics also change vascular compliance and pressures, the exact reason for the beneficial response is uncertain. Nevertheless, our improved understanding of how airway obstruction can promote the development of pulmonary edema led to the present therapeutic strategy of giving only maintenance, or less than maintenance fluids, to patients after they have had their deficits replaced. In the more distant past, it had been customary to advocate increased fluid intake for patients with asthma and bronchiolitis in the false hope that the increased fluid would loosen secretions and facilitate their expectoration; this has never been established, but it is certain that the increased amounts of fluid will promote the development of pulmonary edema.

Cardiac failure and pulmonary edema are also rarely seen in obstructive sleep apnea; in children, this condition is most frequently associated with hypertrophied tonsils and adenoids.[53,54] At the bedside, one can see severe intercostal retractions during inspiration. Indeed, this inspiratory pattern is similar to a Müller maneuver (i.e., a strong inspiration against a closed glottis or obstructed upper airway). The negative pressures would, in addition to promoting edema, also surround and restrain the left ventricle and create an increased afterload to the left ventricle (left ventricular afterload is equal to the mean aortic pressure minus the pleural pressure).

REEXPANSION PULMONARY EDEMA

Reexpansion pulmonary edema is seen in some patients who have rapid lung reexpansion after drainage of a large pneumothorax or pleural effusion. Rarely, it causes systemic hypovolemia and shock, as large volumes of fluid move from the vascular space to airspaces of the rapidly reinflated lung.

The reported incidence of reexpansion pulmonary edema varies considerably, and it has been speculated that the different incidence rates result from various factors. These include the duration of the atelectasis, characteristics of the collapsed lung, and the rate of evacuation of the pleural air or fluid. For example, in many of the case reports, the lung collapse had been present for some time before reexpansion. A prospective study revealed that 20% of adult patients treated with closed thoracostomy drainage for a spontaneous pneumothorax developed classic reexpansion pulmonary edema.[55] In contrast, another report found that the evacuation of pleural fluid was rarely associated with reexpansion pulmonary edema.[56] Regardless of the true incidence, it is irrefutable that this phenomenon does occur. Thus, caution must be exercised when draining large collections of fluid from the pleural space when there is associated collapse of a lobe or lung.

One of the mechanisms responsible for the syndrome is the sudden marked lowering of the interstitial fluid pressure. In addition, experimental studies of reexpansion pulmonary edema in rabbits[57] provide evidence that there is increased vascular permeability to protein. Although the mechanism for injury of the alveolar-capillary membrane is not known, there are at least two possibilities. The first is that there is increased and excessive stretch or tension of the alveolar septal walls during reexpansion of lungs that have been collapsed for several days. Stress-related pulmonary endothelial injury[20] has been described in other experimental conditions, and overexpansion of lungs during positive-pressure ventilation is associated with increases in alveolar-capillary permeability.[18,19] Other mechanisms, such as reperfusion lung injury from reactive oxygen intermediates, also may play a role in the increased alveolar-capillary membrane permeability. Indeed, it has been shown that collapsed lung tissue has decreased mitochondrial superoxide dismutase (SOD) and cytochrome oxidase[58]; these changes could enhance oxygen free radical production.

NEONATAL RESPIRATORY DISTRESS SYNDROME

Studies in humans[38,39] and primates[40] prove that neonatal RDS (nRDS) in premature infants is associated with widespread airspace edema and that the well-described reduction in FRC results more from the excess fluid than from atelectasis.[40]

A number of factors contribute to airspace fluid in patients with nRDS. First, there is the fluid that had been secreted into the developing fetal lungs' airspaces during normal fetal lung development. This fluid must be cleared at birth so that effective gas exchange can occur, and clearance of airspace fluid results from active transepithelial Na^+ transport (see Fig. 36.2). Impaired clearance of this fetal lung liquid arising from inadequate epithelial sodium transport[59,60] combined with an immature surfactant system,[61] results in nRDS.[62] Second, pulmonary edema fluid is generated during the course of nRDS by several mechanisms. These include the high pulmonary vascular pressures and blood flow, especially if there is a patent ductus arteriosus; low interstitial pressures, in part the result of high alveolar surface tension; low plasma protein concentration (and hence low plasma osmotic pressure)[63]; increased epithelial permeability[43]; lung endothelial injury from inflammation and, as a result of therapy, high airway pressures and high inspired oxygen concentrations.

NEUROGENIC PULMONARY EDEMA

Any acute cerebral insult, and rarely cervical spinal cord injury, can lead to neurogenic pulmonary edema (NPE).[64,65] Most frequently, it is seen with head trauma, subarachnoid hemorrhage, brain tumors, status epilepticus, and meningitis. The mechanisms responsible for pulmonary edema following lesions of the brain are not fully understood but appear to result from a combination of hemodynamic and permeability-altering factors. The hemodynamic response arises from a sympathetic storm that causes intense brief vasoconstriction from mediators such as norepinephrine, neuropeptide Y, and endothelin. Vascular permeability is also increased. This might occur by two mechanisms: pressure induced damage to the vascular bed or from the release of factors, such as tumor necrosis factor (TNF)-α, interleukin-1β, and interleukin-6, from astrocytes and microglial cells, which may gain entry into the systemic circulation. These along with inflammatory processes arising from the sympathetic storm may induce a systemic inflammatory response.

The clinical signs of NPE are those of acute pulmonary edema, without evidence of left ventricular failure. There is no specific biologic marker for NPE, and it may develop acutely over minutes to hours or may be delayed. Evaluation of edema fluid suggests that patients may either have predominately high pressure or high permeability pulmonary edema.[66] In the treatment of NPE, it is important to remember that positive ventilatory pressures, especially positive end-expiratory pressure (PEEP), should be administered cautiously because they can interfere with cerebral venous return, thus promoting further cerebral edema. Depending on the severity of the primary result, NPE may resolve within the first 2–3 days and overall outcome relates to the neurologic outcome.

ACUTE LUNG INJURY AND THE ACUTE RESPIRATORY DISTRESS SYNDROME

ALI and its most severe form, ARDS, frequently occur in critically ill patients. Regardless of the inciting event, the clinical and pathologic manifestations of ARDS are similar, indicating a final common pathway ultimately leading to severe endothelial and epithelial inflammatory injury. This causes a compromise of barrier and transport functions, which leads to high permeability pulmonary edema that is often compounded by increases in microvascular pressure from concomitant pulmonary hypertension and pulmonary venoconstriction.

An initiating event, such as sepsis, shock, head injury, or trauma triggers a systemic inflammatory response that promotes sequestration of polymorphonuclear leukocytes (PMN) within the lung. Histologically, ARDS is characterized by large numbers of PMN in the vascular, interstitial, and alveolar space in association with endothelial and epithelial injury. This, combined with the potential of PMN to induce tissue injury in diverse experimental systems, has led to the widely held concept that these potent phagocytes are central to the pathogenesis of ARDS, a notion supported by numerous human and animal studies. The clinical presentation, pathogenic mechanisms, and approaches to therapy are discussed in detail in Chapter 38.

HIGH ALTITUDE PULMONARY EDEMA

High-altitude pulmonary edema (HAPE) can occur when climbers are exercising intensively in hypoxic environments as they ascend to high altitudes. What are the relative contributions of exercise and hypoxia? Although pulmonary edema can occur during marathons conducted near sea level[67] or in elite swimmers,[68] it is extraordinarily rare for normoxic exercise to be associated with pulmonary edema. Similarly, moderate hypoxia by itself is not sufficient for the development of edema. Athough approximately one-third of nonexercising children who rapidly ascend to modest elevations (from 568 to 3450 m) develop acute mountain sickness (AMS), clinically obvious cerebral or pulmonary edema do not seem to occur.[69] Studies have shown that these symptoms of AMS can be prevented by the administration of acetazolamide, but not the herbal supplement ginkgo biloba, just before and during ascent.[70] Although exposure to even more modest hypoxia (equivalent to 2438 m altitude) is associated with small decreases in arterial saturation, it is not associated with AMS.[71]

Clinically important and severe HAPE may affect some sea-level dwellers soon after arriving at a high altitude. Arterial blood gas analyses suggest that there may be subclinical HAPE, or diffusion defect, even in asymptomatic climbers ascending Mt. Everest.[72] HAPE also may occur in some highlanders who return home after a brief stay at sea level.

Much of our initial understanding of HAPE came from observations of Indian soldiers transported to high altitudes during the Indo-China war of the past century.[73] Subsequent work has shown that the incidence of HAPE and AMS is increased when the rate of ascent is rapid and subjects have little opportunity for acclimatization, whereas gender or previous altitude exposure have no effect.[74] Relevant to the previous discussion regarding pulmonary vascular recruitment, the incidence of HAPE is increased in children and young adults[75] and in subjects with only one pulmonary artery.[76] Fatigue, dyspnea, cough, and sleep disturbances are common and may progress rapidly to severe tachypnea, shock, and death unless rapid descent to a lower altitude or administration of oxygen occurs.

The mechanisms leading to HAPE are still incompletely understood. Nonprimate animal studies show that although hypoxia increases PA pressures, it does not by itself increase vascular permeability to solutes.[15] However, the best available evidence suggests that HAPE is initiated by an excessive increase in Pmv. The cause of the Pmv is unknown, although the two favored hypotheses are an unequal pulmonary vasoconstriction with resultant overperfusion of remaining lung microvessels or an abnormal vasoconstriction of the pulmonary venules. Prospective studies suggest that first there is a noninflammatory leakage of fluid across the alveolar-capillary membrane followed by a secondary inflammatory reaction[77] as the disease progresses.[78] Some researchers have assumed that in addition to a constitutional predisposition of some individuals to pulmonary hypertension with hypoxia, nonuniform increases in precapillary resistance are responsible for the very high pressures seen in at least some pulmonary capillaries. The observations that prophylactic administration of the calcium channel blocker nifedipine can diminish the incidence of HAPE[79] and that inhalation of nitric oxide (NO) decreases PA pressures and improves oxygenation[80,81] in such patients support the speculation that HAPE is due in part to an inappropriate pulmonary vasoconstrictive response. The observation that salmeterol diminishes the frequency of HAPE[82] is intriguing; potential mechanisms include its effect on vascular resistance and the augmentation of lung epithelial Na$^+$ transport.

INHALATION OF TOXIC AGENTS

Toxic lung injury can be induced by a wide variety of agents,[83] but only three examples are discussed here. The most common agent is smoke from fires, the toxicity of which will vary with the nature of the combustible product (e.g., plastics vs. wood). In victims of fires, the auscultatory evidence of pulmonary edema resulting from inhalation of smoke with damage to the distal lung unit, including the alveolar capillary membrane, is manifest within 24 hours and usually precedes roentgenographic changes.[84]

Chlorine gas inhalation is an example of a toxic gas that can cause severe lung injury. It is most frequently seen in industrial accidents but can occur following exposure to fumes from liquid chlorine used in swimming pools. Pulmonary edema is frequently seen; however, if the patient survives, there are no long-term sequelae.[85]

The inhalation of phosgene gas may occur following industrial accidents or as a gas generated during fires involving plastics or other chemicals and solvents containing chlorine. Although symptoms may be mild at first, with apparent initial recovery, delayed onset noncardiogenic pulmonary edema may ensure. Accordingly, patients should be admitted to hospital for at least one day for observation.[86]

INTRAVENOUS AGENTS

Infusion of any compound that can act as a microembolic agent can result in high-permeability pulmonary edema as demonstrated in animal models of lung injury[17] and humans who have accidentally suffered from air microembolism.[87]

NARCOTIC-INDUCED AND MEDICATION-INDUCED PULMONARY EDEMA

Heroin and other narcotics also have been associated with pulmonary edema.[88,89] Pulmonary capillary Pw has been elevated in some patients but has been normal in others. Whether hypoxia and acidosis or NPE, as the result of cerebral edema, plays a role is not known. Clinical and roentgenographic signs of pulmonary edema have occurred following the intravenous administration of paraldehyde[90]; although a direct toxic action on the pulmonary vascular bed has been proposed, the cause remains obscure.

Salicylates also have been associated with the development of pulmonary edema in adults[91] and children.[92] Experimental studies in sheep suggest that salicylate pulmonary edema is not due to increased vascular pressure but rather to increased vascular permeability.[93] Insofar as these studies can be applied to the human, the researchers suggest that acetylsalicylic acid can cause pulmonary edema in doses considered therapeutic for some diseases. Although the mechanisms responsible for the altered vascular permeability remain unknown, at least two effects of salicylates could affect vascular integrity: alterations in platelet function and inhibition of prostaglandin synthesis.

Therapy

It is not only biologically reasonable to maintain the postnatal airspace air-filled, and not fluid-filled; there is a substantial

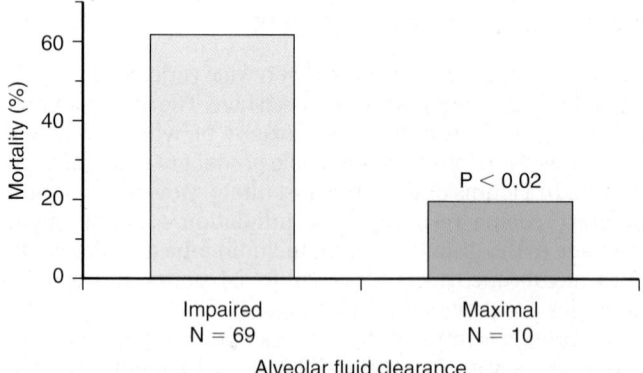

Fig. 36.7 Plot of hospital mortality of two groups of patients with acute lung injury or the acute respiratory distress syndrome: those with maximal alveolar fluid clearance (≥14% per hour) and those with impaired or submaximal alveolar fluid clearance (<14% per hour). Columns represent percent of hospital mortality in each group. Hospital mortality of patients with maximal alveolar fluid clearance was significantly less ($P < .02$). *N* = number of patients. (Reproduced from Ware LB, Matthay MA. Alveolar fluid clearance is impaired in the majority of patients with acute lung injury and the acute respiratory distress syndrome. *Am J Respir Crit Care Med.* 2001;163:1376-1383.)

body of research that suggests that reduction or attenuation of pulmonary edema improves patient outcome. Decreasing PA Pws[94] or avoiding positive fluid balances[95] are both associated with improved survival. EVLW correlates with mortality in adults (see Fig. 36.6).[47,48] Similarly, a randomized study has shown that conservative fluid management improves lung function and shortens the duration of mechanical ventilation in ALI.[96] Indirect assessments of the distal lung epithelium's ability to actively transport Na^+, with Cl^- and water following, from the airspace has been shown to correlate with survival and clinical outcome in both high-pressure and high-permeability pulmonary edema (Fig. 36.7).[24,97]

Therapy should be guided by the pathophysiologic consequences of the edema and the best method to decrease further movement of fluid into, and promote liquid clearance from, the airspace.

REVERSING THE HYPOXEMIA

The first step is to reverse the hypoxemia. If pulmonary edema is mild and predominately interstitial in nature, then increasing the FiO_2 will treat the low V/Q ratios ($0 < V/Q < 1$) arising from airway dysfunction. However, most patients in acute pulmonary edema have significant airspace pulmonary edema, which results in shunt ($V/Q = 0$), and requires an increase in transpulmonary pressures as the therapeutic approach. Positive airway pressures in general, and PEEP, in particular, are beneficial for several reasons: (1) the recruitment (opening) of fluid-filled airspaces[35,36] so that they become partially filled with air and can then participate in gas exchange, (2) a reduction in the fluid filtration within the lung by impeding systemic venous return and therefore decreasing pulmonary vascular volume and pressure, and (3) the prevention of airway collapse, thus enhancing gas exchange. It is important to note that studies have shown that PEEP does not directly decrease lung water content[98] or lung lymph flow.[99]

An increase in transpulmonary pressures may be achieved using both noninvasive and invasive approaches. Although out of favor in the more distant past, it is now known that noninvasive ventilation can be effective in cardiogenic pulmonary edema.[100,101] Similarly, CT imaging has proven that when patients with ALI are placed in the prone position, there is recruitment of edematous lung units.[37] However, most frequently, intubation and assisted ventilation are required both for efficacy and to minimize potential side effects such as overdistention of the stomach and potential aspiration. Mechanical ventilation also reduces the oxygen consumption by reducing the work of breathing.

REDUCE THE RATE OF FLUID FILTRATION

The second step is to reduce the rate of fluid filtration into the lung. Treating the disorder creating the pulmonary edema, for example CHF, is self-evident. Several therapeutic approaches are useful in treating the CHF-induced elevation of pulmonary microvascular pressures. They include measures that (1) improve cardiac contractility and allow the heart to achieve an increased stroke volume at a lower filling pressure (e.g., use of oxygen, digoxin, dopamine, or dobutamine), (2) reduce preload, including the sitting position and positive-pressure ventilation, (3) reduce both preload and afterload by relieving anxiety (e.g., use of morphine), (4) decrease plasma volumes with concomitant reduction of pulmonary microvascular and LA pressures (e.g., administration of diuretics), (5) decrease systemic or pulmonary vascular pressures, or both, using vasodilators such as prostacyclin, nitroprusside, or inhaled nitric oxide, and (6) reduce excessive salt and water intake.

Small changes in lung microvascular pressures can have profound effects on lung water accumulation[16] and leakage of fluid from the microvascular bed (Fig. 36.8) when there is increased permeability of the alveolar-capillary membrane. Similarly, when there is increased permeability of the alveolar-capillary membrane, an increase in cardiac output, with minor changes in LA pressures, has a marked effect on lung lymph flow.[17] In humans who have undergone lung transplantation, echocardiographic evidence of diastolic dysfunction increases the risk of primary graft dysfunction, a condition characterized by increased alveolar capillary membrane permeability.[102]

A reduction in the rate of fluid leakage from the vasculature can also be achieved using other strategies based on the Starling equation (see Factors Responsible for Fluid Movement). For patients suffering from ARDS and its associated high permeability pulmonary edema, our goal is to return the permeability of the alveolar-capillary membrane back to normal levels. Regrettably, despite decades of research, there is no proven way to modulate alveolar-capillary membrane permeability, although low-dose corticosteroids[103] or activated protein C in the subset of ARDS patients with sepsis[104] may be beneficial to some degree in altering the course of the overall disease. A randomized double-blind clinical trial that excluded patients with sepsis showed that the administration of protein C did not improve clinical outcomes in ALI.[105]

Starling's equation indicates that altering intravascular osmotic pressure would lessen the flow of fluid out of the microvasculature. However, an increase in colloid osmotic

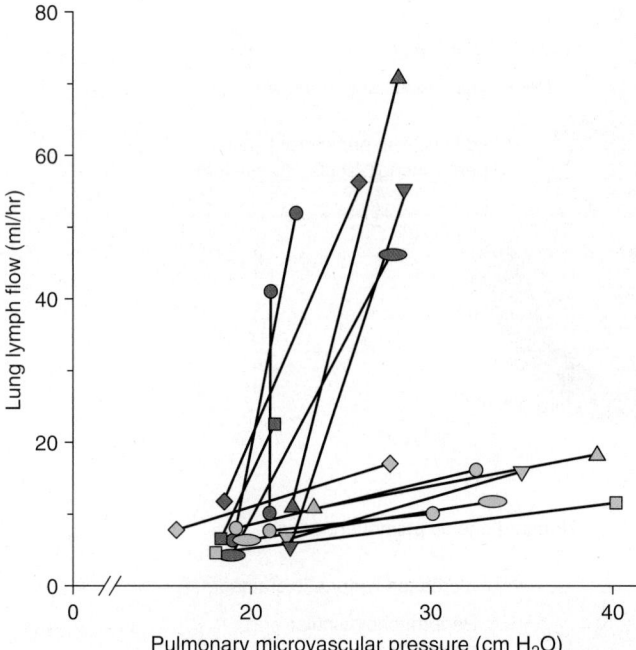

Fig. 36.8 Relation of lung lymph flow to pulmonary microvascular pressures during hemodynamic edema *(green symbols)* and during permeability edema produced by infusion of *Pseudomonas (blue symbols).* For a given reduction in vascular pressures, there is a much greater reduction in lung lymph flow in permeability edema than in hydrostatic edema. (From Brigham KL, Wolverton WC, Blake LH, Staub NC. Increased sheep lung vascular permeability caused by *Pseudomonas bacteremia. J Clin Invest.* 1974;54:792.)

pressure resulting from an infusion of colloid also would augment microvascular pressure, as vascular volume is increased secondary to the movement of water from the systemic tissues to the vascular compartment and may undermine this effort. Indeed, studies in animals with high permeability pulmonary edema have shown that increasing colloid osmotic pressure had no effect on lung water content.[16]

Lowering systemic vascular pressures by use of diuretics and drugs that reduce vascular resistance or afterload are both advantageous for reasons previously described. However, diuretics such as furosemide are beneficial in pulmonary edema because of their ability to increase systemic venous capacitance and not because of the induced diuresis. Evidence for this statement includes the improvement in the patient's status, which is usually seen a few minutes after administering the diuretic before the diuresis. Similarly, furosemide can be beneficial in anuric patients suffering from pulmonary edema. It should be noted that the lung represents only 1% of the total body weight, so even a 1 L diuresis would only remove 10 mL from the lungs, with the remaining fluid coming from the remainder of the body. This 10 mL is trivial compared with the liters of fluid present in the airspaces of adult patients with florid alveolar edema (see Anatomic Considerations).

MINIMIZE TREATMENT-RELATED LUNG DAMAGE

It is important to prevent or minimize treatment-related damage to the lung. This can occur through the use of very

high concentrations of oxygen or the suboptimal use of mechanical ventilation with resultant distention of the lung and damage to the lung's epithelium and endothelium,[18,19] thereby increasing the permeability of the alveolar-capillary membrane to water and solutes. Attention to treatment of the underlying condition combined with excellent supportive care using "lung-protective" ventilatory strategies to minimize treatment-related lung damage have contributed to improved clinical outcomes.[106] This subject is discussed in greater detail in Chapters 34, 37, and 38.

AUGMENT THE RATE OF CLEARANCE OF AIRSPACE FLUID

The fourth step is to augment the rate of clearance of the airspace fluid. It has now been demonstrated that intact active fluid absorption from the airspaces correlates with improved survival and various important clinical parameters such as the length of assisted ventilation and oxygen requirements, regardless of whether the patients suffer from acute CHF-induced or ARDS-induced pulmonary edema (see Fig. 36.7).[24,97] Only 75% of patients with CHF-induced pulmonary edema have demonstrable alveolar fluid clearance, with approximately 40% being capable of achieving maximal clearance rates.[24] The situation is even more grave for patients with ALI and ARDS, because only 13% of these patients can achieve maximal rates of active airspace fluid clearance.[97] Active clearance of airspace fluid is impaired more frequently in men and when there is associated sepsis.[97]

Exogenous catecholamines augment fluid clearance from the airspaces in animals,[107] and a single center randomized controlled study showed that 7 days of intravenous salbutamol therapy is associated with a decrease in EVLW and ventilator pressures.[108] Consistent with these findings, aerosolized β agonists can decrease EVLW and improve clinical parameters in patients undergoing elective lung resections[109] and prevent HAPE in susceptible individuals.[82] However, studies in humans have not shown any correlation between the levels of circulating catecholamines and the rates of fluid clearance,[24,97] and a multicenter trial did not show a beneficial effect of aerosolized albuterol in ALI.[110] The lack of response in the multicenter study may have indicated the inadequate delivery of the aerosolized salbutamol to the airspace, that the epithelium is unresponsive, or that more efficacious strategies may be required to augment airspace fluid clearance. A clinical trial using an intravenous infusion of salbutamol was discontinued when it became apparent that it did not improve patient outcomes and was associated with an increase in mortality.[111] These clinical trials indicate that salbutamol should only be used to treat airway obstruction and not to increase the clearance of fluid from the alveolar spaces. New approaches are needed so that pulmonary edema fluid clearance can be increased without adverse side effects. Perhaps this may be developed from work showing that pulmonary edema fluid itself can modulate Na^+ and fluid transport by distal lung epithelium[112] or other studies where either mesenchymal stem cells (MSCs) or media conditioned by MSCs can restore effective Na+ and water transport by injured human lung lobes.[113] Fig. 36.9 provides a schematic overview of the distal lung unit during health and during high-pressure and high-permeability pulmonary edema.

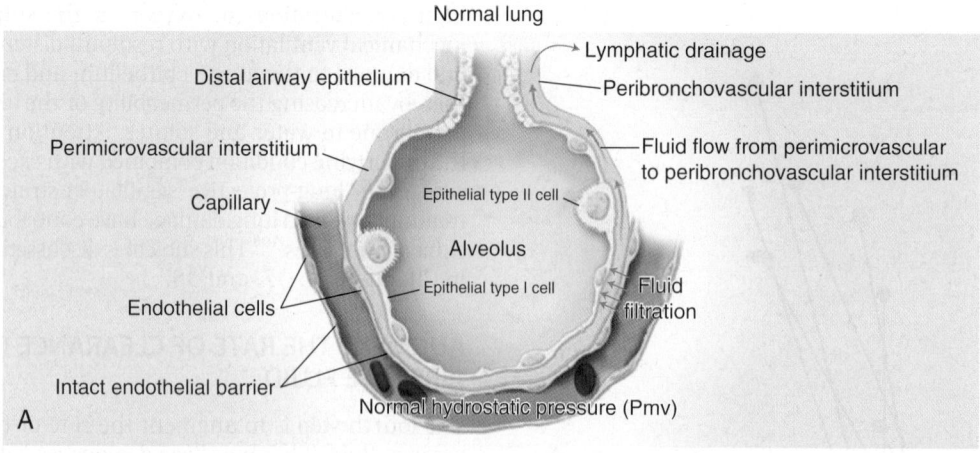

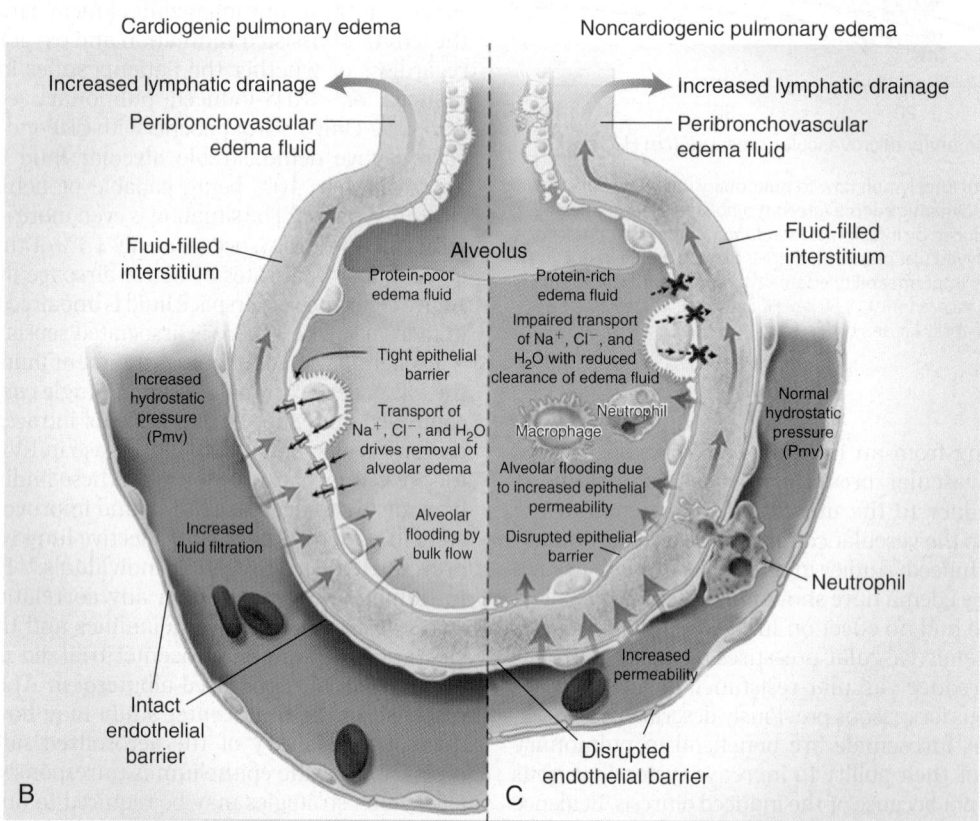

Fig. 36.9 (A) In the normal lung, fluid moves continuously outward from the vascular to the interstitial space according to the net difference between hydrostatic and protein osmotic pressures and to the permeability of the capillary membrane. (B) When transvascular hydrostatic pressure increases in the microcirculation, the rate of fluid filtration rises. Since the permeability of the capillary endothelium remains normal, the filtered edema fluid leaving the circulation has a low protein content. The removal of edema fluid from the air spaces of the lung depends on active transport of Na^+ and Cl^-, with water following across the alveolar epithelial barrier. (C) High-permeability pulmonary edema occurs when the permeability of the microvascular membrane increases because of direct or indirect lung injury, such as the acute respiratory distress syndrome, resulting in a marked increase in the amount of fluid and protein leaving the vascular space. The pulmonary edema fluid has a high protein content because the more permeable microvascular membrane has a reduced capacity to restrict the outward movement of larger molecules such as plasma proteins. In edema due to acute lung injury, alveolar epithelial injury commonly causes a decrease in the capacity for the removal of alveolar fluid, delaying the resolution of pulmonary edema. (Reproduced from Ware LB, Matthay MA. Clinical practice. Acute pulmonary edema. *N Engl J Med.* 2005;353[26]:2788-2796.)

References

Access the reference list online at ExpertConsult.com.

Suggested Reading

More detailed information is available in the 113 references contained within the electronic version of this chapter, earlier versions of this book for classic references and review articles up to the mid-1980s that underpin some of the commentary within this chapter, and the following three recent review articles:

Matalon S, Bartoszewski R, Collawn JF. Role of epithelial sodium channels in the regulation of lung fluid homeostasis. *Am J Physiol Lung Cell Mol Physiol*. 2015;309:L1229–L1238.

Matthay MA. Resolution of pulmonary edema. Thirty years of progress. *Am J Respir Crit Care Med*. 2014;189:1301–1308.

West JB. High altitude medicine. *Am J Respir Crit Care Med*. 2012; 186:1229–1237.

37 Respiratory Complications of Intensive Care

HAMMAD A. GANATRA, MD, and BRIAN MICHAEL VARISCO, MD

History of Pediatric Intensive Care

The first pediatric intensive care unit (PICU) was established in 1955 at Children's Hospital of Göteborg in Sweden, followed by the emergence of PICUs in the United States in the late 1950s and early 1960s. These units originated to meet the medical needs of critically ill children who were undergoing increasingly extensive and complicated surgical procedures or recovering from complex medical problems.[1,2] In these early PICUs, anesthesiologists continued to provide the cardiorespiratory support and pain control that these patients required in the operating room. During the 1970s and 1980s, care teams involving surgeons, anesthesiologists, and pediatric subspecialists evolved, with the leader of that team being the pediatric intensivist. In the early years, these intensivists were largely derived from the ranks of pediatric anesthesiologists with the percentage of pediatricians becoming intensivists steadily increasing through the late 1980s and early 1990s. The Society of Critical Care Medicine (SCCM), which originated as an adult intensive care society, recognized pediatric critical care medicine as a discrete entity and created a separate section of pediatric critical care within the SCCM in 1981. Within 2 years, the section created guidelines defining the minimal requirements for pediatric ICUs. The American Board of Pediatrics sponsored the first pediatric critical care board exam in 1991. Although the majority of pediatric intensivists have completed a pediatrics residency prior to entering the field, many critical care divisions remain within departments of anesthesiology.[1–3]

Indications for Intubation and Mechanical Ventilation

Mechanical ventilation of acutely ill children remains one of the principal therapies provided in PICUs throughout the United States. Available data from the Pediatric Health Information System (PHIS) database and other sources suggests that 20%–30% of all children admitted to PICUs across the United States receive invasive mechanical ventilation.[4,5] While respiratory disease in children is a major indication for endotracheal intubation and ventilation, these patients comprise only one-fifth of PICU admissions,[4] and there are numerous nonrespiratory indications for mechanical ventilation, including postoperative care and pain management, neurological and neuromuscular pathology, congenital heart disease, cardiomyopathy, and shock (Table 37.1).

There has recently been increasing emphasis on the use of noninvasive mechanical ventilation (NIV) in the form of continuous positive airway pressure (CPAP) and bilevel positive airway pressure (BIPAP) to delay or avoid endotracheal intubation and invasive mechanical ventilation. Noninvasive mechanical ventilation is commonly used among adults with cardiogenic pulmonary edema, chronic obstructive pulmonary disease (COPD) exacerbation, and neuromuscular disorders.[7,8] Among preterm neonates with respiratory distress syndrome, noninvasive CPAP use is common and reduces the need for invasive mechanical ventilation.[9,10] No clear indications exist for the use of noninvasive modalities as a standard therapy among infants and children in PICUs. However, data suggest that its use is rapidly increasing, and more pediatric ICUs are adopting the use of NIV for managing mild to moderate acute respiratory failure[11] and in children with chronic conditions such as neuromuscular weakness (e.g., Duchenne's muscular dystrophy and spinal muscular atrophy) or restrictive lung disease. Acute conditions that are transient and self-limiting in nature may be amenable to noninvasive mechanical support and include upper airway obstruction (e.g., croup, postextubation upper airway edema), lower airway obstruction (e.g., asthma, bronchiolitis),[12,13] and lung parenchymal diseases such as bronchiolitis, pneumonia, or pulmonary edema. NIV does not afford a secure airway, and masks may impede airway clearance in the event of vomiting. NIV should therefore be used with caution in patients with poor neurologic function or with potential for rapid deterioration. Examples include severe trauma, cardiomyopathy, and septic shock. Underlying anatomical or airway anomalies that prevent the proper fitting of noninvasive interfaces also preclude the use of NIV.[8] Similarly, patients with respiratory failure following gastrointestinal tract surgeries or disruption of the integrity of the airway are rarely suitable candidates, as positive pressure could disrupt the surgical sites.

Ventilation Strategies

CONVENTIONAL VERSUS OSCILLATORY VENTILATION

PICUs worldwide use a wide variety of ventilation modes. Conventional ventilation modes cycle air or oxygen enriched gas mixtures through the respiratory tract by bulk airflow. Commonly employed modes include pressure control (PC), volume control (VC), or VC modes with decelerating flow that minimizes peak inspiratory pressures. These breaths are cycled using synchronized intermittent mandatory ventilation (SIMV) typically with pressure support for breaths above the set respiratory rate or assist control (AC) in which each breath above that rate is a controlled breath. Most modern ventilators also incorporate one or more support-modes or autoweaning support modes with embedded algorithms to

Table 37.1 Common Indications for Mechanical Ventilation

Primary Category	Primary Pathophysiologic Mechanism	Clinical Example
Respiratory causes	Restrictive pathology (Decreased lung and/or chest wall compliance, low FRC)	Pneumonia Acute respiratory distress syndrome Atelectasis Large pleural effusion or ascites Severe scoliosis
	Obstructive pathology—upper airway	Croup Epiglottitis
	Obstructive pathology—lower airway	Bronchiolitis Asthma
CNS pathology	Poor or absent respiratory drive	Encephalitis Encephalopathy Ingestion of medications Electrolyte disturbance
	Inability to maintain airway	Poor or absent gag/cough
	Increased intracranial pressure	Traumatic brain injury
Neuromuscular pathology	Severe weakness	Electrolyte disturbance Spinal muscular atrophy Myasthenia gravis Guillain-Barré syndrome Tick paralysis Spinal cord injury
	Weakness with inability to protect airway	Infants disproportionately affected
	Diaphragmatic paralysis	
	Flail chest	
Cardiovascular dysfunction	Severe shock	
	Severe myocardial dysfunction	

CNS, Central nervous system.
Reprinted by permission of Edizioni Minerva Medica from Prabhakaran P, Sasser W, Borasino S. Pediatric mechanical ventilation. *Minerva Pediatr.* 2011;63(5):411-424.)[6]

ensure patient safety. Ventilators have traditionally synchronized breaths to patient effort using flow or pressure triggers. A newer innovation, neurally adjusted ventilator assist (NAVA) uses diaphragmatic electrical activity to initiate and terminate breath deliver and modulate flow.[14] Selection of a particular conventional ventilation mode is often not targeted specifically to the underlying disease but rather is determined by the intensive care physician's experience, local PICU policy and protocols, or outcomes of studies in adults.[15]

Less commonly used and unconventional modes of ventilation include high-frequency ventilation (HFV) and airway pressure release ventilation (APRV). High-frequency oscillatory ventilation (HFOV) is the predominant method of HFV used in the PICU setting, other methods being high-frequency jet ventilation, and high-frequency percussive ventilation (HFPV). High-frequency jet ventilators (HFJVs) contain flow interrupters that disrupt high velocity streams of gas, generating high-pressured jets that deliver small tidal volumes at supraphysiologic frequencies. HFPV delivers a series of high-frequency subtidal volumes in combination with low-frequency breathing cycles. HFPV may be defined as a time-cycled pressure-controlled ventilator coupled with a high-frequency flow generator. Most trials comparing HFV to conventional ventilation only assessed the role of oscillators; therefore, we only discuss the use of HFOV in further detail in this chapter.

During HFOV, airway pressure is maintained by constant gas flow (bias flow) through a valve that can be adjusted to increase or decrease mean airway pressure (MAP). Pressure waves are generated by a bellows that oscillates at supraphysiological ventilatory frequencies between 3 and 15 Hz

(180–900 breaths per minute); the pattern of ventilation is akin to panting in dogs.[16,17] The oscillator creates both inspiratory and expiratory pressure waves, because the bellows is actively driven in both directions. Therefore, expiration is also active, which differentiates HFOV from conventional ventilators, HFJV and HFPV, where expiration is passive and dependent on the elastic recoil of the respiratory system. Active expiration may be beneficial in preventing hyperinflation and enhancing CO_2 elimination.[16] Tidal volumes generated with HFOV are smaller than the anatomic dead space. Therefore, unlike conventional ventilation, which relies principally upon bulk flow of gas to the alveoli, ventilation during HFOV is accomplished largely by enhanced gas mixing within the lung. The numerous mechanisms that account for the ability to achieve adequate ventilation with HFOV are outlined in Fig. 37.1, and include bulk convection, cardiac oscillations, Taylor dispersion, asymmetric velocity profiles, pendelluft, and diffusion.[17] For a detailed discussion on mechanical ventilation modes, please refer to Chapter 34, *Principles of Mechanical Ventilation.*

Use of HFOV in the PICU was largely driven from positive studies on its use in the neonatal intensive care unit (NICU)[18]; however, recent large randomized control trials in adults have failed to show benefit.[19–21] Randomized controlled trials evaluating HFOV among children are lacking. A recently published retrospective observational study[22] and a propensity score matched secondary analysis of another pediatric RCT[23] compared early HFOV (initiated within 24–48 hours of intubation) to conventional mechanical ventilation and/or late HFOV. While the studies suggested increased duration of mechanical ventilation and mortality in HFOV groups, patients treated with HFOV also had poorer oxygenation than

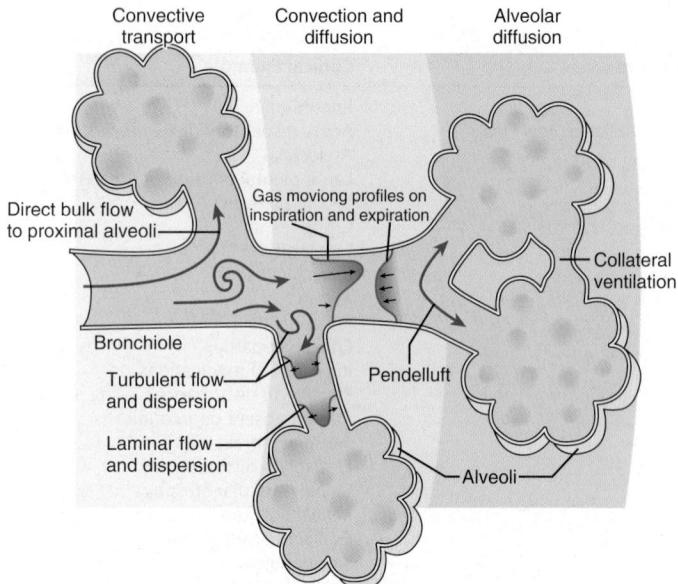

Fig. 37.1 Gas-Transport Mechanisms during High-Frequency Ventilation (HFOV). There are several ways in which gas is transported during HFOV. These include (a) turbulent flow in larger airways, (b) bulk airflow in proximal alveolar units, (c) Pendelluft between adjacent alveolar units, (d) diffusion within alveolar units, (e) continuous streaming of gas into and out of alveolar units due to varying gas movement profiles on inspiration and expiration, and (f) Taylor Dispersion, the collateral ventilation of alveolar units through Pores of Kohn. (From Jean-Christophe Bouchut, M.D.; Jean Godard, M.D.; Olivier Claris, M.D. High-frequency Oscillatory Ventilation. Anesthesiology. Wolter's Kluwer 2014.)

non-HFOV groups. Thus, the decision as to whether and when to initiate HFOV in the PICU is based more upon clinical experience than empiric evidence.

EXTRACORPOREAL MEMBRANOUS OXYGENATION

Some PICU patients cannot be adequately oxygenated or ventilated using conventional ventilators or HFV. These PICU patients may be candidates for extracorporeal membrane oxygenation (ECMO). The ECMO circuit consists of a venous cannula situated in a large central vein or right atrium, a pump, an oxygenator, an arterial cannula with its tip in the aorta (for venoarterial ECMO) or right atrium (for venovenous ECMO); a bridge that permits flow to bypass the patient; connective tubing; ports for patient and circuit access; and continuous monitors of flow, oxygenation, hemoglobin, and other parameters.

As a rule, ECMO is considered only in patients with a reversible disease causing intractable hypoxemia or severe respiratory acidosis or who require an increase in cardiac output to achieve adequate end organ perfusion. The use of ECMO for severe hypercarbia without severe acidosis, for the prevention of ventilator induced lung injury, or for heart failure as a bridge to a ventricular assist device or heart transplant, is common but is perhaps less well accepted.

ECMO comes with its risks and complications. The ECMO circuit requires systemic anticoagulation, and the most common complication of ECMO remains hemorrhage, which can be from cannulation sites, surgical sites, sites of previous

surgical procedures, or in the form of pulmonary and intracerebral hemorrhage.[24] Thromboembolism, infections, and disseminated intravascular coagulopathy are some other commonly encountered problems. Due to the high potential for associated morbidity, the threshold for cannulation in the setting of acute respiratory failure is relatively high. Oxygenation Index (OI) is a valuable measure of mechanical support required to maintain adequate oxygenation, and is measured by:

$$OI = \frac{\text{mean airway pressure (cm } H_2O) \times FiO_2\,(\%)}{PaO_2\,(\text{mm Hg})}$$

Recommendations from ECMOnet and Extracorporeal Life Support Organization (ELSO) recommend an OI > 30 or OI > 40, respectively, as indications for initiating ECMO support.[25] If OI is lower than 30 or 40, ECMO may be indicated in the setting of refractory air leak syndromes.[25] While a more extensive discussion of ECMO is beyond the scope of this chapter, suffice it to say, ECMO may be used to provide only gas exchange support (venovenous) or gas exchange and circulatory support (venoarterial). The pediatric pulmonologist should be aware that venovenous ECMO provides only partial gas exchange support and no circulatory support. Thus, oxyhemoglobin saturation values are typically in the 80%–90% range. Venoarterial ECMO can achieve complete cardiorespiratory support and oxyhemoglobin saturations typically are normal, but pulse oximetry may be unreliable, since pulsatile blood flow may be minimal or absent. Bronchoscopy is often required prior to ECMO discontinuation to perform bronchoalveolar lavage and clear mucus plugs that may accumulate while the child is on rest ventilator settings. While anticoagulation certainly increases the risk of bleeding during invasive procedures, successful weaning off ECMO often requires one or more bronchoscopies.

Complications of Mechanical Ventilation

MUCUS PLUGGING

A common problem encountered among mechanically ventilated patients is secretion management. Multiple factors in the ICU place mechanically ventilated children at an increased risk for retained secretions. The inflated endotracheal tube (ETT) cuff causes significant depression of tracheal mucus velocity and disrupts the mucociliary escalator.[26] Furthermore, defects in ciliary function are likely underappreciated and are probably a greater contributor to respiratory failure in the PICU than commonly appreciated (see Chapter 71, *Primary Ciliary Dyskinesia*). The relative immobility and muscular weakness associated with prolonged ICU admissions contributes to weakened cough and pooling of secretions, and depression of spontaneous breathing through the use of sedatives and paralytics compounds the problem by impairing mucociliary clearance and cough reflexes. Fluid restriction and aggressive diuresis also contribute to thickened secretions.[27] Smaller airways in children are especially prone to obstruction by thick, immobile secretions, contributing to ventilation-perfusion (V/Q) mismatch and further worsening of respiratory failure. Acute decompensation can occur if endotracheal tubes or tracheostomy tubes become obstructed with mucus, and suctioning or ETT exchange may be required. Strategies to minimize and treat mucus plugging include humidification, the use of mucolytics, and mechanical disruption of mucus.

Perhaps the simplest and most intuitive medicinal therapy is to ensure adequate humidification of the ventilator circuit. There is clear evidence that drying of the mucosal surface causes mucus adhesion to the epithelium,[28] and heating and humidifying cool medical gases has now become a standard of care during mechanical ventilation.[29] However, the optimum degree of humidification is frequently debated and there are no straightforward or agreed upon methods for monitoring the adequacy of humidification.[30] Secretion volume and consistency, frequency of ETT occlusion, changes in ETT diameter and/or resistance, and suction frequency are often used as surrogate markers for adequate humidification. However, none of these variables are very reliable as they are easily influenced by underlying disease process or concurrent therapies.

Along with standard methods of humidification, nebulization with hypertonic saline (HS, 3% or greater) is frequently used for airway clearance in the setting of thick tenacious secretions that are difficult to suction. Use of hyperosmolar agents such as HS and mannitol was initially studied in patients with cystic fibrosis (CF) and bronchiectasis and showed significant benefit in that population,[31,32] leading to wider use among mechanically ventilated patients in pediatric ICUs. Theoretically, inhaled HS generates transient osmotic gradients on airway surfaces, drawing water from the submucosal space onto the airway surface.[28] This increased water in the airway lumen reduces the entanglements of the mucin network, thus facilitating mucociliary clearance. Furthermore, in sputum studies, a reduction in the viscoelastic properties, surface tension, and spinability and an increase in the hydration of mucus have been measured in response to HS.[31]

Other adjunctive agents used to treat or prevent mucus plugging include mucolytic agents such as N-acetylcysteine (NAC) and recombinant human deoxyribonuclease (rhDNase). NAC disrupts disulfide bonds that link mucin oligomers and has antioxidant and antiinflammatory properties.[33] NAC was first described as a mucolytic agent in 1963.[34] Several clinical studies were undertaken following the discovery and its use became widespread, particularly among the CF population. Several subsequent trials have failed to show any benefit of using NAC among patients with acute respiratory distress syndrome, ARDS (as well as CF) and a recent meta-analysis of ARDS trials concurred.[35] However, in the setting of mucus hypersecretion and plugging among mechanically ventilated children, its use as a rescue therapy continues due to the lack of clear evidence disproving its efficacy.

DNase is a recombinant endonuclease that cleaves DNA. Its use in the PICU is generally restricted to conditions with purulent respiratory secretions[33] and its use is currently US Food and Drug Administration (FDA) approved in the United States for the treatment of CF lung disease. Multiple studies have evaluated the use of DNase in critical care settings for treatment of atelectasis secondary to mucus plugging in mechanically ventilated patients. Most of these are small

underpowered studies, and their findings seem mixed.[36–39] A recent meta-analysis also recognized the low quality and quantity of existing data,[40] and like NAC, it continues to be used in select patients with thick purulent secretions.

Several mechanical airway clearance techniques are commonly used in the PICU: chest physiotherapy (CPT), intermittent percussive ventilation (IPV), and mechanical insufflation-exsufflation. CPT has been advocated in the field of pediatrics for many years now and is the traditional first-line therapy for secretion management and atelectasis.[41] Several CPT techniques are described and used in mechanically ventilated children: (1) manual percussion with cupping of hand or with a facemask, (2) vibration of the chest wall transmitting energy through the chest wall to loosen or move bronchial secretions, and (3) postural drainage using gravity to move secretions from peripheral airways to the larger bronchi.[42] Despite its historical status and widespread use, evidence for CPT remains weak or absent,[43] and it is not recommended as a routine treatment by the American Association of Respiratory Care.[44]

IPV involves application of high-frequency oscillations to the airways, enhancing secretion clearance when interfaced with conventional mechanical ventilation. The mechanism by which IPV may promote pulmonary secretion clearance is its asymmetrical flow pattern, whereby expiratory flow exceeds inspiratory flow to propel secretions forward.[45] It can be an effective tool in mechanically ventilated patients with refractory atelectasis secondary to mucus plugging. In a small randomized controlled trial, use of IPV in mechanically ventilated pediatric patients produced more clinically important improvement in atelectasis than was observed in children receiving CPT.[46]

Mechanical insufflation-exsufflation, more commonly known as cough-assist, was first introduced in the 1950s, but its use became more widespread in the 1990s. It functions by mechanically inflating the lungs with positive pressure, followed by the rapid application of negative pressure that stimulates a cough. Similar to IPV, cough-assist devices create shear forces in the airway that help mobilize secretions. Typically, positive and negative pressure swings of 30–40 cm H_2O are applied in repetitions of 3–5 maneuvers to mobilize secretions.[45] This therapy has been used primarily to promote pulmonary hygiene in patients with neuromuscular diseases and is one of the few therapies that are recommended by the American Association of Respiratory Care.[44] It should be used with caution in PICU patients prone to lung derecruitment.

ATELECTASIS

Atelectasis occurs when airway pressure declines below the critical closing pressure of a given terminal respiratory unit. In a healthy lung, this closing pressure is below atmospheric pressure, but in disease states, it becomes elevated. To reverse atelectasis, airway pressure must be raised higher than the critical opening pressure. This pressure is again elevated in many disease states. Since lung disease in many PICU patients is heterogeneous, maintaining recruitment of one lung region may result in overdistension or injury to another. Mucus plugging may also contribute to atelectasis and should be treated as discussed in the previous section.

The atelectasis present in many PICU patients compromises oxygenation and ventilation secondary to V/Q mismatching. Additionally, pooling of secretions in atelectatic lung segments may also predispose the patient to nosocomial pneumonia.[47] Mucus plugging is probably the commonest cause of atelectasis as discussed above. Other causes of atelectasis include foreign body aspiration, aspiration of secretions or gastric contents, and the regional atelectasis that occurs as a consequence of ARDS.

Nonpulmonary factors often contribute to atelectasis. In the supine patient, abdominal contents push in a cephalad direction, decreasing the functional residual capacity. Complete or partial closure of alveoli in the dependent lung zones results in reduced compliance and increased risk of atelectasis. The most common segment of the lung to develop atelectasis is the left lower lobe, possibly due to compression by the heart in the supine position and its poor drainage.[48] In such cases, atelectasis frequently responds to judicious use of positive end-expiratory pressure (PEEP) that overcomes the closing pressure of smaller airways and thus "stents" them open. PEEP titration studies can be employed at the bedside to determine optimal PEEP that produces maximal lung recruitment and minimizes dead space ventilation.[49] Similarly, recruitment maneuvers can be employed to expand atelectatic lung segments. These maneuvers involve application of elevated airway pressure to increase transpulmonary pressure transiently. This could be through sustained inflation, intermittent sighs, or stepwise increases of PEEP or airway inspiratory pressure. Several studies have demonstrated improvements in oxygenation, lung mechanics, and lung reaeration after application of recruitment maneuvers, but the optimum method of recruitment and the impact on clinical outcome remains under discussion.[50]

The pediatric pulmonologist is commonly consulted in PICU patients with refractory atelectasis due to mucus plugging who may need therapeutic bronchoscopy. Numerous case series have shown fiberoptic bronchoscopy to be moderately effective in recruiting atelectatic lung segments by suctioning secretions under direct visualization.[47] However, it must be recognized that ICU patients might be too unstable from a hemodynamic or respiratory standpoint to undergo bronchoscopy. A significant decrease in PaO_2 and elevation in $PaCO_2$, as well as increased auto-PEEP leading to reduced venous return and cardiac output, can be seen during bronchoscopy, and this decline is more pronounced as the duration and amount of suctioning is increased.[47,51] Hypoxemia eventually returns to baseline but takes up to 15 minutes in patients with healthy lungs and several hours in those patients with parenchymal disease.[47,51] Studies have also shown elevations in intracranial pressure (ICP) with bronchoscopy despite heavy sedation and paralysis. Decisions regarding bronchoscopy in patients with intracranial pathologies should be made with this information in mind. Importantly, the cause of atelectasis should be established before proceeding with bronchoscopy. While mucus plugging may be amenable to bronchoscopic intervention, atelectasis from other causes (e.g., bronchial compression due to an enlarged cardiac chamber, diaphragmatic dysfunction, and pleural effusion) would not benefit from bronchoscopy. Additionally, while bronchoscopy may temporarily improve atelectasis in patients with severe bronchomalacia or restrictive lung disease, the procedure should be part of a larger respiratory care plan aimed at maintaining lung recruitment. Refer to Chapter 9, *Bronchoscopy and Bronchoalveolar Lavage in Pediatric Patients*, for further details.

VENTILATOR-INDUCED LUNG INJURY

Although mechanical ventilation is essential for supporting many patients, it may itself cause lung damage, particularly in disease states such as acute respiratory distress syndrome ARDS, leading to ventilator-induced lung injury (VILI). The development of VILI is triggered by regional overdistension of the alveoli (volutrauma), high airway and alveolar pressures (barotrauma), cyclic opening and collapse of terminal respiratory units (atelectrauma), and inflammatory cell recruitment due to high shear (biotrauma). Barotrauma can manifest as air leaks causing pneumothorax, pneumomediastinum, interlobular emphysema, or subcutaneous emphysema of the face, neck, or chest wall.[52] Barotrauma was the first widely recognized component of VILI and remained unquestioned until the 1980s when Dreyfuss et al. showed that application of high tidal volume and not airway pressure was the major determinant of VILI, introducing the concept of volutrauma.[53] Additionally, heterogeneity of lung compliance in conditions such as ARDS can aggravate the development of VILI as repeated opening and closing of short time constant lung units renders adjacent zones susceptible to shear stresses, creating a vicious cycle of VILI, both at high and low tidal volumes (atelectrauma). A relatively newer concept is that of biotrauma, which suggests that even in the absence of overt tissue injury, such as that caused by barotrauma, unphysiological shear or stress can promote release of proinflammatory cytokines and recruitment of white cells, with resulting lung inflammation.[54]

The application of generous PEEP can be useful in keeping lung segments well recruited and thus avoid atelectrauma. The optimum PEEP level remains unclear and likely varies between individual patients, but several randomized controlled trials and meta-analyses have failed to demonstrate any mortality benefit of using higher levels of PEEP (>12 cm H_2O).[52] The term "open lung ventilation" is often used to describe the strategy of using higher PEEP to prevent atelectrauma. HFV also offers the advantage of open lung ventilation; continuous and relatively high mean airway pressures keep the alveoli patent at all times as small tidal volumes are administered. As a general rule, pediatric intensivists titrate PEEP or MAP so that at end inspiration the lung is inflated to the approximate volume of the patient's baseline functional residual capacity.

An understanding of the above mechanisms has led to evidence-based efforts to reduce VILI and produced recommendations for "lung-protective" ventilation strategies, including the use of low tidal volumes and generous PEEP, limiting plateau pressures, and using permissive hypercarbia. The use of lower tidal volumes reduces end-inspiratory stress/strain and theoretically prevents volutrauma. The landmark ARDSnet trial of 2000 compared mechanical ventilation with low tidal volume (6 mL/kg) versus high tidal volume (12 mL/kg) ventilation among adults and successfully established the benefits of lower tidal volume resulting in decreased mortality and an increased number of ventilator-free days.[55] Refer to Chapter 38, *Acute Respiratory Distress*

Syndrome for further discussion on ARDS and lung protective strategies.

It is important to realize that children in the ICU may have disease processes (pulmonary or otherwise) that prevent optimal ventilation. In such scenarios, escalation of inspiratory pressures would likely improve gas exchange but would also induce barotrauma in the process and prove harmful in the long run. In these situations, it is advisable to limit plateau pressures to 30–35 cm H_2O and accept higher carbon dioxide levels. While practicing "permissive hypercarbia," care must be taken to avoid severe respiratory acidosis, particularly in hemodynamically unstable children. Ventilator management in PICU patients commonly involves tradeoffs not necessary outside of the PICU, and strategies are dependent upon careful risk-benefit analysis considered in the context of each patient.

AIR LEAK SYNDROMES

Pneumothorax, pneumomediastinum, and subcutaneous emphysema are common air leak syndromes observed in the PICU. One of the commonest causes is aggressive mechanical ventilation and resulting barotrauma or volutrauma with breach of airway integrity. Mechanical ventilation of children with obstructive lung physiology (e.g., asthma, or bronchiolitis obliterans) can also pose challenges with inadequate expiratory flow and resulting hyperinflation, which can cause air leaks. This can occur with both invasive and noninvasive mechanical ventilation. Other causes of air leak include trauma, necrotizing infection, surgical procedure, or endoscopic tracheal and esophageal procedure (Fig. 37.2).

While subcutaneous emphysema can be cosmetically disconcerting, it does not have any life-threatening implications. Adult studies have evaluated the use of subcutaneous fenestrated catheters or fenestrated angiocatheters for treatment,[56] but there is a significant risk of infections associated with these invasive devices and the management strategy in pediatric ICUs is conservative, with treatment of the underlying disease process and possibly chest tube placement.

Similarly, pneumomediastinum is rarely clinically significant. It is generally considered a benign entity of little clinical importance with a good prognosis.[57] There are only rare reported cases of severe pneumomediastinum causing vessel or tracheal obstruction and inducing the symptoms and signs of tamponade and decreased venous return. Management, therefore, is mainly conservative and primarily involves limiting airway pressures.[57]

Pneumothorax, if large enough, can cause respiratory and hemodynamic compromise and is commonly the cause of pneumomediastinum and subcutaneous emphysema. Treatment of pneumothoraces may involve urgent needle thoracostomy (most safely performed in the second intercostal space in the midclavicular line) and chest tube placement. Measures should be made to prevent further alveolar injury by limiting airway pressures, allowing spontaneous healing of injured alveoli and resolution of air leak. A large unilateral air leak may make ventilation of the healthy lung difficult and require selective mainstem bronchus intubation, typically performed with bronchoscopic guidance. Refractory air leak can be treated with temporary bronchial occlusion using fibrin glues or complete lung rest using ECMO. Persistent but medically manageable air leak may be treated with

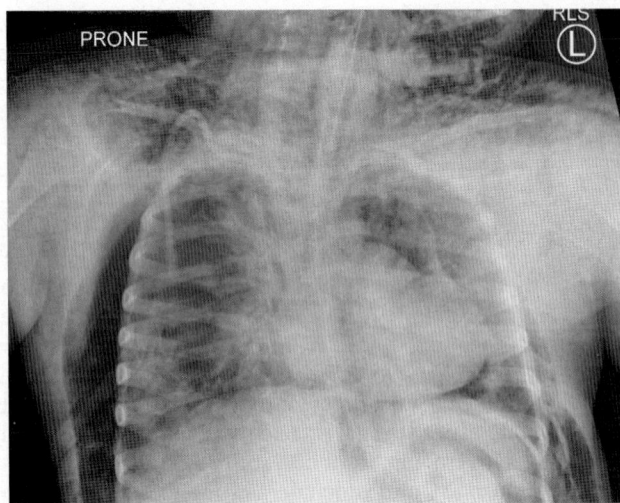

Fig. 37.2 Chest x-ray of a mechanically ventilated child with pneumomediastinum, and severe subcutaneous emphysema of the chest wall and neck.

pleurodesis and persistent difficult to manage air leak may require lobectomy.

VENTILATOR-ASSOCIATED PNEUMONIA

In recent years, ventilator-associated pneumonia (VAP) has gained significant attention due to the associated mortality and morbidity, and it is now believed to be the second most common hospital acquired infection in PICUs, with some studies reporting incidences as high as 20%.[58] There has also been an increasing recognition of the financial and socioeconomic burden from prolonged mechanical ventilation and extended hospital stays associated with VAP, and the Centers for Disease Control and Prevention (CDC) report the average attributable patient cost of VAP ranging from $11,897[59] to $25,072.[60]

Pathogenesis of VAP remains unclear: it is likely the result of microaspiration, but in immunocompromised patients or patients with mucosal breakdown (e.g., burn patients), it may be secondary to lung infiltration from the bloodstream. Entry of bacteria to the lung may also be facilitated directly through the ETT during disconnection from the ventilator circuit. Most of the bacteria found in the endotracheal aspirates of patients suffering from VAP are also found in the naso-oropharynx and even in gastric secretions. Most commonly implicated organisms include *Staphylococcus aureus*, *Streptococcus pneumoniae*, *Haemophilus influenzae*, *Pseudomonas aeruginosa*, *Acinetobacter sp.*, *Stenotrophomonas maltophilia* and enteric gram-negative bacilli including *Enterobacter sp.*, *Klebsiella sp. and Citrobacter sp.*[58,61]

Diagnosing VAP can be challenging, as universally accepted criteria are lacking, and the definition and surveillance published by CDC remain the most commonly accepted approach. It is defined as a pneumonia occurring after the patient has been intubated and received mechanical ventilation for at least 48 hours. The initial diagnosis is based on clinical suspicion and the presence of at least one of the following on two or more serial chest radiographs: new or progressive radiographic infiltrates, consolidation, cavitation, and pneumatoceles in an infant 1-year-old or above. Additionally, the standard diagnostic criteria include at least two or three (applicable only for the under 12-year-olds) of the following: fever of greater than 38°C or hypothermia of less than 36.5°C; change in sputum volume or character, or increased suctioning requirement; new onset or worsening cough, dyspnea, tachypnea or apnea; rales, bronchial breath sounds, wheezing or rhonchi.[58] Other criteria for diagnosis of VAP include worsening gas exchange or increased ventilator demand after a period of stability and the use of serum biomarkers such as C-reactive protein (CRP) or procalcitonin to narrow the diagnostic margin.[62]

Caution must be exercised when diagnosing VAP. The above-mentioned signs and symptoms may also be present in conditions other than VAP (e.g., presence of increased secretions with tracheobronchitis, or radiographic findings with atelectasis). There is debate as to whether to include cultures of endotracheal secretions, since a positive culture result may represent colonization rather than true infection, potentially leading to inappropriate antibiotic use with the ever-present risk of selection of antibiotic-resistant, particularly Gram negative, bacteria.

Efforts to minimize VAP in children have focused on preventive strategies that include hand hygiene, mouth care with antiseptic solution, elevating the head of the bed by 30–45 degrees, changing ventilator circuits only as needed, minimizing patient-ventilator disconnections with in-line suctioning, frequent drainage of ventilator condensate away from the ETT, ETT cuff pressure maintenance, monitoring of gastric residuals to prevent aspiration, and minimizing ventilator days by adopting sedation holidays and weaning protocols. Since VAP pathophysiology is multifactorial, strategies for prevention are commonly implemented in bundles and not with each individual preventive measure in isolation.[58] Table 37.2 reviews key studies that have studied and shown success with pediatric VAP bundles.

Clinical suspicion for VAP mandates early antimicrobial treatment. If the initial choice of antibiotics is inappropriate, or there are significant delays in initiation of therapy, there may be significant morbidity or mortality associated with the VAP episode.[61,63] Pediatric intensivists and pulmonologists should collaborate with infectious disease experts within their own hospitals to develop specific algorithms for treating VAP based on hospital bacterial resistance patterns. While debate continues on the duration of antibiotic therapy for VAP, data suggest that shorter therapies may be equally effective as prolonged antibiotic courses.[64] Fig. 37.3 presents a simplified algorithm for treatment of VAP. Early bronchoalveolar lavage should be considered to help direct VAP treatment. Protected specimen brush culture can also be useful for diagnosis. While endotracheal cultures may represent either ventilator-associated tracheitis or VAP, protected

---

Table 37.2   What Key Interventions Have Been Used for Pediatric VAP Bundle?

Brierley et al.[104]	■ Head up tilt (target 45°, but achieved 20°–30°) ■ Mouth care with oral antiseptic every 4 hourly OR 12 hourly toothbrush ■ Clean suctioning practice ■ Gastric ulcer prophylaxis: Ranitidine ■ Chest x-ray interpretation ■ Documentation to be completed 4 hourly ■ Indication of VAP compliance, to be documented each shift	Prebundle VAP was 5.6/1000 ventilator days. Postbundle VAP was 0/1000 ventilator days over 12-month period.
Bigham et al.[105]	■ Prevention of bacterial colonization of oropharynx, stomach and sinuses ■ Change ventilator circuits and in-line suction catheters only when visibly soiled ■ Drain condensate from ventilator circuit at least every 2–4 h (use heated wire circuits to reduce rainout) ■ Store oral suction devices (when not in use) in nonsealed plastic bag at the bedside; rinse after use ■ Hand hygiene before and after contact with ventilator circuit ■ When soiling from respiratory secretions is anticipated, wear gown before providing care to patient ■ Follow unit mouth care policy every 2–4 h	The VAP rate was reduced from 5.6 to 0.3 infections per 1000 ventilator days after bundle implementation.
Rosenthal et al.[106]	■ Prevention of aspiration of contaminated secretions ■ Elevate HOB 30°–45° unless contraindicated and by written order ■ Always drain ventilator circuit before repositioning patient ■ When possible, for children > 12 years old, use endotracheal tube with dorsal lumen above endotracheal cuff to help suction secretions above the cuff ■ Adherence to hand hygiene guidelines ■ Semirecumbent position 30°–45° ■ Daily assessment to wean and use of weaning protocols ■ Use of noninvasive ventilation whenever possible, minimizing the duration of ventilation ■ Preference of orotracheal intubation over nasotracheal intubation ■ Maintenance of endotracheal cuff pressure of at least 20 cm H_2O ■ Removal of condensate from ventilator circuits, keeping the ventilator closed during condensate removal ■ Changing of the ventilator circuit only when visibly soiled or malfunctioning ■ Avoidance of gastric over distension ■ Avoidance of histamine-receptor 2-blocking agents and proton pump inhibitors ■ Use of sterile water to rinse reusable respiratory equipment	VAP rate was 11.7/1000 ventilator days during baseline period and 8.1/1000 ventilator days during the intervention period (31% reduction in VAP rate).

Review of key studies and interventions that have been used for pediatric VAP bundles. Table modified from Chang I, Schibler A. Ventilator associated pneumonia in children. *Paediatr Respir Rev.* 2015;20:10-16, with permission.

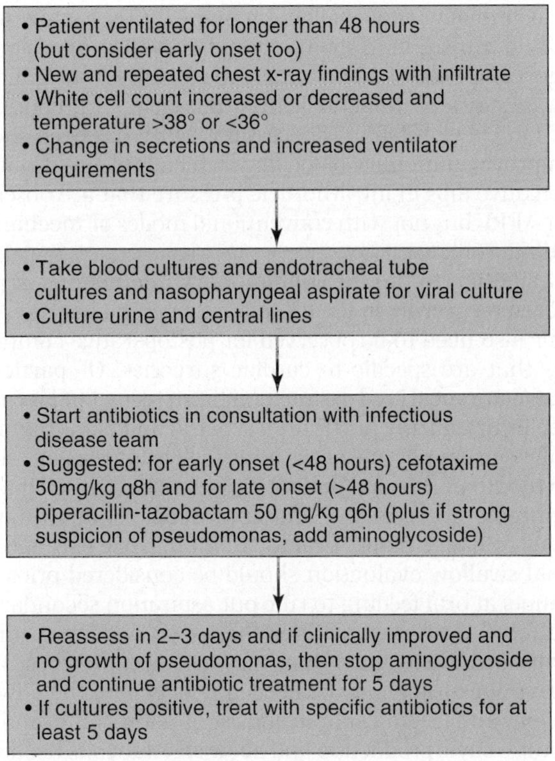

- Patient ventilated for longer than 48 hours (but consider early onset too)
- New and repeated chest x-ray findings with infiltrate
- White cell count increased or decreased and temperature >38° or <36°
- Change in secretions and increased ventilator requirements

↓

- Take blood cultures and endotracheal tube cultures and nasopharyngeal aspirate for viral culture
- Culture urine and central lines

↓

- Start antibiotics in consultation with infectious disease team
- Suggested: for early onset (<48 hours) cefotaxime 50mg/kg q8h and for late onset (>48 hours) piperacillin-tazobactam 50 mg/kg q6h (plus if strong suspicion of pseudomonas, add aminoglycoside)

↓

- Reassess in 2–3 days and if clinically improved and no growth of pseudomonas, then stop aminoglycoside and continue antibiotic treatment for 5 days
- If cultures positive, treat with specific antibiotics for at least 5 days

Fig. 37.3 Suggested approach to diagnose and treat VAP. (Modified from Chang I, Schibler A. Ventilator associated pneumonia in children. *Paediatr Respir Rev.* 2015;20:10-16, with permission.)

specimen brush cultures are only consistent with VAP.[65] However, there is a lack of data in children that would support the routine use of protected specimen brush.

SPECIAL PULMONARY CONSIDERATION IN PEDIATRIC PATIENTS WITH NEUROMUSCULAR DISORDERS

Children with neuromuscular diseases (e.g., muscular dystrophy and spinal muscular atrophy) have limited respiratory system reserve at baseline and are at elevated risk of respiratory failure. Relatively benign upper respiratory tract infections can progress to increased secretion retention, secondary bacterial infection, and an acute respiratory deterioration. Because of their fragile respiratory status, postoperative ICU admission should be considered when children with neuromuscular disease undergo elective surgery.[66,67]

As a general rule, patients with neuromuscular disorders admitted to the ICU with or in anticipation of respiratory compromise should have early or preventative institution of airway clearance and NIV to maintain lung recruitment and minimize retained secretions. Evidence suggests that noninvasive positive pressure ventilation (PPV) in patients with neuromuscular weakness can improve tachypnea, dyspnea, and work of breathing; increase alveolar ventilation; help reexpand the lung bases; and provide respiratory muscle rest.[68] As the patient improves, these therapies can be weaned.

Noninvasive PPV support may be inadequate in the setting of severe respiratory failure. Patients with neuromuscular disorders may require invasive respiratory support for the first

few days of critical illness, but the goal should always be to extubate at the earliest opportunity. Aggressive airway clearance should be continued, and early bronchoscopy should be pursued in the event of persistent infiltrates or atelectasis. As a general rule, patients with neuromuscular disease should be extubated directly to continuous NIV, even if their pulmonary function parameters suggest a high likelihood of successful extubation.[66] Before proceeding with trial of extubation in spinal muscular atrophy patients, it is advisable to ensure that these patients are afebrile and do not require supplemental oxygen, and their chest radiograph should not demonstrate atelectasis or infiltrates.[69] These weaning criteria are unique to this group of patients; in no other group is there the stringent requirement for normal gas exchange in room air before extubation. Since pediatric pulmonologists often have long-standing relationships with these patients and their families, early and frequent discussions regarding extubation criteria are essential. Patients with lesser degrees of muscle weakness can be extubated while they still have increased respiratory support requirements.

PULMONARY HEMORRHAGE

Severe pulmonary hemorrhage is a rare but dramatic reason for ICU admission. The causes can be varied, and include infections, CF, bronchiectasis, trauma, congenital heart disease, arteriovenous collaterals, pulmonary hypertension, pulmonary embolism, tumors, idiopathic pulmonary hemosiderosis, and vasculitides such as systemic lupus erythematosus (SLE), Goodpasture's syndrome, Wegener's syndrome, and Henoch-Schonlein purpura.[70] Definitive diagnosis may require extensive studies such as serology, echocardiogram, computed tomography (CT) scan with contrast, and tissue biopsy via transbronchial biopsy, thoracotomy, or video assisted thoracoscopic surgery (VATS). Many of these patients may present with severe hypoxemic respiratory failure and require resuscitation and stabilization. Once mechanical ventilation is initiated, it is common practice to maintain high MAP and high PEEP to "tamponade" bleeding from smaller and relatively compressible capillaries. Use of HFOV can also be useful in this circumstance to deliver a constant elevated MAP. If there is strong suspicion of vasculitic disorders, evidence suggests early use of high-dose corticosteroids.[71–73] Diffuse alveolar hemorrhage in children is discussed further in Chapter 61.

INTENSIVE CARE UNIT NEUROMYOPATHY

Neuromyopathy in the ICU has been widely recognized and researched among adults but often remains underdiagnosed among children.[74] Both critical illness and its associated treatments lead to muscle and nerve injury.[75] Prolonged immobility and bed rest is common in pediatric ICUs and leads to disuse atrophy secondary to decreased muscle protein synthesis and increased muscle catabolism.[76,77] Furthermore, the interaction of critical illness with immobility may lead to even greater muscle loss,[78] likely secondary to protein catabolism and neurotoxicity induced by proinflammatory cytokines.[75]

A common iatrogenic cause of neuromyopathy in the PICU is the concomitant use of corticosteroids and muscle relaxants (particularly curare derivatives such as rocuronium and vecuronium), which are agents that are commonly administered together in children with severe protracted ARDS or status asthmaticus. Aminoglycoside antibiotics have also been associated with neuromyopathy in the ICU, but the evidence remains mixed.[79]

The implications for children with ICU acquired neuromyopathy can be quite serious. The resultant muscular weakness, particularly involving the respiratory muscles, can lead to prolonged or failed weaning from mechanical ventilation. Acquired ICU neuromyopathy can prolong hospitalization and necessitate continued mechanical ventilation during rehabilitation.[75,79] Ambulation while still receiving mechanical ventilation, in-bed exercise, and early physical therapy are becoming more common in adult ICUs[80,81] and may soon gain acceptance in PICUs as a means to minimize this complication of ICU care. Rehabilitation and conditioning associated with early ambulation can also have positive implications for patients awaiting lung transplantation, as shown among children on ECMO support.[82]

SPECIAL PULMONARY CONSIDERATIONS IN PEDIATRIC PATIENTS WITH CONGENITAL HEART DISEASE

Management of children with congenital heart diseases or heart failure in the PICU can pose special challenges for intensivists and pulmonologists due to the unique cardiopulmonary interactions at play. Of particular interest are children who have undergone palliative surgery for single ventricle physiology. The goal of palliation in single ventricle congenital heart disease is to reduce ventricular work and maintain a balanced pulmonary and systemic circulation by transitioning the heart from dual circulation (pulmonary and systemic) to single circulation physiology. To achieve this, the superior vena cava (Glenn procedure) or superior and inferior vena cava (Fontan procedure) drain into the pulmonary artery with the main pulmonary artery disconnected from the pulmonary trunk. For details on how this is achieved in different congenital heart lesions, we refer the reader to an excellent textbook.[83] Negative intrathoracic pressure during spontaneous ventilation facilitates venous return, leading to increased pulmonary blood flow and cardiac output.[84] Conversely, positive pressure ventilation impedes venous return and decreases cardiac output. In the setting of passive blood flow to the lungs, pulmonary vascular resistance (PVR) is also an important factor limiting pulmonary blood flow and cardiac output. Permissive hypercarbia may increase PVR. The need to both maintain lung recruitment and pulmonary blood flow should be considered when providing mechanical ventilatory support in the ICU to children with single ventricle physiology. The MAP, tidal volume, and minute ventilation need to be adequately titrated so as to offset the effects of hypercarbia, hypoxemia, and reduced lung volumes that may increase PVR and impede pulmonary blood flow.[85] However, if the MAP is maintained too high, the elevated intrathoracic pressure can impede venous return and lung overdistension can increase PVR, both leading to decreased pulmonary blood flow and decreased cardiac output. Negative pressure ventilation via use of a cuirass has also been shown to improve pulmonary blood flow and cardiac output in patients with single ventricle physiology;[84,86,87] however,

this technology is not available in many PICUs. Early extubation and transition to spontaneous ventilation after Fontan surgery has been shown to improve outcomes and length of hospital stay and should be actively pursued.[88,89] If continued mechanical ventilation is necessary, APRV has been shown to improve pulmonary blood flow, which is likely secondary to negative dips in intrathoracic pressure that are observed with APRV but not with conventional modes of mechanical ventilation.[90]

In addition to the cardiopulmonary interactions at play, children recovering in the ICU after congenital heart disease repair also need to be observed for postoperative complications that are specific to cardiac surgeries. Of particular concern are vocal cord dysfunction (from recurrent laryngeal nerve injury during aortic arch repairs) and diaphragmatic paralysis (from phrenic nerve injury). For this reason, failure to extubate in this population should always raise concern for phrenic nerve injury, and fluoroscopic studies may be needed to assess diaphragmatic motion. Once extubated, a formal swallow evaluation should be considered prior any attempts at oral feeding to rule out aspiration secondary to vocal cord dysfunction. Chylothorax secondary to intraoperative thoracic duct injury may also occur in these children. A chest tube may be needed to evacuate the chylous effusion, and feeding should consist of a low-fat formula to minimize chyle production and allow spontaneous healing.[91] Octreotide is another common but unproven therapy for chylothorax. Successful use of octreotide has been reported in several case reports, but no randomized controlled trials have been conducted to date.[92]

SPECIAL PULMONARY CONSIDERATIONS IN PEDIATRIC PATIENTS WITH MALIGNANCY OR HEMATOPOIETIC STEM CELL TRANSPLANTATION

Acute respiratory failure secondary to acute lung injury is a common indication for PICU admission after hematopoietic stem cell transplant (HSCT). Depending on the HSCT center involved, 20%–30% of children receiving HSCT may require intubation and mechanical ventilation,[93,94] and among these patients, mortality is as high as 60% during PICU admission and 74% at 180 days after PICU discharge.[95] Table 37.3 shows that the causes of lung injury in the posttransplant setting can be broadly divided into infectious vs. noninfectious and early (within 100 days of transplant) vs. late (more than 100 days following transplant). Advances in preemptive and prophylactic therapy to prevent respiratory infections during the immune deficient state following HSCT have resulted in a decreasing incidence and proportion of infectious versus noninfectious respiratory complications,[96] but vigilance and timely initiation of therapy remains the key.

Clinical studies have established a strong association between graft-versus-host disease (GVHD) and noninfectious lung injury. The acute inflammation and cellular infiltration into the lung parenchyma during acute GVHD has been implicated in development of restrictive lung disease and idiopathic pneumonia syndrome (IPS) pathogenesis,[97] whereas chronic GVHD has been linked to progressive obstructive lung disease and bronchiolitis obliterans.[98] In a subset of HSCT patients, extensive pulmonary vascular disease secondary to transplant-associated thrombotic microangiopathy (TA-TMA)

Table 37.3 Causes of Lung Injury and Respiratory Failure After Stem Cell Transplant

Early (Day 0–100)	Late (Day 100+)
NONINFECTIOUS CAUSES	**NONINFECTIOUS CAUSES**
Pulmonary edema	Bronchiolitis obliterans
Periengraftment respiratory distress syndrome	Bronchiolitis obliterans organizing pneumonia
Diffuse alveolar hemorrhage	Delayed pulmonary toxicity syndrome
Acute interstitial pneumonitis	Chronic GVHD
TA-TMA	—
TRALI	—
INFECTIOUS CAUSES	**INFECTIOUS CAUSES**
Bacteria: Gram-negative rods and Gram-positive cocci	Bacteria: Encapsulated bacteria, Gram-negative rods and Gram-positive cocci
Virus: HSV, CMV, adenovirus, HHV6, RSV, influenza, parainfluenza, rhinovirus, human metapneumovirus	Virus: adenovirus, CMV, VZV, Epstein-Barr virus
Fungi: Candida, aspergillus, pneumocystis	Fungi: Candida, aspergillus, pneumocystis

CMV, Cytomegalovirus, *HHV6*, human herpesvirus type 6; *HSV*, herpes simplex virus, *RSV*, respiratory syncytial virus; *TRALI*, transfusion related acute lung injury; *VZV*, varicella zoster virus.

Modified from Chima RS, Abulebda K, Jodele S. Advances in critical care of the pediatric hematopoietic stem cell transplant patient. *Pediatr Clin North Am.* 2013;60(3):689-707, with permission.

may be observed, with resulting pulmonary hypertension and hypoxemic respiratory failure.[99] Therefore, TA-TMA should be suspected in patients with reassuring imaging studies that present with unexplained hypoxemia.

Viral, bacterial, and fungal cultures should be performed to identify potential infections, and bronchoalveolar lavage should be considered early during ICU admission. In addition to simple chest radiographs, detailed imaging in the form of CT scan and echocardiography may provide diagnostic clues. Specific therapeutic options to address lung injury after HSCT are limited. Given the paucity of specific therapies to address dysregulated inflammation in the lung, corticosteroids remain the mainstay of therapy, and once initiated, should be tapered slowly. Given the role of tumor necrosis factor (TNF)α in GVHD, etanercept (a soluble TNFα-binding protein) has also shown benefit when combined with corticosteroids.[100]

Supportive care for this population of patients includes early initiation of broad-spectrum antimicrobial coverage, including antiviral and antifungal agents.[96,100] Fluid overload among children undergoing HSCT is associated with worse outcomes[101] and should be aggressively managed with diuretic therapy or renal replacement therapy. Early renal replacement therapy can be beneficial, and studies in children have suggested both short-term oxygenation and survival benefits.[102,103] Mechanical ventilation should be initiated early in these patients, but debate continues whether noninvasive or invasive mechanical ventilation should be the initial modality. Prospective trials are lacking, but a recent multicenter retrospective study showed higher mortality among children placed on noninvasive ventilation prior to intubation when compared to those who were intubated without such a trial (odds ratio, 2.1; 95% CI, 1.2–3.6; $P = .01$). Potential explanations for the worse outcome of noninvasive ventilation include it being employed too late to be of benefit or continued too long resulting in a detrimental delayed intubation.[95] Additionally, limitations such as body habitus, skin breakdown, and the presence of mucositis might make noninvasive ventilation an unfeasible modality in these patients. If evidence of pulmonary hypertension is noted, pulmonary vasodilator therapies such as inhaled nitric oxide, sildenafil, and bosentan may be useful.[100]

Conclusion

Pediatric pulmonologists are commonly consulted to aid in the diagnosis and management of patients admitted to the PICU. A thorough knowledge of the physiology and potential pathology in these complex patients is required to minimize the risk of pulmonary complications and optimize outcomes in this high-risk population.

References

Access the reference list online at ExpertConsult.com.

Suggested Reading

Bateman ST, et al. Early high-frequency oscillatory ventilation in pediatric acute respiratory failure. A propensity score analysis. *Am J Respir Crit Care Med.* 2016;193(5):495–503.

Birnkrant DJ, Pope JF. Eibe RM, Management of the respiratory complications of neuromuscular diseases in the pediatric intensive care unit. *J Child Neurol.* 1999;14(3):139–143.

Branson RD, Gomaa D, Rodriquez D Jr. Management of the artificial airway. *Respir Care.* 2014;59(6):974–989, discussion 989-990.

Brower RG, Matthay MA, Morris A. Ventilation with lower tidal volumes as compared with traditional tidal volumes for acute lung injury and the acute respiratory distress syndrome. The Acute Respiratory Distress Syndrome Network. *N Engl J Med.* 2000;342(18):1301–1308.

Chang I, Schibler A. Ventilator associated pneumonia in children. *Paediatr Respir Rev.* 2015;20:10–16.

Gattinoni L, Protti A, Caironi P, et al. Ventilator-induced lung injury: the anatomical and physiological framework. *Crit Care Med.* 2010;38(10 suppl):S539–S548.

Godfrey S. Pulmonary hemorrhage/hemoptysis in children. *Pediatr Pulmonol.* 2004;37(6):476–484.

Guillamet CV, Kollef MH. Ventilator associated pneumonia in the ICU: where has it gone? *Curr Opin Pulm Med.* 2015;21(3):226–231.

Haddad IY. Stem cell transplantation and lung dysfunction. *Curr Opin Pediatr.* 2013;25(3):350–356.

Hashem MD, Parker AM, Needham DM. Early mobilization and rehabilitation of the critically ill patient. *Chest.* 2016;150(3):722–731.

Jolley SE, Bunnell A, Hough CL. Intensive care unit acquired weakness. *Chest.* 2016;150(5):1129–1140.

Kallet RH. Adjunct therapies during mechanical ventilation: airway clearance techniques, therapeutic aerosols, and gases. *Respir Care.* 2013;58(6):1053–1073.

Prabhakaran P, Sasser W, Borasino S. *Pediatric mechanical ventilation. Minerva Pediatr.* 2011;63(5):411–424.

Schroth MK. Special considerations in the respiratory management of spinal muscular atrophy. *Pediatrics.* 2009;123(suppl 4):S245–S249.

Slutsky AS, Drazen JM. Ventilation with small tidal volumes. *N Engl J Med.* 2002;347(9):630–631.

38 Acute Respiratory Distress Syndrome

ALIK KORNECKI, MD, and RAM N. SINGH, MBBS, FRCPC

Epidemiology

The available epidemiological studies are based on the former North American European Consensus Conference Committee (AECC) definition of acute respiratory distress syndrome (ARDS) from 1994.[1] The incidence of ARDS in children is 3–12.8/100,000 per year,[2,3] which is about 5–8 times less than in adults,[4] and constitutes 2%–10% of all pediatric intensive care unit (PICU) admissions per year.[3,5,6] Approximately 80% of children with mild ARDS will progress to moderate and severe ARDS, and two-thirds of them will require early invasive mechanical ventilation.[7] About 60% of pediatric patients with ARDS are less than 4 years of age and 30%–70% of them suffer from a significant underline disease (e.g., prematurity, genetic or neurologic abnormality, cardiac disease).[2,3,6,8] ARDS affects males and females equally.

Etiology

A variety of heterogeneous direct (*pulmonary ARDS*) or indirect (*extrapulmonary ARDS*) insults to the lungs may provoke a similar cascade of inflammatory reactions, which leads to ARDS (Box 38.1). In case of *pulmonary* ARDS, the insult is direct in the lungs, and in the case of *extrapulmonary* ARDS, the insult is indirect and the pulmonary lesions are caused by circulating mediators released from extrapulmonary foci into the blood (e.g., sepsis, pancreatitis; Box 38.1). Data provided by Flori and colleagues[8] from a large epidemiological study suggest that pneumonia (bacterial or viral; 35%) and aspiration pneumonia (13%) are the most common causes for direct ARDS, whereas sepsis (13%) is the most common cause for indirect ARDS.

Outcome

The mortality from ARDS among children has decreased significantly from the 65% to 80% reported in the 1980s.[9,10] This reduction can be attributed to the establishment of dedicated pediatric critical care units with improved general management, including the reduction in the administered tidal volumes (V_T) during mechanical ventilation.[11] However, in the last two decades the mortality has remained unchanged.[5]

A recent large meta-analysis of 32 studies reported a mortality rate of 33.7% in children with ARDS when defined according to the previous AAEC definition of ARDS.[5] It should be noted that studies performed in western countries reported mortality to be between 4.3%[12] and 30.5%,[13] and studies from Asia reported mortality as high as 61%.[14] The differences in mortality among centers are mainly attributed to patient mix and local resources. In general, mortality is higher among children with underlying immune deficiency, malignancy, status post bone marrow transplantation,[15,16] and with comorbidities (e.g., nonpulmonary organ dysfunction, central nervous system dysfunction)[8]; it is minimal among children with bronchiolitis (<3%). In general, it is perceived that the mortality in children is lower than in adults, and the overall mortality is 27%–45%.[17]

Only one study thus far has reported mortality using the New Berlin definition of ARDS (see below). This European multicenter study reported mortality rates of 13.9% for mild, 11.3% for moderate, and 25% for severe ARDS; however, it was limited to young children aged 1–18 months.[18]

In contrast to adults and premature infants where the quality of life after respiratory failure was studied,[19] the long-term quality of life and lung morbidity among children who recover from ARDS has not been studied. However, we believe that children without underlying lung or cardiac disease recover from a single episode of ARDS without significant mechanical or functional sequelae to the lungs.

Definition and Diagnosis

ARDS is a form of acute respiratory failure characterized by a diffuse, progressive inflammatory lung disease that was first reported in 1967 by Ashbaugh and colleagues in a cohort of 12 surgical patients.[20] They noted that the patients exhibited "acute onset of tachypnea, hypoxemia and loss of compliance." Further reports of patients with ARDS altered the acronym to indicate *adult* respiratory distress syndrome, to differentiate it from the respiratory distress syndrome of neonates, even though Ashbaugh's original description included an 11-year-old child. It was not until 1980 that regular reports[9] of ARDS in children established that it was also a pediatric syndrome, and the 1994 North American–European Consensus Conference Committee (NAECC) recommended that the acronym "ARDS" revert to its original meaning (i.e., acute).[1] Most studies in ARDS published until 2014 used the AECC definition of ARDS. The diagnostic criteria have been modified in the Berlin ARDS Conference in 2012 (Table 38.1).[21] The Berlin four-point definition eliminated the group of acute lung injury (ALI) and created three ARDS entities—mild, moderate, and severe—according to the severity of hypoxemia extrapolated from the PaO_2/FiO_2 (P/F) ratio. The new definition, like the previous AECC, focuses on adult patients and does not consider different risk factors, epidemiology, and pathophysiology in children. In addition, the adult definition requires arterial blood gases to calculate the P/F ratio, which are not always available in children.

Box 38.1 Common Etiologies for Acute Respiratory Distress Syndrome

Pulmonary (Direct)	Extrapulmonary (Indirect)
Pneumonia (viral, bacterial)	Sepsis
Aspiration pneumonia	Nonthoracic trauma
Bronchiolitis	Transfusion of blood products
Near drowning	Pancreatitis
Lung contusion	
Toxic inhalation	

Table 38.1 Acute Respiratory Distress Syndrome

Timing	Within 1 week of known clinical insult or new or worsening respiratory symptoms
Chest imaging	Bilateral opacities—not fully explained by effusions, lobar/lung collapse, or Nodules
Origin of edema	Respiratory failure not fully explained by cardiac failure or fluid overload
	Need objective assessment (e.g., echocardiography) to exclude hydrostatic edema if no risk factor present
Oxygenation	—
Mild	PaO_2/FIO_2 201–300 mm Hg with PEEP or CPAP ≥ 5 cm H_2O[a]
Moderate	PaO_2/FIO_2 101–200 Hg with PEEP ≥ 5 cm H_2O
Severe	PaO_2/FIO_2 ≤ 100 mm Hg with PEEP ≥ 5 cm H_2O

[a]This may be delivered noninvasively in the mild acute respiratory distress syndrome group.
CPAP, Continuous positive airway pressure; *FIO₂*, fraction of inspired oxygen.

Table 38.2 Pediatric Acute Respiratory Distress Syndrome

Age	Exclude patients with perinatal lung disease			
Timing	Within 7 days of known clinical insult			
Origin of edema	Respiratory failure not fully explained by cardiac failure or fluid overload			
Imaging	Chest imaging findings of new infiltrate(s) consistent with acute pulmonary parenchymal disease			
Oxygenation	Noninvasive MV	Invasive MV		
	CPAP ≥ 5 cm H_2O[a]	Mild	Moderate	Severe
	P/F ≤ 300	4 ≤ OI < 8	8 ≤ OI < 16	OI ≥ 16
	SpO_2/FiO_2 ≤ 264[b]	5 ≤ OSI < 7.5[b]	7.5 ≤ OSI < 12.3	OSI ≥ 12.3

[a]For nonintubated patients treated with supplemental oxygen on nasal modes of noninvasive ventilation.
[b]Use PaO_2 when available; if not available, wean the FiO_2 to maintain SpO_2 97% to calculate the OSI or SpO_2/FiO_2.
OI, Oxygen index; *OSI*, oxygen saturation index.

In 2015 a panel of investigators proposed adaptation of the Berlin definition to children, the pediatric ARDS (PARDS; Table 38.2).[22] The PARDS definition uses the P/F ratio or SpO_2/FiO_2 ratio for noninvasive ventilated children and the oxygenation index (OI) or the oxygenation saturation index (OSI), when arterial blood is not available, for ventilated children. The request for bilateral pulmonary infiltrates was eliminated, and a better definition for children with underlying congenital heart disease or chronic lung disease was offered.

The classical histological description of ARDS was published in 1976 by Katzenstein and colleagues[23] as diffuse alveolar damage (DAD) associated with the presence of hyaline membranes, interstitial edema, cell necrosis with proliferation, and fibrosis. The validity of the Berlin definition has been tested against lung histopathologic findings in adults undergoing autopsy following clinical ARDS. Among all patients who met clinical criteria for ARDS, DAD was found in only 45%. The proportion of DAD depended on the severity of ARDS, and was more frequent in severe ARDS (58%). Using DAD as the reference standard, the sensitivity and specificity of the diagnosis in adults were 89% (95% confidence interval [CI], 84%–93%) and 63% (95% CI, 59%–67%),[24] respectively. There has been no similar study in children. However, we may expect similar findings, as a comparable study that was performed with the old NAECC definition reported a sensitivity of 81% and a specificity of 71%.[25] The main limitation of these studies was selection bias because they were limited to patients who died; survivors may have had different pathophysiologic findings.

Over the years, various single specific biomarkers or panels of biomarkers, such as surfactant proteins, cytokines, and markers of pulmonary epithelial and endothelial injury, have been investigated for the early diagnosis of ARDS or pending ARDS.[26] However, all these attempts failed because of low sensitivity and specificity. We are still in the search for the "troponin of ARDS."[27]

Pathophysiology

ARDS arises because of an inflammatory process at the alveolar-capillary interface in the lung. The resultant endothelial and epithelial disruption leads to increased alveolar-capillary permeability and flooding of the alveoli with protein-rich edema fluid. Alveolar gas exchange is impaired and surfactant function is disrupted.[9] In addition, there is uncontrolled activation of coagulation along with suppression of fibrinolysis. Classically, ARDS is described as a progressive clinical condition characterized by four stages, although these are rarely identified in pediatric cases. ARDS is triggered by an acute *direct* injury (e.g., aspiration) or *indirect* lung injury (e.g., sepsis), resulting in the onset of an *acute exudative* phase characterized by pulmonary edema, cytokine release, and activation of neutrophils. The acute exudative stage is associated with increased intrapulmonary shunting, increase in dead space, reduced functional residual capacity (FRC), and a decrease in lung and chest wall compliance.[28] Before the advent of computerized tomography (CT), the acute exudative stage was synonymous with the radiologic finding of bilateral homogenous parenchymal disease; however, pulmonary CT imaging changed our outlook on ARDS, revealing heterogeneity in the extent of regional lung injury, with the coexistence of severely injured (dependent) lung and less injured lung and healthy lung regions. Gattinoni and Pesenti[29] suggested that the lung in ARDS be conceptualized as three functional regions: (1) fully aerated normal (usually nondependent) region(s); (2) poorly aerated injured but recruitable lung; and (3) nonaerated consolidated/atelectatic lung. This group also introduced the term *baby lung* to describe the small volume of normal aerated tissue in the nondependent lung regions of the lung that exhibits normal compliance.

During the acute phase of inflammation, abnormalities in coagulation contribute to the development of small vessel occlusion. In rare cases, pulmonary hypertension, due to vascular obstruction and complicated by right ventricular failure, has been described.[30] The *acute exudative phase* may resolve within hours or days, and some patients do not progress to the subsequent *fibroproliferative early repair phase*. Unfortunately, "repair" may not result in disease resolution in all patients, but may presage the development of *fibrosing alveolitis* characterized by increased alveolar dead space, hypoxia, and reduced lung compliance; progression to this third stage is associated with worse outcome. The fourth stage, the *recovery stage*, occurs within 10–14 days, with gradual improvement in lung compliance and oxygenation. The mechanism of resolution of the acute inflammatory process and fibrosis is not well established, and the rate of recovery is not well characterized; however, a return to normal lung function in those patients without underlying chronic lung disease, is the norm.

Thille and coworkers[31] examined the histopathological changes in a large adult population with clinical ARDS who demonstrated DAD at autopsy examination. The histological findings closely correlated with the duration of evolution of ARDS. The exudative changes were observed in 90% of patients with ARDS of less than 1-week duration, and decreased over time. The occurrence of proliferative changes increased over time and peaked between the second and third week (78%). Fibrosis was noted rarely in the first week (4%) and after 3 weeks it was noted in 61% of patients. Fibrosis occurred more frequent in ARDS of primary pulmonary origin (direct) than that of nonpulmonary origin (indirect).

A somewhat different approach to the pathophysiology of ARDS was proposed by Albert[32] who suggested that ARDS was mainly iatrogenic and not the result of a primary inflammatory process. He proposed that it is a form of ventilation-induced lung injury where the primary problem is atelectasis induced by surfactant abnormalities, and that mechanical ventilation initiates the inflammatory process. If the proposed scenario is correct, at least some instances of ARDS might be prevented by routinely administering a protective strategy of ventilation with sigh breaths, low V_Ts, and positive end-expiratory pressure (PEEP), avoiding supine positioning, increasing the frequency of repositioning, using prone or semi-prone positioning, and limiting the use of sedation.

PULMONARY (DIRECT) VERSUS EXTRAPULMONARY (INDIRECT) ACUTE LUNG INJURY/ACUTE RESPIRATORY DISTRESS SYNDROME

In the initial description of ARDS, Ashbaugh and colleagues[20] observed that different insults appeared to induce a similar injury to the lung; therefore they postulated that a common mechanism of injury must exist. However, careful observation of the clinical progression and histological lung appearance in patients with ARDS suggested that the pattern of lung injury might depend on the etiology. In 1994, the AECC made a distinction between a direct or pulmonary injury (ARDSp), such as might occur following aspiration pneumonia, and contrasted this pattern with indirect or extrapulmonary (ARDSexp) injury associated with a systemic inflammatory response, such as sepsis or acute pancreatitis (Table 38.3).[1]

Data provided by Flori and colleagues[8] suggest that ARDSp constitutes 60% of pediatric ARDS cases, like the reported incidence of ARDSp in adults (47%–75%). The same authors also reported sepsis as the major cause (13%–21%) of ARDSexp in children. Others have reported a higher incidence of sepsis (70%).[2]

The differences between ARDSp and ARDSexp may be most apparent in the acute exudative phase of the disease. ARDSp is characterized by a primary injury to the alveolar epithelium resulting in intra-alveolar edema, and reduced lung compliance with preservation of the chest wall compliance.[33–35] In ARDSexp, the primary insult is systemic and the major injury is to the capillary endothelium; here the edema is predominantly interstitial, and a greater reduction of compliance occurs in the chest wall. That was recently demonstrated in a study conducted in adults where patients with ARDSp had a significantly higher level of a biomarker of lung epithelial injury (surfactant protein D) and significantly lower levels of biomarkers of endothelial injury (angiopoietin-2, von Willebrand Factor) and inflammatory biomarkers (interleukin [IL]-6 and IL-8) than those with ARDSexp.[36] The gross pathology of the lung in ARDSp suggests predominantly consolidation, and in ARDSexp the striking finding is atelectasis. One of the earliest attempts to characterize ARDS based on the mechanism of injury (i.e., direct vs. indirect), was made by Gattinoni and colleagues,[34] who reported differences in respiratory system mechanics. Subsequently, histologic[35] and morphologic[37] evidence supported the distinction between direct and indirect lung injury. These differences may impact the response to treatment and outcome; indeed, a study in children reported that ARDSexp had a greater mortality than ARDSp.[3] Such differences in functional pathology may explain why in ARDSp there is a greater incidence of refractory hypoxemia and resistance to recruitment maneuvers and prone positioning,[38] but a better response to surfactant administration[39] and inhaled nitric oxide (iNO).[40] In the majority of patients, clinical differentiation between ARDSexp and the ARDSp is simple but of uncertain importance, while in other situations it can be more complex (e.g., trauma complicated by sepsis).

Table 38.3 Pulmonary Versus Extrapulmonary Acute Respiratory Distress Syndrome

	Direct (Pulmonary)	Indirect (Extrapulmonary)
Morphology	Consolidation	Atelectasis
Histology	Epithelial injury, alveolar edema	Endothelial injury, interstitial edema
Respiratory mechanics	Reduced lung compliance	Reduced chest wall compliance
RESPONSE TO THERAPY		
Inhaled NO	↑PaO₂	→PaO₂
Prone position	↑PaO₂	→PaO₂
Surfactant	Possible improved outcome	No effect on outcome
Recruitment	→PaO₂	↑PaO₂

NO, Nitric oxide

SEVERITY SCORE

Blood gas analysis, specifically oxygenation, is regarded as the standard for assessment of severity of ARDS. While the P/F ratio provides the threshold value for the definition of ARDS, the (A–a) O_2 difference (difference between "alveolar" vs. arterial PO_2) can express the degree of hypoxemia. Both indices should be used with caution because neither incorporates any measure of the respiratory system mechanics nor the *ventilatory* assistance being provided to the patient. In this regard, the OI = [(mean airway pressure × FiO_2) × 100]/PaO_2 attempts to correct that deficiency. However, even this may mislead if the ventilation strategy employed is not optimized, such as inappropriately high or low airway pressures or FiO_2 in the case of an intrapulmonary shunt, which is minimally responsive to altered FiO_2 or airway pressure.

Although death in ARDS is usually attributable to multi-organ failure[41] rather than persistent hypoxemia, the severity of oxygenation failure, expressed as the OI,[42] or to a lesser extent as the P/F ratio[43] does correlate with the duration of mechanical ventilation and with mortality in children. In contrast to oxygenation, the ventilation index[44]: [$PaCO_2$ × peak airway pressure × respiratory rate]/1000 has been employed to reflect the difficulty involved in clearing CO_2, (i.e., the pulmonary dead space). The magnitude of dead space in the first days of ARDS has been shown to predict outcome in adults[45] and recently in children.[46]

GENETIC MODIFIERS OF ACUTE RESPIRATORY DISTRESS SYNDROME

Other than confirmation that high-pressure, high-volume ventilation is injurious to the lung, the history of ARDS research is replete with interventions that failed to demonstrate clinical benefit.[47] These disappointments often occurred against a background of sound physiologic reasoning and encouraging results from animal studies. It appears that part of the problem has been considering ARDS as a homogeneous disease process. It is already known that only a minority of patients exposed to recognized risk factors develop the ARDS syndrome.

Increasingly, there is recognition that heterogeneity exists in ARDS regarding the development and course of the disease, which is dependent on the interaction of the individual and the inciting event. Consideration of patient-derived factors likely to influence the manifestation of an inflammatory process leads inevitably to scrutiny of the genome. In 2002, Marshall and colleagues[48] were the first investigators to describe a preliminary association between a gene variant and ALI mortality. This group described the increased incidence of a high producer polymorphism of the angiotensin converting enzyme gene in patients with ARDS. Since this report, similar candidate gene studies have revealed a growing number of gene polymorphisms associated with the susceptibility to ALI/ARDS or its clinical course, for example, gene encoding: pulmonary surfactant-associated protein B (SFTPB),[49] IL-6, IL-10, tumor necrosis factor (TNF), angiotensin-converting enzyme,[50] coagulation factor V (F5) and others. It is anticipated that an enhanced knowledge of the role of polymorphisms in ALI/ARDS will permit appropriate grouping of patients for investigation and will facilitate personalized therapy.[51,52]

DIFFERENCES BETWEEN CHILDREN AND ADULTS

Compared to adults, children demonstrate a spectrum of lung and chest wall development as maturation of the lung continues until 8 years of age. Infants and young children have fewer alveoli compared to adults (approximately 20 million alveoli after birth compared to 300 million alveoli by the age of 8 years; the size of each individual alveolus is also smaller in children (150–180 μm vs. 250–300 μm diameter).[53] Together, these two anatomic differences markedly decrease the surface area available for gas exchange. This anatomic variation is prevalent until approximately 8 years of age. The mechanical properties of the lungs of children and infants are also different from those of adults. The infant lung has low inherent elastic recoil, which may protect against lung collapse, so lower PEEP levels may be required to maintain lung recruitment. In contrast, the chest wall of an infant is more compliant, providing less opposition to the natural recoil (deflating tendency). The ribs in infants are more horizontally aligned compared to adults and, in combination with a more compliant chest, it is more difficult to generate negative pressure in the presence of poor lung compliance. Chest wall compliance is inversely related to age, and with pressure preset ventilation, higher chest wall compliance may increase delivered V_T and thereby increase the risk for ventilator-associated lung injury (VALI) in young children.[54] The ratio of lung volume to body weight is greatest in the first 2 years of life, and this suggests that indexing the V_T to body weight may result in a smaller fraction of lung volume being inflated in the young infant compared with the older child. Experimental data indicate that for a given level of inflation, the inflammatory response to either sepsis or high V_T, as well as the propensity to structural injury, might be less in infant versus adult lungs. These physiologic differences are important because adult guidelines for lung protective ventilation are predicated on the behavior of a respiratory system that is very different to that of the infant and young child.

Treatment

Multiple clinical trials for ARDS have been performed in the last three decades, nearly all of them in adults; however, only sporadic trials have shown beneficial effects on mortality. Tonelli and coworkers[47] examined 159 randomized, controlled trials (RCTs) and 26 meta-analyses and found a significant effect on mortality in only two trials for two interventions (low V_T, and prone positioning). Moreover, it was difficult to consistently replicate these results in other trials. This does not mean that clinical strategies do not affect the outcome of the patients, but it emphasizes the difficulties faced in studying ARDS.[52] The two main factors that explain this are the heterogeneity in study populations and the lack of standardization of outcome measures.

CONVENTIONAL MECHANICAL VENTILATION

Since the introduction of new definitions of ARDS and PARDS, no good epidemiological data are available regarding the requirement for invasive mechanical ventilation among children with PARDS. Based on older studies, we estimate that about 30% of patients with PARDS do not require invasive mechanical ventilation at the onset of the disease, However, almost half of the patients eventually require intubation and mechanical ventilation for disease progression, and almost all children with severe PARDS require invasive mechanical ventilation.[8]

Substantial clinical evidence indicates that the injudicious use of mechanical ventilation can initiate or exacerbate lung injury and contribute to the mortality associated with ALI/ARDS. Studies in animal models have demonstrated that mechanical ventilation may induce lung injury through physical disruption of the alveoli (barotrauma); overdistension of the lung (volutrauma); recruitment and derecruitment of collapsed alveoli (atelectrauma); activation of the inflammatory process (biotrauma); and possibly, toxicity from high levels of oxygen.[55] Such factors may produce histologic damage and increased permeability of the alveolar-capillary interface, which is indistinguishable from the lesions seen in other forms of ALI.

The ventilation factors associated with this iatrogenic lung injury are elevated levels of end-inspiratory airway pressure, large tidal volumes, low levels of end-expiratory airway pressure, and possibly high FiO_2. Understanding the roles of elevated levels of inspiratory pressure and V_T from laboratory[56] and clinical[57] studies led to the design of two important outcome studies that compared lower versus higher tidal volumes in patients with ARDS.[58,59] These studies demonstrated a clear association between higher V_T (or inspiratory pressures) and worse outcome. This approach, along with the belief from laboratory and clinical trials[59] that higher levels of PEEP were protective, led to a gradual adoption of the idea that lung protective ventilation, lower tidal volumes, recruitment, and higher levels of PEEP would ensure sufficient gas exchange while minimizing lung injury. Hence, we now employ lower V_T, up to 10 mL/kg; lower inflation pressure (<30 cm H_2O plateau pressure); higher PEEP (~5 to 15 cm H_2O), and lower FiO_2 than two decades ago.[22] It should be noted that the plateau pressure limitations do not consider differences in chest wall compliance between patients. To take this variable into account, one would need to measure the transpulmonary pressure (esophageal pressure). The physiologic goals of mechanical ventilation are not to attempt to achieve normal blood gases values without regard for the V_T, FiO_2, or inflation pressures delivered to the patient. Mechanical ventilation is employed with consideration of a risk/benefit estimation for each patient. If the achievement of normal pH, $PaCO_2$, and PaO_2 levels requires respiratory support strategies that may injure the lungs, then lower pH, PaO_2, and higher $PaCO_2$ (permissive hypercapnia) are tolerated. Despite the lack of data regarding the effect of relative hypoxia on human organ systems in general, and on the developing infant brain, the maintenance of SaO_2 >90% (PaO_2 60–80 mm Hg) using the lowest oxygen concentration necessary to achieve that result is considered by most pediatric intensivists as an optimal approach. Because the likelihood of lung injury is greater if the airway pressure, V_T, and concentration of inspired oxygen are elevated, many clinicians will reduce the target SaO_2 (85%–88%) if necessary. Permissive hypercapnia ($PaCO_2$ 60–80 mm Hg) with a pH >7.2 appears to be well tolerated by most children (although it is avoided in the presence of raised intracranial pressure or

pulmonary hypertension). The "protective" approach has not been validated in children, and the mechanical ventilation strategies used in children mirror the recommendations of the adult critical care community. This approach is physiologically sound, but given the increasingly recognized heterogeneity of ARDS, it is likely that some subtle disease features peculiar to pediatrics have been ignored.

Few studies of mechanical ventilation have been performed in children, and, as a result, no specific approaches have been proven superior to others. Indeed, most approaches for mechanical ventilation in children have been extrapolated from adult studies. Currently there are no data to support the superiority of one mode of ventilation over another (e.g., pressure control vs. volume control). However, advocates of pressure control ventilation argue that it is more physiologic because of the decelerating flow, and that the V_T generated during each breath better reflects dynamic lung characteristics. Interestingly, two surveys reported that clinicians demonstrate a preference for pressure targeted ventilation and pressure regulated volume control (PRVC) ventilation when treating children.[6,60]

OTHER MODALITIES OF VENTILATION

Noninvasive Ventilation

To limit complications associated with endotracheal intubation, noninvasive ventilation (NIV) has been gaining increasing attention in the last few years and it is the focus of several studies.[61] NIV may be administered with positive or negative pressure ventilation and, more recently, through high-flow nasal cannula (HFNC). Since no data are available on the role of negative pressure ventilation in PARDS; we focus here on the use of noninvasive positive pressure ventilation (NIPPV) and HFNC.[62] The role of NIPPV in the pediatric population is not fully characterized and only one RCT in children with acute respiratory failure has been published.[63] In that study of 50 children with acute hypoxemic respiratory failure, NIPPV was compared with standard care. The authors found that the frequency of intubation was significantly lower in the group that received NIPPV (28% vs. 60%). A trial of NIPPV may be attempted in any child with early respiratory failure and mild to moderate PARDS; especially in children with immunodeficiency who are at greater risk of complications from invasive mechanical ventilation. However, one should not persist with its use if there is no clinical benefit within a short time. It appears that patients who are hemodynamically unstable, have a greater severity of illness, or have moderate to severe PARDS are less likely to benefit from NIPPV.[64] Almost any ventilator may be used to provide NIPPV in volume, pressure modes, or a bilevel controlled or continuous positive pressure (CPAP) device can be used. Recently it was reported that the use of neurally adjusted ventilator assist (NAVA) mode[65] resulted in a dramatic reduction in patient-ventilator asynchronies and in trigger delay compared with the pressure control mode of ventilation in infants with severe bronchiolitis. NIPPV may be administered using facial, oronasal or nasal masks. Compared with oronasal masks, nasal masks are better tolerated in younger children. However, nasal interfaces are associated with significant more air leaks and patient-ventilator asynchrony. In contrast, the full facemask is less tolerated and increases the risk of aspiration. In addition, both interfaces do not permit pressures greater than 20 cm H_2O on an ongoing basis.

In the last 5–10 years, HFNC replaced the traditional nasal cannulas for oxygen administration and the "conventional" NIPPV. The old nasal cannulas used flows of 0.5–4 L/min of dry unheated gas. In contrast, HFNC consists of an air–oxygen blender, which delivers heated humidified gas through nasal prongs with flows as high as 60 L/min. It has been proposed as an alternative to CPAP and "conventional" NIPPV.[66,67]

Most of the studies on the use of HFNC in infant and children are small observational studies, which have shown beneficial effects in bronchiolitis.[68,69] Other studies show that the system is well tolerated, safe,[70] and reduces the breathing effort.[71] However, the potential benefit in reducing the rate of intubation in PARDS has not been studied. In a recent RCT trial in adults with acute hypoxemic respiratory failure, treatment with high-flow oxygen, standard oxygen administration, or conventional NIV did not result in significantly different intubation rates.[72]

The mechanism of action of HFNC is not well understood and includes (1) the washout of nasopharyngeal dead space, resulting in increased FiO_2 and reduced carbon dioxide in the dead space; (2) the reduction of inspiratory resistance; and (3) the reduction of the metabolic cost of gas conditioning by providing air with 100% relative humidity and providing an end-expiratory positive pressure.[73]

High-Frequency Oscillatory Ventilation

A variety of high-frequency ventilation devices are available for clinical use; however, high-frequency oscillatory ventilation (HFOV) has achieved the greatest acceptance in neonatal, pediatric, and adult critical care practice. According to several studies, between 5% and 52% of children with acute respiratory failure are ventilated using HFOV at some stage during their disease.[3,6,74] HFOV achieves effective gas exchange while avoiding high peak airway pressures and the inflation–deflation cycles characteristic of conventional ventilation. Lung volume (and hence oxygenation) is maintained by the application of a high continuous mean airway pressure. CO_2 removal is achieved despite small tidal volumes (2–4 mL/kg) by imposing a breath frequency of 300–900 (5–15 Hz) per minute, resulting in large minute volumes. Therefore HFOV involves the application of the open lung strategy accompanied by small swings in pressure and volume in the distal airways and alveoli.[75] Hence, the cyclical application of high distending airway pressures (barotrauma) and the associated cyclical delivery of large tidal volumes (volutrauma) are avoided. In animal models of ALI/ARDS, HFOV has demonstrated comparable or superior gas exchange when compared with conventional ventilation while producing less lung injury.[76] HFOV would appear to represent an optimal lung protective ventilatory device; however, with the progress in protective conventional mechanical ventilation (CMV), it is being deployed only when CMV fails. Although there are no established criteria to define CMV failure, in general HFOV is considered when, despite a plateau pressures of 30–32 cm H_2O and $FiO_2 > 0.6$, there is inadequate oxygenation and/or significant hypercapnia. Two studies comparing HFOV to CMV in children with respiratory failure were published recently. The first study was a secondary analysis of a sedation study, compared the early (24–48 hours) application of HFOV in 181 children to 883 children that received CMV and/or late application of HFOV.[77] The early application of HFOV was associated with a longer duration of mechanical ventilation, but the mortality was similar in the two groups. The second study was a retrospective study that included 1764 patients in 98 hospitals. It showed that early or late application of HFOV was associated with increased mortality (17.3% vs. 8.4%), increased duration of mechanical ventilation, and increased length of stay in the intensive care unit (ICU).[78] The results of these studies are similar to two recently published RCTs in adults, where the early application of HFOV in unselected etiologies of ARDS showed no effect,[79] or an increase in mortality (47% vs. 35%).[80] A different study in adults, in a selected group of patients with severe pulmonary ARDS, hypercapnia, and acidosis, showed a rapid and persistent reduction in CO_2 without adverse effect.[81]

This supports the argument that a trial of a therapeutic intervention in a heterogeneous disease like ARDS should be examined only in selected, well-defined groups of patients.

Airway Pressure Release Ventilation

Airway pressure release ventilation (APRV) is a ventilator modality characterized by cyclical alternation between two levels (high and low) of positive airway pressure, while permitting spontaneous breathing activity at both levels of pressure support. Typically, 80%–95% of the ventilatory cycle is accounted for by the higher pressure (P_{high}, usually 15–30 cm H_2O) and is only briefly interrupted by drops to a lower level of airway pressure (P_{low}, usually 0–15 cm H_2O). The duration of both the P_{high} and P_{low} periods are time cycled and continue even when spontaneous breathing is not detected. In such a case, APRV will resemble inverse (inspiratory: expiratory) ratio pressure-control ventilation with a very long inspiratory time. APRV, facilitates an open lung ventilatory approach, avoids cyclical recruitment and derecruitment of alveolar units, permits homogenous gas distribution during inspiration, minimizes overdistension of healthy lung (volutrauma), and reduces the risk of low-volume lung injury (atelectrauma).[82] There have been few studies of the role of APRV in pediatric and adult ARDS. It has been shown that in children with mild to moderate lung disease, APRV provides good efficacy in ventilation and oxygenation compared with conventional ventilation with significantly lower peak and plateau airway pressures.[47] Despite the potential benefits of APRV, it is not a common modality of ventilation in children. A recent survey of the daily practice of mechanical ventilation among 18 medical centers in Italy reported that less than 4% used APRV.[83]

Neurally Adjusted Ventilatory Assist

Patient-ventilator dyssynchrony is a major issue in the delivery of mechanical ventilation to patients capable of spontaneous breathing. More than 25% of adult ventilated patients exhibit dyssynchrony.[84] Key considerations in patient-ventilator synchrony include signaling of the onset of the patient's inspiratory effort, the pressure/flow profile of gas delivery during the breath, and mechanisms to signal termination of the patient's inspiratory effort. NAVA is a relatively recent innovation to improve such synchrony in invasive[85,86] and, more recently, in noninvasive ventilation.[87] The NAVA system utilizes the electrical activity of the diaphragmatic (right crural) muscle to signal the initiation of patient inspiratory effort. The signal is detected using electrodes embedded in the distal end of a gastric tube that is positioned astride the esophageal hiatus of the diaphragm. Because muscle electrical activity is proportional to the strength of the phrenic signal (which itself reflects the respiratory demands of the patient), the NAVA system offers both improved triggering and variable ventilatory support proportionate to the patient's respiratory demands. This is an improvement over circuit pressure or gas flow triggering systems and the use of a fixed amount of ventilatory support with each breath. There are only few reports of NAVA use in either adults or children.[86,88] It has been demonstrated that NAVA prevents excessive lung distension, efficiently unloads respiratory muscles, and improves, but does not completely abolish, patient-ventilator dyssynchrony. The penetration of this modality of ventilation in pediatric critical care units is unknown; however, we speculate that it is very low, as most surveys do not mention it.[6]

ADJUVANTS TO MECHANICAL VENTILATION

Prone positioning, surfactant, and nitric oxide administration have all been employed as adjuvant therapies in ventilated patients with ALI/ARDS. To date, none of these interventions has demonstrated an ability to improve patient outcome except for prone positioning in adults when employed as a routine part of care.[47]

Corticosteroids

The use of corticosteroids for the treatment of ARDS was suggested by Ashbaugh in 1967.[20] Almost 50 years and several clinical trials later, it is still the subject of debate.[89,90] ARDS is characterized by inflammation that may resolve within a short period; alternatively, it may progress to the unresolving inflammatory (i.e., fibroproliferative) stage. The antiinflammatory properties of corticosteroids and the potential inhibition of both fibroblast proliferation and collagen deposition make corticosteroids an attractive option.

The use of corticosteroids has been examined (in adult patients) in different disease stages, including prophylactically (before development of ALI/ARDS),[91] during the early stages of disease (<7 days),[92] and in later stages of the disease (>7 or 14 days).[93] Corticosteroids have been used for different durations and at different doses. Early studies focused on the prevention of ARDS after events that are known to potentially lead to ARDS (e.g., sepsis). High doses (≥30 mg/kg/day) of corticosteroids for a short period of time (≤24 hours) either had no impact on mortality[91] or, in one case, increased mortality.[94] A relatively recent study of early low-dose corticosteroids (1 mg/kg/day) for 25 days demonstrated a treatment benefit with improvements in lung injury score, days of ventilation, and mortality.[92] However, methodological issues provoked significant controversy. Several studies that examined the role of corticosteroids late in the course of the disease (>7 days) reported contradictory results,[93,95] and there is some evidence that steroids introduced after 2 weeks of illness may result in increased mortality.[95] An examination of adult patients with sepsis-induced ARDS who were nonresponders to adrenocorticotropic hormone (ACTH) stimulation testing demonstrated improved lung function

and decreased mortality with low-dose steroid use in early disease. This study underscores the importance of selecting groups likely to benefit from steroids when studying their potential use in ARDS.[96] A recent analysis of patient data from four randomized trials demonstrated that early and prolonged glucocorticoid treatment accelerated resolution of ARDS and decreased mortality without increasing the risk of infection.[97] In children, only a few case series are available. Recently, it was reported in an observational single study that corticosteroid exposure (>24 h) in children with PARDS is associated with fewer ventilation-free days after adjustment for key potential confounders, including severity of illness, OI, immunocompromised status, and number of organ failures.[98]

In summary, current evidence from clinical trials does not support the use of corticosteroids in any phase of ARDS in adults. Further investigations are required to address the paucity of data in children and to specifically identify potential responders among the population of ARDS patients.

Clinicians should remain vigilant for steroid-responsive diseases, such as acute eosinophilic pneumonia, hypersensitivity pneumonitis, diffuse alveolar hemorrhage from vasculitis, nonspecific interstitial pneumonitis and others, which may present as PARDS.

Prone Positioning

Prone positioning is safe and has been reported to produce a rapid and sustained improvement in arterial oxygenation in 90% of children with PARDS.[99] This response rate was superior to that reported in adults (60%). However, the improvement in oxygenation did not translate into a reduction in days of ventilation or patient mortality in children. Prone positioning is best reserved for patients with persistent refractory hypoxemia when acceptable oxygenation cannot be achieved within the parameters of a lung protective ventilatory strategy. However, where it does not improve oxygenation, it should be discontinued. A multicenter comprehensive study reported that 17.6% of children with ALI/ARDS receive prone positioning as part of their management at some time during their disease.[6]

Inhaled Nitric Oxide

Nitric oxide is a potent short-acting selective pulmonary vasodilator. It has been shown to result in short-term improvements in oxygenation in some patients with ARDS/ALI, but it has no substantial impact on the duration of ventilator support or mortality when used as a routine part of care. Currently, only a minority (12%) of children with ALI receive iNO during the disease.[6] The routine use of iNO is not recommended, but it may be considered in a selected group of patients with pulmonary hypertension or significant right ventricular dysfunction.[22] In addition, it may be considered for patients with refractory hypoxemia, with FiO_2 >0.6, and in whom a trial of iNO demonstrated benefit. Where inhaled iNO is being used, some recommend that a daily trial be conducted to ensure that the minimal effective dose is being used, because it has been shown that the iNO dose can be reduced during the course of the disease.[100]

A recent RCT in adults with moderate to severe ARDS demonstrated significantly better pulmonary function tests 6 months after treatment among adult patients treated with a low dose of iNO (5 PPM) compared to similar patients who received placebo.[101] The potential long-term protective role of iNO in patients with ARDS or PARDS should be explored.

Surfactant

The potential role of surfactant dysfunction in the pathogenesis of ARDS was suggested by Ashbaugh.[1] The concept of surfactant administration to patients with ARDS is very attractive, especially when seen in the context of its benefits in infant respiratory distress. However, at this stage, routine surfactant administration is not recommended. Comparison of results among studies is complicated by the differences in surfactant preparations and delivery methods. Walmrath and colleagues[102] reported improvement in oxygenation when a high dose of bovine surfactant was administered to patients with ARDS and sepsis. Spragg and colleagues[103] reported transient improvement in oxygenation when recombinant surfactant was administered to adult patients with ARDS in a phase III trial; in a post hoc analysis, they also reported a potential improvement in mortality in ARDSp but not in "extrapulmonary" ARDSexp. In children, a relatively small RCT reported a reduction in mortality (19% in the surfactant vs. 36% in the placebo group) following administration of natural calf surfactant[104]; however, there was an unequal distribution of immunocompromised patients among the groups, and controlling for immunocompromised state in multifactorial analysis rendered no difference in mortality between the two treatment groups. Furthermore, there was no effect on ventilator-free days or length of hospitalization. In summary, the routine administration of surfactant in children with PARDS is not recommended. Whether the lack of effect on outcome is a matter of surfactant preparation, patient selection, or method of administration is unclear. However, the transient improvement in oxygenation associated with surfactant administration is tempting, and a survey from 59 centers indicated that more than 50% of intensivists administer surfactant to selected patients with PARDS.[6]

Neuromuscular Blocking Agents

In contrast to paralyzed patients, where it has been shown that most of the tidal breath is delivered directly to the nondependent regions,[105] during spontaneous ventilation, tidal breathing is directed to the dependent better perfused regions,[106] thus reducing dead space and shunt. Therefore until recently, maintaining spontaneous breathing has been recommended in ventilated patients with ARDS. A relatively recent RCT in adults with severe ARDS reported that continuous neuromuscular blockade (NMB; with cisatracurium besylate) during the first 48 hours of ventilation in severe ARDS significantly reduced mortality.[107] Mortality at 90 days in the NMB group was 32% compared with 41% in the controls. This followed earlier mechanistic studies demonstrating that administration of NMB for the first 48 hours of ventilation improved oxygenation and lowered inflammatory markers (IL-8 and IL-6) in the lung bronchoalveolar lavage [BAL]) and serum of patients with ALI/ARDS.[108]

The mechanism of benefit from NMB is speculative. Paralysis of ventilated patients may facilitate protective ventilation through optimization of patient/ventilator synchronization through more accurate adjustment of V_T, or by reduction in inspiratory plateau pressure (because of the reduction in chest wall compliance). Moreover, the use of NMB may reduce the oxygen consumption, which, in turn, will reduce cardiac output and lung perfusion, and may reduce lung injury.

A recent study in 23 children with respiratory failure reported that short-term NMB resulted in a significantly improved OI in all patients while the distribution of V_T and regional lung filling characteristics were unaffected.[109] No data are available regarding the prevalence of use of neuromuscular blocking agents among children. Until more pediatric data are available, the use of NMB should be reserved for patients in whom sedation alone is inadequate to achieve effective mechanical ventilation.

Beta-Adrenergic Agonists

Alveolar edema in ALI/ARDS is mainly due to increased permeability and, to a lesser extent, to increased capillary hydrostatic pressure. The resolution of alveolar edema is critical to recovery from lung injury. β_2 agonists may reduce alveolar edema by several mechanisms. Alveolar fluid clearance is enhanced through upregulation of Na^+ transport in the alveolar epithelial cells by β_2 agonists. In addition, pulmonary vasodilatation and the resulting reduction of pulmonary vascular pressure results in lowered capillary hydrostatic pressures, and β_2 agonists may independently decrease endothelial permeability.

An RCT in a small number (40) of adult patients[110] demonstrated that intravenous (IV) salbutamol (albuterol) reduced the extravascular lung water content and, perhaps as a result, lessened the inspiratory airway pressures required for ventilation. An observational review of children with ARDS suggested that inhaled bronchodilators were associated with a lower mortality.[8] Whether inhaled or IV treatment may affect outcome in patients with ARDS is still to be established in an RCT. However, the current evidence discourages the use of β_2 agonists in ALI/ARDS patients.[111]

Extracorporeal Life Support in Pediatric Acute Respiratory Distress Syndrome

Although pediatric extracorporeal life support (ECLS) is predominantly employed for cardiovascular support,[69] it may have an important role in some pulmonary cases, especially where ARDS results from trauma. For pure respiratory failure in the absence of cardiovascular compromise, venovenous cannulation is appropriate. This provides oxygenated blood into the right ventricle, but does not augment cardiac output. In contrast, venoarterial cannulation, providing oxygenated blood into the aorta under pressure, effectively augments the cardiac output while concomitantly increasing systemic oxygenation.

The survival rate (60%) for ECLS in ARDS has not substantially changed in the last 15 years,[112] in contrast to the improved outcomes associated with conventional management. Because of the improvement in outcomes associated with conventional ventilation, and because ECLS is used only when conventional ventilation has "failed," the efficacy of ECLS may be progressively underestimated because of "referral bias" of progressively more futile cases. Currently, there are no nationally agreed criteria for ECLS in PARDS, and its use is mainly decided by the center. The two potential major criteria for severity of PARDS and ECLS criteria are OI and the P/F ratio. The consensus at this stage is that ECLS may be considered in severe PARDS with persistent inadequate gas exchange (mainly hypoxia), and where the cause of respiratory failure is potentially reversible.

Tracheostomy

Ventilation via a tracheostomy tube has many purported benefits in facilitating weaning from mechanical ventilation: it improves patient comfort, reduces the work of breathing, facilitates bronchopulmonary toilet, reduces the incidence of pneumonia, and improves airway security. In addition, it may reduce the length of stay in the hospital or ICU, and reduce hospital costs, but most importantly, a tracheostomy facilitates patient weaning from mechanical ventilation and lowers patient mortality.[113] For these reasons, tracheostomy has become almost routine in adult critical care, with around 8%–25% of all ventilated adult patients undergoing the procedure during their stay.[114] Considering tracheostomy in an adult patient who is expected to require prolonged ventilation (>14 days) is recommended.[115] In contrast, there is no literature describing the preemptive use of tracheostomy in children in whom prolonged ventilation is anticipated. The prevalence of tracheostomy among children requiring prolonged mechanical ventilation was reported in a limited number of studies and varied from less than 1.5%–2%.[116–118] The differences in prevalence between adult and children may be explained by the faster resolution of ARDS in children compared with adults, as well as the introduction of a percutaneous dilatational tracheostomy technique, which is performed at the bedside in adults.[119] However, this technique is not suitable for children younger than 12 years of age, and tracheostomy is perceived as an aggressive procedure with high complication rates in children. A recently published study revealed a significant risk for morbidity and mortality among children under the age of 2 years undergoing tracheostomy.[120]

Summary/Conclusion

ARDS is a form of acute respiratory failure characterized by a diffuse and progressive inflammatory lung disease. It is caused by a variety of heterogeneous pulmonary or extrapulmonary insults to the lungs that provoke a cascade of inflammatory reactions leading to an increase in the permeability of the alveolar-capillary barrier, which, in turn, leads to alveolar edema and surfactant deactivation. ARDS presents with pulmonary infiltrates on chest radiographs, moderate to severe hypoxemia, ventilation abnormality, reduction in the respiratory system compliance (chest wall, lungs or both) and increased work of breathing in the absence of evidence for cardiogenic pulmonary edema. The diagnostic criteria have evolved from the older European and American consensus definition to the novel Berlin definition,[21] which is exclusively based on clinical criteria with some minor changes in children (PARDS).[22] There is no specific treatment for ARDS except for symptomatic support and treatment of the underline causes (e.g., sepsis, pneumonia). Mechanical ventilation, invasive or noninvasive, is provided to reduce the work of breathing until resolution of the disease has occurred. With the improvements in mechanical ventilation and lung protection that have been developed in the last two decades, the outcome has improved and is generally good with a mortality rate of 7%–35%, unless the patient has underlying chronic lung disease or is immunocompromised. The goals of mechanical ventilation are not to attempt to achieve normal blood gases values without regard to the V_T, FiO_2, or inflation pressures delivered to the patient, but it is employed with regard to a risk/benefit estimation performed for each patient.

References

Access the reference list online at ExpertConsult.com.

Suggested Reading

Ashbaugh DG, Bigelow DB, Petty TL, et al. Acute respiratory distress in adults. *Lancet*. 1967;2:319–323.

De Luca D, Piastra M, Chidini G, et al. The use of the Berlin definition for acute respiratory distress syndrome during infancy and early childhood: multicenter evaluation and expert consensus. *Intensive Care Med*. 2013;39:2083–2091.

Gattinoni L, Pesenti A. The concept of "baby lung". *Intensive Care Med*. 2005;31:776–784.

Jouvet P, Thomas NJ, Wilson DF, et al. Pediatric acute respiratory distress syndrome: consensus recommendations from the Pediatric Acute Lung Injury Consensus Conference. *Pediatr Crit Care Med*. 2015;16:428–439.

Ranieri VM, Rubenfeld GD, Thompson BT, et al. Acute respiratory distress syndrome: the Berlin definition. *JAMA*. 2012;307:2526–2533.

Zimmerman JJ, Akhtar SR, Caldwell E, et al. Incidence and outcomes of pediatric acute lung injury. *Pediatrics*. 2009;124:87–95.

39 Pulmonary Disease Associated With Congenital Heart Disease

WILSON KING, MD, and KENNETH O. SCHOWENGERDT, JR., MD

Introduction

Both acute and chronic pulmonary disease may be present in the setting of various forms of congenital heart disease. Postoperative atelectasis, pulmonary edema, or pleural effusions are commonly seen after cardiac surgery, particularly when cardiopulmonary bypass is required. Atelectasis with resultant ventilation-perfusion mismatch, pulmonary edema, and pulmonary hypertension (not specifically in association with congenital heart disease) are discussed elsewhere within the text, and this chapter will focus on more specific pulmonary conditions that may be encountered in association with congenital heart disease.

Airway Compression Due to Vascular Rings and Slings

BACKGROUND

Pulmonary vascular rings are congenital vascular conditions in which the trachea and esophagus are encircled by vascular structures, as first reported and surgically repaired by Dr. Robert Gross in 1945.[1] Vascular rings are considered rare and thought to represent only approximately 1% of all congenital heart conditions.

Vascular rings develop secondary to abnormalities of embryological vascular development as described below.[2] During normal fetal development, the aortic sac gives rise to six paired vascular branchial arches that connect to the right and left dorsal aortae (Fig. 39.1).[3] The dorsal aortae give rise to intersegmental arteries at each segmental level that connect to the vertebral arteries. Part of the aortic sac becomes the ascending aorta, and the distal portions of the right and left dorsal aorta fuse to become the descending aorta. The proximal left-sided dorsal aorta remains patent and becomes the proximal descending aorta, and the proximal right-sided dorsal aorta regresses. The third, fourth, and sixth branchial arches contribute primarily to the development of the aortic arch and proximal head and neck vessels. The third branchial arches become the common carotid arteries. The right fourth branchial arch becomes the proximal right subclavian artery, and the left fourth branchial arch becomes the transverse aortic arch. The seventh right intersegmental artery becomes the distal right subclavian artery, and the seventh left intersegmental artery becomes the left subclavian artery. The proximal right sixth branchial arch becomes the right pulmonary artery, and the distal right sixth branchial arch regresses. The proximal left sixth branchial arch becomes the left pulmonary artery, and the distal left

sixth branchial arch becomes the patent ductus arteriosus that eventually becomes the ligamentum arteriosum upon closure.

The most common type of vascular ring is the double aortic arch (Figs. 39.2 and 39.3). The ascending aorta gives rise to left-sided and right-sided aortic arches with symmetrical takeoff of carotid and subclavian arteries before connecting with the proximal descending aorta. This occurs if the right-sided dorsal aorta and right fourth branchial arch, which normally regress, persist. The normal left-sided dorsal aorta and left fourth branchial arch also persist. In this situation, the trachea and esophagus are completely encircled by left and right aortic arches.

The second most common type of vascular ring is when there is a right aortic arch in association with an aberrant left subclavian artery (Figs. 39.4 and 39.5). The head and neck vessel branching order is as follows: left carotid artery, right carotid artery, right subclavian artery, and aberrant left subclavian artery that takes a retroesophageal course. This occurs when the right-sided dorsal aorta and right fourth branchial arch persist, the left-sided dorsal aorta and left fourth branchial arch regress, but the left dorsal aorta remains patent. The trachea and esophagus are completely encircled by the right aortic arch and left ligamentum arteriosum which spans the proximal left pulmonary artery and the distal transverse aortic arch near the insertion of the left subclavian artery. Dilation of the proximal left subclavian artery or Kommerell diverticulum is often seen in the setting of a right aortic arch with an aberrant left subclavian artery. This can also cause tracheal and esophageal compression. In addition to double aortic arch and right aortic arch with aberrant left subclavian artery, there are additional complete vascular and incomplete vascular rings such as circumflex aorta, persistent fifth aortic arch, and cervical aortic arch. However, these are less common.

Although not a true vascular ring, a pulmonary artery sling is a condition when the left pulmonary artery connects directly to the right pulmonary artery instead of connecting to the pulmonary trunk (Figs. 39.6 and 39.7). The left pulmonary artery then courses posterior to the trachea and anterior to the esophagus causing tracheal compression. Pulmonary slings can be associated with primary tracheal stenosis with extended segments of complete tracheal rings.[4,5]

Tetralogy of Fallot with absent pulmonary valve is a particular variation of this condition that can be associated with significant respiratory compromise (Fig. 39.8). In addition to presence of a ventricular septal defect, overriding aorta, pulmonary stenosis, and right ventricular hypertrophy, a thick ring of tissue at the pulmonary valve annulus in place of a pulmonary valve results in significant pulmonary

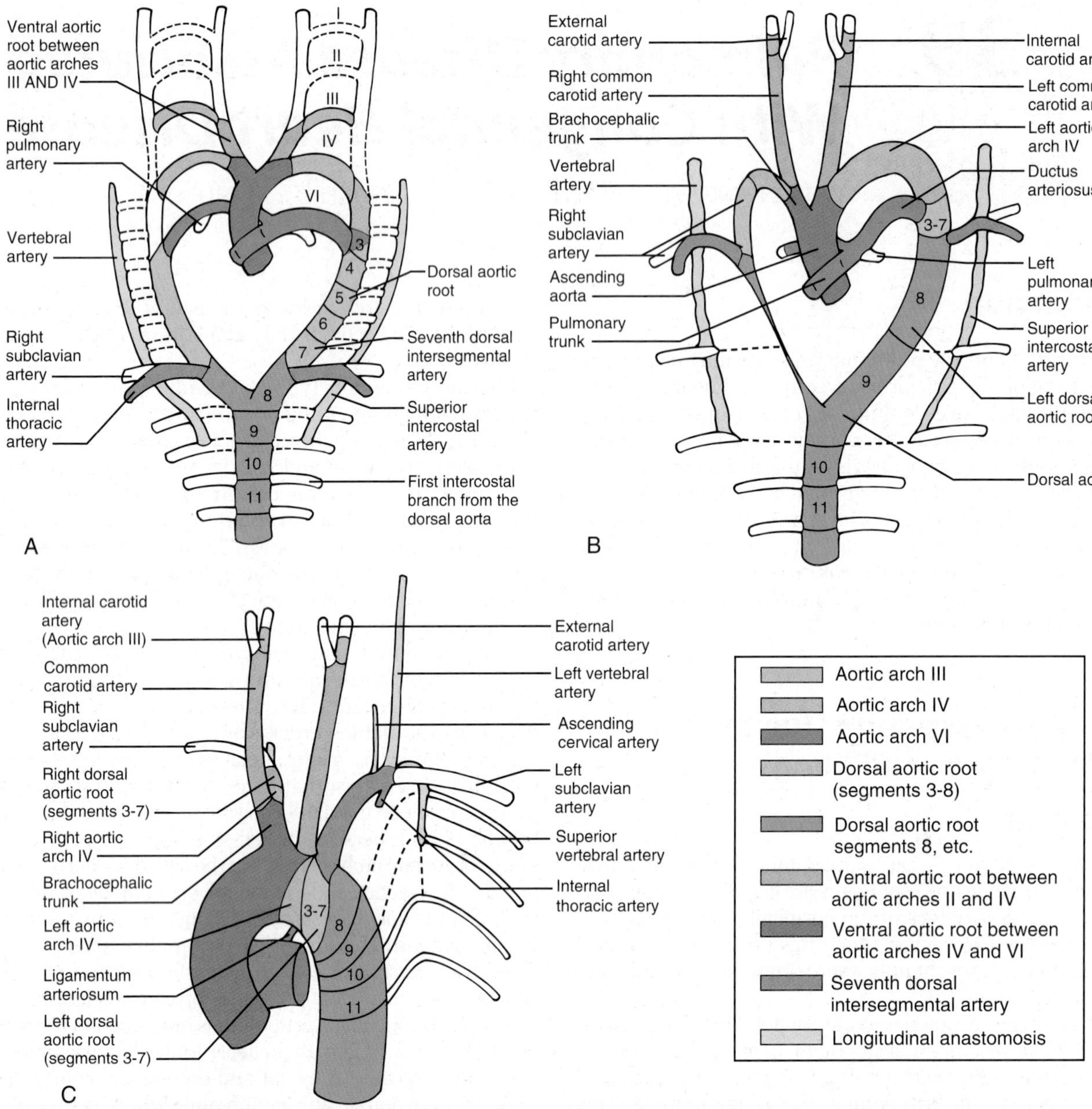

A

Ventral aortic root between aortic arches III AND IV

Right pulmonary artery

Vertebral artery

Right subclavian artery

Internal thoracic artery

I
II
III
IV
VI

3
4
5
6
7
8
9
10
11

Dorsal aortic root

Seventh dorsal intersegmental artery

Superior intercostal artery

First intercostal branch from the dorsal aorta

B

External carotid artery

Right common carotid artery

Brachiocephalic trunk

Vertebral artery

Right subclavian artery

Ascending aorta

Pulmonary trunk

Internal carotid artery

Left common carotid artery

Left aortic arch IV

Ductus arteriosus

3-7

Left pulmonary artery

8

9

10

11

Superior intercostal artery

Left dorsal aortic root

Dorsal aorta

C

Internal carotid artery (Aortic arch III)

Common carotid artery

Right subclavian artery

Right dorsal aortic root (segments 3-7)

Right aortic arch IV

Brachiocephalic trunk

Left aortic arch IV

Ligamentum arteriosum

Left dorsal aortic root (segments 3-7)

External carotid artery

Left vertebral artery

Ascending cervical artery

Left subclavian artery

Superior vertebral artery

Internal thoracic artery

3-7
8
9
10
11

Legend:
- Aortic arch III
- Aortic arch IV
- Aortic arch VI
- Dorsal aortic root (segments 3-8)
- Dorsal aortic root segments 8, etc.
- Ventral aortic root between aortic arches II and IV
- Ventral aortic root between aortic arches IV and VI
- Seventh dorsal intersegmental artery
- Longitudinal anastomosis

Fig. 39.1 Aortic arch arteries and their derivatives (Gray's anatomy) http://clinicalgate.com/development-of-the-head-and-neck/ (Gray's Anatomy: The Anatomical Basis of Clinical Practice, Expert Consult—Online and Print, 40th ed. Chapter 35.)

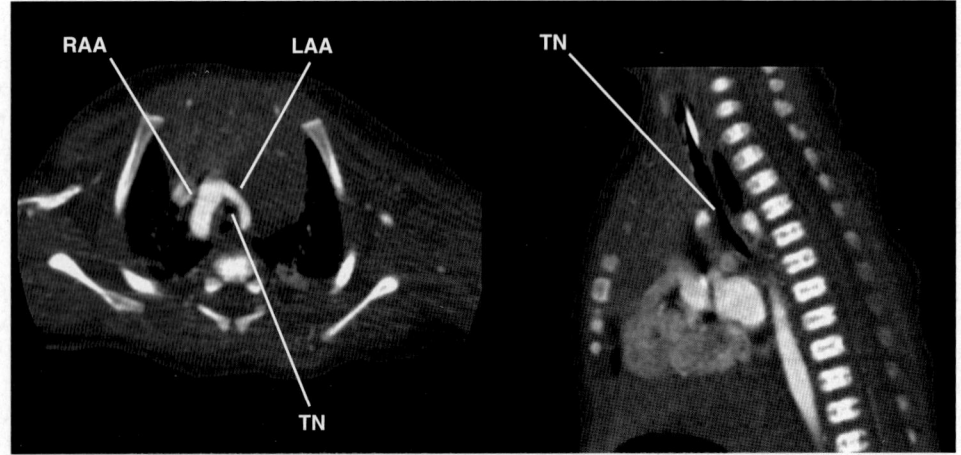

Fig. 39.2 Double aortic arch with axial and coronal oblique planes from computed tomography angiography. Note right dominant aortic arch and discrete tracheal narrowing at the level of the vascular ring. *LAA*, Left aortic arch; *RAA*, right aortic arch; *TN*, tracheal narrowing.

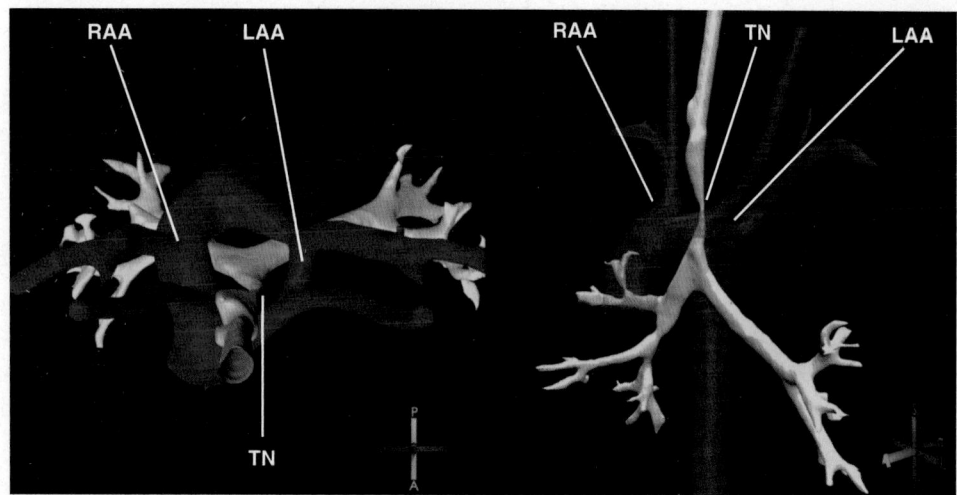

Fig. 39.3 Double aortic arch reconstruction from axial and sagittal oblique projections. Note discrete tracheal stenosis adjacent to the right dominant arch. *LAA,* Left aortic arch; *RAA,* right aortic arch; *TN,* tracheal narrowing.

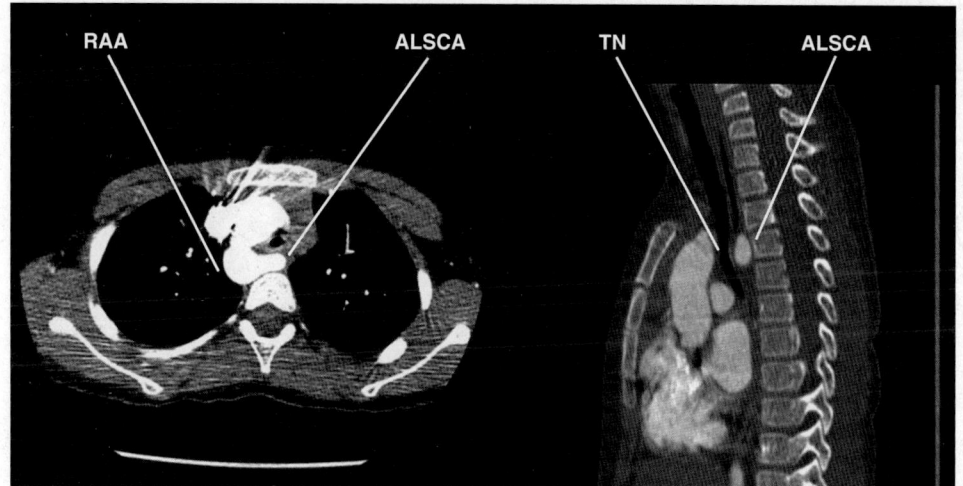

Fig. 39.4 Right aortic arch with retroesophageal aberrant left subclavian artery with axial and sagittal planes from computed tomography angiography. Note tracheal narrowing adjacent to proximal aberrant subclavian artery. *ALSCA,* Aberrant left subclavian artery; *RAA,* right aortic arch; *TN,* tracheal narrowing.

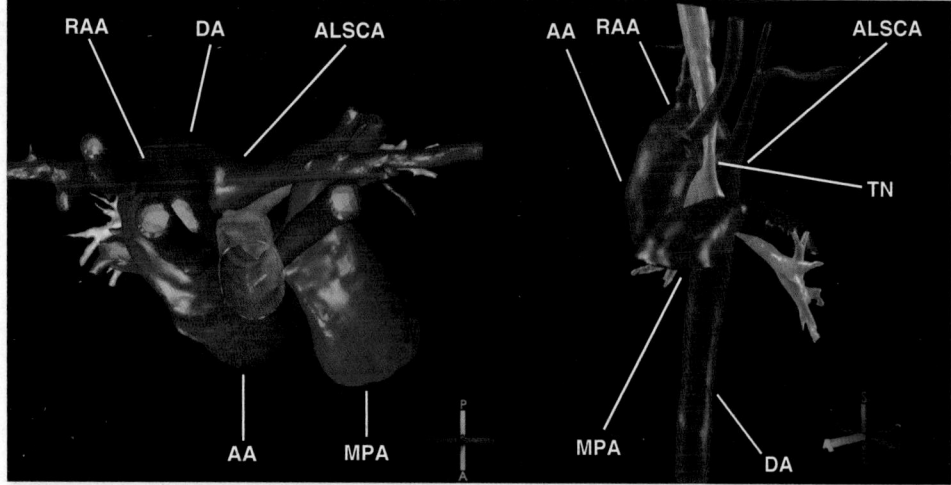

Fig. 39.5 Right aortic arch with aberrant left subclavian artery reconstruction with axial and sagittal oblique projections from computed tomography angiography. The ligamentum arteriosum connects the main pulmonary artery to the aorta at the takeoff of the aberrant left subclavian artery. *AA,* Ascending aorta; *ALSCA,* aberrant left subclavian artery; *DA,* descending aorta; *MPA,* main pulmonary artery; *RAA,* right transverse aortic arch; *TN,* tracheal narrowing.

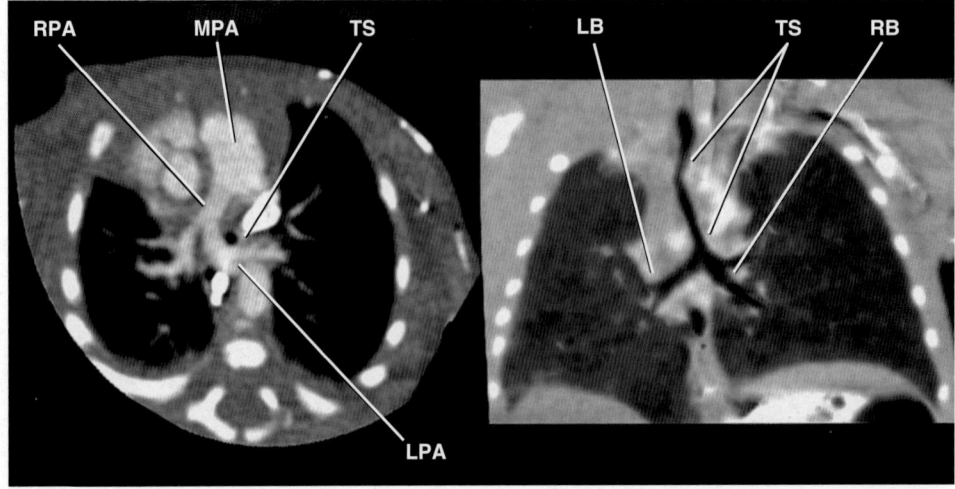

Fig. 39.6 Pulmonary sling in a neonate with axial oblique and coronal oblique planes from computed tomography angiography. Note that the right pulmonary artery gives rise to the left pulmonary artery, the long segment tracheal stenosis, cardiac dextroposition, and thoracic situs inversus. *LB,* Left bronchus; *LPA,* left pulmonary artery; *MPA,* main pulmonary artery; *RB,* right bronchus; *RPA,* right pulmonary artery; *TS,* long segment tracheal stenosis.

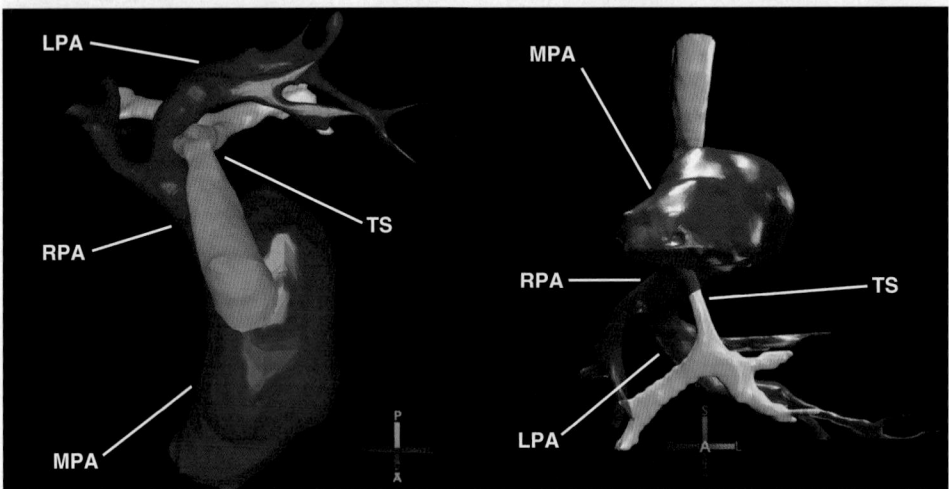

Fig. 39.7 Pulmonary sling reconstruction from a axial and coronal oblique projections. Note that the left pulmonary artery courses posterior to the trachea. *LPA,* Left pulmonary artery, *MPA,* main pulmonary artery, *RPA,* right pulmonary artery, *TS,* long segment tracheal stenosis.

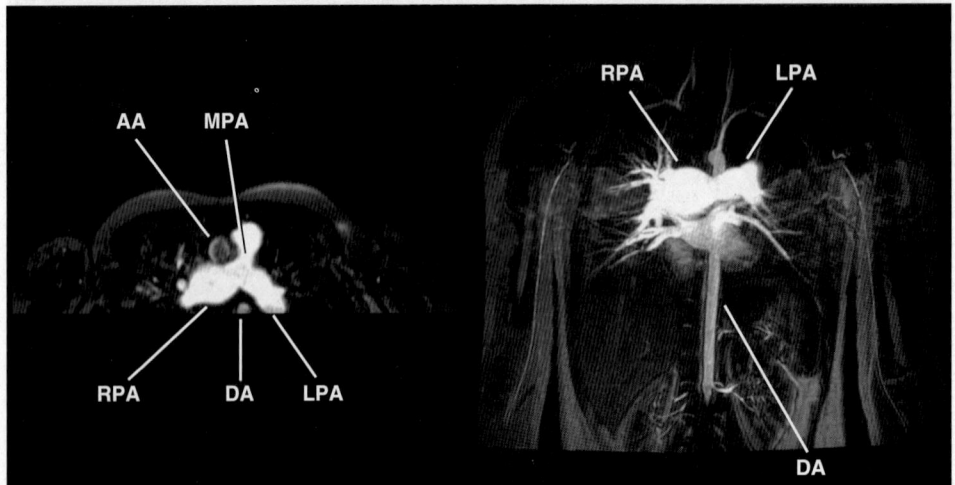

Fig. 39.8 Tetralogy of Fallot absent pulmonary valve syndrome from magnetic resonance angiography from an axial reformat and coronal reformat with maximal intensity projection showing extremely dilated left and right pulmonary arteries in contrast to normal-sized ascending aorta and descending aorta. *AA,* Ascending aorta, *DA,* descending aorta, *LPA,* left pulmonary artery, *MPA,* main pulmonary artery, *RPA,* right pulmonary artery.

stenosis and regurgitation.[6,7] Massive dilation of the main and branch pulmonary arteries can result in significant compression of the trachea and bronchi.

CLINICAL PRESENTATION

Pulmonary vascular rings typically present with respiratory or gastrointestinal symptoms.[4,9] Respiratory signs and symptoms may include noisy breathing, barking cough, wheezing, frequent upper respiratory infections, apneic episodes, or intermittent cyanosis. Gastrointestinal symptoms typically do not present until patients begin eating solid foods. The symptoms may include a sensation of food being stuck in the throat, slow eating, or hyperextension during feedings. Typically, patients with double aortic arches tend to present earlier in life with more profound symptoms than patients with right aortic arch and an aberrant left subclavian artery. Backer et al. reported a series of patients with double aortic arch typically presenting before one month of age and those with right aortic arch and aberrant left subclavian artery generally between 1 and 6 months of age.[4] Patients having a pulmonary artery sling may also have associated "ring-sling" complex in which the trachea is not only compressed by the posterior left pulmonary artery, but the presence of complete tracheal rings that also create further narrowing of the airway. The ring-sling complex is associated with significant respiratory symptoms with high morbidity and mortality. Patients with tetralogy of Fallot with absent pulmonary valve syndrome present with significant respiratory distress during the neonatal period in slightly less than half of all cases. They are often cyanotic initially, although this seems to improve with time.

DIAGNOSIS

Chest x-ray can often suggest the diagnosis of a vascular ring from the position of the aortic knob, apparent tracheal narrowing, and/or unilateral hyperinflation of the lung. Barium swallow has also been used to diagnose vascular rings based on patterns of esophageal compression. Echocardiography may be used to diagnose a vascular ring by delineating the course of the aorta and proximal and neck vessels. A secondary imaging modality is usually required since the airway cannot be evaluated by ultrasound. Echocardiography is nonetheless recommended in patients diagnosed with vascular rings as many have associated congenital heart abnormalities.

In the current era, pulmonary vascular rings are now typically evaluated by tomographic imaging, either computed tomography (CT) with contrast or magnetic resonance imaging (MRI) with or without contrast. Computed tomography allows the airway and vascular anatomy to be evaluated rapidly, oftentimes without the need for sedation. MRI provides excellent evaluation of the blood vessels with the advantage of avoiding ionizing radiation. The airway can be evaluated using spin echo techniques. However, longer acquisition times often require sedation in younger patients.

Bronchoscopy is an important technique in evaluating some patients with vascular rings. Direct observation of the airway can be very useful in determining the both the degree and mechanism of airway obstruction.

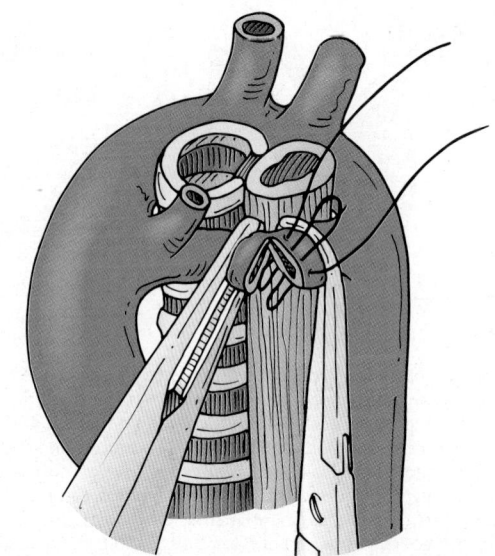

Fig. 39.9. Surgical division of a double aortic arch. (From Backer CL, Mavroudis C. Vascular rings and pulmonary artery sling. In: Mavroudis C, Backer CL, eds: *Pediatric Cardiac Surgery*, 4th ed, Oxford. UK: Blackwell Publishing; 2013:234-255).

TREATMENT

Patients with a vascular ring who are symptomatic are treated surgically. In the case of double aortic arch, the vascular ring is typically relieved by resection of the smaller non-dominant arch, often through a thoracotomy (Fig. 39.9). Patients with a right aortic arch and aberrant left subclavian artery are treated by division of the associated ligamentum arteriosum. Patients with a right aortic arch and aberrant left subclavian artery may have dilation of the proximal left subclavian artery, which is called a Kommerell's diverticulum. The Kommerell's diverticulum can cause direct compression of the airway or the esophagus. Resection of the Kommerell's diverticulum and reimplantation of the left subclavian artery may be required (Fig. 39.10).[10] Pulmonary vascular slings often require translocating the anomalous left pulmonary artery coming from the right pulmonary artery onto the main pulmonary artery. If complete tracheal rings are also seen in the presence of the pulmonary vascular sling, a slide tracheoplasty may be required (Fig. 39.11).[4,11] Patients with tetralogy of Fallot with absent pulmonary valve syndrome who develop respiratory distress during the neonatal period may benefit from prone positioning and often require mechanical ventilation.[8] Airway compression can be addressed surgically. Standard strategies include reducing the size of the pulmonary arteries and repositioning the pulmonary arteries anteriorly (LeCompte maneuver). There is not currently a consensus as to the best approach.[12–16]

Pulmonary Hypertension and Postoperative Pulmonary Hypertensive Crisis

BACKGROUND

Pulmonary hypertension occurring during the postoperative period for congenital heart surgery is a serious condition

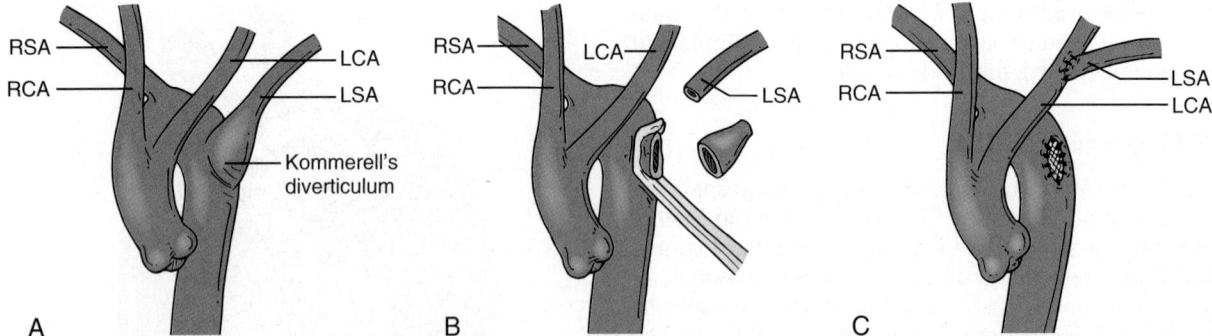

Fig. 39.10 (A) Anatomy of a patient with a right aortic arch, retroesophageal left subclavian artery, and a large Kommerell diverticulum. The Kommerell diverticulum is an embryologic remnant of the left fourth aortic arch. (B) Resection of a Kommerell diverticulum through a left thoracotomy. There is a vascular clamp partially occluding the descending thoracic aorta at the origin of the Kommerell diverticulum. The Kommerell diverticulum has been completely resected. The clamp on the distal left subclavian artery is not illustrated. (C) The completed repair. The orifice where the Kommerell diverticulum was resected is usually closed primarily. The left subclavian artery has been implanted into the side of the left common carotid artery with fine running polypropylene suture. *LCA,* Left common carotid artery; *LSA,* left subclavian artery; *RCA,* right coronary artery; *RSA,* retroesophageal left subclavian artery (From Backer CL, Hillman N, Mavroudis C, Holinger LD. Resection of Kommerell's diverticulum and left subclavian artery transfer for recurrent symptoms after vascular ring division. *Eur J Cardiothorac Surg.* 2002;22(1):64-69.)

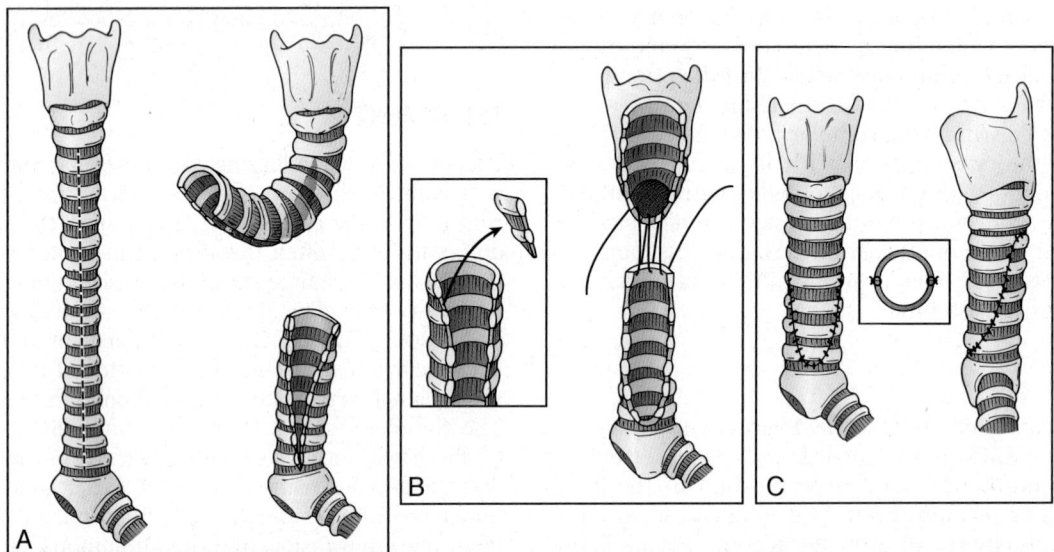

Fig. 39.11 Slide tracheoplasty in a patient with an absent right lung. (A) The patient has been placed on cardiopulmonary bypass with mild hypothermia to 32°C. The trachea is transected in the mid-portion of the tracheal stenosis. This site is determined either by external examination or by internal bronchoscopic findings. The inferior portion of the trachea is incised anteriorly, and the superior portion of the trachea is incised posteriorly. (B) The ends of the trachea are beveled as shown in the small inset. The anastomosis is performed with running 6–0 polydioxanone suture. The suture line is started superiorly (parachute technique) and finished inferiorly just above the carina. (C) Completed slide tracheoplasty. The everting running suture line helps to avoid the "figure of 8" configuration problem after the completed repair. (Reproduced with permission from Backer CL, Popescu AR, Rastatter JC, Russell HM. Vascular rings and slings. In: daCruz E, Ivy DD, Jaggers J, eds. *Pediatric and Congenital Cardiology, Cardiac Surgery and Intensive Care,* vol. 4, London: Springer-Verlag; 2014:2219-2238.)

resulting in significant morbidity and mortality.[17] Mortality related to postoperative pulmonary hypertension was reported to be as high as 20% during prior eras.[18] With a better understanding of the risk factors related to pulmonary hypertensive crises, surgical repair of congenital heart defects at younger ages, and the development of more effective treatments, the incidence of this condition has decreased significantly, with the current incidence estimated to be 2%–7%.[18]

RISK FACTORS

Patients undergoing surgical repair of certain types of congenital heart disease are at higher risk of developing postoperative pulmonary hypertension. These include total anomalous pulmonary venous return, truncus arteriosus, transposition of the great arteries, ventricular septal defect (particularly with late repair), complete atrioventricular canal (with moderate to large ventricular septal defect component), and hypoplastic left heart syndrome.[18] Preexisting pulmonary hypertension as well as the presence of certain chromosomal abnormalities (trisomy 21, trisomy 18, trisomy 13) may also increase the risk of developing postoperative pulmonary hypertensive crises.[19] Cardiopulmonary bypass itself increases the risk of pulmonary hypertension because of endothelial injury, impaired production of nitric oxide, release of endothelin and thromboxane, and release of microemboli.[20,21] Pulmonary hypoxia and ischemia during cardiopulmonary bypass and subsequent pulmonary reperfusion injury may also contribute to a state that may favor development of pulmonary hypertensive crises.[21]

PATHOPHYSIOLOGY

Pulmonary hypertensive crises are particularly dangerous, since they lead to both pulmonary as well as cardiac dysfunction. Increased pulmonary arterial pressure and resistance result in right ventricular dilation and right ventricular dysfunction. Right ventricular dilation leads to right-to-left shift of the interventricular septum and resultant compression of the left ventricle. Left ventricular compression decreases left ventricular compliance and therefore causes a decrease in pulmonary venous return and cardiac output.[21,22] Distention of the pulmonary arteries and resultant pulmonary edema leads to decreased lung compliance and hypoxia, hypercapnia, and respiratory acidosis.

EVALUATION AND MONITORING

Pulmonary hypertensive crises may begin with nonspecific findings such as tachycardia and systemic hypotension.[21] Subsequent progression to bradycardia and poor perfusion may signal impending cardiac arrest. Unless there is an intracardiac shunt present, oxygen saturations may often be normal or near normal until profound clinical deterioration occurs. Several modalities are useful in detecting clinically significant pulmonary hypertension. Presence of an increased gradient between the arterial pCO_2 from a blood gas, and end-tidal CO_2 from capnography may indicate decreased pulmonary blood flow. Direct hemodynamic monitoring using intravascular catheters are also useful in the critical care setting. A right atrial line can assess right ventricular filling pressures and measure mixed venous oxygen saturations to estimate oxygen delivery. Pulmonary arterial lines can directly measure pulmonary arterial pressures.

Echocardiography is another important noninvasive tool to evaluate pulmonary arterial pressure. The systolic pulmonary arterial pressure can be estimated by measuring the peak systolic velocity of the tricuspid regurgitation jet from spectral Doppler. Similarly, mean pulmonary arterial pressures can be estimated measuring the end-diastolic velocity of the pulmonary insufficiency jet by spectral Doppler. Right ventricular size, right ventricular systolic function, and interventricular septal contour and position can all be assessed qualitatively using two-dimensional echocardiography.

TREATMENT

Pulmonary hypertensive crises can be minimized through careful monitoring and treatment by several means. Appropriate sedation and pain control is extremely important to minimize pulmonary vascular resistance.[21] Fentanyl may be particularly useful in this setting, and paralysis is also used. Appropriate oxygenation and ventilation is important in maintaining low pulmonary vascular resistance, as both hypoxia and acidosis may cause pulmonary vasoconstriction. Although alkalosis promotes pulmonary vasodilation, high tidal volumes over time can damage alveoli and result in pulmonary edema. Conversely, inadequate tidal volumes can lead to alveolar collapse and resultant hypoxia.[22]

Current pharmacologic treatment of pulmonary hypertension involves the alteration of three mechanisms of pulmonary vasodilation: the nitric oxide/cyclic guanosine monophosphate (cGMP) pathway, the prostacyclin (PGI2)/cyclic adenosine monophosphate (cAMP) pathway, and the endothelin-1 pathway (see Chapter 35).[22] Inhaled nitric oxide is a selective pulmonary vasodilator, which has rapid onset of action. Inhaled nitric oxide has been used to treat postoperative pulmonary hypertension in patients who have undergone repair of obstructed total anomalous pulmonary venous return, mitral stenosis, and nonrestrictive ventricular septal defects. It has also been shown to be beneficial in single ventricle patients with Glenn and Fontan circulations by improving pulmonary blood flow, oxygen saturations, and central venous pressures.[24,25] Sildenafil has also been used as an adjunct to therapy when transitioning from inhaled nitric oxide to prevent rebound pulmonary hypertension.[26] Inhaled prostacyclin has also been shown to be effective in treating pulmonary hypertension in the postoperative setting.[27,28] Although bosentan therapy may be initiated in the intensive care setting, its effect on pulmonary hypertension is not rapid, so it is not effective in treating a pulmonary hypertensive crisis.

In addition to the pulmonary vasodilators mentioned previously, treatment of heart failure is critical in the management of patients with postoperative pulmonary hypertension. Milrinone infusion, in addition to decreasing pulmonary and systemic vascular resistance, improves left ventricular contractility and diastolic function. Systemic vasodilation may require initiation of a secondary agent. Norepinephrine, phenylephrine, and vasopressin may also be helpful in supporting cardiac function in the setting of pulmonary hypertensive crisis.[21,22]

Pulmonary Vein Stenosis

BACKGROUND

Pulmonary vein stenosis is a rare entity associated with significant morbidity and mortality. Patients with significant pulmonary vein stenosis of multiple vessels have mortality reported as high as 47%.[29,30] Typically, pulmonary vein stenosis is seen in young children, often in the setting of congenital heart disease but occasionally occurring in association with normal intracardiac anatomy.[29,31] There is a reported association of acquired pulmonary vein stenosis with necrotizing enterocolitis in premature infants.[32] Pulmonary vein stenosis often progresses in severity within a short period of time, and a neoproliferative process is believed to drive rapid progression of the disease.[29,31] A form of pulmonary vein stenosis is now also being noted in some adults who have undergone electrophysiologic ablation procedures in the region of the pulmonary vein(s) for treatment of atrial fibrillation.

Focal pulmonary vein stenosis arising near the connection with the left atrium was first described in 1952, and this anatomic type is thought to represent approximately 60% of cases of pulmonary vein stenosis as determined in one multicenter study.[31,33,34] Diffuse stenosis of a longer segment from the junction of the left atrium can also be seen, as well as involvement of the entire pulmonary vein.[29] This process may represent a progression from limited involvement to more diffuse involvement of the pulmonary vein(s) over time. It is estimated that approximately 60% of patients have unilateral disease, of which most stenoses involve the left pulmonary veins. Approximately 40% of patients have bilateral pulmonary vein disease.[30]

PRESENTATION

Pulmonary vein stenosis can often present in the first few days to first few months of life. Symptomatically, it may present with tachypnea, failure to thrive, or repeated lower respiratory infections.[35] An accentuated second heart sound, right ventricular heave, and a short holosystolic murmur of tricuspid regurgitation may be present on physical exam.[34] Despite attempts at catheter-based or surgical intervention, pulmonary vein stenosis often progresses. The number of pulmonary veins involved influences the overall prognosis. Involvement of one or two pulmonary veins often suggests a good prognosis, whereas involvement of three or four pulmonary veins leads to a poor prognosis. Significant progression may result in severe pulmonary vein stenosis and even pulmonary vein atresia. Clinically, this results in worsening hypoxia, pulmonary edema, potential for pulmonary hypertensive crises, and hemoptysis, which may be life threatening.

IMAGING

Chest x-ray typically shows a reticular pattern of central pulmonary venous congestion. Echocardiography is useful in imaging the proximal pulmonary veins, and pulmonary stenosis is present by spectral Doppler if pulmonary venous flow velocities are greater than 1.6 m/second and do not return to baseline (Figs. 39.12 and 39.13). Noninvasive tomographic imaging modalities such as CT and MRI can directly visualize the narrowed pulmonary vein(s), although CT may offer advantages from faster acquisition, higher spatial resolution, and simultaneous evaluation of the lung parenchyma. Cardiac catheterization and angiography is the preferred imaging approach due to the ability to obtain selective pulmonary vein opacification with high resolution, as well as the ability to obtain hemodynamic measurements (Fig. 39.14).[29,35]

TREATMENT

Stenotic pulmonary veins can be addressed surgically and in the cardiac catheterization laboratory, but outcomes remain suboptimal with current therapy. Surgical methods for repairing pulmonary veins include a standard patch repair versus a sutureless pericardial wall technique.[36] Restenosis or mortality was present in over half of patients, and there was no significant difference based upon the surgical technique used.[30,37] Conventional balloon angioplasty, use of cutting balloons, and placement of intravascular stents can improve the stenosis acutely, but repeated interventions are typically needed and are often not curative.[29,38]

Reperfusion Pulmonary Edema in Children Undergoing Procedures for Tetralogy of Fallot, Pulmonary Atresia and Multiple Aortopulmonary Collateral Arteries

Tetralogy of Fallot with pulmonary atresia represents a complex and variable form of congenital heart disease, with anatomic classification based upon the source and distribution of pulmonary blood flow. Sources of pulmonary blood flow may range from the presence of true intrapericardial pulmonary arteries (with varying degrees of hypoplasia) supplied by a patent ductus arteriosus to pulmonary arteries in conjunction with major aortopulmonary collateral arteries (MAPCAs) or to MAPCAs alone. Not surprisingly, patients in the latter two groups present a particular challenge with regard to surgical palliation and complete repair.[39–41] The

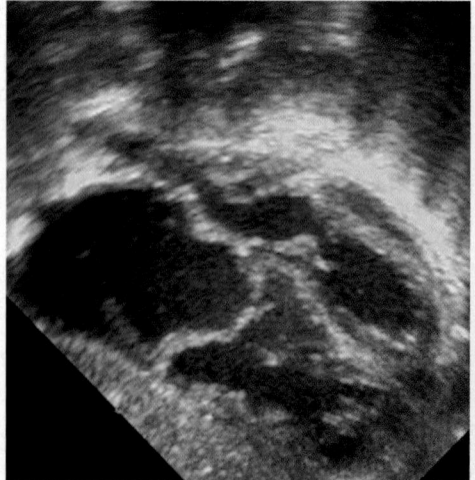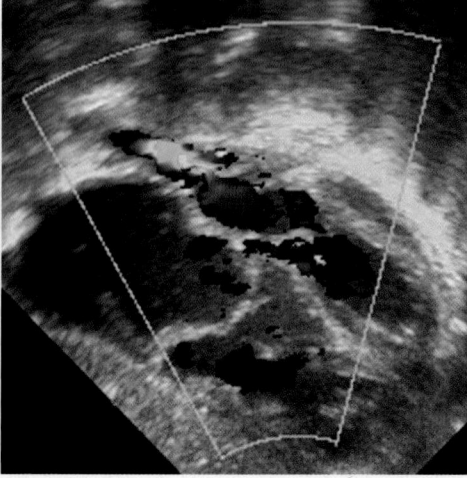

Fig. 39.12 Discrete right pulmonary vein stenosis from apical four-chamber view by 2D and color Doppler echocardiography. The 2D picture shows a dilated right heart and discrete pulmonary vein stenosis. The color Doppler picture shows high-velocity flow at the level of pulmonary vein stenosis.

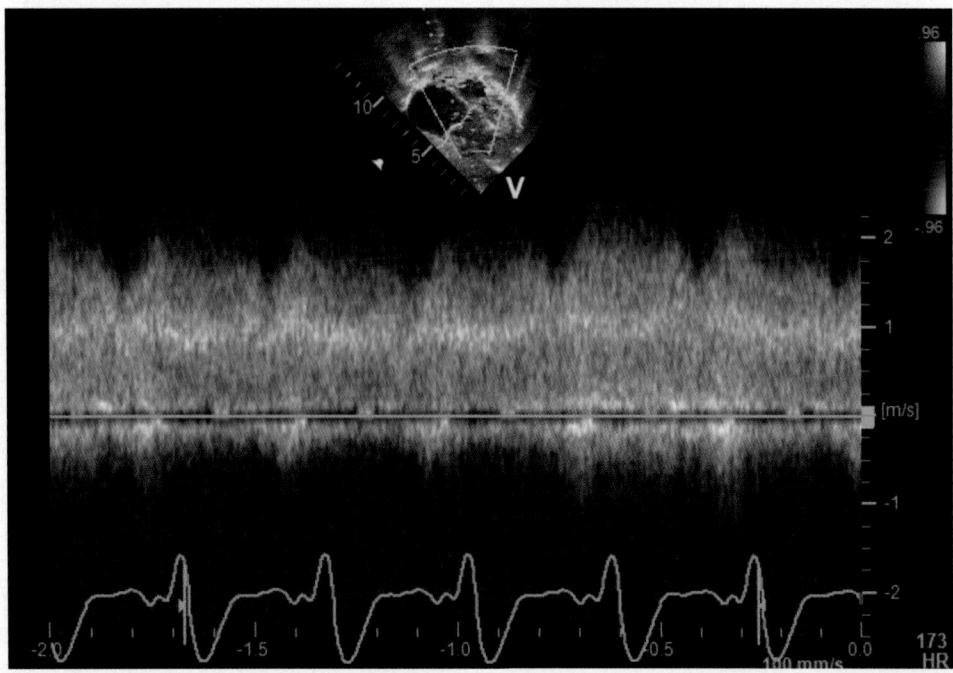

Fig. 39.13 Spectral Doppler echocardiography demonstrates continuous high-velocity flow at the site of discrete pulmonary vein stenosis.

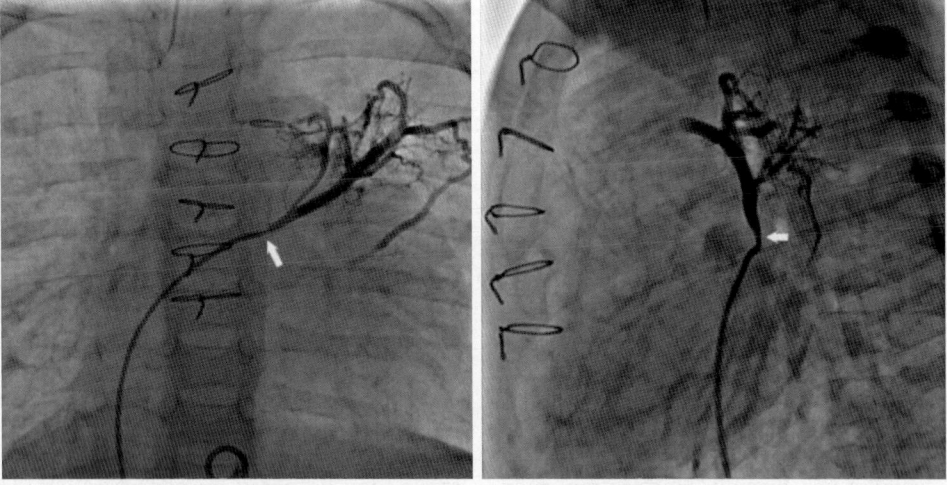

Fig. 39.14 Discrete pulmonary vein stenosis of the left upper pulmonary vein with posteroanterior and lateral projections from biplane fluoroscopy. Left pulmonary vein is directly opacified by catheter. *Arrow* demarcates discrete narrowing of the pulmonary vein.

goal of surgical repair in the presence of MAPCAs supplying a significant portion of the pulmonary blood flow is to incorporate MAPCAs into the true pulmonary arteries by a "unifocalization" procedure, establish adequate pulmonary blood flow, and ultimately separate the systemic and pulmonary circulations by closure of the ventricular septal defect, if possible. In favorable situations, this may be performed as a single procedure but often requires multiple staged procedures.[39,40,42,43]

Inflammatory injury related to reperfusion of ischemic tissue is a well-recognized phenomenon. Pulmonary reperfusion injury occurring after balloon angioplasty of significant pulmonary artery stenosis or treatment of chronic thromboembolic disease has been described, presumably related to

rapid improvement of blood flow to previously underperfused regions of the lung, and manifesting as localized pulmonary edema.[44,45] Maskatia and coworkers evaluated pulmonary reperfusion injury after unifocalization procedures for tetralogy of Fallot, pulmonary atresia, and MAPCAs and noted reperfusion injury to be common in this setting (65% of procedures). Risk factors in this patient population included bilateral unifocalization and severity of stenosis. There was not an association between presence of reperfusion injury and time to tracheal extubation.[46]

Asija and coworkers examined potential pathophysiologic mechanisms of this phenomenon in a similar group of patients by postoperative measurement of plasma biomarkers of alveolar injury and inflammation, including the receptor for advanced glycation end products (RAGE), intercellular adhesion molecule 1 (ICAM-1), and interleukin 6 (IL-6).[47] In this study, 50% of patients developed clinical evidence of reperfusion pulmonary edema. There were no significant differences however in levels of RAGE, ICAM-1, or IL-6 between patients with and those without reperfusion pulmonary edema measured at various time points, suggesting that the process does not appear to be associated with significant alveolar or vascular injury.[47]

Based upon our current knowledge, the entity of reperfusion pulmonary edema is common in certain conditions as described above, is self-limited, and does not appear to significantly alter postoperative course.[46]

Pulmonary Disease Associated With the Fontan Repair of Single Ventricle Physiology

PATHOPHYSIOLOGY

The Fontan operation for single ventricle physiology,[48] which has undergone a series of surgical refinements and modifications over the years,[49,50] involves directing systemic venous return to the pulmonary circulation, thus allowing the functional single ventricle to serve exclusively as the systemic ventricle. Because blood flow to the lungs in this situation is "passive" and nonpulsatile, several situations may lead to impaired cardiopulmonary function and the so-called failing Fontan. These may include elevated central venous pressure, systolic and/or diastolic ventricular dysfunction, and significant atrioventricular valve regurgitation leading to elevated atrial and therefore pulmonary venous pressure, and/or elevated pulmonary vascular resistance.

In an attempt to minimize the occurrence of these complications, contemporary versions of the Fontan-type operation have included the creation of an intraatrial tunnel placing the inferior vena cava in direct continuity with the superior vena cava and right pulmonary artery (via end-to-side anastomosis of the superior vena cava to the right pulmonary artery),[49] or, more recently, placement of an extracardiac conduit directing caval flow to the pulmonary arteries.[50] In patients felt to be of higher risk, a small "fenestration" may be created between the Fontan circuit and the adjacent atrium, providing a source of right to left shunting to augment cardiac output and reduce systemic venous pressure.[51]

Despite these refinements, complications related to Fontan physiology do occur and may be cardiopulmonary in nature. As mentioned earlier, fenestration of the Fontan baffle may result in persistent cyanosis and resultant fatigue and exercise intolerance. Restrictive lung function and reduced aerobic capacity has been described in adult patients who have undergone the Fontan procedure.[52] As a result of post-Fontan physiology with passive pulmonary blood flow, augmentation of cardiac output during exercise is limited, and peak oxygen consumption is reduced.[53,54]

Venovenous collateral vessels and pulmonary arteriovenous malformations may also contribute to chronic cyanosis. Pulmonary arteriovenous malformations are commonly seen in situations where the hepatic venous drainage has not been incorporated into the Fontan circuit.[55]

CLOTTING ABNORMALITIES

Patients with Fontan-palliated single ventricle physiology may manifest clotting abnormalities related to deficiencies in protein C, protein S, antithrombin III, or increased platelet reactivity.[56,57] In the setting of nonpulsatile flow to the pulmonary arteries, the presence of prosthetic material in the Fontan circuit (intraatrial baffle, extracardiac conduit), decreased cardiac output, and presence in some patients of a baffle fenestration create a risk of thrombus formation that is not insignificant. This may lead to acute or chronic pulmonary emboli or systemic emboli. Chronic pulmonary microemboli may contribute to increased pulmonary vascular resistance and impaired Fontan physiology. Prophylactic antithrombotic regimens, particularly in patients with a Fontan fenestration, vary by specific patient characteristics and by center and may include low-dose aspirin and/or warfarin therapy.

PULMONARY VASCULAR RESISTANCE

As noted earlier, optimal Fontan physiology is dependent upon the presence of low pulmonary vascular resistance. Sildenafil, a phosphodiesterase type 5 (PDE5) inhibitor, acts as a pulmonary vasodilator and has been demonstrated to improve myocardial performance and exercise capacity after the Fontan operation.[58,59] Bosentan, an endothelin receptor antagonist, as well as inhaled prostacyclins, have also been shown to improve exercise capacity in Fontan patients.[60,61]

PLASTIC BRONCHITIS

Plastic bronchitis is a rare, potentially life-threatening entity that is seen most commonly in patients who have undergone the Fontan procedure; it usually occurs in children.[62–64] A recent single-center review of Fontan patients at the University of Michigan estimated a prevalence of this condition ranging from 4%–14%.[65] The disease is characterized by the presence of large, dense mucus and fibrin plugs in the tracheobronchial tree with resultant cast formation. Depending on severity, patients may manifest cough, fever, dyspnea, wheezing, and symptoms of pulmonary obstruction. The casts may be noted on expectoration. They are classified histologically either as inflammatory casts composed of fibrin and eosinophilic infiltrates (type 1) or acellular casts containing mucin and fibrin without inflammatory infiltrate (type 2).[66] Type 2 (noninflammatory) casts are typically seen in the post-Fontan patient who has developed plastic bronchitis. Treatment of this condition can be extremely challenging. Pulmonary lymphatic abnormalities may contribute to this condition, and thoracic duct ligation or embolization have been reported as a potential treatment.[67–69] Treatment with aerosolized tissue plasminogen activator has also been utilized with reported benefit.[70,71]

HETEROTAXY SYNDROME

In some patients, single ventricle anatomy may be seen in association with heterotaxy syndrome. Airway disease related to ciliary dysfunction should be evaluated in this setting due to the increased prevalence of ciliary abnormalities in patients with heterotaxy syndrome.[72] Ciliary dysfunction of the respiratory system is discussed in detail in Chapter 71.

Pulmonary Complications Related to Cardiac Surgery and Cardiopulmonary Bypass

A number of factors may contribute to impaired pulmonary function after cardiac surgery and cardiopulmonary bypass. These may include the presence of postoperative atelectasis, pulmonary edema, and/or pleural effusions. Additional factors that may affect lung function may also be present, such as alterations of chest wall mechanics due to sternotomy, or impaired respiratory effort due to postoperative pain. Although uncommon, hemidiaphragmatic paresis or paralysis is an associated risk when surgical correction of congenital heart disease involves proximity to the phrenic nerve.

The period of ischemia to the pulmonary vascular bed followed by reperfusion after cardiopulmonary bypass promotes an inflammatory response that may lead to lung injury. Production of oxygen free radicals and activation of neutrophils, macrophages, and endothelial cells contribute to this process, leading to increased capillary permeability, pulmonary edema, impaired oxygenation, and increased pulmonary vascular resistance.[73,74] The entity of systemic inflammatory response syndrome (SIRS) also contributes to cardiopulmonary bypass related lung injury via complement activation and cytokine release.[75,76]

The administration of blood products during cardiac surgery and cardiopulmonary bypass may result in an inflammatory response and transfusion-related acute lung injury (TRALI). This syndrome is characterized by acute respiratory changes, hypoxemia, bilateral pulmonary infiltrates, fever, and hypotension temporally related to recent transfusion. In a multicenter study reported by Vlaar and coworkers patients who received transfusion during cardiac surgery with cardiopulmonary bypass demonstrated increased pulmonary capillary permeability compared to those patients who were not transfused. This finding was associated with packed red blood cell transfusion but not fresh frozen plasma or platelets.[77] In addition, Koch and coworkers found that patients undergoing cardiac surgery who received packed red blood cells or fresh frozen plasma developed more postoperative respiratory complications.[78] However, avoidance of blood product administration for cardiac surgery requiring cardiopulmonary bypass is generally not possible in the pediatric population due to small patient size/blood volume and associated limitations on hemodilution relative to the priming volume required for the cardiopulmonary bypass circuit.

Conclusion

The pulmonary and circulatory systems are highly interdependent. Rare entities such as vascular rings and pulmonary vein stenosis must be considered in patients with respiratory symptoms that do not follow the expected clinical course. Pediatric cardiac surgery places patients at risk for reperfusion injury, pulmonary inflammation, and pulmonary hypertension. Single ventricle physiology can result in significant pulmonary dysfunction. Developing novel therapies to optimize pulmonary function under abnormal circulatory conditions will be critical in improving clinical outcomes.

References

Access the reference list online at ExpertConsult.com.

Suggested Reading

Backer CL, Monge MC, Popescu AR, et al. Vascular rings. *Semin Pediatr Surg.* 2016;25:165–175.

Brown D, Geva T. Anomalies of the pulmonary veins. In: Allen H, Shaddy R, Penny J, et al, eds. *Moss and Adams' Heart Disease in Infants, Children, and Adolescents.* 9th ed. Philadelphia: Wolters-Kluwer; 2016:881 910.

Collins P. Early embryonic circulation. In: Standring S, ed. *Gray's Anatomy: The Anatomic Basis of Clinical Practice.* 41st ed. London: Elsevier; 2016:200–205.

Ezon D, Penny J. Aortic arch and vascular anomalies. In: Allen H, Shaddy R, Penny D, et al, eds. *Moss and Adams' Heart Disease in Infants, Children, and Adolescents Including the Fetus and Young Adult.* 9th ed. Philadelphia: Wolters Kluwer; 2016:833–870.

Oishi P, Fineman JR. Pulmonary hypertension. *Pediatr Crit Care Med.* 2016;17:S140–S145.

Roche S, Greenway SRA. Tetralogy of Fallot with pulmonary stenosis, pulmonary atresia, and absent pulmonary valve. In: Allen H, Shaddy R, Penny J, et al, eds. *Moss and Adams' Heart Disease in Infants, Children, and Adolescents.* 9th ed. Philadelphia: Wolters Kluwer; 2016:1029–1052.

40 Lung Injury From Hydrocarbon Aspiration and Smoke Inhalation

ADA LEE, MD, and MICHAEL BYE, MD

Epidemiology

In 2014, in the United States, 31,903 total hydrocarbon exposures were reported to poison control centers, and 9546 of these occurred in children less than 5 years old. There were 118,207 exposures to household cleaning substances in children less than 5 years old, resulting in the third leading cause of poisoning deaths in this age group in the United States.[1] The highest morbidity and mortality result from accidental ingestion in children less than 5 years of age.

Etiology

Hydrocarbon toxicity resulting from the ingestion of petroleum solvents, dry-cleaning fluids, lighter fluids, kerosene, gasoline, and liquid polishes and waxes (mineral seal oil) continues to be a common occurrence in small children. This is in addition to the potential harm from additives such as heavy metals, pesticides, and camphor, all of which have potential systemic toxicity.[2–4] Kerosene heaters, cleaning fluids, furniture polishes, and liquid floor waxes are present in homes, too frequently within the easy reach of toddlers, and they account for the persistence of hydrocarbon poisoning. In one series of hydrocarbon ingestions, the material was stored in a standard beverage container almost one-third of the time.[5] The most commonly ingested materials are household cleaning products, solvents, and fuels; in some areas, kerosene ingestion is more common. In 2001, the US Consumer Product Safety Commission required child-resistant packaging for products with low viscosity and a significant concentration of hydrocarbons (>10% by weight).[6] Similar attempts were made by the European Union in 1997. Unfortunately, these regulations do not seem to have had a significant impact on the frequency of such poisonings.[7]

Although central nervous system (CNS) abnormalities (e.g., weakness, confusion, and coma), gastrointestinal irritation, cardiomyopathy, and renal toxicity all occur, the most common and the most serious complication is pneumonitis. Deaths from hydrocarbon poisoning are almost always from respiratory insufficiency.

Pathology

Lung pathology in fatal cases includes necrosis of bronchial, bronchiolar, and alveolar tissue, atelectasis, interstitial inflammation, hemorrhagic pulmonary edema, vascular thromboses, necrotizing bronchopneumonia, and hyaline membrane formation.[8]

Experimental studies in rats reveal an acute alveolitis that is most severe at 3 days, subsides at 10 days, and is followed by a chronic proliferative phase that may take weeks to resolve.[9] Rats develop hyperemia and vascular engorgement of both large and small blood vessels within 1 hour of aspiration.[10] At 24 hours, there is a focal bronchopneumonia with microabscess formation. By 2 weeks, the process largely resolves, although some vascular engorgement and rare peribronchial inflammation persist. In humans, chest roentgenographic abnormalities persist for some time after physical findings have cleared, suggesting a similar prolonged recovery.

Dogs show different responses,[11] which also vary with the amount of kerosene ingested. A low dose causes destruction of alveolar epithelium, resulting in emphysema but insignificant airway involvement. More intense airway obstruction is seen in the high-dose group. At 1 hour after high-dose ingestion, intraalveolar edema and hemorrhage occur most prominently in the subpleural air spaces and those adjacent to large bronchi, suggesting induced interstitial inflammation. By 24 hours after ingestion, many airways show severe destruction and desquamation of the lining epithelium, resulting in near complete obliteration of the airways. The lumens are filled with degenerating neutrophils and scattered macrophages and lymphocytes. The surrounding lung parenchyma and the interstitia of the blood vessels show intense infiltration by macrophages and neutrophils, with microabscesses in the lung parenchyma. While most of the findings heal within a week, scattered areas of bronchiolitis obliterans may persist. By 2 weeks, much of the lung tissue has returned to normal, with rare areas of bronchiolitis obliterans. The severity of these dose-related changes can be explained by two characteristics of kerosene. First, it is a solvent that can dissolve cell walls and/or lipid lining layers, resulting in the desquamation of cells and fluid influx into the airways. Second, as a foreign substance that can penetrate the interstitium, it can provoke an intense inflammatory reaction. Since there are dose-related responses to kerosene with interspecies differences, accurate prediction of the process in humans is difficult.

Pathophysiology

The risk for aspiration varies with the inherent properties of the hydrocarbon. Aspiration is much more likely to occur

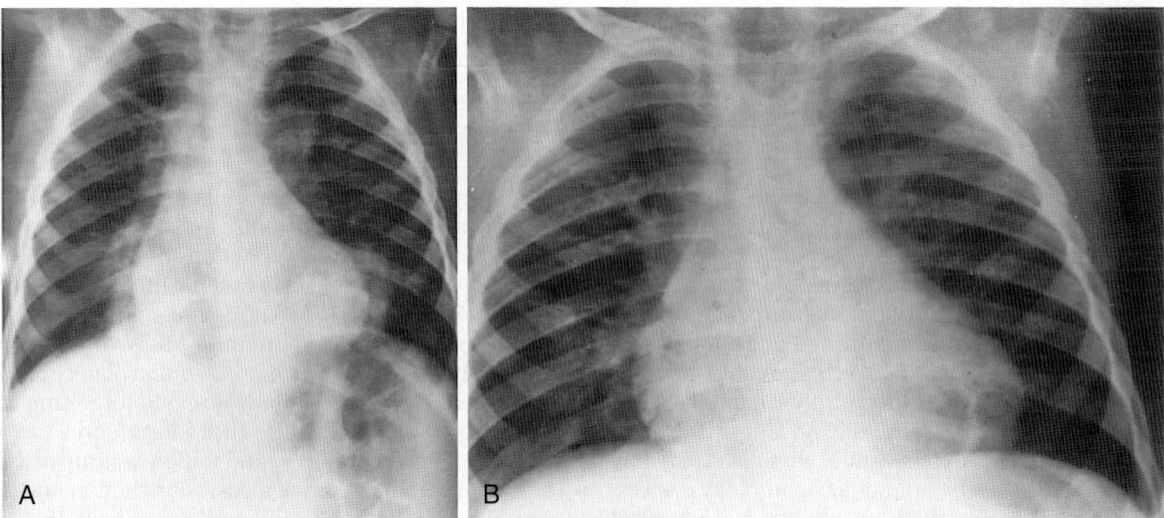

Fig. 40.1 Hydrocarbon pneumonia. (A) Confluent sequential infiltrate is present in the left lower lobe. (B) Three weeks later, pneumatoceles are apparent; the large pneumatocele in the left lower lobe is at the site of the previous infiltrate. (From Felman AH. *Radiology of the Pediatric Chest.* New York: McGraw-Hill, 1987.)

with a substance that has low surface tension, low viscosity, and high volatility, and low surface tension allows the substance to spread throughout the tracheobronchial tree. Low viscosity allows the substance to spread more readily and to seep deeper into the tissues. High volatility increases the likelihood of CNS involvement, presumably due to more rapid absorption into the bloodstream; highly volatile substances may also rapidly spread to the alveoli and immediately interfere with gas exchange.

Hydrocarbons increase surface tension by inhibiting surfactant,[12] which predisposes to alveolar instability and atelectasis. The instillation of artificial surfactant into the trachea of sheep following kerosene exposure resulted in significant improvement in oxygenation and mortality.[13] There is one case report of a 17-month-old child with ARDS from hydrocarbon aspiration who survived after treatment with surfactant.[14]

Pulmonary lesions are believed to be caused by direct aspiration of the hydrocarbon into the airways. This may occur either during the initial ingestion or during subsequent emesis. Small amounts of aspirated hydrocarbons may produce more serious disease than larger amounts in the stomach. Evidence that hydrocarbons are removed by the first capillary bed they encounter[15,16] reinforces the notion that pulmonary damage occurs from aspiration. Indeed, the liver and the lungs filter out sufficient amounts of kerosene to help prevent CNS damage.[15] Fatalities are rarely attributed to CNS involvement per se.

Clinical Findings

Cough may appear within 30 minutes of aspiration or may be delayed for hours. Initially, auscultation of the chest may be normal or may reveal only coarse or decreased breath sounds. When severe injury occurs, hemoptysis and pulmonary edema develop rapidly, and respiratory failure may occur within 24 hours. Radiographic signs of chemical pneumonitis, when present, will develop within 2 hours after ingestion in 88% of cases and within 6–12 hours in 98%.[17,18] The

findings vary from punctate, mottled densities to pneumonitis or atelectasis and tend to predominate in dependent portions of the lung (Fig. 40.1A). Air trapping, pneumatoceles, (see Fig. 40.1B),[19] and pleural effusions may also develop. The radiographic abnormalities reach their peak within 72 hours and then usually clear within days. A review of 16 children showed that children whose chest radiographs were to become abnormal did so by 24 hours after the ingestion, and most cleared within 2–3 weeks.[20]

Occasionally, the radiographic findings persist for several weeks. There is a poor correlation between clinical symptoms, physical findings, and radiographic abnormalities. In general, the radiographic changes are more prominent than the findings on physical examination and persist for a longer period. When pneumatoceles occur, they are likely to do so after a patient has become asymptomatic. They require several months for spontaneous resolution.

Blood gas studies reveal hypoxemia without hypercapnia, suggesting ventilation-perfusion mismatch or diffusion block. Destruction of the epithelium of the airways together with bronchospasm adds to the ventilation-perfusion abnormalities, and displacement of alveolar gas by the hydrocarbon vapors adds to the hypoxemia.

Diagnosis and Differential Diagnosis

Diagnosis is elucidated from the history of hydrocarbon exposure. Differential diagnoses include bronchopneumonia, atelectasis, salicylate overdose, and other toxins.

Management and Treatment

Initial management should comprise a history, physical examination, and chest radiograph. Because hydrocarbons do less damage when swallowed than when aspirated into the lungs, it is important to avoid emetics or gastric lavage. Some toxicologists recommend nasogastric lavage through a large bore tube in patients with a large amount of hydrocarbon with the potential for systemic toxicity if the patient presents within 1 hour of ingestion.[21,22] If the child had no symptoms at the scene or in the emergency room and has a normal chest radiograph, observation for 6–8 hours is important. If no symptoms develop, the child may be safely discharged home.[18] If an abnormality is detected by history, examination, or radiography, arterial blood gas analysis should be performed. Even if no symptoms develop, a repeat chest radiograph at 24 hours is a prudent measure. If results of examination and radiography are normal at 24 hours and the child has no further symptoms, discharge can occur after providing education and reassurance. Supplemental oxygen must be given if the child is hypoxemic. Adequate hydration should be maintained, but excessive fluid administration may be counterproductive, as the pulmonary pathology evolves. Case reports of rapid recovery of lung function and beneficial effects of lung mechanics and gas exchange were noted after early administration of intratracheal surfactant as early as initial presentation to the emergency room.[23,24] In animal studies, nebulized β2-agonist administered to sheep with combined smoke inhalation and burn injury resulted in improved lung function, airway clearance, and reduced pulmonary edema.[25] Although clinical data in humans is lacking on the use of β2-agonist in inhalation injury, some have suggested a trial of bronchodilators if respiratory symptoms progress. Hypoxemic respiratory failure should be treated with mechanical ventilation and positive end-expiratory pressure. If the child fails conventional mechanical ventilation, both extracorporeal membrane oxygenation (ECMO)[26] and high-frequency jet ventilation[27] have been successful in improving oxygenation and allowing survival.

Although superimposed bacterial infection is a potential concern, there is no evidence that this is a common occurrence. Because leukocytosis and fever are common after hydrocarbon aspiration, it is often difficult to detect bacterial superinfection. One thoughtful review concluded that bacterial complications are rare.[28] Until there is further evidence to the contrary, antimicrobial therapy should be reserved for patients who are severely compromised by malnutrition, debilitation, or an underlying disease or in whom the pneumonia is especially severe. Evolving evidence of infection on serial Gram stains of secretions from the endotracheal tube could be an indication for antimicrobials. Because airway closure and collapse are a significant part of the disease, continuous distending airway pressure is desirable to maintain functional residual capacity (FRC) and to keep the concentration of inspired oxygen in safe ranges. Studies in animals and humans show no therapeutic or prophylactic role for corticosteroids.[29–31]

Prevention

Prevention of the accidental ingestion of products containing hydrocarbons must be a high priority. Educating parents to keep potentially toxic materials out of the reach of young children seems obvious. Education about storage of such materials and avoiding containers that children associate with potable liquids must be stressed. Prevention of nonintentional poisonings includes clearly labeling containers that contain hydrocarbons. If kerosene heaters are used in the home, the kerosene must be kept out of the reach of children.

Prognosis

Prognosis and clinical improvement depends on the type, volume, and pH of the substance aspirated. Long-term follow-up studies of pulmonary function in patients with hydrocarbon pneumonitis indicate residual injury to the peripheral airways. A study of 17 asymptomatic children 8–14 years after a hydrocarbon pneumonitis showed abnormal lung function in 14 (82%). The most common abnormalities were an elevated ratio of residual volume to total lung capacity, an increased slope of phase III, reduced forced expiratory volume in 1 second (FEV_1) and a high volume of isoflow[32]; these results indicate small airway obstruction and gas trapping. When radiographic changes accompany the ingestion of hydrocarbons, this same pattern of abnormal lung function is detected 10 years later, even in otherwise asymptomatic subjects. However, the frequency of airway reactivity appears to be normal.[33] Most children survive without serious complications, but some may progress to respiratory failure and death.

Hydrocarbon "Sniffing"

Deliberate inhalation of volatile hydrocarbons to induce a state of euphoria is common among adolescents. It is estimated that 13% of adolescents have used inhalants at one time or another.[34] Unlike other forms of drug abuse, this is more common among those in the seventh to ninth grades.[35,36] The euphoria of mild intoxication may be accompanied by mild nausea and vomiting. Prolonged exposure may lead to violent excitement followed by CNS depression, unconsciousness, and coma. Large doses of halogenated hydrocarbons, especially when combined with exertion, excitement, and hypercapnia, may be associated with dysrhythmias and death. Medullary depression and respiratory paralysis are generally accepted as the mechanism of death in most gasoline inhalation fatalities. Strong psychological dependence may develop in some sniffers. Acute hypoxemia at the time of inhalation and shortly thereafter is not uncommon as a result of displacement of alveolar gas by the inhaled substance. However, this is usually transient and not significant. Lung injury per se from hydrocarbon sniffing has not been described. A toluene embryopathy has been described in infants born to mothers who sniffed toluene,[37] although the "polypharmacy" often used by the mothers may confound the data.[38]

Respiratory Complications of Smoke Inhalation

EPIDEMIOLOGY

In 2014, there were 494,000 structural fires in the United States; of these, 386,500 were residential structural fires.[39] Death from fire is the seventh leading cause of unintentional injury death in the United States in 2014.[40] The United States ranks 10th out of 24 developed countries in fire deaths.[41]

Those at greatest risk are children younger than 4 years of age; African-American and Native American males; those over 85 years of age, and the poor.[42] In 2014, 3275 civilians died in fires in the United States.[39] A great deal of the morbidity and mortality in victims of fires results from pulmonary injuries due to smoke inhalation.[43] The severity of the lung injury depends on (1) the nature of the material involved in the fire and the products of incomplete combustion that are generated and (2) whether the victim has been confined in a closed space. The subject's minute ventilation also plays a role. The deeper and more rapidly the victim breathes, the greater the amount and degree of deposition of toxic materials into the airways and alveoli. The decreased inspired oxygen concentration that results from the fire stimulates compensatory hyperapnea in humans.

ETIOLOGY

Fire-related injuries and death occur as a result of structural and outside fires. Isolated smoke inhalation injury can occur but may be complicated by thermal or chemical burns to the airways.

PATHOGENESIS

The pathogenesis of lung injury from smoke inhalation includes thermal and chemical factors. Because the upper airway is such an effective heat exchanger, most of the heat from inhaled smoke is dissipated before the inhaled material reaches the carina. Direct thermal damage, therefore, primarily affects the supraglottic airways. Only with steam, which is unusual in most fires, or with prolonged exposure to high ambient temperatures, will there be thermal injury to the intrathoracic airways.

Depending on the material involved in fires, a wide variety of noxious gases may be generated. These include the oxides of sulfur and nitrogen, acetaldehydes, hydrocyanic acid, and carbon monoxide (CO). Irritant gases such as nitrous oxide or sulfur dioxide may combine with lung water to form corrosive acids. Aldehydes from the combustion of furniture and cotton materials induce denaturation of protein, cellular damage, and pulmonary edema. The combustion of wood generates considerable quantities of CO and carbon dioxide. Plastics, if heated to sufficiently high temperatures, may be the source of very toxic vapors. Thus, chlorine and hydrochloric acid may be generated from polyvinyl chloride; hydrocarbons, aldehydes, ketones, and acids from polyethylene; and isocyanate and hydrogen cyanide from polyurethane.[44] Although the particulate matter carried in the smoke (soot) probably does not in itself produce injury, toxic gases may be absorbed on the surface of the carbon particles and carried into the lungs; the soot particles may also be responsible for inducing reflex bronchoconstriction.

CARBON MONOXIDE POISONING

CO poisoning is an especially serious complication of smoke inhalation that occurs soon after exposure. While smoke inhalation is the most common cause of inadvertent CO poisoning, other causes include poorly functioning home heating systems; inadequate ventilation for fuel burning systems (e.g., gas grills, kerosene heaters, and camp stoves);

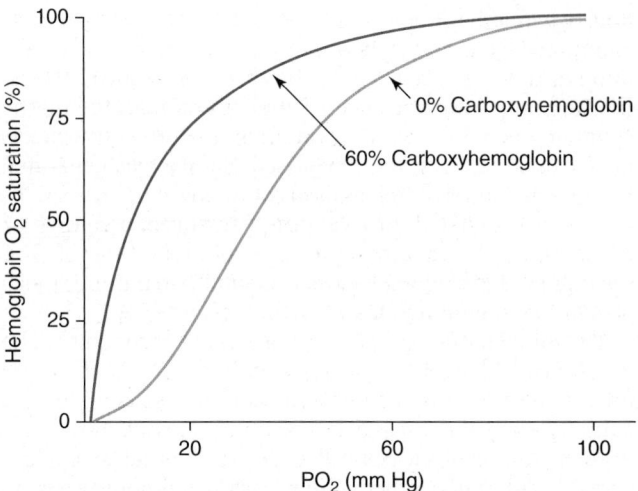

Fig. 40.2 Oxygen–hemoglobin dissociation curve. The presence of carboxyhemoglobin shifts the curve to the left and changes it to a more hyperbolic shape. This results in a decrease in oxygen-carrying capacity and impaired release of oxygen at the tissue level. (From Ernst A, Zibrak J. Carbon monoxide poisoning. *N Engl J Med.* 1998;339:1603-1608.)

and motor vehicles idling in poorly ventilated areas. Some of these can also be the sources for intentional poisoning. The toxicity results from the combination of CO with hemoglobin to form carboxyhemoglobin (COHb), leading to severely impaired tissue oxygenation. The CO displaces oxygen from hemoglobin, reducing the delivery of oxygen to the tissues. CO not only has a higher affinity for hemoglobin than oxygen but also shifts the oxyhemoglobin dissociation curve to the left (Fig. 40.2).[45] For this reason, the toxicity of CO poisoning is greater at high altitude and in the presence of anemia. It is critical to remember that although the oxygen content of the arterial blood is low in CO poisoning, the partial pressure of oxygen in arterial blood (PaO_2) is not reduced. Because the carotid body responds to PaO_2, ventilation may not be stimulated until acidosis develops. Together with the fact that COHb is bright red, this makes the clinical diagnosis very difficult. The bright red color of the blood also makes the currently available oximeters unreliable. If there is a suspicion of CO poisoning, an ***arterial*** blood gas ***must*** be obtained along with COHb levels. CO also binds to myoglobin, resulting in anoxia of muscle cells. With prolonged exposure, CO binds to cytochrome oxidase, impairing mitochondrial function and reducing production of adenosine triphosphate. Both of these actions impair normal cellular function.

PATHOLOGY

Various pathologic lesions are found in smoke inhalation. Part of the variability in pathology may be attributed to differences in the toxic products generated in fires. However, many of the pulmonary changes may not result simply from the direct chemical injury to the respiratory tract. Rather, they may reflect secondary circulatory, metabolic, or infectious complications of surface burns or may be induced by the administration of oxygen, mechanical ventilation, and the administration of excessive volumes of intravenous fluids.

Animal models of the pathology have been of limited value, because steam rather than pure smoke was usually used, and the modifying effects of the upper air passages were eliminated by using tracheal cannulas. Experimental evaluation of the response to smoke has been performed in anesthetized and intubated sheep, kept light enough to breathe spontaneously. Even in these animals, any protective effects of the upper airway were bypassed. Smoke was generated by burning material such as dyed cotton toweling. The smoke was then insufflated into the lungs. In sheep, a volume of 20 cc/kg for 12 breaths and an inspiratory time of 3–4 seconds produced physiologic effects similar to natural smoke inhalation, including mean COHb levels of 45%.[46]

The initial pathologic changes are tracheobronchitis. The greater the tidal volume of the insufflated smoke, the more intense the tracheobronchitis. With sufficient smoke quantity, denudation of the tracheal epithelium occurred, most likely from disruption of the cell-cell and the cell–basal layer adhesions.[47] With much larger volumes, acute pulmonary edema caused by increased pulmonary vascular permeability occurred within 30 minutes.[48] The degree of atelectasis also correlated with the amount of smoke insufflated. Subsequent airway edema only occurred in those animals given large tidal volumes of smoke.[46] The degree of hypoxemia over the 24 hours studied did not correlate with the tidal breath size but was constant for a given total smoke exposure. This suggests that the gas exchange deterioration was based more on the airway pathology than on the alveolar atelectasis or edema.

A group of infants studied postmortem after accidental exposure to smoke in a newborn nursery[49] was found to have necrosis of bronchial and bronchiolar epithelium with vascular engorgement and edema together with the formation of dense membranes or casts that partially obstructed the large and small airways. Bronchiolitis and bronchopneumonia were present in some, as were interstitial and alveolar edema. There was carbonaceous material in the alveoli with alveolar hemorrhage.

Electron microscopic studies of 10 fatal cases of smoke inhalation following a hotel fire revealed interstitial and alveolar edema as well as engorgement of alveolar vessels.[50] Carbon particles were seen within alveolar macrophages. Type I pneumocytes showed more injury than was seen in the pulmonary endothelial cells. Patients who died after severe surface burns have had necrotizing bronchitis and bronchiolitis with intraalveolar hemorrhage, hyaline membrane formation, and massive pulmonary edema. In these patients, it is difficult to know how much to attribute to direct pulmonary injury from smoke or to the complex metabolic, infectious, chest wall, and circulatory derangements that complicate surface burns and result in acute respiratory distress syndrome (ARDS). However, sheep exposed to surface burns plus smoke inhalation sufficient to raise the COHb levels to 25%–30% fared much worse than the sheep exposed to surface burns alone. The burn/inhalation group had greater amounts of lung lipid peroxidation products in bronchoalveolar lavage and at autopsy even without evidence of pulmonary infection or ARDS.[51]

PATHOPHYSIOLOGY

Severe damage to the upper air passages leads to stridor with increased extrathoracic resistance. Upper airway obstruction usually occurs within 24 hours of injury. This increases the work of breathing and can lead to alveolar hypoventilation. Inflammatory changes in the airways lead to ventilation/perfusion mismatch, exaggerating the hypoxemia. Depending on the severity and distribution of the airway obstruction, there may be atelectasis or air trapping. The latter is especially likely with premature closure of the small airways. Altered surfactant function predisposes to atelectasis. Although reflex bronchoconstriction may contribute to the increase in airway resistance, it is difficult to assess the magnitude of its contribution, because airway resistance is already high as a result of bronchial and bronchiolar edema and inflammation.

Smoke is a mixture of gases and particulate matter generated from burning substances. The toxic effects of smoke are primarily seen when animals are exposed to whole smoke. When the particle phase of the smoke was filtered out, there were neither acute nor delayed toxic effects on lung function or gas exchange.[52] Since many of the oxidants are in the gas phase as well in whole smoke, it is possible that only those toxins carried on the smoke particles remain in the airway long enough to elicit an inflammatory response.

Pulmonary edema plays a prominent role in the pathophysiology of lung injury from smoke inhalation.[44] Studies in adults demonstrate increased extravascular lung water without a concomitant increase in pulmonary capillary wedge pressure. Studies in sheep reveal increased lung lymph flow and an increase in the lymph/plasma ratio of protein, suggesting increased permeability of the alveolar capillary membrane.[53] Increased bronchial circulation contributed to the pulmonary edema. Nitric oxide at extremely elevated levels acts as a free radical and potentiates the inflammatory response. Inhibition of inducible nitric oxide synthase reverses the loss of hypoxic pulmonary vasoconstriction and attenuates acute respiratory distress syndrome.[54,55]

Other products of combustion increase the damage. In dogs, acrolein found in herbicides and cigarette smoke results in delayed-onset pulmonary edema. Pure smoke, and smoke with added hydrochloric acid, did not have the same effects.[56] An animal model showed increased pulmonary vascular resistance and decreased cardiac output concomitant with increased secretion of leukotrienes C4, D4, and E4. Pretreatment with a leukotriene antagonist markedly attenuated and delayed those cardiovascular changes.[57] Additional studies in sheep suggest that the acrolein-induced pulmonary edema and pulmonary hypertension are mediated by cyclooxygenase products, because pretreatment with cyclooxygenase inhibitors blocks the cardiorespiratory changes.[58] The acute pulmonary edema associated with very high-dose cotton smoke exposure in sheep is blocked by a combined cyclooxygenase and leukotriene antagonist, but not by indomethacin, a cyclooxygenase inhibitor. Both agents block the elevated airway resistance and hypoxemia that presumably occur as a result of acute bronchoconstriction. Prolonged exposure to acrolein in a kitchen resulted in severe respiratory distress in a previously healthy 27-month-old child who developed bronchiectasis 18 months after the initial exposure.[59]

Oxidants directly from the products of combustion also contribute to airway damage, closure, and atelectasis.[60] Early therapy with aerosolized deferoxamine-pentastarch in sheep exposed to cotton smoke attenuated these findings.[61] It is not clear whether the deferoxamine was acting directly as an antioxidant or reducing the free iron released in the airway.

Neutrophil-mediated proteolytic activity has been implicated in the airway pathology. Sheep treated intravenously with the synthetic protease inhibitor gabexate mesilate after insufflation with cotton smoke had a significant reduction in transvascular fluid and protein flux and were able to maintain better gas exchange than a vehicle-treated control group.[62] Impaired chemotactic and phagocytic function of the alveolar macrophage after smoke inhalation increases the risk for pulmonary infection several days after the acute event.

Any inhaled cyanide binds to the intracellular cytochrome system, inhibiting cell metabolism and the production of adenosine triphosphate. While all cells contain the enzyme rhodanese, which can convert hydrocyanide to thiocyanate, this capability is outstripped by continued or high levels of cyanide. The thiocyanate is excreted in the urine, assuming normal renal blood flow and urine output.[63]

CLINICAL FINDINGS

The initial respiratory assessment of a victim of a fire should focus on hypoxemia. Patients may have facial burns, singed nasal hairs, carbonaceous sputum, or soot in the proximal airway. Blistering or edema of the oropharynx, hoarseness, stridor, and upper airway mucosal lesions may be evident. Symptoms include tachypnea, dyspnea, cough, and cyanosis. Chest retractions may be present, and auscultation may reveal wheezing, crackles, or rhonchi. Oxygen should be administered while arterial blood gas studies, including CO levels, are drawn. The clinical manifestations of CO poisoning vary with the level of COHb. Mild intoxication leads to headache, diminished visual acuity, irritability, and nausea. COHb levels greater than 40% produce confusion, hallucination, ataxia, and coma. CO may increase cerebral blood flow, the permeability of cerebral capillaries, and the cerebrospinal fluid pressure. CO may also have long-term effects on the CNS, and myocardial dysfunction and irritability can result directly from CO, as well as from hypoxemia.

Patients assessed immediately at the scene of a fire have elevated blood cyanide concentrations, and the cyanide levels of victims who die because of smoke inhalation are significantly higher than the levels of survivors. Blood cyanide levels correlate with CO levels, and plasma lactate levels were better correlated with cyanide levels than with CO level. A plasma lactate concentration above 10 mM in the emergency department is a sensitive indicator of cyanide poisoning.[64]

Maximum inspiratory and expiratory flow-volume curves and flexible fiberoptic nasopharyngoscopy or bronchoscopy have been helpful in the early assessment of the extent of supraglottic or tracheobronchial injury and the likelihood of subsequently developing airway obstruction.[65] Although there may be some delay in the clinical evidence of respiratory tract injury resulting from smoke inhalation, manifestations of respiratory disease will usually develop within 12–24 hours. Absence of roentgenographic pulmonary disease is not very helpful in early diagnosis, because abnormal findings may lag several hours or more behind auscultatory or physiologic evidence of damage.

Respiratory insufficiency may also occur as the result of airway obstruction anywhere from the supraglottic airways to the alveoli. It may be difficult to localize the level of obstruction; therefore, whenever there is clinical evidence of severe obstruction, the upper airways should be assessed by direct laryngoscopy before swelling of the head, neck, or oropharynx make this examination difficult. Fiberoptic bronchoscopy may be very useful to evaluate the extent of mucosal damage, but intense vasoconstriction in hypovolemic patients may mask the findings.[66]

Acute CO poisoning is also associated with acute myocardial injury and a delayed neuropsychiatric syndrome, which in children will lead to cognitive defects and sometimes to focal deficits. However, the mechanism of action of these complications has not been elicited.

DIAGNOSIS AND DIFFERENTIAL DIAGNOSIS

Diagnosis of smoke inhalation injury is largely based on history of smoke exposure in a closed space. Facial burns, singed nasal hairs, soot in the nasopharynx, or voice changes may help support the diagnosis. Patients with smoke inhalation with superimposed altered mental status require a careful evaluation for hypoxia secondary to either pulmonary injury or impaired oxygen utilization at the cellular level. Differential diagnoses include acute respiratory distress syndrome, aspiration pneumonitis, pneumonia, asthma, pulmonary embolism, and cyanide poisoning.

MANAGEMENT AND TREATMENT

The initial treatment should focus on reversing CO poisoning, if present, by the administration of high concentrations of humidified oxygen. CO levels may be reduced by half in about an hour when the patient breathes 100% oxygen. If severe CO poisoning is suspected, it is helpful to administer oxygen by nonrebreathing mask at flow rates higher than the victim's minute ventilation to achieve concentrations close to 100%. If results of clinical examination or arterial blood gas studies suggest alveolar hypoventilation, mechanical ventilation is necessary. Subsequently, the administration of oxygen may be important because of the hypoxemia resulting from bronchiolitis and alveolitis with premature closure of small airways. Constant positive distending airway pressure may also be necessary to maintain reasonable levels of PaO_2 without using excessively high and potentially toxic concentrations of inspired oxygen for prolonged periods of time.

Controversy exists regarding the importance of, and need for, hyperbaric oxygen in the management of CO poisoning. Hyperbaric oxygen at 2–3 atmospheres markedly hastens the decline of COHb levels, reducing the half-life of COHb to 20–25 minutes. However, the advantages of hyperbaric oxygen therapy may be offset by complications during transfer to the hyperbaric chamber. While some clinicians claim that all patients with significant COHb levels should be sent to a hyperbaric chamber, there is scant evidence for this approach.[63] There are no clear guidelines on the use of hyperbaric oxygen therapy in the treatment of CO poisoning. One review suggests using hyperbaric therapy for children with COHb levels of 25% or greater if symptomatic and for any with levels of 40% or higher.[67] The potential risks of the hyperbaric chamber include oxygen toxicity to the lung, the fact that patients are not amenable to appropriate observation and intervention while they are in the chamber, and the need for tympanotomy. More data are necessary to adequately assess the risks and benefits of hyperbaric oxygen in the therapy of CO poisoning in children related to fires.[68] Systematic reviews have not established whether hyperbaric oxygen therapy given to adult patients with CO poisoning reduces the incidence of adverse neurological outcomes[69]; consequently, its use in children remains controversial.

Endotracheal intubation may be necessary for a patient with any of the following conditions: (1) severe burns of the nose, face, or mouth, because of the likelihood that nasopharyngeal edema and obstruction will develop; (2) edema of the vocal cords with laryngeal obstruction; (3) difficulty handling secretions; (4) progressive respiratory insufficiency requiring mechanical ventilation; and (5) altered mental status that decreases minute ventilation and diminishes the protective reflexes of the airway. Regardless of whether the glottis is bypassed by endotracheal tube or tracheostomy tube, constant positive airway pressure or positive end-expiratory pressure helps minimize edema and improve oxygenation. Noninvasive positive pressure ventilation may be attempted in patients with acute respiratory decompensation who are otherwise hemodynamically stable, conscious, and without extensive and deep facial burns or trauma. This mode of ventilation has been reported to be effective in avoiding intubation/reintubation in a group of patients with burn-associated acute respiratory failure.[70] However, the risk of upper airway obstruction must be taken into account when selecting patients for noninvasive ventilation.

In addition to the increased airway resistance resulting from edema in and around the walls of airways, it is likely that some reflex bronchoconstriction occurs from irritation of airway receptors. This is more likely to occur in subjects with preexisting lung disease such as asthma or cystic fibrosis or in cigarette smokers. For this reason, it may be reasonable to administer inhaled bronchodilators.

Airway obstruction by cast material containing fibrin often accompanies smoke inhalation injury. In sheep with acute lung injury following burn and smoke inhalation injury, a combination of nebulized heparin and recombinant antithrombin has been demonstrated to improve pulmonary gas exchange and lung compliance, with decreased pulmonary edema, and airway obstruction.[71] In children with burn and smoke inhalation injury, nebulized heparin and N-acetylcysteine significantly decreased incidence of reintubation for progressive pulmonary failure, decreased incidence of atelectasis, and reduced mortality.[72] Similarly, in adults with smoke inhalation injury, nebulized heparin and N-acetylcysteine reduced lung-injury scores.[73]

Coagulation factors should be monitored as significant coagulopathy with prolonged partial thromboplastin time (PTT) has been associated with aerosolized heparin and N-acetylcysteine therapies for inhalation injury.[74] As in many other respiratory conditions, the role of chest physiotherapy is poorly defined. Nevertheless, mucociliary clearance is clearly impaired. The encouragement of deep breathing and cough, or gentle endotracheal suction in the presence of endotracheal intubation, coupled with postural drainage would seem to be reasonable. Using a cough-assist device might be considered.

Although corticosteroids are frequently advocated in the hope of suppressing inflammation and edema, most controlled studies fail to demonstrate a significant effect. Thus, it is difficult to marshal strong support for their use. Furthermore, long-term steroid therapy in victims of fires increases the susceptibility to infection. Until further evidence is available, the empirical use of corticosteroids is discouraged. One review suggests using corticosteroids only for evidence of peripheral airway obstruction, other illnesses requiring steroids, or recent use of steroids.[67] At the experimental level, ibuprofen (but not indomethacin) when given immediately after smoke inhalation injury prevented the development of pulmonary edema.[75] As animal studies further elicit the basic mechanisms of the events occurring within the airways and parenchyma, specific agents may become available to correct the pathophysiology.

Available evidence indicates that antimicrobial agents do not prevent subsequent infection and may only predispose to infection with resistant organisms. Because fever, elevated white blood cell count, and increased erythrocyte sedimentation rate may all result from smoke inhalation and because the chest roentgenogram may show nonspecific opacities that represent either atelectasis or edema, it may be extremely difficult to establish the presence of an infection in the absence of positive blood cultures or a positive Gram stain of airway secretions. It would seem preferable to reserve antimicrobial therapy for patients in whom there is clinical deterioration despite supportive therapy. Changes in the amount, nature, or color of the secretions should raise the suspicion of a bacterial superinfection, which should be confirmed by Gram stain or culture. Because the prevention of infection is clearly an important part of the therapy in victims of fires, aseptic care of the trachea and humidifying equipment is essential. In addition, in a retrospective analysis of children, high-frequency percussive ventilation was associated with a lower incidence of pneumonia.[76]

While dogs benefited from surfactant after smoke exposure,[77] rabbits did not.[78] To our knowledge, there are no data in human subjects. Smoke-exposed sheep did worse with ECMO support than with conventional mechanical ventilation. The ECMO was associated with pulmonary sequestration of leukocytes, increased pulmonary thromboxane B_2, increased blood-free wet/dry lung weight ratios, and more significant hypoxemia at 24 hours after identical degrees of smoke exposure.[79] Two children with inhalation injury and resultant respiratory failure refractory to conventional mechanical ventilation were successfully treated with ECMO.[80]

The Relationship of Pulmonary Injury From Smoke Inhalation to the Pulmonary Complications of Surface Burns

Pulmonary damage from smoke inhalation generally declares itself during the first 24 hours. Individuals with widespread surface burns may develop pulmonary complications after several days, but these late complications are not the result of direct chemical or thermal injury. It is more likely that late pulmonary injury is attributable to metabolic, infectious, or circulatory derangements complicating the surface burns.[65]

Surface burns may be directly and indirectly related to pulmonary pathophysiology. The large amounts of intravenous fluids usually given to counteract ongoing surface and "third-space" losses in the tissues may increase pulmonary edema through two mechanisms. First, there may be pulmonary vascular engorgement from diminished myocardial function due to CO poisoning, the initial hypoxia, and other toxins involved in the fire. Second, the diffuse inflammation within the airways increases vascular permeability with fluid leak into the areas of gas exchange, worsening the hypoxemia and causing additional pulmonary edema. Careful monitoring of fluid balance is critical in these children.

A second indirect relationship between the surface burns and the lung exists in the infection area. Clearly, the postburn lung is at risk for pneumonia. Organisms may also enter the body through the skin at the burn site, and scrupulous attention to the burn sites is necessary to reduce this possibility. The lung can be directly infected in pneumonia or as part of the sepsis syndrome.

The skin surface and lung may be directly related with severe skin burns of the thorax or upper abdomen. Chest wall edema or eschar formation, in addition to the pain at the skin site, increase the risk for hypoventilation and atelectasis.[81] Attention must be directed to skin manifestations (e.g., eschars) and pain control. Pain control with narcotics may increase the risk for hypoventilation, but this can be easily monitored, and adequate pain control is important for children with burns.

PREVENTION

Prevention is paramount when discussing smoke inhalation. Strategies for reducing fire-related injuries include increasing public fire safety education aimed at encouraging homeowners and property managers to install and maintain use of smoke alarms. Carbon monoxide detectors should be utilized in locations at risk for carbon monoxide exposure. Finally, families should develop and practice fire escape plans.

PROGNOSIS

Children with acute pulmonary injury from smoke inhalation generally recover once supported though the initial phase of illness. The severity of pulmonary parenchymal injury depends on the duration and type of inhalant exposure. The impact of smoke inhalation on long-term lung function in children may be dependent upon their stage of lung development at the time of injury as well as confounding lung injury sustained from acute respiratory distress syndrome, pneumonia, or acute lung injury. There are limited studies of the effect on lung function in children with smoke inhalation injury. Obstructive and mixed obstructive and restrictive defects have been reported in children 8 years following thermal injury.[82] Long-term sequelae of tracheal stenosis, bronchiectasis, interstitial fibrosis, and bronchiolitis obliterans may rarely be observed.

References

Access the reference list online at ExpertConsult.com.

Suggested Reading

Eade NR, Taussig LM, Marks MI. Hydrocarbon pneumonitis. *Pediatrics.* 1974;54:351–357.

Haponick E, Summer W. Respiratory complications in burned patients. Pathogenesis and spectrum of inhalation injury. *J Crit Care.* 1987;2:49–54.

Horoz OO, Yilizdas D, Yilmaz HL. Surfactant therapy in acute respiratory distress syndrome due to hydrocarbon aspiration. *Singapore Med J.* 2009;50:130–132.

Lewander WJ, Aleguas A. Petroleum distillates and plant hydrocarbons. In: Shannon MW, Borron SW, Burns MJ, eds. *Haddad and Winchester's Clinical Management of Poisoning and Drug Overdose.* 4th ed. Philadelphia: Saunders Elsevier; 2007:1343.

Ruddy RM. Smoke inhalation injury. *Pediatr Clin North Am.* 1994;41:317–336.

Scharf SM, Prinsloo I. Pulmonary mechanics in dogs given different doses of kerosene intratracheally. *Am Rev Respir Dis.* 1982;126:695–700.

Vale JA, Kulig KAmerican Academy of Clinical Toxicology, European Association of Poison Centres and Clinical Toxicologists. Position paper: gastric lavage. *J Toxicol Clin Toxicol.* 2004;42:933–943.

Van Gorcum TF, Hunault CC, Van Zoelen GA, et al. Lamp oil poisoning: did the European guideline reduce the number and severity of intoxications? *Clin Toxicol (Phila).* 2009;47:29–34.

Weaver LK, Hopkins RO, Chan KJ, et al. Hyperbaric oxygen for acute carbon monoxide poisoning. *N Engl J Med.* 2002;347:1057–1067.

41 *Drowning*

CHRISTOPHER J. L. NEWTH, MD, FRACP, FRCPC, JÜRG HAMMER, MD, and
ANDREW H. NUMA, MBBS, FRACP, FCICM

Definitions

A uniform definition of drowning was agreed upon during the World Congress on Drowning in Amsterdam, The Netherlands, in 2002.[1] Drowning is now defined as "a process resulting in primary respiratory impairment from submersion/immersion in a liquid medium." The term "drowning" now encompasses both fatal and nonfatal outcomes of immersion, and "near-drowning" is no longer used.

Epidemiology

Drowning occurs in all age groups and is responsible for approximately 4000 deaths per annum in the United States, with a mortality frequency of 12–18 deaths per million person years.[2,3] The highest mortality rates of approximately 30 deaths per million person years have been observed in the 0–4 and 15–19 year age groups,[2,3] although there is some evidence that both mortality and hospitalization rates have declined over the last 2 decades.[4] In the first year of life, drowning mortality in the United States is 63 per 100,000 live births.[3] Worldwide, drowning is the 11th most frequent cause of death in the 0–4 years age group, the third most frequent cause of death in children aged from 5 to 14 years,[5] and the second leading cause of injury-related death in childhood.[6] The vast majority of drowning deaths occur in non-Western countries; in Bangladesh, more children in the 1–4 years age group die from drowning than from diarrhea or respiratory infection.[7] Even in a well-developed country such as Australia, where drowning accounts for less than 1% of all reported deaths, there is a disproportionate rate of death in children. The rate of drowning is 4.6 per 100,000 per year for children under 5 years of age, three times the rate for adults.[2] In addition, worldwide, drowning episodes are believed to occur around 3–10 times more frequently than drowning.[8–12]

As with the majority of accidental deaths, there is a strong male preponderance with male-to-female incidence ratios ranging from 2:1 to 10:1.[2,3,6,11] Approximately one in three drowning fatalities occur in accomplished swimmers.[13] Children can and do drown in any receptacle containing water, from buckets to bathtubs to the ocean. The majority of drowning events occur in swimming pools (usually the child's home pool) for children aged under 4 years and in open water for older children.[2,8,14]

Drowning is most frequently a primary event. However, the presence of underlying disease such as epilepsy or cardiac arrhythmia should always be considered along with the possibility of drug or alcohol intoxication in older children. Approximately 6%–10% of drowning victims have a previous history of a seizure disorder,[2,15] and it has been estimated that children with epilepsy have a relative risk for drowning of 96 in the bathtub and 23.4 in a swimming pool compared to nonepileptic subjects.[15] A primary arrhythmia such as prolonged QT syndrome should always be considered, particularly in subjects who are capable swimmers.[16] Approximately 30%–50% of adolescents who drown are intoxicated with drugs or alcohol.[4,14,17]

Drowning Sequence

Based upon studies in animals,[18] the sequence of events in drowning has been reported as follows:

1. Immediate struggle
2. Suspension of movement with frequent swallowing
3. Violent struggle
4. Convulsions and spasmodic inspiratory efforts
5. Death

Loss of consciousness is thought to be related to hypoxia rather than hypercarbia.[13] Some observers have reported that human victims stop moving suddenly after swimming underwater and then float motionless on the surface of the water and subsequently disappear quietly.[12] The scenario of drowning without a struggle is probably due to a primary loss of consciousness secondary to other factors such as hypothermia[19] or cardiac arrhythmia.[8]

Sequelae of Submersion/Immersion Events

The drowning sequence has both pulmonary and nonpulmonary sequelae.

PULMONARY INJURY

The majority of drowning victims aspirate water (salt or fresh) at the time of drowning. However, in about 10% of cases, laryngospasm prevents the entry of water into the lungs.[11,20,21] The quantity of fluid aspirated is usually less than 22 mL/kg,[22] a volume that approximates the functional residual capacity (FRC). In cases where aspiration occurs, local insult arises secondary to infection, surfactant depletion, aspiration of debris, and fluid shifts that depend on the relative tonicity of body fluids and aspirated fluid. While radiological pulmonary edema is the most common finding, the incidence and degree appear to be the same irrespective of saltwater or freshwater immersion, although the mechanisms may be different. Seawater aspiration results in an osmotic gradient with fluid shifts into the alveolar spaces,[23–25] whereas aspirated freshwater is rapidly absorbed into the systemic circulation.[26,27] Pulmonary edema may arise in both seawater and freshwater aspiration secondary to neurogenic causes, forced inspiration against a closed glottis, and altered surfactant or pulmonary capillary permeability.[13,28]

Animal data suggests that 0.225% and 0.45% saline solutions are least injurious to the lungs in terms of gas exchange, possibly because they are rapidly absorbed from the alveolar spaces into the circulation along an osmotic gradient.[9,29–31] Freshwater will also be rapidly absorbed but causes rapid inactivation of surfactant and is probably the most injurious fluid to aspirate, followed closely by seawater, which is approximately 3% saline.[9] The presence of chlorine at 1–2 ppm in freshwater (typical of chlorinated domestic pools) does not affect the pulmonary injury.[9]

Although it has been postulated that drowning in hypertonic fluid may lead to hypovolemia secondary to fluid shifts into the alveolar spaces,[24] animal data indicates that hemodynamic changes following drowning are entirely attributable to hypoxia and are independent of the tonicity of the aspirated fluid.[9,29]

Sepsis may occur, including with unusual and or atypical organisms,[32] and significant allergic reactions to aspirated materials have been described.[33] The incidence of pneumonia in adult patients requiring mechanical ventilation, as deduced from a retrospective study in the Netherlands, is around 50%.[34]

Pathological findings are inconsistent and nonspecific. The most common finding in cases where the drowning medium has entered the lungs is the presence of reactive edema, with hyperinflation of the lungs and increase in lung weight *(emphysema acquosum);* however, these findings may also be seen in deaths from other causes including asphyxia and drug overdose.[35] Even where no water has been aspirated into the lungs, neurogenic pulmonary edema can occur.[28]

In severe cases of immersion/submersion accidents (with or without aspiration of fluid), some patients will develop pneumonia and pediatric acute respiratory distress syndrome (PARDS).[36] The management of this disorder is discussed elsewhere in this textbook (see Chapter 38). However, of the patients admitted to the Intensive Care Unit at Children's Hospital Los Angeles over the past 30 years after drowning events, less than 10% developed this serious complication. Figs. 41.1 and 41.2 show the typical radiological course of pulmonary injury in a drowning patient.

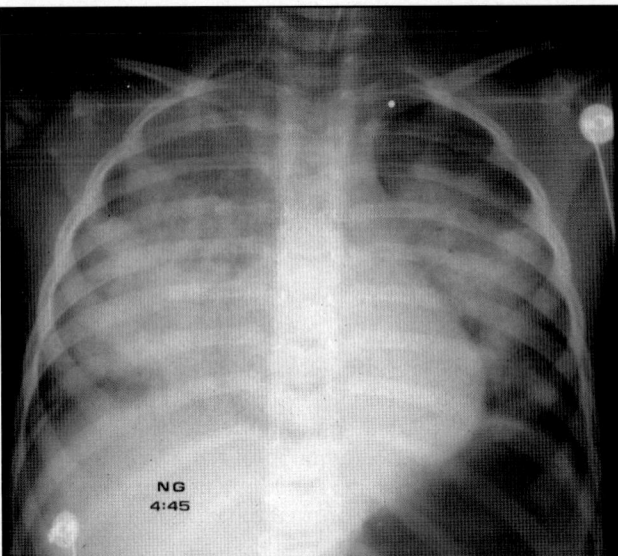

Fig. 41.1 Initial chest radiograph of a drowning victim. The patient has an endotracheal tube in place and a right subclavian venous line going up into the internal jugular vein. Moderate pulmonary edema and some aspiration pneumonitis are seen, especially on the right.

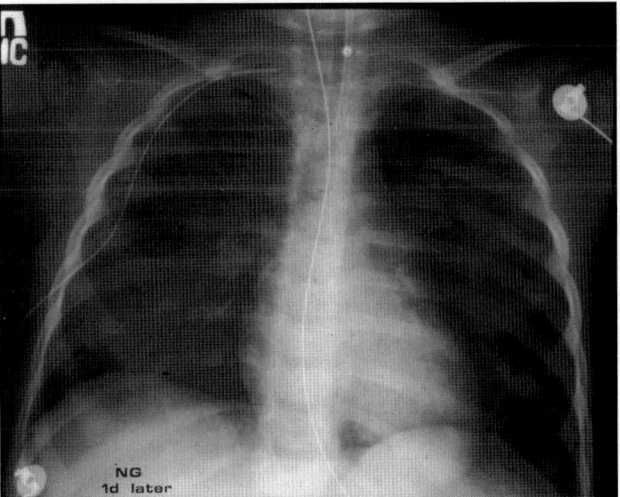

Fig. 41.2 Chest radiograph of the drowning victim shown in Fig. 41.1 taken 1 day after the event. The patient is still intubated and has a nasogastric tube into the stomach. The lung fields are almost clear again, but there is a chest tube on the right side that has drained a pneumothorax subsequent to right-sided aspiration pneumonia.

NONPULMONARY SEQUELAE

Hypothermia

Hypothermia is a common manifestation of drowning in water of almost any temperature, and there is anecdotal evidence that rapid hypothermia in a submersion incident is neuroprotective, particularly in children. Conductive losses through the skin are compounded by rapid heat exchange across the pulmonary capillaries if a significant volume of water is inhaled. In a canine model, dogs breathing water at 4°C demonstrated a decrease in carotid artery blood temperature of 8°C within 5 minutes.[19] Cooling occurs most rapidly in small infants who have a relatively large surface area.[37] In cases of extreme hypothermia, rewarming will be essential to allow return of cardiac function.[38,39] Hypothermia

can also play a major role in facilitating aspiration in immersion victims. As the core temperature drops below 35°C, muscular incoordination and weakness occur, which can interfere with swimming. As the core temperature decreases further, obtundation develops. At core temperatures below 30°C, unconsciousness can occur and the myocardium becomes irritable. Atrial fibrillation can occur, and at temperatures below 28°C, ventricular fibrillation is likely.

Electrolyte Imbalances

Electrolyte imbalances may arise if a significant amount of nonisotonic water is aspirated, although this is unusual in regular seawater.[40] Although freshwater immersion victims have decreased serum sodium, and saltwater immersion victims have elevated serum sodium and chloride levels,[20] these are rarely substantial or clinically significant. Even in the Dead Sea, which has electrolyte concentrations approximately 10 times higher than seawater, immersion victims rarely have severe abnormalities of sodium or chloride, although hypercalcemia and hypermagnesemia are common.[41,42] Hemolysis due to aspiration of hypotonic or hypertonic fluids appears to be an extremely infrequent complication.

Trauma

Traumatic injuries resulting from a fall into water must be considered but are generally of lesser importance than the immersion itself. Cervical spine injuries are the most critical to consider but are uncommon, occurring in only 0.5% of all nonfatal drowning cases, and only then in cases with a clear history of diving, motorized vehicle crash, or fall from a height.[43]

Hypoxic-Ischemic Damage

All organs are susceptible to hypoxic-ischemic injury following prolonged low cardiac output, and inadequate oxygenation and multiorgan failure is an almost inevitable consequence of severe submersion/immersion injury. Clinically, the brain is particularly susceptible, with the liver and the gastrointestinal tract being the most resistant.

MANAGEMENT

Management of the pulmonary injury will usually require supplemental oxygen, diuretic administration for pulmonary edema, and the most severe cases will require support with intubation and mechanical ventilation. Many of these serious immersion accidents occur in relatively isolated locales, and often children are intubated in the field or in outside facilities where there may be little experience managing children. Endotracheal tube sizes can be too large and sufficient to cause significant damage to the larynx if not recognized and promptly downsized after arriving at the receiving pediatric institution. In addition, with severe cases, the lung injury will comprise all the features of PARDS. The management of this disorder is addressed in Chapter 38.

Instillation of surfactant has been reported[44–46] and is an appealing therapeutic intervention given that the majority of victims aspirate a quantity of fluid that will denature and wash out existing surfactant. However, the temptation to administer surfactant should be considered in the context of recent randomized controlled trials demonstrating a lack of efficacy of surfactant in PARDS.[47–50] Administration of steroids appears to be effective in animal models of seawater aspiration,[51] and there is evidence to support the use of steroids in PARDS,[52] although this is by no means universally accepted.[53]

Broad-spectrum antibiotics should be administered to treat likely bacterial contamination of the lungs, such as after drowning in stagnant water.[36] The incidence of neurological infection is stated to be high, with a number of case reports in children.[54]

Most drowning victims will be hypothermic at the time of presentation. In cases of extreme hypothermia, rewarming will be essential to allow return of cardiac function,[38,39]

and if the core temperature is below 26°C–28°C, or the patient is in cardiac arrest, rewarming is probably best achieved using cardiopulmonary bypass.[55] Given the potential benefits of hypothermia on hypoxic CNS injury, it is our view that modest hypothermia (core temperature 32°C–34°C) should be maintained immediately following the injury until the patient reaches the receiving hospital if there is any suspicion of the patient having sustained a hypoxic brain injury. While duration of submersion, but not water temperature, is reported to be more associated with drowning outcome,[56] excellent neurological outcomes have been reported after prolonged immersion in very cold water, with several case reports indicating full neurological recovery after periods of up to 66 minutes in near-freezing water.[38,57,58] Children lose body heat more rapidly than adults, and if significant brain cooling occurs prior to cessation of circulation, then some degree of neuroprotection may occur. It has been estimated that brain temperature needs to fall by at least 3°C within the first 5 minutes of immersion for cerebral protection to be effective.[37]

The role of induced hypothermia for neuroprotection following drowning remains less certain. Some recent studies have highlighted the beneficial effects of hypothermia on a variety of hypoxic CNS injuries in humans.[59,60] However, these studies had control arms of "usual care," and some patients became hyperthermic with potential harmful effects and made the hypothermia group outcomes appear better.[61,62] In a Canadian trial using hypothermia in drowned children to reduce intracranial pressure and limit brain injury,[63] the death rate in the hypothermic group was higher than in the normothermic group, with most deaths attributed to neutropenic sepsis. However, this trial was relatively small, and the hypothermia group was also managed with hyperventilation and high-dose phenobarbitone, which may have influenced the outcomes. A randomized, controlled trial of therapeutic hypothermia versus normothermia after cardiac arrest outside of the hospital has been undertaken by 38 pediatric centers in the United States and Canada under the auspices of the National Institutes of Health. This study showed no benefit of hypothermia over rigorously controlled normothermia in either mortality or neurodevelopmentally in the 1-year follow-up of 295 survivors.[64] However, this study excluded patients with cardiac arrest secondary to drowning in ice water who had a core temperature of ≤32°C on presentation. In a subsequent report of the subset of the 74 pediatric cardiac arrest patients due to drowning from this study, it was concluded that hypothermia did not result in a statistically significant benefit in survival with good functional outcome or mortality at 1 year, as compared to normothermia.[65] Current Pediatric Advanced Life Support guidelines no longer recommend consideration of cooling to 32°C–34°C for 12–24 hours in comatose children following cardiac arrest, but support rigorous temperature control to avoid heating.[66]

OUTCOME OF PULMONARY INJURY

Routine tests of pulmonary function have been reported as normal in adults[67] following a drowning accident. However, in a series of 10 functionally normal children[68] studied 6 months to 8.5 years (mean 3.3 years) after the submersion incident, only one had completely normal pulmonary function. Seven had abnormal methacholine challenges demonstrating a high incidence of bronchial hyperreactivity, and five had clear evidence of peripheral airways disease. Whether these abnormalities were related solely to aspiration inherent in the drowning episode or further related to PARDS was not addressed.[69,70] It is possible these children are at risk for developing chronic lung disease, especially if exposed to further airway or parenchymal irritants.

OUTCOME PREDICTION OF NEUROLOGICAL INJURY

The best prognostic indicators are observed in the field. The strongest predictor of good outcome is duration of immersion. Poor outcomes are observed in 60%–100% of subjects immersed for greater than 10 minutes, compared to 0%–30% of those immersed for ≤5 minutes.[56] Good outcomes are also associated with the presence of sinus rhythm, reactive pupils, and neurologic responsiveness at the scene.[71] The presence of a detectable heartbeat and hypothermia (<33°C) on arrival to the Emergency Department discriminates intact survivors from those with persistent vegetative state or death.[72,73] Predictors of poor outcome include the presence of cardiac (as opposed to respiratory) arrest and the need for prolonged resuscitation (more than 20–25 minutes) or the requirement for more than two doses of epinephrine.[72–74]

The prediction of the neurologic outcome of those children who survive the initial resuscitation event and arrive in the intensive care unit in a comatose state is highly relevant for parents and caregivers. It is difficult to provide early and accurate prognostic information on comatose children, especially if brainstem functions are intact. Severity of illness scores such as the Pediatric Index of Mortality (PIM) and Pediatric Risk of Mortality (PRISM) scores were developed to predict the risk of death in groups of patients and not individuals. However, PRISM has recently been applied to individuals, and it enables the prediction of either absence or presence of serious neurological impairment or death in pediatric drowning patients if they present at extreme values on this scale. In patients with intermediate PRISM scores, though, it is not possible to establish a reliable prognosis.[75] Electrophysiological investigations, such as brainstem auditory evoked potentials and short-latency somatosensory evoked potentials (SSEP), are helpful to assess the likelihood of a permanent vegetative state or a higher level of cognition. The bilateral absence of SSEP is an established predictor for a worse clinical outcome after cerebral hypoxia.[76,77] Diffusion-weighted magnetic resonance imaging (DWI) provides a quick and reliable tool to detect early tissue injury in acute cerebral ischemia, because it is sensitive to water shifts between the extracellular and intracellular compartments, which conventional MRI often cannot detect. Preliminary results suggest that the extent of diffusion-weighted MRI pathology may serve as a reliable predictor for neurological outcome after cerebral hypoxia (Fig. 41.3).[78] Magnetic resonance spectroscopy also shows promise as a diagnostic and prognostic tool in hypoxic/ischemic cerebral injury, with reduced N-acetyl aspartate (NA) and elevated lactate both associated with poor neurological outcomes (Fig. 41.4).[79,80] Although computed tomography (CT) is not a sensitive test for ischemic injury, the presence of any CT abnormalities suggestive of ischemia (typically loss of gray-white differentiation and/or basal ganglia edema or infarction) within the first 3 days of drowning is strongly correlated with poor neurological outcome, and the presence of CT abnormalities in the first 24 hours is associated with a very high risk of mortality.[81]

PREVENTION

Drowning disproportionately affects children, and the majority are preventable. Drowning causes significant mortality

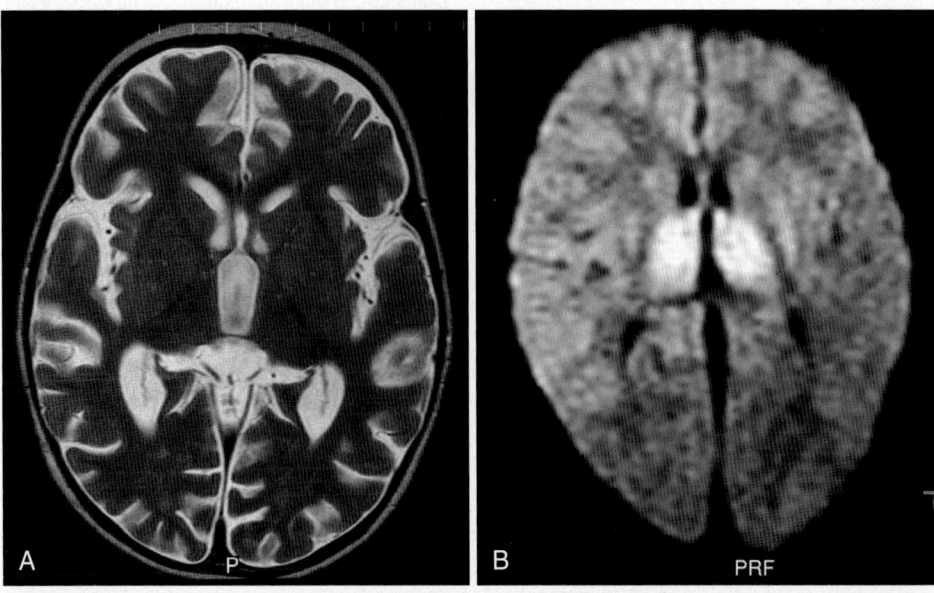

Fig. 41.3 Magnetic resonance imaging (MRI) of the brain of a 3-year-old child 36 hours after a drowning accident. The child remained in a persistent vegetative state. (A) The T2-weighted conventional MRI revealed no signs of hypoxia. (B) Diffusion-weighted imaging shows hyperintensity bilaterally in the basal ganglia.

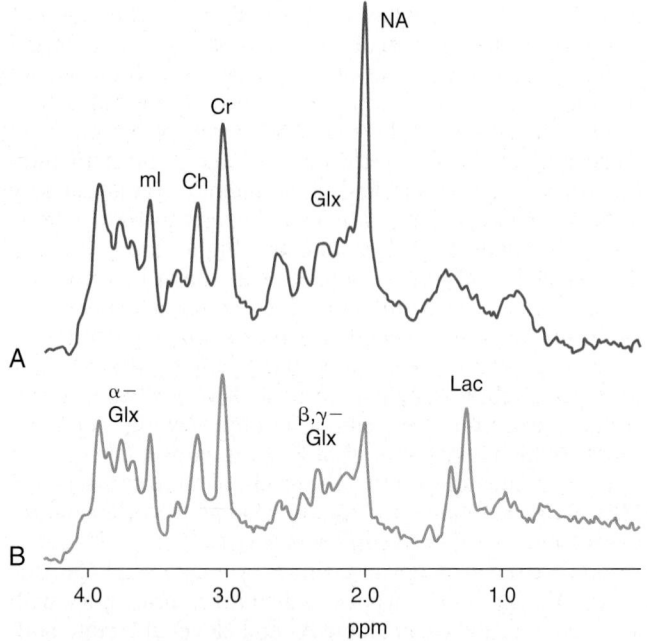

Fig. 41.4 Cerebral ¹H-MR spectra of occipital GM in a 3-year-old boy 48 hours after a severe immersion injury (B) compared with a control spectrum of a healthy age-matched subject (male, 4 years) in (A). The spectrum of the patient who died 70 hours after injury is characterized by a dramatic loss of NA (2.0, 2.6 ppm), a decrease in Cr (3.0 and 3.9 ppm), a large increase in Lac (1.3 ppm), and change in the resonances of Glu and Gln (3.75, 2.0–2.5 ppm). (From Kreis R, Arcinue E, Ernst T, Shonk TK, Flores R, Ross BD. Hypoxic encephalopathy after drowning studied by quantitative 1H-magnetic resonance spectroscopy. *J Clin Invest.* 1996;97:1145.)

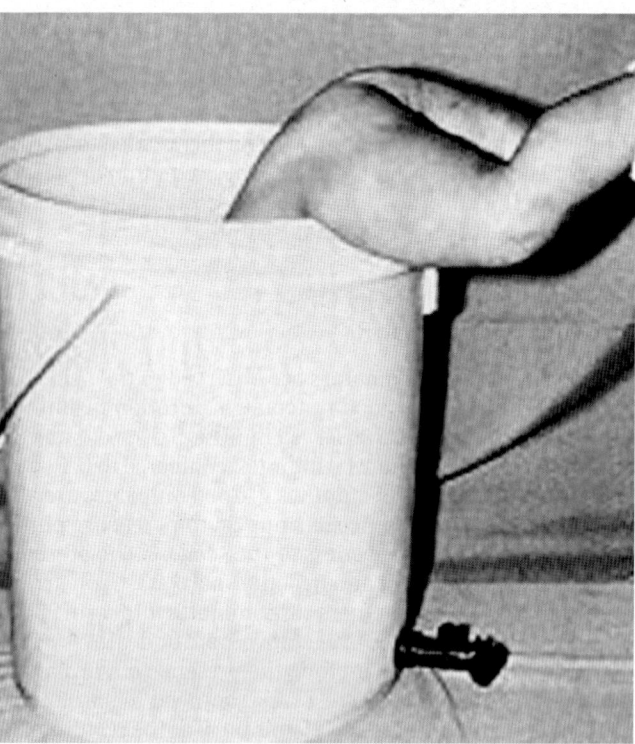

Fig. 41.5 The body of a small child who had tipped headfirst into a bucket of water. The upper segment (torso and head) of a child is longer and heavier than the lower segment (unlike an older child or adult), and he could not extract himself. (From Moon RE, Long RJ. Drowning and near-drowning. *Emerg Med.* 2002;14:378.)

and morbidity throughout the world, although modest decreases in the overall rates have been reported recently in the United States.[82] Factors that appear to have reduced the number of those drowned each year are legislative and public health interventions such as pool fencing and public education campaigns that have improved awareness of the dangers of leaving children unattended in bathtubs and of large commercial-type buckets into which smaller children can fall but not extricate themselves (Fig. 41.5). Participation in formal swimming lessons has been demonstrated to be an effective preventative strategy in younger (1–4 years old) but not older children.[83] So far, improvements in postresuscitation care have not been shown to alter outcome significantly if there has been an out-of-hospital cardiac arrest.

References

Access the reference list online at ExpertConsult.com.

Suggested Reading

Bowman SM, Aitken ME, Robbins JM, et al. Trends in US pediatric drowning hospitalizations, 1993–2008. *Pediatrics.* 2012;129:275–281.

Idris AH, Berg RA, Bierens JJ, et al. Recommended guidelines for uniform reporting of data of drowning. The "Utstein Style." *Circulation.* 2003; 108:2565–2574.

Laptook A, Tyson J, Shankaran S, et al. Elevated temperature after hypoxic-ischemic encephalopathy: risk factor for adverse outcomes. *Pediatrics.* 2008;122:491–499.

Moler FW, Hutchison JS, Nadkarni VM, et al. Targeted temperature management after pediatric cardiac arrest due to drowning: outcomes and complications. *Pediatr Crit Care Med.* 2016;17:712–720.

Quan L, Bierens JJ, Lis R, et al. Predicting outcome of drowning at the scene: a systematic review and meta-analyses. *Resuscitation.* 2016; 104:63–75.

Rafaat KT, Spear RM, Kuelbs C, et al. Cranial computed tomographic findings in a large group of children with drowning: diagnostic, prognostic, and forensic implications. *Pediatr Crit Care Med.* 2008;9:567–572.

Asthma

42 *The Epidemiology of Asthma*

ALEXANDER JOHN HENDERSON, MD, FRCP, FRCPCH, FRCPEd

Overview

Asthma is one of the most common noncommunicable chronic diseases of childhood. It creates a major public health and economic burden on society through its impact on mortality, morbidity, lost school days for children, lost workdays for parents, quality of life (QoL), and costs of health care. Epidemiologic studies have tracked changes in asthma prevalence across time and place and have provided insights into some of the environmental influences that might influence asthma onset, severity, persistence, and outcome. Longitudinal cohort studies have pointed to early life factors, including genetic predisposition, as being critically important in the development of asthma; however, its cause remains elusive. Recent advances in understanding the genetics of asthma and the application of more robust causal epidemiologic models to the consideration of modifiable exposures associated with asthma onset and natural history have started to get around some of the traditional problems of bias and confounding in epidemiology that hamper the identification of the true causes of disease. This chapter will review asthma epidemiology with particular emphasis on how technological and methodological progress can help unlock the potential of the considerable recent growth of asthma epidemiologic studies around the world.

Epidemiologic Approaches to the Study of Asthma

The goal of epidemiology is to identify modifiable factors that influence disease in populations, thus leading to interventions that will prevent disease from occurring or alter its natural history, either by cure or other reduction in the burden of disease. There are several different study designs that have been used in epidemiology to achieve these aims, of which the randomized control trial (RCT) provides the highest level of evidence for a causal relationship between a risk factor and the disease outcome. This is because covariables associated with the risk factor of interest could themselves influence the disease outcome; for example, many environmental exposures are strongly socially patterned and therefore associated with other variables that are influenced by socioeconomic factors. An illustration of this is that people who work in low-income jobs tend to live in disadvantaged, urban areas where they are exposed to poor housing conditions (damp, molds) and more traffic-related pollution, and their lifestyles are more likely to include higher tobacco and alcohol consumption and less physical exercise. Therefore, in a well-designed RCT where subjects are randomly assigned to an intervention ("risk" factor) or comparison (control) group, their additional environmental and lifestyle factors will also be randomly assorted between the intervention and comparison groups. This means that it can be reasonably inferred that any differences in outcome between the two groups is due solely to the intervention being studied.

In all other conventional epidemiologic study designs, these factors remain as possible explanatory variables that confound the relationship between exposure and outcome. A cross-sectional study samples a population at a point in time, collecting information on exposures and outcomes contemporaneously. It is a relatively quick and resource-effective study design, but suffers from uncertainty about the direction of associations between risk factors and disease. (Did A cause B or did B cause A, or did an unknown C cause both?) A case-control study recruits established cases of disease and draws comparable subjects from a suitable source, such as health care settings, electoral rolls, etc. Exposure history is ascertained retrospectively and therefore subject to problems of recall; differential recall of exposure between cases and controls will introduce bias. This design can consider many different exposures for the disease of interest and is relatively quick to perform as the outcome is already known. The other major study design for epidemiologic purposes is the cohort study, which follows a population sample that is disease-free at recruitment to ascertain disease outcome after a period of time. Exposures are ascertained prospectively so the direction of association between exposure and outcome can usually be reasonably inferred. A particular type of cohort study, the birth cohort in which infants are recruited at birth and followed for many years, has been instrumental in shaping our understanding of the evolution of asthma during childhood and the exposures in early life, including before birth, that influence the onset and the natural history of asthma throughout childhood and beyond. Although it is helpful to establish temporal associations between exposure and disease, as with all study designs the sources of bias and error need to be minimized. A particular issue with cohort studies is loss to follow-up of the initial sample. Where a factor, such as continued participation in a cohort study or recruitment of a clinic sample, is affected by exposure status and outcome, conditioning analysis on this factor, for example, complete-case analysis, can introduce spurious (noncausal) associations between the two variables on which it depends, a form of collider bias described by Berkson[1] and referred to as Berkson bias or paradox. Another variation of the cohort design is an historical cohort study, where an exposure has been measured previously in a disease-free population and that population is contacted at a later date so that outcomes can be ascertained. A good example of this comes from historical records of birth weight in a population of adult males that were traced, and in whom cardiovascular and respiratory outcomes were measured in old age. These showed strong associations between low birth weight and increased risk of cardiovascular disease, low lung function and chronic obstructive pulmonary disease (COPD) and were instrumental in formulating the concept of the developmental origins hypothesis of health and disease throughout the life course.[2] Finally,

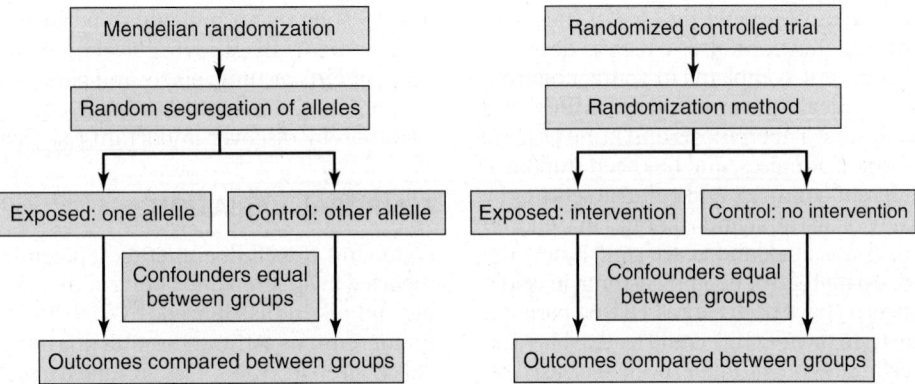

Fig. 42.1 Comparison of design of Mendelian randomization studies and randomized controlled trials. (From Davey Smith G, Ibrahim S. What can Mendelian randomisation tell us about modifiable behavioural and environmental exposures? *BMJ.* 2005;330:1076. doi:10.1136/bmj.330.7499.)

an ecological study can be conducted by ascribing exposures and/or outcomes to groups of individuals defined geographically, for example, by country of residence, or temporally. Exposures and outcomes are averaged across populations and thus cannot be ascribed to individuals within these population groups.

Confounders can be taken into account in analyses that control for their influence, but it is seldom the case that all possible confounders can be accounted for, either because they were not measured or in some cases could not be measured, giving rise to residual confounding. One of the difficulties of investigating asthma epidemiology is the huge range of potential explanatory variables that might influence population disease risk, and, hence, confound the associations between risk factors and asthma outcomes. A further complication is the heterogeneity of asthma, which varies in several domains, such as age of onset, frequency and severity of symptoms, response to treatment, association with allergy, and natural history over the life course of the individual. It is conceivable that different types of asthma manifest as phenotypic variation (*phenotypes*) underpinned by variation in biological pathways (*endotypes*) that may, in turn, be influenced by different risk factors. If this is the case, modest associations between risk factors and asthma in a population may mask large effects in a subpopulation with a specific phenotype. An example of this might occur with occupational exposures, such as wheat flour causing "baker's" asthma, which applies to only a limited proportion of a population and results in a specific type of asthma that could be missed without a proper occupational history and its temporal relationship to symptoms. In this instance, modification of the risk factor will likely have no detectable benefit in the population unless it is restricted to those with the risk phenotype. The problem of residual confounding has beset observational epidemiology from its outset and, although criteria have been developed to help strengthen the evidence for casualty, there are many examples in the literature of strong epidemiologic associations that were not confirmed by RCT evidence; indeed, in some cases, associations were discovered to be in the opposite direction. Technological advances that are applicable to population studies enabling large-scale genotyping have led to the discovery of genetic variants (single nucleotide polymorphisms [SNPs]) that influence exposures that themselves may be risk factors for disease, for example, birth weight and smoking behavior. Because

genotype is randomly allocated at meiosis, a situation analogous to the RCT can be constructed (with certain constraints) using genetic instruments as an unconfounded proxy for exposure in the mendelian randomization design (Fig. 42.1).[3] As genetic knowledge increases, it is hoped that this approach will allow better inference of casual relationships between exposures and asthma, thus enabling targeting of intervention studies to variables that have stronger prior evidence of causing disease.

Defining Asthma in Epidemiologic Studies

To the majority of clinicians, the diagnosis of asthma appears to be relatively straightforward. A combination of a clinical history of the cardinal symptoms of cough, wheeze, and breathlessness varying over time and associated with identifiable triggers supplemented by measures of airflow obstruction that varies spontaneously or in response to short-acting bronchodilators provides a high prior probability of asthma in children. National and international evidence-based guidelines have been developed to assist pediatricians and primary care physicians in making a diagnosis of asthma and directing its management: http://www.nhlbi.nih.gov/health-pro/guidelines/current/asthma-guidelines; https://www.brit-thoracic.org.uk/guidelines-and-quality-standards/asthma-guideline/; http://ginasthma.org/.

Of course, although the diagnosis of asthma is often straightforward and treatment effective, there are exceptions when the diagnosis is in doubt, particularly in infants and preschool children, or treatment does not produce the expected reduction in symptoms. Great efforts have been made to avoid underdiagnosis and undertreatment of asthma, which was a perceived problem in the past, but recent concerns have been raised in high-income countries (HICs) that asthma may now be overdiagnosed in some settings, highlighting some of the uncertainties that remain in clinical recognition of the condition. The continued recognition of avoidable asthma deaths in children, however, emphasizes the importance of maintaining a balance that appropriately recognizes and treats children at risk. In epidemiologic studies, which are carried out at population rather than individual level, it is usually impracticable to clinically examine every participant to identify cases of asthma, so different methods need to be employed. The most frequently used of these has been the written asthma questionnaire, which is designed to be self-completed or parent-completed in young children. This evolved from the Medical Research Council (MRC)[4] and International Union against Tuberculosis and Lung Disease (IUTLD)[5] respiratory questionnaires, and has been standardized for use across different countries and cultural settings by the International Study of Asthma and Allergies in Children (ISAAC) survey (http://isaac.auckland.ac.nz/) and is now the most commonly reported method of defining asthma in epidemiologic studies. Concerns have been expressed that parental understanding of the term "wheezing" could lead to bias and misclassification in estimates of asthma prevalence based on questionnaire surveys. Parents' perception of wheezing has been found to be imprecise compared with clinical findings,[6] different wording of questionnaires can affect prevalence estimates,[7] and clinician-confirmed compared with parent-only reported wheezing was associated with measured airway obstruction in young children,[8] suggesting misclassification of asthma in the latter group. Understanding of the term "wheeze" may also differ between ethnic groups, leading to overestimation or underestimation of its prevalence. The development of a video questionnaire for adolescent children by the ISAAC team (http://isaac.auckland.ac.nz/phases/phasethree/videoquestionnaire.html) sought to address the linguistic and sociocultural differences in questionnaire interpretation. This has been validated against bronchial hyperresponsiveness (BHR) in a number of settings with some variation but generally satisfactory agreement. Comparison of the video with the written questionnaire suggests that their agreement is moderate, although the latter may underestimate the prevalence of asthma symptoms in 10- to 12-year-olds.[9] In contrast, an earlier study in a different setting, while suggesting generally good agreement in 13- to 14-year-olds reported that the video questionnaire identified fewer cases than the written questionnaire.[10] A UK cohort study linked responses to asthma questionnaires in a longitudinal birth cohort to primary care diagnoses in electronic patient records and reported that questions about wheezing had high sensitivity but low specificity for a diagnosis of asthma, and BHR was only found in 50% with a primary care diagnosis.[11] Therefore, it is important to be aware of the possible sources of error and bias in epidemiologic estimates of asthma prevalence, particularly when comparing changes over time, or variations across different study settings. It is equally important to recognize that a population of children with asthma identified through an epidemiologic survey will differ from a clinic population, usually through the inclusion of a greater proportion with less severe asthma, and with a greater chance of misclassification, whatever methods are used. Supplementing responses to a written questionnaire with an objective test, such as bronchial responsiveness to a chemical or physical challenge, is likely to increase specificity but reduce sensitivity of identifying asthma cases.

The Prevalence of Asthma

The prevalence of asthma varies by time, place, and person (population). Asthma is generally accepted to occur as a consequence of genetic factors interacting with the environment and lifestyle of an individual, perhaps at critical stages of development. By studying variations of prevalence across the domains of time, place, and person, it is possible to gain insight into the factors influencing asthma in different settings and thereby discover important risk factors for the disease.

TEMPORAL VARIATION

Following a well-documented epidemic of asthma deaths reported in children and young adults (5–34 years) in several, but not all, industrialized HICs in the 1960s, Burr reported an increase in asthma hospital discharges of 5- to 14-year-old children in Wales. This prompted a series of cross-sectional surveys at intervals, which demonstrated a doubling in the prevalence of ever having asthma in children in South Wales from 6% in 1973 to 12% in 1988; 15 years later. A similar trend was seen in 6–11-year-old children in the US National Health and Nutrition Examination Survey (NHANES) between the early and late 1970s, and in a number of other countries over a comparable epoch from the early 1970s through the 1990s, including the UK, Scandinavia, Israel, New Zealand, and Australia. These mainly relied on parental report of wheeze and/or asthma in repeat cross-sectional surveys of parents in the same geographical setting. By 2000, there were indications that the rising prevalence in childhood asthma in high-income, developed countries was coming to an end. A Swiss study based on national surveillance data suggested that this reversal of the previous trend could be explained by fewer consultations for allergic asthma.[12] One of the longest running surveys of asthma and allergy symptoms started in Aberdeen, UK, in 1964, and has used the same methods in repeat studies of the same age group of children in an economically stable environment with low levels of migration in studies spanning a 50-year period. The original surveys showed contemporaneous rises in the prevalence of asthma, eczema, and rhinitis in this age group of children, pointing to a common etiology mediated through influences on allergic mechanisms. However, later studies, which confirmed a "flattening" of the previous trend for increased prevalence of these conditions similar in magnitude and direction to results from comparable HICs, showed a continued rise in the lifetime prevalence of eczema and hay fever, thus throwing doubt on a common etiology of these conditions.[13] Therefore, the summation of evidence, largely from repeat surveys using identical methodology in different settings, suggests that reported asthma prevalence and the prevalence of asthma symptoms showed an increase from the early 1990s until around the end of the 20th century. However, there are a number of considerations that need to be taken into account before accepting this as evidence for a true increase in disease prevalence. These include changes over time in diagnostic coding, such as changes in the International Classification of Diseases (ICD) definitions; diagnostic preference, such that wheezing illnesses may or may not be labeled as asthma; increased population awareness leading to more presentations to health care with asthmalike symptoms; and systematic bias in questionnaire responses. Although repeat surveys were carried out in comparable groups from similar strata of society, they were not the same individuals or families, so they may have differed in their responses without there being a true change in symptoms. Subsequent analyses have suggested a diagnostic shift explaining part of the observed increase in prevalence, but there is still evidence that at least part of the rise in asthma prevalence was real. The ISAAC study has provided a global perspective of these changes in symptoms over time through incorporation of a repeat survey in the third phase of the study (ISAAC phase III), which was designed to describe time trends and factors associated with these in the centers that completed phase I, which established baseline estimates and their geographical variation. Phase III followed the initial phase by at least 5 years with an average interval of 7 years. The study gathered data from over 190,000 6- to 7-year-olds in 37 countries and over 300,000 13- to 14-year-olds in 56

countries. These showed that between 1992 and 1998, and 1999 and 2004, centers were about equally distributed between substantial increases and decreases in the prevalence of asthma symptoms, whereas in 6- to 7-year-olds more centers showed an increase than a decrease in prevalence (Fig. 42.2). Analysis of the relationship of time trends between asthma, eczema, and rhinitis showed that the strongest correlation was between eczema and rhinoconjunctivitis, and the weakest between eczema and asthma. However, the relationships overall showed consistency across the study period, suggesting that similar factors are affecting them at a global level,[14] and there was no strong association with

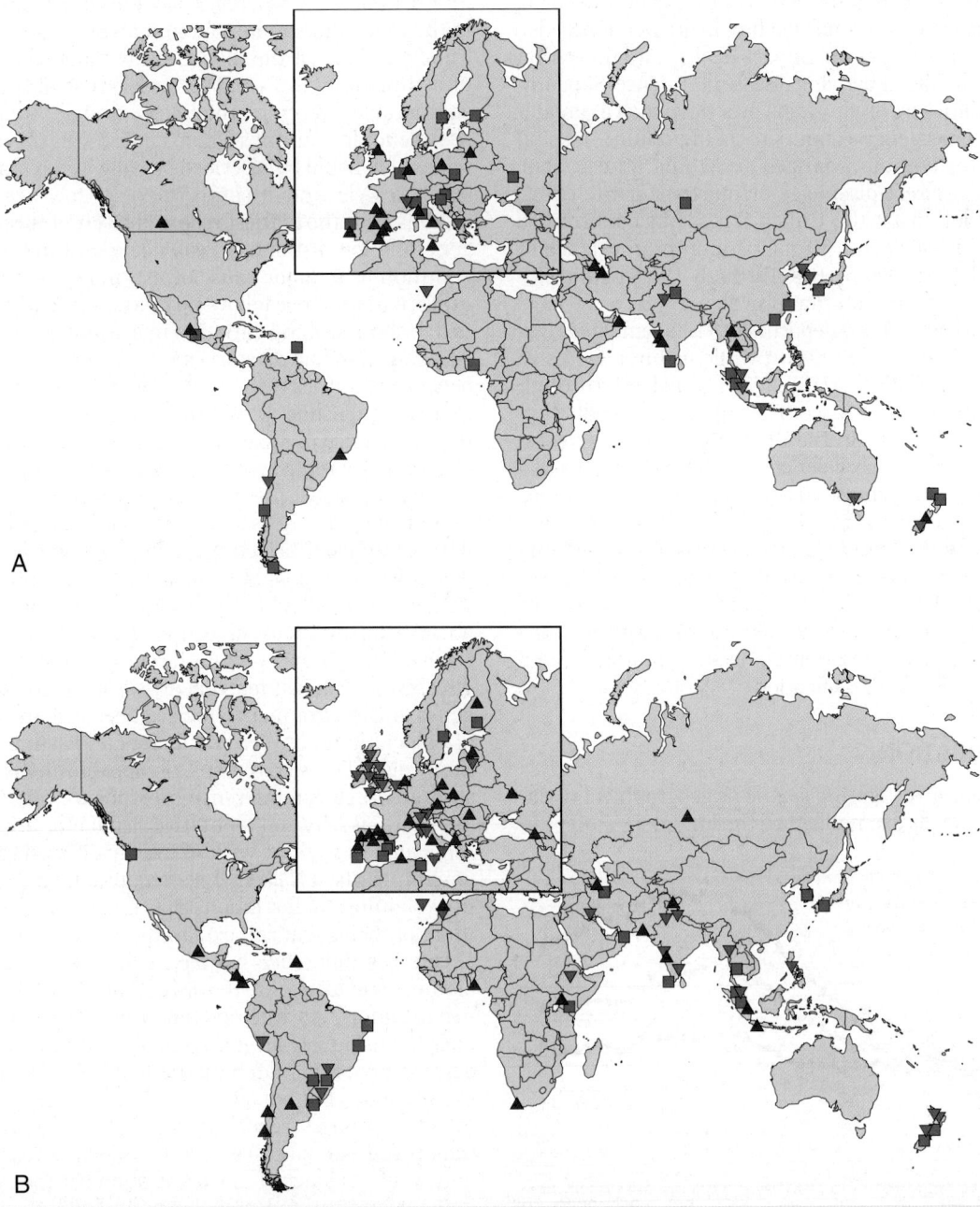

Fig. 42.2 World map showing the direction of change in the prevalence of asthma symptoms for the 6- to 7-year age group (A) and 13- to 14-year age group (B). Each symbol represents a center. *Blue triangle* = prevalence reduced by ≥1 Standard Error per year. *Green square* = little change (<1 Standard Error). *Red triangle* = prevalence increased by ≥ 1 Standard Error per year. (From Asher MI, Montefort S, Björkstén B; ISAAC Phase Three Study Group. Worldwide time trends in the prevalence of symptoms of asthma, allergic rhinoconjunctivitis, and eczema in childhood: ISAAC Phases One and Three repeat multicountry cross-sectional surveys. *Lancet*. 2006;368(9537):733-743.)

gross national income across the low-income countries to HICs comprising the study centers, despite differences in the proportion of atopic and nonatopic asthma between high- and low-to-middle income countries; nonatopic asthma is more prevalent in the latter.[15]

To address the question of whether reported increases in the prevalence of reported symptoms of asthma represent a true underlying change in disease incidence and/or natural history, it is instructive to consider other markers of disease activity that may indicate whether the figures reflect a change across all grades of asthma severity or the inclusion of a greater proportion of milder disease; the latter could represent diagnostic shift to include milder cases or a true change in asthma severity or its management. For example, better drug treatments or behavioral shifts leading to greater adherence to asthma medication, could impact health care utilization without affecting the underlying disease prevalence. Similarly, changes in health care organization over time, such as greater emphasis on emergency room care, could reduce hospital admission rates without changes in asthma attack rates, perhaps due to direct discharge of more moderate cases. Surveillance data from the United States has confirmed a 4.6% annual increase in asthma 12-month prevalence in children (<17 years) from 1980 through 1995 with a stabilization of current asthma prevalence since 1997.[16] Asthma-related emergency department visits remained relatively stable between 1992–2006 while asthma deaths in US children increased by 3.2% per year from1980 through 1996 and have since decreased. These data are broadly supported by similar trends in the UK[17]; children (<14 years) had increased reported prevalence of asthma symptoms and about an eight-fold increase in primary care consultations for asthma between the 1970s and mid-1990s. This was accompanied by increased hospital admissions for asthma until 1990, since when they declined (Fig. 42.3). The evidence of increased prevalence of asthma of all grades of severity during the last few decades of the 20th century support a true increase in disease prevalence rather than a broadening of disease classification.

SPATIAL VARIATION

The potential of investigating spatial or geographical variations in asthma was exemplified by the landmark studies in

Germany following its reunification in 1990. The distinct advantages of this setting were the shared genetic ancestry of the populations of East and West Germany coupled with the contrasting lifestyles and environments of the German Democratic Republic in the East and the Federal Republic of Germany in the West. Thus, it was possible to investigate different environmental influences in two genetically similar groups. At the time, the contemporaneous increase of asthma prevalence in the West and the marked increases in road traffic densities had indicated traffic-related pollution as a possible contributor to asthma etiology. It was reported that the prevalence of atopic sensitization, hay fever, and asthma was higher in children born in the West, where traffic-related pollution dominated, whereas bronchitis prevalence was higher in the East, where industrial sources of pollution persisted.[18] The first phase of the ISAAC study mapped the prevalence of asthma in 6- to 7- and 13- to 14-year-old children using comparable survey methodology, and showed the highest prevalence in countries where English was the first language and which could be described broadly as having a "Westernized" lifestyle, and in Latin America. However, some of the regions with the highest reported levels of air pollution had generally low asthma prevalence, pointing away from air pollution as a major cause of asthma onset (as opposed to exacerbations). The follow-up phase 3 ISAAC report continued to show striking variation in asthma prevalence (http://isaac.auckland.ac.nz/story/methods/maps.php#mapMenu) between countries with similar regional patterns to the phase 1 study published 11 years earlier, and was mirrored by the prevalence of symptoms of severe asthma; high prevalence was associated with HICs. Intercountry comparisons of asthma prevalence present an opportunity for ecological analyses of the differences in lifestyles and exposures associated with asthma in these settings. Although such approaches can give clues about possible etiologic factors, population genetic differences could influence the environmental exposures that are instrumental in asthma onset in different populations. This is particularly important in the study of complex, polygenic diseases, such as asthma, that arise from interactions between genes and environment. However, because the confounders of associations between risk factors and asthma almost certainly differ between regions, an opportunity is presented to strengthen causal inference of exposure-outcome links. If associations between a putative risk factor and asthma are replicated in settings with markedly different lifestyles and environments, it is likely that confounding plays a lesser role in explaining such relationships, making the risk factor the more probable (causal) explanation.

One key difference between countries with contrasting asthma prevalence in the ISAAC studies is the degree of urbanization. An attempt has been made to address this question using satellite images to estimate the extent of urban development and matching these to ISAAC study centers.[19] Despite some, but not all, regional studies, mostly set in low-income countries, reporting links between increased urbanization and asthma prevalence, this global perspective showed only weak evidence of any association between urban development and asthma prevalence, including severe asthma symptoms, in children. Considering asthma prevalence in HICs, there is clear evidence from the United States that asthma prevalence is higher in urban areas with a high proportion of ethnic minority populations, and this is reflected

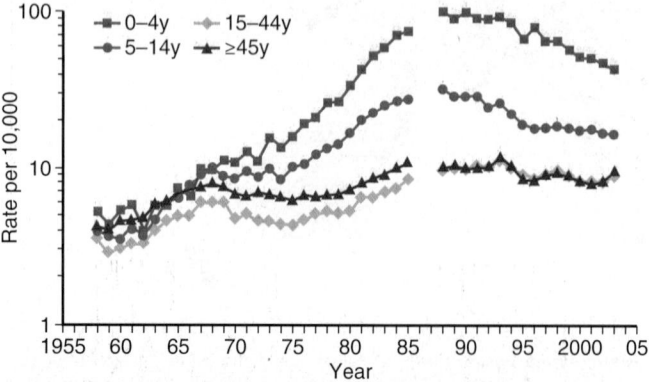

Fig. 42.3 Hospital admissions for asthma by age, England and Wales 1958–2003. (From Anderson HR, Gupta R, Strachan DP, Limb ES. 50 years of asthma: UK trends from 1955 to 2004. *Thorax* 2007 Jan;62(1):85–90.)

in higher indicators of morbidity and mortality in children of Hispanic and African-American origin. Many possible explanatory factors for this observation have been suggested, including genetic predisposition and environmental exposures associated with social disadvantage, such as outdoor and indoor air pollution, allergens, infectious agents, and diet. These will be considered further under etiologic factors associated with asthma. A further ecologic association arising from the ISAAC studies is the low prevalence of reported asthma in countries where a high proportion of the population lives in rural areas with reliance on subsistence farming. These observations are consonant with studies from rural communities, mainly in middle Europe, but replicated in other settings, where the prevalence of asthma and allergy has been reported to be lower in children growing up on farms and exposed to livestock and other factors, such as drinking unpasteurized milk. The common mediating factor of this protective effect is now believed to be early life exposure to microorganisms and their cellular constituents, including endotoxins. Higher levels of endotoxin in dust collected from farms has been associated with lower prevalence of sensitization and allergic diseases, although later exposure from household dust can exacerbate asthma symptoms in urban settings.[20,21] Recent evidence suggests that the protective effect of endotoxin exposure in early life is mediated through induction of an enzyme (A20) in the pulmonary epithelium that modifies interactions between the epithelium,[22] antigen-presenting cells, and the innate immune system.[23]

Of particular interest in the geophysical variation of asthma prevalence is the effect of migration between settings with widely varying rates of asthma. Migrants from countries with low asthma prevalence to high prevalence countries have acquired the rates of asthma in the local population, with the effect dependent on the time spent in the adopted country. There is also evidence that the younger age at which migration occurred in these circumstances, the higher the prevalence of later asthma, lending support to the early origins hypothesis that environment in infancy and early childhood is critical for the development of diseases through the life course. The ISAAC study group has recently analyzed data on migration and reported that being born outside the country of study was associated with a lower prevalence of asthma in both 6- to 7- and 13- to 14-year-old children. This protective effect was restricted to affluent countries and was not evident in low-income settings with low asthma prevalence. It was also lost with increasing time spent in the host country, and points to environmental factors as opposed to genetic factors being important in the variation of the prevalence of asthma between countries.[24,25]

VARIATION BY GENDER AND ETHNICITY

Asthma prevalence is disproportionately higher in black and ethnic minority populations than in white children of European ancestry. The explanations for such disparities are likely to be multifactorial and include genetic and environmental influences, urban living, poverty, and access to health care.[26] Although asthma has high heritability, racial and ethnic minorities are underrepresented in genetic studies of asthma (see: http://www.ebi.ac.uk/gwas/home for a catalog of genome wide association studies [GWAS]) and the current commercially available chips for genome wide, SNP screens were derived from populations of mainly European descent. In Southern California, a study using genetic markers of ancestry in Hispanic children showed that those with a lower proportion of African ancestry were at a lower risk for asthma than those who had major contributions from European or Amerindian ancestries.[27] In common with many other developed, Anglophone countries, asthma prevalence in children in the United States approximately doubled from the early 1980s until the late 1990s. At the beginning of this period, there was little disparity between white and black children, whereas by 2010, the prevalence in African-American children was twice that of their white peers.[28] During the period from 2000 onwards, when the previous increase in asthma prevalence in US children has plateaued, the disparity between asthma in black and white children also stopped increasing. This was largely due to a slowdown in the increasing prevalence of non-Hispanic black children, although asthma prevalence in some groups continued to rise, including those from a deprived socioeconomic background.[29] In addition to higher asthma prevalence, African-American and Hispanic children in the United States were reported previously to have increased rates of hospitalization, emergency department use, and mortality due to asthma than their white counterparts, although a national analysis of in-patient data has reported increased mortality only for Native American children and not for other racial or ethnic groups.[30] In the same study, the length of hospital stay after admission for an asthma attack was related to indicators of social deprivation but was shorter in Asian than in white children. In the UK Leicester Respiratory cohort, which has a high proportion of South Asian participants, a higher prevalence of ever having wheezed was reported in Asian compared with white children, but current symptoms of wheeze and night cough at age 6 years were similar between the two groups.[7] In this study, associations with risk factors were also similar between white and South Asian children. Others have reported racial disparities in some associations, including body mass index (BMI), which was more strongly associated with asthma in US children who were male, non-Hispanic black, and living in deprived neighborhoods,[31] traffic-related air pollution (TRAP), which was associated with hospital readmission in white but not African-American children,[32] and possibly airway inflammatory responses to environmental tobacco smoke (ETS) in adolescents.[33] Intriguingly, racial differences in treatment responses in severe, therapy-resistant asthma have been reported, with poorer fractional exhaled nitric oxide (FeNO) responses in black than white children to intramuscular steroid injections.[34] The mechanism of this has yet to be discovered, although differences in genes affecting pharmacologic responses are likely to be important and could pave the way to personalized approaches to treatment.[35]

Asthma is more common in males in early childhood but a gender switch in asthma prevalence occurs around the time of puberty, so asthma prevalence in young adults is higher in females than males; although reporting bias in favor of asthma in young males has been suggested to explain at least part of the apparent gender switch.[36] The ISAAC study reported a higher prevalence of asthma in males at 6–7 years and a higher prevalence in females at 13–14 years with considerable variation between centers. In the UK longitudinal Isle of Wight cohort, males had a higher prevalence of asthma up to 10 years, which had reversed to higher female prevalence by 18 years, with more wheezing females gaining an asthma diagnosis between 10 and 18 years.[37] Some cross-sectional studies have suggested that the sex discordance in asthma observed through the peripubertal period has become less exaggerated in recent years. There is some uncertainty about the precise age at which the gender switch occurs and its relation to the onset and timing of puberty. Symptom severity has been reported to be greater in boys in early childhood, transitioning through 7–9 years to be greater in females from 10 to 17 years, with a marked influence of puberty on symptom progression.[38] Early menarche in girls has been associated with an increased risk of incident asthma.[39,40] These observations have implicated estrogenic effects as potential mediators of the increased prevalence and severity of asthma in females around the time of puberty. Estrogen receptors are expressed on many cell types, including airway smooth muscle. Their expression in immune cell lines is associated with enhancement of allergic inflammation through Th2 skewing of immune responses, isotype switching of B cells to immunoglobulin E (IgE) production and mast cell degranulation. On the other hand, some evidence points away from estrogenic effects, such as fluctuations in bronchial responsiveness through the menstrual cycle being associated with alterations in serum testosterone concentrations, and it is probable that multiple factors, including sex differences in biological and lifestyle variables, are associated with the changes in asthma prevalence that occur during transition to early adulthood.

OUTCOMES OF CHILDHOOD ASTHMA

A high proportion of asthma presents with symptoms in early childhood, when recurring, intermittent wheeze is very common, affecting 30%–50% of infants and young children. A substantial number of children with early onset wheezing will have symptom remission during childhood, especially those with milder symptoms and an absence of severe attacks requiring hospital admission. Prospective longitudinal studies of asthma have been of vital importance to understanding the outcomes of asthma in childhood. These avoid the inevitable pitfalls of recall bias whereby adults with asthma are more likely to report symptoms in childhood than those whose asthma has resolved.[41] The Melbourne Children's Asthma Study is one of the longest-running studies of asthma in childhood, having recruited 7-year-old children with asthma and wheeze in 1964, with a supplemental recruitment of those with more severe disease at the age of 10 years. Outcomes from this seminal study have now been reported through 50 years of age and have shown that a number of factors in childhood; asthma severity, female sex, and coexistent hay fever were associated with asthma presence in mid-adulthood.[42] Furthermore, severe asthma and asthma in childhood, compared with wheezing bronchitis and healthy controls, were associated with lower forced expiratory volume in 1 second (FEV_1) and the ratio of FEV_1 to forced vital capacity (FEV_1/ FVC) in adults; severe asthma was strongly associated with COPD despite a high proportion of this cohort being never smokers.[43] The lung function differences seen at age 50 years were not explained by between-group differences in the rate of FEV_1 decline in adulthood, suggesting that these differences

were established in childhood and persisted ("tracked") to adult life. This observation is consistent with results of a large comparative study of adult cohorts,[44] which showed that low FEV_1 in early adulthood followed by physiological rates of decline was associated with COPD in a substantial proportion of participants, and supports accumulating evidence about the early life origins of COPD.[45] Another long-running cohort study of asthma in children from Dunedin, New Zealand, also showed evidence of low lung function in adults with persistent wheezing from childhood and had previously reported allergic sensitization, airway hyperresponsiveness, female sex, and smoking as risk factors for the persistence of symptoms in early adulthood and showed similar tracking of low lung function from recruitment at age 9 years.[46] In the UK, a follow-up at 50 years of children recruited in 1964 confirmed associations of childhood asthma with COPD in the absence of accelerated decline of FEV_1 during adulthood.[47] A report from the Childhood Asthma Management Program (CAMP) research group categorized children on the basis of trajectories of repeat lung function measurements and showed that children with persistent asthma with reduced lung function growth were at risk for fixed airflow obstruction and possible COPD in early adulthood.[48] This subject is discussed in more detail in Chapter 15.

Severity and Mortality

HOSPITALIZATION

As asthma prevalence increased in children in the early 1980s, there was a parallel increase observed in asthma hospitalization rates in the same countries, suggesting that the increased prevalence was not wholly explained by the increased recognition of milder cases. However, since the 1990s, hospital admission rates for asthma in children stabilized or decreased in many developed countries. In a US survey, the rates of one or more asthma attacks in the past 12 months in children remained stable over the period 2001–2010.[49] However, these trends were not replicated in all settings. A recent Scandinavian study analyzed hospital discharge codes over a 35-year period and concluded that the asthma admission rate for children had remained stable in the time period 1977–2012 at around 1 per year per 1000 children at risk.[50] The rate of admission for asthma in children in Spain fell from 20.5 to 18.8 per 100,000 from 2002 to 2012,[51] while during an almost contemporaneous period in neighboring France (2002–2010) the age standardized rate of admission in children increased by 2.5% per year.[52] Therefore, variations in time trends of hospital admission rates for asthma likely depend on factors other than the background prevalence of severity. Neighborhood deprivation was associated with increased odds for hospitalization even after taking account of maternal socioeconomic indicators in a Swedish study that included over 17,500 children admitted to hospital with asthma.[53] In a US study of geographical access to care in two states, severe asthma outcomes including emergency department visits and hospitalization differed in their associations with access to care according to a number of factors, including which outcome measure was used.[54]

Many factors have been identified that are associated with increased risk of hospitalization for asthma in children. A recent systematic review of ETS exposure concluded that children with asthma exposed to tobacco smoke were nearly twice as likely to be hospitalized for asthma.[55] The introduction of smoke-free legislation in Scotland in 2006, prior to which asthma admissions were rising at around 5% per year, was associated with a decline of 18.2% per year in both preschool and school-aged children and was independent of socioeconomic status.[56] Similar findings were reported from England when national legislation was adopted in 2007.[57]

Poor adherence to treatment has been identified as a risk for severe asthma outcomes and may be manifested by increased reliance on reliever medications. A US study used a controller-to-total asthma medication indicator in children and found that a ratio of less than 0.5 was associated with increased risk for subsequent hospitalization or emergency department attendance.[58] Psychological stress induced by the death of a close relative was associated with increased risk of asthma hospitalization in adolescents.[59] Acute exposures to environmental factors can trigger transient increases in hospitalizations for asthma. These include extremes of weather conditions,[60,61] seasonal factors, including allergen exposure and respiratory infections,[62] and air pollution.[32,63,64] Genetic factors may also increase the risk of severe asthma exacerbations in relation to specific exposures. A polymorphism of the β-2 receptor has been associated with an increased risk of hospitalization, emergency care, or intensification of treatment in children prescribed long-acting sympathomimetic bronchodilators,[65] and genetic variants in endotoxin signaling pathways can interact with indoor endotoxin exposure to increase the risk of hospitalization in children with asthma.[66]

SEVERE ASTHMA

Although the majority of children with asthma have mild-to-moderate disease that can be managed effectively with appropriate controller medications, a proportion have severe and/or therapy-resistant disease. International consensus guidelines on the definition, evaluation, and management of severe asthma in children have been published[67] and its heterogeneity has been documented using cluster analysis in a US study.[68] A recent European study has used a case-control design to identify features of severe asthma in children compared with those with persistent but nonsevere disease. In a multivariate analysis, severe asthma was characterized by sensitization to food allergens (previously reported as a risk factor for life-threatening asthma), hospitalization and emergency visits for asthma, symptoms in response to physical activity, and lower lung function, although half the cases had FEV_1 within the normal range.[69] Interestingly, the cases could not be distinguished from controls by the home environment (apart from tobacco smoke exposure), parental education, or adherence to treatment.

ASTHMA DEATHS

An epidemic of reported asthma deaths was observed in some, but not all, industrialized HICs in the latter half of the 20th century, beginning in the 1960s.[70] Registered causes of death of 5- to 34-year-olds were analyzed from 1959 to 1979 and found to increase in New Zealand, Australia, England, and Wales, but not in the United States, Canada, or West Germany. As with all temporal trends, it is important to consider changes over time in disease classification, the way death certificates are completed and recorded, and a shift in diagnostic preferences. Of note, the return to pre-epidemic death rates was slower in New Zealand than in other countries, and New Zealand experienced a "second epidemic" in the 1970s, suggesting specific geographical factors in asthma management. This led to speculation that inhaled sympathomimetic drugs were implicated, supported by ecological evidence of higher sales of these (and other) asthma drugs in New Zealand, and some evidence that regular corticosteroids were underused. Further evidence from case control studies implicated the potent β-sympathomimetic drug, fenoterol in deaths due to asthma. A recent Cochrane review of another β-sympathomimetic drug implicated in asthma deaths, formoterol, considered 20 studies in adults and 7 studies in children and adolescents. All deaths occurred in adults, and the authors concluded, on the basis of low-quality evidence, that there was weak evidence of increased adverse events associated with regular use of formoterol in children[71] However, two recent multicenter RCTs comparing combination corticosteroids/long-acting bronchodilators in adults and adolescents (>12 years) using budesonide/formoterol[72] and in children (4–11 years) using fluticasone/salmeterol[73] showed noninferiority of combination treatment compared with inhaled corticosteroid alone in relation to serious asthma-related adverse events. Deaths from asthma in childhood are relatively uncommon in HICs, having declined since the 1990s. National surveillance surveys have been used to attempt to identify factors associated with increased risk of asthma mortality. In New South Wales, Australia, 20 children died from asthma over the 10-year period, 2004–2013 (http://www.ombo.nsw.gov.au/news-and-publications/publications/annual-reports/nsw-child-death-review/nsw-child-death-review-team-annual-report-2013). Risk factors for death included older age, low socioeconomic status, psychosocial problems, and Asian or Pacific Island racial background. A high proportion of those who died had a record of hospitalization in the previous 12 months; other factors identified were lack of follow-up care after admission, poor adherence to medication, and suboptimal asthma control.[74] The Royal College of Physicians in the UK led a national confidential enquiry into all asthma deaths occurring in the year commencing February 2012 (https://www.rcplondon.ac.uk/projects/national-review-asthma-deaths). Of 195 people that died, the majority had asthma diagnosed as adults and only 28 deaths were in people younger than 19 years.[75] Of all those who died, important factors identified were previous hospital admissions, attendance at an emergency department in the 12 months prior to death, failure to seek medical assistance during the final attack, and lack of specialist follow-up care. A low proportion of patients had personal asthma action plans or had received an asthma review in primary care in the year before death. Avoidable factors were identified in almost two-thirds of asthma deaths, including smoking and exposure to tobacco smoke, poor adherence to medications, psychosocial problems, and nonattendance at review appointments. In children and young people, poor recognition of the risk of adverse outcome was found to be of particular relevance.

Quality of Life and Economic Impact of Asthma

There is little doubt that asthma impacts on the QoL of both children and their caregivers. Several factors may impact on the QoL of a child with asthma, including asthma control and health care visits, asthma attacks, medication routines, family factors, socioeconomic status, and caregiver QoL. A systematic review of the magnitude of QoL impairments in 7- to 18-year-old children with asthma compared with healthy controls found lower overall QoL and lower scores in the domains of physical, psychological, and social functioning.[76] An attempt to quantify the impact of a range of 20 chronic childhood conditions using standard health economic methods reported that asthma and allergies were the most prevalent, but had the least impact in terms of loss of quality adjusted life years (QALYs).[77] A range of asthma QoL instruments, which may be self-reported or, for younger children, parent or caregiver reported, has been developed and validated.[78] An example of a commonly used suite of questionnaires can be accessed at: https://www.qoltech.co.uk/index.htm. QoL in children with asthma is linked to poor symptom control[79] and reduced lung function.[80] However, children with equivalent measures of asthma control can have marked differences in QoL scores measured using standardized instruments, which relate, in part, to psychological and family factors, including anxiety and depression.[81,82] Recent evidence has shown that the age of a child moderates the association between asthma severity and QoL, with older children reporting a greater impact on QoL as asthma severity increased.[83] QoL impacts in childhood asthma extend to caregivers and families; in the former case, there is an interrelationship between parent/caregiver QoL and that of the child, including measures of asthma control.[84] Parents of children with poorly controlled asthma report impaired QoL for emotional and family activities.[85] There is evidence for racial disparities in the impacts on QoL of parents of children with asthma, with black and Hispanic caregivers perceiving a greater burden of their children's asthma. However, this may depend on the extent of cultural and psychological adaptation (acculturation) of these families, with less acculturation being associated with an apparent protective role in reducing the burden of asthma on urban, African-American families.[86]

In the US, the Centers for Disease Control and Prevention (CDC) has estimated the proportion of schooldays missed by children aged 5–17 years due to asthma to be equivalent to 13.8 million schooldays with slightly higher rates reported in black and Hispanic children, and in those from poorer social strata (http://www.cdc.gov/asthma/asthmadata.htm). In addition, lost productivity due to parental absence from work to care for their children with asthma accounts for a substantial proportion of the indirect costs of asthma.

As well as impacts on individuals' and families' QoL, asthma carries an economic cost to society, which can be accounted through direct health care resource costs, including emergency care, hospitalizations, physician visits and medication costs, and indirect costs incurred through loss of productivity. Many of the attempts to quantify the economic burden of asthma have been carried out in rich countries and various country-specific estimates have been published (see http://www.globalasthmareport.org/burden/economic.php).   In

Europe, for example, the total costs attributed to asthma in adults and children amounted to almost €34 billion ($38 billion; £26 billion) at 2011 values (ERJ White Book: http://www.erswhitebook.org/)[87] of which almost 60% was accounted for by the direct costs of health care including medications. The equivalent costs in the US are estimated to be $56 billion (€50 billion; £39 billion), of which the greatest portion is attributed to direct health care costs (https://www.epa.gov/asthma/2016-asthma-fact-sheet). Although severe phenotypes of asthma account for a small proportion of the total disease burden, they make a disproportionately high contribution to the economic costs of asthma (GINA report Global Strategy for Asthma Management and Prevention, 2015 update at: www.ginasma.it). The mean monthly costs of children with very poorly controlled asthma compared with not-well-controlled, or well-controlled disease, have been estimated to be more than twice as high.[88]

Phenotypic Variation

TEMPORAL PROGRESSION OF SYMPTOMS

In a seminal paper from the Tucson Children's Respiratory Study based on wheezing history from birth to 6 years, three discrete phenotypes were described with varying associations with lung function, allergic sensitization, and outcome.[89] This study was instrumental in establishing the concept of transient early wheezing in the first few years after birth as a condition distinct from asthma and most likely to arise as a consequence of an airway developmental disorder with low airway function measured soon after birth, a lack of association with allergic sensitization, and loss of symptoms by 6 years of age. Subsequently, in recognition of the phenotypic heterogeneity of asthma and wheezing illnesses in children, several groups have taken various approaches to classifying wheezing from early childhood by temporal progression of symptoms. Most have used statistical approaches that involve clustering symptom patterns using either a single cardinal symptom (wheeze) or several symptoms combined. These methods are generally regarded as data driven with no prior stipulations about the number or characteristics of the phenotypes derived. In a large, population-based study in the UK, latent class analysis was used to derive five different temporal patterns of wheezing from birth to 7 years.[90] The important point to note here is that latent classes are not observable, so individual subjects cannot be assigned to a specific phenotype, but instead have a set of probabilities of belonging to one or several classes. Latent structures in the data are simply a way of describing variations that may have distinct underlying biological pathways (endotypes) with discoverable and preventable risk factors. Therefore, these methods are not directly translatable to the clinic but can be regarded as hypothesis-generating approaches. Replication studies in several different cohorts using latent class analysis or variants of this method confirmed the general description of these temporal classes or phenotypes.[91–94] Wheezing phenotypes that started early (within 6–18 months after birth) and persisted through mid-childhood were particularly associated with a family history of asthma, evidence of allergic sensitization, and reduced airway function in later childhood.[95] Similar associations with lung function outcomes have been reported in a Scandinavian cohort using simple categorization to different wheezing patterns; early persistent wheeze was associated with low FEV_1 at age 16 years and with evidence of small airway dysfunction.[96] Although all wheezing phenotypes compared with children who never wheezed show some decrement in measures of airway function in later childhood, persistent wheeze has also been associated with low growth of FEV_1 through adolescence.[97] Extended latent class analysis of wheeze to age 16 years has recently been reported in a UK birth cohort with similar outcomes associated with persistent wheezing phenotypes; increased bronchodilator responsiveness, lower FEV_1/FVC, and higher FeNO levels (Fig. 42.4).[98] Using a similar statistical approach, but including multiple data dimensions in the Leicester cohorts in the UK enabled identification of three wheezing phenotypes and two of chronic cough. These have subsequently been replicated in an independent, population-based cohort with two distinct phenotypes showing consistency between the discovery and replication samples; atopic persistent wheeze and transient viral wheeze.[99] The overall synopsis of this series of studies is that wheeze that begins in early childhood and becomes persistent is associated with a poorer prognosis than other wheezing patterns. However, the original premise to identify factors influencing different phenotypes has not materialized; known associations of transient early wheezing and low airway function in early childhood with exposure to tobacco smoke during pregnancy and factors associated with a lower incidence of lower respiratory infections in early childhood have emerged from association studies with derived phenotypes, but there were few exposures that showed clear differentiation between different patterns of wheeze.[100,101] The derived phenotypes have been shown to have external validity in a German comparison of latent class-derived and clinical phenotypes and comparison between these two enabled the

discovery of a previously unrecognized clinical phenotype of intrauterine tobacco smoke exposure, decreased lung function, increased genetic risk for asthma, but without an established asthma diagnosis or treatment associated with unremitting wheeze.[94] A joint modeling approach has also been applied to data in a cohort from Manchester, where the availability of links to clinical records allowed latent class analysis of parent reported and physician-confirmed wheezing. This enabled the separation of children with persistent wheezing into those with mild, controlled disease and those with "persistent troublesome wheeze" with the latter displaying reduced lung function, increased airway responsiveness, and a marked increase in exacerbations and hospitalizations compared to the other classes.[102]

Translating evidence from preschool wheeze in epidemiologic studies to a clinically useful phenotypic definition led the European Respiratory Society Task Force to propose discrimination between episodic viral wheeze (EVW) and multitrigger wheeze (MTW), the latter being more likely to be associated with the development of asthma, and should be treated with inhaled corticosteroids.[103] However, these phenotypes are not stable over time[104] and a bronchoscopic study including children with EVW and MTW compared with nonwheezing controls showed no differences in age of onset, symptom duration, prevalence of atopy, or markers of airway inflammation (eosinophils, epithelial loss, and basement membrane thickness) between the two wheezing phenotypes, suggesting they were part of the same spectrum of disease rather than distinct pathological subtypes of asthma.[105] In contrast, invasive studies have shown differences in bronchoalveolar lavage and endobronchial biopsy cellularity between EVW, predominantly neutrophilic, and MTW, classically eosinophilic, and there is evidence that EVW has less severe airway obstruction and impairment of gas mixing and lower FeNO

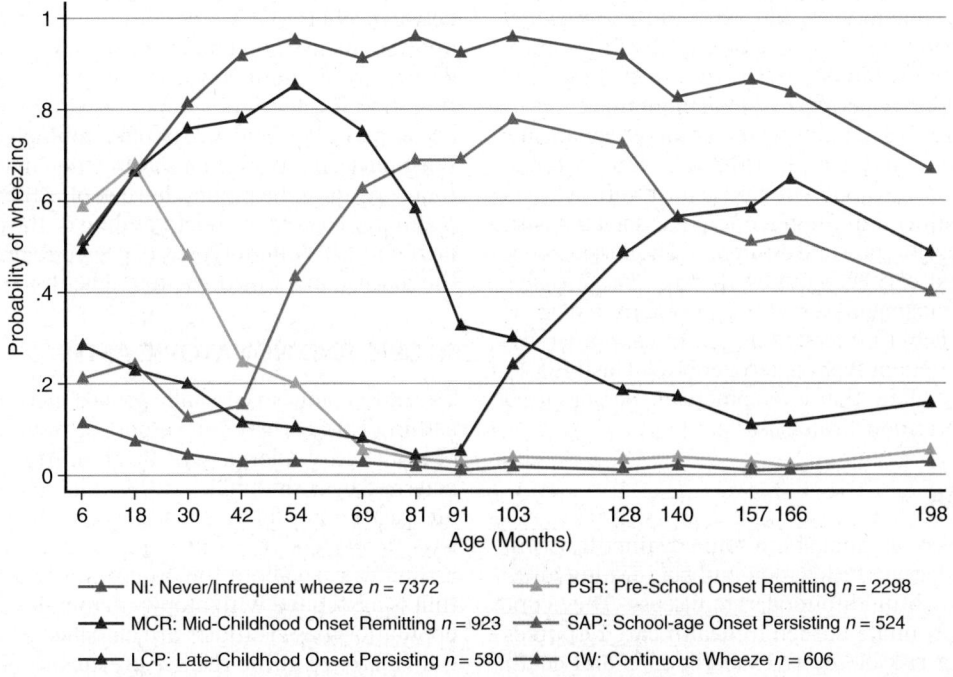

Fig. 42.4 Estimated prevalence of wheezing at each time point from birth to 16 ½ years for each of the six wheezing phenotypes identified by using latent class analysis in 12,303 children. (From Granell R, Henderson AJ, Sterne JA. Associations of wheezing phenotypes with late asthma outcomes in the Avon Longitudinal Study of Parents and Children: a population-based birth cohort. *J Allergy Clin Immunol.* 2016;138(4):1060-1070.e11.)

compared with MTW.[106] In practice, these features may be difficult to establish clinically, and a review of the previous Task Force guidance acknowledges greater uncertainty in the distinction between early life wheezing phenotypes and their responses to pharmacological treatment,[107] although the presence of eosinophilia is likely to be associated with a beneficial response to inhaled corticosteroids.

INFLAMMATORY SUBTYPES

The classification of asthma in adults has evolved around observed biomarkers of disease, including histopathological examination of airway mucosal inflammatory subtypes. Similar approaches in children have largely been limited to specific groups that have either been sampled opportunistically during anesthesia for unrelated conditions, or have presented with diagnostic challenges or severe disease that mandated bronchoscopic investigation. Thus, such approaches have mainly been applied to the classification of more severe disease phenotypes. Less invasive markers of airway inflammation are available, including the measurement of FeNO, the assessment of inflammatory cells in induced sputum, and the measurement of inflammatory markers in exhaled breath condensate. These biomarkers have largely been evaluated in the context of asthma control or responses to specific interventions, although application to different phenotypes of asthma in children has yielded some interesting findings. Sputum examination in a subset of the UK Isle of Wight cohort showed eosinophilia in adolescent-onset disease, which was not seen in persistent asthma from the age of 10 years,[108] although the significance of this was not clear. As expected, sputum eosinophilia was greater in atopic compared with nonatopic asthma in this population. However, one of the potential pitfalls of using sputum cell counts to categorize asthma is that they may not be stable over time.[109] Raised FeNO has been associated with longitudinal wheezing phenotypes, but only those associated with allergic sensitization[110]; therefore, it has little utility in adding to the understanding of the nature of these phenotypes. Examination of peripheral blood mononuclear cells has revealed differences in immune regulatory mechanisms between nonallergic and allergic asthma,[111] and cytokine expression patterns in response to house dust mite extracts have displayed distinct immunophenotypes associated with house dust mite sensitization and asthma.[112] The development of biomarkers that can be acquired through less invasive means and their implementation through systems biology is likely to lead to a better understanding of disease processes underpinning the phenotypic heterogeneity of asthma in children and may allow the development of personalized treatments or prevention strategies.[113]

SEVERE ASTHMA

Children with severe asthma share some distinct features, including more allergic sensitization and poorer lung function than those with mild-to-moderate disease. They contribute a disproportionate burden to health care resources and are at greater risk of severe exacerbations and death from asthma.[114] As with other forms of asthma, there is recognized phenotypic heterogeneity in this group as well. Cluster analysis of children in the US Severe Asthma Research

Program (SARP) identified four different phenotypes that were characterized largely by differences in age of onset and lung function,[68] which have been combined with adult clusters from the same study to form a composite theoretical model of severe asthma phenotypes.[115] However, even within the adult clusters based on clinical variables, there was evidence of substantial heterogeneity in sputum inflammatory cell populations. Clusters identified in the SARP were replicated in an independent cohort,[116] and a separate cluster analysis of children with persistent asthma enrolled in the CAMP identified five clusters that were differentiated on the basis of the atopy, airway obstruction, and exacerbation history.[117] There was also evidence of differential responses to inhaled corticosteroids between clusters. Five clusters of severe asthma were also identified in 6- to 11-year-old children participating in the Epidemiology and Natural History of Asthma: Outcomes and Treatment Regimens (TENOR) study, in this case characterized by atopy, sex, ethnicity, and exposure to tobacco smoke.[118] Similar approaches to disaggregating different phenotypes of severe asthma have been applied to European populations. In a French study, two severe and one milder phenotype of asthma were identified by cluster analysis in 6- to 12-year-old children.[119] The two severe clusters included children who were highly atopic with mild lung function deficits and with poor control despite high-dose inhaled corticosteroids in one cluster, and slightly older children with severe airway obstruction in the other. Although no airway inflammatory markers were included, the former group had high peripheral eosinophil counts while the latter featured a more neutrophilic pattern. The predominant inflammatory cell type identified in the airways of children with severe asthma is the eosinophil, which has been identified in the airways of children with severe wheeze in the preschool age group.[120] In contrast with adults, neutrophilic inflammation does not appear to predominate in severe asthma in children.[121] There appears to be some consistency between phenotypes emerging from unsupervised cluster analyses focused on children with severe asthma and those derived from latent structures in population-based data in that the persistence of symptoms with severe exacerbations accompanied by evidence of often multiple allergic sensitization and decrements of airway function marks those children that constitute the highest burden of asthma in the pediatric population. Greater understanding of the endotypes associated with this phenotype is expected to lead to advances in the management of this often difficult to treat group.

ATOPIC AND NONATOPIC ASTHMA

The most common clinically applied method to phenotyping asthma is to classify it as atopic or nonatopic on the basis of evidence of allergic sensitization. Atopic asthma is characterized by eosinophilic airway inflammation, and is associated with other allergic disorders, such as eczema and hay fever,[122] and tends to be more severe than nonatopic asthma.[123] Estimates vary about the proportion of asthma in children that is associated with atopy; up to half of asthma cases in population-based studies are classified as nonatopic. There is a difference in the relative prevalence of atopic and nonatopic asthma between countries. The population-fraction of asthma attributable to atopy has been reported to be about twice as high in affluent compared with nonaffluent countries, and in Latin America, only a small proportion of asthma is associated with atopy.[124] In children living in a poor area of Ecuador, the population-attributable fraction of recent asthma symptoms was only 2.4%, with heavy parasitic infestation strongly inversely associated with atopic wheezing.[125] Therefore, asthma prevalence in countries with high microbial and parasitic exposure may be explained by different factors than those identified in affluent countries, where atopic asthma is more likely to predominate. It has been speculated that microbial load could be a risk factor for nonatopic asthma. There is certainly evidence that microbial exposure, even in affluent settings, can be differentially associated with asthma severity in children with atopic and nonatopic asthma.[126] However, whether this mechanism is a critical pathway for asthma inception in less affluent countries remains to be conclusively determined. Associations with other putative risk factors for asthma have also been shown to have differential effects depending on the atopic phenotype. These are considered under the various categories of exposures below. It might be supposed, given the differences in exposures associated with increased risk of either atopic or nonatopic asthma, that these phenotypes would associate with clear differences in airway inflammation.

A cross-sectional study of sputum inflammatory cells and chemokines from children with atopic or nonatopic asthma based on the presence or absence of a positive skin prick test or specific serum IgE response showed that those with atopic asthma had a higher proportion of eosinophils than nonatopic asthma or nonasthma controls; however, there were no differences in sputum neutrophil percentages between the three groups, although the children with nonatopic asthma had higher total neutrophil numbers. Sputum cytokine concentrations were consistent with these findings, with atopic asthma (rather than nonatopic asthma) being associated with higher levels of interferon-gamma (IFN-γ), interleukin (IL)-2, IL-4, and IL-5, and both asthma groups having higher concentrations than the controls.[127] Although this study seems to confirm eosinophilic airway inflammation as the typical inflammatory phenotype of atopic asthma, others have reported neutrophilic inflammation in induced sputum to predominate in nonatopic asthma.[128] However, in a bronchoscopic study, no differences were reported in eosinophils and eosinophil cationic protein levels between children with atopic or nonatopic asthma, and there were no differences in neutrophils or related Th1 mediators IL-8 and tumor necrosis factor (TNF)-α between the asthma and the control groups.[129] Therefore, there remains uncertainty about the inflammatory endotype underpinning asthma phenotypes in children differentiated by the presence of evidence for allergic sensitization. Additionally, concepts of allergy are changing with recognition that different patterns of sensitization are associated with different manifestations of asthma (see section "Allergy, Asthma, and the Allergic March," p. 663 for more details).

The Genetics of Asthma

GENETICS

Changes in the prevalence of asthma over time in the latter part of the 20th century in many affluent countries have been ascribed to likely changes in environment and lifestyle; these were thought to be too rapid to be due to genetic shifts in the population, although asthma is a highly heritable disease. Twin studies were the classic design to apportion disease inception to nature (genetics) or nurture (environment and lifestyle). Monozygotic twins share the same DNA, whereas dizygotic twins will share approximately 50% of their genes on average. In the majority of cases, their early life environment will also be shared, so comparing disease outcomes between the two biological categories of twins it is possible to estimate what proportion of disease is heritable. Using this approach, a large number of twin studies have been carried out to estimate the contribution of heritable factors to asthma, and heritability estimates have generally been high, ranging from 50% to 90%. A study of over 20,000 Danish twin pairs recently not only confirmed the importance of heritable factors for asthma in childhood, but also that the importance of this diminished through the life course into late adulthood. They also reported that different genes influenced the liability to asthma in males and females, although the proportion of asthma explained by genetic factors did not differ between the sexes.[130] A Swedish study of over 25,000 twin pairs recently reported a heritability estimate for childhood asthma of 82%.[131] Therefore, it is clear that genetic factors are important in the development of childhood asthma. This does not negate the importance of environment in explaining temporal trends in asthma prevalence but it does highlight the roles of gene–environment interactions in asthma, and the influence of environment on gene expression through epigenetic mechanisms.

Methods used for the discovery of asthma genes have evolved over time,[132] driven—to a large extent—by advances in genotyping technology that have scaled up throughput and reduced costs to make it feasible to apply these technologies to population studies. The earliest studies used a candidate gene approach, which is usually applied to a case-control study, to look for enrichment of a marker for a gene of interest in cases compared with controls, either without disease or from a general population sample. In this approach, the function of the gene is known *a priori* and, unsurprisingly, genes in immune pathways have featured large in candidate gene studies of asthma. Although this is a way to test hypotheses about association of genes with asthma, it does not have any utility for gene discovery. Many candidate gene studies for asthma have been published and extensively reviewed with particular focus on those that have been replicated in more than a handful of studies.[133] Next came genome-wide approaches, initially through family linkage studies looking for cosegregation of genes with disease in family members, and positional cloning followed by GWAS in which the idea is to tag all common variations in the human genome and perform a hypothesis-free analysis of association of these SNP tags with disease. This has been made possible by high throughput genotyping platforms that type over 1 million SNPs. Through the HapMap project (the database has been retired by The National Center for Biotechnology Information) and the 1000 Genomes study (http://www.1000genomes.org/), it is possible to impute SNPs that were not directly typed. Due to of the number of tests being carried out, the false discovery burden of GWAS means that very large sample sizes are needed to have statistical power to detect "significant" associations. One of the limitations of GWAS is that it will detect only common risk variants and most results from GWAS studies in asthma to date have yielded risk alleles that together account for a small proportion of the genetic risk, leading to the so-called "hidden heredity" of asthma. Resequencing studies are now being done to investigate rare variants in asthma susceptibility.[134] Rare variants with large effects have been postulated to contribute to the hidden heritability of asthma, although recent evidence suggests that this may not be as important as previously thought.[135] A meta-analysis of 20 genome-wide linkage studies identified two regions (2p21-p14 and 6p21) with evidence of linkage to asthma in European families.[136] Large GWAS of asthma in children and adults have identified SNPs associated with asthma at genome-wide levels of significance, which have been replicated in independent populations.[137,138] The association of asthma with SNPs in the 17q21 region was shown to be primarily with asthma of childhood origin.[139,140] This has been confirmed in a recent GWAS of age of asthma onset with additional regions (9p24 and 17q12-q21) which was also associated with the earlier onset of asthma.[141] Other asthma phenotypes have been considered, and GWAS have discovered associations with the asthma, hay fever/rhinitis phenotype,[142,143] and childhood asthma with severe exacerbations.[144] In the latter case, the susceptibility locus *CDHR3* was subsequently found to mediate binding and replication of human rhinovirus (HRV) C.[145]

GENE–ENVIRONMENT INTERACTIONS

Knowledge that environmental factors and the timing of exposure are important associations of asthma onset in early childhood has focused attention on interactions between genetic and environmental influences explaining variations in asthma risk. One consequence of assembling the very large consortia needed for GWAS studies is that they tend to come from widely varying geographical distributions and hence a very heterogeneous exposure background, which could reduce the chances of detecting genetic associations in GWAS. Most gene–environment interaction studies to date have taken a candidate gene approach, seeking to find evidence that genetic variation in known biologic pathways or with known associations with asthma modifies the effect of an exposure on asthma outcomes. These have included interactions with infectious agents, notably genetic variants in the *CD14* gene and endotoxin exposure,[146] and interaction between HRV infection and *17q21* genetic variants, a risk locus discovered in a GWAS of asthma.[147] Following the discovery that 17q21 SNPs were associated specifically with childhood onset asthma, an interaction between variants at this locus and tobacco smoke exposure was reported.[139] A number of other candidate gene studies of genetic interactions with tobacco smoke exposure on the risk of asthma or asthma exacerbations have been published.[148] These have shown interactions of various genetic regions with prenatal and/or postnatal tobacco smoke exposure and asthma risk. Gene–environment interaction can also be used in a non-targeted way to identify new genetic associations with asthma. A genome-wide interaction study (GEWIS) of interactions with tobacco smoke exposure in a European consortium of birth cohorts found evidence for interaction between *in utero* and early childhood exposure with novel genetic variants.[149] Interestingly, this approach did not identify interactions with

variants in genes previously reported to interact with tobacco smoke exposure in the etiology of asthma, including *TNF,*[150] *GSTP1,*[151] and *ADAM33.*[152] Another GEWIS of children from farming communities in Europe, where endotoxin exposure has been associated with protective effects on asthma and allergy, found no strong evidence for new or previously reported polymorphisms interacting with farm exposure on asthma risk. This included SNPs that had previously been reported in association with asthma or had shown interaction with farming exposure.[153] As with GWAS, which are essentially hypothesis free, there is a high statistical penalty for multiple testing; therefore, large studies are required to have sufficient power to detect interactions, especially for polymorphisms that have a low minor allele frequency.

Other exposures for which evidence of gene–environment interactions related to asthma risk have been found in candidate gene studies include the outdoor environment with genes in antioxidant and inflammatory pathways pollutants.[154-156] In the indoor environment, interactions between gas cooking and glutathione-S-transferase M1 *(GSTM1)* null mutations were described in relation to bronchial responsiveness in adults.[157] A study of indoor mold exposure found no evidence of interactions with *GSTP1* mutations in childhood asthma.[158] (See Table 42.1 for details of candidate genes implicated in gene–environment interactions.)

EPIGENETICS

Epigenetics refers to changes in the way genes are expressed as opposed to changes in their structural sequence. This provides a mechanism by which the ability of cells to read a genetic code can be open or silenced, effectively controlling whether genes are active or dormant in a cell. A number of modifications determine gene expression, including DNA methylation, chromatin remodeling, histone modification, and the action of noncoding RNAs. Of these, the most studied to date is DNA methylation, which is technically the most straightforward to assay using current technology. Therefore, epigenetic modification is a phenotype, which can indicate responses to environmental exposures or stressors, providing a link between exposure and gene expression, and which can be transmitted to daughter cells making such modifications potentially heritable across generations (transgenerational epigenetic inheritance). Studies of DNA methylation of relevance to asthma include those which have studied epigenomic changes in association with pertinent exposures, such as tobacco smoke exposure and air pollutants, and intergenerational studies linking ancestral exposures to disease in subsequent generations. Tobacco smoke exposure during pregnancy has been associated with global DNA methylation and gene-specific effects in neonatal or cord blood,[159-161] which can persist into childhood.[162-164] Air pollution exposure has been associated with effects on DNA methylation in infants' cord blood, which was dependent on the type of pollutant and timing of exposure during pregnancy.[165] In inner-city children with asthma, DNA methylation of specific gene loci in peripheral blood differed from control children from the same environment.[166] Mammalian cell DNA methylation is reprogrammed on a global scale at two points in the life cycle: at fertilization of the zygote and in primordial germ cells[167]; however, there is still uncertainty about the heritability of epigenetic marks between generations. There have

Table 42.1   Genes and Gene Regions Cited in Gene–Environment Interaction Studies of Childhood Asthma

Gene or Region		Gene Name	Location	Function
CD14		Cluster of differentiation 14	Chr5	Encodes a surface antigen that is preferentially expressed on monocytes/macrophages and acts a coreceptor for bacterial lipopolysaccharide
17q21	ORMDL3	ORM1-like protein 3	Chr17	The ORM genes are a conserved gene family that act as negative regulators of sphingolipid synthesis
	GSDMB	Gasdermin B		Encodes a member of the gasdermin-domain containing protein family, which are implicated in the regulation of apoptosis in epithelial cells,
TNF		Tumor necrosis factor	Chr6	Encodes a multifunctional proinflammatory cytokine that belongs to the TNF superfamily
ADAM33		A disintegrin and metalloproteinase domain 33	Chr20	Encodes a member of the ADAM family of membrane bound proteins involved in cell–cell and cell–matrix interactions.
GLUTATHIONE-S-TRANSFERASES				
GSTM1		Glutathione-S-transferase Mu 1	Chr1	GSTs are a family of enzymes that play an important role in detoxification by catalyzing the conjugation of many hydrophobic and electrophilic compounds with reduced glutathione
GSTP1		Glutathione-S-transferase Pi 1	Chr11	
GSTT1		Glutathione-S-transferase Theta 1	Chr22	

been studies of the relationships of grandparental exposures with outcomes in second-generation offspring. Grandmothers' smoking during pregnancy has been associated with asthma in her grandchild, even when the mother did not smoke during pregnancy.[168] In a UK cohort, this association was limited to paternal grandmothers' smoking, and was stronger for female than for male descendants.[169] The DNA methylation in the grandchildren was not measured in either of these observational studies, but in the Norwegian Mother and Child Cohort, grandmothers' smoking when pregnant with the mother was not associated with altered grandchild cord-blood DNA methylation at loci, which was previously reported to be associated with maternal tobacco smoking during pregnancy.[170] The availability of high throughput arrays will shortly enable epigenome-wide association studies (EWAS) to be carried out in large case control studies of children with asthma using a similar hypothesis-free approach to GWAS.

Environmental Influences on Asthma

PREGNANCY AND CHILDBIRTH

Maternal Factors

The heritability of asthma has long been recognized, but there has also been a parent-of-origin effect described with a stronger association of maternal than paternal asthma with offspring asthma.[171] This could be explained by genetic imprinting, maternal exposures during pregnancy, immune interactions between the mother and fetus, or a shared postnatal environment. In the prospective, population-based UK Isle of Wight cohort, a sex-dependent parent-of-origin effect was reported; maternal allergy was associated with asthma only in girls, and paternal allergy was associated with asthma only in boys.[172] This led the authors to speculate that epigenetic programing might be important in determining the differential effect of parental allergic disease on the risk of asthma in their offspring.

There has been increasing recognition of the role of early life factors in the etiology of asthma, extending to the intrauterine environment. This reach has extended yet further to influences prior to conception, particularly with the recognition of the potential for epigenetic marks to be both heritable and responsive to environmental challenge.[173] Maternal obesity before pregnancy was reported to be associated with an increased risk for offspring asthma independent of gestational weight gain in the Danish national birth cohort,[174] and similar observations were seen in the Generation R study for preschool wheeze.[175] The mechanisms of these observations have still to be explained, but there are suggestions that they may operate through nonallergic pathways as the excess risk appears to be associated with nonatopic asthma. Part of the association, but not all, can be explained by the association between maternal and offspring BMI and the relationship between the latter and asthma.[176] Younger maternal age also has been associated with increased asthma risk in their offspring in populations of white, European descent although the obverse of this relationship was recently reported in US Latino populations.[177] Although evolving interest in preconceptual influences and transgenerational effects is likely to continue, there is considerable literature on maternal exposures during pregnancy and the risk of subsequent asthma in their offspring.

The health of a mother during pregnancy can have important effects on the health and development of her fetus. Some maternal diseases and complications of pregnancy have been associated with an increased risk of asthma in the offspring. These include hypertension and preeclampsia,[178] anemia,[179] and the use of a number of drugs used to treat mothers during pregnancy. Antibiotic prescription during pregnancy has been associated with an increased risk of offspring asthma, although this may be confounded by shared familial factors.[180] Acetaminophen use by women during pregnancy also has been associated with an increased risk of asthma and wheezing in their offspring. A meta-analysis of published observational studies found a positive association between asthma and any use of acetaminophen in the first trimester, but noted a high degree of heterogeneity between studies, and an attenuation of the association when adjusting for respiratory tract infections.[181] Recent analysis of a large Scandinavian cohort study with detailed information on the indication for use of acetaminophen, reported associations between prenatal use and asthma in children, which could not be completely explained by confounding by indication.[182] Additionally, this study was able to consider maternal use outside pregnancy and paternal use of acetaminophen, neither of which was associated with offspring asthma, suggesting unmeasured confounding was having little influence on these associations. To date, these observational studies have not been confirmed by experiment and there has been sufficient uncertainty to deter any change in guidelines for the use of acetaminophen during pregnancy.

Maternal Lifestyle and Environment

Exposure to maternal smoking during pregnancy is associated with increased asthma risk in the offspring. A systematic review of 43 studies concluded that prenatal tobacco smoke exposure was associated with an increased risk of asthma and wheeze, particularly in younger children, but could not separate out the effect of postnatal exposure due to the limited number of studies of children only exposed after birth.[183] Another systematic review found evidence that not only active smoking but also passive exposure of pregnant women to tobacco smoke was associated with an increased risk of asthma and wheezing in their offspring.[184] A collaborative study based on 15 European birth cohorts comprising nearly 28,000 children has found evidence that both active smoking and passive exposure of pregnant women, and the exposure of infants to maternal smoking postnatally, were associated with an increased risk of offspring wheeze in early life. The highest risk was associated with combined active maternal and passive exposure in the prenatal period.[185] Pregnant women's exposure to air pollution has also been shown to be associated with asthma in their offspring in a Chinese study of traffic-related nitrogen dioxide (NO_2) exposure with evidence of trimester-specific effects.[186] Similar findings regarding fine particulate ($PM_{2.5}$) exposure in mid-gestation were reported from a US population, where high levels of exposure from weeks 16 to 25 of gestation were associated with the development of asthma.[187]

Maternal diet during pregnancy has been studied extensively after observational associations suggested a link between dietary constituents and the occurrence of wheeze and asthma in the offspring. This body of research has culminated in RCTs of interventions in pregnancy as a strategy for the primary prevention of asthma. In prospective observational studies, vitamin deficiency has been elicited as having a strong association with increased asthma risk. Several studies based on estimated dietary intake of vitamin D of women during pregnancy consistently reported increased rates of asthma and allergic diseases in the offspring, although the results of studies using measurements of vitamin D status at various points during pregnancy were less conclusive.[188–191] In the long-running Aberdeen SEATON study, low intake of both maternal vitamin D and E during pregnancy have been associated with asthma outcomes during childhood up to 10 years of age, and low maternal α-tocopherol levels in early pregnancy were confirmed to be related to a higher risk of asthma.[192] The observational evidence that vitamin deficiency and particularly that of vitamin D, which has several bioregulatory functions that are in plausible asthma etiologic pathways, led to the development of supplementation trials in pregnant women. Although they used different dose regimens of vitamin D supplements, two RCTs have reported a lower incidence of wheezing illnesses in early childhood

and physician-diagnosed asthma to the age of 3 years.[193,194] Short-term differences in sensitization to aeroallergens have also been reported following vitamin D supplementation during pregnancy.[195] The longer-term effects on confirmed asthma outcomes are awaited.[196,197] Vitamin E supplementation in pregnancy has been suggested to reduce the risk of preeclampsia, although the evidence from RCTs of this intervention do not support benefit in either maternal preeclampsia or neonatal outcomes.[198] A dietary intervention has been proposed to optimize vitamin E intake with the objective of reducing asthma in the offspring;[199] however, although a pilot study was completed (ClincalTrials.gov NCT01661530 https://clinicaltrials.gov/), the results of a definitive trial are yet to be published. A follow-up of offspring from a high-dose vitamin C and E supplementation trial for preeclampsia found no differences in respiratory outcomes of infants to the age of 2 years.[200] In addition to antioxidant vitamins, there is longstanding interest in the role of long-chain polyunsaturated fatty acids (PUFAs) in the etiology of allergic diseases, including asthma. A systematic review of dietary exposure to or supplementation with PUFAs during pregnancy found that the majority of observational studies reported a beneficial effect of increased n-3 long-chain PUFA or fish intake (a rich source of these) on lower rates of allergen sensitization or atopic eczema in infancy.[201] However, an RCT of fish oil supplementation during pregnancy that followed the offspring through 6 years did not find evidence to support a reduction of IgE-mediated sensitization in the supplemented population.[202] There is no current evidence to support n-3 PUFA supplementation in pregnancy, or during breast-feeding after birth, to reduce the occurrence of asthma or wheeze in the offspring.[203] The gradient in asthma prevalence in Europe (http://www.globalasthmareport.org/burden/burden.php) has raised the prospect that a Mediterranean diet could be protective against asthma and thus contribute to the lower prevalence seen in countries in Southern compared with Northern Europe. However, a systematic review of dietary patterns and asthma did not find strong evidence to support that a Mediterranean diet in pregnancy reduces the risk of asthma in children.[204] There is currently no trial evidence to support a Mediterranean diet in pregnancy as a primary prevention strategy for asthma in the offspring.

There is good evidence in mammalian species that prenatal stress has biological effects on the evolving neuroendocrine system,[205,206] and may lead to dysregulated immune development and allergic diseases in the offspring. A recent systematic review of published studies reported that the majority showed positive associations between prenatal maternal stress and asthma or wheezing in the offspring.[207] However, the authors pointed out several methodologic caveats, including the use of self-reported instruments for exposure and outcome assessments, and the potential information bias arising from women with higher stress levels possibly reporting more asthma symptoms in their children.

Fetal Growth and Birth Size

Size at birth has been extensively studied in relation to subsequent history of asthma and allergies in childhood. Low birth weight (<2.5 kg) is reported to be a risk factor for wheezing[208] and asthma[209,210] in childhood. Conversely, increased neonatal size (weight, length, and head circumference) has been found to be positively associated with asthma, but not allergic sensitization in children. In a US study, low birth weight was associated with a specific asthma phenotype that manifested in mid-childhood and persisted to adolescence.[211] The sometimes conflicting evidence about birth size and asthma can, in part, be attributed to the definitions used to categorize birth size, including whether gestational age at birth was used to stratify low birth weight. Preterm delivery is associated with asthma symptoms,[212] and, in a large European collaborative meta-analysis, this largely explained the association of low birth weight with asthma.[213] In the Dutch Generation R study, antenatal growth measures were available from repeat fetal ultrasound estimates during pregnancy. In an analysis of preschool asthma symptoms, no associations were found with predefined restricted or accelerated fetal growth, although accelerated weight gain in the first 3 months after birth was associated with asthma symptoms suggesting postnatal growth may be more important than fetal growth in the development of asthma.[214] An alternative explanation is that rapid postnatal growth acts as a marker of intrauterine growth restraint, which is associated with developmental effects on lung growth, which, in turn, may manifest as early asthma symptoms. In studies that have measures of lung function shortly after birth, evidence of airway obstruction in infancy has been shown to be associated with the subsequent development of asthma and wheezing.[215–217] In the Generation R cohort, lower gain of fetal weight and length between the second and third trimester of pregnancy were associated with higher airways resistance and physician-diagnosed asthma in mid-childhood, providing a mechanism by which fetal growth restriction could influence the etiology of asthma symptoms in children.[218]

Mode of Delivery

In concert with the rise in asthma prevalence experienced in many developed countries in the late 20th century, there was a rise in the rates of births by cesarean section, including in low-risk pregnancies (http://www.cdc.gov/nchs/fastats/delivery.htm). Knowledge that cesarean delivery was associated with differences in microbial colonization of the newborn gut led to speculation that this could influence postnatal immune development and increase the risk of asthma and allergy.[219–221] A substantial number of studies compared asthma risk in children born by cesarean section compared with children delivered vaginally, and, although not all confirmed a positive association between the mode of delivery and asthma, two meta-analyses in 2008[221a,221b] and a more recent one have reported a consistent overall increased risk of asthma in children born by cesarean section of about 20%.[222] A study from Denmark suggested that this association was more pronounced in children who were delivered by cesarean section before membrane rupture.[223] However, there remains doubt about the proposed biological mechanisms for this association. Increased asthma risk has been associated with emergency, but not elective, cesarean section delivery, suggesting that factors associated with the indications for emergency delivery may be more important than early gut colonization.[224] Association between cesarean section delivery and directly measured outcomes are not entirely consistent with the increased risk of reported asthma and wheezing. Although cesarean section delivery was associated with persistent preschool wheezing in the Dutch Generation R study, there was no association with airway resistance and only elective, but not emergency, cesarean section was associated with raised FeNO levels.[225] A follow-up to adolescence of a German study of healthy term newborns found no increased risk of asthma and no difference in lung function at age 15 years according to the mode of delivery.[226] However, recent population-based studies based on linkage data report a small increased risk of hospital admissions for asthma in children born by cesarean section compared with vaginal delivery,[227–229] suggesting that there is a true but modest association that remains to be explained biologically.

EARLY CHILDHOOD

Breast-Feeding Diet

Dietary intake could affect asthma development in many ways, through ingestion of allergens, modification of the gut microbiota, rate of growth and development of obesity, or specific nutrients acting directly on immunological and pulmonary development. Patterns of breast-feeding infants vary between HICs and low- and middle-income countries (LMICs); with both the rate of initiation of breast-feeding and the duration of exclusive breast-feeding being lower in HICs than LMICs.[230] The coincidence of low breast-feeding rates with high asthma prevalence in HICs has suggested breast-feeding as a possible protective influence on asthma and allergic diseases. Many observational studies have considered the association between asthma risk and breast-feeding in infancy. They have used different metrics of exposure, including ever-versus-never breast-feeding and the duration of any, more, or exclusive breast-feeding, studied either general or high-risk populations and comprised a combination of prospective cohort, case-control, and cross-sectional study designs of varying methodological quality. Two key considerations in evaluating these studies are confounding; breast-feeding is strongly socially patterned and is therefore prone to confounding by other lifestyle and environmental variables and bias; parents with personal or family histories of asthma or allergies may be more or less likely to adopt breast-feeding in the belief that it will prevent disease in their offspring. A systematic review identified 42 reports of asthma and wheezing at 5–18 years of age in association with breast-feeding, with the majority of these being from high-income settings. Pooled odds ratios from a meta-analysis showed evidence of a protective effect on asthma risk of any breast-feeding compared with no breast-feeding, and more breast-feeding compared with less breast-feeding, with both effects being stronger in LMICs than HICs.[231] A separate systematic review and meta-analysis using different search criteria identified 117 studies reporting asthma outcomes (asthma ever, recent asthma, and recent wheezing illness) in association with breast-feeding history. This also reported evidence to support a protective effect of breast-feeding on asthma risk for all three outcomes considered.[232] Age-stratified analyses showed that this effect was strongest in young children aged 0–2 years when asthma is difficult to differentiate from other causes of wheezing illness and diminishes with time. It is possible that the effect observed resulted from protection against early respiratory infections and associated wheezing in early life. In contract with the results of the meta-analyses cited above, a large population-based study of Hong Kong

Chinese children found no association between exclusive or partial breast-feeding and hospitalization for asthma[233] In contrast with many lifestyle choices that are not conducive to randomized trials to strengthen the evidence base, there has been an innovative cluster-randomized trial of breast-feeding promotion carried out in Belarus: the PROBIT trial,[234] which successfully increased the rates of breast-feeding exclusivity and duration in the intervention arm. Despite this, there were no differences in rates of asthma or skin prick sensitization assessed by pediatricians at a follow-up clinic when the children were 6 years old.[235] Thus, it appears likely, on the basis of current evidence, that the apparent protective effects of breast-feeding on asthma could be explained by a combination of confounding and variation in phenotypic definition of the outcome, which includes infection-associated wheeze in preschool children. Breast milk could be a source of dietary allergen ingestion by the infant. Trials of allergen restriction in the diets of pregnant and lactating mothers showed little evidence of a beneficial effect on asthma in their offspring, and observational studies of high- compared with low-allergen-containing diets produced conflicting results.[236] There has been a recent shift in thinking about allergen avoidance in early life, including lactation, as a means of primary prevention of food sensitization in particular. Publication of the results of the LEAP study[237] provided robust evidence that tolerance to peanut sensitization could be induced by the consumption of peanut allergen by infants. However, a randomized trial of the introduction of allergenic foods to breast-feeding mothers did not show a reduction in food allergies in a population-based sample of infants.[238] Therefore, current evidence does not support modification of maternal diet during lactation and breast-feeding, either by allergen reduction or supplementation, but there is a lack of data on asthma outcomes from well-conducted clinical trials.

Childhood Diet. Interest to date in the relationship between diet and asthma in children has centered on the potential modifying effects of dietary constituents on oxidant-antioxidant balance and their role in regulating airway inflammation.[239] Much of the evidence to date comes from observational studies, many cross-sectional, of dietary intake of foods, such as fruit and vegetables, dietary patterns, including the Mediterranean diet, and specific nutrients, such as vitamins and trace elements. One of the difficulties of interpreting this evidence arises from the methods used to categorize the intake of various nutrients, usually relying on food frequency questionnaires or diet diaries. Therefore, the epidemiologic evidence needs to be viewed with caution. In the cardiovascular literature, there are examples of evidence from randomized trials going in the opposite direction of effect from associations seen in observational studies[240]; that is, the vitamin intake that was "protective" in observational studies was associated with increased cardiovascular and all-cause mortality in trials of supplementation. There are currently few randomized trials of nutritional interventions in relation to children's asthma, and the evidence from trials of supplementation with specific food items in adults have been generally disappointing.[241,242] A synthesis of systematic reviews of diet and asthma in children and adults was undertaken under the auspices of the European Academy of Allergy and Clinical Immunology. This limited its search strategy to foods and diets but not nutrient supplements in relation to asthma outcomes, and identified seven systematic reviews that met quality criteria.[243] The synthesis of evidence from these reviews concluded that there was a beneficial effect of a high intake of antioxidant vitamins C, D, and E, and fresh fruit and vegetables, and of adherence to a Mediterranean dietary pattern in reducing the risk of asthma, with most of the beneficial effects being observed in children.[244,245] A meta-analysis of vitamin D supplementation in children with asthma found some evidence to support this supplementation to reduce asthma exacerbations, but the evidence was of low quality and not consistent for other indicators of asthma control.[246] However, vitamin D supplementation for the primary prevention of asthma rather than to improve asthma control is currently limited to prenatal interventions. In contrast to the evidence that the traditional diets, including the Mediterranean diet, may be protective for asthma, there has been concern that the introduction of highly processed "fast food" into the Western diet could be implicated in the rising prevalence of childhood asthma. In the ISAAC phase 3 study, a consistent association was found between questionnaire-reported frequency of fast food intake and asthma in children and adolescents.[247] However, on the basis of the current state of knowledge, there are no dietary interventions beyond pregnancy and early infancy that can be recommended specifically to lower the risk of developing childhood asthma. The role of the Mediterranean diet comprising a high proportion of fruit, vegetables, grains, and fish with olive oil contributing the chief source of fats, remains a topic of intense interest as there is observational evidence of a beneficial association between adherence to this dietary pattern and a number of health-related outcomes, including metabolic syndrome, cardiovascular disease, and type 2 diabetes as well as asthma. There is accumulating evidence that such benefits could result from immunomodulatory effects of the diet mediated through the gut microbiome.[248] The microbiome is the combined genetic material of all microorganisms in a particular environment and access to this information has been facilitated by modern, rapid DNA sequencing technology. According to the Gut Microbiome Project, the number of genes represented in the gut microbiome probably exceeds the number of human genes by at least two orders of magnitude (http://genome.wustl.edu/projects/detail/human-gut-microbiome/). Therefore, a complex interplay exists between nutrients and their metabolites, gut microbiota, and human immune cells. Adherence to a largely plant-based Mediterranean-type diet has been associated with a more favorable gut microbiome.[249] Targeted interventions to restore the healthy human microbiome may become an effective strategy to reduce the burden of asthma and allergic disease.[250]

Obesity

In parallel with the increased prevalence of asthma experienced in many developed countries in recent decades, there has been a large increase in childhood obesity in these countries. In the United States, childhood obesity has more than doubled over the last 30 years,[251] but the rate of increase has been even higher in developing countries (http://www.who.int/end-childhood-obesity/facts/en/). According to the World Health Organization (WHO) there will be a global increase to 7 million overweight or obese infants and young children by 2025. However, the contemporaneous increase in the prevalence of two conditions does not necessarily infer a direct relationship between them, far less a casual one. The epidemiologic evidence does support a positive association between overweight or obesity and asthma in children, and there is some evidence from adult studies of a temporal order of association with overweight/obesity preceding incident asthma.[252] Obesity is defined in adults as a BMI $\geq$ 30 kg/m^2 and overweight as a BMI $\geq$ 25 kg/m^2; age-specific values have been derived by the International Obesity Task Force, but different definitions have been used in the literature. A recent systematic review synthesized the evidence for the relationship between overweight and obesity with asthma in 38 studies that included over 1.4 million children. There was a positive relationship between increased BMI and asthma with some evidence of a "dose-response" with obesity having a stronger association than the overweight category, although there was substantial heterogeneity between studies.[253] Both asthma and obesity are complex polygenic diseases, and a number of possible explanations have been advanced to explain their coexistence. These include a common genetic background, mechanical changes in lung function associated with high body weight, changes in physical activity and diet, increased insulin resistance, and systemic inflammation, but evidence is still lacking to support a direct causal link.[254,255] So, the question remains whether high body mass causes asthma, potentially through the inflammatory influence of adipokines,[256] or that asthma and obesity share common etiologic pathways. Other possibilities are that this is a stochastic (random) association between two highly prevalent entities or that it is spurious and due to increased respiratory symptoms experienced by the obese, which are misinterpreted as asthma. Shared genes underpinning obesity and asthma were first suggested by linkage studies pointing to the β-adrenergic receptor, TNF-α, glucocorticoid receptor-β, and leptin genes, but none of these loci was associated with asthma in a GWAS, which indicated *DENND1B* variants to be associated with BMI in children with asthma.[257] A large number of genetic variants have now been identified from GWAS of obesity. A genetic risk score for BMI in children based on 32 of these SNPs was used in a Mendelian randomization study of BMI and asthma in children. This showed that higher BMI predicted from the genetic risk, and this, unconfounded by lifestyle and environment, was associated with an increased risk of asthma, lending some support to the existence of a true causal relationship.[258] This is further supported by intervention studies of weight-loss programs in obese patients with asthma, which have reported improvements in asthma control, bronchial responsiveness, and markers of airway inflammation.[259] A small RCT of diet-induced weight loss in obese children with asthma has confirmed some of these findings with reported improvement in asthma control, but without any observed changes in markers of airway or systemic inflammation.[260] Another trial of a multifactorial intervention that achieved weight loss in obese children with asthma also reported improvements in asthma control and lung function measures, although airway inflammation was not assessed.[261] These results mirror those in adult studies, which suggest that the mechanism of improvement in asthma control associated with weight loss are mediated through factors other than reduction in airway inflammation.[262]

INFECTIONS

Viral wheezing illness in early life is common, and affects around one-third of infants and young children. Viruses are also well recognized as the most frequent triggers of asthma in both adults and children. The two virus species that have received the most interest in relation to asthma development in early life are respiratory syncytial virus (RSV) and HRV. The growing interest in HRV infection is associated with modern molecular techniques of viral identification as it grows poorly in standard viral culture. RSV is a common cause of hospitalization for bronchiolitis during infancy and has long been recognized to be associated with postbronchiolitic wheezing. Serological evidence suggests that the vast majority of young children have encountered RSV infection by 2–3 years of age. So the question has been whether continued wheezing illnesses and subsequent diagnosis of asthma after bronchiolitis in infancy indicates a causal role for RSV in asthma development, or that hospitalization for RSV bronchiolitis is selective of those infants with either or both airway and immunological developmental features that already predispose them to later wheezing and asthma. A series of follow-up studies of a Swedish case control study of infants who were hospitalized with severe RSV bronchiolitis in their first year has shown an increased risk of asthma and allergic sensitization in the bronchiolitis group compared with healthy controls. This cohort has now been followed to age 18 years and the early findings have persisted.[263] Young adults who were hospitalized for RSV in infancy compared with controls had increased prevalence of asthma and allergic sensitization, lower FEV$_1$/FVC, and increased airway responsiveness. Shorter-term cohort studies have also reported an increased risk of wheezing, asthma, and lower FEV$_1$ following hospitalization for RSV bronchiolitis in infancy.[264,265] In an observational study of a randomized trial of montelukast after bronchiolitis, a family history of asthma, aeroallergen sensitization, and the severity of RSV infection were predictors of asthma at age 6 years.[265] It is possible that differences in outcomes from previous cohort studies that followed children hospitalized for bronchiolitis in infancy, but reported no increased risk of asthma, could be explained by the inclusion of a greater proportion of milder cases in population-based samples compared with clinical samples. The familial association of asthma with severe RSV bronchiolitis has recently been explored in genetic epidemiologic studies, showing a number of shared genes associated with the severity of response to RSV infection and asthma risk.[266] This evidence provides a plausible causal link between a severe RSV lower respiratory infection in infancy and an increased asthma risk in later childhood. Empirical evidence of differences in immune responses to RSV infections and subsequent asthma has also been provided by studies of blood and airway chemokines and cytokines during infection in relation to subsequent asthma. Gene variants in *ILRL1*, an asthma-associated gene, and ILRL1-a expression in the upper airway have been reported in association with severe RSV bronchiolitis.[267] Increased expression of CCL5 (RANTES) in the upper airway at the time of severe RSV bronchiolitis, in addition to the development of aeroallergen sensitization, has been linked to an increased risk of subsequent asthma.[268] Thus, there is a shifting focus to innate and adaptive host responses and their dysregulation in the etiology of asthma,[269] and therefore the therapeutic potential of immunomodulatory interventions, such as vaccines in primary prevention.[270,271] Meanwhile, trials of therapeutic interventions with antiinflammatory medications after bronchiolitis have been generally disappointing. Treatment with long-term, high-dose inhaled corticosteroids following hospitalization for RSV bronchiolitis has not been shown to influence respiratory outcomes.[272,273] Systematic reviews of leukotriene inhibitors after bronchiolitis in young children show that they may reduce symptoms of postbronchiolitic wheezing, but there is no evidence of a beneficial effect on the longer-term outcomes of recurrent wheezing or the use of inhaled corticosteroids for asthma.[274,275] The macrolide antibiotic azithromycin has been shown to reduce neutrophilic airway inflammation in a murine model of viral bronchiolitis[276] and has been shown to reduce the risk of subsequent severe lower respiratory infections in children with a history of such infections.[277] In a proof-of-concept trial, 14 days treatment with azithromycin after bronchiolitis was shown to reduce upper airway levels, but not serum IL-8 levels, and to reduce respiratory symptoms in the succeeding 12 months after illness.[278] Immunoprophylaxis for RSV with palivizumab is currently restricted to infants at high-risk of severe RSV bronchiolitis, so results may not be generalizable to the general population. Short-term reductions in

the frequency of wheezing symptoms have been reported in palivizumab-treated preterm infants[279,280] and, although suggestions of lower asthma prevalence in association with better adherence to palivizumab were reported in a retrospective analysis of an eligible cohort, this evidence needs to be confirmed in further studies[281] and in term infants at high risk for asthma.

A complex interplay between early life viral infection, host immune responses, and interactions with allergic sensitization in the genesis of asthma has also emerged from studies of the relationships between HRV infection and subsequent asthma risk. HRV is the most common virus identified in early life wheezing illnesses.[282] The association of early HRV-associated severe respiratory illnesses and subsequent wheezing and asthma was initially reported in a Finnish observational cohort study followed to 11 years of age. Prospective birth cohort studies have since confirmed this association.[283,284] The Childhood Onset of Asthma (COAST) study in the US has been instrumental in uncovering the mechanisms underlying this strong association (http://www.medicine.wisc.edu/coast/family). A recent follow-up of this high-risk birth cohort has shown a strong positive association between HRV and not RSV with regard to wheezing in the first 3 years and asthma at age 13 years (Fig. 42.5).[285] There was also evidence that the presence and timing of aeroallergen sensitization was

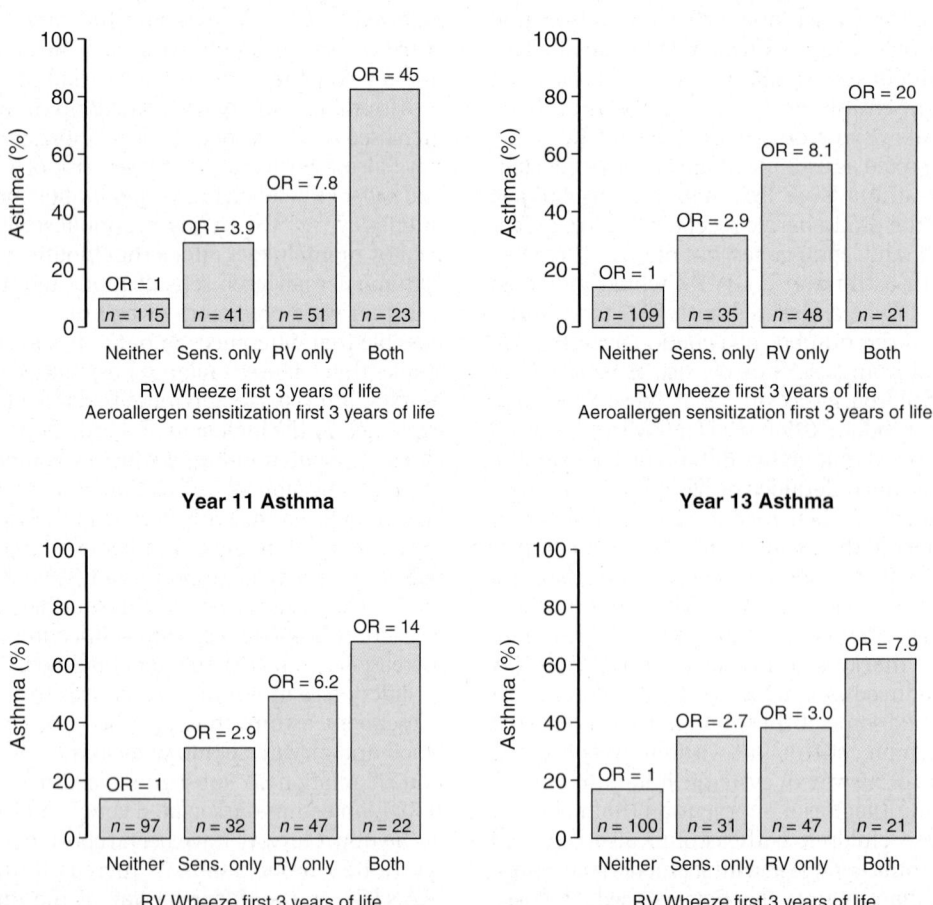

Fig. 42.5 Both aeroallergen sensitization and rhinovirus (RV) wheezing illnesses in the first 3 years of life increased asthma risk. The effects are additive and those children with both risk factors had the highest risk between the ages of 6 and 13 years. (From Rubner F, Jackson DJ, Evans MD, et al. Early life rhinovirus wheezing, allergic sensitization, and asthma risk at adolescence. *J Allergy Clin Immunol.* 2017;139(2):501-507.)

associated with subsequent asthma in this cohort; 65% of those sensitized in the first year compared with 40% sensitized by 5 years but not in the first year and 17% not sensitized by age 5 years, had asthma at 13 years and there was an additive effect with HRV wheezing illnesses. Furthermore, a temporal analysis of the association between allergic sensitization and viral wheezing illnesses in the COAST study has shown that allergic sensitization increases the risk of wheezing illnesses caused by HRV; however, the converse, HRV wheezing preceding allergic sensitization, was not supported.[286] This suggests a causal role for allergic sensitization in the biological pathway of asthma development following respiratory infection, particularly with HRV. Blunting of the seasonal increase of asthma exacerbations associated with viral infections by pretreatment with omalizumab provides additional support for the pivotal role of allergic sensitization in modifying the response to viral infections in the asthmatic airway.[287] The risk of subsequent asthma following HRV infection has also been found to be enhanced by genetic variants at the 17q21 locus, an asthma associated locus in the GWAS of asthma in children, and with expression of two of the genes at this locus, *ORMDL3* and *GSDMB* in the COAST and the Copenhagen Study on Asthma in Childhood (COPSAC) birth cohorts.[147] It is likely that dysregulated immune responses to viral infections of the airway play an important role in asthma inception. Candidate genes selected for their role in antiviral responses have been identified in association with viral-induced asthma exacerbations and childhood asthma phenotypes.[288] Impaired innate immunity with deficient interferon responses to respiratory viral infections has been previously reported. Studies of airway epithelial cells from children with asthma compared with cells from healthy controls have shown increased susceptibility of the former to HRV infection with increased viral replication, reduced production of interferons, and impaired apoptotic responses,[289] although it is conceivable that the presence of asthma alters cellular immune responses rather than arising as a direct consequence of immune dysregulation.

The almost exclusive focus on the role of viral pathogens in the respiratory tract in the development of asthma has recently been broadened to the consideration of the role of airway colonization with bacteria.[290] Bacterial colonization of the upper respiratory tract in asymptomatic infants with the pathogenic bacteria, *Streptococcus pneumonia*, *Haemophilus influenzae* or *Moraxella catarrhalis* was reported to be associated with increased risk for asthma at age 5 years in the COPSAC study.[291] Subsequent evaluation of the mucosal inflammatory response associated with bacterial colonization of the infant airway demonstrated an inflammatory mediator profile indicating a mixed T-helper cell response.[292] Using molecular genetic techniques (*16sRNA* sequencing), the lower airway microbiome, which comprises a very high proportion of organisms that cannot be cultured using conventional methods, has been investigated in adults and children with and without asthma. These showed that the density of bacterial genomes in the lower airways was equivalent to the upper intestine and there were marked differences in the bacterial phyla and genera between asthmatic and healthy airways (Fig. 42.6).[293] The phylum Proteobacteria was overrepresented in asthmatic airways and contains the pathogens, *Haemophilus* spp. and *Moraxella* spp., which were identified in association with asthma in infant airways in the COPSAC

study. A number of exposures that could potentially perturb the composition of the airway microbiome have been associated with increased asthma risk in observational studies. These include cesarean section birth (baby not exposed to vaginal microflora), exposure to tobacco smoke,[294] and treatment with antibiotics during early life.[295] However, the causal association of the airway microbiome with asthma inception has yet to be established. Although perturbation of the microbiome offers a plausible explanation for these associations, confounding is an alternative explanation for all observational associations. In the case of antibiotic use, both erroneous treatment of early asthma symptoms with antibiotics (reverse causation) and confounding by indication, where antibiotic use is associated with an independent factor, which is itself associated with increased asthma risk, could explain the observed association.[296]

Helminth infestations are common in many low-income countries where asthma prevalence and morbidity in children is low.[297] It has been suggested that modulation of the host-immune response by helminth infection, which is mediated through Th2 responses, could be protective for the development of asthma and allergies in children.[298] However, although there is some evidence to support a reduction in prevalence of allergic sensitization associated with specific helminth infections,[299–301] there also have been reports of positive associations between IgE sensitization to helminths and increased risk of asthma in children.[302–304] A recent study of coinfection with helminths in poor, urban children in Latin America showed a dose-dependent reduction in aeroallergen sensitization, but no influence on asthma risk.[305]

FARMING STUDIES

In contrast with studies suggesting a causal role of infections in the etiology of asthma in early childhood, following Strachan's formulation of the hygiene hypothesis in 1989 based on his observations of an inverse association between family size in childhood and subsequent hay fever,[306] there has been interest in the possible protective effect of early infections on the risk of asthma and allergies in children. Farming studies from central Europe and other settings, reported a reduced prevalence of asthma, hay fever, and allergic sensitization in children growing up on farms.[307] The main environmental factors associated with reduced risk of asthma and allergy were contact with farm animals and their foodstuffs, and the consumption of unpasteurized milk, with the strongest effects for exposure during pregnancy and early life. Environmental studies based on the analysis of dust samples from farm residences suggested that increased diversity of microbial exposure compared with reference populations could be the mechanism for the observed protective effect of farm living on asthma in children.[308] Endotoxin, a lipopolysaccharide constituent of gram-negative bacterial cell walls had previously been shown to be inversely associated with allergy in children living on farms, but there were inconsistencies in associations reported between endotoxin exposure and asthma in other settings, including urban environments. A recent study of Hutterite and Amish children in the United States has shed further light on the mechanisms of microbial exposure in farming environments. The Hutterite and Amish share common European ancestry and lifestyles, but have markedly different farming practices; the former living on

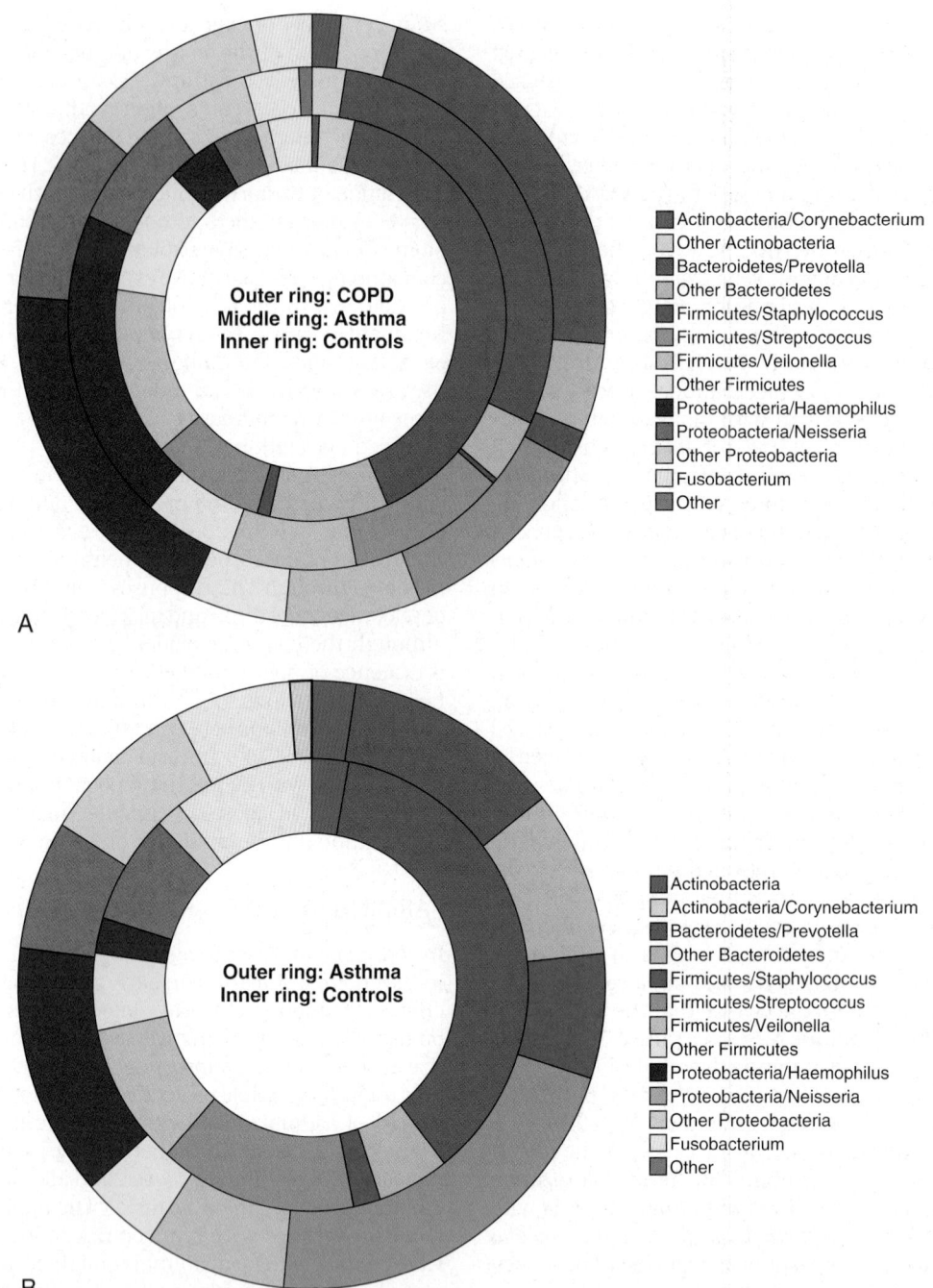

Fig. 42.6 (A) Distribution of the phyla from sheathed bronchoscopic brushings of the left upper lobe for patients with asthma and COPD, and normal subjects, subdivided into the seven most frequent genera. *(Corynebacterium, Prevotella, Staphylococcus, Streptococcus, Veilonella, Haemophilus, and Neisseria.)* (B) Distribution of the phyla from broncho-alveolar lavage in children with difficult asthma and controls. *COPD,* Chronic obstructive pulmonary disease. (From Hilty M, Burke C, Pedro H. Disordered microbial communities in asthmatic airways. *PLoS One.* 2010;5(1):e8578.)

large-scale, communal, industrialized farms and the latter following more traditional farming practices. They also have striking differences in the prevalence of asthma and allergic sensitization in their children, being around four times higher in the Hutterite than Amish communities.[309,310] This study showed markedly higher endotoxin levels in dust from Amish homes accompanied by differences in innate immune profiles between the two populations, suggesting that microbial exposure in the Amish acted through innate immune targets to decrease asthma risk in this population.[23]

PHYSICAL ACTIVITY

Exercise is well recognized as a common trigger for wheeze in children with asthma but the relationship between habitual levels of physical activity and asthma inception is less clear. There is also a complex relationship between physical activity, obesity, and asthma.[311] The contemporaneous rise in asthma prevalence and the move to more sedentary leisure pursuits in children has led to a suggestion that low levels of physical activity or changes in breathing patterns associated with long periods of sitting could influence asthma development.[312] Some studies have reported associations of low levels of physical activity in children with asthma, but the measurement of exposure is problematic; self-report diaries of physical activity are notoriously inaccurate although they remain the dominant instrument in epidemiologic surveys. Objective measurements of heart rate and movements have their own problems, including participant burden, suitability for all forms of physical activity, such as swimming and cycling, and interpretation of the resulting metrics.[313] It is likely that some of these problems inherent in measuring physical activity will be overcome in future with developments in smart technology. One form of physical activity that has received particular attention is swimming, due to the putative risk associated with exposure to products of water chlorination for disinfection.[314] Although there is some evidence to suggest an increase in new-onset asthma in children exposed to chlorinated pools, swimming training for children with asthma appears to be well-tolerated and is not associated with the worsening of asthma control.[315] Physical training has been suggested to reduce airway inflammation in asthma and therefore to be of potential therapeutic benefit. A systematic review of studies that measured airway inflammatory markers after a period of physical training noted generally small sample sizes and substantial heterogeneity in the prescribed interventions and in the methods used to measure airway inflammatory responses.[316] Therefore, although there was some evidence to support a beneficial effect of physical training on airway inflammation, it was inconclusive. A further systematic review of exercise training in children with asthma concluded that it was well tolerated, but there was no evidence to support beneficial effects on asthma control, bronchial responsiveness, and airway inflammation.[317] There is no current evidence that physical training improves lung function in children with asthma, but it does increase aerobic capacity and may be associated with overall benefits in health-related QoL.[318] One caveat to the potential benefits of exercise in childhood asthma is the observation from the Southern California Children's Health Study (CHS) that asthma incidence associated with air pollution (ozone) exposure was modified by physical exercise; and children that participated in more team sports and spent more time outside had higher asthma incidence, but only in areas of high ozone exposure.[319]

AIR QUALITY

Outdoor Air Pollution

Since the seminal report of increased asthma and allergies in West German children compared with their peers from East Germany after reunification in 1990,[18] there has been a great deal of interest in the concept that air pollution, particularly from traffic-related sources of fossil fuel combustion, could contribute to the development of asthma in children. Like many observational associations, an argument has raged over whether traffic-related pollutants are causal risk factors for asthma or triggers for asthma symptoms, compounded by the problems of socioeconomic confounding, as children in deprived urban neighborhoods are likely to be exposed to higher levels of air pollution than those in more affluent areas.[320] Advances in geospatial modeling methods with greater resolution have added considerably to the ability to study longitudinal exposure to air pollution at an individual rather than an ecological level in large, unselected population cohorts[321] in which some of the problems of confounding and effect modification can be addressed. Technological advances will soon facilitate meaningful personal exposure monitoring and the ability to incorporate individual activity patterns to modeled estimates of microenvironmental exposure levels. Evidence is now beginning to emerge that air pollution exposure is causal in the development of asthma in childhood.[322] A report by the British Royal College of Physicians has reviewed the evidence for long-term effects of air pollution on health throughout the life course with an emphasis on exposure during the early years of life (https://www.rcplondon.ac.uk/projects/outputs/every-breath-we-take-lifelong-impact-air-pollution),[323] and a detailed review of the evidence of the health effects of air pollution has been published by the WHO with a focus on the impact on policy making in Europe (http://www.euro.who.int/en/health-topics/environment-and-health/air-quality/publications/2013/review-of-evidence-on-health-aspects-of-air-pollution-revihaap-project-final-technical-report).[324] Also, there is evidence that the exposure of pregnant women to air pollution can be associated with increased asthma risk in children (see section "Maternal Lifestyle and Environment," p. 654) and with low lung function in the newborn, which, in turn, increases the risk of early respiratory symptoms and is associated with later asthma.

Traffic-related air pollution comprises a range of toxic gases and particulate matter (PM). Due to the cost and bulk of personal exposure monitoring for several components contemporaneously, the majority of epidemiologic research has relied on modeled estimates of exposure, which is often linked to the residential addresses of study participants.

Results of these observational studies have been heterogeneous. A systematic review of TRAP exposure in birth cohort studies found evidence that increased longitudinal exposure to $PM_{2.5}$ and black carbon was associated with an increased risk of asthma. Different methods were used to estimate exposures, the most common being land-use regression (LUR) but including dispersion models, passive sampling, and the distance of the residence to the main roads. These results were consistent with a recent US study showing that long-term exposure to TRAP from birth to 7 years estimated from LUR models was associated with asthma.[325] However, a large, European, multicenter collaboration that modeled six traffic-related pollutants (NO_2, nitrogen oxides [NOx], PM_{10}, and $PM_{2.5}$, coarse particulates and $PM_{2.5}$ absorbance) also using LUR in five birth cohorts found no associations with asthma prevalence for any of the pollutants considered.[326] The Pollution and the Young (PATY) project in Europe and North America found no associations of annual average PM_{10} concentrations[327] or NO_2 levels[328] with asthma or lung function. The ISAAC study also found no strong evidence of associations between modeled annual, city-level estimates of PM_{10} exposure and asthma outcomes in children, although it was acknowledged that these exposure estimates were likely to be imprecise.[329] In contrast, the US and Puerto Rican GALA II and SAGE II studies, using fixed monitoring sites to measure annual average exposures to ozone, NO_2, sulfur dioxide (SO_2), PM_{10} and $PM_{2.5}$ reported early-life exposure to NO_2 was associated with asthma risk in Latin and African-American populations.[330] Also, using fixed monitoring sites, a Chinese study has shown that early life exposure to NO_2 and SO_2 was associated with increased asthma risk in children.[331] Clearly, there are differences in both the methods of estimating pollution exposures and in the populations and settings in which these studies were conducted. Gene–environment interaction studies have recently been done to attempt to identify populations at risk of air pollution effects. The traffic asthma and genetics (TAG) study found an association between NO_2 exposure and asthma risk in children with minor alleles in the *GSTP1* gene.[154] A meta-analysis of 19 studies of TRAP exposure in children reported that high levels of NO_2, nitrous oxide (N_2O), and carbon monoxide (CO) were associated with an increased risk of prevalent asthma in childhood, and NO_2 was associated with new-onset asthma.[332] Taken together, there is certainly evidence to support early life exposure to TRAP being associated with new-onset respiratory symptoms and asthma in children, although there remains some doubt about whether there is a specific component of relevance with evidence of positive associations for both gaseous and particulate exposures. Recent evidence suggests that exposure to diesel exhaust particles (DEP) results in accumulation of TH2/TH17 cells in the airways, providing an environment that predisposes towards the development of allergic asthma.[333] Exposure to DEP has also been associated with early sensitization to aeroallergens in children,[334] which may interact with viral respiratory illnesses in the developmental pathway of asthma. An increase in the proportion of diesel vehicles in Europe, although not in the United States or Japan, combined with technological difficulties in reducing their real-world emissions of PM and NO_2, has meant that urban levels of these pollutants have not fallen as quickly as hoped, to meet European clean air legislation standards.

The effect of exposure to gaseous pollutants, CO, SO_2 and NO_2 measured at the closest monitoring site to residential address was studied in children with asthma in the US CAMP study and was found to be associated with worsening lung function and increasing bronchial responsiveness.[335] There is also evidence for increased systemic markers of inflammation in children with asthma exposed to high levels of NO_2 in two German cohorts.[336] Living close to main roads was associated with an increase in the risk of asthma attacks in an Italian study[337] and TRAP exposure from LUR model estimates was associated with hospital readmissions for asthma or wheezing in a US cohort, but only in white American, not African-American, children.[32] The association between asthma hospital encounters and ambient levels of ozone and $PM_{2.5}$ were stronger in areas with higher-than-median traffic-related sources of pollution in a US study.[338] The evidence that traffic-related exposures could exacerbate asthma symptoms prompted a study in the UK to investigate the effects of an intervention designed to reduce urban air pollution exposure—the London Low Emission Zone (LEZ). However, during its first 3 years of operation, there was no evidence that the LEZ had led to a reduction in either ambient air pollution levels or the prevalence of respiratory symptoms in 8- to 9-year-old school children.[339]

Although traffic-related pollution is a major concern in HICs, the rise in asthma prevalence in rapidly industrializing LMICs has been accompanied by an increase in the contribution to ambient pollutant levels of industrial processes,[340] including fossil-fuel-fired power stations, waste incineration, and agricultural emissions, plus a greater reliance on coal combustion, which is a major emitter of gaseous and particulate pollution.[341] A cross-sectional study in Brazil found increased respiratory symptoms in children living downwind of a petrochemical plant, despite ambient levels of several pollutants being consistently lower than regulatory limits.[342] Similar results have been reported for children living near a petrochemical plant in Spain.[343] Therefore, industrial sources of air pollutants remain an important consideration for asthma inception in industrializing nations and contributing to asthma morbidity worldwide. Industrial sources also contribute to indoor air pollution in developing countries.[344]

There is increasing interest in the relationship of the built environment with human health and residential green space, and increased biodiversity has been suggested as a possible health benefit, although previous studies of asthma have been conflicting. In a Spanish study, green space was associated with a lower prevalence of obesity but not of asthma, although, conversely, living close to a park was associated with asthma but not with obesity.[345] In a population-based cohort of preschool children in British Columbia, residential access to green space was associated with a lower risk of incident asthma, which was enhanced in models that included air pollution exposure.[346] In contrast, a Lithuanian study found that residential greenness was associated with a small increase in asthma risk in 4- to 6-year-old children.[347] A multicenter study of five cohorts from Europe and North America reported differential associations between centers of residential greenness with aeroallergen sensitization by 10–12 years and with no strong evidence of an overall effect.[348] Therefore, the evidence for a beneficial or harmful effect of residential green space on asthma and allergy risk in children remains to be determined; it has potential benefit through increased biodiversity, but also can increase seasonal aeroallergen exposure in the immediate environment.

Indoor Air Quality. Young children spend a large part of their time indoors, especially in temperate and cold climate countries. The contribution of air quality to asthma risk and asthma control has tended to focus on the outdoor environment, but the realization that early life exposure is such a critical period for the development of asthma and related illnesses makes the indoor environment an important factor in asthma inception. The most well-established risk factor for asthma in young children is exposure to tobacco smoke with a major contribution coming from exposure in the prenatal period.[185] Second-hand smoke (SHS) exposure in the postnatal period is associated with increased asthma morbidity. A meta-analysis of 25 studies showed that children exposed to SHS were almost twice as likely to be hospitalized for asthma and suffered more emergency room and urgent care visits than nonexposed children with asthma.[349] The introduction of smoking bans in many legislatures caused initial concerns that smoke-free workplaces and public spaces might paradoxically increase children's exposure in the home. However, this was not borne out in practice. Smoke-free legislation has been associated with a reduction in SHS and improved indices of asthma morbidity in adults[350] and children.[351] Hospital admissions for asthma in English children fell after the introduction of national smoke-free legislation[57] and a systematic review of the impact of smoke-free legislation on children's health, including studies in Europe and

North America, showed an overall reduction in hospital attendances for asthma of around 10%.[352] In a Chinese study of multiple factors in the home environment in early childhood in relation to new-onset asthma, smoking was identified as a risk factor, although this may have been linked to prenatal exposure that was not assessed. Other features of the home environment in the first 2 years that were associated with later asthma were molds and poor air quality as judged by questions on dryness and odor of the indoor air.[353] Residential indoor molds and dampness have been associated with increased asthma risk in meta-analyses and with asthma exacerbations in both adults and children.[354] However, a Swedish study quantified culturable fungi in dust from the homes of children with asthma and allergies, and healthy controls, and found no associations between fungal concentrations and any health outcomes.[355] A review of other measured microbial factors in the indoor air confirmed only suggestive associations, despite clear observational evidence of an association between asthma and the reported presence of molds and dampness.[354] The ISAAC study also confirmed a link between questionnaire reports of molds and dampness and increased risk of prevalent wheezing in 8- to 12-year-old children in both affluent and nonaffluent countries unrelated to atopy.[356] A recent study used structural inspection of the home at age 5 months in a birth cohort to confirm evidence of moisture damage and found a positive association with asthma at 5 years.[357]

Sources of combustion in the home to provide heat and cooking have been recognized for a long time as emitters of indoor pollutants that might be associated with respiratory symptoms in young children. There is considerable evidence from developed countries that gas stoves used for cooking or heating are associated with an increased risk of asthma in children. Gas stoves are a source of particulate matter and NOx. In a cross-sectional study of participants in the NHANES III Examination, the ventilation characteristics of gas stoves were evaluated. Children in homes that reported using ventilation when the gas stove was in use had a lower risk of asthma and higher lung function values than those where ventilation was either not available or not used.[358] From a worldwide perspective, biomass combustion is a common fuel for cooking and heating in low-income countries, and has a high burden of mortality and morbidity.[359] A systematic review of biomass smoke exposure of women and children found evidence for an increased risk of acute respiratory tract infection, but not asthma, in children.[360] A subsequent cross-sectional study of 5- to 11-year-old children in Nigeria confirmed a lack of association of lifetime asthma risk and evidence of airway obstruction associated with the daily use of firewood compared with a lower frequency of exposure.[361]

A further source of indoor atmospheric pollutants that has been linked to asthma risk is derived from volatile organic compounds (VOCs); a range of chemicals that enter the breathed environment through evaporation from common domestic products, such as cleaning agents, air fresheners, cosmetics, furnishing fabrics, plus paint and floor and wall coverings (https://www.epa.gov/indoor-air-quality-iaq). Most exposure to VOCs occurs indoors as a result of numerous emission sources, low ventilation rates, and the length of time spent indoors, especially in homes.[362] A systematic review of observational and intervention studies of VOCs and the risk of asthma and allergy concluded that the evidence base was of poor quality with inconsistent results.[363] The most frequently studied VOCs in relation to children's asthma are aromatic compounds, such as benzene, toluenes, xylenes, and formaldehyde. A systematic review of formaldehyde exposure and childhood asthma suggested a positive association, but this was largely based on cross-sectional data.[364] Benzene has been suggested to adversely affect respiratory health, including asthma, in children, but the diversity of study design in a systematic review meant that definitive conclusions could not be drawn.[365] Studies of the effects of VOC exposure on asthma symptoms have been beset by similar methodological heterogeneity as the studies of associations of VOCs with asthma prevalence or incidence. For example, a systematic review of exposure to paint fumes in domestic (as opposed to occupational) settings suggested a possible association with wheezing in children, but variations in exposure assignment and study design made it difficult to determine if this particular exposure could cause or exacerbate asthma symptoms.[366] The overall synthesis of evidence, while suggestive of an adverse effect of VOCs on the development and exacerbation of asthma in children needs to be confirmed in well-designed, prospective studies.

Allergy, Asthma, and the Allergic March

Asthma in childhood is commonly associated with allergic sensitization, and in epidemiologic studies, evidence of allergic sensitization, either through skin prick or specific serum IgE testing, is often used to distinguish between atopic and nonatopic asthma. Atopic asthma, particularly when accompanied by evidence of multiple sensitizations, is associated with onset in childhood, increased risk of severe exacerbations, and poorer long-term prognosis.[367] Asthma clusters within families with other diseases that have an allergic basis,[368] including eczema and allergic rhinitis, and the rise in asthma prevalence experienced in industrialized nations towards the end of the 20th century, were accompanied by an increased prevalence of other allergic conditions.[369] These observations gave rise to the notion of the allergic march; a temporal progression of allergic diseases through early childhood.[370] However, despite their shared characteristic of allergic sensitization, much of the circumstantial evidence for the allergic march was derived from repeat cross-sectional studies. Recent analysis of longitudinal data from birth cohorts indicates that the allergic march is the exception rather than the rule in children with early onset of one of these conditions, usually eczema.[371,372] The situation is probably complex as specific genetic associations with the asthma–hay fever phenotype that are distinguishable from GWAS hits for asthma alone have been identified.[142] This fits with emerging evidence that allergic asthma in children is not a single phenotype, but comprises several subphenotypes.[374] Concepts of allergy are also evolving, and the reductionist approach of assigning allergic status on the basis of defined "positive" thresholds of skin or serological tests is now anachronistic. More sensitive and precise methods allow better quantitation of the strength of the allergic response,[375] component resolved diagnostics enable responses to different epitopes to be identified,[376] and new analytical methods that group responses to allergen classes have been developed. Applying a machine learning approach for analyzing longitudinal repeat assessments of allergic sensitization in a birth cohort led to the identification of different latent patterns of allergic sensitization,[377] which were replicated in an independent cohort.[378] Multiple, early sensitization had a substantially stronger association than conventional classification of atopy with asthma and with markers of asthma severity. The evidence that monosensitization and polysensitization carry different risk profiles combined with novel approaches to classification of disease are now being integrated with "-omics" data in systems biology models of disease in a bid to increase the understanding of allergy and its relationship with disease manifestations.[379]

The importance of allergic sensitization to asthma inception inevitably raises the question of whether allergen exposure in early life is an important step in this process. However, although allergen exposure is a prerequisite for sensitization, the evidence from observational and intervention studies suggests a complex interplay between the dose, timing, and route of allergen exposure, the presence of coexposures, and the genetic predisposition of the individual in the development of allergic diseases.[380] Allergen avoidance was shown to be ineffective in reducing respiratory symptoms in children up to 3 years of age, but increased dust mite sensitization in the intervention group in a highly effective dust mite avoidance study in a high-risk population of infants.[381] Therefore, different approaches to primary prevention of allergic sensitization and prevention of progression to asthma are required.[382] These might include the therapeutic application of allergen[383] and the blocking of host responses,[384] some of which have been tested in proof-of-principle studies pending larger scale trials.

Conclusions

Epidemiology has been remarkably successful in tracking change in the prevalence of asthma over time and geography, particularly through collaboration in large-scale international studies, such as ISAAC. These studies, in turn, pointed to variations in the environment and lifestyle that were associated with greater or lesser prevalence of asthma. The recognition of early life events as being fundamental to asthma etiology prompted the development of birth cohorts, some of which were recruited in pregnancy and were well placed to study antenatal as well as postnatal influences. These have been instrumental in developing ideas about phenotypic variation in asthma and in studying the associations of environment on the risk of developing the disease. However, despite enormous efforts, few risk factors were identified that had more than modest evidence of association, and the establishment of causality was not possible, even with stringent attention to the sources of bias, confounding, and measurement error. New approaches to epidemiologic analysis are starting to address some of these problems, but proof of causal association still relies on experiments. The advent of high throughput methods for genomic and other-omic assays moved asthma genetics beyond the field of candidate gene discovery to agnostic genome-wide associations, which have indicated novel genetic regions that are associated with asthma and which have been replicated in independent studies. Attention is now shifting from gene discovery to the investigation of gene–gene and gene–environment interactions, and to the modification of genetic effects through epigenetic mechanisms that form a bridge between the environment and genetic expression. The jury is still out on whether heritable epigenetic marks are important in explaining some of the high heritability of asthma that is seen in twin studies. Recent convergence of two important pathways that have long been recognized as being fundamentally important in the early origins of asthma in children has produced new insights into the interplay between allergic sensitization and viral respiratory tract infections, so we are now on the brink of interventions for primary prevention. Therefore, despite the limitations of identifying causal factors in the development of disease that are inherent to epidemiologic study design, epidemiology has made a major contribution to understanding the phenotypic variation of asthma in children, particularly around the critical time when early life respiratory infections progress to asthma. It has also provided insights into how genetic predisposition influences responses to environmental exposures, and which factors in the environment are likely to be important in asthma inception. The generation of massive amounts of data from technological innovations in assaying genetic variation, biomarkers of disease, and environmental factors—and their integration into systems biology models of disease—present new challenges to developing the analytical tools and interpretative strategies necessary for the translation of this new knowledge into patient benefit.

References

Access the reference list online at ExpertConsult.com.

Suggested Reading

Asher MI. Recent perspectives on global epidemiology of asthma in childhood. *Allergol Immunopathol (Madr)*. 2010;38:83–87.

Chang TS, Lemanske RF Jr, Mauger DT, et al. Childhood asthma clusters and response to therapy in clinical trials. *J Allergy Clin Immunol*. 2014;133:363–369.

Jackson DJ, Gern JE, Lemanske RF Jr. The contributions of allergic sensitization and respiratory pathogens to asthma inception. *J Allergy Clin Immunol*. 2016;137:659–665.

Ober C, Yao TC. The genetics of asthma and allergic disease: a 21st century perspective. *Immunol Rev*. 2011;242:10–30.

Tai A, Tran H, Roberts M, et al. Outcomes of childhood asthma to the age of 50 years. *J Allergy Clin Immunol*. 2014;133:1572–1578.

43 The Immunopathogenesis of Asthma

SEJAL SAGLANI, BSc, MBChB, MD, and CLARE M. LLOYD, PhD

The fundamental pathophysiological features of asthma include airway hyperresponsiveness (which can also manifest as reversible airflow obstruction), inflammation, and structural changes in the airway wall, collectively termed airway remodeling. The development of allergic sensitization is also key to the immunopathology of pediatric disease. The combined clinical effects of these abnormalities result in the manifestation of symptoms which include shortness of breath and wheezing, with or without cough.

A key factor that needs to be considered in the immunopathogenesis of pediatric asthma is the age of the child. Wheezing disorders are common in children aged 5 and under, but not all preschool wheezers will develop asthma and the mechanisms mediating preschool wheeze are likely to be distinct from those that result in progression to asthma and drive asthma in school-aged children. A complex interplay between host susceptibility, the developing airway microbiome, environmental insults such as exposure to allergens and pollution, and respiratory infections results in pulmonary immune responses and the pathophysiological features of asthma (Fig. 43.1). The aim of this chapter is to summarize what is known about the immunology and pathology of allergic asthma in children and to highlight specific situations, such as preschool wheeze, asthma exacerbations, and severe therapy resistant asthma, in which this common immunopathology may not apply. The need to focus on approaches to achieve disease modification and asthma prevention in the future will also be discussed.

Altered Pulmonary Immunity in Asthma Inception

Development of allergic sensitization is a key component of asthma pathogenesis in children. Sensitization may develop to food or aero-allergens and is initiated at mucosal or barrier surfaces where there is an epithelial layer. Respiratory mucosal surfaces (airways) are continuously exposed to inhaled, nonpathogenic foreign particles (antigens, microbes, and pollutants). A key challenge for the healthy respiratory system is therefore to distinguish innocuous antigens from pathological microbes.[1] However, in disease, and with a host underlying susceptibility to allergic disease, an exaggerated immune response is mounted to inhaled allergens. The pulmonary epithelium is the first point of contact and both barrier and immune function of this airway structure is altered in children with asthma.[2,3] The altered bronchial epithelial function results in a "leaky" airway wall and permits entry of antigen (allergen) through the epithelium (Fig. 43.2)[4] with recognition and uptake by the pulmonary antigen presenting cells—dendritic cells (DCs)—that are continuously undertaking surveillance close to the mucosal surface.[5] DC dendrites may protrude through to the airway lumen to undertake antigen recognition via cell surface receptors (see Fig. 43.2). DCs take up the antigen, then migrate to the pulmonary draining (mediastinal) lymph nodes where they present the antigen to naive T cells. The naive T helper (Th0) cells subsequently differentiate to type 2 T helper cells under the influence of inflammatory cytokines such as interleukin (IL)-4. The Th2 cells are then released and migrate back to the pulmonary tissue where, with further allergen exposure, they initiate an allergic reaction characterized by the release of additional allergic inflammatory cytokines including IL-5 and IL-13. In parallel, antigen is presented to B cells in the draining lymph nodes where the antigen (allergen) is processed, and immunoglobulin (Ig)E antibody to the antigen is secreted by B cells and released into the circulation and pulmonary tissue in preparation for a response to future allergen exposure (see Fig. 43.2). IL-4 is necessary to allow the isotype switch of antibody production from IgG molecules to Ig-E molecules in an allergic environment. Allergen sensitization results from the initial allergen exposure, and subsequent allergen exposure results in an allergic reaction. This is characterized by recognition of the allergen (antigen) by Ig-E (antibody), which binds to mast cells and results in mast cell degranulation with release of histamine and leukotrienes and a resulting type 1 immediate reaction (see Fig. 43.2). This is associated with a more chronic allergic reaction that results from induction of Th2 cells and downstream inflammatory mediators including IL-4, IL-5, and IL-13, which are the hallmark of and drive for allergic reactions.

Cells, Molecules, and Cytokines Involved in Pediatric Allergic Asthma

EOSINOPHILS AND INTERLEUKIN-5

Eosinophils are the hallmark feature of the asthmatic immune response in most patients,[6] children in particular. The role of eosinophils in allergic inflammation is summarized in Box 43.1.

Eosinophils contain multiple granule proteins that exhibit an array of toxic and immune-modulatory activities. The granule proteins can be released by different mechanisms, including during an acute allergic insult, and they cascade the proinflammatory, Th2 responses associated with allergic asthma.[8] The cytokines and chemokines released following eosinophil degranulation promote longevity of eosinophils in tissues, which leads to the cyclical nature of signaling, activation, and survival. Additionally, these proteins target any foreign antigen, promote inflammation in the

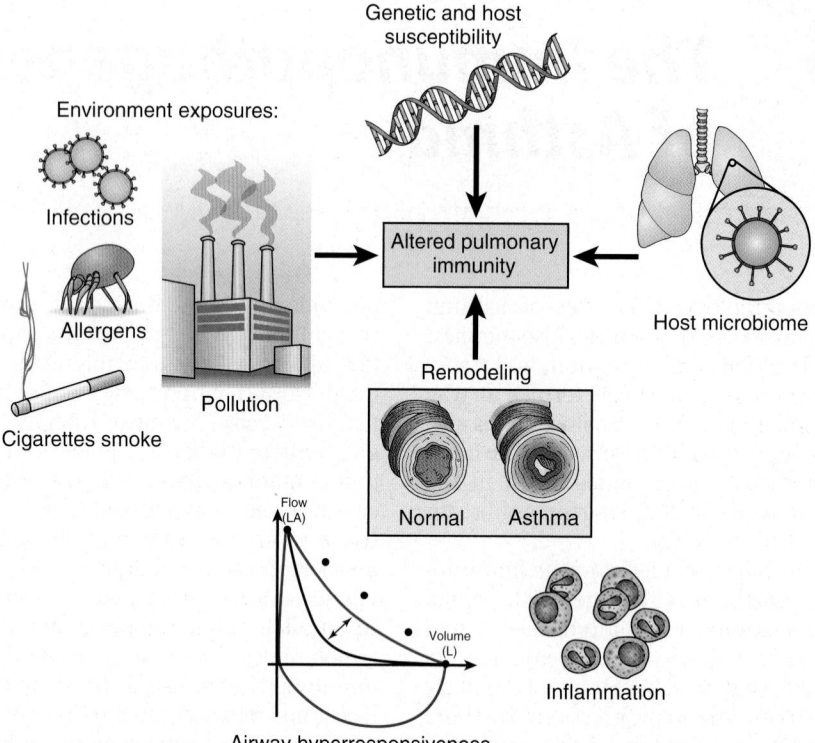

Fig. 43.1 Multiple interactions and factors leading to asthma development. Environmental exposures such as allergens, viruses, cigarette smoke, and pollution, combined with an underlying genetic susceptibility and an altered airway microbiome, result in the development of altered pulmonary immunity and the pathophysiological abnormalities of asthma.

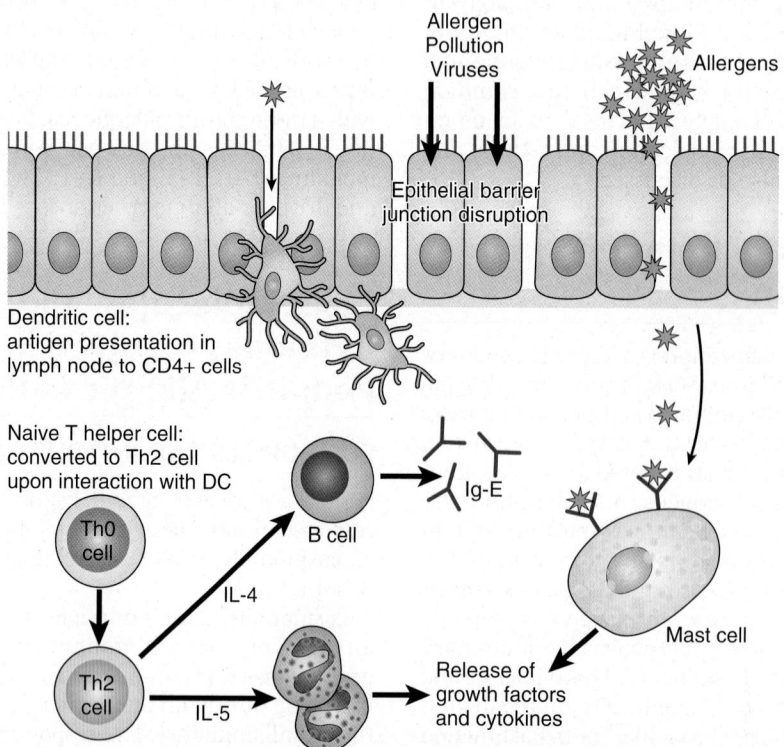

Fig. 43.2 Development of allergic sensitization and asthma. Inhaled exposures cause barrier dysfunction, which makes the epithelium "leaky" and allows entry of allergens through the airway wall, to be recognized by the pulmonary antigen presenting cells (dendritic cells) for subsequent antigen processing and development of allergic sensitization. Immunoglobulin (Ig)-E antibodies are synthesized by B cells and released into the circulation where they recognize antigen. This is followed by binding to mast cells to release growth factors and mediators results in symptoms of allergy and asthma.

Box 43.1   The Role of Eosinophils in the Development of Allergic Inflammation

1. Initiation of events that lead to Th2 inflammation
2. Suppression of Th1 mediated immunity
3. Recruitment of Th2 cells to the lung
4. Release of growth factors that contribute to the development of airway remodeling[7]

Th, T helper.

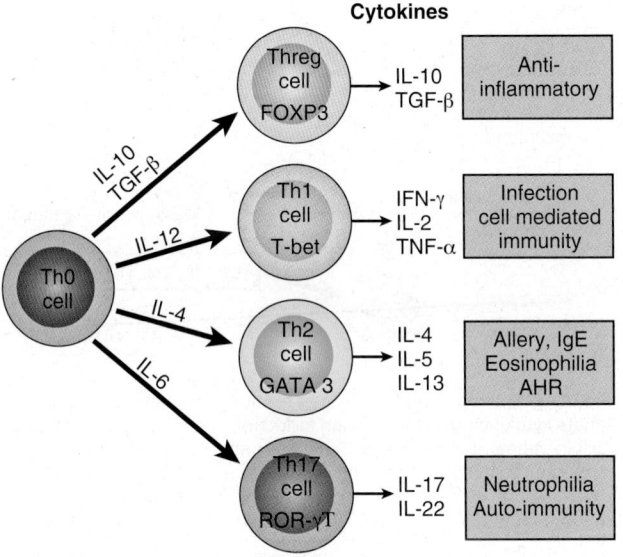

Fig. 43.3 Differentiation of Th0 naïve T cells to specific T helper cell phenotypes under the influence of specific cytokines. Each T helper cell subtype is defined by a unique transcription factor which determines its function and secretion of helper cell specific cytokines. *FOXP3*, Forkhead box P3; *IFN-γ*, interferon gamma; *IL*, interleukin; *TGF-β*, transforming growth factor beta; *Th*, T helper; *Treg*, T regulatory.

area, and may cause considerable damage to surrounding structures.[6]

IL-5 is released by Th2 cells in asthma (Fig. 43.3) and results in the induction and recruitment of eosinophils from the peripheral circulation to the airways. IL-5 also promotes eosinophil differentiation, growth, and survival.[9] The airway eosinophilia that is characteristic of pediatric allergic asthma in children is therefore thought to be mediated by IL-5. However, this is an assumption based on extrapolation from animal and adult studies. Firm evidence for the presence of IL-5 in the airways of children with stable asthma is difficult to find. As airway samples are not easily obtained from children, most studies investigating the mediators of allergic asthma include assessments of peripheral blood, but this is not always a reliable surrogate for the airways.[10] Another issue that affects the detection of Th2 cytokines in asthma is that they are steroid sensitive, so it can be difficult to find elevated levels in patients who are not "steroid naïve" and who have been prescribed maintenance inhaled steroids (which is the case for most children long before referral to hospital). However, it remains certain that the predominant airway inflammatory phenotype of pediatric asthma is eosinophilic, and this is independent of disease severity[11,12] or

duration.[13–15] Therefore modulating eosinophil function or reducing their numbers has been one of the most important therapeutic goals in asthma for many years. The mainstay of treatment for asthma is inhaled glucocorticoid steroids. Glucocorticoids increase eosinophil apoptosis and block the survival effect of interleukin-5, resulting in a reduction in airway eosinophilia with steroid therapy.[16] Assessment of the receptor for IL-5 on peripheral blood eosinophils from healthy, steroid naïve, and steroid treated asthmatic children has shown reduced IL-5 receptor expression in patients treated with inhaled steroids, and this was concomitant with reduced *in vitro* responsiveness to IL-5.[17] This is therefore a potential mechanism by which steroids inhibit IL-5 in children on maintenance therapy for asthma. Interestingly, children with severe asthma, who are on high-dose maintenance inhaled steroids, have a persistent airway eosinophilia in the absence of detectable IL-5, suggesting that alternative mechanisms contribute to the development of eosinophilia as disease becomes more severe.[11] This has obvious implications for the use of anti-TH2 monoclonal therapy.

MAST CELLS IN ASTHMA

The immediate response during an allergic reaction in a patient with asthma results from binding of allergen-specific Ig-E antibodies to mast cells, and following cross-linking of the allergen across two antibody molecules, the resulting degranulation of mast cells results in a release of mediators that cause the symptoms of bronchoconstriction, airway edema, and inflammation (see Fig. 43.2). The predominant mast cell mediators that are released include histamine and cysteine leukotrienes.[18] Despite the obvious role of mast cells in allergic reactions, their importance in asthma pathogenesis remains uncertain,[19] since treatments that have aimed to prevent or reduce mast cell degranulation, such as sodium cromoglycate and other mast cell stabilizers, have been relatively ineffective in children,[20] and there is little evidence of an increase in tissue mast cells in children with severe asthma.[11] Therapies that have targeted mast cell mediators, such as leukotriene receptor antagonists that minimize the downstream proinflammatory effects of leukotrienes,[21] have also been trialed in children with asthma, but again, their efficacy has been disappointing.[22] It may be that the location of mast cells within specific structures in the airway wall is important in determining their pathological effect. Increased numbers of mast cells have been shown to be present specifically within airway smooth muscle in patients with asthma but not those with eosinophilic bronchitis.[23] Moreover, mast cells have been shown to modulate the function of airway smooth muscle[24] and, via release of Th2 mediators such as IL-13, can result in increased airway hyperresponsiveness.[25] It is therefore likely that only therapies targeting tissue-specific mast cells will prove to be beneficial.

LYMPHOID CELLS

T-Lymphocytes

The key inflammatory cell that is central to driving asthma pathogenesis, and is induced following the development of an adaptive immune response to allergen exposure, is the T-helper 2 (Th2) lymphocyte (see Fig. 43.2). These CD4[+] cells express the T-cell receptor and have the capacity to secrete various cytokines depending on their local environment. Th2 lymphocytes are induced following allergen exposure and release hallmark Th2 cytokines including IL-4, IL-5, and IL-13 (see Fig. 43.3), which are considered important in the initiation and development of the pathophysiology of asthma.[26,27] IL-4 is essential for the development of Ig-E and allergic sensitization; IL-5 is an eosinophil growth factor, chemoattractant, and promoter of eosinophil survival; while IL-13 is most closely associated with the development of airway hyperresponsiveness (AHR) and airway remodeling. Although Th2 cells are important in driving allergic airway responses, these are not the only lymphocyte subset involved in asthma pathogenesis. Numerous other T-cell subsets have been implicated in asthma, including Th9 cells and Th17 cells.[26] Effector CD4+ T cells are defined by expression of specific transcription factors, which determine their secreted cytokines. Th2 cells express the transcription factor GATA3 and secrete IL4, 5, 13; while Th17 cells express receptor-related orphan receptor gamma t (ROR-γT) and secrete IL-17 (see Fig. 43.3). However, it is also becoming increasingly apparent that the inflammatory environment is central to determining cellular function. A change in milieu can result in a change in cytokine secretory pattern, which is termed T-cell plasticity.[28] In addition, not all T lymphocytes are proinflammatory and pathogenic. There is a critical balance between regulatory and proinflammatory T-lymphocytes that needs to be maintained to prevent disease, and it is proposed that in asthma an imbalance in favor of Th2 cells with a concomitant reduction in T regulatory (Tregs) cells results in disease manifestation.[29] There are two main types of Tregs in the lung: CD4+ cells that secrete the antiinflammatory cytokine IL-10, and CD4+CD25+ cells that have the transcription factor FoxP3. At present, data relating to the presence of these cells in the airways of children with asthma is scant, but assessment of peripheral blood and bronchoalveolar lavage has shown reduced numbers of CD4+CD25+FoxP3+ cells in asthmatics compared to healthy children[30,31]; however, these results were from steroid naïve patients. It is interesting to note that treatment with inhaled steroids results in higher levels of circulating[32] and airway Tregs, but the cells remain functionally impaired.[31] Children with severe asthma, whose symptoms are not controlled despite high-dose steroid therapy, have significantly lower levels of airway IL-10 and have a significantly reduced capacity for secreting IL-10 from circulating peripheral blood CD4+ T cells,[33] suggesting relatively steroid resistant disease is characterized by a poor induction of IL-10 secretion from CD4+ cells after steroid therapy.

Innate Lymphoid Cells

Until recently, the predominant immune response that was thought to drive allergic asthma was an adaptive response mediated by Ig-E and T lymphocytes. However, it is now apparent that innate immunity plays a significant role in asthma pathogenesis. Murine experimental models have demonstrated the release of innate cytokines from the airway epithelium in response to allergen. These cytokines include IL-33, IL-25, and thymic stromal lymphopoeitin (TSLP).[34] Of these, IL-33 has more specifically been associated with the onset of allergic immune responses by the induction of a group of cells called innate lymphoid cells (ILCs) (Fig. 43.4).[35] ILCs are of comparable size and morphology to T

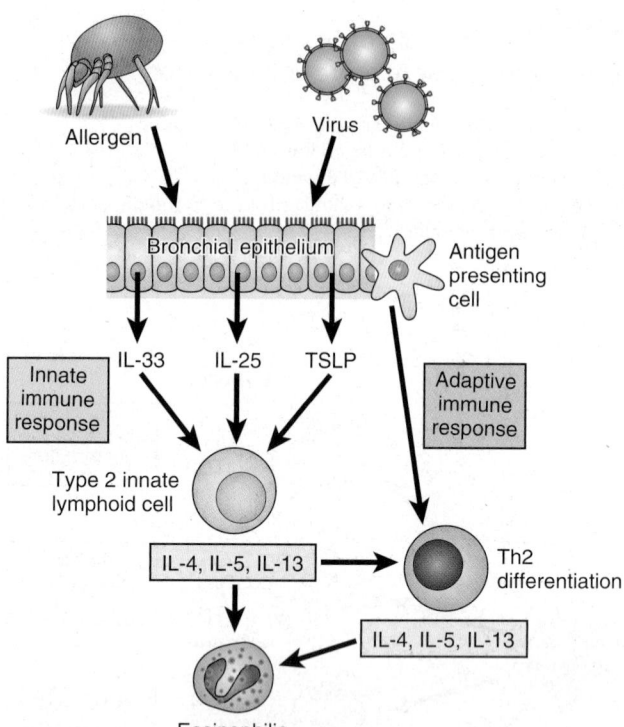

Fig. 43.4 Environmental exposures result in the release of epithelial innate cytokines and downstream induction of type 2 innate lymphoid cells in asthma. In parallel, type 2 adaptive immunity develops via antigen presenting cells such as dendritic cells, which drive T helper 2 (Th2) cell differentiation with secretion of interleukin (IL)-5 and eosinophilic inflammation. *TSLP,* Thymic stromal lymphopoeitin.

Table 43.1 Phenotypic and Functional Comparisons of T Helper 2 Lymphocytes (Th2) Cells and Type 2 Innate Lymphoid Cells (ILC2)

Th2	ILC2
Lineage surface markers	Lineage negative
T cell receptor, CD4+, CD3+	No T cell receptor
Lymphoid morphology	Lymphoid morphology
Intranuclear transcription factor GATA3	Intranuclear transcription factor GATA3
Induced via adaptive immune responses: Ig-E, dendritic cells, lymph nodes	Induced via innate epithelial cytokines: IL-33, IL-25, TSLP
Type 2 cytokine production: IL-4, IL-5, IL-13, IL-9	Type 2 cytokine production: IL-4, IL-5, IL-13

Ig, Immunoglobulin; *IL,* interleukin; *TSLP,* thymic stromal lymphopoeitin.

lymphocytes, but lack the T-cell receptor and surface markers, such as CD3/CD4/CD8 that are the hallmark features of T cells (Table 43.1). The importance of the innate cytokines and ILCs in initiating pediatric asthma remains uncertain, but IL-33 is likely to be important in mediating severe therapy resistant asthma since it promotes airway remodeling and is relatively steroid resistant.[36] Subpopulations of ILCs are induced depending on the stimulus and environment in a similar manner to T cell subtypes.[37] Group 2 ILCs (ILC2s) that secrete the Th2 cytokines IL-4, IL-5, and IL-13 are therefore induced by IL-33 upon allergen exposure. There is evidence for increased numbers of ILC2s in the airways

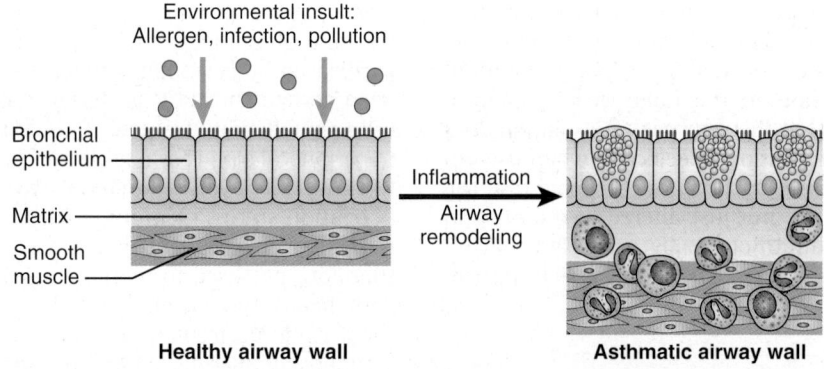

Fig. 43.5 Pathology of allergic asthma: parallel development of airway inflammation and remodeling. Environmental insults including allergens, infection, and pollution result in the pathogenesis of asthma with parallel development of airway inflammation and remodeling. The airway wall structures that are altered in asthma include the airway epithelium, increased thickness of the subepithelial matrix, and increased smooth muscle mass. The predominant inflammatory phenotype is eosinophilia.

of children with severe asthma compared to controls,[38] but their functional role in mediating disease and relative importance compared to T lymphocytes in pediatric disease remains unknown. Importantly, it is becoming increasingly apparent that an equal interplay between both ILCs and T cells is essential in initiation and persistence of disease,[39–41] and it is unlikely that only one cell type is predominant.

NEUTROPHILS

Neutrophils are thought to be important in mediating severe asthma in adults[42] and it is proposed that dampening down neutrophilic inflammation may be beneficial. However, their role in pediatric disease is far less clear. There is no convincing evidence of increased airway mucosal neutrophils in children with asthma during stable disease.[11,43,44] However, neutrophils are increased during exacerbations that are precipitated by infection, suggesting they may not be pathogenic, but an important response in clearing infection. There is recent evidence showing a subgroup of children with severe asthma have increased neutrophils specifically within the airway epithelium, and contrary to expectation, those with intraepithelial neutrophils had better lung function, symptom control, and were on lower doses of maintenance inhaled steroids.[43] Therefore at present, blocking or reducing neutrophils cannot be recommended as an important therapeutic strategy for children with asthma, as they may indeed be beneficial. The role of neutrophils in the specific case of wheezing in preschool disorders is discussed below.

School-Age Allergic Asthma: Pathology and Mechanisms

Asthma is a chronic inflammatory airway disease, which in children is characterized by a predominance of eosinophils in the airway wall and lumen.[45] Evidence of eosinophilia has been confirmed in endobronchial biopsies[13,46] and broncho-alveolar lavage[12] from school-aged children regardless of disease severity.[11] The inflammation is accompanied by the presence of structural airway wall changes, or airway remodeling (Fig. 43.5). These changes are thought to be inappropriate to maintain normal lung function.[47] However,

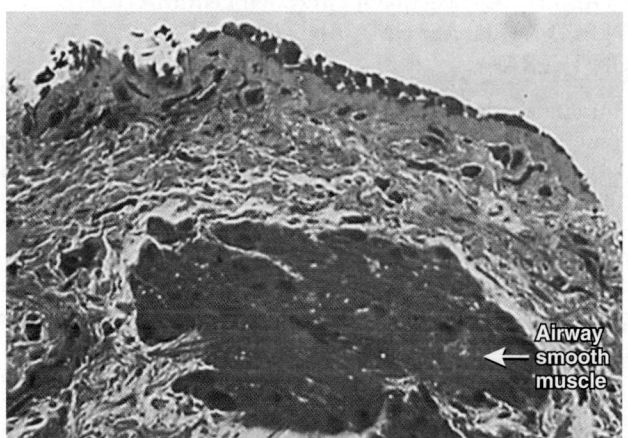

Fig. 43.6 Endobronchial biopsy stained with toluidine blue showing increased airway smooth muscle mass in a patient with asthma.

there is some evidence that certain structural changes, increased thickness of the reticular basement membrane in particular, may be protective as they provide reduced airway collapsibility.[48] The specific structural airway changes present in children with asthma include increased thickness of the sub-epithelial reticular basement membrane (RBM),[13,49] increase in both size and quantity of airway smooth muscle (Fig. 43.6),[11,50] and increased number of vessels (angiogenesis).[13] All of these changes are present by school age regardless of disease severity.[13,49] Certain features, such as thickness of the RBM, are present to the same extent in children as they are in adults with asthma and are therefore also independent of disease duration.

It had been proposed that repeated cycles of inflammation resulting from allergen exposure resulted in the development of structural airway changes,[51] however, experiments using a neonatal mouse model[52] and findings from cross-sectional studies that have investigated asthma pathology in children[53,54] have shown that the key pathophysiological changes of allergic asthma (airway hyperresponsiveness, eosinophilic inflammation, and airway remodeling) develop in parallel (see Fig. 43.5). Importantly, this implies that therapies that only target eosinophilic inflammation may be insufficient to achieve optimal disease control and improved lung function in all patients. Targeting eosinophilic inflammation alone, using inhaled steroids, has resulted in improved symptom control and lung function in the majority of children; however, it is apparent that this approach in isolation does not achieve disease modification, specifically when used in early onset preschool disease.[55] It is now accepted that the airway structural cells are not just altered in quantity in asthma, but they are immunologically active and have a fundamentally altered functional phenotype which contributes to asthma pathogenesis as well.[56]

The Clinical Relevance of Eosinophilic Inflammation in School-Age Asthma

STABILITY OF EOSINOPHILIC INFLAMMATION IN PEDIATRIC ASTHMA AND IMPACT ON THERAPY

Although pediatric asthma is predominantly an eosinophilic condition, the inflammatory profile is heterogeneous between patients. The predominant pattern of airway inflammation has been used to define and subdivide patients with asthma according to inflammatory phenotypes. These include eosinophilic, neutrophilic, pauci-granulocytic (no inflammation), or mixed.[57] However, it is recognized that the inflammatory phenotype may not remain stable over time in the same patient. One reason for a "switch" in inflammatory phenotype is the development of an acute respiratory infection, which may change the profile from predominantly eosinophilic to neutrophilic or mixed. However, intriguingly, in children with asthma, change in airway inflammatory phenotype can be documented over time independently of exacerbations, symptoms, disease manifestation, or alteration in therapy.[58] Therefore a possible explanation for eosinophil directed therapy being unsuccessful in children[59] may be the impact of phenotype switching, or indeed, a less important functional role of eosinophils in causing disease pathogenesis in children compared to adults. The differences between eosinophil targeted therapy in adults and children highlights the importance of investigating disease mechanisms in age appropriate experimental models and not undertaking direct extrapolation of data from studies in adults to children.[60] In addition, these findings question whether novel therapies that are targeted to a reduction in levels of IL-5 (monoclonal antibody to IL-5 or its receptor) and thus a specific reduction in eosinophils will be beneficial in children. Mepolizumab (monoclonal antibody to IL-5) has proven to be effective in reducing exacerbations in adult eosinophilic asthma,[61] but efficacy data in children are awaited, and are mandatory before these therapies are offered to children.

NONINVASIVE BIOMARKERS OF EOSINOPHILIC INFLAMMATION

Much effort has been undertaken to find a noninvasive objective biomarker to assess the efficacy of inhaled steroids in reducing airway eosinophilia as a guide to monitor disease and tailor treatment.[62] Several biomarkers have been investigated in pediatric allergic asthma. One of the first was serum eosinophilic cationic protein (ECP), a mediator that is released by eosinophils when they are activated. It has been shown that ECP is steroid sensitive and therefore is reduced following treatment, and levels are closely related to peripheral blood eosinophils,[63,64] but there is little evidence to show ECP levels relate to airway eosinophil numbers or activation status, meaning serum ECP adds little as a biomarker over peripheral blood eosinophil counts, and it is therefore not used to monitor disease. Another issue that complicates the use of eosinophil biomarkers measured in the peripheral circulation and not in the airways in asthma is that other allergic conditions may also be associated with elevated levels. For example, children with atopic dermatitis, whether or not they have asthma, may have elevated ECP, and blood eosinophils. It is therefore important to interpret results, specifically of peripheral blood biomarkers, with some caution.[10]

A biomarker that has been extensively investigated more recently is exhaled nitric oxide (FeNO). It is associated with airway eosinophilia in children with difficult asthma[10,65] and therefore considered a better noninvasive marker than serum ECP or total eosinophils. Reference values for normal levels are also available for children of all ages.[66] FeNO is useful to support a diagnosis of asthma in steroid-naïve patients, although it can be elevated in atopic, nonasthmatics.[67] It is very steroid sensitive, and in children it has been repeatedly shown to be no better than clinical parameters alone to monitor disease control.[68,69] A recent systematic review of the accuracy of currently available noninvasive biomarkers to detect airway eosinophilia has shown only moderate diagnostic accuracy of exhaled nitric oxide in correctly detecting airway eosinophils, so the use of this alone as a biomarker would lead to a significant number of false positives and false negatives.[70] In addition, longitudinal relationships between FeNO and sputum eosinophils vary over time within the same patient regardless of clinical status.[71] The steroid sensitivity of FeNO can be used as a very reliable surrogate assessment of adherence to inhaled steroids, whereby a significant fall in FeNO was observed in all previously nonadherent patients after a period of directly observed therapy.[72]

Essential Role of Structural Airway Cells in Pulmonary Immunity and Asthma Pathogenesis

PULMONARY EPITHELIUM

Until recently, it was thought that the function of the airway epithelium was simply to act as a passive barrier to prevent the entry of particles such as allergens, pathogens, or pollution into the airway wall. However, it is now known that the pulmonary epithelium is not just a barrier, but is also immunologically active and is central to the development of immune responses involved in the pathogenesis of asthma.[73] Cultured primary bronchial epithelial cells from children with asthma have dysregulated functional capacity to repair wound injury.[3] In addition, responses to rhinovirus infection of epithelial cells from children with asthma are impaired, whereby production of the antiviral cytokine interferon-β is reduced and epithelial repair following infection is delayed.[74,75] There are significant differences in release of mediators from bronchial epithelial cells following exposure to a range of proinflammatory stimulants including IL-1β, IL-4, and IL-13 between children with and without asthma.[76] The functional importance of the airway epithelium is also reflected in findings from genome wide association studies (GWAS) of asthma susceptibility genes. The majority of genes that are associated with a high risk for asthma, specifically in children, such as interleukin-33, protocadherin, and CDHR3, are expressed in the pulmonary epithelium.[77] This suggests that altered airway epithelial function is central to asthma pathogenesis. Several SNPs in the ORMDL3 gene located on chromosome 17q have been shown repeatedly to be associated with asthma that develops following recurrent infection with rhinovirus in the preschool years.[78,79] Thus, future studies that manipulate pulmonary epithelial function by altering the expression of these susceptibility genes may uncover novel therapeutic targets that may allow restoration of epithelial function in patients with asthma.

An important immunological function of the airway epithelium in asthma and other chronic inflammatory airway diseases is its ability to secrete cytokines in response to various stimuli. The role of the innate epithelial cytokines in initiating allergic airway responses and in the pathogenesis of asthma is currently being extensively investigated as a pathway that may lead to novel therapies. Exposure of the bronchial epithelium to allergens, infections, and pollutants in patients with asthma is thought to result in the direct release of three key innate cytokines, IL-33, IL-25, or TSLP (see Fig. 43.4). The actual cytokine released is determined by the environmental exposure and the host susceptibility.[34] The airway epithelium thus provides an innate mechanism of initiating immune responses, without the need for adaptive immunity via antigen-presenting cells, allergen sensitization, and Ig-E production. The downstream effects of the innate cytokines are to induce ILCs, which have the capacity to function in the same way as T helper 2 cells with secretion of the type 2 cytokines IL-4, IL-5, and IL-13 (above). This key role in disease initiation has put the pulmonary epithelium at the center of asthma pathogenesis and it is a key tissue whose function is being extensively investigated to allow the discovery of novel therapeutic targets.[56]

AIRWAY SMOOTH MUSCLE

In an analogous manner to the epithelium, it is known that stimulation of airway smooth muscle does not simply result in contraction, as it is an immunologically active component of the airway wall. There is extensive cross-talk and interaction specifically between mast cells and the airway smooth muscle in asthma (see above section on mast cells). Although the function of airway smooth muscle has been investigated in adult asthma, very little is known about its function in children with asthma. This is an important area for future research since significant evidence suggests that early alterations in smooth muscle function is one of the best predictors of development of asthma from preschool wheeze (see Fig. 43.6).[80]

Preschool Wheeze: A Unique Maturing Immune Environment

PHENOTYPES OF PRESCHOOL WHEEZE AND RESPONSE TO CURRENTLY AVAILABLE ANTIINFLAMMATORY THERAPIES

An important clinical phenotype that is very distinct and unique to children is that of wheezing in preschool children. Cohort studies have shown that there are several clinical phenotypes of wheezing in preschool children with different outcomes by school age.[81] However, these phenotypes can only be applied retrospectively after the child is 6 years old. Prospective clinical phenotypes have therefore been defined by the European Respiratory Society.[82] These include viral episodic wheeze, which is characterized by wheezing in discrete episodes with no symptoms in between, and multiple trigger wheeze in which children have symptoms both during and in between acute episodes. Little is known about immunopathogenesis and molecular mechanisms that specifically mediate viral episodic wheeze, but what is known is that usual therapies that are effective in allergic asthma at school age are rarely beneficial in preschool children with viral wheeze. Specifically, during exacerbations, there is no evidence for efficacy of systemic corticosteroids on any clinical outcome measure.[83–86] In addition, leukotriene receptor antagonists confer little benefit during exacerbations of viral induced preschool wheeze.[87,88] These data imply the inflammatory process during acute viral wheezing episodes in preschool children is very different to that in allergic asthma. Recently, it has become apparent that similar numbers of wheezing episodes in preschool children are associated with bacterial infections as with viral infection.[89] The term episodic viral wheeze may therefore be better represented as infection associated wheeze. Furthermore, bronchoscopy studies have shown that the airway inflammatory profile of episodic wheezers during stable disease is either similar to nonwheezing controls[46] or it is predominantly neutrophilic,[90,91] and may be associated with positive bacterial cultures, despite the absence of symptoms.[92] There is therefore increasing data to suggest the pathogens that cause acute episodes of wheezing in preschool children are distinct from those in allergic asthma, and that the underlying immune and inflammatory mechanisms mediating disease are also distinct.

AIRWAY INFLAMMATION IN INFECTION ASSOCIATED PRESCHOOL WHEEZE EXACERBATIONS

In view of the evidence for bacterial infections being associated with preschool wheezing episodes, two recent clinical trials have been undertaken to determine the efficacy of the macrolide azithromycin to treat acute exacerbations. Although both have shown a benefit for their primary outcome,[93,94] the use of azithromycin for acute preschool wheeze cannot be recommended in routine clinical practice, since both trials have significant limitations.[95,96] Neither showed benefit in the most relevant clinical outcome measure of hospitalizations, or need for oral steroids, and neither investigated the mechanism of action of the azithromycin. The efficacy of the macrolide therapy in both trials seemed more likely due to the antiinflammatory effects of azithromycin than the antibacterial effects. Importantly, and worryingly, the trial by Bacharier et al. showed a significant increase in macrolide resistance over the short trial duration.[93] A much clearer picture of the airway inflammatory profile during both stable disease and exacerbations in preschool wheezers is therefore needed, with an aim to targeting specific inflammatory and infective phenotypes to achieve more effective treatments.

AIRWAY PATHOLOGY IN PRESCHOOL WHEEZERS WITH SYMPTOMS DURING AND IN BETWEEN EXACERBATIONS

Preschool wheezers with persistent symptoms present both during and in between exacerbations (multiple trigger wheeze), and have a distinct airway inflammatory profile compared to those who wheeze only during acute respiratory infections.[46] Preschool confirmed wheezers, with interval wheeze symptoms, have evidence of eosinophilic airway inflammation (Fig. 43.7).[54] Children with this phenotype tend to have a good response to treatments for allergic asthma; in particular they have reduced symptoms and exacerbations if treated with maintenance low-dose inhaled steroids.[97] Although the inflammatory profile is eosinophilic, numbers of mast cells are similar in wheezers and nonwheezers. Little is known about the cytokines driving preschool persistent wheeze, although increased expression of IL-4 in the submucosa has been reported in preschool multiple trigger wheezers.[46] Since leukotriene-receptor antagonists have variable benefit, there are few other therapeutic targets currently available for those with severe preschool wheeze that persists despite high-dose inhaled steroids. It is known that

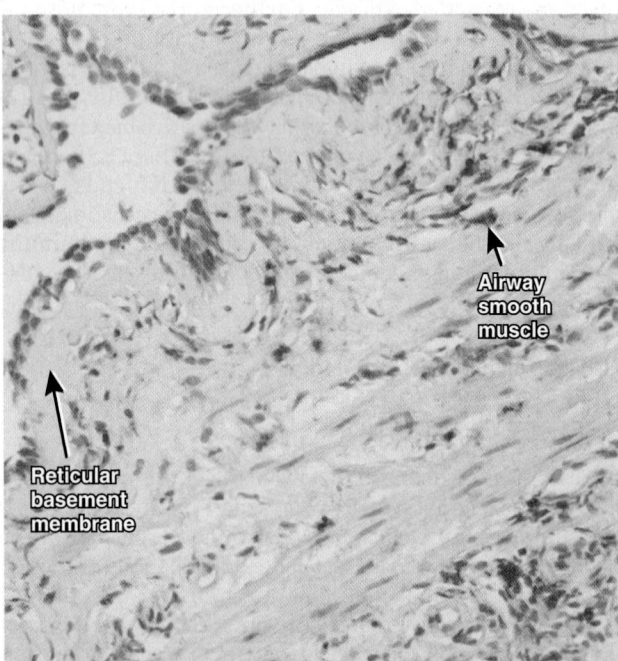

Fig. 43.7 Endobronchial biopsy from a preschool wheezer showing eosinophilic inflammation and increased thickness of the reticular basement membrane—the hallmark pathological features of asthma in children.

in addition to eosinophilia, features of airway remodeling, specifically increased thickness of the reticular basement membrane, are already present in children with persistent, severe wheeze.[46,54] However, neither of these features is predictive of asthma development by school age. The only pathological abnormality that predicts future asthma is airway smooth muscle,[80] but at present there are no known biomarkers that represent smooth muscle function in preschoolers, so this feature cannot be used to identify future asthmatics. In any event, we lack interventions to prevent the evolution of preschool wheeze to asthma.

IMPACT OF EOSINOPHILIC INFLAMMATION ON DISEASE INCEPTION

Evidence for the direct effect of eosinophilic inflammation on clinical disease/symptom manifestation is hard to find in children. Interestingly, murine models of house dust mite induced allergic airway disease have shown the pathophysiological manifestation of disease (airway hyperresponsiveness, total leukocytic inflammation, and airway remodeling) in mice that are deficient in eosinophils is the same as that in wild-type mice,[98] suggesting little role for eosinophils alone in disease inception. In support of this conclusion, clinical trials that have used antiinflammatory therapies targeted to eosinophils (inhaled steroids) to prevent asthma development from preschool wheeze have failed. Inhaled steroids were used in double-blind randomized controlled trials in children with preschool wheeze from several large birth cohorts in the UK,[99] America,[55] and Denmark,[100] but none of these have shown any benefit in terms of secondary prevention. Although preschoolers may benefit symptomatically while taking the treatment, there was no sustained benefit from the inhaled steroids once treatment was stopped.

EOSINOPHILIC INFLAMMATION AND DISEASE PERSISTENCE

In contrast to disease inception, the role of eosinophils in maintaining disease once it has developed is undoubtedly of importance. The mainstay of treatment for asthma, inhaled glucocorticoids, targets eosinophils and they are of huge benefit in established disease. However, glucocorticoids have several mechanisms of action. They reduce airway eosinophils via IL-5, but they also reduce levels of the other Th2 cytokines that drive asthma, so an isolated reduction in eosinophils may not be as effective as the global reduction in allergic Th2 mediators that is achieved by steroid therapy.

Studies in adults have shown that adjusting the dose of maintenance inhaled steroids according to the presence or absence of airway eosinophils (in induced sputum) is significantly better at reducing number of acute exacerbations compared to therapy tailored to clinical disease manifestation (symptoms/lung function).[101] In contrast, directing therapy to sputum eosinophils in school-age children with moderate–severe asthma did not affect exacerbation rate, asthma control, or lung function.[59] In children, no relationship could be demonstrated between airway hyperresponsiveness and FeNO (a noninvasive surrogate marker for airway eosinophilia).[102] In younger preschool children with persistent wheezing, use of inhaled steroids results in an improvement in symptoms and exacerbations,[97] but impact on lung function is less certain. Currently there is significantly more evidence for therapy targeted to airway eosinophilic inflammation in adult patients than there is in children,[103] with the overall documented benefit of reducing eosinophilic inflammation being a reduction in acute exacerbations but not daily asthma control.[104]

IMPACT OF IMMUNE MATURATION AND THE DEVELOPING AIRWAY MICROBIOME ON PRESCHOOL WHEEZE—MECHANISTIC STUDIES

The importance of the changing immune environment in influencing the development of disease in early life is being increasingly recognized. Since mechanistic studies are very difficult in children because of the very limited airway samples that can be obtained, experimental studies that use age appropriate models are being undertaken increasingly to understand the pathogenesis of preschool wheeze and early-onset asthma. A neonatal murine model using intermittent inhaled allergen exposure, with one of the commonest perennial aero-allergens to which children are sensitized, house dust mite (HDM), has been developed. Pups from day 3 of life are exposed to inhaled HDM and assessments of lung function, inflammation, and remodeling made weekly. This model closely mimics the findings in preschool children with multiple trigger wheeze, since there is evidence of airway hyperresponsiveness, eosinophilia, and remodeling.[52] Importantly, it has shown that all pathological and physiological abnormalities develop in parallel in early life, and questions the hypothesis that repeated cycles of inflammation result in structural airway changes. More recently, use of this model has shown that there is a critical time window in early life during which allergen exposure results in exaggerated eosinophilia and AHR. If pups are exposed to allergen in the first week, the degree of airway inflammation and AHR is significantly higher than if allergen exposure starts in adult mice (aged 6–8 weeks). Importantly, the underlying mechanism for this is the relative lack of T regulatory cells in the first 2 weeks of life, which are present subsequently and protect from severe inflammation and AHR. The development of the T regulatory cells is determined by the relatively immature airway microbiome in the first 2 weeks, which develops and becomes increasingly diverse with maturity. The more diverse microbiome results in an appropriate immune environment for the protective T regulatory cells.[105] Other studies in neonatal mice have shown that the first two weeks of life are a critical window of immune maturation, an essential period that determines the type of immune response that develops to either infection or allergen. Infection of neonatal mice with respiratory syncytial virus (RSV) results in a significant increase in T helper 2 cytokine production with compromised function of T regulatory cells.[106] This has highlighted a mechanism by which viral infection targets a host-protective mechanism in early life and increases susceptibility to allergic disease. It is becoming increasingly apparent that environmental exposures during a critical window of immune maturation in early life contribute to susceptibility to long term allergic disease.[107,108] Although the first 3 years seem the likely period of susceptibility in children, we are still unable to identify an intervention that can be used to alter susceptibility and provide protection from the development of allergic responses.

GENE–ENVIRONMENT INTERACTIONS: THE DEVELOPING MICROBIOME AND PROTECTION FROM PRESCHOOL WHEEZE

Wheezing and asthma occur because of the interplay of genetic susceptibility and environmental influences on the developing lungs and immune maturation. Therefore identification of environmental risk factors is as important as deciphering genetic susceptibility in determining mechanisms of disease onset and to find therapeutic interventions. The most striking data showing an environmental effect on asthma outcome is from studies that have very convincingly and repeatedly shown that growing up on a farm has a protective effect on asthma development.[109,110] Specifically, the microbial and endotoxin components of the inhaled products from farmyards are thought to impact the mucosal epithelial innate immune system to skew away from asthma and type 2 immunity and towards a T regulatory cell phenotype.[111] The specific farm environmental effect has recently been shown in a comparison of two populations with similar genetic ancestry, but different farming practices. The Amish practice traditional farming, while the Hutterites practice Westernized industrialized farming. Despite similar lifestyles, the prevalence of asthma was approximately sixfold lower in Amish children compared to the Hutterites.[112] There was a significantly higher endotoxin load in the dust samples from Amish homes and the proportion, phenotype, and function of innate immune cells were significantly different between the two, whereby the Amish had a more robust innate immune response. This study has shown the importance of a specific environmental factor that can influence the onset of wheeze; however, to translate to the clinic, the specific underlying mechanisms need to be investigated. But, this work does demonstrate the importance of the components of inhaled dust and the likely impact they have on shaping the airway microbial profile and immune maturation. The interactions between genetic susceptibility, immune responses, and the airway microbiome are central to understanding the factors that determine the onset of preschool wheeze and how we may prevent progression to asthma.

GAPS IN KNOWLEDGE AND THOUGHTS FOR THE FUTURE

Preschool children make up the majority of acute admissions for wheezing in children,[113] and we know that they respond poorly to systemic steroids during exacerbations, and there are few effective maintenance therapies available; but we still have very little knowledge of the mechanisms mediating wheezing in preschoolers. We cannot extrapolate from adult studies,[114] nor from studies in older children with allergic asthma as these are very different diseases. An important focus for future research is therefore to understand the inflammatory and immune pathways that contribute to the development of wheezing in preschool children to allow us to find effective therapies.

Currently, management of preschool wheeze is based predominantly on the clinical phenotype. However, a lack of phenotype stability over time has been acknowledged as a significant factor that limits the effective use of clinical phenotypes alone to manage disease.[115] A limitation of our current approach to managing preschool wheeze is that the underlying presence of airway inflammation or infection is not incorporated in the management plan, only the clinical symptom pattern is used. However, the treatments used, such as inhaled steroids, target eosinophilic inflammation, and could worsen infection by inducing topical immunosuppression. In addition, if eosinophils are not present, then it is unlikely that inhaled steroids will work. Use of objective biomarkers that will identify steroid responders will avoid the inappropriate use of steroids in young children, and importantly will prevent unwanted side effects. It has therefore been suggested that blood eosinophils could be utilized as an attractive biomarker to guide therapy for preschool wheeze.[116] Interestingly, although induced sputum following nebulized hypertonic saline can be obtained safely from preschool children,[117] the relationship between sputum and BAL inflammation is poor in this age group. However, a very close relationship between blood and BAL eosinophils is apparent,[117] confirming blood eosinophils as an important biomarker that needs to be investigated in future studies to determine which preschool wheezers may benefit from inhaled steroids. Interestingly, a recent clinical trial in children aged 1–5 years has shown that the probability of response to daily inhaled steroids was highest in those who had both aeroallergen sensitization and the presence of a blood eosinophilia (defined as >300/μL),[118] suggesting blood eosinophils are a promising biomarker for response to therapy in this age group.

SEVERITY AND FREQUENCY OF ACUTE WHEEZING EPISODES AND PROGRESSION TO ASTHMA

A key aspect of preschool wheeze for which we lack knowledge is trying to predict which child will progress to asthma. This is important because we know from cohort studies that those preschoolers who do develop asthma have an early and sustained reduction in lung function.[119] Although several clinical indices have been developed to aid prediction, such as the modified Asthma Predictive Index,[120] most have a good negative predictive value, but few have a positive predictive value much above 50%, making accurate prediction of disease development very difficult. One of the factors to be considered is that an assessment of just the presence or absence of atopy is insufficient. The severity and degree of sensitization is important in predicting wheeze persistence. The subgroup of children with sensitization to multiple allergens and the presence of allergic sensitization at an early age (multiple early atopy) is much more likely to result in disease persistence and progression to asthma.[121]

Until recently, it was thought that symptom pattern might be useful for prognosis, whereby episodic wheeze was much less likely to progress to asthma than multiple trigger wheeze. However, it is now apparent that children with acute attacks of wheeze, especially when severe and frequent, are likely to progress to asthma, regardless of whether they wheeze in between the episodes.[115] Therefore the long-held belief that "viral" wheeze, or transient wheeze is benign and short lived is increasingly challenged. This reinforces the urgent need to investigate the mechanisms mediating wheezing in preschool children so that objective biomarkers other than clinical wheeze pattern or symptoms can be used to more accurately determine acute management and disease progression.

Specific Clinical Scenarios for Consideration

IMMUNOLOGY OF ASTHMA EXACERBATIONS

Acute exacerbations are an important feature of pediatric asthma. The most common precipitant of exacerbations, even in patients with allergic disease, is respiratory infection, usually caused by viruses, the most common pathogen being rhinovirus.[122] The airway inflammatory profile present during exacerbations is significantly different to that during stable disease. Children with asthma have altered immune responses to virus compared to nonasthmatic controls. There is a defect in production of antiviral interferons[74] accompanied by an exaggerated Th2 response during viral induced asthma exacerbations. The airway inflammatory infiltrate during exacerbations is composed of neutrophils and eosinophils, with a prolonged duration of inflammation being associated with the viral load.[123] The current approach to treatment is based predominantly on targeting airway eosinophils with the use of systemic steroids. In addition, the most significant clinical effect of newer therapies that are directed to eosinophils, including the anti-IL-5 antibody mepolizumab, is on reduction in exacerbations, suggesting that a surge in Th2 inflammation and eosinophilia is responsible for most exacerbations,[124] and that the associated neutrophilic inflammation may be beneficial and necessary to fight the infection. However, most data related to the airway inflammatory profile present during acute exacerbations comes from studies in adults. This is because it is very difficult to obtain lower airway samples from children during exacerbations when bronchoscopy would be unsafe. A possible avenue that could be pursued to try to obtain some information about acute disease would be to undertake bronchoalveolar (or blind) lavage in children with very severe exacerbations requiring intubation and ventilation.

SEVERE THERAPY RESISTANT ASTHMA: A UNIQUE PULMONARY IMMUNE ENVIRONMENT

The immunopathogenesis of allergic asthma in children with controlled, mild–moderate disease is a Th2 driven eosinophilia, which is treated effectively in most patients with maintenance inhaled steroid therapy. However, there is a small group of children with very severe disease who remain poorly controlled, with frequent exacerbations despite maximal doses of inhaled steroids, and in some cases, despite maintenance systemic steroids. These children, who are known to be adherent to their prescribed therapy, and in whom all modifiable factors that contribute to poor control such as persistent allergen exposure, have been addressed, have severe therapy resistant asthma (STRA).[125] Most pediatric asthma studies that have assessed airway inflammation and pathology have been undertaken in children with STRA, and so a significant amount is known about the airway inflammatory profile of these patients during stable disease. As a group, they have an airway eosinophilia, but no increase in tissue mast cells

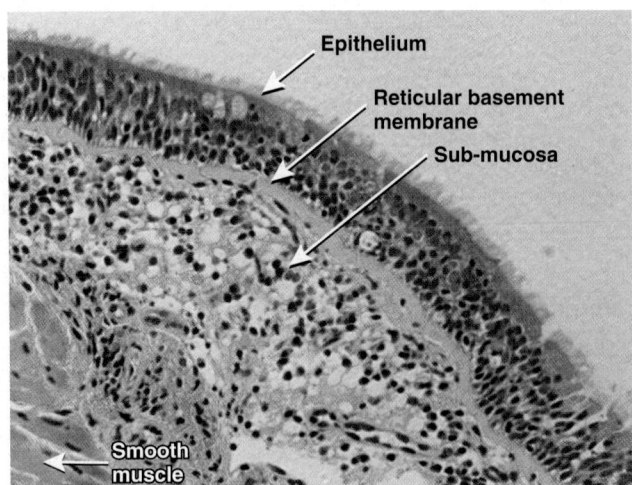

Fig. 43.8 Endobronchial biopsy stained with hematoxylin and eosin showing the key structural airway features that are altered in childhood asthma.

or airway neutrophils.[11] They also have very significant and marked sensitization to multiple allergens, and those with concomitant food allergy appear have the most severe disease.[126] The most interesting finding about these patients is the relative paucity of the expected Th2 cytokines in the airways. However, it is known from animal models that the Th2 cytokines are steroid sensitive, so they are likely to be driven down in these patients by high-dose steroids. Their overall pathological profile as a group is therefore one of a steroid resistant eosinophilia and airway remodeling (see Figs. 43.7 and 43.8).[11] However, it must be remembered that even though they are a small group, there remains marked molecular phenotypic heterogeneity between patients.[43,127] The innate immune system may be important in driving and maintaining very severe asthma in children, since they have increased IL-33 positive cells in the airway walls, which has been shown to be relatively steroid resistant.[36] Moreover, children with STRA have increased airway ILC2 cells, and a subgroup with the most severe allergies, including sensitization to fungal allergens, have the highest levels of IL-33. Although significant steps have been made towards determining some of the mechanisms underlying STRA in children, and it is apparent that this has a different immunopathogenesis to severe asthma in adults, we still have no clinical trials that are targeted to the molecular pathways that drive the disease in children. At present, and disappointingly, novel molecular targets that are being tested are targeted against the Th2 cytokines IL-5 and IL-13, extrapolated from studies in adults.[128,129] However, recruitment of children to these trials is proving difficult because most children can achieve good control if they take their maintenance inhaled steroid treatment regularly. It will not be surprising if efficacy is disappointing, since the molecular phenotype of children is one of eosinophilia with infrequent detection of Th2 cytokines. A feature lacking from our current data relating to the immunology of STRA in children is adequate transcriptomic profiling of airway samples to determine molecular targets and signatures that will allow phenotyping of these patients and achieve personalized treatment.[130] However, unbiased cluster analyses of children with severe asthma have been

undertaken and have shown that the overwhelming finding is that children with severe asthma are an extremely heterogeneous group. It is therefore difficult to find a common pathophysiological mechanism that explains disease in all patients, but the identification of subphenotypes is the only way that targeted therapies are likely to be effective.[131] A factor that determines severity and is common to both adult and pediatric patients is that early age of onset and allergen sensitization predict increased severity. A specific feature that defines relative steroid resistance and more severe allergic disease is the presence of fungal sensitization. Severe asthma with fungal sensitization (SAFS) is a recognized subphenotype of severe asthma in both children and adults. However, until recently, the mechanisms mediating this subphenotype were unknown. It is now apparent that SAFS in children is characterized by very high levels of serum Ig-E, worse aero-allergen sensitization, and the need for increased doses of steroids. Use of a neonatal mouse model with inhaled exposure to the fungal allergen *Alternaria alternata* has shown increased levels of the innate cytokine IL-33 compared to HDM exposure, and that the *Alternaria* model is more resistant to steroids than the HDM model. Airway samples from children with SAFS also show higher levels of IL-33 on BAL and biopsy compared to children without SAFS, suggesting this subphenotype is mediated by IL-33 and is more resistant to steroid therapy than severe asthma without fungal sensitization.[132]

Another factor that may contribute to the relative steroid resistance seen in children with severe asthma is low levels of serum vitamin D. Children with severe asthma have significantly lower serum vitamin D levels than those with mild–moderate asthma, or nonasthmatic controls.[133] Furthermore, the low vitamin D levels are associated with lower lung function, increased symptoms, and increased frequency of exacerbations.[133] Mechanistically, in a neonatal murine model, vitamin D deficiency has been associated with increased eosinophilia, Th2 cells, and fewer CD4+IL-10+ T regulatory cells.[134] Moreover, children with severe asthma have lower BAL levels of the antiinflammatory cytokine IL-10, and reduced capacity for IL-10 secretion from peripheral blood mononuclear cells.[33] However, addition of both steroids and vitamin D results in significantly increased IL-10 secretion and thus improved steroid sensitivity.[33] In addition, ensuring vitamin D sufficiency in severe asthma is important because it has been shown to inhibit IL-33 by enhancing the production of the soluble decoy receptor for IL-33, soluble ST2.[135]

Analyses of severe asthma in adults have repeatedly shown that early (childhood) onset disease is eosinophilic, associated with the most severe atopy, and the worst lung function.[136] Moreover, longitudinal studies that have followed children with asthma to adulthood show that an early loss in lung function is apparent by school age, is greatest in children with severe disease, and is irreversible and tracks to adulthood. Up to 50% of children who had severe asthma at school age had evidence of persistent airflow limitation and COPD by adulthood.[131] These data confirm the life-long impact of severe asthma on adult lung health and highlight the urgent need for future studies to focus on specific mechanisms that mediate severe pediatric asthma so that appropriate disease modifying interventions can be identified to minimize the long-term morbidity from pediatric severe asthma.

Summary

Interactions between host factors (genes, immune maturation, lung development) and environmental exposures (tobacco smoke, pollution, infection, allergens) and the timing of these interactions are key in the immunopathogenesis and development of disease manifestation in childhood asthma. Currently, we can achieve asthma control in most children with inhaled steroid therapy, but there are specific subgroups for whom we have little to offer. These include preschool wheezers and children with very severe asthma for whom detailed molecular characterization to identify therapeutic targets is urgently needed. At present, our understanding of the mechanisms mediating childhood asthma is very limited, but if we want to progress from the basics of symptom management (our current status) towards disease modification and cure, we must address the need for more detailed understanding of the molecular pathways driving the disease, in different phenotypes, and in children of different ages.

References

Access the reference list online at ExpertConsult.com.

44 Asthma in the Preschool Age Child

JONATHAN GRIGG, MD, and FRANCINE M. DUCHARME, MD, MSc

Epidemiology and Burden

Preschool asthma (i.e., wheeze in children 5 years of age and younger) is a common condition. Indeed, a UK study reported that between 1990 and 1998, there was an increase in the prevalence of parent-reported preschool "wheeze ever" (from 16% to 29%), "current wheeze" (from 12% to 26%), "diagnosis of asthma" (from 11% to 19%), and "admission for wheeze" (from 6% to 10%).[1] This high prevalence of wheeze in preschool children results in a high burden of disease. For example, US National Surveillance of Asthma statistics[2] report the highest average annual asthma physician office visits, hospital outpatient department visits, emergency department visits, and hospitalizations in the preschool period than other age groups (Fig. 44.1)—a pattern also found in other countries.[3]

Episodes of preschool wheeze are frequently associated with signs of an upper respiratory tract infection (URTI).[4] A wide range of infectious agents triggers these episodes (exacerbations). In a prospective cohort study done in Copenhagen, both respiratory viruses (e.g., picornaviruses, respiratory syncytial virus [RSV], and coronavirus) and bacteria (*Streptococcus pneumoniae*, *Haemophilus influenzae*, and *Moraxella catarrhalis*) were isolated from the hypopharynx in just over half of preschool wheeze episodes. Bacteria alone were isolated in just over a third of wheeze episodes, and respiratory viruses alone were isolated in 10% of episodes.[5] In preschool children with clinically severe wheeze, human rhinovirus species C (HRVC) is often isolated, especially in those admitted to hospital.[6,7] While an increased virulence of HRVC has been suggested for this association,[8] there is accumulating evidence that gene-environment interaction is important. For some children this may be due to genetic susceptibility.[9] In other children, allergy may be important, potentially because of impaired innate immune response leading to increased viral replication.[10]

Diagnosis

Asthma is considered an inflammatory disease presenting with episodic or persistent respiratory symptoms associated with variable airflow obstruction to endogenous or exogenous stimuli.[11] However, preschool children with wheeze do not always have airway inflammation between wheezing episodes. As in adults and older children, asthma in preschool is based on recurrent (i.e., two or more) episodes of airflow obstruction and reversibility with appropriate inhaled medication. The diagnosis should be considered in children aged 12 months and older with no suspicion of another condition.[12] Wheeze is the most specific sign of airflow obstruction; it refers to the presence of a continuous musical tone or squeaking commonly heard on auscultation in early expiration or at the end of inspiration. Accompanying signs of obstruction include cough, tachypnea, accessory muscle use, hypoxemia, and, in severe cases, alteration of the mental state. Significant clinical improvement with bronchodilators or corticosteroids is required to document reversibility or, alternatively, fluctuation of symptoms spontaneously over time.

In infants, there is some inconsistency about the diagnostic label applied for wheeze heard on auscultation. A frequent condition in this age group is bronchiolitis—a condition that is associated with signs of a respiratory infection, predominantly, but not exclusively, associated with primary RSV infection of the lower respiratory tract. Infants with bronchiolitis typically do not display significant reversibility, either to bronchodilators or other asthma medications, and in this condition a therapeutic trial is not indicated.[13,14] Although the diagnosis of bronchiolitis is clinical, its varied definition results in diagnostic confusion. In Canada and the United States, a diagnosis of bronchiolitis is a first episode of wheezing in children up to the age of 1 and 2 years, with lower respiratory signs that include wheeze. By contrast, in the United Kingdom and South Africa, the diagnosis of bronchiolitis is mainly limited to infants under 6 months of age, typically with fine crackles but without wheezing.[15] Consequently, wheeze in children, particularly those between 6 months and 2 years, with a first or second episode of respiratory difficulty, and no observed clinical response to asthma medication falls into a clinically unclear area, and is thus frequently labeled as "preschool wheeze" while awaiting a firm diagnosis. However, preschool wheeze is not a diagnosis, but only a symptom underlying an, as yet, poorly defined pathological entity. By careful observation including, when indicated, a therapeutic trial—clinicians should aim to make a definitive, if not at least a presumptive, diagnosis to apply appropriate therapy. In this regard, a therapeutic trial of asthma medication (bronchodilators with oral corticosteroids [OCS], in case of a moderate or severe exacerbation) would be indicated in children aged 12 months and older to document reversibility.

The diagnosis of preschool asthma (defined previously) is best made on the observation of a trained health care professional (or alternatively a convincing parental history) of two or more episodes with signs of airflow obstruction and reversibility. A thorough history and examination is essential to make a presumptive or conclusive diagnosis of asthma and to exclude alternative diagnoses that may cause respiratory symptoms in infancy and early childhood. There are two important caveats to parent-reported wheeze: the

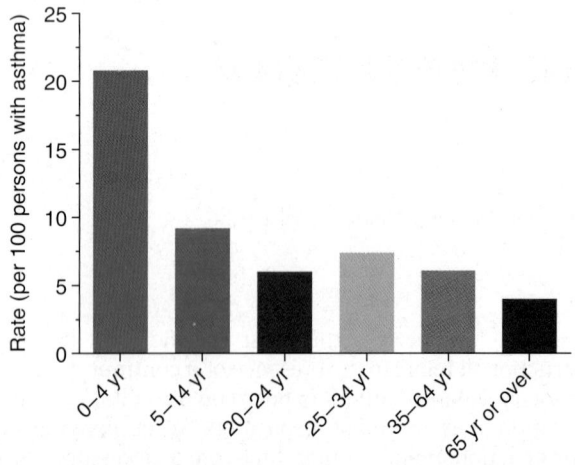

Fig. 44.1 Emergency department visits for acute wheeze (risk-based) for the United Sates. (Data are the age-specific average annual rates for 2007–2008, from the U.S. National Surveillance of Asthma report [2]).

Table 44.1 Differential Diagnosis of Preschool Wheeze

Diagnosis	Clinical Features
Aspiration syndromes (e.g., gastroesophageal reflux, H-type fistula)	Vomiting, poor weight gain, coughing during feeding, and abdominal distension with H type fistula
Inhaled foreign body	Prior episode of coughing or choking (this may be absent), chronic cough
Immune deficiency	Wheeze with infections that are severe, persistent, unusual, or recurrent
Cystic fibrosis	Cough in first weeks of life, poor weight gain
Primary ciliary dyskinesia	Rhinorrhea in first weeks of life, term respiratory distress, with or without situs invertus
Bronchomalacia	Harsh, monophonic expiratory sound
Bronchopulmonary dysplasia/ chronic lung disease of prematurity	Premature birth, home oxygen
Cardiac abnormality	Tachycardia, hepatomegaly, pulmonary crackles
Post infectious obliterative bronchiolitis	History of previous viral infection (especially adenovirus), tachypnea

Table 44.2 American Thoracic Society Recommendations for the Diagnostic Evaluation of Infants With Recurrent of Persistent Wheeze Despite Appropriate Inhaled Treatment

Investigation	Recommendation	Quality of Evidence
Fiberoptic bronchoscopy	Should be done	Very low
Bronchoalveolar lavage	Should be done	Very low
24-hour esophageal pH monitoring	Should be done	Very low
Gastroesophageal scintigraphy instead of pH monitoring	Not preferred to pH monitoring	Very low
Swallowing function study	Should be done	Very low

Ren CL, Esther CR, Debley JS, et al. Official American Thoracic Society Clinical Practice Guidelines: diagnostic evaluation of infants with recurrent or persistent wheezing. *Am J Respir Crit Care Med.* 2016;194:356-373.

accuracy of the vocabulary and the lower sensitivity of ears compared with a stethoscope. When taking a history, wheeze should be separated from other respiratory sounds by asking about "a high-pitched whistling or squeaking sound from the chest, not the throat." Parental reporting of wheeze cannot be regarded as the gold standard. For example, in a large population-based study, 17% of families did not define wheeze as a whistling noise, despite being given a description of wheeze in a questionnaire.[16] Showing parents a video of common respiratory signs and then asking them to identify the closest match help distinguish wheeze from other sounds such as stridor and upper airway rattles.[17] However, direct observation of signs of airflow obstruction and reversibility during an exacerbation by a trained health care professional remains the preferred approach. In a child with a prior documented exacerbation or a convincing history of an exacerbation, who does not present with clinical signs of airflow obstruction, an alternative approach is to document reversibility with a 12-week trial of maintenance inhaled corticosteroids (ICS), with parent-reported change in the frequency and severity of chronic and acute symptoms. This treatment should be discontinued if there is no benefit; many would want to exclude the possibility that the child had in fact recovered spontaneously by having a trial period of stopping treatment.

Parents should be asked about the nature and duration of symptoms, exacerbating factors, family history, and presence of atopy, rhinitis, and smoking in the home or car. History and examination should focus on eliminating the other important diagnoses that may cause respiratory symptoms in infancy and early childhood. Alternative diagnoses include structural abnormalities, gastroesophageal reflux, congenital heart disease, foreign body, chronic aspiration, chronic airway infection, and the consequences of extreme prematurity. Red flags for alternative diagnoses include prominent upper airway symptoms, symptoms from the first day of life, sudden onset of symptoms, chronic moist cough, symptoms worse after meals, and weight loss (Table 44.1).[18] Examination should pay attention to clubbing, wasting, severe tonsillar hypertrophy, severe chest deformity, fixed monophonic or asymmetrical wheeze, and cardiac murmurs. A 2016 review of the diagnostic evaluation of infants with recurrent or persistent wheezing (despite adequate inhaled asthma therapy) by the American Thoracic Society recommends flexible bronchoscopy, pH monitoring, and a swallowing study; however, the evidence to support these recommendations was found to be of low quality (Table 44.2).[19]

Investigations should be tailored to the medical history, physical examination, and suspected diagnosis. For the majority of wheezy preschool children, no investigations are needed. For the minority of children with clinically very severe wheeze (and no red flags on history and examination), it is reasonable to perform a chest radiograph and assess the possibility of sensitization to outdoor and indoor allergens as contributing factors. Exposure to cigarette smoke should be ascertained for all children,[20] with a firm recommendation for a smoke-free environment.

Natural History

The first complete picture of the natural history of preschool wheeze originated from the Tucson Children's Respiratory Study.[21] Retrospective analysis of this longitudinal dataset from 1246 newborns assessed at both 3 years and 6 years revealed distinct temporal patterns of wheeze that were associated with different factors. First, there are "transient infant wheezers" (the majority of wheezers in this cohort) who wheezed occasionally during the first 3 years of life and then did not wheeze after the age of 3 years. This pattern was not significantly associated with markers of atopy, such as blood eosinophilia or high levels of serum immunoglobulin E (IgE), but was associated with lower lung function (measured in infants prior to their first episode of wheezing) and maternal smoking during pregnancy. Although many of these preschoolers probably met the definition of preschool asthma (obstruction and reversibility with asthma therapy), this pattern was not significantly associated with parent-reported ongoing asthma symptoms at and beyond 6 years of age, suggesting a transient asthma phenomenon. Second, there were "nonatopic wheezers" who begin wheezing at 3 years, but whose wheeze resolved by 6 years. Third, there are "atopic wheezers," whose preschool wheeze continued as allergic asthma after 6 years of age. Similar trajectories of preschool wheeze have subsequently been reported in other longitudinal cohorts, albeit with subtle differences. For example, an analysis of longitudinal data from the Leiccstershire and Avon Longitudinal Study of Parents and Children (ALSPAC) cohorts found patterns consistent between the two cohorts. Those children with persistent wheeze and chronic cough, associated with atopy, have reduced lung function and a poorer prognosis, whereas those with early-onset nonpersistent whcczc have a more favorable prognosis.[22] To date, however, these important epidemiological studies have not produced a clinically useful method for predicting which preschool children will develop asthma symptoms at school age. Indeed, a systematic review of 12 asthma prediction models, including the asthma predictive index (API), found that although some models were better at predicting ongoing asthma at 6 years, and other models were better at ruling it out, no single model could accurately do both.[23] Thus the prediction of whether preschoolers with asthmalike symptoms will continue to have asthma at 6 years, from contemporaneously obtained information, cannot be achieved with sufficient precision in a large proportion of preschool children with wheeze. One main reason is that most children have symptoms only in preschool years and "outgrow" symptoms before the age of 6 years, although, unfortunately, some still have residual lung function impairment.[24] Another reason is the different prevalence of disease in various settings, such as the general population, a family physician practice, or a specialist clinic. When discussing outcomes with parents, clinicians therefore should make it clear that (1) wheezing is very common in the first few years of life, (2) there is a good chance that wheeze will resolve by school age and only a minority of affected children will become lifelong asthmatics, and (3) there is an increased chance of exhibiting ongoing asthma symptoms at school age if wheeze continues beyond 3 years of age, and particularly if it is associated with allergies, although accurate prediction of outcome is not possible.

As the pattern of wheeze changes over time, the subgroup of children who become persistent or recurrent wheezers needs careful follow-up and treatment (or at least a therapeutic trial) to improve symptoms and reduce the frequency and severity of exacerbations. Importantly, as a group, preschoolers with wheezing (confirmed or suspected asthma) are at an increased risk of attenuated lung function growth,[25] and those with more frequent or severe exacerbations appear to be most affected.

ENVIRONMENTAL FACTORS

Exposure to air pollution is associated with an increased risk of developing preschool wheeze. A longitudinal study of US children found that increased exposure to traffic-derived pollution at birth was associated with both preschool wheeze that subsequently resolved by 7 years (transient) and with wheeze that continued to 7 years (persistent).[26] In this study, exposure to traffic-derived air pollution from birth to 1 year of age and from 1 to 2 years of age were both associated with persistent wheeze.[26] There is emerging evidence that prenatal exposure to chemicals, especially bisphenol A and phthalates, increases risk of preschool asthma. For example, a recent study reported that metabolites of these compounds in the urine of pregnant Spanish women are associated with increased risk of wheeze in their offspring during the first 4 years of life.[27]

CLINICAL PATTERNS OF WHEEZE

There have been several attempts to classify preschool asthma by pattern of symptoms, with a view to better targeting treatment (e.g., intermittent treatment for episodic symptoms). A classification suggested by a European Respiratory Society Task Force is to divide children into those with multiple-trigger wheeze, defined as episodes of wheeze associated with one or more triggers (including but not limited to URTIs and interval symptoms), versus those with episodic wheeze, defined as discrete episodes of wheeze (usually triggered solely by URTI) but without interval symptoms.[28] In cross-sectional surveys, episodic wheeze predominates in children younger than 3 years old.[1,29,30] Whether wheeze patterns are clinically useful remains unclear, as these are unstable over time in the same child, and there is a high variation in the categorization of patterns between pediatricians.[29,31]

Pathology

Increased bronchial airway smooth muscle (ASM), subepithelial eosinophilia, and increased reticular basement membrane thickening (a pattern found in adult atopic asthma) are reported in a highly selected group of preschool children with severe recurrent wheeze.[32] Furthermore, increased ASM, but not the latter two features, was associated with an increased risk of having ongoing asthma at school age.[33] There are no reported data from bronchial biopsies in children with less severe disease. However, transient increases in urinary cysteinyl leukotriene metabolites and urinary eosinophil activation markers are reported during acute wheeze[34,35]— whether these indirect markers reflect airway inflammation is unclear.

Treatment

Compatible with the management objectives for older children and adults, the goals of children presenting with preschool asthma are to achieve good control of symptoms, maintain normal activity levels, and minimize future risk—that is, the prevention of future exacerbations, impaired lung growth and function, and side effects.[36] A diagnosis, at least a presumptive one, is essential to achieve this goal, as treatment varies according to the condition. In reviewing the treatment of preschool asthma, this chapter focuses on children who wheeze after 1 year of age and those younger than 1 year with recurrent wheeze. Treatment recommendations do not apply to infants less than 1 year presenting with a first episode of wheezing where bronchiolitis is suspected. The management of preschool wheeze and asthma includes both non-pharmacological and pharmacologic approaches.

TREATMENT—NONPHARMACOLOGICAL

All preschool children with suspected or confirmed asthma should have preschool asthma education, with an explanation of the condition, the role of relief and controller medication, and adequate inhalation technique.[11] They should be provided with a self-management plan with written instructions on how to achieve and maintain asthma control ("green zone"), how to manage deterioration ("yellow zone"), and when to consult the physician in case of an asthma attack ("red zone"). While shown effective in all age groups,[37] the only randomized trial that tested an educational guided self-management approach exclusively in preschoolers did not show a significant difference from usual care.[38] However, the authors recognized substantial contamination between groups, with close to half of control patients recalling that they received the same verbal instructions as those in the intervention; further, they acknowledged the absence of documented effectiveness of their recommended intervention—namely preemptive home administration of oral steroids in viral-induced wheezing. Given these study limitations, asthma self-management education remains indicated in preschoolers.[11]

Avoidance of exposure to cigarette smoke and other irritants, and if sensitized, to aeroallergens, should be recommended. Although respiratory illnesses are the most frequent triggers, there is currently no proven, effective approach to avoid the common cold, other than reduced exposure to infected individuals. This is a difficult task when children are placed in childcare during the first years of life or in the presence of numerous siblings.

TREATMENT—PHARMACOLOGICAL

Challenge to Personalizing Therapy

Despite the worldwide move toward personalized medicine, most, if not all, preschool trials have failed to show convincing evidence that a particular approach is more beneficial for some children than others. Specifically, there is little evidence that children with positive and negative asthma predictive scores respond differently to therapeutic approaches.[39,40] This is probably due in part to poor stability of these phenotypes within the same child over time and high between-physician variability.[29,31] Clearly, significant progress in personalized medicine hinges on the future identification of accurate, precise, and reproducible determinants of response, such as preschool lung function, inflammatory markers, genotype, metabolomics, and other "omics" obtainable in preschool children. Stratification on these determinants must then be proven to be associated with differential treatment response, in randomized clinical trials.

Until then, the therapy shown most effective for the majority of preschoolers with asthma in a rigorously designed trial should dictate the best management. The therapeutic section of this chapter is informed by a literature search that identified systematic reviews of randomized controlled trials and randomized controlled trials of children aged 1–5 years described as having preschool wheeze and/or asthma; trials related to wheeze arising from alternative diagnoses (as discussed previously) were specifically excluded whenever feasible. The pharmacological approach is presented by sections corresponding to the "green zone" (maintaining control) and "yellow zone" (managing deterioration) of a self-management plan and for the initial management of an exacerbation in the acute care setting.

Preventive Management—"Green Zone"

The evidence supporting therapy in preschool children is derived from randomized controlled trials and systematic reviews of trials, which included children with either asthma or preschool wheezing with specific or a variety of wheezing phenotypes (Fig. 44.2).

Daily Preventive Monotherapy

All identified trials pertained to the use of ICS or montelukast, as the leukotriene receptor antagonist (LTRA). With regard to first-line monotherapy, clearly the strongest evidence relates to the use of daily ICS. In a meta-analysis of children with preschool wheeze and asthma by Castro-Rodriguez and Rodrigo,[41] daily ICS was associated with a 41% reduction in the risk of exacerbations of all severity (RR 0.59, 95% CI 0.52–0.67), risk of withdrawals due to exacerbations (RR 0.52, 95% CI 0.43–0.63), symptoms (standardized mean difference [SMD] 0.93, 95% CI 0.49–1.37), and β2-agonist use (SMD 0.63, 95% CI 0.30–0.63), and with a significant improvement in forced expiratory volume in one second (FEV$_1$) (weighted mean difference [WMD] 0.06L, 95% CI 0.05–0.09). A second meta-analysis of trials not included in the Castro-Rodriguez and Rodrigo review (noted previously) done by Ducharme et al[42] pertained to a mixed population of preschoolers with or without atopy (or a positive API); again, daily ICS was found to reduce the risk of moderate exacerbations (i.e., exacerbations needing rescue OCS) by more than 40%, compared with placebo (RR 0.57, 95% CI 0.40–0.80) and was associated with a significantly greater percentage of asthma-free days (mean difference [MD] 5.52 days, 95% CI 2.22–8.81). However, daily ICS therapy is not curative and must be sustained to maintain benefit. For example, during the 1-year period after the cessation of ICS in the Prevention of Early Asthma in Kids (PEAK) trial, there was a similar frequency of symptoms in ICS- and placebo-treated children.[43]

Only two pediatric trials have compared daily LTRAs to placebo in preschoolers. While daily montelukast was

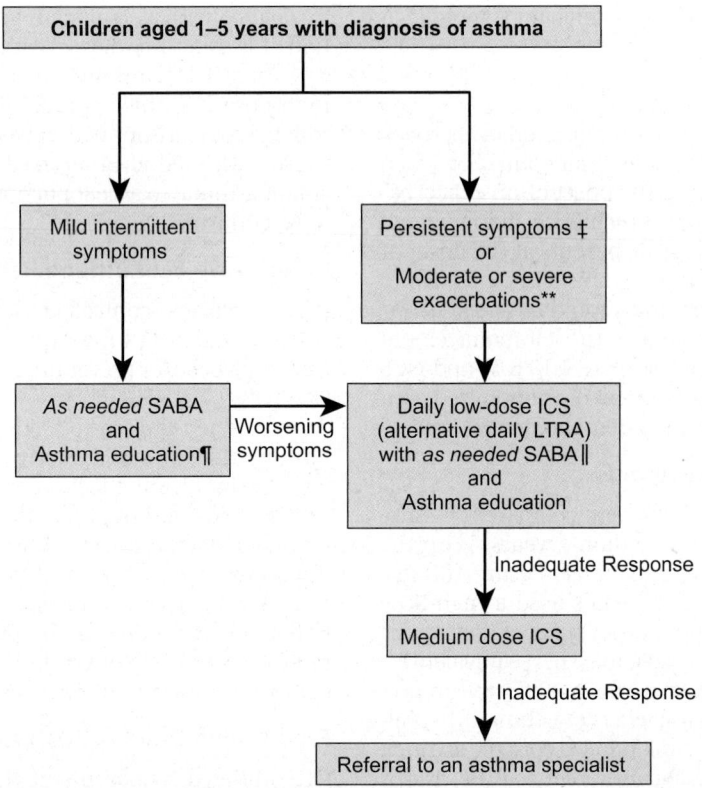

Fig. 44.2 Diagnostic algorithm for treatment of wheeze in preschool children (1–5 years of age). *ICS,* Inhaled corticosteroids; *OCS,* oral corticosteroids; *SABA,* inhaled short-acting β2-agonists. ¶, Asthma education including environmental control and a written self-management plan; ‡, eight or more (≥8) days/month with symptoms, ≥8 days/month with use of SABA, ≥1 night awakening due to symptoms/month, any exercise limitation/month or any absence from usual activities to asthma symptoms; **, episodes requiring rescue oral corticosteroids or hospital admission; ‖, ICS are more effective than LTRA. (Figure adapted from Ducharme FM, Dell SD, Radhakrishnan D, et al. Diagnosis and management of asthma in preschoolers: a Canadian Thoracic Society and Canadian Paediatric Society position paper. *Can Respir J Vol.* 2015;22:135-143 and reproduced with permission).

associated with a reduction in the number of overall exacerbations in one trial,[44] it was not associated with a reduction in exacerbations requiring rescue oral steroids,[44] or in asthma-free days.[44,45] When data were reanalyzed after including only children with an apparent episodic (viral-triggered) wheeze or episodic asthma phenotype, no statistically significant group reduction in the number of episodes requiring rescue OCS was associated with daily montelukast versus placebo (OR 1.20, 95% CI; 0.70–2.06).[46]

What Is the Best Preventive Strategy for Specific Wheezy Children?

In the absence of head-to-head trials comparing daily ICS to daily montelukast, the best strategy may only be gauged at present by the size of the effect of each monotherapy compared with placebo. Children showed a greater magnitude of response with ICS than with montelukast. Compared with placebo, potential markers of the best ICS responders were explored. A subgroup analysis of the systematic review by Castro-Rodriguez and Rodrigo[41] suggested a stronger effect for reducing exacerbations in children with a clinical diagnosis of asthma than in those with wheezing (RR 0.50 vs. 0.65, $P = .04$), with no apparent effect of other patient characteristics such as age, atopy, or treatment characteristics such as specific ICS, delivery mode, or duration of therapy.

In contrast, in a post hoc analysis of the PEAK trial, preschoolers with a health care utilization in the preceding year, those with aeroallergen sensitization, boys, and Caucasians were better responders to ICS compared with placebo.[47] These apparent conflicting determinants attest to the need for replication.

In the future, the identification of consistent and strong determinants of response is needed to better identify responders, with a confirmatory trial of different therapies, stratified on the presence/absence of determinants (as noted previously) to validate their discriminative ability, will be required. Until then, given the strength of the evidence supporting ICS as opposed to LTRA over placebo, the preferred daily monotherapy should be ICS.

Adjunct Therapy

To date, there are no published trials exploring adjunct therapy to ICS in this age group.[48]

In summary, the best daily management for preschoolers with repeated wheezing episodes or persistent symptoms is daily low-dose ICS, although it appears slightly more effective in those with a clinical diagnosis of asthma than yet undiagnosed children (i.e., preschool wheezers). The evidence for montelukast is less compelling, partly because of the paucity of trials and apparent lesser efficacy. In view of the difficulty in the recognition of specific phenotypes, initiation of therapy with daily ICS in any child with clinically significant symptoms is reasonable.

Preemptive Therapy—Yellow Zone

For children with apparent episodic asthma, another approach is the preemptive initiation of an asthma controller when exposed to a known trigger or at the onset of an exacerbation (i.e., intermittent therapy). Preemptive management refers to the initiation of therapy by parents at the onset of an exacerbation. Short-acting β2-agonists are effective in children aged 1 year and over, and should be the first-line relief medication in the yellow zone of the self-management plan.[49] Preemptive administration of ICS, LTRA, and OCS has been formally tested in the context of randomized controlled trials and summarized in systematic reviews.[42,48]

Preemptive Inhaled Corticosteroids

Six trials, identified by systematic review, compared preemptive ICS to placebo in children less than 6 years. With the exception of one trial in infants and toddlers using 400 μg/day of nebulized budesonide,[50] all trials used a high-dose ICS over 5–10 days (i.e., 1500 μg/day or greater of budesonide or beclomethasone in hydrofluoroalkane [HFA] equivalent).[42] Preemptive low-moderate ICS dose was not effective in preschoolers with mild episodic viral wheeze/asthma.[50] In children with moderate-to-severe viral induced episodic asthma, preemptive high-dose ICS significantly reduced the risk of exacerbations requiring rescue OCS by more than 30% (RR 0.68 [95% CI; 0.53–0.86]; Fig. 44.3A), but was not

associated with a significant group difference in the proportion of asthma-free days.[42] Although children with moderate to severe URTI/viral-induced asthma respond to preemptive high-dose ICS, this approach has not been tested in head-to-head comparisons with other groups of children, including those with mild viral-induced asthma and those with persistent asthma, so a clear phenotype-specific response remains to be confirmed.

Preemptive Leukotriene Receptor Antagonists

In three placebo-controlled trials,[40,45,51] the effect of preemptive montelukast (4 mg) was not significantly different from that of placebo for preventing exacerbations requiring rescue OCS (OR 0.77, 95% CI; 0.48–1.25), or reducing asthma-free days.[42] When limited to a subgroup of children with only viral-induced wheezing derived from a single study,[52] there was no significant effect on exacerbations requiring rescue oral steroids, although a small but statistically significant reduction was observed in unscheduled medical attendances due to wheeze (RR 0.83, 95% CI; 0.71–0.98).[46] With only one 3-arm placebo-controlled trial[40] comparing preemptive LTRA to preemptive high-dose ICS in preschoolers with moderate-to-severe intermittent wheezing, neither was associated with less rescue OCS or more episode-free days.

Preemptive Oral Corticosteroids

OCS initiated by parents at the onset of URTI symptoms, or after not responding to a first dose of bronchodilator, were tested in two trials of children aged 1–5 years with

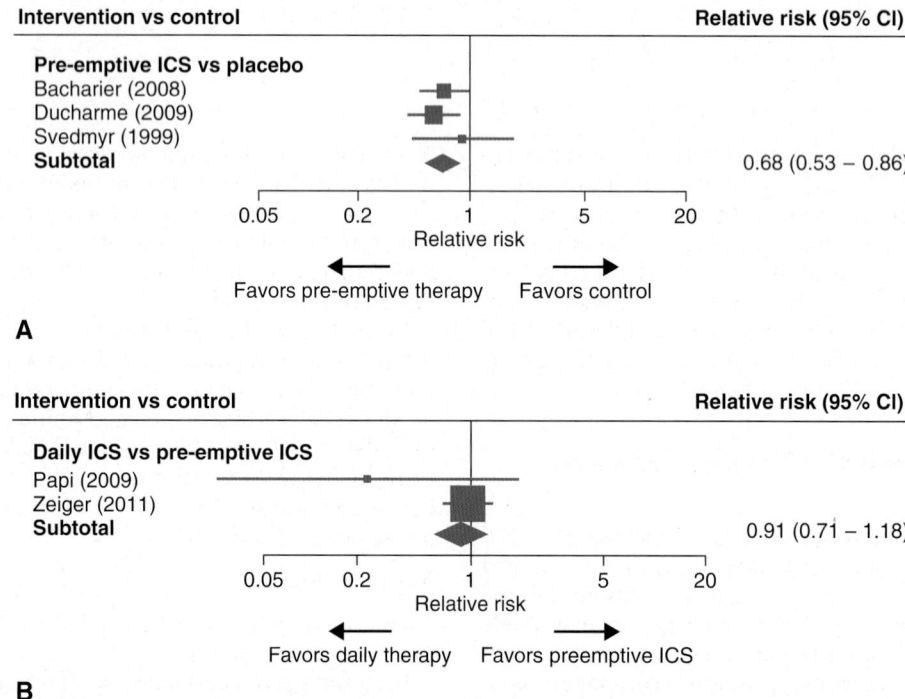

Fig. 44.3 (A) Comparison of preemptive inhaled corticosteroids (ICS) with preemptive placebo. In preschool children with moderate-to-severe viral induced episodic asthma, preemptive high-dose ICS reduced the risk of exacerbations requiring rescue oral corticosteroids. In these studies, prescription of oral steroids is used as a marker for clinically severe wheeze. (B) Comparison of daily ICS with preemptive high-dose ICS. Results are described as pooled relative risk of preschool children with wheeze or asthma experiencing exacerbations treated with rescue oral corticosteroids. The wide confidence interval underlines the lack of power to draw firm conclusions about the relative efficacy of daily low-dose ICS versus preemptive high-dose ICS. (Figure adapted from Ducharme FM, Tse SM, Chauhan B. Diagnosis, management, and prognosis of preschool wheeze. *Lancet.* 2014;383:1593-1604 and reproduced with permission).

recurrent viral-induced wheeze.[53,54] There was no statistically significant group difference with regard to symptoms, emergency department visits, or hospital admission. The absence of a benefit of preemptive OCS on symptoms during episodes was subsequently confirmed by a post hoc analysis of two randomized controlled trials testing other preemptive strategies.[55]

Step-Up of Daily Therapy Dose at the Onset of an Exacerbation

There are no identified trials with preschoolers on daily ICS exploring the strategy of increasing the ICS dose at the onset of an exacerbation compared with maintaining the usual dose. Since no beneficial effect was observed in school-aged children and adults,[56] this strategy does not appear promising.

Which Preemptive Strategy Is Most Effective?

There are no published trials comparing the use of preemptive OCS with either of the two other strategies. Only one trial compared preemptive nebulized budesonide to preemptive montelukast or placebo: there was no statistically significant group difference, despite a nonsignificant trend favoring ICS over LTRA for rescue oral steroids and symptom-free days.[40] Consequently, there is insufficient evidence to firmly conclude on the equivalence or superiority of any of these three preemptive options.[42] However, in view of the absence of a significant effect of preemptive LTRA or OCS on episode-free days, rescue OCS, health care utilization, or symptom severity compared with placebo, the strength of the evidence clearly supporting preemptive high-dose ICS over placebo for reducing exacerbations requiring rescue OCS would support this latter strategy over the former two in preschoolers with episodic moderate to severe viral induced asthma.

Daily Versus Preemptive Asthma Controller: What Is the Best and Safest Approach?

With regard to efficacy, two trials of preschool children with recurrent moderate to severe episodic viral-induced wheeze or asthma, with and without a positive API, compared daily low-dose ICS with preemptive high-dose ICS: there was no statistically significant group difference with regard to the need for rescue OCS (0.91 [0.71–1.18]).[42] In these two trials, initiation of OCS therapy was used as a marker for clinically severe wheeze. The wide confidence interval (see Fig. 44.3B) underlines the lack of power to draw firm conclusions about the relative efficacy of daily low doses versus preemptive high-doses of ICS.[42] However, daily ICS trials included a variety of children with interim symptoms, atopy, or recurrent viral-induced asthma, such that this approach appears as the most effective first-line therapy irrespective of apparent phenotype and is recommended as such by most national and international guidelines.[12,36,57,58] By contrast, preemptive high-dose ICS was tested in younger preschool children with moderate or severe viral-induced wheezing with no or minimal interim symptoms, such that this approach may be best reserved to those with two or more exacerbations requiring an emergency department visit or rescue OCS, who failed to respond to daily ICS.[12] Because of the risk of ICS overuse by parents and physicians, the preemptive high-dose

ICS strategy should be reserved for preschool children who remain poorly controlled, despite good compliance with a medium dose of daily ICS, under the supervision by asthma specialists with close monitoring of potential side effects and follow-up of efficacy.

Safety Profile. Clinical trials conducted in preschoolers have seldom documented potential adverse effects systematically (specifically growth), and impact on adrenal function has been insufficiently studied. Concerning the former, only two trials were identified in a systematic review of randomized controlled trials. In the subgroup of toddlers or infants (n = 903), the change in the baseline of height (cm) during 1 year of ICS (MD −0.58, 95% CI; −0.55 to −0.20, P = .003) was of similar magnitude than that observed in prepubertal school-aged children (MD −0.46, 95% CI; −0.75 to −0.16, P = .004).[59] In another trial, daily ciclesonide up to 200 µg/day for 24 weeks was not linked with any detectable impairment in growth or adrenal function in children less than 6 years.[60] This systematic review, including mostly prepubertal school-aged children, showed a significant molecule- and dose-dependency in the magnitude of growth suppression associated with ICS.[59] Compared with placebo, repeated intake of preemptive high-dose ICS has been associated with a group difference of 0.6 cm, equivalent to a 4 percentile point difference in growth,[30] analogous to that reported with daily low ICS dose.[43] The potential for overuse of preemptive high-dose ICS by both parents and physicians has led to calls for caution in the use of this strategy. In the absence of solid data for preschool children, the selection of the safest molecules and careful monitoring of growth seems to be the most prudent approach for any child receiving daily or preemptive ICS.

TREATMENT—INITIAL MANAGEMENT OF EXACERBATIONS IN THE ACUTE CARE SETTING

As for older children and adults, the initial step is to assess asthma severity and apply severity-specific management. Several signs suggest increasing severity of airflow obstruction, namely accessory muscle use, wheezing, oxygen saturation at or below 92%,[12] decreased air entry, agitation, or apathy.[61] Use of validated standardized clinical scores, such as the 12-point pediatric respiratory assessment measure (PRAM, Fig. 44.4),[62] has been shown to be effective and practical to apply guidelines and reduced hospital admissions.[63,64]

Bronchodilators

Short-acting β2-agonists are the most effective bronchodilators, with a significant bronchodilator effect documented in children aged 1 year and over.[49] In a meta-analysis of children aged 1–18 years, with moderate or severe airflow obstruction, the addition of ipratropium bromide to β2-agonists has been shown to be superior to β2-agonists alone.[65] The administration of salbutamol by metered dose inhaler with a spacer was more cost-effective and associated with fewer side effects than by nebulizer in young children (1–4 years) with moderate and severe acute asthma.[66] In these patients, repeating the dose of β2-agonists at 20 minutes, the time of peak action, led to better and more sustained bronchodilation.[67] Supplemental oxygen should be provided for children with hypoxemia.

PRAM scoring table

Criterions	Description	Score
O₂ saturation	95%	0
	92-94%	1
	< 92%	2
Suprasternal retration	Absent	0
	Present	2
Scalene muscle contraction	Absent	0
	Present	2
Air entry*	Normal	0
	↓ at the base	1
	↓ at the apex and the base	2
	Minimal or absent	3
Wheezing§	Absent	0
	Expiratory only	1
	Inspiratory (± expiratory)	2
	Audible without stethoscope or silent chest (minimal or no air entry)	3
	PRAM score: (max. 12)	

Score	0-3	4-7	8-12
Severity	Mild	Moderate	Severe

© Ducharme 2000

Fig. 44.4 The pediatric respiratory assessment measure (PRAM) scoring table. *, In case of asymmetry, the most severely affected (apex-base) lung field (right or left, anterior or posterior) will determine the rating of the criterion. §, In case of asymmetry, the two most severely affected ausculation zones, irrespective of their location (right upper lobe, right middle lobe, right lower lobe, left upper lobe, left lower lobe), will determine the rating of the criterion. (Reproduced with the permission of Francine M. Ducharme. Reprinted from The Journal of Pediatrics, Vol. 137, Issue 6. Chalut DS, Ducharme FM, Davis GM. The Preschool Respiratory Assessment Measure (PRAM): A responsive index of acute asthma severity. Pages 762-768, Copyright © 2000, with permission from Elsevier.)

Oral Corticosteroids

National and international guidelines recommend the addition of OCS in preschoolers with moderate or severe airflow obstruction and in those with poor responses to bronchodilators. This view is consistent with a systematic review of randomized controlled trials, confirming a 25% reduction in hospital admission rate in children treated with systemic corticosteroids compared with placebo in pediatric trials that collectively included about 50% preschoolers[68]; one trial included only preschoolers,[69] whereas the other four pediatric trials included both preschool and school-aged children.[70-73] The efficacy of OCS was challenged by a 2009 placebo-controlled trial in children aged 10 months to 5 years, with viral-induced wheezing showing no apparent effect on the duration of hospital stay; young age and viral infection were suspected explanations for the negative findings.[74] By contrast, a recent cohort study conducted in children aged 1–17 years presenting with a moderate or severe asthma exacerbation and treated with a severity-specific treatment protocol with β2-agonists, ipratropium bromide, and OCS reported a very low treatment failure rate of 17%.[75] After adjusting for baseline severity (i.e., PRAM score and oxygen saturation), the presence of symptoms between exacerbations, viral detection, and fever were significant predictors of failure of emergency management. Of note, age was not significantly associated with treatment response. These data suggest that a higher rate of respiratory infections, rather than age, may explain the apparent higher treatment failure observed in preschoolers presenting with acute asthma.

In summary, the evidence specific to preschoolers to support the efficacy of OCS in those with repeated episodes of airflow obstruction and who meet the criteria for asthma is scarce; consequently, it remains debated whether one should restrict or liberalize its use in preschool children with ongoing wheeze, despite an initial adequate dose of inhaled bronchodilator therapy. By contrast, children who are younger than a year, with a first episode of wheezing, who do not meet the operational definition of asthma (obstruction and reversibility with asthma medication) are unlikely to benefit from OCS, irrespective of severity or setting. In children falling between these two extremes, OCS should be used sparingly and on an individual trial basis only.

Inhaled Corticosteroids

A systematic review of eight randomized controlled trials of children (and an unspecified proportion of preschoolers) presenting to the emergency department with an acute asthma exacerbation concluded that there was a beneficial effect of ICS alone in reducing the rate of hospital admission. Although there was no significant group difference in hospital admission rate between groups, the power was insufficient to conclude regarding the equivalence between ICS versus OCS for preventing hospital admission, relapse, and the need to rescue OCS. Although promising, the evidence is thus insufficient to recommend replacing oral steroids by high-dose ICS therapy (which is also more costly), either in emergency management, or upon discharge from the emergency department.[76]

Magnesium Sulfate

Treatment with intravenous magnesium sulfate showed a significant benefit in children and adults with acute severe asthma, but not in those with milder severity.[77] Several pediatric trials are ongoing and will help confirm the best route (nebulized vs. intravenous) and indication for magnesium sulfate in children, including preschoolers.

Antibiotics

The observation that bacterial colonization of the hypopharynx is common during episodes of preschool wheeze (discussed previously) led researchers to assess the efficacy of azithromycin. In a randomized placebo controlled trial that recruited infants from the COPSAC cohort, Stokholm et al[78] found that a course of azithromycin started 3 days into an episode reduced the mean duration of subsequent troublesome lower respiratory symptoms by about 4 days. Since improvement of symptoms with azithromycin may be due to an improvement in (clinically trivial) bronchitic cough, and not wheeze,[79] azithromycin cannot be recommended at this time.

FUTURE DIRECTIONS

As most of the airflow obstruction reported by 7 years of age in children with asthma is not attributable to prenatal or perinatal programming, there is a window of opportunity for interventions in the preschool years to prevent early airway remodeling. This may imply finding novel strategies to prevent key triggers such as viral infections, to reduce the frequency and severity of viral-induced exacerbations, and to improve the monitoring of preschool lung function to identify "unrecognized" persistent airway obstruction. Although there are no long-term trials to determine if sustained controller therapy introduced early could prevent lung function impairment in school-aged children with asthma symptoms, it seems prudent to initiate controller therapy early.

Until determinants of a differential response to therapy are identified, the best approach for preschool children with recurrent or chronic wheeze is the administration of daily-ICS at the lowest effective dose. A proven effective alternative for children with moderate and severe viral-induced exacerbations is preemptive high-dose ICS, with safeguards to prevent overuse by parents and physicians. Future advances in objective markers of phenotype would enable major advances in personalized therapy. Trials are needed to clarify the role of adjunct therapy and immunotherapy in this young age group. Meanwhile, careful regular reassessments remain the cornerstone of an appropriate follow-up to ensure an adequate response and enable timely reduction to the minimal effective dose.

References

Access the reference list online at ExpertConsult.com.

Suggested Reading

Ducharme FM, Dell SD, Radhakrishnan D, et al. Diagnosis and management of asthma in preschoolers: A Canadian Thoracic Society and Canadian Paediatric Society position paper. *Can Respir J.* 2015;22(3):135–143. [Epub 2015 Apr 20].

45 Wheezing in Older Children: Asthma

CAROLYN M. KERCSMAR, MS, MD, and KAREN M. MCDOWELL, MD

Introduction

Wheezing is a musical, high-pitched, largely expiratory sound, typically made through the partially obstructed larger airways, most commonly caused by asthma in school-age children. Nevertheless, wheezing can also be generated by narrowing in the distal trachea and by glottic closure. A number of other conditions can cause both acute and chronic wheezing in children, but many causes are associated with other symptoms that generally distinguish them from asthma (Box 45.1). The major focus of this chapter will be on the diagnosis and treatment of asthma in children beyond the preschool years.

As defined in the National Heart, Lung, and Blood Institute (NHLBI) guidelines, asthma is characterized by variable, reversible obstruction of air flow (but not completely so in some patients), which may improve spontaneously or may subside only after specific therapy.[1] Airway hyperreactivity, defined as the inherent tendency of the trachea and bronchi to narrow in response to a variety of stimuli (e.g., allergens, nonspecific irritants, or infection), is also a prominent feature. Both the airway obstruction and hyperreactivity may be associated with chronic, dysregulated airway inflammation that involves many cell types (e.g., eosinophils, lymphocytes, neutrophils, epithelial cells, airway smooth muscle, fibroblasts) and mediators (e.g., cytokines, chemokines, enzymes, growth factors, IgE). Symptoms of wheeze, cough, and shortness of breath are episodic in most patients but may occur daily in some. Asthma is now viewed as an "umbrella term" for a complex, heterogeneous disorder with numerous phenotypes and endotypes that differ in children and adults. Although all asthma phenotypes demonstrate airway obstruction, the pathophysiological processes, genetics, natural history, and response to treatment differ widely.

Although there has been an increased awareness of the prevalence of childhood asthma, substantial physical, psychological, and socioeconomic morbidity continue to occur. Among the 7 million children younger than 18 years of age in the United States with asthma, it is estimated that each year more than 10 million school days are lost, 3 million sick visits are made to health care providers, and more than 450,000 hospitalizations occur.[2] The annual direct and indirect health care costs for treatment of asthma were recently estimated at over $50 billion per year in the United States. Poor, disadvantaged minority children who reside in central urban areas have both the highest prevalence and greatest morbidity. Nevertheless, both acute health care utilization and mortality rates from asthma appear to have stabilized and for some groups, declined slightly in recent years, following a steady rise in the period from 1980 to the mid-1990s.[2] Mortality remains rare and is declining, and less than 150 children and adolescents younger than 15 years of age in the United States die annually from asthma.

Pathology

Examination of postmortem lung specimens of patients who died from asthma shows marked hyperinflation with smooth muscle hyperplasia in the bronchial and bronchiolar walls, thick tenacious mucous plugs often completely occluding the airways, markedly thickened basement membrane, and variable degrees of mucosal edema and denudation of bronchial and bronchiolar epithelium (Fig. 45.1).[3] Eosinophilia of the submucosa and secretions is often prominent whether or not allergic (IgE-mediated) mechanisms are present. Airway smooth muscle mass is also increased in the airways by school age and may begin in the preschool years. Mucous plugs contain layers of shed epithelial cells and eosinophils, as well as neutrophils and lymphocytes. Although the exact role of airway eosinophils in causing and perpetuating the asthma phenotype remains controversial, eosinophil products (e.g., major basic protein and other proteases) may play an important role in the destructive changes observed. The mucosal edema with separated columnar cells and stratified nonciliated epithelium, which replaces ciliated epithelium, results in abnormal mucociliary clearance. Mast cells are increased in airway smooth muscle of asthmatics. In addition, there is increased mast cell degranulation, which is often worse in those with more severe asthma. Submucosal gland hypertrophy and increased goblet cell size are not constant features of asthma, but mucous metaplasia caused by increased synthesis and stores frequently occurs across all ranges of asthma severity. The thickened basement membrane caused by submucosal deposition of type IV collagen and various other materials is a striking feature of asthma and has been reported even in mild asthmatics. Basement membrane thickening is thought to occur early in the disease, but its pathologic significance remains to be determined. All of these findings have been observed in symptom-free asthmatic individuals who died accidental deaths, as well as in endobronchial biopsy specimens from research subjects (Fig. 45.2). Significant basement membrane thickening in airway mucosal biopsies taken from pediatric patients with severe asthma has been observed in the absence of active eosinophilic or neutrophilic infiltrates.[4,5] Moreover, normal lung function as measured by forced expiratory volume in 1 second (FEV_1) can be achieved by patients with severe airway remodeling. These observations call into question the role of inflammation and remodeling in asthma that is difficult to control. Although an occasional patient may show localized bronchiectasis and small focal areas of alveolar destruction, these are not characteristic of asthma, and there is little evidence that asthma leads to destructive emphysema. However, the incomplete reversibility of air flow limitation seen in some asthmatics suggests that a phenotype exists that may be considered a form of chronic

Box 45.1 Causes of Wheezing in Older Children

α1-antiprotease deficiency (adolescent, young adult)
Anatomic lesion or airway compression
Angioedema
Aspiration/gastroesophageal reflux
Asthma
Bronchiectasis
Bronchogenic or pulmonary cyst
Congestive heart failure
Cystic fibrosis
Eosinophilic bronchitis
Exercise-induced asthma
Foreign body aspiration
Granulation tissue in intrathoracic airway
Hypersensitivity pneumonitis
Immotile cilia syndrome

Immune deficiency
Infection
Inflammation of lower airway
Irritant inhalation (smoke, illicit drugs, cocaine)
Lymph nodes (mediastinal, paratracheal)
Mycoplasma
Pertussis
Postinfection
Sarcoidosis
Tumor (carcinoid, lymphoma)
Vascular ring
Vasculitis (Wegener granulomatosis, other)
Virus (adenovirus, respiratory syncytial virus [RSV], human
 metapneumovirus, parainfluenza, influenza)
Vocal cord adduction/dysfunction

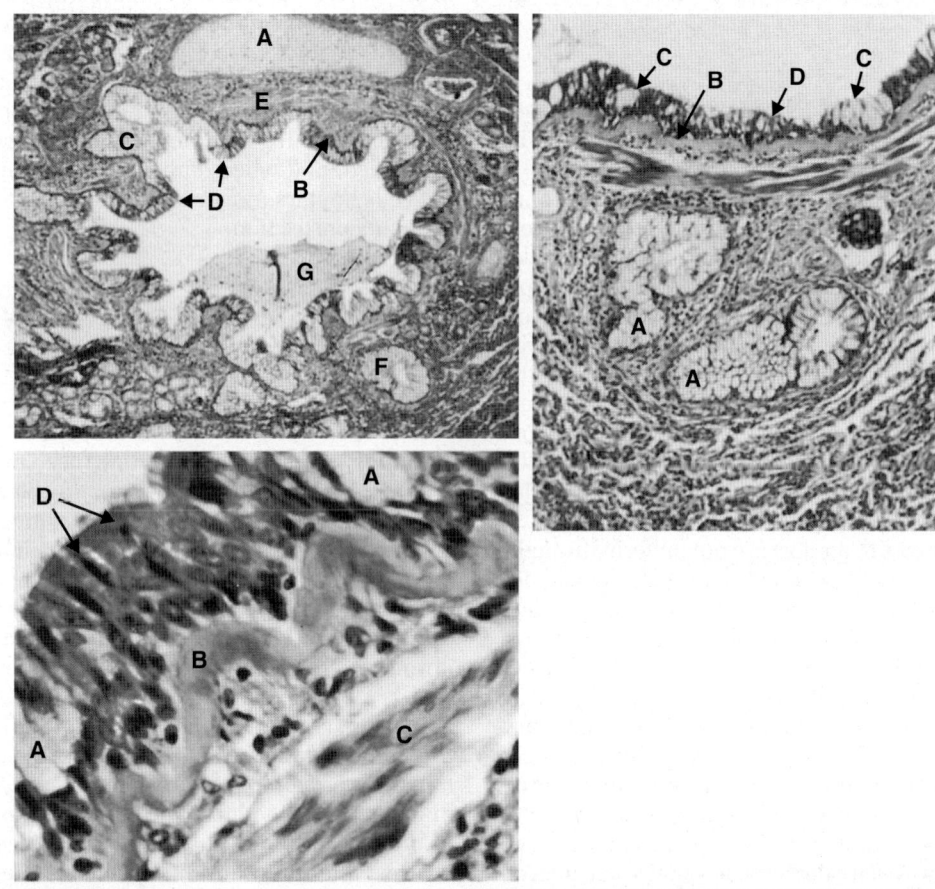

Fig. 45.1 Sections of asthmatic lung. *Top left,* Cross-section of bronchus (original magnification ×66) showing cartilage *(A),* thickened basement membrane *(B),* epithelium containing many goblet cells *(C),* area of many ciliated epithelial cells *(D),* connective tissue *(E),* mucous gland *(F),* and mucous plug *(G). Top right,* Bronchial epithelium (original magnification ×136) showing mucous glands *(A),* hyaline basement membrane *(B),* goblet cells *(C),* and ciliated cells *(D). Bottom left,* Bronchial epithelium (original magnification ×700) showing goblet cell *(A),* basement membrane *(B),* connective tissue *(C),* and ciliated respiratory epithelial cells *(D).*

obstructive pulmonary disease (COPD), the so-called overlap syndrome.[6]

Pathophysiology

Air flow limitation in asthma results from a combination of obstructive processes, principally mucosal edema, bronchospasm, loss of alveolar tethering points, and mucous plugging. The relative roles of these processes in producing obstruction may differ, however, according to the age of the child, the size and anatomy of various portions of the airway, the type of agent precipitating obstruction, and the duration and severity of asthma. An example of acute bronchoconstriction following bronchial lavage with normal saline in a child with asthma can be viewed in the video clip.

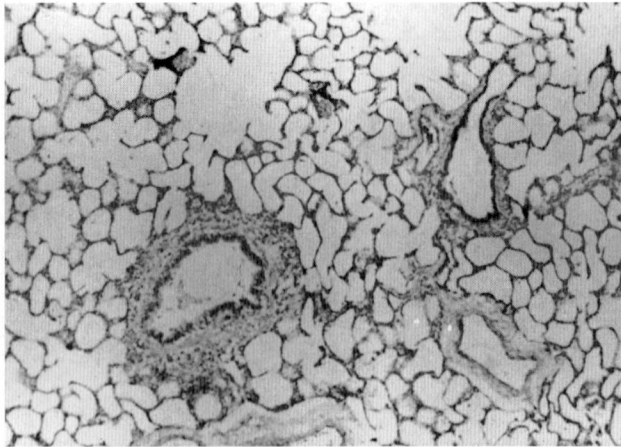

Fig. 45.2 Autopsy specimen from an asthmatic child who died from toxic ingestion. Note the infiltration of cells around the bronchus with sloughing of epithelial cells into the bronchial lumen. The alveoli all appear normal.

Note the furrowing of the bronchial mucosa prior to lavage, which is associated with smooth muscle hypertrophy in the airway (Video 45.1).

Airway obstruction results in increased resistance to air flow through the trachea and bronchi and in decreased flow rates due to narrowing and premature closure of the smaller airways. These changes lead to a decreased ability to expel air and result in hyperinflation. Although pulmonary overdistention benefits respiration by helping to maintain airway patency, the work of breathing increases because of the altered pulmonary mechanics. To a certain extent, increasing lung volumes can compensate for pulmonary obstruction, but compensation is limited as tidal volume approaches the volume of pulmonary dead space, with resultant alveolar hypoventilation.

Changes in resistance to air flow are not uniform throughout the tracheobronchial tree, and because of regional differences in this resistance, the distribution of inspired air is uneven, with more air flowing to the less resistant portions. In most patients with asthma, both larger and smaller airways are obstructed, but some patients may have small airway obstruction primarily, or even exclusively.[7] The pulmonary circulation also is affected by hyperinflation, which induces increased intrapleural and intraalveolar pressures and uneven perfusion of the alveoli. The increased intraalveolar pressure, decreased ventilation, and decreased perfusion (the last through hypoxic vasoconstriction) lead to variable and uneven ventilation-perfusion relationships within different lung units. The ultimate result is early reduction in blood oxygenation, even though carbon dioxide is eliminated effectively because of its ready diffusibility across alveolar capillary membranes. Thus, early in acute asthma, hypoxemia occurs in the absence of CO_2 retention. The hyperventilation resulting from the hypoxemic drive causes a fall in partial pressure of carbon dioxide in alveolar gas ($PaCO_2$). However, as the obstruction becomes more severe and the number of alveoli being adequately ventilated and perfused decreases, a point is reached at which CO_2 retention occurs.

Alterations in pH homeostasis result from respiratory and metabolic factors. Early in the course of acute asthma, respiratory alkalosis may occur because of hyperventilation.

Metabolic acidosis can occur because of the increased work of breathing, increased oxygen consumption, and as a result of excessive β-adrenergic agonist treatment. The metabolic acidosis usually results from lactic acid accumulation, which most commonly occurs as a result of high and frequent doses of β-adrenergic agonist use. In such cases, the acidosis resolves as the β-agonist use is tapered. The mechanism of β-adrenergic agonist induced lactic acid production is somewhat controversial, but most likely results as a consequence of the increased plasma glucose concentration (caused by both beta-agonist and systemic glucocorticoid administration) and its conversion via glycolysis to pyruvate, which is then converted to lactate.[8] When respiratory failure is superimposed, respiratory acidosis may result in a precipitous decrease in pH.

In short attacks of acute asthma, bronchospasm, mucosal edema, or both can occur. In a minority of asthmatics, acute severe episodes are characterized by neutrophilic, not eosinophilic infiltration, and bronchospasm occurs with little mucus secretion. These episodes may have an abrupt onset and cause severe or life-threatening symptoms. Mucous secretions become far more important as a cause of obstruction as the inflammation becomes more intense and prolonged, and when damage to and sloughing of epithelial cells impairs mucociliary function and increases reflex bronchoconstriction.

Inflammatory Cell Biology and Asthma Etiology and Pathophysiology

Although tremendous strides have been made in the cellular and molecular biology of asthma in the past two decades, a complete understanding of the causative factors and those responsible for perpetuating the asthmatic state remain inadequately explained. Current data support the hypothesis that inflammation underlies the pathophysiology of asthma, and the airway epithelium, inflammatory leukocytes, multiple immune cells, and other airway structural cells all play a role.[9,10] The mechanisms producing airway inflammation are legion, cross-talk among various pathways occurs, and the predominant mechanisms responsible for cellular dysfunction vary among asthma phenotypes. The cell–cell communications that initiate and perpetuate asthma likely result from inhaled stimuli such as inhaled allergens, respiratory viruses, and air pollutants (particulate and gaseous) that cause airway epithelial cells to secrete cytokines, interleukins, and other mediators. In turn, these proinflammatory agents act on resident cells in the subepithelial layer, (e.g., dendritic cells, mast cells, and lymphoid cells, including lineage negative innate lymphoid cells) to recruit other leukocytes and the release of Th2 cytokines such as IL-4, IL-5, and IL-13. Biologically active neuropeptides and acetylcholine can also be released from afferent nerves in the epithelium by similar environmental triggers/irritants. The ongoing recruitment of T lymphocytes and release of other mediators, such as IL-17 and IL-33, further enhances the inflammation and dysfunction of the epithelium and airway smooth muscle.

The propensity to develop IgE-mediated sensitization to environmental allergens, particularly in association with rhinovirus infection, coupled with subsequent exposure, is one of the strongest predictors for the development of childhood asthma. The persistence and chronic activation of mast cells, dendritic cells, eosinophils, and lymphocytes in the airways as a result of Th2 cytokine-mediated events (e.g., recruitment of circulating inflammatory cells, interruption of apoptosis) may be important in producing chronic asthma. In addition, innate immune responses modulated by Toll-like receptor recognition and Th17 cells also may be operative in some asthma phenotypes, such as those with more severe disease and neutrophilic predominance in the airways.[11] Impaired production of natural airway defense mediators such as lipoxins, resolvins, and protectins (all important in the active resolution of airway inflammation) may also promote a proinflammatory state in the asthmatic airway. Prolonged or recurrent episodes of inflammation are associated with progressive structural and functional changes in the airway epithelium, musculature, and connective tissue. The continued dysregulation of the cytokine networks perpetuates inflammation in what now may be the structurally altered airways of chronic asthma. Several specific effector mechanisms (e.g., IgE, arachidonic acid metabolites, mast cell proteases, numerous cytokines, thymic stromal lymphopoietin [TSLP], nitric oxide [NO], the β-adrenergic receptor [BAR], growth factors, the airway microbiome, and intrinsic muscular abnormalities) appear to play key roles in airway inflammation and are discussed further in Chapter 7.

Natural History and Prognosis

Knowledge of the natural history of asthma remains incomplete, but several longitudinal studies have added substantial insight. The widespread notion that most children "outgrow" their asthma in adolescence is only partially true. Between 30% and 70% of children with episodic asthma have less severe or absent symptoms by late adolescence, and some features of childhood presentation and course seem to predict clinical outcome. The presence of allergic sensitization, female sex, and severe or persistent asthma in early childhood are predictors of asthma in adulthood. Data from the Melbourne Asthma Study suggested that mild asthma or infrequent wheezing associated with viral infections in childhood was not likely to progress to severe disease in adulthood. In this longitudinal cohort of approximately 500 subjects, data have been collected on the symptoms, growth, and lung function for more than 50 years.[12] Subjects were entered in the study at 7 years of age and were classified as never wheezed (controls), mild wheezy bronchitis, wheezy bronchitis, and asthma; a cohort with more severe asthma was added 3 years later. The loss of lung function seen in the groups with asthma and severe asthma by 10–14 years of age did not worsen over time. The rate of loss of lung function as measured by FEV$_1$ had the same rate of decline up to age 50 in all the groups, even after adjusting for smoking history. Moreover, asthma remission, defined as no symptoms and no medical treatment for 3 years, occurred in 64% of those with intermittent childhood asthma, 47% of those with persistent childhood asthma, and 15% of those with severe childhood asthma. Data from the Childhood Asthma Management Program (CAMP) also indicate that outcomes in children initially diagnosed with moderate asthma vary and are predicted by certain features.[13] During a 7- to 10-year follow-up period of 909 children initially enrolled in a 4-year-long clinical trial of placebo versus budesonide (BUD) versus nedocromil, 6% remitted, 39% had periodic asthma, and 55% had persistent disease. Prestudy factors associated with disease remission included lack of allergen sensitivity and exposure to indoor allergens, milder asthma, older age, less airway responsiveness (methacholine PC$_{20}$), and higher prebronchodilator FEV$_1$. Moreover, there was no effect on disease outcome by treatment. These results also highlight the lack of current antiinflammatory treatments' ability to alter disease natural history.

Studies of children with asthma based both on history and on assessment of pulmonary function indicate that many children who lose overt symptoms have persistent airway obstruction. Nonspecific airway hyperreactivity associated with asthma is present in formerly asthmatic patients who are free from clinical asthma.[14] Individuals who had asthma as children have a significantly lower FEV$_1$, more airway reactivity, and more frequent persistence of symptoms than those with infection-induced wheezing or the controls. In addition, 88% of the adults with childhood asthma who had persistent symptoms had positive methacholine challenge test results, as did 42% of the asymptomatic former asthmatics. The recurrence of overt asthma after years of freedom from symptoms is not unusual. Thus asthma is often a lifelong disease with periodic exacerbations and remissions, although laboratory evidence of decreased pulmonary function, airway inflammation, and airway hyperresponsiveness may persist, even when symptoms are quiescent.

In children and adolescents, asthma is frequently a completely reversible obstructive airways disease, and indeed no abnormalities in pulmonary functions can be detected in many asthmatic patients when they become symptom-free. However, recent studies that examine not only symptoms and pulmonary function but also indices of airway inflammation and bronchial hyperresponsiveness suggest that airway inflammation may persist in the absence of symptoms. In a study of 54 young adults (18–25 years of age) with atopic asthma or asthma in clinical remission (absence of symptoms for at least 12 months, median duration 5 years), subjects in remission were found to have evidence of airway inflammation and remodeling.[14] When compared with normal healthy controls, the subjects in remission had increased epithelial and subepithelial major basic protein and reticular basement membrane thickness; values were close to those of subjects with active asthma. Peripheral eosinophil counts were also elevated in the remission patients, and there was a significant correlation between basement membrane thickness, exhaled NO, and hyperresponsiveness to adenosine monophosphate. These findings indicate that the airways of some asymptomatic asthmatics, seemingly in clinical remission, may still show significant abnormalities and evidence of active inflammation. It is unclear that continued treatment in the face of absent symptoms will alter the natural history of the disease in these patients.

Asthma does appear to progress to chronic obstructive disease in some individuals, and features of asthma can be found in some adult patients with COPD (the so-called overlap syndrome).[6] The functional and structural causes of this irreversible airway obstruction variant of asthma are not understood. A process referred to as *airway remodeling* is often suggested as the cause of chronic obstruction and severe asthma, but data to conclusively support this hypothesis are lacking. It is believed that chronic mucous plugging, tracheobronchial ciliary dysfunction, smooth muscle and goblet cell hyperplasia, and collagen deposition in the lamina reticularis of the basement membrane occur as a consequence of persistent inflammation. Genetically determined dysregulation of inflammatory mediator production with or without repeated exposure to certain environmental stimuli may also play a role. Data from animal models demonstrate that even when inflammation is suppressed and changes consistent with remodeling are reduced markedly, airway hyperresponsiveness persists.[15] These data suggest that airway remodeling alone is probably not responsible for severe, irreversible airway obstruction or bronchial hyperresponsiveness.

The natural history of childhood asthma and the effects of aggressive long-term management on outcomes remain incompletely understood, but a great deal of data have come from the CAMP study.[16] CAMP was a well-designed comprehensive longitudinal study in which the primary objective was to compare the effects of long-term treatment (4 years) with an inhaled steroid (BUD) and a nonsteroidal treatment (nedocromil) to placebo in school-age children ($n = 1041$) with mild to moderate asthma. The hypothesis was that treatment with an inhaled steroid would result in better lung growth compared with no or lesser treatment. Primary outcome was postbronchodilator FEV_1, but a wealth of other data on atopy, airway reactivity, symptoms, exacerbations, and linear growth was obtained. After a brief improvement in FEV_1 in the BUD group, there was no difference in FEV_1 between the groups over the last 3 years of the study. However, patients in the BUD group had decreased hospitalizations and urgent care visits compared with the placebo group. Patients in the nedocromil group also had fewer emergency visits but not hospitalizations, and both groups had less oral prednisone use. There was a small, transient decrease in growth velocity in the BUD group compared with the placebo and nedocromil groups. These data suggest that long-term treatment with inhaled steroids in school-aged asthmatics does not alter pulmonary function over time, even though the symptom control and airway reactivity improved. Failure to alter the natural history of asthma, as measured by lung function, in the CAMP study was thought in part to be caused by beginning treatment too late after the onset of disease. However, subsequent studies of inhaled steroid treatment (Fluticasone 88 μg twice a day) in younger children (2–3 years of age) who had recurrent wheezing and were at very high risk for developing asthma showed improvement in clinical symptoms and exacerbations compared with those receiving placebo. However, the treatment did not prevent clinical symptoms or alteration in lung function (measured by impulse oscillometry) in the subsequent year when treatment was stopped.[17] These data again indicate the inability of inhaled corticosteroids (ICSs) to modify the long-term disease state.

Asthma Mortality

Despite the relatively high prevalence of asthma, mortality rates for childhood asthma are extremely low and have stabilized and actually decreased over the past decade.[2] This is evident when adjusting outcome metrics for the population at risk rather than the overall population.[18] Overall, fewer than 4000 individuals (of whom fewer than 150 are children) die of asthma in the United States each year. However, death rates are significantly higher in African Americans of all ages. Analyses of causes of death in children with asthma suggest that the major causes are the failure of the physician, parent, or patient to appreciate the severity of asthma, which results in inadequate or delayed treatment, poor access to health care, and the use of inappropriate medications (e.g., overreliance on β-adrenergic agonists and avoidance of use of corticosteroids). In fact, recent data from Costa Rica demonstrated that a 129% increase in the prescription of ICSs over a 7-year period was associated with an approximately 80% reduction in deaths due to asthma.[19] Labile asthma, regardless of severity, is also a risk factor, as are respiratory infections, nocturnal asthma, history of respiratory failure, and marked diurnal variation in air flow limitation. Some patients cannot perceive severe air flow obstruction, especially when it occurs gradually, and a small number may have sudden profound bronchospasm, which can be fatal. Other factors, such as exposure to allergens (mold), psychosocial disadvantage, poverty, previous episodes of respiratory failure, history of hypoxic seizure, previous admission to an intensive care unit, and psychological factors in both the patient and family have been implicated in deaths from asthma.

Diagnosis of Asthma

An asthma diagnosis requires demonstration of episodic symptoms of air flow obstruction, which must be at least partially reversible, and alternative diagnoses should be excluded. Although airway hyperresponsiveness is an almost universal feature of asthma, it is not unique and therefore cannot be used as a defining characteristic. The methods to establish the diagnosis include a detailed medical history, a physical examination with a focus on the respiratory system, and performance of spirometry in children who are 5 years of age or older. A number of ancillary tests (e.g., allergy skin tests, inhalation or exercise challenge tests, home peak flow monitoring) may also be useful and, in some cases, necessary.

Although patients with asthma may present in a variety of ways, most have certain common historical features, such as intermittent or recurrent wheezing, an expiratory, musical, high-pitched, whistling sound produced by air flow turbulence in the large airways below the thoracic inlet. Many parents and even older children cannot accurately describe wheezing and may actually report stridor (from upper airway obstruction), stertor, snoring, or rhonchorous breathing. Careful explanation or even demonstration of wheezing is often necessary to obtain an accurate history. Wheezing can also be generated by adduction of the vocal cords and forceful inspiration and expiration. Inspiratory wheezing per se is not characteristic of asthma and suggests obstruction in the laryngeal area, such as that induced by croup or vocal cord dysfunction (VCD). However, wheezing also occurs during inspiration when asthma worsens and may disappear altogether as obstruction becomes more severe and air flow is limited. Asthma can occur without wheezing if the obstruction involves predominantly the small airways. Coughing or shortness of breath may be the only complaint. However, so-called cough-variant asthma may be overdiagnosed. Probably no more than 5% of asthmatic children have cough as the only or primary symptom, and the cough should resolve with appropriate asthma medications and recur when the medications are stopped. Older children often complain of a "tight" chest with colds, recurrent "chest congestion," or bronchitis. Usually, symptoms are more severe at night or in the early morning and improve throughout the day. A history of symptomatic improvement after treatment with a bronchodilator suggests the diagnosis of asthma, but a failure of response does not rule out asthma. When asymptomatic, many asthmatic children will have normal lung function (FEV_1). Reduction of the FEV_1/FVC is considered to be a more reliable indicator of airway obstruction in children. An inhalation challenge test (e.g., methacholine or mannitol) should be performed when asthma is suspected but spirometry is normal or near-normal.

Family history is often positive for asthma or allergy (allergic rhinitis, eczema) in a first-degree relative. A history of personal allergy is found in more than two-thirds of children with asthma.

PHYSICAL EXAMINATION

The physical examination should focus on overall growth and development; the condition of the entire respiratory tract including the upper airway, ears, and paranasal sinuses as well as the chest; and other associated signs of allergic disease. Although severe asthma can adversely affect linear growth, this is not a common feature, and its presence should suggest evaluating for alternative causes of growth failure.

Unless acutely ill, examination of the lungs is frequently normal in children who are ultimately diagnosed with asthma. In some cases, particularly during periods with acute symptoms, auscultation reveals coarse crackles or unequal breath sounds, which may clear at least partly with coughing. If they persist, particularly during clinical stability, the possibility of another diagnosis should be considered. Although wheezing can often be elicited with a forced expiratory maneuver, occasionally there is only prolongation of expiration without wheezing. The older child or adolescent may resist exhaling forcefully to induce latent wheezes, because such a maneuver may induce coughing, which can increase bronchospasm. Some patients with severe asthma do not wheeze because too little air is moving to generate the sound. Wheezing from the lower respiratory tract should be differentiated from similar sounds that can emanate from the laryngeal area in even nonasthmatic children with sufficient forced expiration.

A variety of extrapulmonary signs indicating the presence of complicating factors or alternative diagnoses (e.g., allergy or cystic fibrosis) should be sought in all children being evaluated for asthma. Nasal polyps occur rarely in the child with uncomplicated asthma, and their presence suggests cystic fibrosis. However, nasal polyps can occur in highly allergic adolescents or those with aspirin sensitive asthma. Digital clubbing is not a feature of asthma; although clubbing may be a nonpathologic familial trait, its presence suggests cystic fibrosis, congenital heart disease, inflammatory bowel disease, or another chronic lung disorder. The conjunctivae should be examined for edema, inflammation, and tearing, suggesting allergy. Flexor creases and other areas of the skin should be examined for active or healed atopic dermatitis.

Hyperventilation and VCD syndrome should be considered in the differential diagnosis of the child with asthma that is apparently refractory to all therapy, especially if there are no symptoms during sleep. Both conditions are more likely to occur in adolescence or later childhood and may be mistaken for asthma, or may coexist with it. Typically the patient with hyperventilation is anxious and complains of marked dyspnea and difficulty getting enough air to breathe in spite of excellent air exchange on auscultation and an absence of wheezing. Often there are associated complaints of headache and tingling of the fingers and toes. Pulmonary function tests (PFTs) are helpful in differentiating hyperventilation syndrome from asthma; a normal spirogram during or around the time of symptoms is inconsistent with asthma. Immediate therapy consists of giving reassurance and having the patient rebreathe into a paper bag to elevate $PaCO_2$. VCD is another condition that must be differentiated from true asthma.[20] In these patients, wheezing is often a prominent feature, may occur on inspiration and expiration, and is typically loudest over the trachea or central, anterior chest. This condition is more common in older children, adolescents, and females, and it may also be seen in elite athletes. Most patients with VCD cannot voluntarily induce an episode, although in many patients, including highly trained athletes, exercise can precipitate an attack.[20,21] Although VCD was originally described in adults with psychiatric disorders, in children it is not usually associated with serious psychological disturbances and should not be labeled as such. The etiology in children remains poorly understood. The mechanism involves holding the anterior third of the vocal cords in a position of relative adduction during inspiration, but also in expiration. There may also be inward deflection of the supraglottic structures as well; this condition is sometimes called exercise-induced laryngomalacia (EILO). A recent study suggested that EILO in adolescence may be related to a diagnosis of clinically significant congenital laryngomalacia in infancy.[22] The result is loud, monophonic wheezing in a patient who has normal oxygen saturation and responds poorly to inhalation of a bronchodilating aerosol. Patients may appear comfortable or anxious in the face of loud wheeze. Pulmonary function testing may reveal a pronounced flattening of the inspiratory loop; however, since some patients with VCD also have true asthma, there may be evidence of large and/or small airway obstruction on the expiratory loop as well (Fig. 45.3). An increase in the mid–vital capacity expiratory/inspiratory flow ratio from the normal value of about 0.9 to a value of greater than 2 indicates extrathoracic obstruction consistent with VCD. It should be noted that most patients with VCD will have normal pulmonary function testing when asymptomatic. The diagnosis is confirmed by direct observation of paradoxical vocal cord movement via flexible laryngoscopy during an acute episode. Upper and lower airway examination with a flexible bronchoscope should be considered in patients with atypical reports of wheeze, dyspnea on exertion, or stridor to identify anatomic lesions such as cysts, hemangiomas, or laryngotracheomalacia. Older children with both VCD and asthma often can distinguish the "site" of the wheezing when the source of the problem is explained to them. The absence of nocturnal

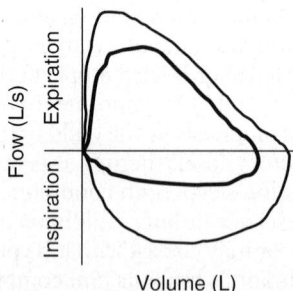

Fig. 45.3 Flow-volume curve from a patient with vocal cord dysfunction. The thin line represents the flow at normal baseline. The thick line represents the flow during an obstructive episode and depicts a slight decrease in expiratory flow and a marked decrease in and flattening of the inspiratory loop.

symptoms may also be a diagnostic clue that VCD is the diagnosis rather than asthma. Effective treatment consists of appropriate asthma medication (when an asthma diagnosis has been confirmed), treatment of aggravating conditions (reflux, rhinitis), and referral to a speech therapist or psychologist specializing in behavior modification in order to learn relaxation techniques and alternative breathing strategies. The vast majority of patients will improve with this treatment.

ASTHMA TRIGGERS

Many older children will identify more than one precipitating factor responsible for asthma. Moreover, patterns of reactivity may change. Thus exercise-induced asthma (EIA) may not be viewed as a problem in many adolescents or adults with asthma who have learned in childhood that exercise induces symptoms and have developed a lifestyle that avoids exercise. Allergic factors that precipitated asthma in childhood may no longer cause symptoms in adolescence or adulthood, even though the patient continues to have asthma. Patterns also may change with treatment or the institution of environmental control measures. The use of quality-of-life questionnaires can help uncover latent symptoms and provide information that may be useful in identifying more subtle triggers.

ALLERGENS

In the majority of children with asthma, it is possible to induce an asthmatic reaction to substances in which IgE-mediated reaction is involved. Allergens that can induce asthma symptoms include animal allergens, mold spores, pollens, insects (cockroach), infectious agents (especially Mycoplasma and fungi), and occasionally drugs and foods. Cockroach and rodent allergens appear to be potent factors, particularly in inner-city children, and have been associated with increased health care utilization in children who are both sensitized and exposed to the allergens.[23] Allergic reactions may induce bronchoconstriction directly, may increase tracheobronchial sensitivity in general, and may be obvious or subtle precipitating factors. Bronchoconstrictor responses to allergens via IgE antibody–induced mediator release from mast cells generally occur within minutes of exposure, last for a relatively short period of time (20–30 minutes), and

resolve. Such reactions are termed *early antigen* or *asthmatic responses.* It is the "late asthmatic response" (which occurs 4–24 hours after antigen contact) that results in more severe and protracted symptoms (lasting hours) and ultimately contributes to the chronicity and severity of the disease. The late response is due to inflammatory cell reactions and the release of multiple mediators, including IL-4, IL-5, and IL-13. Such allergen-induced dual responses can only be demonstrated in approximately half of all asthmatics challenged in a laboratory setting.

IRRITANTS

Numerous upper and lower respiratory tract irritants have been implicated as precipitants of asthma. These include paint odors, hairsprays, perfumes, chemicals, air pollutants, diesel particulates, tobacco smoke, cold air, cold water, and cough. Some allergens may also act as irritants (e.g., molds). Some irritants such as ozone and industrial chemicals may initiate bronchial hyperresponsiveness by inducing inflammation, yet they do not produce a late-phase response. Active and passive exposure to tobacco smoke, in addition to acting as a precipitant and aggravator of asthma, can also be associated with an accelerated irreversible loss of pulmonary function.

WEATHER CHANGES

Atmospheric changes are commonly associated with an increase in asthmatic activity. The mechanism of this effect has not been defined but may be related to changes in barometric pressure and alterations in the allergen or irritant content of the air. Grass pollen, which in its native state is too large to enter the lower airways, fractionates into numerous small starch granules bearing allergen when exposed to water, such as during storms. These small particles, along with fungal spores (*Alternaria* or *Cladisporium*) and PM 2.5 particles readily enter the lower airways and can trigger severe acute asthma in susceptible individuals; the risk is particularly high when grass pollen counts exceed 20–50 grains/m^3. A recent outbreak of asthma deaths in Melbourne, Australia, following thunderstorms during periods of high grass pollen counts was attributed to this mechanism.[23a,23b]

INFECTIONS

By far, the most common infectious agents responsible for precipitating or aggravating asthma are viral respiratory pathogens. It is estimated that up to 85% of asthma exacerbations in school-aged children are due to viral infections, and rhinovirus has emerged as a prominent pathogen in causing acute asthma.[24] Among the three serotypes of rhinovirus, infection with hRV-C is more likely to be associated with acute asthma exacerbations than infection with hRV-A or hRV-B. In addition, there is some evidence that rhinovirus, detected in nasal lavage, can cause an increase in daily asthma symptoms apart from significant exacerbations.[25] In some instances, bacterial infections (e.g., pertussis or mycoplasma) and, more rarely, fungal infections or colonization (e.g., bronchopulmonary *Aspergillosis*) and parasitic infestations (e.g., *Toxocariasis* and *Ascariasis*) can be triggers. The mechanisms of viral-induced exacerbations are incompletely understood, but probably involve some direct respiratory epithelial injury caused by infection, alteration of host inflammatory responses driven by the infection, and influence of other cofactors (concomitant allergen exposure or mediator production). For instance, it is clear that children who have significant respiratory viral–induced wheezing are more likely to have elevated IgE and allergen sensitization.[26] In addition, asthmatics may have decreased production of interferons type I, II, and III, which can be associated with decreased airway function.

EXERCISE

Strenuous exercise (i.e., exercise sufficient to cause breathlessness and hyperventilation) may induce bronchial obstruction in as many as 90% of individuals with persistent asthma; this phenomenon is termed *exercise-induced bronchospasm (EIB)*. In addition, exercise can cause significant bronchospasm in up to 40% of individuals with allergic rhinitis who do not have persistent asthma. When otherwise normal individuals develop bronchoconstriction in response to exercise with hyperventilation, it is often termed *EIA;* this may occur in 10%–13% of the general population. Symptoms induced by exercise range from subtle (mild dyspnea) to significant coughing, wheezing, and excessive breathlessness. Symptoms typically begin after 5–10 minutes of vigorous activity and are most prominent after activity ceases (by contrast with VCD/EILO, in which symptoms come on during exercise). The mechanisms underlying EIA remain somewhat uncertain. Recent data indicate that hyperventilation of cold, dry air causes heat and water loss from the airways, producing a hyperosmolar lining fluid and injuring the airway epithelium. Induced sputum obtained from individuals with EIB demonstrates columnar epithelial cells, eosinophils, and increased concentrations of leukotrienes. There is also cytokine release from neutrophils.[27] Cooling of the airways has also been described to result in vascular congestion and dilatation in the bronchial circulation. The subsequent mucosal swelling as a result of vascular congestion and edema produces airway narrowing. Symptoms of EIB usually resolve spontaneously within 1 hour after ceasing exercise, but may require treatment with a short-acting β agonist (SABA) for complete resolution. There is typically a refractory period of 1–3 hours following an episode of EIA/EIB, during which further exercise will not cause significant bronchospasm. Although studies are conflicting, there is generally not a late-onset response (8–12 hours postexercise) following the immediate reaction. A recent study of a cohort of Swedish adolescents, aged 13–15 years, who underwent exercise challenge tests and continuous exercise laryngoscopy testing showed that the prevalence of EIB was 19.2%, the prevalence of EILO was 5.7%, and 5% had both conditions. Of note, 49.4% of those who complained of exercise-induced dyspnea had neither condition.[28] EIA may be both underdiagnosed when symptoms are subtle, or it may be overdiagnosed or misdiagnosed due to a number of masquerading conditions (e.g., VCD, EILO, poor conditioning, or cardiac dysfunction).

EMOTIONAL FACTORS

Emotional upsets clearly trigger asthma in some individuals; however, there is no evidence that psychological factors are the basis for asthma. Coping styles of patients, their families, and their physicians can intensify or lead to more rapid amelioration of asthma. Conversely, denial of asthma by patients, parents, or physicians may delay therapy to the point that reversibility of obstruction is more difficult. Psychological factors have been implicated in deaths from asthma in children. The influence of psychosocial factors on compliance is yet another important factor related to treatment failure or success. Asthma itself can strongly influence the emotional state of the patient, the family, and other individuals associated with the patient. In addition, some studies indicate that psychosocial stressors, both internal (lack of parental support) and external (witnessing violence), may modulate immune responses, increase inflammation, or decrease steroid responsiveness, leading to poorer asthma control.[29,30]

GASTROESOPHAGEAL REFLUX

Reflux of gastric contents into the tracheobronchial tree can aggravate asthma in children and is one of the causes of nocturnal asthma. Typical symptoms of gastroesophageal reflux (GER)—heartburn, chest pain, regurgitation, sour brash—may be absent in many children with asthma; estimates are that reflux may be "silent" in more than 50% of asthmatic patients. Pediatric studies have reported a prevalence of GER between 19% and 80%, with a mean of about 22%.[31] However, due to methodological flaws and absence of longitudinal studies, a clear association between GER and asthma symptoms in children remains unclear. Although the exact extent to which reflux exacerbates asthma remains controversial, it is clear that acid (or even nonacid) reflux of gastric contents into the distal esophagus can lead to cough and bronchospasm, presumably via increased vagal activity. Aspiration of gastric contents in even micro amounts is also presumed to cause bronchial irritation and bronchospasm. Data from a large double-blind clinical trial in children did not show benefit to improving any aspect of asthma control with treatment with proton pump inhibitor (PPI) in asthmatic patients who did not have symptoms of GER.[32] In addition, the data support possible adverse effects in the form of increased respiratory infections and symptoms in some children with asthma treated with lansoprazole.[33]

ALLERGIC RHINITIS AND SINUSITIS

Acute or chronic sinusitis can be associated with aggravation of asthma and can be a cause of recalcitrant asthma. In some patients, asthma and sinusitis occur at the same time; the nasal symptoms from the sinusitis may make cough and other symptoms of asthma worse and less responsive to bronchodilator therapy alone. The upper airway may be viewed to some extent as a continuum of the lower airway; inflammatory mediator release in the lower airway may be triggered as a response to sinus infection. This subject is discussed in more detail in Chapter 47.

Nonallergic Hypersensitivity to Drugs and Chemicals

Aspirin and nonsteroidal antiinflammatory drugs (NSAIDs), such as ibuprofen, can exacerbate asthma in selected individuals by increasing production of 5-lipoxygenase metabolites, including leukotrienes. The typical aspirin-sensitive asthmatic has nasal polyps, urticaria, and chronic rhinitis. Aspirin ingestion may diminish pulmonary function and produce wheeze, cough, rhinitis, conjunctivitis, urticaria, and angioedema in 10%–20% of adults with asthma.[34] Although more common after the third decade of life, the prevalence in children (as determined by a decrease in FEV_1 of at least 20% from baseline following aspirin or NSAID ingestion) has been reported to be as high as 5% when determined by direct challenge testing. Although aspirin in particular is rarely given to children and adolescents because of the risk of Reye syndrome, there is a very high cross-reactivity to common NSAIDs in aspirin-susceptible patients. High-dose acetaminophen may also cause wheezing in a small portion (<2%) of aspirin-sensitive asthmatics. Some (but not all) studies suggest that early-life use of acetaminophen may increase the risk of developing asthma, and one large trial found a reduced risk of an acute care visit for asthma following treatment with ibuprofen compared with treatment with acetaminophen.[35] However, the data are more compelling for prenatal exposure to acetaminophen and development of asthma. Moreover, some studies are "confounded by indication," and when adjusted for the incidence of respiratory tract infection, the risk of developing asthma is greatly attenuated.[35,36] The absence of a history of increased symptoms following NSAID ingestion in asthmatic children is generally sufficient to warrant safe use of NSAIDs as needed. A recent trial comparing acetaminophen use with ibuprofen in children aged 1–5 years found no difference in the incidence of asthma exacerbations.[37] However, aspirin/NSAID sensitivity should be considered in children and adolescents with severe or difficult-to-control asthma, who also have chronic rhinitis, urticaria, and nasal polyps.

Metabisulfite has been reported as a precipitant or aggravator of asthma, both by allergic and nonallergic mechanisms. Sensitive individuals should avoid foods containing or preserved using sulfites (e.g., shrimp, dried fruit, beer, and wine).

ENDOCRINE FACTORS

Aggravation of asthma and increased pulmonary function variability occurs in some adolescent and adult women in relation to the menstrual cycle, beginning shortly before menstruation and ending shortly after the onset of menses.[38] Whether this reflects changes in water and salt balance, irritability of bronchial smooth muscle, or other factors is unknown. The use of the oral contraceptive pill has been reported to both aggravate and ameliorate premenstrual asthma. Hyperthyroidism has been reported to worsen or precipitate asthma in an occasional patient, and treatment of hyperthyroidism usually ameliorates the asthma.

Vitamin D deficiency has gained increasing attention as a possible contributor to both the development of asthma and a contributor to its control. Data from the National Health and Nutrition Examination Survey (NHANES) study indicated a direct relationship between serum vitamin D concentration and FEV_1/FVC. In addition, several studies demonstrate lower vitamin D levels in African Americans, Hispanics, and obese individuals, all groups with increased risk for higher asthma morbidity. Among asthmatic children, vitamin D insufficiency

(defined as serum concentration ≤30 ng/mL) occurs in approximately one-third of those studied.[39] Among 1024 participants in the CAMP study, 35% were vitamin D insufficient at study entry. This group had an increased risk of severe asthma exacerbation (OR 1.5, 1.1–1.9, $P = .01$) during the 4 years of the study, after adjusting for numerous factors (i.e., age, sex, body mass index [BMI], and treatment group). Those in the BUD treatment group had an even greater effect (OR 1.8, 1.0–3.2, $P = .05$). These results are similar to those described for a cohort study ($n = 616$) of asthmatic Costa Rican children, 28% of whom were vitamin D insufficient. Serum vitamin D was inversely associated with serum IgE and peripheral eosinophil count. In addition, higher vitamin D levels were associated with a significant decrease in risk of hospitalization in the previous year, a decrease in the use of antiinflammatory medicines, and borderline decreased airway hyperresponsiveness. The mechanisms by which vitamin D influences asthma expression remain unclear, but there are many possibilities. Vitamin D suppresses bronchial smooth muscle mass and goblet cell hyperplasia, and serum concentrations are inversely associated with the frequency of viral respiratory infections. Vitamin D treatment of T reg cells from steroid-resistant asthmatics resulted in increased production of the antiinflammatory cytokine IL-10 with steroid stimulation and also reduced IgE production from human peripheral B cells.[40] Moreover, it has also been speculated that polymorphisms in the vitamin D receptor play a role in asthma, but data are inconsistent. Several clinical trials to demonstrate efficacy of vitamin D in asthma treatment have been performed in children and adults. In a study of vitamin D_3 supplementation in adults with persistent asthma vitamin D insufficiency, the rate of first treatment failure or exacerbation was not reduced.[41] Data in children are more mixed, with some studies showing modest effect on exacerbation reduction but little effect on other clinical outcomes.[42] Further research is needed to substantiate the role of vitamin D in asthma pathophysiology.

NOCTURNAL ASTHMA

There is a circadian variation in airway function and bronchial hyperresponsiveness in most patients with asthma. In individuals with a normal sleep-wake cycle, the worst peak expiratory flow rate (PEFR) and the most pronounced reactivity occur at approximately 4 a.m., and the best occur at 4 p.m. Nocturnal asthma is a risk factor for asthma severity and even death in some asthmatics. Although nocturnal asthma may result from late-phase reactions to earlier allergen exposure, GER, or sinusitis in some patients, these conditions are not present in most patients with severe nocturnal asthma. Another explanation is an increase in inflammatory cell infiltrate as an exaggerated normal circadian variation. Abnormalities in central nervous system control of respiratory drive, particularly with defective hypoxic drive and obstructive sleep apnea, as well as physiologic increases in airway parasympathetic tone, reduction in lung volume, and airway smooth muscle unloading may also be present in some patients with nocturnal asthma. Recent work suggests that those with African ancestry who are obese and have lower lung function may be at increased risk for nocturnal asthma and reported a twofold increase compared to European Caucasian counterparts.[43]

Laboratory Diagnosis

A number of laboratory studies may be useful in confirming the diagnosis of asthma, and objective measures of pulmonary function are among the most important.

Lung Function Tests

PFTs, particularly spirometry, are objective, noninvasive, and extremely helpful in the diagnosis and follow-up of patients with asthma. Examination of the forced vital capacity (FVC), FEV_1, and forced expiratory flow rate over 25%–75% of the FVC (FEF_{25-75}) is a reliable way to detect baseline airway obstruction. Examination of the volume-time curve and shape of the flow-volume loop provides an estimate of the adequacy of the patient effort in performing the test. A PFT should be attempted on all children older than 5 years of age when considering the diagnosis of asthma. However, there is some controversy regarding the value of repeated measures of lung function compared with symptom report in improving asthma outcomes.[44] Nevertheless, attempting to achieve and maintain normal or near normal lung function is a goal for all asthmatic children.

In children, measurement of FEV_1 alone may miss airway obstruction; the FEV_1/FVC has been proposed as a more sensitive measure of obstruction. FEF_{25-75} has been proposed as a more sensitive indicator of airway obstruction, in the small airways in particular, and a better indicator of a response to bronchodilators and airway hyperresponsiveness than either FEV_1 or FVC. However, recent data indicate that this information is not entirely accurate. The FEF_{25-75} is a highly variable measure that is readily influenced by expiratory time and change in FVC. Examination of large data sets including children with asthma and cystic fibrosis indicates that less than 3% of the test results showed a reduced $FEF_{25-75}\%$ with both FEV_1/FVC and FVC within the normal range.[45] Documentation of reversibility of air flow obstruction following inhalation of a bronchodilator is central to the definition of asthma. If obstruction is demonstrated on a baseline PFT, a bronchodilating aerosol (albuterol) should be administered and the PFT repeated in 10–20 minutes. An improvement of at least 12% and 200 mL in the FEV_1 is considered a positive response and is indicative of reversible air flow obstruction; however, in children, an improvement of 10% may be adequate to indicate significant improvement. A 10% improvement in the percent predicted FEV_1 is also considered a positive response.

Use of a peak flow meter in the office setting may provide some useful information about obstruction in the large central airways, but the test should not be used to diagnose asthma. PEFR is extremely effort-dependent and is only reflective of obstruction in the large central airways.

Although standard spirometry has long been considered the gold standard for use in diagnosing and monitoring change in airway function in patients with asthma, other modalities may have particular application in both younger and older children. Forced oscillation capitalizes on the resonant oscillation properties of the airways to measure conductance and reactance and, indirectly, airway resistance.[46] The technique requires only tidal breathing on a mouthpiece for 30 seconds in order to obtain a measurement; response

to a bronchodilator can also be detected. In some studies, area of reactance (AX) as measured by forced oscillation was able to discriminate those with asthma, even when FEV_1 was not different between the two groups.[47] Widespread adoption of forced oscillation techniques has not occurred largely due to lack of reliable normative values.

Bronchial Challenge Tests

Airway hyperreactivity to substances such as methacholine, histamine, hypertonic saline, adenosine monophosphate, or mannitol forms the basis of an adjunctive diagnostic test for asthma (Video 45.2). However, the sensitivity and specificity of the tests vary widely, and bronchoprovocation testing cannot serve as the sole determinant of an asthma diagnosis. Methacholine and histamine are considered direct bronchoprovocation agents because they act directly on smooth muscle. Direct bronchoprovocation challenge testing with methacholine is very sensitive and has a better negative than positive predictive value. As such, it is generally more helpful in excluding than diagnosing asthma because positive results may be seen in disorders such as cystic fibrosis, COPD, chronic bronchitis, allergic rhinitis, and even in some normal individuals. FEV_1 is the primary measure used to assess response, and the concentration of methacholine at which a 20% decrease in FEV_1 occurs is recorded (PC_{20}); other methods use the cumulative dose (PD_{20}). A PC_{20} of ≤ 4 mg/mL is considered a positive test result indicative of airway hyperreactivity. However, there is no universally accepted threshold PC_{20} value that is considered diagnostic of asthma (Table 45.1). Accurate interpretation must account for degree of baseline obstruction (if any), the pretest probability of asthma, the presence of current symptoms, and the degree of recovery in postchallenge FEV_1. Mild transient adverse effects (i.e., cough, wheezing, chest tightness, and dizziness) are uncommon and occur in less than 20% of patients receiving either histamine or methacholine challenge. Delayed or prolonged reactions are extremely rare, and fatalities after methacholine have not been reported. However, methacholine (or any bronchoprovocation test) should not be performed if the baseline FEV_1 is low (generally less than 60% predicted).[48]

Indirect bronchoprovocation agents (i.e., hypertonic saline, adenosine monophosphate [AMP], mannitol) act by inducing release of inflammatory mediators in the airway, which then cause bronchoconstriction. In addition, indirect testing is well correlated with the degree of airway inflammation. Inhalation testing with dry-powder mannitol has good validity, and a commercial kit is approved for use in Europe, Australia, and

Table 45.1 Interpretation of Methacholine Challenge Test Results

PC_{20} (mg/mL)	Suggested Interpretation
<1.0	Moderate to severe reactivity (asthma likely)
1–4	Mild reactivity
4–16	Borderline reactivity
>16	Normal (no significant reactivity; asthma unlikely)

Assumes that there is no baseline airway obstruction and that postchallenge improvement to baseline forced expiratory volume in 1 second occurs.

the United States. Mannitol has the advantage of being safe and easy, and it requires no special equipment apart from a spirometer. A cut point of 15% decrease in FEV_1 from baseline had a specificity of 98% but a sensitivity of only 58%.[49] Other agents such as allergens and occupational sensitizers have been used for inhalation challenge tests, but such challenges may pose significant risk and should only be performed by experienced physicians and investigators in the context of specific clinical or research settings. Indeed, bronchial challenge tests with any inhaled agents should only be performed in certified pulmonary function laboratories under the direct supervision of a trained specialist.

Exercise Challenge Test

In individuals 6 years of age through adulthood, a treadmill or bicycle ergometer exercise test provides useful information about the presence of EIB or EIA. In children with histories suggestive of EIB, an exercise challenge test is a more useful diagnostic aid than a methacholine challenge test (Video 45.3). The inhaled air should be dry, and the child should exercise at maximal level for 4–6 minutes and for a total time of 6–8 minutes. Maximal exercise is usually determined by heart rate (80%–90% of age maximum) or maximum voluntary ventilation ($FEV_1 \times 35$); the target should be reached relatively quickly. Pulmonary function should be measured 5 minutes before exercise. Following exercise, serial pulmonary function measurements should be obtained for at least 20 minutes (at 5, 10, and 20 minutes postexercise) to determine the presence and severity of EIA. A decrease in FEV_1 of more than 10% is diagnostic of exercise-induced bronchoconstriction; some sources suggest a threshold of 15% decrease.[48]

Other Tests

COMPLETE BLOOD CELL COUNT

Often the complete blood cell count is normal and offers little information in the diagnosis or management of asthma and may be most useful when searching for other complicating conditions (e.g., immunodeficiency states) rather than as a primary diagnostic aid.

However, eosinophilia, if present, most commonly suggests asthma, allergy, or both. Although there are other causes of peripheral eosinophilia in children (i.e., gastrointestinal or systemic eosinophilic disorder, parasitic infection, malignancy, and human immunodeficiency virus infection), asthma and allergy are the most likely causes. There has been renewed interest in using peripheral eosinophil count to both suggest an asthma diagnosis as well as to assign asthma phenotype.[50] Elevated blood eosinophil counts are not always associated with atopy, but there are data to support that eosinophil counts of 400/μL and above are more strongly associated with atopic asthma.[51]

CYTOLOGIC EXAMINATION OF SPUTUM

Obtaining induced sputum by inhaling hypertonic saline aerosols generated by an ultrasonic nebulizer is a useful technique for helping identify active inflammation in the airways characteristic of asthma. The presence and number of eosinophils and other inflammatory cells can provide useful information about disease phenotype, activity, and response to therapy.[52] Improved asthma control and reduced exacerbations were noted when there were less than 3% eosinophils in the induced sputum of adult asthmatics, but results in children are not consistent.[53,54] Neutrophilic inflammation predominates in some patients, while others have a paucity of inflammatory cells. Using cluster analysis in a study of adults enrolled in the Severe Asthma Research Program, over 80% of those in clusters with more severe asthma refractory to treatment with high-dose inhaled steroids and those with lower lung function had sputum neutrophilia.[55] Those in clusters with mild to moderate atopic disease had either eosinophilia or minimal inflammatory cells of any type. However, data from a small study of children with more severe asthma showed that the absence of blood eosinophilia did not predict absence of eosinophils in induced sputum or bronchoalveolar lavage (BAL).[56] Although the technique of obtaining induced sputum is relatively simple, it does require trained personnel, use of an established protocol, and specimen processing and is usually only successful in children that are at least 8 or 9 years of age. However, a recent report demonstrated success in obtaining induced sputum samples in children as young as 7 months using physical activity (or crying) followed by oropharyngeal suctioning to obtain the sample; 96% of 72 children aged 7–76 months were able to produce a sample.[57]

EXHALED NITRIC OXIDE

NO is an important and widespread regulatory molecule that has diverse biological functions. NO is synthesized from L-arginine by three different forms of the enzyme NO synthase (NOS): constitutive forms—endothelial NOS (eNOS) found in endothelial cells and nNOS in neuronal tissue—and an inducible form, iNOS. Although the precise role of NO in the asthmatic airway remains uncertain, NO can function as a bronchodilator, has antimicrobial properties, has antiproliferative action on fibroblasts, and is involved in regulation of ciliary beat frequency and epithelial ion transport.[52] Fractional exhaled NO (FeNO) monitoring has been proposed as a biomarker useful in asthma diagnosis, monitoring control and adjusting treatment, and predicting exacerbations. In many but not all asthma patients, high exhaled NO concentrations, compared with the nonasthmatic, coupled with a reduction with inhaled steroid treatment suggest an active or counterregulatory role in the development or persistence of asthma. Most data support direct correlation between clinical markers of eosinophilic airway inflammation or atopy and FeNO, including the degree of airway hyperresponsiveness as measured by methacholine challenge.[52,58,59] Other measures (e.g., FEV_1, bronchodilator response, and symptom report) correlate only weakly with FeNO. In a study of 128 school-aged children with asthma and allergic sensitization, mean FeNO levels were significantly different between those children with no sensitization and those children with 1–3, 4–5, and ≥6 positive skin prick tests.[60] In addition, those sensitized to cat, mouse, dust mite, rat, and cockroach had FeNO levels that were significantly higher compared with those who were not sensitized. After adjustment for age, sex, ICS use, and asthma control level, cat and rat allergen

Table 45.2   Range and Interpretation of Fractional Exhaled Nitric Oxide Values in Adults and Children. Symptoms Refer to Cough and/or Wheeze and/or Shortness of Breath

	FeNO < 25 ppb (<20 ppb in Children)	FeNO 25–50 ppb (20–35 ppb in Children)	FeNO > 50 ppb (>35 ppb in Children)
	DIAGNOSIS		
Symptoms present during past 6 + weeks	Eosinophilic airway inflammation unlikely Alternative diagnoses Unlikely to benefit from ICS	Be cautious Evaluate clinical context Monitor change in FeNO over time	Eosinophilic airway inflammation present Likely to benefit from ICS
	MONITORING (IN PATIENTS WITH DIAGNOSED ASTHMA)		
Symptoms present	Possible alternative diagnoses Unlikely to benefit from increase in ICS	Persistent allergen exposure Inadequate ICS dose Poor adherence Steroid resistance	Persistent allergen exposure Poor adherence or inhaler technique Inadequate ICS dose Risk for exacerbation Steroid resistance
Symptoms absent	Adequate ICS dose Good adherence ICS taper	Adequate ICS dosing Good adherence Monitor change in FeNO	ICS withdrawal or dose reduction may result in relapse Poor adherence or inhaler technique

FeNO, Fraction of exhaled nitric oxide; *ICS,* inhaled corticosteroid.
Reprinted with permission of the American Thoracic Society. Copyright 2016 American Thoracic Society. *The American Journal of Respiratory and Critical Care Medicine* is an official journal of the American Thoracic Society. See reference 53.

remained significant independent predictors of elevated FeNO.

Although FeNO has proved of value in some situations and patient populations, a number of limitations exist.[61] Weaknesses include poor ability to identify noneosinophilic inflammation and lack of specificity for asthma. Elevated FeNO also occurs in individuals with allergic rhinitis, eosinophilic bronchitis, COPD, and lung allograft rejection.

The determination of clinical cutoff points for diagnosing asthma, adjusting treatment, and predicting exacerbations remains controversial. FeNO levels are affected by many factors, including, race, age, ingestion of nitrate rich foods (raises), and tobacco smoke exposure (lowers). If other clinical conditions associated with elevated FeNO are excluded, a FeNO higher than documented clinical cutoffs (Table 45.2) can be useful in supporting a diagnosis of asthma.[62] The common presence of atopy in children apart from asthma limits FeNO as an accurate diagnostic tool.

A number of studies have used FeNO to adjust treatment with inhaled steroids with mixed results.[63–65] A large trial conducted in largely black and Hispanic children compared adding FeNO to usual care (Expert Panel Review [EPR] 2 guideline) in children aged 12–20 years.[63] All participants improved during the run-in period, probably related to the use of guideline care by specialists and the direct provision of medication to the child. In the intervention period, using symptom days and exacerbations as outcomes, no differences between usual care and FeNO groups were noted; but the use of FeNO resulted in higher doses of ICSs.

In a relatively small study done in seven Belgian hospitals, children aged 5–14 years with allergic asthma were randomized to a group managed with symptoms and FEV1 or FeNO.[64] In the FeNO group, a single target value of 20 ppb was used to increase treatment (>20 ppb) or lower treatment (≤20 ppb). In a 1-year follow-up period, there was no difference between the groups in the primary outcome of symptom free days, but there was a significant decrease in exacerbations. However, the exacerbations were largely related to an increase in symptoms and unscheduled medical contact; there was no difference in emergency visits or hospitalizations. A recent

meta-analysis suggested that using FeNO to guide treatment decisions has little clinical benefit, although this may result in a decrease in asthma exacerbations.[65]

Commercial devices are available that permit the rapid, noninvasive, and easy measurement of eNO (in parts per billion, ppb) and are priced in the same range as a desktop portable spirometer.[61,67] Although somewhat easier to perform than standard spirometry, children younger than 6 or 7 years of age are not consistently able to perform an online FeNO measure; however, offline collection methods using tidal breathing and Mylar collection bags have been used in younger children and infants.

A number of studies have demonstrated the presence of a variety of inflammatory mediators in the liquid condensate from cooled exhaled air collected over a number of minutes. Cytokines, leukotrienes, nitrates, and other substances have all been reported in exhaled breath condensate (EBC), and in some but not all studies, they correlate with asthma disease activity.[68] In addition, an acid pH in the EBC has also been reported to be a marker of airway inflammation. More recently, devices that measure volatile organic compounds in exhaled breath, so-called electronic noses, have been used to discriminate airway and lung disease states, including asthma. These devices capitalize in part on measuring metabolomic airway products that provide a selective "breath print" that identifies asthma phenotypes.[69] However, there is still great controversy over standardization of the technique, the derivation of the measured substances (sampling of airway lining fluid rather than volatilized molecules), and the measurement of mediators. EBC has yet to prove useful as a noninvasive measure of airway inflammation, and it is currently a research tool.[70]

SERUM TESTS

Determining quantitative levels of immunoglobulin G (and subclasses), M, and A is useful only to rule out immunodeficiency syndromes in children with recurrent or chronic infection. In children with asthma, IgG levels usually are normal, IgA levels are occasionally low, and IgM levels may be elevated. Systemic steroids, however, can depress IgG and perhaps IgA levels. Total serum IgE is often elevated in the child with asthma, atopy, or both; however, a normal IgE does not rule out asthma as a cause of symptoms. Although a rare condition in pediatric patients, in the child with shifting pulmonary infiltrates, a marked elevation of serum IgE (>1000 IU/mL) should prompt tests for both IgG and specific IgE antibody to *Aspergillus* to evaluate for allergic bronchopulmonary aspergillosis (see Chapter 65).

SWEAT TEST

A sweat test (determination of chloride concentration in sweat) should be considered in children with chronic, otherwise unexplained, respiratory symptoms, including recurrent wheezing, to rule out cystic fibrosis, even in areas where newborn screening for the disease is carried out (discussed later). Associated signs and symptoms that should prompt a sweat test include poor weight gain and short stature, steatorrhea, nasal polyps, pansinusitis, hemoptysis, and digital clubbing. Newborn screening for cystic fibrosis is now universal in the United States, and most cases of cystic fibrosis are diagnosed in infancy or the preschool years, but screening does have a false negative rate of approximately 5%, depending on the cutoff values and the methods chosen. Mutations conferring pancreatic sufficiency, and other rare mutations are typically associated with milder pulmonary disease and may present much later than infancy (see Chapter 50).

RADIOGRAPHS

Most children with suspected asthma should have a chest radiograph at some time to rule out parenchymal disease, congenital anomaly, and (direct or indirect) evidence of a foreign body, particularly if the asthma diagnosis is questionable. However, a normal chest radiograph does not rule out other diagnoses, particularly a retained airway or esophageal foreign body. A chest radiograph should be considered for the child admitted to a hospital with asthma, particularly if there are localized findings on physical examination (i.e., crackles, egophony, diminished breath sounds), fever, or persistent hypoxemia. Radiographic findings in asthma may range from normal to hyperinflation with peribronchial interstitial markings and atelectasis (Fig. 45.4A); infiltrates, atelectasis, pneumonia, or a combination of the three (see Fig. 45.4B); and pneumomediastinum (see Fig. 45.4C), often with infiltrates. Pneumothorax occurs rarely (see Fig. 45.4D).

Paranasal sinus radiographs or screening sinus computed tomography can also be considered for children with persistent nocturnal coughing, nasal symptoms, and headaches. Although acute and chronic rhinosinusitis have long been associated with an increase in symptoms in children with asthma, a recent study indicates that long-term treatment with nasal corticosteroids did not improve asthma control.[71] In a 24-week placebo controlled trial of daily intranasal mometasone, children with asthma and symptoms of rhinosinusitis did not show improvement in asthma control or reduction in exacerbations compared to placebo. Nasal symptoms did improve, but the study results argue against treating nasal symptoms to improve asthma control.

ALLERGY TESTING

Allergy testing (skin testing or in vitro serum allergen-specific IgE measure) is indicated in patients in whom specific allergic factors are believed to be important and in all children with severe asthma. Numerous allergic factors that might contribute significantly to the asthma (e.g., pollen, mold, dust mite, cockroach, or dander from domestic animals) occur in the home or at school. After taking a detailed environmental history, skin testing should be performed (usually percutaneous or scratch), limited to the most likely allergens, as suggested by the history.

Skin test results may vary with age, drug therapy, and inherent skin factors. Drugs that affect skin test results include H_1 antihistamines (which may inhibit skin reactions for up to 72 hours or longer), tricyclic antidepressants, and some histamine (H_2) blockers. Topical and systemic corticosteroids or montelukast do not affect skin reactions. Positive (histamine) and negative (saline) control tests should be included to detect inherent skin factors that may affect the reaction to allergen, such as dermatographism and extensive dryness or eczema.

The in vitro measure of allergen-specific IgE (s-IgE) makes use of the affinity of serum IgE antibody for antigen that has been bound to a solid phase substrate. The s-IgE is no more specific than the antigen employed, but it can produce a quantitative result, thus allowing the degree of sensitization to be measured. The s-IgE test is significantly more expensive than skin testing, but it can be performed in commercial laboratories and is useful for situations in which skin tests are impractical (e.g., for the patient with generalized dermatitis or dermatographism, or if the patient must continue to receive medications with antihistaminic activity) or to better quantify the degree of allergic sensitization (higher value of s-IgE).

Therapeutic Considerations

Both the most recent US guidelines for the diagnosis and management of asthma (Expert Panel Report 3) and the international Global Initiative for Asthma (GINA) guidelines stress the importance of asthma control as compared with severity.[1,72] Asthma severity refers to the intrinsic intensity of the disease and is typically assigned prior to beginning treatment with controller medications, and is also reassessed at intervals after treatment to determine degree of responsiveness to treatment. As a result, severity becomes defined by the level of treatment necessary to achieve and maintain adequate control. Identifying children and adolescents with severe or therapy resistant asthma is important because the need for close monitoring and aggressive treatment will be significant. For most other patients, accurate assessment of control is more important than severity assignment in order to adequately manage asthma.

Asthma control is divided into two components: impairment or symptom control and risk. The *impairment* domain refers to daytime and nighttime symptoms (i.e., cough, wheeze, exercise limitation), the need for rescue medication (SABA) for the treatment of symptoms, deviation from normal levels of activity (i.e., playing, sleeping, attending work or school), preserving normal or near-normal lung function,

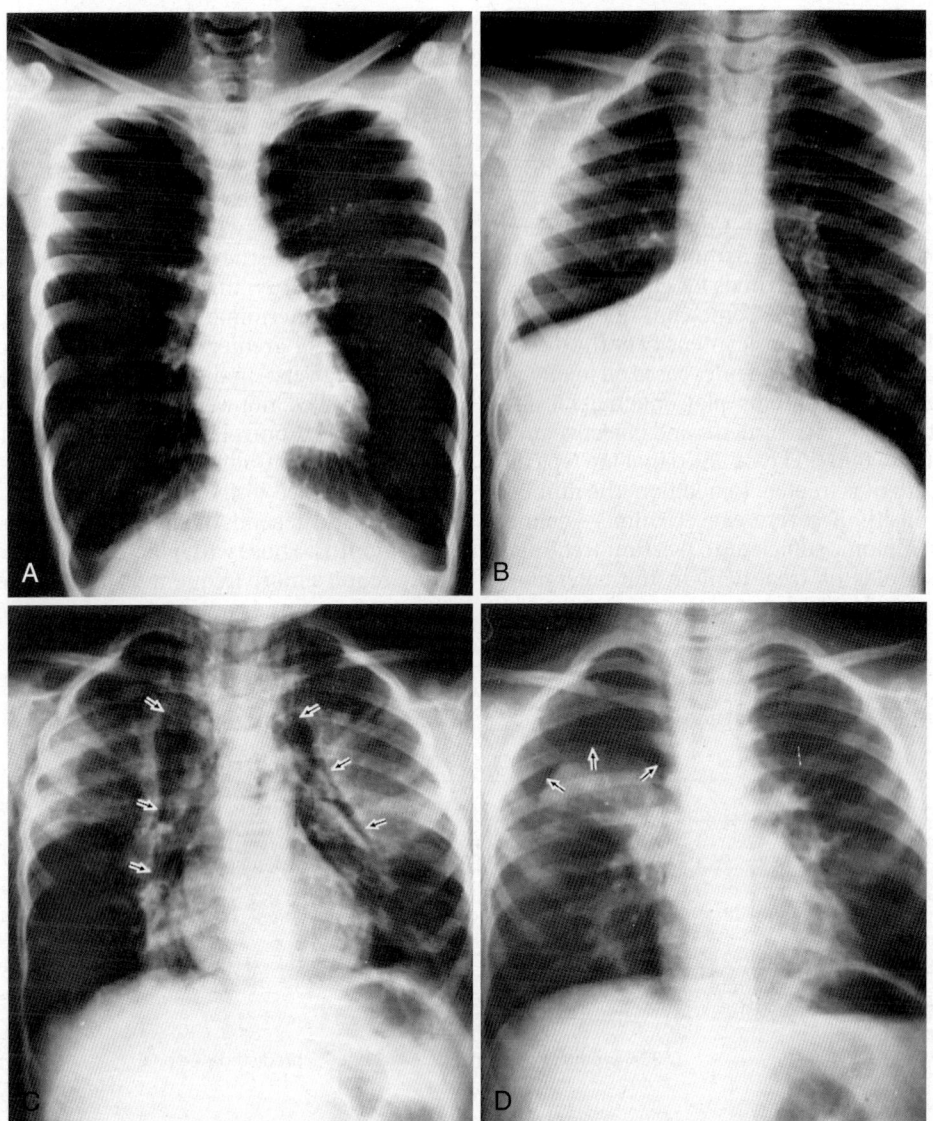

Fig. 45.4 Radiographic findings in asthma. (A) Hyperinflation with increased bronchial markings. (B) Atelectasis involving a complete lobe. (C) Massive pneumomediastinum complicating asthma. (D) Pneumothorax secondary to paroxysmal coughing in asthma. *Arrows* mark air in (C), lung margin in (D).

and meeting patient and parent expectations. The *risk* domain refers to preventing severe exacerbations that require medical attention, such as prescription of systemic steroids, emergency medical treatment or hospitalization, loss of lung function or impairment of normal lung growth, and adverse effects caused by medication use. This strategy draws attention to the management of current symptoms and functional impairment, as well as the future effects of asthma and its treatment on lung function and severe exacerbations. It also highlights the very important observation that asthma treatment strategies that improve symptoms may not always result in the prevention of significant exacerbations.

Asthma is best managed in a continuous fashion by forming a partnership with a knowledgeable physician or other health care provider. The concept of expecting a near symptom-free lifestyle (for all but the most severely affected patients) should be instilled in patients and their families. Unnecessary restrictions of the child's and family's lifestyles should be avoided. Participation in recreational activities, sports, and school

attendance should all be expected. Psychosocial factors such as the child's behavior, social adjustments in the family and at school, and attitudes toward managing asthma should also be addressed. Parents should understand that asthma is a chronic disease with acute exacerbations that with currently available treatments can be controlled, but not cured. As better characterization of the inflammatory processes and pathways that affect the airway in specific patients and development of real-time noninvasive monitoring techniques occurs, more precise control of asthma symptoms or even primary or secondary disease prevention may become a realistic goal of asthma management.

Classification of Asthma

Over the past decade, increasing awareness has been focused on the broad heterogeneity of asthma, both with respect to its causes, manifestations, and response to treatment.

Identification of specific asthma phenotypes is expanding, and the use of biomarkers, molecular phenotyping, and cluster analysis based on symptoms, lung function, and comorbidities can help identify specific subtypes. Age of onset of symptoms, lung function, inflammatory cell types and mediators in induced sputum, and atopic versus nonatopic are all markers used to characterize disease severity, symptom pattern, and response to treatment. Considerable research is still needed to accurately identify asthma phenotypes and to determine clinically useful methods for classification.

Although the clinical utility is somewhat questionable, asthma severity refers to the intrinsic intensity of the disease and may be classified into broad categories based on frequency of daytime and nighttime symptoms, play or activity limitation, need for rescue/reliever treatment, and objective measures of pulmonary function (PEFR or FEV$_1$) that are typically present *before* the patient is treated. In addition, the number, frequency, and intensity of severe exacerbations—defined as an increase in symptoms sufficient to warrant treatment with oral corticosteroids or treatment in the emergency department or inpatient hospital unit—are considered. Some patients who have relatively well-controlled symptoms and good functional status may have frequent or intense exacerbations. Although the correlation between the number and intensity of exacerbations with severity levels is less clear, the greater the number and severity (e.g., need for hospitalization, intensive care treatment), the higher the severity. However, the degree of severity of asthma often changes in a given individual with time, response to treatment, airway injury or growth, the development of newly acquired allergic sensitivities, or change in exposure to recognized triggers. As a result, determination of *control* after treatment has been instituted is of greater significance than assigning a severity level. Using very similar criteria, asthma is determined to be well controlled, not well controlled, or very poorly controlled (Table 45.3). Control is determined at every visit, and appropriate treatment adjustments are made. The frequency of physician office visits for assessment of asthma control is variable and depends on disease activity but typically is every 1–6 months. Those with poor control or recent exacerbation may require more frequent visits for treatment monitoring of response and adjustment and monitoring of lung

Table 45.3   Assessing Asthma Control and Adjusting Therapy in Children 5–12 Years of Age

Components of Control		CLASSIFICATION OF ASTHMA CONTROL (5–11 YEARS OF AGE)		
		Well Controlled	Not Well Controlled	Very Poorly Controlled
Impairment	Symptoms	≤2 days/week but not more than once on each day.	>2 days/week or multiple time on less than 2 days/week	Throughout the day
	Nighttime awakenings	≤1×/month	≥2×/month	≥2×/week
	Interference with normal activity	None	Some limitation	Extremely limited
	Short acting beta-agonist use for symptom control (not prevention of EIB)	≤2 days/week	>2 days/week	Several times per day
	Lung function FEV$_1$ or peak flow	>80% predicted/personal best	60%–80% predicted/personal best	<60% predicted/personal best
	FEV$_1$/FVC	>80%	75%–80%	<75%
Risk	Exacerbations requiring oral systemic corticosteroids	0–1/year	≥2/year (see note)	
		CONSIDER SEVERITY AND INTERVAL SINCE LAST EXACERBATION		
	Reduction in lung growth	Evaluation requires long-term follow-up		
	Treatment related adverse effects	Medication side effects can vary in intensity from none to very troublesome and worrisome. The level of intensity does not correlate to specific levels of control but should be considered in the overall assessment of risk.		
	Recommended action for treatment (See Fig. 45.1B for treatment steps)	Maintain current step Regular follow-up every 1–6 months Consider step down if well controlled for at least 3 months	Step up at least 1 step and Reevaluate in 2–6 weeks For side effects consider alternative treatment options	Consider short course of oral systemic corticosteroids Step up at least 1 step and Reevaluate in 2–6 weeks For side effects consider alternative treatment options

The stepwise approach is meant to assist, not replace, the clinical decision making required to meet individual patient needs.

The level of control is based on the most severe impairment or risk category. Assess impairment domain by patient's/caregiver's recall of previous 2–4 weeks and by spirometry/or peak flow measures. Symptom assessment for longer periods should reflect a global assessment such as inquiring whether the patient's asthma is better or worse since the last visit.

At present, there are inadequate data to correspond frequencies of exacerbations with different levels of asthma control. In general, more frequent and intense exacerbations (e.g., requiring urgent, unscheduled care, hospitalization, or ICU admission) indicate poorer disease control. For treatment purposes, patients who had ≥2 exacerbations requiring oral systemic corticosteroids in the past year may be considered the same as patients who have persistent asthma, even in the absence of impairment levels consistent with persistent asthma.

Before step up in therapy:

Review adherence to medications, inhaler technique, environmental control, and comorbid conditions.

If alternative treatment option was used in step, discontinue it and use preferred treatment for that step.

EIB, Exercise-induced bronchospasm; *FEV$_1$*, forced expiratory volume in 1 second; *FVC*, forced vital capacity.

From NIH Expert Panel Report 3.[1]

function. Since asthma is a chronic disorder that may become clinically obvious only periodically—one in which the severity of airway obstruction, intensity of symptoms, and degree of impairment is frequently underestimated by physicians and patients alike, the use of a standard, validated questionnaire can help overcome this discrepancy.

There are several short, self-administered instruments (e.g., the Asthma Control Test [ACT], Asthma Control Questionnaire, Asthma Therapy Assessment Questionnaire) that provide a score indicative of well-controlled, not well-controlled, and poorly controlled asthma.[1] These tools do not assess the risk domain, which must also be factored into treatment decisions. A newer measure, the Composite Asthma Severity Index (CASI), incorporates symptoms, treatment level, exacerbations, and lung function into a measure that shows better responsiveness than the ACT or symptom measure alone.[73] Further validation will be necessary to determine its clinical utility.

The most recent NHLBI guidelines classify asthma as either *intermittent* or *persistent* and within the persistent category as *mild*, *moderate*, or *severe*.[1,74,75]

The use of cluster analysis techniques shows promise in further stratifying severe asthma phenotypes into more discrete subtypes that will help with prospective identification and long-term follow-up and treatment.[76] See Chapter 46 for a detailed discussion of severe asthma.

OTHER MEASURES FOR ASSESSING ASTHMA SEVERITY AND CONTROL

Biomarkers that provide more information on disease activity and severity could better guide asthma treatment and improve control or reduce exacerbations. However, currently available tests are limited in both availability and utility or practicality. Older models using degree of airway reactivity based on methacholine responsiveness or proportion of eosinophils contained in induced sputum, and then adjusting treatment to decrease airway reactivity or eosinophil counts were shown to achieve better pulmonary function and fewer exacerbations than monitoring symptoms and pulmonary function alone in adults.[1] However, repeated methacholine challenge testing or sputum induction is expensive, time-consuming, and generally impractical in the clinical setting, especially in the pediatric population. As discussed earlier, FeNO has been proposed as an easily obtainable measure of eosinophilic airway inflammation and could therefore be used to titrate treatment to achieve better control. Although in steroid-naïve asthmatics FeNO is elevated and in most patients the levels decrease within 1 week of instituting inhaled steroid treatment, FeNO remains essentially unchanged in as many as 30%, even when clinical improvement occurs.[59] Moreover, a number of large randomized, controlled trials that used either daily home or intermittent in-office FeNO measures to adjust treatment failed to find a difference in improvement in the number of symptom-free days or a reduction in ICS dose when compared with standard treatment using symptom report and pulmonary function measures.[77,78] It has been suggested that FeNO may be useful when there is discordance between patient-reported symptoms and airway inflammation.[63] However, data from one prospective study using ACT and FeNO to monitor asthma control and adjust treatment in school-aged children did not support added benefit from FeNO measurement.[79] In addition, nearly a third of the patients switched from a concordant to discordant phenotype over the course of 4 weeks in the trial. Although symptom-free days improved over a year in those with unstable phenotype, there was no difference in those in the FeNO group compared with those without FeNO monitoring. In spite of its limitations, FeNO may be useful in some settings, such as a diagnostic aid for asthma, identification of steroid-responsive patients, and (to a lesser extent) adjusting the dose of controller medications and predicting relapse during medication taper.

Recently there has been substantial interest in the airway microbiome, with several lines of evidence supporting a role for the bacterial ecosystem of the upper and lower airway in both maintaining pulmonary health and causing chronic conditions, such as asthma. Although there are data that suggest the airway microbiome may differ in those with asthma and healthy controls, as well as differences between degrees of asthma severity,[80,81] further research is needed to determine causation and influences of microbiome on immune dysregulation in the airways. Moreover, it is likely that there are "fungal-biomes" and "viral-biomes" that may also influence development and severity of airway disorders, but little data are currently available.

Pharmacologic Management of Asthma in Children Older Than 5 Years of Age

The medical treatment of asthma involves the administration of controller medications designed to prevent asthma symptoms and the use of rapid-acting reliever medications that quickly abort acute exacerbations. Controller medications are administered to all asthmatics other than those with intermittent disease and are typically, but not uniformly, antiinflammatory in nature (Table 45.4A). Reliever medications are SABA or anticholinergics. Several immunomodulatory drugs are currently available for treatment of severe persistent asthma and a number of other such biologics are under development, discussed in Chapter 48.

Reliever Medications: Short-Acting β Agonists

Short acting β_2-adrenergic agonists (SABAs) constitute the most potent bronchodilators currently available for treatment of asthma[1] and are used to relieve bronchospasm and its attendant symptoms of cough, wheezing, and shortness of breath. SABAs bind to the widely distributed BAR (primarily those located on the bronchial smooth muscle, airway epithelial cell, and mast cell) and result in the intracellular conversion of adenosine triphosphate (ATP) to adenosine 3', 5' cyclic monophosphate. The result is relaxation of airway smooth muscle and improved air flow. Onset of action is generally within a few minutes, peak action occurs at approximately 30 minutes, and duration of action is from 4 to 6 hours.[1] The preferred route of administration is by inhalation, because this method results in the most rapid onset and duration of action while minimizing adverse

Table 45.4A   Usual Dosages for Long-Term Controller Medications

Medication	Youth >12 Years	Child Dose
SYSTEMIC CORTICOSTEROIDS		
Methylprednisolone (chronic control)	7.5–60 mg Once daily or every other day as needed for control	0.25–2 mg/kg[1]
Prednisolone, prednisone (short-course for exacerbation)	40–60 mg Administer for 3–10 days once or in 2 divided doses	1–2 mg/kg maximum 60 mg/day
Dexamethasone	10–16 mg Give oral or IM for 1–2 days	0.6 mg/kg, maximum 16 mg
LONG-ACTING INHALED β-2 AGONISTS[a]		
Salmeterol 50 µg/puff	50 µg q 12 h	50 µg q 12 h
Formoterol 12 µg/capsule	1 capsule q 12 h	1 capsule q 12 h
COMBINATION MEDICATION		
Fluticasone/Salmeterol		
DPI 100, 250, 500 µg/50 µg	1 inhalation bid	1 inhalation bid
MDI 45/21, 115/21, 230/21 µg	2 inhalations bid	1–2 inhalations bid
Budesonide/formoterol	1–2 inhalations bid	1–2 inhalations bid
MDI 80/4.5; 160/4.5 µg		
Mometasone/formoterol	1–2 inhalations bid	1–2 inhalations bid
MDI 100/5 µg; 200/5 µg	Adjust dose strength to achieve control	
LEUKOTRIENE MODIFIERS		
Montelukast	5 mg daily (6–14 years) 10 mg daily (>14 years)	4 mg daily (2–5 years) 5 mg daily (6–14 years)
Zafirlukast	20 mg twice daily	10 mg twice daily (7–11 years)
Zileuton	1200 mg bid	
Methylxanthines		
Theophylline, sustained release	300 mg daily Adjust dose to serum concentration 5–10 mg/mL	10/mg/kg daily, max 300 mg

[a]Should not be used for symptom relief or for exacerbations. Use with inhaled corticosteroids.
DPI, Dry-powder inhaler; *IM*, intramuscular; *MDI*, metered-dose inhaler.

Table 45.4B   Adjunct Medications for Severe Episodes

Medication	Child (<12 years)	Adolescent
MAGNESIUM SULFATE		
Intravenous (IV)	Bolus: 50 mg/kg per dose (25–75 mg/kg per dose; max 2 g) Administer over 20 min	
SYSTEMIC (INJECTED) β₂ AGONISTS		
Epinephrine		
Intramuscular (IM) 1:1,000 (1 mg/mL)	0.01 mg/kg (max 0.3–0.5 mg) every 20 min for 3 doses	0.3–0.5 mg every 20 min for 3 doses
Terbutaline		
Intravenous (IV) Subcutaneous (SQ) (1 mg/mL)	0.01 mg/kg bolus (max 0.4 mg) over 10 min 0.01 mg/kg (max 0.25 mg) May repeat every 15 min for 3 doses	0.01 mg/kg bolus (max 0.75 mg) over 10 min 0.01 mg/kg (max 0.25 mg) May repeat every 15 min for 3 doses

No advantage has been found for higher-dose corticosteroids in severe asthma exacerbations.[1]
There is no advantage for intravenous administration over oral therapy, provided gastrointestinal function is intact.
Therapy following a hospitalization or emergency department visit is typically 5 days but may last from 3 to 10 days. Studies indicate that there is no need to taper the systemic corticosteroid dose when given up to 10 days. Dosages in excess of 1 mg/kg of prednisone or prednisolone have been associated with adverse behavioral effects in children, whereas 1 mg/kg provides equivalent pulmonary benefit without the adverse effects in most cases.

effects. Inhalation of SABAs can be accomplished with the use of a small-volume jet nebulizer, metered-dose inhaler (MDI; usually and ideally with a spacer), or dry-powder inhaler (DPI).

Several selective SABAs are available for treating acute asthma, such as terbutaline and albuterol. Racemic albuterol, the predominant bronchodilator in current use, is a 50:50 mixture of (R)-enantiomers and (S)-enantiomers. Levalbuterol, the (R)-albuterol isomer, has a 100-fold more potent β₂ receptor binding than (S)-albuterol, and it is responsible for the bronchodilator effects of the racemate. In vitro, (S)-albuterol has been demonstrated to increase intracellular Ca²⁺ to stimulate eosinophil recruitment and degranulation and recruit other inflammatory cells. The in vivo effects of (S)-albuterol remain unproven; however, it has no bronchodilator activity and has a prolonged plasma half-life, but it does not cause bronchoconstriction or interfere with the binding of (R)-albuterol to its receptor. When administered in equivalent doses based on the concentration of (R)-albuterol, there does not appear to be any consistent clinical advantage to using levalbuterol versus racemic albuterol as measured by improvement in clinical symptoms, pulmonary function testing, or adverse effect profile. Since levalbuterol is typically more expensive than the racemic drug, the routine use of levalbuterol is generally not recommended.

Typical adverse effects of SABAs include muscular tremor, tachycardia, irritability, and with very high doses, hypokalemia, hypertension, and tachyarrhythmia. Adverse effects are greater with systemic administration (oral, intravenous [IV], intramuscular [IM]) compared with the inhaled route. Moreover, the dose delivered by an MDI is substantially less than that from a small-volume nebulizer, and since most of the inhaled dose is swallowed and absorbed by the gastrointestinal tract, annoying side effects are best minimized by using an MDI with an appropriate spacer.

The clinical significance of serious adverse events that develop as a result of the chronic administration of inhaled SABAs is, in most instances, probably less than was once believed. The current recommendation is for the as-needed use of a SABA for relief of symptoms or for protection against EIA. A retrospective review of prescription records in patients in Canada found an increased risk for asthma death or near-death in patients who used more than one canister of a SABA per month. However, an association with the use of a number of other asthma medications was also noted, suggesting that disease severity might actually be more causative than overuse of SABAs alone.[82] Nonetheless, SABA overuse is a worrying marker of future risk.

Reports have suggested that repeated use of a SABA may result in an increase in airway hyperresponsiveness or a decrease in protection from allergen-induced bronchospasm. The reduction in beneficial effects of SABA following chronic use may result in part from receptor desensitization, uncoupling of the receptor from its signaling G protein, inactivation of receptors, or reduction in receptor number caused by increased degradation or decreased synthesis. A well-designed randomized double-blind placebo-controlled study performed in adults with mild asthma examined the effects of regularly administered albuterol versus intermittent administration compared with placebo. There was no significant difference in any outcome measures between the groups, including exacerbations, treatment failures, lung function, symptoms, or methacholine responsiveness.[83] However, regular use of albuterol was also not beneficial to the patients. Finally, there may be specific subgroups of patients who are at risk for developing adverse effects, as measured by worsening pulmonary function with chronic use of SABAs, and this may be related to genetic variability in the BAR. Nine polymorphisms in the *BAR* gene have been described, and several of the more frequent types may have biological significance. One involves the beta 2AR-16 region, with replacement of arginine (Arg16) for glycine (Gly16). In a study involving bronchodilator response in children, those with the *Arg/Arg* polymorphism had the highest prevalence (60%) of bronchodilator response to a single dose of albuterol, whereas fewer than 30% of those with the *Arg/Gly* polymorphism responded and only 13% of those with the *Gly/Gly* polymorphism were responders.[84] In contrast, data from a prospective study of chronic albuterol administration to patients segregated by BAR genotype found that those with the Arg16 homozygous polymorphism had steadily declining PEFR as compared with those receiving intermittent treatment or treatment with ipratropium.[85] This effect did not occur in those with the *Gly/Gly* genotype. Chronic administration of ipratropium to the *Arg/Arg* group did not result in PEFR deterioration. In addition, recent studies point to other polymorphisms not associated with the BAR but related to smooth muscle proliferation that are associated with differential responsiveness to short acting beta-agonists.[86-88] Lastly, rare genetic variants that are associated with ethnicity are also likely contributors to the variability in response to SABA. A study in Latino children described a number of such rare genetic variants in genes associated with membrane ion transport, vascular smooth muscle adhesion, and TGF-beta pathways.[89] These data indicate the importance of understanding ethnic and ancestral background in identifying genetic risks for SABA responsiveness.

Anticholinergic Agents

Ipratropium bromide is a quaternary ammonium congener of atropine and is an anticholinergic compound approved for use as a bronchodilator. Anticholinergic agents produce bronchodilatation by antagonizing the activity of acetylcholine at the level of its receptor, particularly those found on airway smooth muscle in the large, central airways. The onset of action of ipratropium is relatively slow (20 minutes), and the peak effect occurs at 60 minutes.[1] Ipratropium, unlike atropine, is poorly absorbed across mucous membranes and has little toxicity at the usual doses. In particular, ipratropium does not inhibit mucociliary clearance. Data from several studies conducted in children presenting to the emergency department for treatment of acute asthma indicate that when combined with a β-adrenergic agonist, ipratropium improves pulmonary function and relieves symptoms better than either drug alone.[1] The effect is modest and appears to be most evident in those who present with the most severe airway obstruction; this may be a marker for patients who have increased cholinergic tone in the large central airways. Ipratropium has not been shown to be effective in the treatment of children hospitalized with acute asthma, particularly if ipratropium failed to induce improvement when administered in the emergency department.[90]

Controller Medications

INHALED CORTICOSTEROIDS

ICSs are currently considered the most effective controller medication available for the treatment of chronic asthma. Most ICSs have a high topical potency and relatively low systemic effects, either as a result of poor absorption or rapid and effective metabolism to inactive compounds. However, all ICSs are absorbed through the respiratory epithelium to some degree, resulting in the potential for systemic effects.

Table 45.5 Estimated Comparative Daily Dosages for Inhaled Corticosteroid in Older Children and Adults

Drug	Low Daily Dose		Medium Daily Dose		High Daily Dose	
	5–11 years	>12 years	5–11 years	>12 years	5–11 years	>12 years
Beclomethasone HFA 40 or 80 µg/puff	80–160 µg	80–240 µg	>160–320 µg	>240–480 µg	>320 µg	>480 µg
Budesonide suspension for nebulization dry powder (90, 180, or 200 µg/inhalation)	0.5 mg 180–400 µg	180–600 µg	1.0 mg 400–800 µg	>600–1200 µg	>2.0 mg >800 µg	>1200 µg
Flunisolide HFA 80 µg/puff	160 µg	320 µg	320 µg	320–640 µg	≥ 640 µg	>640 µg
Fluticasone dipropionate HFA/MDI: 44, 110, 220 µg/puff	88–176 µg	88–264 µg	>176–352 µg	264–440 µg	>352 µg	>440 µg
DPI: 50, 100, 250 µg/puff	100–200 µg	100–300 µg	200–400 µg	300–500 µg	>400 µg	>500 µg
Fluticasone furoate 100, 200 µg/puff	NA	100 µg/day	NA	200 µg/day	NA	400 µg/day
Mometasone DPI 110, 220 µg/puff	110 µg	220 µg	110–220 mcg	440 µg	>440 µg	>880 µg
Ciclesonide MDI 80, 160 µg/puff	NA	160 µg	NA	320 µg	NA	640 µg

DPI, Dry-powder inhaler; *HFA,* Hydrofluoroalkane; *NA,* not approved for this age group; *MDI,* metered-dose inhaler.
Adapted from NAEPP Expert Report 3.[1]

The ideal ICS should demonstrate excellent clinical efficacy and minimal to no toxicity in combination with a convenient and easy-to-use inhaler device. To achieve such a profile, an ICS should have the following properties: a high affinity for and potency at the glucocorticoid receptor (GR); prolonged retention in the lung; a high level of serum protein binding for the systemically absorbed fraction; a high volume of distribution; minimal or no oral bioavailability; and rapid, complete systemic inactivation (e.g., high first-pass hepatic inactivation, or inactivation in the lung before systemic absorption).[91] Together these properties confer a higher therapeutic index with prolonged antiinflammatory activity in the lung and relatively few systemic adverse effects. Pharmacologic properties alone are not sufficient for optimum clinical effect. The delivery devices should provide maximal deposition in the lung in both large and smaller airways, with little to no deposition or absorption in the oropharynx or gastrointestinal tract. Once-daily administration is also likely to improve patient adherence. Inhalation devices should be simple to use, should be acceptable to a wide age range, and should deliver a consistent dose throughout the life of the inhaler.

FLUTICASONE PROPIONATE

Fluticasone propionate (FP) is a potent and poorly orally absorbed topically active corticosteroid that is extensively metabolized in the liver to an inactive compound. This highly lipophilic drug demonstrates an extremely high affinity for lung GRs compared with beclomethasone (BDP) and shows a slow rate of dissociation from its receptor. As a result, FP has a negligible oral bioavailability, and the topical-to-systemic activity ratio is exceptionally favorable and better than most currently available ICSs. However, FP is readily absorbed through the respiratory mucosa and can enter the systemic circulation in this fashion (without hepatic metabolism). FP is more likely to produce sore throat and hoarseness than other ICS. In addition, there have been reports of adrenal suppression in children younger than 12 years of age who receive more than 400 µg/day of FP, but the data are inconsistent. FP is therefore considered a high-potency ICS, with the potential to effectively control symptoms and improve lung function, but at higher doses it has greater potential to cause adverse effects. In vivo, FP appears at least twice as potent as BDP and BUD on a milligram-per-milligram basis.

Comparative trials indicate that fluticasone at half the dose of BUD and BDP results in a slight improvement of some pulmonary function measures, such as morning PEFR and end-of-treatment trial FEV_1.[92] FP is currently available in MDI and DPI form in three strengths (Table 45.5); it is approved in the United States for use in children 4 years of age and older.

Fluticasone furoate is a new formulation of fluticasone that has an extended half-life and can be taken once daily. It is available in the United States as a dry powder inhaler in doses of 100 µg or 200 µg of fluticasone administered once per day and approved for children and adolescents 12 years of age and older. The dose response curve is similar to other ICS formulations.[93] Fluticasone furoate is also available with a fixed dose of 25 µg of the long-acting beta-agonist, vilanterol per inhalation. At the current time, the combination inhaler has been approved for use only in adults with COPD and asthma.

BUDESONIDE

BUD has been widely studied and used clinically for many years. It has moderate potency in vitro and in vivo, with well-documented clinical efficacy and safety. In addition, the presence of a free C21 hydroxy group on the BUD molecule results in formation of esters with long-chain fatty acids. This results in an inactive depot of drug within the airway epithelial cells that is released slowly into an active state. BUD is currently available in a dry powder inhaler and a nebulizer suspension. BUD is approved in the United States for use in children 1 year of age and older. It is available in combination with formoterol in an MDI form, which is approved in the United States for use in children age ≥12 years.

BECLOMETHASONE

Although clearly less potent than FP and slightly less so than BUD, BDP is effective in reducing symptoms and improving pulmonary function. However, BDP is readily absorbed from the gastrointestinal tract, and the parent compound (BDP) is metabolized to the more potent monopropionate. As a result, BDP has a less favorable topical-to-systemic potency ratio. However, concerns about its ability to cause adverse effects such as growth and adrenal suppression have not been substantiated. BDP is currently available as a fine-particle aerosol dispensed by a hydrofluoroalkane propellant. This propellant system permits greater deposition into the lower and smaller airways and a reduction in the effective dose. The clinical advantage of these properties remains to be clarified. BDP is approved in the United States for use in children 5 years of age and older. In low- and middle-income countries, the low cost of BDP makes it a very attractive medication.

MOMETASONE

Mometasone is a potent, highly topically active steroid that has long been used to treat allergic rhinitis and dermatologic disorders. It has the advantage of poor systemic absorption and has been shown to be effective in improving lung function and controlling symptoms in children with asthma who were previously treated with other ICSs and SABAs. Mometasone is similar to FP in its high receptor affinity and half-life. It appears to have a similar safety profile to other ICSs. Mometasone is approved in the United States for use in children 4 years of age and older. It is available in both DPI and MDI forms for treatment of asthma and is labeled for once-a-day dosing.

CICLESONIDE

Ciclesonide is a prodrug that must be metabolized to active form in the lung, where its metabolite has approximately 100 times greater receptor affinity. It has essentially no oral bioavailability and is tightly bound to plasma proteins. Ciclesonide is converted at the airway epithelial cell into its active metabolite, des-ciclesonide (Des-CIC); the enzyme responsible for the conversion is only found in the lower respiratory tract. A recent meta-analysis concluded that ciclesonide was probably as effective as fluticasone, BUD, and BDP in equivalent doses at improving pulmonary function and controlling mild symptoms. Incidence of oral candidiasis was lower in groups treated with ciclesonide. A single long-term (12-month) safety study in children compared two doses of ciclesonide to placebo and concluded that there was no significant effect on linear growth or adrenal suppression.[94] The study was somewhat flawed in that there was no active comparator, no clinical effect of drug was seen, and adherence was indirectly measured. Further studies in children are necessary to assess dose responsiveness and safety. Ciclesonide is approved in the United States for use in children 12 years of age and older.

Other Inhaled Corticosteroids

Flunisolide is an older, relatively less potent steroid that, while effective, is less commonly used. It must be given in fairly high microgram amounts, resulting in a bitter unpleasant taste.

MECHANISM OF ACTION AND CLINICAL USE

There are several pathways through which corticosteroids decrease inflammation. The action of corticosteroids begins as passive diffusion across the cell membrane and into the cytoplasm where binding to the GR occurs. The GR exists in the cytoplasm as a large heterodimeric complex that includes two 90-kD heat shock protein (HSP) molecules. After hormone binding, the HSPs are shed, the receptor-steroid complex is translocated to the nucleus, and then binds as a dimer to a glucocorticoid response element (GRE) on steroid-responsive genes. The GR acts to regulate transcription of target genes either directly or indirectly by interaction with other transcription factors. The binding of the GR complex to GRE results in either induction or repression of a gene. The number of GREs and the proximity to transcriptional start sites affects the steroid inducibility of the gene. Activation of inflammatory genes is achieved by histone acetylation of the transcription complex. At low doses, steroids suppress inflammation by recruiting histone deacetylase-2 (HDAC2) to inactivate transcription of these genes. GRs may also act independently of binding to GRE by coactivating other transcription factors (e.g., STAT5). At higher doses, glucocorticoids control inflammation by increasing histone acetylation of the transcription complex of antiinflammatory genes.[95]

A major mediator of corticosteroid action on genes is the nuclear transcription factor NFκB (nuclear factor kappa-light-chain-enhancer of activated B cells). Corticosteroids block NFκB signaling by preventing it from binding to DNA, which decreases transcription of proinflammatory cytokines. Corticosteroids may also inhibit NFκB by directly increasing production of its cytoplasmic inhibitor protein IκB. IκB proteins bind to NFκB and keep it anchored in the cytoplasm. In this manner, corticosteroids inhibit the transcription of a number of cytokines and chemokines implicated in the pathogenesis of asthma, such as interleukin-1 (IL-1) through IL-6, tumor necrosis factor alpha (TNFα), granulocyte-macrophage colony-stimulating factor, IL-13, IL-8, released on activation, normal T cell expressed and secreted (RANTES), and eotaxin. Steroids may also inhibit the synthesis of some cytokine receptors, such as the IL-4 receptor, intracellular adhesion molecule (ICAM), and vascular cell adhesion molecule (VCAM). In addition to the action on cytokines, steroids also inhibit the inducible form of NO synthase, cyclooxygenase, phospholipase A2, and endothelin, all important factors in the inflammatory cascade relevant to asthma. Corticosteroids also increase the synthesis of BAR by increasing gene transcription.[75,95]

Because topical steroids can also cause rapid effects (e.g., skin blanching), it is likely that there is also a rapid cellular mechanism of action with transient vasoconstriction in the microcirculation, which is independent of the genomic mechanism.[96] This action could involve the generation of vasoconstrictive mediators either at the point of glucocorticoid (GC) binding to certain membrane receptors or at the time of dissociation of the HSP from the cytoplasmic receptor complex.

ICSs are currently recommended as first-line therapy for children with persistent asthma. ICSs are the most effective chronic treatment for asthma and reduce airway reactivity, reduce acute symptoms and exacerbations, attenuate the late allergen response, and decrease the need for rescue bronchodilators. In addition, ICSs decrease deposition of collagen and extracellular matrix glycoproteins, or tenascins, in the subepithelial basement membrane. For these reasons, ICSs alone should be used as the initial treatment for persistent asthma; it is not appropriate, in the vast majority of cases, to use a fixed-dose combination of ICS plus a long-acting β-agonist as initial treatment. Withdrawal of ICS treatment is usually accompanied by a rapid return of airway hyperresponsiveness and decreased symptom control within several weeks.

A small but not insignificant proportion of patients do not have a significant response to ICS. Children and adolescents who are obese, smoke cigarettes, and have significant and continuous exposure to certain allergens are relatively refractory to the beneficial effects of ICSs on symptoms and lung function. The mechanisms of this relative steroid resistance are not yet fully understood. Recent data suggest that vitamin D deficiency is associated with worse asthma control, and the mechanism may involve induced steroid resistance.[97] Vitamin D deficiency is associated with increased oxidative stress and enhanced expression of inflammatory mediators such as TNFα and NF-κB in patients with asthma exacerbations.[98] Vitamin D also prevents the conversion of CD8 T lymphocytes to those that produce IL-13 by affecting activity of CYP11A1, a steroidogenic enzyme.[99,100] Studies to further examine the role of vitamin D in steroid resistance are ongoing. Oxidative stress also results in reduced expression and activity of HDAC2; consequently, transcription of inflammatory genes is not inactivated and inflammation becomes resistant to the antiinflammatory actions of glucocorticoids.[95]

The dose-response curve for ICS treatment reaches a plateau at a fairly low dose in most patients, and there is little added benefit to pulmonary function or airway reactivity when doses are as much as quadrupled. A study performed in adults to evaluate the efficacy and safety of escalating doses of ICS demonstrated that, for the majority of patients, maximal improvement in FEV_1 and methacholine responsiveness occurred at low to moderate doses of FP and BDP, with no added benefit of extremely high doses.[101] However, a substantial linear increase in cortisol suppression was seen as ICS dose increased. Therefore in the majority of patients, the most clinical benefit with the least risk will occur at low to medium doses of ICS. However, higher doses of ICS may be required to effectively decrease serious exacerbations. Patients receiving higher ICS doses require more careful monitoring for both response to therapy and emergence of systemic side effects.

ADVERSE EFFECTS OF INHALED CORTICOSTEROIDS

Local adverse effects, such as oral candidiasis and dysphonia, are the most common but least severe complications of ICS treatment. They are dose-related with some variability depending on steroid type, and they only occur in a small minority of patients (1%–3%). Reducing the dose, using a spacer device, and rinsing the mouth with water after use may minimize both these side effects. The more serious systemic adverse effects for children include adrenal suppression and depression of linear growth. A meta-analysis of 15 studies comparing low to medium dose ICS with placebo or nonsteroidal drugs in a total of more than 5700 children for at least 3 months found a mean reduction in linear growth velocity of 0.48 cm per year and a decrease of 0.6 cm from predicted height over 12 months in children who received ICS. There were no differences in growth velocity between placebo and ICS groups over subsequent years in the few studies that reported growth for longer than 1 year.[102] Thus the effect of ICSs on linear growth in most patients is minimal, even after long-term administration of low-dose ICSs. Most of the decrease in growth velocity appears in the first few months after initiating steroid treatment. The specific ICS molecule given was more important than age, delivery device, or dose in determining the magnitude of the effect.[102–104] However, head-to-head comparisons among ICS molecules are needed to provide more definitive data. Data on the growth of children in the 4-year-long CAMP trial demonstrated that there was indeed a significant decline in growth velocity over the first year of the study, but the growth rate returned to normal thereafter. Children in the BUD group were on average 1.1 cm shorter than those in the placebo and nedocromil groups at the end of the 4-year treatment period.[16] In addition, Agertoft and Pedersen showed that there was no reduction in final predicted adult height in a group of 142 children treated with a mean dose of 400 μg/day of BUD for an average of 9.2 years.[105] These longer-term studies of chronic low-dose ICSs point to an excellent safety profile and the potential to reach final predicted adult height, in spite of short-term decline in height velocity.

Adrenal suppression has been extensively studied, although the results are often difficult to interpret owing to flawed design, previous use of oral corticosteroids, or inappropriate tests used to assess adrenal function. Nonetheless, adrenal suppression is unlikely in children receiving less than 400 μg/day of inhaled BUD, or fluticasone 200 μg/day, even after long-term use.[1,16]

Adrenal suppression indicated by impaired adrenocorticotropic hormone stimulation tests can be demonstrated in children receiving higher doses; however, in most patients, even these impairments are of no or uncertain clinical significance when the patient is well. A significant stress (e.g., major illness, surgery) could warrant administration of exogenous corticosteroids to prevent an Addisonian response.[106]

Since there is variability among individual clinical response to corticosteroids and the predisposition to develop adverse effects, careful monitoring of each patient's growth during ICS treatment should be performed, and the dose should be adjusted to the lowest necessary to achieve good symptom control.

Systemic Corticosteroids

The therapeutic benefits of systemic corticosteroids when used as chronic therapy are marred by their potential adverse effects, which include excessive weight gain, hypertension, osteoporosis, decreased linear growth, metabolic derangement, and cataracts. Adverse effects from long-term steroid therapy may be reduced, but not eliminated, by using steroids with shorter half-lives (e.g., prednisone, prednisolone, methylprednisolone) at the lowest possible dose administered in the morning in a single dose and given every other day.

LONG-ACTING β AGONISTS

β-adrenergic agonists that have a prolonged duration of action (8–24 hours) occupy a unique niche in the asthma treatment armamentarium, somewhere between that of a controller and a reliever medication. There are currently two long-acting β agonists (LABAs) available on the US market and approved for use in children: salmeterol (approved for patients 4 years of age and older) and formoterol (approved for patients 12 years of age and older); others, such as indacaterol and vilanterol, both ultralong acting β_2 agonists with a 24-hour duration of action, are available but not approved for use in children. Indacaterol is approved only for treatment of COPD, and vilanterol is only approved to treat *adults* with asthma.

Formoterol and salmeterol differ in structure, potency, efficacy, and selectivity for the beta receptor. Salmeterol is a partial agonist, has a relatively slow onset of action (10–30 minutes), and has extremely high selectivity for the β_2 receptor. Salmeterol is more than 10,000 times more lipophilic than albuterol, and it also has three to four times the affinity for the β_2 receptor of albuterol. However, salmeterol diffuses out into the cell membrane somewhat slowly to approach the β_2 adrenoceptor active site, which results in a slower onset of action. Salmeterol has a long side chain that interacts with an exosite domain of the β_2 receptor. This side chain attachment allows association and dissociation with the active receptor site for a prolonged time period and results in the long duration of drug action (9–12 hours).[107,108] Salmeterol is available as both a dry powder in a Diskus device and in combination with fluticasone as a MDI in the United States.

Formoterol is a moderately lipophilic, highly effective full agonist with a very different molecular structure from salmeterol. It is taken up into the cell membrane to form a dose-dependent depot, from where it progressively diffuses out to interact with the active site. It has a rapid onset of action (~5 minutes) comparable to albuterol, but duration of activity is 12 hours. Formoterol is dispensed as a DPI or MDI in the United States and is also available in combination with BUD or mometasone in the United States.

The continued use of LABAs can lead to an alteration in their biologic effects. Although the mechanisms of tolerance to the bronchoprotective effect are unclear, downregulation of beta-receptor number or lack of receptor sensitivity are possibilities. Following a single dose of salmeterol (25–50 µg), there is sustained improvement in bronchodilatation for at least 12 hours, as well as a bronchoprotective effect to the bronchoconstriction caused by both methacholine and exercise. However, after repeated doses, within a few days or weeks there is a loss in the degree of bronchoprotection to methacholine and exercise. However, the loss of bronchoprotection is greater for exercise than in the response to methacholine, but it is unclear if this is clinically significant. When used as monotherapy (which is medical negligence in children), protection from EIB persists after daily dosing for 2–4 weeks, but in several studies the duration of action decreases from 9 to 12 hours to as little as 1 hour. The bronchodilator effect is less likely to decrease than the bronchoprotective effect following repeated dosing, and the decline is usually most apparent after a few days of use, followed by stabilization. Formoterol is likely to behave in a fashion similar to salmeterol.[108] Long-term use of LABAs has been shown to decrease responsiveness to SABA via β_2 adrenoreceptor downregulation. Similar to the decrease in bronchoprotection, the clinical significance of the reduction in response to albuterol after continued use of LABAs is unclear.[109–112] At least one study has demonstrated no loss of asthma control in patients using LABAs, even when a decrease in bronchoprotection is confirmed.[113]

The LABAs are not generally considered antiinflammatory agents, but studies show that salmeterol has either no effect on airway inflammation or reduces inflammatory cells in the airway mucosa. It has also been proposed that LABAs may enhance the actions of ICSs, and the mechanism has been linked to regulator of G-protein signaling 2 (RGS2) expression, which inhibits the intracellular influx of Ca^{2+} triggered by spasmogens.[114]

Past and recent concerns persist about the use of LABAs as monotherapy and the risk of adverse events. A study performed by the Asthma Clinical Research Network demonstrated that the combination of triamcinolone and salmeterol was effective in controlling asthma in patients 12–65 years of age.[115] However, complete withdrawal of the ICS and continuation of the LABA caused significant deterioration in asthma control, as measured by asthma exacerbations, deterioration in pulmonary function, and the need for oral corticosteroid treatment. These data and those from similar studies all suggest that LABAs cannot be used as a replacement for ICSs and should never be used as monotherapy for treatment of chronic asthma. Deaths have also been reported in patients chronically using inhaled salmeterol. It remains uncertain if there is a direct link between medication use and death, or if the increase in deaths is a reflection of inappropriate use of a LABA (e.g., attempt to use it as an acute bronchodilator or in place of a controller medication). A large trial (>26,000 enrollees) compared the safety of daily salmeterol or placebo added to usual treatment for chronic asthma over a 28-week period.[116] The Salmeterol Multicenter Asthma Research Trial (SMART) trial was stopped early when an interim analysis showed futility in reaching the required enrollment numbers as well as an association between salmeterol use and severe or fatal asthma. The risk for asthma-related death, albeit small (13 of 13,174) in the salmeterol group, was significantly greater than that in the placebo group (4 of 13,179); RR = 4.37 (95%, CI 1.25–15.34) for combined asthma deaths or life-threatening experiences. This translates into a death rate of 1.98 per 1000 person-years and is significantly greater than the expected death rate in the United States asthmatic population of 0.48/1000 person-years. Importantly, the increased risk for death was stronger in African-American subjects. The African-American participants were also more likely to have more severe asthma and less likely to be treated with an ICS. However, the study was not designed or powered to accurately examine the effects of race or concomitant use of an ICS on modulating the effect of salmeterol. Although there were a number of flaws in this trial, the data resulted in a "black box" warning being placed on the salmeterol package insert advising of the potential risk of life-threatening asthma. The results of several subsequent pooled analyses of adverse effects of LABA have also supported the conclusion that unopposed LABA use is associated with asthma deaths. As a result, the US FDA now recommends that (1) LABA not be used as monotherapy, (2) LABA not be used in patients whose asthma is well-controlled on ICS alone, (3) LABA be used in combination with another controller medication, and (4) LABA be discontinued as soon as possible after asthma control is achieved. In addition, a recent meta-analysis that used reports of events provided by the drug manufacturers to the FDA suggests that there is an increased risk of death with LABA use even with the use of an ICS.[117] Reassuring results were obtained in a recent multicenter trial of 11,679 adolescents and adults where there was no increased risk for an asthma related adverse event when LABA was added to ICS therapy and delivered by a single inhaler.[118] These data remain controversial, and further large-scale trials are planned to determine the actual risk.

Some of the risk attributable to chronic LABA use may be attributed to polymorphisms in the *BAR* at the 16 position. Similar to the results obtained with chronic administration of SABA to those with the *Arg/Arg* polymorphism, it was suspected that deterioration in pulmonary function and symptom control might occur with LABA use, even when given in conjunction with an ICS. In a prospective randomized crossover 18-week study of ICS treatment plus LABA or placebo in adult patients stratified by *BAR 16* polymorphisms (*Arg/Arg* or *Gly/Gly*), there was no difference in the degree of improvement in PEFR or FEV_1 with the addition of LABA, regardless of genotype. However, those with the *Gly/Gly* polymorphism had a higher PC_{20} with LABA treatment compared with placebo; there was no difference in PC_{20} in the *Arg/Arg* group between placebo and LABA.[119] No difference in adverse effects was seen in either group. These data suggest that chronic use of LABA in combination with an ICS is safe in patients with either genotype. However, longer-duration treatment and larger-scale studies will be necessary to determine continued efficacy and safety.

A major benefit of LABAs is use in combination with an ICS to improve asthma control without increasing the steroid dose. A number of studies that included older children and adults have demonstrated that the addition of a LABA to a regimen that includes an ICS results in better asthma control and improved pulmonary function compared to doubling the dose of ICS.[120] More importantly, the ICS dose can often be reduced by as much as 50% and still maintain asthma control when the LABA is added. Although the data are striking and consistent in studies on adults, there are fewer pediatric studies. An early study suggested that addition of a LABA to an ICS in pediatric patients may not have the same steroid-sparing effect or enhancement of steroid effect as that seen in adults and found the addition of a LABA or higher-dose ICS conferred no further benefit, but growth suppression occurred at the higher ICS dose.[121] A more recent large multicenter trial (VIAPAED) compared the effect of salmeterol 50 mg plus fluticasone 100 μg combination (given in a single inhaler) compared with fluticasone 200 μg given twice daily for 8 weeks in 441 children 4–16 years of age whose asthma was not well-controlled while taking an ICS alone.[122] Children in the salmeterol plus fluticasone group had significantly greater improvement in morning PEFR (improvement of 30.4 ± 34.1 L/min combination vs. 16.7 ± 35.8 L/min fluticasone) and a longer duration of asthma control (~1 week longer, favoring combination). A meta-analysis of 10 studies examining high-dose ICS compared with low-dose ICS and LABA concluded that the addition of LABA to ICS allowed a 37%–60% reduction in inhaled steroid dose without loss of asthma control.[120]

A study conducted by the Childhood Asthma Research and Education Network in asthmatic children 6–17 years of age who were not well controlled on ICS alone examined the response to the addition of LABA, increasing the dose of ICS, or adding the leukotriene receptor antagonist (LTRA) montelukast.[123] Using a double-blind randomized triple-crossover design and a composite of three outcomes (exacerbations, asthma-control days, and FEV_1), this study demonstrated a differential response to the treatment steps in 161 of the 165 children enrolled. The response to LABA step-up was most likely to be the best option compared with LTRA (1.6 relative probability) or increasing the ICS dose (1.7 relative probability). White race or Hispanic ethnicity predicted a better response to LABA; African Americans were as likely to respond to LABA as to ICS step-up therapy and least likely to respond to LTRA. Although all step-up options provided good symptom control during the trial, none of the step-up options eliminated acute asthma flares. The duration of this trial was relatively short (16 weeks), and issues of safety or long-term maintenance of effect remain unanswered. Although some would argue that increasing the dose of ICS may be safer and less expensive than adding a LABA or LTRA, the more important issue is to carefully and frequently monitor the patient with poorly controlled asthma who requires any step-up therapy to ensure both safety and efficacy. Failure to improve or the development of any adverse effect or medication intolerance warrants further medication adjustment and reevaluation.

Overuse (or possibly any use) of LABA could also be detrimental to some patients, as suggested by a systematic review of adverse events associated with LABA plus ICS use.[124] However, more recent meta-analyses and systematic reviews have shown that there is no increased risk for adverse asthma-related events in patients receiving a combination of inhaled steroid and LABA compared with those receiving inhaled steroid alone in studies examining both salmeterol and formoterol.[125,126] Similar reassuring results were obtained in a recent multicenter trial of 11,679 adolescents and adults, which found there was no increased risk for asthma-related adverse events when LABA was added to ICS therapy and delivered by a single inhaler.[118] Finally, a multicenter international pediatric study including over 6200 children age 4–11 years found no increase in safety events (hospitalizations, intubation, or death) or decrease in efficacy (time to exacerbation requiring oral steroids) for fluticasone-salmeterol fixed-dose combination compared with fluticasone alone over 26 weeks.[127] There were no deaths or asthma-related intubations for any enrollees in the study regardless of treatment group; however, children with very severe or unstable asthma were not included in the study. Both of these large-scale prospective studies examining safety and efficacy of ICS and LABA provide further evidence that ICS and LABA combinations are safe for use in the pediatric population.

There are currently four fixed-dose combination-inhaled steroid and LABA medications available: fluticasone proprionate/salmeterol, BUD/formoterol, mometasone/formoterol, and fluticasone furoate/vilanterol. The dosing interval for all but one is every 12 hours (fluticasone furoate plus vilanterol is once a day). It is also possible to administer each medication separately from individual inhalers; however, this is less convenient for the patient, may be more expensive, and runs the risk of inadvertent overuse, or even sole use, of LABA. Although use of separate inhalers does allow more flexibility in adjusting the dose of ICS, this strategy is not recommended because of the risks associated with unopposed LABA use. Salmeterol is combined with fluticasone in a DPI or MDI; the dose of salmeterol is 50 μg per inhalation in the DPI and 21 μg per inhalation in the MDI, while the fluticasone component is available in three different concentrations to allow for flexibility in dosing the ICS while avoiding excessive LABA use. A combination of formoterol and BUD or mometasone is also available in DPI or MDI forms. Salmeterol is a partial agonist of the β receptor compared with formoterol, which results in a flatter dose response curve and a weaker protective effect against methacholine-induced airway reactivity for salmeterol.

When the LABA combined with an ICS is formoterol, a different dosing strategy is possible because of the rapid onset of action of formoterol. When formoterol is taken in combination with an ICS for relief of symptoms at the first sign of deterioration, the additional dose of ICS helps prevent serious exacerbation. This strategy was examined in a large multicenter trial that evaluated 2760 asthmatics 4–80 years of age who were randomized to treatment with BUD 320 mg twice daily and terbutaline as reliever, BUD/formoterol 80/4.5 mg twice daily and terbutaline as reliever, or BUD/formoterol 80/4.5 mg twice daily both as maintenance and reliever. The child treatment arm (4–11 years of age) was dosed at once a day.[128,129] Both adults and children in the BUD-formoterol as maintenance and reliever arm had significantly reduced risk of exacerbation compared to the other two treatment arms. The child study showed a significant reduction in severe exacerbations (defined as sustained fall in morning PEFR, need for oral corticosteroid, acute care visit or hospitalization); 14% of those in the combined maintenance plus reliever group had a severe exacerbation, compared with 38% in the BUD/formoterol plus SABA group and 26% in the BUD plus SABA group. In addition, the overall exposure to oral corticosteroids and exacerbations requiring medical attention was also significantly reduced in the maintenance plus reliever group. Moreover, linear growth over the year was approximately 1 cm greater in the groups receiving BUD/formoterol compared with the higher-dose BUD group. Although this treatment approach has found acceptance in Europe, Australia, and Canada (but not in the United States), some concerns remain about safety and long-term effectiveness. Overuse of the BUD/formoterol combination can occur, leading some patients to mask progressing symptoms or delay seeking medical attention.

Leukotriene Antagonists

Leukotrienes are lipid mediators produced by the metabolism of arachidonic acid via a complex cascade, including the action of phospholipase A_2. The enzyme 5-lipoxygenase catalyzes the production of leukotrienes, LTB_4 and the cysteinyl members LTC_4, LTD_4, and LTE_4, from arachidonic acid. Arachidonic acid can also be a precursor for the cyclooxygenase pathway and results in the production of prostaglandins and thromboxane. However, it is the cysteinyl leukotrienes (cysLTs) that are the potent mediators which induce smooth muscle constriction, vascular permeability, mucus hypersecretion, edema formation, and inflammatory cell recruitment into the airways. Elevated levels of cysLTs are recovered from bronchoalveolar lavage fluid, and urinary LTE_4 levels are elevated following airway allergen challenge in atopic asthmatics. CysLTs are produced by a number of cell types found in the airways, including mast cells, eosinophils, basophils, macrophages, and neutrophils. Corticosteroids do not directly inhibit the synthesis or block the action of leukotrienes.

Two basic strategies targeting cysLTs include inhibition of 5-lipoxygenase and leukotriene receptor antagonism. Because of the nature of the lipoxygenase synthetic cascade, interruption at an early level (e.g., at the 5-lipoxygenase) could diminish overall cysteinyl LT and LTB_4 production, both of which are generally elevated in biological fluids (i.e., blood, bronchoalveolar lavage fluid, urine) from symptomatic asthmatics. The 5-lipoxygenase inhibitor zileuton blocks the bronchoconstriction response to inhaled allergen or cold air challenge, exercise, and aspirin ingestion in sensitive individuals. However, because the drug can cause hepatic injury, which is usually reversible, regular liver enzyme monitoring is necessary. Although previously the drug required 4 times daily dosing, an extended release form that permits twice a day dosing is now available.

There are two clinically available LTRAs: zafirlukast and montelukast. When administered orally, zafirlukast resulted in significant reduction in daytime and nighttime symptoms and the need for SABA compared with placebo. Zafirlukast has modest efficacy at best, must be given twice daily, and in some patients also results in elevated hepatic enzymes. Montelukast is a LTD_4 receptor antagonist and is administered once daily. It has been shown in a number of studies to decrease urinary excretion of LTE_4, reduce both circulating and sputum eosinophil counts, and decrease exhaled NO.[1] Clinical effects include improvement in FEV_1 and protection from EIB and allergen-induced bronchospasm. Improvement in pulmonary function can be detected after the first dose and reaches a peak after a few weeks of treatment. However, the montelukast effect on asthma control is not as great as that from an ICS, as measured by improvement in FEV_1, symptom control, and reduction in inflammatory markers.[130] Trials in children with slightly more severe disease based on lower FEV_1 also showed significantly greater improvement in pulmonary function measures, symptom reduction, and need for rescue SABA with fluticasone compared with montelukast.[131]

Predicting which patients will have a more favorable response to montelukast versus ICSs has proven difficult. However, a study examining the rate of response of children with mild asthma to ICS, montelukast, or both demonstrated that 23% responded to fluticasone alone, 5% responded to montelukast alone, 17% responded to both, but 55% responded to neither drug.[132] Children who are older, have had asthma for a longer duration, have a parental history of asthma, have a higher exhaled NO, and have a lower PC_{20} are more likely to respond favorably to ICS treatment compared with LTRA treatment.[133]

Montelukast may provide improved asthma control when combined with other controller medications, such as inhaled steroids. Although study results are somewhat conflicting, most show that the addition of montelukast to an ICS results in modest improvement that is not quite as efficacious as adding an LABA, particularly on pulmonary function outcomes. One pediatric trial demonstrated a small improvement in FEV_1 (6.0% montelukast, 4.1% placebo, $P < .01$) and in the need for rescue bronchodilator use (1.65 puffs/day montelukast, 1.98 puffs/day placebo, $P < .013$) when montelukast was added to a regimen of low-dose BUD.[134]

Adverse effects of montelukast have been relatively minor and mainly consist of headache, abdominal pain, vivid dreams, and sleep disruption. Reports of behavioral changes (e.g., moodiness, depression) and an unsubstantiated association with a suicide report have led to a label change including behavioral changes as a possible side effect of treatment with montelukast. There are several case reports of adults developing Churg-Strauss syndrome when treatment with montelukast was instituted and ICS treatment withdrawn. Since the majority of these patients had what was considered to be severe steroid-dependent asthma, it is believed that the development of systemic vasculitis was actually the emergence of an underlying disease as a result of steroid withdrawal and less likely a result of the direct action of montelukast. Care should be taken, however, if montelukast is used in an attempt to decrease or discontinue oral steroids in a patient with presumed severe asthma.

Long-Acting Muscarinic Antagonists

Short-acting quaternary anticholinergic medications such as ipratropium bromide have been used for decades as bronchodilators in the treatment of asthma. Tiotropium, a long-acting muscarinic receptor antagonist with a duration of action of 24 hours, which has been a mainstay of COPD treatment, has recently been approved for use in patients with severe persistent asthma not controlled with ICS. There are five subtypes of muscarinic receptors, three of which are found in human airways (M_1, M_2, M_3). All three types of muscarinic receptors mediate neurally induced bronchoconstriction. Tiotropium has a high affinity for M receptors but dissociates very slowly from type M1 and M3 receptors, resulting in prolonged prevention of bronchoconstriction and a 24-hour bronchodilatation effect.[96]

Although there is a paucity of studies compared to those examining glucocorticoids, the available data have consistently shown that tiotropium, when added to ICS or ICS and LABA, resulted in improved lung function, which was maintained even after ICS dose reduction and LABA discontinuation.[135,136] In fact, when used in combination with low-dose ICS, tiotropium is more effective at improving lung function than doubling the ICS dose and is noninferior to LABA as measured by decrease in symptom days, improvement in quality of life, and asthma control score.[136–138] When added to medium-dose ICS, tiotropium continued to result in improvement in lung function[135,136,138,139] The effect on lung function is comparable to that of salmeterol, and there may also be acute bronchodilatation in patients with poorly controlled symptoms.[137,140,141] In addition, tiotropium in combination with ICS and LABA decreased the risk of severe exacerbations, and extended the length of time to the first exacerbation.[139,142]

Most studies of tiotropium in asthma have been conducted with adults, however more recently there have been trials with children that show similar benefits and an excellent safety profile.[138,139,143,144] Tiotropium has been added as recommended therapy for children aged ≥ 12 years in steps 4 and 5 of the most recent version of the GINA guidelines.[72] Tiotropium is available in two doses via soft mist MDI (Respimat), 2.5 µg and 1.25 µg per actuation. Two puffs of the 1.25 µg dose administered once daily has been approved in the United States for children with asthma, although higher doses have been approved for use in COPD.[145] Peak effect on FEV_1 occurs within 1–3 hours after dosing. Other anticholinergic agents such as umeclindinium and aclinidium are currently used in treatment of COPD but have not yet been adequately studied in asthma.

METHYLXANTHINES: THEOPHYLLINE

Although methylxanthines have been used for the treatment of asthma since the early part of the 20th century, their role in managing acute and chronic asthma has become very restricted. Theophylline is now considered a second- or third-line medication, largely because it is a poor acute bronchodilator; it has a narrow therapeutic index and significant adverse effects, and antiinflammatory drugs have replaced it. It does have the advantage of being inexpensive and can be administered in a long-acting oral formulation. Theophylline is a phosphodiesterase inhibitor that causes smooth muscle relaxation and bronchodilatation. However, theophylline can also act centrally as a respiratory stimulant and may also increase diaphragmatic contractility and help prevent diaphragmatic fatigue. In addition, more recent data suggest that it blocks histone deacetylation, which may be important to the action of corticosteroids and modulation of inflammatory mediators; further work is necessary to confirm the clinical relevance of this action. Low-dose theophylline (amounts sufficient to cause a serum level of 5–10 mg/mL) may be helpful in some patients for chronic management. The addition of theophylline to ICSs may have a steroid-sparing effect in some patients, but it is less effective than adding a long-acting β agonist.[146–149] However, adverse effects, such as tremor, gastric irritation, gastrointestinal hemorrhage, agitation, and convulsions, may occur at even relatively low serum concentrations. Also, many commonly used medications can interfere with theophylline metabolism, resulting in clinically significant elevation (e.g., some macrolide and fluoroquinolone antibiotics) or lowering (carbamazepine) of serum concentrations. Febrile viral illnesses may also substantially increase serum concentrations. Careful monitoring of serum concentration is mandatory when doses above 10 mg/kg per day are administered to children and adolescents.

BIOLOGIC THERAPY FOR ASTHMA

Several novel approaches to asthma therapy involve immune modulation, which may be useful for both the prevention and treatment of asthma. Use of a humanized monoclonal anti-IgE antibody (omalizumab) to complex with and lower the circulating concentration of IgE has demonstrated efficacy in select patients. This drug is approved by the US Food and Drug Administration for use in patients 6 years of age and older. Mepolizumab, a monoclonal antibody to IL-5, resulted in a significant reduction in exacerbations and improvement in quality of life for patients with severe eosinophilic asthma. It is approved in the United States for patients aged 12 years and older. Reslizumab, also an anti-IL-5 antibody, is available in the United States for those asthmatics ≥ 18 years old who have eosinophilic disease. Biologic therapies for asthma are discussed in more detail in Chapter 48.

Management of Chronic Asthma

The effective management of chronic asthma should focus on (1) identification and elimination of exacerbating or aggravating factors, (2) pharmacologic therapy, and (3) education of the patient and family about the disease and the management skills necessary to avoid and treat acute exacerbations. The goals of management of chronic asthma in children include minimizing symptoms and exacerbations, maintaining normal activities of daily living, maintaining normal or near-normal pulmonary function, and avoiding adverse effects from asthma medications. To achieve these goals, a combination of pharmacologic and nonpharmacologic modalities must be utilized.

Successful asthma management includes appropriate grading of disease control (see Table 45.3). Asthma severity, or the intrinsic intensity of the disease, should be distinguished from asthma control. Patients may have relatively mild asthma that is poorly controlled due to multiple factors, such as inadequate treatment, impaired adherence, or excessive exposure to allergens or irritants. Once appropriate medical and environmental measures are instituted, the asthma may become "mild" in terms of absence of symptoms and normalization of pulmonary function while taking low doses of a controller medication. Patients who demonstrate a progressive decline in pulmonary function, frequent exacerbations, and persistent or recurrent symptoms in spite of regular use of controller medication and environmental controls have more severe disease.

The emphasis in most guidelines is now placed on establishing asthma control, which includes minimizing impairment (symptoms) and avoiding risk of serious exacerbations, medication adverse effects, loss of lung function, and (in the case of children) reduction in lung growth. As discussed earlier in the chapter, other biomarkers of airway inflammation (eNO, sputum, or peripheral blood eosinophils) may add additional useful data for grading asthma severity and guiding treatment to improve control. Several brief, validated questionnaires can be used in most clinical or community settings to provide a rapid assessment of asthma control (see the section on "Other Measures for Assessing Asthma Severity and Control" earlier in the chapter). Although the utility of the scores as a single measure is established, the responsiveness to change over time, collection of data in relation to recent exacerbations, and seasonal variability all need further evaluation.

The risk domain of control includes exacerbations that are severe enough to warrant treatment with oral corticosteroids, emergency medical care, or hospitalizations. There are limited data that are useful in predicting future exacerbations; however, there is an inverse relationship between FEV_1 and the risk of developing an exacerbation in the subsequent year. In addition, having one severe exacerbation is a strong risk factor for a subsequent episode in the same year. Data are lacking to accurately correlate the number and severity of exacerbations with degree of asthma control. More than one exacerbation per year indicates asthma control is inadequate and the frequency and severity of exacerbations increases with worsening control. Patients should start treatment at the step most appropriate to the initial severity grading (or control level for those already receiving treatment) of their asthma.

The most recent National Asthma Education and Prevention Program (NAEPP) guidelines continue to list four severity classifications: intermittent, mild, moderate, and severe persistent, but have expanded the stepwise treatment algorithm to six steps while the GINA guidelines have five steps (Fig. 45.5). Immunotherapy continues to be recommended for children who are at steps 2–4, have documented allergy, and have persistent symptoms. However, immunotherapy is most likely to be effective for those with single allergen sensitization, and this evidence for efficacy is strongest for animal dander, house dust mites, and pollen. The two added treatment steps for adolescents and adults are aimed at those who are allergic, have refractory symptoms in spite of high-dose ICSs, plus another antiinflammatory controller. At these steps 5 and 6, recommended additional treatment includes oral corticosteroids and omalizumab for those older than 12 years of age who are also allergic. Mepolizumab, which was not available at the time of publication for the NAEPP guidelines, should now be considered for patients 12 years of age and older who have eosinophilic asthma and are not well controlled, with high-dose ICS and another controller. The GINA guidelines for asthma management have included tiotropium as add-on therapy for patients requiring step 4 or step 5 therapies in the 2015 revision.[72] The treatment steps are used in conjunction with control levels. Patients who achieve good control are maintained at the lowest step level possible. Those with not well-controlled or poorly controlled asthma receive step-up treatment until control is achieved. Step-down to a lower treatment level should be attempted once control is maintained for at least 3 months and no other contraindications for reducing medication exist (e.g., persistent allergen exposure, entry into high-risk season). Patient education, environmental controls, and management of comorbid conditions are stressed at all steps. In addition, it is critical that all patients and their adult caregivers be thoroughly trained in the appropriate use of the specific medication delivery devices and monitoring tools prescribed (e.g., MDI, DPI, nebulizer, PEFR meter). In addition to obtaining spirometry at the time of initial assessment, at least annual monitoring of lung function in children age 5 years and older is recommended for all levels of asthma severity; however, spirometry is more likely to be of value for those with more severe disease and low lung function at baseline. Spirometry should also be obtained during periods of progressive or prolonged loss of asthma control.[1]

Intermittent Asthma

Children with intermittent asthma or EIA have brief episodes of wheeze or cough that are easily relieved with SABA treatment and occur no more frequently than once or twice per week. Treatment is with the as-needed use of an inhaled SABA agonist.[1] The usual dose of inhaled racemic albuterol is 2–6 puffs (90 µg/puff) every 3–4 hours or 0.15 mg/kg (usual dose 2.5 mg, maximum 5 mg) nebulized from a small-volume nebulizer in 2 mL of saline. Other SABAs (e.g., levalbuterol and terbutaline) may also be used, and it is unlikely that there is any significant difference in efficacy among the drugs. Numerous studies have demonstrated that administration of albuterol by MDI is equally effective as that given by nebulizer.[1,65] Moreover, use of an MDI by older

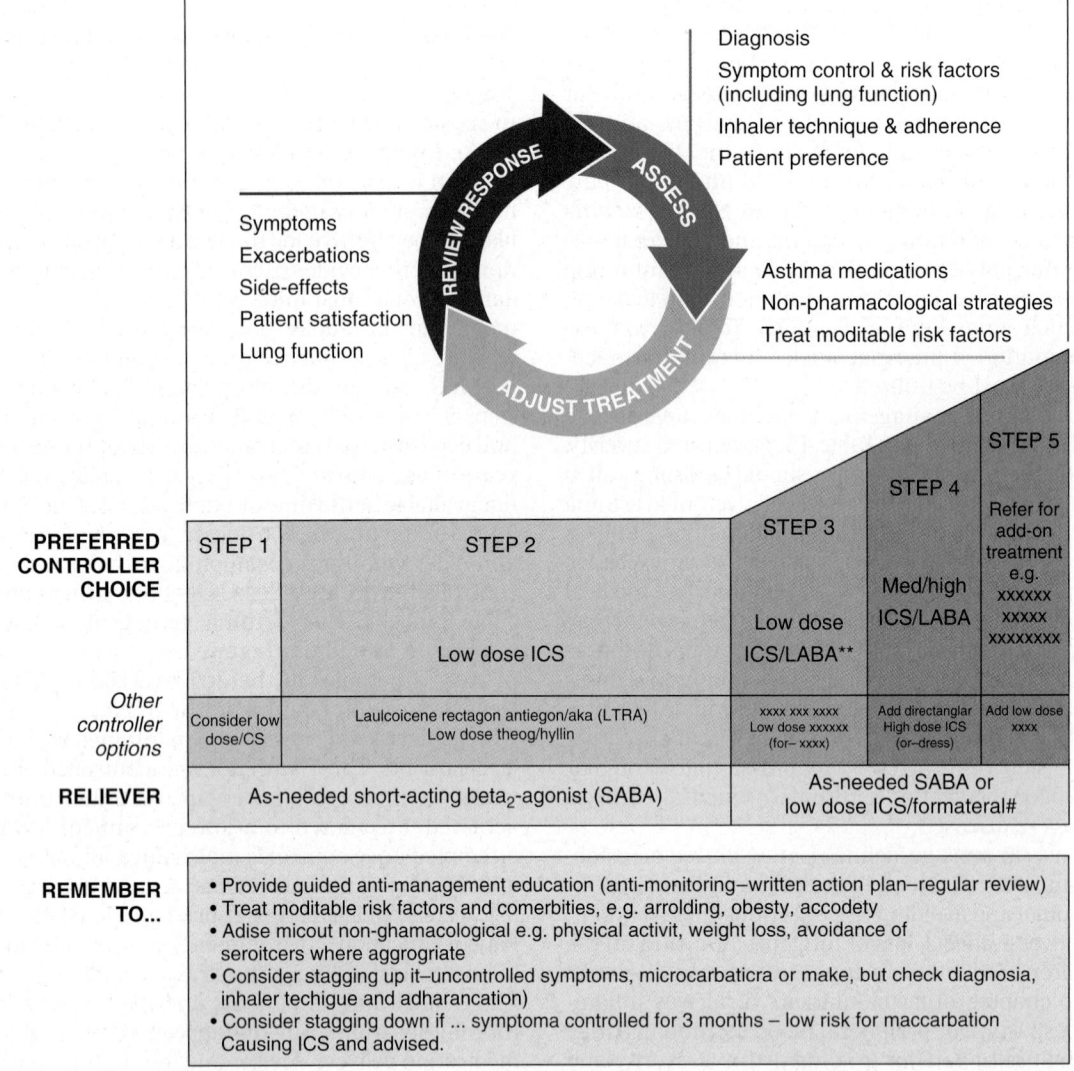

Fig. 45.5 Stepwise treatment algorithm for chronic treatment of children and adolescents with asthma. *ICS,* Inhaled corticosteroids; *LABA,* long-acting β agonists. (Figure reproduced with permission from 2016 GINA Report, Global Strategy for Asthma Management and Prevention, www.ginasthma.org.)

children (with or without a valved holding chamber [VHC]) is far more convenient and less expensive than a nebulizer. EIA may be prevented to a large extent with inhalation of albuterol (or formoterol) 5–20 minutes before exercise. Montelukast taken 1–2 hours before exercise may also help prevent EIB.

Mild Persistent Asthma

The majority of asthmatics are classified as having mild persistent asthma, based on symptoms that occur several times per week, but not daily; infrequent nocturnal symptoms; and normal pulmonary function. The primary treatment of mild persistent asthma is a low-dose ICS. Data from multiple studies support the superior efficacy of ICSs compared with other treatments in improving pulmonary function, reducing symptoms and need for rescue medications, and improving bronchial hyperreactivity. As outlined previously, the safety profile for ICSs given at low dose is excellent. There are few data to suggest that one type of ICS will offer

significantly greater benefit than the others, but the dose equivalency and ranges for low, medium, and high doses differ (see Table 45.5). BDP, fluticasone, and BUD have been extensively studied in children for many years, are available in easy-to-use devices (MDIs or DPIs), are well tolerated by most patients, and the adverse event profile is well understood. Large comparative effectiveness trials, particularly in children, are sparse. However, a retrospective observational study that used a large general practice research database in the United Kingdom examined asthma control in newly treated asthmatics 5–60 years of age. Using a matched cohort analysis, more than 2600 patients, including 773 children age 5–12 years of age who were prescribed HFA BDP, or FP, were followed for 2 years. Although more than 80% of the patients in each group achieved control, patients who were treated with or received step-up treatment with BDP were more likely to be controlled (adjusted odds ratio 1.30; 95% CI, 1.02–1.65).[150] However, the control measure used was a composite of largely risk domain elements (i.e., exacerbation, oral steroid use, hospitalization) and probably missed impairment domain measures (symptoms). Older inhaled steroids (e.g., flunisolide, triamcinolone) with lower topical potency are used less frequently. Newer inhaled steroids, such as mometasone and ciclesonide, are currently labeled for use in the United States for children 12 years of age and older.

Although chronic daily dosing of ICS is the general recommendation to maintain good asthma control, other strategies have been investigated and hold promise as valid alternatives. There are a few studies that have compared chronic daily inhaled steroid use with intermittent treatment. There was no difference in morning PEFR or asthma exacerbations between those that used daily inhaled steroids and those that used them as needed, but daily use of inhaled steroids resulted in better asthma control based on symptom days, asthma control scores, FeNO, and eosinophils.[151,152] This strategy appears to benefit the risk domain more than the impairment (daily symptom) domain; therefore if daily symptom burden reduction is more important than infrequent and mild exacerbation reduction, a daily treatment strategy may be preferable.

Implications for pediatric asthma management with intermittent steroid use may be even greater, since the risk of growth suppression is higher in children. A recent study compared daily with as needed use of BDP in children with mild asthma who were previously well controlled while taking daily low-dose ICS. In this multicenter study, children ages 5–18 were randomly assigned to one of four treatment groups: placebo twice daily with albuterol plus placebo as rescue, placebo twice daily with albuterol plus BDP as rescue, BDP twice daily with albuterol plus placebo as rescue, or BDP twice daily with BDP plus albuterol as rescue. Children who received inhaled steroids daily had fewer exacerbations than children who used no inhaled steroids and albuterol alone as rescue (28% vs. 49%, $P = .03$). Children who received BDP daily and as a rescue (with albuterol) or as rescue (with albuterol) only had fewer exacerbations than the placebo group, but the results did not reach statistical significance (31% for BDP daily and as rescue with albuterol, $P = .07$; 35% for BDP as rescue only with albuterol, $P = .07$). Notably, linear growth was over 1 cm lower in both groups who received inhaled steroids daily compared with the group which received no ICS ($P < .0001$). There was no difference in growth between the placebo group (no ICS) and those who received BDP only as a rescue medication ($P = .26$).[153] These data suggest that some patients with mild asthma of relatively new onset may achieve adequate control with intermittent ICS use after a period of stabilization with continuous ICS treatment, and with less risk of minor growth suppression. However, daily use of an ICS, even when tapered to low dose, provides the best overall control, particularly in the exacerbation risk domain.

An alternative treatment is an LTRA, such as montelukast. This drug has the advantage of once-a-day oral administration and only uncommon mild adverse effects (i.e., nausea, headache, vivid dreams). However, numerous comparative studies indicate that ICSs provide superior asthma control.[133,154] Although the current NAEPP guidelines still list cromolyn, nedocromil, and theophylline as alternative treatments, nedocromil and cromolyn have limited availability (neither is available for inhalation in the United States) and efficacy, while theophylline is less well tolerated.

Moderate Persistent Asthma

Children who have daily symptoms, nocturnal symptoms more than weekly, and mild obstruction on pulmonary function have moderate persistent asthma. Children who continue to experience symptoms or exacerbations while being treated with low-dose ICSs should have a step up in treatment. Current recommendations for treatment include increasing the ICS dose to the moderate range, or continuing the low-dose ICS and adding a second controller drug with a complimentary mechanism of action. As discussed earlier in the chapter, the dose response curve for ICSs reaches a plateau at relatively modest doses, as determined by pulmonary function and bronchial hyperreactivity measures. However, certain patients may derive benefit in both the impairment and risk domains when the ICS dose is increased to the moderate range. LABAs are the current add-on drugs of choice because of the large body of evidence from randomized controlled trials that indicate efficacy and effectiveness. In older children and adults, the addition of a LABA to a low-dose ICS results in greater improvement in pulmonary function and reduction in symptoms than a further increase in steroid dose. The availability of a fixed-dose combination of fluticasone and salmeterol or BUD and formoterol in a single inhaler make this combination attractive. An alternative is to raise the dose of the inhaled steroid alone to the medium range; this is the current recommended strategy for children younger than 4 years of age,[1] but is a secondary option in older children. When concerns exist about the use of LABA or medium-dose ICSs, the addition of an LTRA (e.g., montelukast) should be considered. Although the additive effect of LTRA is more limited, the safety profile may be viewed as more favorable. LTRA, when added to inhaled BUD in one study, resulted in a modest improvement in PEFR and a reduction in need for SABA.[134] Low-dose theophylline is another low-cost add-on medication that may also help improved symptom control. Data indicate that the latter two add-on medications are also effective in improving asthma control, but less so than the addition of a LABA. Use of theophylline as a single daily dose of a time-release preparation can be well tolerated and is typically less expensive than using a LABA or LTRA. Any patient who has deterioration of lung function while using a LABA chronically should have an alternative medication prescribed. Whatever combination of medications is used, attempts should be made at regular intervals to decrease the ICS dose to the lowest level that adequately controls symptoms and maintains normal pulmonary function. Children in this category will benefit from referral to a pulmonologist and may also require ongoing specialty care.

Severe Persistent Asthma

Approximately 5%–10% of patients will have severe persistent asthma as described by persistent daily symptoms, frequent nocturnal awakenings, and a moderate or severe obstructive pattern on pulmonary function testing. These symptoms may occur in spite of treatment with high-dose ICSs, LABAs, and/or a LTRA or low-dose theophylline. Patients with the most severe disease have inadequate response to even high doses of ICS in combination with other available controller medications. If there is no response, oral corticosteroids are the

Table 45.6   Directions for Use of a Metered-Dose Inhaler, With and Without a Spacer

MDI Use Without Spacer Device	MDI Use With Spacer Device
1. Shake canister for 5 s.	1. Shake canister for 5 s.
2. Position finger on top of canister for support.	2. Attach canister to spacer.
3. Patient exhales normally (to FRC).	3. Patient exhales normally (to FRC).
4. Place mouthpiece 2 cm in front of open mouth around tube (may place in mouth if coordination is a problem).	4. Place mouthpiece in mouth and close lips.
5. Begin slow inspiration.	5. Activate canister.
6. Activate canister.	6. Begin slow inspiration.
7. Complete inhalation over several seconds.	7. Complete inhalation over several seconds.
8. Hold breath for 10 s.	8. Hold breath for 10 s.
9. Wait 30–60 s, and repeat steps 2–8 for prescribed number of inhalations.	9. Wait 30–60 s, and repeat steps 2–8 for prescribed number of inhalations.

FRC, Functional Residual Capacity; *MDI,* metered-dosed inhaler.

next recommended treatment step. It may be necessary to administer a short course (<10 days) of daily dosing (40–60 mg/day) and then a longer every-other-day course at the lowest effective dose (0.5 mg/kg every other day). Before instituting such therapy, a thorough search for remediable exacerbating factors or comorbid conditions (e.g., sinusitis, persistent allergen exposure, poor compliance, GER, VCD) should be sought. As soon as symptoms are controlled, the lowest possible oral steroid dose at which symptom control is maintained should be administered. Although a single morning dose is generally preferred to minimize systemic side effects, some patients with severe or refractory symptoms may benefit from twice-daily dosing. Children receiving chronic oral corticosteroid therapy should be carefully monitored for development of adverse effects, such as hypertension, cataract formation, hyperglycemia, loss of bone mineral content, and impaired linear growth. Systemic corticosteroids may be given in the presence of acute viral infections, otitis media, or pneumonia and will not result in worsening infections. However, patients who develop varicella while taking systemic corticosteroids, or who take the medication during the incubation period, should have the steroid dose reduced to the minimum tolerable to control the asthma and should also be provided adrenal replacement. In addition, consideration should be given to administering acyclovir for 5–7 days, and the patient should be carefully observed for signs of severe or disseminated disease. If there has been a significant exposure to varicella identified within the previous 96 hours, passive immunization with varicella zoster immune globulin can be offered. Children with persistent asthma should receive varicella vaccine if they have not previously contracted the disease.

A proportion of severe asthmatics may be steroid resistant; in one series of patients with refractory asthma, 25% were determined to be steroid resistant. Such patients may have altered steroid metabolism or receptor dysfunction. A careful evaluation and specialized pharmacokinetic and cellular studies may be needed to ascertain the etiology of the defect. Patients deemed to be steroid resistant may be candidates for alternative therapies, such as omalizumab, mepolizumab, or other immune modulator treatments. Children with severe asthma should receive routine care from a specialist. Frequent visits to assess symptom control, pulmonary function testing, quality of life, patterns of medication use, presence of comorbid conditions, adverse effects caused by treatment, and adherence to treatment regimen are essential. Severe asthma is discussed in more detail in Chapter 46.

Holding Chambers and Spacer Devices

A number of studies indicate that as many as 80% of patients use MDIs incorrectly, even after appropriate instruction, and many residents, physicians, and nurses are unable to teach patients correctly. Proper steps are given in Table 45.6. Although there is a relatively small difference in the amount of medication that reaches the lower respiratory tract from a properly used MDI alone compared with an MDI plus a VHC (10% for MDI alone, 15% for MDI plus holding chamber), a VHC helps ensure that the maximum possible dose reaches its target. The holding chamber also minimizes deposition of the medication in the mouth and oropharynx, a particularly important feature when ICSs are prescribed. There are several important points to remember when using a VHC. The child should take a slow deep inspiration and try to hold his or her breath for 5–10 seconds after inhalation of the medication. Only one medication should be dispensed into the chamber at a time, although the same chamber may be used for other medications. A holding chamber that is of at least 150 mL volume and that accommodates the MDI canister in its original boot is preferable to one that requires the canister to be inserted into an adapter. The latter chambers may not result in accurate dispensing of medication because of a mismatch between the adapter and the actuator. Newer holding chambers are made of antistatic plastics or metal that minimizes static charge, which can cause excessive retention of medication in the chamber. Washing the chamber with a mild detergent and air drying can also help prevent static charge. See www.cdc.gov/asthma/inhaler_video/default.htm for a video demonstrating proper VHC (spacer) device use.

Peak Expiratory Flow Rate Monitoring

Home monitoring of PEFR has been advocated for optimal management of the patient with moderate to severe persistent asthma, but the utility remains somewhat limited. PEFR is only moderately correlated with FEV_1, and other measures such as FEF_{25-75}, FEF_{50}, or mid-maximal expiratory flow (MMEF) that can be used as a valid measure of obstructive ventilatory defect. The degree of diurnal and day-to-day PEFR variability has been proposed for years as a marker of asthma severity and airway hyperreactivity. However, the correlation between PEFR variability and airway hyperreactivity is only moderate. Moreover, the correlation of PEFR variability with other clinical markers of asthma disease activity or severity remains unclear. PEFR probably has its greatest value when used repeatedly to indicate severity of an acute asthma exacerbation and the subsequent response to treatment. Normal PEFR ranges are determined by the patient's age, sex, and height, and are readily available. Some patients have PEFR readings well above, or in some cases below, published standards. For this reason, an individual patient's personal best reading is often used as a target. It is important that the personal best be determined only when efforts have been made to ensure that asthma is optimally managed at the time the measure is made; this may require short courses of oral corticosteroids and other antiinflammatory medications.

Small portable handheld PEFR devices can provide an objective measure of lung function in the home or school setting. Currently available devices record measurements electronically and some also measure FEV_1 and FEV_6. Patients may use the PEFR reading to alter medications according to a predetermined plan. Patients and families must know when and how to use the PEFR meter, how to interpret the measurement and respond to the reading, and when to communicate with their physician. Some of these steps can be obviated with the use of a commercial system that uses a recording PEFR meter capable of transmitting a longitudinal report via phone line or the Internet to the managing physician. Although earlier guideline recommendations were that all patients with asthma use a PEFR-driven asthma action plan, studies suggest that routine use of PEFR monitoring is more likely to benefit those with more severe or unstable disease and is more likely to be used intermittently (around the time of increased symptoms or seasonally), rather than continuously.[1,72]

After determining the target, normal, or personal best PEFR reading, a care plan incorporating the measure can be made. Sample plans may be obtained from readily available sources (Fig. 45.6).[1]

The zones are generally defined as follows:

Green: PEFR 80%–100% predicted/personal best; all clear, no symptoms.
Yellow: PEFR 50%–80% predicted/personal best; indicates worsening airway obstruction or an impending attack. Symptoms include slowed play, intermittent cough, wheeze, and dyspnea.
Red: PEFR less than 50% predicted/personal best; indicates significant airway obstruction and need for immediate medical attention. Symptoms include severe dyspnea, retractions, continuous wheeze, or cough.

There are limitations to PEFR monitoring efficacy. The PEFR is effort-dependent, and some children learn how to deliberately adjust the reading artificially high or low by the effort used. In addition, PEFR only measures obstruction in the large central airways; many asthmatics have a normal or near-normal PEFR, but significant obstruction in the small airways or as measured by FEV_1 or FEV_1/FVC. Moreover, it is unclear that long-term PEFR use as part of an asthma action plan results in better outcomes than monitoring symptoms without PEFR and adjusting therapy accordingly.[13] Symptom-based asthma action plans are equally effective as those based on peak flow monitoring.

Nonpharmacologic Measures

Nonpharmacologic interventions necessary for successful management include formation of an effective partnership with a knowledgeable health care provider, frequent monitoring of asthma symptoms and response to therapy, objective measures of pulmonary function, and avoidance of asthma triggers. Trigger avoidance is important, yet patients are often unaware of specific triggers or how to put environmental controls in place. Environmental exposures (e.g., diesel particulates, ozone, and sulfur dioxide) are likely to be more pronounced in those living near highways, on bus lines, or near certain industrial plants. For the indoor environment, dust mites, cat and dog dander, mold, and, in the inner city, cockroach antigen have all been strongly linked to asthma exacerbations and morbidity. Removal of these allergens can result in reduced symptoms and airway hyperresponsiveness. However, it is difficult to reduce indoor allergen burden below the threshold likely to induce symptoms without a multifaceted approach. The use of room air filters and special cleaning agents have some appeal but are not as effective as keeping ambient humidity low (30%–40%), putting plasticized covers on pillows and mattresses, washing bedding weekly in hot water, and removing carpeting. A recent study suggested that application of dust covers alone is not effective in improving airway function. Removing pets from the bedroom and ideally from the household is also desirable. Exterminating roaches is difficult, but the use of integrated pest management strategies and eliminating water sources can be effective. For all asthmatics, avoidance of passive exposure to cigarette smoke is of paramount importance.

The Inner-City Asthma Study utilized a multidimensional environmental intervention that instructed families on providing a "safe sleeping zone" for the asthmatic child. Pets, dust, and other irritants were barred from the sleeping area, and HEPA room filters and vacuums were provided to all. In addition, specific strategies to reduce mold and roaches were implemented in households where dust sampling revealed high levels. This integrated and individualized strategy resulted in significant allergen reduction and improvement in symptom-free days over the yearlong intervention and beyond.[155] Another trial optimized asthma medical care and control and then provided a mold and moisture remediation program that removed existing mold and repaired construction defects and leaks that promoted the mold problem. Compared with those who lived in homes not remediated, the children in the intervention group had more symptom-free days and fewer serious exacerbations.[156] A multicenter study in Europe demonstrated that use of a device that provides temperature controlled, laminar air flow to reduce inhalant allergen exposure is associated with improved quality of life (as measured by the Asthma Quality of Life Questionnaire) and decreased FeNO level.[157]

Use of ancillary personnel (e.g., a social worker who can conduct formal risk assessment of psychosocial, economic, and school-related risks) may be of great benefit in improving asthma control. Social determinants of chronic disease management often relate to, or operate through, poverty.

ASTHMA ACTION PLAN

PLAN FOR: _____ Date: _____ Nurse: _____ Doctor: Dr. _____

Hospital/Emergency Phone Number: _xxx-xxx-xxxx/ 911_ Doctor's Phone: _xxx-xxx-xxxx_ (weekdays) / _xxx-xxx-xxxx_ (night and weekend)

GREEN ZONE: Doing Well

Take these control medicines every single day. They work to keep your lungs healthy and prevent asthma symptoms.

- No cough, wheeze, chest tightness, or shortness of breath during day or night

- Can do usual activities

PEAK FLOW between _____ and _____

(80%–100% of my best)

Medicine	How much to take	When to take it

Before running or sports:

☐ _____ ☐ 2 puffs ☐ 4 puffs ☐ 1 aerosol ☐ 5 to 20 minutes ☐ 60 minutes before exercise

YELLOW ZONE: Asthma Getting Worse

- Cough, wheeze, chest tightness, or shortness of breath, or
- Waking at night due to asthma, or
- Can do some, but NOT all activities

PEAK FLOW between _____ and _____

(50%–80% of my best)

<u>First</u>: Add quick-relief medicine: Albuterol, ventolin, proventil, maxair, or xopenx

Inhaler ☐ 2 to 4 puffs   OR   ☐ **aerosol machine** (1 vial) once

Next: AFTER 1 hour

• <u>IF</u> your symptoms return to the GREEN ZONE:
  ☐ Take the quick-relief medicine every 6–8 hours for 1–2 days

• <u>IF</u> your symptoms **DO NOT** return to the GREEN ZONE:
  ☐ Repeat quick-relief medication NOW and then every 4–6 hours for 1–2 days
  ☐ ADD/DOUBLE inhaled steroid: _____ puffs/vial twice daily for 7–10 days
  ☐ **Advair**: stop 100/50 and <u>start higher strength</u> preparation: 250/50 or 500/50
  ☐ Add _____
  ☐ Call doctor for more advice

<u>Remember</u>: **Continue all green zone medications.**

RED ZONE: Medical Alert!

- Very short of breath, or
- Quick-relief medicines have not helped, or
- Cannot do usual activities, or
- Symptoms are the same or worse after 24 hours in the yellow zone

PEAK FLOW less than _____

(less than 50% of my best)

Add this medicine (In addition to green and yellow zone medicines):
☐ **Albuterol or** _____
☐ Repeat albuterol or _____ ☐ 4 puffs   or   ☐ aerosol machine
  _____ in **20 minutes if NOT better**

☐ **Oral steroid: one dose a day for 3–5 days**
  Take _____ pills (_____ mg) prednisone **OR** Take _____ cc/mL Prelone or Orapred

Then: • **Call your asthma doctor (xxx-xxx-xxx) or pediatrician** *NOW.*
  • Go to the hospital or call an ambulance if your child is still in the RED ZONE after 20 minutes **AND** you have not reached the doctor.

Fig. 45.6 Sample treatment plan form for management of chronic asthma. Instructions may use peak expiratory flow rate monitoring in addition to symptoms to assess the need for additional treatment.

Substandard housing, limited access to high-quality medical care, and transportation and child care barriers can all contribute to poor asthma control in patients from lower socioeconomic groups. Impaired maternal mental health, lack of social supports, and child behavior problems may all contribute to poor adherence and asthma control.

Adherence to a treatment regimen is key to successful asthma management. Adherence differs from compliance, in that adherence stresses the role of the patient and family in helping develop a treatment program and contributing to the strategies necessary to utilize the treatment plan. Compliance implies that a patient must utilize a plan derived by the physician; failure to do so indicates that the patient is at fault and irresponsible. The factors that contribute to adherence are complex and incompletely understood. It is difficult to predict which patients will have good adherence, and it is not well correlated with race, gender, or intelligence. Moreover, many patients overreport good adherence in an attempt to please the physician. Adherence to suggested medical treatment for asthma often ranges from 30% to 70% use of prescribed medicine. Families should be encouraged to identify areas of a treatment regimen that might offer difficulty, concerns they have about medications, and lifestyle issues that might impair adherence. Physicians must be willing to provide suitable alternatives (e.g., medications, dose schedules). Regularly scheduled office visits should be conducted to evaluate the success of the treatment plan and offer the patient the opportunity to voice concerns and ask for help. When a child or the parents fail to adhere, the physician should try to find out the reasons and to work out a practical solution that is acceptable to the patient and family. Use of motivational interviewing techniques and shared decision-making strategies can often provide better results than direct reminders.

Patients must be given ready access to medical advice (e.g., over the telephone), including how to deal with school-related asthma management and behavior problems. Other technologies, such as text messaging, email, videoconferencing, and social networking, are also gaining popularity as ways to communicate with patients. Most importantly, parents and patients must learn that frequent symptoms and limitation of lifestyle due to illness should not be accepted; a symptom-free existence should be the goal.

Management of an Acute Episode

Acute asthma in children can occur as a mild illness that responds promptly to bronchodilators, or it can develop into a medical emergency over a matter of a few hours or days. Failure to respond to aggressive home treatment mandates further evaluation and treatment in the physician's office or a hospital emergency department. Use of treatment algorithms and guidelines provide useful infrastructure on which to base treatment, referral, and admission decisions (Fig. 45.7).

For mild acute asthma (cough, wheeze without dyspnea; PEFR between 50% and 80% predicted), treatment can begin at home or in the physician's office, and the drug of choice is an inhaled SABA, most commonly albuterol, 0.15–0.3 mg/kg per dose (or 2.5–5 mg) given once from a small-volume nebulizer, or preferably, 2–6 puffs (90 μg/puff) of albuterol (using a VHC if necessary) every 20 minutes for 1 hour. A recent study of 226 adults found that use of albuterol plus ipratropium via MDI as rescue medication on an as needed basis for symptoms provided better bronchodilatation, as measured by FEV1, than albuterol via MDI ($P < .0001$).[158] If symptoms resolve, PEFR (if used) improves, and the patient remains well for 3–4 hours, the short-acting bronchodilator can be repeated as necessary, routine medications continued, and contact with the physician considered. Doubling the dose of inhaled steroids at the onset of an exacerbation is no longer recommended, because most studies have not found a clear benefit. Higher (quadruple) doses of inhaled steroids for acute exacerbations may benefit some patients, but the data are limited thus far.[159] Initiating ICSs as a chronic treatment for a steroid-naïve patient during an acute episode is appropriate, but other treatment with a SABA and systemic corticosteroids should still be used as necessary. If symptoms persist and PEFR improves little after the administration of albuterol, the dose of inhaled albuterol should be repeated and a dose of oral steroid (1–2 mg/kg, maximum 60 mg prednisone) should be given. Physician contact is necessary at this point. For the patient with progressive symptoms in spite of all of the listed measures, care should be sought in a medical facility.

In the emergency department, further administration of nebulized albuterol (2.5–5.0 mg) or 4–6 puffs every 20 minutes may be continued for another hour, and an oral corticosteroid dose may be given if not done earlier. Oral steroids commonly administered for acute asthma exacerbations include prednisone and prednisolone. A body of evidence supports the use of dexamethasone. Its longer half-life allows for fewer doses of medications, thereby facilitating patient adherence.[160,161] There is no benefit to giving IV steroids unless the patient cannot tolerate or will not take the oral form. Ipratropium (250 or 500 μg) should also be given every 20–30 minutes by nebulizer for three doses; this may most likely benefit patients with more severe exacerbations of airway obstruction. A subcutaneous (SQ) injection of epinephrine (or terbutaline) can be given if the patient is in severe distress and unable to comply with aerosol therapy. Studies of continuous albuterol nebulization (10–15 mg/hour) have yielded mixed results, although most favor continuous nebulization over intermittent administration. Significant adverse side effects during continuous nebulization protocols in severe acute pediatric asthma are rare, suggesting that this mode of delivery is safe, if not necessarily more effective, and may be more convenient for patient and staff. A study compared continuously nebulized levalbuterol to racemic albuterol and found no significant efficacy or safety advantage, using pharmacologically equivalent doses.[162] These finding were confirmed in a more recent meta-analysis.[163]

Other treatments that may be used in the acute hospital setting include IV magnesium sulfate ($MgSO_4$) and heliox. $MgSO_4$ can act as a smooth muscle relaxant, possibly by blocking calcium-mediated contraction, decreasing acetylcholine release from neuromuscular junctions, and reducing histamine-induced airway spasm. $MgSO_4$ has been utilized for patients who fail to improve significantly following administration of inhaled SABA and systemic corticosteroids. Several studies demonstrate improved pulmonary function, decreased symptoms, and decreased rate of hospitalization following

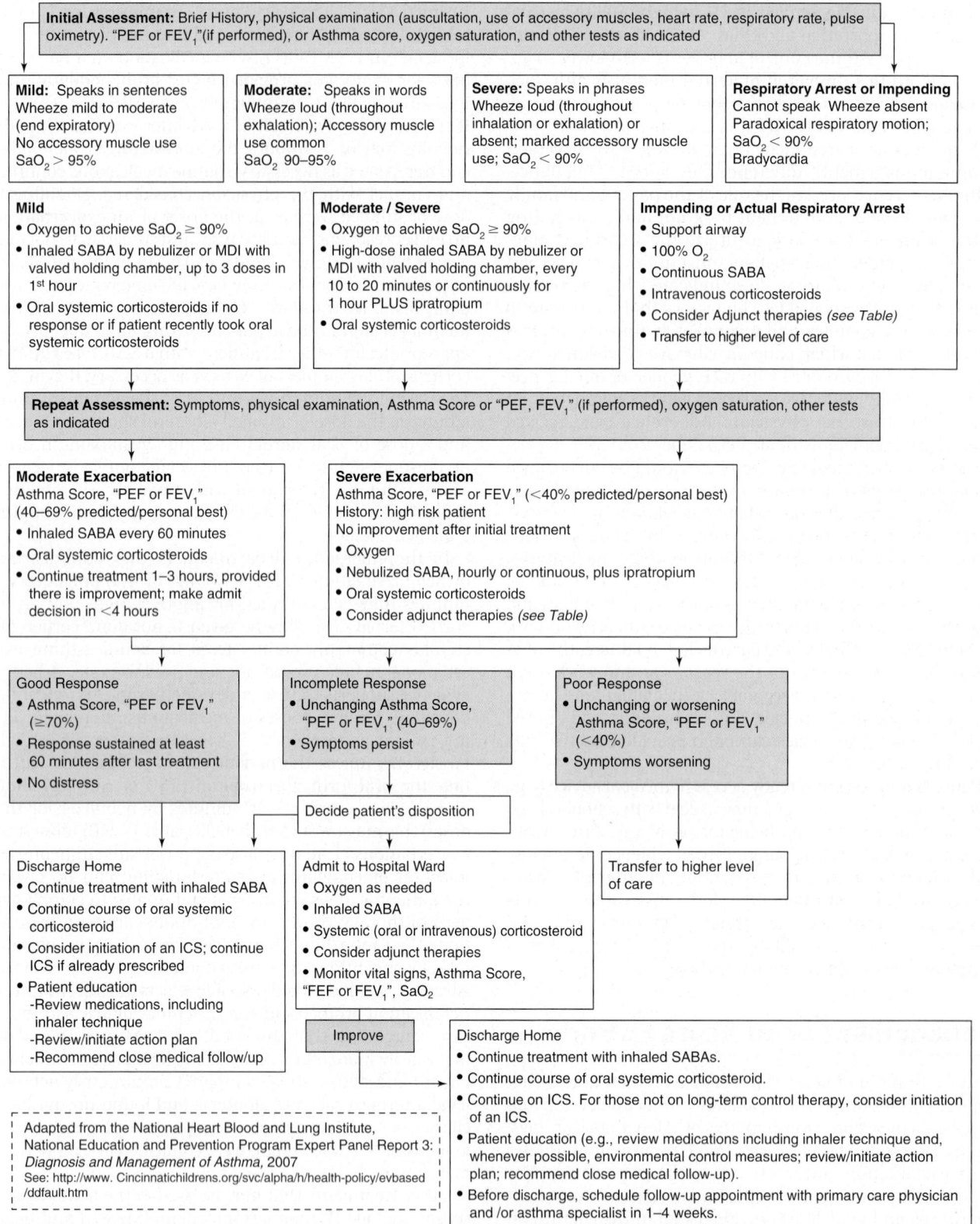

Fig. 45.7 Treatment algorithm for medical facility management of acute asthma. *FEV₁,* Forced expiratory volume in 1 second; *ICS,* inhaled corticosteroid; *MDI,* metered-dosed inhaler; *PEF,* peak expiratory flow; *SABA,* short-acting β agonist; *SaO₂,* oxygen saturation in arterial blood.

a single infusion of 40–75 mg/kg (maximum 2 g) over a 20-minute period. $MgSO_4$ should strongly be considered in severely ill patients who are in a monitored unit in an emergency department and are failing conventional therapy. Adverse events include flushing, headache, decreased blood pressure, and weakness; the more significant effects are infrequent unless the serum magnesium level rises above twice normal.

Heliox, a mixture of helium (80%) and oxygen (20%), is a specialty gas that is less dense than nitrogen. When administered to the acutely ill asthmatic, heliox can decrease airway resistance by restoring laminar flow in obstructed airways where flow has become more turbulent. Work of breathing is decreased, and the patient is less likely to fatigue. However, there is no direct curative action of heliox, and its effect occurs only while in use. It may also be used to drive a small-volume nebulizer to deliver albuterol, but this requires a specialized closed delivery system. Current data do not support the routine use of heliox in the emergency department. Heliox may be a useful bridge therapy for the severely ill patient in the intensive care unit who is tiring. It becomes less effective if concentrations lower than 70% helium are used, making it less useful in significantly hypoxic patients.

Montelukast administered intravenously or orally as an adjunct treatment for status asthmaticus, in addition to standard treatment with a SABA and systemic corticosteroids, has not proven useful in improving symptoms, pulmonary function, or need for hospital admission in children.[164] The routine use of montelukast for treatment of status asthmaticus cannot be recommended at this time.

Failure to clear symptoms (particularly dyspnea, chest wall retractions, or use of accessory muscles); persistent hypoxemia (O_2 saturation < 92% while breathing room air); and improve air exchange and (if measured) PEFR to above 40% to 50% predicted are some indicators for hospital admission.

Hospital Management of Asthma

Status asthmaticus, or acute severe asthma that is resistant to appropriate outpatient therapy, is a significant medical emergency that requires prompt, systematic, and aggressive management in the hospital. The initiation of early appropriate therapy shortens hospitalization and reduces complications for the vast majority of acutely ill patients. In spite of improved efforts at diagnosing and treating asthma, status asthmaticus continues to be the one of the most common discharge diagnoses from children's hospitals, accounting for 15%–30% of all admissions. The increase in hospitalizations for asthma reported in all age groups during the last decade now appears to have slowed.

General Treatment

A physician, nurse, respiratory therapist, and consultant pulmonologist team should manage the child with status asthmaticus in a closely monitored inpatient unit. Although the management of each child with status asthmaticus must be individualized, certain general principles apply to all patients with this diagnosis.

Humidified oxygen should be administered (2–3 L/min by nasal cannula or 30% fraction of inspired oxygen [F_{IO_2}] by facemask) to maintain oxygen saturation in arterial blood (SaO_2) greater than 93% at sea level. The appropriate use of oxygen helps relieve dyspnea, aids in bronchodilatation, supports the myocardium, and helps prevent arrhythmias. Failure of improvement in hypoxemia with modest amounts of oxygen suggests either severe airway obstruction and impending respiratory failure or a complicating factor, such as pneumonia, atelectasis, or another diagnosis besides asthma. IV infusion of fluids is generally not required unless the patient is unable to take or tolerate oral fluids or requires IV access for steroids or antimicrobials (if needed for concomitant infection). PFTs (FEV_1 or PEFR) may be performed at the bedside if the child can cooperate; however, most acutely ill children cannot do acceptable spirometry. Pulse oximetry (or arterial or capillary blood gas if hypercarbia or acidosis is suspected) should be measured as soon as possible and repeated as the patient's condition warrants. Although not needed on all asthmatics, a chest radiograph provides information on other pulmonary problems that might complicate management in patients who do not respond rapidly to treatment (e.g., pneumonia, atelectasis, pneumomediastinum, or pneumothorax).

Details about the acute illness (its duration, progression, manifestations, and initiating factors), information on the duration and the reports of previous acute episodes, and level of functional morbidity and medication use at the patient's stable baseline should be noted. The patient's medication (including the names, dosages, and exact time of all medications administered within 24 hours) and any systemic corticosteroid drugs administered within 12 months should be documented. These data will be useful in constructing a treatment plan upon hospital discharge.

On physical examination, the general appearance and level of activity, respiratory effort, presence or absence of wheezing, tachycardia, tachypnea, air exchange, adventitious breath sounds, use of accessory muscles, dyspnea, and color are important clinical parameters that provide information about pulmonary dysfunction.

Although the number of pharmacologic agents for treatment of status asthmaticus is relatively limited, management strategies are inconsistent among and within institutions (see Table 45.4A and B). Evidence-based practice is often replaced by physician personal experience and preference. Elimination of treatment that adds risk and cost but does not improve quality of care should be a primary goal. Status asthmaticus readily lends itself to treatment by the standardized clinical pathway, and several published studies have demonstrated shortened hospital stays using such care paths.[165] Administration of oral corticosteroids within 75 minutes of arriving in the emergency department decreases the need for admission.[166]

Medical management of the hospitalized asthmatic should include aggressive use of inhaled bronchodilators, most commonly albuterol, and systemic corticosteroids. The frequency of treatment should be guided by the patient's condition. In most inpatient, nonintensive care unit settings, inhalations may be administered as frequently as every 1–2 hours. In some settings, where close monitoring is available outside the intensive care unit, consideration may be given to administering albuterol continuously (10–15 mg/hour) for short time periods (1–4 hours). Treatments should be administered only if the patient's respiratory status indicates need; studies have shown that such assessment-driven administration of SABAs is as effective as scheduled treatments. Moreover, patients who are treated on an "as-needed" basis are likely to receive fewer treatments at less cost. If the patient cannot tolerate oral therapy, IV administration of corticosteroids should be ordered. Methylprednisolone, 1–2 mg/kg (maximum 125 mg) may be given daily. Failure to improve significantly after a maximum of 12 hours of such therapy should prompt a search for other complicating factors and impending respiratory failure, and indicates a need for more aggressive monitoring and treatment. If at any time the patient's condition deteriorates, consideration should be given to administering immediate intensified treatment, such as SQ epinephrine (0.01 mL/kg, maximum 0.3 mL), terbutaline, or 500 µg aerosolized ipratropium with 5 mg albuterol. If a favorable response is observed, the aerosol treatment may be repeated every 20 minutes over the next hour. Patients who fail to sustain improvement after such treatment should be transferred to the intensive care unit.

The asthmatic child requiring intensive care should be monitored carefully for the development of respiratory failure. Physical findings such as severe dyspnea, inability to lie flat, poor air exchange, severe wheezing, and use of accessory muscles of respiration are all indicators of impending respiratory failure. Continuous cardiorespiratory monitoring and pulse oximetry with intermittent determination of arterial or venous blood gas measurement to assess oxygenation, ventilation, serum electrolyte, and acid-base status are necessary. Treatment should consist of continuously nebulized albuterol (0.15 mg/kg per hour, maximum 15 mg), ipratropium 500 µg nebulized every 4–6 hours, and methylprednisolone 1–2 mg/kg (maximum 125 mg) every 24 hours. Serum potassium concentration should also be closely monitored, because frequent SABA administration may cause hypokalemia.

A few studies suggest that IV aminophylline may result in the more rapid resolution of symptoms compared with placebo, although overall intensive care length of stay was not affected. For the patient who fails to respond, treatment with a bolus and possible continuous IV infusion of a β-adrenergic agonist (e.g., terbutaline) can be considered (IV albuterol [salbutamol] is not available in the United States). Delivery of the medication via the circulation may provide relief of bronchospasm in areas not receiving medication via the inhaled route due to severe airway obstruction. However, most studies do not report significant improvement compared with use of continuous nebulized SABA treatment. The starting dose of terbutaline is 5 µg/kg, followed by a continuous infusion of 0.4 µg/kg per minute. The dose is increased by 0.2 µg/kg per minute to a maximum dose of 12–16 µg/kg per minute, although higher doses have been used. Baseline and twice-daily cardiac isoenzymes and continuous electrocardiograms must be monitored because myocardial toxicity has been reported. Although every effort should be made to avoid intubation and mechanical ventilation, a small percentage of severely ill patients (<10%) may require invasive ventilatory support. It is difficult to mechanically ventilate an asthmatic, and the complication rate may exceed 30%. Indications for intubation have become more conservative and should be reserved for patients who have

apnea, unstable vital signs, impaired level of consciousness, severe acidosis, extreme fatigue, and failure of noninvasive ventilation. A trial of noninvasive ventilation using continuous positive airway pressure (CPAP) or bilevel positive airway pressure (Bi-Pap) may be successful in some patients. Low levels of H_2O pressure (5–10 cm) may be helpful in reducing work of breathing and improving oxygenation over a several-hour trial. Some patients become anxious using the tight-fitting facemask necessary for effective CPAP and may require a modest dose of a short-acting benzodiazepine to comply with treatment. Risks include gastric distention, vomiting, aspiration, or air leak.

A skilled intensivist or anesthesiologist using rapid-sequence induction anesthesia should perform intubation when necessary. It is important to make certain the patient is adequately hydrated prior to intubation and not given excessive positive pressure bag ventilation immediately after. Asthmatic patients are at risk for significant hypotension following intubation because of extreme hyperventilation leading to auto-PEEP, which impedes systemic venous return; this can be further exacerbated by volume depletion and application of aggressive positive pressure ventilation. Continuous sedation is usually required during mechanical ventilation. High peak inspiratory pressures are often noted, and efforts should be made to reduce them to less than 45 mm Hg. Use of selective hypoventilation (permissive hypercapnia) must be practiced, and attempts to immediately normalize ventilation should be avoided. Relief of hypoxemia, respiratory distress, and muscle fatigue are the goals. Volume ventilation with a square wave form and the lowest volume and flow to minimize peak pressure and volume damage while maximizing expiratory time is usually recommended, but there are reports of successful use of pressure-controlled ventilation. Relatively low respiratory rates (8–10/min), low tidal volumes (6–8 mL/kg), and prolonged expiratory time should be tried as ventilator strategies. Decreasing the minute ventilation can maximize expiratory time; this can be best accomplished by using a lower respiratory rate or tidal volume. Shortening the inspiratory time by increasing the inspiratory flow rate can work, but it may be less effective and may contribute to airway injury caused by high shear forces. As long as metabolic acidosis is not present, a pH as low as 7.2 can be tolerated. IV infusion of sodium bicarbonate for more profound acidosis is controversial and generally not recommended. All medications should be continued while the patient is mechanically ventilated. Delivery of aerosolized bronchodilators through the endotracheal tube using an MDI and spacer device should be continued as well. Extubation should be considered and attempted using standard criteria, such as normoxemia with an FIO_2 of less than 0.40, spontaneous tidal volume greater than 5 mL/kg, vital capacity greater than 15 mL/kg, maximum inspiratory pressure (MIP) greater than 25 cm H_2O, and the ability to protect the airway and handle secretions. Most patients can be successfully weaned and extubated within 72 hours.

Several other therapies for the severely ill asthmatic have been tried, but they are still considered unproven or experimental. IV $MgSO_4$ should be tried, particularly if not administered previously. Heliox has been reported to decrease pulsus paradoxus and improve air flow in acutely ill, nonintubated asthmatic children, and can also be administered during mechanical ventilation. However, this therapy is unproven, and the less-dense gas alters ventilator function, requiring careful ventilator adjustment and a knowledgeable respiratory therapist. Administration of inhaled general anesthetic agents (e.g., enflurane and sevoflurane, which are bronchodilators) has also been used with some success; however, reports are anecdotal, and no controlled trials have been conducted. These agents are also myocardial irritants and may precipitate serious arrhythmias in the acidotic, hypoxemic asthmatic. Ketamine infusions can be considered for sedation of the intubated patient, since the drug also has some bronchodilator properties. However, the adverse psychoactive effects of ketamine can be problematic in older children and may only be partially obviated by the concomitant administration of a benzodiazepine.

Of note, most patients who develop life-threatening asthma and respiratory failure do so outside the hospital or shortly after arriving at a medical facility. Most asthma deaths occur prior to reaching an intensive care unit and institution of successful airway management. Once successfully stabilized in an intensive care unit that is familiar with the management of acute severe asthma, patients who have not experienced respiratory arrest or prolonged hypoxia are likely to survive intact.

References

Access the reference list online at ExpertConsult.com.

Suggested Reading

Bunyavanich S, Schadt EE. Systems biology of asthma and allergic diseases: a multiscale approach. *J Allergy Clin Immunol.* 2015;135:31–42.

Martinez FD, Chinchilli VM, Morgan WJ, et al. Use of beclomethasone dipropionate as rescue treatment for children with mild persistent asthma (TREXA): a randomised, double-blind, placebo-controlled trial. *Lancet.* 2011;377:650–657.

Pruteanu AI, Chauhan BF, Zhang L, et al. Inhaled corticosteroids in children with persistent asthma: dose-response effects on growth. *Evid Based Child Health.* 2014;9:931–1046.

Reddel HK, Bateman ED, Becker A, et al. A summary of the new GINA strategy: a roadmap to asthma control. *Eur Respir J.* 2015;46:622–639.

46 *Severe Asthma*

ANDREW BUSH, MB BS(Hons), MA, MD, FRCP, FRCPCH, FERS[a], and
LOUISE FLEMING, MB ChB, MRCP, MRCPCH, MD

Most children with asthma can be easily treated with low-dose inhaled corticosteroids (ICS) if these are regularly and correctly administered. Hence, refractory asthma probably accounts for less than 5% of all pediatric asthma.[1] It may be becoming less common over time, possibly because of more effective modern treatments and likely also improved management.[2] However, this group accounts for an enormous amount of morbidity and health care costs, and even mortality, and so although rare, it is important. Here, our practice approach to the child with apparent refractory asthma is described. Severe preschool wheeze is not discussed here.

Overarching Principles

The cardinal sin in asthma management is to continue to escalate asthma therapy in a child who is not responding, without asking, "Why is simple prescribed treatment not working?" We know that most children with asthma will respond very well to low-dose ICS, sometimes also requiring a second controller, such as long-acting beta-2 agonists (LABA), or a leukotriene receptor antagonist (LTRA).[3] So, faced with the child with apparently refractory asthma, the pediatrician should not reach again for the prescription pad, but go through a rigorous protocol to determine what it is about this child and his or her asthma that means the anticipated response is not happening. The overall aim of the protocols discussed below is to determine whether the individual child is truly a candidate for "beyond guidelines" therapy or can, in fact, be managed with standard approaches.

Definitions

The conventional developed world definition of severe asthma[4,5] is that the patient requires treatment with guideline-suggested medications for GINA (Global Initiative for Asthma) steps 4–5 asthma (high-dose ICS, conventionally 800 μg/day beclomethasone equivalent for 5- to12-year-olds; >1600 μg for children aged >12 years; and LABA or leukotriene modifier/theophylline) for the previous year; or systemic corticosteroids (CS) for ≥50% of the previous year to prevent it from becoming "uncontrolled"; or which remains "uncontrolled" despite this therapy; or controlled asthma that worsens on tapering of these high doses of ICS or systemic CS (or additional biologics). Uncontrolled asthma is currently defined as one or more or of:

1. *Poor symptom control:* Asthma Control Questionnaire (ACQ) consistently >1.5, Asthma Control Test (ACT) <20 (or "not well controlled" by NAEPP [National Asthma Education and Prevention Program]/GINA guidelines).
2. *Frequent severe exacerbations:* two or more bursts of systemic CS (>3 days each) in the previous year.
3. *Serious exacerbations:* at least one hospitalization, intensive care unit (ICU) stay or mechanical ventilation in the previous year. However, objective evidence of the severity of the attack should be obtained. In theory, the treatment of an asthma attack is based on objective evidence of current severe airflow obstruction. In practice, especially in emergency situations dealt with by the inexperienced, the previous history may unduly influence practice. It is essential to determine what (if any) objective assessments were carried out before instituting treatment, and whether in fact the child was overtreated because of a "severe asthma" label. One child under our care was actually started on intravenous albuterol despite being fully saturated on room air! In fact she had dysfunctional breathing and vocal cord dysfunction.
4. *Airflow limitation:* after withholding bronchodilators for 4 hours (short acting) or 12 hours (long acting) first second forced expired volume (FEV_1) <80% predicted (in the face of reduced FEV_1/forced vital capacity (FVC) defined as less than the lower limit of normal); however, it should be noted that normal spirometry does not exclude severe asthma in children[6]; unlike in adults, spirometry is poorly discriminatory between different levels of asthma severity and is not a good end-point in pediatric asthma trials.[7–9]
5. *Fixed airflow limitation:* FEV_1 <80% predicted (in the face of reduced FEV_1/FVC defined as less than the lower limit of normal) despite a trial of systemic steroids and acute administration of short-acting beta-2 agonists (SABA).
6. *Disconnect symptoms:* perhaps strictly the child presenting with a multitude of symptoms with no objective evidence of uncontrolled disease may belong in a separate disease category, and certainly is not placed conventionally in severe asthma guidelines, but the means of addressing this scenario are so very similar that this is pragmatically justified. The reverse scenario, the underreporting of symptoms, is also considered below.

Inherent in this definition is that basic management, including adherence, has been optimized, a process described in more detail below.

It can be argued that the level of ICS dose has been set too high. The Best Add-on Therapy Giving Effective Responses (BADGER) study[10] shows that for most children, there is no benefit from increasing ICS above 100 μg bid (200 μg beclomethasone); a child not responding to this level of ICS plus one additional controller medication definitely merits a careful review.

---

[a]Andrew Bush is a National Institute for Health Research (NIHR) Senior Investigator and additionally was supported by the NIHR Respiratory Disease Biomedical Research Unit at the Royal Brompton and Harefield NHS Foundation Trust and Imperial College London.

722

Furthermore, the WHO has defined three types of severe asthma[11]:

1. *Untreated:* due to undiagnosed asthma or the unavailability of therapy (this being the most common worldwide)
2. *Difficult-to-treat:* due to adherence issues, inappropriate or incorrect use of medicines, environmental triggers or comorbidity
3. *Treatment-resistant:* this includes asthma for which control is not achieved despite the highest level of recommended treatment, or asthma that is controlled only with the highest level of recommended treatment.

Clearly, each of these categories merits a different response. The lack of availability of therapy needs to be tackled at a public health level, ensuring that each and every child with asthma has access to the basics; namely, inhaled beclomethasone and albuterol, prednisolone, and a plastic bottle spacer. Biologicals have no place in this setting. For those with treatment-resistant severe asthma, on the other hand, deploying novel therapeutics may be transforming.

An overlapping approach, which is also a useful conceptual framework, is to define risk by considering domains of asthma severity. Conventionally, these are:

1. Level of prescribed treatment
2. Level of baseline asthma control over the previous month
3. Level of underlying airway eosinophilia (in adults, possibly children, also)
4. Burden and nature of exacerbations over the last 6–12 months
5. Risk of future complications, including the failure of normal airway growth (for which there is increasing evidence); the risk of either or both of future loss of control and exacerbations; the risk of medication side effects.

It could certainly be argued that the conventional definition fails to focus on domains that the patients and families find important, such as quality of life, the impact on school attendance, and the time away from work for the carers. Perhaps what we mean by "control" needs a broader perspective. Furthermore, the recent UK review of asthma deaths[12] suggests that we need to refocus our definitions: around 60% of those who died from asthma were classified as "mild to moderate." Since it is difficult to imagine a more severe outcome than dying, it is obvious that our definitions need to be reconsidered. These patients could be placed in the difficult to treat category, but patient factors (Box 46.1) need to be added to the conventional definitions of risk.

This underscores that difficult-to-treat asthma can be just as serious as treatment-resistant severe asthma, and merits a response that is just as focused if we are to impact deaths from asthma.

A New Approach: Airways Disease Deconstructed and Placed in Context

A new framework has been suggested for the assessment of airway disease.[13] The problem is multicomponent, and is best considered under three headings: airway disease itself, extrapulmonary disease (comorbidities), and environmental/

Box 46.1 Lessons From the UK NRAD— What Makes a Patient a High Risk for Death From Asthma?

- A single severe exacerbation
- Recent discharge from hospital after an acute asthma attack
- Use of hospital urgent care facilities in the previous year
- Utilization of more than six canisters of SABA/year
- Failure to attend follow-up appointments

SABA, Short-acting beta-2 agonists.

Box 46.2 What May Lie Under the "Problematic Severe Asthma" Umbrella?

1. *Not asthma at all:* the diagnosis is wrong.
2. *Asthma plus:* there are associated comorbidities that need to be addressed.
3. *Difficult asthma:* accounts for about 90% of those in whom the first two categories have been excluded. This comprises children who need to get the basic steps of asthma management correct; the percentage of difficult asthma compared with severe, therapy-resistant asthma has risen over the years as we have become more expert in assessing these children, in particular adherence issues.
4. *Severe, therapy-resistant asthma:* these children appear to have ongoing problems with asthma despite the optimization of all basic steps of asthma management; such children are candidates for "beyond guidelines" therapy, and account for around 10% of referrals.

---

lifestyle factors. The initial assessment of problematic severe asthma focuses on the last two, because generally, the first is easily managed (above), and therefore the focus is on potential confounding factors. If the problem remains, the nature of the airway disease is ascertained invasively. The protocol used is discussed in more detail below.

Initial Evaluation: Problematic Severe Asthma

Problematic severe asthma is the umbrella term when a referral of a child meeting one or more of the above criteria is received in a specialist respiratory center (Box 46.2). A full history and physical examination is the essential first step. The nature of the symptoms should be determined. The word "wheeze" is used very imprecisely, often being used to describe many nonspecific respiratory sounds, and even stridor[14-18]; until a physician has heard wheeze with a stethoscope, it should be considered as "possible."[19] Most children who have a cough as their sole symptom (particularly an isolated dry cough) do not have a disease.[20]

Physiological tests are mandatory at this point. It should be noted that spirometry is often normal in children with severe asthma, which is different from adults. Testing for airway hyperresponsiveness is not routine, and may be risky in these severe asthma patients. In any event, the relationship between PC_{20} to methacholine and asthma severity is poor. The most common use of this test is in a child with normal spirometry who is reporting a multiplicity of symptoms; a normal methacholine challenge excludes asthma as a cause of these symptoms. Airflow obstruction, which changes over time or with treatment, must be documented and consideration given to determining whether the child is atopic and has airway eosinophilia. Nonatopic asthma does occur in childhood, but is uncommon, and if skin prick tests or specific immunoglobulin E (IgE) are negative, the diagnosis should be reevaluated. Blood eosinophilia may give a guide to airway eosinophilia, but an elevation may be due to other atopic disease, for example eczema. Fractional exhaled nitric oxide (FeNO) measured at a flow rate of 50 mL/s ($FeNO_{50}$) has been used as a diagnostic tool for asthma, but it should be noted that a low $FeNO_{50}$ does not exclude asthma, and elevation is seen in atopic children with no respiratory disease.[21] An induced sputum cytospin will give more direct evidence of airway eosinophilia, but is not available in most centers. Although evidence of airway inflammation is not a mandatory diagnostic test for asthma, and a child already on treatment with ICS may be inflammation free, the absence of any evidence of airway inflammation in a child supposedly symptomatic with asthma should prompt a diagnostic review. Finally, the diagnostic process should not end at this stage; the possibility of a wrong diagnosis should be at the forefront throughout, and further testing should be considered in the presence of a surprising finding, such as airway neutrophilia (see later).

It may be thought inappropriate to be discussing basic asthma diagnosis in a chapter on severe asthma, but wrong diagnosis, often due to failure to perform objective tests, is an all-too-common reason why treatment fails.

The suggested flow chart for evaluating children with asthma who are not responsive to treatment is shown in Fig. 46.1. The low level of ICS used to trigger evaluation may raise the specter of tertiary services being drowned in referrals, but this is not necessarily the case. Furthermore, this framework can be modified and adapted to all health care settings. Given (1) the plateau of the ICS dose response curve being low[10]; and (2) the generally poor response to LTRAs,[22] time should not be wasted by increasing ICS doses ever higher, and adding in more and more different controllers. Rather, one should ask, "why is this child not responding to low-dose ICS and one controller?" Simple checks can easily be done in primary care. A diagnostic review is mandatory: are the symptoms in fact due to no more than repeated viral upper respiratory infections? Is the child using the medication delivery device correctly? Are there adverse environmental factors, such as tobacco smoke exposure (passive or active)? Nonadherence can easily be checked by examining prescription records. In one study, only one in six children was having enough prescriptions filled to take their prophylactic medication.[23] Even patients referred to us with apparently severe asthma collect less than half of their prescriptions.[24] Of course, picking up a prescription does not mean the medication has actually reached the lower airways (below)!

Referral may also be indicated even if the primary pediatrician is confident that the child has difficult asthma, but repeated interventions have failed to reduce the risk factors for asthma death. The possibility of diagnostic error still remains, and the use of a multifaceted intervention may be able to reduce risk.[25,26]

Problematic Severe Asthma: Not Asthma at All

The differential diagnosis of problematic severe asthma is summarized in Table 46.1. There is a wide differential diagnosis of asthma, the nature of which varies across the world. Important red flags, which should prompt investigation, include neonatal onset of symptoms, chronic productive cough for more than 8 weeks continuously (not recurrent acute cough with complete resolution between episodes), and evidence of systemic disease. The nonatopic child with apparently severe asthma should always be carefully reassessed, and alternative diagnoses sought. We do not routinely perform a chest high-resolution computed tomography (HRCT) in all children referred with problematic severe asthma, reserving this investigation for those with atypical features; there is no evidence in children to set against this selective approach. Specifically, HRCT cannot differentiate obliterative bronchiolitis from asthma,[27] and severe asthma; HRCT phenotypes such as those known in adults[28,29] have not been described in children. In general, testing should be focused to eliminate specific conditions, rather than taking a scattergun approach.

Airway Disease in Context: Asthma Plus (Extrapulmonary Comorbidities)

A so-called comorbidity may (1) worsen asthma; (2) be a coincidental fellow traveler; (3) obscure the assessment of asthma; or (4) be an example of Berkson fallacy. This last is a special example of selection bias. This occurs when, for example, the combination of exposure and disease under study increases the risk of hospital admission, thus leading to a higher exposure rate among the hospital cases than the

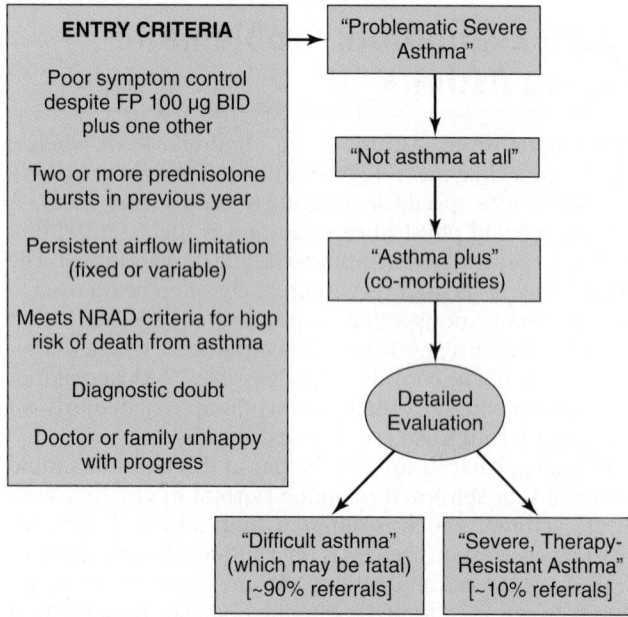

Fig. 46.1 Modified diagnostic protocol for investigation of severe asthma. *BID,* Twice daily; *NRAD,* National Review of Asthma Deaths.

Table 46.1 Differential Diagnoses of Severe Asthma

Class of Diagnosis	Examples
Defects of host defense	Cystic fibrosis, primary ciliary dyskinesia, persistent bacterial bronchitis The effects of high dose inhaled steroids should be considered
Systemic immunodeficiency	Any, including B-cell and T-cell dysfunction
Intraluminal bronchial obstruction	Foreign body, carcinoid, other tumor
Intramural bronchial obstruction	Bronchomalacia, complete cartilage rings, intramural tumor In low- and middle-income countries, bronchiectasis due to severe infection in an otherwise healthy child is particularly important
Extraluminal bronchial obstruction	Vascular ring, pulmonary artery sling, congenital lung cyst, enlarged lymph nodes due to tumor or tuberculosis, other mediastinal masses In low- and middle-income countries, tuberculosis is a particularly important cause
Direct aspiration	Bulbar or pseudobulbar palsy; laryngeal cleft; laryngeal neuropathy or myopathy
Aspiration by direct contamination	H-type fistula, which may not present until adult life
Aspiration secondary to reflux	Any cause of gastro-esophageal reflux, including hiatus hernia and esophageal dysmotility (e.g., achalasia or after neonatal repair of tracheoesophageal fistula)
Complications of prematurity	Bronchomalacia, stricture secondary to intubation, vocal cord palsy secondary to surgery for patent arterial duct
Congenital heart disease	Bronchial compression from enlarged cardiac chambers or great vessels; pulmonary edema
Interstitial lung disease	Any not presenting with neonatal respiratory failure
Dysfunctional breathing	Vocal cord dysfunction, hyperventilation syndromes (usually a comorbidity in a known asthmatic, but may present in isolation)

hospital controls; and is a frequent cause of manuscripts being rejected! The clinical significance of the first three categories is obviously different: (1) and (3) are important as "treatable traits," whereas (2) is not. Furthermore, it may be easy to identify a treatable trait, such as obesity, but in practice, treatment may be difficult. The ethics of escalating treatment with expensive and potentially hazardous drugs under these circumstances are debatable.

OBESITY

The relationships between asthma and obesity are difficult to assess, and too many studies merely report associations that are difficult to disentangle. Obesity may cause breathlessness and "wheeze" especially on exercise without evidence of asthma, leading to inappropriate treatment. Obesity may be associated with a pauci-inflammatory form of asthma, at least in adults, although it is sometimes unclear whether this is true asthma[30]; asthma with raised sputum interleukin (IL)-5 and airway wall eosinophilia[31]; or steroid resistance.[32] Obesity is a proinflammatory state,[33] as is obstructive sleep apnea (see later).[34] Asthma (via reduced exercise performance)

and its treatment (prednisolone bursts or long-term therapy) may cause or contribute to obesity. Hence, particular care is necessary before escalating therapy for "asthma" in the obese child with respiratory symptoms; an exercise-induced asthma test may be enlightening. A normal methacholine challenge also may be useful to exclude asthma as a cause of symptoms. In asthmatic adults, bariatric surgery improved distal airway function (impulse oscillometry, systemic inflammation [serum high sensitivity C-reactive protein, adiponectin, and leptin] and airway inflammation [decrease in mast cell numbers]).[35] In summary, obesity hits all three mechanisms of comorbidity: it may worsen asthma, obscure the assessment of asthma, and be a fellow traveler. Weight reduction is always beneficial in the obese child, but is often difficult to achieve, and its contribution to the clinical picture must be assessed on an individual basis.

GASTROESOPHAGEAL REFLUX

The relationship between respiratory disease and gastroesophageal reflux is also complex. Reflux can cause symptoms either by direct contamination of the lower airway, or indirectly by an esophago-bronchial reflex[36–38]; respiratory disease may lead to abnormal pleural pressure swings or altered configuration of the diaphragm—the latter reducing the efficiency of the lower esophageal sphincter; and reflux may be present but noncontributory. However, irrespective of any symptoms suggestive of reflux, therapy with, for example, a proton pump inhibitor does not improve severe asthma,[39–41] which is certainly our experience. This does not exclude the possibility that nonacid reflux may be contributory, although there is also no positive evidence for this. So, reflux is a potentially treatable trait, and the symptoms of reflux may mimic or coexist with asthma, and thus complicate the assessment of asthma.

FOOD ALLERGY

Atopy is almost inevitable in severe pediatric asthma, and indeed "non-atopic asthma" merits the most careful diagnostic review. However, food allergy is reported more commonly than expected in severe asthma.[42,43] Whether food allergy is causative of the problem or a marker is unclear; certainly anaphylaxis enters the differential diagnosis of acute, severe asthma, and should always be considered because it is treatable. Exercise-induced anaphylaxis must be differentiated from other causes of breathlessness on exercise (see later) by a careful history. Food allergy should always be documented with a double-blind challenge unless there is overwhelming evidence for the diagnosis if exclusion diets are proposed; however, blind dietary exclusions are frequently tried and inevitably useless in our experience.

RHINOSINUSITIS

Upper airway disease worsens the quality of life, and should be treated on its own merits in any context.[44–46] There is increasing evidence that treating rhinosinusitis may be beneficial at least in mild-to-moderate asthma.[47–49] The mechanisms of any benefit remain conjectural.[50] Upper airway symptoms may complicate the assessment of asthma; for example, causing night waking, which may be mistaken for uncontrolled asthma. In our series, significant rhinosinusitis is unusual in severe asthma, but in the **U-BIOPRED** (**U**nbiased **BIO**markers for the **PRED**iction of respiratory disease outcomes) cohort,[51] two-thirds had a diagnosis of allergic rhinitis. An assessment of the respiratory tract is incomplete without consideration of the nose.

SLEEP DISORDERED BREATHING

There is an increasing amount of literature on asthma and obstructive sleep apnea (OSA).[52] Although the literature reports associations in at least mild-to-moderate asthma, in our patients, OSA is very rare in severe asthma, except in the presence of concomitant obesity. We do not routinely perform polysomnography on children with severe asthma who are not obese. OSA has been reported to cause sputum neutrophilia rather than eosinophilia in one study[53]; this inflammatory pattern rarely, if ever, occurs in true severe, therapy-resistant asthma, and if seen, it should prompt a diagnostic reevaluation. As with rhinosinusitis, disturbed sleep due to OSA may be misdiagnosed as uncontrolled asthma.

SYNDROMES OF VOCAL CORD DYSFUNCTION AND OTHER FUNCTIONAL BREATHING ISSUES

Dysfunctional breathing is common in some,[54] but not all,[55] asthma cohorts. The symptoms are easily confused with uncontrolled asthma, leading to inappropriate treatment escalation. There is much less work in children than in adults.[56–58] Of the children investigated in our protocol, 15% had evidence of dysfunctional breathing,[24] including hyperventilation and vocal cord dysfunction. Clues include the absence of symptoms at night, and often stridor rather than expiratory noises. Spirometry is frequently not reproducible, and there may be attenuation of the inspiratory curve during attacks.

Breathlessness on exercise may be challenging to evaluate, with a wide differential diagnosis (Box 46.3). Exercise induced laryngeal dysfunction (EILO) may be particularly challenging to diagnose. There are important points on the history: exercise-induced bronchoconstriction is common in asthma, and is characterized by symptoms usually more than 5 minutes after exercise, a feeling of difficulty breathing out, and a good response to pretreatment with SABA. By contrast, EILO (which often complicates asthma) is characterized by

---

Box 46.3   Differential Diagnosis of Exercise-Induced Breathlessness

- Exercise-induced bronchoconstriction
- VCDEILO
- Deconditioning (which may have resulted from asthma)
- Obesity (which may also be the consequence of asthma and its treatment)
- Exercise-induced anaphylaxis (a detailed history of food intake prior to exercise is essential)
- Pulmonary hypertension (consider especially in children who "faint" during exercise)

EILO, Exercise-induced laryngeal obstruction; *VCD,* vocal cord dysfunction.

---

symptoms during exercise in which breathing in, not out, is difficult, and is accompanied by an inspiratory noise, which are not helped by asthma medications. A video during an attack of exercise-induced breathlessness may be very informative; in older children, direct laryngoscopy during an exercise test enables direct demonstration of the problem.

A large community-based questionnaire study in 3838 adolescents reported a prevalence of exercise-induced bronchoconstriction of 19.2%, with 5.7% reporting EILO.[59] A sub-sample ($n = 99$ with exercise dyspnea; $n = 47$ without) underwent standard treadmill exercise-induced asthma and EILO (direct laryngoscopy) tests. A total of 39.8% had exercise-induced bronchoconstriction, 6% EILO, and 4.8% had both on objective testing. Thus, nearly 50% had neither condition, but many were being prescribed treatment for asthma. The cause of breathlessness in this group could not be determined, but they were not the obese. This important manuscript underscores the importance of objective assessment of breathlessness on exercise.

If dysfunctional breathing is suspected, an experienced respiratory physiotherapist should be asked to assess the breathing pattern. Treatment with breathing exercises may be helpful, although currently there is no randomized, controlled trial evidence of benefit.[60] The services of a sports psychologist may also be useful.

EILO also may be related to laryngomalacia in the newborn period.[61] A total of 20/23 (87%) of infants hospitalized for laryngomalacia (half with an unconfirmed clinical diagnosis) were followed up at a mean age of 11 years and compared to a group of matched controls. A respiratory symptom questionnaire, and spirometry and laryngoscopy at rest and during exercise were performed, and the exercise laryngoscopy findings scored blind. EILO was found on exercise in 14/20 (compared with 2/20 controls) and at rest in 9 (none in controls). Thus a neonatal history is an important part of the evaluation of suspected EILO, and laryngomalacia in infancy may be a less benign condition than previously thought.

A further problem is that the perception of dyspnea has been little studied in severe pediatric asthma,[62] but in adults, severe asthmatics do not become as dyspneic as mild during bronchoconstriction.[63] The possibility of poor symptom perception as a cause of an apparent sudden catastrophic deterioration should be borne in mind.

Airway Disease in Context: Environmental/Lifestyle (Difficult Asthma)

When, as far as possible, a correct diagnosis has been ensured, and comorbidities dealt with, a detailed nurse-led assessment is performed (Table 46.2). We evaluate allergic sensitization by both skin prick tests (SPTs) and sIgE tests, because there is imperfect concordance (76%–83%) between them.[64,65] Because it is so labor intensive, we are increasingly using electronic monitoring to screen out the nonadherent before going on to a detailed work-up, which is led by the specialist asthma nurse and often involves the clinical psychologist and respiratory physiotherapist. This includes both a hospital outpatient visit and a community assessment, which includes

Table 46.2 Nurse-Led Assessments in Problematic Severe Asthma (Hospital, Home, and School Visit)

Issue to Be Addressed	Tests Performed
Symptom pattern	■ Asthma control test (≥12 years), or Childhood Asthma Control Test (6–11 years), prednisone bursts, unscheduled visits ■ Obtain records of objective assessments of the severity of asthma attacks ■ Asthma plan reviewed and updated
Psychosocial factors	■ Questionnaires (PI-ED; we also use the Hospital Anxiety and Depression Scale [HADS] to assess the main care giver); this is readdressed during the home visit, and it is after this that most issues come to light
Lung function	■ Spirometry before and after bronchodilator

Allergic sensitization
■ Aeroallergens
■ Food allergens
■ Fungi
	■ Skin prick tests, specific IgE
	  ■ grass and tree pollen, house dust mite, cockroach, cat and dog, and any others suggested by the clinical history
	  ■ peanut, milk, egg and any others suggested by the clinical history
	  ■ See Box 46.7

Airway inflammation	■ FeNO50 (multiple flow rates are not routinely used) ■ Induced sputum with hypertonic saline if FEV1 >70% predicted
Tobacco exposure	■ Urine or salivary cotinine ■ Exhaled CO for active smoking
Medication adherence	■ Serum prednisolone and theophylline levels if prescribed ■ Serum ICS levels if available ■ Prescription uptake ■ Electronic monitoring
Home visit	■ Environmental exposures, particularly pets and tobacco smoke ■ Psychosocial issues reassessed ■ Asthma education and plan reassessed ■ Medication availability and accessibility addressed
School visit or contact by telephone	■ School attendance ■ School assessment of level of disability ■ School concerns about any psychosocial issues

CO, Carbon monoxide; *FeNO₅₀,* fractional exhaled nitric oxide at expiratory rate 50 mL/s; *FEV₁,* forced expiratory volume first second; *ICS,* inhaled corticosteroids; *IgE,* immunoglobulin E; *PI-ED,* pediatric index of emotional distress.

a home visit and at least a telephone call to the school by the nurse specialist.[24]

The nurse-led home visit is a pivotal key part of the work-up of problematic, severe asthma[24]; doctors sitting in the clinic know little or nothing of what is really happening at home. Five areas are explored: adherence, tobacco smoke, allergens, psychosocial issues, and asthma education. If the patient has been referred from a distant center, the home visit may be performed by a local specialist nurse after discussion with our own team. This approach may not be feasible everywhere, but in our hands, it allows the identification of significant and potentially reversible factors in more than half of those referred with problematic severe asthma. It is absolutely clear that relying purely on a hospital-based assessment by a pediatrician will lead to many mistakes.

ADHERENCE

Physician estimates of adherence are notoriously inaccurate, adherence is often poor, and parents overestimate how much medication is being administered. In our hands, questionnaires that rely on self-report, such as medication adherence rating scale (MARS)[66] are not useful.[67] There are multiple reasons for poor adherence.[68,69] The Practicalities and Perceptions Approach (PAPA) helpfully divides these into intentional (e.g., doubts about need for medications, their efficacy, and side effects) and unintentional (e.g., regime impractical because too complex) reasons; clearly different strategies are needed to deal with these. The biggest adherence studies are in children in the community and adult severe asthmatics, rather than severely asthmatic children.[23,70–73] Medication issues are the commonest cause of failure of response to treatment in our severe asthma clinic.

Prescription Records

We found that less than half the patients had picked up more than 80% of the required prescriptions, and nearly one-third had picked up less than 50% (24), similar to other work.[74] Although those who have not collected prescriptions by definition cannot be using them, electronic monitoring (see later) has shown no relationship in prescription uptake and medication use even in those who do collect prescriptions.[75] We also determine the number of refills forSABA, which have been represcribed; collecting ≥6/year is associated with a poor outcome.[76]

The Home Visit

Medications were commonly found to be past the expiration date, and 25% could not produce a complete set of in-date medications during the visit. Other issues identified were total inaccessibility of any medications, and medications unopened in their original wrapping, both suggesting nonadherence.[24]

Parental Supervision

In one study, even young children (20% of 7-year-olds, 50% of 11-year-olds) were left to take asthma medications unsupervised.[77] Often parents think they are supervising treatment, but in fact are actually not directly witnessing the therapy being taken by the child; they are merely calling reminders when the child is upstairs. This situation requires sensitive exploration. When parental supervision is not working, we have used directly observed therapy (DOT) at school, on the basis that 5 days' treatment is better than none. However, this founders if the child does not attend school. Even if the child goes to school, school staff often fail to appreciate that DOT means closely watching the child take the medication with their full attention, not carrying on with other tasks while the child "takes" the medication standing behind their back.

Use of Inhaler Devices

These are often wrongly used. Regular teaching sessions may lead to improvements,[78,79] but do not guarantee good technique in the long term. However, all the children in our series had had repeated instruction in specialized centers, and yet still had a poor technique. A common adolescent issue is using pressurized metered-dose inhalers without spacers, because spacers are thought to be babyish; however, without a spacer, drug deposition in the lower airway will be minimal.

Electronic Monitoring: Towards a Definitive Test

We increasingly use electronic monitoring inhalers to assess adherence. We always tell the families that they are being monitored in this way. Our current technology records the time and number of actuations, but not whether the child actually inhaled; this last is a weakness, which means that adherence may still be overestimated. The first lesson we have learned is that all the above methods are inadequate to determine adherence; they can, of course, determine a definitely nonadherent group. Electronic monitoring allows us to divide children who are apparently not responding to treatment into one of three groups requiring different management strategies:

1. The child starts with poorly controlled asthma, often with a reduced FEV_1 and $FeNO_{50}$), and is adherent during monitoring. During this time, and despite no change in treatment, asthma control improves, FEV_1 rises, and $FeNO_{50}$ falls (Fig. 46.2). This group was clearly previously nonadherent, and when they took the medication they responded well. The treatment is left unchanged, and the findings and ways to maintain adherence are discussed with the child and family.
2. The child remains poorly controlled, and does not take the medication during monitoring. There is no point in escalating treatment, and the reasons for nonadherence are explored.
3. The child adheres to treatment well, but the condition remains poorly controlled. The possible explanations include activation of the inhaler without inhalation; environmental factors (below) driving asthmatic inflammation to override the effects of treatment; and true steroid resistance. These different factors are teased out on an individual basis.

On the basis of our experience, we believe that access to electronic monitoring is essential for the proper management of many children presenting with problematic severe asthma.

ENVIRONMENTAL FACTORS

Allergen Exposure

Denial of the importance of allergen exposure is common. At a level insufficient to cause acute deterioration, allergen exposure leads to increased airway inflammation, bronchial responsiveness,[80] and steroid resistance via IL-2 and IL-4 dependent mechanisms[81,82] in adults. Allergen exposure in the home, combined with evidence of sensitization, synergizes with viral infection to cause asthma attacks.[83] The relationships between allergen exposure, allergen sensitization, and symptoms, are complex, and may vary from antigen to antigen.[84] Indeed, an allergen may lead to symptoms even without evidence of specific IgE-mediated sensitization.[85,86] Nonetheless, in a child with significant symptoms of asthma, and in particular with severe asthma attacks, it seems reasonable to try to reduce environmental allergen exposure, since neither sensitization nor viral infection can be modulated.

Home Exposure. The aeroallergens likely most susceptible to intervention are pets, cockroaches, molds, and house dust mites (HDM)—with the latter being a controversial area.[87–89]

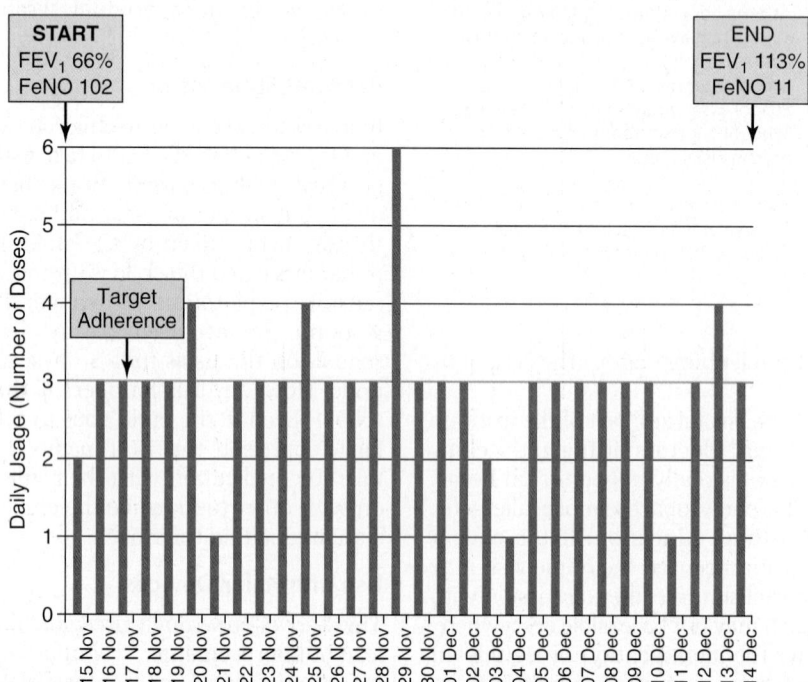

Fig. 46.2 Electronic monitoring. The adherence is good, and despite no change in treatment, first second forced expired volume *(FEV₁)* has risen, and fractional exhaled nitric oxide *(FeNO)* has fallen, both becoming normal. The child was clearly nonadherent prior to monitoring. (Courtesy Dr A Jochmann.)

Ideally, we would use environmental dust sampling to determine exposures and any response to avoidance measures. Exposure is common in asthmatics of all severites.[90–92] Pet and cockroach sensitization may be a marker for high morbidity[89,90]; although whether the latter can be separated from the effects of low socioeconomic status is arguable.[93] Passive smoking may increase the likelihood of pet sensitization.[92] The use of synthetic bedding may be associated with severe wheeze.[94] In our study,[24] 17 of 30 children who owned furry pets were sensitized to that pet on SPT, and only two had any allergen avoidance precautions in place. A total of 31 children were clinically thought to have significant HDM exposure; 5 were using comprehensive allergen avoidance measures, 15 partial, and 11 none. Reduction of mold exposure may be particularly important if severe asthma with fungal sensitization (SAFS) is suspected. This is discussed in more detail below.

School Exposure. Allergen exposure in school may also be important,[84] but difficult to change. Exposure to cat allergen on the clothes of classmates at school is sufficient to cause deterioration of asthma with a pattern similar to occupational exposure; namely, worsening during the week and improving at weekends, assuming there is no cat in the home.

Passive and Active Smoking. Active smoking by adult asthmatics causes steroid resistance,[95–98] and passive smoke exposure likely has the same effect. This is common in asthmatic children,[99–101] being 25% in our series[24]; the prevalence of active smoking as well as other risk-taking behaviors is also likely to be high in children and young people.[102] The mechanisms of tobacco smoke-induced steroid resistance have been researched mainly in adults[103]; the phenotype is neutrophilic. In a pediatric study,[104] we found that parental smoking reduced histone deacetylase protein expression and activity, and reduced the *in vitro* inhibitory effects of dexamethasone on tumor necrosis factor-α-induced IL-8 release from alveolar macrophages in severe, therapy-resistant asthma. Bronchoalveolar lavage (BAL) had higher IL-8 concentrations and neutrophil counts and the children had lower ACT scores compared with nonpassive smoke-exposed children, which are findings supported by adult data. Additionally, it is likely that symptoms are exacerbated by a direct irritant effect of smoke. Other environmental irritants sometimes encountered include incense or joss sticks, and the extensive use of air fresheners and other aerosol sprays. Environmental pollution is also important, but difficult to modulate except at the level of public health.

PSYCHOSOCIAL MORBIDITY

The relationships between asthma and the brain are complex. Acute and chronic stress may trigger asthma exacerbations.[105–107] Stress has been shown to amplify the airway eosinophilic response to allergen challenge.[108] Functional magnetic resonance imaging scanning has identified asthma neurophenotypes in circuits that process emotional information, with greater anterior insular activation with asthma-related psychological stimuli, and associated more profound airway inflammatory response and increased disease severity, although which was cause and which was consequence could not be established.[109] We, and others,[24,110]

have shown that psychosocial issues are common, especially anxiety and depression. Most issues only emerged during discussions between the nurse and the family in the home. Altogether, about half the families were referred to clinical psychology for a more detailed assessment. It is not productive to try to determine whether anxiety and depression are the cause or result of severe asthma; both are treated on their individual merits.

Asthma Education

Some adherence issues relate to basic misunderstandings of asthma and the purpose of treatment, and this is also addressed. If the child does not have a detailed asthma plan, this is put in place and communicated to the school. It is hoped that this will have been done previously, but the asthma plan is always reassessed in detail.

Safeguarding Issues: Symptom Reporting

We have safeguarding concerns in around 10% of children with "severe" asthma. Much relates to symptom overreporting; parents not reporting asthma severity accurately may be the underlying problem, and this is extremely difficult to detect. This is separate from the effect of understandable parental anxiety leading to exaggeration of symptoms. Motivation may include access to financial and other benefits as a result of having a "sick" child, right up to deliberate fabrication of symptoms, or Munchausen by proxy. Unfortunately, diagnosis is often long delayed because a basic tenet of pediatrics is to believe the mother. In such circumstances, contact with the school can be illuminating. Teachers are an important resource; they are experienced in assessing children, and spend many hours each day with them. One child allegedly suffering from severe asthma was, in fact, the captain of sports and was nicknamed "the Greyhound." The school did not know that the child had a diagnosis of asthma, and had no short-acting β-2 agonist in case of emergency. The lesson here is that early discussion with the safeguarding team is essential if there are any concerns, and that no pediatric referral center for severe asthma can function without access to a really good safeguarding service.

Increasingly Important in the Assessment Process: A Hospital Admission

We find that an admission to hospital for assessment over 2 weeks is valuable when symptoms are thought to be overreported.[111] A detailed plan is worked out in advance (Box 46.4), including regular measurement of lung function and FeNO$_{50}$; there is a regular program of exercise; all medications are supervised; and no short-acting β-2 agonist is given unless the child has first been assessed. The usual outcome is that the child is well and active without additional rescue medication; their lung function improves; and importantly, the FeNO$_{50}$ falls. This last point cannot be attributed to lack of exercise in hospital. On occasion, the admission serves to rehabilitate the child and demonstrates that exercise is not prevented by asthma; and restored confidence is maintained after discharge. Often, it is clear that the problem is either nonadherence to medication or an adverse home

Box 46.4   Sample Admission Plan

The purpose of this admission is to allow a period (usually 2 weeks) of observation and assessment in a controlled and safe environment. As far as possible, normal activities, including attending the hospital school and participating in physical activity, should continue. This is intended as an opportunity to adjust and hopefully reduce some asthma medications.

Admission plan

- To remain resident on the ward during the period of the admission and only leave the ward for short periods with the permission of ward staff or longer trip supervised by a nurse
- Attend school on school days. Our school staff will liaise with the child's school to ensure that appropriate work and, if necessary, assessments are undertaken
- Review by the physiotherapists at the beginning of the admission and a program of physical activity agreed
- Psychology review early on in the admission and further input as decided following the initial consultation
- All medications (including inhalers) are to be kept by the nursing staff and directly observed as per ward policy
- If albuterol is requested, to be assessed by a doctor first and peak flow readings recorded before and after albuterol (and documented in the case notes)
- Morning and evening peak flows every day
- Ward spirometry with bronchodilator reversibility on admission and thereafter on Tuesdays and Fridays
- Exhaled nitric oxide measurements on admission and thereafter on Tuesdays and Fridays
- ACT to be completed at the beginning of the admission
- Paediatric Asthma Quality of Life Assessment to be completed at the beginning and the end of admission
- Regular review by one of the Respiratory Clinical Nurse Specialists. The Difficult Asthma Team will liaise closely with the attending medical team throughout the admission
- Urine cotinine on admission
- Prednisolone level and random cortisol on the day of admission for all children prescribed prednisolone. If not on prednisolone, blood tests including total IgE, specific IgEs, FBC, and other clinically indicated tests can be performed during the first few days of the admission
- Other tests, including histamine challenge, cardiopulmonary exercise test, induced sputum and cardiorespiratory polygraphy, as indicated by the clinical team

ACT, Asthma control test; *FBC,* full blood count; *IgE,* immunoglobulin E.

environment, or both, which needs addressing rather than escalating prescribed treatment.

Difficult Asthma: Summary

This assessment process generates a huge amount of detailed information, and this is reviewed in a dedicated, multidisciplinary team meeting, where we attempt to place the child in one of two categories: (1) difficult asthma, in which comorbidities and environmental/lifestyle factors are responsible for the poor response to treatment; and (2) severe, therapy-resistant asthma, in which atypical airway disease is the cause of the problem. This latter is addressed below. Even though we have shown that many children who are identified as having difficult asthma do well in the medium term with better asthma outcomes and reduction in prescribed medication,[112] it should not be assumed that, just because

the child does not need a monoclonal antibody, all will be well. In particular, children from families who continue to exhibit the risk factors identified by National Review of Asthma Deaths (NRAD) (see Box 46.1) are at high risk of severe asthma attacks and death and should be very carefully monitored.

Severe, Therapy-Resistant Asthma: Deconstructing the Airway Disease

If extrapulmonary and environmental/lifestyle have been excluded, attention switches to the nature of the underlying airway disease. It should be noted that this evaluation cannot separate the consequences of treatment of severe asthma from the nature of the disease itself, for obvious reasons. So the use of high-dose ICS are locally immunosuppressive,[113] and their use in adults has been associated with an increased risk of pneumonia in chronic obstructive pulmonary disease patients,[114] as well as tuberculosis and atypical mycobacterial infection.[115,116] So the finding of bacterial infection or changes in the airway microbiome using molecular techniques cannot be assumed to be causal in severe asthma. There are potentially six components of airway disease (Box 46.5). In most cases of severe asthma, abnormal airway contents (mucus) are a secondary phenomenon, although they are occasionally sufficiently severe as to merit treatment with mucolytics. Likewise, a cough is a secondary phenomenon, and the treatment is of the underlying cause.

There are a number of differences between the typical severe, therapy-resistant asthmatic child and the picture in adults. In our series, there was no female predominance; a strong atopic history was common (85% atopic with a total median IgE of 386 [range: 115-1286]).[117,118] Also, the children were not obese. U-BIOPRED is a large Pan-European study recruiting adults and children with severe asthma and comparing them to mid-moderate controls. Although the adult severe asthmatics had significantly worse lung function and higher FeNO than the controls, these were not significantly different in the pediatric cohorts. In both adults and children, asthma-related quality of life was significantly worse in the severe groups.[51,119]

The main focus of the evaluation is on fixed and variable airflow obstruction, and airway inflammation and infection; four key questions are answered (Box 46.6).

PROTOCOL: INVASIVE INVESTIGATION OF SEVERE, THERAPY-RESISTANT ASTHMA

We assess symptoms (ACT), recent steroid bursts, spirometry, and acute response to bronchodilator, sputum induction, and FeNO$_{50}$. The same day, the child undergoes a bronchoscopy under a general anesthetic, with BAL and endobronchial biopsy.[118,120] When the samples have been obtained, and at the end of the procedure, we administer a single dose of intramuscular triamcinolone (40 mg if the child's weight <40 kg, otherwise 80 mg). The child is discharged the next day and is reviewed 4 weeks later, when all the noninvasive measurements are repeated (Fig. 46.3).

The key requirement for the safe performance of bronchoscopy in these children is a skilled anesthesiologist. The child may be premedicated with SABAs, and adverse events

Box 46.5   Components of Airway Disease, Their Underlying Cause and Management

AIRWAY CHARACTERISTIC	UNDERLYING CAUSE	TREATABLE CHARACTERISTIC
Fixed airflow obstruction	■ Extramural: loss of alveolar tethering ■ Intramural: circumferential narrowing, from antenatal or postnatal exposure to pollutants, postnatal viral infection, or airway remodeling	■ Avoid increasing the doses of medications, which will be ineffective
Variable airflow obstruction	■ Extramural: loss of alveolar tethering ■ Intramural: increased airway smooth muscle, airway edema, any cause of circumferential narrowing ■ Intraluminal: mucus	■ SABA, LABA (potentially long-acting muscarinic antagonists) for bronchospasm ■ Airway clearance, mucolytics
Airway inflammation	■ Present or absent ■ Beneficial (combating infection) or adverse ■ Cell based description: eosinophilic, neutrophilic, mixed cellularity ■ Pathway based description: Type 2 or innate cytokines, other	■ Do not use antiinflammatories if airway not inflamed ■ Do not suppress if beneficial ■ Specific biologicals will increasingly be deployed in the future
Airway infection	■ Bacterial, viral, fungal ■ Luminal or latent within airway wall	■ Antibiotics and antifungals as appropriate
Abnormal airway contents	■ Too wet: increased airway surface liquid or mucus; aspiration syndromes ■ Too dry: increased airway surface liquid absorption	■ Airway clearance, treat any reflux, assess swallowing ■ Rehydrate with hypertonic saline aerosols
Abnormal cough reflex	■ Increased cough sensitivity ■ Reduced sensitivity	■ No licensed pediatric therapies as yet

LABA, Long-acting beta-2 agonists; *SABA,* short-acting beta-2 agonists.

Box 46.6   The Four Key Questions Answered by Invasive Investigation of Children With Severe, Therapy-Resistant Asthma

1. Is there phenotype discordance, namely a disconnect between symptoms and eosinophilic airway inflammation? Antiinflammatory medication is not escalated if the airway is not inflamed, and should be intensified in an exacerbating child if there is airway inflammation when the child is asymptomatic.
2. Is the airway inflamed at all, and if so, what is the pattern of inflammation? (Usually neutrophilic) inflammation may be a beneficial response to infection.
3. Is the child partially or totally steroid responsive, or steroid resistant, according to our multidimensional framework?
4. Does the child have persistent airflow limitation? Therapy for airflow obstruction is not escalated if the child has reached the plateau of the dose-response curve in terms of spirometry.

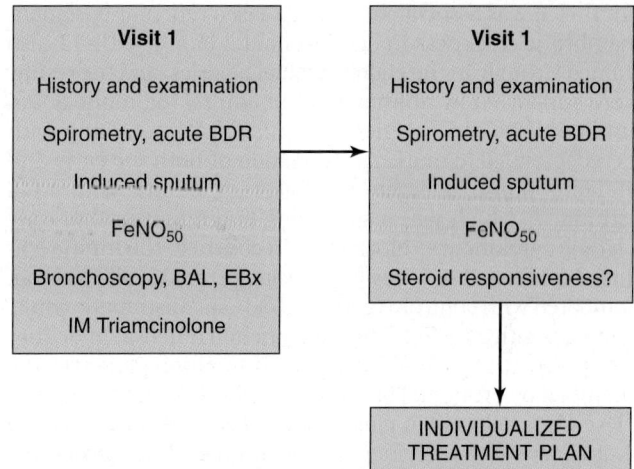

Fig. 46.3 Invasive investigation of putative severe, therapy-resistant asthma. *BAL,* Bronchoalveolar lavage; *BDR,* bronchodilator responsiveness; *EBx,* endobronchial biopsy; *FeNO50,* fractional exhaled nitric oxide at expiratory rate 50 mL/s; *IM,* intramuscular.

are very rare. We saw an acute severe bronchospasm on one occasion, which rapidly responded to treatment. Close post-procedure monitoring of the child is essential.

ASSESSMENT OF AIRWAY INFLAMMATION

We do not see submucosal neutrophilic inflammation in children with severe asthma,[118] unlike in adult severe asthma. Interestingly, intraepithelial neutrophils are associated with *better* markers of asthma control, which underscores that possibly some forms of inflammation may be beneficial.[121] Instead, induced sputum, BAL, and the bronchial submucosa are eosinophil dominated, although there are marked variations between individuals in the extent of eosinophilia, including their complete absence. A neutrophilic submucosa should prompt reconsideration of the diagnosis of asthma. Although the findings in induced sputum and BAL are concordant, airway wall histology is discordant.[122] It is not clear which is most relevant to disease pathophysiology.

However, as an increasing array of monoclonal antibodies are coming on the market, we need to move from cell-based descriptions to pathway based, if these expensive resources are to be targeted properly. Given the marked eosinophilic phenotype, a T_H2 cytokine profile would be expected, and is indeed found in adult asthma, but two pediatric severe asthma studies have failed to confirm this. We studied both induced sputum and BAL using both the Luminex and the Cytometric Bead Array platforms, and performed immunohistochemistry on endobronchial biopsies. We found scant evidence of the T_H2 signature cytokines IL-4, IL-5, and IL-13.[118] The Severe

Asthma Research Program group also failed to find evidence of T_H2-driven inflammation.[123] They compared severe, therapy-resistant asthma with mild-moderate disease and showed that the cytokines that best discriminated between the two groups were GRO (CXCL1), RANTES (CCL5), IL-12, IFN-γ and IL-10. They concluded that pediatric severe, therapy-resistant asthma was neither a T_H1- nor a T_H2-driven disease. We do not know if some eosinophilic children are T_H2 high, and the noneosinophilic group corresponds to T_H2 low adult disease.[124] It should be noted that periostin, a useful serum biomarker in adults for the T_H2 high phenotype, is not useful in children because it is released from growing bone. The other two discriminatory genes, CLCA1, and SERPINB2, have not been evaluated in children.

The findings of these two large studies do not necessarily show that T_H2 cytokines are unimportant in the early stages of severe asthma. All these children were prescribed high-dose ICS, which may have controlled the T_H2 component of their disease. What it does mean is that the factors driving ongoing severe disease are different, and are, as yet, unknown. There is increasing evidence that the epithelial-derived cytokines (IL-25, IL-33, and TSLP) may be implicated, as well as lineage-negative innate lymphoid cells.[125] We have shown that IL-33 is steroid resistant and promotes collagen synthesis from fibroblasts from pediatric severe asthma patients.[126] We also showed that increased cellular expression of IL-33, but not IL-13, was associated with increased reticular basement membrane thickness in endobronchial biopsies. IL-33 also stained strongly in the endobronchial biopsies, and the results were supported by animal data. In adults, the monoclonal antibody AMG 157, which prevents TSLP interacting with its receptor, led to marked attenuation of both the early and the late phase allergen responses in adults with mild asthma,[127] which was a surprising finding given that only a single cytokine was blocked.[128] In contrast, the innate epithelial cytokine IL-25 may be more important in mild asthma. Compared with controls, corticosteroid-naïve asthmatic adults stained positive for IL-25 in the bronchial mucosa; in neither group was TSLP or IL-33 detected. IL-25 high patients were identified by bronchial brushing IL-25 transcript levels, and these were reflected in plasma IL-25 levels. A raised plasma IL-25 correlated with increased sputum and endobronchial biopsy eosinophils and a better response to ICS.[129]

The T_H17 pathway has been studied in adults, but it would probably drive a neutrophilic phenotype, and thus is an unlikely candidate in children. However, in animals at least, IL-17 is also an eosinophil chemoattractant.[130,131] A recent adult trial of the monoclonal anti-IL-17 receptor antibody brodalumab was negative,[132] perhaps because neutrophilic asthma was not an entry criterion. Further work is clearly needed in order to delineate the proinflammatory mechanisms driving pediatric severe, therapy-resistant asthma.

There is certainly a pressing need to define these pathways. Studies of anti-T_H2 cytokine strategies, such as mepolizumab (anti-IL-5),[133] lebrikizumab (anti-IL-13),[134] and dopilumab (IL-4 receptor alpha chain)[135] have often recruited children aged 12 and over, and trials are largely dominated by adult participants. It is essential that promising results in these trials are not uncritically extrapolated to children. It may be justified to perform a therapeutic n of 1 trial in a child doing badly on all therapies. Further trials in children are needed, including measurements of T_H2 cytokines, before

wide usage in pediatric severe, therapy-resistant asthma can be recommended.

ASSESSMENT OF STEROID RESPONSIVENESS

It is likely that steroid responsiveness is a continuum; true steroid unresponsiveness is likely confined to rare cases of mutations in the corticosteroid receptor. The widely accepted adult definition of steroid response[136,137] is ≥15% predicted increase in FEV_1 in patients with a bronchodilator reversibility (BDR) ≥12% from baseline and an abnormal FEV_1 (≤80%) prior to the trial. There is no accepted definition in children, and the adult definition cannot be applied to around half of our severe, therapy-resistant asthmatics, mainly because their baseline spirometry is not sufficiently abnormal prior to the trial[118]; and indeed, spirometry is often a poor reflection of asthma severity in children (above). Furthermore, there is no consensus on the dose and duration of CS for the trial. We opted to use triamcinolone intramuscularly to ensure adherence. We use a multimodality definition of steroid responsiveness (Table 46.3).[6,138] Most children are partial responders; about 10% are total nonresponders, and 10% completely responsive in all domains (complete responders). Some children who were nonresponsive using the adult definition were partial responders in the multidomain assessment. We have also shown that additional doses of triamcinolone do not change the category of responsiveness (unpublished). While the clinical utility of this approach has yet to be confirmed, it might serve as a useful template for current research; so, for example, an intervention with an antiinflammatory medication might be expected primarily to affect the inflammatory domain. Indeed, we have shown that steroid response in the inflammatory domain is predictive of a therapeutic response to omalizumab.[139]

Assessment of Persistent Airflow Limitation

The definition of persistent airflow limitation (PAL) is relatively easy, FEV_1 <80% (or better, −1.96 Z [standard deviation]

Table 46.3 Multidomain Definition of Steroid Responsiveness

Domain	Response Pattern 4 Weeks After Intramuscular Triamcinolone
Spirometry (FEV_1)	Increase in FEV_1 (% predicted) to normal (≥80%) or by ≥15% over baseline
Symptoms (ACT)	Increase to normal or by ≥50% or by ≥5 points
FeNO	Normalizes (<24 ppb)
Sputum eosinophils	Normalizes (<2.5%)

Response may be complete (all domains), partial (≥1 domain) or absent (no domains), of which partial is much the commonest.
ACT, Asthma control test; *FeNO*, fractional exhaled nitric oxide; *FEV_1*, first second forced expired volume.
From Bossley CJ, Fleming L, Ullmann N, et al. Assessment of corticosteroid response in pediatric patients with severe asthma by using a multidomain approach. *J Allergy Clin Immunol*. 2016. pii: S0091-6749(16)00309-2. doi: 10.1016/j.jaci.2015.12.1347. [Epub ahead of print] and Bossley CJ, Saglani S, Kavanagh C, et al. Corticosteroid responsiveness and clinical characteristics in childhood difficult asthma. *Eur Respir J.* 2009;34:1052-1059.

scores) despite a trial of systemic steroids and acute administration of SABA. However, as above, the dose, duration, and route of administration of steroids are still not agreed on, nor is the dose of SABA. We have shown that neither 40 mg prednisolone for 2 weeks[140] nor a single dose of triamcinolone combined with 1 mg albuterol inhaled from a large volume spacer[141] is adequate to determine whether the child has PAL, but it is doubtful whether a higher or longer duration of systemic steroids can be justified. So we have taken the pragmatic decision that PAL will be at least provisionally diagnosed after a single dose of triamcinolone and albuterol, as above. Using this definition, approximately 25% of our severe cohort have PAL.

Treatment of Severe, Therapy-Resistant Asthma

The treatment options, with the exception of the use of omalizumab, are largely anecdote based.[142] The following scheme is suggested.

1. *Is omalizumab indicated?* Much of the omalizumab evidence is inevitably in less severe asthma,[143–153] but if the child meets national guidelines for asthma, AND has been assessed in detail as above, AND been found to have persistent eosinophilic airway inflammation on bronchoscopy, AND every effort has been made to reduce the allergen burden in the environment, then we recommend a 16-week trial of omalizumab, with detailed monitoring of the response. Although guidelines mandate aeroallergen sensitization, omalizumab may be trialed in the rare nonatopic child with IgE in the range where omalizumab is indicated.[148] If, after 16 weeks, there is no benefit, we discontinue therapy. Steroid-responsive inflammation may predict a good response to omalizumab (above).[139]

2. *Should standard medications be used in novel ways?* The options are high-dose ICS, fine-particle ICS, oral prednisolone, intramuscular triamcinolone, and the SMART regime. The latter is a single combination ICS and LABA device (usually a Symbicort turbohaler); and low-dose theophylline (antiinflammatory dose). For all but the SMART regime, the demonstration of ongoing eosinophilic airway inflammation is essential (the exception is theophylline, which may benefit neutrophilic asthma, at least in adults[154]); and steroid total nonresponders who have eosinophilic or neutrophilic inflammation should only be considered for low-dose theophylline, and not the steroid-based regimes.

   ▪ *High-dose ICS:* for most children, the plateau of the ICS dose-response curve is 100 µg twice daily of fluticasone,[10] and escalation of dosing risks increased side effects. However, a small minority of asthmatic children may benefit from increasing the dose as high as 2000 µg/day.[155] However, if there is no response to dose escalation, it is essential that it is promptly stepped down to the lowest possible dose.

   ▪ *Fine-particle ICS:* there is evidence from adult studies that some asthmatics may have very distal inflammation, shown on transbronchial biopsy (TBB).[156–158] These studies have not been performed in children because of fears of the risks of TBB. There is also physiological

evidence from C_{alv} nitric oxide measurements of distal airway inflammation in adult asthmatics, with responses both symptomatically and physiologically to fine-particle ICS or systemic steroids.[159,160] There is too much variability in C_{alv} for it to be used as a biomarker in individual children[161]; and there is no evidence for this approach in severe, therapy-resistant asthma. However, a trial of fine-particle ICS may be worth considering, and discontinuing if there is no benefit. Finally, it is interesting to speculate whether the distal airway inflammation is related to the poor peripheral deposition of ICS, and might respond to low-dose oral prednisolone, delivering the steroid by the blood rather than the airway.

   ▪ *Oral prednisolone:* the nonevidence-based starting dose is 0.5 mg/kg, tapering down to the lowest dose needed to control the disease. If this is at the price of unacceptable side effects, then a steroid-sparing agent (see later) should be considered.

   ▪ *Intramuscular triamcinolone:* there is no evidence that this offers any advantage other than assuring adherence, which is an insufficient reason for using it other than for a steroid trial (see earlier). Indeed, if it is used as a "quick fix" for nonadherence, there is a risk that this will lead to long-term use with severe steroid side effects.

   ▪ *SMART regime*[162–164]: we use this approach particularly in adolescents, to try to keep the regime simple. We also consider its use in the child with symptoms and ongoing peak flow variability, but without evidence of eosinophilic airway inflammation. It could be argued that a LABA, as a single inhaler added to the child's base medications, would be more logical, but given the risks of LABA as a single agent, we prefer the compromise of the additional ICS. The risk of this strategy is that it relies on adequate symptom perception, which may not always be the case in children with severe asthma (see earlier).

   ▪ *Low-dose theophylline:* there is laboratory evidence and data from adult studies, that theophylline in a dose attempting serum levels of 5–10 µg/mL may have significant antiinflammatory effects, and restore steroid responsiveness—the latter making it attractive particularly in steroid complete nonresponders.[165–172] The lower serum levels reduce but do not eliminate the risk of drug interactions and other side effects. Despite the strong theoretical background, this approach has rarely been successful in our hands.

3. *Does the child meet criteria for SAFS?* The fungi that are implicated in this condition are listed in Box 46.7 and the definition of SAFS[173] is given in Table 46.4. The results of trials of antifungal therapy in adults conflict with itraconazole[173] but not voriconazole,[174] showing benefit. Fungal sensitization in children may be associated with a more severe phenotype,[175] but there are no randomized, controlled trials of treatment. Our approach is to minimize environmental fungal exposure in the home, including checking any nebulizer the child may have for fungal contamination, and banning visits to stables (by analogy with management of allergic bronchopulmonary aspergillosis [ABPA] in cystic fibrosis). If antifungals are to be used, it is essential to remember that there is an interaction

Box 46.7   Fungi Implicated in Severe Asthma With Fungal Sensitization

- *Aspergillus fumigatus*
- *Cladosporium herbarum*
- *Penicillium chrysogenum (notatum)*
- *Candida albicans*
- *Trichophyton mentagrophytes*
- *Alternaria alternata*
- *Botrytis cinerea*

From Denning DW, O'Driscoll BR, Powell G, et al. Randomized controlled trial of oral antifungal sensitization. The fungal asthma sensitization trial (FAST) study. Am J Respir Crit Care Med 2009;179:11-18.

Table 46.4   Diagnostic Criteria for Severe Asthma With Fungal Sensitization in Adults and the Proposed Modification in Children

Adults	Children

- Sensitization (positive skin prick test or specific IgE) to one or more fungi in Box 46.7, with IgE <1000 and with negative IgG Aspergillus serology AND
- Therapy with:
  - 500 µg FP/day, or
  - Continuous oral CS, or
  - 4/6 Pred bursts in 12/24 months
	- Severe, therapy-resistant asthma as defined in the text, with any pattern of symptoms
	- Fungal sensitization as defined by adult criteria
	- BUT, no IgE criteria since allergic bronchopulmonary aspergillosis is rarely if ever seen in children

CS, Corticosteroids; *FP*, fluticasone propionate; *IgE*, immunoglobulin E; *IgG*, immunoglobulin G.
From Denning DW, O'Driscoll BR, Powell G, et al. Randomized controlled trial of oral antifungal sensitization. The fungal asthma sensitization trial (FAST) study. *Am J Respir Crit Care Med.* 2009;179:11-18 and Castanhinha S, Sherburn R, Walker S, et al. Pediatric severe asthma with fungal sensitization is mediated by steroid-resistant IL-33. *J Allergy Clin Immunol.* 2015;136:312-322.

with ICS, such that iatrogenic Cushing syndrome may be seen.[176–179] Anecdotally, antifungals have been successful in some children. Recent evidence suggests that the innate epithelial cytokine IL-33 may be implicated in the pathogenesis of SAFS[180]; however, as yet, there is no clinically approved monoclonal that can be used.

4. *Should nonstandard medications be used?* The possible approaches are macrolide antibiotics, immunosuppressives, intravenous Ig as an immunomodulator, and a continuous subcutaneous infusion of terbutaline.
   - Macrolide antibiotics are the safest option, and might be indicated for the rare child with a neutrophilic phenotype, or if an atypical infection is suspected.[181,182] One study comparing azithromycin with montelukast as add-on therapy ended in futility,[183] as only 55 of 292 of those who were symptomatic while prescribed ICS and LABA could be randomized; most of the rest were nonadherent or did not have asthma at all, which underscores the need for detailed evaluation of these patients before uncritical acceptance of the diagnosis "severe asthma." However, in the small group actually studied, the results were not encouraging. In an adult study, azithromycin reduced asthma attacks only in noneosinophilic patients. Data in children with severe asthma but no airway eosinophilia are awaited.

   - *Ig infusions:* the evidence is scanty in adults, and it is anecdotal and conflicting in children.[184–187] As with immunosuppressives (see later) they are used only in children with evidence of ongoing airway inflammation, which is either steroid resistant or only responsive at the cost of major side effects. One small study in steroid-dependent teenage asthmatics showed a reduction in maintenance oral steroids, steroid bursts, and hospitalizations for asthma. They suggested that the mechanism may be a synergistic interaction with dexamethasone in suppressing lymphocyte activation and significant improvement in the glucocorticoid receptor binding affinity.[188] In view of how tightly Ig use is controlled, it would be difficult to justify this approach to regulatory bodies.
   - Immunosuppressives are used in children on the basis of small case series (methotrexate,[189,190] cyclosporine[191]) or zero published evidence (azathioprine). Nebulized cyclosporine might be an attractive way of getting benefits while avoiding systemic toxicity, but it has only been used after lung transplantation.
   - Subcutaneous terbutaline infusions may be considered in children with ongoing documented labile airflow obstruction and no underlying airway inflammation.[192] This is a rare group, and the evidence base is a small case series. We now perform a double blind n of 1 therapeutic trial, but rarely find any benefit.

5. *What about other biological agents?* The differences in pathophysiology between childhood and adult severe asthma have been highlighted above. Nonetheless, in a child who has persistent eosinophilic inflammation with ongoing symptoms, either totally steroid responsive or suffering major steroid side effects—in particular in the rare child in whom T_H2 activation can be documented—a trial of one of the monoclonal T_H2 strategies (above) could justifiably be sought on compassionate grounds.

6. *Physical methods?* There is no evidence to recommend bronchial thermoplasty in children; indeed, the potential long-term consequences of the procedure on the growing airway are worrying.

A DIFFICULT SPECIFIC PROBLEM: TREATMENT OF THE EXACERBATING PHENOTYPE

Acute asthma exacerbations cause considerable morbidity, sometimes death; however, they are not a feature of all children with asthma. Asthma lung attacks (a term we favor over "exacerbations") have been associated with an accelerated decline in lung function in children not prescribed ICS. Acute asthma lung attacks cannot be abolished completely. Acute asthma lung attacks and loss of baseline control are not the same thing; loss of baseline control is characterized by wide diurnal peak expiratory flow variation, while acute asthma lung attacks are characterized by a steep decline in peak flow, with no increased variability.[193] Children may have good control, but still have attacks,[194] and increasing the interval medications merely increases the risk of side effects. However, poor control[195] and previous severe attacks[195,196] both predict a high risk of future acute attacks.

In older children, the combination of respiratory viral infection, and both sensitization and exposure in the home to high allergen levels, is strongly predictive of asthma lung attacks.[83]

They are typically characterized by mixed eosinophilic and neutrophilic, or pure neutrophilic inflammation.[197–199] At the other extreme, really high-dose allergen exposure can cause acute asthma lung attacks (e.g., thunderstorm asthma,[200] and the Barcelona soya bean epidemic asthma[201]); thunderstorm asthma at least is characterized by airway eosinophilia.[200]

In school-aged children with multiple asthma lung attacks, we aim to increase the baseline dose of ICS to abolish interval sputum eosinophilia, the effects of which are best shown through the proof of concept anti-IL5 studies.[202,203] LABAs also reduce asthma lung attacks.[204–206] Allergen sensitization is identified, and avoidance measures advised. High-dose ICS[207] or LTRAs[208] may be considered at the first sign of a viral asthma lung attack. However, none of these measures will completely obviate the need for oral CS. Finally, if asthma lung attacks are of very sudden onset with rapid deterioration over minutes, we provide the child with a source of injectable adrenaline (Epipen). The hospital treatment of acute asthma lung attacks is beyond the scope of this chapter.

Monitoring the Child With Severe, Therapy-Resistant Asthma on Treatment

MONITORING TREATMENT BENEFIT

On the basis of work in adult asthmatics, it may be thought that monitoring therapy in the inflammatory phenotypes would be beneficial in children,[209,210] but the only trial in children with severe, therapy-resistant asthma using induced sputum every 3 months was negative.[211] A *post-hoc* analysis did suggest a reduction in acute asthma attacks in the month after the sputum measurement; however, currently, there is insufficient evidence to recommend induced sputum or FeNO$_{50}$ to monitor severe asthma. Two studies may help explain the reasons. In the first, the variability of sputum phenotype longitudinally was determined in children with either mild/moderate or severe asthma, and spontaneous phenotype changes were common in both groups, and not predictable. This is in marked contradistinction to adult results in which they appeared much more stable over time.[212] A second study reported the relationship between sputum eosinophil count and FeNO$_{50}$ in severe therapy-resistant asthma. A total of 148 samples were concordant (eosinophil positive, FeNO$_{50}$ positive = 77; both negative = 71) and 49 (25%) were discordant (eosinophil positive, FeNO$_{50}$ negative = 25; eosinophil negative, FeNO$_{50}$ positive = 24). Fifty-nine children produced at least two sputum samples. Of these, 31 (53%) were consistently concordant, 24 (41%) were discordant in one sample but concordant on at least one other occasion (one showed discordance in both directions and concordance in a third sample), and only 4 (7%) demonstrated consistently discordant levels.[213] Thus, these two markers cannot be used interchangeably, and neither can currently be recommended for monitoring children with acute severe asthma.[214]

MONITORING SIDE EFFECTS

In addition to standard monitoring for both asthma and systemic steroid therapy, the question of adrenal insufficiency must be considered. Clearly, adrenal suppression is inevitable if the child is on all but the lowest dose of oral steroids. Most would recommend a Synacthen test for children on high-dose ICS, but the dose of adrenal corticotrophin, the sampling protocol, and the frequency that the test is performed are still controversial. Our current recommendation is for an annual standard Synacthen test.

THE ROLE OF AN ANNUAL ASSESSMENT

There is a strong case to be made for a structured annual assessment in all children with severe, therapy-resistant asthma. This would include a reevaluation of adherence (see earlier) and allergen exposure, as well as at least screening questionnaires for psychological morbidity. Spirometry and acute bronchodilator responsiveness, sputum induction, and at least FeNO$_{50}$ should be part of the evaluation too. This would also be the opportunity to evaluate side effects with measurements of height and weight, blood pressure, urinalysis, and the performance of a short Synacthen test. We do not routinely refer for ophthalmology examination. Following this reassessment, a multidisciplinary planning meeting is held. An annual review should not replace a much more frequent and regular review of treatment and progress.

Summary and Conclusions

Severe asthma continues to be one of the most challenging problems in the whole of pediatrics. The need to get the basics right is and will remain the bedrock of management. Children are not small adults, and pediatric asthma is not a watered-down version of adult asthma. With the advent of the new era of monoclonals, we need pediatric biomarkers and clinical trials to define who will benefit from which monoclonal. Recent lessons learned the hard way are:

- Unless you are doing electronic adherence monitoring, you are clueless about whether the patient is adherent to therapy; this has become pivotal in severe asthma clinics.
- It is also increasingly clear that child abuse will present as severe asthma, and many so-called severe asthmatics are in fact no such thing; this is an instance where believing the mother may not always be the right approach. Always talk to the school; always get the details of what objective evidence there is for "severe" asthma attacks; and, if in doubt, admit the child for observation and objective monitoring.

Without doubt, there will be more painful lessons to learn in the coming years.

References

Access the reference list online at ExpertConsult.com.

Suggested Reading

Bel EH, Souza A, Fleming L, et al. Diagnosis and definition of severe refractory asthma: an international consensus statement from the Innovative Medicine Initiative (IMI). *Thorax*. 2011;66:910–917.

Bousquet J, Mantzouranis E, Cruz AA, et al. Uniform definition of asthma severity, control, and exacerbations: document presented for the World Health Organization Consultation on Severe Asthma. *J Allergy Clin Immunol*. 2010;126(5):926–938.

Bush A, Fleming L, Saglani S. Severe asthma in children. *Respirology.* 2017;22:886–897.

Bush A, Saglani S. Management of severe asthma in children. *Lancet.* 2010;376:814–825.

Cates CJ, Karner C. Combination formoterol and budesonide as maintenance and reliever therapy versus current best practice (including inhaled steroid maintenance), for chronic asthma in adults and children. *Cochrane Database Syst Rev.* 2013;(4):CD007313.

Chipps BE, Lanier B, Milgrom H, et al. Omalizumab in children with uncontrolled allergic asthma: review of clinical trial and real-world experience. *J Allergy Clin Immunol.* 2017;139:1431–1444.

Chung KF, Wenzel SE, Brozek JL, et al. International ERS/ATS guidelines on definition, evaluation and treatment of severe asthma. *Eur Respir J.* 2014;43:343–373.

Cook J, Beresford F, Fainardi V, et al. Managing the pediatric patient with refractory asthma: a multidisciplinary approach. *J Asthma Allergy.* 2017;10:123–130.

Martin Alonso A, Saglani S. Mechanisms mediating pediatric severe asthma and potential novel therapies. *Front Pediatr.* 2017;5:154.

Pavord I, Beasley R, Agusti A, et al. The Lancet Commissions. After asthma: redefining airways diseases. *Lancet.* 2017;389:embargoed until 11 Sept.

Petsky HL, Kew K, Chang AB. Exhaled nitric oxide levels to guide treatment for children with asthma. *Cochrane Database Syst Rev.* 2016. doi:10.1002/14651858.CD011439.pub2.

Petsky HL, Li A, Chang AB. Tailored interventions based on sputum eosinophils versus clinical symptoms for asthma in children and adults. *Cochrane Database Syst Rev.* 2017;8:CD005603. doi:10.1002/14651858. CD005603.pub3. [Epub ahead of print.].

Puranik S, Forno E, Bush A, et al. Predicting severe asthma exacerbations in children. *Am J Respir Crit Care Med.* 2017;195:854–859.

Ramratnam S, Bacharier L, Guilbert T. Severe asthma in children. *J Allergy Clin Immunol Pract.* 2017;5:889–898.

Saglani S, Fleming L. How to manage a child with difficult asthma? *Expert Rev Respir Med.* 2016;10:873–879.

47 The Influence of Upper Airway Disease on the Lower Airway

JONATHAN CORREN, MD

During the past century, practicing clinicians have frequently observed that allergic rhinitis, sinusitis, and asthma coexist in the same patients. Despite a wealth of data supporting an association between the upper and lower airways, not until recently have reliable data emerged that suggest that upper airway disease is a risk factor for the development of asthma and that experimentally induced nasal dysfunction causes asthma to worsen. In addition, there is a growing body of literature demonstrating that appropriate treatment of nasal allergy and chronic sinus disease results in improvements in asthma symptoms and lower airway function. In this chapter, data from a variety of epidemiologic, clinical, and laboratory studies will be highlighted to help clarify our understanding of these complex and important relationships.

Allergic Rhinitis and Asthma

THE EPIDEMIOLOGIC RELATIONSHIP BETWEEN ALLERGIC RHINITIS AND ASTHMA

The first population-based studies that explored the relationship between allergic rhinitis and asthma were cross-sectional surveys, which demonstrated that rhinitis and asthma commonly occur together. Many of these studies reported that nasal symptoms occur in 28%–78% of patients with asthma[1] as compared with approximately 5%–20% of the general population.[2] Generally, these data were drawn from a variety of epidemiologic studies and clinical settings in which patients were not interviewed in a standardized fashion and insensitive instruments were used for detecting rhinitis. In a study that utilized a standardized and detailed questionnaire in 478 patients across all age groups, rhinitis was found to be a nearly universal phenomenon in patients with allergic asthma, occurring in 99% of adults and 93% of adolescents.[3] Conversely, asthma has been shown to affect up to 38% of patients with allergic rhinitis,[1] which is substantially higher than the 11.9% global prevalence noted in unselected children.[4]

While these studies demonstrate that rhinitis and asthma frequently occur in the same patients, longitudinal studies are required to accurately assess the actual risk for developing asthma in patients with rhinitis alone.

Settipane and colleagues[5] published the first prospective study regarding the relationship between allergic rhinitis and the development of asthma. In a study that spanned 23 years from entry to completion, 690 adolescents who had allergic rhinitis (without chest symptoms) developed asthma 3 times more often (10.5%) than individuals without rhinitis (3.6%). In another prospective study, Burgess and coworkers[6] enrolled 8583 children, beginning at 7 years of age, and evaluated them at 13 and 43 years of age. Children diagnosed with allergic rhinitis at the beginning of the study had a twofold to sevenfold increased risk of developing asthma at both 13 and 43 years of age. In the most recent study, Rochat and colleagues[7] followed 1314 healthy children from birth to 13 years of age. Allergic rhinitis present at 5 years of age was found to be a significant predictor for developing wheezing between 5 and 13 years of age, with an adjusted relative risk of 3.82. These longitudinal studies, taken together, strongly support the role of allergic rhinitis in childhood or adolescence as a risk factor for developing subsequent asthma.

In children younger than 2 years of age, it has been more difficult to prospectively assess the progression of allergic rhinitis to asthma, in part due to the high prevalence of viral upper respiratory tract infections in this age group. In the study by Rochat,[7] children with allergic rhinitis diagnosed by 2 years of age were not at increased risk of developing wheezing between 5 and 13 years of age. The authors noted that rhinitis at 2 years of age is usually not a persistent condition and will often remit as the child grows older.

Studies dating back over 20 years have demonstrated that adults and adolescents with allergic rhinitis are more likely to have increased bronchial hyperresponsiveness (BHR) than children without rhinitis.[8] More recently, airway hyperresponsiveness has also been shown to be increased in children who have allergic rhinitis but no asthma. Choi and colleagues.[9] performed bronchial methacholine challenges in a group of 115 nonasthmatic children, 4–6 years of age. BHR, assessed as a methacholine dose required to produce wheezing or oxygen desaturation of <8 mg/mL, was significantly more common in children with allergic rhinitis compared with nonrhinitis children (32.5% vs. 9.4%, respectively). Among children with allergic rhinitis, serum total IgE, the number and pattern of skin-prick test responses, blood eosinophil markers, and parental history of allergic rhinitis and atopic dermatitis were not different between the BHR-positive and BHR-negative groups, whereas the persistent type of rhinitis and parental history of asthma were more frequent in the BHR-positive group than in the BHR-negative group.

While nonspecific BHR appears to be more common in children with allergic rhinitis, a second and equally important question is whether this characteristic predisposes them to the development of asthma. A 12-year follow-up study of 291 randomly selected children and adolescents (7–17 years of age) examined a number of historical and laboratory features, including bronchial responsiveness to inhaled histamine.[10] Increased airway responsiveness to histamine was a powerful independent predictor of future lower airway disease, with an approximate fourfold increased risk of developing symptomatic asthma during this period of observation. In a second study, Ferdousi and colleagues[11] followed up a much smaller group of children (*n* = 28) for only 2 years.

Sixteen of the 28 children were found to have an increase in BHR (assessed by isocapnic hyperventilation of cold air or inhaled methacholine challenge), and 8 of these 16 developed asthma after 2 years.

These studies support the theory that bronchial hyperreactivity may represent an intermediate phase between nasal allergy and symptomatic asthma and may help identify children and adolescents at highest risk for developing asthma.

Pharmaco-economic studies from the past decade have attempted to correlate the presence of rhinitis with asthma severity and health care costs attributable to asthma. In an analysis of a database of 1261 children with asthma, Huse and colleagues[12] compared patients with significant nasal allergy with those who had mild or no symptoms of nasal disease. These investigators noted that patients with more severe rhinitis were much more likely to have nocturnal awakening caused by asthma (19.6% vs. 11.8%, respectively), "moderate to severe asthma" as defined by the National Asthma Education Program (60.2% vs. 51.2%, respectively), or work loss related to asthma (24.1% vs. 21.1%, respectively). Similarly, Halpern and coworkers[13] observed that patients with symptomatic rhinitis used more asthma medications, particularly more inhaled and supplemental oral corticosteroids. Judging from these recent investigations, one can postulate that allergic rhinitis may also be related to increased asthma severity and the use of more potent anti-asthma medications. Although these data suggest that rhinitis may be contributing to asthma, an alternative explanation for this association may be that nasal inflammation is a marker for increasing dysfunction of the entire respiratory tract. The possibility of a cause-and-effect relationship is better addressed by therapeutic studies of rhinitis therapy in patients with asthma.

It has been speculated that allergic rhinitis may add a significant burden of disease to patients with asthma. A survey of approximately 800 parents of children with asthma attempted to determine the impact of nasal disease upon their quality of life.[14] In three-quarters of children, rhinitis symptoms preceded the diagnosis of asthma. The concomitant presence of nasal allergy and asthma disrupted the ability to get a good night's sleep (79%), to participate in leisure and sports activities (75%), to concentrate at work or school (73%), and to enjoy social activities (51%). Importantly, parents (79%) reported worsening asthma symptoms when nasal symptoms were most active, and many (56%) avoided the outdoors during the allergy season because of worsening asthma symptoms. The majority of the parents (60%) indicated difficulty in effectively treating both conditions, and 72% were concerned about using excessive medication. Information collected from this study and other similar data indicate that allergic rhinitis does impose a significant additional symptomatic burden on patients with asthma.

COMMON IMMUNOPATHOLOGY OF ALLERGIC RHINITIS AND ASTHMA

During the past decade, we have learned that the immunologic processes leading to allergic rhinitis and atopic asthma are the same. A large number of studies have examined the composition of inflammatory cell infiltrates in the nasal and bronchial mucosa of patients with allergic rhinitis and asthma. Critical cells that have been consistently identified in both upper and lower airway tissue include both resident (epithelial cells, mast cells, dendritic cells) and infiltrating cell types (eosinophils, Th 2 cells).[15,16]

Allergen provocation studies have also demonstrated striking similarities between immunopathologic processes in the nasal and bronchial mucosa, including allergen-induced infiltration by inflammatory cells, cellular activation, and cytokine and chemokine expression or production.[17] In addition, the development of early- and late-phase reactions and the acquisition of airway hyperresponsiveness have been convincingly demonstrated in both the nasal and the lower airways after allergen provocation.[18]

Histologic studies of individuals with allergic rhinitis and no evidence of clinical asthma consistently demonstrate abnormalities of the bronchial mucosa, including thickening of the lamina reticularis and mucosa eosinophilia. These abnormalities are generally less pronounced than those of asthmatic patients,[19] but sometimes, the findings in subjects with rhinitis are indistinguishable from those in subjects with mild asthma.[20] A recent investigation of this phenomenon confirmed that airway inflammation in allergic rhinitis is midway between normal controls and asthmatics and that asthmatics have much lower levels of interferon gamma than these other two groups, indicating that this cytokine may be an important regulator of the asthma phenotype.[21] Findings from these and other histologic studies demonstrate that both the upper and lower airways are histologically and functionally abnormal in patients with rhinitis and no asthma and that select cytokines may determine which patients manifest clinical signs and symptoms of asthma.

EFFECTS OF RHINITIS THERAPY ON ASTHMA

Physicians often note anecdotally that treatment of allergic nasal disease results in improvements in asthma symptoms and pulmonary function. However, there have been relatively few well-controlled, large-scale clinical trials that have attempted to quantify this effect.

Intranasal Corticosteroids

Intranasal corticosteroids (INS) are widely recognized as the most effective pharmacotherapy for allergic rhinitis, with potent effects on symptoms, nasal physiology, and upper airway mucosal inflammation. Given the important pairing of nasal disease and asthma, it therefore stands to reason that treatment of rhinitis with INS might have a salutary effect on the lower airways. During the past 25 years, a large number of clinical trials have been conducted to determine the effects of INS on asthma outcomes. A recent systematic review and meta-analysis examined all prior studies of INS in patients with allergic rhinitis and concomitant asthma and identified a total of 18 randomized, controlled studies with 2162 patients for inclusion in the analysis.[21a] Asthma outcomes consisted of pulmonary function (including first second forced expired value (FEV_1) and domiciliary peak expiratory flow rate), measures of nonspecific bronchial responsiveness, asthma symptoms scores, asthma-specific quality of life, and rescue bronchodilator use. Statistical analysis of a subgroup of studies that compared INS with placebo demonstrated significant improvements in all the above parameters, including FEV_1 (standardized mean difference [SMD] = 0.31, 95% CI, 0.04–0.08) and asthma symptoms (SMD = −0.42, 95% CI, −0.53 to −0.30). Importantly, there were no significant changes in asthma outcomes when INS were added to orally inhaled corticosteroids, suggesting that the impact of INS on chronic lower airways symptoms may be strongest in patients who are not receiving adequate asthma therapy. While these data are helpful in assessing the effects of INS on daily asthma outcomes, such as lung function and symptoms, the studies included in the meta-analysis were not designed to examine the effects of nasal therapy upon asthma exacerbations.

In addition to the above-randomized studies, clinical data from large populations has been employed to assess the relationship between INS use and asthma exacerbations and asthma-related resource utilization.[22,23] A nested case-control study was performed using claims records from 215,000 members, age 6 years and older, of a managed care organization in the United States.[22] Patients with both allergic rhinitis and asthma were identified and assessed for types and numbers of prescriptions for these conditions along with hospital-based care (emergency room visits and hospitalizations) for asthma. Patients who had used INS had a significantly lower risk for both asthma-related emergency room treatment and hospitalization (adjusted odds ratios: ER, 0.75, 95% CI, 0.62–0.91; hospitalization, 0.56, 95% CI, 0.42–0.76). These data suggest that use of INS may have an effect on major exacerbations of asthma, although it is uncertain whether this is a direct effect of rhinitis therapy or may reflect better overall care of the asthmatic patient.

Both the randomized trials and large database analyses indicate the potential importance of INS in reducing both daily assessments of asthma control (symptoms, beta-agonist use, and pulmonary function in patients not receiving inhaled corticosteroids [ICS]) and asthma exacerbations. As most of the INS preparations that were used during the above studies have very limited systemic availability, it is unlikely that these effects were due to systemic effects of the glucocorticoids.

Antihistamines. The presence of histamine in the lower airways has been correlated with bronchial obstruction,[24] and histamine has long been thought to play a role in bronchial asthma. However, early studies of first-generation antihistamines in adolescents and adults showed minimal improvements in bronchial asthma, and initial small trials of second-generation antihistamines yielded mixed results.[25,26] However, two recent large-scale clinical studies using an antihistamine alone and an antihistamine-decongestant combination both resulted in significant improvements in asthma control. Grant and colleagues[27] demonstrated that seasonal symptoms of rhinitis and asthma were significantly attenuated in patients treated with cetirizine 10 mg once daily in a large group of adolescents and adult patients. In a second study using loratadine 5 mg plus pseudoephedrine 120 mg twice daily in patients with seasonal allergic rhinitis and asthma, Corren and colleagues[28] demonstrated that asthma symptoms, peak expiratory flow rates, and FEV_1 were all significantly improved in patients taking active therapy. In reviewing data from these and similar trials, it is difficult to determine whether the salutary effects of antihistamines in asthma can be attributed to direct effects on lower airway physiology or to improvements in rhinitis. Because many of the currently available agents appear to have weak or

transient effects on resting airway tone, benefits to the lower airway may be due to modulation of upper airway function.

In the nested case-control study of rhinitis therapy and asthma outcomes, the use of second-generation oral antihistamines was associated with a nonsignificant trend toward lower risk of asthma-related emergency room visits and hospitalization.[21] However, there appeared to be a possible additive effect between second-generation antihistamines and INS in further lowering the probability of a major asthma-related event.

These studies demonstrate that treatment of rhinitis may result in improvements in a number of asthma outcomes and suggest that nasal disease contributes to the pathophysiology of asthma. Based on the data in these studies, treatment of rhinitis may reduce symptoms of mild asthma to such an extent that the requirement for asthma therapy may be reduced or even eliminated. While population-based analyses have also shown that major asthma exacerbations resulting in hospital care may be reduced by INS, these findings reflect an important association but do not prove cause and effect.

PATHOPHYSIOLOGIC CONNECTIONS BETWEEN ALLERGIC RHINITIS AND ASTHMA

Although there is increasing evidence that allergic rhinitis may influence the clinical course of asthma, the mechanisms connecting upper and lower airway dysfunction are not entirely understood. A variety of theories have been invoked, including both direct and indirect effects of nasal dysfunction on the lower airways.

Systemic Effects of Nasal Inflammation on the Lower Airways

Research over the past few years has demonstrated that several inflammatory mediators produced during allergic reactions may enter the systemic circulation. Experimental nasal allergen challenge has been shown to induce both peripheral blood eosinophilia[29] and activation of peripheral blood leukocytes.[30] It has been postulated that the net result of these various factors on the systemic circulation is the promulgation of inflammation in other sites. Braunstahl and colleagues performed a nasal provocation study, suggesting a link between systemic inflammation and changes in airway inflammation and function.[29] Prior to and 24 hours after the nasal challenge, bronchial mucosal biopsies were performed that demonstrated that the number of eosinophils in the lower airway mucosa, as well as the expression of adhesion molecules, increased after nasal allergen challenge. Further supporting this interaction between the upper and lower airways, Braunstahl and colleagues[31] also found increased inflammatory markers in the nasal mucosa following the instillation of allergen into the lower airways of subjects with allergic rhinitis. Given this emerging evidence, it is likely that systemic factors do play a critical role in the interaction between the upper and lower airways.

Impaired Mucosal Function

It has been shown that allergic inflammation in the respiratory mucosa results in impairment of the barrier function of

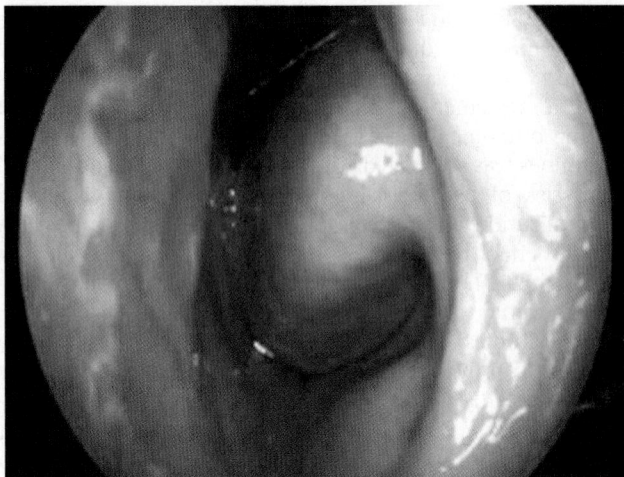

Fig. 47.1 Pale mucosa and clear secretions in child with allergic rhinitis.

the epithelium.[32] It has been hypothesized that this alteration in epithelial integrity might then lead to increases in allergen uptake, synthesis of IgE, and ultimately involvement of the lower airways. Alternatively, impaired nasal mucosa may be more susceptible to viruses, resulting in an increase in allergic sensitization and subsequently more asthma (Fig. 47.1).[33]

Nasal-Bronchial Reflex

Early mechanistic studies investigated the effects of several mucosal irritants on lower airway function in normal human subjects. In 1969, Kaufman and Wright[34] applied silica particles onto the nasal mucosa of individuals without lower airway disease and noted significant, immediate increases in lower airway resistance. Bronchospasm induced by nasal silica was blocked by both resection of the trigeminal nerve[35] and systemic administration of atropine. Fontanari and coworkers[36] recently reevaluated the possibility of a neural connection between the upper and lower airways by using cold, dry air as the nasal stimulus. These investigators demonstrated that nasal exposure to very cold air caused an immediate and profound increase in pulmonary resistance that was prevented by both topical nasal anesthesia and cholinergic blockade induced by inhalation of ipratropium bromide. Both these studies strongly suggest the presence of a reflex involving irritant receptors in the upper airway (afferent limb) and cholinergic nerves in the lower airway (efferent limb).

Subsequent studies used challenge materials considered to be more biologically relevant to allergic rhinitis, including histamine, whole pollen particles, and allergen extracts. Yan and Salome[37] performed nasal histamine challenges in subjects with perennial rhinitis and stable asthma and observed that FEV_1 was reduced by 10% or more immediately after provocation in 8 of 12 subjects. Importantly, radiolabeling studies were performed as part of this study that demonstrated that histamine was not deposited into the lower airways. However, other studies that used histamine[38] or allergen[39] failed to demonstrate bronchoconstriction after nasal provocation. This discrepancy in results may be partly explained by the type of patients who participated in these studies. Whereas Yan and Salome[37] investigated subjects with perennial, symptomatic nasal disease, the majority of other studies examined asymptomatic patients outside their pollen season. Certainly, a substantial degree of heterogeneity exists between patients in their lower airway response to nasal stimulation.

In addition to neurally mediated bronchospasm, it has been postulated that a nasal allergic reaction might result in an alteration in lower airway responsiveness. Corren and colleagues[39] investigated the effects of nasal allergen provocation on nonspecific bronchial responsiveness to methacholine. Ten subjects with seasonal allergic rhinitis and asthma were selected for study; all patients related worsening of their asthma to the onset of hay fever symptoms. Nonspecific bronchial responsiveness was significantly increased 30 minutes after nasal challenge and persisted for 4 hours.

Because radionuclide studies demonstrated no evidence of allergen deposition into the lungs, it seems unlikely that these increases in airway reactivity can be attributed to direct effects of allergen. In addition, the rapidity with which these changes occurred suggests the possibility of a reflex mechanism.

Mouth Breathing Caused by Nasal Obstruction

Nasal blockage resulting from tissue swelling and secretions may cause a shift from the normal pattern of nasal breathing to predominantly mouth breathing. Previous work has shown that mouth breathing associated with nasal obstruction resulted in worsening of exercise-induced bronchospasm, whereas exclusive nasal breathing significantly reduced asthma after exercise.[40] Improvements in asthma associated with nasal breathing may be the result of superior humidification and warming of inspired air before it reaches the lower airways.[41] Similarly, it would be expected that airborne allergens and pollutants would also be less likely to enter the lungs during periods of normal nasal function.

Postnasal Drip of Inflammatory Material

Patients frequently complain that postnasal drip triggers episodes of coughing and wheezing. Early studies investigating the possibility of aspiration of nasal secretions demonstrated that substances placed in the upper respiratory tract could later be recovered from the tracheobronchial tree.[42] More recently, Huxley and colleagues[43] investigated pharyngeal aspiration during sleep both in healthy subjects and in patients with depressed sensorium. With the use of a radiolabeled marker that was intermittently released into the nose, pulmonary aspiration was detected in a significant number of both the normal and the ill subjects. In a more recent and definitive investigation, however, Bardin and colleagues[44] were unable to document significant aspiration of radionuclide in a study of 13 patients with chronic rhinosinusitis (CRS) and asthma.

It is difficult to determine which of these experimental mechanisms is most important in linking the nose to the lower airways. In all likelihood, however, several of these phenomena may contribute in some way to alterations in lung physiology in patients with allergic rhinitis and asthma.

DIAGNOSTIC AND THERAPEUTIC IMPLICATIONS

Diagnosis

The previously discussed data suggest that all patients with asthma be evaluated to determine the presence of concomitant chronic rhinitis. The patient should be questioned regarding types of symptoms, focusing on the presence of nasal congestion, sneezing, itching, discharge, and postnasal drip. Other associated symptoms (e.g., snoring, poor sleep quality, and ear congestion or popping) should also be investigated and considered when choosing therapy. The upper airway should then be carefully examined, with an emphasis on the size and vascularity of the nasal turbinates, type and presence of nasal secretions, tonsillar size, and color and elasticity of the tympanic membranes.

While allergic rhinitis is the most common form of chronic rhinitis in children (older than 2 years of age) and adolescents, a smaller number of patients will have chronic nonallergic rhinitis or CRS without allergy as the cause of their symptoms (Table 47.1). Some children with CRS have concomitant allergy and may have symptoms and signs of both conditions. Much less likely is the possibility of a structural problem resulting in obstruction. In children, this is most likely to be a foreign body, such as a peanut or small piece of toy, which is inserted into the nose and causes unilateral nasal blockage and discharge with sneezing; occasionally, this is followed by a secondary sinus infection. Bony or cartilaginous problems (such as a deviated nasal septum) are unusual and most likely the result of trauma.

Regarding diagnostic testing in patients with persistent rhinitis and asthma, allergy skin tests or *in vitro* measures of specific IgE should be performed using a panel of common airborne allergens. At a minimum, these should include house dust mites (*Dermatophagoides farinae* and *D. pterynissinus*), cockroaches, animal dander types (cat and dog), indoor and outdoor molds (*Penicillium, Aspergillus, Cladosporium, and Alternaria*), and regional pollens. This information is critical in differentiating allergic rhinitis from nonallergic disease or CRS and establishing an appropriate program of environmental control measures. Other tests, including total serum IgE level, microscopic analysis for nasal cytology, and total circulating blood eosinophils, have not proven helpful in either differentiating allergic rhinitis from other nasal disorders or in assessing the severity of the problem.

Allergen Avoidance

Once allergy testing is complete, the physician may devise a comprehensive program of allergen avoidance. The effects of environmental control strategies have been most heavily studied regarding dust mites and furry pets (Box 47.1).[45] Compliance with these measures may be difficult, but they will certainly be helpful in many patients with hypersensitivity to these allergens.

Pharmacotherapy

While carefully designed allergen avoidance strategies may reduce symptoms to varying degrees, most patients will still require pharmacotherapy. In patients with persistent symptoms, particularly if nasal congestion is present, INS should be considered as first-line therapy. A large number of studies have established that there are no differences in efficacy between all the available compounds,[46] and most compounds (including budesonide, mometasone furoate, and fluticasone propionate) have been shown to have no significant effects on linear growth velocity in young children. These drugs should be used on a regular basis in patients with daily symptoms, or as long as symptoms dictate in children with intermittent problems.

Oral H_1 antihistamines have long been a mainstay of therapy for allergic rhinitis and are most effective in relieving sneezing, itching, and rhinorrhea, with minimal effects on nasal congestion. For this reason, they are often combined with oral decongestants, such as pseudoephedrine. Oral antihistamines that cause minimal or no sedation have been approved for use in young children, including cetirizine, fexofenadine, and loratadine.[47] Because they are available

---

Table 47.1 Differential Diagnosis of Chronic Nasal Symptoms in Children

	Allergic Rhinitis	Nonallergic Rhinitis	Chronic Rhinosinusitis
Nasal congestion	Mild-severe	Usually severe	Mild-severe
Sneezing	Mild-severe	None	None
Pruritis	Mild-severe	None	None
Watery discharge	Mild-severe	Mild-severe	None
Purulent discharge	None	None	Mild-severe
Eye symptoms	Mild-severe	None	None
Periorbital darkening	Mild-severe	Mild-severe	Mild-severe
Headache/ pressure	None-mild	None-mild	Mild-severe

Box 47.1   Allergen Avoidance Strategies for Allergic Rhinitis

House Dust Mites

Weekly washing of all bedding in hot water (>130°F)
Weekly vacuum cleaning of all floor surfaces, using high-efficiency particulate air (HEPA)-type vacuum cleaner or standard vacuum cleaner with double-thickness reservoir bag
Removal of carpeting, or treatment of carpeting every 2–3 months with acaricidal spray or powder

Animal Danders (Any Furry Pet)

Optimal—Removal of the animal from indoor environment, followed by replacement of carpeting and aggressive housecleaning
Possibly effective—Keeping the cat indoors and instituting the following measures: Noncarpeted floors
Plastic or leather furniture
Frequent vacuum cleaning of floors
High-flow air filtration
Frequent cat bathing

Indoor Mold

Thorough eradication of infestation
Repair of source of water intrusion

Cockroach

Appropriate handling and storage of food and garbage

in a number of different formulations (i.e., tablets, rapidly dissolving pills, and liquids), patient preference may dictate choice of medication.

Montelukast, a leukotriene D_4 receptor antagonist, is also used for allergic rhinitis in children.[48] Montelukast has been shown to reduce all the symptoms of rhinitis, including nasal congestion. Because montelukast also has been shown to be effective in treating concomitant asthma, this medication may be very effective as a solo treatment for children with mild persistent allergic rhinitis and concomitant asthma.

Specific Allergen Immunotherapy

Many children will continue to have persistent symptoms of rhinitis despite employing environmental control measures for indoor allergens and a combination of drugs, often including an intranasal corticosteroid with an antihistamine or montelukast. Occasionally, children may experience adverse effects that necessitate discontinuation of some or all their rhinitis medications. In these children, specific allergen immunotherapy should be strongly considered. Studies performed over the past decade have demonstrated that subcutaneous specific allergen immunotherapy to a wide range of allergens, including dust mites; cat dander; selected outdoor molds; and numerous grass, tree, and weed pollens; have had a high rate of clinical efficacy, with approximately 75% of children manifesting a good clinical response. Other studies have documented multiple salutary immunologic effects of immunotherapy, including a reduction in allergen-induced early- and late-phase allergic responses and attenuation of cytokine (e.g., Interleukin-4) production. An important potential benefit of immunotherapy is its effect on progression of allergic airway disease. A recent large prospective study in children with seasonal allergic rhinitis demonstrated that a 3-year course of subcutaneous immunotherapy (SCIT) reduced the development of asthma symptoms and improved bronchial responsiveness compared with an open control group.[49] In a follow-up of this group 7 years after stopping SCIT, 24 of 53 (45%) children treated with a placebo had developed asthma, compared with 16 of 64 (25%) who received active immunotherapy, representing a 44% reduction in asthma cases.[50] Regarding duration of treatment, once initiated, SCIT should be continued for at least 3 years.

More recently, investigators have turned their attention to other modes of administering allergen immunotherapy to both children and adults, particularly sublingual immunotherapy (SLIT). In a meta-analysis of clinical trials of SLIT in children with allergic rhinitis and asthma, SLIT caused a significant reduction in both symptoms (SMD −1.14; 95% CI, −2.10 to −0.18; $P = 0.02$) and medication use (SMD −1.63; 95% CI, −2.83 to −0.44; $P = .007$).[51] SLIT does have advantages compared with SCIT, including the absence of a buildup phase, fewer systemic reactions, and the convenience of home administration. However, it is unknown whether SLIT is as effective as SCIT, whether the effects are sustained after stopping treatment, and whether it can prevent the development of lower airway disease. Future trials will be essential in answering these questions.

Given the ability of SCIT to cause long-term modifications in nasal allergic disease as well as reduce the risk of developing asthma, allergen immunotherapy should be a strong consideration in all children with moderate to severe allergic rhinitis.

SUMMARY

Allergic rhinitis is virtually ubiquitous in children with asthma that is frequently underidentified and undertreated. In adolescents, allergic rhinitis may in fact serve as a risk factor for developing asthma. INS appear to significantly modulate lower airway reactivity and have been shown in a number of small studies to have beneficial effects on mild asthma. Current research suggests that the upper and lower airways are most importantly connected via the systemic circulation, which likely distributes products of inflammation throughout the respiratory tree. Allergic rhinitis should always be considered in patients with asthma and should be treated aggressively once it has been identified. Immunotherapy may be particularly useful in children with allergic rhinitis and new-onset asthma, because it may modify the long-term prognosis of their airway disease.

Chronic Rhinosinusitis and Asthma

EPIDEMIOLOGIC RELATIONSHIP BETWEEN CHRONIC RHINOSINUSITIS AND ASTHMA

Since the early 20th century, physicians have noted that CRS and asthma frequently coexist in the same patients. In 1925, Gottlieb[52] noted that 31 of 117 adolescent and adult patients with asthma suffered from severe symptoms of CRS. Other investigators reported similar findings in both children and adults during the next decade, with an incidence of symptomatic CRS as high as 72% in patients with asthma.[53] Conversely, a large retrospective study of pediatric, adolescent, and adult patients with CRS noted a 12% incidence of asthma,[54] and only one-third of the patients with both sinus disease and asthma in this study reported that CRS preceded their lower airway symptoms.

Attempts to define the incidence of sinus disease in patients with asthma again lay dormant until the early 1970s. These more recent reports have emphasized the role of radiography in diagnosing CRS. Several studies have demonstrated that 31%–53% of asthmatics across all age groups have abnormal sinus radiographs, with 21%–31% of patients demonstrating significant findings (defined as opacification of one or both maxillary sinuses, air-fluid levels, or mucosal thickening >5 mm).[55-58] In a more recent study that examined the utility of sinus computed tomography (CT) scanning in children with asthma, 58% of the children studied had varying abnormalities of all of the sinuses (Table 47.2).[59]

Although the incidence of radiographic sinus abnormalities is universally high in asthmatics, others have questioned whether these changes have clinical significance. Fascenelli[60] prospectively performed sinus radiography on 411 asymptomatic normal adolescent and adult male volunteers and noted a 28% incidence of maxillary sinus abnormalities. Most of these changes, however, consisted of minimal thickening, and only 5% of the group demonstrated significant thickening (>5 mm) of the maxillary antrum. In a similar prospective study of young children, Kovatch and colleagues[61] noted that 8 of 22 (36%) asymptomatic children younger than 1 year of age demonstrated either thickening greater than 4 mm or opacification of the maxillary sinuses. Only

Table 47.2 Prevalence of Radiographic Sinusitis in Asthmatics

Study	Sample Size	Age Range (Years)	Total Abnormalities (%)[a]	Significant Abnormalities (%)
Berman et al.[55]	52	19–80	62	NA
Rachelefsky et al.[56]	70	3–16	52	27
Schwartz et al.[57]	217	9–70	47	21
Zimmerman et al.[58]	138	6–19	31	31
Chen et al.[59]	53	4–14	58	NA

NA, Not assessed.

[a]Opacification, air-fluid level, or >5 mm mucosal thickening.

2 of 31 (6%) children older than 1 year of age, however, demonstrated these same changes. These two studies demonstrate that it is unusual to detect significant radiographic abnormalities of the maxillary sinuses in normal, healthy individuals older than 1 year of age. Significant abnormalities of sinus radiographs are much more common in patients with asthma than in healthy, nonasthmatic individuals, suggesting that these radiographic findings most likely reflect pathologic changes of the sinus tissue rather than radiologic artifact.

UNIQUE FEATURES OF CHRONIC RHINOSINUSITIS IN ASTHMATICS

Clinical Features

CRS in children is often an indolent illness, usually characterized by the following cardinal symptoms: nasal congestion, purulent anterior or posterior nasal drainage, and cough.[62] Several other symptoms are reported by patients with CRS, including fatigue, malaise, cough, sleep disturbance, ear pain or pressure, dizziness, halitosis, dental pain, dysphonia, or nasal or throat irritation. However, none of these is specific enough to be clinically useful in diagnosis.

Although headache and facial fullness may also be prominent complaints in adults, it is uncommon in children with CRS. While fever may occasionally be observed in patients with acute sinusitis, it is rarely seen in chronic disease. Because cough may be the most prominent presenting symptom of CRS in children, the physician must maintain a high index of suspicion regarding this possibility. Therefore, any child with symptomatic asthma and cough who has responded poorly to conventional asthma treatment (e.g., inhaled corticosteroid plus a long-acting β_2 agonist, a leukotriene D_4 receptor antagonist, or both) and has persistent nasal symptoms should be evaluated thoroughly for chronic sinus disease.

Physical findings usually include nasal swelling, dried purulent secretions, and occasionally shiners (periorbital darkening) (Figs. 47.2 and 47.3).

Chronic Rhinosinusitis With Nasal Polyps. Nasal polyps (NP) represent inflammatory masses that originate in the paranasal sinuses of patients with CRS and evaginate into

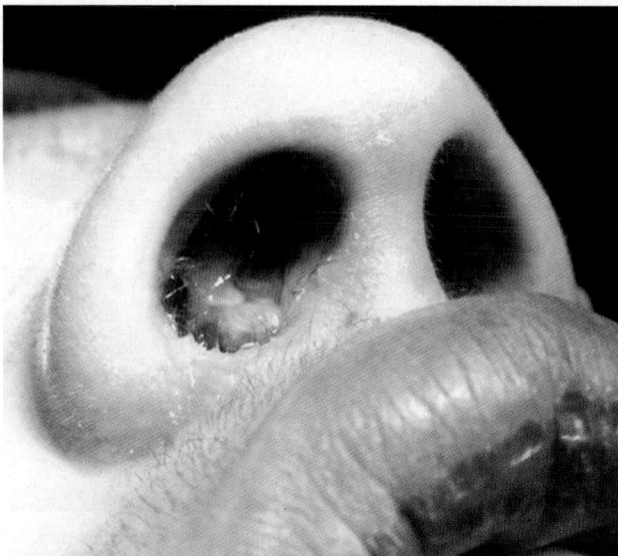

Fig. 47.2 Purulent secretions in child with chronic rhinosinusitis.

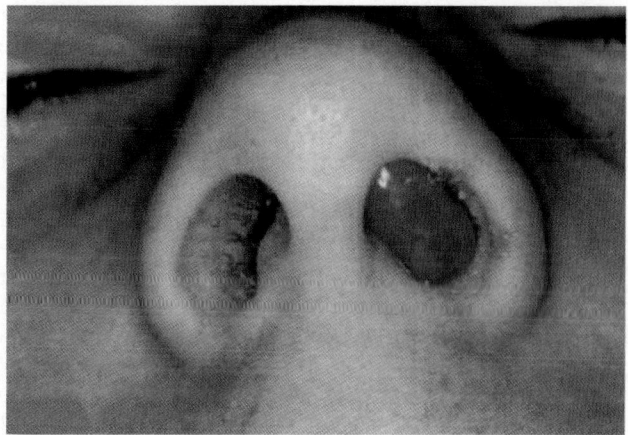

Fig. 47.3 Nasal polyp in child with chronic rhinosinusitis.

the nasal airway. CRS with NP (CRS/NP) is seen most commonly in adult patients and is unusual in young children. NP are present in approximately 0.1% of unselected children in the United States,[63] but the vast majority are diagnosed in children with cystic fibrosis[64] and allergic fungal rhinosinusitis. In children with asthma, the exact prevalence of NP is not known, but in patients diagnosed with NP, roughly one-third have concomitant asthma.[65] Therefore, when polyps are visualized in children, the clinician should suspect that the patient may also have asthma and should always consider the possibilities that the child may have underlying cystic fibrosis or allergic fungal sinusitis (AFS) (Fig. 47.4).

Histopathology

Most studies of sinus histopathology have historically been performed in adult patients, and only in the past 20 years have investigators carefully examined the sinus mucosa of children with CRS. A study of children with CRS were compared regarding the concomitant presence of asthma (*n* = 13), cystic fibrosis (*n* = 10), or neither (*n* = 11).[63] More

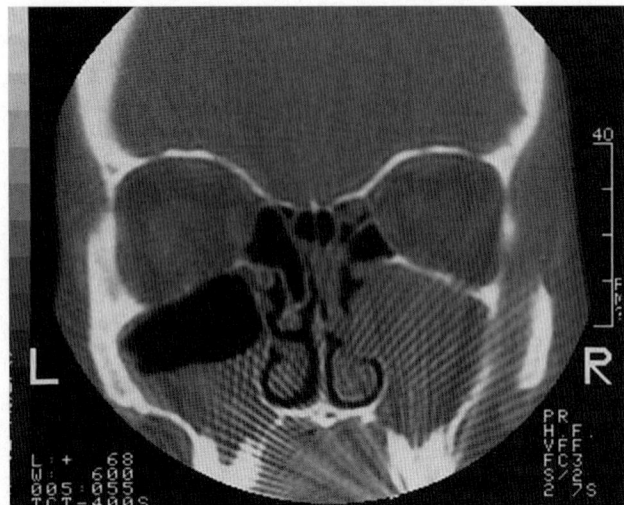

Fig. 47.4 Sinus computed tomography of child with chronic rhinosinusitis.

eosinophils were counted in the sinus tissues of patients with asthma and cystic fibrosis compared with patients without concomitant disease, but this did not reach statistical significance, most likely as a result of very small sample sizes. In addition, allergy status (as defined by skin testing) did not affect the degree of tissue eosinophilia. A small number of other studies confirm that children with CRS but without asthma have low numbers of sinus mucosal eosinophils. The above studies suggest that the sinus mucosa in children with CRS and asthma may have a similar histologic profile to the sinuses of adult patients with CRS and asthma and that eosinophils play a potential role in the pathogenesis of both their sinus and lower airway diseases.

Microbiology

In 1974, Berman and colleagues[55] studied 21 adolescent and adult patients with asthma and radiographic abnormalities of the maxillary sinuses. Bacterial cultures of sinus aspirates demonstrated positive bacterial growth in only 5 of 25 aspirates. Eighty percent of the subjects in this study, however, had minimal evidence of sinusitis (mucosal thickening <2 mm and no sinus polyps). Therefore, conclusions from this study are most relevant to patients with mild sinusitis and may not be applicable to individuals with evidence of more severe disease. In children with asthma and CRS, several bacteriologic studies have been conducted. In 1983, Adinoff and colleagues[67] published a report regarding 42 asthmatic children with sinusitis. Only 12% of maxillary sinus aspirates had positive bacterial cultures; however, many of the studies involving children showed only mild radiographic abnormalities with <5 mm mucosal thickening. Friedman and colleagues[68] in 1984 and Goldenhersh and colleagues[69] in 1990 performed maxillary aspirates in groups of 8 and 12 asthmatic children, respectively, with significant radiographic evidence of sinusitis (i.e., opacification, air-fluid levels, or mucosal thickening >5 mm). These two groups demonstrated that 60% and 75% of these children, respectively, had positive bacterial cultures, and the organisms were the same as those found in acute sinusitis, including *Streptococcus pneumoniae*, *Haemophilus influenzae*, and *Moraxella*

catarrhalis. Taken together, the above studies demonstrate that the majority of children with sinusitis and asthma appear to have a chronic inflammatory disease of the sinus mucosa that is prone to persistent infection with predominantly aerobic bacteria. Data from the radiographic studies also suggest that minor degrees of mucosal inflammation observed on sinus radiograph are usually not associated with active bacterial infection.

Allergic Fungal Sinusitis

An unusual type of chronic sinusitis in children is caused by an allergic reaction to fungi, referred to as AFS. A recent retrospective review characterized 20 children and adolescents (7–18 years of age) with AFS and determined that 90% had NP, 55% had a prior history of asthma, and 50% had proptosis. Laboratory analyses revealed that all patients had abnormal sinus CT findings and positive skin tests to fungi, 90% had an elevation of total IgE, and 70% had peripheral eosinophilia.[70] Surgical specimens demonstrated allergic-type mucin in 55% of patients and positive fungal cultures in 85%. Importantly, relapse was seen in 55% of patients at 1-year follow-up.

EFFECTS OF SINUS THERAPY ON SEVERITY OF ASTHMA

For the past century, otolaryngologists have cataloged the effects of sinus therapy on asthma symptoms. Because most of the earliest data were based on postsurgical observations, these studies are reviewed first.

Surgical Treatment

In the early 20th century, physicians observed that surgical treatment of nasal and sinus disease resulted in variable improvements in asthma symptoms. In 1936, Weille[71] published his study of 500 asthmatic patients of varying ages, 72% of whom had chronic sinus disease. Following sinus surgery in 100 of the patients, 56 reported that their chest symptoms were improved, and 10 experienced complete resolution of asthma. Improvement in asthma symptoms, however, also occurred in 40% of the patients who did not undergo sinus surgery. In 1969, Davison[72] reported that 23 of 24 adolescent and adult patients with CRS and asthma experienced a 75% or greater improvement in asthma symptoms after surgical drainage of the sinuses. Werth[73] presented the results of sinus surgery in children, noting that 20 of 22 pediatric patients with severe asthma and sinusitis experienced a marked improvement in asthma after sinus surgery.

To date, there have been no randomized, controlled trials examining the effects of sinus surgery on lower airway symptoms or function. The study by Weille indicates that asthma symptoms may improve spontaneously in the absence of surgical intervention. Collectively, however, these reports suggest that long-term control of asthma symptoms may improve after surgical sinus procedures.

Medical Treatment

During the past decade, multiple investigators have studied the effect of medical therapy for CRS on asthma symptoms, primarily in children. In 1981, Businco and colleagues[74] reported that 10 of 12 children with chronic asthma had an improvement in lower airway symptoms after medical therapy, although no objective measures of pulmonary function were performed. In 1983, Cummings and colleagues[75] performed a double-blind, placebo-controlled study of sinus therapy in asthma. Active treatment (i.e., antimicrobials, nasal steroids, and oral decongestants) of children with opacification or marked thickening of the maxillary sinuses resulted in significantly fewer asthma symptoms and a reduced requirement for inhaled bronchodilator and oral steroid therapy. Neither pulmonary function results nor measures of bronchial reactivity were significantly improved with active treatment. In 1984, Rachelefsky and colleagues[76] studied 48 children with a 3-month or longer history of sinusitis and wheezing. After 2–4 weeks of antimicrobials with or without antral lavage, 38 of the patients were able to discontinue daily bronchodilator therapy, and 20 of 30 patients demonstrated normalization of pulmonary function tests. More recently, Tsao et al. treated a group of 41 children with CRS and mild asthma with oral antibiotics (amoxicillin-clavulanate) for 6 weeks versus nasal saline irrigations for 6 weeks in an unblinded crossover trial.[68] Children treated with antibiotics experienced significant improvements in signs and symptoms of CRS. While FEV$_1$ did not change following antibiotic therapy, methacholine PC$_{20}$ increased significantly after treatment with amoxicillin-clavulanate for 6 weeks.

Similar to the surgical observations, these studies suggest that medical treatment of sinusitis may result in improvement of bronchial asthma. Although only one randomized, placebo-controlled trial has been performed, the literature shows that both chest symptoms and lower airway function improve after medical therapy.

PATHOPHYSIOLOGIC LINKS BETWEEN CHRONIC SINUSITIS AND ASTHMA

As noted in the section entitled Allergic Rhinitis and Asthma, a number of potential mechanisms may help explain the connection between upper and lower airway dysfunction. Specifically, with respect to the relationship between sinus inflammation and asthma, an animal model has provided some promising insights into this interaction. Brugman and colleagues[77] created an experimental model of sinus inflammation in rabbits using complement fragment C5a. Although induction of sterile sinus inflammation in rabbits caused no changes in baseline lung function, bronchial responsiveness to inhaled histamine was significantly increased. Because these changes could be prevented by strategies that blocked drainage of inflammatory exudates beyond the larynx, the researchers postulated that postnasal drip was most likely responsible for the alteration in airway reactivity. Importantly, however, there was no evidence of lower airway inflammation by either histologic examination or bronchoalveolar lavage. This association of hyperresponsiveness with morphologically normal airways is difficult to explain but again suggests the possibility of a neurally mediated response.

DIAGNOSTIC AND THERAPEUTIC IMPLICATIONS

In children with moderate to severe asthma, chronic sinusitis should always be considered as a possible provocative factor. The clinical history and physical examination, however, are neither sensitive nor specific for chronic sinus disease.

Therefore, we evaluate all children with poorly controlled or steroid-requiring asthma with a Waters' view (occipitomental) sinus radiograph, which is primarily useful for examining the maxillary sinuses. Although CT of the paranasal sinuses has proven to be considerably more sensitive than plain radiographs in detecting subtle mucosal disease,[78] plain radiographs maintain an important role as an initial imaging study. First, plain radiographs are simple, convenient, and relatively inexpensive to perform. Second, in contrast to CT imaging, plain radiographs do not require sedation in infants or young children. Finally, the significance of subtle sinus CT changes is unclear because such abnormalities may be present in up to 50% of children[79] who have no clinical evidence of either sinusitis or asthma. We reserve CT imaging of the sinuses for patients with clinical histories strongly suggestive of sinusitis who have normal plain radiographs and patients with persistent, severe sinus disease before surgical intervention.

Flexible fiberoptic rhinoscopy has been suggested as an alternative to plain radiographs because purulent drainage may be visualized in the vicinity of the middle and superior meatus.[80] This procedure does require sedation in young children, limiting its practical application in patients below the age of 8 years unless deemed medically necessary. In addition, there are diagnostic limitations of the procedure. The absence of visualized pus during the rhinoscopic examination does not rule out active infection, since sinus drainage may be obstructed by ostial edema or obstructing lesions of the nasal airway. Additionally, rhinoscopy will not detect significant hyperplastic changes in the sinuses, which may play an important pathogenic role in CRS.

Patients with well-defined symptoms of CRS or who demonstrate significant radiographic abnormalities of the maxillary sinuses (i.e., opacification, air-fluid levels, or thickening >5 mm, or more than 50% of the maxillary antrum) are treated with medical therapy. We classify medical treatment modalities for CRS into three categories: antimicrobials to eliminate possible concomitant infection, medications to reduce swelling, and measures to thin and evacuate secretions (Box 47.2).

Because up to 25% of the bacterial isolates found in chronic sinusitis are β lactamase producers, we prescribe amoxicillin-clavulanate potassium as a first-line antimicrobial for a period of no less than 3 weeks. In children who are allergic to penicillin, clarithromycin is employed as an alternative. For nasal swelling, we often use topical decongestants (e.g., oxymetazoline) for the initial 3 days of therapy and continue oral decongestants (either phenylpropanolamine or pseudoephedrine) for an additional 7–10 days. If nasal swelling does not respond to these measures, we prescribe a 5- to 7-day tapering course of oral corticosteroids. All patients are also started on a topical nasal corticosteroid, which is usually continued on a long-term basis. We have found that evacuation of secretions, particularly dried crusts, is enhanced by performing nasal irrigations with saline or increasing humidification using a freestanding humidifier or hot shower. Nasal saline irrigations have been evaluated in a number of clinical trials, and a recent Cochrane review concluded that this treatment modality is helpful to patients with chronic sinusitis, either when used alone or as an adjunct to other treatments.[81] If patients fail to respond adequately to the aforementioned regimen, we obtain a sinus CT and refer them to an

Box 47.2   Pharmacotherapy for Allergic Rhinitis

EXAMPLES	2–5 YEARS	6–11 YEARS
Loratadine	5 mg QD	10 mg QD
Cetirizine	2.5–5 mg QD	5–10 mg QD
Fexofenadine	30 mg BID	30 mg BID
Beclomethasone (40 µg/sp)	1 sp QD	1 sp QD
Budesonide (32 µg/sp)	NA	2 sp QD
Fluticasone propionate (50 µg/sp)	1–2 sp QD	Same
Fluticasone furoate (27.5 µg/sp)	1 sp QD	Same
Mometasone furoate (50 µg/sp)	1 sp QD	Same
Triamcinolone (55 µg/sp)	NA	2 sp QD

NA, Not applicable.

Box 47.3   Medical Treatment of Chronic Sinusitis in Asthmatics

Antimicrobials

Amoxicillin-clavulanate potassium for 21 days (or clarithromycin in penicillin-allergic patients)

Medications to Reduce Swelling

For severe swelling, topical oxymetazoline for 3 days
If swelling persists, continue with oral pseudoephedrine on a regular basis for 7–10 days or longer if needed
Intranasal corticosteroid spray for 3–6 weeks; consider long-term use
If swelling is severe and does not respond to above measures, prednisone 0.5 mg/kg body weight for 5 days, tapered over 3–5 days

Measures to Enhance Evacuation of Secretions

Saline irrigations twice daily
Consider hot steam inhalations if mucus is tenacious and difficult to irrigate out of nose

otolaryngologist for consideration of an endoscopically obtained sinus culture or possible surgery.

Regarding surgery for CRS in children, most experts suggest adenoidectomy for children with CRS and adenoidal enlargement who have not responded adequately to medical treatment (Box 47.3). The efficacy of adenoidectomy in this group of patients is uncertain but has been recommended by a 2014 consensus statement on CRS in children developed by an expert panel.[82] Favorable results are seen in some children in observational studies, but there are currently no available randomized trial data regarding the efficacy of adenoidectomy on either CRS or concomitant asthma.

If adenoidectomy is not helpful in reducing chronic nasal obstructive symptoms and reducing recurrent or chronic symptoms of sinusitis, endoscopic sinus surgery may be considered.[82]

SUMMARY

A great deal of data supports an association between chronic sinusitis and asthma. We have developed a better understanding of the pathogenesis of sinus disease in asthmatic patients and now realize that eosinophilic sinus infiltration plays a direct role in chronic mucosal inflammation that may predispose the paranasal sinuses to recurrent or chronic bacterial infection. Long-term blinded, placebo-controlled trials need to be completed before we can reliably predict the effect of

sinus therapy on clinical asthma. Until then, we recommend that sinus disease be considered in all patients with moderate to severe asthma and treated aggressively when it is identified.

References

Access the reference list online at ExpertConsult.com.

Suggested Reading

Braunstahl G-J, Overbeek S, Kleinjan A, et al. Nasal allergen provocation induces adhesion molecules expression and tissue eosinophilia in upper and lower airways. *J Allergy Clin Immunol.* 2001;107:469–476.

Burgess JA, Walters EH, Byrnes GB, et al. Childhood allergic rhinitis predicts asthma incidence and persistence to middle age: a longitudinal study. *J Allergy Clin Immunol.* 2007;120:863–869.

Jacobsen L, Niggemann B, Dreborg S, et al. Specific immunotherapy has long-term preventive effect of seasonal and perennial asthma: 10-year follow-up on the PAT study. *Allergy.* 2007;62:943–948.

Kusel MM, de Klerk NH, Kebadze T, et al. Early-life respiratory viral infections, atopic sensitization, and risk of subsequent development of persistent asthma. *J Allergy Clin Immunol.* 2007;119:1105–1111.

Platts-Mills TA. Allergen avoidance. *J Allergy Clin Immunol.* 2004; 113:388–391.

48 Modern Molecular Therapies for Application in Managing Childhood Asthma

HEATHER ELLEN HOCH, MD, WILLIAM CARL ANDERSON III, MD, and
STANLEY JAMES SZEFLER, MD[a]

Introduction

Attention in asthma management is now being directed toward the development of immunomodulators, medications that can potentially stimulate or impair features of the immune system. Based on current therapeutic strategies, the available medications, such as inhaled corticosteroids (ICS), long-acting β-adrenergic agonists, and leukotriene modifiers, have been shown to reduce asthma symptoms and exacerbations but have not been shown to alter the natural history of asthma. This review will focus on the class of immunomodulators, beginning with allergen immunotherapy (AIT) in its subcutaneous and sublingual forms, followed by experience with anti-IgE (omalizumab), and subsequently by recent experience with the introduction and evaluation of anti-IL5 and anti-IL4/13. Aside from AIT, the other immunomodulators have limited data in children. However, all of these agents hold promise in the possibility of altering the course of asthma, and further studies will be needed to assist the clinician in selecting these medications and the appropriate time for introduction in the management of children with asthma.

Allergen Immunotherapy

INDICATIONS AND PATIENT SELECTION

AIT remains the only treatment modality available that can alter the natural course, and potentially have a curative approach in some patients, for asthma and other allergic conditions through its sustained disease-modifying effects.[1-3] The therapeutic preparation for AIT is extracted from source materials, such as pollen and animal pelts.[4] Two forms of AIT administration are currently in wide-scale clinical practice: subcutaneous immunotherapy (SCIT) and sublingual immunotherapy (SLIT). SLIT has been increasing in use over the last two decades, especially in Europe.[1,2] AIT is addressed both by the Global Initiative for Asthma (GINA) and National

Institute of Health National Heart, Lung, and Blood Institute Expert Panel 3 (NIH NHLBI EPR-3) guidelines for the management of asthma when there is clear evidence between symptoms and exposure to an allergen to which the patient is sensitized.[5,6]

AIT should be reserved only for patients who have both documented evidence of sensitivity to an allergen, either through immediate hypersensitivity skin testing or in vitro testing for serum specific IgE antibodies, and symptoms that correlate with exposure to said allergen.[4] Skin-prick testing has been shown to have greater sensitivity than serum-specific IgE measurements based on nasal and bronchial challenge test results.[4] Patient-specific factors to consider when deciding whether to start AIT include the patient's preference, adherence, current medication requirements, level of asthma disease control, seasonality of disease, response to avoidance measures, medication adverse effects, coexisting allergic rhinitis, cost, impact on quality of life, and geographic location.[1,4,6] Patients whose symptoms are not well controlled by medications or avoidance measures, who are requiring multiple medications or high doses of medications to maintain asthma control, who may be experiencing side effects from their medications, or who wish to avoid long-term pharmacotherapy could be appropriate candidates for AIT.[4,6]

ADMINISTRATION

SCIT may be administered via a conventional, cluster, or rush schedule. In conventional SCIT, the allergen is administered via once-weekly injections at increasing concentrations until a maintenance dose is achieved, followed by injections typically at 4-week intervals.[2,4] In a cluster schedule, multiple injections, usually 2–3, are administered on nonconsecutive days, while in a rush protocol, multiple injections are administered on consecutive days, allowing the patient to reach maintenance typically in 1–3 days.[2] As opposed to SCIT, SLIT's safety profile allows it to be administered with either a shortened or absent build-up phase.[2] A typical course of immunotherapy is 3–5 years in duration,[2,4,6] as studies with SCIT have demonstrated prolonged remission after 3–4 years of treatment.[7] Three years of SCIT may be sufficient in asthmatic children, as a prospective study did not show a significant clinical benefit, including change in asthma symptoms, ICS dose, quality of life, and bronchial hyperreactivity, from an additional 2 years of SCIT.[8] SLIT has a similar course, with its use for allergic rhinitis from house dust mites showing sustained remission for 7 and 8 years

[a]Stanley James Szefler has consulted for Aerocrine, Astra Zeneca, Boehringer-Ingelheim, Daiischi Sankyo, Glaxo Smith Kline, Genentech, Merck, Novartis, and Roche and has received research support from the National Institutes of Health, the National Heart, Lung and Blood Institute, the National Institute for Allergy and Infectious Diseases, the National Institute for Environmental and Health Sciences and the Environmental Protection Agency, the Colorado Cancer, Cardiovascular and Pulmonary Disease Program, and Glaxo Smith Kline.

after 3 and 4–5 years of treatment, respectively.[9] The decision to stop or continue immunotherapy is based on the severity of the disease, benefits sustained from treatment, and convenience of treatment.[4]

MECHANISM OF ACTION

The goal of AIT is to induce immune tolerance to specific allergens via downregulation of T_H2-mediated responses, through both induction of allergen-specific T regulatory (T_{reg}) cells and an ultimate shift toward a T_H1-mediated response (Fig. 48.1).[1,3,4,10]

Very early into the course of AIT desensitization, mast cells and basophils bearing the high-affinity IgE receptor, FcεRI, decrease their susceptibility to degranulation in response to the specific allergen.[1,10] With continued AIT desensitization, the proportion of IL-4-secreting T_H2 cells decreases, while T_{reg} cells for the same allergic epitope increase in number and function.[1,4,10] These inducible CD4+CD25+ T_{reg} cells secrete IL-10 and transforming growth factor beta (TGF-β), regulatory cytokines that function to mediate allergen-specific peripheral T-cell tolerance.[1,10,11] IL-10 directly inhibits T-cell cytokine production, including IL-4 and IL-5 by T_H2 cells, through suppression of the CD28 costimulatory pathway.[4,11] Cytokine production is also inhibited by IL-10 through the inhibition of the costimulatory molecules CD80 and CD86 on antigen-presenting cells, which eliminates the ability of these cells to provide the accessory signals necessary for T helper cell activation.[11]

IL-10 has regulatory effects on B-cells, mast cells, and eosinophils. IL-10 acts on B-cells to decrease antigen-specific IgE production and undergo class switching with IgG4 production.[1,4,10] Allergen-specific IgG4 competes with allergen-specific IgE for allergen binding, thus preventing the IgE-mediated release of inflammatory mediators from mast cells and basophils.[1,4,10] The binding of allergens to IgG4 also inhibits IgE-facilitated allergen presentation to T-cells.[1,4] In addition to the IgG4 isotype switching, TGF-β produced by T_{reg} cells will induce the production of IgA at mucosa surfaces, which will also compete with IgE for allergen binding.[1,4,11] Allergen-specific IgE levels often transiently increase after AIT but then gradually decrease with continued treatment late into the AIT course, likely secondary to IL-10 and T_{reg} cells.[1,4] Acting on mast cells, IL-10 and T_{reg} cells modulate the threshold for mast cell activation, decrease IgE-mediated histamine release, and inhibit FcεRI-dependent mast cell degranulation.[1,4] IL-10 also downregulates eosinophil function, proinflammatory cytokine release, and activity.[1,4,10]

IMPACT ON ASTHMA CONTROL

Meta-analyses of randomized controlled trials using SCIT to treat asthma in children and adults have demonstrated a significant reduction in asthma symptoms, asthma medication use, and allergen-specific and nonspecific bronchial hyperreactivity.[12,13] The effect on lung function has been mixed in these studies, with one meta-analysis showing no consistent effect on lung function,[12] while another showed an improvement in peak expiratory flow rates.[13] Specific individual studies in children have demonstrated similar results with improvement in asthma symptom-medication scores with the use of SCIT,[14] medication use,[15] decreased allergen-specific bronchial hyperreactivity when used in combination with ICSs,[14,16] and improvement in peak expiratory flow rates.[17]

Meta-analyses of randomized controlled trials examining the impact of SLIT on the treatment of asthma in children and adults have been limited in their ability to draw such significant conclusions as seen with SCIT, primarily secondary

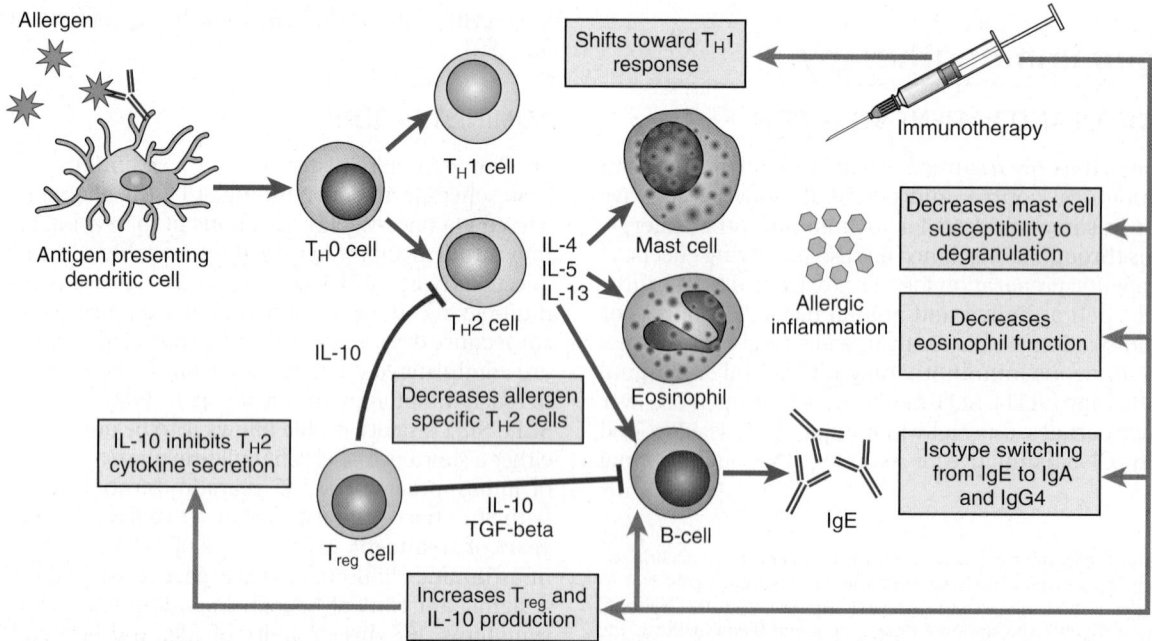

Fig. 48.1 The impact of immunotherapy on allergic inflammation. Immunotherapy shifts the immune response to an allergen from a T_H2 to a T_H1 pathway. Through the induction of immunosuppressive T_{reg} cells producing IL-10 and TGF-beta, immunotherapy inhibits T_H2 cell cytokine secretion. Ultimately these changes decrease downstream induction of T_H2-mediated inflammation. *IL*, Interleukin; *TGF*, transforming growth factor.

to wide but varied use of largely unvalidated symptom and medication scores, and significant heterogeneity between studies.[3,4,18,19] Meta-analyses examining symptom and medication scores in both pediatric and adult patients with both asthma and comorbid allergic rhinitis treated with SLIT have demonstrated a consistent reduction in combined asthma and allergic rhinitis symptom and medication scores, but differing results regarding its ability to impact asthma symptoms and medication use alone.[19,20] There is evidence that the benefit of SLIT for asthma may be more impactful in the pediatric than adult population. A meta-analysis investigating the use of SLIT exclusively in pediatric patients with allergic asthma as young as 3 years old showed a significant reduction in both asthma symptom scores and rescue medication use compared with placebo.[21] In a real-life randomized open controlled trial of SLIT in patients with allergic rhinitis with or without asthma, the use of SLIT compared with conventional medical therapy alone showed a significantly more pronounced reduction in combined rhinitis and asthma symptoms scores in patients less than 18 years of age than in adults.[22] Studies in children and adults have demonstrated a decrease in the number of patients with a positive methacholine challenge in those treated with SLIT in addition to standard medical therapy, versus those without SLIT.[22,23]

Most important would be SCIT and SLIT's ability to reduce ICS doses, especially in a pediatric population. Randomized trials of adults, adolescents, and pediatric patients with mild and moderate persistent allergic asthma have demonstrated that the addition of house dust mite SCIT and SLIT to ICSs resulted in a reduction in ICS dose while still maintaining asthma control.[17,24] Post hoc analysis of adolescent and adult patients treated with house dust mite SLIT with more severe disease, represented by only partly controlled asthma and higher ICS dose, demonstrated a greater significant impact on asthma control, ICS reduction, and quality of life than the less severe population.[25] In a trial of adults with house dust mite allergy–related asthma poorly controlled on ICSs or combination therapy, the addition of house dust mite SLIT increased the time to first moderate or severe asthma exacerbation during an ICS reduction period compared to placebo.[26]

PERSISTENT CLINICAL EFFECTS AFTER DISCONTINUATION

AIT's ability to have persistent effects on asthma control or even resolution of the disease (stemming from its alteration of the underlying immunological response long after discontinuation of therapy) separates it uniquely from other therapies. A prospective study using house dust mite SCIT in asthmatic children showed that 3 years after discontinuation of SCIT, more than 50% of treated patients had remission of their asthma, compared with 3.3% of controls.[8] Patients treated with SCIT had significantly reduced doses of ICSs, lower asthma symptom scores, higher quality-of-life scores, less bronchial hyperreactivity, and higher forced expiratory volume in 1 second (FEV_1) compared with controls at the 3-year time mark.[8] Some of the impact of SCIT in childhood persists into adulthood, as demonstrated by a retrospective study that showed 9 years after the discontinuation of therapy, that asthmatic children who were not treated with SCIT had a three times higher risk of frequent asthma

symptoms than those treated with house dust mite or grass pollen SCIT.[27] This study, however, did not show any difference in lung function or medication use between the groups 9 years after discontinuation of SCIT.[27] Similar findings have been demonstrated with the use of house dust mite SLIT in asthmatic children, with a reduction in the presence of asthma, number of patients using asthma medications, use of bronchodilator, and peak expiratory flow rate 5 years after the discontinuation of SLIT compared with controls.[28]

PREVENTION OF ASTHMA AND ALLERGIC SENSITIVITY DEVELOPMENT

Perhaps the most profound effect of AIT is its ability to prevent progression of allergic sensitization and the development of asthma in children with allergic rhinoconjunctivitis.[4] Treatment with both SCIT[15,29,30] and SLIT[23] against house dust mite, grass, and birch in monosensitized children with allergic rhinoconjunctivitis with or without asthma for 3 years has been shown to prevent or reduce the development of new aeroallergen sensitizations. The preventative effects of SCIT in the development of new aeroallergen sensitizations has been observed even 12 years after the discontinuation of therapy.[31]

The use of SCIT in children with seasonal allergic rhinoconjunctivitis to grass and/or birch pollen without asthma for 3 years in a randomized open trial resulted in significantly fewer patients developing asthma or having asthma symptoms after 3 years of treatment compared with controls,[32] with the preventative effect persisting at 2 years[33] and 7 years[34] after discontinuation of SCIT. Similar prevention of the development of asthma in children with allergic rhinoconjunctivitis has been demonstrated with the use of SLIT to dust mites, grasses, or birch for 3 years in addition to standard medical therapy, compared with medical therapy alone.[23,35] Those children who had bronchial hyperresponsiveness with allergic rhinoconjunctivitis[34] or who were younger[35] at baseline were most at risk of developing asthma, suggesting a potential benefit of the initiation of AIT in these groups for the prevention of asthma.

SAFETY

According to the GINA, the benefits of AIT compared with other pharmacologic and avoidance options must be weighed against several factors, including the risk of adverse events.[2,5] SCIT carries the risk of localized injection site reactions, large local reactions, anaphylaxis, and even death.[36] Annual survey reports show the rate of a severe reaction of any severity is 11.8 reactions per 10,000 injection visits, with the rate of a severe life-threatening reaction being 0.1 reactions per 10,000 injection visits.[36] Overall, 95% of reactions were only mild to moderate in severity.[36] SCIT meta-analysis data estimated the risk of a near-fatal injection was once per 1 million injections and a fatal injection to occur once per 2.5 million injections.[12] Patients with severe or uncontrolled asthma are at increased risk for systemic reactions to SCIT, including fatal and near-fatal reactions, secondary to bronchoconstriction.[36,37] As such, poorly controlled asthma is a major contraindication to AIT.[2,4] Given the risk of these reactions, practice parameters recommend that SCIT only be administered in a supervised medical facility by a professional trained in the prescribing and administration of SCIT and patients be monitored for 30 minutes following the injection, as the risk of a life-threatening anaphylactic reaction after 30 minutes is rare.[1,4]

Unlike SCIT, the safety of SLIT is far superior, with no confirmed reports of SLIT-related fatalities to date, but anaphylactic reactions have been reported.[1,2,4,38] A comprehensive review showed the risk of a severe reaction to SLIT was 1.4 events per 100,000 doses.[39] The most common adverse reactions for SLIT are typically localized oral-mucosal pruritis or mild local edema, which occur within the first 30 minutes of administration, resolved spontaneously, and did not persist with continued therapy.[1,4,19] SLIT's favorable safety profile allows administration outside of a supervised medical setting.[2]

Clinical Application. AIT offers the potential for remission of disease activity but requires careful consideration for benefit-risk assessment, especially for the SCIT form of administration and for those with moderate to severe asthma. Experience with SLIT is more limited in terms of allergens currently approved for administration, but it does offer the benefit of a safer form of AIT administration.

Omalizumab

MECHANISM OF ACTION

Omalizumab is the best studied of the new class of biologic medications for asthma. IgE is known to be important in the T_H2-related asthma response[40–46] and binds to high-affinity receptors on basophils, mast cells, and neutrophils,[40] leading to the release of inflammatory mediators, which are part of the allergic cascade that leads to asthma-related symptoms (Fig. 48.2).

Eosinophils also contain a high-affinity IgE receptor.[41] IgE also has the ability to facilitate antigen presentation to T cells, allowing small amounts of antigen to provoke a T_H2-related asthma response.[40] Omalizumab is a humanized, anti-IgE-specific form of IgG for the treatment of asthma.[41] It binds to circulating IgE, preventing it from binding with both high- and low-affinity receptors on effector cells, leading to a reduction in the release of allergic mediators.[42] Importantly, it does not cross-link bound IgE, which could amplify the allergic cascade and increase the risk of anaphylaxis.[43] IgE levels are decreased in the airway mucosa, as well as in the blood after 16 weeks of treatment, indicating good penetration to the affected tissues.[44] Reports have shown that treatment with omalizumab reduces cellular activation, leading to basophil and mast cell degranulation,[45] as well as modifying dendritic cell antigen presentation mechanisms.[46] In addition, there is early evidence that omalizumab may also downregulate bronchial smooth muscle proteins, indicating a possible role in disease-modifying remodeling.[47] There is evidence that omalizumab actually decreases IgE production over time, indicating that indefinite treatment may not be required.[48] One evaluation of shorter-term therapy showed that after 7 months of treatment, withdrawing omalizumab led to a recurrence of symptoms.[49] One study recommended a minimum duration of treatment of 12–16 weeks to fully assess treatment response.[50] Another study evaluated

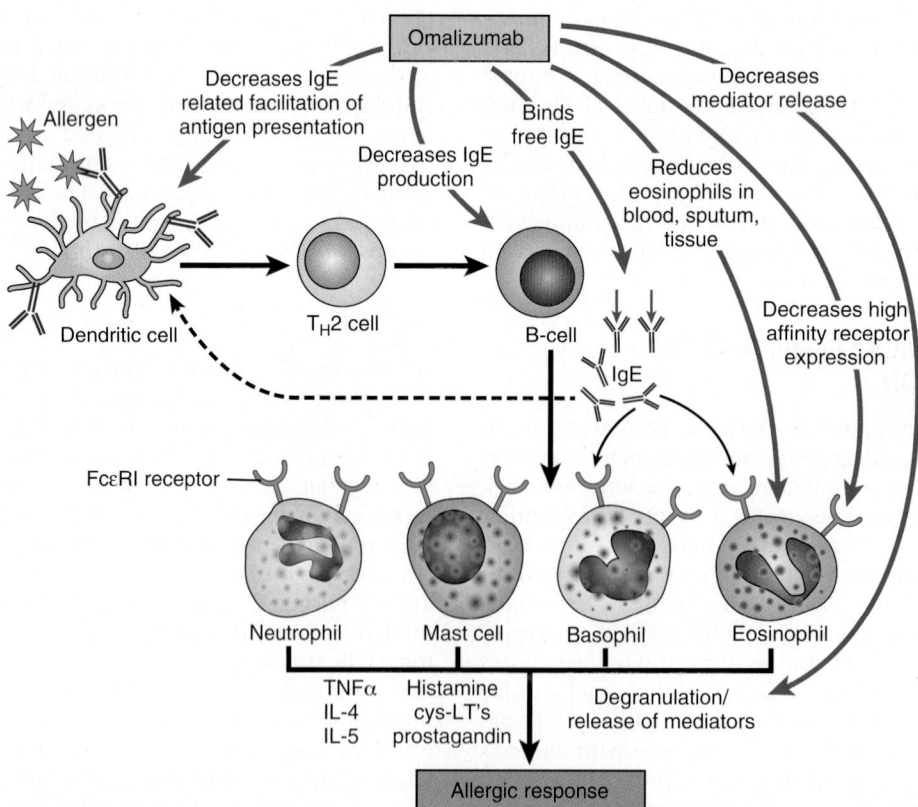

Fig. 48.2 Omalizumab binds to free IgE, inhibiting its ability to bind with the high affinity FcεRI receptor on mast cells, basophils, neutrophils, and eosinophils, therefore decreasing degranulation and release of mediators of allergic inflammation. *FcεRI,* High affinity IgE receptor; *IL,* interleukin; *LT,* leukotriene; *TGF,* transforming growth factor; *TNF,* tumor necrosis factor.[41]

patients 3 years after the discontinuation of omalizumab therapy (which they had received for 6 years), and found that most patients continued to have reduced asthma symptoms at that time.[51]

PHARMACOLOGY

Pharmacodynamics

In vitro allergen-stimulated basophil histamine release is reduced by approximately 90% in treated subjects.[52] Serum-free IgE values are reduced within 1 hour of the first dose, and this is maintained between doses, and immediately after treatment discontinuation, IgE levels return to pretreatment levels without any evidence of rebound.[52]

Pharmacokinetics

Bioavailability. After subcutaneous administration, average bioavailability is approximately 62%.[52] It is absorbed slowly and reaches peak serum concentrations after approximately 7–8 days. Pharmacokinetics are linear at doses greater than 0.5 mg/kg.[52]

Distribution. Omalizumab forms complexes of limited size with IgE, without evidence of precipitation of these complexes.[52] The apparent volume of distribution following subcutaneous administration is approximately 78 ± 32 mL/kg.[52]

Elimination. Clearance occurs via IgG elimination processes as well as via complex formation with IgE.[52] Liver elimination occurs via degradation in the reticuloendothelial system and endothelial cells, and intact IgG is excreted in bile.[52] Serum elimination half-life averages 26 days, clearance averages 2.4 ± 1.1 mL/kg per day, and the doubling of body weight doubles clearance.[52] There is no evidence for a need for dose adjustment, due to factors such as age (above 6 years), race/ethnicity, gender, and there is no available data at this time regarding dosing in renal or hepatic impairment.[52]

MODE OF ADMINISTRATION

Omalizumab is administered via subcutaneous administration every 2–4 weeks, depending on the weight and IgE level of the patient.[42] Clinicians should not administer more than 150 mg per injection site, and be prepared and equipped to identify and treat anaphylaxis should this occur.[6] Observation for 2 hours postinjection for the first three injections and 30 minutes postinjection thereafter has been recommended.[53,54]

DOSING STRATEGIES

Dosing tables exist, based on a combination of total IgE and weight, to guide omalizumab dosing, and reducing doses below those recommended has been shown to increase free IgE and thus could cause a reduction in asthma control.[49] European guidelines specify a maximum dose of 600 mg every 2 weeks and do not support dosing in IgE levels above 1500 IU/mL.[52] US guidelines specify a maximum dose of 300 mg for every 4-week dosing or 375 mg for every 2-week dosing, and do not support dosing in IgE levels above 700 IU/mL if administered every 4 weeks, 1300 IU/mL

if administered every 2 weeks.[55] Country-specific dosing tables are available and should be consulted to determine patient-specific dosing. Unfortunately, a significant proportion of asthmatic children and adolescents that may benefit from omalizumab therapy may not qualify due to elevated IgE levels,[56] and though current dosing tables are close to optimal, it may be possible to treat patients with higher baseline IgE levels than currently recommended.[57] This area will need to be continually studied in order to fully optimize treatment for all asthmatic children and adolescents.

CLINICAL STUDIES

Adult Studies

Omalizumab has been shown to be effective in the adult population across a wide range of clinical outcomes, including asthma exacerbations,[58–64] ED (emergency department) visits/hospitalizations,[63,65,66] exhaled nitric oxide,[58] asthma control test (ACT),[60] quality-of-life scores,[58,61,64,67] unscheduled physicians visits,[58] decreasing ICS requirements,[67] and airway wall thickness.[58] Omalizumab has also been shown to be effective in nonatopic asthmatic adults,[68] though not all data supports its use in this population.[69]

Child Studies

The studies described previously were largely conducted on adolescents and adults 12 years of age or older. The remainder of the literature in children focuses on the 6–18-year-old population. Omalizumab has also been shown to improve exacerbation rates,[56,70–74] decrease inhaled and oral corticosteroid doses,[70,72,73,75] and improve asthma-related quality-of-life scores,[75–77] ACT,[75] asthma control,[72] and lung function.[70] Omalizumab has also been found to be a potential alternative to treatment in patients who have poor adherence to ICSs.[78] In addition, omalizumab has been shown to improve interferon alpha (IFN-α) responses to rhinoviral infection in children.[71]

SAFETY

Early concerns with the use of omalizumab included concerns of anaphylaxis, serum sickness, and even risk for malignancy. Omalizumab has a mostly good safety and tolerability profile[79] and no significant development of omalizumab specific antibodies,[80] although urticaria is a potential side effect.[81] One meta-analysis of 2749 patients receiving omalizumab therapy showed similar rates of minor adverse effects in treatment and placebo groups and a slightly lower incidence and profile of serious adverse effects in the omalizumab groups.[82] The safety and tolerability of omalizumab in children remains stable over longer time frames (52 weeks) as well.[81] Anaphylaxis does remain a risk with omalizumab injection (see the notes on monitoring given previously), however, and clinicians should be aware that it may be characterized by delayed onset (>2 hours after dose) and protracted progression of symptoms[83]; patients should be trained in the recognition of anaphylaxis and use of epinephrine autoinjector use, and be sent home with an epinephrine autoinjector.[54] Pain and swelling at the injection site occurs in 5%–20% of patients.[6] The EXCELS study evaluated 7857 patients, of whom 5007 were treated with omalizumab, and found that omalizumab was not associated with any increased risk of malignancy.[84] However, there is evidence that omalizumab may increase the risk of cardiovascular and cerebrovascular events.[84a]

CLINICAL APPLICATION—CURRENT AND FUTURE CONSIDERATIONS

Age

Currently omalizumab is approved in the US and Europe in children greater than 6 years of age, adolescents, and adults. Further study is needed to determine safety and efficacy in children younger than 6 years of age.

Biomarkers

Omalizumab has effects on several biomarkers. It is known to decrease serum free IgE,[44,85] and it also reduces sputum and tissue eosinophils and airway lymphocytes[44] and reduces basophil numbers.[86]

Target Response Expected

There is evidence that patients with high baseline levels of fractional exhaled nitric oxide (FeNO), eosinophils, and serum periostin have the greatest improvement in exacerbation frequency with omalizumab compared with placebo.[62] In addition, the response to inhaled allergens in asthma is diminished by omalizumab, and this decrease is paralleled by a reduction in eosinophils and IgE bearing cells.[87] However, it is important to recognize that monitoring IgE alone does not predict clinical response in omalizumab treated patients.[85]

Other Diseases

Omalizumab has been studied in various other diseases as well, has been shown to be effective in allergic rhinitis and allergic bronchopulmonary dysplasia (ABPA), and has been found equivocal in nasal polyposis.[69] In addition, it has been utilized successfully for the treatment of chronic urticaria.[88]

Cost Effectiveness

Omalizumab currently remains a high-cost therapy for asthma treatment. Studies have shown it to be cost effective with regard to decreasing exacerbations and improving health-related quality of life when used in severe asthmatic adults.[89,90] The selection of patients to receive omalizumab therapy should focus on those children who have severe allergic asthma in order to maximize cost efficiency.

Mepolizumab

MECHANISM OF ACTION AND TARGET EFFECTS

Mepolizumab is a humanized murine monoclonal IgG1κ antibody directed against interleukin-5 (IL-5).[91–93] The IL-5 receptor is composed of the IL-5Rα chain, which binds IL-5, and the common β chain (βc), which mediates the signal transduction (Fig. 48.3).[94–97] Mepolizumab binds to IL-5, preventing its interaction with the IL-5 receptor and subsequent signaling.[92]

IL-5 is predominantly synthesized by CD4+ T_H2 lymphocytes but also is produced in smaller amounts by mast cells, eosinophils, basophils, NK T cells, group 2 innate lymphoid cells, and CD34+ progenitor cells.[91,94–97] The presence of the IL-5 receptor, along with CD34 and CCR3, designate stem cells for eosinophil development.[98,99] IL-5 is responsible for eosinophil hematopoiesis, proliferation, maturation, and terminal differentiation in the bone marrow and mobilization of the eosinophils from the bone marrow into circulation.[91,93–97] IL-5 enhances chemotaxis and adhesion of eosinophils to the vascular wall in the circulation and increases eosinophil activation, degranulation, and cytotoxicity in tissues.[91,95,97] The presence of locally generated IL-5 promotes the survival of eosinophils in tissues, and in vitro studies have demonstrated that the absence of IL-5 results in

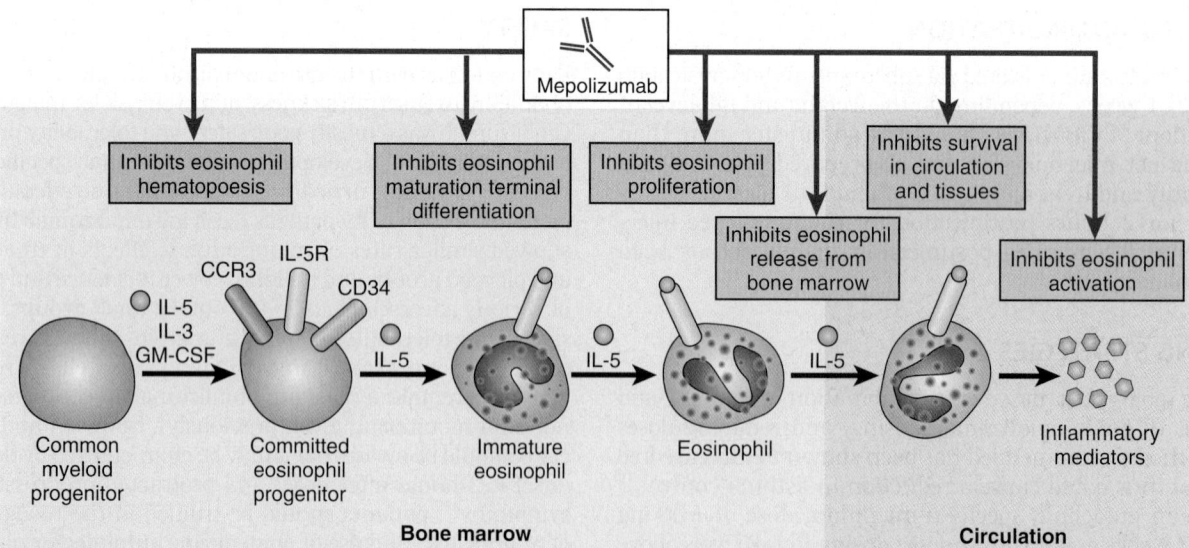

Fig. 48.3 The impact of mepolizumab on IL-5 in eosinophil development and function. Mepolizumab binds to IL-5 inhibiting its ability to bind with the IL-5 receptor. By blocking IL-5, mepolizumab inhibits eosinophil hematopoiesis, maturation, differentiation, and proliferation in the bone marrow as well as eosinophil migration into circulation. In the tissue and circulation, mepolizumab prevents IL-5-mediated eosinophil survival and activation. *CCR3,* C-C chemokine receptor type 3; *GM-CSF,* granulocyte macrophage colony-stimulating factor; *IL,* interleukin.

spontaneous cellular apoptosis.[91,93,94] Patients with asthma have increased IL-5 in their bronchoalveolar lavage fluid and bronchial biopsies at baseline, with an upregulation in bronchial mucosa IL-5 mRNA and serum IL-5 after allergen provocation.[94,97,100]

The inhibitory effect of mepolizumab on eosinophils through suppression of IL-5 has been well demonstrated. In both asthmatics as well as patients with eosinophilic syndromes, mepolizumab reduced, but did not completely deplete, peripheral blood,[100–106] airway/sputum,[100,103–105,107] and bone marrow[98,100,107] eosinophil counts, with the greatest effect being reduction of blood eosinophil counts. Mepolizumab also decreased eosinophil precursors, including eosinophil myelocytes and metamyelocytes, in the bone marrow, inducing partial maturational arrest of the eosinophil lineage.[98] In patients with eosinophilic syndromes, mepolizumab did increase serum IL-5 levels, IL-5Rα expression, and percentage of CD4+ and CD8+ T cells, producing intracellular IL-5.[102]

PHARMACOLOGY

Pharmacodynamics

Mepolizumab has been studied in intravenous and subcutaneous forms. The route of administration has been found not to affect the exposure-response relationship.[108] Utilizing an indirect pharmacological response model, mepolizumab demonstrated a maximal decrease in peripheral eosinophil counts of 85% from baseline, with a half-maximal inhibitory concentration (IC_{50}) of 0.045 µg/mL.[92] A nonlinear inhibition I_{max} model based on blood eosinophil levels after 12 weeks of therapy identified subcutaneous mepolizumab doses of 11 mg and 99 mg, provided 50% and 90% of maximal blood eosinophil inhibition, respectively.[108] Studies using intravenous (IV) mepolizumab have demonstrated a dose-dependent decrease in blood[105,108] and sputum[105] eosinophil levels. In a study of adult patients administered mepolizumab every 4 weeks for 8 weeks, there was a pronounced reduction as early as day 3 (first postdose measurement), with a return to baseline from day 70 (2 weeks postlast dose) to day 140 (last day of follow-up).[108] A sustained decrease in blood eosinophilia has been observed even 3 months after the final infusion in 76% of patients with eosinophilic syndromes.[102] An observational study demonstrated that following discontinuation of mepolizumab, there were significant increases in serum eosinophil counts, with a return to baseline over 6 months.[109] Sputum eosinophil counts increased over 3 months after discontinuation of mepolizumab, but not thereafter.[109]

Mepolizumab induces an increase in blood IL-5 levels, likely secondary to circulating IL-5/mepolizumab complexes precipitating with protein A/G.[102,108] In the aforementioned study of adults treated with mepolizumab, IL-5 increased until day 28 of treatment and remained constant up to the last day of follow-up, at day 140.[108] Upon discontinuation of mepolizumab, however, patients did not have a rebound phenomenon in their eosinophil counts secondary to this increased IL-5 during treatment.[109] No relationship was found between levels of serum total IL-5 and mepolizumab plasma concentrations.[108] Patient response to mepolizumab is not related to baseline plasma IL-5 levels.[102]

Pharmacokinetics

Pharmacokinetics for mepolizumab are dose proportional and time-independent.[92] Mepolizumab has an absolute bioavailability of 64%–75% following subcutaneous injection[92,108] and 81% following intramuscular injection.[92] The median time to maximal concentration (t_{max}) is 6–8 days postdosing, with subcutaneous administration compared with 0.5 hours with intravenous administration.[108] The steady-state volume of distribution ranges from 49 to 93 mL/kg.[92] The exact route of elimination for mepolizumab is unknown but is believed to be similar to that of other IgG1 antibodies.[92] Mepolizumab is eliminated slowly with a terminal half-life of 20 days,[92] with another study showing a range of 22–28 days for subcutaneous and IV administration, respectively.[108] Mepolizumab plasma clearance ranges from 0.064 to 0.163 mL/h/kg.[92] There is no available data regarding dosing in renal or hepatic impairment.[92]

MODE OF ADMINISTRATION AND DOSING

Early studies of mepolizumab trialed multiple doses with a progression from an intravenous to a subcutaneous formulation.[103–107,110] Mepolizumab is currently administered as a 100 mg subcutaneous injection every 4 weeks.[111]

BIOMARKERS TO DIRECT USE

Initial studies of mepolizumab that recruited patients on the basis of asthma severity but not markers of eosinophilia showed a reduction in sputum and blood eosinophilia but failed to show an improvement in any clinical endpoints compared with placebo, including exacerbations, symptom scores, FEV_1, quality of life, or β2-agonist use.[107] Subsequent studies explored mepolizumab use in patients with eosinophilic asthma, defined as either a sputum eosinophil percentage greater than 3%,[103–105] FeNO of 50 ppb or greater,[105] or a peripheral eosinophil count of 300 cells/µL or greater in the previous year or at least 150 cells/µL at screening.[105,106,110] Directing the therapy toward patients with this eosinophilic phenotype demonstrated an improvement in clinical outcomes, outlined later. In particular, exploratory modeling of baseline characteristics indicated that those patients with a higher eosinophil count, including greater than 300 cells/µL, and a higher number of exacerbations in the previous year, were most predictive in achieving a reduction in asthma exacerbations with mepolizumab.[105]

CLINICAL STUDIES

Mepolizumab was initially studied in adults, with only recent studies enrolling adolescents as young as 12 years old, thereby limiting insight into pediatric use.[112] In patients with eosinophilic asthma with recurrent severe exacerbations in the past 12 months despite the use of high-dose ICSs, with or without a long-acting beta-agonist or maintenance oral corticosteroids, mepolizumab reduced the number of severe exacerbations,[103–106,110] reduced exacerbations requiring emergency room visits or hospital admission,[105,106] and delayed the time to first exacerbation,[105] compared with placebo.

In patients with severe eosinophilic asthma with refractory symptoms requiring daily oral corticosteroids, mepolizumab allowed a reduction in their oral corticosteroid dose while improving asthma control compared to placebo.[104,110] Initial studies with mepolizumab in eosinophilic asthmatics failed to show an improvement in FEV_1,[103,105] asthma control, or symptom scores,[103,105] with subsequent studies demonstrating an improvement in these parameters[104,106,110] compared with placebo. Mixed results have been observed on the effect of mepolizumab on quality of life, with some studies showing improvement[103] and others showing no change.[105] Following discontinuation of therapy, there was a significant increase in severe asthma exacerbations over a 12-month observation period in those previously treated with mepolizumab, with the exacerbation rate at the end of the 12-month period being similar between subjects whose mepolizumab was discontinued and subjects originally treated with placebo.[109]

SAFETY

Overall, mepolizumab has a favorable safety profile, with most adverse events being reported as mild or moderate in intensity and no fatalities reported.[108] The most frequently reported adverse event was injection site reaction,[108] with other common adverse events, including upper respiratory infections, asthma, headaches, rhinitis, bronchitis, sinusitis, viral infection, injury, back pain, nausea, and pharyngitis.[107] Given mepolizumab's impact on eosinophils, it is recommended that patients with preexisting helminth infections be treated before the initiation of therapy.[111] In clinical trials, two serious adverse reactions of herpes zoster occurred in patients on mepolizumab, prompting a consideration for varicella vaccination if medically appropriate before starting therapy.[111]

Clinical Application. Mepolizumab is currently approved for the treatment of eosinophilic asthma in the United States for patients 12 years of age and older. The experience in adolescents is admittedly with a comparatively smaller number of adolescents than adults. Based on less experience, it could be a consideration for patients who do not qualify for omalizumab therapy or an alternative to omalizumab in the distinctly eosinophilic phenotype.

Other Biologics

RESLIZUMAB

Reslizumab is a monoclonal antibody directed against IL-5, differing from mepolizumab by being a humanized rat IgG4κ antibody.[113,114] Given its target of IL-5, reslizumab also decreases sputum[113] and peripheral blood eosinophils.[113,114] Following discontinuation of therapy, patients on reslizumab had a return of their eosinophil counts to baseline by 90 days.[113] Similar to mepolizumab, reslizumab has been studied in eosinophilic asthma, defined as a sputum eosinophil count greater than 3%[113] or a peripheral serum eosinophil count of 400 cells/µL or greater,[114] which is higher serum eosinophil cutoff than that used for mepolizumab.[112] When used in patients with poorly controlled eosinophilic asthma despite the use of at least medium-dose ICSs and another controller medication, reslizumab reduced asthma exacerbations, increased time to first exacerbation, and improved FEV_1, quality-of-life scores, and asthma control scores,[114] compared with placebo.

BENRALIZUMAB

Benralizumab is a monoclonal afucoslylated IgG1κ antibody directed against the IL-5Rα chain.[115,116] Afucosylation of IgG1 increases its affinity for FcγRIIIa, which is expressed on natural killer cells, macrophages, and neutrophils.[116] This results in enhanced antibody-dependent cell-mediated cytotoxicity of eosinophils through the interaction of benralizumab and with FcγRIIIa.[116] Benralizumab reduces peripheral blood eosinophil counts in a dose-dependent fashion, with a marked reduction in peripheral blood,[115,117,118] sputum,[117] airway mucosa,[117] and bone marrow[117] eosinophil counts. In a phase 2b dose ranging study of adults with uncontrolled asthma with recurrent exacerbations despite the use of medium- or high-dose ICSs and long-acting beta-agonists, benralizumab reduced exacerbation rates in those patients with a peripheral blood eosinophil count of at least 300 cells/µL.[119] Those patients with eosinophilic asthma had improvement in both FEV_1 and asthma control scores.[119] In adult asthmatic patients with a prior exacerbation in the 12 months presenting to the ED with an acute asthma exacerbation, a single administration of benralizumab reduced asthma exacerbation rates and exacerbations, resulting in hospitalization over the following 12 weeks, compared with placebo.[118] This may present a unique application of this therapy in managing acute asthma and calls for further studies in children and adults in relation to dose and timing.

DUPILUMAB

Dupilumab is a monoclonal antibody to the interleukin-4 receptor α subunit, which should inhibit both IL-4 and IL-13 downstream signaling.[120] Dupilumab has been shown to be effective in moderate to severe adult asthmatics who were already being treated with ICS and LABA medications, with fewer exacerbations upon withdrawal of these medications in dupilumab treated patients,[120] and phase II trial in adults showed that it was effective in improving lung function and reducing exacerbations.[121] Further study is needed to determine the efficacy of this drug in children.

Conclusion

As indicated in this review, there is good evidence that AIT has the capacity to induce at least a temporary remission in asthma symptoms after 3 years of administration, but alteration on progression of disease, especially in relation to irreversible loss of pulmonary function associated with disease progression, has not been evaluated. Similarly, the new immunomodulators, including omalizumab, have shown promise in reducing asthma exacerbations with variable effects on other features of the disease, such as symptoms and pulmonary function. However, studies to date have not shown that these medications can alter the course of the disease and lead to remission after discontinuation. Aside from omalizumab and mepolizumab, the effects of the other new agents in adolescents have not been reported. In addition, omalizumab and mepolizumab are not approved for use in children less than 12 years of age in the United States. As experience is obtained in adults and adolescents, and safety profiles established, there will be a gradual progression of studies in younger children. Hopefully, one or more of these agents will be successful in altering the course of the disease, as it often presents in early childhood. It will be necessary to define the effect of the various immunomodulators, and the profile of the child most likely to benefit, to establish the cost effectiveness of this line of treatment. Future studies may determine that combination immunomodulators may be needed to obtain the full effect on altering the early onset and progression of asthma.

References

Access the reference list online at ExpertConsult.com.

Suggested Reading

Bousquet J, Wenzel S, Holgate S, et al. Predicting response to omalizumab, an anti-IgE antibody, in patients with allergic asthma. *Chest.* 2004; 125:1378–1386.

Global Initiative for Asthma. Global Strategy for Asthma Management and prevention, 2016. Available from: http://www.ginasthma.org/. Accessed July 11, 2016.

Gouder C, West LM, Montefort S. The real-life clinical effects of 52 weeks of omalizumab therapy for severe persistent allergic asthma. *Int J Clin Pharm.* 2015;37:36–43.

Jutel M, Agache I, Bonini S, et al. International Consensus on Allergen Immunotherapy II: Mechanisms, standardization, and pharmacoeconomics. *J Allergy Clin Immunol.* 2016; 137:358–368.

Lowe PJ, Renard D. Omalizumab decreases IgE production in patients with allergic (IgE-mediated) asthma; PKPD analysis of a biomarker, total IgE. *Br J Clin Pharmacol.* 2011;72:306–320.

Mauri P, Riccio AM, Rossi R, et al. Proteomics of bronchial biopsies: galectin-3 as a predictive biomarker of airway remodelling modulation in omalizumab-treated severe asthma patients. *Immunol Lett.* 2014;162:2–10.

Nopp A, Johansson SG, Adedoyin J, et al. After 6 years with Xolair; a 3-year withdrawal follow-up. *Allergy.* 2010;65:56–60.

Pereira Santos MC, Campos Melo A, Caetano A, et al. Longitudinal study of the expression of FcepsilonRI and IgE on basophils and dendritic cells in association with basophil function in two patients with severe allergic asthma treated with Omalizumab. *Eur Ann Allergy Clin Immunol.* 2015;47:38–40.

Slavin RG, Ferioli C, Tannenbaum SJ, et al. Asthma symptom re-emergence after omalizumab withdrawal correlates well with increasing IgE and decreasing pharmacokinetic concentrations. *J Allergy Clin Immunol.* 2009;123:107–113.e3.

Xolair powder and solvent for solution for injection: summary of product characteristics. http://www.ema.europa.eu/docs/en_GB/document_library/EPAR_-_Product_Information/human/000606/WC500057298.pdf. Accessed February 1, 2016.

Cystic Fibrosis

49 Genetics and Pathophysiology of Cystic Fibrosis

GARRY R. CUTTING, MD, JOHN ENGELHARDT, PhD, and
PAMELA LESLIE ZEITLIN, MD, PhD

The genetic basis of cystic fibrosis (CF) has been recognized by the medical community since the 1940s.[1] A genetic etiology and autosomal-recessive inheritance was suggested by the recurrence of CF in siblings and the absence of the illness in parents. Genetic linkage analysis confirmed that a single locus was responsible for classic CF.[2,3] In 1989, technical breakthroughs allowing identification of disease-causing genes on the basis of position rather than function enabled Tsui and colleagues to clone the gene responsible for this disorder.[4] The identified gene was aptly named the cystic fibrosis transmembrane conductance regulator *(CFTR)*.[5] During the past three decades, our understanding of the molecular basis of CF has exploded. We now recognize that deleterious variants in *CFTR* give rise to a range of phenotypes, extending from classic CF to single-organ pathology. The successful use of therapies directed at the complications of CF has raised the question as to the potential efficacy in disease phenotypes that mimic CF, including idiopathic bronchiectasis,[6,7] chronic *Pseudomonas aeruginosa* airways colonization in tracheostomy patients,[8] or chronic obstructive pulmonary disease.[9] The assumption that all carriers of a single disease-causing variant in *CFTR* are asymptomatic also has been questioned. The consequences of many variants on the function of the encoded protein have been determined, allowing correlation of altered function of *CFTR* with CF pathophysiology.[10] Two variant-specific *CFTR* modulator therapies are approved by the Food and Drug Administration (FDA) in the United States.[11,12] Additional investigational molecules capable of repairing several different classes of *CFTR* variants are in clinical trials in North America, Europe, and Israel, potentially increasing the number of patients eligible for drugs directed at the primary cause of CF.

CFTR Gene

STRUCTURE

The *CFTR* gene resides on the long arm of human chromosome 7 and encompasses approximately 189,000 base pairs of DNA.[13] The coding portion of the gene is divided into 27 exons that are transcribed into a messenger RNA (mRNA) of approximately 6500 base pairs.[5] The exon and intron structure of the *CFTR* gene is well conserved among mammals and evolutionarily distant species such as amphibians (Xenopus) and fish (killifish and dogfish).[14]

Transcription of *CFTR* is initiated 80 base pairs upstream from the start site of translation.[15,16] The *CFTR* gene demonstrates exquisite temporal and spatial differences in expression. For example, specific cell types within the human lung express high levels of *CFTR*, while surface epithelial cells

have a very low level of *CFTR* expression.[17] *CFTR* expression is also regulated during organ development.[18,19] Despite considerable evidence that the expression of *CFTR* is highly selective, the precise elements that regulate *CFTR* expression have not been identified. Sequences immediately upstream of the transcriptional start site of *CFTR* generate low-level expression in most tissues. This pattern of expression is consistent with the presence of basal promoter elements.[20,21] A cyclic adenosine monophosphate (cAMP) response element has been identified within this region of *CFTR*, but this element does not appear to account for the spatial and temporal expression patterns.[22] Assays that search for binding of protein to DNA have identified several regions elsewhere in the *CFTR* gene that may be involved in transcriptional regulation.[23] Strain-specific differences in *CFTR* expression in mice have been mapped to sequences about 700 base pairs upstream of the *CFTR* gene, indicating the existence of regulatory elements in this region.[24] Epigenetic mechanisms such as methylation do not appear to play a major role in regulating *CFTR* expression.[25,26] However, there is growing evidence that microRNAs (miRNA) modulate the level of *CFTR* mRNA transcripts.[27,28] Thus, despite extensive efforts to locate transcriptional elements, the molecular mechanisms regulating *CFTR* expression are not completely understood.

SPLICING

Variations in *CFTR* splicing patterns have been identified by the reverse transcription-polymerase chain reaction technique.[29,30] There are relatively few alternatively spliced transcripts that create functional isoforms of *CFTR*.[31] RNA transcripts resulting from alternative splicing of exon 5 *CFTR* create a functional form of *CFTR* in the rabbit heart but have not been identified in other species or organs. Transcripts missing a portion of exons 13 and 14a encode a functional isoform of *CFTR* expressed in mouse and human kidney.[32] Neither the heart nor the kidney appears to be primarily involved in CF pathophysiology; thus the role of these alternatively spliced forms of *CFTR* is unclear.

In contrast to alternative splicing, many aberrantly spliced versions of *CFTR* have been identified. Aberrantly spliced *CFTR* RNA transcripts do not produce functional *CFTR*. Aberrant splicing occurs as a result of variation in intronic or exonic sequences required for normal splicing of *CFTR*. The aberrant splicing of exon 10 (legacy exon 9) is a notable example.[33,34] Variation in the length of the polythymidine tract, an element in the 3' splice site of intron 9, is correlated with the amount of properly spliced *CFTR* mRNA.[35] Longer versions of this tract called 9T and 7T are common in the population and are associated with high levels of normally

757

spliced *CFTR* mRNA. A shorter version of this tract called 5T is associated with a substantial reduction in full-length *CFTR* RNA.[36] While abbreviated polythymidine tracts in 3′ splice sites do not usually cause mis-splicing of the subsequent exon, it appears that a special situation occurs in the *CFTR* gene. Sequence surrounding exon 9, including unusual variation in splice sites surrounding exon 9 and splice-silencing sequences in intron 9, appear to make exon 9 vulnerable to mis-splicing.[37–39] Thus alterations in secondary splicing signals of this exon such as the polythymidine tract have an exaggerated effect on splicing. The splicing efficiency of *CFTR* genes bearing 5T also varies by tissue. The vas deferens splices *CFTR* genes bearing the 5T variant less efficiently than respiratory epithelia, which explains the existence of congenital bilateral absence of the vas deferens (CBAVD) without other symptoms.[40,41]

Individuals carrying the 5T variant in their other *CFTR* gene manifest a variety of phenotypes, ranging from healthy to nonclassic CF (discussed later). The latter phenomenon is due to the variable effect that 5T has on the splicing of *CFTR* exon 9. This splicing variability is caused by variation in the number of TG dinucleotides adjacent to the polythymidine tract.[42] The role of the TG tract in splicing of 5T alleles is controversial. It may serve as a site for binding of a splicing repressor, or the RNA may form a secondary structure such as a hairpin that affects gene expression.[43,44] Either way, there is a robust correlation between the length of the TG tract and the phenotypes associated with a 5T variant.[45]

Many other *CFTR* transcripts derived from aberrant splicing of exons 9 through 12 have been reported, yet none appear to be correlated with phenotype.[30,46–49] Another example of aberrant *CFTR* splicing involves exons 23 and 24, resulting in a prematurely truncated *CFTR* protein that is nonfunctional.[50] The many variants that affect *CFTR* splicing and result in disease are summarized in the following section.

DNA VARIANTS

More than 2000 variants in the *CFTR* gene associated with disease have been reported to the Cystic Fibrosis Genetic Analysis Consortium (http://www.genet.sickkids.on.ca/cftr/). The Consortium website has implemented variant nomenclature according to Human Genome and Variome Society (HGVS) guidelines. Variants are now provided in legacy and HGVS format (http://www.genet.sickkids.on.ca/cftr/). Legacy names are used in this chapter, and the HGVS nomenclature is provided with the first mention of a variant. The vast majority of *CFTR* variants reported to be associated with disease involve only one or a few nucleotides. Nearly 50% of variants change an amino acid, while variants that affect splicing or introduce a nonsense codon account for approximately 25%. Deletion and insertion variants that alter the reading frame and usually result in the introduction of a premature termination codon account for about 20%. Deletions and insertions involving multiples of three nucleotides are much less common (2%). The latter variants do not shift the reading frame, so a protein missing one or more amino acids is usually produced (e.g., *CFTR* with the F508del [HGVS p.Phe508del] variant). Most of the remaining disease-associated variants (3%) involve the deletion of larger regions of DNA involving hundreds to thousands of base pairs. Finally, a few variants

(1%) have been purported to occur in sequences thought to be involved in transcriptional regulation of the *CFTR* gene, although a convincing case has been made in only a few instances.[51] In addition to the disease-associated variants, almost 270 variants in *CFTR* have not been associated with disease. There are some variants in *CFTR* (e.g., *M470V* HGVS p.Met470Val) that may affect phenotype.[42,52] Variants that are "silent" (that do not change an encoded amino acid or known splicing signal) are not predicted to alter *CFTR* function. However, the elucidation of intronic and exonic signals that enhance or repress exon splicing raises the possibility that some "silent" changes may affect *CFTR* splicing.[53–55]

The distribution of disease-associated variants in the *CFTR* gene among human populations has been extensively reviewed.[56,57] One variant, a deletion of three nucleotides that leads to loss of a single phenylalanine residue at codon 508 (F508del), accounts for approximately 70% of CF alleles in Northern European Caucasians. The frequency of the F508del variant varies on the European continent from less than 50% of CF alleles in Southern Europe to as high as 88% of CF alleles in Denmark. The F508del variant is quite rare in native Africans and native Asians. However, the F508del variant is found in racially admixed populations. For example, 30% of the *CFTR* genes in American CF patients of African descent have the F508del variant.[58] On the other hand, the second most common variant in African Americans with CF (3120 + 1G>A; HGVS c.2988 + 1G>A) appears to be a common CF allele in native Africans.[59,60] Deleterious CF alleles also have been found in CF patients of Asian ancestry.[61,62] These variants have not been observed in Caucasians or native African populations. Thus rare deleterious variants in the *CFTR* gene occur in all human populations. However, it is the frequency of the F508del variant in Europeans that accounts for the high incidence of CF in Caucasians.

In addition to F508del, only about 25 other variants occur, with a frequency of 0.1% or greater in the Caucasian CF population.[58,63] Other variants are seen with some frequency in African Americans.[59] Finally, some ethnic groups have one or more variants that reach a frequency of ≥1% that are rare in the general population. The higher frequency of the latter variants is probably the consequence of a founder effect.[64] The remainder of the reported variants (~1000) has been reported in only a small number of individuals. Screening for the F508del variant and 22 variants that have a frequency of greater than 0.1% detects about 85% of variants in Caucasian CF patients.[65] Variant screens involving 50–100 CF variants produce a minimal increase in detection rate in the general CF population (1%–3%). Because there are so many rare variants, in order to achieve a detection rate for classic CF over 95%, screening of the entire coding region of the *CFTR* gene is required.[66,67]

CFTR Protein

CHARACTERISTICS

The *CFTR* protein is composed of a linear stretch of 1480 amino acids that form an integral membrane glycoprotein. A comparison of the nucleotide sequence across available databases places this protein as a member of the ABC transporter superfamily. The topology of the protein contains the common features of twofold symmetry with six transmembrane domains and an intracellular nucleotide-binding fold. The *CFTR* is unique in the presence of a central intracellular R domain enriched in phosphorylation sites used by the protein kinases A and C. Although most members of the superfamily are transporters (e.g., the multidrug resistance transporter (MDR) transports chemotherapy agents), the *CFTR* is a cAMP-regulated chloride and bicarbonate channel that must function for the outwardly rectifying chloride channel (ORCC) to transport chloride. Functional *CFTR* also downregulates the epithelial sodium channel (ENaC) in those cells in which both reside. More controversial functions have been reported, including transport of nucleotides and fatty acids.

BIOGENESIS

The *CFTR* polypeptide is translated from the mRNA in the endoplasmic reticulum (ER) as a linear chain of amino acids with hydrophilic (water-soluble) and hydrophobic (lipid-soluble) domains. The nascent polypeptide is assisted by interactions with chaperone proteins within and outside the ER, to assume a tertiary or folded structure that buries the membrane-spanning domains in the ER membrane. The process is relatively slow, taking approximately 10–15 minutes to complete, and is followed by two different fates. Depending on the cell type making the *CFTR*, the wild-type (WT) chain could be ubiquitinated and sent to the proteasome for degradation,[68] or it could continue along the trafficking pathway to the Golgi apparatus. Chloride transport through the *CFTR* can be detected in the ER using patch-clamping techniques, but it is not known whether the immature functional channel is the one protected from proteasomal degradation. The successful *CFTR* is packaged into vesicles for transport.[69] Adequate anion channel transport through cell surface *CFTR* depends not only on the characteristics of the channel pore or degree of phosphorylation and ATP hydrolysis but also on numbers of *CFTR* proteins and residence time at the surface. *CFTR* is actively recycled from the plasma membrane, and some mutants are much less stable than WT-*CFTR*.[70]

FUNCTION

The three-dimensional topology of *CFTR* is under investigation. The two nucleotide binding domains (NBDs) and the R domain probably interact such that phosphorylation of the R domain is required for chloride channel opening and probably affects the affinity of the NBDs for adenosine triphosphate (ATP).[71] ATP hydrolysis at NBD1 is associated with opening the channel, but hydrolysis at NBD2 is associated with closure. The chloride pore is formed by transmembrane domains, and the single-channel conductance is low, at 6–10 picosiemens. The current-voltage relationship is linear, meaning that it is just as easy for chloride to leave as to enter the cell, depending on the direction of the voltage applied across the membrane. This bidirectionality is possible because ATP is the ligand that is hydrolyzed to gate the channel.

The most common variant in *CFTR*, the F508 deletion of the code for phenylalanine at position 508, has two consequences. First, the channel has a low open time for chloride—about 10% of normal.[72,73] Second, the newly translated *CFTR*

is unstable in the ER, leading to premature proteolysis and a reduced half-life in the cell. The variant appears to affect intermolecular interactions within *CFTR* rather than NBD1 folding.[74,75]

CELLULAR DISTRIBUTION AND FUNCTION

Developmental Expression and Function

CFTR mRNA is detectable in many fetal tissues in the first trimester. Data have been collected for fetal lung, intestine, pancreas, and kidney from humans, rats, rabbits, and mice. During early mammalian embryonic tissue development, *CFTR* may be more important as a regulator of other ion channels rather than as a pathway for chloride transport.[76] *CFTR* protein becomes detectable in the second trimester, still quite early in development. *CFTR* expression declines in postnatal lung, and this decline begins even earlier in the rat, during the last trimester. There is a bronchial centrifugal expression gradient and a developmental shift from nonpolar localization to apical localization, with a timing that matches that of *CFTR* regulation of the ENaC. In other words, since ENaC function is required to resorb fetal lung fluid at birth as an adaptation to air-breathing, *CFTR* expression, a downregulator of ENaC function, declines and ENaC expression increases.

Postnatal Expression and Function

Regulated airway fluid and ion composition become more important for the air-breathing mammal than they were during lung development. CF lungs are morphologically normal at birth, in part because there are sufficient alternative chloride transport pathways in fetal lung to support tissue expansion and differentiation.[76] After birth, airway mucociliary clearance is affected by the depth and characteristics of the periciliary fluid layer, which in turn is dependent on ENaC function.[77–79] Over time, the human infant with pancreatic-insufficient CF is increasingly vulnerable to infection and inflammation in the airways, which lead to the classic lung phenotype of airways obstruction.

TISSUE DISTRIBUTION

Absent or reduced function of *CFTR* can be measured quantitatively in the sweat duct, where the reabsorptive coil is designed to conserve chloride, sodium, and water to protect the mammal from dehydration. The diagnostic sweat test takes advantage of the cholinergic pathway for generation of sweat by the sweat gland coil. *CFTR* is only responsible for at most 1% of sweat generation but is required for chloride reabsorption in the duct, thus leading to elevated sweat chloride concentrations.

CFTR plays a vital role in several other organs, tissues where epithelial proteins are secreted along with electrolytes. The most important organs are the airways, bile ducts, pancreatic ducts, and vas deferens. Interestingly, although *CFTR* is highly expressed in the kidney, its absence is not detrimental. The simplified scheme in which *CFTR* plays an electrophysiologic role to control the ion and water content of luminal secretions is insufficient to explain the nature of CF lung disease. In CF lungs, additional abnormalities of fluid are associated with chronic inflammation and infection.

Genotype-Phenotype Correlations

MOLECULAR CONSEQUENCES OF VARIANTS

The implementation of newborn carrier screening for CF and the development of *CFTR* targeted therapies has brought renewed interest in the clinical and functional consequences of variants in *CFTR*. To increase the sensitivity and specificity of genetic testing for CF, a project entitled the Clinical and Functional Translation of *CFTR* or *CFTR2* was undertaken. In its first phase, *CFTR2* coordinated the collection of clinical data on almost 40,000 individuals with CF from 25 countries. These individuals carried 1,036 unique *CFTR* variants. Comprehensive clinical and functional analysis of 159 variants that achieved a frequency of 0.0001 (0.01%) revealed that only 127 (80%) could be definitively assigned as CF-causing.[10] Of the remaining 32 variants, 12 (7.5%) lacked clinical and functional evidence to be CF-causing, while the remaining 20 could not be assigned. The latter group consisted of variants that had varying clinical consequence (VCC) and a few variants of uncertain significance (VUS) that lack sufficient clinical or functional evidence to be assigned. The *CFTR2* project has undertaken a second round of data collection, thereby increasing enrollment to almost 90,000 individuals with CF from 40 countries, of which 69,745 were alive in 2015. The additional clinical data, along with more extensive functional analysis of variants that affect *CFTR* splicing, have allowed for the assignment of disease status to 306 variants (272 CF-causing, 19 VCC, non-CF causing, and 3 VUS as of August 2016; http://www.cftr2.org).

The functional consequences of CF-causing variants have historically been grouped into five (or six) classes that are described as follows.[80,81] Variants that have consequences that do not fall into one of the five classes are discussed at the end of this section. This scheme has proven useful for relatively coarse correlation with disease severity in the lung, pancreas, and sweat gland.[82–85] However, a number of variants, including F508del, display effects on *CFTR* that fall into two or more of these classes.[86] Recognizing that variants can have multiple effects is important for optimizing *CFTR*-targeted treatments.[12]

Class I variants cause changes in the synthesis of *CFTR* by affecting *CFTR* transcription. These variants manifest their effect within the nucleus and usually involve the processing of transcripts. In most cases, the introduction of a premature termination codon, whether by a change of a codon to a nonsense variant or by frameshift, results in degradation of the transcript by a nonsense-mediated mRNA decay mechanism.[87] G542X (HGVS p.Gly542X) is an example of this type of variant.[88] In some cases, the premature termination codon does not lead to nonsense-mediated decay, and a truncated but nonfunctional protein is produced (e.g., R1162X [HGVS p.Arg1162X]).[89,90] A third consequence of nonsense variants is that they can cause skipping of the exon in which they occur.[91] An example of this phenomenon is seen with the R553X (HGVS p.Arg553X) variant.[92] Variants in the highly conserved splicing signals 5′ and 3′ of exons invariably lead to a loss of full-length transcript due to exon skipping.[93] Loss of exons can also cause a shift in the reading frame, leading to the introduction of a premature termination codon and subsequent RNA degradation. In each case, these types of variants lead to complete, or almost complete, loss of functional *CFTR* protein and produce a classic form of CF (Fig. 49.1). Some of the nonsense variants in *CFTR* have been shown to be rescued in cell lines with application of aminoglycoside antibiotics that can induce read-through of premature termination codons. Atalauren (PTC124), an investigational drug reported to suppress termination codons in some studies but not others,[94,95] is in phase III clinical trials in CF worldwide. The premature termination codon mutants are relatively frequent in Israel, where early phase clinical trials with Atalauren have shown some promise,[96,97] whereas a double-blind placebo controlled phase III study did not show improvement in lung function.[98]

The second class of variants involves those that affect the processing of *CFTR* (see Fig. 49.1).[99] A prime example of a class II variant is F508del. Loss of the phenylalanine residue at codon 508 within the first nucleotide-binding fold leads to a misfolding of *CFTR*.[100] Misfolded *CFTR* is recognized by chaperones that shunt the misfolded protein to degradation pathways.[101] The folding defect can be partially overcome by reduction in temperature. Cells grown at 21°C instead of 37°C can produce properly folded *CFTR*.[102] Folded *CFTR* bearing F508del is functional in the cell membrane, but it is not stable and is more rapidly removed from the membrane than its WT counterpart.[103] Because F508del is found in at least 70% of CF patients, the mechanisms underlying *CFTR* degradation have been studied intensively, in hopes of finding approaches that permit *CFTR* bearing the F508del variant to evade degradation (see Chapter 53). Other class II variants have been found that reduce folding efficiency, resulting in a small amount of properly folded functional *CFTR* at the cell membrane.[104,105] Two new molecules have been developed for correction (lumacaftor) and potentiation (ivacaftor) of the F508del mutant protein.[106,107] Phase III clinical trials demonstrated that the two drugs in combination produce improvement in lung function, decrease in pulmonary exacerbations, and increase in body mass index in CF patients homozygous for the F508del variant.[12,108,109]

Disease-associated variants in class III affect the regulation of *CFTR* (see Fig. 49.1). Binding of ATP to the NBDs is required to activate *CFTR*. Variants that affect *CFTR* interaction with ATP have been shown to alter its function.[72,110] An example is the G551D (HGVS p.Gly551Asp) variant, in which the glycine (G) at codon 551 is substituted with aspartic acid (D). The G551D variant severely affects interaction with ATP, creating a form of *CFTR* that is properly folded and inserted in the cell membrane, yet unable to be activated.[100,111] Multiple clinical trials of individuals carrying at least one *CFTR* gene with the G551D variant show that the novel drug ivacaftor (Vertex compound VX770) is safe and produces substantial improvements in lung function, reduction in sweat chloride concentration and infection with *P. aeruginosa*, and increase in body mass index.[112–118] Since G551D affects the gating behavior of *CFTR*, variants that have similar function effects on *CFTR* have been tested for response to VX770. A group of "gating" variants that respond to VX770 in cell-based studies showed significant clinical response in vivo.[119] These results suggest that the hundreds of *CFTR* variants without current approved treatment might be grouped according to functional effect and

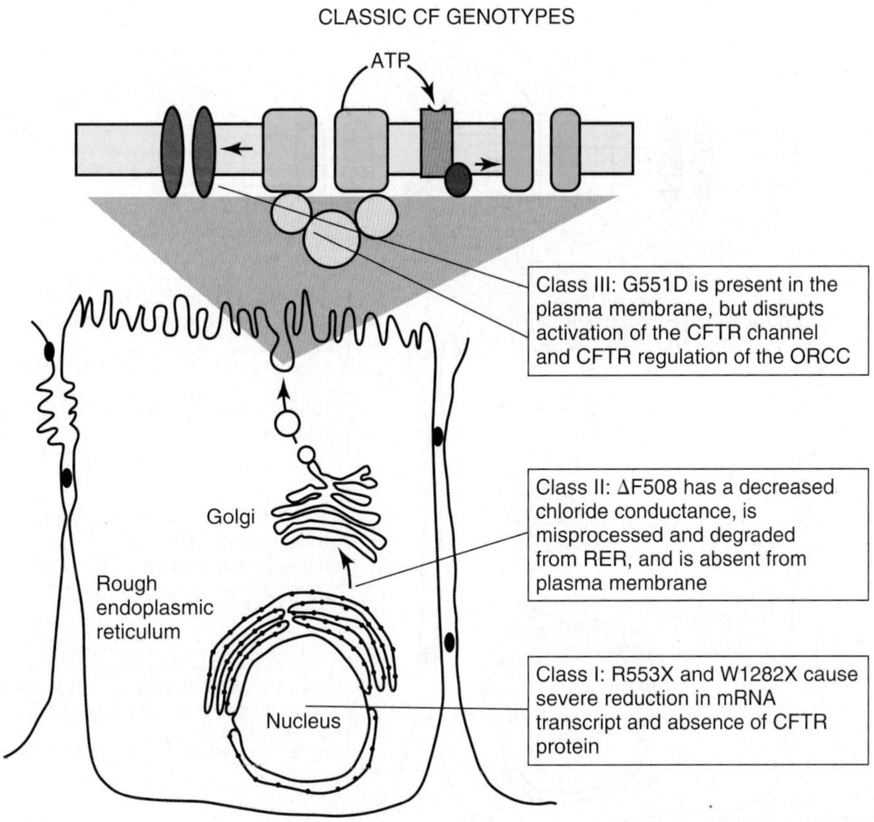

CLASSIC CF GENOTYPES

Fig. 49.1 Functional consequences of severe classic variants leading to pancreatic insufficiency. *ATP,* Adenosine triphosphate; *CFTR,* cystic fibrosis transmembrane conductance regulator; *mRNA,* messenger RNA; *ORCC,* outwardly rectifying chloride channel; *RER,* rough endoplasmic reticulum.

cellular response to drugs, so-called theratypes.[120] Such an approach could expedite the use of approved drugs for the many *CFTR* genotypes carried by CF patients.

Class IV variants alter the chloride conduction properties of *CFTR,* and in some cases affect the magnitude and the ion selectivity of the channel pore.[121,122] Most class IV variants occur in the transmembrane domains. Since class IV variants may reduce but do not eliminate the flow of ions, some *CFTR* function is preserved (Fig. 49.2), which in turn leads to a milder phenotype or a nonclassic form of CF. However, by the same token, it is recognized that altering this property of *CFTR* produces CF. Thus loss or alteration of the chloride channel function of *CFTR* is key to the development of the CF phenotype, demonstrating that a defect in chloride transport is the primary abnormality in cells of CF patients.

Class V variants are also associated with a milder form of CF, because they can also result in the production of a reduced amount of normally functional protein (see Fig. 49.2). An example of the latter type of variant is 3849 + 10 kbC > T (HGVS c.3717 + 12191C > T). This variant occurs within intron 22 (legacy intron 19), approximately 10 kilobases from the nearest splice site of exon 22, and leads to the aberrant splicing of *CFTR,* a nonfunctional protein.[123] However, the aberrant splicing mechanism is incomplete, and a small amount of normally spliced *CFTR* transcript is made, leading to the synthesis of some normal *CFTR* and a CF phenotype that is moderate in severity.

CF-causing variants have been shown to affect other functions of *CFTR.* *CFTR* regulates other ion channels, such as the ENaC and the ORCC.[124] Variants in the first NBD have been shown to variably affect *CFTR* regulation of these channels.[125,126] Variants in the N terminus or in the C terminus of *CFTR* can affect the trafficking, membrane insertion, or stability of *CFTR.*[127,128] These genotypes are sometimes classified as class VIA or VIB. Finally, variants in ENaC have been shown to cause cases of atypical CF.[129,130]

CLINICAL CONSEQUENCES OF VARIANTS

Correlation of the *CFTR* genotype with the CF phenotype has been investigated using three methods. In genotype-driven studies, patients are grouped according to genotype, and clinical features are compared. When patients who were homozygous for the F508del variant were compared with patients who carry one copy of F508del and a different CF variant, it was shown that a number of the less common variants produce the same degree of disease severity as the F508del variant.[131] Some variants cause less severe organ disease, or disease in a subset of organ systems affected in classic CF, resulting in a "nonclassic" CF phenotype.[132] The *CFTR* genotype demonstrates a consistent association with the severity of pancreatic disease.[133] A less consistent correlation has been noted with abnormalities in sweat chloride concentration.[134] However, only one variant, A455E (HGVS p.Ala455Glu), has been unequivocally correlated with severity of lung disease.[135,136] A few other variants, particularly those in class IV and V, may associate with less severe lung disease.[137] In the phenotype-driven method, *CFTR* variants are identified in patients grouped according to disease severity.

NONCLASSIC CF GENOTYPES

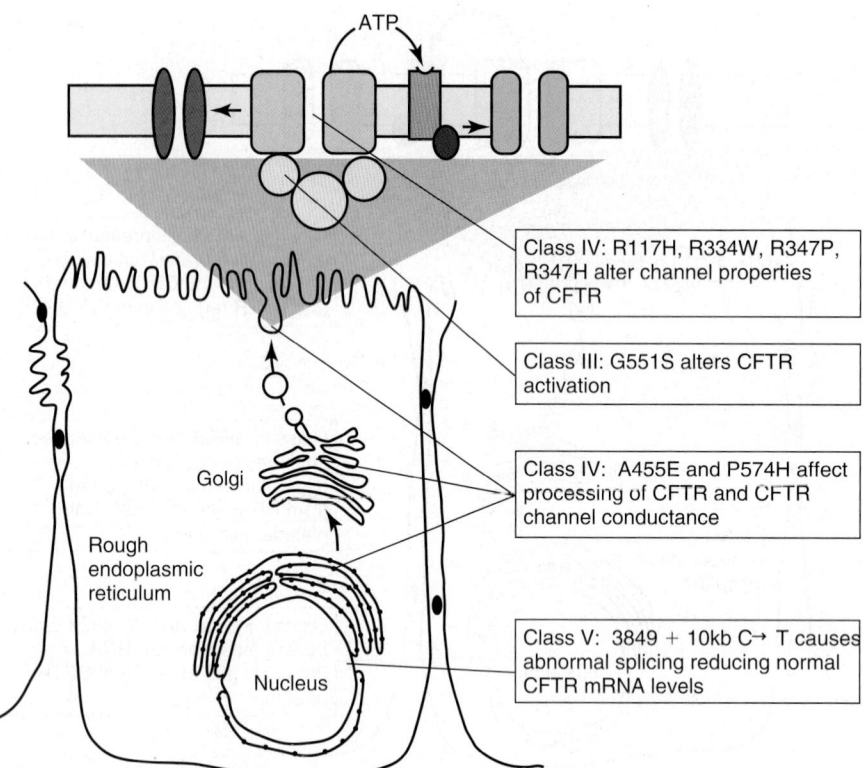

Fig. 49.2 Functional consequences of variants leading to nonclassic (mild) forms of cystic fibrosis. *ATP*, Adenosine triphosphate; *CFTR*, cystic fibrosis transmembrane conductance regulator; *mRNA*, messenger RNA.

This approach has identified relatively uncommon variants that are associated with nonclassic forms of disease.[138–141] A third approach has been to correlate the class of variant with the severity of disease. Those who carry variants that cause a complete or nearly complete loss of function, such as class I, II, and III variants, usually manifest classic CF. Variants that permit some residual function, such as those in classes IV and V, have been associated with milder phenotypes usually associated with pancreatic sufficiency.[134,137,142] However, it is important to recognize that many exceptions exist. For example, *CFTR* containing A455E affects the processing of *CFTR* (class II) but is associated with pancreatic-sufficient CF and milder lung disease.[104,105]

Diagnosis of atypical forms of CF can be difficult, especially when one or more alleles fails to demonstrate a disease causing variant.[143,144] Sweat chloride may be normal in some combinations of CF genotypes, making the test less reliable for nonclassic CF. Standardization of protocols to measure nasal epithelial chloride and sodium transport has proven useful in the diagnosis of CF.[145,146] The nasal potential difference (NPD) test can detect both classic and nonclassic forms of the disease,[147] and has been a secondary outcome measure in clinical trials of ataluren, VX809, and VX770.

Pathophysiology

CF is caused by the reduction or dysfunction of the *CFTR*, a cAMP-regulated chloride and bicarbonate channel and a master regulator of other ion channels that coexist in the apical membranes of cells lining the airways, sweat glands, hepatobiliary system, and reproductive tracts. In the absence of disease, *CFTR* activity downregulates or tempers the sodium absorption through ENaC.[148,149] In CF, the combination of a reduction in chloride transport and unregulated excessive sodium transport leads to the classic ion and water hydration defects that occur in the pancreas and vas deferens in utero, and the airways, biliary tract, intestines, reproductive tracts, and sweat glands after birth. *CFTR* is also expressed in other organs that do not succumb to disease, such as the heart and kidneys. Abundant alternative channels exist in those tissues to compensate for lack of *CFTR*-mediated chloride transport.[33,150,151]

AIRWAYS DEHYDRATION AND DISRUPTION OF MUCOCILIARY CLEARANCE

Airway surface liquid (ASL) bathes the cilia of the upper airway, and the depth and composition of this fluid is regulated by *CFTR* and ENaC. In CF, the ASL height is reduced and cilia are less efficient at moving particles and mucus.[152] Secondary effects of *CFTR* dysfunction include abnormal mucus secreted by the submucosal glands and epithelial cells. The blanket of airway surface mucus becomes excessive, but does not help eradicate bacteria that colonize and inflame the CF airways.

CFTR controls both the ENaC and the ORCC. When *CFTR* is absent, the ORCC cannot secrete chloride, amplifying the secretion defect.[153] The calcium-activated chloride channel (CaCC) and the pH-activated ClC-2 coexist and are independent of *CFTR*.[154–160] The latter are therapeutic targets in CF. A phase III program testing aerosolized denufosol, which activates the CaCC through binding to P2Y2 receptors and increasing intracellular calcium, failed to improve lung function over 1 year. It is yet unclear whether activation of an alternative chloride secretion pathway will be sufficient to overcome the defects associated with classic CF.

CF airways quickly become colonized with bacteria after birth. Defective mucociliary clearance likely plays a major role, but additional defects in bacterial clearance related to the importance of *CFTR* in the lipid raft region of the plasma membrane are emerging.[161–164] Inflammation in response to bacterial colonization is excessive and ineffective.[165,166] The ASL becomes infiltrated with neutrophils that respond to IL-8 secretion. As the neutrophils die, they liberate their DNA, which contributes to the viscosity of the mucus. Aerosolized DNase thins this mucus and improves lung function. Aerosolized hypertonic saline also facilitates clearance and improves lung function by a different mechanism.

Cystic Fibrosis Animal Models

CF research is perhaps the only field that benefits from having five mammalian genetic animal models, including the mouse,[167] rat,[168] rabbit, ferret,[169] and pig.[170–171] While the phenotype of the CF rabbit model has not been published, scientists have learned much from the differences and similarities between species. Broadly speaking, phenotypes can be broken down into lung, gastrointestinal (intestine, pancreas, liver, and gallbladder), and reproductive (vas deferens).

LUNG PHENOTYPES

With more than two decades of research on CF mice of various *CFTR* genotypes, the general consensus is that they have a negligible or mild lung phenotype[172–174] Early research implicated a CaCC in the airways of mice as compensating for the lack of *CFTR*.[175] More recent research has suggested that *CFTR* counterbalances H+ secretion through the H+/K+ exchanger ATP12A, which acidifies ASL and impairs innate immunity in CF humans, but not mice, due to the differential expression of this exchanger.[176] Despite the lack of a robust lung phenotype in CF mice, there is evidence that they have a hyperinflammatory phenotype when challenged with pseudomonas-laden agarose beads.[177] While the CF rat model is relatively new, it does not develop a spontaneous bacterial colonization phenotype in the lung, despite having a reduced ASL volume and a reduction in submucosal gland mass.[168]

The lung phenotype in CF ferrets[178,179] and pigs[180] is considerably more robust than in CF rodents and clearly demonstrates similarities to the CF human phenotype.[181] When challenged with bacteria, both newborn CF pigs and ferrets have impaired antibacterial killing in comparison to non-CF animals.[180,182] Interestingly, impaired innate immunity in newborn CF ferrets appears to be selective for *P. aeruginosa*,[182] despite the fact that other species of bacteria colonize the lung later in life.[178] Studies in CF pigs have suggested that the lack of *CFTR*-dependent bicarbonate secretions leads to a reduced ASL pH, and that this impairs bacterial killing at

the airway surface.[183] By contrast, impaired antibacterial killing of ASL from CF ferrets is unaltered by bicarbonate.[182] Unlike CF pigs, the lungs of newborn CF ferrets are rapidly colonized by bacteria after birth and die within the first week of life if not reared on antibiotics.[179] These differences in early innate immunity between CF pigs and ferrets may be due to the fact that ferrets postnatally develop submucosal glands and ciliated cells, whereas pig airways are fully developed at birth. By a week of life, mucociliary clearance rates decline in CF as compared with non-CF ferret airways as ciliogenesis increases.[182] There remains a debate as to whether the ASL is dehydrated in these CF models with supporting evidence in the ferret[182] and pig[184] models using microoptical coherence tomography and other refuting evidence in the pig model using histologic endpoints.[185]

Inflammation in the CF lung is thought to be an important component of the disease process, with evidence in CF mice for a hyperinflammatory phenotype.[177] While inflammation is not observed in the newborn CF pig lung,[180] newborn CF ferret lungs have elevated IL-8 and TNFα and reduced IL-1β in the bronchoalveolar lavage fluid (BALF), despite having no differences in bacterial load as compared with non-CF animals.[182] While sterile BALF harvested from breathing C-sectioned ferrets lacked genotype-specific differences in these cytokines, IL-8 induction in the BALF of naturally born as compared with C-section animals was only observed in CF animals,[182] suggesting that first bacterial exposure to the lung induces IL-8 in the absence of *CFTR*. Interestingly, proteomics analysis of CF and non-CF newborn and C-section BALF suggests that certain pathways that control immunity and inflammatory (including the complement system, macrophage functions, mammalian target of rapamycin signaling, and eukaryotic initiation factor 2 signaling) are repressed in the naive CF ferret lung, and that these pathways are accentuated at birth following exposure to bacteria[182] Similarly, gene expression array studies on 15-day-old CF ferret lungs demonstrate significant elevations in IL-8-mediated inflammatory pathways.[186] More recent transcriptome analysis of newborn CF pig lungs challenged with heat-killed bacteria also suggests dysregulation of acute inflammatory responses, as compared with non-CF littermates.[187]

GASTROINTESTINAL PHENOTYPES

The intestine, pancreas, liver, and gallbladder are all adversely affected in CF, although the penetrance of clinically apparent disease varies for each of these organs. All CF animal models have intestinal disease that manifests either in utero (ferret and pigs) or at weaning (mice and rats). Meconium ileus, an in utero complication of gut obstruction, is observed in ~15%–20% of CF patients.[188] The incidence of meconium ileus is higher in CF ferrets (75%)[179] and pigs (100%),[189] while CF mice and rats generally manifest gut obstruction at weaning.[168,172] Genetic modifiers of meconium ileus have been identified in CF humans,[190] and this also appears to occur for meconium ileus in CF ferrets[179] and gut obstruction at weaning in CF mice.[191] Juvenile CF ferrets also present with other intestinal CF phenotypes, including rectal prolapse and distal intestinal obstruction syndrome (DIOS).[192]

Exocrine pancreatic disease has a significant impact on the health of CF patients, with ~85%–90% being pancreatic-insufficient within the first 2 years of life.[193] CF animal models have a diverse range of exocrine pancreas phenotypes.[194] CF rodents (mice and rats) generally lack apparent disease in the exocrine pancreas,[168,172–174] and in mice this is thought to be due to an alternative CaCC that compensates for the lack of *CFTR*.[175] Disease of the exocrine pancreas begins in utero in CF pigs, with significant acinar cell atrophy and pancreatic remodeling by birth.[195] In contrast, CF ferrets are born with minor abnormalities of pancreatic histopathology[179] but have progressive loss of acinar cells within the first month of life.[192] While nearly all CF ferrets are born pancreatic-insufficient, with impaired growth and a lack of fecal elastase in the stool, a small percentage of CF ferrets have been found to be pancreatic-sufficient with normal growth and fecal elastase present in the stool.[192] Such findings suggest that genetic modifiers of pancreatic disease also exist in this species. However, it has not been possible to capture this pancreatic-sufficient phenotype through breeding to date, suggesting that multiple genetic modifiers may be responsible. The progression of exocrine pancreatic disease in CF ferrets occurs within the first several months of life and is associated with a robust inflammatory and fibrotic response that transitions to adipogenic remodeling by 3 months of life.[192,196,197]

Liver abnormalities are not uncommon in CF patients and are characterized by biliary cirrhosis (25%), hepatic steatosis (30%), and clinical cirrhosis (5%).[198–200] These disease processes are considerably more variable in CF animal models. Both CF mice and rats lack major pathologies in the liver,[168,172–174] and CF ferrets also lack signs of liver disease at birth.[179] However, with age, ferrets develop variable signs of steatosis, necrosis, biliary hyperplasia, and biliary fibrosis in ~39% of animals.[192] Newborn CF pigs demonstrate evidence of focal biliary cirrhosis[189,201] and a reduced pH of bile collected from the biliary ducts.[202]

Gallbladder disease occurs in ~30% of CF patients.[203] While both the CF mouse and ferret gallbladder lack cAMP-inducible chloride currents indicative of *CFTR*,[173,204] they have grossly different histopathology. In CF mice, the extent of gallbladder disease is quite variable, with some backgrounds showing evidence of decreased size and inflammatory infiltrates.[173] Although newborn CF ferrets demonstrated little gallbladder pathology,[179] as CF ferrets age, they develop significant mucous plugging and mucosal proliferation (~80%–90%).[192] CF pigs have the most severe gallbladder disease, presenting with a microgallbladder at birth.[189,201] Interestingly, rats lack a gallbladder, and thus CF-associated disease in this organ is irrelevant in this species.

VAS DEFERENS PHENOTYPE

Nearly all male adults with CF suffer from infertility caused by bilateral absence of the vas deferens.[205] While CF male mice have normal fertility,[173] newborn CF rats,[168] ferrets,[179] and pigs[206] lack a vas deferens bilaterally and thus appear to model this component of the human disease.

CYSTIC FIBROSIS-RELATED DIABETES

Cystic fibrosis-related diabetes (CFRD) is a common complication of CF and affects 20%–25% of adolescents and 40%–50% of those older than 30 years of age[207,208] There have been several reports suggesting that *CFTR* plays a functional role within the beta-cell to facilitate insulin secretion.[209–211] Furthermore, chemical-induced killing of beta-cells in CF mice exacerbates islet cell dysfunction and leads to an altered inflammatory response.[212,213] By contrast, other findings have suggested that CF mice harboring the F508del-*CFTR* variant do not have an intrinsic beta-cell secretory defect, but rather acquire insulin resistance and a reduced beta-cell mass with age.[214] Interestingly, lung bacterial clearance in diabetic CF mice, following streptozotocin (STZ)-induced beta-cell injury, is significantly diminished compared with nondiabetic CF mice.[215]

While CF mice appear to have some abnormalities that affect glucose metabolism, their lack of significant exocrine pancreatic disease is likely the reason they do not develop classical CFRD seen in humans. Both CF ferrets and pigs are born with impaired glucose tolerance (IGT).[197,216] IGT in newborn CF pigs appears to be due to a reduced glucose-stimulated insulin secretion.[216] By contrast, IGT in newborn CF ferrets appears to be due to a lack of first phase insulin secretion despite a greatly accentuated later phase.[197] However, the poorly regulated insulin secretion in newborn CF ferrets does not appear to be due to insulin resistance.[197] These early differences in glucose tolerance between the two models are likely due to the more severe exocrine pancreatic damage and islet remodeling at birth in the CF pigs, as compared with CF ferrets.

The CF ferret model has been most extensively studied in terms of CFRD pathogenesis. Isolated islets from newborn CF ferrets have reduced glucose-stimulated insulin secretion due to a heightened level of insulin secretion in the presence of low glucose,[197] demonstrating that islet-intrinsic defects in insulin secretion exist in CF ferrets. This dysregulated insulin secretion by CF ferret islets appears to mirror that seen in nursing newborn CF ferrets and is thought to be a result of the emerging inflammation at birth in the pancreas. Recently, rising pancreatic inflammation in juvenile CF ferrets has been shown to significantly reduce beta-cell mass and lead to spontaneous diabetic-level hyperglycemia at 1–2 months of age, a time at which proinflammatory cytokines (IL-1β, TNFα, IL-6, CXCL10) peak in the pancreas.[196] Interestingly, at 2–3 months of age, CF ferrets undergo a rapid recovery in their ability to regulate blood glucose following a meal with a coincident increase in beta-cell mass and islet cell function.[196] This novel finding of productive islet remodeling following peak exocrine inflammation in the CF ferret pancreas was associated with a fibrotic to adipogenic transition, marked by elevation in PDX1, PPARγ, and adiponectin. Such findings suggest that the early CF pancreas has a remarkable ability to repair damaged islets, although formal proof of regenerating beta-cells is still lacking.[196] Despite this unique "honeymoon" period observed in CF ferrets following glycemic crisis, with age they go on to develop the more classically studied CFRD phenotype in CF patients with impaired insulin secretion in response to hyperglycemic clamp and to arginine. However, insulin sensitivity was normal, as measured by using a euglycemic hyperinsulinemic clamp.[196] An interesting clinically relevant observation from this study was that mixed meal tolerance was impaired at all ages in CF ferrets, while oral glucose intolerance was not detected until 4 months.

Characteristics of Systemic Disease

AIRWAYS, UPPER AND LOWER

Lung disease remains the major expression of morbidity and mortality in CF. Infants with CF are born with normal lungs, and pulmonary disease develops over a variable time course. The earliest lesion is obstruction of the small airways by abnormally viscous airway mucus. A secondary bronchiolitis with plugging of the airways invariably follows and develops into bronchiectasis as the respiratory epithelium becomes chronically infected. A striking feature of CF lungs is that the parenchyma is virtually untouched for much of the course, while the airways are severely afflicted. The airways become a reservoir for chronically infected mucopurulent secretions, first by *Staphylococcus aureus* and *Haemophilus influenzae*, and later by a distinctive mucoid form of *P. aeruginosa*. Once mucoid *P. aeruginosa* colonizes the lungs, it is virtually impossible to eradicate. Emergence of methicillin-resistant strains of *S. aureus* (MRSA) is increasing and a cause for concern.[217] Respiratory failure is the major cause of death, with the median life span now increased to 41.6 years in the United States (Cystic Fibrosis Foundation Registry Data, 2015).

The respiratory disease is usually progressive, with superimposed acute exacerbations. Cough is an early symptom and may be nonproductive and mistaken for asthma. Production of sputum develops and is an indicator of chronic inflammation and infection. A typical course is characterized by intermittent acute pulmonary exacerbations, in which there is an increased volume of sputum, a change in the color of sputum, decreased exercise tolerance, and weight loss. Digital clubbing is a universal finding with progression of the lung disease. The chest radiograph becomes abnormal early in the course of the disease and demonstrates hyperinflation (Fig. 49.3) and patchy atelectasis (Fig. 49.4). The chest computed tomography (CT) scan is even more sensitive to changes (Fig. 49.5) and may be preferred over the chest radiograph for a quantitative assessment of progression of lung disease.[218] Bronchiectasis develops from progressive chronic infection and destruction of the airways (Fig. 49.6). Pulmonary function tests early in the disease reflect small airways obstruction but then progress toward a decrease in the forced expiratory volume in 1 second (FEV_1) and increases in residual volume, functional residual capacity, and the ratio of residual volume to total lung capacity. The vital capacity is eventually reduced. With treatment of the acute exacerbations, variable improvements in some of these lung functions can be documented.

The upper airway is also severely affected in CF. Chronic pansinusitis is found in more than 99% of patients with CF, due in part to mucous gland hyperplasia, abnormal chloride ion transport by the sinus epithelial cells, and colonization with bacteria. Chronic sinusitis may contribute to infection of the lower respiratory tract by acting as a reservoir of infection. CT scans of the sinuses are useful in assessing the extent of sinus involvement and in the selection of patients who might benefit from a surgical drainage procedure.

Sinus involvement is complicated by nasal polyposis in 6%–40% of patients. Nasal polyps should be suspected if

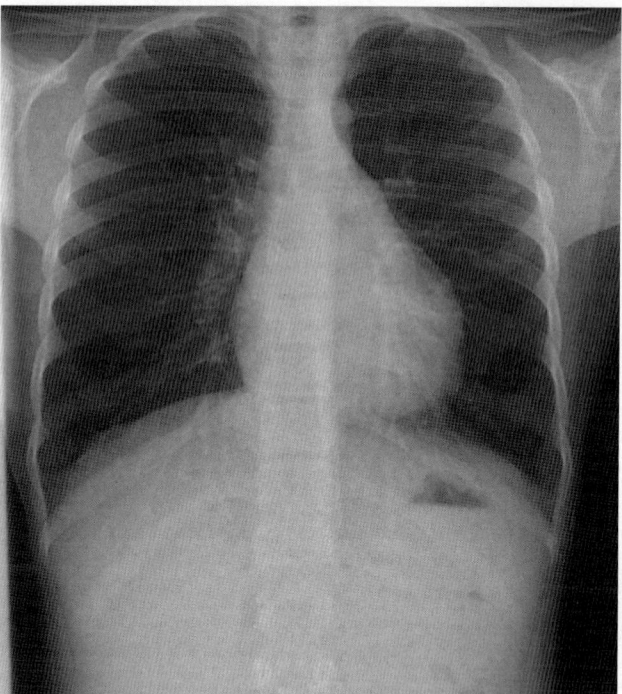

Fig. 49.3 Chest radiograph of a 10-year-old female with cystic fibrosis (genotype F508del homozygous) who complained of increasing cough and sputum production. Both lung fields are hyperinflated, and there are increased lung markings. Expectorated sputum culture grew nonmucoid *Pseudomonas aeruginosa*.

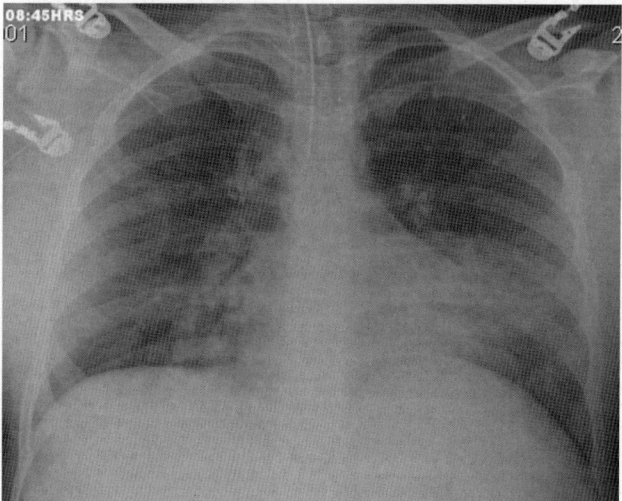

Fig. 49.4 Chest radiograph at bronchoscopy of an adolescent female with cystic fibrosis (genotype F508del/621 + 1G) who complained of sudden and transient chest pain on the left side, followed by an increase in cough. There are lingular, right lower, and right middle lobe infiltrates and atelectasis. Lung fields improved after 14 days of intravenous antibiotics directed against the *Staphylococcus aureus* and mucoid *Pseudomonas aeruginosa* that grew from bronchoalveolar lavage fluid cultures.

nasal airflow is obstructed, the nasal bridge widens, or there is persistent epistaxis, loss of taste, or loss of appetite. Polyps appear in childhood and often recur after initial resection. If the disease is left untreated, serious bony erosions can occur. Medical management consists of topical glucocorticoids,

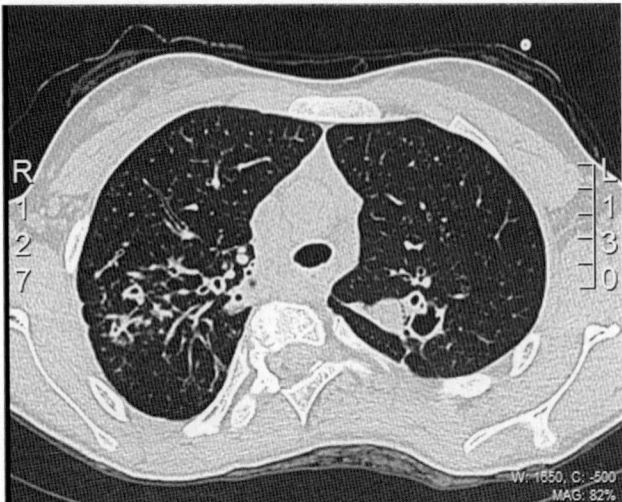

Fig. 49.5 Spiral chest computed tomography scan of an adolescent female with cystic fibrosis (genotype F508del homozygous) and a slight decline in forced expiratory volume in 1 second. There is bilateral upper lobe bronchiectasis. Her sputum cultures grew *Pseudomonas aeruginosa* and methicillin-resistant strains of *Staphylococcus aureus* (MRSA).

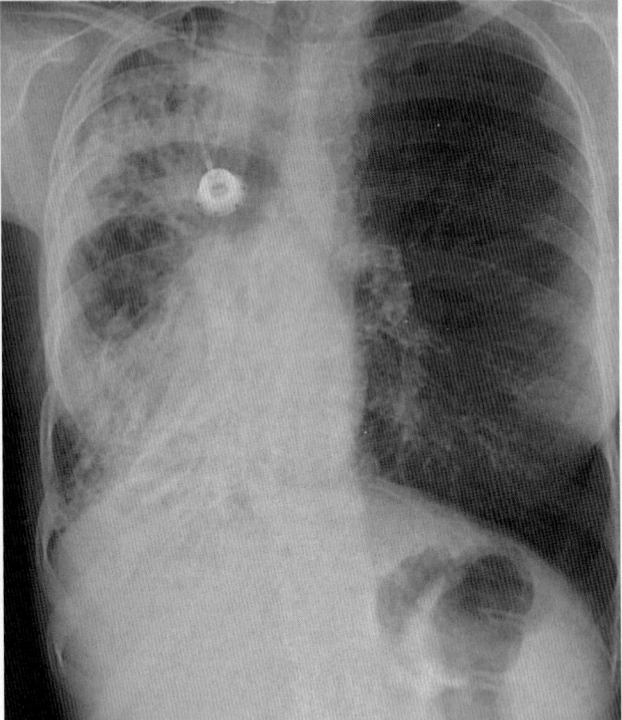

Fig. 49.6 Chest radiograph of a 16-year-old female with cystic fibrosis (genotype F508 homozygous) and recurrent pulmonary exacerbations. The left lung shows hyperaeration and bronchial wall thickening. The right lung shows decrease in volume, bronchial wall thickening, and bronchiectasis. Sputum cultures grew *Achromobacter xylosoxidans*.

macrolide antibiotics for their antiinflammatory action, antibiotics to cover the organisms in the sinuses, and surgical approaches.[219]

Inflammation

A particularly intense inflammatory state appears early in the CF airways. Konstan and colleagues[220] demonstrated that the inflammatory infiltrate is predominantly neutrophilic.

BALF studies in infants suggest that inflammation may even precede colonization with bacteria, although this is controversial.[221,222] If inflammation is both a primary defect related to dysfunctional *CFTR* and a result of infection, then antiinflammatory therapy may be helpful.

Immune-mediated inflammation contributes significantly to the lung damage present in patients with CF. Specific antipseudomonal antibiotics do not eradicate the organism permanently. Despite aggressive intravenous therapy with large doses of increasingly more potent agents, colonization proceeds. Chronic infection then elicits recruitment and activation of neutrophils in the airways. The neutrophils release proteases such as granulocyte elastase and cathepsin G. This protease burden has been associated with both destruction of the lung matrix and cleavage and inactivation of a variety of opsonins. There is also evidence of immune complex formation in CF patients that correlates with disease severity and prognosis.

Infection

Nonencapsulated *H. influenzae* often colonizes the oropharynx of the young child with CF. Although it is not considered a serious pathogen, rising antibody titers to *H. influenzae* have been detected.[223] *S. aureus* is the most frequent organism detected initially on oropharyngeal cultures, and it is still debated whether chronic antibiotic prophylaxis against this organism is useful. The acquisition of MRSA is increasing and emerging as a potential pathogen in communities of both CF and healthy children. Nonmucoid *P. aeruginosa* is acquired at varying times after birth, and transformation to a mucoid phenotype is associated with increased inflammatory burden and sputum volume. Early intervention strategies and chronic antibiotic protocols are aimed at eradicating or reducing the infection for as long as possible. *Burkholderia cepacia* complex (composed of nine different species) is particularly feared. Genomovar III is highly virulent and transmissible, and can be associated with a sepsislike condition that markedly reduces survival. Transient colonization with a *B. cepacia* spp. is becoming more common.

With more aggressive antibiotic strategies in place and frequent sputum and oropharyngeal cultures, a number of multiply resistant organisms are being identified. *Stenotrophomonas maltophilia*, *Alcaligenes xylosoxidans*, and nontuberculous mycobacteria alone or in combination with *P. aeruginosa* or *S. aureus* are challenging clinicians.[224] The complexity of microbial communities suggests that diversity is lost with aging in CF, but traditional culture methods are inadequate to completely catalog the totality of microbes. Antibiotic exposures shift microbial composition, and recovery postexposure may be incomplete.[225] Efforts in antibiotic stewardship are ongoing to prevent increasingly resistant organisms.

Additional details pertaining to bacterial, viral, and fungal pathogens in CF are discussed in Chapter 51. An extremely important message to learn from this work is that infection control strategies in the acute care setting, ambulatory clinics, and the home are mandatory if we are to contain the spread of transmissible organisms.[226]

GASTROINTESTINAL DISEASE

Gastrointestinal disease begins in utero in the pancreas, where dysfunctional *CFTR* produces a deficiency in exocrine pancreatic secretions because of progressive plugging of the pancreatic ducts by viscous secretions. The combination of the in utero deficiency of proteolytic enzymes with secretion of abnormal mucoproteins by the goblet cells of the small intestine leads to obstruction of the distal ileum by inspissated, tenacious meconium. About 15% of infants with CF are born with intestinal obstruction called meconium ileus. There are associated intestinal complications including small bowel atresia, volvulus, perforation, and peritonitis; alternately, there may simply be delayed passage of meconium and distal colonic obstruction secondary to the meconium plug syndrome.

The loss of pancreatic enzyme activity leads to intestinal malabsorption of fats, proteins, and, to a lesser extent, carbohydrates after birth. Pancreatic function is lost incrementally until complete loss is seen in 85% of patients. Infants manifest poor or absent weight gain, chronic abdominal distention, absence of subcutaneous fat and muscle tissue, steatorrhea, and rectal prolapse. Paradoxically, the untreated child may have a voracious appetite, but the caloric intake is insufficient to meet daily needs.

In older individuals, intestinal mucous gland hyperplasia is associated with abnormal mucins and slowing of intestinal transit time. If pancreatic enzyme replacement is inadequate, fecal impaction or DIOS can result.

Children, adolescents, and adults with residual pancreatic function may develop recurrent episodes of pancreatitis. Serum and urine amylase and serum lipase are elevated. Attacks can be precipitated by a fatty meal, alcohol, or tetracycline. Patients with one or more class IV or V variants tend to have residual pancreatic function and to be at risk.

Liver disease can result from biliary tract obstruction and inflammation. Normally, *CFTR* is found on the apical membranes of biliary tract cells where chloride transport facilitates bile flow. In CF, focal biliary cirrhosis appears in 10%–20% of infants by 1 year and in up to 80% of adults.[227,228] Little is known about the pathogenesis of liver failure in CF, or why some individuals escape significant injury. Therapeutic intervention is limited to dietary bile salts to reduce biliary sludging.

SWEAT GLAND EFFECTS

The gold standard for diagnosis of CF for many years has been the demonstration of elevated chloride and sodium in sweat collected by quantitative pilocarpine iontophoresis. Although no histopathologic changes can be found in the CF sweat gland, the function is abnormal as a result of inadequate reabsorption of salt by the distal collecting duct. The CF sweat is isotonic with plasma, and the skin of affected infants has been described as tasting "salty." Heavy exercise in hot, humid climates can lead to increased salt losses and profound clinically significant dehydration.

Sweat production occurs in all individuals, primarily by cholinergic stimulation. Cyclic AMP-mediated sweat secretion is insignificant, which is why sweat can be produced in CF individuals through the cholinergic pathway. Sweat chloride concentrations can sometimes be normal or borderline in people with a mild *CFTR* variant. Thus genetic variant analysis or NPD testing may be required to make the diagnosis.

REPRODUCTIVE TISSUES

The male reproductive tract is exquisitely sensitive to defects in *CFTR* function. Even carriers of one CF gene can present with isolated male infertility. Azoospermia results from an atretic or absent vas deferens that begins in utero. Most males with CF are infertile because of this mechanism.

Other Disorders Related to the Cystic Fibrosis Transmembrane Conductance Regulator

CONGENITAL BILATERAL ABSENCE OF THE VAS DEFERENS

Male infertility due to obstructive azoospermia is a consistent feature of CF, and it has been estimated that 98% of all males with CF have this condition.[229] One notable exception has been males who carry the 3849 + 10 kbC > T variant, as a substantial fraction are fertile.[230] Male infertility is due to malformation of structures derived from the Wolffian duct reproductive tract, manifesting as atrophy of the vas deferens. The seminal vesicles and associated structures also can be involved.[231] Abnormal development of the male reproductive tract begins in utero and continues in the first year of life.[232] On occasion, only one of the vas deferens is destroyed, while the other remains patent. This reduced-fertility condition is termed *unilateral absence of the vas deferens*. Males with CF produce sperm, although spermatic morphologic abnormalities have been reported.

CBAVD also has been reported in healthy males as an isolated cause of male infertility.[233] It has been estimated that approximately 1 in 5000 males are affected with this condition. Because of the phenotypic overlap between CBAVD and male infertility seen in CF males, investigators analyzed the *CFTR* genes in males with isolated CBAVD and discovered that a high proportion carried CF variants.[234] More recent studies with extensive analysis of the *CFTR* gene indicate that approximately 86% of CBAVD patients carry at least one deleterious variant.[235] F508del is the most common variant, occurring in approximately 44% of the cases.[235] The second most common *CFTR* variant in CBAVD males (32%) is the 5T polymorphism of the intron 9 splice acceptor.[236] The frequency of 5T in the general population (10% carrier rate) posed a question as to how it could be associated with male infertility. Pedigree studies revealed that 5T is inconsistently associated with CBAVD, suggesting that other factors contribute to the disease. The dinucleotide TG tract immediately adjacent to the T tract (see earlier) determines whether the 5T variant produces male infertility in an individual who carries a variant in his other *CFTR* gene.[42,45] The variant R117H (HGVS p.Arg117His) is also quite common in males with CBAVD. Approximately 10% of CBAVD males carry this variant, yet less than 1% of CF patients carry this variant. The 5T variant in intron 8 also plays a role in this phenomenon. The R117H variant has occurred at least twice in human evolution—once in association with the 5T variant and once in association with the more common 7T variant.[237] Males and females who have a CF variant paired with R117H and the 5T variant invariably have a CF phenotype, while those males who have R117H with the 7T variant usually develop CBAVD, although some cases of CF have been observed.[235,237] Notably, females with this combination of variants have presented with pancreatitis and with a normal phenotype.[238,239]

PANCREATITIS

Pancreatitis is a rare presenting sign of CF in patients with residual pancreatic function.[240] Isolated pancreatitis does not present with similar clinical features to CF. However, the concept that *CFTR* dysfunction may play a role in idiopathic pancreatitis is supported by two observations. First, sweat electrolyte concentrations have been found to be elevated in a subset of chronic pancreatitis patients.[241] Second, *CFTR* is known to be expressed in pancreatic ducts, a major site of disease in pancreatitis. Two studies of patients with idiopathic pancreatitis found an increased frequency of variants in the *CFTR* gene.[238,242] In both studies, the frequency of *CFTR* variants in the patients with pancreatitis was significantly higher than in the control population and higher than the expected frequency in the general population. Several other reports have since confirmed that CF variants occur at a higher frequency in patients with isolated pancreatitis.[243–246] However, it appears that additional genetic or environmental influences are required for the development of pancreatitis.[247] Variants in other genes known to give rise to monogenic forms of pancreatitis, such as the secretory trypsinogen inhibitor gene *ST8SIA4 (PST1)*, can combine with *CFTR* variants to increase the risk of developing pancreatitis.[243,244] While nonalcoholic chronic pancreatitis has been associated with CF variants, it is not clear that the risk of developing pancreatitis in the case of alcohol abuse is increased in the presence of *CFTR* variants.[248]

SINUSITIS

Chronic sinusitis is a consistent feature of CF.[240] In addition, some males with CBAVD and *CFTR* variants also have chronic rhinosinusitis.[249,250] Because the sinus epithelium is reliant on *CFTR* function for fluid and electrolyte transport, alterations in *CFTR* could play a role in isolated cases of chronic rhinosinusitis. Indeed, patients who presented with chronic rhinosinusitis to an otorhinolaryngology clinic were found to have a higher frequency of CF variants than disease-free control populations, suggesting that deleterious variants in *CFTR* predispose to the development of sinusitis.[52] Two other studies have found that patients with chronic rhinosinusitis have an increased frequency of CF variants,[251,252] while one study did not find this association.[253] More recently it has been demonstrated that the prevalence of chronic rhinosinusitis in CF carriers is approximately twice the population prevalence.[254] Thus reduction of *CFTR* function by approximately 50% appears to increase the risk of developing chronic forms of sinus disease.

References

Access the reference list online at ExpertConsult.com.

50 Diagnosis and Presentation of Cystic Fibrosis

COLIN WALLIS, MD, MRCP, FRCPCH, FCP, DCH

A diagnosis of cystic fibrosis (CF) has lifelong implications for affected individuals, their families, and their acquaintances. This important step needs to be taken accurately and early on. A late diagnosis is often preceded by a catalogue of doctor's visits, family anguish, and anger associated with a delay in the initiation of treatment that may have an impact on long-term outcome. Equally disturbing is a small but increasingly documented experience of children, diagnosed as having CF, whom on review—often years later—are found not to fulfill diagnostic criteria.

Many countries have now introduced newborn screening programs for the diagnosis of CF. This has changed the experience of diagnosing CF for both parents and pediatricians.[1,2] Appropriate monitoring of the child's condition and early therapy are introduced, often before the emergence of signs and symptoms traditionally associated with CF.[3,4] Apart from the advantages of early detection through newborn screening, new challenges have arisen from the screening program, including:

1. Uncertainties about the diagnostic label in some infants who, following a positive screening result, do not fulfill all the criteria for a CF diagnosis[5,6];
2. The recognition of an ever-widening phenotype for an individual with two cystic fibrosis transmembrane conductance regulator (CFTR) mutations, ranging from a traditional CF phenotype, a spectrum of atypical disease forms, and even individuals with no discernible CFTR dysfunction at all and no evidence of end organ disease at the time of assessment[7,8];
3. The recognition that a CF phenotype can emerge and change over time, presenting de novo in adulthood or moving from "atypical" forms to a more classical CF[7,9];
4. The need for pediatricians and adult physicians to remain vigilant in order to diagnose those individuals who may have been missed by the screening process or did not undergo screening.

In this chapter, we will describe the diagnostic criteria for CF, the diagnostic techniques available for assessing the CFTR function, the screening process, and the need to identify and label atypical cases—both screened and clinically detected.

Diagnostic Criteria for Cystic Fibrosis

In more than 90% of cases, the diagnosis of CF in an unscreened patient arises from a clinical suspicion supported by a test of CFTR function, the sweat test, with genetic testing for CFTR mutation used as confirmatory testing. A Cystic Fibrosis Foundation (CFF) Consensus Panel (United States)

synthesized diagnostic criteria for CF.[10] The key features are summarized in Box 50.1. The basic premise of the consensus statement is that CF is a clinical and not a genetic diagnosis, although acknowledging that genetic testing may have a role in sorting out atypical clinical situations. Any such document must be considered a work in progress to accommodate new developments[11,12] and acknowledged shortcomings.[13] The latest version of the consensus guidelines from the CFF is now available online (https://www.ncbi.nlm.nih.gov/pubmed/28129811).

Making the Diagnosis of Cystic Fibrosis

A clinician may need to confirm a diagnosis of CF in various settings such as when

1. A patient has one or more suspicious clinical features;
2. A newborn screening program has identified a child at risk for CF;
3. An individual is being examined after the diagnosis of CF in a family member; or
4. Postnatal confirmation is required when an antenatal test has proven suspicious for CF.

CLINICAL SUSPICION

The majority of unscreened children with CF present with a history of bulky fatty stools, failure to thrive, and recurrent chest infections.[14] Shortly after birth, 10%–15% will present with intestinal obstruction as meconium ileus. However, there is a wide range of less common presenting features (Box 50.2). Any children or adults presenting with suspicious features of CF should be investigated further, even if they have undergone newborn screening. A possible diagnosis of CF in a child with suggestive clinical findings should not be discounted just because the child appears too well or is thought to be too old. Although the diagnosis is established in most children by the age of 1 year—and earlier if screened—in approximately 10% of children the diagnosis is delayed until after 7 years of age.[15] Patients with pancreatic sufficiency and non-Caucasian patients are particularly vulnerable to delays in diagnosis.[16,17]

THE SWEAT TEST

The sweat test was first described in 1959 and remains a gold standard for the diagnosis of CF.[18] In the appropriate clinical setting, whether the child has entered the diagnostic algorithm via clinical suspicion or newborn screening, a positive sweat chloride test is diagnostic of CF. There are a number of other rare conditions (sometimes single case

Box 50.1 Diagnostic Criteria for Cystic Fibrosis (Cystic Fibrosis Foundation Consensus Panel)

One or more characteristic phenotypic features consistent with cystic fibrosis (CF):
 Chronic sinopulmonary disease
 Gastrointestinal and nutritional abnormalities
 Salt loss syndromes
 Male urogenital abnormalities resulting in obstructive azoospermia
 OR
A history of CF in a sibling
 OR
A positive newborn screening test result
 AND
an increased sweat chloride concentration
or identification of two disease causing CF mutations
or demonstration of abnormal nasal epithelial ion transport.

Box 50.2 Clinical Features of CF at Diagnosis in Unscreened Populations— Grouped According to Age and Approximate Order of Frequency

0–2 Years

Failure to thrive
Steatorrhea
Recurrent chest infections including bronchiolitis/bronchitis
Meconium ileus
Rectal prolapse
Edema/hypoproteinemia/"kwashiorkor" skin changes
Severe pneumonia/empyema
Salt depletion syndrome
Prolonged neonatal jaundice
Vitamin K deficiency with bleeding diathesis

3–16 Years

Recurrent chest infections or "asthma"
Clubbing and "idiopathic" bronchiectasis
Steatorrhea
Nasal polyps and sinusitis
Chronic intestinal obstruction, intussusception
Heat exhaustion with hyponatremia
CF diagnosis in a sibling

Adulthood (Often Considered CFTR-Related Disorder)

Azoospermia/congenital absence of the vas deferens
Bronchiectasis
Chronic sinusitis
Acute or chronic pancreatitis
Allergic bronchopulmonary aspergillosis
Focal biliary cirrhosis
Abnormal glucose tolerance
Portal hypertension
Cholestasis/gall stones

CF, Cystic fibrosis.

Box 50.3 Examples of Noncystic Fibrosis Causes of a Positive Sweat Test

Adrenal insufficiency or stress
Anorexia nervosa
Ectodermal dysplasia
Eczema
Fucosidosis
G6PD deficiency
Glycogen storage disease type 1
Human immunodeficiency virus infection
Hypoparathyroidism
Hypothyroidism
Malnutrition from various causes
Nephrogenic diabetes insipidus
Pseudohypoaldosteronism
Chronic arsenic exposure

accredited laboratories. Localized sweating is stimulated by the iontophoresis of pilocarpine into the skin. Sweat is collected on filter paper, gauze, or in microbore tubing[19] over a controlled period of time to ensure that the rate of sweating and the total sweat collected are sufficient and standardized. Guidelines for sweat testing procedures and precautions are available in published[20–23] and electronic format (http://www.acb.org.uk/docs/sweat.pdf).

Chloride is the analyte of choice.[24,25] The sodium levels and osmolality of sweat are less reliable and should never be used in isolation. A sweat chloride concentration of more than 60 mmol/L is considered positive, and levels below 30 mmol/L are likely to be in the normal range. This lower limit of 30 mmol/L was previously set at 40 mmol/L in children older than 6 months, but recent consensus guidelines have revised to a chloride level of less than 30 mmol/L for all age groups.[12,26] Results between 30 and 60 mmol/L have traditionally been considered intermediate and require further evaluation. A high proportion of patients with chloride concentrations in this intermediate range will have two CFTR mutations—usually one at least that is not defined as disease causing, a situation found with increasing frequency with the advent of more detailed CFTR mutation testing.[27,28]

Following the introduction of newborn screening (NBS) for CF, sweat tests are increasingly performed on infants. It is recommended that sweat chloride testing in asymptomatic newborns with a positive NBS test be performed when the infant is older than 2 weeks of age and more than 2 kg.[29,30] The vast majority of affected infants will have a chloride level greater than 60 mmol/L. A sweat chloride value between 30 and 59 mmol/L should be considered intermediate and trigger further patient evaluation, including repeat testing when older.[31] Certain CFTR mutations (such as R117H, R334W, 3849+10kbC>T) associated with a milder CF phenotype may also demonstrate a normal sweat chloride.

Some normal adolescents and adults can have sweat chloride values in the intermediate range, and sweat chloride levels alone may be insufficient to diagnose CF in the older adolescent.[32] A false-positive sweat test in the severely malnourished child or the critically ill child in intensive care needs cautious interpretation and follow-up.

Research continues to explore the development of an easier sweat test. Collecting systems such as the Macroduct[33] and

reports) that have been associated with a positive sweat test, but these are usually clearly distinguishable by their clinical features (Box 50.3).

The standard sweat test (Gibson and Cooke technique) requires skill and care, and should be undertaken by

Nanoduct[19] simplify collection and are now in routine practice. The role of sweat conductivity as a diagnostic tool in CF is debated.[34] In one large trial, the best conductivity cutoff value to diagnose CF was ≥90 mmol/L, and the best conductivity cutoff value to exclude CF was less than 75 mmol/L.[35] However, most clinicians and laboratories will chose to confirm a positive sweat conductivity result with a formal measurement of chloride concentration.

MUTATION ANALYSIS

The 1989 identification of the CF gene[36] and the characterization of its protein product (CFTR) held the promise that the diagnostic dilemmas for the condition were over. If you had two CFTR mutations, you had CF—if not, you did not. Unfortunately it has not worked out that simply. Even though the presence of two mutations is very supportive of the diagnosis of CF in the appropriate clinical setting, two alterations in the gene that encodes CFTR does not necessarily mean that you will develop classic CF disease, as outlined later.

There are more than 2000 different CF gene mutations documented, although the clinical impact of these mutations is frequently uncharacterized. A valuable online resource lists identified mutations at http://www.genet.sickkids.on.ca/app.

Clinically available techniques do not routinely allow a full screen of the entire CF genome, and most laboratories will only search for the most common mutations within their geographical region—focusing on those known to be disease causing. Examples of disease-causing CFTR mutations are listed in Table 50.1, highlighting the dominance of the ΔF508 mutation (present in >70% of CF alleles in Caucasian populations). Customizing mutation panels to match the patient's ethnic background and clinical presentation can enhance the sensitivity of DNA testing in CF.

Second, there is a range of mutation types that have been classified into classes according to the functional impact on the CFTR.[37,38] The final protein product may be incomplete, complete but incorrectly packaged and processed, or a final CFTR molecule that is unstable or incapable of reaching the cell surface in sufficient quantity to be physiologically effective. This is discussed further in Chapter 49.

In addition to the "disease-causing" mutations, there are also recognizable polymorphisms that do not necessarily result in a clinical phenotype but may influence the structure of the final protein product when associated with another mild mutation. The thymidine run in intron 8 is a well-described example where the 5T allele leads to a substantial reduction in functional protein compared with the 9T allele; the 7T allele is intermediate in its effect. The clinical phenotype associated with two CFTR mutations is far broader than previously anticipated (Box 50.4). Caregivers should avoid making prognostic predictions based on genotype alone.[39] Examples of the potential clinical impact of selected CFTR mutations[39] is shown in Table 50.2 and can also be researched on the CFTR2 website (http://www.cftr2.org/), which also regularly updates the growing list of disease causing mutations.

Failure to find two CF mutations from a selective or extended search does not exclude the diagnosis of CF. There are also rare reports of patients with classical CF symptoms and signs and a positive sweat test who do not appear to have any mutations in the CFTR gene—even when the entire gene

Table 50.1 Common Mutations That Cause Cystic Fibrosis Listed According to Frequency[a]

Traditional Name	HGVS[b] Nomenclature	Frequency (%)
ΔF508	p.Phe3508del	75.0
G551D	p.Gly551Asp	3.4
G542X	p.gly542X	1.8
R117H	p.arg117His	1.3
621+1G>T	c.489+1G>T	1.3
ΔI507	p.Ile507del	0.5
N1303K	p.Asn1303Lys	0.5
R560T	p.arg560Thr	0.4
Q493X	c.1477C>T	0.3
R1162X	p.Arg1162X	0.3
R533X	p.Arg553X	0.3
W1282X	p.Trp1282X	0.3
3659delC	c.3527_3528delC (p.Lys1177Serfs)	0.3
1154insTC	c.1021_1022dup (p.Phe342HisfsX28)	0.3
E60X	p.Glu60X	0.2
G85E	p.Gly85Glu	0.2
P67L	c.200C>T (p.Pro67Leu)	0.2
R347P	p.Arg347Pro	0.2
V520F	p.Val520Phe	0.2
1078delT	c.946_947delT (p.Phe316Leufs)	0.1
2184delA	c.2052_2053delA (p.Lys684Asnfs)	0.1
A455E	p.Ala455Glu	0.1
R334W	p.Arg334Trp	0.1
S549N	p.Ser549Asn	0.1
2789+5G>A	c.2657+5G>A	0.1
3849+10kbC>T	c.3717+10kbC>T	0.1
711+1G>T	c.579+1G>T	0.1
1717-1G>T	c.1585-1G>A	0.6
1898+1G>T	c.1766+1G>A	0.6

[a]In Caucasian populations—variations in frequency occur between different ethnic groups and geographic regions.
[b]Human Genome Variation Society nomenclature.

Box 50.4 Examples From the Range of Clinical Features That Can Be Associated With Two Mutations in the CF Gene

"Classical CF" with pancreatic insufficiency
Sinopulmonary disease, pancreatic sufficiency and positive sweat test
Sinopulmonary disease and male infertility with a normal sweat test
Severe sinusitis and congenital bilateral absence of the vas deferens
Male infertility only
Chronic pancreatitis only
Allergic bronchopulmonary aspergillosis
Sclerosing cholangitis
Positive sweat test only
No clinical features including normal sweat chloride.

---

has been sequenced—screening all 27 exons and the intron-exon boundaries.[40] These findings suggest that, on these very rare occasions, CF may be caused by mutations within the promoter region of the CFTR gene, in one of the introns, or even in a distant controlling gene from an unrelated locus.[41] This highlights the fact that despite advances in molecular diagnostics, CF remains a clinical diagnosis supported by a functional test of CFTR dysfunction.

Table 50.2 Examples of *CFTR* Mutations With Regard to Their Clinical Consequences

Mutation Group	Examples
A. CF-causing	F508del, R553X, R1162X, R1158X, 2184delA, 2184insA, 3120+1G>A, I507del, 1677delTA, G542X, G551D, W1282X, N1303K, 621+1G>T, 1717-1G>A, A455E, R560T, G85E, R334W, R347P, 711+1G>T, 711+3A>G[a], 1898+1G>A, S549N, 3849+10kbC>T, E822X, 1078delT, 2789+5G>A, 3659delC, R117H-T5[a], R117H-T7[a], D1152H[a], L206W[a], TG13-T5[a]
B. CFTR-related disorders associated	R117H-T7[a], TG12-T5[a], R117H-T5[a], D1152H[a], TG13-T5[a], S997F, R297Q[a], L997F, M9521, D565G[a], G576A[a], TG11-T5[b], R668C-G576A-D443Y, R74W-D1270N
C. No clinical consequences	I148T, R75Q, 875+40A/G, M470V, E528E, T854T, P1290P, 2752-15G/C, I807M, I521F, Γ508C, I560V, TG11-15[b]
D. Unknown or uncertain clinical relevance	Mainly missense mutations[c]

[a]Mutations that may belong either to Group A or to Group B.
[b]Mutations that may belong either to Group B or to Group C.
[c]Certain common sequence (missense) variants with subclinical molecular consequences (e.g., M470V) may cosegregate on the same chromosome and exert more potent, cumulative phenotypic effect. Such polyvariant haplotypes could be potentially disease causing.[56]

An unintended consequence of the newborn screening programs has been the detection of infants who have a high immunoreactive trypsin and, on further assessment, have a normal or borderline sweat test, and in whom the genotyping reveals one or two mutations of uncertain clinical consequence. These children have no clinical features at the time of detection and present a difficult diagnostic conundrum. The classification of the various "types" of CF is discussed at the end of this chapter.

ASSESSMENT FOR ORGAN INVOLVEMENT

To determine the presence of specific organ disease in a patient with the genetic predisposition to develop CF disease, but in whom there are few clinical indicators, may require more detailed and targeted assessment.[42] Examples include the following:

1. Computed tomography scanning of the lungs can be used to evaluate subtle pulmonary changes such as bronchial wall thickening, small airway disease, and air trapping not readily visible on plain radiography.
2. Computed tomography can also be used to evaluate the sinuses, which are invariably opacified in CF patients.
3. Testing for pancreatic function testing can involve sophisticated tests of pancreatic enzyme measurements from endoscopic sampling or 3-day stool collections for fecal fat analysis. A simple test for quantification of fecal elastase 1 to diagnose pancreatic sufficiency[43,44] has shown considerable sensitivity and reliability and is not contaminated by exogenous enzyme administration.[45] Caution is required in the interpretation of early-life stool samples, especially in the premature infant or newborn within the first few days of life.[46]

4. Sputum, bronchoalveolar lavage fluid, oropharyngeal swabs, or sinus aspirates can be cultured for known CF pathogens. *Staphylococcus aureus* or *Pseudomonas aeruginosa*, although not unique to CF, may support a possible CF diagnosis.
5. Congenital bilateral absence of the vas deferens (CBAVD) is a common finding in many males with CF. Postpubertal males can have semen analysis for azoospermia, or younger males can be assessed with ultrasound for CBAVD.[47]
6. Valuable information can be obtained with spirometry, including assessment of small airway function even in young children, using validated techniques such as the multiple breath washout test.[48]
7. An ultrasound examination of the pancreas can show atrophy or cystic changes in many patients with CF. Tests for abnormal glucose tolerance may also demonstrate CF pancreatic involvement.

TRANSEPITHELIAL POTENTIAL DIFFERENCE MEASUREMENTS

In rare instances where the diagnosis of CF remains unclear or the evidence is equivocal, additional tests of CFTR function can be utilized. Patients with CF demonstrate defective chloride secretion and sodium hyperabsorption, and nasal potential difference (PD) measures the voltage created by chloride and sodium as they move across the epithelium. Nasal PD can be measured in the mucosa or the inferior turbinates by placing an exploring electrode on the respiratory epithelium and a reference electrode into the subcutaneous tissue of the forearm or an area of abraded skin. Baseline PD is more negative in patients with CF. Diagnostic accuracy is assured by documenting a bioelectric profile of change to the basal reading in the presence of amiloride application (becoming less negative in CF) with the addition of a chloride-free solution and isoproterenol (little or no response in CF; Fig. 50.1).[49,50] Results are influenced by recent viral infections, the presence of rhinitis, the precise anatomic localization of the measuring catheter, as well as polyps and the genotype. The test requires precise perfusion rates and duration of the chloride-free solution and the addition of isoprenaline. Not infrequently, atypical forms of CF with borderline sweat chloride levels produce a nasal PD that is also equivocal.[11,51] PD measurements are difficult to perform, especially in young children, and the technique is generally confined to specialist centers.[52,53] A video featured on the following website demonstrates the technique: http://www.rbht.nhs.uk/patients/condition/cystic-fibrosis/patient-information/films/#NPD.

Alternatively to NPD and independent of the patient's age, intestinal current measurements can be done on rectal mucosal biopsy specimens ex vivo in an Ussing chamber.[54] This technique is not yet widely available and limited to a few centers.[55,56]

Antenatal Testing for Cystic Fibrosis

Parents with an increased risk of having a child with CF, either because their own carrier status is known or because

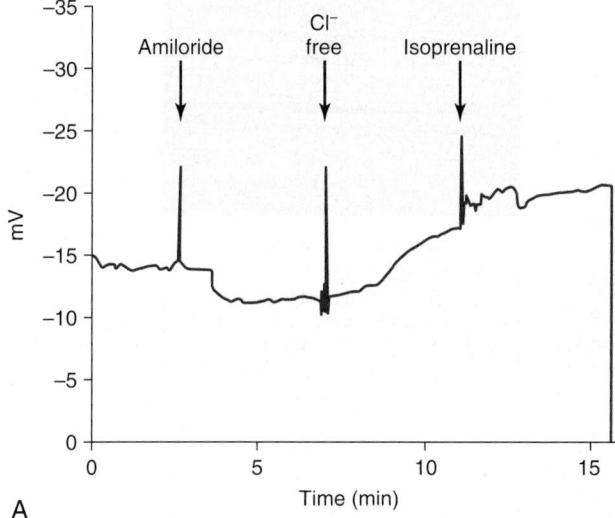

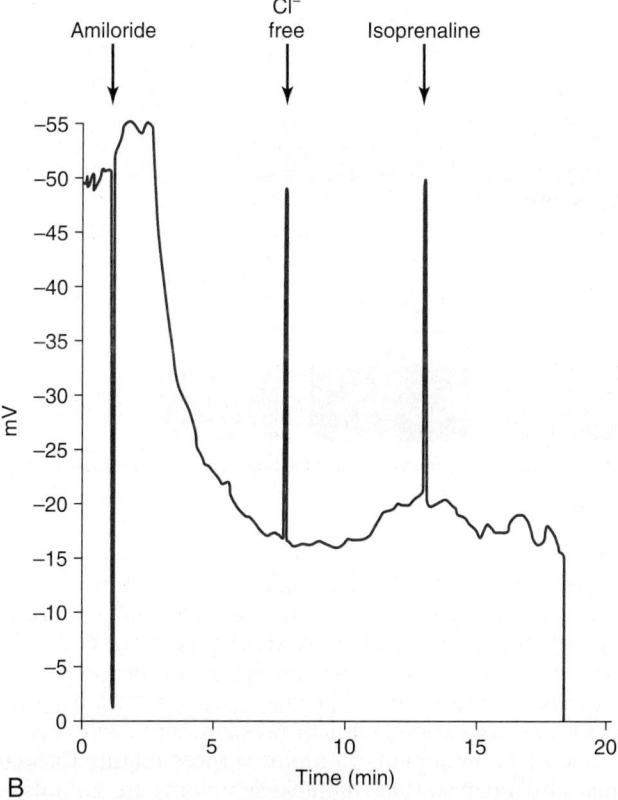

Fig. 50.1 Nasal potential difference (PD) in a normal subject (A) and a cystic fibrosis patient (B), illustrating the difference in baseline PD, response to perfusion with amiloride, followed by the addition of a chloride-free solution and then isoproterenol. Note that the spikes on the trace associated with the perfusion of solutions are artefactual and do not represent mucosal voltage changes. (With thanks to Dr. N. Simmonds for the trace.)

they already have an affected child, may request antenatal testing. The diagnosis can be confirmed or excluded, with a high degree of accuracy by direct mutation analysis performed on fetal cells obtained by chorionic villus sampling (10 weeks gestation) or cultured amniotic fluid cells (15–18 weeks gestation).

Preimplantation diagnosis is an alternative for at-risk couples. After in vitro fertilization, a cleavage-stage biopsy is carried out on day 2 or 3, and normal or carrier embryos are then transferred to establish pregnancy. Further postnatal confirmation is still recommended.

Occasionally, routine fetal anomaly scans may detect a suspicion for meconium ileus by abnormal bowel echogenicity or evidence of perforation. Although such findings are usually discovered too late into the second trimester to enable decisions on the fate of the pregnancy, a positive scan will help provide optimal facilities for the delivery and subsequent medical and surgical care. Hyperechoic bowel often occurs as a benign variant and is distinguished by spontaneous resolution, usually before the third trimester.[57]

Neonatal Screening for Cystic Fibrosis

Although CF is not an ideal condition for a newborn screening program, as there is no highly specific or sensitive biomarker and there is no cure at this stage, the ability to identify CF in infants as early and accurately as possible has advantages that outweigh any potential disadvantages.[4,58,59] Over the last decade, newborn screening for CF has been widely adopted by many regions and countries and is now emerging as the commonest route to the diagnosis of CF, sharply altering the traditional diagnostic paradigm of symptom-led investigations described previously for the pediatrician. A range of screening algorithms has been developed, often to suit local resources and conditions.[31,60,61]

The first step of CF neonatal screening is usually based on the immunoreactive trypsin assay (IRT), which is relatively inexpensive to perform on the newborn heel prick sample (Guthrie test).[62] Increased IRT concentrations can be raised transiently in healthy newborns, but in newborns with CF IRT remains raised for weeks to months in both pancreatic sufficient and insufficient CF individuals. A repeat IRT 2 weeks after birth further improves the specificity of the screening algorithm.[63] Infants with raised or persistently raised IRT above a locally devised cutoff point proceed to further testing. This may consist of a panel of common CFTR mutations for the region performed on the same blood sample or a sweat test.[64,65] An example of the algorithm currently adopted by the United Kingdom is illustrated in Fig. 50.2.

Screened babies may have early manifestations of pulmonary or gastrointestinal disease at the time of diagnosis, but may also be completely asymptomatic, even though they have two disease-causing mutations and a positive or intermediate sweat test. CF teams have had to acquire special skills in conveying information to the families of these seemingly well children.[66]

The CF screening program is primarily designed to pick up all cases of classical CF in newborns who have two disease-causing mutations and a positive sweat test who will benefit from early therapy, and to exclude healthy carriers. However, all newborn screening programs will also identify infants with an equivocal diagnosis where the screening results are neither clearly diagnostic nor normal. This has led to some confusion about this group—both in terms of nomenclature and subsequent clinical follow-up and management. For example, infants identified with hypertrypsinogenemia

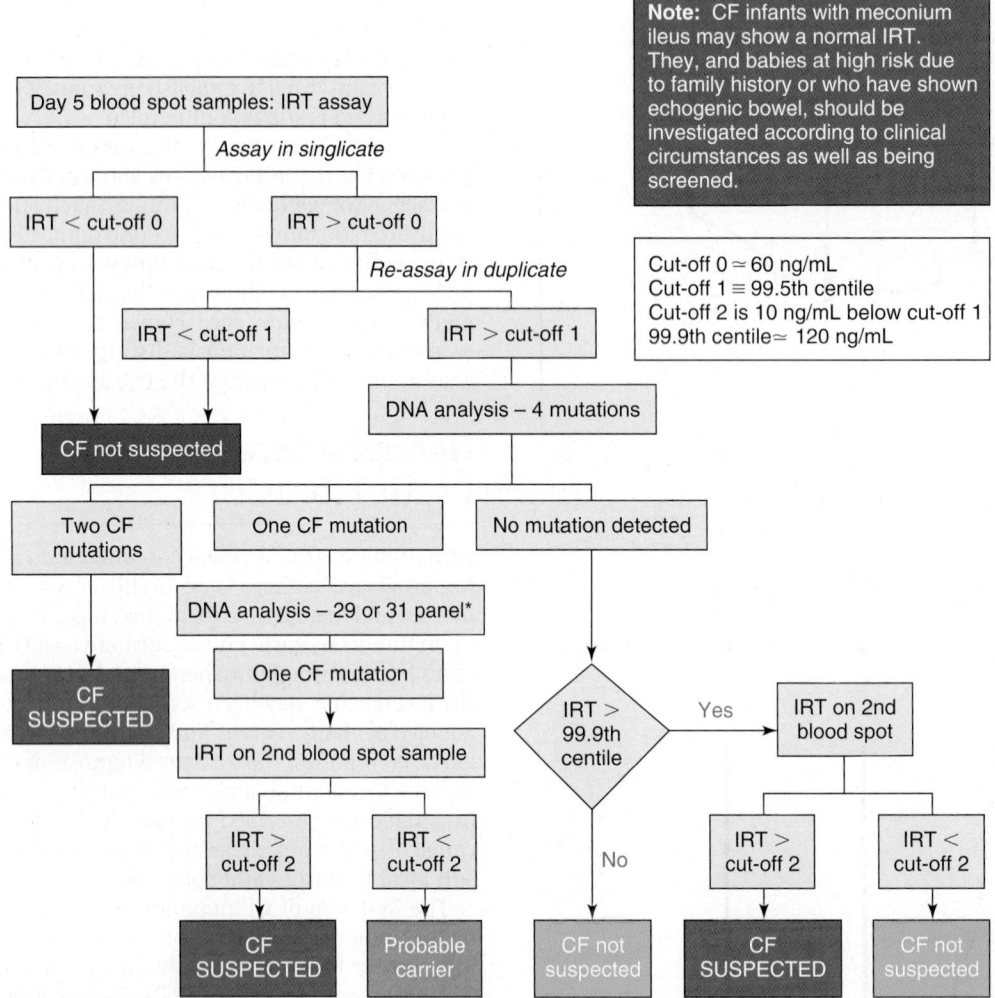

Note: CF infants with meconium ileus may show a normal IRT. They, and babies at high risk due to family history or who have shown echogenic bowel, should be investigated according to clinical circumstances as well as being screened.

Cut-off 0 ≈ 60 ng/mL
Cut-off 1 ≡ 99.5th centile
Cut-off 2 is 10 ng/mL below cut-off 1
99.9th centile ≈ 120 ng/mL

Fig. 50.2 An example of a newborn screening algorithm using an IRT/IRT/DNA protocol. *CF,* Cystic fibrosis. *, In some areas this mutation analysis has been extended to include 50 CFTR mutations.

on NBS may have sweat chloride values less than 60 mmol/L (or even normal levels of <30 mmol/L) and up to two CFTR mutations, at least one of which is not clearly categorized as a "CF-causing mutation."[6,67] These infants do not fulfill all the diagnostic criteria for CF, are pancreatic sufficient, and have no or nonspecific clinical symptoms at the time of presentation to the clinicians. There has been significant debate on what to call such infants who do not have a disease and how to monitor them longer term for the emergence (if ever) of end organ changes that require intervention and control. The term CFTR-related metabolic syndrome (CRMS) has been proposed to describe these atypical cases in the United States—in an attempt to provide a label rather than a diagnosis but satisfy the need for funding to provide care.[6] Consensus documents outline possible management protocols. A collaborative European effort preferred the term "Cystic Fibrosis Screen Positive, Inconclusive Diagnosis" (CFSPID), which is used in most other parts of the world to describe this group of children and included a suggested follow-up plan.[5,69] The natural history of these children with CRMS/CFSPID is unknown. They may grow up to become adults who, in the prescreening era, would have been diagnosed with "CFTR–Related Disorders"—presenting with predominantly single-organ disease such as male infertility, sinusitis, pancreatitis, or allergic bronchopulmonary aspergillosis (ABPA). Equally they may enjoy trouble-free lives and never develop a disease at all or potentially emerge over time into a more classical CF phenotype.[70,71] Pediatric teams, with expertise in CF and its various clinical presentations, will need to develop follow-up plans to monitor these infants through their childhood so that treatable symptoms are not missed but unnecessarily burdensome treatments are spared.

The Phenotypic Spectrum of Cystic Fibrosis— Influencing Factors

Although two disease causing CFTR mutations are likely to be associated with both a positive sweat test and the presence of disease manifestations in the lung, pancreas, and other organs, the road from genotype to phenotype is not easily predictable. As described in Chapter 49, mutations can be categorized as mild or severe, but the spectrum of phenotype is broad, even for a given CFTR mutation.[39,72] Different organs appear to have different thresholds for CFTR functioning. The vas deferens, for example, requires a relatively higher level of functioning CFTR and appears to be particularly sensitive.

There are four major contributing factors that influence the path from genotype to end-organ involvement and an individual's eventual phenotype[7,73]:

1. The severity of the individual CFTR mutations: "Mild" mutations may cause milder phenotypic effects, but when there is a mixture of mild and severe mutations, the final impact is less predictable. Similarly, coexistent polymorphisms hitchhiking within the CFTR gene may influence the final protein product—such as the polythymidine run (5T/7T), in conjunction with the R117H mutation.

2. Modifying genes: Genes other than CFTR lying elsewhere in the genome can have significant impact on the CFTR protein's clinical influence. These genes and their protein products can correct or exacerbate influencing pathological processes such as the biochemistry of the cell surface liquid, the innate and acquired immunity of the lungs, and may even influence the predisposition to meconium ileus.[74] Each individual with CF has an orchestra of modifying genes and proteins unique to themselves and influential in their clinical outcome in concert with their CFTR genotype.[75,76]

3. Environmental factors: The environment in which a patient with CF lives and grows has central bearing on the outcome of their disease. Poor access to treatment or nonadherence to therapy, social circumstances and diet, exposure to infections such as pseudomonas, or viral infections in infancy can produce a sustained negative influence on the clinical course.

4. The passage of time is an important influence on outcome. CF is not necessarily an all-or-nothing disease. A clinical phenotype can emerge with time, for example, in those children initially designated as CRMS/CFSPID. Effective therapies and adherence to treatment can help stall the disease progression. Patients with documented pancreatic sufficiency in childhood can become pancreatic insufficient later in life. Some but not all patients with CF may, over time, develop diabetes, liver disease, and osteoporosis.

Cystic Fibrosis Phenotypes

While CFTR dysfunction clearly causes a clinical spectrum of disease, three phenotypes can be distinguished:

CLASSICAL CF

Most children with classical CF in current times are likely to be picked up through newborn screening programs and confirmed by the finding of two CF-causing mutations and a positive sweat test. They may be clinically well at the time of detection through the CF screening program but are highly likely to develop CF symptoms that require early intervention. Some children will be missed through screening, but no racial group is exempt from the disorder, and children of ethnic minorities or mixed heritage are at greatest risk of a delayed or missed diagnosis.[77] The clinical features of recurrent chest infections, malabsorption with pancreatic

---

> **Box 50.5 Conditions That May Be Associated With an Increased Incidence of Cystic Fibrosis Transmembrane Conductance Regulator (CFTR) Mutations and Partial Evidence for CFTR Dysfunction But Insufficient Evidence to Fulfill a Cystic Fibrosis Diagnosis**
>
> Pancreatitis—acute or recurrent
> Disseminated bronchiectasis
> Isolated obstructive azoospermia
> Allergic bronchopulmonary aspergillosis
> Diffuse panbronchiolitis
> Sclerosing cholangitis
> Rhinosinusitis
> Heat exhaustion

insufficiency in the majority (but not all), salt-losing syndromes, or infants presenting with meconium ileus or rectal prolapse require investigation. Appropriate therapy should be introduced without delay.

CFTR-RELATED DISORDERS

The terms "CFTR-related disorders" or "atypical CF" or "non-classic CF" or "delayed CF" have all been used to describe individuals—often with single organ disease, and often picked up later in life—who have symptoms and signs reminiscent of those found in CF, but in whom the full diagnostic criteria are not met.[78–80] Sweat testing can be normal, intermediate, or positive, and mutation analysis may reveal one or two CFTR mutations whose clinical significance is uncertain. Examples of such conditions are listed in Box 50.5. Most of these individuals are currently detected in later childhood or as adults. Caregivers have recognized that it is inappropriate to label individuals with these atypical forms as having classic CF.[81] Both the diagnostic labeling and management needs to be tailored to the patient's individual phenotype and requirements.[67] The introduction of arduous therapies aimed at the patient with classical CF may not be appropriate or beneficial. The negative connotations of a CF label can be avoided with a more considered approach to diagnostic categorization.

The concept of classical and atypical forms has been useful in countering the "all-or-nothing" approach to the diagnosis of CF. Equally, however, it should be recognized that careful monitoring and timely management are crucial for all affected children—even those with atypical forms. Terms such as "atypical" or "mild" should not lead to complacency in care and follow-up.

It is likely that some of the children currently detected through newborn screening and labeled as CRMS/CFSPID (described later) may emerge over time to develop single organ disease and move into the CFTR-related diagnostic category.[70,71]

CFSPID/CRMS

As discussed previously, the newborn screening program can detect NBS infants with hypertrypsinogenemia subsequently identified with one or two CFTR mutations of uncertain clinical significance and a normal or equivocal sweat test. As such, they do not fit the criteria for a CF diagnosis. The term "cystic fibrosis screen positive, inconclusive diagnosis" (CFSPID) was considered preferable for these children in a European consensus study. Like the acronym, CRMS, it is a label, not a diagnosis. These children do not have clinical symptoms, and there is no evidence for end organ CF disease. Before the advent of widespread screening programs, this scenario was rarely encountered and considered a form of genetic "pre-CF."[83] Currently this group can comprise between 10%–40% of the CF screen–positive infants—and even more depending on the local cutoff levels for IRT.[84,85] There is the potential that clinical features may emerge with time, but there is insufficient evidence to label these asymptomatic infants as CF or even atypical CF. Most clinicians would advise a program of careful surveillance, including repeating the sweat test during the first 2 years of life.[69] The role of prophylactic therapy such as physiotherapy or antibiotics is unclear, and the need for regular surveillance respiratory cultures is debated. The natural history for this group of children is likely to emerge with greater clarity over the next decade.[8,86] The decision to reclassify children designated as CRMS/CFSPID will need to take into account functional assessment of CFTR (sweat chloride, nasal PD), CFTR genetic analysis, and evidence for organ disease, as assessed by an experienced CF team.

References

Access the reference list online at ExpertConsult.com.

Suggested Reading

Borowitz D, Parad RB, Sharp JK, et al. Cystic Fibrosis Foundation practice guidelines for the management of infants with cystic fibrosis transmembrane conductance regulator-related metabolic syndrome during the first two years of life and beyond. *J Pediatr.* 2009;155(6 suppl):S106–S116.

Castellani C, Southern KW, Brownlee K, et al. European best practice guidelines for cystic fibrosis neonatal screening. *J Cyst Fibros.* 2009;8(3):153–173.

De Boeck K, Wilschanski M, Castellani C, et al. Cystic fibrosis: terminology and diagnostic algorithms. *Thorax.* 2006;61(7):627–635.

Farrell PM, White TB, Ren CL, et al. Diagnosis of cystic fibrosis: consensus guidelines from the cystic fibrosis foundation. *J Pediatr.* 2017;181S: S4–S15.

Gonska T, Ratjen F. Newborn screening for cystic fibrosis. *Exp Rev Respir Med.* 2015;9(5):619–631.

Goubau C, Wilschanski M, Skalicka V, et al. Phenotypic characterisation of patients with intermediate sweat chloride values: towards validation of the European diagnostic algorithm for cystic fibrosis. *Thorax.* 2009; 64(8):683–691.

Green A, Kirk J. Guidelines for the performance of the sweat test for the diagnosis of cystic fibrosis. *Ann Clin Biochem.* 2007;44(Pt 1):25–34.

LeGrys VA, Yankaskas JR, Quittell LM, et al. Diagnostic sweat testing: the Cystic Fibrosis Foundation guidelines. *J Pediatr.* 2007;151(1):85–89.

Levy H, Farrell PM. New challenges in the diagnosis and management of cystic fibrosis. *J Pediatr.* 2015;166(6):1337–1341.

Levy H, Nugent M, Schneck K, et al. Refining the continuum of CFTR-associated disorders in the era of newborn screening. *Clin Genet.* 2016;89(5):539–549.

Mayell SJ, Munck A, Craig JV, et al. A European consensus for the evaluation and management of infants with an equivocal diagnosis following newborn screening for cystic fibrosis. *J Cyst Fibros.* 2009;8(1):71–78.

Munck A, Mayell SJ, Winters V, et al. Cystic Fibrosis Screen Positive, Inconclusive Diagnosis (CFSPID): a new designation and management recommendations for infants with an inconclusive diagnosis following newborn screening. *J Cyst Fibros.* 2015;14(6):706–713.

Sermet-Gaudelus I, Mayell SJ, Southern KW. Guidelines on the early management of infants diagnosed with cystic fibrosis following newborn screening. *J Cyst Fibros.* 2010;9(5):323–329.

Solomon GM, Konstan MW, Wilschanski M, et al. An international randomized multicenter comparison of nasal potential difference techniques. *Chest.* 2010;138(4):919–928.

Southern KW, Merelle MM, nkert-Roelse JE, et al. Newborn screening for cystic fibrosis. *Cochrane Database Syst Rev.* 2009;(1):CD001402.

51 Pulmonary Disease in Cystic Fibrosis

PETER MICHELSON, MD, MS, ALBERT FARO, MD, and THOMAS FERKOL, MD

Epidemiology

While present in all races and ethnicities, cystic fibrosis (CF) is the most common, life-shortening inherited disease of Caucasians. An autosomal recessive defect, occurring in approximately 1 in 3500 live births based on data from neonatal screening, the life expectancy of a child born with CF has gradually improved and now exceeds 40 years in the United States.[1] The predominant morbidity and mortality from CF continues to result from progressive pulmonary involvement. The CF lung is susceptible to infection; endobronchial infection induces an intense inflammatory response that leads to bronchiectasis and eventually respiratory failure, thus shortening the life of the patient. In this chapter, we will build on earlier sections and relate the pulmonary manifestations and complications of CF lung disease to its pathophysiology, and describe current and emerging therapies to address this progressive lung disease.

Etiology and Pathogenesis

CF is caused by defects in the CF transmembrane conductance regulator (CFTR), a cyclic adenosine monophosphate (cAMP)-regulated chloride channel expressed on the surface of airway epithelial cells and the serous cells of the submucosal glands (discussed in more detail in Chapter 49).[2] CFTR is functionally linked to other apical chloride channels, such as the calcium-dependent chloride channels (ClCa), and the epithelial sodium channel (ENaC), which reabsorbs sodium in the airways (Fig. 51.1). Aberrant expression or function of CFTR in the airway leads not only to reduced chloride conductance but also upregulation of ENaC activity. Failure of chloride secretion and sodium hyperabsorption result in dehydration of the airway surface. The reduced airway surface liquid and desiccated secretions obstruct the airways and reduce mucociliary clearance, permitting bacterial infection to become established and allowing the inflammatory response to be amplified.[3–5] The mucus secreted by submucosal glands in the CF airway is also abnormal, possibly related to altered CFTR anion transport, and hinders bacterial clearance.[6] Gaps in innate airway defenses contribute to bacterial persistence and chronic infection in the CF airway. Altered bicarbonate secretion in the CF airway impairs the activity of airway epithelial antimicrobial proteins and thus interferes with innate airway defenses resulting in chronic infection (Fig. 51.2).[6–8]

Respiratory infections are not a consequence of altered or abnormal pulmonary development. The lungs of neonates with CF appear histologically normal with the exception of plugging and distension of submucosal gland ducts. Bacterial cultures of respiratory secretions from infants often fail to yield a specific pathogen. Early in life, the airways are not chronically infected, although various bacteria may be found intermittently. As intrabronchial mucus stasis evolves, the respiratory tract becomes persistently infected with common patterns of bacterial species (Fig. 51.3). Bacterial infection is highly localized to the airway.[9–12]

Initially, *Staphylococcus aureus* and *Haemophilus influenzae* are isolated from patients with CF. *S. aureus* is often found in the respiratory tract of infants and young children with CF and the prevalence of methicillin-resistant *S. aureus* strains has greatly increased.[13] There is mounting evidence that methicillin-resistant *S. aureus* contributes to pulmonary deterioration and poorer survival.[14,15] The significance of *H. influenzae* in the progression of CF lung disease is uncertain, although it is a recognized and often treated pathogen in other forms of bronchiectasis.[9,16]

Pseudomonas aeruginosa emerges as the predominant organism over time but the percentage of children with chronic lung infection with *P. aeruginosa* has declined, with less than 50% of patients transitioning to adult care centers testing positive for *P. aeruginosa*.[1] Early *P. aeruginosa* isolates have planktonic, motile, nonmucoid phenotypes. Most patients eventually become chronically infected with mucoid *P. aeruginosa* that survives in the lung as biofilms, and these anaerobic, sessile communities of bacteria contribute to antibacterial resistance in the CF airway.[9,17,18] Approximately 70% of CF adults in the United States are chronically infected with mucoid *P. aeruginosa*[1] and the isolation of mucoid strains from the lungs of a patient is characteristic but not pathognomonic for CF.[19] Isolation of mucoid strains of *P. aeruginosa* from the lungs of a patient is associated with a poorer prognosis. Encouragingly, studies have reported that persistent infection with *P. aeruginosa* can be delayed or avoided with antibiotic treatment, which may lead to slower decline in pulmonary function.[20–22]

Antibiotic-resistant strains of *P. aeruginosa* are found increasingly in CF respiratory secretions. Other resistant, gram-negative bacteria, *Stenotrophomonas maltophilia* and *Achromobacter xylosoxidans*, are opportunistic organisms that may appear later in life; recent cohort data suggest some impact on disease progression with *Stenotrophomonas*, but further analysis is warranted.[23–25] Alternatively, *Burkholderia cepacia* complex can have profound effects on the clinical course of the disease and be associated with rapidly progressive necrotizing pneumonia and greater mortality.[26,27] The prevalence of *B. cepacia* complex varies markedly between care centers with a nationwide prevalence of about 2%.[1] Most *B. cepacia* complex infections are caused by genomovar II *(B. multivorans)* and genomovar III *(B. cenocepacia)*. These

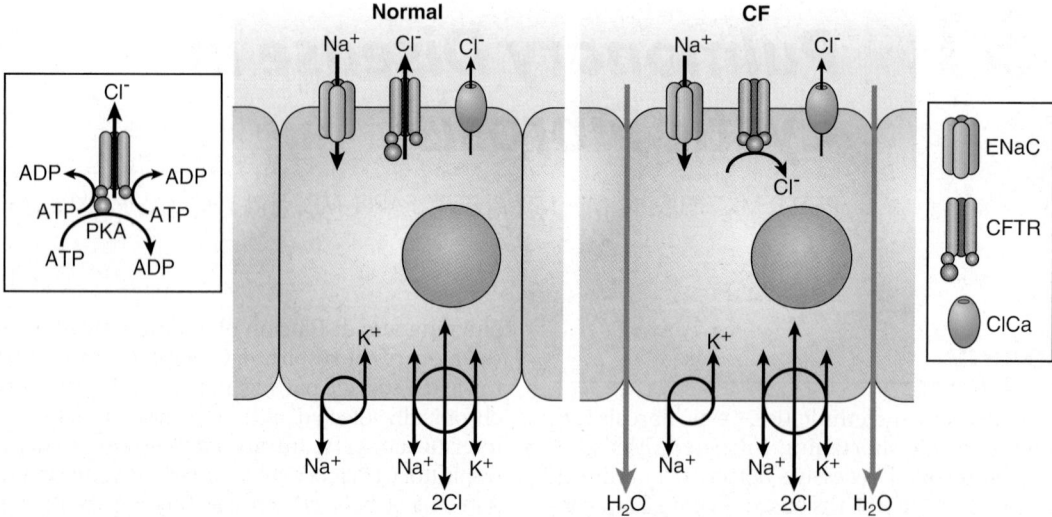

Fig. 51.1 Schematic diagram depicting cystic fibrosis *(CF)* epithelial channel defects, characterized by impaired chloride secretion, massive sodium absorption, and movement of water through the epithelium, leading to a dehydrated airway surface. *ADP,* Adenosine diphosphate; *ATP,* adenosine triphosphate; *CFTR,* cystic fibrosis transmembrane conductance regulator; *ClCa,* alternative chloride channel; *ENaC,* epithelium sodium channel; *PKA,* protein kinase A.

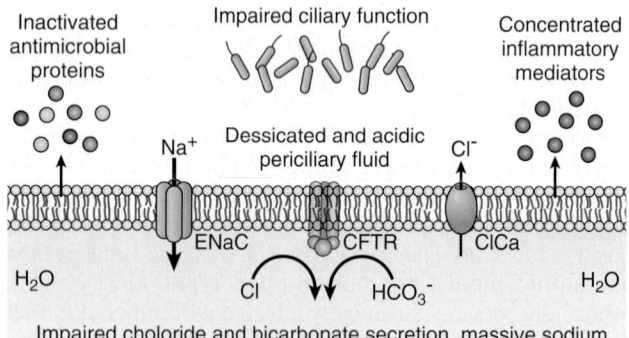

Impaired choloride and bicarbonate secretion, massive sodium absorption, and dehydration of the apical surface fluid that leads to reduced periciliary fluid volume and pH

Fig. 51.2 Schematic diagram showing cystic fibrosis pathophysiology in the airway epithelium, characterized reduced periciliary fluid volume and pH, which interferes with mucociliary clearance and innate defenses, resulting in chronic infection. The decreased periciliary fluid volume also concentrates inflammatory mediators at the immediate epithelial surface. *CFTR,* Cystic fibrosis transmembrane conductance regulator; *ClCa,* alternative chloride channel; *ENaC,* epithelium sodium channel. (Modified from Pittman JE, Ferkol TW. The evolution of cystic fibrosis care. *Chest.* 2015;148:533-542.).

organisms are transmissible, and infection control policies are critical to limiting exposure and spread. Epidemic infections have been linked to *B. cenocepacia,* but other genomovars have been associated with severe disease.[28,29] To prevent bacterial transmission between CF patients, infection control guidelines have been developed and applied to patients in both clinical settings and during social activities.[30]

Invasive fungal infections are rare. Nontuberculous mycobacteria, typically *M. avium-intracellulare* complex or *M. abscessus,* can infect the CF lung. About 13% of patients in the United States harbor nontuberculous mycobacteria in their lungs.[31] Therefore CF patients should be screened at least annually for mycobacterial colonization.

In patients with respiratory symptoms refractory to antibiotic therapy, viral infections should be considered. Indeed, there is evidence indicating that viruses play a significant role in the pathogenesis of pulmonary exacerbations and are associated with progressive clinical deterioration.[32] Respiratory viruses have the potential for injuring or altering the airway and can induce secretion of inflammatory mediators from respiratory epithelium. Moreover, viral infections result in a damaged epithelial barrier, leading to acquired ciliary dyskinesis, disruption of cell-cell connections, and cell death.[33] A breach in the airway epithelium potentially allows pathogens to reach the basolateral surface, provoking a greater inflammatory response.[34] Viral infections can affect airway surface fluid levels in CF epithelial cell cultures, which could further impair mucociliary clearance.[35] In particular, influenza can complicate CF disease, but immunization and chemoprophylaxis have lessened its clinical impact.

Although pulmonary infection contributes to the morbidity of patients with CF, an intense host inflammatory response hastens the progressive, suppurative pulmonary disease. Inflammation in the CF lung is primarily contained in the airway lumen, while the alveolar space is relatively spared (Fig. 51.4). The airway is filled with mucopurulent secretions. Large numbers of neutrophils are found in the airway, even in children with mild disease.[36,37] Bronchoalveolar lavage (BAL) fluid from CF patients has remarkably high concentrations of proinflammatory mediators.[38,39] Infection and local mediators stimulate epithelial cell secretion of IL-8, a potent neutrophil chemoattractant and activator that perpetuates airway inflammation. Complement-derived chemoattractants and leukotriene B_4 also contribute to neutrophil influx.[40,41] Both IL-1β and TNF-α are macrophage-derived cytokines that contribute to the local inflammatory response in the CF airway by mediating neutrophil chemoattraction and degranulation. IL-17 pathways have also been identified to contribute to the proinflammatory gene expression in the

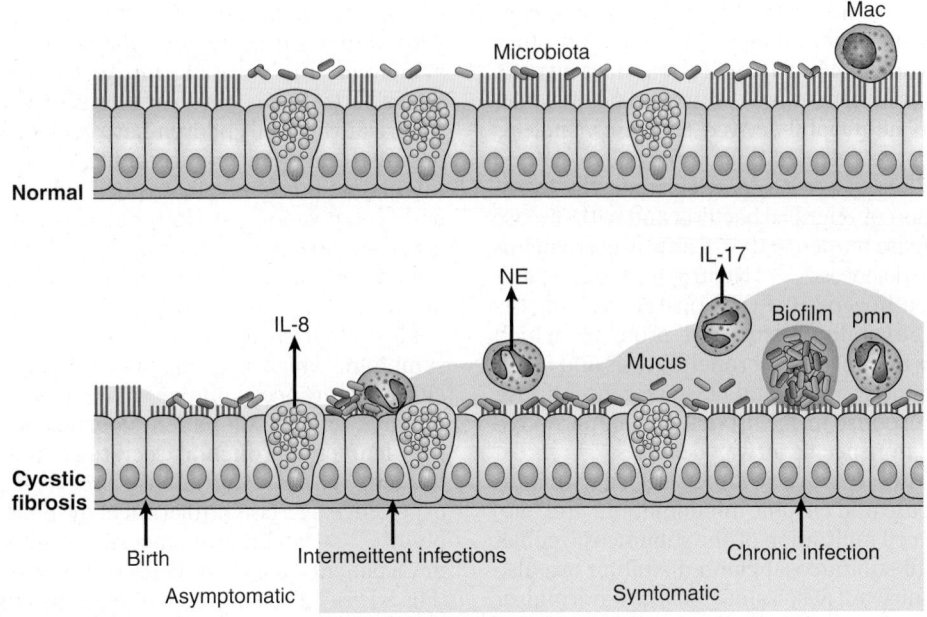

Fig. 51.3 Schematic diagram showing for the progression of disruption of mucociliary clearance leading to intermittent, then chronic infection and inflammation in the lungs of patients with cystic fibrosis. *IL*, Interleukin. (Modified from Pittman JE, Cutting G, Davis SD, Ferkol T, Boucher R. Cystic fibrosis: NHLBI Workshop on the Primary Prevention of Chronic Lung Diseases. *Ann Am Thorac Soc.* 2014;11(suppl 3):S161-S168.)

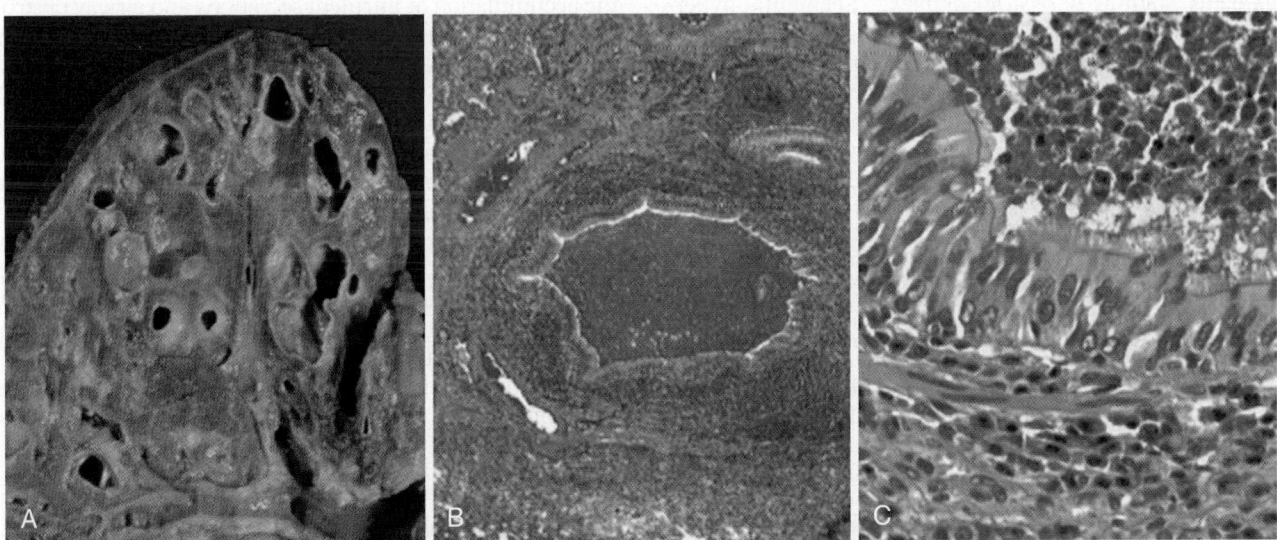

Fig. 51.4 Pathology of cystic fibrosis lung disease. (A) Photograph of lung explant from an adolescent cystic fibrosis (CF) patient showing bronchiectatic changes and mucus plugging, primarily involving the upper lobe (image generously provided by Carlos Milla, MD, Stanford University). (B and C) Photomicrographs of a section of CF lung explant (40× and 400×, magnification), demonstrating intense endobronchial and peribronchial inflammation with plugging of airways by exudate, degenerating neutrophils, bacteria, and mucus.

airway and are especially involved in established CF lung disease.[42,43]

Inflammation in the CF lung is primarily driven by local stimuli, mediators, and chemoattractants and is not a local effect of a systemic inflammatory reaction. Systemic indicators of inflammation are often normal or only modestly increased, even during acute illnesses. Several lines of evidence suggest that airway inflammation in CF may be excessive to the threat posed by bacteria, possibly mediated through dysregulation of the transcription factor nuclear factor kappa-light-chain-enhancer of activated B cells (NF-κB) or

other signal transduction molecules.[44–49] Although not a universal finding, infants and children with CF have high levels of proinflammatory cytokines and neutrophils in BAL fluid, even in the absence of detectable infection.[10,11] It is possible that inflammation may occur independent of infection or that a relatively minor infection may induce a robust inflammatory reaction in the CF lung that does not subside. However, not all experimental models and clinical studies have demonstrated an exaggerated inflammatory response in the CF airway,[50–52] and this phenomenon may be related to reduced apical surface fluid volume.[53]

The inflammatory response in the CF airways is characterized by a massive influx of neutrophils across the respiratory epithelium, even in individuals with mild pulmonary involvement. The phagocytic system affords protection against bacterial invasion, and neutrophil-derived proteases, such as neutrophil elastase, are released during phagocytosis and neutrophil death. These proteases participate in the intralysosomal degradation of engulfed bacteria and with disease progression the protease burden in the CF airway overwhelms existing antiprotease defenses.[37,54,55] Neutrophil elastase plays several roles in the pathogenesis of CF lung disease. It digests diverse substrates, including structural proteins, which weakens the airway and results in bronchiectasis and bronchomalacia. Uninhibited neutrophil elastase can enhance the inflammatory response in the bronchi[56] and, paradoxically, interfere with nonspecific airway defenses.[57,58]

As disease progresses, the airway lumen is filled with neutrophil exudates, acute and chronic inflammation, and bacteria. Mononuclear cell infiltration of the submucosa, goblet cell hyperplasia, and submucosal gland dilatation are also features of the CF airway. Respiratory cilia are normal or have nonspecific changes secondary to epithelial injury. Bronchiectasis is the predominant pathological feature, more severe in the upper lobes. Despite high bacterial concentrations in the CF lung, bacteremia and sepsis are rare. Tissue invasion is uncommon, and usually associated with particular organisms, such as *B. cepacia* complex.[29] Segmental hyperinflation or atelectasis results from airway obstruction. Lung overinflation, postinflammatory blebs, and bronchiectatic cystic lesions increase susceptibility to pneumothorax. Over time, bronchial arteries become hypertrophied and can cause pulmonary hemorrhage. Chronic alveolar hypoxia and inflammatory changes contribute to pulmonary hypertension and cor pulmonale.[59]

Clinical Features

SYMPTOMS AND PHYSICAL FINDINGS

The onset and progression of clinical manifestations of CF lung disease is highly variable and detecting the presence of disease in infants and children can be challenging. Although it is unusual for neonates to manifest respiratory symptoms, the work of the Australian Respiratory Early Surveillance Team for Cystic Fibrosis (AREST CF) has shown that relatively well children have evidence of CF lung disease during the first few months of life.[60,61] Viral illnesses in older infants can precipitate tachypnea, wheezing, and cough, but early colonization with lower airway pathogens, specifically *S. aureus* and *P. aeruginosa*, may be associated with pulmonary inflammation, early-onset bronchiectasis, and an associated decline in lung function.[62]

Most children will present with cough as their primary symptom, which becomes increasingly productive. Mucociliary clearance is impaired throughout the conducting airways, and the CF patient depends on cough to mobilize purulent endobronchial secretions and reduce bacterial burden. As the lung disease progresses, CF patients can experience exercise intolerance, dyspnea, and shortness of breath.[63] Typically, bronchiectasis begins in the upper lobes in CF patients and then progresses to involve the whole lung (Fig. 51.5).[64] The treatment of bronchiectasis is the treatment for the CF lung disease. Lobar resection is seldom indicated but may be considered in instances of severe hemoptysis or bronchiectasis that are not responsive to conservative management.[65,66]

Atelectasis often coexists with bronchiectasis because of the accumulation of purulent secretions and airway obstruction. Atelectasis also generates negative intrapleural pressure and dilates the associated bronchus that has been already weakened by the lytic enzymes released from neutrophils in the purulent material in the airway. Typically, treatment for atelectasis involves airway clearance techniques, inhaled recombinant DNAse (dornase alfa), or other mucolytic agents, plus antimicrobials.

Altered balance between airway pathogens and local host defenses leads to acute changes in respiratory signs and symptoms; this phenomenon is termed a *pulmonary exacerbation*.[67] Clinically, a pulmonary exacerbation is manifested as increased respiratory symptoms such as cough, dyspnea, and sputum production, often accompanied by systemic symptoms such as fatigue, anorexia, and weight loss.

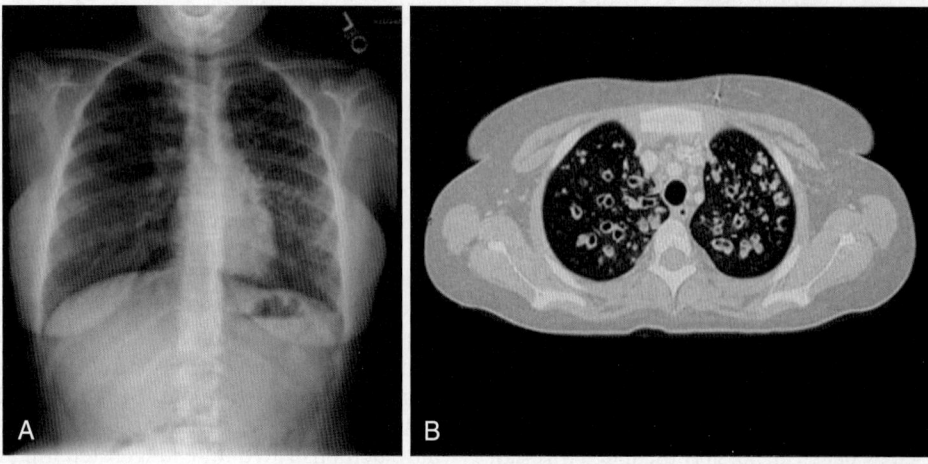

Fig. 51.5 Chest imaging of a cystic fibrosis patient. Standard posteroanterior radiograph (A) and high-resolution computerized tomography (B) of the chest show lung overinflation, bronchiectasis, and airway wall thickening.

Pulmonary function values usually decrease during exacerbations, and a therapeutic goal is to restore the best baseline of pulmonary function, regardless of the patient's symptoms. Exacerbations are treated with aggressive airway clearance techniques and antibiotic therapy based on bacterial isolates from sputum or oropharyngeal cultures.[67,68]

CF patients have chronic upper respiratory tract involvement, clinically manifested as nasal congestion and rhinorrhea. Pansinusitis is almost universally present in affected individuals. If upper airway symptoms worsen, systemic antibiotic therapy may be indicated. The percentage of CF patients who have features consistent with clinical sinusitis varies widely.[69,70] Bacteria isolated from the paranasal sinuses parallel those found in the lower respiratory tract, although distinct strains may colonize different anatomic sites in the CF airway.[71-73] Occurring in 7%–56% of CF patients, nasal polyposis is a common complication leading to nasal obstruction and congestion, which can require surgical intervention.[74] Surgical management usually results in symptomatic improvement, but sinusitis and polyps often recur.[75]

Digital clubbing is a sign of long-standing pulmonary involvement and eventually develops in virtually all CF patients. Hypertrophic pulmonary osteoarthropathy, a syndrome characterized with clubbing, long bone periostitis, and synovitis that usually flares during acute pulmonary exacerbations, has been described infrequently in CF patients and is usually associated with more advanced lung disease.[76]

As airway disease progresses, there is an increased likelihood of respiratory complications, including hemoptysis and pneumothorax. Pneumothorax is a late and worrisome complication of CF lung disease resulting from severe obstructive airways disease and/or the rupture of overexpanded apical blebs. Approximately 3% of CF patients will experience pneumothorax during their lifetime, and the average annual incidence of pneumothorax is 0.6%.[77] Pneumothoraces are usually associated with more severe disease (75% occur in patients with a forced expiratory volume in one second [FEV_1] of less than 40%)[78,79] and can be associated with fatalities. Although small pneumothoraces can be treated conservatively, evacuation of intrapleural air is often necessary to reexpand the lung. With recurrence rates ranging 50%–90%,[80] chemical or mechanical pleurodesis may be indicated, depending on the clinical scenario; even with pleurodesis, the risk for recurrent pneumothorax remains high.[79] Whereas pleurodesis was previously considered an absolute contraindication for lung transplant referral, that is no longer universally applied.[81]

Hemoptysis is common in older CF patients, particularly during pulmonary exacerbations, and is usually treated with antibiotics and, depending on the volume, withholding airway clearance. As CF lung disease progresses, bronchial arteries or collateral vessels enlarge and may rupture into an inflamed airway, producing massive hemoptysis, defined as more than 240 mL in 24 hours. This is a medical emergency, and roughly 4% of all patients with CF will suffer massive hemoptysis in their life.[77] These episodes can be fatal. Although many episodes spontaneously remit, hemoptysis can be worsened by coagulopathy secondary to hypovitaminosis K or underlying CF liver disease. Although patients can be stabilized with intravenous vasopressin, selective bronchial artery embolization is the definitive treatment.[82] Recurrent hemoptysis does occur, and repeated embolization may be indicated.

Airway hyperreactivity is often diagnosed in patients with CF, as evidenced by routine treatment with inhaled albuterol and corticosteroids. Roughly half of CF children and adults have a bronchodilator response, even if they do not have asthmalike symptoms, and the degree of airway hyperresponsiveness may change over time.[83,84] In different studies, airway hyperresponsiveness to exercise, histamine, or methacholine were found in 22%–54% of CF children.[85,86]

The defect in airway clearance associated with CF may also allow for endobronchial fungal growth and the development of allergic bronchopulmonary aspergillosis (ABPA).[87,88] ABPA is an inflammatory complication, clinically manifested by wheezing and cough refractory to standard therapies. Bronchiectasis with mucus impaction and atelectasis should also prompt consideration of ABPA.[89,90] ABPA is an intense immunologic response to surface colonization with the fungus *Aspergillus fumigatus*, which is characterized by (1) clinical deterioration that is not explained by other etiologies, (2) elevated serum quantitative immunoglobulin (Ig) E concentrations (>500 IU/mL), (3) positive skin prick test to *Aspergillus fumigatus* or elevated *in vitro Aspergillus*-specific IgE levels, and (4) *Aspergillus*-specific IgG levels or precipitins. Fulfilling these diagnostic criteria complicates the diagnosis and results in varying prevalence rates. Features that should raise concerns for the diagnosis include high-resolution computed tomography (HRCT) findings of mucus impaction, central bronchiectasis, tree-in-bud opacities, and centrilobular nodules.[88,91] Serum quantitative IgE concentrations should be measured annually to monitor for this complication. Once the diagnosis is made, patients are treated with extended courses of high-dose corticosteroids. Antifungal therapy is a therapeutic option to reduce the antigen burden in the lung, but few studies have shown that this strategy reduces the duration of corticosteroid treatment or improves outcome.[92]

Cor pulmonale is a complication of hypoxemia that is most commonly seen in older patients with advanced disease. Aggressive treatment of the underlying lung disease is indicated in early pulmonary hypertension, combined with oxygen supplementation. With disease progression and volume overload, diuretics are indicated to treat the right-sided heart failure.[93] With more advanced disease, the presence of pulmonary hypertension significantly reduces life expectancy.[94]

IMAGING AND LABORATORY STUDIES

The United States Cystic Fibrosis Foundation (CFF) has established Clinical Practice Guidelines that outline standards for routine monitoring and intervention to slow progression of lung disease. Evaluations include regular radiologic examinations, pulmonary function testing, and microbiologic cultures of airway secretions. Clinical evaluations are also essential and include monitoring for weight loss, anorexia, exercise tolerance, and school attendance, which are indirect measures of pulmonary morbidity. Indeed, the child's nutritional health is relevant to pulmonary outcomes. Younger children who have maintained their body weight had better pulmonary function at age 6 years, showing the relationship between nutrition and lung disease.[95]

MONITORING LUNG DISEASE

Chest imaging studies are useful tools to assess disease progression. Standard chest radiographs are often normal early in life, but as lung disease evolves, hyperinflation, peribronchial thickening, mucus plugging, and atelectasis develop. The progressive bronchiectasis, characteristic of CF lung disease, is usually a later finding on plain chest films. HRCT of the chest is more sensitive and provides greater anatomic detail, showing abnormalities well before detection on plain radiographs or changes in pulmonary function. HRCT can be performed on infants and small children, and it may reveal unsuspected airway wall thickening, segmental overinflation, and early bronchiectasis.[61,96-98] Although scoring systems to measure the extent and progression of CF lung disease have been developed, there are still no consensus guidelines regarding the use of computerized tomography, and the long-term consequences of radiation exposure remain concerns.[99-101]

Pulmonary function testing is routinely used to assess lung disease in children and adolescents with CF. Spirometric measurements permit assessment of progression of airway disease and are routinely used to diagnose pulmonary exacerbations and response to antibiotic therapy. Most CF children are able to perform reproducible spirometric maneuvers by age 6 years. The FEV_1, or more accurately, the rate of FEV_1 decline, is a useful index of disease severity. Deteriorating FEV_1 is a key marker for disease progression.[102-104] Pulmonary function decline varies greatly between patients, but in this decade, the average annual reduction in FEV_1 is approximately 2% per year in the United States. Although first described more than 25 years ago, CF patients with a baseline FEV_1 30% of predicted for age, still have a 2-year mortality rate of 50%.[102] Blood gas measurements are remarkably normal until late in the course of disease, but may reveal gas exchange abnormalities related to worsening ventilation-perfusion inequalities in patients with more advanced lung disease or clinical deterioration. Finally, infant pulmonary function testing can be a useful tool to assess infants and young children, but its value is limited by its ability to predict later disease severity. Recent testing in preschool children, including the multiple breath washout test or lung clearance index (LCI), has promise as an objective outcome measure in CF.[105]

Since progression of CF lung disease is inextricably linked to airway infection, regular comprehensive microbiological assessments of specimens from the lower respiratory tract, for example, sputum, are important.[9] Younger patients may not be able to expectorate, and in those cases, respiratory secretions can be collected using posttussive oropharyngeal swabs or BAL. Investigations have shown that negative oropharyngeal cultures may exclude lower airway infections, but a positive culture is not reliable to make the diagnosis of *P. aeruginosa* endobronchitis.[106] It is essential that respiratory cultures are processed and performed in laboratories with expertise in the handling of CF specimens and that recognize the difficulties in speciation of infecting pathogens. The CFF has established guidelines for handling and processing of respiratory tract specimens and supports reference laboratories for confirmatory identification of certain organisms such as *B. cepacia* complex.

Hypertonic saline has been used to induce sputum for lower airway sampling for both microbiological and inflammatory markers in older pediatric patients.[107] Cytokines, chemokines, oxidation species, and neutrophil products are elevated in the CF lung and may also be increased in the sputum and BAL fluid during exacerbations. However, such measures can have significant interpatient and intrapatient variability, even in those with seemingly stable lung disease. It is unclear whether these markers reflect disease progression, although the presence of detectable neutrophil elastase in lavage fluid early in life predicts development of bronchiectasis.[108] Inflammatory markers in the blood, such as peripheral leukocyte counts and C-reactive protein levels, have not been useful in the assessment of lung disease.

Management and Treatment

Treatment for CF lung disease is evolving, incorporating the newer therapies developed over the last two decades.[63,109] Current management of CF incorporates antibiotics, inhaled mucolytics, vigorous airway clearance, nutritional support, antiinflammatory agents, and, increasingly, small molecule potentiators and correctors in an attempt to forestall progression (Fig. 51.6).[110-112] Indeed, early intervention and primary prevention of CF lung disease may be possible.[113]

AIRWAY CLEARANCE

Effective airway clearance is a critical component of CF therapy.[114] To maintain lung health, physical removal of airway secretions is needed to not only relieve airway obstruction but also to reduce infection and airway inflammation.[115] Numerous airway clearance therapies (ACT) have been utilized and remain one of the most fundamental therapies for individuals with CF.[116] Additionally, novel agents aimed at restoring airway surface liquid and changing mucus viscosity have provided new opportunities to clear mucus and sustain normal lung function.[117]

There are many passive and active methods of ACT used in CF care. Active ACT includes positive expiratory pressure, active-cycle-of-breathing technique, and autogenic drainage.[116,118] No specific ACT has been definitively shown to be superior in changing long-term clinical outcomes, although this may be attributable to the challenges of performing randomized controlled trials in this area and the resultant paucity of data. An individual's choice should be based on age, experience, apparent effectiveness, and adherence.[63,119]

As an adjunct to airway clearance techniques, one must consider the benefit offered by aerobic exercise to mobilize secretions. In a systematic review of exercise for children with CF, both improved pulmonary function and aerobic fitness were demonstrated.[120] In addition to increased aerobic fitness, exercise programs may confer both short and long-term protection against pulmonary function decline.

Any discussion of ACT would be incomplete without discussing the advances in agents aimed at rehydrating secretions.[121] Reduced mucus viscosity and increased mucociliary clearance is achieved by improved airway surface hydration offered by these agents.[122,123] Hypertonic saline acts directly as an osmotic agent and may increase airway surface liquid volume. In older CF patients, hypertonic saline resulted in reduced frequency of pulmonary exacerbations and enhanced airway clearance.[124] A similar beneficial effect was not seen

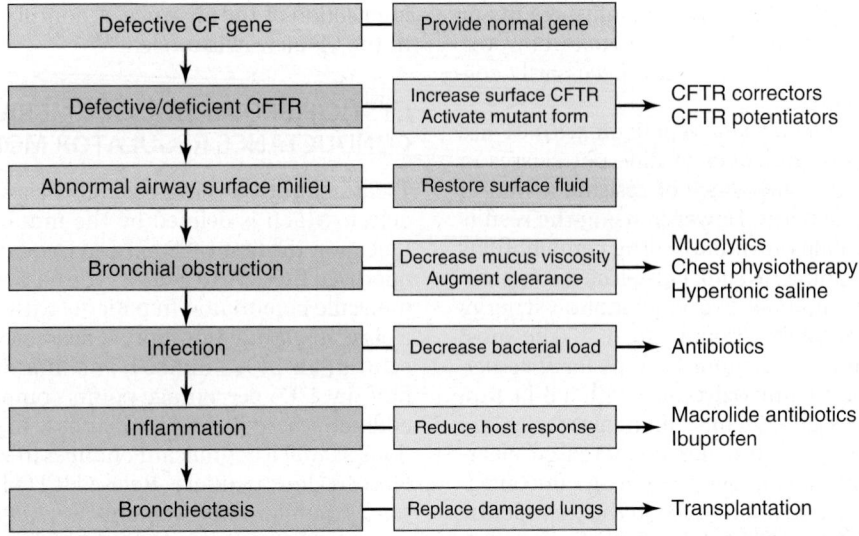

Fig. 51.6 Pathophysiological cascade leading from mutant cystic fibrosis transmembrane conductance regulator *(CFTR)* to bronchiectasis in the cystic fibrosis *(CF)* lung, interventions, and current treatment strategies.

in children between 4 and 60 months of age.[125] However, in a small, pilot, single-center sub-study of young children, the lung clearance index (LCI) was significantly decreased in the group that received hypertonic saline.[105] As a result, a larger, multicenter investigation is ongoing. Working as a surface-acting osmotic agent, inhaled mannitol has been shown to improve lung function over 52 weeks in a placebo-controlled trial.[126] In addition, trials are underway to study the effect of ENaC inhibitors to rehydrate the CF airway. Finally, inhaled bronchodilators are often used before ACT to maintain airway patency and facilitate mucus removal.[127]

INHALED MUCOLYTICS

Aerosolized mucolytics facilitate airway secretion clearance. The inspissated secretions in CF are predominately composed of pus with high concentrations of DNA from degraded neutrophils. Inhaled recombinant DNAse treats CF lung disease[128] by reducing sputum viscosity and increasing mucus clearance. Regular administration leads to improvement in lung function in some individuals with CF and is widely used. N-acetyl-L-cysteine is an alternative mucolytic agent, as it hydrolyzes disulfide bonds in mucins, and it has a long history of use in CF[129]; however, few data support its effectiveness other than as an airway irritant that induces cough.[130] Other mucolytics remain under investigation as potential therapeutic agents.[128]

ANTIBIOTIC THERAPY

During the past two decades, antibiotic use in CF care has evolved in both indications for usage and modes of delivery. Antibiotics continue to be utilized in the setting of acute infections and pulmonary exacerbations, but they are now also routinely used to eradicate organisms in otherwise asymptomatic young children or to reduce the bacterial burden in chronically infected patients.

CF patients acquire bacterial pathogens in an age-dependent manner that will chronically colonize their airways over time. Chronic infection with *P. aeruginosa* portends a poorer prognosis and, once established, is virtually impossible to eradicate.[9,18,19] However, studies treating initial acquisition of *P. aeruginosa* have shown that the organism can be eradicated with aggressive antibiotic therapy.[20,21,131] Although patients reacquired the organism later, the realization that early *P. aeruginosa* infection can be effectively eradicated led to a change in how antibiotics are prescribed in CF. No longer are antibiotics solely used to treat symptomatic disease; now they are used to treat early positive *P. aeruginosa* cultures, even in the absence of symptoms. Although effective in reducing reacquisition of *P. aeruginosa*, the impact of early eradication on later lung function remains obscure.[132] Potential confounders include the frequent use of antibiotics for pulmonary exacerbations and the need for longer follow-up of the two groups (those who achieved eradication and those who did not). In addition, there is insufficient evidence to support whether one antibiotic regimen is superior to another in achieving eradication.[22,133,134]

Although there is no consensus as to what defines a pulmonary exacerbation, most clinicians would agree that increase in cough, increase in sputum production, decline in lung function, shortness of breath, weight loss, and new adventitious sounds on auscultation warrant further investigation or therapy. Antibiotic treatment during an exacerbation, depending on the circumstance, may be delivered intravenously, orally, or by nebulization. The severity of the symptoms and the patient's available resources will assist the clinician in determining the appropriate course of therapy. Antibiotic therapy is typically guided by the findings of previous sputum or deep oropharyngeal culture and the susceptibility testing of the identified organisms. These cultures typically reflect the airway flora in older children and adolescents, but that may not be the case in infants.[106] BAL fluid cultures may be necessary to more accurately direct therapy. Antibiotics may be changed during the course of treatment based on more recent culture and susceptibility results or the patient's clinical response. It is important to note, however, that susceptibility testing in vitro does not necessarily correlate with clinical response.

Infections caused by *P. aeruginosa* in patients with CF are usually treated with two antibiotics of different classes in an attempt to prevent the emergence of resistance and in the hopes of achieving synergy. However, using the results from testing for susceptibility to multiple drug combinations does not confer any advantage to clinician-selected combinations of antibiotics, and multiple drug combination synergy testing is no longer routinely recommended.[135] The most common combination of intravenous therapy for *P. aeruginosa* involves the use of an aminoglycoside with a β-lactam antibiotic. Higher doses of systemic aminoglycosides are required in patients with CF because of increased clearance and altered pharmacokinetics[136] so drug concentrations must be monitored and maintained in the therapeutic window. For CF patients with multidrug-resistant *P. aeruginosa*, colistin may be used intravenously, but its use requires close monitoring for neurological symptoms and renal toxicity. Concurrent intravenous aminoglycoside therapy should be avoided with intravenous colistin. Oral fluoroquinolones are frequently used, but *P. aeruginosa* can develop resistance rapidly.[118] Inhaled antibiotics can be used in conjunction with either intravenous or oral therapy depending on antibiotic sensitivities.

Length of antibiotic therapy is determined by resolution of symptoms and return of lung function to its previous baseline or to a new plateau. Concern for emergence of resistant organisms limits extending courses beyond these endpoints. Complete eradication of organisms in the chronically infected patient is not achievable in most patients. Typically, return of lung function to baseline and resolution of symptoms can be achieved with 10–21 days of therapy with the majority of patients receiving 2 weeks of antibiotics, although little data is available that precisely defines adequate length of therapy.[131,137]

Suppressive or maintenance therapy with inhaled antibiotics is appropriate for the majority of patients who are chronically infected with *P. aeruginosa*. Inhaled tobramycin administered on an alternate month basis led to a significant improvement in lung function.[120] Additionally, emergence of tobramycin resistance is low when employing this strategy. Similar improvement in FEV$_1$ was described with inhaled aztreonam.[138] Aerosolized colistin has been used and this route minimizes the risk of systemic toxicity.[139]

Infection with nontuberculous mycobacteria is a growing concern.[140] Finding "atypical" mycobacteria presents a perplexing problem for the CF clinician trying to determine whether this organism is colonizing the airway or is acting as a pathogen; many of the presenting symptoms and radiographic findings can be explained by the more commonly isolated bacteria. In addition, therapy for nontuberculous mycobacteria involves prolonged treatment with multiple antibiotics, each of which has associated toxicities and variable tolerability. The recommended approach is to first treat the other organisms found on culture and closely monitor the patient's response to this therapy. When nontuberculous mycobacteria are cultured from a patient with CF, it is recommended that routine macrolide therapy be discontinued to prevent the emergence of resistance. The long-term implication of the presence of nontuberculous mycobacteria in the CF airway is unclear.[141]

CYSTIC FIBROSIS TRANSMEMBRANE CONDUCTANCE REGULATOR MODULATORS

Treatment of CF is increasingly based on the specific CFTR defect, which is defined by the mutation class (Fig. 51.7). Ivacaftor, the first US Food and Drug Administration (FDA)-approved therapy to address the basic defect in CF, is a small molecule potentiator. In patients with the G551D mutation, a class III gating mutation, it decreased sweat chloride concentrations by 48 mmol/L and improved percent predicted FEV$_1$ by 10.6 percentage points compared to placebo.[110] In addition, there was a 55% decrease in pulmonary exacerbations as well as significant changes in weight gain and Cystic Fibrosis Questionnaire–Revised (CFQ-R) respiratory domain scores. Similar improvements were documented in a subsequent trial of patients with most other class III mutations.[111] However, when studied in patients with the R117H mutation, a class IV mutation, the results were mixed. Improvement was documented in both sweat chloride concentrations and CFQ-R scores, while FEV$_1$ percent predicted improved significantly only in subjects older than 18 years of age, but not in children.[142]

For class II mutations, such as the common ΔF508, lumacaftor, a small molecule corrector designed to chaperone the defective CFTR protein, was combined with ivacaftor. This combination therapy reduced the number of pulmonary exacerbations and hospitalizations but demonstrated only a modest, albeit statistically significant, improvement in FEV$_1$.[112] This combination therapy appears to destabilize the corrected ΔF508 CFTR *in vitro*.[143] Similar decreases in plasma membrane density of ΔF508 CFTR with concomitant loss of chloride conductance were seen when ivacaftor was combined with VX-661, another corrector.[144]

Class I mutations are nonsense mutations resulting in the absence of CFTR production; several agents allow the ribosome to read through the premature stop codon but not through normal termination codons. A phase III study using a candidate drug (PTC124) did not demonstrate significant improvement in lung function or in the number of pulmonary exacerbations compared to placebo. However, post hoc subgroup analysis showed that in those subjects not using chronic inhaled tobramycin, there was an improvement in both of those measures.[145] A follow-up multinational, multicenter study in subjects not treated with inhaled tobramycin is underway.

ANTIINFLAMMATORY THERAPY

Several decades ago, CF caregivers noted that patients with CF who were hypogammaglobulinemic tended to have less severe lung disease than those with elevated serum IgG concentrations,[146] which supported the hypothesis that an overzealous immune response in patients with CF may be deleterious and provided rationale for early trials with antiinflammatory therapy. Two studies using systemic corticosteroids demonstrated an improvement in lung function over placebo.[147,148] However, excessive side effects were noted during the larger second study, including diabetes, cataracts, and growth failure, even during alternate-day dosing. Multiple studies

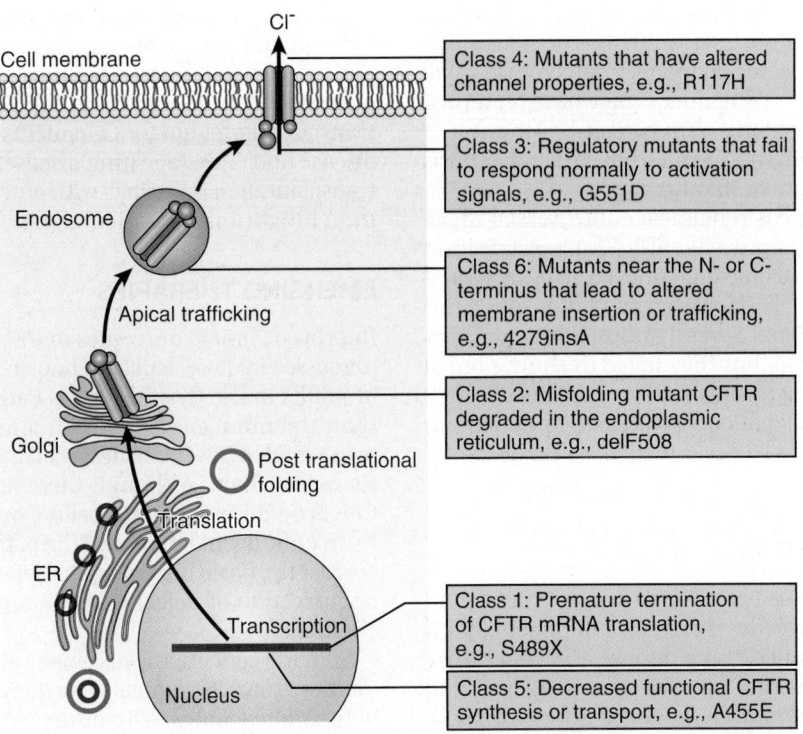

Fig. 51.7 Schematic diagram showing the classes of cystic fibrosis transmembrane conductance regulator (CFTR) mutations. *ER,* Endoplasmic reticulum. (Modified from Pittman JE, Ferkol TW. The evolution of cystic fibrosis care. *Chest.* 2015;148:533-542.)

have examined the potential use of inhaled corticosteroids in patients with CF, but they failed to show benefit.[149]

High-dose ibuprofen slows the annual rate of decline in lung function with the greatest effect seen in school-age children.[150] Even though the risks associated with its use, gastrointestinal hemorrhage and renal failure, are small, they are so dramatic that few CF centers have adopted this treatment.

Azithromycin is known to possess antiinflammatory effects, but its exact mechanism of action in CF is unclear. Studies in CF patients over 6 years of age infected with *P. aeruginosa* in whom azithromycin was administered thrice weekly demonstrated better lung function, weight gain, and fewer pulmonary exacerbations compared to placebo.[151] A recent study in patients not chronically infected with *P. aeruginosa* failed to demonstrate a difference in lung function, but they did show a 50% reduction in pulmonary exacerbations compared to placebo.[152] Adverse effects have been minimal, and this agent has gained widespread acceptance; however, data analysis from a recent study not designed for this specific question has raised concerns that azithromycin may antagonize the beneficial effects of inhaled tobramycin.[153] A study to test this hypothesis is underway.

Other novel approaches include addressing the depletion of antioxidants in the neutrophils and airway surface liquid in patients with CF. N-acetlycysteine, a glutathione prodrug, given orally in high doses did not decrease sputum elastase activity in patients with CF, but it did stabilize lung function compared to placebo.[154] A large multicenter study to better evaluate this agent is presently underway.

Antiinflammatory therapy in CF patients must be approached cautiously, since the immune system does contain

infection within the lung. A clinical trial with a leukotriene B4 antagonist was terminated early because the treatment group had more pulmonary exacerbations requiring hospitalizations.[155] Another trial examining the efficacy of nebulized interferon γ1B also increased hospital admissions.[156] Identifying a safe and effective antiinflammatory treatment will continue to be an active area of research in CF, and three antiinflammatory agents with different mechanisms of action are in phase 2 trials.

PREVENTATIVE CARE

Prevention of complications remains a priority for CF clinicians. The adoption of newborn screening in the United States has had a significant impact on care and has expanded traditional prophylaxis to include presymptomatic identification of nutritional and respiratory complications. While prevention of illness with immunization remains a significant focus, avoiding nutritional deficiencies and eradication of *P. aeruginosa* have become active areas of both research and quality improvement.

Routine immunization is an important component of CF care. Although systematic reviews have failed to demonstrate long-term benefit of immunization, the impact of influenza can be substantial, and yearly vaccination continues to be recommended.[157,158] Similarly, respiratory syncytial virus infection is associated with more severe respiratory complications, thus prevention using palivizumab should be considered in all children less than 2 years and it is recommended in high-risk patients.[159]

Nutritional interventions have resulted in improved outcomes. Better growth parameters at age 3 are associated with improved lung function at 6 years of age.[95] Whereas earlier recognition by newborn screening has demonstrated improved growth and improved pulmonary outcomes in small single-center cohorts,[160,161] confounders may have prevented the demonstration of any long-term benefit.[162] However, a reduced treatment burden may result from earlier diagnosis with an overall improvement in outcome.[163]

Antibacterial prophylaxis remains a controversial topic. A trial with cephalexin to prevent early *S. aureus* infection did not improve health outcomes and unexpectedly increased *P. aeruginosa* infection.[164,165] However, the latter effect has not been reported elsewhere. Several antipseudomonal vaccines have been developed, but they failed to show clinical effectiveness in protecting against *P. aeruginosa* infection.[166] Although its benefit to CF patients is unclear, antipneumococcal vaccination should be performed as a routine childhood immunization.[167]

LUNG TRANSPLANTATION

Although we have witnessed great improvements in median survival over the past decade, there are still patients with CF who progress to advanced lung disease and respiratory insufficiency at a very young age. For these children and adolescents, replacement of their damaged lungs with new lungs is their only hope to prolong survival and improve their quality of life. In 2014, a total of 205 adults and children with CF underwent bilateral lung transplantation in the United States. Unfortunately, the benefits of lung transplantation remain limited, with 5-year survival rates remaining at approximately 50%.[168,169] While there are many factors associated with success, if lung transplantation is to truly extend life, appropriate timing of the procedure is paramount. For more than 20 years, transplant referrals have been made when FEV_1 reaches 30% predicted for age; although several alternative models have been proposed to predict survival with CF, none are substantially better than others.[102,170]

Transplant physicians grasped the importance of these predictor models early in determining the appropriate time to list patients for transplantation. Before 2005, the lung allocation system in the United States was based on time spent waiting on the list. Since then, donor lungs have been allocated using the lung allocation score,[171] derived from variables that include forced vital capacity, body mass index, age, renal function, diabetes, supplemental oxygen, and assisted ventilation. Since implementation, CF patients 12 years and older have organ allocation based on their clinical status and not time on the wait list. Nevertheless, despite this more equitable system of organ distribution, the supply of donors is limited, and patients still die waiting for donor lungs.

Contraindications to lung transplantation for CF vary based on individual center experience or emergence of new information. Because of poor posttransplant outcomes, some centers will consider the presence of *B. cenocepacia* or *B. dolosa* as absolute contraindications. The need for invasive positive pressure ventilation before transplant is no longer considered an absolute contraindication to transplantation at many centers. Short-term outcomes regarding morbidity and mortality are worse in patients requiring ventilatory support, but long-term outcomes do not appear to be impacted.[172] Rather than maintaining a patient in respiratory failure on mechanical ventilation, many transplant centers now opt for ambulatory extracorporeal support to maximize the patient's rehabilitation potential and improve posttransplant outcomes. Multiorgan failure is a contraindication to lung transplantation, but for CF patients with both advanced liver disease and end-stage lung disease, simultaneous liver-lung transplantation is feasible, with outcomes as good if not better than lung transplantation alone.[173]

EMERGING THERAPIES

Improved clinical outcomes in CF patients are encouraging (discussed in more detail in Chapter 53). In 2015, the number of adults in the Cystic Fibrosis Patient Registry was greater than the number of children, a testament to the progress being made with the widespread institution of conventional therapies alone. Although there are many therapies in the CFF drug development pipeline, our focus in this section is to describe agents that have the potential to more proximally correct the basic ion transport defect, including modulation or correction of defective CFTR and activation of other ion channels.

Somatic gene therapy is a potential strategy for correcting CF. More than 20 clinical gene therapy trials were conducted in the United States, with disappointing results. Many obstacles to airway gene therapy need to be overcome, including airway obstruction that prevents vector delivery to the epithelial or submucosal gland cells, incitement of acute inflammatory and immune responses that interfere with repetitive dosing, and inefficiency of gene delivery to the airway epithelium. A consortium in UK recently examined the efficacy of a nonviral, liposomal gene transfer vector in CF adolescents and adults in a randomized, double-blind, placebo-controlled, phase 2b trial and found a modest difference in FEV_1, which may be related to a marked decline in pulmonary function measures in the placebo group.[174] In addition, the absence of evidence showing CFTR transgene delivery or expression raises questions about the success of the trial. Nevertheless, this research continues.

More recently, newer forms of gene editing, such as clustered regularly interspaced short palindromic repeats (CRISPR), which relies on Cas9 nucleases to recognize and cut genetic elements or insert desired sequences, has been widely used for genomic engineering in vitro,[175] but their application to the treatment of CF lung disease is still premature. These approaches have the same delivery limitations as gene therapy.

Prognosis

Survival of patients with CF has improved dramatically since it was first described over 70 years ago. While gastrointestinal signs and symptoms tend to predominate early, sinopulmonary manifestations increase with age. The progressive lung disease leads to considerable morbidity and respiratory failure and accounts for the vast majority of CF deaths.[109] In the United States, the predicted survival has steadily increased and now exceeds 40 years.[1,176] This improvement is related to advances in monitoring and better, more aggressive treatment strategies. Thus, routine surveillance studies are recommended in the care of children with CF, which include regular spirometry to monitor lung function, chest radiographs, and sputum or oropharyngeal cultures to assess lower respiratory tract flora.

Factors that negatively affect prognosis include malnutrition,[177] diabetes mellitus,[178] infection with *P. aeruginosa*,[179,180] *B. cepacia* complex,[26,181] and the frequency of pulmonary exacerbations.[179] There is a gender gap in CF, and males tend to do better than female counterparts.[182,183] Socioeconomic status can influence survival of CF patients, and environmental factors, such as exposure to tobacco smoke and airborne pollutants, have detrimental effects.[184,185] Conversely, patients with atypical or pancreatic-sufficient forms of the disease have slower decline in pulmonary function when compared to those with classical CF; their prognosis and long-term survival are better.[186]

As the benefits of CF newborn screening become more widely evident, we expect that the progression and extent of nutritional failure and lung disease can be slowed. Preliminary small-cohort studies support that early recognition and nutritional intervention results in not only more rapid growth recovery but also in associated respiratory benefit.[187–189]

Conclusions

Pulmonary disease in CF is the consequence of defective function of apical ion channels and impaired mucociliary clearance, which renders the airway susceptible to endobronchial bacterial infection and induces an intense inflammatory response that leads to bronchiectasis and ultimately respiratory failure. Children with CF born today have greater potential to live longer, primarily because of earlier diagnosis and multidisciplinary, center-based care, where children can benefit from treatments for downstream consequences of defective ion transport, such as inhaled mucolytics, antibiotics, antiinflammatory agents, and airway clearance techniques. More recently, newer therapeutics have emerged that target the basic defect and have shown promise in early clinical trials. If successful, these treatments are poised to profoundly change the course of CF lung disease.

References

Access the reference list online at ExpertConsult.com.

Suggested Reading

Ferkol T, Rosenfeld M, Milla CE. Cystic fibrosis pulmonary exacerbations. *J Pediatr*. 2006;148:259–264.

Flume PA, O'Sullivan BP, Robinson KA, et al. Cystic fibrosis pulmonary guidelines: chronic medications for maintenance of lung health. *Am J Respir Crit Care Med*. 2007;176:957–969.

Gibson RL, Burns JL, Ramsey BW. Pathophysiology and management of pulmonary infections in cystic fibrosis. *Am J Respir Crit Care Med*. 2003;168:918–951.

Knowles MR, Boucher RC. Mucus clearance as a primary innate defense mechanism for mammalian airways. *J Clin Invest*. 2002;109:571–577.

Pittman JE, Ferkol T. The evolution of cystic fibrosis care. *Chest*. 2015;148:533–542.

Stoltz DA, Meyerholz DK, Welsh MJ. Origins of cystic fibrosis lung disease. *N Engl J Med*. 2015;372:351–362.

52 Nonpulmonary Manifestations of Cystic Fibrosis

AMY MICHELLE GARCIA, MD, MS, and JILL DORSEY, MD, MS

Although lung disease continues to be the main cause of morbidity and mortality, gastrointestinal complications have become increasingly important in the care of individuals with cystic fibrosis (CF). Thus it behooves caregivers to become familiar with the effects of CF outside of the lungs. This chapter presents a summary of the current knowledge of the extrapulmonary manifestations of CF with focus on the gastrointestinal and endocrine systems.

Pancreatic Disease

PATHOBIOLOGY

The pancreas is composed of endocrine cells that secrete hormones, exocrine cells that make digestive enzymes, and duct cells that secrete bicarbonate and water. The exocrine pancreas consists of cells organized into acini and a duct system that leads to the small intestine. The pancreatic juice secreted from the duct cells is clear, colorless, and nearly isotonic. In both animals and humans, bicarbonate seems to drive fluid secretion by the pancreatic ducts.[1] Bicarbonate allows the highly concentrated proteins that are secreted by the pancreatic acinar cells to remain in a soluble state. Moreover, bicarbonate is important for neutralizing gastric acid to create the optimal pH for pancreatic enzymes, bile acids, and micelles. The adult pancreas normally secretes 1–2 L of a bicarbonate-rich fluid each day. The basis of the bicarbonate secretion relies on the exchange of luminal chloride for bicarbonate, but the exact mechanism is still not fully understood. The CF transmembrane conductance regulator (CFTR) protein is located in the apical membrane of the epithelial cells of the pancreatic ducts. The apical Cl^-/HCO_3^- exchanger is dependent on the expression of CFTR,[2] which functions as the apical Cl^- channel.[3] Most likely, the apical anion exchanger in the pancreatic duct cells is a member of the SLC26 family.[4] A physical association between SLC26A6 and CFTR has been suggested due to the presence of a PDZ domain at the C terminus of SLC26A6, which is identical to that of CFTR.[5] Furthermore, they both bind through the PDZ motif to scaffolding proteins. It is possible that SLC26A6 and CFTR interact through these scaffolding proteins, allowing CFTR to stimulate the apical anion exchange.[2] However, the classic proposal of a 1:1 exchange of Cl^-/HCO_3^- cannot explain the large sustained secretion of bicarbonate. Two of the members of the SLC26 family, SLC26A3 and SLC26A6, have been proposed to work in conjunction to achieve normal bicarbonate secretion. SLC26A3 secretes $Cl^-:HCO_3^-$ in a ratio of 2:1, whereas the ratio by SLC26A6 is 1:2. This information, combined with the location of SLC26A6 at the proximal ducts and SLC26A3 at the distal ducts, may explain the high bicarbonate concentration found in normal pancreatic juice.[6]

However, it does not appear that the combination of the two exchangers are able to reach the necessary concentration of luminal bicarbonate.[7] Alternatively, the activation of the WNK1-OSR1/SPAK (protein kinase with no lysine 1-oxidative stress response kinase 1/sterile20-related, proline-alanine rich kinase) pathway causes CFTR to become permeable to HCO_3^-, which allows for the generation of the necessary concentration of 140 mmol/L of HCO_3^- of normal pancreatic juice.[8]

Dysfunction of CFTR, as in CF, results in impaired electrolyte transport and thus a reduction in fluid secretion. Thus the pancreatic juice in individuals with CF is significantly more concentrated then controls.[9] These thickened secretions then lead to obstruction of the pancreatic ducts, as well as inflammation and injury (Fig. 52.1).

PANCREATIC INSUFFICIENCY

Pancreatic insufficiency (PI) occurs when the amount of digestive enzymes delivered to the intestine is inadequate for nutrient digestion. Steatorrhea, the presence of excess fat in the stool, then occurs. Infants with PI at diagnosis often have decreased weight gain, minimal fat stores, and reduced serum albumin and blood urea nitrogen (BUN) levels.[10] Children with PI may present with growth failure, weight loss, abdominal bloating, foul-smelling stools, edema, or diarrhea. Parents of children who are toilet-trained may report that the stools appear to be floating due to the high fat content of the stool, although stools may float due to increased air content, and this is seen in other conditions as well. It is possible that with mild PI, stools appear normal. Imaging of the pancreas will show atrophy with replacement by fatty tissue in individuals with PI.

CF is the most common cause of PI in childhood. Approximately two-thirds of children with CF are pancreatic insufficient at birth, and approximately 90% will develop PI by 1 year of age.[10] Individuals with two mutations from class I, II, or III CFTR mutations typically have severe pancreatic disease resulting in PI.[11] In patients with severe disease, the obstruction and destruction of exocrine function begins in utero. The damage to the pancreas that occurs in utero forms the basis for newborn screening for CF disease. Serum immunoreactive trypsinogen (IRT) is a precursor to trypsin that is elevated in the blood of infants with CF.[12] When pancreatic dysfunction is present, release of pancreatic enzymes is impaired, and IRT accumulates in the blood stream. Therefore most infants with CF have elevated blood levels of IRT. It has been shown that children who develop PI and those diagnosed with PI in early infancy have similar patterns of IRT levels.[13] One study found that IRT determinations alone were not sufficient to demonstrate differences between mild and severe disease in the first year of life, suggesting ongoing pancreatic damage, and thus elevated IRTs, in both groups.[14]

NORMAL ACINAR AND DUCTAL SECRETION

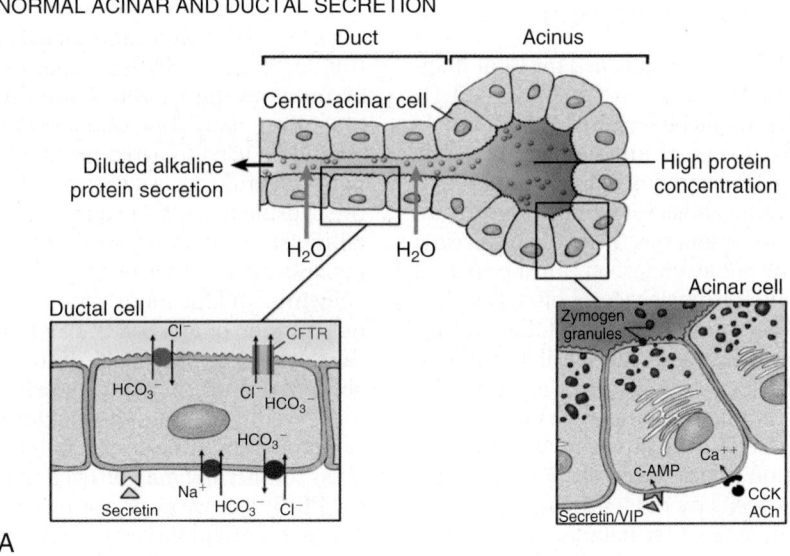

CYSTIC FIBROSIS

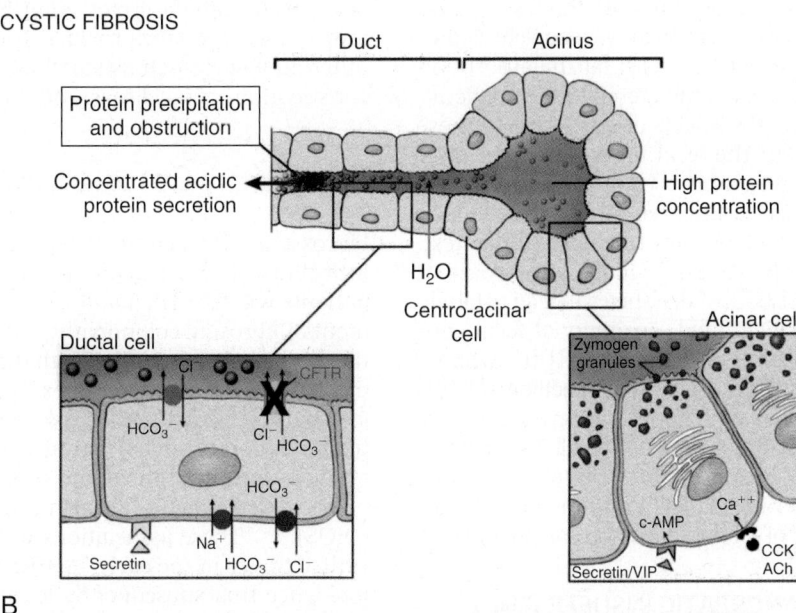

Under normal circumstances (A) Cl⁻ and HCO₃⁻ secretion provides a driving force for the movement of fluid into the lumen of the duct, which maintains the solubility of secreted proteins in a dilute, alkaline solution. In CF (B), impaired anion transport results in decreased secretion of more acidic fluid, which leads to precipitation of secreted proteins. Intraluminal obstruction of the ducts then causes progressive pancreatic damage and atrophy.

Fig. 52.1 Pathophysiology of pancreatic disease in cystic fibrosis.

PANCREATIC SUFFICIENCY

Approximately 10%–15% of individuals with CF produce sufficient amounts of pancreatic enzymes to prevent malabsorption of nutrients and are considered to be pancreatic sufficient (PS). These individuals tend to have at least one of the CFTR mutations that are associated with mild pancreatic disease (class IV or V).[15] However, if only one mild CFTR mutation is present, then this does not exclude the possibility of developing PI in the future.[16] On average, sweat chloride levels are lower in individuals with PS as compared with those with PI. Individuals with PS also tend to have less severe lung disease and better nutritional status than those who have PI. With milder disease, the diagnosis of CF tends to occur later in childhood or early adulthood. Twenty percent of individuals with CF who are PS will develop pancreatitis.[17] The diagnosis of pancreatitis may, in some cases, precede the diagnosis of CF.[18]

ASSESSMENT OF PANCREATIC FUNCTION

Every individual with CF should be screened for PI at diagnosis. In addition, individuals with at least one severe CFTR mutation (class I, II, or III) should be screened at least annually for PI. Evaluation of pancreatic function can be made by direct or indirect testing. Direct testing requires stimulation of the pancreas (with secretin, cholecystokinin, or both) and collection of pancreatic fluid for analysis. To obtain pancreatic fluid for direct testing, a tube or an endoscope must be placed in the small intestine, which is invasive and often requires sedation. In children who require long-term follow-up for their PI, repeated invasive testing is not feasible. Indirect tests are noninvasive and less costly, so they are typically preferred. However, with mild pancreatic exocrine dysfunction, indirect testing can be less sensitive and specific.[19] In contrast, direct stimulation of the pancreas with secretin has high sensitivity and specificity in identifying PI.[20]

The 72-hour quantitative fecal fat balance method has been used as an indirect test to diagnose PI. If fecal fat excretion is more than 15% of total fat intake in infants less than 6 months of age, and 7% in older infants, then malabsorption is present. Compliance remains an issue with this test because it requires a 3- to 5-day stool collection and a complete dietary history. In addition, most patients with fat malabsorption have diarrhea, which makes complete collection difficult, especially in infants with absorbable diapers. Due to these limitations, alternatives to the fecal fat balance test have been sought. The most commonly used of the indirect tests is fecal pancreatic elastase-1. Children do not have to stop pancreatic enzyme supplementation to complete this test. However, the presence of intestinal villous atrophy, as in celiac disease, or acute episodes of diarrhea can lead to falsely low values.[21,22] The specificity and sensitivity of fecal pancreatic elastase-1 in a pediatric CF cohort is 100% when a value of less than 100 µg/g is used.[23] The specificity of this test was lower in individuals with non-CF pancreatic disease (e.g., Shwachman-Diamond syndrome). Overall, the negative predictive value was 99%. An empiric trial of pancreatic enzyme replacement therapy (PERT) in an individual with a strong clinical history of PI could also be considered.

MANAGEMENT OF PANCREATIC INSUFFICIENCY

In CF, treatment for PI focuses on optimizing PERT to promote absorption of nutrients and fat-soluble vitamins. In 1991 the US Food and Drug Administration (FDA) mandated that all pancreatic enzymes be approved; prior to the enactment of FDA standards in 2010, PERT was not regulated. Currently, six approved products are available. Each product includes a combination of lipase, protease, and amylase. These enzymes are in the form of granules or microspheres with a pH-sensitive coating to allow release in the alkaline environment of the small intestine. Dosing for PERT is based on the lipase component. Because of this, it is not advisable to use an unregulated generic or nonproprietary preparation because the amount of lipase can potentially vary even in the same product. More importantly, enzyme dosage should not exceed 2500 lipase units/kg per meal or 4000 lipase units/g fat per day (10,000 lipase units/kg/day total) to avoid fibrosing colonopathy.[24] Fat-based dosing of PERT relies more on the number of fat grams per meal or snack than the person's

weight. This method may be more applicable for infants ingesting around the same amount every day and individuals with tube feedings or reliance on packaged foods. The dose should be no more than 2500 lipase units/kg per feeding, with a maximum daily dose of 10,000 lipase units/kg.[24] Caution should be used to avoid prolonged contact of the enzymes with the oral mucosa because this may cause ulceration. If the capsule needs to be opened, the microspheres should be administered with a food that can be swallowed whole (like applesauce, gelatins, or pureed bananas that do not require chewing) and the mouth should be inspected after to ensure no retention of any beads. PERT should be taken just prior to the start of a meal or snack. If the individual continues to have abnormal stools, bloating, or belly pain, despite PERT, dosing may be adjusted until the maximum daily dose is reached. If symptoms continue despite maximum dosing, then acid suppression therapy may be tried to help the enteric coating of the PERT dissolve by providing a more alkaline environment. The provider should keep in mind the significant potential side effects of these medications (tachyphylaxis with H2 receptor antagonists; increased susceptibility to pneumonia, increased susceptibility to *Clostridium difficile*, and possible impact on bone health with the proton pump inhibitors). If clinical symptoms persist, then the provider should investigate further for other etiologies such as small bowel bacterial overgrowth, constipation, celiac disease, or chronic giardiasis.

Fibrosing Colonopathy

Fibrosis and thickening of the colon wall in a circular and intramural fashion is another unique clinical problem of patients with CF. The pathophysiology behind this development of fibrosing colonopathy remains uncertain, although there is a noted correlation with the use of high PERT dosing, most especially if the dosing exceeds 50,000 lipase units per kilogram per day.[25] Other risk factors associated with this phenomenon include a young age (between 2 and 7 years), previous history of intestinal surgery, meconium ileus (MI), or prior occurrence of distal intestinal obstruction syndrome (DIOS).[25,26] These associations were brought to light in the United States in the early 1990s, as there was an increased incidence that subsequently led to a review of these cases and the CF patient registry.[25] The colonic wall thickening results in decreased motility and narrowing of the lumen that can sometimes lead to stricture. Clinical symptoms may vary though the most common include abdominal pain with concern for colonic obstruction that may or may not involve emesis. Other clinical signs may include constipation, diarrhea, hematochezia, anorexia, and failure to gain weight as expected. Abdominal ultrasound, barium enema, magnetic resonance scans, and endoscopies can all be used to help make this diagnosis.[26]

TREATMENT OF FIBROSING COLONOPATHY

Antiinflammatory treatments including prednisone pulses and antibiotics have been used with varying success.[26] In extreme cases the use of balloon dilation or surgical resection of the fibrosed portion of the colon may be necessary.[25,26] There is consensus on limiting doses of PERT to 2500 lipase units per meal or 10,000 lipase units per kg per day.[24,25]

Pancreatitis

Acute pancreatitis requires the presence of preserved pancreatic tissue. Thus pancreatitis tends to occur in 20% of PS individuals with CF and is rare in those with PI. It typically occurs in adolescence and young adulthood and may be the first manifestation of CF.[17,27] A two-hit model has been proposed to explain the development of pancreatitis in CF. CFTR dysfunction leading to ductal obstruction and inflammation makes up the first hit, whereas acinar damage from alcohol, drugs, or hypercalcemia leads to the second hit. It has been shown that there is decreased bicarbonate flow through pancreatic ducts in patients with CF and PS with preserved pancreatic mass.[28] Furthermore, a study demonstrated that during alcohol-induced pancreatitis, CFTR expression is decreased on pancreatic ductal epithelial cells.[29]

The diagnosis of acute pancreatitis can be made when two of the three following criteria are met: epigastric abdominal pain that may radiate to the back, an increase in amylase or lipase that is greater than 3 times the upper limit of normal, and typical findings on imaging. If possible, nutrition should be maintained during treatment and follow-up.

Hepatobiliary Disease

CFTR is found on the apical membrane of intrahepatic and extrahepatic bile ducts, as well as the gallbladder, but not on the hepatocytes.[30] How CFTR mutations lead to liver fibrosis is unclear. It has been proposed that the dysfunctional CFTR leads to thickened secretions and obstruction of intrahepatic bile ducts. This would allow for the accumulation of toxic bile acids that may activate hepatic stellate cells, via monocyte chemotaxis protein-1, which then produce increased periductular collagen.[31,32] This focal portal fibrosis is the pathognomonic histopathologic liver lesion in CF.

Cystic fibrosis liver disease (CFLD) encompasses a number of different liver disorders, from elevated liver enzymes to multilobular cirrhosis (advanced liver disease). Only approximately 5%–10% of individuals with CF will develop multilobular cirrhosis (Fig. 52.2).[33] Thus the vast majority has clinically insignificant hepatobiliary disease. In fact, 40%–50% of individuals with CF have intermittent elevations in their aspartate aminotransferase (AST), alanine aminotransferase (ALT), or gamma-glutamyl transferase (GGT) that can be up to 2.5 times the upper limit of the reference range but do not predict the presence or development of significant liver disease. Interestingly, these same blood tests may be normal in the setting of multilobular cirrhosis.[34]

CFLD occurs most commonly in individuals with class I, II, or III mutations on both alleles,[35] although there does not appear to be a strong correlation between genotype and phenotype. Perhaps additional genetic factors (modifier genes) and environmental factors play a role in the development of significant liver disease.[34] For example, an increased risk of cirrhosis was found in those carrying a single copy of the SERPINA1 Z allele (the PiZ heterozygote state for alpha-1 antitrypsin).[36] CF patients who are carriers of the Z allele have an increased population attributable risk of 7% for multilobular cirrhosis, but this only accounts for approximately 9% of CF patients with cirrhosis.

A history of MI was thought to be a risk factor for the development of CFLD. However, more recent studies have not confirmed this association.[37,38] Male gender and PI have also been thought to be associated with CFLD.[39]

CLINICAL PRESENTATION OF LIVER DISEASE

Liver disease in CF is often subclinical and the majority of individuals are asymptomatic until the development of advanced disease. Advanced CFLD typically develops around 10 years of age and is often slowly progressive.[40] CFLD accounts for 2.8% of overall mortality in the CF population.[41] Physicians should remain vigilant for signs of advanced liver disease such as splenomegaly or thrombocytopenia.

A thorough physical examination should be completed with every visit because the most common clinical finding in CFLD is hepatomegaly on routine physical examination. The liver may be felt 2–3 cm below the right costal margin or the xyphoid, with enlargement potentially limited to the right or left lobe. The examiner may note that the liver is firm and nodular. If the liver feels smooth, the hepatomegaly may be the result of fatty infiltration of the liver, which is felt to be a benign condition. However, given the recent studies of the progression of nonalcoholic steatohepatitis to cirrhosis, the implications of hepatic steatosis in CFLD may change.[42] It also should be noted that a cirrhotic liver tends to be small and therefore no hepatomegaly may be found on abdominal examination. Even without hepatomegaly, the physician could still be guided towards the diagnosis of significant liver disease by the presence of splenomegaly, resulting from portal hypertension, a late complication of cirrhosis.

Besides hepatosplenomegaly, other signs of liver disease are less common on physical examination. Spider nevi, palmar erythema, jaundice, edema, distension of abdominal wall veins, and ascites can be seen with chronic liver disease. These manifestations are found in more advanced disease with the exception of jaundice in early infancy. Cholestasis, or elevation in the conjugated bilirubin, tends to be the earliest manifestation of liver involvement in CF occurring in 2% of infants with CF. Cholestasis generally resolves within 3 months but occasionally can mimic biliary atresia.[43]

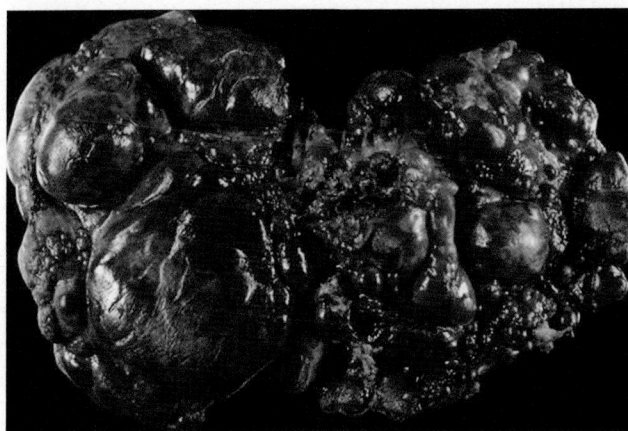

Fig. 52.2 Liver explant from an individual with cystic fibrosis demonstrating multilobular cirrhosis.

DIAGNOSIS OF LIVER DISEASE

Early diagnosis of CFLD remains problematic even with published guidelines for the management of liver and biliary tract disease in CF.[44] Unfortunately, there are no tests currently available to identify individuals with CF who are at high risk of developing liver cirrhosis. In general, the combination of physical examination findings, biochemical results, and imaging are used to make the diagnosis of CFLD.

Routine annual blood work may reveal an elevation in AST, ALT, or GGT. As mentioned earlier, intermittent elevations in these values are common and do not necessarily indicate significant liver disease. Normal values may even be found in the setting of multilobular biliary cirrhosis.[34] However, persistent elevation of AST, ALT, or GGT greater than three times the upper limit of normal is rare.[45] Elevation of AST and ALT, with normal GGT, may indicate hepatic steatosis. The possibility of hepatic steatosis should prompt further testing for deficiencies in essential fatty acid, carnitine, and choline, as well as assessment for malnutrition. However, hepatic steatosis can also be present in individuals with adequate nutritional status.[46] Elevation of alkaline phosphatase without an elevation in GGT can be found in growing children and does not indicate liver disease.[47,48]

The AST to platelet ratio index (APRI) has been studied in the setting of non-CF–related liver disease as a noninvasive marker of liver fibrosis and cirrhosis. More recently, investigators looked at APRI as a predictor of liver fibrosis in individuals with CF. They found that APRI correlated well with severe fibrosis but tended to overestimate earlier stages of fibrosis.[46]

In general, further evaluation should be considered if an individual's ALT or GGT remain elevated for 6 months or more.[45] At that time, it would be prudent to evaluate for other causes of liver disease such as alpha-1 antitrypsin deficiency, celiac disease, autoimmune disease, Wilson disease, chronic viral hepatitis, primary sclerosing cholangitis, drug toxicity, and toxins. Evaluation of liver synthetic function should also be checked with albumin, prothrombin time (PT), international normalized ratio (INR), and glucose. However, only approximately 10% of individuals with CF and cirrhosis will develop synthetic failure.[49]

Doppler ultrasound of the liver should be ordered when CFLD is suspected. This noninvasive modality provides information about the appearance of the liver without any radiation exposure, which is preferred in this CF population, which is often exposed to chest x-rays and computed tomography (CT) scans of the chest. A homogeneous pattern is typically associated with hepatic steatosis.[50] However, it is important to keep in mind that periportal steatosis and focal fibrosis have a similar appearance on ultrasound.[44] Individuals with heterogeneous parenchyma of the liver found on ultrasound are thought to be at increased risk for development of cirrhosis.[51] A pattern indicative of cirrhosis of the liver, including heterogeneous echogenicity and coarse echo texture of the liver parenchyma accompanied by nodularity of the liver contour, can also be found. Surprisingly, 3.3% of individuals with CF, not known to have cirrhosis, were found to have a cirrhotic pattern on ultrasound in a prospective, multicenter study of using ultrasound to predict hepatic fibrosis. The investigators found that an abnormal ultrasound liver pattern was associated with CF-related diabetes, whereas a normal

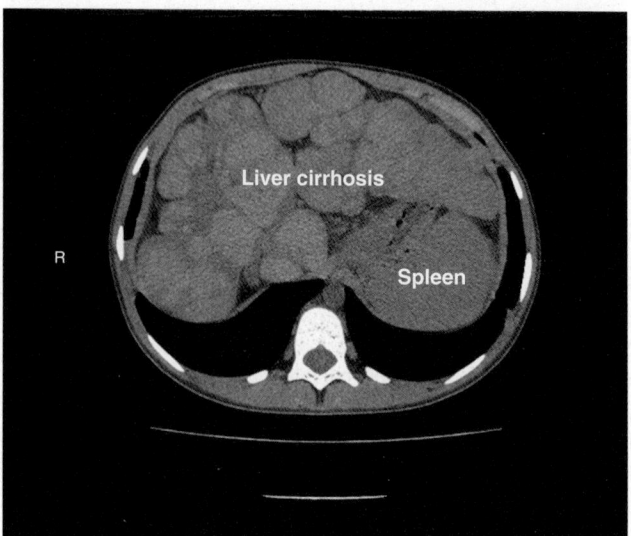

Fig. 52.3 Computed tomography scan of an individual with cystic fibrosis demonstrating cirrhosis of the liver.

ultrasound was associated with early *Pseudomonas aeruginosa* infection.[52] However, a normal liver ultrasound does not preclude significant liver fibrosis.[53]

The liver Doppler ultrasound also provides information about CFLD by documenting the flow patterns of the vasculature, as well as the presence of dilatation. Hepatofugal flow (away from the liver) in the portal vein, as well as recanalization of the umbilical vein, suggests advanced portal hypertension. Ultrasound can also detect thrombosis of the portal or splenic veins which leads to splenomegaly. Finally, increased right heart pressure leading to hepatomegaly may be suggested by dilated hepatic veins.[44]

Magnetic resonance imaging (MRI) and abdominal CT both provide useful information regarding hepatic steatosis versus fibrosis. Because MRI does not require radiation, it is generally preferred over CT. Even though CT is not the test of choice, the liver is often seen on unenhanced CT of the chest (Fig. 52.3). Transient elastography (FibroScan) is another noninvasive technique that uses ultrasound, rather than radiation, to quantify liver stiffness which correlates with liver fibrosis. Furthermore, magnetic resonance cholangiography (MRCP) allows evaluation of the intrahepatic and extrahepatic bile ducts. Thus a beaded appearance to the intrahepatic ducts, suggestive of sclerosing cholangitis, or choledocholithiasis can be seen with MRCP.

Liver biopsy is viewed as the gold standard for the diagnosis of a variety of non-CF–related liver diseases. However, in CFLD, the disease tends to be patchy and sampling error is possible.[47] Obtaining two cores, or dual pass, has been advised for evaluation because it improves detection of fibrosis by 22% compared with a single core.[54] Liver biopsy tends to be helpful when there is a question of an additional or alternative disease process, for determining the extent of fibrosis, or for identifying the predominant liver lesion (steatosis or focal biliary cirrhosis [FBC]).[44,46] The liver biopsy can demonstrate focal portal fibrosis and inflammation, cholestasis, and bile duct proliferation in FBC, which is primarily a histologic diagnosis that is often clinically silent.[55] FBC is the pathognomonic histopathologic liver lesion in CF and may rarely progress to multilobular cirrhosis.

MANAGEMENT OF LIVER DISEASE

Unfortunately, a therapy to slow down or reverse fibrosis in CFLD has not been identified. Current management focuses on supportive care and addressing complications of advanced liver disease. Prevention of concomitant liver disease by ensuring complete vaccination against hepatitis A and hepatitis B is also essential to the treatment of individuals with CFLD.

The use of ursodeoxycholic acid (UDCA) in CFLD remains controversial. The proposed benefits include improved bile flow, displacement of toxic hydrophobic bile acids, cytoprotection, and stimulation of biliary bicarbonate secretion. UDCA is typically well tolerated, although the side effect of diarrhea has been reported. Typical dosing of UDCA is 20 mg/kg per day divided into two doses.

However, a 2014 Cochrane review did not find sufficient evidence to recommend routine use in individuals with CF. Specifically, this review underlined the paucity of randomized controlled trials evaluating the effectiveness of UDCA in CF. The available studies did not assess prevention of liver disease in individuals with CF, portal hypertension, liver transplantation, or survival.[56] Furthermore, a study evaluating high-dose UDCA (28–30 mg/kg per day) in primary sclerosing cholangitis was terminated due to an increase risk of death or liver transplantation in the group receiving UDCA.[55] Thus the role of UDCA in CF remains unclear.

In the CF population, for which nutrition already remains an important focus of care, the development of liver disease exacerbates this issue. It has been recommended that individuals with CF receive 150% of the recommended daily allowance (RDA) for calories by increasing dietary fat as opposed to carbohydrate supplements due to the risk of developing CF-related diabetes mellitus. The requirements of fat-soluble vitamins (A, D, E, and K) are also increased in CFLD and higher doses are often needed. Fat-soluble vitamin levels should be monitored closely and the doses adjusted accordingly. Pancreatic enzymes should be optimized to allow maximal absorption of long-chain triglycerides and essential fatty acids.[57]

Recognizing the development of portal hypertension is essential to the care of individuals with CFLD. Signs of this CFLD complication include splenomegaly, leucopenia, and thrombocytopenia. Reversal of, or abnormal, portal vein flow can be identified on liver Doppler ultrasound. Other complications associated with portal hypertension include variceal bleeding, low oxygen saturations due to hepatopulmonary syndrome, or abdominal distension due to ascites.

The greatest concern with portal hypertension is the life-threatening complication of variceal bleeding from either esophageal or gastric varices. An individual with an acute variceal bleed may present with hematemesis or passage of maroon-colored or melanotic stools. In children with portal hypertension, unlike in adults with portal hypertension, screening for the presence of varices is not recommended because there is no evidence-based therapy that is safe and effective to prevent the first variceal bleed (also known as primary variceal prophylaxis).[58] However, recent expert opinion has suggested that adult guidelines can be followed after puberty for variceal screening at the discretion of the treating physician.[59] Unfortunately, there is a paucity of literature in dealing with primary prophylaxis for varices in pediatrics; there are several case studies but only one randomized clinical trial. In one retrospective study of 38 children with CF and liver cirrhosis, variceal bleeding occurred in 50%; two of the children had exposure to salicylates prior to the bleed.[60] Thus salicylic acid and nonsteroidal antiinflammatory drugs (NSAIDs) should be avoided to minimize the risk of bleeding from esophageal or gastric varices.[47]

Once a variceal bleed has occurred, the child is at high risk of recurrence of bleeding. The prevention of a second bleeding episode is called secondary prophylaxis. In adults the preferred method for secondary prophylaxis is the use of a long-term nonselective β blocker with serial endoscopic variceal ligation (EVL) until the obliteration of the varices is complete.[61] The use of a nonselective β blocker has not been adequately studied in children for secondary prophylaxis. Furthermore, the pulmonary side effects of nonselective β blockers would most likely preclude their use in children with CF. Thus EVL is the preferred method of secondary prophylaxis in pediatrics.[58] EVL is not possible in infants weighing less than 12 kg due to the size of the equipment needed for EVL, so endoscopic sclerotherapy is used as secondary prophylaxis in these patients.

Gastric varices tend to be technically more difficult to address in pediatrics than in adults. In the adult literature, EVL can be performed with gastric varices that extend onto the cardia on the lesser curvature of the stomach.[62] Injection of cyanoacrylate glue is another option for treatment of gastric varices.[63] In children with difficult to control gastric varices or recurrent variceal bleeding, caregivers may consider the options of surgical portosystemic shunt or bypass procedure, transjugular intrahepatic portosystemic shunt (TIPS), or liver transplantation. Hepatic encephalopathy has occurred after portosystemic shunting; treatment includes lactulose and nonabsorbable antibiotics.

The decision on when to proceed with liver transplantation in the CF population has been controversial. Proposed indications include progressive hepatic dysfunction (decreasing albumin level and coagulopathy not correctable with vitamin K), development of ascites or jaundice, variceal bleeding not amenable to standard therapy, hepatopulmonary syndrome, unresponsive severe malnutrition, deteriorating quality of life, and deteriorating pulmonary function (Tiffeneau-Pinelli index $FEV_1/FVC < 50\%$).[47] Relative contraindications to liver transplant include colonization with multidrug resistant *P. aeruginosa* or *Burkholderia cepacia* due to the high risk of postoperative infection, which may be lethal.[64] The database for the United Network for Organ Sharing (UNOS) showed that 148 children with CF underwent liver transplantation alone, with a 5-year unadjusted survival of 86%. In an adjusted analysis the CF liver transplant recipients had inferior survival rates in long-term follow-up as compared with recipients with other indications for liver transplantation.[65] A higher incidence of anastomotic biliary strictures requiring creation of a Roux-en-Y portoenterostomy has been reported in CF liver transplant recipients, possibly due to their underlying CF-related bile duct disease.[66] Most of the CF liver transplant recipients will develop diabetes, but 60% of untransplanted individuals with CF-related portal hypertension will develop diabetes as well.[67]

Other than the development of diabetes, CF liver transplant recipients do not have increased mortality from other complications from CF (pulmonary failure, infections).[68] Some advocate for isolated liver transplantation prior to deterioration of lung function because combined liver-lung transplantation carries a worse prognosis.[69] However, it has been reported that outcomes for isolated liver transplantation and combined liver-lung transplantation in CF recipients are comparable.[64]

Gallbladder Disease

Gallstones occur in approximately 15%–30% of individuals with CF. These affected individuals are more likely to carry at least one Gilbert syndrome–associated UGT1A1 mutation which results in increased levels of unconjugated bilirubin.[70] This unconjugated bilirubin combines with calcium, which results in the calcium bilirubinate stones that are found in individuals with CF.[71] Unfortunately, these stones do not respond to UDCA. Thus cholecystectomy is considered in symptomatic individuals with cholelithiasis. Elevation in GGT and conjugated bilirubin with right upper quadrant abdominal pain should prompt urgent evaluation for gallstones.

Microgallbladder has been found in approximately 30% of individuals with CF on autopsy.[72] Some have proposed that this is the result of atresia or stenosis of the cystic duct.[73] In general, no treatment is required for microgallbladder.

Infertility

In addition to the airway and digestive tract, CFTR is found in the male and female reproductive tract. CFTR mutations have been associated with congenital bilateral absence of the vas deferens (CBAVD) and congenital absence of the uterus and vagina (CAUV), suggesting that CFTR may play a role in the development of both the female and male embryogenic reproductive tracts.[74] In men with CF, 98% are infertile.[75] Typically, infertility is due to obstructive azoospermia.[76] However, less than 2% of men with CF will remain fertile, especially those with a class V CFTR mutation.[77] Sperm harvest techniques including microsurgical epididymal sperm aspiration (MESA), percutaneous epididymal sperm aspiration (PESA), and testicular sperm aspiration are possible options for treatment. Although the number of pregnancies after these procedures is small, the outcomes are similar to those in men without CF.[74]

In contrast, approximately 50% of women with CF are able to conceive a child naturally.[78] Typically, the reproductive anatomy for females with CF is normal. Even with a normal cervix, the abnormal CFTR function leads to thickened and dehydrated tenacious cervical mucus that interferes with cervical penetration by sperm.[78] Menarche is delayed in females with CF by almost 2 years on average regardless of nutritional status, especially among those with abnormal oral glucose tolerance test (OGTT) and those who are homozygous for ΔF508.[79] Treatment involves medication like clomiphene citrate to help stimulate ovulation, intrauterine insemination (IUI), in vitro fertilization (IVF), or intracytoplasmic sperm injection (ICSI) in more complicated cases.[74]

Cystic Fibrosis Transmembrane Conductance Regulator Actions in the Small Bowel

Typical gastrointestinal (GI) physiology follows the entrance of acid pH chyme from the stomach into the duodenum, triggering a host of gut hormone release from the duodenum that has an effect on the pancreas and duodenal cells to secrete bicarbonate and stimulates release of pancreatic enzymes in the zymogen form. Those enzymes are converted into a functioning form when contact is made with activating enzymes on the bowel luminal surface followed by a self-activation cascade. These pancreatic enzymes work optimally in a neutral pH environment and aid in the breakdown of protein and fat into digestible components. The gut hormone release from the duodenum also stimulates the gallbladder to excrete bile that begins the emulsification of lipids thus activating fat digestion. There are still other brush border enzymes that aid in carbohydrate metabolism and also work best in a neutral pH environment. CFTR is found on the apical surface of the intestinal crypts and villi and, in the pancreas, contributes to the release of bicarbonate into the bowel lumen. Without proper function of this protein channel there is an impaired bicarbonate secretion that results in a duodenal pH that is 1–2 units lower in CF patients than in healthy controls.[80] This more acidic pH has an adverse effect on the pancreatic enzyme function, micelle formation, and brush border enzyme function, thus affecting the digestion of all macronutrients.[80–82] The use of ivacaftor, the CFTR potentiator, has been shown to normalize the buffering capacity in patients with the G551D CFTR mutation.[80,81] Fluid secretion into the small bowel also appears linked to bicarbonate secretion via CFTR.[80]

MECONIUM ILEUS

MI is nearly pathognomonic for CF, although there can be other clinical causes. MI is one of the earliest signs of CF and occurs in 15%–20% of the CF population.[83,84] The occurrence of MI has been linked to CFTR gene mutations and thus clinical severity, which together can be used to further delineate CF phenotypes. Those with class I, II, or III mutations, in that order, are more likely to present with MI.[83] Nearly half the patients that present with MI will have at least one additional GI complication that could include ileal atresia, intestinal volvulus, bowel necrosis, bowel perforation with meconium peritonitis, or giant meconium pseudocyst; any of these additional complications confer the designation of a complicated MI case[84] (Fig. 52.4).

Nonoperative management of MI can include the use of a water-soluble radiopaque solution (Gastrografin) that hydrates and softens the meconium mass when used via careful rectal instillation. While being therapeutic, it can also help to define the extent of the ileus and the size of the colon (often a microcolon). The goal of a Gastrografin enema is to have the solution reflux into the terminal ileum to relieve the obstruction. The Gastrografin also allows for observation of the bowel movements and can be repeated every 12–24 hours.[84] Other enema solutions that can be considered as supplementation to Gastrografin include warm saline with

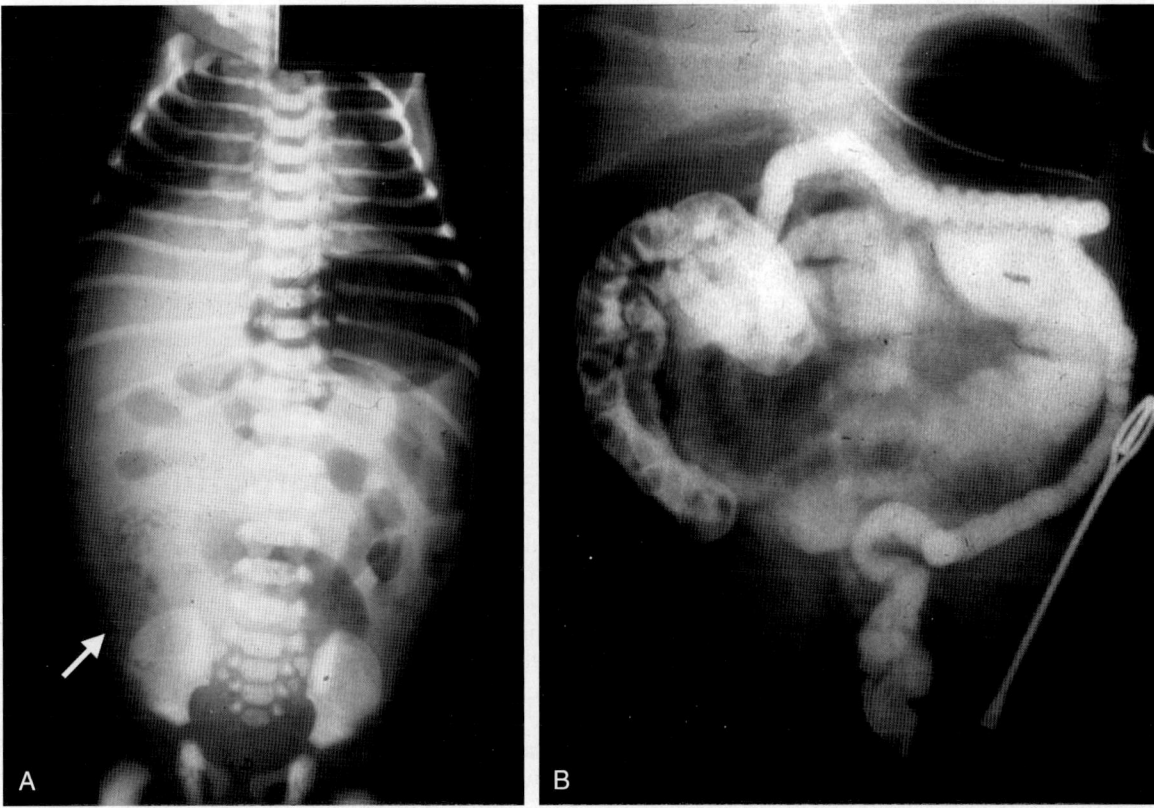

Fig. 52.4 Meconium ileus. (A) Abdominal x-ray showing air-fluid levels in the small bowel and granular material in the right lower quadrant with an absence of air in the colon. (B) Barium enema showing the presence of inspissated material in the small bowel and a microcolon.

1% N-acetylcysteine. The risks of hypertonic enemas can include severe bowel distention with perforation, hypovolemic shock due to fluid shifting, and bowel ischemia from over-distention and hypoperfusion.[84,85] These potential complications can be anticipated and require monitoring and rapid response to the fluid needs of the neonate. Success rates of nonsurgical management for simple MI have typically been reported near 80%, although more recent review of the literature reports closer to 40% success, citing less aggressive enema management and lower osmolarity of enema solutions as the reason for a faster conversion to surgical management.[84,85] In using this approach the complication rates have also decreased.[85]

Operative management remains an option, although it is typically reserved for complicated MI or MI that has not been responsive to the nonoperative approach. Over the years there have been many different surgical approaches with and without enterostomies but most with a resection of part of the affected bowel along with some instillation of irrigants.[84] A strong effort to minimize the amount of bowel resected can help with clinical management in the postoperative period. Following surgery some providers continue to instill 4% N-acetylcysteine via an ileostomy to help solubilize any residual meconium. It is recommended that stomas be closed as soon as possible to help avoid further fluid and electrolyte disturbances.[84] Most patients undergoing surgical management of MI require nutritional supplementation with parenteral nutrition (PN) for a short period of time. The longevity of PN dependence will vary from patient to patient, and early use of enteral nutrition is encouraged. The enteral nutrition

could be breast milk or routine infant formula, although some cases may require partially hydrolyzed or elemental formula supplementation depending on the amount of bowel resected and patient's response to enteral feeding. When enteral feeding is initiated, it is important to also begin the use of PERT and vitamins.[84] Early involvement of your local pediatric gastroenterologist and CF dieticians who can help guide through the finer aspects of nutritional management is advised.

Constipation

Constipation is defined as a decreased frequency of bowel movements from one's baseline bowel habits with increased consistency (hardening) of the stool or pain with defecation with or without abdominal distention. This is a common problem among patients with CF and thought to be in part due to the increased viscosity of the fluid secreted in the GI tract. Defective CFTR leads to reduced chloride and fluid secretion into the bowel lumen while also upregulating the epithelial sodium channel (ENaC), leading to increased absorption of sodium and fluid from the luminal mucus.[86] Newer treatments with CFTR channel activators have shown some improvement of fluid secretion in the intestinal lumen as measured by a wet to dry ratio in mice.[87] Treatment of constipation can be achieved with medications to increase the osmolality of the chyme so as to effectively pull in more water and keep the stool soft. Other treatments that may sometimes be necessary include stimulant laxatives and colonic lavage if osmotic laxatives alone are not successful.

Distal Intestinal Obstruction Syndrome

Inadequate hydration of the chyme/stool can lead to a unique issue in patients with CF known as DIOS in which the chyme of the small bowel is inspissated and thick enough to activate the ileal brake, effectively causing a partial or complete bowel obstruction at the transition of the small bowel to the colon. In 2010 the European Society for Paediatric Gastroenterology Hepatology and Nutrition (ESPGHAN) CF working group defined two distinct types of DIOS.[88] First, there is complete DIOS, which is a complete intestinal obstruction with confirmatory clinical or radiographic findings, fecal mass seen or felt in the ileocecal area, and abdominal pain or distention or both. Second, there is incomplete DIOS that has days of abdominal pain or distension with a fecal mass in the ileocecal area without clinical or radiographic signs of obstruction.[88]

In either complete or incomplete DIOS the clinical presentation of these patients includes an acute onset of abdominal pain, typically in the right lower quadrant, that can be mistaken for appendicitis by those unfamiliar with the care of CF patients. There is an estimated prevalence range for the occurrence of DIOS of 5–12 episodes per 1000 patients per year.[89] Munck and colleagues prospectively studied 102 patients (both pediatric and adults) with at least 1 episode of DIOS in 10 countries for 1.6 years and found a recurrence of DIOS in nine patients for a total of 112 episodes of DIOS recorded. Using a multivariate analysis they found some association with comorbid conditions including MI, PI, CF-related liver disease, CF-related diabetes, and *P. aeruginosa* colonization.[90]

DISTAL INTESTINAL OBSTRUCTION SYNDROME MANAGEMENT

DIOS is treated with the goal of moving the bowel contents forward through the colon. Often this involves the use of oral osmotic laxatives along with oral hydration. Oral lavage with polyethylene glycol is commonly used at a dose of 2 g/kg per day, with a maximum of 80–100 g/day.[89] Gastrografin administered orally or via enemas is another effective treatment, it is diluted to various concentrations depending on the age of the patient and the route of administration.[88,89,91] Aggressive management of constipation with appropriate hydration and optimization of pancreatic replacement therapy is thought to help minimize the occurrence of DIOS, although this remains anecdotal.[88-91] In extreme cases with persistent obstruction or ischemia surgical management may be necessary.

Rectal Prolapse

Rectal prolapse occurs in 3.5% of patients with CF, and we also know that 3.6% of patients who have rectal prolapse will be found to have CF.[92] Rectal prolapse can occur at any age, although it is most common younger than 3 years of age and generally resolves spontaneously without need for surgical intervention. Management of constipation and adequate PERT may help to lessen the frequency of prolapse occurrences.

Gastric Emptying and Small Bowel Motility

Gastric emptying studies have not been consistently abnormal in CF patients. Prolonged intestinal transit time has been shown in adult and pediatric patients with CF when compared with healthy controls by breath testing.[93,94] Orocecal transit time has been shown to be greater than 7 hours in 80% of the CF patients compared to 12% of the healthy controls with the velocity of small bowel transit slowing in the distal small bowel, using radiopaque markers and magnet-based motility tracking.[95,96]

Small Intestine Bacterial Overgrowth

Delayed small bowel motility along with frequent administration of antibiotics, a high-fat/high-carbohydrate diet and use of acid suppression may predispose patients with CF to small intestinal bacterial overgrowth (SIBO). SIBO is described as one or more types of bacteria that have overgrown their "normal" amount within the small bowel. Symptoms can include increased gas and bloating, with or without abdominal distention, and sometimes diarrhea. In particular the use of low-dose azithromycin has been implicated in SIBO in the CF community.[97] Diagnosis for SIBO may be clinical, or for older patients the use of a hydrogen breath test or methane measurement could be diagnostic.[97,98] Consequences of SIBO include a further exacerbation of malabsorption of nutrients and micronutrients if diarrhea is present. There is a decreased association of SIBO in patients with CF if they are regularly using laxatives.[97] Treatment can include a therapeutic trial of oral antibiotics (metronidazole, rifaximin, or ciprofloxacin). In CF patients with an exacerbation and also diagnosed with SIBO via hydrogen-methane breath test, oral treatment with ciprofloxacin was far superior to intravenous treatment with ceftazidime and amikacin for the resolution of SIBO.[99] There was also significant improvement in fat digestion and absorption in the ciprofloxacin group during this treatment.[99]

MICROBIOME

In the past several years there has been a focus on both the intestinal and respiratory microbiome of CF patients. The microbial colonization of both the respiratory and intestinal tracts occur early in the life of an infant and is likely influenced by many factors, such as mode of delivery, contact with environment, feeding practices, and early antibiotic exposure. Infants followed from birth to 3 years of age with regular interval evaluation of the GI and respiratory microbiota were monitored for onset of CF exacerbations and were found to have a significant decrease in normal GI flora consisting of *Bacteroides* and *Bifidobacterium* just prior to onset of CF pulmonary exacerbations.[100] There was also a suggestion that increased GI microbial diversity and breast feeding were protective against CF exacerbations,[100] although more studies will be needed to evaluate this further. There has also been demonstration of an early dysbiosis in the microbiota of CF patients linked to malabsorption of dietary fat that therefore selects for a proinflammatory GI microbiome.[101]

The use of newer metagenomic sequencing and taxonomic profiling methods has led to a rapidly expanding field that is defining not only which bacteria are present but in what quantity and is starting to allow us to define relationships to the health of CF patients. We anticipate a swift application and expansion of these techniques in the years to come.

GI Cancers

Although the underlying pathobiology of GI carcinogenesis in CF patients remains speculative, both adenocarcinoma of the small bowel and colon have been found to be prevalent in this population. An increase in GI cancer incidence in CF patients compared with the general population with an odds ratio of 6.5 has been described with most of these cancers occurring in the third decade of life.[102] Registry data assessed over a 10-year period found that in the nontransplanted group there was a predominance of small bowel, colon, and biliary cancers that were diagnosed at a mean age of 39 years, with the highest risk group being patients homozygous for the 508del mutation.[103] In the transplanted cohort, small bowel and colon cancers remained the bowel cancers of note.[103] Adenomatous polyps as a precursor of adenocarcinoma have been described in 30- to 39-year-old patients. Risk factors associated with the formation of polyps include: homozygosity for the 508del mutation, CFRD, being a male, and lung transplantation.[102–104] Indications for colonoscopy include persistent diarrhea, iron deficiency anemia, hematochezia, and abdominal pain. At this time there are no consensus guidelines for colonoscopy screening in the CF population, although we expect such guidelines to emerge in the next few years.

Nutrition

In the 1980s there were several published articles illustrating the link between nutritional status and CF pulmonary disease. One study demonstrated that increasing the caloric intake with night feeds stabilized pulmonary decline compared with standard of care.[105] Other studies linked improved nutrition with enhanced exercise performance.[106] One of the most convincing articles was a retrospective review at two respected CF centers that noted no difference in pulmonary treatment/care, but one of the centers had adopted an aggressive approach to the use of PERT and caloric intake in their patients and that resulted in significantly improved survival.[107,108] There have been several newer studies that have linked good nutritional status as measured by nutritional indices such as height growth, weight gain, and body mass index (BMI) early in life with improved survival and preserved pulmonary function.[109–112] Nutrition has become a major clinical focus in recent years. There is also an association of poor nutrition with decreased health related quality of life in children age 9–19 years.[113]

Given all these supporting data, several clinical nutrition guidelines have been published recently, including the European Society for Clinical Nutrition and Metabolism (ESPEN), European Society for Paediatric Gastroenterolgy Hepatology and Nutrition (ESPGHAN), and the European Cystic Fibrosis Society (ECFS) guidelines[114] and the clinical practice guidelines

from the CF foundation.[115] These guidelines give structure to screening nutritional status and recommend obtaining height and weight at every visit so that a weight for length or BMI can be calculated. Goal weight for length, on the World Health Organization growth curves given the same age population, is the 50th percentile during the first 2 years of life.[114,115] From age 2–18 years on the Centers for Disease Control and Prevention growth curves, the BMI goal is 50th percentile of the same age population.[114,115] For adults greater than 18 years, the female goal for BMI is 22 kg/m^2 and for males 23 kg/m^2.[114]

Given these aforementioned BMI goals, the guidelines also focus on recommended caloric intake goals. It is estimated that an infant with CF has caloric needs closer to 150 kcal/kg than the standard of 100–120 kcal/kg.[116] Breast milk is still considered best for patients with CF because it offers colonization with mother's microbiome, passive antibody transmission for increased immunity, and nutrients that are easy to digest.[24,116] Although the concentration of breast milk can vary, it is rarely higher than 20 kcal/ounce. Some mothers can overcome the increased caloric intake needs by increased volume production. Otherwise, these needs can be met by increasing the caloric density of the feeds with supplementation or fortification of breast milk.[24,116] We would highly recommend breast-feeding unless the child is losing weight or failing to gain weight. After solid foods are introduced, the simultaneous introduction of high-calorie, high-fat foods will help to address the increased caloric need. Finding healthy ways to enrich foods with additional calories and fats is encouraged from an early age.[114–116] Supplements of additional oils, especially medium chain fatty acids (no transport needed for absorption) are often started early.

The caloric goals of a toddler/preschool child with CF is closer to 90–110 kcal/kg per day, with a protein goal that increases from 13 g/day at ages 2–3 years to 19 g/day for children aged 4–5 years.[115] For older children and adults it is estimated that patients with CF require from 120% to 150% of the energy needs of a healthy population (Fig. 52.5).[114]

Consuming adequate calories for a patient with CF can be difficult given their increased needs due to malabsorption, along with chronic and recurrent infections, and exacerbations. If patients are having difficulty gaining weight, optimization of PERT and consideration of acid suppression to enhance PERT efficacy should be considered.[112,114,115] Other therapies to consider include promotility agents and appetite stimulants.[112] Dietary supplements should be considered, although the evidence for this remains low and there is a strong recommendation to individualize care in this arena; there may be need for behavioral interventions as well.[114] If there is a continued struggle to gain weight, care providers may need to consider tube feedings via nasogastric tubes (NGTs) or gastrostomy tubes (G-tubes), to provide nutritional supplements either during the day or at night.[114,115] The preschool guidelines offer algorithms to consider when analyzing the utility of G-tubes.[115] PN is not generally recommended except for specific cases where enteral feedings are not possible.[114]

Another aspect of nutrition involves the micronutrient requirements of CF patients. These markers of nutritional status are monitored via biochemical or laboratory measurements of serum or plasma. The general recommendation is to obtain these markers yearly for screening and more frequently

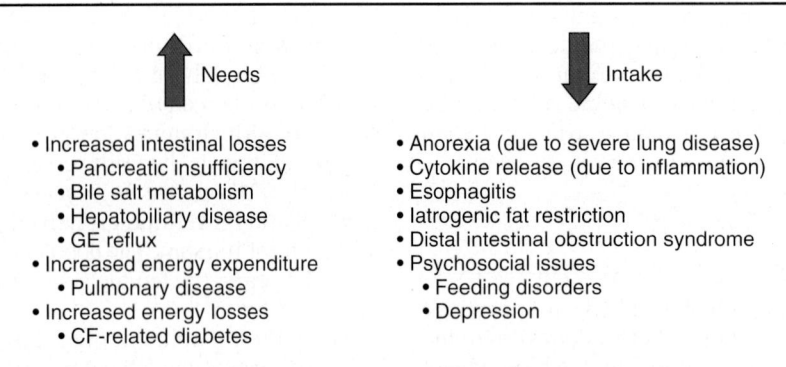

Fig. 52.5 Model for the development of energy imbalance in cystic fibrosis.

Table 52.1   Fat-Soluble Vitamins

	Pathophysiology	What to Measure	Signs of Deficiency	How to Treat Deficiency
Vitamin A	Cofactor in pathways for vision, growth and immune development and regulation	Serum vitamin A level	Night blindness	Oral supplementation **can have toxicity
Vitamin D	Bone/calcium homeostasis	25-OH vitamin D	Osteoporosis is a late finding but can be monitored with DEXA scans	Oral supplementation with cholecalciferol and weight-bearing exercise
Vitamin E	Antioxidant throughout the body	α-tocopherol/cholesterol ratio or total serum lipid ratio	Peripheral neuropathy with loss of reflexes or hemolytic anemia	Oral supplementation
Vitamin K	Cofactor for many proteins in the clotting cascade	PT/INR	Coagulopathy with a prolonged PT/INR	Oral, IV, or IM supplementation

DEXA, Dual-energy x-ray absorptiometry; *IM*, intramuscular; *IV*, intravenous.

if abnormalities arise and adjustments are being made.[114–117] The recommended markers include a red blood cell count, iron status, fat-soluble vitamin levels, electrolyte levels, zinc, transaminases (AST/ALT), biliary tree measurements (bilirubin and GGT) and "liver function tests."[114,115] There are some special circumstances when B_{12}, folic acid, vitamin C, or selenium are monitored, but these are not routinely recommended. Patients with CF are at increased risk of some micronutrient deficiencies; in particular they are at risk of fat-soluble vitamin deficiencies given the higher rates of fat malabsorption in patients who are pancreatic insufficient. Specific fat-soluble vitamin formulations are available commercially and are typically used to supplement the fat-soluble vitamin intake, although there are times when individual vitamin supplementation should be considered, especially if there are specific deficiencies (Table 52.1).

Zinc and sodium are other micronutrients that also require monitoring in CF patients.[24,112,114,115] Zinc is an enzymatic cofactor used in many growth and immune function pathways. Measurement of a serum zinc level can be followed over time. Clinical symptoms of deficiency include diarrhea, dermatitis, and poor weight gain. Oral zinc supplements can be used to replace stores. Sodium is a cation that is prevalent in the extracellular fluid and is used in many regulatory processes throughout the body. It is measured routinely as a serum electrolyte, and patients with CF are at an increased risk of depletion due to their excessive salt loss through the skin. Higher dietary requirements or supplements may need to be considered especially in summer months or early in life when growth is rapid.[24,112]

Cystic Fibrosis–Related Diabetes

CFRD has an age-dependent incidence that ranges from 5% in 10–14 year olds to 13% in 15–19 year olds and near to 50% in patients 30–50 years of age.[118] The pathophysiology of CFRD appears quite complex, with multiple possible contributors. It has characteristics of both type I and type II diabetes but is in fact a unique type. Exocrine pancreas destruction from chronic pancreatitis with progressive fibrosis leading to islet disruption and loss of alpha and beta cells is the generally accepted explanation.[118,119] Therefore insulin insufficiency, as in type I diabetes, is the main contributor to the pathophysiology, although there is some thought that a fluctuating level of insulin resistance is also contributing to the pathophysiology. The insulin resistance may work through other factors including autoantibodies, inflammation, infection, malnutrition, genetic susceptibility, and impaired insulin sensitivity.[118,119] The use of A1C testing in not recommended for CFRD, instead early detection is reliant on an OGTT.[118–120] It is recommended that annual screening is started with an OGTT at age 10 years.[118–120] There are also recommendations to monitor patients receiving antibiotics, glucocorticoids, and enteral tube feedings and to monitor women prior to, during, and post pregnancy.[120] Medical nutrition therapy with a reduction in carbohydrate load and insulin are the mainstays of treatment.[118–120] According to a recent Cochrane review, there is no advantage to using oral hypoglycemic agents compared with insulin in CFRD.[121] There are current clinical care guidelines for CFRD that address the specifics of diagnosis, treatment, and management.[120]

Conclusion

There has been substantial advancement in the knowledge of CFTR function outside the pulmonary system and its relation to disease manifestations and progression. This has led to a rapid expansion of necessary care team members on both the pediatric and adult side, including specialists in gastroenterology, endocrinology, fertility, and women's health. The role of CFTR corrector and potentiator therapies is just starting to be addressed in these other organ systems, which will continue to lead to a better overall understanding of pathophysiology related to CFTR.

References

Access the reference list online at ExpertConsult.com.

53 Molecular Therapies for Cystic Fibrosis

GWYNETH DAVIES, MBChB, MSc, PhD, MRCPCH, UTA GRIESENBACH, PhD,
ERIC ALTON, BA Cantab, MBBS, MRCP, MD, MA, FRCP, FMedSCI, and
JANE C. DAVIES, MB ChB, FRCPCH, MD

Introduction

The impressive improvement in life expectancy in cystic fibrosis (CF) over recent decades has been achieved by treatments that are aimed at the downstream consequences of absent or dysfunctional CF transmembrane conductance regulator (CFTR) activity (including aggressive treatment of infection, airway clearance and nutrition) rather than by targeting CFTR directly. In contrast, novel approaches using CFTR modulators or gene therapy aim to target the root cause of the disease, replacing/repairing the CFTR gene or addressing the underlying defects responsible for defective CFTR channel function, intracellular processing, or production. Ultimately, the aim is to fully correct the defective CFTR and restore normal function. There is already some evidence that CFTR modulation can affect the disease trajectory in CF.[1]

This chapter describes the therapeutic strategies for CF which are based on targeting CFTR, either at the gene or protein level. We will provide updates on small molecule CFTR modulators and gene therapy, focusing on clinical development and evaluation. The challenge for the field is to find drugs or combinations of drugs capable of restoring CFTR function, applicable to patients with any genetic mutation.

Small Molecule Cystic Fibrosis Transmembrane Conductance Regulator Modulators

The focus of this section is on CFTR modulators licensed for clinical use or in clinical trials at the time of writing. The wave of CFTR modulators currently in the initial stages of development or under evaluation in clinical trials will inevitably mean that for the reader to remain up to date, information in this chapter will need to be reviewed in conjunction with new evidence as it becomes available. Table 53.1 lists the drugs targeting CFTR, which are at clinical stages of testing. Clinical trials are registered on the US National Institutes of Health ClinicalTrials.gov website (https://clinicaltrials.gov/). The US Cystic Fibrosis Foundation also has an interactive drug development pipeline on its website that takes the reader to an overview of evidence to date from clinical trials and trials currently in progress (https://www.cff.org/Trials/Pipeline).

IDENTIFYING CANDIDATE DRUGS

Drug development typically starts with identification of a therapeutic target, which may be site-, cell-, or receptor-specific. Candidate compounds are then investigated for their ability to modulate this target. These can be either selectively or randomly chosen; the latter clearly requires high-throughput screening techniques—automated assays that allow high numbers of potential compounds to be screened quickly. "Lead" compounds showing potential undergo further preclinical assessment (further information at http://www.cftr.info/drug-research-development/pre-clinical-development/pre-clinical-validation-of-cftr-therapies/). Optimization to improve selectivity of the desired target, pharmacokinetics, and preclinical toxicology follows. The agents that are considered promising at the end of this process may proceed to clinical trials. Both traditional and high-throughput screening processes have been used to identify potential compounds that target defective or absent CFTR. Understanding functional manifestations at the protein/molecular level of a particular disease-causing mutation in CF allows the use of assays in high-throughput screening that can identify any impact on CFTR function (e.g., assays measuring anion conductance across cell membranes act as a "readout" for CFTR function).

IMPACT OF CYSTIC FIBROSIS TRANSMEMBRANE CONDUCTANCE REGULATOR MUTATIONS ON PROTEIN EXPRESSION, MATURATION, OR FUNCTION

A basic understanding of CFTR structure and function is important to understand the rationale for CFTR modulators. CFTR is a 1480–amino acid protein belonging to the adenine nucleotide binding cassette (ABC) transporter superfamily, expressed at the apical membrane of specialized epithelial cells.[2] It has multiple functions, but its role as a chloride and bicarbonate transporter is best characterized.[3] A detailed description of the consequences of absent or dysfunctional CFTR in CF is described in Chapter 49.

More than 2000 mutations in the *CFTR* gene have been identified (http://cftr2.org), although the number determined as definitely disease causing is currently less than 200. The single residue deletion of phenylalanine at codon 508 (Phe-508del) is the commonest mutation globally, present in almost 90% of CF alleles. Of the remaining mutations, 159 occur at a prevalence >0.01% in the CF population.[4] Six main classes of CFTR mutation have been defined, categorized

Table 53.1 New Drugs in the Therapeutic Pipeline

Class of Drug	Agents	Current Status
Gene replacement therapy	pGM169/GL67A (UK CF Gene Therapy Consortium)	Primary end point met in phase IIb clinical trial (59)
mRNA repair	QR-010 (ProQR Therapeutics)	Trials of nasal delivery and nebulization underway
Read-through agents	Ataluren (PTC124; PTC Therapeutics)	Recent announcement of 2nd phase III trial failure http://ir.ptcbio.com/releasedetail.cfm?releaseid=1015471
Amplifier	PTI-428 (Proteostasis Therapeutics Inc)	Early-phase trials of oral agent underway
Correctors (+/−potentiator)	Lumacaftor/ivacaftor (Orkambi, Vertex)	Licensed for F508del homozygous patients
	Tezacaftor (VX661)/ivacaftor (Kalydeco; Vertex)	Phase III program in F508del homozygous and heterozygous patients underway
	Next-generation triple component drugs (Vertex)	Early-phase trials underway with several agents administered with 661/ivacaftor
	Riociguat (Bayer)	Phase II trial underway
	GLPG2222 and GLPG2737 (Galapagos)	Early-phase trials underway
	FDL169 (Flatley Discovery Labs)	Phase II trial to commence 2017
Potentiator	Ivacaftor (Kalydeco; Vertex)	Licensed for patients with gating mutations aged 2 years and older and R117H
		A component of all Vertex's combination drugs
	GLPG1837 (Galapagos)	Phase II trial data awaited
	QBW251 (Novartis)	Phase II study results awaited
	GLPG2451 (Galapagos)	Early-phase trials as mono and in combination with GLPG2222
	GLPG3067 (Galapagos)	In phase I trial
	Deuterated ivacaftor (CTP-656, Concert)	In phase II trial of patients with gating mutations
Stabilizer	Cavosonstat (N91115; Nivalis Therapeutics)	Recent announcement of failed phase II trial http://ir.nivalis.com/press-releases/detail/60
ENaC inhibitor	VX-371 (Vertex)	In phase II trial in patients on Orkambi (also being tested in primary ciliary dyskinesia [PCD])

The authors accept no responsibility for content on external sites.

according to effects on CFTR production, intracellular processing, and function (Fig. 53.1).

In class I mutations, a premature termination codon prevents full-length CFTR protein from being produced; these are present in approximately 10% of CF patients worldwide, although they are very much more common in certain populations such as the Ashkenazi Jewish population. Class II mutations (Phe508del being the commonest) result in CFTR being misfolded within the epithelial cell. As a result the protein cannot be transported to its site of action in the cell membrane, instead being prematurely degraded by the ubiquitin-proteasome system. In class III mutations, CFTR is produced and sited within the cell membrane, but there is infrequent opening ("gating") of the chloride ion channel; these mutations are present in approximately 5% of CF patients worldwide, with the commonest by far being Gly551Asp (G551D). Class IV mutations (e.g., Arg117His) result in reduced ion conductance. Class V are splicing mutations, which result in reduced protein expression, and class VI mutations impact the turnover of CFTR at the cell membrane due to a reduced half-life. Despite these distinctions, it is important to recognize that the functional impact of the mutation may traverse several classes; for example, Phe508del (predominantly considered to be a class II mutation) also impacts the function of any CFTR that does reach the cell membrane (such as abnormal gating and reduced half-life).[5,6]

TARGETING CYSTIC FIBROSIS TRANSMEMBRANE CONDUCTANCE REGULATOR PROTEIN WITH SMALL MOLECULE DRUGS

The small molecule drugs that target CFTR dysfunction are commonly referred to according to their mechanism of action.

They include ribosomal read-through agents, "potentiators," and "correctors." Agents capable of "reading-through" a prematurely placed stop codon aim to produce a full-length functional protein. Potentiators are aptly named as they potentiate CFTR function but rely on appropriate placement within the cell membrane in the first instance. Correctors aim to rectify protein misfolding and thereby facilitate trafficking to the cell membrane.

Therapeutic candidates using one or more of these approaches have been evaluated in clinical trials, and a small number have now progressed through licensing to the clinic. They tend to be administered via the enteral route (possible due to their low molecular weight), which means multiorgan effects may be achieved (Fig. 53.2), and once commenced, the duration of treatment is potentially lifelong.

Read-Through Agents

Stop codons are nucleotide triplets in messenger RNA (mRNA) that serve a key role in signaling the end of protein coding sequences (e.g., UAG, UAA, UGA). Premature stop codons are those that occur within the normal coding sequence due to a mutation. This means that the message to create the protein of interest is incomplete; thus only truncated protein is formed. Molecules that allow the read-through of premature stop codons, thus enabling the production of full-length protein, are being evaluated for several diseases including class I mutation CF.

The aminoglycoside gentamicin was initially shown to possess such capabilities,[7] but concerns over the adverse safety profile of this group of agents (renal toxicity and sensorineural deafness) led to a search for other potential candidates. The one that has been most extensively investigated

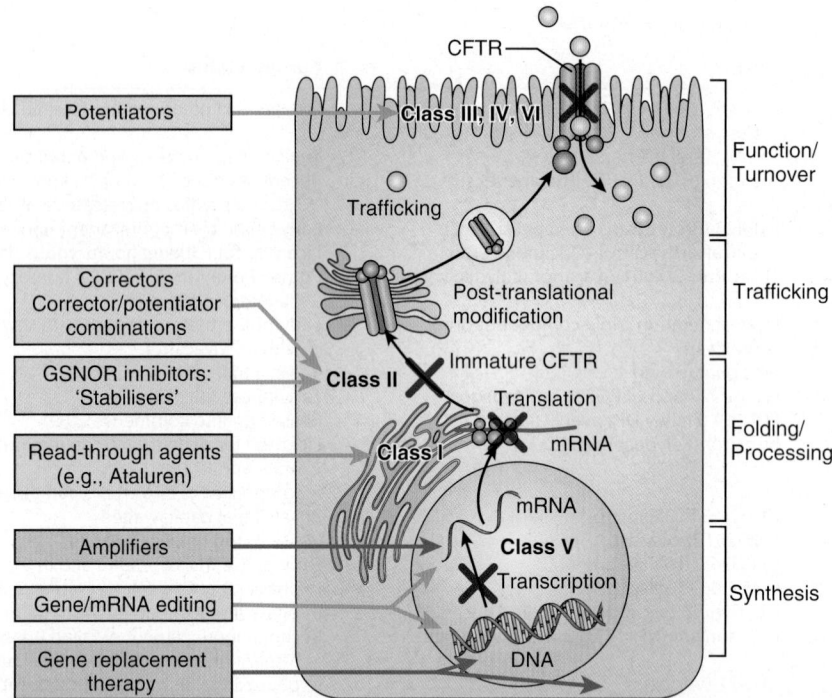

Fig. 53.1 The many mutations in CFTR can be broadly grouped into classes depending on the effect the mutation has on the CFTR protein. Many drugs are being developed that target specific classes or individual mutations (examples shown in *green*), whereas other approaches could be considered mutation agnostic *(blue)*. Reused with permission from www.cftrscience.com. *CFTR,* Cystic fibrosis transmembrane conductance regulator; *GSNOR,* S-nitrosoglutathione reductase; *mRNA,* messenger ribonucleic acid.

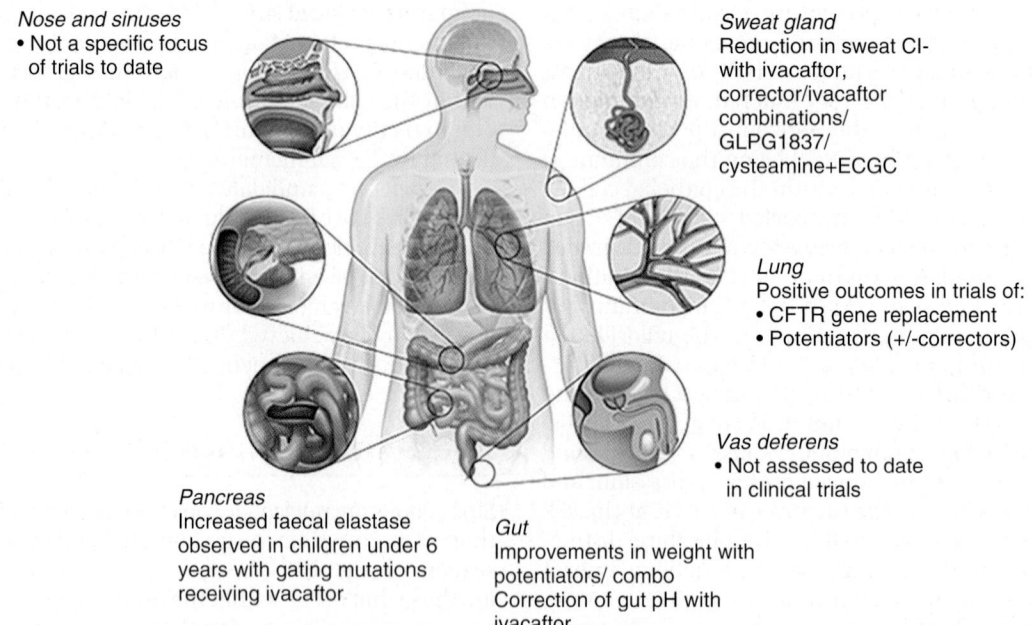

Nose and sinuses
• Not a specific focus of trials to date

Sweat gland
Reduction in sweat Cl- with ivacaftor, corrector/ivacaftor combinations/ GLPG1837/ cysteamine+ECGC

Lung
Positive outcomes in trials of:
• CFTR gene replacement
• Potentiators (+/-correctors)

Vas deferens
• Not assessed to date in clinical trials

Pancreas
Increased faecal elastase observed in children under 6 years with gating mutations receiving ivacaftor

Gut
Improvements in weight with potentiators/ combo
Correction of gut pH with ivacaftor

Fig. 53.2 The multiorgan manifestations of CF and the changes that have been reported in trials of new therapies. Adapted with permission from www.cftrscience.com. *CF,* Cystic fibrosis; *CFTR,* cystic fibrosis transmembrane conductance regulator.

is the oral small molecule drug ataluren (Translarna, formerly PTC124. PTC Therapeutics; http://www.ptcbio.com/en/pipeline/ataluren-translarna/). This was identified by a high-throughput screening process involving more than 800,000 compounds. In *CFTR* knockout mice expressing human G542X mutant *CFTR,* ataluren increased CFTR

expression at the apical surface of epithelial cells and restored cyclic adenosine monophosphate (cAMP)-stimulated chloride currents to approximately 25% of wild type.[8] Ataluren has been evaluated in both adults and children older than 6 years with at least one CFTR nonsense mutation. Changes toward normal in nasal potential difference (nPD) measurements (a bioelectrical test of CFTR function) were observed in most adults[9] and in approximately half of children in early phase trials.[10] An increased proportion of airway epithelial cells expressing CFTR detected by immunofluorescence was also seen.[10] These phase II trials involved CF patients from Israel (adults) and Europe (children). The results were in contrast to the lack of efficacy seen in a phase II trial of PTC124 in the United States.[11] The phase III randomized controlled trial (RCT) that followed involved 238 patients with a nonsense CFTR mutation. Patients were randomized to receive ataluren in a 3 times daily dosing regimen (10 mg/kg morning and midday; 20 mg/kg evening) or placebo for 48 weeks.[12] Although neither the primary outcome of forced expiratory volume in one second (FEV_1) nor the secondary outcome of a reduction in pulmonary exacerbations were met, on *post hoc* analysis these outcomes were statistically significant for patients who were not receiving concurrent inhaled tobramycin as part of their routine CF management.[12] This has led to a further phase III trial (NCT02139306) specifically for patients not on inhaled aminoglycosides, as it has been suggested that the lack of response in patients receiving aminoglycosides may be due to competition with ataluren at the ribosomal binding site; at the time of writing, the results of this second trial have not been published, but a sponsor's press release describes it as having failed to achieve its outcomes (http://ir.ptcbio.com/releasedetail.cfm?releaseid=1015471). Drugs such as ataluren targeting premature stop codons have the potential for broader applicability than being limited to a single disease. For example, ataluren has been granted a conditional marketing authorization by the European Medicines Agency, based on the results of a phase IIb study in boys with Duchenne muscular dystrophy in conjunction with an unmet need for disease-modifying therapies in this condition.[13,14]

Potentiators

The clinical trials of ivacaftor (Kalydeco, VX-770 Vertex Pharmaceuticals; http://www.kalydeco.com/how-kalydeco-works) undertaken to date have represented an important milestone in the proof of concept for drugs aiming to target the underlying molecular defect in CF. Identified through high-throughput screening, ivacaftor potentiated CFTR in human bronchial epithelial cells from compound heterozygotes with the commonest class III mutation Gly551Asp/Phe508del *in vitro*.[15] It was then evaluated in patients with at least one copy of this mutation; early-phase studies demonstrated evidence of functional improvement in CFTR with nPD and sweat chloride measurements. Phase III placebo controlled studies followed with impressive results. Efficacy was demonstrated on a regimen of ivacaftor 150 mg twice daily in adults and adolescents (STRIVE),[16] and children aged 6–11 years (ENVISION).[17] In both trials a significant improvement in lung function was seen on active treatment with absolute improvements in FEV_1 of 10.6% and 12.5%, respectively. The improvement in lung function was evident by week two of treatment with ivacaftor and was sustained through 48 weeks. In parallel, there were also significant reductions in sweat chloride concentrations, and improvements in quality of life and weight.[16,17] The pulmonary exacerbation frequency was significantly reduced in adults receiving ivacaftor.[16]

A key question for any therapy which can potentially affect the natural history of a disease course is whether efficacy can be demonstrated in patients with mild disease (i.e., before irreversible changes within the airway occur). The use of more sensitive outcome measures has helped to move this area forward in patients with normal lung function as assessed by FEV_1, the historically favored primary outcome. In patients with mild CF lung disease ($FEV_1 \geq 90\%$ predicted) aged 6 years and older with the Gly551Asp mutation, a clinical trial in patients demonstrated significant improvements in lung clearance index (LCI).[18] LCI has also been used to demonstrate efficacy in those with advanced disease ($FEV_1 < 40\%$ predicted).[19]

Following the clinical trial that demonstrated that improvement in LCI was observed in those with preexisting normal FEV_1, it became important to consider if the CFTR modulator ivacaftor could be given in the early years of life because CFTR modulation therapy might have the greatest potential to prevent organ damage at that stage. Outcome measures for lung efficacy are a challenge in this population, and therefore a clinical trial in preschool children was primarily undertaken using outcomes for safety and pharmacodynamics (sweat chloride). This open label study (KIWI) involved ivacaftor (50 mg or 75 mg twice daily) in preschool children with any *CFTR* gating mutation and found it was well-tolerated and safe, although an elevation in liver function tests (transaminases) warrants close monitoring in the clinic.[20] A notable finding in the KIWI study was the effects of ivacaftor on growth and pancreatic function. Increases in fecal elastase and decreases in serum immunoreactive trypsinogen on treatment were suggestive of partial improvement of exocrine pancreatic function. As a systemically administered therapy, small molecule CFTR modulators have the potential to affect nonpulmonary disease manifestations. At the time of writing, efficacy outcomes (LCI and computed tomography [CT] scans) are being further explored in a trial in 3–5 year olds (NCT02742519) and a trial in infants less than 24 months of age (NCT02725567) is assessing safety, pharmacokinetic, and pharmacodynamic outcomes.

Although initially restricted to patients with the commonest mutation in the class III group, *in vitro* evidence of efficacy in other *CFTR* gating and residual function mutations[15,21,22] led to the investigation of ivacaftor in non-Gly551Asp gating mutations and the Arg117His (R117H) class IV mutation. Efficacy was successfully demonstrated in non-Gly551Asp gating mutations in the KONNECTION study,[23] although for patients with Arg117His (KONDUCT),[24] efficacy was limited to patients older than 18 year. The authors suggested that ivacaftor may therefore be beneficial for patients with the Arg117His mutation who have established CF disease. The lack of effect in children may reflect the inclusion of this mutation in many CF newborn screen testing algorithms and its known phenotypic variability with milder variants being detected and thus skewing the population included in such clinical trials.

Key to the success of CFTR modulation is in the ability to alter the disease trajectory in CF. There is already some evidence that ivacaftor can achieve this,[1] and as the proportion of patients for whom this drug becomes part of routine CF care increases (in terms of mutation class and younger age), long-term pharmacovigilance will be eagerly awaited. The open label extension study of patients enrolled in the STRIVE and ENVISION trials (PERSIST; NCT01117012) reported absolute change in FEV_1 at week 96 (i.e., total duration of ivacaftor 144 weeks) of 9.4% and 10.3% in adults/adolescents and children, respectively, in those receiving ivacaftor in the original phase III trials.[25] A longitudinal study of ivacaftor in the postapproval setting reported improvements in several clinically relevant markers, including lung function, body mass index, mucociliary clearance, hospitalization rate, and *Pseudomonas aeruginosa* burden.[26]

The successes of the ivacaftor clinical trials have sparked heightened interest in the search for more efficacious CFTR potentiators. Several companies are conducting early-phase clinical trials at the time of writing. This includes Galapagos NV with GLPG1837[27] in patients with the Gly551Asp mutation (NCT02707562) and the S1251N gating mutation (NCT02690519), as well as two other molecules. Novartis Pharmaceuticals have undertaken a trial of their CFTR potentiator, QBW251, in patients with CF (NCT02190604).[28]

Concert Pharmaceuticals, Inc. have conducted a phase I trial of deuterated ivacaftor. Their strategy is based on selectively replacing hydrogen atoms with deuterium (a heavy isotope of hydrogen), with the aim of stabilizing carbon bonds within a compound. Their deuterium-modified ivacaftor (CTP-656) had a superior pharmacokinetic profile to standard ivacaftor (Kalydeco) in healthy volunteers.[29]

As a single agent therapy, the patients benefiting from potentiator therapies are limited to a minority of the CF population with class III and IV mutations. In patients with the class II mutation Phe508del, the *in vitro* data suggesting small potentiating effects of ivacaftor in bronchial epithelial cells from Phe508del homozygotes[15,30] did not translate into clinically detectable benefit.[31] Strategies for tackling Phe508del are discussed in the next section.

Correctors

Drugs that target class II mutations in CF (e.g., Phe508del) in which a misfolding of CFTR leads to failure of its trafficking to the apical cell membrane are referred to as *correctors*. Because this class of mutations represents the greatest proportion of mutations within the CF population, an effective CFTR modulator in this group would have a profound impact. The furthest developed drug in this class is the oral small molecule drug lumacaftor (VX-809, Vertex Pharmaceuticals). *In vitro* studies demonstrated that in cell culture of bronchial epithelial cells homozygous for the Phe508del mutation, lumacaftor increased chloride secretion to approximately 14% of wild-type CFTR,[32] through its mechanism of action on the processing of CFTR in the endoplasmic reticulum. Functional evidence of efficacy as assessed by sweat chloride was demonstrated in adult CF patients homozygous for the Phe508del mutation, although these were small in magnitude and were not associated with significant clinical changes.[33] The single drug approach may be limited by the complexity required to restore CFTR function in patients with Phe508del.[34]

There are several other drugs being investigated that may have a novel mechanism of action in modulating CFTR. The nitric oxide pathway may be a possible CFTR corrector strategy (either via the direct or indirect pathways).[35] Examples in early-phase clinical trials include N91115 (Nivalis Therapeutics, Inc.), which the company describes as a first-in-class CFTR "stabilizer." N91115 is an S-nitrosoglutathione reductase inhibitor. The aim is to stabilize CFTR both from within the cell and on the apical surface of the airway epithelial cells. Following a phase Ib clinical trial investigating N91115 monotherapy in adults homozygous for the phe508del mutation (NCT02227888), a phase II trial of safety and efficacy in patients receiving lumacaftor/ivacaftor (i.e., as a triple approach) (NCT02589236) has recently completed. Most recently, Nivalis Therapeutics have commenced a further phase II trial of N91115 in adult patients heterozygous for F508del-CFTR and a gating mutation receiving ivacaftor treatment (NCT02724527); results have not been published in a peer-reviewed journal, but at the time of writing, the company's press release indicates a safe but ineffective drug (http://ir.nivalis.com/press-releases/detail/60). Also involving the nitric oxide pathway, the drug riociguat (BAY63-2521, Adempas, Bayer), with existing approval for the treatment of chronic thromboembolic pulmonary hypertension, has been found to have CFTR corrector function and is currently being investigated in a phase II study (NCT02170025) assessing safety, tolerability, and efficacy of the orally administered drug in adult patients homozygous for phe508del. Phosphodiesterase inhibitors including sildenafil, vardenafil, and tadalafil may also prove useful in CF caused by class II mutations. Using an inhaled preparation, these drugs have been shown to induce changes toward normality in nPD measurements in p.Phe508del mice,[36] but it has been suggested that high doses may preclude this as a therapeutic approach in humans.[37]

Combination Therapy

Given the lack of clinical efficacy of lumacaftor alone in patients homozygous for Phe508del, the addition of a potentiator to maximize the function of any CFTR reaching the cell surface is an attractive option. Most research to date has been with the combination of ivacaftor and lumacaftor, the potentiator and corrector described in previous sections. *In vitro* studies showed that addition of ivacaftor to lumacaftor-exposed Phe508del homozygous cells further increased chloride transport to 25% of wild type,[32] in keeping with prior observations of defective gating in addition to defective processing of Phe508del CFTR.

Subsequently, two large phase III RCTs (TRAFFIC and TRANSPORT) studied patients aged 12 years and older homozygous for Phe508del. They showed relatively small but significant improvement in lung function of the magnitude of 3%–4% predicted FEV_1, on a regimen of lumacaftor (either 400 mg twice daily or 600 mg daily) and ivacaftor 250 mg twice daily.[38] More impressive was the reduction in the rate of pulmonary exacerbations (30%–39% reduction). Although the lumacaftor-ivacaftor was generally well tolerated, trial discontinuation was higher in the active arm, and the adverse events occurring more frequently in the active treatment group tended to be respiratory in nature (e.g., bronchospasm and dyspnea). The combination therapy lumacaftor-ivacaftor has now been licensed by the US Food and Drug Administration (FDA) (lumacaftor/ivacaftor, Orkambi, Vertex Pharmaceuticals, Inc.), and is available clinically in several countries, although reimbursement is not approved worldwide.

The magnitude of the improvement in lung function with ivacaftor and lumacaftor in Phe508del homozygotes was lower than that observed with ivacaftor in class III mutations.[38] *In vitro* assays on Phe508del human bronchial epithelial cells treated with lumacaftor/ivacaftor have shown that ivacaftor may be destabilizing CFTR that has been transported to the cell membrane by lumacaftor, and this may help to explain the relatively limited efficacy observed with this combination of drugs *in vivo* in clinical trials. This destabilization has been shown to cause a reduction of CFTR on the apical cell membrane and a reduced half-life resulting from increased turnover.[39,40]

As described for CFTR modulation with ivacaftor, one of the key aims is to be able to instigate therapy before irreversible changes resulting from CF lung disease occur. Therefore the tolerability, safety profile, and efficacy in children and those with mild disease are important. A phase III trial in younger children (6–11 years) to assess the impact of Orkambi in earlier disease (NCT02514473), using LCI as the primary outcome, is in progress.

Lumacaftor is the only CFTR corrector to have progressed to licensing (as the combination formulation); however, other candidates are being investigated. The corrector VX-661 in combination with ivacaftor (Vertex Pharmaceutical, Inc.) showed promising results in early-phase trials[41,42] and is currently undergoing evaluation in a number of large, phase III clinical trials in Phe508del homozygotes (NCT02347657) and Phe508del heterozygotes with a second mutation (1) which has been shown to be responsive to ivacaftor (NCT02412111), (2) with residual function (NCT02392234), and (3) likely unresponsive to VX661 or ivacaftor (NCT02516410). Following participation in these trials, patients may elect to roll over into a longer, open-label trial (NCT02565914). Interestingly the compound VX-661 does not appear to destabilize ivacaftor in the same way reported for the lumacaftor/ivacaftor combination and thus may be suited to the combination therapy approach.

Other companies are also developing drugs for a triple therapy approach with existing combinations of CFTR modulation. Proteostasis Therapeutics, Inc. have developed PTI-428 as a CFTR amplifier, which aims to increase an immature form of CFTR protein to provide additional substrate for other CFTR modulators. A safety and pharmacokinetic study involving adult patients with CF is being undertaken at the time of writing (NCT02718495). Flatley Discovery Labs have a combination of modulators from which encouraging *in vitro* data have recently been reported.[43]

Autophagy, a major mechanism used by cells in protein turnover within the cytoplasm, has been shown to be abnormal in CF cells with the F508del mutation related to depletion of the essential autophagy-related protein Beclin 1 (BECN1). A phase II trial of two proteostasis regulators (cysteamine and epigallocatechin gallate [EGCG]) for the autophagy-dependent rescue of CFTR reported improvements in sweat chloride, inflammatory markers, and FEV_1 in patients with Phe508del or other class II homozygotes or compound heterozygotes.[44,45] The authors reported that patients in this trial whose primary nasal brushed cells did not respond to cysteamine plus EGCG *in vitro* also exhibited deficient therapeutic responses *in vivo*.[45]

Other Noncystic Fibrosis Transmembrane Conductance Regulator–Based Approaches

Small molecule drugs targeting the epithelial sodium channel ENaC are emerging as an active field of research. For example, Vertex Pharmaceuticals, Inc. have, at the time of writing, commenced a phase II clinical trial of a triple therapy approach with VX-371 (P-1037) in combination with Orkambi (NCT02709109) in patients aged 12 years and older homozygous for the F508del CFTR mutation.

Cystic Fibrosis Gene Therapy

The successful development and licensing of Kalydeco and Orkambi have provided proof of concept that correction of CFTR function can improve CF. Gene therapy defined as the addition of *CFTR* DNA into cells, which is transcribed and translated into CFTR protein, has been developed since identification of the disease-causing gene more than 25 years ago, and important milestone studies are shown in Box 53.1.

Box 53.1   Gene Therapy Milestone Studies

- Three years after cloning of *CFTR*, Rosenfeld et al. provided evidence of successful CFTR mRNA and protein expression after adenovirus-mediated *CFTR* cDNA transfer into cotton rats[95]
- Four years after cloning of *CFTR* Hyde et al. showed that nonviral *CFTR* cDNA transfer could partially correct the chloride transport in tracheal epithelium of CF knockout mice[96]
- In the same year, Zabner et al. performed the first, albeit small and not placebo-controlled, CF gene therapy trial in three patients. A first-generation adenoviral vector carrying the *CFTR* cDNA was administered to the nasal epithelium and shown to partially restore cAMP-mediated chloride transport[97]
- Five years after cloning of *CFTR*, Crystal et al. performed the first phase I dose-escalation CF gene therapy study. This was first and foremost a safety study and showed transient inflammatory responses only at the highest dose (2×10^9 plaque forming units [PFUs]/patient)[98]
- Six years after cloning of *CFTR*, Caplen et al. provided first evidence that a nonviral gene transfer agent (DC-Chol:DOPE) complexed with *CFTR* cDNA could partially correct cAMP-mediated chloride transport in the nasal epithelium of CF patients[99]
- Ten years after cloning of *CFTR*, the first of six AAV2 trials was published.[100] These trials initially looked encouraging[101] but ultimately were discontinued due to lack of efficacy
- The same year, Alton et al. demonstrated that a nonviral gene transfer agent (GL67A) complexed with a plasmid DNA carrying the *CFTR* cDNA could partially correct cAMP-mediated chloride transport in the lungs of CF patients[53]
- Twenty-six years after cloning of *CFTR*, Alton et al. demonstrated that repeated administration of GL67A complexed with a plasmid DNA carrying the *CFTR* cDNA significantly, albeit modestly, stabilized lung function in CF patients[59]

CF, Cystic fibrosis; *CFTR,* cystic fibrosis transmembrane conductance regulator.

The combination of (1) CF being a single gene disorder, (2) the comparatively easy, noninvasive access to the lung, (3) the fact that gene therapy does not require detailed information about the patient's genotype or to which of the six mutation classes these might belong, and (4) lack of understanding of the disease pathophysiology led to unrealistic expectations by academia, industry, and patients in early phases of the program. It quickly became clear that CF gene therapy was considerably more challenging than initially anticipated. However, over the past two decades significant progress has been made, including identification of suitable gene transfer agents (GTAs), understanding limitations of molecular surrogate markers, and optimization of clinical trial design.

The older literature related to CF gene therapy has been reviewed in many publications (e.g., see Griesenbach et al.),[46] and therefore we will provide a brief description and discussion of the key lessons learned and focus on more recent progress in the field.

VIRAL VERSUS NONVIRAL GENE TRANSFER AGENTS

Vectors that carry nucleic acids into cells fall broadly into two categories; viral and nonviral vectors. In general, viral vectors are more efficient because they have evolved to infect cells and therefore carry suitable proteins to overcome at least some of the barriers described later. Adenoviruses and adeno-associated viruses (AAVs) have a natural tropism for the lungs and seemed obvious choices for early CF gene therapy trials.[46] However, preexisting and induced immune responses to the viral vector limit their usefulness for the treatment of a lifelong disease such as CF. To date, we have not seen convincing evidence in either preclinical models or clinical trials to demonstrate that repeated administration of adenoviral or AAV vectors to immune-competent lungs without loss of efficacy is feasible.

In contrast to viral vectors, the simpler structure of nonviral formulations that generally do not contain proteins make them less likely to induce immune responses. Between 1999 and 2004 nine CF gene therapy trials used nonviral GTAs.[46] Combined, these studies presented a scattered picture with some trials detecting vector-specific mRNA and some partial correction of the chloride transport defect, whereas others did not. Proof of concept for efficacy (based on detection of mRNA and partial correction of chloride transport on nPD) of repeated administration (three doses delivered to the nasal epithelium) of a nonviral vector was only assessed in one study.[47]

LUNG IS A CHALLENGING TARGET ORGAN

Potent intracellular and extracellular barriers that have evolved to protect the human host from viruses, bacteria, and other inhaled particles also "protect" against inhalation and uptake of inhaled GTAs. Among the intracellular barriers, the nuclear membrane presents a significant hurdle, particularly for nonviral GTAs. Furthermore, there are extracellular barriers, including airway mucus, mucociliary clearance, and mucopurulent CF sputum,[48–50] as well as humoral and cellular immune responses (see Xia et al.[51] for more detailed discussion).

RECENT PROGRESS IN THE FIELD

The UK CF Gene Therapy Consortium (GTC; http://www.cfgenetherapy.org.uk/; https://www.youtube.com/watch?v=JiO23xq8LJA) was founded in 2001, consisting of the three groups in Edinburgh, London, and Oxford that had previously conducted CF gene therapy trials. The explicit aim was to share expertise and knowledge in a translational program to assess whether gene therapy could lead to clinical benefit. It is generally considered inappropriate for authors to devote a considerable proportion of a review to their own work. However, the GTC is currently the only group conducting CF gene therapy trials and recently completed a pivotal phase IIb multidose trial. In brief, the GTC has:

a. Following an extensive screening program, determined that the cationic lipid formulation GL67A, first used in the 1990s, remained the most potent nonviral GTA for airway gene transfer some two decades later.[52]

b. Identified that first-generation plasmids used in previous trials contained many immune-stimulatory CpG dinucleotides that may have contributed to the mild "flu-like" symptoms noted in previous single dose lung trials.[53,54] We improved the plasmid (termed pGM169) by removing the CpG islands, codon-optimized the CFTR cDNA, and generated the novel regulatory element, hCEFI, consisting of the elongation factor 1α promoter coupled to the human cytomegalovirus (CMV) enhancer.[55]

c. Undertaken regulatory-compliant multidose toxicology studies in mice[55,56] and sheep,[56,57] supporting progression into a multidose clinical trial. Interestingly, repeated aerosolization of pGM169/GL67A to mice led to cumulative dose-related expression on repeat dosing, reaching 94 ± 19% of endogenous murine CFTR levels after 12 deliveries. These data further supported progression into a multidose clinical trial.

d. Shown in a single dose, dose-escalation (5, 10, and 20 mL of pGM169/GL67A) phase I/IIa safety trial, that despite CpG-depletion of the plasmid, patients receiving the 10- and 20-mL dose still developed mild "flu-like" symptoms including a fever.[58] The likely explanation is that both the volume administered to the lung and the lipid contribute to the inflammatory response (in addition to CpG sequences). The 5 mL dose (containing approximately 13 mg plasmid DNA) was chosen for the multidose trial.

e. Undertaken a double-blind, placebo-controlled multidose trial. Patients (12 years or older with moderate or mild lung disease) received 5 mL of nebulized pGM169/GL67A or 5 mL 0.9% saline every month for 12 months. The primary end point was a change in lung function measured as a relative change of % predicted FEV_1. Efficacy data from 116 patients (who received nine or more doses) were analyzed.[59] The treatment was well tolerated, and the trial met its primary end point, showing a significant, albeit modest, treatment effect in the pGM169/GL67A group versus placebo at 12 months' follow-up (3.7%, 95% confidence interval [CI] 0.1–7.3; $P = .046$; Fig. 53.3A). Prespecified subgroup analysis showed that patients with more severe lung disease at the start of treatment responded better than those with milder lung disease at the start of treatment (see Fig. 53.3B and C). Reasons for

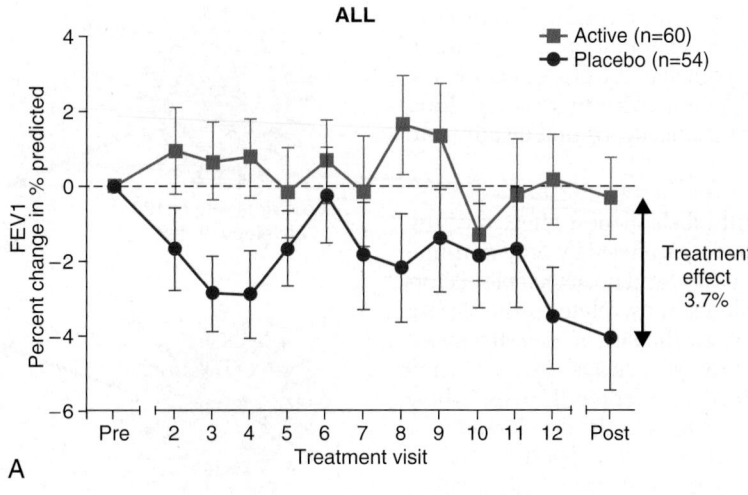

A

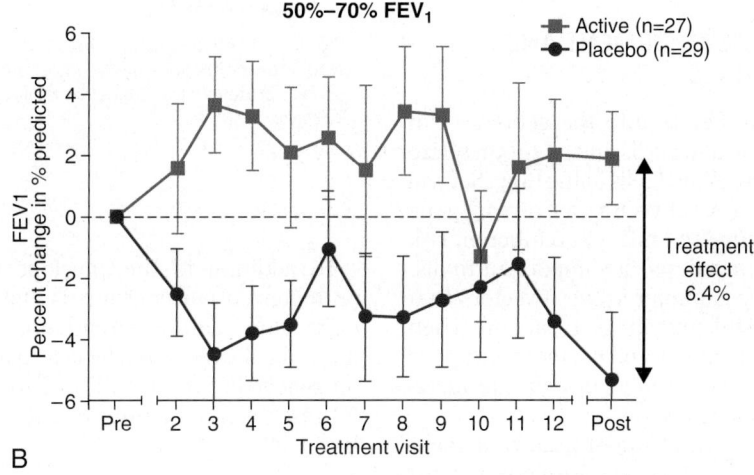

B

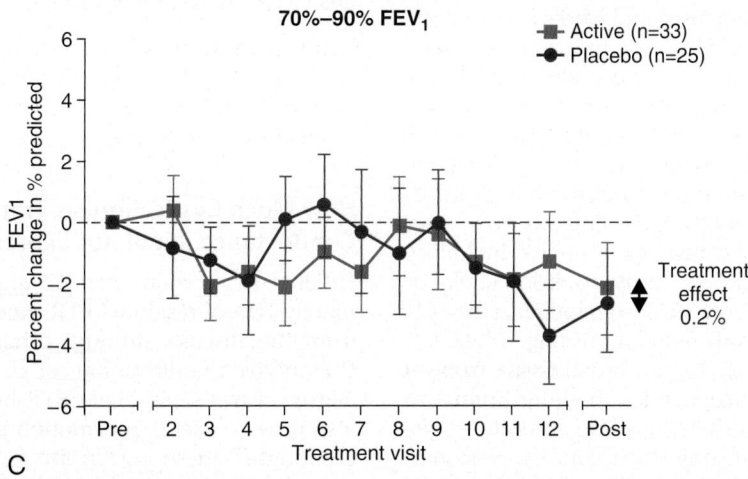

C

Fig. 53.3 Change in the primary outcome ($FEV_1\%$ predicted) over a 12-month period of a phase 2b RCT (59) of nonviral CFTR gene therapy *(blue)* or placebo *(red)*; (A) within the whole group there was stabilization of the actively treated arm which was significantly ($P < .05$) different than placebo, (B) subjects with baseline $FEV_1 < 70\%$ who demonstrated a pronounced effect, and (C) subjects with baseline $FEV_1 > 70\%$ in whom little effect was seen. *CFTR,* Cystic fibrosis transmembrane conductance regulator; *FEV_1,* forced expiratory volume in 1 second; *RCT,* randomized controlled trial. (Modified from Alton EW, Armstrong DK, Ashby D, et al. Repeated nebulisation of non-viral CFTR gene therapy in patients with cystic fibrosis: a randomised, double-blind, placebo-controlled, phase 2b trial. *Lancet Respir Med.* 2015;3(9):684-691.)

this are currently unknown, and various hypotheses should be tested. One simple explanation may relate to the amount of material deposited in the proximal airways, which is likely higher in patients with more severe lung diseases due to sputum-restricted deposition distally into the smaller airways.

The statistically significant albeit modest effect on lung function shown in this trial was paralleled by only minimal changes in the ion transport assays and no detectable vector-specific mRNA. This discordance may relate to the timing and/or sensitivity of the assays, the site of measurement, and/or the relatively small area of airways assessed when using molecular assays and further questions the use of these assays as "go/no-go" decision points in the development of CF gene therapy. The results have raised questions about dose, dose interval, and suitability of placebo, which will be taken into consideration for future studies.

MORE RECENT VECTOR DEVELOPMENT AND UPCOMING CLINICAL TRIALS

Lentiviral vectors, which integrate into the genome, can transduce dividing and nondividing cells and might therefore be suitable for targeting differentiated cells in the lung. Several groups have investigated lentiviral vectors for airway gene transfer. Although integrating vectors have an inherent risk of inducing insertional mutagenesis, it is important to discriminate between the early gamma retroviral vectors that have been shown to cause leukemia in some patients when used for bone marrow transduction[60] and the more advanced lentiviral vectors, which have not shown evidence of insertional mutagenesis in clinical trials.[61-63]

Lentiviral vectors have no natural lung tropism and therefore require pseudotyping with appropriate envelope proteins to facilitate lung gene transfer. The vesicular stomatitis virus G (VSV-G) protein is commonly used and works well for bone marrow transduction *ex vivo*. However, for transduction of airway epithelium, it is necessary to precondition the tissue with detergents that damage the epithelium and allow access to the basolateral membrane via intercellular spaces.[64] This approach raises safety concerns for translation into clinical trials, particularly in CF patients with chronic lung infections. As a result, several groups, including our own, have investigated the use of other envelope proteins, including the baculovirus protein GP64,[65] proteins from Ebola or Marburg filoviruses,[66] the HA protein from influenza virus,[67] and the F and HN protein from Sendai virus (Fig. 53.4),[68-70] which are viruses that either have a broad tissue tropism (baculovirus) or a natural tropism for the lung (influenza and Sendai virus). We and others have shown that a single dose of lentivirus leads to lifelong stable gene expression in the murine lung (~2 years; Fig. 53.5) and that repeated administration of the vector (10 daily doses or 3 times one monthly doses) is feasible.[65,69,70] To date, there has been no report of insertional mutagenesis or other untoward toxicity in lungs of mice. A direct comparison between the lead nonviral vector GL67A that was used in the recently completed phase IIb CF gene therapy trial (see earlier) and the F/HN-pseudotyped lentiviral vector indicates that the virus is several log orders more efficient in transducing airway epithelial cells, which are the target cells for CF gene therapy.

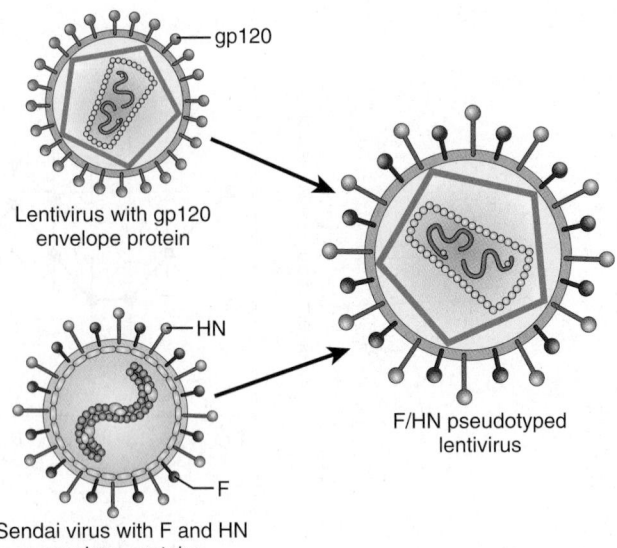

Fig. 53.4 Lentivirus, which does not possess natural tropism for the respiratory epithelium, has been pseudotyped to express the *F* and *HN* surface proteins of Sendai virus facilitating effective gene transfer to airways.

In addition to the envelope proteins, optimization of promoter/enhancer elements that drive recombinant protein expression require careful optimisation.[71] The efficiency, duration of expression, lack of toxicity, and, uniquely, efficacy on repeated administration support progression of the F/HN-pseudotyped lentivirus into a first-in-human phase I/IIa CF clinical trial.

OUTSTANDING QUESTIONS

Many of these questions, although raised in the context of gene therapy, also relate to the small molecule modulator field; certainly, lessons learned from one approach may have implications for others.

How Much Cystic Fibrosis Transmembrane Conductance Regulator Expression Do We Need?

Patients with certain "mild" CF mutations who retain approximately 10% of residual CFTR expression per cell do not suffer from lung disease, although other organs may be affected.[72] Phenotypic manifestations of CFTR dysfunction reflect the degree of transepithelial CFTR function *in vivo*, which may also provide useful information in guiding the "how much is enough?" question.[73] *In vitro* cell mixing experiments have shown that approximately 10% of non-CF cells restore CFTR-mediated chloride secretion when mixed with 90% of CF cells in a monolayer.[74] In a separate study, it was shown that CFTR must be expressed in at least 25% of cells grown in a monolayer to restore mucus transport.[75] However, these studies do not address whether complete correction of CFTR expression in 10% cells is equivalent to a low level (approximately 10%) of CFTR expression in all cells. We currently also do not know whether the various forms of genetic medicines are more likely to achieve the former or the latter.

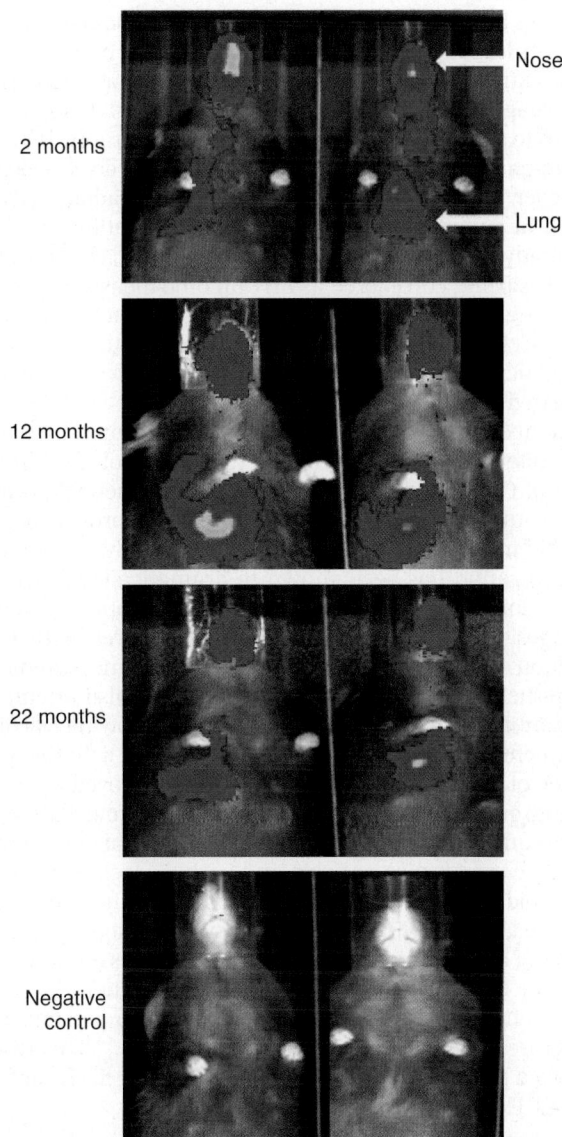

2 months Nose

Lung

12 months

22 months

Negative control

Fig. 53.5 Bioluminescent imaging demonstrates luciferase expression out to 22 months in the nose and lungs of mice dosed with the pseudotyped lentivirus vector. (Reused with permission from Griesenbach U, Inoue M, Meng C, et al. Assessment of F/HN-pseudotyped lentivirus as a clinically relevant vector for lung gene therapy. *Am J Respir Crit Care Med.* 2012;186(9):846-856.)

Which Cells Do We Need to Target for Restoration of Cystic Fibrosis Transmembrane Conductance Regulator Function?

CFTR is expressed in various cell types in the lung, including submucosal glands, ciliated epithelial cells, and goblet cells. It is currently unknown which cells express the CFTR transgene following gene transfer. To correct submucosal glands, any agents applied topically to the airways, such as gene transfer vectors and oligonucleotides, will need to negotiate ducts filled with mucus; this barrier may be substantial. It has been postulated that CFTR is also expressed in macrophages and neutrophils. Whether this leads to an intrinsic defect in host defense in the CF lung is still widely debated[76] and needs to be resolved before deciding whether these cell types are suitable targets.

Should Studies in Cystic Fibrosis Models Form a "Go/No-Go" Decision Point Before Progression Into Clinical Trials?

CF mice do not acquire spontaneous airway infections or develop CF lung disease, but the nasal epithelium shows the characteristic CF chloride and sodium transport defects.[77] However, the relevance of measurement of CFTR function in the murine nose (via *in vivo* potential difference) has been called into question by Ostrowski et al. who showed that expression of human CFTR under the transcriptional control of a cilia-specific promoter did not correct ion transport in CF knockout mice.[78] In addition, Grubb et al. have suggested that the olfactory, rather than the respiratory, nasal epithelium mainly contributes to the ion transport defect in CF mice.[79] Thus the CF mouse has been of limited value as a steppingstone to human gene therapy trials[80] and, in our opinion, should not be used as a go/no-go decision point for progression into gene therapy clinical trials. Whether correction of lung disease in CF knockout pigs or ferret is a better model to predict clinical success remains to be seen. Currently, these animals die shortly after birth due to intestinal disease and therefore are not yet available in large enough numbers to conduct clinically meaningful studies. In addition, it is currently unclear whether the CF-like pathology is a suitable enough mimic of human disease to be used as a critical decision point for therapeutic development.

Are There Other Genetic Medicine-Based Approaches?

In addition to the *"classical"* gene therapy described previously, mRNA as a template for CFTR gene supplementation has long been appealing as an alternative to DNA-based gene delivery because it avoids the rate-limiting step of nuclear entry into nondividing airway epithelial cells, being translated rapidly and efficiently directly in the cytoplasm[81] and chemical modifications made to enhance efficacy of mRNA therapy have been successful.[82] Proof of concept for the efficacy of repeated pulmonary delivery of chemically modified mRNA has been established in a murine model of surfactant protein B deficiency,[83] but due to a comparatively long transcript the development of CFTR mRNA therapy is more complex and has not been reported yet.

In addition to gene and mRNA therapy, *correction* of the genetic defect in the genome (gene editing) or in the mRNA (mRNA repair) are being developed. Genome editing using zinc finger nucleases, TALENS, or the CRISPR/Cas9 system are revolutionizing research and therapeutic strategies for many diseases.[84] In the context of CF, genome editing has been used to repair CFTR mutations and restore protein function in cell lines,[85] intestinal organoids,[86] and CF patient–derived induced pluripotent stem cells (iPS) *in vitro*.[87,88] This technology will be very useful for developing mutation-specific cell lines for drug screening.

Wong et al. have developed protocols to allow differentiation of human pluripotent stem cells into mature airway epithelium expressing functional CFTR protein,[89] which may lead to speculation that genome-edited iPS cells could be differentiated into airway epithelial cells or airway progenitor cells, which could then be used to replenish cells in the CF lung. However, there are currently no successful reports of cell therapy in the lung due to the structural complexity of the organ.

The technology may also lead to proposals for genome editing of airway epithelial cells *in vivo*. However, there are several flaws with this. First, genome editing *in vivo* will require the delivery of the genome-editing molecules, as well as appropriate wild-type CFTR sequences, required for homologous recombination-based repair of the mutant CFTR, which is yet more complex than standard gene therapy. Second, current thinking is that airway epithelial cells are terminally differentiated and do not undergo homologous recombination. Third, one might argue that *in vivo* genome editing of airway progenitor cells is an alternative. However, these cells are buried beneath the surface epithelium and difficult to access with gene therapy vectors. In addition, airway progenitor cells divide very slowly, again making homologous recombination inefficient. The development of alternative gene editing strategies may, in the future, be able to overcome these current problems.

Different strategies have been suggested to *"repair"* mutations in the CFTR mRNA. Small molecule drugs such as ataluren, which bypass premature stop mutation, are being assessed in clinical trials (described in detail previously). Alternative strategies are based on direct repair of the mRNA using a short RNA oligonucleotides. QR-010, developed by ProQR Therapeutics, targets the Phe508del mutation and is currently being assessed in early phase clinical trials (NCT02532764, NCT02564354).

Evaluating Therapies Targeting the Basic Defect in Clinical Trials

There has never been a more crucial time to be able to identify suitable end points for clinical trials in CF. Clinical trials of CFTR modulators have already provided us with a wealth of information about trial design and end points, which will guide those in the future. The potential to modify a disease course (as reported for ivacaftor reducing the decline in lung function over time in older subjects) means that questions such as when to start therapy or the severity of disease for which they are recommended are important, particularly in areas of the world where prohibitive cost of drugs may impact on access to patients. It is likely that those with the greatest to gain from such treatments will be those with mild disease (i.e., before the onset of irreversible structural change and established infection). Although FEV_1 is well established by the regulatory authorities as an acceptable outcome on which to evaluate efficacy in clinical trials, other measures remain in relative infancy. The role of pulmonary outcome measures such as LCI, as a more sensitive marker than FEV_1, is a continued area of development, and standardized protocols now exist to promote quality control (e.g., via the US Cystic Fibrosis Foundation Therapeutic Development Network or European CF Clinical Trials Network). Proof that LCI could be used to demonstrate efficacy in the ivacaftor trial involving patients with normal spirometry was important to the field—LCI is now also the primary outcome in the lumacaftor/ivacaftor combination therapy trial in those with mild disease. Pulmonary efficacy outcome measures for very young children may be more challenging to capture in multicenter studies; however, it is also of note that the regulatory

agencies have accepted extrapolated efficacy data from older patients for ivacaftor, in the presence of data on safety outcomes and markers of CFTR function (e.g., sweat chloride) in this age group.[20] There may be a role for radiologic outcomes (e.g., high-resolution computed tomography [HRCT]) in late-phase clinical trials in young children to detect efficacy; however, there are concerns over additional radiation exposure[90] in patients for whom a degree of radiation exposure is already a standard component of their CF care. However, HRCT is being considered as an outcome measure for trials in young children. Imaging modalities without radiation exposure may offer an alternative in the future, including magnetic resonance imaging (MRI)[91] with or without hyperpolarized gas (helium or xenon).[92]

Sweat chloride concentrations and/or nPD measurements have often been included in the trial protocols for clinical trials of CFTR modulators and for the latter, gene therapies. These outcomes are of interest because they provide organ-specific information about CFTR function. Sweat chloride concentration has been shown to dramatically reduce following initiation of CFTR small molecule therapies, although changes within patients do not correlate well with lung function outcomes.[93] Within the airway, nPD measurements of epithelial CFTR chloride transport have also attempted to quantify CFTR activity. Changes in nPD following ivacaftor treatment were relatively small in comparison with the magnitude of lung function and nutritional improvement seen, raising questions about the degree of "normalization" of nPD required to demonstrate CFTR functional efficacy; the measurement is also variable and perhaps lacks sensitivity. Organoids, hollow structures formed *ex vivo* from epithelia obtained from, for example, rectal suction biopsies, are an evolving area of interest because these models allow assessment of CFTR function at the individual patient level (an approach that may be particularly relevant for patients with very rare or uncategorized CFTR mutations).[94] This would enable a personalized approach to predicting likely efficacy of a CFTR modulator.

Challenges for the Field

Aside from the technical challenges associated with discovering novel agents and testing them as sole or combination agents *in vitro* or *in vivo*, there are other significant challenges to consider. These include managing patient expectations and designing future clinical trials in the limited number of CF patients worldwide, particularly with powering late-phase clinical trials appropriately when effect sizes may be expected to be small. In comparison with the early trials of CFTR modulators when comparison was made with placebo, as these drugs become standard care for an increasing proportion of the CF population, this will no longer be appropriate. Adding new molecules onto these "standards of care," particularly if combined effects are sought, will require careful consideration of trial design and effect size. The field is still in its infancy, and as CFTR modulators become established as part of routine care in CF, the long-term impact on outcomes will become clear. National and international CF registries will be able to play an important role in capturing this impact at the population level in the real-world setting. In an era where treatment options are becoming personalized according to genotype, ensuring that such information is known for each patient is important for treatment options and eligibility for clinical trials.

The CFTR modulators licensed for use are associated with high per-patient drug costs—which is particularly relevant for treatments that are likely to be taken on a lifelong basis. The impact of this cost from a patient perspective will vary across the globe and according to whether there is an insurance-based or national health care system.

Summary

It is difficult to underestimate the impact of CFTR modulators over recent years and the momentum driving investigation into further-refined treatments targeting the underlying molecular defect in CF. The impressive results of the clinical trials in patients with class III mutations may be difficult to follow, and it will be important not to set the therapeutic bar too high based on these data, but increased understanding of the abnormalities in the structure and function of CFTR protein will help to better understand the approach or approaches required for normalizing function and in doing so help to rationalize the design of clinical trials. In addition, to identify progressively more efficacious drugs, determining the appropriate patient population for each approach will be key. Long-term follow-up to understand not only potential impact on disease modification but also the safety profile of these novel agents is paramount. In the context of such success with certain of these small molecule approaches, questions are sometimes raised about the relevance of gene therapy and other genetic approaches, which are, undeniably, some way behind. We perceive three major benefits of this approach: (1) gene replacement is completely mutation agnostic, so applicable to all classes of mutations including those that are incompletely understood; (2) the potential for long duration expression translating into infrequent treatment, and (3) topical application reducing the potential for drug-drug interactions. The latter are substantial for current, systemically absorbed CFTR modulators. Furthermore, we consider that there could be substantial synergy by combining gene-based and small molecule approaches, to build on the potential of each.

Overall, we are enthusiastic about the potential for therapies targeting the basic defect. Maybe future optimal approaches will harness the benefits of more than one of these approaches and lead to considerable synergy.

Declaration of Interests

GD, UG, and EA have no interests to declare. JCD has served on advisory boards, undertaken educational activities, and lead clinical trials for which Imperial College London has received fees, for the following companies relevant to this chapter: Vertex, PTC, AlgiPharma, Novartis, Galapagos, Bayer, Chiesi. JCD, GD, UG, and EA are part of the UK CF GTC, which has received funding from the UK Cystic Fibrosis Trust and the National Institute for Health Research (NIHR).

Acknowledgments

Work conducted by EA, JCD, and UG is supported by the NIHR Respiratory Disease Biomedical Research Unit at the Royal Brompton and Harefield NHS Foundation Trust and Imperial College London. GD is supported by a NIHR Academic Clinical Lectureship at University College London and by the NIHR Biomedical Research Centre at Great Ormond Street Hospital for Children NHS Foundation Trust.

References

Access the reference list online at ExpertConsult.com.

Interstitial Lung Disease

54 New Concepts in Children's Interstitial and Diffuse Lung Disease

ROBIN DETERDING, MD

The field of children's interstitial and diffuse lung disease (chILD) has undergone tremendous development over the past decade, driven by new genetic discoveries, improved techniques in imaging and lung biopsy, and organized efforts to better define clinical phenotypes (Table 54.1).[1] This progress has resulted in recognition of new disorders, the definition of a diffuse lung disease pediatric classification system, and formation of the chILD Foundation [http://child-foundation.org/(USchILD); http://www.childlungfoundation.org/(UKchILD)] and chILD research networks around the world. Research networks in the USA and the European Union now have prospective multicenter registries. Chapters in this section have been organized to align with these new developments and to provide the reader with a new framework to care for these children.

The cliché that "children are not little adults" is a good paradigm to explain the confusing early literature on children with ILD.[1,2] Although adult patients with desquamative interstitial pneumonitis (DIP) were found to have a good prognosis, children with DIP had high mortality.[3,4] DIP in children is now a recognized pathologic phenotype, which is consistent with congenital surfactant mutations that have significant mortality.[5,6] Conversely, children with severe ILD were frequently labeled as cases of idiopathic pulmonary fibrosis (IPF),[7,8] which is synonymous histologically with usual interstitial pneumonia (UIP), a leading cause of mortality in adult ILD.[9] However, on further review, the histologic diagnostic criteria for UIP characterized by fibroblast foci have not been seen in infants and young children, and have been seen in only one older adolescent.[10] New disorders in young children less than 2 years of age—not previously described in adult patients—were also reported. There were disorders, such as neuroendocrine cell hyperplasia of infancy (NEHI),[11,12] pulmonary interstitial glycogenosis (PIG),[13] and alveolar capillary dysplasia with misalignment of pulmonary veins (ACDMPV).[14] The differences in diagnosis highlighted the fact that forcing children with ILD into adult classification systems did not serve their interests and signaled the need to reorganize thinking in this area, and to create a pediatric-specific diffuse lung disease classification system.[6,9]

New Concepts, Terminology, and Classification

The field of diffuse lung disease is large and includes commonly recognized pediatric diseases. For example, diffuse lung diseases, such as cystic fibrosis, chronic lung disease of prematurity, and pulmonary infections have recognized clinical presentations and diagnostic testing. However, once these more recognized disorders have been ruled out, some children remain undiagnosed and are labeled with the general term ILD, as if this were a final diagnosis, or they are listed as having unknown lung disease. The concept of chILD syndrome was created to further define this subset of poorly diagnosed children with diffuse lung disease.[15] chILD syndrome is defined as a child who has three to four of the following findings without a known underlying lung disease to fully explain the clinical condition: (1) respiratory symptoms, such as coughing, rapid breathing, or exercise intolerance; (2) physical signs, such as crackles, adventitial breathing sounds, digital clubbing, or intercostal retractions; (3) a low blood oxygen tension or hypoxemia; and (4) diffuse parenchymal abnormalities on chest imaging.[16] chILD syndrome is a constellation of findings that should signal the clinician that further diagnostic evaluation is indicated to reach a definitive diagnosis. Using this definition, Van Hook reviewed two large data sets of young children with biopsy-proven diffuse lung disease and found this definition to be sensitive to make the diagnosis of chILD syndrome.[17] Furthermore, if a child with a known diagnosis has symptoms out of proportion to the recognized disease, they may still have chILD syndrome and require further evaluation for a secondary diagnosis. This is an important nuance, as some chILD diseases occur in conjunction with other known conditions, such as congenital heart disease and chronic lung disease of prematurity or PIG.[6] (See Chapter 56 for further discussion.)

The designation of a pediatric-specific classification system for diffuse lung disease was essential. Based on the expertise of Dr. Claire Langston and her extensive experience reviewing lung biopsies in children with diffuse lung disease, a new clinical and pathologic classification system was proposed, which incorporated features unique to children, especially the category "disorders more common in infancy" (see Table 54.1).[5] A landmark study, published in 2007, reported on the application of this classification system by a multidisciplinary cooperative that reviewed more than 180 lung biopsies over a 5-year period in children less than 2 years of age at 11 children's hospitals in North America.[6] This review further established that the Langston classification system could realistically be applied, and was appropriate, for infants and young children. Chapters in the chILD section are organized loosely around these categories, and should provide a diagnostic framework for children with diffuse lung disease. The Europeans have used a similar classification with minor differences.[18] Refinements of this classification system are evolving and will continue to evolve as more genetic disease

Table 54.1   Diffuse Pediatric Lung Disease Classification

Classification Category	Specific Disorders	Common Age Presentation
Disorders More Common in Infancy		
Developmental Disorders	Alveolar capillary dysplasia with misalignment of pulmonary veins	Birth
Growth Abnormality Disorders (alveolar simplification)	Pulmonary hypoplasia, chronic neonatal lung disease associated with chromosomal disorders, associated with congenital heart disease	Birth
Specific Conditions of Unknown Etiology	Neuroendocrine cell hyperplasia of infancy (NEHI), pulmonary interstitial glycogenosis (PIG)	Birth—1 month (PIG) Infancy—24 months (NEHI)
Surfactant Dysfunction Mutations	Surfactant protein B (*SFTPB*), surfactant protein C (*SFTPC*), ATP-binding cassette A3 (*ABCA3*); NKX2.1 (thyroid transcription factor 1); and histology consistent with a surfactant mutation	Birth (*SFTPB*) Birth—Adulthood (*SFTPC, ABCA3 NKX2.1*)
Disorders Related to Systemic Disease	Immune-mediated collagen vascular disease, storage disease, sarcoidosis, and Langerhans cell histiocytosis.	Childhood—Adolescence
Disorders of the Normal Host/Environment Exposure	Infectious or postinfectious process, hypersensitivity pneumonitis, aspiration, eosinophilic pneumonia.	Infancy—Adolescence
Disorders of the Immunocompromised Host	Opportunistic infections, transplantation and rejection, therapeutic interventions	Infancy—Adolescence
Disorders Masquerading as Interstitial Lung Disease	Pulmonary hypertension, cardiac dysfunction, veno-occlusive disease, lymphatic disorders	Birth—Adolescence
Unknown	Pulmonary biopsy tissue that cannot be classified	

associations are identified with the increased use of exome and genome sequencing for the diagnoses of unknown disease.

Retrospective studies in North America and Europe illustrate that children with chILD syndrome are overly represented in infants and younger children.[5,6] The application of the Langston classification system and an adapted version in Europe also demonstrated that over half the patients reviewed could be classified in the category "disorders more prevalent in infancy."[6,18] It is less clear if the Langston pediatric classification system is appropriate for older children. A recently published review of more than 180 lung biopsies in children older than 2 years of age at multiple centers in North America, using the same methodologies as the previous under 2 years of age retrospective review, suggests that the classification system does work well for these older children.[19] Biopsies in older children were rarely classified in the category "disorders more common in infancy"; older children had significantly more biopsies classified in the categories "disorders related to system disease" (see Chapters 57 and 58) and "disorders related to the immunocompromised host" (see Chapter 64).[19] This is further illustrated in the chapters that deal with these categories.

General Diagnostic Approach

The evaluation of chILD can be complicated, expensive, and associated with a risk for significant morbidity. To address these concerns, clinical guidelines focused on infants and young children have been published.[20]

Any newborn or child presenting with diffuse lung disease should have a complete history and physical (H&P) performed.[20,21] Although most diagnoses are not established with an H&P, specific clues can be uncovered that may be suggestive. Important history questions should include: birth history, a complete family history for use of oxygen or pulmonary deaths in any age family member to suggest genetic disease, previous pulmonary infections to suggest lung injury, family history of autoimmune disease, and a thorough environmental history to evaluate for hypersensitivity pneumonitis.[20,22] A complete physical examination should evaluate for nutritional indices, sinopulmonary disease, chest wall deformities, skin rash, clubbing, and neurologic disorders.

Other noninvasive testing should then be completed to rule out known causes of lung disease, such as cystic fibrosis, primary ciliary dyskinesia, aspiration, immunodeficiency, hypersensitivity pneumonitis, pulmonary infections, or autoimmune disease. An echocardiogram should be obtained to rule out masqueraders of lung diseases, such as congenital heart disease and pulmonary vein abnormalities, and to identify the presence of pulmonary hypertension, which may require more aggressive treatment, and may be associated with a worse prognosis.[23,24]

Imaging is often ordered to determine the pattern of diffuse lung disease. Chest radiographs are nonspecific and not helpful for specific diagnoses. Volume-controlled inspiratory and expiratory high-resolution computerized topography (HRCT) has been the most helpful way to obtain quality images for children with chILD syndrome, and may suggest bronchiolitis obliterans, pulmonary alveolar proteinosis, hypersensitive pneumonitis, or neuroendocrine cell hyperplasia.[25,26] The lowest amount of radiation possible should always be used. In children less than 4 years of age, or in those neurologically impaired, HRCTs will likely require sedation for optimal scans unless newer fast scanners are used, and some children may require prone positioning if atelectasis is seen posteriorly.[20,27] Though HRCT scanning is available at most hospitals around the country, it is highly recommended that scans in newborns, infants, and young children be completed at centers with expertise and protocols developed to optimize HRCTs for children with chILD using the lowest radiation dose possible. Newer imaging modalities are also emerging, such as hyperpolarized 3He ventilation magnetic resonance imaging (MRI), which may be more sensitive for early lung disease and is done without radiation.[28]

Infant pulmonary function testing is currently used to evaluate children with cystic fibrosis and chronic lung disease of prematurity. Limited, but important, data exist for children with chILD syndrome. Infant pulmonary functions can be completed reliably in children with NEHI at centers experienced in these techniques, and may be helpful because a classic pattern of airway obstruction and gas trapping has been reported in infants and young children.[29] Data suggest that the severity of small airway obstruction may correlate to the prominence of bombesin staining (a marker for neuroendocrine cells) in the lung tissue,[30] and that measures of small airway obstruction also may trend toward correlation with lower weight.[29] Some experienced chILD centers currently use infant pulmonary function data in conjunction with other testing (HRCT imaging, bronchoscopy, and clinical findings) to determine the need for a diagnostic lung biopsy in a child with classic findings for NEHI. The American Thoracic Society (ATS) consensus guidelines address the ideal timing and use for infant pulmonary function tests (PFTs).[20] New techniques with a lung clearance index have not yet been tested in children with chILD.

Genetic testing has emerged as a significant consideration in the evaluation of children with chILD, especially for inborn errors of surfactant metabolism. Any child with chILD syndrome without a clear etiology, and especially those who present with a family history of infant deaths, prolonged oxygen use, or family members with IPF, should have testing for abnormalities in surfactant metabolism.[31] Clinical testing is available through clinical laboratory improvement amendments (CLIA)–certified laboratories. A useful site for genetic information and laboratory testing is GeneTests (https://www.genetests.org/). The type of genetic testing is related to clinical presentation, so that those who present immediately in the newborn period with respiratory failure and pulmonary hypertension may be more likely to have surfactant protein B *(SFTPB)* and ATP-binding cassette A3 *(ABCA3)* mutations, while those who present later may be more likely to have surfactant protein C *(SFTPC)* mutations.[32] Genetic testing for (ABCA3) mutations has become very important for prognosis, as mutations that are null/null are associated with death or transplant at 1 year.[33] For those infants who present with respiratory failure and congenital hypothyroidism, investigations for mutations in the *NKX2.1* or thyroid transcription factor-1 *(TTF-1)* gene should be performed because this is a more recently recognized gene that regulates surfactant proteins.[34] NKX2.1 can also present with the complete triad of "Brain, Thyroid, Lung Syndrome" or a combination of any two organs. Children with chorea should be checked for NKX2.1[35] and evaluated for lung disease. As the time to sequence these genes has decreased and test results can become available in weeks (instead of months), many centers wait for test results before proceeding to lung biopsy if the child's clinical status is stable. If test results are unclear or if testing is negative, a lung biopsy may be indicated. There is still a great deal to learn about both genetic and environmental modifiers for these genes. Chapter 57 provides a more detailed discussion of disease associated with abnormal surfactant metabolism. Recently, the forkhead box transcription factor *(FOXF)* gene has been associated with familial cases of children with ACDMPV, and testing may be indicated for this fatal disorder.[36] Finally, more genetic mutations are likely to be found in children with chILD, such as NEHI, which has been shown to occur in families,[37] and some surfactant genetic abnormalities may be important modifiers of more common diseases such as respiratory distress of the

Table 54.2 New Genetic Mutations Associated With Diffuse Lung Disease

Disease	Genetic Defect
Lethal cystic lung disease	FLNA (filamin A, alpha) mutations
Severe pediatric PAP	MARS (methionyl-tRNA synthetase) mutations
Autoimmunity with arthritis, vasculitis, and chILD	COPA (Coatomer subunit alpha) mutations
Immunodeficiencies with monocytopenia, infections, lymphatic abnormalities, chILD, and PAP	GATA-2 transcription factor mutations
Immune-mediated lung disease— GLILD/CVID-like	LRBA (lipopolysaccharide-responsive and beigelike anchor protein) mutations
Immune-mediated lung disease— GLILD/CVID-like	CTLA 4 haploinsufficiency

CVID, Common variable immunodeficiency; *GLILD,* granulomatous-lymphocytic interstitial lung disease; *PAP,* pulmonary alveolar proteinosis.

newborn,[38,39] and adult diseases, such as chronic obstructive pulmonary disease (COPD).[40–42] Exome and whole genome technologies are becoming more available in a timely manner and at more reasonable price points. Also, there are pulmonary genetic panels that examine many genes. Genetics will clarify how many unknown chILD conditions exist and allow better mechanistic understanding of the disease. Many new diseases are being defined, and this will only grow with enhanced genetic techniques. Table 54.2 provides a list of recently described serious chILD diseases with genetic causes, such as mutations in filamin A (FLNA),[43] coatomer subunit alpha (COPA),[44] GATA-2 transcription factor,[45] Methionyl-tRNA synthetase (MARS),[46] lipopolysaccharide-responsive and beigelike anchor protein (LRBA)[47] and CTLA4.[48]

Bronchoscopy and bronchoalveolar lavage (BAL) remain important diagnostic tools in the evaluation of children with chILD syndrome. This is particularly true in children who have pulmonary hemorrhage, or who are immunocompromised to diagnose infection.[49–51] Bronchoscopy also may be important to rule out anatomic abnormalities and to suggest alveolar proteinosis,[52] pulmonary histiocytosis,[53] sarcoidosis,[54] and Niemann-Pick disease.[55] Active research is currently underway to identify diagnostic BAL biomarkers that may aid diagnosis, provide prognostic information, and shed insight into the pathophysiology of chILD syndrome.[56] More specific information about the use of bronchoscopy and BAL is addressed in the following chapters.

Lung biopsy remains the gold standard for diagnosis when the less invasive testing is negative or inconclusive.[20,57] The pediatric classification system relies heavily on histologic diagnosis, and the application of this classification system to lung biopsies is likely to provide a classification category or the diagnosis of the chILD syndrome.[6] At this time, only lung biopsies can accurately establish a diagnosis of pulmonary hemorrhage with diffuse capillaritis,[50] pulmonary interstitial glycogenosis,[6,13] alveolar simplification,[6] and ACDMPVs.[5] Lung biopsies also will likely provide the final diagnosis for infections in the immunocompromised patient, NEHI, unclear genetic testing for surfactant mutations, hypersensitivity, follicular bronchiolitis, and other lymphocytic disorders in chILD syndrome.[6,58,59] Newer techniques are emerging to evaluate tissue with advanced staining techniques for many protein markers simultaneously, to better define disease mechanisms.

When weighing the decision to pursue a lung biopsy, many factors that relate to the severity of illness, the progression of disease, and the skill of the surgical and pathology team should be considered. Any surgical approach should be the least invasive approach, and most centers now consider this to be a video-assisted thoracoscopy (VATS).[60] Centers experienced in chILD and VATS have shown that a chest tube may not be needed outside the operating room and may be pulled in the operating room if a simple lung biopsy was performed in a child who does not require positive pressure ventilation postoperatively.[61] Removing the chest tube early may also decrease pain, radiation, length of stay, and cost of care.[62] This is particularly important in chILD syndrome where splinting and pain may create scenarios that derecruit lung and prolong the hospital course. Selecting and processing the tissue is critical to making the correct diagnosis, and this must include selecting the best site for the biopsy, inflating the lung tissue for fixation, saving tissue for electron microscopy, and freezing tissue for future evaluation. Choosing a biopsy location is frequently aided by an HRCT, and a recent study in NEHI suggests that more than one biopsy site may be required to make this diagnosis.[30] Guidelines for tissue handling have been published by the chILD research pathology working group and should be followed.[63] Because experience reviewing the lung tissue in these rare conditions is limited, sending the slides for expert review is sometimes indicated.

Resources for Families and Physicians

The pursuit of improved care and cures for children with rare diffuse lung disease requires partnerships between families, clinicians, and foundations. Private foundations frequently provide advocacy and resources for family education and support, as well as funding, to move these fields forward through research.

References

Access the reference list online at ExpertConsult.com.

Suggested Reading

Deutsch GH, Young LR, Deterding RR, et al. Diffuse lung disease in young children: application of a novel classification scheme. *Am J Respir Crit Care Med.* 2007;176:1120–1128.

Fan LL, Dishop MK, Galambos C, et al. Diffuse lung disease in biopsied children 2–18 years of age: application of the chILD classification scheme. *Ann Am Thorac Soc.* 2015;12(10):1498–1505.

Kurland G, Deterding RR, Hagood JS, et al. An official American Thoracic Society clinical practice guideline: classification, evaluation, and management of childhood interstitial lung disease in infancy. *Am J Respir Crit Care Med.* 2013;188:376–394.

Langston C, Patterson K, Dishop MK, et al. A protocol for the handling of tissue obtained by operative lung biopsy: recommendations of the chILD pathology co-operative group. *Pediatr Dev Pathol.* 2006;9:173–180.

Nadlonek NA, Acker SN, Deterding RR, et al. Intraoperative chest tube removal following thoracoscopic lung biopsy results in improved outcomes. *J Pediatr Surg.* 2014;49:1573–1576.

55 *Rare Childhood Lung Disorders*

DANIEL LESSER, MD, LISA R. YOUNG, MD, and JAMES S. HAGOOD, MD

Introduction

Although some respiratory diseases occur rarely in the pediatric population, knowledge of these disorders is valuable from a number of perspectives. Timely diagnosis and treatment of rare disorders can be made only if the practitioner is familiar with the entity in question. Furthermore, elucidation of the pathophysiology underlying rare disorders can be applied to understanding both normal respiratory physiology and related but more prevalent disorders. Many rare lung disorders are covered in other chapters. This chapter characterizes both selected disorders with a primary respiratory component and respiratory disease occurring secondary to systemic disorders, with emphasis on interstitial lung disease. The diseases covered may present predominantly during childhood, such as respiratory disorders of the lymphatic system, or primarily during adulthood but with implications for pediatric patients, such as pulmonary alveolar microlithiasis (PAM) and alpha-1 antitrypsin (AAT) deficiency. Foundations provide invaluable information, support, and advocacy to families and patients affected by rare diseases and also function as important resources for practitioners. This chapter therefore directs the reader to selected disease-specific groups.

Respiratory Disorders of the Lymphatic System

A number of rare disorders related to dysregulation of lymphatic development occur in pediatric patients from infancy to adolescence. The normal pulmonary lymphatic system is composed of two interconnected pathways: one drains the subpleural space and outer surface of the lung, while the other follows bronchovascular bundles to drain the deeper portions of the lung (see Chapters 6 and 36).[1] In humans, the pulmonary lymphatic system begins to form approximately 6 weeks into embryonic growth with sprouting of distinct endothelial cells directly from the developing venous system.[2] A number of growth factors that direct development of the lymphatic vasculature have been identified,[3] and the pathophysiology leading to lymphatic dysfunction varies among the disorders described in this section. For example, disordered embryonic development has been hypothesized to play a role in pulmonary lymphangiectasia (PL), a disorder that often presents in the neonatal period. In disorders that present outside of the neonatal period, such as lymphangiomatosis, disease is associated with abnormalities of lymphatic growth. Furthermore, a significant number of children with pulmonary lymphatic disorders also manifest lymphatic involvement of other organ systems, congenital cardiac disease, and chromosomal disorders. This section describes disorders associated with lymphatic dysfunction affecting the respiratory system. The reader is referred to Chapter 69 regarding congenital chylothorax.

PULMONARY LYMPHANGIECTASIA

Epidemiology

PL is characterized by dilatation of pulmonary lymphatic vessels and disordered drainage, leading to the accumulation of lymph within the lungs and a spectrum of respiratory disease. Although its exact incidence is not known, it has been estimated that 0.5%–1% of neonates who die in the neonatal period have PL.[1] The majority of reported cases occur sporadically, and most present in the neonatal period or during infancy. However, cases of PL have also been described to occur during childhood and into adulthood.[4]

Etiology and Pathogenesis

One commonly used classification system for PL distinguishes between disease caused by a primary developmental defect and that occurring secondary to an obstructive process impeding normal lymph drainage.[3] It has been hypothesized that primary PL occurs secondary to failure of normal regression of the large lymphatic vessels, observed in the embryo at 9–16 weeks of gestation.[3] A recently described murine model of PL was generated by expressing vascular endothelial growth factor (VEGF)-C on a lung-specific promoter.[5] Lymphatic growth is regulated in part by the lymphangiogenic receptor VEGFR3, and mice lacking this gene die shortly after birth from failure of lung inflation.[6] Some infants with primary PL present with disease that seems confined to the respiratory system, while others display more generalized symptoms characterized by lymphedema and extrathoracic involvement.[3] Recent studies in families with inherited isolated forms of lymphedema have identified eight genes causing lymphedema (i.e., *FLT4* [encoding VEGFR3] [MIM 153100], *FOXC2* [MIM 153400], *SOX18* [MIM 607823], *HGF* [MIM 142409], *MET* [MIM 164860], *CCBE1* [MIM 235510], *PTPN14* [MIM 603155], and *GJC2* [MIM 608803]).[7] Secondary causes of PL usually involve congenital cardiac diseases associated with obstructed pulmonary venous flow. Thus hypoplastic left heart syndrome, congenital mitral stenosis, and pulmonary vein atresia have all been associated with PL.[3,8] In addition to cardiac disease, thoracic duct agenesis and infection may also block lymphatic drainage and cause PL.

Clinical Features

A number of chromosomal disorders are associated with PL, including Noonan syndrome, Hennekam syndrome, yellow nail syndrome, and Down syndrome.[1,3] Children with PL associated with chromosomal disorders are more likely to present with generalized lymphangiectasia. These patients may display a less severe pulmonary component and may have a better prognosis when compared with those who present with primarily pulmonary disease during the neonatal period.[1]

At birth, infants with PL often present with respiratory distress that progresses rapidly to respiratory failure.[1] Chylous pleural effusions may be prominent, but a significant number of children with PL do not present with effusions.[1] Individuals who first develop symptoms later in infancy or during childhood usually display less severe disease when compared with those with neonatal onset. In later-presenting forms, initial symptoms include chronic tachypnea, recurrent cough, and wheezing.[4] PL in these individuals has been associated with chylothorax, chylopericardium, and chylous ascites.[3] These patients have frequent respiratory exacerbations, possibly related to lower respiratory tract infection that leads to transient worsening of lymphatic drainage.[1,4]

Imaging

The diagnostic workup of the child with suspected PL includes plain chest radiography, high-resolution tomography of the chest (HRCT), and lung biopsy. Chest radiography often reveals interstitial infiltrates and hyperinflation, with or without pleural effusion.[1] HRCT shows thickening of peribronchovascular septa and septa surrounding lobules (Fig. 55.1).[3] Lung biopsy, the "gold standard" for diagnosing PL, is characterized by the appearance of dilated lymphatic vessels located in the interlobular septa, near bronchovascular bundles and/or within the pleura.[8] Dilated lymphatic vessels may occasionally appear cystic.[2] In addition to lymphatic findings, lung biopsy may also show thickening and widening of interlobular septa.[2] The risk of worsened lymphatic leak should be considered in the decision to proceed with lung biopsy. Because lymphangiectasia may be part of a systemic dysplasia, consideration should also be given to careful evaluation for extrapulmonary disease manifestations, such as gastrointestinal involvement, bone disease, or skin lesions from draining lymphatics.

Management

There is no known cure for PL, and treatment is primarily supportive. Respiratory failure in a significant number of neonates with PL is refractory to conventional positive-pressure ventilation and high-frequency oscillation. In these cases, inhaled nitric oxide and extracorporeal membranous oxygenation (ECMO) have been used with variable success.[8] Therapy for older children with PL includes supplemental oxygen, judicious use of antibiotics for bacterial respiratory infection and treatment for recurrent wheezing or cough.[4] A number of medications have been reported to be effective for the management of PL and chylothorax in case reports and small series, but none have been tested in randomized clinical trials.

Prognosis

Although the natural course of PL is variable among individuals, the disease has historically carried a high mortality rate when diagnosed in the neonatal period. One report suggests improved survival with aggressive interventions and modern neonatal intensive care.[4] Subsequently, however, Mettauer et al. have reported survival in only one of seven children referred to their tertiary center.[8] The authors concluded that although the prognosis for PL is poor, the condition is survivable with aggressive intervention.[8] Furthermore, those who survive the neonatal period seem to eventually

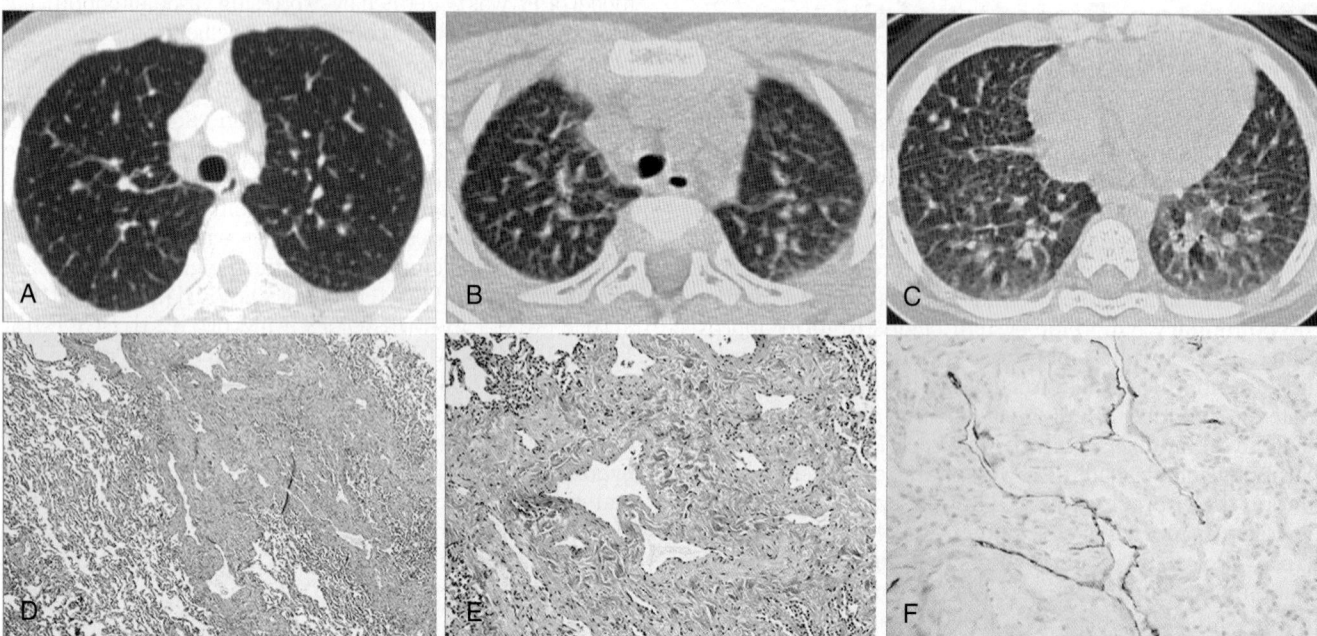

Fig. 55.1 Chest high-resolution computed tomography from an 8-year-old (A) and a 2-year-old (B and C) with lymphangiectasia. Imaging shows variable intensity of interlobular septal thickening. Both children presented with nonspecific respiratory symptoms and recurrent pneumonia without identification of pathogens; neither had overt extrapulmonary manifestations of lymphatic dysplasia. Lung biopsy shows septal widening with prominent and muscularized lymphatics (D and E, hematoxylin and eosin), as illustrated by D240 immunostaining highlighting the lymphatic endothelium (F). (Cases provided by Lisa R. Young, MD, Cincinnati Children's Hospital Medical Center, Susie Millard, MD, Helen DeVos Children's Hospital and Michigan State University, and Gail Deutsch, MD, Seattle Children's Hospital.)

experience improvement of their disease.[4,8] Clearly a spectrum of severity exists. With further delineation of the molecular mechanisms controlling development of the lymphatic system, it is likely that new methods of classifying and ultimately treating PL will become available.

Lymphangioma, Lymphangiomatosis, and Gorham-Stout Disease

Abnormal proliferation of lymphatic vessels distinguishes lymphangioma, lymphangiomatosis, and Gorham-Stout disease from other lymphatic disorders of the lung. Whereas lymphangioma refers to a solitary malformation, lymphangiomatosis refers to the presence of multiple lymphangiomas and is less common than the occurrence of a single lymphangioma. Gorham-Stout disease is a related syndrome characterized by chylothorax and bone cysts, with lymphangioma seen on biopsy.

Lymphangiomatosis is a severe disease characterized by the occurrence of numerous lymphangiomas, often affecting multiple organs. Involvement of the liver, soft tissue, spleen, bones, mediastinum, and lungs may occur.[2,9] The disease is reported more frequently in children than adults, and a significant percentage of these cases present during infancy.[9] Lymphangiomatosis involving the thorax can manifest in the mediastinum, pleural space, chest wall, lungs, or pericardium. Individuals with thoracic involvement may present with cough, chest pain, dyspnea, or wheezing.[9] Chylous effusions are often a prominent component of the clinical disease pattern of lymphangiomatosis.[2,9] Chest radiography reveals interstitial infiltrates, chest masses, effusions, or bone lesions.[2] In addition to multiple lymphangiomas, HRCT of the chest may exhibit smooth thickening of interlobular septa and bronchovascular bundles, ground-glass attenuation, or effusions.[9] Biopsies of lymphatic lesions are characterized by increased numbers of dilated lymphatic channels lined by endothelium.[2]

The natural history of lymphangiomatosis entails progressive growth of lymphangiomas, which eventually compress vital structures. Both young age and respiratory involvement predict a particularly poor outcome.[9] However, successfully treated cases of lymphangiomatosis with thoracic involvement have been reported.[10] Therapy for severely symptomatic pleural effusions may include thoracentesis or pleurodesis. When lymphangiomas are diffuse, complete surgical resection may not be possible. Medical therapy for lymphangiomatosis using sirolimus or interferon alpha-2b has been reported, with the aim of halting the lymphatic proliferation that is the hallmark of the disease.[10,11]

Gorham-Stout disease is characterized by the proliferation of vascular structures within bones, leading to osteolytic lesions evident on radiography.[12] Chylothorax is associated with the disease, possibly related to dysplasia of lymphatic vessels at the pleura.[12] Children are more commonly affected than adults, and presenting symptoms may include cough, dyspnea, and pain.[13] The presence of chylothorax is associated with worsened prognosis in this severe disease.[12] Similar to what is reported in lymphangiomatosis, there are case reports describing approaches to medical therapy.[12–14] Ongoing efforts to improve the classification and phenotyping of lymphatic dysplasias, including PL and lymphangiomatosis, may lead to improved diagnostic strategies, molecular understanding, and targeted therapeutic considerations. The Lymphangiomatosis and Gorham Disease Alliance advocates on behalf of patients and families and provides education and support (https://www.lgdalliance.org/).

Lymphangioleiomyomatosis

Lymphangioleiomyomatosis (LAM) is characterized by abnormal smooth muscle proliferation and cystic destruction in the lung. This disorder typically presents in women of childbearing age with recurrent pneumothoraces, progressive dyspnea, and/or multiple lung cysts evident on HRCT.[15] Although lymphatic involvement is not always a prominent feature, some patients may develop chylous effusion.[15] Despite the similar-sounding terminology, LAM is distinct from lymphangiomatosis and is differentiated based on the presence of lung cysts and distinct immunohistochemistry.[15] LAM may occur sporadically, without a known inheritance pattern, or it may be associated with tuberous sclerosis complex (TSC), an autosomal dominant disease with variable penetrance.[15] Rarely, cystic pulmonary disease can occur in children with TSC (Fig. 55.2).[16] Although at least 40% of adult women with TSC have lung cysts compatible with LAM, symptomatic

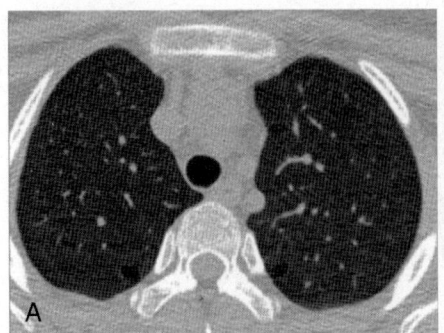 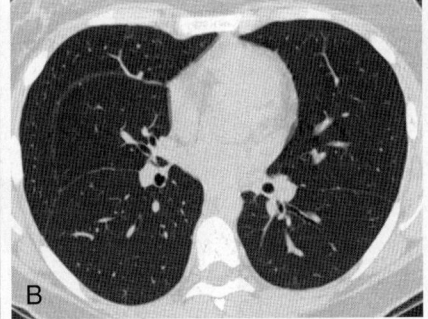 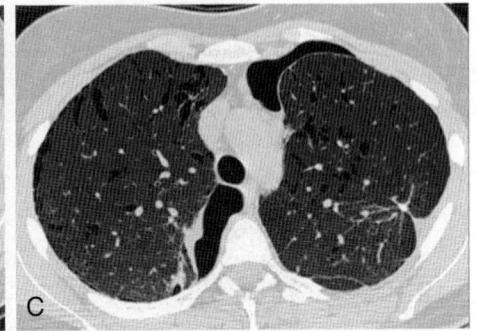

Fig. 55.2 (A) Chest high-resolution computed tomography (c-HRCT) image from a 16-year-old female with tuberous sclerosis complex (TSC), showing a few radiolucent thin-walled cysts bilaterally. These findings, which are consistent with very mild early lymphangioleiomyomatosis, were detected on screening c-HRCT in this asymptomatic teenager. (B) c-HRCT demonstrates only a few tiny cysts in this 17-year-old female with TSC; however, she subsequently experienced unusually rapid progression, including bilateral pneumothoraces. (C) Subsequent c-HRCT (age 18.5 years) shows diffuse cystic lung disease and residual bilateral pneumothoraces. (Case provided by Lisa R. Young, MD, Cincinnati Children's Hospital Medical Center.)

pulmonary disease is rare in girls with TSC.[17–19] One study from a single referral center reported age-dependent risk of LAM in females with TSC, with a prevalence of 26% in females with TSC below 21 years of age and 81% in those above 40 years of age.[20] Consensus guidelines published in 2013 recommend LAM screening in females with TSC starting at age 18 years.[21] The Tuberous Sclerosis Alliance (www.tsalliance.org) and LAM Foundation (www.thelamfoundation.org) offer information, resources, and a worldwide network to those affected.

Pulmonary Alveolar Microlithiasis

EPIDEMIOLOGY

PAM is an autosomal recessive disease characterized by the deposition of calcium phosphate calculi within alveoli. Although the majority of reported cases of PAM historically describe adults, increased numbers of children with the disorder have been identified more recently. A few cases report diagnosis during infancy and early childhood.[22] Tachibana et al. report 52% of a series of 111 patients identified before the age of 15 in Japan.[23] In Turkey and Italy, the mean age of diagnosis was 27 and 30 years, respectively.[23]

ETIOLOGY AND PATHOGENESIS

A gene linked to PAM has been identified, and the cause of the disease has been linked to disordered phosphate transport in the alveolar space.[24] *SLC34A2* encodes a type IIb sodium-dependent phosphate transporter and is expressed in type II alveolar cells.[24] Mutations most often lead to a loss of function or premature termination.[22] One of the functions of type II alveolar cells involves degradation of surfactant. Phosphate is a waste product of this degradation and will build up in cells unless properly removed. Saito et al. showed that epithelial deletion of the SLC34A2 gene product NPT2b sodium-dependent phosphate cotransporter in mice results in a PAM phenotype.[24] Mice with this deletion develop

microlith accumulation in alveoli, typical radiographic findings, and pulmonary fibrosis, strongly suggesting that dysfunction of NPT2b causes PAM.[24]

CLINICAL FEATURES

Individuals with PAM, especially in the pediatric population, are usually asymptomatic at the time of diagnosis.[23] Remarkably, this absence of symptoms occurs despite impressive radiologic changes evident on chest imaging. Mariotta et al. reviewed the literature to describe 576 cases of the disorder and reported the presence of symptoms (including dyspnea, cough, and chest pain) in only about half of those affected.[25]

Patients may also present with digital clubbing or, less commonly, pneumothorax.[22] The micronodules evident on chest radiography often appear denser at the lung bases and can obscure the borders of the cardiac silhouette and diaphragm.[23] HRCT may reveal micronodules, ground-glass opacities, subpleural interstitial thickening, and interlobular septal thickening.[22] In pediatric patients, ground-glass opacification can predominate over the nodular calcific densities classically ascribed to the disease in adults (Fig. 55.3).[26] At diagnosis, pulmonary function testing may be normal or show slightly decreased vital capacity or diffusing capacity.[23] Decline of pulmonary function and occurrence of respiratory insufficiency occur over decades.[23,25]

DIAGNOSIS AND DIFFERENTIAL DIAGNOSIS

PAM is distinguished from other pulmonary diseases by its "sandstorm" appearance on plain chest film, representative of calcium-phosphate micronodules. This finding is considered by some to be pathognomonic for the disease. Sarcoidosis, tuberculosis, histoplasmosis, and idiopathic pulmonary hemosiderosis can be considered in the differential diagnosis.

MANAGEMENT AND PROGNOSIS

PAM usually progresses, at varying rates, to pulmonary fibrosis, pulmonary hypertension, and respiratory failure

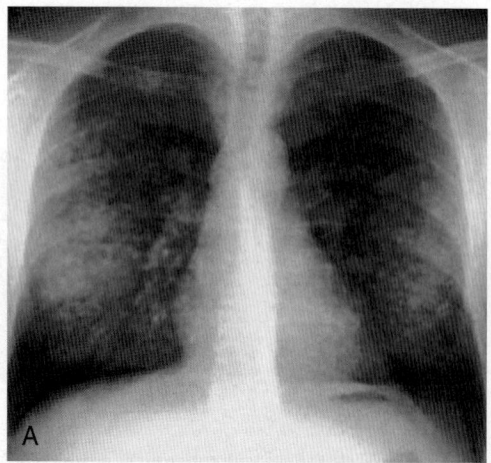
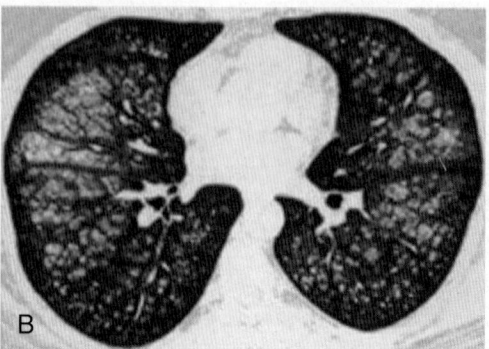

Fig. 55.3 Radiographic features of pulmonary alveolar microlithiasis. (A) Posteroanterior chest radiograph showing the classic "sandstorm" appearance of pulmonary alveolar microlithiasis, including diffuse, patchy, bilateral sharp micronodular disease. (B) High-resolution computed tomographic scan of the chest showing micronodular densities. (From Brandenburg VM, Schubert H. Images in clinical medicine. Pulmonary alveolar microlithiasis. *N Engl J Med.* 2003;348:1555.)

over several decades following diagnosis.[22] Although various therapies have been tried, there is currently no cure for PAM. Corticosteroids and whole-lung lavage have not shown efficacy.[22] Lung transplantation has been performed successfully.[22] It is hoped that new therapies directed at correcting the disease-causing Npt2b-dependent phosphate transporter will halt or slow the formation of microliths and prevent the severe lung disease associated with PAM.

Ataxia Telangiectasia

Ataxia telangiectasia (AT) is an autosomal recessive, progressive multisystem disorder caused by homozygous or compound heterozygous mutations in the gene ATM (ataxia-telangiectasia mutated; 11q22.3).[27] Disease manifestations occur in early childhood, with progressive cerebellar ataxia and later conjunctival telangiectases, progressive neurologic degeneration, immune deficiency, and malignancies. The molecular pathogenesis is complex but involves abnormal DNA damage responses leading to a high rate of intrachromosomal recombination and genomic instability. Respiratory manifestations include recurrent infections related to immunodeficiency, chronic aspiration due to swallowing dysfunction, ineffective airway clearance, and interstitial lung disease. Most patients die young of respiratory causes or malignancies, with a disparately higher mortality rate among African Americans historically.[28] As is true for most rare lung diseases, there are few controlled trials to guide management. The European Respiratory Society (ERS) recently published a thorough statement on the multidisciplinary management of the respiratory manifestations of AT.[29]

Immunodeficiency in AT is variable, with both humoral and cellular abnormalities. Patients with recurrent respiratory infections and poor vaccine responses are candidates for immunoglobulin replacement therapy. Immunodeficiency does not seem to progress over time in AT.[30] Bronchiectasis develops in many patients in the first decade of life. Neuromuscular involvement, discoordinated swallowing, and impaired mucociliary clearance should be evaluated and managed, as for many patients susceptible to these disorders. Lung function measurement can be challenging because of neurologic abnormalities but can be useful to define bronchodilator response and to monitor lung function over time. A recent study of children and young adults with AT demonstrated an inverse relationship between serum interleukin (IL)-6 levels and vital capacity, suggesting that systemic inflammation is correlated with lower lung function in AT, although the mechanism is uncertain.[31] In a large retrospective series, approximately one fourth of AT patients with chronic respiratory symptoms were found to have ILD, which has a unique histopathologic pattern and may be responsive to steroids if treated early in the course.[32] Because of the known cellular and chromosomal sensitivity to ionizing radiation in AT, effort should be made to limit diagnostic radiation as much as possible. A recent study showed that inspiratory muscle training improved ventilatory pattern, lung volume, respiratory muscle strength, and the health and vitality domains for quality of life in patients with AT.[33] A coordinated, multidisciplinary approach to monitoring and managing respiratory involvement in AT will likely result in improved respiratory health for these patients.

Gaucher Disease

EPIDEMIOLOGY, ETIOLOGY, AND PATHOBIOLOGY

The most common lysosomal storage disease, Gaucher disease is an autosomal recessive disorder caused by a mutation in the glucocerebrosidase gene, resulting in an abnormal buildup of glucocerebroside. This accumulates within macrophages and is identified pathologically as Gaucher or foam cells. In the lung, infiltration of Gaucher cells may occur within alveoli, interstitial spaces, around airways, or within pulmonary vasculature.[34,35]

CLINICAL FEATURES

Some patients with type 2 and type 3 Gaucher disease display a pattern of alveolar consolidation related to Gaucher cells, whereas others manifest a pattern of interstitial disease with associated fibrosis, usually seen in type 3 disease.[36] In addition to parenchymal lung disease, type 1 Gaucher disease may be complicated by pulmonary vascular disease, including pulmonary arterial hypertension and hepatopulmonary syndrome.[36] Although clinical pulmonary disease is uncommon, a significant number of patients have abnormal pulmonary function testing.[37] Chest radiography may display reticulonodular changes, and HRCT shows ground-glass consolidation, interstitial involvement, alveolar opacities and bronchial wall thickening (Fig. 55.4).[38]

MANAGEMENT, TREATMENT, AND PROGNOSIS

Whereas enzyme replacement therapy for Gaucher disease decreases organomegaly and improves hematologic parameters, it may not reverse severe pulmonary parenchymal disease.[34] However, this therapy may in some cases slow or prevent a progressive decline in lung function.[35,39] Most cases of clinically significant pulmonary vascular disease have been described in adults.[36] The severity of pulmonary arterial hypertension does not correlate with the severity of Gaucher disease in other organ systems and may improve or stabilize with the initiation of enzyme replacement therapy and medical therapy for pulmonary hypertension.[36] Hepatopulmonary syndrome in Gaucher disease is associated with more severe liver disease and also may improve with the initiation of enzyme replacement therapy.[36] The National Gaucher Foundation (www.gaucherdisease.org) seeks treatments and a cure for Gaucher disease.

Niemann-Pick Disease

EPIDEMIOLOGY, ETIOLOGY, AND PATHOBIOLOGY

Niemann-Pick disease (NPD) is a rare, autosomal recessive lysosomal storage disorder characterized by a deficiency of acid sphingomyelinase, leading to the accumulation of sphingomyelin within cells and tissues. In the lung, buildup of foam cells containing sphingomyelin occurs within alveoli, alveolar walls, lymphatic spaces, and the pleural space.[40]

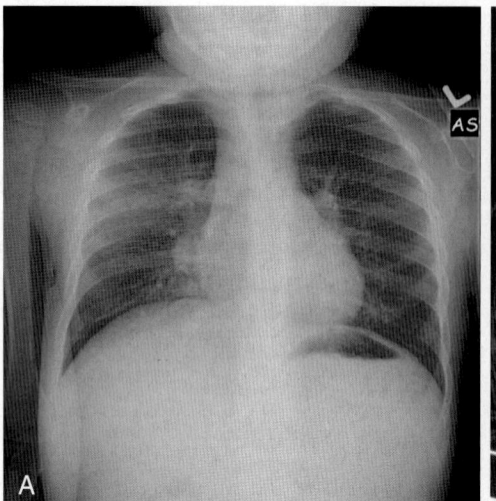
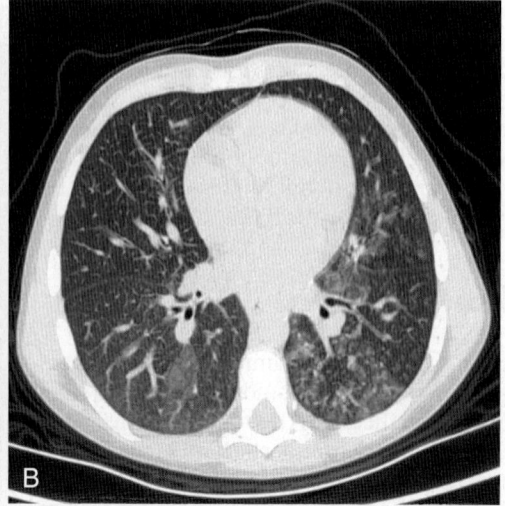

Fig. 55.4 (A) Chest radiograph of a 3-year-old female with Gaucher disease who had received enzyme replacement therapy since infancy reveals reticulonodular changes and areas of consolidation. (B) Computed tomography of the chest with mosaic pattern and areas of septal thickening. Bronchoalveolar lavage revealed numerous foam cells *(not pictured)*. (Images provided by Roberta Kato, MD, Children's Hospital, Los Angeles.)

CLINICAL FEATURES

Whereas type A NPD manifests as a severe neurodegenerative disorder, individuals with type B NPD have little or no neurologic involvement and often survive into adulthood.[41] Pediatric patients with type B NPD present with hepatomegaly, splenomegaly, thrombocytopenia, and dyslipidemia. Respiratory involvement can be seen in all forms of NPD but has been seen most frequently in type B.[41] Individuals may present with recurrent cough, exercise intolerance, or recurrent respiratory infections.[41] Pulmonary function abnormalities are common and are characterized by decreased FVC, FEV$_1$, and diffusing capacity.[42]

A significant number of individuals with type B NPD exhibit chest imaging and lung histopathology consistent with interstitial lung disease (ILD).[42] Rarely, a severe form of ILD due to NPD may present in infancy or early childhood. Radiographic abnormalities of HRCT observed in NPD include ground-glass appearance, reticulonodular densities, thickening of interlobular septa, and a crazy-paving pattern.[41,42] The severity of radiologic findings has not been found to correlate with pulmonary function testing.[41,42] Bronchoalveolar lavage is characterized by Niemann–Pick cells, which appear as multivacuolated histiocytes with blue-staining granules.[41] Histopathology shows infiltration of the interstitium, alveoli, lymphatics, and subpleural space.[41]

MANAGEMENT, TREATMENT, AND PROGNOSIS

Although no specific treatment for NPD exists, research into bone marrow transplantation, enzyme replacement therapy, and gene therapy is ongoing. Whole-lung lavage has been tried for the most severe cases, with varying success.[40] In many cases ILD is indolent and associated with survival well into adulthood.[41] However, some cases of ILD due to NPD can be rapidly progressive and lead to respiratory failure during childhood.[41] It is hoped that therapies aimed at correction of the underlying disease will contribute to stabilization or improvement of lung disease associated with NPD. The National NPD Foundation (www.nnpdf.org) provides

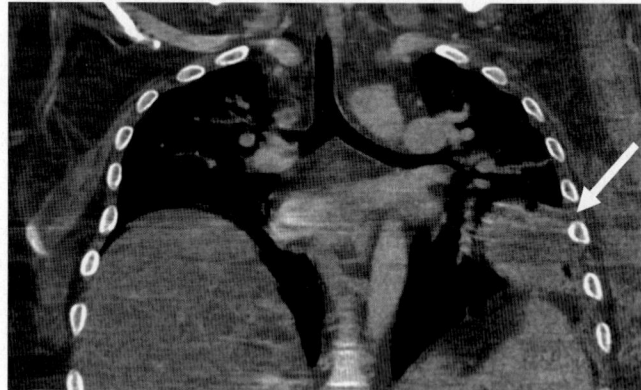

Fig. 55.5 Computed tomography sagittal section of a 21-year-old with neurofibromatosis type I, demonstrating a soft tissue mass abutting the left chest wall with adjacent atelectasis. Biopsy of the mass was consistent with neurofibroma.

support services for individuals and families affected by the disorder.

Neurofibromatosis

Neurofibromatosis type 1 (NF-1) is an autosomal dominant disorder characterized by neurofibromata, café au lait spots, pigmented hamartomas of the iris, skeletal dysplasia, and optic glioma. Thoracic involvement in NF-1 mainly entails the presence of neurofibromata, often plexiform, that may arise from the chest wall or posterior mediastinum (Fig. 55.5).[42] Plexiform neurofibromata have multiple nerve roots and can surround vital structures, making resection complex.[43] As malignant transformation may occur, biopsy of these masses should be considered.[43] In addition to tumors and bony abnormalities affecting the thorax, NF-1 is also associated with ILD.[44] The ILD associated with NF-1 appears radiographically as large, apical thin-walled bullae and basilar fibrosis.[44] Diffuse lung disease associated with neurofibromatosis mainly occurs

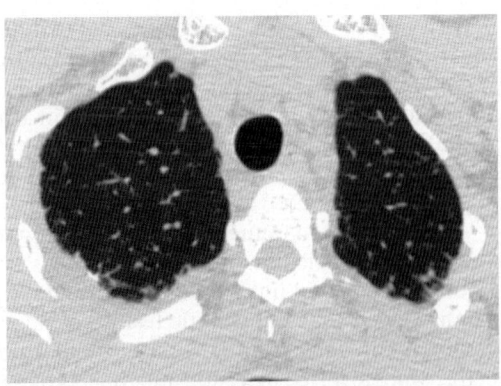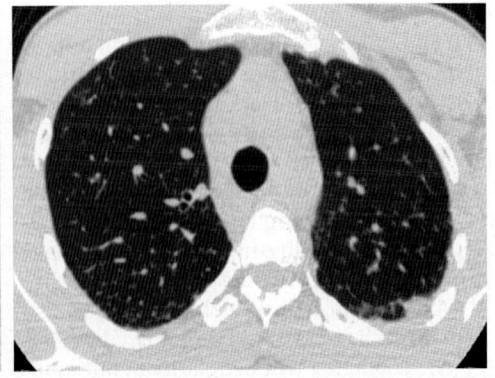

Fig. 55.6 Chest high-resolution computed tomography images demonstrating subpleural-predominant thickening of the secondary interlobular septa, consistent with early pulmonary fibrosis in this 18-year-old patient with dyskeratosis congenita. (Case provided by Lisa R. Young, MD, and Ronald Bokulic, DO, Cincinnati Children's Hospital Medical Center.)

in adult patients and has not yet been reported in children.[44] The Children's Tumor Foundation (www.ctf.org) is dedicated to improving the health and well-being of individuals and families affected by NF.

Dyskeratosis Congenita

Dyskeratosis congenita (DC) is a form of ectodermal dysplasia characterized by skin hyperpigmentation, nail dystrophy, oral leukoplakia, and bone marrow failure.[45,46] A number of mutations in genes coding for proteins that function to maintain telomeres have been identified in patients with DC.[45] Whereas a minority of those with DC manifest pulmonary involvement such as fibrosis, the disease can have significant morbidity (Fig. 55.6).[46] Owing to the high percentage of children with DC receiving bone marrow transplants, characterization of the etiology of lung disease when it occurs after transplant can be difficult. However, a number of pulmonary complications, including pulmonary fibrosis and hepatopulmonary syndrome, have been described after bone marrow transplantation.[46–48] Therefore it is likely that at least in some cases, development of pulmonary fibrosis is either due to or exacerbated by the telomerase dysfunction known to occur in DC.[48]

Hermansky-Pudlak Syndrome

Hermansky-Pudlak syndrome (HPS) is an autosomal recessive disorder characterized by oculocutaneous albinism, bleeding diathesis, and pulmonary fibrosis.[49] Notably, the disease has an especially high prevalence in a section of Puerto Rico. The underlying disorder in HPS involves disturbed formation or trafficking of intracellular vesicles. This perturbation results in dysfunction of lysosome-related organelles within a number of cell types, including macrophages and type II pneumocytes.[50,51] Clinically, lung disease has been reported only in individuals with subtypes HPS-1, HPS-2, and HPS-4; it usually manifests in the third or fourth decades of life, although pediatric onset has been reported.[51–53] Pulmonary function testing reveals restrictive lung disease, and HRCT indicates pulmonary fibrosis.[53] Disease may progress to death in the fourth or fifth decade of life.[53] Lung transplantation

has been successfully performed in a number of individuals with HPS, although consultation with a hematologist is advised to assist in the management of potential bleeding complications. The HPS Network (www.hpsnetwork.org) is a support group for people and families dealing with the disorder. Ongoing investigation of the cellular mechanisms responsible for disease as well as medications targeted against pulmonary fibrosis will contribute significantly to the care of patients with HPS.

Alpha-1 Antitrypsin Deficiency

Although alpha-1 antitrypsin (ATT) deficiency is not a rare disorder per se, pulmonary manifestations of AAT deficiency occur very rarely, if ever, in children. Familiarity with the disorder is of value to pediatric pulmonologists since pediatric practitioners are responsible for educating patients and families regarding genetic testing and providing anticipatory guidance for those who carry the diagnosis.

EPIDEMIOLOGY

AAT deficiency is one of the most common inherited diseases worldwide, and its diagnosis often goes delayed or unrecognized.[54] It is estimated that only about 5% of individuals in the United States with the disorder are actually diagnosed.[55] AAT deficiency is inherited in a codominant manner, and over 100 variants of the AAT protein have been identified. Various AAT phenotypes are associated with different levels of the protein, and the serum level of AAT determines the risk of emphysema. The PiZZ genotype is the most prevalent disease, causing phenotype in populations of Northern European descent.[56]

Much of the available knowledge regarding the epidemiology of AAT deficiency in children stems from a birth cohort that identified 184 individuals in Sweden, where AAT screening of 200,000 newborns occurred from 1972 to 1974.[57] These studies found lung function testing to be normal in adolescents up to age 18 with PiZZ.[57] However, when compared with those who do not smoke, Piitulainen and Sveger (1998) found 18-year-olds with either PiZZ or PiSZ genotypes who smoked to have a lower FEV_1 and FEV_1/FVC.[57] Thus the authors concluded that the first signs of lung disease in

AAT-deficient smokers occur in adolescence.[57] At the age of 22 years, pulmonary function testing, although still within the normal range (mean FEV$_1$ 98% predicted), was found to have significantly declined (mean 1.2% annual decline) when compared with testing done at 16 and 18 years.[58] Furthermore, 29% of individuals reported wheezing and 15% had been diagnosed with asthma.[58] Thus the authors speculated that respiratory symptoms in young adults with PiZZ may be misidentified as asthma, contributing to a delay in diagnosis for those with symptoms of AAT deficiency.[58] Exposure to environmental tobacco smoke during childhood has also been associated with an earlier onset of symptoms.[59] Families of children with AAT deficiency will benefit from anticipatory guidance regarding the dangers of exposure to tobacco smoke.

ETIOLOGY AND PATHOBIOLOGY

AAT inhibits the activity of a number of proteolytic enzymes, the most important of which is neutrophil elastase.[54] Lung disease in AAT deficiency occurs primarily secondary to loss of function, resulting in an imbalance between levels of AAT relative to the amount of neutrophil elastase. Neutrophil elastase degrades elastin and extracellular matrix elements located within the lower respiratory tract that normally function to maintain the structural integrity of the lung.[56]

Considering that not all at-risk individuals develop disease, other environmental and genetic components modulate the development of emphysema. For instance, a relationship between smoking, AAT deficiency, and the development of emphysema has been well established. In addition to cigarette smoking, exposure to kerosene heaters, employment in agriculture, and exposure to other pollutants from biomass fuel sources have all been implicated in the development of emphysema.[55,56]

CLINICAL FEATURES

It should be emphasized that AAT deficiency has not been shown to cause clinical lung disease in the pediatric population. The vast majority of children with AAT deficiency present with liver disease. The mean age of presentation of lung disease in AAT deficiency is 32 to 41 years, and presentation before 25 years is rare.[56] Relatively early onset of symptoms usually occurs in smokers or those with a history of smoking. In addition to liver disease, AAT deficiency has also been associated with bronchiectasis, necrotizing panniculitis and multisystem vasculitis.[56]

DIAGNOSIS

Decreased serum levels of AAT indicate disease and necessitate further workup. Genotyping by polymerase chain reaction (PCR) or isoelectric focusing (phenotyping) identify AAT variants and are used to confirm the diagnosis.[56]

Predispositional testing, or the testing of asymptomatic individuals at risk for developing disease, has relevance to the pediatric population. Concerns exist regarding the psychological ramifications of being diagnosed during childhood with a disease that may not manifest for decades, if at all.[55,56] It has been speculated that knowledge of the illness may have a negative impact on a child's self-image or relationship with family members and peers.[56] Furthermore, concerns exist regarding the ability to secure health insurance and employment.[55] However, pediatric patients diagnosed with AAT deficiency can be counseled against tobacco use and the dangers of other relevant environmental exposures, and such counseling may be more effective when initiated at a younger age.[55,56]

Guidelines recommend testing of siblings of an individual with AAT deficiency, and genetic testing should be discussed for siblings of an individual who is heterozygous.[56] It is recommended that the genetic testing of adolescents proceed only if the adolescent is sufficiently mature to understand the issues involved in testing and that both assent and parental permission have been obtained.[56]

MANAGEMENT AND TREATMENT

Treatment of respiratory manifestations of AAT deficiency centers on therapy for airways obstruction and hypoxemia, antimicrobials for secondary infection, and replacement enzyme (augmentation) therapy.[56] Although the benefit and cost-effectiveness of augmentation therapy remain controversial, many experts recommend treatment for selected individuals.[54,56] Future therapies seek to address the misfolding of AAT or use small fragment homologous replacement therapy to correct the gene defect of AAT deficiency.[54] The Alpha-1 Association (www.alpha1.org) and Alpha-1 Foundation (www.alpha-1foundation.org) provide resources, support, education, and advocacy.

Summary

Rare lung disorders influence the care of children with respiratory diseases in a number of fundamental ways. Understanding of normal biologic function is often facilitated via characterization of the disrupted pathways occurring in rare diseases. This knowledge can then be applied to related diseases that occur with higher prevalence. Most importantly, the respiratory practitioner's ability to identify and care for pediatric patients with diseases that occur uncommonly will have a significant impact on the lives of those affected.

References

Access the reference list online at ExpertConsult.com.

Suggested Reading

Bellini C, Boccardo F, Campisi C, et al. Congenital pulmonary lymphangiectasia. *Orphanet J Rare Dis.* 2006;1:43.

Bhatt JM, Bush A, van Gerven M, et al. ERS statement on the multidisciplinary respiratory management of ataxia telangiectasia. *Eur Respir Rev.* 2015;24(138):565–581.

Castellana G, Castellana G, Gentile M, et al. Pulmonary alveolar microlithiasis: review of the 1022 cases reported worldwide. *Eur Respir Rev.* 2015;24(138):607–620.

Faul JL, Berry GJ, Colby TV, et al. Thoracic lymphangiomas, lymphangiectasis, lymphangiomatosis, and lymphatic dysplasia syndrome. *Am J Respir Crit Care Med.* 2000;161(3 Pt 1):1037–1046.

Stoller JK, Aboussouan LS. A review of α1-antitrypsin deficiency. *Am J Respir Crit Care Med.* 2012;185(3):246–259.

von Ranke FM, Pereira Freitas HM, Mançano AD, et al. Pulmonary involvement in Niemann-Pick disease: a state-of-the-art review. *Lung.* 2016;194(4):511–518.

56 Childhood Interstitial Lung Disease Disorders More Prevalent in Infancy

LISA R. YOUNG, MD, and GAIL H. DEUTSCH, MD

Overview

While there are areas of overlap, childhood interstitial lung diseases (ILD) frequently include differing entities and histologic patterns than those described in adult ILD. The areas of distinction are particularly apparent for ILD in infants and young children; therefore this chapter reviews specific forms of childhood ILD that are "more prevalent in infancy."

One factor prompting the need for distinct consideration of childhood ILD in infants is that prominent case clustering occurs in infancy. In a series reported by Fan et al., the median age of onset was 8 months.[1] Two subsequent large multicenter studies have also shown a predominance of cases in young children. In the European Respiratory Society task force survey of chronic ILD, children under age 2 years comprised 31% of cases.[2] Because this study's inclusion criteria required symptom duration of at least 3 months, neonates with a rapidly progressive course would have been excluded, and the proportion of cases in young children is likely underestimated. In studies utilizing lung biopsy ascertainment, the Children's Interstitial Lung Disease Research Network (ChILDRN) has identified that approximately 50% of lung biopsies for diffuse lung disease are performed in children less than 2 years of age.[3,4] Furthermore, within the cohort of young children, infants represent a large proportion of cases. Of 187 cases reviewed in the ChILDRN infant study, 30% underwent biopsy by 3 months of age and 52% underwent biopsy by 6 months of age.[3]

As detailed in a 2013 American Thoracic Society Clinical Practice Guideline, it is useful to separately consider the clinical differential diagnosis of ILD in an infant versus an older child.[5] Certain entities are either not seen in older children or clearly have symptom onset in infancy. Finally, there is high variability in morbidity and mortality associated with infant ILD disorders, emphasizing the critical need for accurate diagnosis. This chapter highlights several disorders that present in infancy or within the first year of life, including Alveolar Capillary Dysplasia with Misalignment of Pulmonary Veins (ACDMPV), Pulmonary Interstitial Glycogenosis (PIG), and Neuroendocrine Cell Hyperplasia of Infancy (NEHI). Additionally, while bronchopulmonary dysplasia is discussed in Chapter 20, lung growth abnormalities are included in this chapter, because they manifest in infancy and their clinical and radiographic presentation frequently overlaps with other forms of infant ILD. Disorders of surfactant production and homeostasis, more prevalent in infancy but also present in older children, are discussed separately in Chapter 57.

Alveolar Capillary Dysplasia With Misalignment of Pulmonary Veins

EPIDEMIOLOGY

Alveolar capillary dysplasia with ACDMPV is a rare and generally lethal developmental disorder of the lung that typically causes very early postnatal respiratory distress.[6,7] The disorder is named based on distinctive abnormalities of the pulmonary vasculature and is also variably termed *alveolar capillary dysplasia* and *congenital alveolar capillary dysplasia*. As definitive diagnosis currently depends on histologic examination of the lung on biopsy or at autopsy, the true prevalence is unknown; over 200 cases of ACDMPV have been reported in the literature to date. While the majority of cases are sporadic, approximately 10% are familial with affected siblings,[8–12] and no sex predilection has been identified.

ETIOLOGY AND PATHOGENESIS

Heterozygous inactivating point mutations and microdeletions involving *FOXF1* and its upstream interval on chromosome 16q24.1 have been found in a large number (~50%) of sporadic and familial cases of ACDMPV and concurrent anomalies.[8,13] Among deletions in which parental origin can be determined, all arose de novo on the maternal chromosome consistent with *FOXF1* being paternally imprinted.[12,14,15] The ability to noninvasively test for this gene has recently uncovered that patients with *FOXF1* mutations can have a variable phenotype, including milder symptoms with long-term survival.[16,17] This variability may be because of somatic mosaicism, partial imprinting, or modifier genes.[17] The frequently associated cardiac and gastrointestinal anomalies in patients with ACDMPV are thought to be due to haploinsufficiency for the neighboring FOXC2 and FOXL1 genes in the Forkhead box (FOX) transcription gene cluster.[13]

FOXF1 in mice is regulated by hedgehog and bone morphogenetic protein (BMP) signaling and encodes a transcription factor expressed in the lung mesenchyme and involved in murine vasculogenesis and lung development.[18,19] Mice with reduced levels of pulmonary Foxf1 die of pulmonary hemorrhage with deficient alveolarization and vasculogenesis, but they do not have malposition of pulmonary veins.

Mechanisms linking the abnormal lung vasculature with severe hypoxemia and pulmonary hypertension in ACDMPV remain to be fully explained. It is currently unclear whether the prominent arterial and lobular abnormalities in this disorder are primary or secondary to the vein misalignment. Medial hypertrophy of small pulmonary arteries may result from deficient lobular development with poor gas exchange and resultant hypoxemia, and intrapulmonary right-to-left shunts through bronchial veins have been demonstrated by three-dimensional image reconstruction of lung from infants who died from ACDMPV.[20]

CLINICAL FEATURES AND PRESENTATION

Infants with ACDMPV are usually born at term, and, in the majority of cases, the onset of cyanosis and respiratory failure occurs within 48 hours after birth.[10] Delayed onset by weeks or even months has been described rarely, but this is becoming more recognized as genetic testing for *FOXF1* mutations and deletions are now available.[21–24] The initial presentation is indistinguishable from persistent pulmonary hypertension of the newborn, and echocardiogram typically demonstrates suprasystemic right ventricular pressures and right-to-left shunting through a patent ductus arteriosus or patent foramen ovale. Approximately 80% infants with ACDMPV have additional malformations with cardiac (commonly hypoplastic left heart), gastrointestinal (intestinal malrotation and atresias), and renal abnormalities (hydronephrosis) being the most frequent.[11,13,25,26]

Radiologic Findings

The initial chest radiograph is often normal with subsequent development of diffuse hazy opacities, and the findings are also dependent on concurrent anomalies. Pneumothoraces are frequently reported, which may be a consequence of abnormal lung architecture or aggressive ventilation. Computed tomography (CT) or magnetic resonance lung imaging of patients with lethal ACDMPV have not been described, although a long-term survivor (36 months) had bilateral widespread ground glass opacities with relatively less affected areas on chest CT.[16]

HISTOLOGIC FINDINGS

ACDMPV is defined by a characteristic constellation of features, of which anomalously situated pulmonary veins running alongside small pulmonary arteries is essential (Fig. 56.1A–D).[3] Normally, pulmonary veins are in the interlobular septa, arising from small veins that drain pulmonary lobules. In addition to aberrant placement of the veins in ACDMPV, there is reduction or absence of veins in interlobular septa. Muscularization of small pulmonary arteries and arterioles is often striking, and there is reduced capillary density in alveolar walls (see Fig. 56.1E and F). Simplification of the lobular architecture with lymphangiectasia is variably present.

DIAGNOSIS AND DIFFERENTIAL DIAGNOSIS

The diagnosis of ACDMPV should be considered in infants who present with severe hypoxemia and pulmonary hypertension for which no anatomical cause can be established. Historically lung biopsy or autopsy was required to confirm the diagnosis. Currently, genetic testing for disruption of FOXF1 may obviate the need for a tissue diagnosis. On histologic examination, the characteristic constellation of findings may be subtle, particularly when the lung sample is limited with few bronchovascular bundles for evaluation. Patchy distribution has rarely been reported,[24] and multiple lung sections may be required for confirmation.

The presentation of ACDMPV with persistent pulmonary hypertension of the newborn overlaps with other etiologies of severe idiopathic neonatal lung disease, including genetic abnormalities in surfactant metabolism (particularly *SFTPB* and *ABCA3 mutations*), diffuse PIG, and lymphangiectasia. Histologically, ACDMPV should be distinguished from other disorders that demonstrate a similar arrest in lung development, including congenital alveolar dysplasia and advanced pulmonary hypoplasia. While these disorders also demonstrate lobular simplification and frequently vascular changes (hypertensive changes of the pulmonary arteries and reduced capillary density within alveolar walls), they do not have malpositioned veins in the lobules.

MANAGEMENT AND TREATMENT

Standard therapy is supportive and includes mechanical ventilation, inhaled nitric oxide, and extracorporeal membrane oxygenation (ECMO). These therapies prolong life by days to weeks but have rarely led to long-term survival, and lung transplantation has rarely been attempted.

PROGNOSIS

Historically initial presentation of ACDMPV in the neonatal period denoted a grim prognosis. However, variable phenotypes and longer survival are now increasingly reported. The clinical presentation should be considered in determining on a case-by-case basis.

Lung Growth Abnormalities Presenting as Childhood Interstitial Lung Diseases

EPIDEMIOLOGY

The epidemiology of lung growth abnormalities is best considered in the context of their associated conditions including prematurity, oligohydramnios, congenital heart disease, and Trisomy 21. While only a small portion of cases undergo lung biopsy, it is important to acknowledge that lung growth abnormalities are a principal cause of diffuse lung disease in young children that prompts surgical lung biopsy. In the ChILDRN study, lung growth abnormalities represented the primary diagnostic category, with 25% of lung biopsies from children less than age 2 being classified in this category. Furthermore, this was the leading diagnostic category for five of the eleven participating centers.[3]

ETIOLOGY AND PATHOGENESIS

Lung growth is a continual process that occurs well into the postnatal period. As such both prenatal and postnatal insults can impact lung maturation and growth. Distension

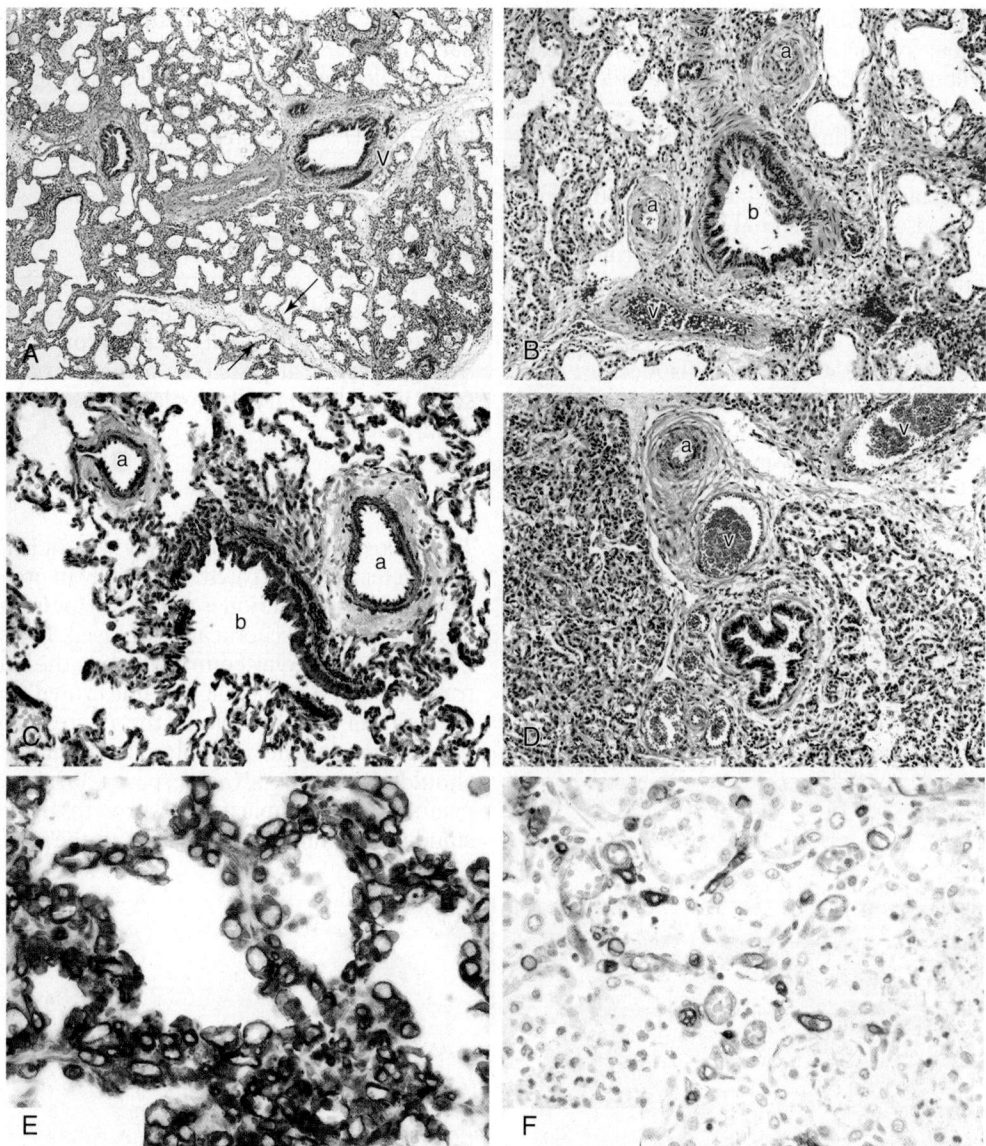

Fig. 56.1 Alveolar capillary dysplasia with misalignment of pulmonary veins. (A, B, and D) Pulmonary veins (v), which are normally in the interlobular septa *(arrowheads)*, are malpositioned and accompany pulmonary arteries (a) and bronchioles (b). There is lobular maldevelopment with no alveoli and interstitial widening (A, H&E, ×40); (B, H&E, ×100); (D, 10×, Movat pentachrome stain). (C) Normal airway for comparison (Movat pentachrome stain, original magnification 100×). (E and F) The marked decrease in alveolar wall capillaries is highlighted by the endothelial cell marker CD31 (×400).

of the lung with liquid and fetal respiratory movements is required for normal fetal lung growth, so any mechanism that interferes with these processes can result in a prenatal growth disorder. Prenatal onset pulmonary hypoplasia ranges from mild to severe, depending on the mechanism of hypoplasia and timing of the insult in relation to the stage of lung development. Early insults that occur before 16 weeks gestation (renal anomalies, congenital diaphragmatic hernia) may interfere with airway branching as well as acinar development, while later events (premature rupture of membranes) will exclusively impact acinar development. Postnatal onset growth abnormalities impact late alveolarization, most evident in the subpleural space. Multiple factors likely lead to deficient alveolarization in infants with congenital heart disease, including hypoxia and abnormal pulmonary blood flow.

In addition to chromosomal disorders, single gene disorders are also associated with abnormal lung growth, particularly deficient alveolarization. For example, while mutations or deletions in *NKX2.1* may present with a phenotype of surfactant dysfunction, alveolar simplification may be the predominant finding.[27] Mutations in *FLNA* (filamin A), which cause X-linked periventricular nodular heterotopia, have also been associated with severe diffuse lung disease with alveolar simplification, lung cysts, and pulmonary hypertension.[28–31]

CLINICAL FEATURES AND PRESENTATION

While not traditionally considered a classic form of ILD, abnormalities of lung growth represent a prominent proportion of cases that undergo lung biopsy to define the nature of the diffuse lung disease.[3] Furthermore, the features of tachypnea, retractions, hypoxemia, and often diffuse radiologic abnormalities overlap with other forms of childhood ILD.

Although lung growth abnormalities are traditionally considered in the context of prematurity and prenatal onset pulmonary hypoplasia, they also occur in the setting of congenital heart disease, chromosomal abnormalities (particularly Trisomy 21), and in otherwise normal-term infants with early postnatal lung injury (Table 56.1). While difficult

Table 56.1   Conditions Associated With Deficient Lung Growth

Factors limiting prenatal lung growth
- Oligohydramnios (e.g., premature rupture of membranes, bladder outlet obstruction)
- Restriction of thoracic volume from space-occupying lesions or thoracic deformities
- CNS, neuromuscular disorders and other agents resulting in decreased fetal breathing

Prematurity-related chronic lung disease (classically termed *bronchopulmonary dysplasia*)

Congenital heart disease
- Disorders with poor pulmonary blood flow (e.g., tetralogy of Fallot)
- Cyanotic heart disease impairing postnatal alveolarization

Genetic defects
- Trisomy 21 with deficient postnatal alveolarization
- Other chromosomal abnormalities
- *Nkx2.1* disruption
- *FLNA* disruption

to objectively define, most infants diagnosed with lung growth abnormalities by lung biopsy were reported to have clinical severity deemed out of proportion to their known comorbidities or circumstances.[3] In other words, typically an additional form of ILD is suspected, leading to the decision to pursue surgical lung biopsy in these patients.

Radiologic Findings

Radiologic findings are variable based on the etiology, age of the infant, and severity of the growth abnormality (Fig. 56.2). Subpleural cysts may be present and are frequently seen in pulmonary hypoplasia associated with Down's syndrome.[32]

HISTOLOGIC FINDINGS

The ratio of lung weight to body weight is the most reliable parameter of lung growth, especially in preterm infants.[33,34] Obviously, this criterion is not useful for lung biopsies; therefore microscopic criteria are employed. The simplest method is the radial alveolar count, which is the number of alveoli transected by a perpendicular line drawn from the center of a respiratory bronchiole to the nearest septal division or pleural margin. The radial alveolar count in a full-term infant should average five alveolar spaces. While a valuable tool to evaluate lung complexity and growth, this method requires standardized inflation of the lung, as the radial alveolar count

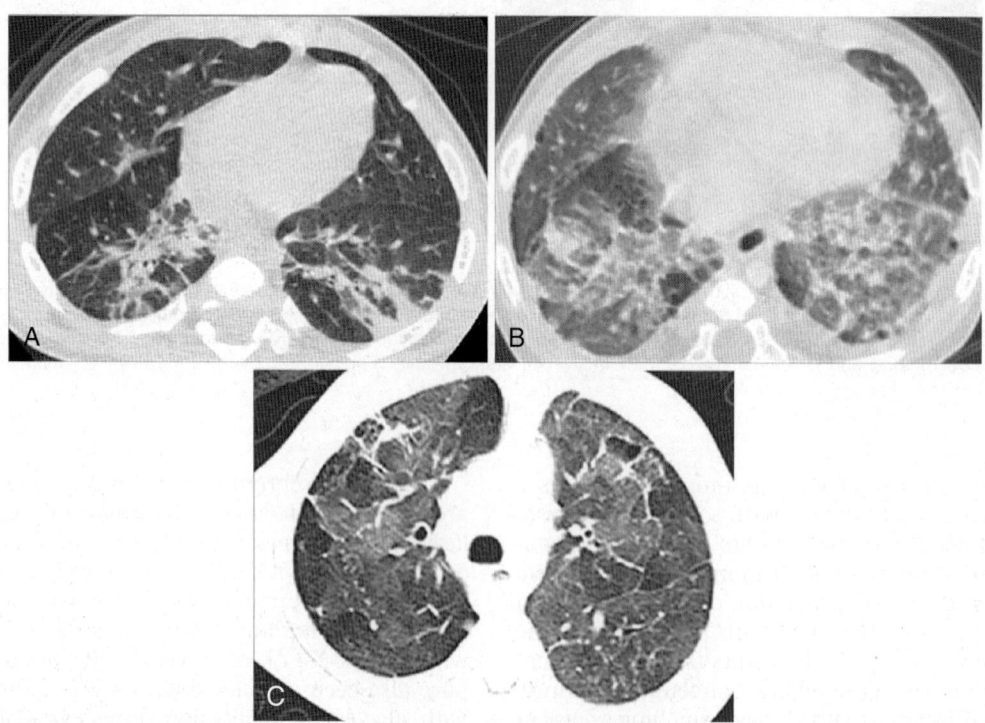

Fig. 56.2 Imaging appearance of lung growth abnormalities. (A) Chest HRCT from a 22-month-old shows thickened irregular scarlike densities bilaterally, most pronounced in the lower lobes. Other findings (not shown) included mild airspace consolidation, mild air-trapping, and peribronchial cuffing without definite bronchiectasis. These findings were felt consistent with bronchopulmonary dysplasia in this former 27-week preterm infant with a history of prolonged need for ventilatory support. (B) Chest HRCT from a 5-month-old, former 32-week preterm infant with Trisomy 21 and AV canal shows diffuse irregular opacities, architectural distortion, septal thickening, and numerous small subpleural cysts. (C) Chest HRCT from a 3-year-old former 30-week preterm infant shows mosaic appearance with irregular ground-glass opacities and geometric areas of hyperlucency, which are predominately peripheral in location and consistent with dilated secondary pulmonary lobules. Other findings included scattered small cysts, few dilated bronchi, and air-trapping on the expiratory images (not shown).

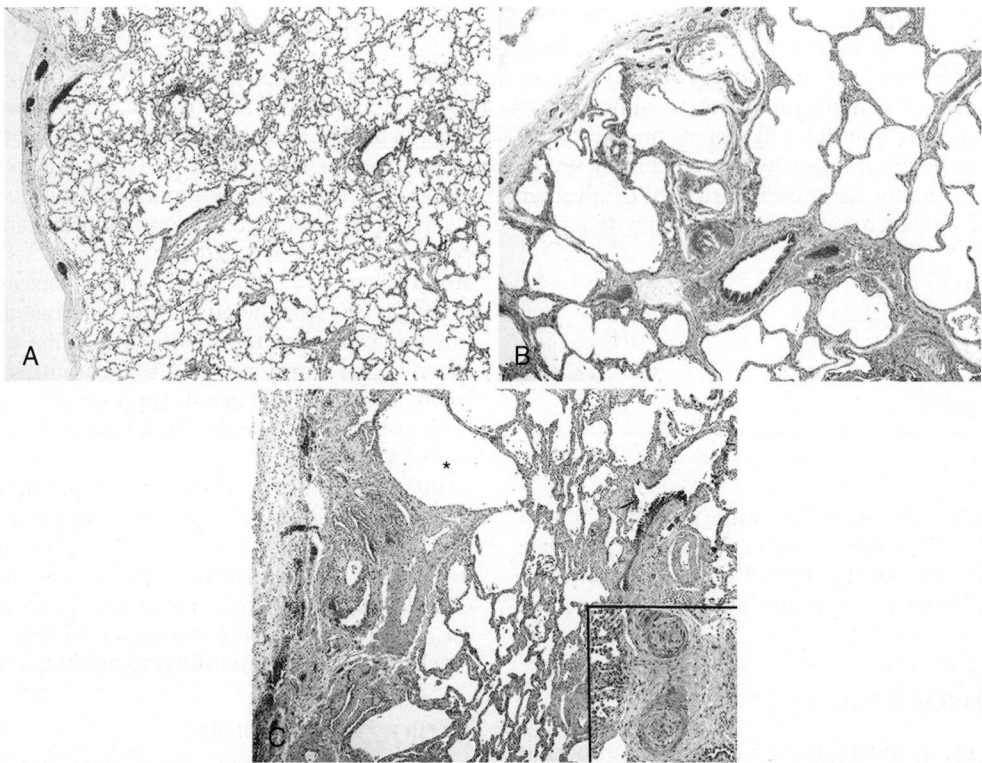

Fig. 56.3 Abnormal lung growth. Lung biopsy from a 3-year-old former 32 week preterm infant (B) (H&E, ×40) demonstrates the characteristic abnormalities of impaired postnatal alveolarization, with reduced and markedly enlarged airspaces; compare with a normal-term infant at the same magnification (A). In Down syndrome (C) deficient lung growth is often most prominent in the subpleural space with cystic dilatation of alveoli *(asterisk)* and often accompanied by prominent hypertensive changes of the pulmonary vasculature *(inset)*.

is substantially reduced in uninflated lungs.[35,36] In prenatal onset pulmonary hypoplasia, there is a reduction of number of alveolar spaces for gestational age, which is often accompanied by prominence of the bronchovascular structures and a widened interstitium. Lobular simplification with alveolar enlargement, often accentuated in the subpleural space, characterizes deficient alveolarization of postnatal onset (Fig. 56.3A and B). Following the widespread use of surfactant replacement and other therapies, the histology of "new bronchopulmonary dysplasia (BPD)"/chronic neonatal lung disease is characterized by less fibrosis and more uniform inflation than the classic form of BPD.[37] Hypertensive changes of the pulmonary arteries are commonly seen and are especially prominent in infants with a severe lung growth abnormality or Trisomy 21 (see Fig. 56.3C).[3,38] As discussed below, PIG is a frequent histologic finding in biopsies demonstrating impaired lung growth.

DIAGNOSIS AND DIFFERENTIAL DIAGNOSIS

Clinical context provides high pretest probability of this diagnosis, and consideration of the clinical setting may obviate the need for lung biopsy in many cases. Infant pulmonary function tests may suggest pulmonary hypoplasia, but they do not exclude concurrent processes. For infants with respiratory morbidity out of proportion to their clinical context, lung biopsy may still be required for diagnosis and to exclude alternative diagnoses. Proper tissue handling is essential, and expert pathologic review may be required.[39]

The clinical differential diagnosis is broad and may include other abnormalities in lung development such as lymphangiectasia, ACDMPV, PIG, and genetic disorders of surfactant production and metabolism. From a pathology perspective, the presence of alveolar enlargement and simplification is often misinterpreted as emphysematous change or a consequence of lung remodeling after injury. However, in lung growth abnormalities, there is no evidence of a destructive process in a lung growth abnormality. Without proper orientation and handling, alveolar simplification may be overlooked or difficult to recognize. Indeed, in the ChILDRN study, the majority of lung growth abnormality cases were not suspected clinically or recognized histologically at the initial institution, especially when occurring outside the setting of prematurity.[3]

MANAGEMENT AND TREATMENT

Management is focused largely on supportive care and underlying conditions. Recognition of this category of diagnosis may have important clinical implications, particularly as corticosteroids may not be indicated in this setting.

PROGNOSIS

Lung growth and maturation are key determinants of postnatal outcome, especially in premature infants or those with chromosomal or congenital abnormalities. Lung growth abnormalities are associated with considerable morbidity and mortality when compared to other causes of diffuse lung disease. In the ChILDRN study, mortality was 34% for lung growth abnormality cases, a proportion similar to the entire study cohort. However, among lung growth abnormality cases, prematurity and pulmonary hypertension were independent clinical predictors of mortality. On lung biopsy, severe lung growth abnormality, as judged by degree of alveolar enlargement and simplification, was associated with a high mortality (80%).[3]

Pulmonary Interstitial Glycogenosis

EPIDEMIOLOGY

PIG is a form of childhood ILD unique to neonates and young infants.[3,40] Although the incidence and prevalence of PIG are unknown and it is rare, PIG occurs more frequently and in a broader clinical spectrum than previously recognized.

ETIOLOGY AND PATHOGENESIS

The etiology of PIG is incompletely understood, although clearly related to lung development. Expert pathologic review of lung biopsies from the multiinstitutional ChILDRN study found that patchy PIG was present in over 40% of cases classified as having a lung growth abnormality.[3] This included not only chronic neonatal lung disease due to prematurity but also pulmonary hypoplasia and lung growth abnormalities in the setting of Trisomy 21 and congenital heart disease. Patchy PIG was also present in 22% of cases classified as vascular disorders masquerading as ILD.[3] Published and personal experience indicates that it is very unusual to observe PIG in lung biopsies beyond 6 months of age.

In their original report, Canakis and colleagues speculated that PIG reflects a delay or aberration in the maturation of pulmonary mesenchymal cells that do not normally contain abundant glycogen.[40] Others have suggested that PIG might reflect a nonspecific feature of several conditions that transiently alter lung growth and development in the neonatal period.[41] Recently, the presence of interstitial lipofibroblasts, cells reportedly seen only during prenatal lung development, were demonstrated in PIG biopsies.[42] Pulmonary lipofibroblasts are known to play critical roles in lung maturation through stimulating alveolarization during the period of septation and in lipid homeostasis by mediating lipid transfer to type 2 alveolar epithelial cells for surfactant phospholipid synthesis. Furthermore, these mesenchymal cells have been demonstrated to have transient proliferative capacity,[43] which is similar to interstitial fibroblasts in animal models of lung development and injury.[44-46] Within these models, coordinated control of fibroblast proliferation and apoptosis is necessary for septation of the distal airspaces during alveolarization.[47] Collectively, this evidence including the presence of lipofibroblasts in PIG strongly suggests that aberrant lung development is a critical component of PIG.

CLINICAL FEATURES AND PRESENTATION

Most infants with PIG are symptomatic in the first days to weeks of life, which may follow an initial period of well-being after birth. The clinical presentation can be variable, ranging from indolent tachypnea and hypoxia to neonatal acute respiratory failure and pulmonary hypertension. The initial report of PIG included seven neonates, and five of whom presented in the first 24 hours of life.[40] In the ChILDRN study,[3] six cases (3.2% of infant lung biopsies) were identified in which PIG was the only significant histologic finding. All but one case presented with hypoxemia at birth, and the mean age at biopsy was 1.3 ± 0.4 months. There is clinical and pathologic evidence to support that PIG is often a self-limited disorder, and the diagnosis is typically made by 6 months of age.[3,40,43]

PIG can occur in either term or premature infants and may be an isolated disorder or a component of other congenital conditions. PIG commonly occurs in the setting of lung growth abnormalities (see earlier) and has also been observed in infants with congenital heart disease, Trisomy 21, pulmonary hypertension, meconium aspiration, and rarely other developmental anomalies.

RADIOLOGIC FINDINGS

Case series have reported that chest radiographs have diffuse infiltrates or hazy opacities, but no common high-resolution CT (HRCT) scan pattern has been identified (Fig. 56.4A–D).[3,48-51]

HISTOLOGIC FINDINGS

Formally known as cellular interstitial pneumonitis and histiocytoid pneumonia,[52] the term *PIG* was coined by Canakis et al. based on the histologic finding of increased glycogen-laden mesenchymal cells in the alveolar interstitium.[40] Lung biopsy shows a patchy or diffuse expansion of the alveolar walls by bland spindle-shaped cells with pale or bubbly cytoplasm (see Fig. 56.4E and F). Patchy distribution is frequent when there is a concomitant lung growth abnormality,[3] and associated inflammation or fibrosis in the interstitium is absent. The cells are strongly immunopositive for vimentin, a mesenchymal marker, and periodic acid–Schiff (PAS) stain may demonstrate PAS positive diastase labile material within the cytoplasm of the cells (see Fig. 56.4G and H). As the preservation of glycogen is influenced by using aqueous fixatives (i.e., 10% formalin), the presence of PAS positivity may be difficult to demonstrate on routine sections. Electron microscopy is considered the best approach to reveal the accumulation of monoparticulate glycogen in these interstitial cells, and treating ultrathin sections with tannic acid enhances visualization of glycogen.[40]

DIAGNOSIS AND DIFFERENTIAL DIAGNOSIS

Currently, lung biopsy is the only way to diagnose PIG. The diagnosis may be suspected in the context of a neonate with respiratory compromise, particularly when the severity is disproportionate to the degree of coexisting conditions, including prematurity and congenital heart disease.

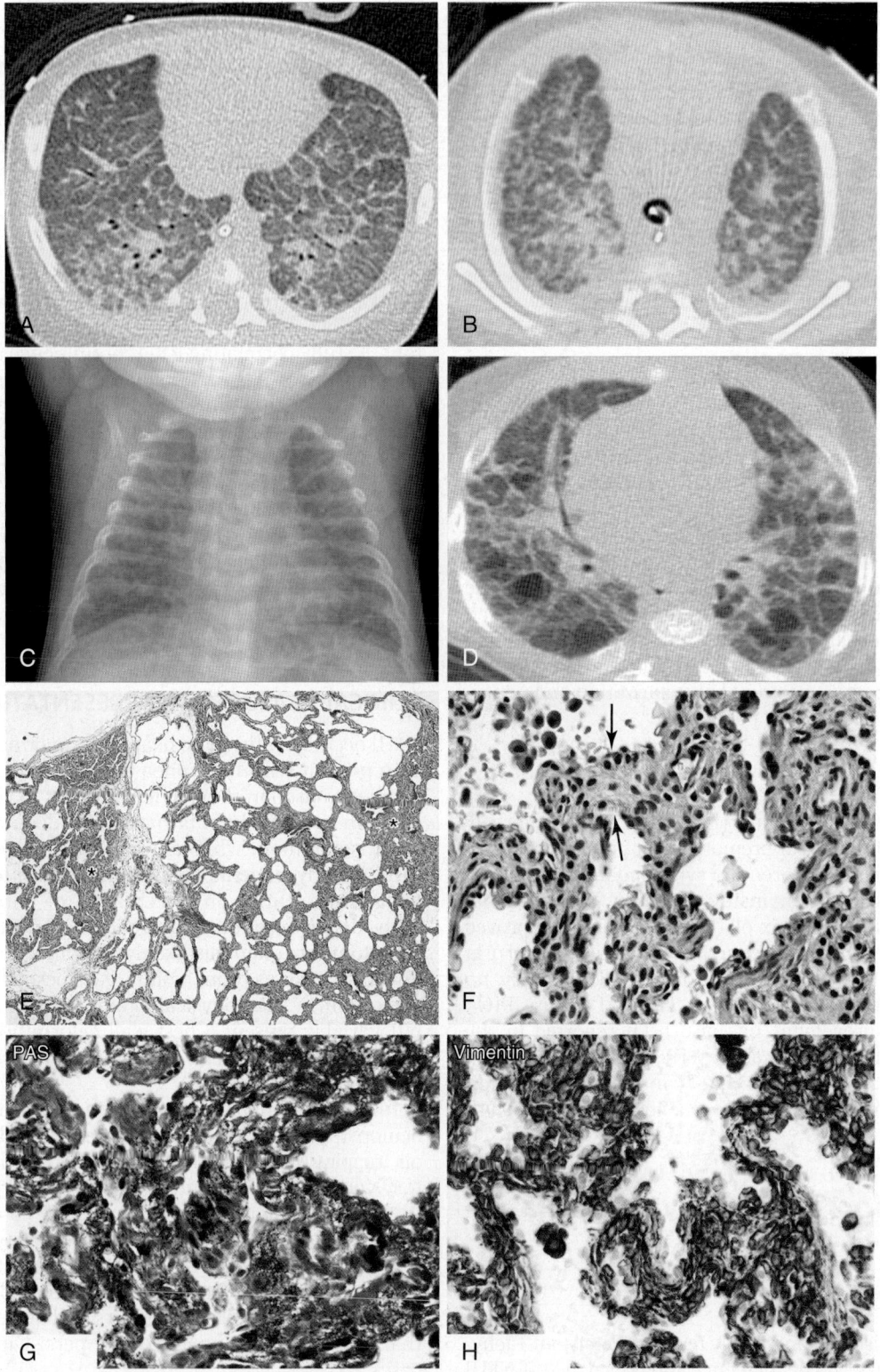

Fig. 56.4 Imaging and histologic findings in pulmonary interstitial glycogenosis. Chest HRCT (A and B) from a 2-week old infant shows diffuse interstitial markings and interlobular septal thickening present bilaterally throughout all lung zones. This 38-week estimated gestational age infant had no respiratory difficulties at birth but required supplemental oxygen in the first days of life, intubation on day of life 5, and nitric oxide for severe pulmonary hypertension. Chest radiographic (C) and HRCT (D) images from a 5-month-old, former 34-week preterm infant show diffuse coarse interstitial and parenchymal abnormalities including architectural distortion and cystic change. This infant had persistent tachypnea and hypoxemia without need for mechanical ventilation; lung biopsy (E) (H&E, ×40) performed at 5 months of age showed patchy pulmonary interstitial glycogenosis *(asterisks)* and moderate deficient alveolarization, which is consistent with a lung growth abnormality. (F) On higher power (H&E, ×200), the bland spindled cells of pulmonary interstitial glycogenosis are seen to widen the alveolar septae *(arrows)*. These cells contain glycogen (G) (periodic acid Schiff stain, ×200) and show strong immunoreactivity with vimentin (H) (×200).

Disorders to be considered in the clinical differential diagnosis include sepsis, congenital heart disease, lung developmental disorders (e.g., alveolar capillary dysplasia with misalignment of the pulmonary veins), pulmonary hypoplasia, pulmonary vascular disease, lymphangiectasia, and genetic disorders of surfactant production and metabolism. Primary ciliary dyskinesia (PCD) could also mimic milder cases of PIG due to the frequent occurrence of neonatal tachypnea in PCD.[53] From the perspective of the pathologist, careful attention is required to identify potential concurrent histologic findings, such as lung growth abnormalities or structural alterations of the pulmonary vasculature.

MANAGEMENT AND TREATMENT

Most children will require supplemental oxygen and some will require aggressive support including mechanical ventilation and therapy for pulmonary hypertension. When present, comorbidities such as congenital heart disease or complications of prematurity are often the focus of management.

High-dose intravenous corticosteroids have been reported to have benefit in case reports and case series,[40,43,48,49] but no controlled studies have been performed and there is little evidence to guide therapeutic recommendations. It has been suggested that consideration for use of corticosteroids should be assessed in the context of clinical severity and the potential detrimental impact on postnatal alveolarization and neurodevelopment in this patient population.[51]

PROGNOSIS

The natural history is unknown, but mortality is largely related to complications of prematurity or pulmonary hypoplasia.[3,40,51] Patients may remain symptomatic for months, and supportive care is a mainstay of therapy. In the original report by Canakis et al., six of the seven infants improved over time, with mortality occurring in one infant born at 25 weeks gestation.[40] Similarly, in the ChILDRN study, no mortality occurred among the six cases of diffuse PIG,[3] and clinical improvement has also been reported in the small number of published case reports.[43,48,50] However, high mortality has occurred when significant pulmonary conditions are present along with PIG, particularly lung growth abnormalities.[43,51]

Neuroendocrine Cell Hyperplasia of Infancy

EPIDEMIOLOGY

NEHI is a rare disorder previously termed "Persistent Tachypnea of Infancy."[54,55] The incidence and prevalence of NEHI are unknown, and it is suspected that many cases remain undiagnosed, although cases are increasingly recognized worldwide.[56–61] In the ChILDRN study, NEHI cases represented 10% of all lung biopsies from children less than 2 years of age.[3] A recent study from a large referral center identified 19 cases (14%) from among 138 lung biopsy cases accrued over a 10-year period.[62] The original series of 15 cases had a slight male predominance, which was not observed in a subsequent study.[51,55]

ETIOLOGY AND PATHOGENESIS

The etiology of NEHI is unknown, but genetic mechanisms play a role in at least some cases.[63] In one family, a heterozygous mutation in NKX2.1 (also called thyroid transcription factor 1, or TTF1) was identified in association with familial NEHI.[64] The mutation results in a nonconservative amino acid substitution in the homeodomain in a codon extensively conserved through evolution. To date, NKX2.1 mutations have not been identified in other NEHI cases.

Lung biopsies in NEHI are characterized by prominent pulmonary neuroendocrine cells (PNECs) in the distal airways, but the role of PNECs in NEHI pathogenesis remains uncertain. A study correlating PNEC prominence and the severity of small airway obstruction on infant PFTs in NEHI patients suggests a potential causal role.[62] Based on the role of PNECs and bombesin in oxygen sensing as well as airway and arterial tone, it has been hypothesized that neuroendocrine cells may lead to ventilation/perfusion mismatch within the lung.[55] The physiologic abnormalities observed on infant pulmonary function tests in NEHI suggest that the disorder is not fully explained on this basis. The absence of active neuroendocrine cell proliferation in lung biopsies and lack of correlation with airway injury suggest that PNEC prominence in NEHI is not due to injurious stimuli.

CLINICAL FEATURES AND PRESENTATION

NEHI occurs in otherwise healthy-term or near-term infants who present with tachypnea and retractions, generally of insidious onset, in the first few months to year of life. Rare cases in preterm infants have been documented. Hypoxemia is common, while chronic cough and wheezing are rare.[55] Many patients come to medical attention because of failure to thrive or exacerbation of chronic symptoms with upper respiratory infections. However, respiratory symptoms are often mistakenly attributed to more common disorders such as bronchiolitis, gastroesophageal reflux, or aspiration.[56,60] On physical exam, crackles are prominent but variably present. Chest wall deformity with increased anteroposterior diameter is common, while clubbing has not been reported.

Infant pulmonary function testing (PFT) in NEHI patients demonstrates a mixed physiologic pattern including profound air-trapping and proportionate reductions in the forced expiratory volume in 0.5 seconds (FEV0.5) and forced vital capacity (FVC), with particularly reduced FEF75 and FEF85 and markedly elevated functional residual capacity (FRC), residual volume (RV), and RV/TLC. Pulmonary function testing has not been systematically studied in older children, although limited published data and personal experience suggest that this physiologic pattern can persist in at least some cases.[58,65,66]

RADIOLOGIC FINDINGS

Chest radiographs may be normal or may reveal hyperinflation.[55] HRCT findings are distinctive with geographic ground-glass opacities centrally and in the right middle lobe and lingula (Fig. 56.5A–C). Air-trapping is often demonstrated when expiratory images are performed. Brody et al. evaluated chest HRCT scans from 23 children with biopsy-proven

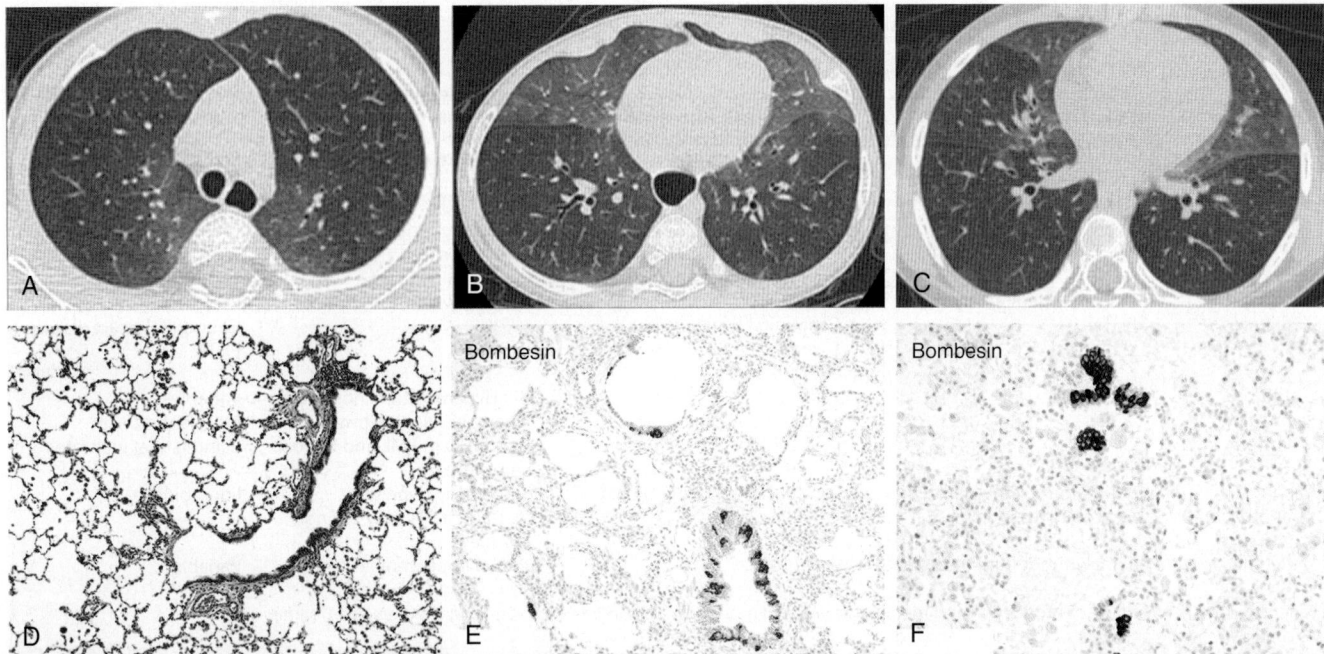

Fig. 56.5 Characteristic radiographic and pathologic findings in neuroendocrine cell hyperplasia of infancy (NEHI). (A and B) A 13-month-old term infant presented at age 6 months with chronic tachypnea, retractions, and hypoxemia, had chronic indolent respiratory symptoms since the first month of life and poor weight gain since 5 months of age. HRCT images obtained at total lung capacity under general anesthesia show well defined regions of apparent ground glass opacity in the medial portions of the upper lobes (A) and in the right middle lobe and lingula (B). Diffuse air-trapping was seen on expiratory images (not shown). (C) HRCT shows a similar pattern of apparent regional ground glass opacity in a 3-year-old with chronic tachypnea, retractions, and crackles since infancy being treated for recurrent pneumonia and refractory asthma. No additional radiographic abnormalities were identified. (D). Lung biopsies from NEHI patients typically show essentially normal histology. Mild nonspecific changes that may be present in the biopsy include mild periairway lymphocytic aggregates and increased alveolar macrophages (H&E, ×100). Increased neuroendocrine cells within bronchioles is best visualized by bombesin immunostaining (E) (×100). (F) Neuroepithelial bodies (NEBs) around alveolar ducts are frequently prominent (×200).

NEHI and 6 children with other forms of ILD. While HRCT specificity for the diagnosis of NEHI was 100% in this study when the CTs were reviewed by two expert radiologists, the sensitivity of HRCT was incomplete, as readers did not suggest NEHI in up to 22% of the cases.[67]

HISTOLOGIC FINDINGS

In contrast to the clinical severity of the disorder, lung biopsies in NEHI often show minimal to no pathologic alterations and may be initially interpreted as normal (see Fig. 56.5D). Patchy mild inflammation or fibrosis (bronchiolitis) may be present, especially following a viral infection, but this not sufficient to support an etiology for the patient's significant symptomatology. Pathologic diagnosis of NEHI rests on finding an increased proportion of neuroendocrine cells within distal airways, best seen by bombesin and serotonin immunohistochemistry.[55,59,61] Neuron-specific enolase, calcitonin, synaptophysin, and chromogranin have been shown to be less reliable in demonstrating this increase in neuroendocrine cell numbers. Immunohistochemical assessment of this disorder requires an adequate biopsy with at least 10–15 airways for evaluation. As wide intra and inter-subject variability in neuroendocrine cell number has been reported, which does not relate to imaging appearance of the region biopsied, more than one biopsy site is recommended. Morphometric quantification of bombesin staining may be required. In general, bombesin immunopositive cells

in NEHI are prominent in the distal respiratory bronchioles and as clusters (neuroepithelial bodies) in the alveolar ducts (see Fig. 56.5E and F). Two individual airways with more than 10% bombesin-immunopositive area or cell number of the airway epithelium is also suggestive of the diagnosis, although may not be present.[59] A minor degree of airway injury does not alter pathologic confirmation of the diagnosis.

DIAGNOSIS AND DIFFERENTIAL DIAGNOSIS

Clinical suspicion is essential in the diagnosis of NEHI. The initial diagnostic approach should be to exclude more common causes of the clinical symptoms such as infection, cystic fibrosis, and congenital heart disease. In the appropriate clinical context, the diagnosis may be made by chest HRCT in a majority of cases and sometimes be supported by data from infant PFTs, which may play a role in supporting the diagnosis of NEHI.[68] At this time, genetic testing is not routinely helpful in making the diagnosis.[64]

Although lung biopsy is the historical gold standard, lung biopsy is not required to make the diagnosis except in patients with atypical clinical or HRCT findings. There are important limitations to lung biopsy. Specifically, the numbers of PNECs are variable and not always seen without sufficient airway sampling. Furthermore, the presence of increased number of neuroendocrine cells on lung biopsy is not sufficient for the diagnosis, as PNEC prominence is associated with a variety

Table 56.2   Forms of Childhood Interstitial Lung Diseases "More Prevalent in Infancy"

Disorder[a]	Alveolar Capillary Dysplasia With Misalignment of the Pulmonary Veins	Lung Growth Abnormalities	Neuroendocrine Cell Hyperplasia of Infancy	Pulmonary Interstitial Glycogenosis
Common age of presentation	Birth	Birth	Infancy with most in first year of life Rare at birth	Early neonatal
Hereditary basis	Yes *FOXF1*; autosomal dominant	Uncertain Frequent in association with chromosomal abnormalities	Suspected Not established	Unknown
Associated features	Other congenital anomalies PHTN	Prematurity Congenital heart disease Trisomy 21 PHTN	None known	Prematurity Congenital heart disease PHTN
Common Imaging Pattern	Uncertain	Variable May include architectural distortion, cystic change	CXR: Hyperinflation, normal, or mild perihilar infiltrates HRCT: GGO in RML and lingual Air-trapping	Variable Frequent diffuse interstitial infiltrates
Diagnostic approach	Lung biopsy; emergence of genetic testing	Clinical context, lung biopsy	Lung biopsy definitive HRCT and iPFTs may strongly suggest	Lung biopsy
Outcome	Fatal without lung transplant[b]	Variable	Gradual improvement (years)	Variable

[a]Genetic disorders of surfactant production and metabolism are also more prevalent in infants and young children. See Chapter 57.
[b]Variable penetrance and phenotype data emerging.
FOXF1, Forkhead Box F1 gene; *GGO*, ground-glass opacities; *iPFT*, infant pulmonary function test; *PHTN*, pulmonary hypertension; *RML*, right middle lobe.

of other pulmonary conditions, including BPD, sudden infant death syndrome, pulmonary hypertension, cystic fibrosis, and follicular bronchiolitis.[59,69–74]

Disorders to be considered in the clinical differential include acute or chronic infection, asthma, and airway injury including bronchiolitis obliterans. In addition, other infant lung disorders such as pulmonary hypoplasia, PIG and genetic disorders of surfactant production, and metabolism should be considered. As discussed previously, neuroendocrine cell prominence on lung biopsy should be correlated with other potential pathologic findings, and other entities associated with increased neuroendocrine cells excluded.

MANAGEMENT AND TREATMENT

There is no known definitive therapy for NEHI, and management largely consists of general supportive and preventative care. Most children will require supplemental oxygen, and many will require nutritional supplementation. Corticosteroids are not helpful in most cases[55]; therefore establishment of the diagnosis of NEHI helps to avoid the complications of long-term steroid therapy. Genetic counseling and family support are important components of care for all families who experience the diagnosis of a rare disease.

PROGNOSIS

While long-term outcomes are not well established for this recently recognized disorder, a diagnosis of NEHI brings a cautious but welcomed prognosis relative to other forms of childhood ILD. There have been no deaths reported, and no patients have required lung transplantation.[3,55] The clinical course is prolonged, but most children demonstrate gradual improvement. The need for supplemental oxygen is variable and may be many years in duration.[55,58] Patients may also

remain symptomatic with respiratory infections or exercise intolerance.[63,75] In one report, six of nine infants developed a phenotype consistent with nonatopic asthma.[58] Exacerbations, with concomitant air-trapping, have also been described.[65] The CT abnormalities may persist into adulthood in at least some cases, but the time course of radiologic resolution in relationship to clinical parameters has not been systematically studied.[64,66]

Summary

Despite overlapping clinical features most forms of ILD have distinct imaging and histologic findings (Table 56.2). Recognition of these disorders informs diagnostic approach, enables timely diagnosis, and has implications for management and prognosis.

References

Access the reference list online at ExpertConsult.com.

Suggested Readings

Brody AS, Guillerman RP, Hay TC, et al. Neuroendocrine cell hyperplasia of infancy: diagnosis with high-resolution CT. *AJR Am J Roentgenol.* 2010;194(1):238–244.

Canakis AM, Cutz E, Manson D, et al. Pulmonary interstitial glycogenosis: a new variant of neonatal interstitial lung disease. *Am J Respir Crit Care Med.* 2002;165(11):1557–1565.

Deterding RR, Pye C, Fan LL, et al. Persistent tachypnea of infancy is associated with neuroendocrine cell hyperplasia. *Pediatr Pulmonol.* 2005;40(2):157–165.

Deutsch GH, Young LR, Deterding RR, et al. Diffuse lung disease in young children: application of a novel classification scheme. *Am J Respir Crit Care Med.* 2007;176(11):1120–1128.

Deutsch GH, Young LR. Pulmonary interstitial glycogenosis: words of caution. *Pediatr Radiol.* 2010;40(9):1471–1475.

Kurland G, Deterding RR, Hagood JS, et al. An official American Thoracic Society clinical practice guideline: classification, evaluation, and management of childhood interstitial lung disease in infancy. *Am J Respir Crit Care Med*. 2013;188:376–394.

Langston C, Patterson K, Dishop MK, et al. A protocol for the handling of tissue obtained by operative lung biopsy: recommendations of the chILD pathology co-operative group. *Pediatr Dev Pathol*. 2006;9(3):173–180.

Stanewicz P, Sen P, Bhatt SS, et al. Genomic and genic deletions of the FOX gene cluster on 16q24.1 and inactivating mutations of FOXF1 cause alveolar capillary dysplasia and other malformations. *Am J Hum Genet*. 2009;84(6):780–791.

Young LR, Brody AS, Inge TH, et al. Neuroendocrine cell distribution and frequency distinguish neuroendocrine cell hyperplasia of infancy from other pulmonary disorders. *Chest*. 2011;139(5):1060–1071.

57 Lung Diseases Associated With Disruption of Pulmonary Surfactant Homeostasis

LAWRENCE M. NOGEE, MD, and BRUCE C. TRAPNELL, MD

Pulmonary surfactant is a mixture of specific lipids and proteins that reduces surface tension at the air-liquid-tissue interface, thereby preventing alveolar collapse at end expiration. This critical function requires tight regulation of alveolar surfactant composition and quantity (i.e., surfactant homeostasis), which is achieved through coordinated expression of multiple genes resulting in balanced production and clearance of surfactant.

The most common lung disorder associated with disruption of surfactant homeostasis is the respiratory distress syndrome (RDS), which occurs mainly in premature infants, principally due to surfactant deficiency from insufficient production by alveolar epithelial cells secondary to immaturity. Another disorder of surfactant homeostasis is pulmonary alveolar proteinosis (PAP), a syndrome (not a disease) characterized by the slow, progressive accumulation of surfactant lipids and proteins within alveoli resulting in displacement of air and impairment of oxygen uptake. The most common cause of the PAP syndrome is an autoimmune disease mediated by neutralizing autoantibodies against the cytokine granulocyte-macrophage colony-stimulating factor (GM-CSF). High levels of GM-CSF autoantibodies block GM-CSF stimulation of alveolar macrophages, which is critical for enabling surfactant clearance by these cells. Although autoimmune PAP occurs most commonly in adults and adolescents, it has been seen in children as young as 3 years old.

Single-gene mutations that disrupt the production of normal surfactant and that impair GM-CSF–dependent surfactant clearance by alveolar macrophages have been identified. These genetic disorders of surfactant homeostasis can be usefully categorized as disorders of surfactant production or surfactant clearance. The clinical presentation and features, pathogenesis, natural history, therapeutic responses, and prognosis of individual disorders of surfactant homeostasis vary widely. Although rare, these disorders are associated with significant morbidity and mortality. A heightened awareness can improve early recognition, accurate diagnosis, and facilitate counseling about prognosis and the risk of disease recurrence in future pregnancies. Understanding the pathophysiology of these disorders provides potential insights into normal surfactant metabolism and how genetic mechanisms contribute to more common diseases, such as neonatal RDS.

This chapter summarizes current knowledge concerning disorders of surfactant production and clearance that cause acute and chronic lung disease. Further advances in the understanding of lung development and surfactant metabolism combined with technological advances and data derived from the human genome project are likely to allow for continued identification of novel genetic mechanisms for neonatal and pediatric lung disease.

Epidemiology

OVERVIEW OF SURFACTANT COMPOSITION AND METABOLISM

Pulmonary surfactant is a complex mixture of phospholipids, neutral lipids, and specific proteins that is produced by the alveolar type II epithelial cell (AEC2), stored in intracellular organelles known as lamellar bodies, and secreted by exocytosis into the alveolar lumen. The major lipid present in pulmonary surfactant is phosphatidylcholine (PC), a large fraction of which contains two palmitic acid side chains that are fully saturated (dipalmitoyl or disaturated phosphatidylcholine, DPPC or DSPC); its presence is critical for surfactant to function in reducing surface tension. ABCA3 is a member of the adenosine triphosphate (ATP) binding cassette family of membrane transporters that is located on the limiting membrane of lamellar bodies and has a key role in the transport of phospholipids into lamellar bodies during the biosynthesis of surfactant. The effective lowering of surface tension also requires the presence of one or both of two extremely hydrophobic surfactant proteins (SPs), SP-B and SP-C. Pulmonary surfactant also contains two larger glycoproteins, SP-A and SP-D, which are members of the collectin family, having both a collagenous domain and a carbohydrate-binding domain. The principal roles for SP-A and SP-D appear to be in local host defense and immunomodulation rather than surface tension lowering.[1,2] The production of ABCA3 and SP-A, SP-B, SP-C, and SP-D is developmentally regulated and increases during gestation. Specific transcription factors that bind to DNA sequences in the promoter regions of each gene are important for the proper expression of each protein, including thyroid transcription factor 1 (TTF-1), which is encoded by the gene *NKX2-1*.[3,4] Mutations in the genes encoding SP-A (*SFTPA1, SFTPA2*) have been associated with the phenotypes of pulmonary fibrosis and lung cancer in adults; disease-causing mutations in the gene encoding SP-D (*SFTPD*) have not yet been reported.[5–7]

After secretion, pulmonary surfactant is both recycled into AEC2s and is cleared by alveolar macrophages. For macrophages to properly mature and efficiently catabolize surfactant, GM-CSF must bind to a specific receptor at the cell

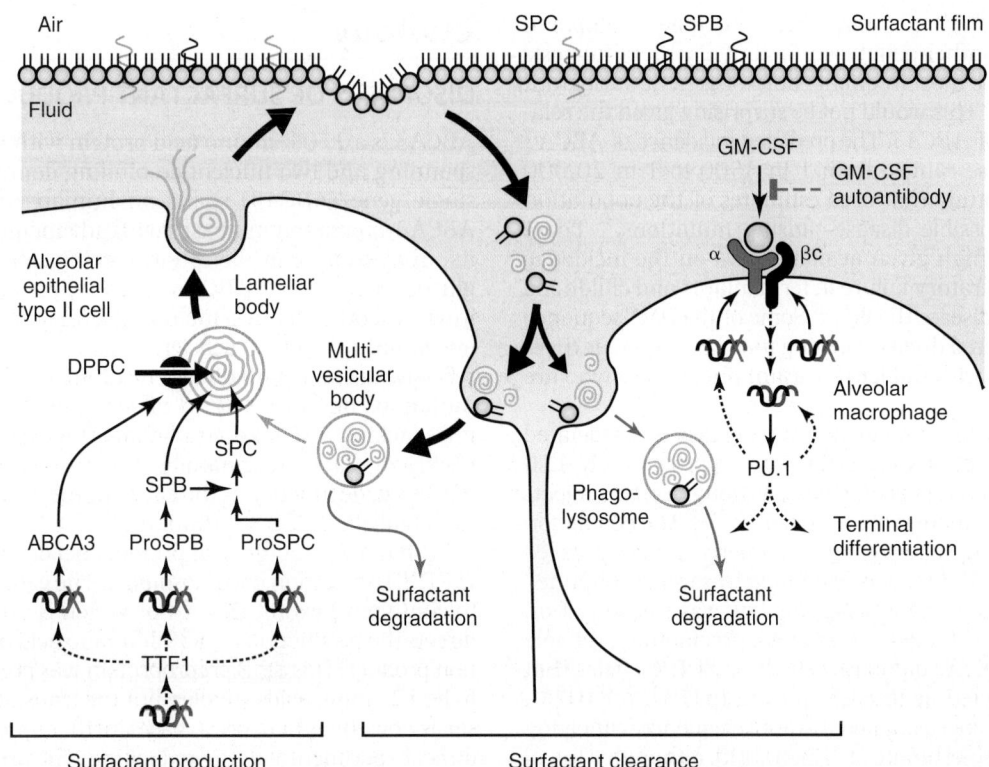

Fig. 57.1 Simplified overview of surfactant production and clearance. Surfactant lipids and proteins are synthesized by alveolar type II cells, with thyroid transcription factor 1 *(TTF-1)* needed for transcription of SP-B, SP-C, and ABCA3. SP-B and SP-C are synthesized as proproteins and processed in lamellar bodies. The lamellar bodies fuse with the apical cell membrane, and the surfactant complex is secreted by exocytosis, with SP-B and SP-C helping enhance adsorption to the air-liquid interface and organize surfactant lipids. Surfactant material is recycled through type II cells by endocytosis and taken up in multivesicular bodies. Surfactant is internalized and its components broken down in the phagolysosomes of alveolar macrophages. Binding of granulocyte-macrophage colony-stimulating factor *(GM-CSF)* to its receptor initiates signaling pathways leading to nuclear binding of the transcription factor PU.1 to regulatory elements in genes needed for macrophage maturation and functions, including clearance of surfactant.

surface and initiate specific signaling events. The receptor is composed of two chains: a specific ligand-binding α chain (CD116) and a β chain (CD131) that enhances affinity and is shared with the receptors for interleukin (IL)-3 and IL-5.[8,9] Binding of GM-CSF to its receptor initiates intracellular signaling cascades and activates the transcription factor PU.1, which regulates multiple alveolar macrophage functions, including the ability to catabolize surfactant components (Fig. 57.1).[10]

EPIDEMIOLOGY OF SURFACTANT PRODUCTION DISORDERS

The precise incidence and prevalence of disorders of surfactant production and clearance are unknown, although both relative and absolute estimates may be made based upon case ascertainment and population-based studies of the frequency of deleterious genetic variants identified in each of the responsible genes *(SFTPB, ABCA3, SFTPC, NKX2-1, CSF2RA, CSF2RB)*. Publicly available databases of genetic variants identified through large-scale exome sequencing of different populations are available, including the 1000 genomes project (www.1000genomes.org), Exome Aggregation Consortium (exac.broadinstitute.org), and Exome Sequencing Project of the US National Institutes of Health (evs.gs.washington.edu/EVS/). However, the potential clinical

significance of most of the variants listed is usually unclear, and thus caution is needed in the interpretation of findings from these databases in inferring the population frequency of potentially deleterious variants.

Hereditary SP-B deficiency was the first recognized genetic abnormality of surfactant production but is probably the rarest.[11] Fewer than 60 cases have been reported in the literature.[12] The carrier frequency of the most commonly encountered mutation in the SP-B gene *(SFTPB)* in the US population was estimated to be approximately 1 in 1000 individuals.[13,14] Combining this finding with the observation that this mutation has accounted for approximately ⅔ of the mutant *SFTPB* alleles identified to date, this would predict a disease incidence of 1 in 1.5 million live births. The relative incidence in other countries and subpopulations may differ: the carrier rate for the same mutation in Denmark was found to be 1 in 560 individuals, which would still predict a very low incidence of disease.[15] This mutation has been found mainly in individuals of Northern European descent, and the incidence of deleterious *SFTPB* mutations in other populations may be even less. SP-B deficiency has not been recognized in Japan, and the prevalence of likely pathogenic mutations in databases obtained from large-scale exome sequencing studies is very low.[16,17]

More than 250 subjects with ABCA3 deficiency have been reported, and the relative frequency with which

ABCA3-deficient infants have been identified compared with those with other genetic surfactant disorders suggests that it may be the most frequent cause of genetic surfactant dysfunction.[18-23] This would not be surprising given the relatively large size of *ABCA3*. The predicted incidence of ABCA3 deficiency disease ranged from 1 in 3500 to 1 in 20,000 live births in a study that used estimates of the population frequency of possible disease-causing mutations.[24] These estimates seem high given available data on the incidence of neonatal respiratory failure in term infants and childhood interstitial lung disease (ILD).[25-27] Some of the DNA sequence variants considered disease causing may be benign, or there may be patients with milder or variant phenotypes who are not recognized.

The incidence and prevalence of lung disease associated with *SFTPC* mutations are unknown. Approximately 170 subjects have been reported to date, although some subjects are represented in more than one report.[22,28-32] The population frequency of the most frequently encountered mutation, called p.Ile73Thr (or p.I73T), was examined in samples obtained from neonatal screening programs but was not found on any of almost 9000 alleles examined, precluding a reliable estimate.[14] The ExAc database lists three *SFTPC* alleles that have been reported as disease causing (p.I73T, p.V102M, p.A112T) out of approximately 120,000 sequenced, implying a minimal disease-estimate of 1 in 40,000, although clinical data on these subjects are not available.

The incidence of lung disease due to *NKX2-1* mutations or deletions is unknown. Almost 200 patients with deleterious *NKX2-1* genetic variants have been reported, but such variants may also cause neurologic symptoms or hypothyroidism in the absence of lung disease, and in approximately $\frac{1}{3}$ of reported cases either a pulmonary phenotype was not recognized or formally investigated.[33-41] Such mutations appear to be a rare cause of congenital hypothyroidism,[42,43] but studies focusing on the frequency of the pulmonary phenotype have not been performed. None of the sequence variants listed in the ExAc database have been reported as disease causing, precluding an estimate of disease incidence using this resource.

EPIDEMIOLOGY OF SURFACTANT CLEARANCE DISORDERS

Autoimmune PAP accounts for approximately 85% of all PAP cases, with an incidence and prevalence, respectively, of 0.42 and 6–7 per million in the general population.[44,45] The disorder affects all races and ethnic groups, is globally distributed, and is more common in men than women, due to the increased frequency of smoking among men. The disease usually presents in the third to fifth decade of life, with progressive dyspnea of insidious onset and diffuse bilateral lung infiltrates on radiologic evaluation. The presentation is similar in younger adults, adolescents, and children as young as 3 years of age. Clubbing is not a feature, although occasionally fever and hemoptysis may be present and usually indicate the presence of a secondary infection.

Approximately 35 people with hereditary PAP due to mutations in *CSF2RA* or *CSF2RB* have been reported to date, and population estimates of the frequency of these disorders are not available.[46-52]

Etiology

DISORDERS OF SURFACTANT PRODUCTION

ABCA3 is a 1704–amino acid protein with two membrane-spanning and two nucleotide-binding domains encoded by single gene *(ABCA3)* spans on human chromosome 16. ABCA3 expression increases with advancing gestation, and its expression can be pharmacologically increased by glucocorticoids.[53-55] ABCA3 is also expressed at low levels in several other tissues, including kidney, intestine, thyroid, and brain.[53-56] ABCA3 deficiency is inherited in an autosomal recessive fashion, with disease resulting from loss-of-function mutations on both *ABCA3* alleles. Genetically engineered mice lacking ABCA3 do not inflate their lungs and die from respiratory failure perinatally, supporting that disruption of ABCA3 gene function is the cause of the findings in children with biallelic ABCA3 mutations.[57-60]

SP-B is a 79–amino acid protein encoded on a single gene *(SFTPB)* on human chromosome 2. The gene is now thought to contain 12 exons, the last of which is untranslated, and directs the production of a 393–amino acid primary translation product. This SP-B preproprotein was previously believed to be 12 amino acids smaller, but the translational initiation site is now thought to be 36 bases further upstream, although direct experimental data are lacking. The proprotein undergoes proteolytic processing to yield the mature, very hydrophobic protein found in the airspaces, which is encoded in exons 7 and 8.[61,62] SP-B is produced primarily by AEC2s, routed to lamellar bodies, and secreted along with surfactant phospholipids into the airspaces. The gene is also expressed within the lung in nonciliated bronchiolar epithelial cells, although only AEC2s fully process the proprotein (proSP-B) to mature SP-B.

SP-B deficiency is inherited as an autosomal recessive disorder due to loss-of-function mutations on both alleles. The first recognized *SFTPB* mutation remains the most frequently identified and involves a net 2-base insertion in what, at the time of its discovery, was thought to be codon 121, and the mutation was thus termed 121ins2.[63] The mutation results in a frameshift and premature codon for the termination of translation; current terminology for this variant is c.397delCinsGAA (p.P133Qfs*95), and a common ancestral origin likely accounts for it being found in multiple unrelated individuals.[64] More than two dozen other SP-B mutations have been identified, as well as a deletion spanning exons 7 and 8.[12,21,65-71] Most of these mutations are unique to a given family, although several mutations have been identified in apparently unrelated families in certain ethnic groups.[65]

SP-C is an extremely hydrophobic 35–amino acid protein encoded by a single gene *(SFTPC)* on human chromosome 8, containing 6 exons, of which the sixth is untranslated. Mature SP-C, encoded in the second exon, is derived from proteolytic processing of a larger precursor protein (proSP-C) of 191 or 197 amino acids, depending upon alternative splicing at the beginning of exon 5. The last 100 amino acids of proSP-C have homology with a group of proteins known as BRICHOS that are mutated in some familial dementias.[72] Proper folding of this domain may provide an important chaperone function in terms of moving the hydrophobic proSP-C protein through the cell.[73,74]

Lung disease resulting from mutations in *SFTPC* is either inherited in an autosomal dominant fashion with variable penetrance, or sporadic disease may occur due to de novo mutations.[28-31,75-86] A mutation on one allele is sufficient to cause disease, although subjects with biallelic mutations have been reported.[16,29,32,77,87-89] One mutation, a predicted substitution of isoleucine for threonine in codon 73 (p.Ilet73Thr or p.I73T), has accounted for 35%-50% of the mutant *SFTPC* alleles reported to date from multiple unrelated families.[28,75-77,86,90-92] This mutation has arisen on genetically diverse *SFTPC* alleles, suggesting recurrent mutation as the mechanism for a common mutation.[77,86] Most other reported mutations are in the region encoding the BRICHOS domain.

TTF-1 is a member of the homeodomain-containing family of transcription factors encoded by a single, three exon gene *(NKX2-1)* on human chromosome 14q13.3.[3,93] NKX2-1 is also expressed in the thyroid, where it is important for development of that gland, and in the central nervous system (CNS) (primarily basal ganglia). In the lung, it is critical for the expression of ABCA3, SP-A, SP-B, and SP-C, along with many other genes.[54,93,94]

Familial lung disease inherited in an autosomal dominant pattern with variable penetrance due to *NKX2-1* mutations and deletions has been recognized, but most reported cases appear to have resulted from de novo events.[34,36,38,40] Unlike disorders due to mutations in *ABCA3*, *SFTPB*, or *SFTPC*, patients with *NKX2.1* mutations or deletions may have extrapulmonary manifestations of hypothyroidism and neurologic findings, and the term "brain-thyroid-lung syndrome" has been used to encompass the constellation of findings.[34,95-97] Approximately 50% of reported patients with *NKX2.1* deletions or mutations had some pulmonary disease, but detailed evaluation of lung function was not necessarily performed in all subjects.[34] Affected individuals need not have abnormalities in all three organ systems and may have normal thyroid function, or chemical hypothyroidism may be present without clinical symptoms. The neurologic findings may be subtle in infants, consisting of nonspecific hypotonia or developmental delay, and attributed to the severity of the lung disease. The more specific finding of chorea may not manifest until later in life.

DISORDERS OF SURFACTANT CLEARANCE

A plethora of different terms have been used to report on PAP, resulting in inconsistent use of overlapping terminology; some brief definitions are useful here. Elucidation of the pathogenic mechanism of the most common PAP-associated disease (idiopathic PAP) was the basis for recommending use of the term "autoimmune PAP."[98] Genetic diseases causing hereditary PAP can be specified by the affected gene (i.e., *CSF2RA* or *CSF2RB*) encoding the GM-CSF receptor α- or β-chains, respectively. These autoimmune and genetic diseases share strikingly similar features, including clinical presentation (although age of presentation may be different), radiographic appearance, histopathology (alveolar filling without marked distortion), pathophysiology, overlapping pathogenesis (loss of GM-CSF signaling), and response to whole lung lavage therapy. Consequently, they are usefully considered together and sometimes called primary PAP, reflecting their occurrence in previously healthy individuals.

PAP occurring because of another underlying disease is referred to as secondary PAP. Diseases associated with the development of secondary PAP include hematologic disorders (e.g., myelodysplasia, hematologic malignancies, aplastic anemia), certain chronic infections (e.g., human immunodeficiency virus [HIV]), toxic inhalation exposures (e.g., silica fibers, metal dusts), and generalized myelosuppression caused by chemotherapy and hematopoietic stem cell transplantation. PAP may be a prominent finding in other genetic diseases not involving disruption of GM-CSF signaling (lysinuric protein intolerance [LPI], mutations in the gene encoding methionyl tRNA synthetase).[45,99-102]

PAP can also occur in disorders of surfactant production, as described previously. Pulmonary surfactant in these disorders is deficient in one or more of its critical components, resulting in deficiency of functional surfactant that causes marked alveolar distortion, a spectrum of acute and chronic ILDs, and varying degrees of accumulation of abnormal surfactant (PAP). The clinical presentation, response to whole lung lavage (which is poor), and therapeutic approaches are quite different from primary PAP in which the primary abnormality is the accumulation of biochemically and functionally normal surfactant without alveolar distortion.

Autoimmune Pulmonary Alveolar Proteinosis

This disease is caused by an immune reaction to GM-CSF that blocks signaling to alveolar macrophages (and other cells), thereby impairing their ability to clear surfactant lipids and proteins. Neutralizing, polyclonal immunoglobulin (Ig) G (primarily IgG1 and IgG2) is associated with the development of PAP when levels exceed a critical threshold required to eliminate GM-CSF signaling in vivo (estimated to be approximately 5 µg/mL). Disruption of GM-CSF signaling blocks the differentiation of alveolar macrophages, impairing surfactant clearance and host defense functions. Loss of GM-CSF signaling also impairs neutrophil host defense functions, which, together with impairment of macrophage host defense functions due to maturational arrest, provide a molecular and cellular explanation for the increased morbidity and mortality from infection seen in this disorder.[103] Impaired pulmonary surfactant clearance caused by alveolar macrophage dysfunction results in a slow net accumulation of surfactant within alveoli, which blocks the entry of air and transfer of oxygen into the blood, eventually resulting in hypoxemia and respiratory insufficiency. Alveolar distortion is not a prominent histopathologic feature in most patients, but lymphocytosis can be present and fibrosis has also been reported.

Pulmonary Alveolar Proteinosis Caused by Autosomal Recessive *CSF2RA* Mutations

In 2008 two groups independently reported children with the phenotype of PAP who had deleterious variants in the gene encoding the α-chain of the GM-CSF receptor *(CSF2RA)*, which is located within the pseudoautosomal regions of the X and Y chromosomes. In one report, two sisters were found to be compound heterozygotes for a complete deletion of the *CSF2RA* locus and a missense mutation that was demonstrated in vitro to produce nonfunctional GM-CSF receptors.[49] The proband developed progressive dyspnea apparent by age 4, was diagnosed with PAP on lung biopsy at age 6, and responded well to whole lung lavage therapy. Her 8-year-old sister had the same genotype and evidence for mild PAP by high-resolution computed tomography (HRCT) but was asymptomatic at the time of the report and had not needed any therapy for PAP. These two genetically similar siblings illustrate the phenotypic variability of this disorder. In another report a child with Turner syndrome (45 XO) was diagnosed with PAP at age 3 years, confirmed on biopsy, and found to have a partial deletion of *CSF2RA* accounting for the lack of receptor expression and GM-CSF signaling.[104] The child died of a respiratory infection following a bone-marrow transplant prior to engraftment.

A subsequent study expanded on these initial observations with the identification of five additional patients with deleterious *CSF2RA* genetic variants from three families of differing ethnicity and geographic origin, indicating that this disorder is not confined to one ethnic group or geographic location.[46] The age of onset of symptoms ranged from 1.5 to 9 years; one patient was asymptomatic. Usual presenting symptoms included dyspnea and fatigue. None of the subjects had autoantibodies to GM-CSF, but all had elevated serum levels of GM-CSF compared with family members and healthy control subjects. A variety of *CSF2RA* genetic defects were identified; CSF2RA protein was absent in all but one patient with a missense mutation, but all affected patients had reduced signaling induced by GM-CSF in isolated mononuclear cells. Symptomatic patients had undergone multiple whole lung lavages with intervals ranging from every several months to more than 2 years. All were alive at the time of the report, ranging in age from 4 to 13 years.[46]

Pulmonary Alveolar Proteinosis Caused by Autosomal Recessive *CSF2RB* Mutations

A genetic defect of the GM-CSF receptor was first suggested as a mechanism for PAP in four infants who had undetectable amounts of the common β-chain (βc) shared with IL-3 and IL-5 receptors, as determined by immunologic methods.[105] Deficient response to exogenous stimulation by GM-CSF was also observed in monocytes obtained from affected infants. However, no convincing genetic mechanism was identified to account for the lack of βc, and the only genetic variant identified in its gene *(CSF2RB)* was subsequently found to be a nondisease causing polymorphism.[51]

Function-altering mutations in *CSF2RB* have since been reported in two unrelated patients.[51,52] Both presented with the typical symptoms and signs of PAP, one at age 9 and the other at age 36. Both had elevated levels of serum GM-CSF, and antibodies to GM-CSF were not detected. One patient was homozygous for a missense mutation that was confirmed in in vitro studies to be nonfunctional; the other was homozygous for a single base deletion in exon 6 and had no detectable βc protein. In contrast to the earlier report involving infants with absent βc protein expression, these reports provided convincing evidence that genetic defects in *CSF2RB* can cause the phenotype of PAP. The mechanism(s) for decreased βc expression in the infants in the earlier study and whether it contributed to the pathophysiology of their lung disease remain unknown. It is interesting that the age at presentation of patients with *CSF2RB* mutations was older than those with *CSF2RA* genetic variants, but additional patients will need to be identified to determine if there is a true difference in age of onset of disease depending upon the gene involved.

Pulmonary Alveolar Proteinosis Syndrome Associated With Other Genetic Disorders. Genetically determined primary defects in GM-CSF production have not been reported as a cause of PAP in humans, although this mechanism is expected based upon observations in experimental animals.[106,107] PAP develops in some but not all children with LPI, a disorder of cationic amino acid transport caused by mutations in the gene *SLC7A7*, a member of the solute carrier family.[100,108,109] The mechanism of PAP in children with LPI is unknown but appears likely to involve macrophage dysfunction rather than surfactant production, because defects are present in mononuclear phagocyte lineage cells.[110] PAP also recurred in a child with LPI who had undergone heart-lung transplantation, consistent with alveolar macrophages and not alveolar epithelial cells comprising the site of pathogenic disruption of surfactant homeostasis.[111]

Biallelic mutations in the gene encoding methionyl tRNA synthetase *(MARS)* have been identified in subjects with a complex multiorgan phenotype in which PAP can be the presenting and/or predominant feature.[99] Liver disease and anemia are common in affected subjects, and ILD was also observed in a child with this condition.[112] The mechanism whereby mutations in this gene result in the phenotype of PAP is unclear. As supplementation with additional methionine augmented function of enzymes in yeast that were homologous to human mutations, difference in dietary methionine intake may influence the severity and course of disease.

Heterozygous mutations in the gene encoding GATA2, a transcription factor important in hematopoietic cell development, have also been associated with the development of PAP. These subjects have a complex phenotype with features of immune deficiency, myelodysplasia, and lymphatic abnormalities, but PAP and diffuse lung disease may be prominent and presenting features.[113,114] The mechanisms underlying PAP are likely related to a role of GATA2 in regulating alveolar macrophage development and phagocytosis.[115]

Pathology/Pathogenesis

DISORDERS OF SURFACTANT PRODUCTION

The lung histopathology findings associated with genetic surfactant production disorders include several characteristic features and collectively have been referred to as surfactant dysfunction. Typical findings include marked AEC2 hyperplasia, interstitial thickening with mesenchymal cells progressing to fibrosis in subjects with late disease, and variable amounts of proteinaceous material and foamy macrophages in distal airspaces (Fig. 57.2). The proteinaceous material may be quite striking, particularly in younger patients, which led to the term congenital alveolar proteinosis initially being associated with SP-B deficiency.[11] However, findings of alveolar proteinosis are not always observed in SP-B deficiency and are also seen in other disorders of surfactant production and surfactant clearance, in which the underlying mechanisms differ. Thus the term congenital alveolar proteinosis is best avoided.

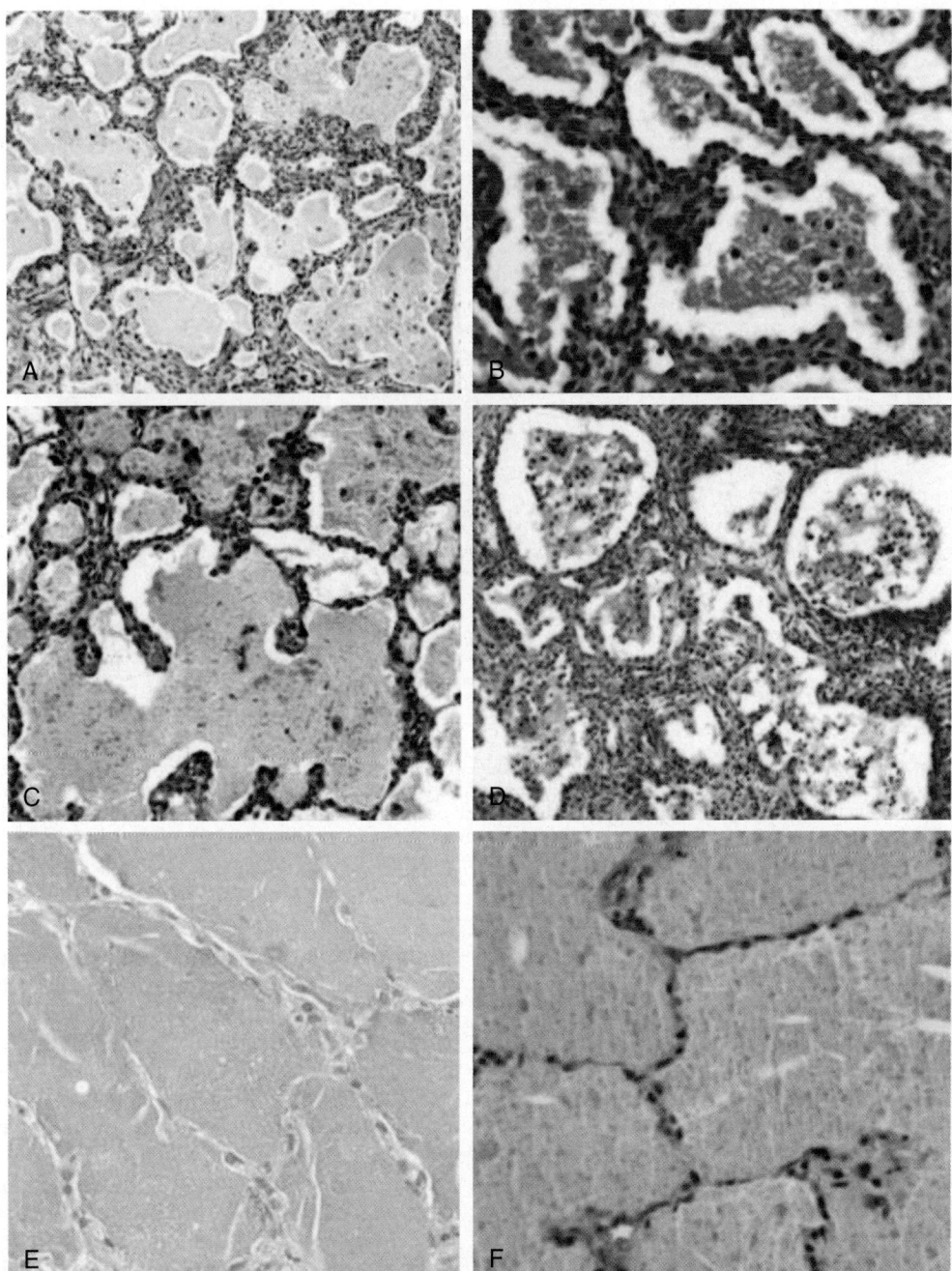

Fig. 57.2 Variable and overlapping histology associated with genetic disorders disrupting surfactant homeostasis. (A) is from an SP-B–deficient infant, demonstrating marked accumulation of granular proteinaceous material with entrapped macrophages filling distal airspaces. (B) Similar pathology is demonstrated in a patient with ABCA3 deficiency and from a patient with an SP-C mutation (C), although with better preservation of the alveolar architecture in C. (D) is from a patient with a different SP-C mutation, demonstrating interstitial thickening and accumulation of foamy macrophages in the airspaces, but with scant amounts of proteinaceous material. (E) and (F) are from patients with *CSF2RA* and *CSF2RB* mutations, respectively. Although the airspaces are totally filled with granular material, the alveolar walls remain thin without thickening by mesenchymal or inflammatory cells or fibrosis. ([A–F] Courtesy Susan Wert, PhD.)

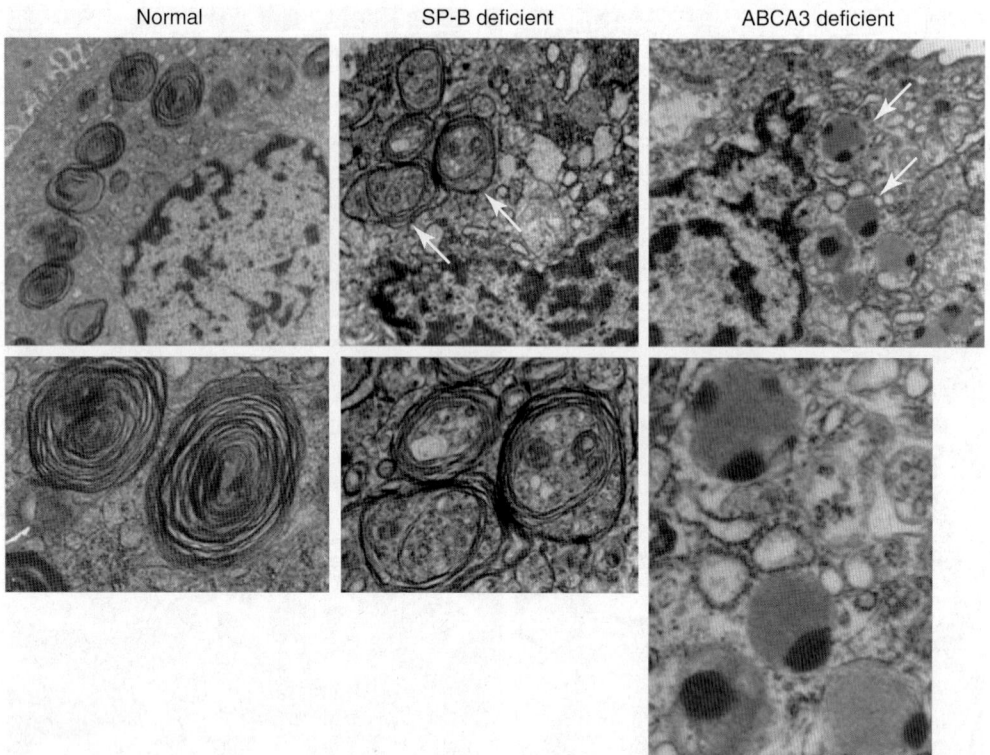

Fig. 57.3 Ultrastructural findings associated with SP-B and ABCA3 deficiency. A portion of a type II cell with normal lamellar bodies is shown in the top left panel. In the top middle panel a type II cell from an SP-B–deficient patient contains abnormally formed lamellar bodies with large whorls and vacuolar inclusions (*arrows*). In the top right panel the lamellar bodies in the type II cells of a patient with ABCA3 deficiency are small and dense, with eccentrically placed inclusions (*arrows*). The bottom panels show higher-power views of normal (*left*), SP-B–deficient (*middle*), and ABCA3-deficient (*right*) lamellar bodies. (Courtesy Susan Wert, PhD.)

The histopathology findings in different genetic lung disorders overlap considerably such that determination of the specific gene defect is not readily discernable from the routine histopathology. Pathology terms that have been used to describe the findings include chronic pneumonitis of infancy (CPI), desquamative interstitial pneumonia (DIP), and nonspecific interstitial pneumonitis (NSIP).[38,78,116,117] Lung pathology findings in children with *NKX2-1* mutations may include those observed with other causes of surfactant dysfunction, as well as alveolar simplification.[97,118,119]

Characteristic ultrastructural features may be seen in lung tissue from SP-B– and ABCA3-deficient infants by electron microscopy (Fig. 57.3).[20,120–125] The lamellar bodies in SP-B–deficient infants (and mice) are poorly organized, with loosely packed lamellae and vacuolar inclusions, having the appearance more of multivesicular or composite bodies. In contrast, absent or small, abnormally formed lamellar bodies have been observed in the lungs of ABCA3-deficient infants.[20,121,123,124,126] Their AEC2s instead contain small, dense-appearing inclusions that upon higher magnification have densely packed membranes. Eccentrically placed electron-dense inclusions within the abnormal lamellar bodies give them a "fried-egg" appearance.[123] Similarly, abnormal lamellar bodies have been observed in genetically engineered ABCA3 null mice.[58,60]

Specific ultrastructural features associated with *SFTPC* or *NKX2-1* mutations have not been consistently observed. Abnormally formed lamellar bodies have been observed in lung tissue from some children with *SFTPC* mutations[79,125] but have been reported as normal in other studies.[127]

Abnormal lamellar bodies like those seen in SP-B–deficient or ABCA3-deficient infants have been observed in lung tissue from children with *NKX2-1* mutations, but a consistent pattern has not emerged.[38] Because TTF-1 is a transcription factor important for expression of both SP-B and ABCA3, the lamellar body phenotype may depend upon the impact of the specific mutation on relative expression of these target genes.

Both human and animal studies support that loss-of-function mechanisms resulting in both deficiency of surfactant components and altered surfactant composition and function are clearly important in the pathophysiology of the acute RDS phenotype observed in SP-B– and ABCA3-deficient infants. Bronchoalveolar lavage fluid (BALF) from ABCA3-deficient infants who underwent lung transplantation in infancy had diminished surface tension–lowering properties and was markedly reduced in DSPC and phosphatidylglycerol (PG) content compared with controls,[128] and similarly altered surfactant lipid and protein profiles were found in lung fluid samples from BALF from ABCA3- and SP-B–deficient subjects in another study.[129,130] Targeted disruption of either *sftpb* or *abca3* in genetically engineered mice resulted in a neonatal lethal respiratory phenotype.[57–60,131] In addition, the phospholipid profiles of *abca3* null mice were markedly abnormal, with very low levels of DSPC and PG.[57,59] These observations support an essential role for ABCA3 in the transport of lipids important for surface tension reduction.

Secondary changes in the metabolism of other surfactant components have been observed in lung tissue and fluid from

SP-B–, and to less extent ABCA3-, deficient infants that likely further complicate the extent of surfactant deficiency. In SP-B deficiency, there is an accumulation of aberrantly processed SP-C peptides that result from incomplete processing of the SP-C precursor (proSP-C) to mature SP-C.[120,122,132] This block in SP-C processing may result in SP-B–deficient infants also being deficient in mature SP-C, and the partially processed proSP-C peptides have reduced surface tension–lowering activity, further contributing to surfactant dysfunction in SP-B–deficient infants.[133] This appearance is consistent with a role for SP-B in membrane fusion of smaller vesicles to pack and organize lipid bilayers into lamellar bodies.[134] The final processing steps for mature SP-C occur in lamellar bodes, and the failure to properly form this intracellular organelle is therefore probably related to the SP-C processing abnormality. The abnormal lamellar body formation in ABCA3 deficiency may also relate to abnormally processed proSP-C intermediates observed in lungs of affected infants, although such peptides have not been as abundant or consistently observed as in SP-B–deficient infants.[135]

The pathophysiology underlying the relatively milder phenotype of some ABCA3-deficient children who do not exhibit findings of neonatal surfactant deficiency and who present later in life with lung disease is less clear. One potential mechanism is that some mutations allow for partial ABCA3 function. A mutation (p.Glu292Val or p.E292V) that has been found in multiple unrelated subjects with a relatively milder phenotype has been shown to cause partially impaired lipid transport compared with wild-type ABCA3 in vitro.[136,137] In addition, children with genotypes that are predicted to completely preclude ABCA3 expression have almost universally had a severe phenotype with neonatal-onset disease and early lethality, whereas children with relatively milder disease have had genotypes in which at least one mutation could allow for some ABCA3 expression and function.[23] Other mechanisms for later lung injury may also be important. Some mutations may also be associated with endoplasmic reticulum (ER) stress and trigger the unfolded protein response (UPR), contributing to AEC2 injury and chronic lung disease, and ABCA3 may have a role in protecting AEC2s from cholesterol toxicity.[138,139] More than 250 ABCA3 mutations scattered throughout the gene have been reported to date.[19–21,23,90,117,121,124,128,135,140–150] Type I mutations are not properly routed to distal cellular compartments, and type 2 mutations result in reduced ATP hydrolysis and/or impaired lipid transport.[136,151,152] This classification scheme does not incorporate nonsense and frameshift mutations, which are likely associated with unstable transcripts, and it is likely to evolve as our understanding of normal ABCA3 cell biology increases.

Although ABCA3 and SP-B deficiency generally are recessive disorders with mutations on both alleles (biallelic) needed to manifest disease, in some circumstances a mutation on just one allele (monoallelic) may contribute to lung disease. Preterm and near-term infants with monoallelic ABCA3 mutations may be at higher risk for developing RDS,[24,153] and heterozygosity for an ABCA3 mutation may modify the course of SFTPC-related diseases.[90,128] Adult carriers for the most common SFTPB mutation appear to be at higher risk for development of obstructive lung disease, particularly in conjunction with smoking exposure.[15] Genetically engineered mice with one null sftpb allele were more susceptible to

pulmonary oxygen toxicity than their wild-type littermates,[154] and mice who were genetically engineered to be able to turn off their SP-B production developed lung disease when their SP-B levels fell to less than 20%–25% of normal adult levels.[155] These observations suggest that a critical level of SP-B is needed for normal lung function and that having a loss-of-function SFTPB mutation on only one allele could thus be a risk factor for the development of lung disease if other factors further reduce SP-B expression.[156,157] Similarly, mice with one inactivated abca3 allele were also observed to be more susceptible to pulmonary oxygen injury.[158] Finally, patients with only one ABCA3 mutation and both severe neonatal lung disease and ILD have been recognized.[159,160] It is possible that these patients had a mutation on the other allele that escaped detection. Alternatively, a single ABCA3 mutation may predispose individuals to lung disease in conjunction with other genetic or environmental mechanisms. There is evidence that ABCA3 expression may be monoallelic at a cellular level, and thus in individuals with heterozygous ABCA3 mutations unequal expression of the abnormal allele within a population of AEC2s could result in abnormal surfactant metabolism and disease.[161]

The pathophysiology of lung disease due to SFTPC mutations is complex and incompletely understood. Lack of mature SP-C could plausibly contribute to the lung disease. Mice unable to produce SP-C due to targeted inactivation of sftpc develop progressive air space enlargement and interstitial inflammation as they age in a strain-dependent fashion.[162,163] The variability depending upon the genetic background of the null mice indicates that genetic modifiers are likely important in the development of SP-C–related lung disease. Mutations in other genes important in surfactant metabolism, such as ABCA3, may modify the severity of lung disease due to SFTPC mutations.[90,91] Human lung disease resulting from null mutations on one or both alleles of SFTPC has not been reported. Familial ILD, associated with markedly reduced SP-C expression in lung tissue and undetectable SP-C in BALF, has been observed, but disease in this family was subsequently found to be due to NKX2-1.[38,164] In support of SP-C deficiency as a mechanism for disease, a lack of both proSP-C and mature SP-C has been observed in the lung tissue of subjects with some SFTPC mutations.[78,165,166] SP-C self-associates in the secretory pathway, and thus a dominant negative effect on SP-C production from the abnormal proSP-C that results from a mutation could account for the lack of mature SP-C.[167] Subsequent studies in which an SFTPC mutation that resulted in the skipping of an entire exon (Δexon4) was expressed in in vitro systems provided support for this mechanism, as the abnormal proSP-C was not processed to mature SP-C, not routed appropriately in the cells, and was rapidly degraded.[165,168,169]

SFTPC mutations may cause lung disease due to toxicity from abnormal proSP-C, a "gain-of-toxic-function" mechanism. All of the SFTPC mutations associated with human lung disease reported to date are predicted to result in the production of an abnormal proprotein, which is likely misfolded.[170] The exposure of hydrophobic epitopes in the misfolded proprotein may be directly toxic to AEC2s, especially if produced in sufficient amounts to be unable to be efficiently degraded through the proteasome pathway. Proteasome dysfunction may also inhibit expression of other SP, further contributing to surfactant dysfunction.[171] Accumulation of misfolded protein within the ER may trigger the UPR and eventually caspase activation and apoptosis of AEC2s.[168,169,172–174] SP-C lung disease may thus represent a conformational disease with accumulation of misfolded protein in the cell causing secondary cellular toxicity.[170] Increased levels of UPR components and caspase activation have also been observed in lung tissue from patients with pulmonary fibrosis not due to *SFTPC* mutations, suggesting that protein misfolding may be a more general mechanism for AEC2 injury.[175,176]

Other mechanisms may also contribute to the pathophysiology of lung injury with *SFTPC* mutations. ProSP-C intermediates are normally routed to lamellar bodies, but with some mutations, particularly those located in the bridging domain between the mature SP-C peptide and the BRICHOS domain, proSP-C is routed to the plasma membrane and then internalized through an endosomal pathway. Accumulation of intermediates and a block in autophagy may then contribute to cellular injury.[165,166,177] With multiple mechanisms that may be dependent upon the location and nature of a specific mutation, different strategies aimed at correcting folding or routing of specific mutations may be needed.

Because TTF-1 is essential for the expression of SP-B, SP-C, and ABCA3, it is not surprising that reductions in the amount of this transcription factor could result in the phenotypes of RDS (surfactant deficiency) and ILD (surfactant dysfunction). Complete loss of function of one *NKX2-1* allele has been demonstrated both by complete gene deletions and *in vitro* studies of mutations demonstrating impaired DNA binding or decreased transcription of reporter genes; a gain-of-function mechanism with overexpression of downstream genes is also possible.[37,95,96] It is unknown whether lung disease results primarily through the reduction of one surfactant component (such as SP-B or ABCA3) below a critical level needed for normal lung function or a combination of reduced levels of more than one protein. Evaluation of SP expression has been evaluated in a limited number of subjects with *NKX2-1* mutations with variable findings. Diminished immunoreactivity for SP-A and ABCA3 but robust staining for SP-B and proSP-C were observed in a subject with a *NKX2-1* deletion.[118] Because SP-A is also regulated by TTF-1, reductions in this pulmonary collectin may account for the observation of recurrent pulmonary infections in some subjects. Severely reduced expression of another pulmonary collectin, SP-D, was observed in a child with a *NKX2-1* mutation who developed respiratory failure after a viral infection.[38] Reduced amounts of both proSP-C and mature SP-C were observed in three members of the same family with a *NKX2-1* missense mutation.[38,164] Intriguingly, a missense variant of *NKX2-1* has been identified that segregated with familial lung disease of a different pulmonary phenotype, that of neuroendocrine cell hyperplasia of infancy (NEHI).[178,179] The lung histopathology and immunostaining pattern in one affected family member were not typical for surfactant dysfunction. Combined with observations of variable expression of SP in lung tissue from other subjects with *NKX2-1* mutations, this observation suggests the hypothesis that the primary pulmonary phenotype due to *NKX2-1* mutations may relate to the downstream target genes whose expression is most affected by the mutated allele. Because TTF-1 is also important for the expression of many other genes in

the lung important in lung physiology (examples include the club cell secretory protein, and the genes encoding the amiloride-sensitive sodium channel), this may explain some of the diverse phenotypic features associated with *NKX2-1* mutations. Finally, the mechanisms for the variable severity of disease associated with *NKX2-1* mutations are unknown but may relate to either genetic variants in *NKX2-1* affecting expression level of the remaining functional allele, or factors controlling the expression and function of the multiple other transcription factors (including GATA6, FOXA2, C/EBPα, NFAT) needed for SP and ABCA3 gene expression.

DISORDERS OF SURFACTANT CLEARANCE

PAP is a syndrome that occurs in a heterogeneous group of diseases and is defined histopathologically by the presence of a finely granular, lipoproteinaceous material filling pulmonary alveoli and terminal airspaces. The accumulated material stains with eosin and periodic acid–Schiff (PAS) reagent has biochemical and ultrastructural features identical to surfactant and frequently contains cholesterol "needles" and cellular debris. Depending on the underlying PAP-causing disease, alveolar distortion and/or fibrosis may or may not be present. The relative proportion of these specific histologic features present varies markedly among the diseases causing PAP (i.e., the histopathologic pattern depends on the pathogenesis involved).

The pathogenesis of PAP remained obscure for nearly four decades after its initial description in 1958 because research was hampered by its rarity and the heterogeneity of diseases causing the syndrome.[45,180] Most cases occur in previously healthy individuals without significant environmental pulmonary exposure other than smoking, referred to as idiopathic or acquired PAP. However, PAP also occurs in association with various underlying diseases, termed secondary PAP (see later). A serendipitous but critical pathogenic clue for the common idiopathic form was the observation that mice deficient in GM-CSF or a component of its receptor developed a phenotype virtually identical to idiopathic PAP in humans.[8,9,106,107] Although PAP caused by GM-CSF deficiency has not yet been reported in humans, a second pathogenic clue was the observation that idiopathic PAP is specifically associated with high levels of neutralizing autoantibodies against GM-CSF.[102,181,182] Passive transfer studies established that GM-CSF autoantibodies cause PAP by blocking GM-CSF signaling to alveolar macrophages,[183] which is required to stimulate surfactant clearance.[183] Additional pathogenic insight was provided by the identification of hereditary PAP in mice and children due to genetic mutations in *CSF2RA* and *CSF2RB*, which block GM-CSF signaling by impairing GM-CSF receptor function.[46,49,51,52,104]

Clinical Features of Surfactant Production Disorders

PRESENTATION, SYMPTOMS, AND PHYSICAL FINDINGS

Two typical clinical presentations are seen in children with surfactant production disorders. The first is a neonatal presentation with diffuse lung disease in a full-term infant that is like that of a premature infant with RDS. Clinical signs include tachypnea, grunting, nasal flaring, retractions, and cyanosis in room air and may develop within minutes to hours after birth. Affected infants rapidly progress to hypoxemic respiratory failure, often needing high-frequency ventilation and support with extracorporeal membrane oxygenation in the past. This is the usual presentation for children with SP-B deficiency and many with ABCA3 deficiency. Children with *NKX2-1* mutations may also present in a similar fashion. Newborns with *SFTPC* mutations may have a similar presentation, but the initial lung disease is usually not as severe as seen in SP-B or ABCA3 deficiencies and most individuals with *SFTPC* mutations present later in life, ranging from early infancy until well into adulthood.

The other clinical presentation of children with surfactant production disorders is with nonspecific respiratory symptoms and signs, which may be acute, subacute, or chronic in onset, and this is typical for children with *SFTPC* mutations. Respiratory symptoms in children (and adults) with *SFTPC* mutations include cough, difficulty breathing, and exercise intolerance, and signs include tachypnea, crackles, digital clubbing, pectus excavatum, failure to thrive, and need for supplemental oxygen and have been summarized in several clinical studies.[29,75,88,184] The age of onset of symptoms is highly variable in individuals with *SFTPC* mutations, with some infants developing very early in life and others remaining asymptomatic well until adulthood.[29,31,78,85,184] Importantly, infants and children with very severe disease who require aggressive supportive measures, including mechanical ventilation, may show steady but gradual improvement over time, although the disease does not resolve.[185] Clinical presentation of lung disease in some children has apparently been triggered or exacerbated by viral infections.[31,184] Cells in culture that stably expressed a *SFTPC* mutation at low levels did not have overt signs of cellular toxicity but died when exposed to respiratory syncytial virus (RSV), providing a potential mechanism for such a genetic-environmental interaction.[186]

Although initial reports of children with ABCA3 deficiency focused on severe neonatal disease, it is now recognized that ABCA3 deficiency may result in milder lung disease and later presentation, including as adults.[117,144–146,187] Affected children may not have exhibited any symptoms or signs of lung disease in the neonatal period or have had apparently transient or mild lung disease in the neonatal period but subsequently developed findings like those of children with *SFTPC* mutations.[19,23,117,144,188]

IMAGING, PULMONARY FUNCTION TESTING, AND LABORATORY FINDINGS

The typical initial chest radiographic findings in neonates with surfactant production disorders resemble those of preterm infants with RDS, with diffuse granular alveolar and interstitial infiltrates, along with air bronchograms. Air leak (pneumothorax, interstitial emphysema) is common. Over time, infiltrates become coarser but do not resolve. In the early phase of the disease, HRCT images show diffuse ground-glass opacities with interlobular thickening. In such infants, if supported with long-term ventilation as a bridge to lung transplantation, later imaging studies may show areas of cystic dilatation and interstitial fibrotic changes.[189]

In older children, radiographic findings depend upon severity of disease, but ground-glass opacities are common, as are peripheral cysts seen on HRCT.[188]

Because most affected infants succumb early in life, there are no reported studies of pulmonary function tests in SP-B–deficient infants. There are limited data on pulmonary function testing (PFT) findings in infants and older children with other surfactant production disorders. Infant PFTS in two children with *SFTPC* mutations demonstrated a restrictive pattern, and a restrictive pattern was also noted in older children with ABCA3 mutations.[144,190] In a population-based study, carriers for the 121ins2 mutation were found to be at risk for reduced lung function as adults, especially in conjunction with smoking.[15]

Currently there are limited data on the utility of other laboratory tests and biomarkers for surfactant production disorders. Serum lactate dehydrogenase (LDH) levels may be elevated reflecting ongoing epithelial cell injury. Serum KL-6, a mucin produced by alveolar epithelial cells, may be a useful serum biomarker, but the availability of clinically available assays is limited.[191]

Diagnosis and Differential Diagnosis

The identification of genetic abnormalities as causes of surfactant production and clearance provides the means for diagnosis of these rare conditions through noninvasive genetic or serologic testing. Although specific therapies may not be available, timely diagnosis is important to provide accurate counseling regarding prognosis, assessment of risk for other family members, and recurrence risk for future pregnancies. Clinical algorithms for a diagnostic approach to suspected genetic causes of surfactant production and clearance have not been formally evaluated, but the typical clinical presentations of each disorder may provide guidance as to which patients to evaluate.[192–194]

Diffuse lung disease in a full-term infant with radiographic features of surfactant deficiency should prompt consideration of a genetic disorder of surfactant production, particularly due to mutations in *SFTPB*, *ABCA3*, and *NKX2-1*. Gestational age less than 38 weeks, male gender, operative delivery (especially elective), and white race are known risk factors for RDS in near-term infants.[26,195] Absence of these risk factors, failure to improve after the first 7–10 days of life, or a family history of severe neonatal lung disease should increase suspicion for a genetic mechanism for the lung disease. Other diagnoses to be considered include infection (both viral and bacterial), cardiac disease (especially total anomalous pulmonary venous return), pulmonary lymphangiectasia, pulmonary hypoplasia, and alveolar capillary dysplasia with misalignment of the pulmonary veins.

The diagnosis of genetic disorders of surfactant production and clearance should be considered in older children and young adults who present with what has been termed "chILD syndrome."[192–194] Criteria for chILD syndrome include three of four of the following: (1) respiratory symptoms, including cough, rapid breathing, shortness of breath, difficulty breathing, or exercise intolerance; (2) respiratory signs, including tachypnea, adventitial sounds, retractions, digital clubbing, pectus excavatum, failure to thrive, or acute respiratory failure; (3) hypoxemia while breathing room air; and (4) diffuse abnormalities on chest imaging. Other both rare and more common causes of lung disease should first be excluded, including cystic fibrosis, infectious causes, immunodeficiency, bronchopulmonary dysplasia, congenital heart disease, primary ciliary dyskinesia, and chronic aspiration.[194] The absence of a family history of lung disease should not preclude evaluation because de novo *SFTPC* and *NKX2.1* mutations may cause sporadic disease and ABCA3 deficiency is inherited as an autosomal recessive disorder. Neurologic findings, including hypotonia or developmental delay, should prompt consideration of an *NKX2.1* mutation or deletion, as should hypothyroidism. Children or adolescents with insidious onset of disease and diffuse alveolar infiltrates after the neonatal period, or who have biopsy findings consistent with alveolar proteinosis, should be evaluated for serum GM-CSF autoantibodies, and/or *CSF2RA* and *CSF2RB* mutations.

GENETIC TESTING

The diagnosis of a surfactant production disorder is made through genetic testing, which is available in certified diagnostic laboratories (www.genetests.org).[22] The availability of panels using next-generation sequencing (NGS) methods allows for simultaneous analysis of multiple other genes that may result in similar phenotypes. Such panels may also detect copy number variants, and entire deletions of *NKX2-1*, as well as large deletions in *SFTPB* and *ABCA3*, have been recognized.[38,70,196,197] For SP-B and ABCA3 deficiencies a diagnosis is established by finding of pathogenic or likely pathogenic mutations on both alleles. Testing of the parents is advisable both to confirm segregation of the variants and determine that they are on opposite alleles when two different mutations are found, or a homozygous mutation is found to confirm that both parents are carriers, as opposed to a rare mechanism such as uniparental disomy, which would alter the recurrence risk.[23,147,197,198] For *SFTPC* and *NKX2-1* a diagnosis is established with the finding of a pathogenic or likely pathogenic mutation on one allele.

There are important limitations to genetic testing. Such testing is not 100% sensitive; functionally significant variants in untranslated regions that affect gene expression or mRNA splicing will not be detected. Gene deletions, insertions, duplications, and rearrangements may be missed unless specific methods are used to look for such variants. In addition, interpretation of results may be difficult, particularly for what are called "variants of uncertain significance" (VUS), where it is unknown whether a variant represents a pathogenic or benign sequence variant. As the number of genes included in NGS panels increase, the likelihood of finding a VUS in one or more genes increases. It also may be difficult to determine whether subjects with recessive disorders in whom only one mutation is identified are affected with a mutation that escaped detection on the other allele or are simply carriers with a pathogenic variant unrelated to the cause of their lung disease. The turnaround time for genetic testing can be several weeks, which may be inadequate in a patient who is unstable or has rapidly progressive disease. Finally, genetic testing is expensive, the costs for such testing may not be covered by insurance, and it may be impractical for patients to pay for the testing out of pocket.

LUNG AND SERUM BIOMARKERS

Levels of mature SP-B protein are usually undetectable in tracheal aspirate (TA) or BALF in children with SP-B deficiency.[66,130] In addition, the presence of aberrantly processed proSP-C peptides in the TA or BALF is a marker for the disorder.[132] However, assays for these proteins in biologic samples are not currently available in diagnostic labs, and there may be overlap in the findings with those of children with other genetic surfactant production disorders, so assays of TA or BAL fluid may not be helpful in making the diagnosis.[130,135]

Serum GM-CSF autoantibody testing is now commercially available (https://www.cincinnatichildrens.org/service/r/rare-lung/professionals/pap-lab) and is particularly useful in identifying individuals with autoimmune PAP and has a sensitivity and specificity approaching 100%. This test is recommended for all adults, adolescents, and older children with the typical history and radiographic findings of PAP. Identification of specific biomarkers in blood or lung fluid could provide useful tools for diagnosis or disease progression.[46,191] For example, increased levels of SP in either lung fluid or serum may provide a simple and useful means to monitor lung disease severity in these disorders. However, such tests are currently available only in research protocols and are of uncertain sensitivity and specificity for surfactant-related lung diseases.[135] In contrast, the finding of an elevated serum GM-CSF level and a negative serum GM-CSF autoantibody level in a patient with hereditary PAP caused by *CSF2RA* or *CSF2RB* mutations appears to be a useful screening diagnostic test for this group of genetic diseases of surfactant homeostasis.

LUNG HISTOPATHOLOGY

Lung biopsy has a potentially important role in the diagnosis of ILDs but has distinct limitations in the differential diagnosis of PAP-causing diseases. Lung histopathology may help to distinguish disorders of surfactant clearance from disorders of surfactant production, based in part on the presence and level of disruption of alveolar architecture. However, lung histopathology does not distinguish the relatively common form of autoimmune PAP from hereditary PAP caused by *CSF2RA* or *CSF2RB* mutations, nor can it distinguish between the latter two. Sampling error can be an important limitation for diagnosis based on lung histopathology even when tissues are obtained based on surgical biopsies. This is particularly true in diseases with a heterogeneous, "geographic" involvement of the lungs. When lung biopsies are indicated, the tissues should be obtained and handled appropriately according to published guidelines to optimize diagnostic yield and should include obtaining electron microscopy and frozen tissue.[199]

Tissue examination can also be used for diagnosis, particularly when immunohistochemistry and electron microscopy augment routine histologic examination. Histologic findings overlap with those of other surfactant dysfunction disorders and include AEC2 hyperplasia, interstitial thickening with mesenchymal cells and fibrosis in advanced stages of the disease, and variable amounts of lipoproteinaceous material accumulating in alveolar macrophages and filling distal airspaces. Absent staining for SP-B is suggestive of SP-B deficiency, but this is not necessarily specific because absent staining for SP-B has also been observed in some cases of ABCA3 deficiency. Intense staining of extracellular material with antibodies directed against amino-terminal epitopes of proSP-C appears to be indicative of SP-B deficiency, but such staining may not be available in many labs. Electron microscopy (EM) findings of abnormal lamellar bodies that are disorganized with multivesicular inclusions have been consistently observed in the lungs of SP-B–deficient infants. Ultrastructural examination of lung tissue obtained at biopsy or autopsy may also be helpful in establishing the diagnosis of ABCA3 deficiency and distinguishing it from other inborn errors of surfactant metabolism if no normal lamellar bodies are observed and only the characteristic small, "fried egg–" appearing organelles are present. A caveat is that most of the reported ultrastructural studies were in children with the most severe form of ABCA3 deficiency, and ultrastructural findings may be more variable in children with milder disease. EM requires proper handling of the tissue because the lipid components of lamellar bodies are extracted with many fixatives and EM is not routinely performed on lung tissue samples. Thus, although tissue examination may be strongly suggestive, genetic testing is needed to establish a definitive diagnosis.

Management, Treatment, and Prognosis

As a common phenotype for surfactant production disorders is that of RDS, such newborns are often treated initially with exogenous surfactant. SP-B– or ABCA3-deficient infants may show some initial improvement after treatment with exogenous surfactant, but in SP-B deficiency the disease is invariably progressive with diminished responses to subsequent doses. The course of children with ABCA3 deficiency is more variable, with some acting similarly to those with SP-B deficiency, whereas others may improve considerably after one or two doses, although the disease does not resolve completely. As surfactant deficiency underlies part of the pathophysiology of NKX2-1 mutations, a trial of exogenous surfactant is not unreasonable in affected infants. With SFTPC mutations, because the pathophysiology of the lung disease depends more upon direct cellular injury as opposed to deficiency of surfactant lipids or proteins, there is less rationale for surfactant augmentation therapy. However, in the absence of a family history, a diagnosis is usually not established at the time surfactant therapy is considered.

Currently there are no specific treatments for children with surfactant production disorders. Thyroid hormone replacement is indicated in those patients with evidence of hypothyroidism, but specific therapies for the lung disease due to NKX2-1 mutations have not been evaluated. ABCA3 gene transcription is increased by glucocorticoids in vitro, providing a rationale for treatment with steroids to augment any remaining gene function, but clinical evidence for the efficacy of steroids for this condition is limited.[19,200] Similarly, rare children with partial SP-B deficiency, which results from mutations that allow for some SP-B production and can be associated with intermediate survival, may show improvement with corticosteroids.[156] Treatment of SFTPC mutations has also included corticosteroids, as well as hydroxychloroquine,

and azithromycin, and these agents have also been used in treating ABCA3 deficiency. Anecdotal reports provide evidence that these drugs may help some patients with these disorders, with worsening of disease observed when the drug was stopped and improvement observed when drug therapy resumed, but not all affected subjects respond.[29,84,184,201–204] The efficacy of these agents is uncertain and complicated by the variability in the natural history of the disease, and the possible mechanisms of action are also unclear.[202] The use of drugs to correct and facilitate protein folding and trafficking within AEC2s may represent a future approach to the treatment of these disorders similarly to current approaches for treating some mutations responsible for cystic fibrosis.[165,205] Advances in gene-editing approaches may represent another novel therapeutic option in the future.[206] The generation of animal models will be important to test both existing and novel therapies.

Lung transplantation has been performed in children with end-stage lung disease from surfactant production disorders, with results comparable to those of similarly age-matched subjects.[207,208] Complete deficiency of SP-B is generally lethal, and the lung disease in ABCA3 deficiency is often severe and invariably progressive. ABCA3 genotypes involving biallelic mutations predicted to completely preclude ABCA3 expression have to date been invariably associated with a poor prognosis.[23] ABCA3 genotype may thus be helpful in deciding upon which ABCA3-deficient children are early candidates for lung transplantation, although caution is warranted because siblings with the same genotype may have very different clinical courses.[187,209,210] In contrast, no consistent association of SFTPC genotype with clinical course has been observed.[29] The variability in the natural history of lung disease due to SFTPC and NKX2-1 mutations complicates the decision for lung transplantation for these disorders, particularly with the potential for considerable improvement with supportive care for SFTPC mutations.[211]

Because SP-B and ABCA3 deficiencies are autosomal recessive conditions, there is a 25% recurrence risk for future children born to the parents of an affected child, and they should be referred for formal genetic counseling. Identification of responsible mutations allows for antenatal diagnosis and potentially even preimplantation genetic diagnosis such that an unaffected child may be born after in vitro fertilization. Because familial disease due to SFTPC or NKX2-1 mutations is inherited in a dominant pattern, there is a 50% recurrence risk should a parent carry the same mutation found in the child. As de novo mutations in both genes may cause sporadic disease, the recurrence risk may be much lower if neither parent is found to carry the mutation, but the risk is not zero, owing to the possibilities of germline mosaicism or nonpaternity. A complicating factor in genetic testing of the parents of children with these disorders, particularly SFTPC, is that an asymptomatic parent may be found to have a mutation, with important implications for their health, reinforcing the need for formal genetic counseling when undertaking such testing.

Whole lung lavage is currently the standard therapy for autoimmune PAP; it works well in most patients and improves survival and quality of life. Occasionally, or possibly late in the course of disease, whole lung lavage therapy can become less effective. Over the past decade, a series of small clinical studies have demonstrated that GM-CSF augmentation can be effective in treating this disease. However, neither the indications for use, route or timing of administration, dosage, or duration of therapy have been evaluated in prospective clinical trials. Thus further studies are needed. Anti-CD20 therapy using rituximab has been reported in a very limited number of patients with this disease and more studies are needed to evaluate the safety and efficacy of this potential therapy.

The number of patients with PAP caused by GM-CSF receptor defects identified to date is small, and therefore information regarding the natural history of these disorder remains unclear. Whole lung lavage has been successfully used to ameliorate the severity of the pulmonary symptoms, but, because the underlying defect remains, in most cases therapy is required on a periodic basis.[46] As serum GM-CSF levels are already elevated and patient macrophages do not respond to GM-CSF in vitro, exogenous GM-CSF seems unlikely to benefit most of these patients because components of the GM-CSF receptor are absent. However, in cases in which impaired GM-CSF signaling is due to decreased GM-CSF binding affinity rather than the absence of the receptor itself, GM-CSF augmentation therapy to increase the GM-CSF concentration may overcome the signaling defect and restore surfactant clearance by alveolar macrophages.[46,49] Clinical trials to evaluate inhaled GM-CSF as potential therapy thus warrant consideration. Because alveolar macrophages are bone marrow derived and based upon experiments in βc receptor–deficient mice, bone marrow transplantation may be curative for this group of disorders.[212] Cell- and gene-transfer–based therapeutic strategies are also in development for these disorders. Transplantation of pulmonary macrophages shows promise in reversing the phenotype of hereditary PAP in a mouse model.[213]

Summary

Single gene defects have been identified that disrupt surfactant production and metabolism (ABCA3, SFTPB, SFTPC, NKX2-1), as well as surfactant clearance (CSF2RA, CSF2RB). The phenotypes of these disorders include acute neonatal respiratory failure, progressive diffuse childhood lung disease, pulmonary fibrosis in adults, and dyspnea and respiratory failure from surfactant accumulation in children, adolescents, and adults. There is considerable overlap in the clinical features and lung pathology findings associated with these disorders, which are summarized in Table 57.1. Genetic testing is needed for specific diagnosis, which may obviate the need for lung biopsy in some patients. Specific therapies for these disorders are not currently available. Lung transplantation has been performed for disorders of surfactant production. Disorders of surfactant clearance result from macrophage dysfunction, and bone marrow transplantation is a potential therapy. Given the complexity of the surfactant system, it is likely that other genetic disorders disrupting surfactant metabolism will be identified as causes of rare lung diseases, providing new insights into normal surfactant metabolism and suggesting candidate genes contributing to the pathogenesis of more common lung diseases such as neonatal RDS.

Acknowledgments

The authors gratefully acknowledge the collaboration and contributions of Jeffrey Whitsett, Susan Wert, Timothy Weaver, and Takuji Suzuki, Cincinnati Children's Hospital and University of Cincinnati College of Medicine, Cincinnati, OH; Jennifer A. Wambach and F. Sessions Cole, St. Louis Children's Hospital and Washington University, St. Louis, MO; Aaron Hamas, Lurie Children's Hospital and Northwestern University School of Medicine, Chicago, IL; and Michael Dean, NCI, Frederick, MD. Supported by grants from the National Institutes of Health, HL-54703 (L.M.N), (HL-085433) (B.C.T), National Center for Research Resources, RR019498 (B.C.T., the Division of Pulmonary Biology, Cincinnati Children's Hospital Research Foundation) (B.C.T.) and the Eudowood Foundation (L.M.N.).

References

Access the reference list online at ExpertConsult.com.

Table 57.1   Features of Hereditary Disorders of Surfactant Production and Clearance

OMIM Name	SP-B Deficiency SMDP1	ABCA3 Deficiency SMDP3	SP-C Dysfunction SMDP2	TTF-1 Haplo-Insufficiency Brain-Thyroid-Lung	Hereditary PAP SMDP4	Hereditary PAP SMDP5
Epidemiology	Extremely rare, <1 in 1 million	Rare; incidence estimate 1 in 3500 to 1 in 20,000	Rare; incidence and prevalence unknown	Rare; incidence and prevalence unknown	Very rare; incidence and prevalence unknown	Very rare; incidence and prevalence unknown
Etiology						
Gene	*SFTPB*	*ABCA3*	*SFTPC*	*NKX2-1*	*CSF2RA*	*CSF2RB*
Chromosomal location	2p11.2	16p13.3	8p21	14q13.3	Xp22.32; Yp11.3	22q13.1
Inheritance pattern	Recessive	Recessive	Dominant or Sporadic 2nd de novo mutation	Sporadic 2nd de novo mutation Dominant	Recessive	Recessive
Pathology features	AEC2 hyperplasia Mesenchymal thickening Proteinaceous material and macrophages in distal air spaces	AEC2 hyperplasia Mesenchymal thickening Proteinaceous material and macrophages in distal air spaces	AEC2 hyperplasia Mesenchymal thickening Proteinaceous material and macrophages in distal air spaces	Altered growth AEC2 hyperplasia Mesenchymal thickening Proteinaceous material and macrophages in distal air spaces	Granular, eosinophilic PAS-positive material filling distal airspaces. Alveolar architecture preserved.	Granular, eosinophilic PAS-positive material filling distal airspaces. Alveolar architecture preserved.
Histologic diagnoses	PAP, CPI, DIP	PAP, DIP, CPI, NSIP	CPI, DIP, NSIP, PAP	CPI, DIP, NSIP, PAP	PAP	PAP
Pathogenesis	Loss of function Impaired processing of proSP-C Abnormal lamellar bodies	Loss of function Surfactant deficiency AEC2 injury Abnormal lamellar bodies	Gain of toxic function Dominant negative ER stress 2nd UPR Impaired autophagy	Haploinsufficiency Altered transcription of downstream genes	Loss of function	Loss of function
Clinical features	Neonatal RDS Very rarely chILD syndrome No extrapulmonary findings	Neonatal RDS chILD syndrome: Tachypnea Exercise intolerance Clubbing Pectus excavatum Failure to thrive No extrapulmonary findings	Neonatal RDS (unusual chILD syndrome) Asymptomatic Adult-onset DLD	Neonatal RDS chILD syndrome Recurrent infection Adult DLD Hypothyroidism Neurologic: Chorea, ataxia Hypotonia Developmental delay	Insidious onset Dyspnea, cough Exercise intolerance	Insidious onset Dyspnea, cough Exercise intolerance
Diagnosis	Genetic testing (NGS) panel most efficient	Genetic testing (NGS) panel most efficient	Genetic testing (NGS) panel most efficient	Genetic testing (NGS) panel most efficient	Genetic testing Serum GM-CSF level elevated	Genetic testing Serum GM-CSF level elevated
Management	Supportive Palliative care Lung transplant	Supportive (nutrition) Steroids, hydroxychloroquine, Azithromycin. Lung transplant	Supportive (nutrition) Steroids, hydroxychloroquine, Azithromycin. Lung transplant	Thyroid supplementation if hypothyroid. Supportive (nutrition) Steroids	Whole lung lavage	Whole lung lavage
Prognosis	Very poor. Usually fatal in first 3 months of life	May be rapidly fatal, predicted null mutations on both alleles associated with early-onset and poor prognosis. Prolonged survival possible.	Highly variable Severe disease in infancy with possible improvement. Asymptomatic for decades. Onset respiratory symptoms and pulmonary fibrosis in adulthood.	Highly variable	Variable	Variable

chILD, Childhood interstitial lung disease; *CPI,* chronic pneumonitis of infancy; *DIP,* desquamative interstitial pneumonia; *DLD,* diffuse lung disease; *ER,* endoplasmic reticulum; *GM-CSF,* granulocyte-macrophage colony-stimulating factor; *NGS,* next-generation sequencing; *NSIP,* nonspecific interstitial pneumonia; *OMIM,* online mendelian inheritance in man; *PAP,* pulmonary alveolar proteinosis; *PAS,* periodic acid–Schiff; *RDS,* respiratory distress syndrome; *UPR,* unfolded protein response.

58 Pulmonary Involvement in the Systemic Inflammatory Diseases of Childhood

SHARON D. DELL, BEng, MD, RAYFEL SCHNEIDER, MBBCh, and RAE S. M. YEUNG, MD, PhD, FRCPC

Overview of Chapter

In this chapter, we will highlight pulmonary manifestations of the systemic inflammatory diseases of childhood. We will focus on the diseases that are either common in the pediatric rheumatology clinic or those that commonly involve the lungs. These include juvenile idiopathic arthritis (JIA), the connective tissue diseases (systemic lupus erythematosus [SLE], scleroderma [SSc], juvenile dermatomyositis [JDM], and mixed connective tissue disease [MCTD]), vasculitides (especially granulomatosis with polyangiitis [GPA]), and sarcoidosis. Clinically significant pulmonary involvement due to systemic inflammatory disease is rare in the pediatric setting. However, it is important for the pediatric pulmonologist to be familiar with this topic for two reasons: (1) pulmonary involvement may be associated with high morbidity and mortality in this population and (2) pulmonary disease may be the predominant initial clinical presentation in a subset of these patients. The systemic inflammatory diseases most frequently encountered by the pediatric pulmonologist include GPA, SLE, SSc, and MCTD. Symptom patterns along with specific autoantibody serological tests are most useful for diagnosing the underlying systemic inflammatory disease (Table 58.1). Pulmonary involvement in these cases can often be a difficult diagnostic dilemma, as lung toxicity due to potent pharmacotherapies and opportunistic infections must be considered alongside the possibility of the lung being a target organ of the underlying inflammatory disease. Lung disease may involve any compartment of the lung (chest wall, pleura, airways, parenchyma, and vasculature), and often more than one pulmonary etiology may be present simultaneously (e.g., pulmonary fibrosis and chest wall restriction). Although there is certainly overlap in the pulmonary manifestations between different diseases, certain patterns are recognized with greater frequency in some entities (Table 58.2). For example, interstitial lung disease (ILD) and pulmonary arterial hypertension (PAH) are characteristic of systemic sclerosis, while pleuritis and pleural effusions are characteristic of JIA and SLE and would be very unusual in the context of JDM. For the purposes of classifying lung disease in this chapter, ILD will be defined as a clinical diagnosis of "pulmonary fibrosis" or a lung biopsy histopathological pattern of nonspecific interstitial pneumonitis (NSIP), usual interstitial pneumonitis (UIP), lymphocytic interstitial pneumonitis (LIP), bronchiolitis obliterans (BO) organizing pneumonia (BOOP, also known as cryptogenic organizing pneumonia), or diffuse alveolar damage (DAD).[1] Treatment of lung disease is specific to the underlying systemic disease

and is often effective at reducing pulmonary morbidity. Prognosis is variable and dependent on the severity of the disease and its response to therapy. Disease progression is monitored by following symptoms, particularly dyspnea, the use of routine pulmonary function and exercise testing, and high-resolution computed tomography (HRCT) imaging. The role of serological biomarkers to detect and monitor progression of ILD, particularly SP-D and KL-6, is an area of active investigation. As the prognosis for the systemic inflammatory diseases improves, increasing emphasis is being placed on early detection and treatment of lung disease.

Juvenile Idiopathic Arthritis

EPIDEMIOLOGY

JIA is the most common chronic rheumatic disease in childhood, with a prevalence of 16–150 per 100,000.[2] The term JIA includes a heterogeneous group of diseases that have in common the following characteristics: arthritis, which begins before the age of 16 years, persists for at least 6 weeks, and for which no specific cause can be found. Overall, girls are affected approximately twice as commonly as boys are, but this varies considerably with the different subtypes. The age of onset ranges from less than 1 year to 16 years, with a peak between 1 and 3 years for the most common subtypes. The onset of JIA in the first 6 months of life is rare and should raise suspicion of another diagnosis. In a large multiethnic cohort of JIA patients, children of European descent had an increased risk of JIA, and there were significant differences in the frequency of different subtypes of JIA in different ethnic groups.[3]

ETIOLOGY AND PATHOGENESIS

The cause of JIA remains unknown, and the pathogenesis has not been clearly elucidated. Given the heterogeneity of the disease phenotypes, it is not surprising that the different subtypes have different genetic predispositions and associations, different autoantibody profiles, and differences in immune dysregulation. JIA is a complex genetic disease, where there are multiple genetic associations. HLA-A2 is associated with early-onset JIA, especially in the oligoarticular subtype. There are strong HLA associations with oligoarticular JIA (HLA-DRB1*08, 11, and 13 and DPB1*02). HLA DRB1*08 is also associated with rheumatoid factor negative polyarticular JIA), and RF-positive JIA is associated with DRB1*04,

Table 58.1 Commonly Requested Serologic Tests for Selected Pediatric Systemic Inflammatory Diseases With Possible Pulmonary Involvement

Autoantibody Serologic Test	Disease Entity	Comments
ANA	Nonrheumatic disease	Present in 10% of normal children; may occur with infection, drug, malignancy
	SLE	Present in virtually 100% of SLE, but not specific
	Oligoarticular JIA	Present in 60%–80%, marker for uveitis
	JDM	Present in 50%–75%
	SSc	Present in 90% systemic sclerosis, 50% of localized scleroderma
	MCTD	Present in 100%, speckled pattern and very high titer
Anti-dsDNA	SLE	Present in 60%–90%; very specific; titer correlates with disease activity
Anti-Sm	SLE	Present in 25%–40%; very specific; correlates with renal disease
Anti-Ro/anti-La	SLE, Sjögren's syndrome	
Anti-RNP	SLE, MCTD, scleroderma	When present in very high titer, suggests MCTD
Anticardiolipin	SLE, Antiphospholipid antibody syndrome	May also occur in infection and malignancy; IgG isotype associated with thrombosis
Anti-Jo-1	Myositis	Rare in children; marker for ILD in adult dermatomyositis
Anti-Scl-70	SSc	Marker for severe lung disease
Anticentromere	Limited SSc	Rare in children; marker for late development of pulmonary hypertension
ANCA	Vasculitides	May also occur with SLE and inflammatory bowel disease
■ PR3 (antiproteinase 3 antibody)	GPA	Sensitive (>90%) and specific for GPA
■ MPO (antimyeloperoxidase antibody	MPA	Sensitive (~70%) and specific for MPA
Rheumatoid factor	RF+ polyarticular JIA	Poor sensitivity and specificity for JIA; when present in patients with JIA it is associated with severe disease (usually adolescent females). Also positive in 50% GPA.

ANA, Antinuclear antibody; *ANCA*, antineutrophil cytoplasmic antibody; *GPA*, granulomatosis with polyangiitis; *IgG*, immunoglobulin G; *ILD*, interstitial lung disease; *JDM*, juvenile dermatomyositis; *JIA*, juvenile idiopathic arthritis; *MCTD*, mixed connective tissue disease; *MPA*, microscopic polyangiitis; *SLE*, systemic lupus erythematosus; *SSc*, scleroderma.

Table 58.2 Summary of Pulmonary Manifestations of Systemic Inflammatory Disease in Children

	JIA	SLE	JDM	SSc	MCTD	Sarcoidosis	GPA	MPA
Frequency at initial presentation[a]	+	++	+	+++	+	+++	+++	+
Frequency during disease course[b]	+	+++	+	+++	+++	+++	+++	++
Chest wall/diaphragm[c]	+	+	+++	+	+	−	−	−
Pleural disease[d]	++	+++	−	+	++	+	+	−
Large airway lesions[e]	−	−	−	−	−	++	++	−
Bronchiectasis	+	+	−	+	−	+	+	−
Acute pneumonitis[f]	+	++	+	−	−	−	−	−
ILD[g]	+	+	+	+++	++	+	−	−
Pulmonary granulomas	−	−	−	−	−	+++	+++	−
Vasculitis/DAH[i]	+	+	−	+	+	−	++	+++
Pulmonary hypertension	−	+	+	++	++	−	−	+
Thrombosis	−	++	−	−	−	−	+	−

[a]Pulmonary involvement at initial presentation of systemic inflammatory disease.
[b]Frequency of pulmonary involvement during disease course.
[c]Includes respiratory muscle weakness and diaphragm dysfunction.
[d]Pleuritis and/or pleural effusion.
[e]Upper airway and endobronchial lesions and/or stenosis visible on bronchoscopy.
[f]A clinical diagnosis with acute onset of fever, tachypnea, hypoxia, and pulmonary infiltrates with or without pleural effusion on chest imaging, in the absence of infection and usually responding quickly to antiinflammatory treatment.
[g]Includes clinical diagnosis of "pulmonary fibrosis" and histopathological diagnosis of usual interstitial pneumonia (UIP), nonspecific interstitial pneumonitis (NSIP), lymphocytic interstitial pneumonitis (LIP), bronchiolitis obliterans organizing pneumonia (BOOP), and diffuse alveolar damage (DAD).
[i]DAH, diffuse alveolar hemorrhage.
GPA, Granulomatosis with polyangiitis; *ILD*, interstitial lung disease; *JIA*, juvenile idiopathic arthritis; *JDM*, juvenile dermatomyositis; *MCTD*, mixed connective tissue disease; *MPA*, microscopic polyangiitis; *SLE*, systemic lupus erythematosus; *SSc*, scleroderma.

DQA1*03, and DQB1*03.[4] There is also a significant association of HLA-B27 with enthesitis-related arthritis (ERA) and juvenile ankylosing spondylitis.[5] A number of polymorphisms have been associated with JIA, including a polymorphism involving the protein tyrosine phosphatase N22 gene (PTPN22).[6] Antinuclear antibodies are frequently found in children with oligoarticular disease and somewhat less frequently seen in polyarticular JIA. The presence of ANA is clearly associated with a higher risk of uveitis, the most common extraarticular manifestation of both oligoarthritis (occurring in 21%) and RF-negative polyarticular arthritis (14%).[7] The systemic subtype is characterized by a lack of autoantibodies and by dysregulation of interleukin-1β production and significant elevations of interleukin-6 (IL-6). Studies using biologic agents that block the actions of IL-6 (tocilizumab) and IL-1β (anakinra, canakinamab, and rilonacept) have proven to be effective in treating patients with active systemic disease. The dysregulation of IL-1β in systemic JIA and the efficacy of IL-1β inhibitors in reversing manifestations of the disease suggest that it is more likely an autoinflammatory disease than an autoimmune disease.

CLINICAL MANIFESTATIONS

The clinical manifestations of JIA depend on the subtype, which is defined by the presenting features within the first 6 months of disease onset (Table 58.3). The most common subtype in Europe and North America is oligoarticular JIA, which primarily affects large joints. This can remain oligoarticular or extend after the first 6 months to involve additional joints. Both oligoarticular and RF-negative polyarticular JIA most commonly affect young preschool age girls. Asymptomatic anterior uveitis occurs in oligoarticular JIA, RF-negative polyarticular JIA, and psoriatic arthritis. If undetected by routine slit lamp examination, uveitis can result in blindness. Rheumatoid factor-positive polyarticular JIA most commonly first manifests in older girls, is phenotypically similar to adult rheumatoid arthritis, where arthritis affects small and large joints in a symmetrical pattern, and is sometimes associated with rheumatoid nodules. ERA typically develops in boys over the age of 8 years and is characterized by predominantly lower limb arthritis in association with enthesitis, inflammation where ligaments, tendons, or joint capsules attach to bone. This may be the forerunner of ankylosing spondylitis in adult life. The heel and knee are the most commonly involved entheses. ERA may be accompanied by symptomatic anterior uveitis with a painful, red eye in a proportion of patients. Arthritis may occur at disease onset but sometimes only develops after weeks or even months. The diagnosis of psoriatic arthritis in children may depend on arthritis associated with psoriatic nail changes, dactylitis, or a family history of psoriasis, since arthritis frequently precedes the development of psoriatic skin lesions by many years. Systemic arthritis is distinct from the other subtypes, both clinically and biologically, since the systemic manifestations of fever, rash, hepatosplenomegaly, lymphadenopathy, and serositis (particularly pericarditis) are usually prominent at onset, and it is thought to have an autoinflammatory pathobiology.

Macrophage activation syndrome (MAS) is a severe, potentially life-threatening complication of JIA, occurring in approximately 10% of children with the systemic subtype. Characteristic clinical features are sustained, high fever, hepatosplenomegaly, lymphadenopathy, and sometimes bleeding, bruising, and encephalopathy. Characteristic laboratory features include a sudden drop in white blood cell count, platelet count, and hemoglobin, with elevated transaminases, LDH, coagulopathy, and very high levels of serum ferritin. Dysregulation of the IL-1β pathway is prominent in both sJIA and MAS. The mortality in a recent large series of patients with systemic JIA and MAS was 8%.[8]

CLASSIFICATION AND DIAGNOSIS OF JUVENILE IDIOPATHIC ARTHRITIS

The International League of Associations for Rheumatology (ILAR) criteria for the classification are widely accepted. The inclusion criteria for the different subtypes are listed in Table 58.3. There are also a number of exclusions for each category[9] that are beyond the scope of this chapter.

Table 58.3   Subtypes of Juvenile Idiopathic Arthritis

Subtype	Subtype Inclusion Criteria (9)	% of All JIA (2)	Sex Ratio (2)
Systemic	Arthritis PLUS fever for 2 weeks, daily for at least 3 days PLUS at least one of the following: ■ Rash ■ Serositis ■ Generalized lymphadenopathy ■ Hepatomegaly or splenomegaly	4%–17%	F=M
Oligoarticular	4 or fewer affected joints within first 6 months Persistent—remain with ≤ four joints Extended—>four joints after 6 months	27%–56%	F≫>M
Polyarticular RF negative	≥Five joints in first 6 months	11%–28%	F≫M
Polyarticular RF positive	≥Five joints in first 6 months	2%–7%	
Enthesitis related arthritis	Arthritis PLUS enthesitis OR Arthritis OR enthesitis PLUS at least 2 of the following: ■ Sacroiliac joint tenderness and/or inflammatory spinal pain ■ Presence of HLA-B27 ■ Family history of HLA-B27-associated disease ■ Anterior uveitis (usually symptomatic) ■ Onset of arthritis in a boy > 8 years	3%–11%	M≫F
Psoriatic arthritis	Arthritis PLUS Psoriasis OR Arthritis PLUS at least 2 of: ■ Dactylitis ■ Nail pitting or onycholysis ■ Psoriasis in a first-degree relative	2%–11%	F>M
Unclassified	Does not meet criteria for one of above OR Meets criteria for >1 of above	11%–21%	

JIA, Juvenile idiopathic arthritis.

PULMONARY INVOLVEMENT IN JUVENILE IDIOPATHIC ARTHRITIS

Pulmonary involvement in JIA is uncommon and significant pulmonary manifestations, except for pleuritis, are sufficiently rare that these warrant thorough evaluation for other conditions such as infections, systemic vasculitis, SLE, and other connective tissue diseases. Pleuritis is a well-reported manifestation of systemic JIA, but it is usually accompanied by pericarditis. One should be particularly careful to exclude the diagnosis of SLE in an older girl who presents with isolated pleuritis and arthritis. There are few reports of pulmonary disease in JIA. One of the earliest studies completed more than 30 years ago found pulmonary disease in 4% of JIA patients. The radiological abnormalities included pneumonitis, interstitial reticular and nodular infiltrates, and pleural effusions. Pathologic correlates of these findings were pulmonary hemosiderosis, lymphoid follicular bronchiolitis, and LIP. Some patients with parenchymal disease developed radiographic evidence of interstitial fibrosis.[10] There are additional reports of pulmonary hemosiderosis in JIA[11,12] and a report of LIP that actually preceded the diagnosis of RF-positive JIA by 10 years.[13] Recently patients with familial JIA-like symptoms and ILD have been described with COPA (coatomer subunit α) gene mutations, which impair vesicular transport and cause endoplasmic reticulum stress.[14] It is possible that some of the extreme phenotypes of lung disease in association with JIA are also inherited monogenic inflammatory diseases that we will discover as our knowledge increases and with improved genetic testing.

Severe pulmonary manifestations, seen predominantly with systemic JIA, are uncommon but may be associated with a high mortality rate. An international series described 25 patients with systemic JIA and PAH ($n = 16$), ILD ($n = 7$), and/or alveolar proteinosis (AP; $n = 5$), with six patients having more than one diagnosis.[15] In comparison to a large cohort of systemic JIA patients in a North American registry, these patients were more likely to be female and to have active systemic disease features, and were more likely to have been treated with biological agents, most commonly IL-1 inhibitors, which were used in two-thirds of patients. There was a striking association of these pulmonary complications with MAS, which was reported in 60% of patients at the time of the pulmonary diagnosis, approximately 6 times the rate at which MAS is reported to occur at any time during the disease course. Symptoms most commonly reported were shortness of breath, exertional dyspnea, cough, and chest pain, but some patients only had digital clubbing. Most concerning is that 17 patients died within a mean period of less than 9 months from the time of the pulmonary disease diagnosis. Since almost all patients developed severe pulmonary complications in the biological era (after the year 2000), biological agents have neither prevented nor effectively treated these complications. Further surveillance studies will help determine whether biological agents may potentially be involved in their pathogenesis.

One systemic JIA patient with PAH in the absence of documented pulmonary parenchymal disease responded well to treatment with cyclosporine and systemic corticosteroids.[16] A 5-year-old girl who developed radiographic features suggestive of progressive pulmonary fibrosis had interstitial and intraalveolar cholesterol granulomas identified on lung biopsy.

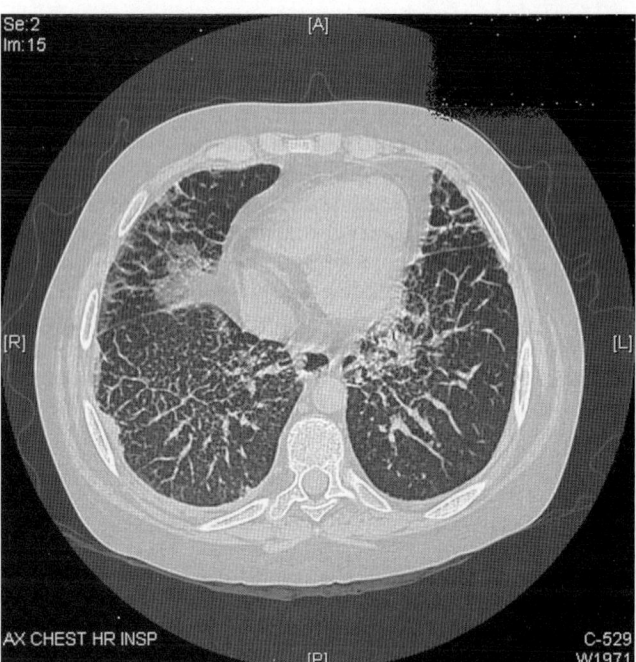

Fig. 58.1 Twelve-year-old child with systemic onset juvenile idiopathic arthritis at age 15 months who developed gradual onset of dyspnea, cough, and crackles on auscultation. High-resolution computed tomography scan showed bilateral diffuse interstitial changes, including thickening of the interlobular septa, nodules, and areas of fibrosis and ground glass densities. A lung biopsy confirmed the diagnosis of endogenous lipoid pneumonia with interstitial and intraalveolar cholesterol granulomas.

Although she appeared to stabilize on immunosuppressive treatment with methotrexate and etanercept, she subsequently succumbed with respiratory failure.[17] We have seen an additional systemic JIA patient with a similarly refractory disease course who developed fatal pulmonary lipoid pneumonia (Fig. 58.1). A 21-year-old male, following a long history of severe systemic JIA with persistent systemic symptoms and damaging arthritis, developed endogenous lipoid pneumonia that was ultimately treated with double lung transplantation.[18]

Pulmonary manifestations of MAS include lung infiltrates, pneumonitis, pulmonary hemorrhage, and pulmonary edema, which may result from myocardial dysfunction associated with the hypercytokinemia typical of MAS. One large series reported pulmonary involvement in 50% of patients, and one-third of all patients required ventilatory support.[19]

BOOP has been described in adults with rheumatoid arthritis,[20] but there are few reports of this complication associated with JIA.[21] BO was described in a 12-year-old girl following treatment of her arthritis with intramuscular gold injections. Despite immunosuppressive treatment and subsequent lung transplantation, the BO was progressive and fatal.[22] BO has also been reported in a patient with JIA whose first symptoms were those related to pneumomediastinum.[23]

Studies of pulmonary function in JIA have detected abnormal pulmonary function tests (PFTs) in more than 50% of asymptomatic patients. Restrictive disease patterns have been more commonly identified than obstructive abnormalities.[24] Results of diffusing capacity of the lungs for carbon monoxide (DLCO) measurements have been more variable with reductions in DLCO reported in 3.7%–45%.[25–27] Reductions of maximum inspiratory and expiratory pressures, suggestive of respiratory muscle weakness, may influence PFTs in these patients, but there may also be a correlation of impaired pulmonary function with disease severity, as measured by the erythrocyte sedimentation rate (ESR) and requirement for treatment with methotrexate. Since methotrexate is the most commonly used second-line drug for the treatment of JIA, it is important to consider whether it has any impact on the development of lung disease. Low-dose weekly methotrexate has been reported to cause an acute pneumonitis associated with fever, cough, and dyspnea. There have also been concerns raised about methotrexate-induced chronic, progressive pulmonary fibrosis.[28,29] However, several studies suggest that methotrexate does not increase the risk of pulmonary disease in children with arthritis.[25,30,31]

TREATMENT

Nonsteroidal antiinflammatory drugs (NSAIDs) and intraarticular corticosteroid injections[32] are considered first-line treatments for children with JIA and may be all that is required to treat oligoarticular involvement or mild disease. Children whose arthritis does not respond adequately, especially those with a polyarticular course, are treated with low-dose weekly methotrexate. The advent of biological agents has dramatically improved outcomes for children whose arthritis is refractory to methotrexate.[33] Tumor necrosis factor alpha (TNFα) inhibitors, such as etanercept,[34] adalimumab,[35] or infliximab, are usually used if there is an inadequate response to methotrexate or if there is intolerance to methotrexate. Newer biological options for polyarticular course JIA include abatacept[36] and tocilizumab.[37] There are different treatment algorithms followed for different subtypes: neither methotrexate nor TNFα inhibitors are particularly effective for systemic JIA. Children who have persistent systemic symptoms and arthritis despite NSAIDs usually respond to systemic corticosteroids. IL-1 antagonists such as anakinra,[38] canakinumab,[39] and rilonacept[40] or the IL-6 antagonist, tocilizumab,[41,42] have proven to be highly efficacious for steroid-dependent systemic JIA. Pediatric rheumatologists are changing the treatment paradigm to treat earlier and more aggressively to try to change the course of the immune response and prevent long-term joint damage in all subtypes of JIA. For example, many treat JIA patients with IL-1 inhibition, even before corticosteroids are used. Acute symptomatic serositis, especially pericarditis, may require intravenous pulsed methylprednisolone. A similar approach is taken for MAS with early use of cyclosporine or IL-1 inhibitors if there is not a rapid response. ERA does not respond as well as other subtypes to methotrexate but may respond to treatment with sulfasalazine.[43] Axial spine involvement may need early institution of TNFα inhibitors.

PROGNOSIS

The mortality in JIA is well below 1%,[44] with a disproportionately higher mortality risk in the systemic subtype, largely because of MAS associated with the disease and infections associated with immunosuppressive therapy. Overall, active arthritis persists on long-term follow-up, even into adult life, in more than 50% of patients. Poor prognostic features of the systemic subtype include persistent systemic symptoms,

marked thrombocytosis, and polyarticular arthritis in the first 6 months of disease.[45] For the other subtypes, positive rheumatoid factor, marked and persistent elevation of inflammatory markers, involvement of the hip joint, and early joint space loss and erosions predict poor outcome.[46,47] Acute pleuritis usually responds well to treatment without sequelae, but the pulmonary manifestations such as PAH, ILD, and AP carry a high mortality.

Systemic Lupus Erythematosus

EPIDEMIOLOGY

SLE predominantly affects young women, but in approximately 15%–20% of individuals, the disease presents prior to the age of 18 years. SLE is relatively rare in children, with an estimated incidence of 10–20 per 100,000 that is considerably higher in black, Hispanic, South and South-East Asian, as well as North American First Nations populations. In postpubertal adolescents, females are clearly more commonly affected than males (~6 : 1), but in the younger age groups, the female predominance is much less marked.[48]

PATHOGENESIS

SLE is the prototypic autoimmune disease, characterized by presence of autoantibodies in virtually all patients. There is substantial evidence of both innate and adaptive immune dysregulation and of immune activation and autoimmunity, resulting from the interaction of lupus-associated genes with environmental triggers. Environmental triggers include ultraviolet radiation, infections, drugs, and chemicals. The activation of the immune system is amplified by lupus autoantibodies and their associated nucleic acids, together with cytokines and chemokines, resulting in inflammation and tissue damage.[49] Autoantibodies can actually be detected many years before the development of clinically symptomatic SLE.[50]

CLINICAL FEATURES

Common presenting symptoms of SLE in children are rash, joint pain, and constitutional symptoms such as fatigue, fever, and weight loss. The most common presenting features in a large cohort of pediatric lupus patients were arthritis (67%), malar rash (66%), nephritis (55%), and central nervous system disease (27%).[51]

The American College of Rheumatology criteria for the classification of lupus in adults appear to apply well to children with SLE (Box 58.1) and have been reported to achieve a sensitivity of 96% and specificity of 100% for the diagnosis of SLE in a pediatric population.[52] Although the classification criteria require that four or more of the 11 criteria are present, there are no published diagnostic criteria, and the diagnosis of SLE in children can certainly be made when fewer than four criteria are present.

PULMONARY INVOLVEMENT

Pulmonary involvement in pediatric SLE has been reported to occur in 18%–40% of patients within the first year of diagnosis and in 18%–81% of patients at any time during

Box 58.1   Classification Criteria for Systemic Lupus Erythematosus

1. Malar rash
2. Discoid rash
3. Photosensitivity
4. Nasal or oral ulcers
5. Arthritis involving at least two joints
6. Serositis
   Pleuritis, or
   Pericarditis
7. Renal disorder
   Proteinuria >0.5 g/day, or
   Cellular casts in the urine
8. Neurologic disorder
   Seizures, or
   Psychosis
9. Hematologic disorder
   Hemolytic anemia, or
   Leukopenia (<4000/mm), or
   Lymphopenia (<1500/mm), or
   Thrombocytopenia (<100,000/mm)
10. Immunologic disorder
    Anti-DNA antibody, or
    Anti-Sm antibody, or
    Antiphospholipid antibody
11. Positive antinuclear antibody

A person is classified as having SLE if at least 4 of the 11 criteria are present serially or simultaneously.

SLE, Systemic lupus erythematosus.

Modified from Hochberg MC. Updating the American College of Rheumatology revised criteria for the classification of systemic lupus erythematosus. Arthritis Rheum. 1997;40(9):1725.

the disease course.[53] It occurs more frequently in Afro-Caribbeans.[54] Studies that report higher rates of pulmonary involvement include abnormal pulmonary function tests or abnormal imaging studies, even in the absence of symptoms. Pulmonary involvement can indeed be very mild, or even asymptomatic, but can also be life-threatening with respiratory failure. Pulmonary lupus has been reported to be more severe when SLE begins within the first 2 years of life.[55] Pleuritis with pleural effusion is the only pulmonary manifestation to be included among the criteria for the classification of SLE[56] and occurs in 9%–32% of patients,[57–59] and may even be the initial clinical manifestation of SLE. In a large cohort of adult lupus patients, pleuritis was found to occur more frequently in patients with a younger age at disease onset, and longer disease duration, who manifested more cumulative disease-related damage, and in those who had positive anti-Sm and anti-RNP antibodies.[60] Pleural effusions are exudative and may be unilateral or bilateral. These must be differentiated from infectious exudative effusions and from transudative effusions related to renal or cardiac disease. SLE is associated with an increased risk of a wide range of infections, including bacterial, viral, mycobacterial, fungal, and parasitic infections, with the respiratory tract as one of the common sites.[61] In addition, immunosuppressive treatments to control the disease confer an increased risk of opportunistic infections such as pneumocystis, cytomegalovirus, and fungal infections. Inflammatory pulmonary lesions may be difficult or even impossible to differentiate from pulmonary hemorrhage or pulmonary infections.

Since infection is the leading cause of death in children with lupus,[62] rigorous exclusion of potential infections is necessary before attributing pulmonary manifestations to disease activity. Cultures of sputum (if obtainable), nasopharyngeal secretions, blood, and pleural fluid should be performed, but bronchoalveolar lavage (BAL) and lung biopsy may be necessary. Children at risk should be carefully evaluated for tuberculosis.

Acute pneumonitis is uncommon in adults with lupus and even less common in pediatric lupus. The presentation includes fever, nonproductive cough, dyspnea, pleuritic chest pain, and tachypnea. Chest radiographic findings are nonspecific, with infiltrates that can mimic infections or hemorrhage and that may be accompanied by pleural effusions (Fig. 58.2). Chronic ILD due to SLE is extremely rare; in a necropsy series of 90 lupus patients, none had acute or chronic pneumonitis.[63] If chronic pneumonitis does occur, Sjögren syndrome (SS), infection, or drug toxicity should be excluded. Chronic ILD can follow acute lupus pneumonitis[64] but can also develop in a more insidious manner with exertional dyspnea, chronic cough, pleuritic chest pain, and basal rales.[65] Patients tend to have multisystem manifestations of SLE. Pulmonary function studies typically follow a slowly progressive course with a restrictive pattern, but may improve or at least stabilize. Histopathology demonstrates alveolar wall thickening, interstitial fibrosis, interstitial lymphocytic infiltrates, and granular deposits of immunoglobulin and complement.

Pulmonary hemorrhage is a rare but potentially life-threatening complication of SLE in children that has been reported to occur at disease onset[66] or during the course of the disease. Significant acute pulmonary hemorrhage is accompanied by severe dyspnea with or without hemoptysis and a sudden drop in hemoglobin, and it may progress rapidly to respiratory failure. Lupus nephritis is present in a high proportion of patients. The mortality resulting from pulmonary hemorrhage in adult series of SLE has been as high as 50%,[67] and one report suggests an even higher mortality in childhood lupus.[68] Chest radiographs show diffuse alveolar opacities indistinguishable from fluid or infection. Lupus patients with acute pulmonary hemorrhage should be carefully investigated for pulmonary infections. In one report,[69] more than 50% of patients had an infection identified within 48 hours of presentation with pulmonary hemorrhage. Infections identified included pseudomonas, cytomegalovirus, and aspergillus. Empiric treatment with antibiotics may improve survival. Thrombotic thrombocytopenic purpura should be ruled out, particularly in the presence of fever, thrombocytopenia, and renal dysfunction, since this may be associated with SLE.

Pulmonary hypertension is rare in children with SLE, but has been reported in 14% of adult patients, followed at a tertiary care center.[70] In a large series of adult patients followed at nontertiary care centers, the prevalence of pulmonary hypertension determined by echocardiography was found to be 4.2%.[71] The presence of a lupus anticoagulant was the only risk factor identified for the development of pulmonary hypertension in this cohort. Raynaud phenomenon occurs more frequently in lupus patients with pulmonary hypertension than in other lupus patients. Potential causes of pulmonary hypertension in SLE include pulmonary vasculitis, pulmonary thromboembolism, ILD, and valvular

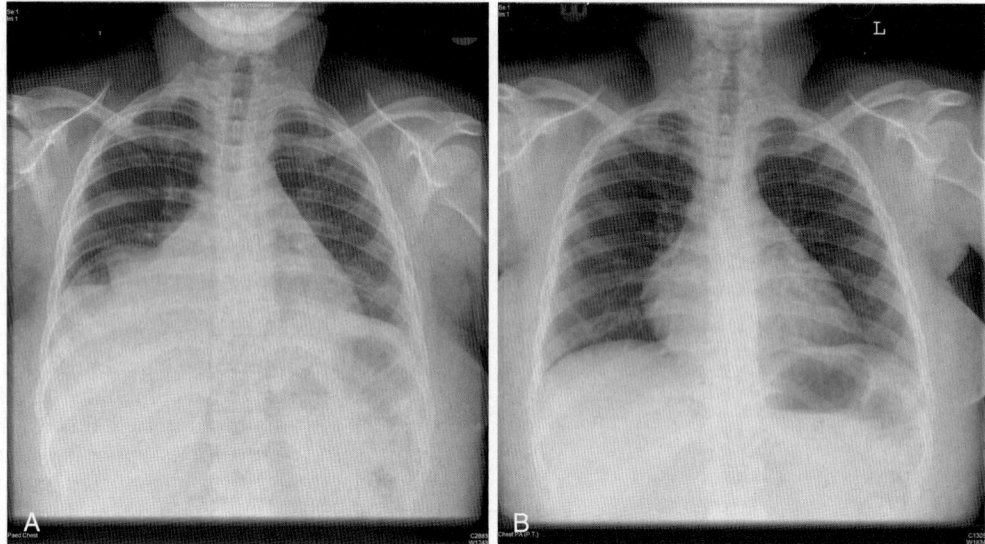

Fig. 58.2 (A and B) Chest radiographs of a 10-year-old girl diagnosed with systemic lupus erythematosus who presented with acute onset of fever, dyspnea, chest pain, malaise, weight loss, malar skin rash, and arthralgias. (A) Initial presentation with pleuritis and acute interstitial pneumonia. Radiograph shows bilateral pleural effusions and lower lobe opacification, worse on right side. (B) Rapid resolution of symptoms and imaging abnormalities after pulse steroid therapy.

heart disease. Serum endothelin levels have been found to be higher in patients with pulmonary hypertension than in other lupus patients, and antiendothelial cell antibodies are elevated in patients with active lupus and pulmonary hypertension.[72]

Antiphospholipid antibodies are found more frequently in SLE than other connective tissue diseases, with a prevalence of 44% for anticardiolipin antibodies, 40% for anti-β2 glycoprotein I, and 22% for the lupus anticoagulant.[73] Anticardiolipin titers correlate with lupus disease activity. Several studies have confirmed a strong association with antiphospholipid antibodies and vascular thromboses in children with SLE. Lupus anticoagulant appears to confer the highest risk of thrombosis, but there is also a clear association of thrombosis with anticardiolipin and anti-β2GPI.[74,75] Pulmonary embolism is the most frequent pulmonary manifestations of the antiphospholipid antibody syndrome, and recurrent pulmonary embolism can result in pulmonary hypertension.[76]

Shrinking lung syndrome occurs predominantly in adults with SLE but has also been reported in children. It typically presents with progressive dyspnea, pleuritic chest pain, and tachypnea. Chest radiographs may demonstrate reduced lung volumes, raised hemidiaphragms, and basal atelectasis (Fig. 58.3); PFTs are usually restrictive. Chest computed tomography (CT) scans do not reveal significant pleural or parenchymal lung disease. The cause of this syndrome in SLE remains unclear, but diaphragmatic dysfunction with poor diaphragmatic movement demonstrable on fluoroscopy has been reported in some pediatric cases.[77] Diaphragmatic dysfunction with subsequent shrinking lung syndrome has been linked to symptomatic pleuritis.[78] Although the optimum treatment is not clear, some patients appear to respond to immunosuppressive therapy.[79]

Studies in pediatric SLE patients without clinically or radiographically apparent lung disease have found PFT abnormalities in at least one-third, with a range of 38%–84%.[80]

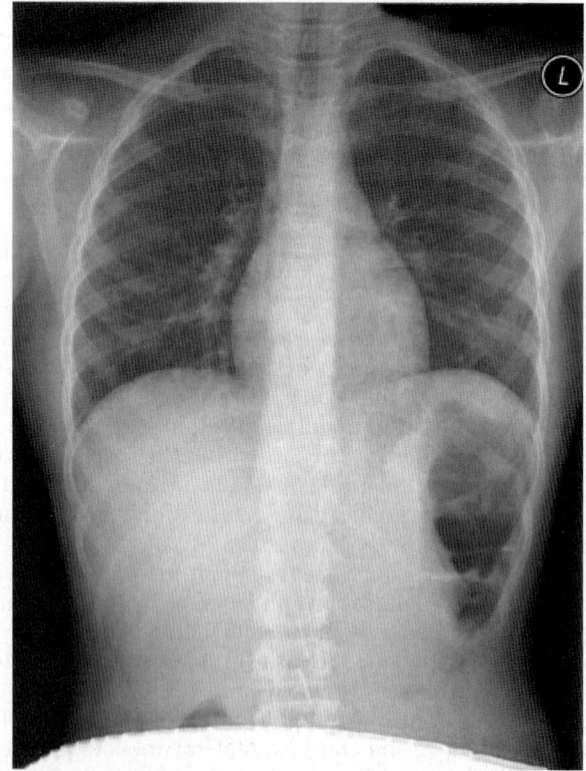

Fig. 58.3 Chest radiograph of an 11-year-old child diagnosed with lupus and "shrinking lung syndrome." Child presented with fever, muscle weakness, weight loss, malaise, and severely restricted pulmonary function tests. Chest radiograph showed an elevated left hemidiaphragm while high-resolution computed tomography scan showed only subtle nonspecific changes out of keeping with pulmonary function. Pulmonary function tests normalized over a period of 6 months with high-dose prednisone treatment.

PFT abnormalities most frequently seen are restrictive with or without a diffusion abnormality. Most studies have not shown any correlation between PFT abnormalities and lupus disease activity. It is important to note that isolated abnormal pulmonary function tests in children with lupus do not predict progressive lung disease.[81]

High-resolution CT imaging in a cohort of 60 Norwegian patients with childhood-onset SLE revealed that 8% had abnormal findings, including micronodules and bronchiectasis, but none had ILD.[82] These findings did not correlate with PFT abnormalities, but a more recent study did show some correlations.[83] Although CT imaging is more sensitive than plain chest radiography, routine screening of asymptomatic pediatric lupus patients with CT is not recommended.

TREATMENT

Since infection is the major cause of mortality in pediatric SLE, children with pulmonary manifestations require rigorous investigation and treatment of infectious complications. It is also important to exclude other causes of pulmonary pathology in SLE, such as thromboembolism, drug toxicity, and the impact of cardiac or renal disease. Corticosteroids are highly effective in treating lupus pleuritis and pleural effusions, and remain the mainstay of treatment for moderate to severe pulmonary manifestations of SLE in children. The majority of children with SLE are treated with hydroxychloroquine, which is particularly effective for cutaneous disease, arthritis, and mild constitutional symptoms, and in reducing the risk of disease flares.[84] Immunosuppressive drugs such as azathioprine[85] and mycophenolate mofetil[86] are frequently used to prevent organ damage and as corticosteroid-sparing agents. There may also be a role for methotrexate[87] and cyclosporine.[88] For the most severe manifestations such as pulmonary hemorrhage, pulse methylprednisolone (30 mg/kg per dose up to 1000 mg) may be administered daily for 3 days or longer, followed by high-dose daily oral systemic corticosteroids. Although there are no controlled clinical trials for the treatment of pulmonary hemorrhage, intravenous pulse cyclophosphamide (CYC) is frequently used[89] and appears to be associated with improved survival.[90] Although plasmapheresis is not of proven benefit, it has been used in life-threatening pulmonary hemorrhage. Certainly, in patients with TTP and catastrophic antiphospholipid antibody syndrome, plasmapheresis can be a life-saving therapy.[91] Rituximab, a B-cell depleting biologic agent, is assuming an increasing role in the treatment of pediatric SLE, but its role in the treatment of pulmonary manifestations remains to be defined.[92,93] Vascular thromboses associated with antiphospholipid antibodies require anticoagulation.

PROGNOSIS

Disease severity is greater in children with SLE than in adults, and the majority of children develop organ damage within 5–10 years of diagnosis. Long-term morbidity includes premature atherosclerosis and osteoporosis.[48] Five-year survival rates in pediatric SLE range from 85% to 95%, but this may be improving, with a recent study reporting a 99.6% survival rate. Renal disease and infections were the most common causes of death.[44]

Juvenile Dermatomyositis

JDM is a rare autoimmune inflammatory myositis in which a capillary vasculopathy causes characteristic cutaneous and muscle manifestations, although other organs can be affected. In children, symptomatic lung involvement is infrequent, which is distinct from adult dermatomyositis (DM), where symptomatic lung involvement occurs in more than half of patients.

EPIDEMIOLOGY

JDM is the most common inflammatory myopathy in children, accounting for approximately 85% of cases[94] and has an incidence of 0.2–0.4 per 100,000 children.[95–98] It is a distinct disease entity from adult DM. Peak incidence occurs from 5 to 10 years of age,[97,98] and females are 2 to 5 times more likely to develop the disease than males.[96,98,99] A case report in monozygotic twins has suggested a genetic predisposition to JDM in some families.[100]

PATHOGENESIS

Although the etiology of JDM is unknown, genetics, environmental exposure, and infections are thought to be related to the disease development.[94,101] No specific causative gene has been found, but certain HLA alleles (HLA-B8, HLA-DQA1*0301, and HLA-DQA1*0501) and polymorphisms in tumor necrosis factor-alpha and interleukin-1 receptor antagonist have been reported as risk factors for the development of JDM and for certain phenotypes.[102,103] There is increased type I interferon gene expression[104] and upregulation of MHC class I expression on the surface of muscle fibers. JDM is characterized by various degrees of vasculopathy with immune complex deposition and the development of calcinosis in the later stages of disease.

CLINICAL MANIFESTATIONS

JDM has a relatively homogeneous presentation in children with mainly cutaneous and muscle manifestations.[99,105] The initial symptoms are usually skin rash (often with heliotrope rash over the eyelids and Gottron's papules over extensor surfaces of joints), fever, and proximal muscle weakness. Characteristic changes in the nail fold capillary bed are common, and measuring the density of capillaries/mm may be a useful tool for monitoring clinical activity in JDM.[106,107] Other disease manifestations include skin ulcerations, soft tissue calcification, arthritis, lipodystrophy, and insulin resistance. Serious gastrointestinal and lung involvement occur only occasionally.

DIAGNOSIS

According to the traditional criteria of Bohan and Peter,[108,109] the diagnosis of JDM is based on the following five criteria: proximal muscle weakness, characteristic rash, elevated muscle enzymes, characteristic myopathic findings on electromyography, and typical muscle biopsy findings. Criteria for definite JDM are the pathognomonic rash and three other criteria, while the diagnosis of probable JDM requires the

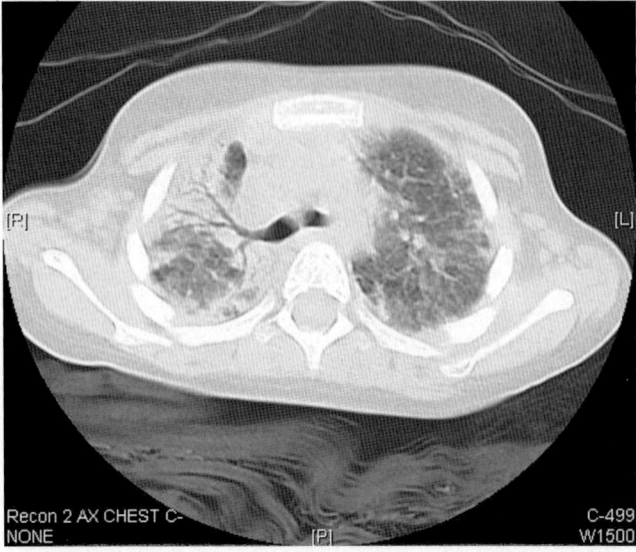

Fig. 58.4 Two-year-old who presented with fever, hypoxia, and persistent chest infiltrates. High-resolution computed tomography showed bilateral patchy airspace consolidation with air bronchograms. A lung biopsy confirmed the diagnosis of bronchiolitis obliterans organizing pneumonia. Six months later the child developed myalgias and heliotrope rash and was diagnosed with juvenile dermatomyositis.

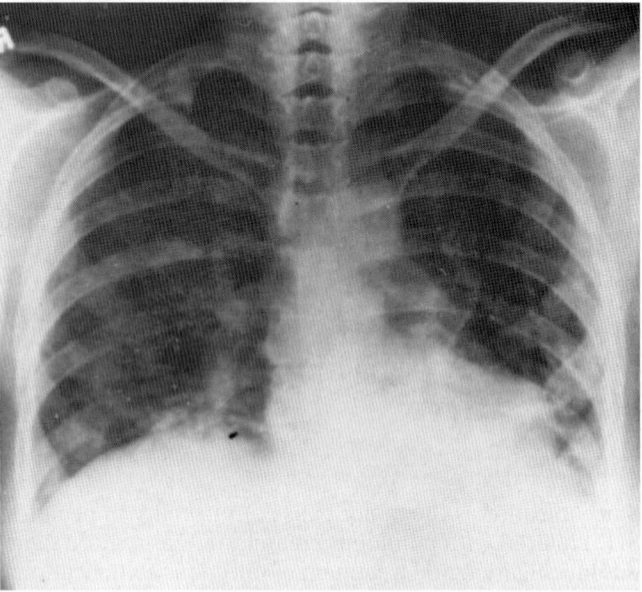

Fig. 58.5 Chest radiograph of a 21-year-old female diagnosed with juvenile dermatomyositis at 12 years of age and onset of slowly progressive pulmonary fibrosis at 18 years of age. The heart is normal in size, and soft tissue calcifications are present in both axillae. Interstitial thickening and cystic changes are bilateral and most pronounced at the bases.

rash and two other criteria.[105] Most children with JDM do have both proximal muscle weakness and rash, and elevated serum muscle enzymes are usually, but not always, present. Newer proposed criteria include the presence of nail fold capillary abnormalities,[106] magnetic resonance imaging that demonstrates the presence of muscle inflammation,[110] calcinosis, and dysphonia.[111] In cases where the diagnosis remains uncertain, the more invasive muscle biopsy may be necessary. JDM must be differentiated from other noninflammatory causes of muscle weakness (muscular dystrophies and metabolic myopathies), transient postviral myositis, and myositis due to other rheumatologic diseases (systemic scleroderma, SLE, MCTD, and systemic JIA). Elevated C-reactive protein and erythrocyte sedimentation rate and the presence of antinuclear antibodies are common but nonspecific findings that have limited diagnostic value. Myositis-specific antibodies, which are commonly associated with adult forms of DM and polymyositis, are uncommon in JDM; hence they are not usually helpful in making the diagnosis.[112,113] However, the presence of anti-Jo-1 and antisynthetase antibodies are associated with ILD in adults[114] and may also be associated with more severe disease in children that more closely resembles adult DM.[102,112]

PULMONARY INVOLVEMENT

ILD is a common cause of morbidity and mortality for adult onset DM and polymyositis, occurring in up to 65% of cases.[115] In adults, ILD may precede, appear concomitantly with, or develop after the onset of skin and muscle manifestations.[115] In contrast, symptomatic pulmonary involvement is infrequent in children with JDM. In the largest case series of JDM presented to date, only 1 of 105 patients (<1%) at the Hospital for Sick Children in Toronto, Canada, developed symptomatic ILD (Fig. 58.4).[105] Other case series have reported higher

rates of ILD detected by pulmonary function testing and HRCT scanning; however, most of these cases were not histologically confirmed.[116,117] Although symptomatic ILD is rare enough that its description is mainly limited to case reports,[118–121] it is important to recognize its onset, as it can be rapidly progressive and fatal (Fig. 58.5).[119–121] A Japanese nationwide collaborative study identified 10 cases of rapidly progressive interstitial lung disease (RP-ILD), seven of whom died.[122] Antimelanoma differentiation-associated gene 5 (MDA5) antibodies, and high serum levels of interleukin 18 (Il-18), Krebs von den Lungen-6 (KL-6), and ferritin were associated with RP-ILD.[122] Pneumomediastinum is a characteristic complication of adult DM with interstitial pneumonitis[123] and has also been reported in JDM (Fig. 58.6).[118–121] Aspiration pneumonia and hypoventilation are also frequently reported pulmonary complications in adult DM.[115] In adult studies, the strongest predictive factor for ILD in patients with myositis is the presence of anti-Jo-1 antibodies.[114]

The most common presenting symptoms of ILD are cough and dyspnea, although ILD has been reported to occur without symptoms. Pulmonary function tests show a restrictive ventilation defect, with decreased lung volumes, reduced diffusing capacity for carbon monoxide and normal or elevated FEV_1:FVC ratio. Decreased DLCO is not specific for ILD, as it may also occur with pulmonary hypertension, which can occur in patients with a variety of connective tissue diseases. Chest radiographs may have changes suggestive of ILD, but HRCT of the lungs is considered the standard procedure for initial evaluation of patients with suspected ILD. The most common pattern observed in adult DM is irregular linear opacities with areas of consolidation and ground-glass attenuation, suggesting active inflammation.[115] Honeycombing occurs uncommonly. The differential diagnosis for ILD always

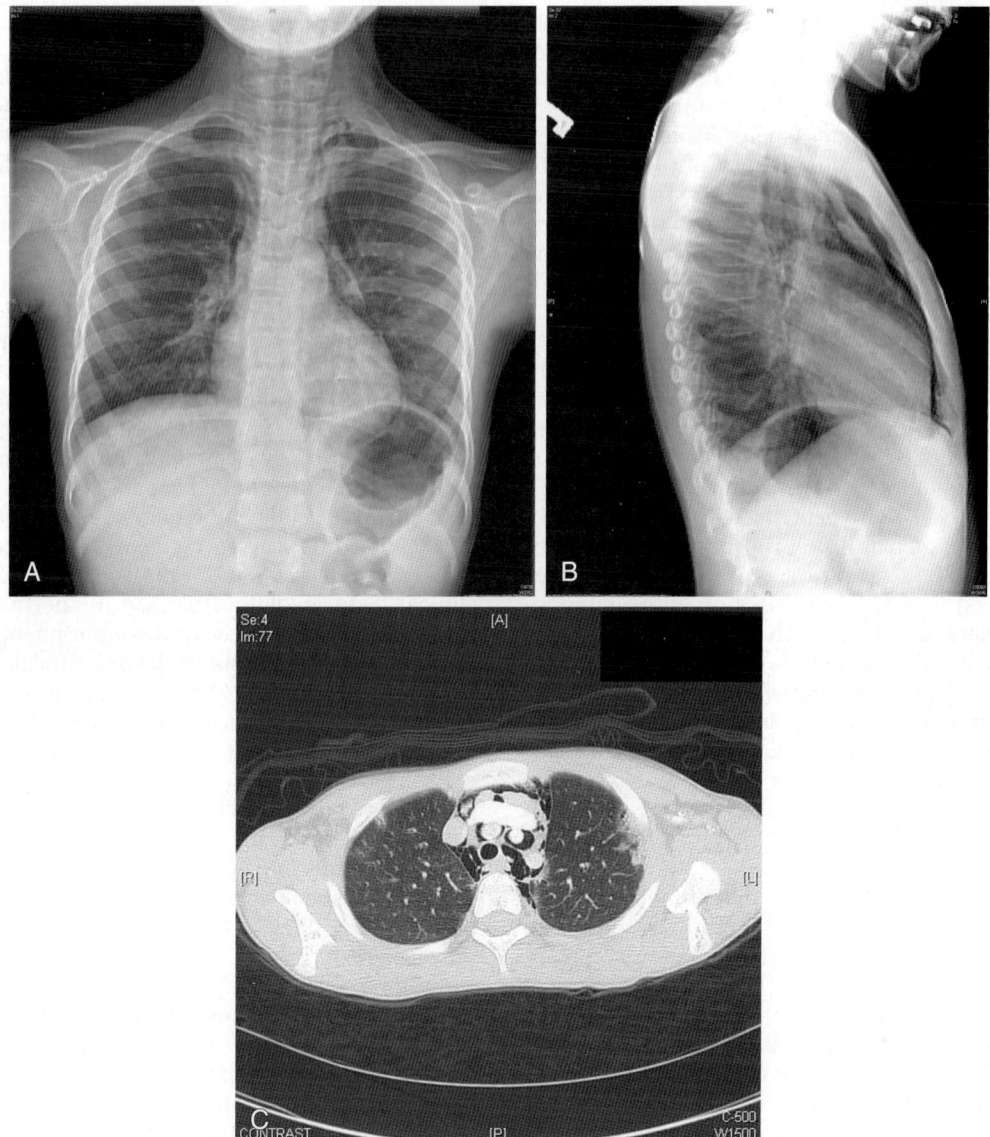

Fig. 58.6 (A) Posterior-anterior (PA) and (B) lateral view of chest radiograph of 9-year-old child presenting with juvenile dermatomyositis showing extensive pneumomediastinum and blunting of right costophrenic (CP) angle. (C) High-resolution computed tomography scan of chest also shows multiple pleural-based wedge-shaped opacities with interstitial thickening and cystic areas consistent with early interstitial lung disease (usually NSIP pattern).

includes infection and drug-induced lung disease. BAL can help rule out infection. Although lung biopsies are not routinely performed in adult DM, in children where ILD is uncommon and there are no data on the role of HCRT in predicting histological patterns, a lung biopsy may be required to obtain a diagnosis. Pulmonary fibrosis,[120] acute interstitial pneumonitis,[119] BOOP[105] (see Fig. 58.4), and DAD[122] have all been reported as lung histological findings in JDM.

Many observational studies have reported asymptomatic pulmonary function abnormalities in 30%–40% of children with JDM.[105] A small longitudinal case series reported pulmonary function abnormalities in 5 of 12 patients with JDM who had no respiratory symptoms, but these abnormalities were generally of a mild nature and nonprogressive, showing a restrictive defect.[124] More recently, a larger case-control study of 59 JDM patients from Oslo showed a restrictive ventilatory defect in 26% compared with 9% of controls.[125] These mild nonprogressive restrictive pulmonary

defects have generally been attributed to respiratory muscle weakness or calcinosis in the chest wall and need to be differentiated from the reduced lung compliance that occurs with ILD. Findings of reduced maximal inspiratory and expiratory pressures, reduced maximal voluntary ventilation, normal DLCO, and increased residual volume without decreased FEV_1:FVC ratio help distinguish respiratory muscle weakness from ILD.

TREATMENT

The mainstay of treatment is high-dose corticosteroids, usually weaned slowly over a 1–2 years period. Intravenous pulse methylprednisolone is frequently used for children with more severe weakness. Immunosuppressive therapy is used to treat JDM, based mainly upon results reported in observational studies and clinical experience.[126] In a single randomized but unblended multicenter trial, 139 children with new-onset JDM were assigned to prednisone alone, prednisone plus methotrexate, or prednisone plus cyclosporine: the two combination arms had better efficacy but more adverse events, particularly infection, compared with prednisone alone.[127] The most commonly used immunosuppressive agent is methotrexate administered weekly. Since reports of the benefits of methotrexate in reducing the duration and cumulative dose of systemic corticosteroids have emerged, in many centers, methotrexate is routinely added to systemic steroids at the initiation of treatment.[128] There are also reports of the efficacy and steroid sparing effects of cyclosporine in JDM,[129] and some clinicians use cyclosporine as initial therapy together with prednisone.[130] Cyclosporine has also been reported to be effective in combination with systemic corticosteroids in the treatment of a small series of children with JDM-associated ILD.[131] Controlled trials of intravenous immunoglobulin in adults,[132] and uncontrolled trials in children, support its use.[133] In patients with severe or life-threatening disease, such as ILD, chronic skin ulceration, or gastrointestinal involvement, intravenous CYC (500–750 mg/m² every 4 weeks) is used in combination with high-dose corticosteroid therapy.[134] Rituximab has been shown to be associated with clinical improvement in two small case series of severe JDM[135,136] and a randomized trial that included 48 children with refractory JDM.[137] Case reports have also suggested improvement in selected refractory JDM patients with infliximab[138] and abatacept.[139]

PROGNOSIS

Mortality rates for JDM declined from more than 30% in the 1960s before routine glucocorticoid therapy was given, to less than 3% in the 2000s with the advent of early combination immunosuppressive therapy.[126] Patients with typical disease who are treated with early immunosuppressive therapy now usually have an excellent prognosis.[140] Long-term morbidity is generally related to disease complications, such as calcinosis and other complications related to drug toxicity, including growth retardation and osteoporosis.[141] Acute onset and rapidly progressive ILD with associated air leak is only very occasionally a cause of mortality in JDM.[119-121] Small defects in pulmonary function should be followed over time to ensure that slowly progressive ILD, which is well described in adult DM, does not develop.

Scleroderma

EPIDEMIOLOGY

Systemic scleroderma, also known as systemic sclerosis (SSc), is a connective tissue disease marked by typical skin thickening and hardening (sclerosis) and multiorgan fibrotic changes. It is rare in childhood. One study of Finnish children found an incidence of juvenile SSc of 0.05 per 100,000,[142] while a 2005–2007 survey in the UK and Ireland found an incidence of 0.27 cases per million children.[143] It has been estimated that up to 10% of adults with SSc have the onset of their disease in childhood.[144] In a large series of children from multiple countries, juvenile SSc was almost four times more common in females and began at a mean age of 8 years.[145]

CLINICAL FEATURES

SSc usually has an insidious onset in children with skin changes in the hands and face and/or Raynaud phenomenon. Other common presenting findings are constitutional symptoms (fatigue, weight loss), arthralgia, muscle weakness and pain, subcutaneous calcifications, dysphagia, and dyspnea. The time interval between onset of symptoms and diagnosis is often prolonged (average 1.9 years).

The skin abnormalities are often heralded by a phase of edema, which is then followed by the development of skin tightening and sclerosis, and as this becomes more prominent, contractures develop. When sclerosis affects the face, loss of wrinkling of the skin results in the pathognomonic expressionless facies. The skin can subsequently atrophy and develop telangiectasia. The vasculopathy is reflected in abnormalities easily seen in the nail fold capillaries with dropout, dilatation, tortuosity, and hemorrhages. Digital ulcers (with resulting digital pitting scars) accompanying Raynaud phenomena is very suggestive of SSc. The most common, nondermatologic clinical features of juvenile SSc in the two largest series reported to date[145,146] were Raynaud phenomenon (72%–84%), followed by musculoskeletal (arthralgias, muscle weakness and pain 64%–79%), gastrointestinal (esophageal dysfunction 65%–69%), and pulmonary (42%–50%) involvement. Cardiovascular (29%–44%), renal (10%–13%), and neurologic disease (3%–16%) occurred less frequently. Calcinosis developed in 18%–27%. The disease tends to be most active during the first 5 years after onset, when skin sclerosis advances rapidly and visceral involvement commonly occurs. After 5 years, constitutional symptoms abate, skin abnormalities often stabilize or even improve, but visceral disease may progress.

Systemic sclerosis can be divided into limited and diffuse forms. Skin involvement is limited to an acral distribution (hands, face, and feet) with limited disease, while diffuse disease has truncal and acral skin involvement and usually early and significant multiorgan disease. More than 90% of children with juvenile SSc have the diffuse form.[145] A higher proportion of children than adults with the disease have features of an overlap connective tissue disease syndrome.[147]

SSc is classified according to the extent of skin and pattern of internal organ involvement. Consensus-based classification criteria for juvenile SSc have been proposed for children whose disease begins before the age of 16 years.[148] These criteria require the presence of the major criterion of proximal sclerodermatous changes and at least two of the minor criteria, which have been expanded to 20 items, including involvement of other organ systems as well as some serological abnormalities (ANA and systemic sclerosis selective autoantibodies).[148] The minor criteria are sclerodactyly, peripheral vascular disease (Raynaud phenomenon, nail fold capillary abnormalities, digital tip ulcers), gastrointestinal (dysphagia, reflux), cardiac (arrhythmia, heart failure), renal (renal crisis, hypertension), neurologic (neuropathy, carpal tunnel syndrome) and musculoskeletal disease (tendon friction rub, arthritis, myositis), respiratory (DLCO of <80% predicted), PAH, and pulmonary fibrosis seen on chest radiography or HRCT and serology (antinuclear antibodies, SSc selective autoantibodies [anticentromere, antitopoisomerase I [Scl-70], antifibrillarin, anti-PM/Scl, antifibrillin, or

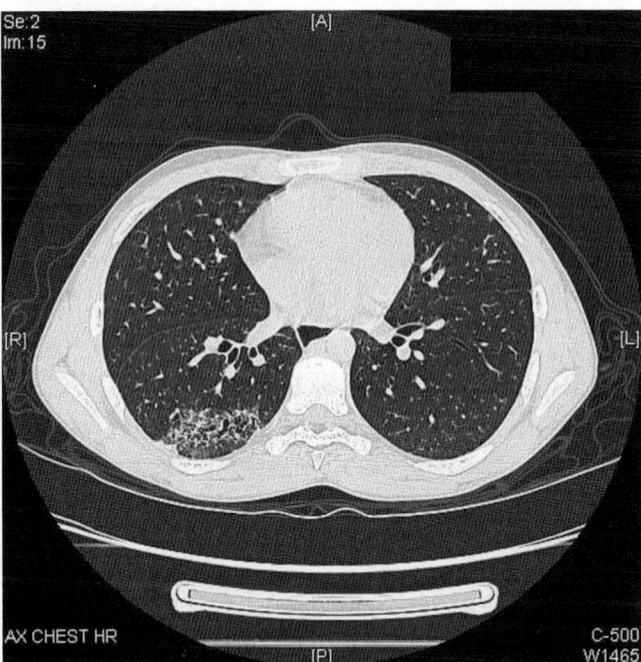

Fig. 58.7 Early interstitial lung disease in teen with scleroderma. High-resolution computed tomography shows typical changes of peripheral interlobular septal thickening with fibrosis and traction bronchiectasis.

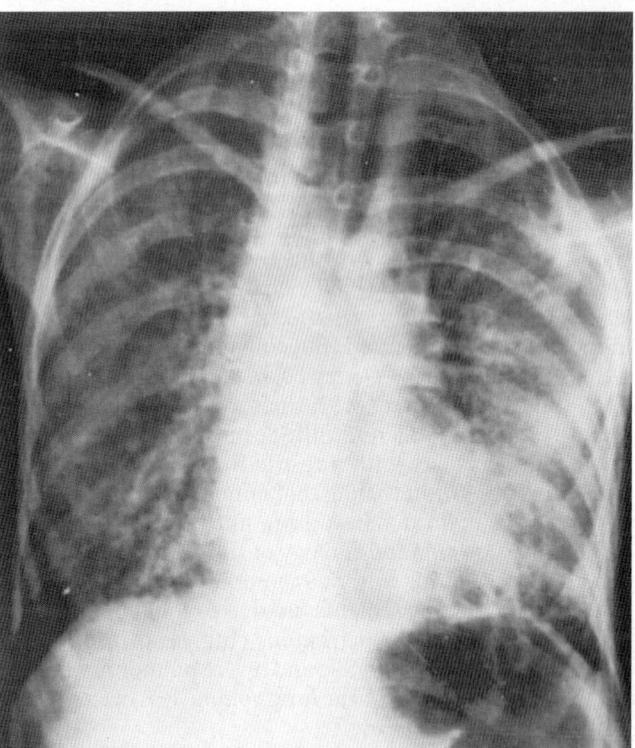

Fig. 58.8 18-year-old female who was diagnosed with scleroderma at 6 years of age and had onset of interstitial lung disease at age 10 years. This chest radiograph shows an advanced case of scleroderma lung with chronic pulmonary fibrosis in a reticulated honeycomb pattern more prominent in the lower lobes. The heart is minimally enlarged, gaseous distention of the proximal and distal thirds of the esophagus is present, and there is a moderate right convex scoliosis.

anti-RNA polymerase I or III]). The 1980 criteria for adult SSc[149] have been widely used for children in the past. These rely on either the presence of the major criterion of sclerodermatous changes proximal to the metacarpophalangeal or metatarsophalangeal joints or the presence of at least two of the following minor criteria: sclerodactyly, digital pitting scars, or bibasilar pulmonary fibrosis.

PATHOGENESIS

SSc is characterized by inflammation, excessive fibrosis and vasculopathy affecting the skin, and multiple organs with evidence of immune, endothelial, and fibroblast dysfunction. While the etiology and exact pathogenetic mechanisms remain elusive, endothelial cell injury appears to be an early and important event. Endothelin-1 has emerged as an important mediator of the vascular changes, and serum levels correlate with disease severity markers.[150] There are features of autoimmunity with the following SSc-selective autoantibodies included in the new proposed minor criteria: anticentromere, antitopoisomerase I (Scl-70), antifibrillarin, anti-PM-Scl, antifibrillin, and anti-RNA polymerase I or III. ANA is found in approximately 80%, ENA in 40%, and anti-Scl-70 in approximately one-third of pediatric patients.[145]

PULMONARY INVOLVEMENT

ILD (Figs. 58.7 and 58.8), PAH, and cardiomyopathy are dreaded organ manifestations associated with mortality in children; initial workup and monitoring should focus on detecting these manifestations. ILD, while relatively common in adults, is rare in children. Hence, most of what we know about the characteristics and risk factors for ILD, prognosis and treatment comes from adult studies. ILD is best detected on HRCT.[151] Dyspnea and dry cough are late symptoms. Pulmonary function tests (FVC and DLCO) correlate with severity of disease. The typical form of ILD (seen in 77.5% of adult cases) has a histological pattern of NSIP, while a few cases have a UIP pattern.[152] When ILD occurs, it usually is detected at initial presentation or within the first 3 years after onset of symptoms. Not all cases of ILD progress; hence decisions on which cases to treat can be difficult.[153]

SSc is also associated with pleuritis, pleural effusions, bronchiectasis, BOOP, and alveolar hemorrhage. Spontaneous pneumothorax with severe fibrosis and aspiration pneumonia associated with esophageal reflux may also be seen.[153] ILD and progressive decline of pulmonary function have been associated with more severe esophageal dysmotility in adults with SSc.[154]

Pulmonary involvement is often asymptomatic. Although dyspnea is the most frequent symptom in children with lung involvement, it only occurs in 10%–26% of children with SSc at presentation or during the disease course.[155] Dry cough is even less frequent. Abnormal chest radiography is seen at presentation in 12% and in 29% during the disease course.[145] Ground-glass opacities are suggestive of ILD, and a reticular pattern and traction bronchiectasis may be seen.[153] High-resolution CT is a more sensitive method of detecting these findings and may find additional abnormalities in addition to ground glass densities, such as subpleural micronodules, linear opacities, and honeycombing appearance.[156,157] Patients with normal HRCT scans on initial assessment are likely to have normal HRCT scans after a follow-up period of 5 years.[158] One study in adults with SSc found that ground-glass opacity was the most common finding on HRCT and was only reversible in a small minority of patients who had sequential scans,[159] suggesting that ground-glass opacity may actually indicate fine fibrosis.

Global disease activity is monitored with a multidimensional disease severity score, the Juvenile Systemic Sclerosis Severity Score (J4S),[160] which includes measures of spirometry, DLCO, HRCT, and oxygen dependency. PFTs are important in the initial assessment and ongoing monitoring of patients with SSc. Reduced DLCO may be an early marker of ILD or PAH and also correlates with the severity of these disease manifestations.[153] Children with SSc most often have reduced forced vital capacity with a restrictive PFT pattern (42%–65%). It is important to note that almost half of those with abnormal PFTs do not have lung imaging abnormalities, calling into question the etiology of the decrements in lung function.[155] It is this author's opinion that some of these unexplained PFT decrements are due to limited chest wall expansion due to sclerodermatous changes of the thorax. Serial PFTs in adults with SSc and severe pulmonary fibrosis demonstrate that most of the lung volume loss occurs in the first 4 years of the disease.[161]

The best way to monitor pediatric SSc patients for the new onset of ILD or progression of ILD is not clear. A study of serial PFTs and HRCT in children with SSc found that PFTs, particularly lung volume studies, correlate with findings on HRCT, suggesting that monitoring with PFTs can identify which patients require follow-up HRCT. The authors acknowledge, however, that PFTs do not completely exclude mild pulmonary involvement, and they therefore entertain the notion of a surveillance low-radiation dose HRCT at some point during follow-up for lung disease.[162] More extensive disease on HRCT correlates with poor prognosis in adult SSc patients.[163]

In adults, anti-Scl-70 antibodies are associated with ILD, while anticentromere antibodies are protective.[164] In children, serum KL-6 has been reported as a potentially useful biomarker of ILD in juvenile SSc and correlates with PFT abnormalities and the severity of ILD.[165] Lung biopsy is generally not required when the clinical features, pulmonary function test results, and imaging findings are typical for ILD. Moreover, pathological findings do not reliably predict disease course and outcome.[152] BAL has not been found to predict disease course reliably or response to treatment.[166]

PAH may occur as an isolated phenomenon or in association with ILD. Right heart catheterization may be the gold standard for identifying PAH, but Doppler echocardiography is effective and noninvasive. Anticentromere antibodies are associated with isolated PAH, and anti-U3 RNP antibodies are associated with PAH in adults with SSc.[167]

TREATMENT

Nonpharmacologic therapy measures include skin care, exercise programs, and corrective splints as needed. Pharmacologic therapy tends to be targeted toward controlling disease in specifically involved organs. There have been no controlled treatment trials in juvenile SSc. Treatment approaches for juvenile SSc–related lung disease have

therefore drawn heavily on reports of successful treatment in adults. Both daily oral CYC[168] and monthly intravenous CYC[169] have demonstrated some degree of efficacy in ILD associated with SSc, with only modest benefits on respiratory function. There are only uncontrolled studies using mycophenolate mofetil, azathioprine, and rituximab in adults. Lung transplantation has been successful in carefully selected patients who have limited involvement of other major organs.[170] Autologous hematopoietic stem cell transplantation has also been shown to stabilize major organ disease and is currently being evaluated in controlled trials.[171]

PROGNOSIS

Prognosis is generally better in childhood-onset compared with adult-onset SSc, likely due to lower rates of ILD and PAH. Survival rates of juvenile SSc at 5, 10, 15, and 20 years after diagnosis are 89%, 80%–87%, 74%–87%, and 69%–82%, respectively.[146,147,172] The mortality risk in adults with SSc is dramatically higher with PAH, and survival is negatively impacted by lung disease, even without PAH.[173] Survival in pulmonary hypertension associated with ILD is significantly worse than isolated PAH.[174] Similarly, in children with a fatal outcome, pulmonary involvement occurs more frequently and earlier in the disease course. Antitopoisomerase I (anti-Scl-70) antibodies and anti-U3RNP antibodies are associated with pulmonary fibrosis and poor prognosis in adults, but not children.[172,175] However, some children with early organ involvement have a rapidly progressive course. Scleroderma-related heart disease is a frequent cause of death among children with SSc.[147] In adults, some risk factors for mortality and progression of SSc associated ILD have been identified, including older age, lower FVC, lower diffusing capacity for carbon monoxide, and extent of disease on HRCT chest imaging.[176] Similar work has not been done in childhood onset SSc and is more difficult due to the rarity of ILD in children. However, one should cautiously and carefully monitor children with ILD, as some do follow a rapidly progressive course.

Mixed Connective Tissue Disease

MCTD is a very rare diagnosis in children but can have life-threatening pulmonary involvement. It is characterized by the presence of high titer anti-U1 ribonucleoprotein (RNP) antibodies in combination with clinical features of SLE, SSc, or DM and was first described as a distinct clinical phenotype in 1972.[177]

EPIDEMIOLOGY AND PATHOGENESIS

MCTD accounts for only 0.1%–0.5% of pediatric rheumatology cases.[178] Median age of childhood onset is approximately 11 years (4–16 years) with girls diagnosed three times more often than boys.[178] More commonly MCTD presents in women in the second to third decade of life, although pediatric onset accounts for 25% of cases.[179]

The etiology of MCTD is unknown. Complex interactions occur between the innate and adaptive immune system, and there is evidence that anti-RNP antibodies are involved in pathogenesis of disease.[180]

CLINICAL MANIFESTATIONS AND DIAGNOSIS

Children usually have an insidious onset of disease, with Raynaud phenomenon, constitutional symptoms (malaise, fatigue, and low-grade fever) and polyarthritis as initial clinical symptoms in combination with a high titer of speckled ANA pattern.[181–184] A high titer of anti-RNP antibodies is a strong predictor of the eventual evolution to MCTD.[185] Classic clinical manifestations of other connective tissue diseases (often the skin rash of SLE or JDM, SSc skin, swollen hands, proximal muscle weakness, esophageal dysmotility, pericarditis, leukopenia, and pulmonary dysfunction) develop sequentially over time but not in any predictable manner or time frame. A clear diagnosis of MCTD may not be evident for years, and the initial presenting syndrome may be referred to as "undifferentiated CTD."

Several sets of diagnostic criteria for MCTD exist; however, Kasukawa's criteria are used most frequently in children and are the most restrictive.[186] Three criteria must be fulfilled for diagnosis of MCTD: (1) Raynaud phenomenon or swollen fingers or hands, (2) anti-RNP antibody positive, and (3) at least one abnormal sign or symptom from two or more of these categories: SLE, SSc, or DM. Almost any organ can be involved in MCTD; however, there are four clinical features that are distinctive for MCTD: (1) the presence of Raynaud phenomenon and swollen hands or fingers, (2) the absence of severe renal or central nervous system disease (differentiates MCTD from SLE), (3) more severe arthritis with insidious onset of pulmonary hypertension (without pulmonary fibrosis), and (4) autoantibodies with specificity to anti-U1 RNP.

PULMONARY INVOLVEMENT

Pulmonary disease is a major source of morbidity and mortality in adults with MCTD, occurring in about 75% of adult patients.[187] Case series of MCTD in children suggest a similar frequency of pulmonary involvement, although pulmonary hypertension seems to be less common and lung disease is generally mild.[184] Pulmonary disease onset is often initially asymptomatic and develops insidiously. Common symptoms include dry cough, dyspnea with exertion, and chest pain. Pulmonary fibrosis, pleural effusions, and PAH are the most common manifestations. Other findings include thromboembolic disease, pulmonary hemorrhage, diaphragmatic dysfunction, and aspiration pneumonitis.[188]

PAH is due to a pulmonary vasculopathy with intimal proliferation and medial hypertrophy of pulmonary arterioles. Unlike SSc, the lung parenchyma is not fibrotic.[179] Although PAH is rare in children with MCTD, it can develop rapidly.[189] One adult case of pulmonary hypertension due to veno-occlusive disease has been reported.[190] PAH should be suspected, with symptoms of exertional dyspnea, increased second heart sound, dilatation of pulmonary arteries on chest imaging, or reduced DLCO on pulmonary function testing.

TREATMENT

No controlled trials are available to guide therapy of MCTD, so that treatment is based on case series experience and conventional therapies that are known to be effective for manifestations of disease common to other CTDs (SLE, SSc, PM/DM). Since the clinical course of disease in MCTD is variable, therapy should be individualized to address specific organ involvement and disease severity. Most clinical manifestations of MCTD, with the exception of Raynaud phenomenon, are steroid responsive. Low-dose glucocorticoids, nonsteroidal antiinflammatory drugs, hydroxychloroquine, or combinations of these medications are used for early nonaggressive disease. Vasodilating drugs are used for Raynaud phenomenon, with nifedipine the most common. High dose systemic corticosteroids, methotrexate, or cytotoxics may be added for more severe disease, particularly organ threatening disease.

PAH may require treatment with the same classes of drugs used to treat idiopathic PAH (prostacyclin analogues, endothelin receptor antagonists, phosphodiesterase type 5 inhibitors—see Chapter 72 for management of PAH). PAH can be fatal but is not always progressive and sometimes resolves.[179,191] Multiple case reports in adults[179,187,192] and children[191,193,194] also report successful treatment of PAH with immunosuppressive therapy (corticosteroid and CYC), considering the PAH as part of a "disease flare." Heart and lung transplantation is an option for end-stage PAH.

PROGNOSIS

MCTD is considered incurable and outcomes are variable depending on organ involvement; however, most children have a favorable prognosis. Ten years mortality is reported to be 16%–28% in adults and 7.6% in children.[191] Deaths are most often due to rapid-onset pulmonary hypertension in adults[179] and infection in children.[191]

Sarcoidosis

Sarcoidosis is a chronic multisystem disorder of unknown etiology affecting mostly young adults and rarely children.[195–197] It is characterized by noncaseating epithelioid cell granulomas, which have a predilection for thoracic lymph nodes and lung tissue. Children with sarcoidosis commonly have disease manifestations similar to adults with sarcoidosis, with bilateral hilar lymph adenopathy (BHL) with or without parenchymal infiltrates. At least half of adult cases will resolve spontaneously within 2 years without any specific therapy. However, progression of lung disease to pulmonary fibrosis and uveitis to blindness are two potential long-term morbidities that call for careful consideration for treatment and follow-up of the sarcoidosis patient.

Early onset sarcoidosis (EOS), with symptom onset at the age of 4 years or younger and a unique phenotype of skin rash, uveitis, arthritis, and absence of lung disease, was previously described to be a rare presentation of sarcoidosis.[198] However, it is now believed that EOS is the sporadic form of Blau syndrome, a familial autoinflammatory disease with autosomal dominant inheritance caused by mutations in the NOD2/CARD15 gene.[199,200] With increasing recognition of EOS, previously unidentified visceral involvement, including interstitial pneumonitis, has now been reported.[201] EOS tends to present to the pediatric rheumatologist and will not be discussed further in this chapter. However, the pulmonologist should consider genetic causes in the differential diagnosis of sarcoidosis in young children and familial cases.

EPIDEMIOLOGY

The incidence of sarcoidosis varies by geographic location, race, and age, but usually develops before the age of 50 years and peaks in incidence between 20 and 39 years. The highest incidence of disease has been reported in northern European countries (5–40 cases per 100,000 people)[202,203] and among black Americans (35.5 cases per 100,000 compared with 10.9 per 100,000 in white Americans).[204] The incidence in children is less well described but is generally felt to be much lower than in adults. Data from the Danish national patient registry show an overall incidence of 0.29 per 100,000 children-years (15 years of age and younger) compared with the overall Danish incidence of 7.2/100,000 person-years.[205] Incidence in children increases with age and peaks at 1.02 per 100,000 in the 14–15-year-old age group.[205] In the two largest American pediatric case series from Virginia[206] and North Carolina,[207] 75% of children with sarcoidosis were black, and most were over the age of 10 years. Males and females are equally affected. There is some familial clustering of cases, but no inheritance pattern has been established.[208,209]

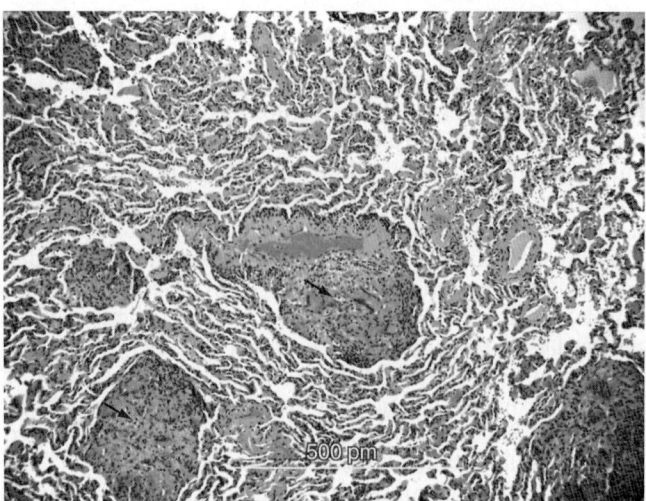

Fig. 58.9 Biopsy of the apex of the left lung from a 15-year-old African-American boy with a history of skin lesions, bilateral ankle swelling, a painful red eye, and lung infiltrate (see Fig. 58.10). Biopsy shows nonnecrotizing interstitial granulomas *(arrows)*. Special stains for acid-fast bacillus and fungi were negative, as were stains for vasculitis. Similar results were found on biopsy of axillary lymph nodes.

ETIOLOGY AND PATHOGENESIS

The etiology of sarcoidosis remains largely unknown; however, a variety of environmental, occupational, and genetic risk factors have been associated with the disease.[197,210] Current models of pathogenesis suggest that an exaggerated TH-1 immune response to unidentified antigen(s) in individuals who are genetically susceptible leads to granuloma formation in many different organs. The mycobacterium tuberculosis catalase-peroxidase protein has been identified as a potential sarcoidosis antigen,[211,212] and several associations of sarcoidosis with MHC-2 alleles have been described.[196]

Granulomatous lesions are the hallmark of sarcoidosis, and they may occur in any organ of the body. These are typically noncaseating, which distinguishes them from the necrotizing granulomatous lesions of tuberculosis and GPA. The granulomas consist of tightly organized collections of predominantly CD4+ T lymphocytes and mononuclear phagocytes (epithelioid cells, macrophages, and multinucleated giant cells). The epithelioid and giant cells may contain Schaumann or asteroid inclusion bodies. In the lung, most granulomas are located in the perilymphatic areas, including near bronchioles, in the subpleural space and the perilobular spaces (Fig. 58.9). In more mature granulomas, fibroblasts and collagen may encase the ball-like cluster of cells. Special stains for fungi and mycobacteria are negative. The granulomatous lesions usually heal with preservation of lung parenchyma; however, in 20%–25% of patients, fibroblasts proliferate at the periphery of the granuloma and produce fibrotic scar tissue.

CLINICAL MANIFESTATIONS

Children older than 8 years of age tend to present with similar clinical manifestations as adults, with pulmonary findings predominating.[213] Granulomatous lesions may occur in any organ, but the lungs, lymph nodes, eyes, skin, and liver are the most commonly involved. Occasionally joints, bone, spleen, central nervous system (neurosarcoidosis), heart, or kidneys are involved. Nonspecific and often minor symptoms of general malaise, weight loss, fatigue, and fever are common. Other symptoms are related to local tissue injury caused by granulomas and hence depend on the organs involved. Cough, dyspnea with exertion, and chest pain are common symptoms of lung involvement.[205,214,215] Common skin lesions include papules, plaques, nodules, changes in old scars, erythema nodosum, hyperpigmented lesions, and hypopigmented lesions. Lupus pernio, erythroderma, and ichthyosis are less common skin lesions in children. Central nervous system involvement may present with headache, seizures, cranial nerve palsies, motor signs, hypothalamic dysfunction, and hydrocephalus.[216] Physical exam findings may include peripheral lymphadenopathy, eye changes, skin rashes, hepatosplenomegaly, abnormal chest sounds, neurologic deficits, and parotid gland enlargement. Cardiac disease is rare but may present with heart block, arrhythmias, or dilated cardiomyopathy. Asymptomatic patients may be identified by routine screening chest radiographs. Löfgren syndrome, a triad of acute arthritis, BHL, and erythema nodosum, is a common presentation in 9%–34% of adults[217] but is less common in children.[205] A diagnosis of sarcoidosis should prompt a slit-lamp exam of the eye to look for asymptomatic uveitis, since blindness is one of the described morbidities of sarcoidosis.

Frequent laboratory abnormalities include increased erythrocyte sedimentation rate, anemia, hypergammaglobulinemia, cutaneous anergy (>40% of adults), hypercalciuria (19%–30%), hypercalcemia (8%–12%), eosinophilia, leukopenia, and increased angiotensin-converting enzyme (ACE; 60%–80%). Rheumatoid factor is occasionally positive (14% of adults).

PULMONARY INVOLVEMENT

Pulmonary involvement occurs in more than 90% of adult[217] and pediatric[218] cases, commonly affecting the intrathoracic

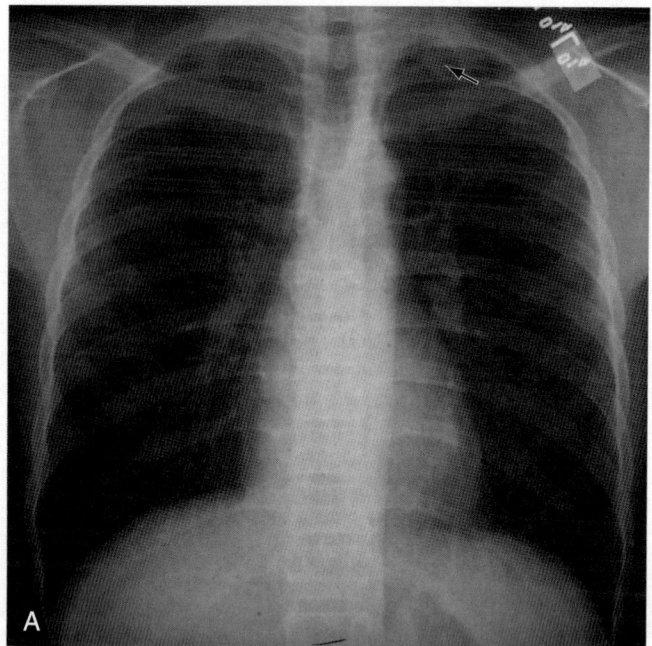

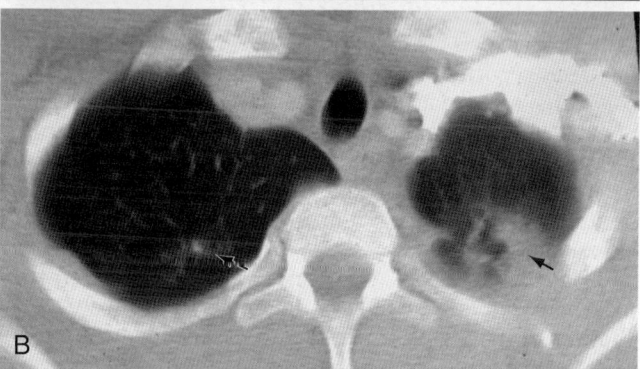

Fig. 58.10 (A and B) Chest radiograph (A) from the adolescent described in Fig. 58.9 that shows an 8-mm density in the left lung apex *(arrow)*. Chest computed tomography image (B) shows parenchymal opacifications in the lung apices *(arrows)* and axillary adenopathy on the right (not shown). The patient was diagnosed with sarcoidosis after lung and axillary lymph node biopsies revealed typical sarcoid granulomas (see Fig. 58.9).

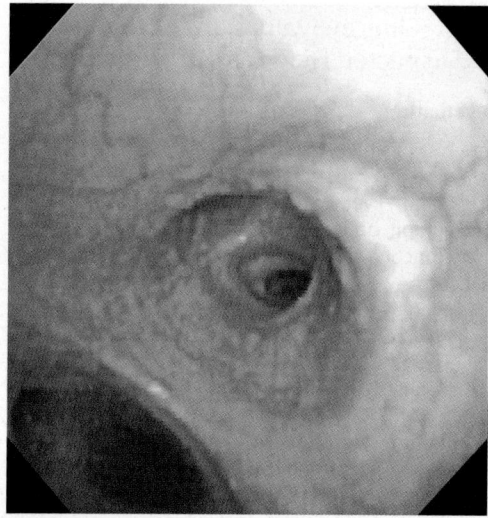

Fig. 58.11 Bronchoscopy picture of sarcoid airway: right upper lobe (RUL) airway involvement with hypervascularity and waxy nodules.

lymph nodes and the pulmonary parenchyma (Fig. 58.10). Presenting symptoms of pulmonary sarcoidosis may include dyspnea, wheezing, and cough. Physical examination of the chest may be normal or include crackles and wheezing. Radiographic findings have classically been categorized as Stage 0 = normal radiograph; Stage I = BHL; Stage II = BHL with parenchymal infiltrates; Stage III = parenchymal infiltrates without BHL. Some authors also define pulmonary fibrosis as Stage IV disease. A population-based Danish pediatric study found that 10% of children present with stage 0 disease, 71% with stage I, 8.3% with stage II, and 8.3% with stage III disease. Parenchymal infiltrates may be nodular, fibrotic, or alveolar, and tend to occur in the upper lobes. Recently, a French multicenter study group demonstrated that parenchymal lung abnormalities occurred on chest HRCT imaging in 95% of children with normal (stage 0) CXR.[213] Classic HRCT parenchymal abnormalities at disease presentation are similar in children and adults,[219] and consist of

widespread micro-nodules and nodules in a perilymphatic distribution (peribronchovascular), with nodular pleural thickening and thickening of interlobular septae, as well as hilar and mediastinal lymphadenopathy. Nodules may coalesce into areas of consolidation with air bronchograms, bronchiectasis, and bronchiolectasis. Areas of ground-glass attenuation may also be present. Pulmonary fibrosis with honeycombing occurs in 20%–25% of sarcoidosis patients, but only after years of disease activity.[195] Pulmonary function tests may be normal, particularly with stage 0 or I disease. The most common abnormality is a restrictive pattern with a reduction in DLCO, and occasionally an obstructive pattern may be seen.[195,213–215]

Airway involvement is well described in adults with sarcoidosis.[220] Airway changes are best appreciated with bronchoscopy: these include specific changes of waxy yellow mucosal nodules and nonspecific changes such as erythema, edema, granularity, and cobblestoning of airway mucosa and bronchial stenosis, typically in the lobar and segmental bronchi. In our experience, these typical airway lesions may also be observed in children with sarcoidosis (Fig. 58.11). Airway hyperreactivity is well documented in adult studies and is associated with the presence of visible airway involvement on bronchoscopy.[221] Pediatric laryngeal sarcoidosis, presenting with symptomatic supraglottic edema, has been described in multiple case reports, including several where the disease was isolated to the larynx.[222]

Progression of granulomatous lung lesions to pulmonary fibrosis and end-stage lung disease may be a fatal complication of pulmonary sarcoidosis. Pulmonary disease may also be complicated with the development of bronchiectasis and chronic infections, including development of an aspergilloma in damaged tissue. Hemoptysis may occur secondary to bronchiectasis or aspergilloma development.[217]

DIAGNOSIS

Box 58.2 describes the clinical evaluation that should be considered for a patient with suspected sarcoidosis. Diagnosis is established when typical clinical features are supported

Box 58.2 Clinical Evaluation for the Patient With a Suspected Diagnosis of Sarcoidosis

Initial Evaluation

Complete history and physical exam, including careful examination of lungs, peripheral lymph nodes, skin, eyes, parotid glands, liver, spleen, nervous system, and joints

Chest radiograph, both posteroanterior and lateral views

Pulmonary function tests, including spirometry, lung volumes, and DLCO

Tuberculin skin test

Biopsy of affected organ, with special stains and culture of specimen

Electrocardiogram

Complete blood count with white cell differential, erythrocyte sedimentation rate, serum calcium, creatinine, alkaline phosphatase, alanine, and aspartate aminotransferases

Serum level of angiotensin-converting enzyme (if elevated, may be useful to monitor patient compliance)

24 hour urine collection for calcium:creatinine ratio

Complete ophthalmologic evaluation (slit-lamp, tonometric and funduscopic)

Other tests as indicated for assessment of involved organs (e.g., MRI with gadolinium and cerebral spinal fluid analysis if central nervous system involvement)

Consider referral to pediatric rheumatologist for comanagement of disease depending on local experience

Consider genetic analysis for CARD15 mutations, especially if young or no pulmonary involvement

Follow-Up Monitoring (Every 3 Months Initially, and for at Least 3 Years After Discontinuation of Therapy)

Assessment for decline in physiologic function based on initial organ involvement (for lung involvement follow chest radiograph and pulmonary function tests)

Tests to monitor side effects of therapy (e.g., bone densitometry and blood pressure for steroid use, semiannual eye exam for hydroxychloroquine use)

Further testing as indicated if new symptoms or physical findings develop

MRI, Magnetic resonance imaging.

Summarized from recommendations in the following publications: (1) Statement on Sarcoidosis. Joint Statement of the American Thoracic Society (ATS), the European Respiratory Society (ERS) and the World Association of Sarcoidosis and Other Granulomatous Disorders (WASOG) adopted by the ATS Board of Directors and by the ERS Executive Committee, February 1999. Am J Respir Crit Care Med. 1999;160:736-755. (2) Pattishall EN, Kendig EL, Jr. Sarcoidosis in children. Pediatr Pulmonol. 1996;22:195-203. (3) Iannuzzi MC, Rybicki BA, Teirstein AS. Sarcoidosis. N Engl J Med. 2007;357:2153-2165.

by a tissue biopsy showing noncaseating granulomas. One must also be careful to exclude other causes of noncaseating granulomas, including immunodeficiency syndromes (especially chronic granulomatous disease and common variable immune deficiency), fungal and mycobacterial infections, berylliosis, ulcerative colitis (UC), and GPA. Any organ that is involved and accessible may be used for a tissue diagnosis. Whole body positron emission-computed tomography (PET-CT) may help localize inflammatory activity and biopsy sites.[223] In children, biopsies are often performed from peripheral lymph nodes, skin lesions, salivary glands, lung lesions, and the liver.[215] It is generally accepted that young adults presenting with Löfgren syndrome do not require a biopsy to confirm the diagnosis.[195] The Kveim-Siltzbach test is no longer used as a diagnostic test in routine clinical practice, and ACE levels have poor sensitivity.

When mediastinal nodes or lung tissue are the obvious site for biopsy, several options for tissue diagnosis exist. Transbronchial lung biopsy (TBLB) has a relatively high yield (40%–90% sensitivity) in adults with at least stage I disease, but there are no data on its utility in children.[195] In one adult study, endobronchial biopsy (EBB) in addition to TBLB was safe and increased the diagnostic yield of bronchoscopy by 20%. When abnormal airway mucosal lesions were visualized, 75% of EBB were positive, while only 30% of EBB specimens were positive in those with normal appearing airways.[224] If TBLB does not yield a diagnosis, which occurs in about 58% of unselected adult patients,[225] surgical biopsy of mediastinal nodes or peripheral lung lesions is the next step.[195] Hilar and mediastinal nodes may be assessed with mediastinoscopy, or alternatively with the newer and minimally invasive technique of endobronchial ultrasound-guided transbronchial needle aspiration (EBUS-TBNA), which has been reported to have a sensitivity of 71%–85% for diagnosing sarcoidosis.[225–227] Although technical issues limit the application of this technique in younger children, EBUS-TBNA has been reported to be successful in the diagnosis of sarcoidosis in a 13-year-old with BHL as well as hypercalcemia, nervous system, and eye involvement.[228] CT-guided transthoracic fine needle aspiration with core needle biopsy may also be used as an alternative to surgical biopsy to access peripheral pulmonary infiltrates in centers with sufficient experience.[229]

BAL cell profiles are not specific for sarcoidosis, but they may help narrow the differential diagnosis. However, BAL shows a lymphocytosis in greater than 85%; neutrophils are normal or low except in late disease; and CD4:CD8 ratio is increased (opposite to findings in ILD associated with connective tissue diseases) in 50%–60%. BAL cell profile is not helpful in monitoring disease progression or response to therapy.[195,215]

TREATMENT

The decision to treat pulmonary sarcoidosis is often difficult, as disease will spontaneously remit in many patients. If therapy is needed, corticosteroids are the mainstay. Efficacy data on treatments for pulmonary sarcoidosis are mainly based on adult data, which are well summarized in two Cochrane reviews.[230,231] Limited observational data from a pediatric cohort suggest similar outcomes of corticosteroid therapy in children.[215] Indications for treatment of lung disease are generally based on data about the natural history of spontaneous remission of different forms of lung disease: stage 1 60%–80%, stage II 50%–60%, and stage III 30% remit.[195,197,217]

The following criteria should prompt consideration for corticosteroid treatment:

1. Pulmonary sarcoidosis: Worsening pulmonary symptoms, deteriorating lung function, progressive radiographic changes (worsening of interstitial opacities, cavitation, progression of fibrosis with honeycombing, development of pulmonary hypertension).

2. Cardiac, neurologic, ocular, renal involvement, or hypercalcemia, even with mild symptoms, because fatal arrhythmias, blindness, and renal failure may develop.
3. Severe debilitating symptoms from any organ involvement.

Therapy is not indicated in asymptomatic children with stage one or two pulmonary disease with normal or mildly abnormal lung function. However, stage 3 disease needs to be followed closely, as adult data suggest that the majority do not resolve, it may progress to pulmonary fibrosis, and most patients will require therapy in the future.[195,230] The limited pediatric data support this concept.[214,215,218]

Corticosteroid therapy is typically started at a relatively high dose (1 mg/kg per day depending on severity of disease) for 4–6 weeks and then tapered. A response to therapy is usually seen within 6–12 weeks of initiation of therapy with improvement in symptoms, pulmonary infiltrates, and lymphadenopathy on imaging, and variable improvement in pulmonary function. Steroid therapy typically needs to be continued for 12–18 months in order to prevent relapse of disease. Relapses are treated with increasing doses of corticosteroids. Alternative immunosuppressive and/or cytotoxic therapies may be added if disease is steroid-resistant or as steroid-sparing agents in relapsing disease; however, data on the efficacy of these agents are very limited.[231] Low-dose methotrexate is the most commonly used alternative therapy, which has been shown to have a steroid-sparing effect in one adult randomized controlled trial[232] and in a small case series of children.[233] Hydroxychloroquine has been reported to be successful in treating patients with hypercalcemia and neurological involvement.[234,235] Infliximab, a tumor necrosis factor inhibitor, has a strong pathophysiological basis for use, but side effects of therapy are a concern, and randomized controlled trials do not support its routine use. It has been shown to have limited efficacy in severe pulmonary disease refractory to steroid therapy.[236] Lung transplantation has been reported to be successful in many young adults with end-stage lung disease[237] and candidate selection criteria specific to sarcoidosis have been published.[238]

PROGNOSIS

In adults, spontaneous recovery occurs in about two-thirds of patients with sarcoidosis within 2 years of diagnosis without therapy. Another one-third to one-half of patients is treated with corticosteroids, and most improve with treatment, but relapse occurs in many when the drug is tapered or discontinued. The clinical course is chronic or progressive in 10%–30%, and fatalities occur in 1%–5% of patients, typically due to progressive pulmonary fibrosis or central nervous system or cardiac involvement.[195] Limited long-term pediatric outcome data from the United States,[239] France,[215] and Denmark[218] suggest that most children with sarcoidosis also have a good prognosis, as most have a complete recovery. Chronic active disease with impaired lung function occurs in a small proportion and there are few deaths (mainly patients with neurosarcoidosis). Population-based data from Denmark is particularly informative for white children with sarcoidosis, showing that in 46 Danish children identified between 1979 and 1994, after a median follow-up time of 15 years, 78% of children showed complete recovery, 11% had chronic active disease with multiorgan involvement and impaired lung function, and 7% died of their disease.[218] Newer cohort data from France, which identified 41 children of mainly Afro-Caribbean and sub-Saharan ethnicity and 1.5–5 years of follow-up, presented a less favorable outcome, with less than half of children in remission at 5 years.[213] The French children had a more severe disease presentation with multiorgan involvement and all but one patient requiring systemic steroid therapy at disease presentation. These observations are concordant with adult data that show that African-American race is a risk factor for more severe disease.[240,241] Pulmonary involvement may lead to progressive pulmonary fibrosis and end stage chronic lung disease; this seems to be more likely with stage III pulmonary disease at the onset in both adults and children.[195,218,239] Eye involvement may lead to blindness.

Löfgren syndrome (i.e., BHL, erythema nodosum, fever, and polyarthritis) has an excellent prognosis with greater than 85% spontaneous remission rates within 6–12 months.[195] Clinical factors associated with a worse prognosis in adults include black race, hypercalcemia, lupus pernio, splenomegaly, pulmonary infiltrates on chest radiograph (stage II and III disease), chronic uveitis, cystic bone lesions, nasal mucosal sarcoidosis, neurosarcoidosis, cardiac involvement, and low family income.[195,241] In children, where prognostic data are much more limited, erythema nodosum has been associated with a good prognosis,[218] while the increased number of organs involved is associated with relapses,[213] and central nervous system involvement has been associated with fatalities.[218]

Childhood Vasculitides

Vasculitis is defined as the presence of inflammation in a blood vessel. Vasculitis syndromes are generally named according to their clinical manifestations, the size and type of blood vessels involved, and the pathologic features found within the vessel walls.[242] Clinical manifestations and epidemiological features are different in childhood vasculitides compared with adult vasculitides.[97] A pediatric classification scheme has been developed by the European League against Rheumatism and the Paediatric Rheumatology European Society, which includes classification criteria for the more common childhood vasculitis syndromes (Table 58.4).[243–245] The clinical presentation of vasculitis depends on the size of the vessel involved. When predominantly large- or medium-sized vessels are affected, arterial insufficiency to the affected organ results in infarction, necrosis, and end organ dysfunction. Smaller vessel (arterioles, venules, capillaries) inflammation may result in leakage of blood into the tissues. In the lung, this causes diffuse alveolar hemorrhage (DAH), which is characterized by diffuse alveolar infiltrates and a drop in hemoglobin with or without hemoptysis. Other clinical features suggestive of vasculitis are associated acute glomerulonephritis, pulmonary-renal syndrome, ulcerating or deforming upper airway lesions, cavitary or nodular disease on chest imaging, tracheobronchial stenosis, palpable purpura, arthritis, uveitis, and systemic symptoms including weight loss, fatigue, and fever.

Pulmonary involvement has been reported in association with most vasculitis syndromes; however, clinically significant pulmonary involvement occurs mainly with vasculitis

Table 58.4   Nomenclature of Childhood Vasculitis and Associated Pulmonary Involvement

Classification Category	Pulmonary Involvement
LVV	
■ Takayasu arteritis	Rare: Pulmonary arteritis[317,318]
MVV	
■ Childhood polyarteritis nodosa	Rare: Isolated case reports of pulmonary arteritis in adults[319,320]
■ Kawasaki disease	■ During acute phase cough is common and chest radiograph changes occur in 15%[321]
	■ Unresolving pneumonia is a rare presentation of disease[322]
SVV	
AAV	
■ GPA (previously Wegener's)[a]	Almost universal: upper and/or lower airways and/or parenchymal (see text)
■ EGPA[a] (previously Churg-Strauss syndrome)	Nonfixed pulmonary infiltrates in 85%; prior history of asthma almost universal (see text)
■ MPA[a]	Pulmonary hemorrhage in 30%–50% and may have clinical presentation identical to idiopathic pulmonary hemosiderosis (see text)
Immune complex SVV	
■ Henoch-Schönlein purpura (IgA vasculitis)	Rarely may have pulmonary hemorrhage[323]
■ Antiglomerular basement membrane disease	Pulmonary-renal syndrome[324] but rare in children[325]
VVV	Infrequent (1%–8%); pulmonary artery aneurysms, hemoptysis, thrombi reported in adults[326]
■ Behçet's disease	
SOV	Isolated pulmonary capillaritis[246,a]
	Isolated pulmonary arteritis case report[327]
Vasculitis associated systemic disease	(SLE, SSc, others—see Table 58.2)
Vasculitis associated with probably etiology (infection, malignancy, and drugs, including hypersensitivity vasculitis)	Rarely may have pulmonary hemorrhage or thrombosis

[a]ANCA associated vasculitides that commonly have pulmonary involvement.
Table includes only childhood vasculitides with reported pulmonary involvement.
AAV, ANCA-associated vasculitis; *EGPA*, eosinophilic granulomatosis with polyangiitis; *GPA*, granulomatosis with polyangiitis; *IgA*, immunoglobulin A; *LVV*, large-vessel vasculitis; *MPA*, microscopic polyangiitis; *MVV*, medium-vessel vasculitis; *SLE*, systemic lupus erythematosus; *SOV*, single-organ vasculitis; *SSc*, scleroderma; *SVV*, small-vessel vasculitis; *VVV*, variable vessel vasculitis.

Table 58.5   Small Vessel Vasculitides With Frequent Pulmonary Involvement

	GPA	MPA	EGPA	IPC
Common presenting features	Epistaxis, saddle nose deformity, dyspnea, cough, pulmonary nodules, constitutional symptoms	Necrotizing crescenteric glomerulonephritis (pauciimmune), marked constitutional symptoms	Severe asthma, chronic rhinosinusitis, peripheral blood eosinophilia, migrating chest infiltrates, constitutional symptoms	Anemia, diffuse alveolar infiltrates with or without hemoptysis
Frequency of pulmonary involvement	>80%	~30%–60%	70%–90%	100%
Typical pulmonary manifestations	Nodules with or without cavities, tracheobronchial stenosis, DAH	DAH	Asthma, patchy pulmonary infiltrates, rarely DAH	DAH
Autoantibody status	85%–90% PR3-ANCA+	50%–75% MPO-ANCA+	0%–25% MPO-ANCA+ in children; 35%–50% MPO-ANCA+ in adults	0–?[a]
Other organ involvement	Kidney, skin, ocular, MSK, nervous system, heart	Kidney, skin, MSK, bowel, cardiac, ocular	Kidney, skin, cardiac, GI, CNS, mononeuritis multiplex, skin	None at initial presentation, but may evolve into MPA with kidney disease

[a]IPC cases (*n* = 12) reported in literature to date all ANCA negative but ANCA+ cases may have been classified as MPA and MPO-ANCA+ idiopathic pulmonary hemosiderosis cases are reported.
CNS, Central nervous system; *DAH*, diffuse alveolar hemorrhage; *EGPA*, eosinophilic granulomatosis with polyangiitis; *GI*, gastrointestinal; *GPA*, granulomatosis with polyangiitis; *IPC*, isolated pulmonary capillaritis; *MPA*, microscopic polyangiitis; *MPO-ANCA+*, myeloperoxidase-antineutrophil cytoplasmic antibody positive; *MSK*, musculoskeletal; *PR3-ANCA+*, proteinase 3-antineutrophil cytoplasmic antibody positive.

associated with antineutrophil cytoplasmic antibody (ANCA).[246] ANCA-associated vasculitis (AAV) syndromes are characterized by necrotizing vasculitis of small vessels, frequent pulmonary and renal involvement, and a paucity of immune deposits in the blood vessel wall. The major clinicopathologic variants of AAV syndromes with frequent pulmonary involvement are GPA (formerly Wegener's), microscopic polyangiitis (MPA), eosinophilic granulomatosis with polyangiitis (EGPA, formerly Churg-Strauss), and isolated pulmonary capillaritis (IPC; Table 58.5). MPA is recognized mainly as a rare pauci-immune small vessel vasculitis of adults involving the skin, joints, kidneys, and lungs, but it may present in childhood and is often (10%–30%) associated with pulmonary hemorrhage.[247,248] It is distinguished from GPA by the presence of high titers of antimyeloperoxidase (MPO)–ANCA and the absence of granulomatous inflammation pathologically. It may present initially to the pulmonologist as a case of idiopathic pulmonary hemosiderosis, which on lung biopsy is proven to be IPC, with the subsequent development of pauci-immune glomerulonephritis.[249] MPA is discussed in detail in Chapter 58. EGPA is a small-vessel vasculitis that is exceedingly rare in children, and most of the published literature is limited to single case reports.[250–252] It is characterized by fever, peripheral eosinophilia, migrating pulmonary infiltrates, and anti-MPO-ANCA antibodies in patients with concomitant severe atopic asthma or allergic rhinitis. Sinusitis, skin, neurologic, and cardiac involvement are also common, while renal disease is uncommon.[253,254] In the largest pediatric case series report of 117 children with new diagnoses of AAV from 30 different North American centers from 2004 to 2008, two children had EGPA compared with 76 with GPA and 17 with MPA.[251]

Stimulator of interferon genes (STING)–associated vasculopathy with onset in infancy (SAVI) is a rare inherited autoinflammatory disease that should be suspected in infants who present with skin vasculitis changes and ILD.[255] The differential diagnosis for DAH and pulmonary-renal syndrome includes ANCA-associated vasculitides, Goodpasture syndrome, SLE, thromboembolic disease, and infections, and is discussed separately in Chapter 61. The remainder of this section will focus on GPA, as this is the most common vasculitis syndrome presenting to the pulmonologist, and it may initially present with isolated airway or lung involvement.

Granulomatosis With Polyangiitis

EPIDEMIOLOGY

Vasculitis is rare in children. One English survey of family clinicians estimated an annual incidence of 53.3 per 100,000 children less than 17 years of age, with Henoch-Schonlein purpura and Kawasaki disease being the most common vasculitides. All other primary vasculitides, including ANCA-associated vasculitides, had an incidence together of 0.24 per 100,000.[97] Population-based studies of GPA from America and Norway specifically suggest that incidence is less than 1 per million in children, and the disease incidence peaks in the fourth to sixth decades of life.[256,257] The multicenter ARChiVe (A Registry for Childhood Vasculitis: e-entry) study suggests that GPA accounts for most (65%) new pediatric AAV cases. The GPA patients had a median age of diagnosis of 14.2 years (range 4–17 years), 69% were Caucasian, and 63% were female.[251]

PATHOGENESIS

The etiology of GPA is largely unknown; however, the almost universal presence of ANCA and response to immunosuppressive therapy provide strong rationale for an autoimmune basis.

Many recent studies examining the effects of ANCA-neutrophil and neutrophil-endothelial cell interactions have provided evidence supporting a pathogenic role for ANCA. ANCA are directed against the neutrophil granule components proteinase 3 (PR-3-ANCA) and MPO-ANCA. ANCA interact with these target antigens on cytokine-primed neutrophils. This causes neutrophil activation and interaction with endothelial cells via multiple signaling pathways. The end result is tissue inflammation and damage as the neutrophils migrate through the endothelial cells and undergo respiratory burst, and degranulation with release of toxic

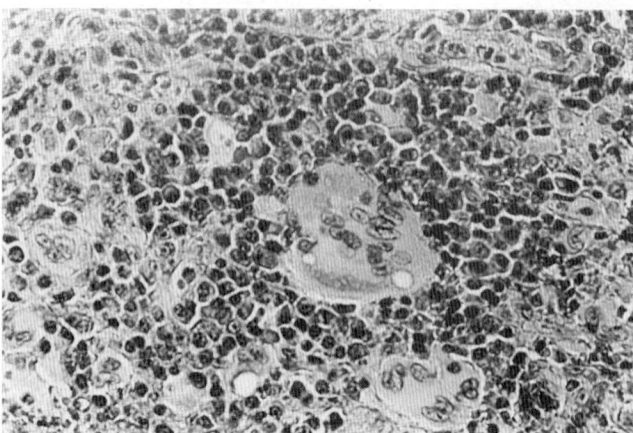

Fig. 58.12 Photomicrograph of a lung biopsy from a patient with granulomatosis with polyangiitis showing a dense pleomorphic infiltrate, numerous mononuclear cells, scattered neutrophils, and several giant cells. This aggregate of cells would be considered a granuloma.

products. Failure of adaptive immune system regulation mechanisms results in a loss of self-tolerance, so that T-helper and B cells also assist in this autoantibody reaction.[258] The histopathology of all AAV is hence marked by necrotizing vasculitis of the small blood vessels without immune complex deposition (i.e., pauci-immune vasculitis). GPA is distinguished among the AAV by the anti-PR-3-ANCA specificity and by the presence of granulomas (Fig. 58.12).

What is still poorly understood is why and how ANCA develop in the first place. It has long been recognized that some drugs and infectious agents may trigger the development of ANCA and a clinical syndrome of secondary vasculitis, which is similar to the clinical presentation of primary vasculitis.[259] Some studies have suggested a triggering role for infections, particularly bacteria colonizing the upper airway such as *Staphylococcus aureus*.[260] This has led to a clinical trial investigating the role of prophylactic cotrimoxazole in preventing GPA relapses.[261] In addition, other autoantibodies have recently been described as having a potential role in the disease pathogenesis, including lysosomal membrane protein 2[262] and antiendothelial cell antibodies.[263]

CLINICAL MANIFESTATIONS

Four large pediatric case series describe the typical clinical presentation of GPA with a triad of upper airway, lower respiratory tract, and renal disease manifestations.[251,264–266] Symptom onset is most often insidious, with dyspnea or chronic cough along with constitutional symptoms, but it may also be dramatic, presenting with pulmonary hemorrhage, upper airway obstruction, or renal failure. The median interval from symptom onset to diagnosis is 2.7 months (range 0–49 months).[251] Most children present with multiorgan involvement. The most frequent presenting features are constitutional (fever, malaise, fatigue, weight loss; 89%); pulmonary (80%); ear, nose, and throat (80%); and renal (75%). Less commonly eyes (37%), skin (35%), gastrointestinal (42%), musculoskeletal (57%), and nervous system (25%) may be involved.[251] In a series of 25 patients from Toronto, Canada, 16% experienced venous thrombosis associated with antiphospholipid antibodies during the disease course.[266]

Case reports describe involvement of the heart, spleen, and pituitary gland. Contrary to the adult experience, limited GPA without renal involvement is uncommon in children. Laboratory abnormalities include elevated white blood cell counts, normochromic normocytic anemia, thrombocytosis, elevated erythrocyte sedimentation rate or C-reactive protein level, abnormal urinalysis with proteinuria, hematuria and red blood cell casts, and elevated serum creatinine. ANCAs are present in 89% of children with cytoplasmic immunofluorescence staining pattern (cANCA) in 86%, and 68% positive for anti-PR3,[251] which is comparable to serology results in adults with GPA.[267]

PULMONARY INVOLVEMENT

Presenting pulmonary symptoms include dyspnea or chronic cough in over half of children.[251,265] Hypoxia requiring oxygen therapy is present in 19%.[251] Hemoptysis may signal necrotizing mucosal airway involvement or DAH. Symptoms of dyspnea with hoarseness and stridor suggest subglottic stenosis. Subglottic stenosis has been reported in one series to occur with higher frequency in pediatric onset GPA compared with adults[264]; hence this feature has been included in the new EULAR/PReS classification criteria.[244,245] Frequent upper airway findings include sinusitis, nasal septal ulceration or perforation, otitis media, mastoiditis, hearing loss, oral ulcers,

and nasal cartilage damage, characteristic of long-standing disease, with resultant saddle-nose deformity (which must be distinguished from the diagnosis of relapsing polychondritis). About half of children will have abnormalities on chest radiographs. The most common findings are nodules followed by fixed infiltrates. Cavitations, mediastinal lymphadenopathy, pleural effusions, and pneumothoraces may also occur. Chest CT is more sensitive in detecting small nodules and ground-glass abnormalities than plain radiography. The largest case series ($n = 18$) of chest CT findings in children with GPA showed pulmonary involvement in 90% of newly diagnosed patients with nodules (90%), ground-glass opacification (52%), and air space opacification (45%), the predominant findings. Nodules tended to be multiple (69% had more than five nodules), greater than 5 mm in diameter, and cavitating in 17% (Fig. 58.13). Air-space opacification usually correlated with clinical evidence of pulmonary hemorrhage.[268] Chest CT findings in children were similar to findings in adults, except that the frequency of identified bronchial narrowing seems to be lower in children (6.7%) compared with adults (59%; Figs. 58.14 and 58.15).[268,269] Sinus CT may be useful to identify upper airway involvement, particularly sinus opacification and bony destruction. Pulmonary function test abnormalities are seen in 42%, and these may show obstructive or restrictive defects, depending on the tissues involved.[251,270]

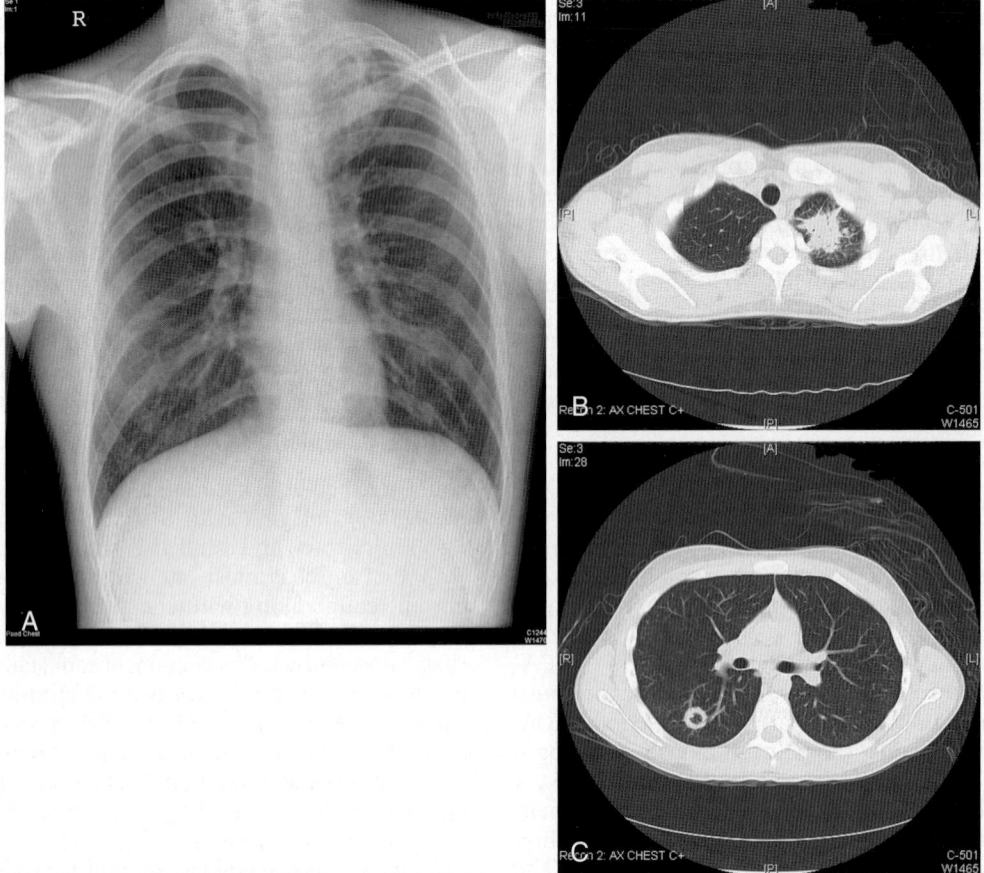

Fig. 58.13 (A–C) Fifteen-year-old teen with granulomatosis with polyangiitis who presented with renal failure, pulmonary infiltrates, and antineutrophil cytoplasmic antibody positive serology. a CXR shows air space infiltrate left upper lobe and near right hilum. (B and C) High-resolution computed tomography scan confirms a cavitating lesion in right lower lobe and multiple bilateral nodules and areas of air space disease.

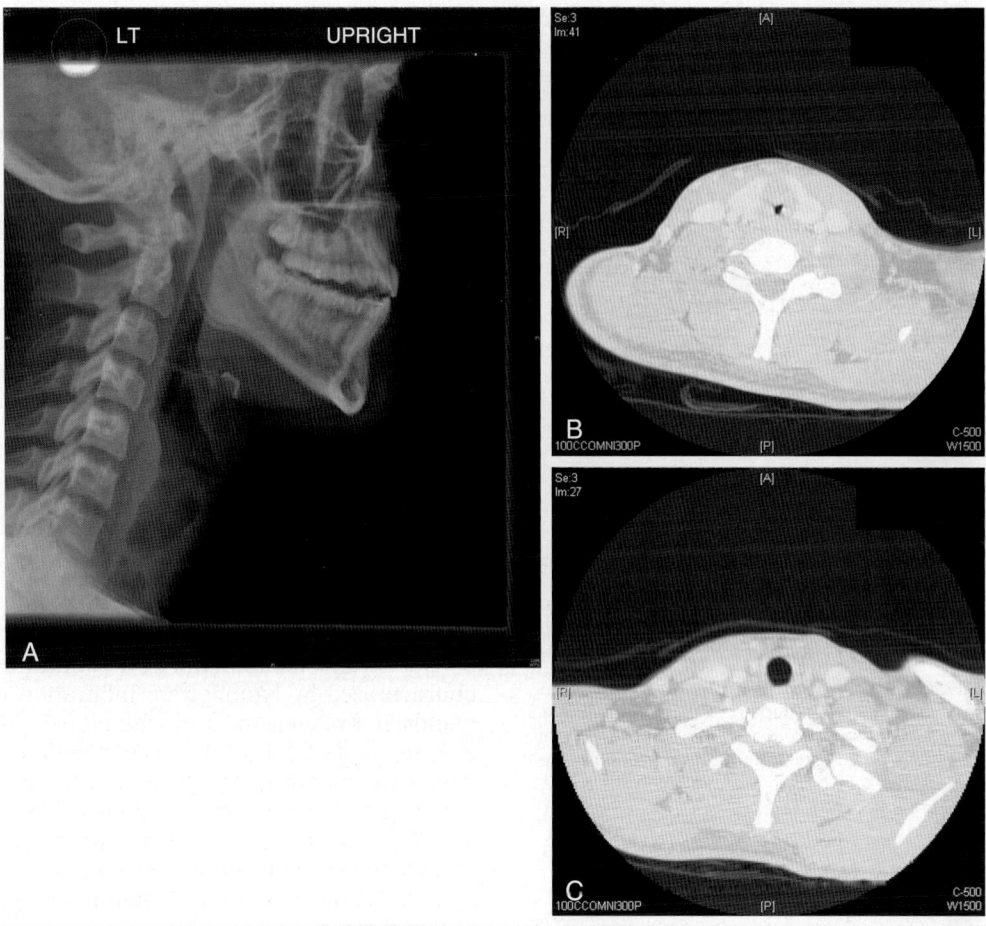

Fig. 58.14 (A–C) Fifteen-year-old teen with GPA presenting with a hoarse voice, hemoptysis, weight loss, and antineutrophil cytoplasmic antibody positive serology. (A) Soft tissue radiograph of neck shows narrowing of trachea at level of seventh cervical vertebrae. (B and C) computed tomography scan of neck shows severe stenosis of the upper trachea (15 mm in length and narrowing to a diameter of 4 mm [B] from 14 mm [C] above the stenotic area) secondary to circumferential soft tissue thickening. Stenosis improved with pulse steroid therapy and local airway laser ablative therapy.

It is important for the pulmonologist to recognize the bronchoscopy findings of GPA, as these may provide the first clue to the diagnosis for a child presenting with nonspecific symptoms of cough (Fig. 58.16). Mucosal erythema, edema, ulceration, hemorrhage, cobblestoning, nodules, polyps, submucosal tunneling, synechial bands, and airway stenosis have all been described in airways from the oropharynx down to the bronchi, in case series that include mostly adults and a few children.[270–273] Endobronchial findings are nonspecific, as similar findings may be encountered with infections and sarcoidosis.

DIAGNOSIS

The diagnosis of GPA is based on a combination of clinical findings (e.g., pulmonary-renal syndrome), supportive serology (i.e., anti-PR-3 ANCA positive), and characteristic histopathology (pauci-immune granulomatous inflammation of predominantly small to medium sized blood vessels or pauci-immune glomerulonephritis). If GPA is suspected, it is important to examine the urine and to obtain chest and sinus imaging to rule out asymptomatic renal or upper and lower respiratory tract disease. The differential diagnosis often includes infections (especially mycobacterial, fungal, or

helminthic infections in addition to common viral and bacterial causes), other causes of pulmonary-renal syndrome (other ANCA-associated vasculitides, SLE, MCTD, Goodpasture syndrome), sarcoidosis, UC with pulmonary involvement, malignancy, and chronic granulomatous disease. Renal biopsy has a high yield for identifying pauci-immune glomerulonephritis if there are urinary abnormalities. Diseased upper respiratory tract tissues (e.g., ears, nose, sinuses, trachea) and endobronchial airway lesions offer relatively noninvasive access for tissue diagnosis, but often have low yields for diagnosis. Lung biopsy yield may also be low, since disease is often patchy, but open lung biopsy procedures may offer a better yield than less invasive fine needle aspiration or transbronchial techniques.

TREATMENT

Historically, standard treatment for GPA at diagnosis is a combination of glucocorticoids and CYC. This therapy has changed GPA from a rapidly fatal disease to a manageable chronic illness with frequent relapses in most adult and pediatric cases.[274,275] CYC may be used as a daily oral therapy or pulse intravenous therapy, which results in a less cumulative dose and is the preferred dosing regimen in children. Disease

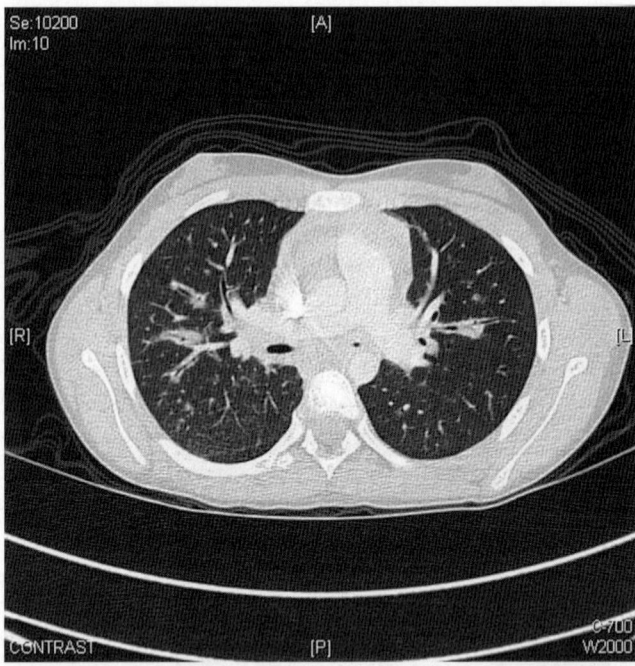

Fig. 58.15 Nine-year-old girl with granulomatosis with polyangiitis presenting with hemoptysis and antineutrophil cytoplasmic antibody+. Computed tomography scan shows pericardial effusion, diffuse bilateral irregular peribronchial soft tissue thickening, and an 11-mm nodular-like mass surrounding the left mainstem bronchus causing pinhole narrowing; no cavitary lesions present.

remission may be maintained, with low-dose weekly methotrexate or daily azathioprine.[276] Methotrexate may also be effective in inducing remission when the disease is localized or has milder manifestations, and renal disease is not a concern.[277] Rituximab, a monoclonal antibody against B cells, has been effectively used for severe refractory disease that does not respond to conventional cytotoxic therapy and has emerged as an excellent option for both induction phase treatment and maintenance phase treatment to prevent disease relapse. Rituximab has been shown to be not inferior to CYC for induction phase treatment for AAV in new onset disease and disease flare, and is superior for those with PR3-ANCA+.[278,279] In maintenance phase treatment, patients on rituximab therapy had fewer major relapses compared with azathioprine.[279]

Obstructing airway lesions, including tracheal and bronchial stenosis, may not respond to cytotoxic therapy. These lesions should be managed by a specialized airway team with expertise in the area. They may require intralesional injections of glucocorticoids, endoscopic dilatation, stent placement, or tracheostomy.[270–273] Intralesional corticosteroids may be most effective when used before other surgical interventions, which may result in scarring.[280]

Patients with GPA are at increased risk of infection due to the immunosuppressive therapy they are receiving, as well as the presence of vulnerable damaged tissues.[281] Prophylaxis against *pneumocystis jiroveci* pneumonia is recommended while receiving CYC[282] and should be considered for children receiving high dose corticosteroids with methotrexate, and those receiving rituximab.[283]

PROGNOSIS

GPA was almost universally fatal in both adults and children at an average of 5 months after diagnosis prior to the advent of cytotoxic therapy.[274,275] With current induction therapy, over 90% of patients are expected to respond partially or completely; however, about half will relapse within 5 years.[274] Fatalities reported in children are due to lung disease or sepsis,[264] while malignancy, renal failure, and cardiac disease are additional reported causes of death in adults with GPA.[274] Long-term morbidity may result from persistent airway obstruction, renal insufficiency, or treatment-related side effects, including cystitis, infertility (due to CPA), cataracts, glaucoma, vertebral compression fractures, and growth effects (due to steroids).[264,266,274]

Other Systemic Inflammatory Diseases With Significant Pulmonary Involvement

SS is a chronic inflammatory autoimmune disorder that is characterized by lymphocytic infiltration of the exocrine glands. It is often associated with other CTD, including JIA, SLE, SSc, and JDM. The classic symptoms are keratoconjunctivitis sicca (dry eyes) and xerostomia (dry mouth), along with a high prevalence of ANA, RF, anti-Ro, and anti-La antibodies. SS is very rare in children, with most major pediatric rheumatology centers only reporting a few cases. There is a lower frequency of sicca symptoms and higher frequency of parotitis with childhood onset compared with adult onset SS.[284–286] Pulmonary involvement occurs in up to 75% of adult patients, but is usually mild and nonprogressive.[287–289] Dryness of the airways resulting in "sicca" cough occurs in up to half of adult patients. Small airways obstructive disease and airway hyperreactivity are also common and are thought to be caused by lymphocytic inflammation around the bronchioles and bronchi (follicular bronchiolitis). ILD occurs infrequently, usually with the histopathological changes of LIP, a finding generally not seen with other CTDs in the absence of SS.[290,291] Chest radiograph changes include diffuse reticular or reticulonodular infiltrates and bronchiectasis, while CT scan may have a variety of additional findings, including ground glass attenuation, subpleural nodules, and cysts.[288] Pulmonary hypertension responsive to steroid and CYC therapy has also been reported in a 9-year-old child with SS.[292] Prognosis is generally very good, but a poor outcome may occur from progression of LIP to lymphoma in adults.[293]

Inflammatory bowel disease (IBD), including Crohn disease (CD) and UC, is commonly associated with extraintestinal manifestations but only very rarely (<1%) associated with clinically significant pulmonary disease.[294,295] Subclinical pulmonary involvement is probably common, as latent pulmonary function abnormalities have been demonstrated in a case series of children with CD[296] and adults with both CD and UC[297,298] who have no respiratory symptoms and normal chest radiographs. The main abnormality is a reduction in DLCO that tends to be worse during active disease. Children with CD have also been demonstrated to have bronchial hyperreactivity.[299] The etiology of these pulmonary function abnormalities is likely secondary to a subclinical airway or

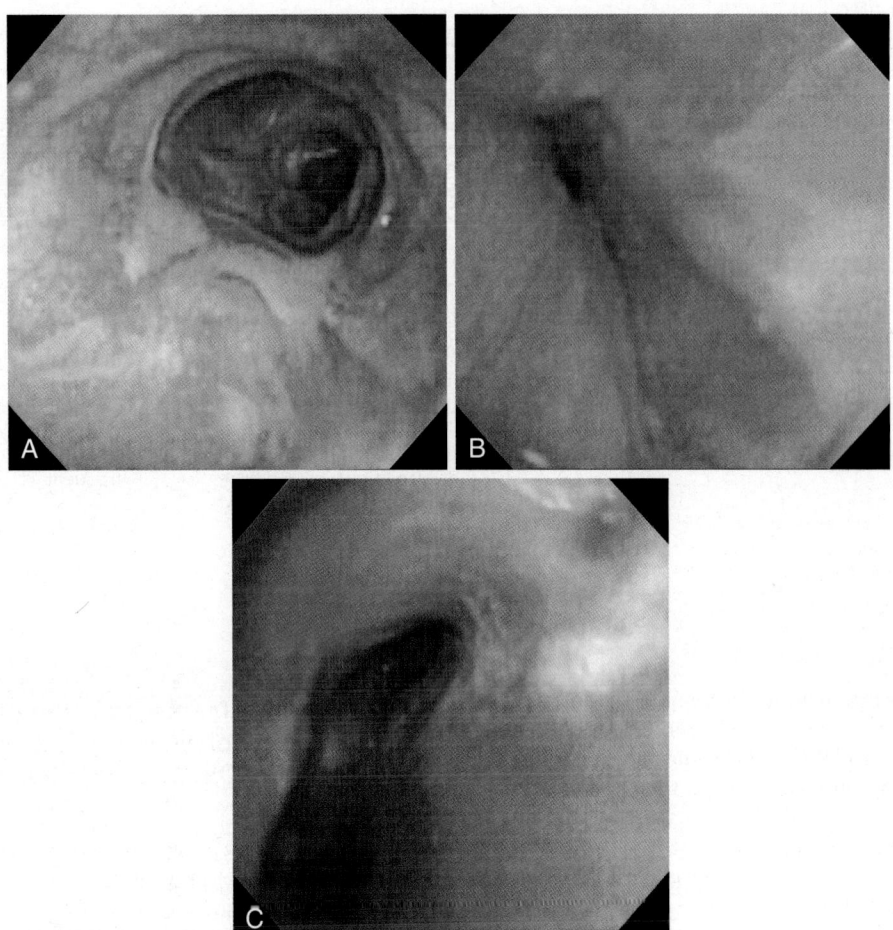

Fig. 58.16 Bronchoscopic photographs of the airways of a 15-year-old teenager diagnosed with granulomatosis with polyangiitis (A) Main carina showing mucosal erythema. (B) Left main stem bronchus showing pinhole stenosis. (C) Left secondary carina showing erythematous friable mucosa.

alveolar inflammatory process, as BAL samples in CD show hypercellularity with lymphocytosis.[300-302]

Symptomatic lung disease associated with IBD has been reported in two large case series[303,304] as well as multiple case reports, and is summarized well in recent reviews.[295,305] Bronchiectasis is the single most common disorder described in adults, although a range of rare pulmonary manifestations have been reported, including tracheal stenosis, colobronchial and ileobronchial fistulae, chronic bronchitis, BO, BOOP, granulomatous pulmonary nodules (including necrobiotic[306]), ILD, pulmonary vasculitis, and pleural effusions.[295,307] Descriptions of pulmonary disease in children with IBD are limited to isolated case reports of granulomatous and necrobiotic nodules, BO, and BOOP in CD,[308-311] and vasculitis, BOOP, and ILD in UC.[312-314] High-resolution CT findings include air trapping with mosaic perfusion pattern, tree-in-bud appearance, bronchiectasis, and multiple pulmonary nodules.[304] Pulmonary involvement in IBD usually responds to corticosteroid therapy, with systemic therapy for more severe or interstitial disease and inhaled therapy for mild airways disease.[305] Infliximab therapy (monoclonal antibody to tumor necrosis factor alpha) has been used successfully in children with granulomatous lung disease.[310] The differential diagnosis for pulmonary manifestations associated with IBD must also include drug induced disease (especially hypersensitivity pneumonitis associated with sulfasalazine[315] and mesalamine[316]), opportunistic infection, malignancy, and thromboembolism. When significant lung disease and IBD coexist, consideration should also be given to distinguishing between CD and sarcoidosis or UC and GPA, as these diseases may have striking similarities; however, management strategies may differ.[295]

Clinical Approach to Diagnosis and Management of Pulmonary Involvement in the Systemic Inflammatory Diseases of Childhood

The clinical presentation of pulmonary involvement is highly variable. The most common presentation for ILD is slowly progressive dyspnea with or without a dry cough. Dyspnea due to ILD must be distinguished from the dyspnea due to muscle weakness, deconditioning, thromboembolic disease, and cardiac causes. Patients may also present with pleuritic chest pain. Infection and drug toxicity must always be considered in the differential diagnosis of pulmonary involvement.

Following a detailed history and physical examination, pulmonary function testing may be very helpful for further elucidating the type of pulmonary involvement. Patterns of

Table 58.6   Patterns of Pulmonary Function and Gas Exchange Impairment in Lung Disease Associated With Systemic Inflammatory Conditions

	Pattern of Ventilatory Impairment	Diffusing Capacity for Carbon Monoxide	Gas Exchange Characteristics
Chest wall restriction (muscle weakness or chest wall deformity)	Restrictive defect with low MIPS/MEPS[a] (especially with associated muscle weakness) and low peak flow in more severe disease	Preserved until severe loss of volume	With severe disease, hypoventilation results in hypercapnia and hypoxia with normal a-A gradient[b]
Pulmonary fibrosis	Restrictive defect	Reduced	With severe disease, hypoxia at rest
Bronchiectasis	Obstructive defect	Preserved until severe end stage disease	With end-stage disease, hypoxia at rest
Diffuse alveolar hemorrhage	Variable—often restrictive	Increased if hemorrhage is recent[c]	During active bleeding, hypoxia, often profound with a wide a-A gradient[b]
Pulmonary vascular disease	Normal pulmonary function tests	Reduced	Hypoxia at rest even with moderate pulmonary hypertension
Mixed disease: Pulmonary fibrosis and muscle weakness	Restrictive defect, often severe	Less reduced than expected for degree of restrictive defect	Hypoxia at rest or with exercise is frequent

[a]MIPS/MEPS = maximal inspiratory pressures and maximal expiratory pressures as measured at the mouth opening.
[b]a-A gradient = alveolar-arterial oxygen gradient.
[c]Within past 24–36 hours.

pulmonary function impairment are suggestive of certain diagnoses (Table 58.6). Abnormal pulmonary function tests are best followed up with HRCT. The anatomical distribution of pulmonary involvement varies with the type of disease (see Table 58.2). Patterns of HRCT findings have been much better described and correlated with pathological changes in the adult literature; however, some generalities can be extrapolated to the pediatric population. Ground glass densities generally correlate with parenchymal lung disease, while peribronchovascular changes and air trapping correlate with airways disease. Pleural inflammation is manifested as pleural thickening with effusion.

Bronchoscopy with BAL may be very helpful for distinguishing autoimmune lung disease from opportunistic infection, alveolar hemorrhage, and cancer. BAL cytology patterns may suggest specific disease etiologies, although the use of BAL for monitoring CTD-ILD is still investigational. There may also be characteristic airway changes of GPA or sarcoidosis noted during bronchoscopy, and EBB may yield additional diagnostic information (see previous disease sections in this chapter).

Lung biopsy is reserved for a small subset of patients where a diagnostic dilemma remains, despite investigation utilizing previously suggested modalities. If lung biopsy is required, it is best to do so expeditiously before clinical deterioration of the patient makes it too risky or even impossible to undertake. It may be needed to rule out an opportunistic infection or to confirm a diagnosis of inflammatory lung disease that will require a change in the management strategy, particularly the addition of a cytotoxic or biologic agent with potential significant side effects.

Occasionally patients present with sudden onset of new respiratory symptoms and progression to respiratory failure can occur rapidly. Multiple etiologies of disease need to be considered as the potential cause of acute respiratory deterioration (Table 58.7). Prompt recognition and treatment of the cause of respiratory symptoms in this scenario may be lifesaving.

End with Key Messages in a box (Box 58.3).

Box 58.3   Key Messages in the Approach to Pulmonary Involvement in the Systemic Inflammatory Diseases of Childhood

Pediatric pulmonologists must work closely with the rheumatologist to diagnose and manage lung disease associated with systemic inflammatory diseases of childhood.

The differential diagnosis of respiratory symptoms includes generalized muscle weakness, deconditioning, cardiac disease, thromboembolic disease, opportunistic infection, and drug toxicity effects, as well as inflammatory lung disease.

Recognize that pulmonary disease may sometimes be the predominant initial presentation of a systemic inflammatory disease.

Specific inflammatory diseases are associated with probable patterns of pulmonary involvement (see Table 58.2).

Pulmonary function testing, including measurement of lung volumes and diffusing capacity for carbon monoxide, are helpful in refining the differential diagnosis, measuring the severity, and following the progression of lung disease (Table 58.6).

Bronchoscopy may reveal recognizable airway abnormalities associated with specific conditions (e.g., granulomatosis with polyangiitis and sarcoidosis).

Bronchoalveolar lavage is helpful in ruling out infection, and the cytology count may also help refine the differential diagnosis of lung disease.

High morbidity and possible mortality are associated with pulmonary involvement of some systemic inflammatory diseases; hence it is important to diagnose and treat early.

Pulmonary involvement may require specific drug therapies for some diseases (e.g., cyclophosphamide for vasculitis).

Most treatment protocols in pediatrics are extrapolated from results of clinical trials in adult patients.

Early identification of pulmonary involvement may lead to application of new therapies, including biologic agents and therapies for pulmonary arterial hypertension.

Table 58.7 Causes of Acute Respiratory Deterioration in Children With Systemic Inflammatory Diseases

Etiology	Distinguishing Features
Infection	Fever, tachypnea, change in cough, increase in sputum volume, change in sputum color, malaise, new areas of consolidation on chest imaging. May be difficult to distinguish from disease flare.
Air leak: pneumothorax or pneumomediastinum	Sudden onset of chest pain or shoulder tip pain and dyspnea, tracheal shift in the presence of tension pneumothorax, absence of fever and cough, more common in dermatomyositis/polymyositis
Upper airway obstruction	Stridor and dyspnea of subacute onset caused by progressive tracheal circumferential soft tissue thickening in GPA
Acute pneumonitis or pleuritis	Fever, new nonproductive cough and/or chest pain, dyspnea, basal coarse crackles on chest exam, hypoxia, diffuse interstitial infiltrates on chest imaging, more common in lupus and JIA
Diffuse alveolar hemorrhage	Anemia, tachypnea and hypoxemia, hemoptysis usually absent, diffuse alveolar infiltrates on chest imaging, more common with ANCA + serology and lupus
Pulmonary embolus	Sudden onset chest pain, dyspnea, hypoxemia, no change in chest radiograph or rounded or wedge shaped opacity with apex directed to hilum, more common with hypercoagulable states like lupus
Progression of chronic lung disease	End-stage lung disease prior to deterioration, absence of fever or viral prodrome, rapid increase in dyspnea and oxygen need over a period of 1–2 weeks, mild (or no) changes on chest imaging out of keeping with severity of symptoms
Cardiac dysfunction	Low blood pressure, poor perfusion, may have wheezing, signs of left or right heart failure, cardiomegaly and/or pulmonary venous congestion on chest imaging, abnormal electrocardiogram

ANCA, Antineutrophil cytoplasmic antibody; *GPA,* granulomatosis with polyangiitis; *JIA,* juvenile idiopathic arthritis.

References

Access the reference list online at ExpertConsult.com.

Suggested Reading

Araujo DB, Borba EF, Silva CA, et al. Alveolar hemorrhage: distinct features of juvenile and adult onset systemic lupus erythematosus. *Lupus.* 2012;21(8):872–877.

Boyer D, Thomson CC, Cohen R, et al. ATS core curriculum 2016: part III. Pediatric pulmonary medicine. *Ann Am Thorac Soc.* 2016;13(6):955–966.

Cabral DA, Uribe AG, Benseler S, et al. Classification, presentation, and initial treatment of Wegener's granulomatosis in childhood. *Arthritis Rheum.* 2009;60(11):3413–3424.

Iannuzzi MC, Rybicki BA, Teirstein AS. Sarcoidosis. *N Engl J Med.* 2007;357(21):2153–2165.

Kimura Y, Weiss JE, Haroldson KL, et al. Pulmonary hypertension and other potentially fatal pulmonary complications in systemic juvenile idiopathic arthritis. *Arthritis Care Res (Hoboken).* 2013;65(5):745–752.

Kobayashi N, Takezaki S, Kobayashi I, et al. Clinical and laboratory features of fatal rapidly progressive interstitial lung disease associated with juvenile dermatomyositis. *Rheumatology (Oxford).* 2015;54(5):784–791.

Levine D, Akikusa J, Manson D, et al. Chest CT findings in pediatric Wegener's granulomatosis. *Pediatr Radiol.* 2007;37(1):57–62.

Nathan N, Marcelo P, Houdouin V, et al. Lung sarcoidosis in children: update on disease expression and management. *Thorax.* 2015;70(6):537–542.

Polychronopoulos VS, Prakash UB, Golbin JM, et al. Airway involvement in Wegener's granulomatosis. *Rheum Dis Clin North Am.* 2007;33(4):755–775, vi.

Watkin LB, Jessen B, Wiszniewski W, et al. COPA mutations impair ER-Golgi transport and cause hereditary autoimmune-mediated lung disease and arthritis. *Nat Genet.* 2015;47(6):654–660.

59 Lung Injury Caused by Pharmacologic Agents

MARIANNA M. HENRY, MD, MPH, and TERRY L. NOAH, MD

Numerous drugs can cause pulmonary or pleural reactions in children. The most frequent offenders are chemotherapeutic agents used in the treatment of childhood neoplasms (Table 59.1), although toxic effects of other agents are increasingly recognized (Table 59.2).[1,2] Diffuse interstitial pneumonitis and fibrosis constitutes the most frequent clinical syndrome. Hypersensitivity lung disease, noncardiogenic pulmonary edema, pleural effusion, bronchiolitis obliterans, and alveolar hemorrhage are also encountered.

Although some drug-induced pulmonary damage is reversible, persistent and even fatal dysfunction may occur. Lung reactions occasionally are temporally remote from exposure to chemotherapeutic agents. Depending on the agent involved, the reaction may or may not be dose related. The mechanism of toxicity is thought to be direct injury to lung cells in most cases, but immunologic and central nervous system-mediated mechanisms seem to play a role in the toxicity of certain agents. Identified risk factors associated with cytotoxic drug therapy vary, but they include cumulative dose, age of patient, prior or concurrent radiation, oxygen therapy, and use of other toxic drugs. Most reactions to noncytotoxic drugs appear to develop idiosyncratically. When patients are treated with combinations of potentially toxic drugs or with a toxic drug plus irradiation to the chest or high concentrations of oxygen, as is common in the treatment of childhood cancers, specific offenders often cannot be identified. There is little if any evidence that children are more susceptible to drug-related pulmonary injury, and in fact, they may be less susceptible to some agents such as bleomycin.

The clinical presentation of drug-induced lung disease often includes fever, malaise, dyspnea, and nonproductive cough. Radiologic studies almost always demonstrate diffuse alveolar and/or interstitial involvement. Segmental or lobar disease, particularly if unilateral, should suggest another diagnosis. Abnormal pulmonary function, indicative of restrictive or obstructive disease, may be found before appearance of roentgenographic lesions. Chest computed tomography (CT) may also provide early evidence of parenchymal abnormalities,[3] and hypoxemia is an early and clinically important functional consequence. Pathologic features do not distinguish between most drugs and most often consist of interstitial thickening with chronic inflammatory cell infiltrates in the interstitial or alveolar compartment, fibroblast proliferation, fibrosis, and hyperplasia of type II pneumocytes, which contain enlarged hyperchromatic nuclei.[4] With hypersensitivity reactions, the interstitial infiltrate includes substantial numbers of eosinophils. Interstitial pneumonitis can be part of the multisystem syndrome known as "drug-induced hypersensitivity syndrome/drug rash with eosinophilia and systemic symptoms" (DIHS/DRESS).[5] Other diagnoses, such as infection, pulmonary hemorrhage, lung disease related to an underlying disorder, and radiation damage must be considered in patients with suspected drug-induced lung injury. Bronchoalveolar lavage (BAL) is increasingly utilized to provide microbiologic and cytologic information essential to differential diagnosis and as a tool to begin to identify disease markers and potential pathogenic mechanisms.[6]

Practical criteria for diagnosing drug-induced lung disease have been suggested by Kubo and colleagues.[7] These include (1) history of ingestion of a drug that is known to induce lung injury, (2) clinical manifestations have been reported to be induced by a drug, (3) other causes of clinical manifestations have been ruled out, (4) improvement of clinical manifestations after drug discontinuation, and (5) exacerbation of clinical manifestations after resuming drug administration.

Cytotoxic Drugs Used in Cancer Therapy

Survivors of childhood cancers have often been exposed to multiple cytotoxic agents with potential lung toxicity, in addition to radiation, and are thus at increased risk for long-term pulmonary complications from these agents.[8] Compared to children without a cancer history, leukemia and lymphoma survivors are at increased risk for hospitalization for pulmonary-related reasons (relative risk [RR], 8.1; 95% confidence interval [CI], 3.9–16.8).[9] A recent review by the Children's Oncology Group Guideline Task Force on Pulmonary Complications recommended that health care providers following such children should receive a standardized cancer treatment summary from their oncologist to assess risk for pulmonary complications and that pediatric cancer survivors who received bleomycin, or who are subsequently undergoing general anesthesia for procedures, should have lung function monitored.[10] A cohort of 5000 survivors of childhood cancers, using the Children's Oncology Group Long-Term Follow-Up (COG-LTFU) Guidelines, underwent rigorous screening with pulmonary function tests (PFT), and abnormalities were present in 84%.[11]

BLEOMYCIN

Bleomycin is a mixture of peptide antibiotics obtained from *Streptomyces verticillus*. Its major use in children is in the treatment of Hodgkin disease and other lymphomas. Because of the high frequency of pulmonary reactions and the utility of bleomycin for generating animal models of lung fibrosis, this agent has been studied more thoroughly than others. Pulmonary damage develops in two distinct patterns, most commonly progressive fibrosis and uncommonly an acute hypersensitivity reaction.

Table 59.1 Cytotoxic Drugs Used in Cancer Therapy

	Incidence (%)	Mortality (%)	Clinical/Pathologic Syndromes
Bleomycin	2–40	1–10	IP/PF, H, P Eff, EP
Cyclophosphamide	≤1	40	IP/PF, PE, B, AH
Chlorambucil	a	≤50	IP/PF
Busulfan	2–43	b	IP/PF, P Eff, AH
Melphalan	a	≤60	IP/PF
Carmustine (BCNU)	10–30	15–90	IP/PF
Methotrexate	8	1	IP/PF, H, PE, P Eff
6-Mercaptopurine	a	b	IP/PF
Cytosine arabinoside	13–28	50	IP/PF, PE, BOOP, DMD
Gemcitabine	a	b	IP, B, PE, ARDS
Fludarabine	9	b	IP/PF
Procarbazine	a	b	H
Hydroxyurea	a	b	H
Paclitaxel	4–9	0	H
Docetaxel	73	0	H, IP, decreased DL_{CO}
Gefitinib	1	33	IP
Imatinib	a	b	P Eff, PE
Cetuximab	1	b	IP
Interleukin-2	>50	0	PE, P Eff
ATRA	5–27	5–29	IP, P Eff, PE, AH

[a]Infrequent case reports.
[b]Unknown.
AH, Alveolar hemorrhage; *ARDS*, acute respiratory distress syndrome; *ATRA*, all-*trans* retinoic acid; *B*, bronchospasm; *BOOP*, bronchiolitis obliterans organizing pneumonia; *DMD*, diffuse micronodular disease; *EP*, eosinophilic pneumonitis; *H*, hypersensitivity lung reaction; *IP*, interstitial pneumonitis; *PE*, pulmonary edema (noncardiogenic); *P Eff*, pleural effusion; *PF*, pulmonary fibrosis.

Table 59.2 Noncytotoxic and Other Drugs

	Recorded Cases or Incidence	Mortality	Clinical/Pathologic Syndromes
Nitrofurantoin	>500 adult >10 pediatric	8% (chronic exposure)	H, IP/PF, B, AH, P Eff, BOOP, GIP
Sulfasalazine	>50 adult	a	H, EP, IP/PF, BOOP, FA, B
Mesalazine	>40 adult 8 pediatric	a	H, EP, IP/PF,G
Diphenylhydantoin	>5 adult >5 pediatric	0	H, B, BOOP
Carbamazepine	>10 adult >10 pediatric	0	H, IP/EP, B, BOOP
Levetiracetam	2 adult 1 pediatric	0	IP
Minocycline	>50 adult and adolescent	a	EP
Penicillamine	>40 adult 1 pediatric	50% (AH, BO)	H, DA, BOOP, AH
Leflunomide	>40 adult	20%	IP, DAD
Azathioprine	>15 adult 1 pediatric	12%	H, AH, IP, DAD, BOOP
Amiodarone	5% 4 pediatric	10% 50% for ARDS	H, EP, IP/PF, BOOP,P Eff, AH, ARDS
HMG-CoA reductase inhibitors (statins)	>15 adult	25%	H, IP/PF
Pegylated interferon	b	7%	IP

[a]Unknown.
[b]Infrequent case reports.
ARDS, Adult respiratory distress syndrome; *AH*, alveolar hemorrhage; *B*, bronchospasm; *BO*, bronchiolitis obliterans; *BOOP*, bronchiolitis obliterans organizing pneumonia; *DA*, diffuse alveolitis; *DAD*, diffuse alveolar damage; *EP*, eosinophilic pneumonia; *FA*, fibrosing alveolitis; *G*, granuloma, nonnecrotizing; *GIP*, giant cell interstitial pneumonia; *H*, hypersensitivity lung reaction; *IP/PF*, interstitial pneumonitis/pulmonary fibrosis; *PE*, pulmonary edema; *P Eff*, pleural effusion.

Pulmonary disease secondary to bleomycin occurs in as many as 40% of patients receiving the drug,[12] and a recent systematic review identified bleomycin exposure (along with alkylating agents) as a significant risk factor for long-term pulmonary toxicity.[13] Forty-one percent of childhood cancer survivors treated with bleomycin had abnormal spirometry (obstructive changes) in a cross-sectional analysis, although only 9% were symptomatic.[14] Multivariate analyses of follow-up data from the multicenter Childhood Cancer Survivor Study indicate that use of bleomycin is significantly associated with lung fibrosis (RR 1.7), bronchitis (RR 1.4), and chronic cough (RR 1.9) ≥5 years postdiagnosis.[15] Bleomycin-induced pneumonitis may be diagnosed years after its use, as reported in a 15-year-old girl who had received bleomycin as an infant for yolk sac carcinoma.[16] Significant lung damage rarely occurs in adults at cumulative doses less than

150 mg. When more than 283 mg/m^2 is administered, 50% of adult patients develop severe pneumonitis.[17] Pulmonary damage is more severe in elderly than in young patients and in those with reduced glomerular filtration rate.[12] Slow intravenous administration results in less lung disease than intramuscular injection or intravenous bolus. The combination of radiotherapy or high inspired oxygen concentrations and bleomycin produces more lung injury than either alone. Pulmonary toxicity associated with relatively small quantities of bleomycin has been reported during combination drug therapy,[18] and pediatric sarcoma or Hodgkin disease patients receiving bleomycin have increased risk for radiation pneumonitis.[19]

Pulmonary injury due to bleomycin occurs by direct injury to cells as well as by secondary immunologic reactions. Direct toxicity may be mediated by oxidant injury, either through the production of reactive oxygen metabolites or through inactivation of antioxidants. Data supporting this mechanism include the findings that pretreatment of rodents with antioxidants, or upregulation of the antioxidant gene transcription factor Nrf2, can reduce subsequent bleomycin-induced pulmonary fibrosis.[20–22] Additionally, bleomycin may directly induce senescence or apoptosis of type II epithelial cells.[23–25] Bleomycin also generates production of inflammatory mediators by lung cells,[26–31] and inflammatory cells may participate in further oxidant and proteolytic damage to lung cells.[32] Bleomycin promptly increases collagen synthesis by fibroblasts, an effect which may be mediated by transforming growth factor-β.[33] Anti-inflammatory agents, antioxidants and, specifically, nebulized heparin or urokinase can inhibit bleomycin-induced lung damage in animal models.[34,35] Gunther and colleagues[36] have reported complete abrogation of bleomycin-induced pulmonary fibrosis in rabbits using nebulized heparin or urokinase.

Bleomycin-induced lung disease can begin insidiously, and asymptomatic patients may have decreases in arterial oxygen saturation and carbon monoxide diffusing capacity (DL$_{CO}$). As the illness progresses, there is a decline in vital capacity and total lung capacity, which is characteristic of restrictive lung disease. In both interstitial pneumonitis and hypersensitivity lung reactions, patients typically present with a dry hacking cough and dyspnea; these signs occur only on exertion in mild cases, but profound respiratory distress accompanies advanced illness. Fever suggests a hypersensitivity reaction. Physical examination reveals tachypnea and fine crackles. Chest radiographs in symptomatic patients most commonly demonstrate diffuse linear densities. A widespread reticulonodular or alveolar pattern may also be seen. Chest CT is more sensitive for detection of early interstitial disease, and in animal models, chest CT findings correlate well with pathologic changes.[37,38] Biopsy specimens usually reveal interstitial pneumonitis, fibrosis, and extensive alveolar damage with hyperplasia of type II cells, which are most prominently in subpleural and basilar regions.

Patients receiving bleomycin should be monitored by serial determinations of DL$_{CO}$. Chest CT may also be useful for monitoring progression of disease, although the radiation exposure from this source cannot be ignored.[38] Therapy of bleomycin-induced pneumonitis consists largely of supportive measures. Withdrawal of the drug at the onset of toxicity must be considered. Careful monitoring of oxygen therapy to avoid excessive exposure is imperative.[39] Although

the inflammatory cell element resolves substantially with therapy, much of the fibrotic damage is irreversible. Treatment with bleomycin is a significant predictor of long-term respiratory symptomatology and pulmonary function decrements in survivors of Hodgkin disease.[40] Use of steroids is controversial, but reversal of severe toxicity has been documented in some patients after use of high-dose steroids.[41] In the few patients exhibiting hypersensitivity reactions or eosinophilic pneumonitis with bleomycin,[42] corticosteroids have a definite role.

ALKYLATING AGENTS

Cyclophosphamide

Cyclophosphamide is widely used in the treatment of leukemias, lymphomas, and nonmalignant illnesses. Although pulmonary toxicity is uncommon, it does produce severe and even fatal lung damage.[43,44] Data from the Childhood Cancer Survivor Study indicate a significantly increased long-term risk for supplemental oxygen requirement, recurrent pneumonia, chronic cough, dyspnea on exertion, and bronchitis.[15] Frankovich and colleagues[45] reported a series of 34 children who underwent autologous bone marrow transplant for relapsing Hodgkin disease and were treated with cyclophosphamide in combination with etoposide and either carmustine, chloroethylcyclohexylnitrosourea, or irradiation. Fifteen of these patients developed lung injury syndromes including interstitial pneumonitis, acute alveolitis, diffuse alveolar hemorrhage, acute respiratory distress syndrome (ARDS), and bronchiolitis obliterans. Four of the patients died of pulmonary complications. In this series, a history of atopy was associated with pulmonary complications.

Cyclophosphamide appeared to result in greater pulmonary toxicity than fludarabine in one pediatric series when either agent was combined with busulfan for prehematopoietic cell transplantation conditioning.[46] Experiments in rodents indicate that, as for bleomycin, both oxidant and inflammatory or immune mechanisms are involved in cyclophosphamide lung toxicity.[47–50] Acute IgE-mediated systemic reactions have been reported, including angioedema and bronchospasm. Cyclophosphamide also may predispose to toxicity when medications such as bleomycin, azathioprine, and carmustine are used subsequently.

Little is known regarding the relationship of dose, duration, and frequency of administration to the appearance of parenchymal disease in humans, although cytotoxicity appears to be dose-related in rats.[48] Pulmonary reactions have occurred following total doses between 0.15 and 50 g. Pulmonary disease may begin during cyclophosphamide therapy or weeks to years after.[51,52] A striking feature in pediatric cases has been chest wall deformity secondary to failure of lung growth during the adolescent growth spurt.[52] Subacute dry cough and dyspnea herald the onset of pulmonary toxicity; and then malaise, anorexia, and weight loss follow.[51,53] Physical examination reveals tachypnea and diffusely diminished breath sounds. Chest roentgenograms may show diffuse bilateral infiltrates, sometimes with pleural thickening, and pulmonary function testing reveals hypoxemia and restrictive lung disease. Biopsy and postmortem specimens show interstitial fibrosis, alveolar exudates, and atypical alveolar epithelial cells.[51,53] Withdrawal of the drug, supportive therapy, and corticosteroids are recommended treatment.

Chlorambucil

Chlorambucil is used in the treatment of leukemias, some lymphomas, nephrosis, and inflammatory conditions such as sarcoidosis.[54] Several reports indicate that the drug produces pulmonary toxicity, albeit rarely. Little is known concerning the dose or duration of therapy necessary to produce lung damage. Patients develop cough, dyspnea, fatigue, and weight loss that appear 6 months to 3 years after initiation of therapy and progressively worsen.[55,56] Physical examination reveals tachypnea and fine bibasilar crackles. Chest roentgenograms demonstrate diffuse interstitial infiltrate, and pulmonary function tests indicate restrictive lung disease accompanied by a defect in DL_{CO}. Histopathologic findings are similar to those associated with busulfan and cyclophosphamide therapy.[55,56] Although improvement with discontinuation of the drug and corticosteroid therapy has been reported,[57] progression of disease may occur.[55]

Other Alkylating Agents

Busulfan (Myleran) is used to treat chronic myelogenous leukemia, which occurs occasionally in childhood, and in some preparative regimens for bone marrow transplantation. Four percent of adult patients undergoing long-term treatment with this drug develop interstitial pneumonitis and fibrosis.[58] Mertens and colleagues[15] reported increased long-term risk for supplemental oxygen requirement and pleurisy after busulfan treatment. As with chlorambucil, pulmonary injury is usually not evident for many months after initiation of treatment, and radiation and previous cytotoxic therapy are risk factors.[59] The clinical syndrome is similar to that produced by the other alkylating agents,[58] and the treatment consists of discontinuation of busulfan. Efficacy of corticosteroids is unproven, but a carefully monitored trial is indicated because of the poor prognosis.

An increase in incidence of alveolar hemorrhage has been reported when *etoposide* (VP-16) was added to a regimen of busulfan and cyclophosphamide for bone marrow transplantation; toxicity in this study was largely confined to patients who had been given prior chest radiotherapy.[60] However, Quigley and colleagues[61] found that in children, preparative regimens for bone marrow transplantation that included busulfan were associated with preservation of pulmonary function compared to regimens using other combination high-dose chemotherapeutic regimens or total body irradiation.

Melphalan is used primarily in the treatment of multiple myelomas and hence is employed infrequently in pediatrics. Although overt toxicity is unusual, frequency of epithelial changes and fibrosis at autopsy may be as high as 50%.[62] Bronchial epithelial cell proliferation has been an unusual finding. Otherwise, the pathologic changes are typical for alkylating agents and may be reversible with discontinuation of the drug.[63]

NITROSOUREAS

Carmustine

Carmustine, also called bis-chloroethylnitrosurea (BCNU), is a synthetic antineoplastic compound, and its major use is in the therapy of lymphomas and gliomas. The incidence of BCNU pulmonary toxicity is quite variable; 20%–30% of treated patients develop some lung disease.[64,65] The total dose administered, duration of therapy, and preexistence of lung disease are the most accurate predictors of pulmonary toxicity. Most patients with symptomatic respiratory disease have received large cumulative doses (>777 mg/m²). When the cumulative dose exceeds 1500 mg/m², there is a 50% probability of lung disease. Patients with toxicity also appear to have received the drug over a shorter period, irrespective of the total dose given. The onset of pulmonary symptoms has been noted between 30 and 371 days after institution of therapy, sometimes after BCNU has been discontinued. Young patients are reportedly at greater risk, but this may be the result of relatively higher doses and increased numbers of therapy cycles because of greater general tolerance. Mertens and colleagues[15] reported a significant risk for supplemental oxygen requirement among children ≥5 years status post BCNU or *lomustine* (CCNU) treatment. A study of 73 children with high-grade glioma treated with the combination of BCNU, cisplatin, and vincristine reported that seven children developed interstitial pneumonitis, which was fatal in six children.[66] Radiation therapy may be synergistic. In adult patients, female gender and combination with cyclophosphamide have been identified as risk factors for pulmonary complications.[65,67]

Patients with BCNU pulmonary toxicity exhibit much the same clinical picture as that described for bleomycin.[64] Histologic findings are also similar. In a study of eight patients who underwent lung biopsy 12–17 years after treatment with BCNU, there was electron microscopic evidence of ongoing endothelial and epithelial damage, suggesting long-term toxic effects of the drug.[68] One of these patients died with pulmonary hypertension due to interstitial fibrosis. The disease is fatal in approximately 15% of those affected.

Therapy is essentially supportive. Corticosteroids are often administered concomitantly with BCNU for brain tumors and afford no protection from subsequent pulmonary toxicity. However, corticosteroids may offer some benefit in the treatment of early stages of acute disease. Thymidine has been used as a biomodulator to protect from BCNU pulmonary toxicity in patients with malignant melanoma and may act via modulation of DNA repair enzymes in normal tissue.[69] In a rat model, metallothionein attenuated BCNU toxicity via antioxidant effects.[70]

ANTIMETABOLITES

Methotrexate

Methotrexate (4-aminopteroylglutamic acid) is a folic acid antagonist used in the treatment of several childhood malignancies, notably leukemias and osteogenic sarcoma as well as nonmalignant conditions such as rheumatoid arthritis and psoriasis.[71,72] The lung inflammation induced by methotrexate appears to be linked to activation of the p38 mitogen-activated protein (MAP) kinase signaling pathway with subsequent cytokine activation.[73] Prevalence rates of 0.3%–11.6% have been reported for pulmonary toxicity due to methotrexate, but ascertainment of its effects is complicated by the frequent use of combination therapy and the tendency of underlying diseases such as rheumatoid arthritis to also cause lung disease.[72] No correlation has been found between lung toxicity and dose of methotrexate, and pneumonitis may occur remotely.

The clinical features of methotrexate lung toxicity are consistent with a hypersensitivity pneumonitis.[74] Disease usually begins with a prodrome of headache and malaise and is then followed by dyspnea and dry cough. Pleuritic pain is rare, and fever may also occur. Physical examination reveals tachypnea, diffuse crackles, cyanosis, and occasionally skin eruptions. Hypoxemia is observed in 90%–95% of patients, and mild eosinophilia has been reported in 41%.[72] Few reports have documented pulmonary function changes but decreased DL_{CO} may occur.[75] Lung function testing in a series of children with juvenile rheumatoid arthritis who received methotrexate showed a similar incidence of abnormal function, including DL_{CO}, to a control population not receiving methotrexate.[76] The most common abnormalities on chest radiographs are bilateral interstitial infiltrates or mixed interstitial and alveolar infiltrates. Lung biopsy in adults reveals interstitial pneumonitis with lymphocytic and sometimes eosinophilic infiltrates, bronchiolitis, and granuloma formation consistent with a hypersensitivity reaction, although type II alveolar cell hyperplasia typical of cytotoxicity has also been found.[77,78] BAL fluids typically show lymphocytosis with variable CD4/CD8 ratios and moderate neutrophilia.[79,80]

Diagnosis of methotrexate-induced pneumonitis is difficult because this condition may mimic other diseases. Pulmonary infection must be excluded, particularly if high-dose methotrexate is used or if the underlying disease is associated with immunosuppression. Therapy consists of withdrawal of the drug and administration of corticosteroids, but the latter has not been analyzed in controlled trials. Treatment with folinic acid (leucovorin rescue) does not prevent methotrexate lung toxicity,[72] and the outcome is usually favorable with clinical improvement preceding radiographic and pulmonary function improvement.[72,81] However, two fatal outcomes in arthritis patients with a history of lung toxicity suggest that retreatment should be avoided after recovery from methotrexate lung injury.[82]

6-Mercaptopurine, Cytosine Arabinoside, and Gemcitabine

Scattered case reports have linked pulmonary dysfunction to *6-mercaptopurine* and *cytosine arabinoside* (also known as Ara-C). In addition, an autopsy study of patients who had leukemia and who received cytosine arabinoside within 30 days of death demonstrated significant pulmonary edema for which there was no obvious other explanation in most instances. An adult patient receiving low-dose cytosine arabinoside ($20\ mg/m^2$ per day) and recombinant human granulocyte-macrophage colony stimulating factor (GM-CSF) developed ARDS on day 12 and died 40 days after initiation of therapy.[83] It has recently been reported that 5 of 22 pediatric patients receiving Ara-C ($1.0–1.5\ g/m^2$ per day) for treatment of acute myelogenous leukemia developed pulmonary insufficiency secondary to noncardiogenic pulmonary edema. The outcome was fatal in 3 of 5 patients.[84] Bronchiolitis obliterans organizing pneumonia (BOOP) developed in an adult patient with chronic myelogenous leukemia after treatment with Ara-C in combination with interferon alpha,

and the condition resolved after discontinuation of these agents.[85] Chagnon and colleagues[86] described a series of six young adults with acute myelogenous leukemia who developed fever and diffuse micronodular lung disease associated with high-dose Ara-C. *Gemcitabine*, a similar drug in structure and metabolism to Ara-C, has been associated with ARDS in three patients.[87] These authors reported that corticosteroids and diuretics were helpful, but two of the three patients died. Gemcitabine has also been associated with dyspnea, bronchoconstriction, and nonspecific pneumonitis, particularly in Hodgkin disease patients also treated with bleomycin.[88] The nucleoside analog *fludaribine*, used in treatment of lymphoma and chronic lymphocytic leukemia, is associated with steroid-responsive interstitial disease in 9% of cases.[89]

OTHER CYTOTOXIC AGENTS

Procarbazine, VM-26, and vinca alkaloids (vinblastine and vindesine) have been associated with pulmonary injury, but in all cases, other agents may have contributed. Three of five young adults treated with a regimen of vinblastine, doxorubicin, bleomycin, and dacarbazine for Hodgkin disease, and granulocyte colony stimulating factor (G-CSF) to increase neutrophil counts developed pulmonary toxicity in one report.[18] G-CSF may thus potentiate the lung toxicity of these agents. Reactions to procarbazine have been of the hypersensitivity type. *Hydroxyurea* has been reported to induce severe, corticosteroid-responsive, hypersensitivity pneumonitis.[90] *Paclitaxel* is a plant-derived taxane agent that has been used against a broad range of tumors, including breast, ovarian, lung, head, and neck cancers; and it has been associated with a high frequency of hypersensitivity pneumonitis reactions. Lung biopsy has shown interstitial pneumonitis, and BAL fluid has shown eosinophilia and lymphocytosis with a depressed CD4/CD8 ratio.[91] In a 5-year review of a series of cancer patients who received monthly paclitaxel infusions, the incidence of hypersensitivity reactions was 4%, and pretreatment with dexamethasone, diphenhydramine, and H_2-blockers was effective in preventing recurrence.[92] Interstitial pneumonitis is more common when paclitaxel is combined with radiation therapy[93] and has been reported in association with a paclitaxel-eluting coronary artery stent.[94] *Docetaxel*, a semisynthetic taxane, has been proposed as a safer alternative but has also occasionally been associated with severe hypersensitivity reactions or corticosteroid-responsive interstitial pneumonitis.[95–97] For example, a series of asymptomatic adult cancer patients who received docetaxel monotherapy for nonlung cancers had a small but significant drop in lung function post treatment.[98] *Oxaliplatin* appeared to cause cryptogenic organizing pneumonitis in a 30-year-old being treated for colorectal cancer and has been associated with fatal diffuse alveolar damage in adults.[99,100]

Epidermal Growth Factor Receptor/Tyrosine Kinase Inhibitors

Gefitinib is an inhibitor of the tyrosine kinase activity of the epidermal growth factor receptor (EGFR), and it inhibits the growth of human cancer cell lines expressing EGFR in preclinical studies. In an irradiated rat model, gefitinib treatment augmented lung inflammation but attenuated fibrotic lung remodeling due to the inhibition of lung fibroblast proliferation.[101] In clinical trials in patients with nonsmall cell lung cancer, gefitinib was associated with development of interstitial lung disease in about 1% of patients, and about one third of cases of gefitinib-associated interstitial lung disease have been fatal.[102,103] Patients presented with acute dyspnea with or without cough or fever at a median of 24–42 days after starting treatment. Another tyrosine kinase inhibitor, *imatinib*, is used in treatment of chronic myelogenous leukemia and has been associated with pleural effusion and pulmonary edema in a small number of cases.[104] *Cetuximab* is a monoclonal antibody that specifically binds to EGFR and inhibits its downstream signaling. In a series of 2006 patients with colorectal cancer in a prospective multicenter registry, ranging in age from 18 to 80 years, 1.2% developed diffuse interstitial pneumonitis due to cetuximab.[105] Such drugs targeting specific molecular pathways are likely to be increasingly used in cancer treatment, as well as pulmonary fibrosis, in the future.[106,107]

Interleukin-2 (IL-2) has been used as an antitumor factor that stimulates lymphokine-activated killer (LAK) cell and natural killer cell activity, and it is sometimes given in combination with LAK cells. Although a number of systemic side effects such as fever and hypotension are seen, its major toxicity appears to be a vascular leak syndrome characterized by fluid retention, peripheral edema, ascites, pleural effusion, and pulmonary edema.[108] This syndrome has been described in children with acute lymphocytic leukemia (ALL) treated with IL-2.[109] Infusion of IL-2 in cancer patients has resulted in increased alveolar-arterial oxygen gradients and decreased forced vital capacity (FVC), forced expiratory volume in 1 second (FEV_1), and DL_{CO}.[110,111] A retrospective review of chest radiographic abnormalities in 54 patients with metastatic cancer receiving IL-2 revealed that 52% developed pleural effusions, 41% developed pulmonary edema, and 22% developed focal infiltrates. While most changes resolved by 4 weeks after therapy, residual pleural effusion was sometimes seen, primarily in patients receiving IL-2 by intravenous bolus rather than by continuous infusion.[112] Lung histopathology in rodents that received high doses of IL-2 showed widespread mononuclear and eosinophilic infiltration of parenchyma, increased lung weight, and endothelial damage.[113] Mechanisms implicated are increased generation of oxygen free radicals, activation of complement by IL-2, and injury mediated by tumor necrosis factor (TNF)-α.[114–116] Rapid recovery from toxic effects of IL-2 followed withholding of treatment in most cases.[111]

All-*trans* retinoic acid (ATRA), a vitamin A derivative with multiple regulatory activities in the lung, is effective as induction and maintenance chemotherapy for acute promyelocytic leukemia (APL). Its major toxicity is a syndrome including fever, weight gain and peripheral edema, respiratory distress, interstitial infiltrates, pleural and pericardial effusions, hyperleukocytosis, intermittent hypotension, and acute renal failure. Chest CT shows small, irregular parenchymal lung nodules and pleural effusions.[117] The incidence of ATRA syndrome was 26% in a large series of APL patients followed prospectively,[118] and among patients developing ATRA syndrome, mortality was 2% including a 4-year-old child. Mean duration of therapy before the syndrome appeared was 11 days with a range of 2–47 days. Nicolls and colleagues[119] reported an 18-year-old with APL

who developed diffuse alveolar hemorrhage 15 days after starting ATRA. Lung histology in patients who died of ATRA syndrome showed differentiation of APL cells, endothelial cell damage, and leukocyte infiltration.[118] ATRA may upregulate TNF receptors on lung cell lines.[120] In a murine model of APL, ATRA increased lung and heart expression of chemokines macrophage inflammatory protein 2 (MIP-2) and keratinocyte-derived cytokine (KC), suggesting that proinflammatory cytokines play a role.[121] Treatment for ATRA syndrome consists of prompt initiation of corticosteroids. Tallman and colleagues[118] used dexamethasone 10 mg/day and found that the syndrome resolved rapidly in most patients, even if ATRA was continued. In addition, these authors suggested that ATRA may be safely restarted in most patients once the syndrome has resolved. The cis-retinoic acids used for the treatment of neuroblastoma have not been associated with lung toxicities.

Noncytotoxic and Other Drugs

NITROFURANTOIN

Nitrofurantoin is an antimicrobial agent used for prophylaxis of urinary tract infections. Significant pulmonary reactions are relatively common, and more than 500 cases have been reported, including children (see Table 59.2).[122–128] Pulmonary reactions occur in two distinct clinical patterns. In the more common acute presentation, patients report abrupt onset of fever, cough, and dyspnea within hours to 2 weeks after initiation of therapy. Alveolar hemorrhage has been described in two patients.[129,130] Rash and flu-like symptoms may occur. Diffuse fine crackles and, rarely, wheezes are noted. Bilateral interstitial or alveolar infiltrates with or without pleural effusions are characteristically present, although chest radiographs may be normal. Physiologic abnormalities include hypoxemia, evidence of a restrictive ventilatory defect, and a reduced DL_{CO}. Eosinophilia, leukocytosis, and an elevated sedimentation rate may accompany the reaction. Symptoms and chest radiographic abnormalities usually resolve within several days after withdrawal of the drug. Pulmonary histopathology of the acute syndrome has not been well defined, as patients improve rapidly, making biopsy unnecessary.

In the less common chronic presentation, patients develop insidious onset of cough, dyspnea, and chest pain after months to years of nitrofurantoin therapy.[131,132] Fever may be present, and a lupus-like syndrome has also been reported.[126] Crackles are heard, and diffuse interstitial infiltrates are present on chest radiographs. Pleural effusion is less common than in the acute reaction. Physiologic abnormalities are similar to those found in the acute reaction but are often more severe. Eosinophilia, positive reactions for antinuclear antibodies, and elevated gamma globulin and hepatic enzymes are often found, and significant concurrent hepatic toxicity has been reported.[133] Pulmonary histopathology typically reveals interstitial pneumonitis with variable fibrosis, and chest CT findings vary but may show ground glass opacities.[131,132] Desquamative interstitial pneumonia, BOOP, and giant cell interstitial pneumonia have also been reported on long-term nitrofurantoin therapy.[128,134–137] Treatment includes withdrawal of the drug and supportive measures. Corticosteroids have been used with apparent benefit; however, controlled studies to evaluate efficacy are not available. Resolution of symptoms, physiologic dysfunction, and radiographic abnormalities require weeks to months and may be incomplete. Approximately 8% of adult cases with the chronic syndrome are fatal.

The findings of eosinophilia, elevation of sedimentation rate, and positive antinuclear antibodies support a role for immunologic mechanisms of injury.[138] The drug may also damage the lungs by promoting production of toxic oxygen species.[139–141]

SULFASALAZINE AND MESALAZINE

Sulfasalazine, a combination of 5-aminosalicylic acid and sulfapyridine, is used primarily in the treatment of inflammatory bowel disease. Adverse reactions occur in approximately 20% of recipients, but pulmonary reactions are uncommon; 50 cases were identified in the most comprehensive review.[142–147] Diagnosis can be challenging, because inflammatory bowel disease is at times associated with lung disorders including bronchitis, BOOP, bronchiectasis, nonspecific interstitial pneumonitis, and granulomatous lung disease.[148–152] Patients experiencing drug-related illness report acute onset of fever, cough, dyspnea, and chest pain 1 month to several years into therapy; and fine crackles are usually present. Hypoxemia, eosinophilia, obstructive and occasionally restrictive pulmonary function patterns, and bilateral alveolar densities have been noted. Cytology from BAL fluid has no consistent pattern of cell predominance. Histopathologic lesions include interstitial pneumonitis with or without fibrosis, eosinophilic pneumonia, fibrosing alveolitis, and bronchiolitis obliterans with or without a component of organizing pneumonia. Discontinuation of the drug usually results in resolution of symptoms and radiographic abnormalities in several weeks to months. Corticosteroids may accelerate improvement, although effectiveness is not well established. At least five fatalities have been reported.[146] The mechanism of toxicity is unknown.

Therapy with mesalazine or 5-aminosalicylic acid, an alternative for inflammatory bowel disease that is related chemically to sulfasalazine, has also been associated with pulmonary toxicity; more than 40 cases have been described, including children.[153–157] Symptoms typically include fever, cough, dyspnea, and chest pain recognized 1–6 months into therapy. Eosinophilia is often present peripherally and may be present in BAL fluid. Bilateral densities are present on chest radiographs, and CT scans may show patchy infiltrates, ground glass opacities, or lung nodules. Eosinophilic pneumonia, interstitial pneumonitis, and nonnecrotizing granulomas have been observed on lung biopsy. Symptoms and radiographic changes usually resolve when therapy is discontinued. Consideration of corticosteroid therapy has been suggested in patients with severe disease and those not responding to discontinuation of the medication.

DIPHENYLHYDANTOIN, CARBAMAZEPINE, AND LEVETIRACETAM

The anticonvulsant agents diphenylhydantoin, carbamazepine, and levetiracetam have been associated rarely with acute pulmonary disease as part of a generalized hypersensitivity reaction, including the syndrome of drug reaction with eosinophilia and systemic symptoms (DRESS).[5,158–164] Clinical manifestations include fever, cough, dyspnea, and rash occurring typically 2–8 weeks after initiation of therapy. Facial swelling and lymphadenopathy may be prominent. Crackles and, rarely, wheezes are heard; bilateral interstitial or alveolar infiltrates, sometimes with hilar adenopathy, are seen on chest radiographs. Associated findings include eosinophilia, elevated liver enzymes, hypoxemia with a restrictive pattern of lung function, and reduced DL_{CO}. Cell counts from BAL fluid reveal lymphocyte predominance, and lung biopsy typically shows interstitial pneumonitis, possibly with mild fibrosis, and rarely BOOP.[165,166] Ventilatory failure has been described.[166] Rapid improvement occurs over days to weeks, following discontinuation of the drug, although manifestations may linger with multisystem involvement. Resolution may be hastened by corticosteroid administration. Carbamazepine hypersensitivity has been associated with transient pan-hypogammaglobulinemia[167] and has been implicated in the occurrence of interstitial pneumonitis/eosinophilic pneumonia in an adolescent with cystic fibrosis (CF) on immunosuppressive therapy following lung transplant.[168] Levetiracetam has been associated with biopsy demonstrated diffuse interstitial lung disease in a child.[169]

MINOCYCLINE

Multisystem hypersensitivity with a prominent component of skin rash has been associated with minocycline, often in a pattern consistent with DRESS. More than 50 cases have involved the lung, often in adolescents and young adults treated for acne.[5,170–175] Eosinophilic pneumonia has been suggested by the finding of excess eosinophils in blood and BAL fluid or on lung biopsy. Minocycline-associated lupus has been well described. Infrequently, significant organ dysfunction with or without lung involvement has been reported including hyperthyroidism or hypothyroidism, renal failure, hepatitis, sometimes in an autoimmune pattern, and, rarely, myocarditis.[176–178] Withdrawal of the drug typically prompts improvement, although resolution may require months. Corticosteroids may accelerate improvement and have been used in combination with immunosuppression for autoimmune hepatitis. Hypersensitivity to doxycycline has been implicated in a single case involving respiratory failure.[179]

PENICILLAMINE

Penicillamine, a chelating agent, is commonly used to treat Wilson disease, cystinuria, and lead poisoning and, occasionally, rheumatoid arthritis and primary biliary cirrhosis. A conclusive association of this agent with lung disease is problematic, because similar lung disorders occur in underlying diseases.[180,181] More than 40 cases of penicillamine-associated lung disease are reported, and these cases are primarily in patients with rheumatoid arthritis.[182,183] Several patterns have been described: diffuse alveolitis, hypersensitivity pneumonitis, alveolar hemorrhage with or without associated acute glomerulonephritis (similar to antiglomerular basement membrane disease [Goodpasture syndrome]), and obstructive airway disease characterized pathologically as bronchiolitis obliterans. Duration of therapy before onset of symptoms tends to be short in patients with hypersensitivity reactions (<2 months), intermediate with diffuse alveolitis and bronchiolitis obliterans (3–19 months), and prolonged with alveolar hemorrhage (7 months to 20 years, but typically 2–7 years). Cough and dyspnea develop progressively over several weeks but may begin abruptly in hypersensitivity reactions with hemoptysis. Crackles and, occasionally, wheezes are present. Elevation of erythrocyte sedimentation rate, increased serum IgE, and eosinophilia may be noted. Chest films show diffuse alveolar or interstitial infiltrate, hyperinflation alone, or no changes. Hypoxemia and severe obstructive lung disease are usually identified in patients with bronchiolitis obliterans or restrictive disease in those with alveolitis or hypersensitivity disease. Discontinuation of the drug and corticosteroid therapy is warranted in most cases. Diffuse alveolitis and hypersensitivity pneumonitis generally improve using this approach, although some patients have residual lung disease. Response to corticosteroids alone has been disappointing in most cases of bronchiolitis obliterans and alveolar hemorrhage. Addition of azathioprine or cyclophosphamide in combination with plasmapheresis has been beneficial in several patients with Goodpasture-like syndrome and in a single patient with bronchiolitis obliterans.[183–186]

LEFLUNOMIDE

Leflunomide, an immunomodulatory drug that inhibits pyrimidine synthesis in activated lymphocytes that is used in treatment of rheumatoid arthritis and other autoimmune disorders, has been associated rarely with significant lung injury.[187–203] Injury appears to be more likely in those with underlying interstitial lung disease.[200–203] Presentation typically includes acute onset of cough and dyspnea 12–20 weeks after its introduction (occasionally after its discontinuation) with crackles on exam and bilateral patchy densities on chest radiograph. Ground glass and reticular/interstitial densities are identified on chest CT. The most common histologic abnormalities are diffuse alveolar injury and interstitial pneumonia. Leflunomide should be stopped when injury related to the drug is suspected. Because of its long half-life, some have advocated treatment with cholestyramine, although the benefit of cholestyramine is uncertain.[203,204] Steroid therapy has been recommended; however, effectiveness is unclear. Mortality of nearly 20% has been described.

AZATHIOPRINE

Azathioprine, an immunosuppressive agent used in a variety of conditions including inflammatory bowel disease, autoimmune disorders, and following solid organ transplant, has been implicated rarely in lung injury.[205–213] Fever, cough, shortness of breath, and hypoxemia typically develop within weeks to months of onset of therapy in association with infiltrates on chest imaging. Hemoptysis and a clinical pattern of ARDS have been described and restrictive lung disease and reduced DL_{CO} observed. Histologic patterns identified in the lung have been consistent with hypersensitivity, interstitial pneumonitis, diffuse alveolar damage, and BOOP. Treatment consists of discontinuation of the drug with or without corticosteroids. Most improve relatively quickly, but progressive deterioration and death have occurred in about 12%.

OTHER IMMUNOMODULATORY AGENTS

Drugs targeting or modifying immune pathways are increasingly used for a variety of chronic inflammatory diseases and after transplantation. Most information on pulmonary toxicities of these agents is from adult literature. *Rituximab*, a monoclonal antibody against CD20 expressed on B lymphocytes has been associated with interstitial pneumonitis, including a fatal case in a 10 year old status-post renal transplant.[214,215] Rituximab-associated lung injury (RALI: ground-glass lesions on CT, negative bronchoscopy with BAL and deficit in DL_{CO}) was described in two adolescents with nephrotic syndrome, 14 and 40 days following a single rituximab infusion.[216] Infusion of *alemtuzumab* (Campath), a humanized monoclonal antibody against CD52 expressed on all lymphocytes, as well as some natural killer (NK) cells and monocytes, was associated with severe bronchospasm responsive to steroids in an adult with chronic lymphocytic leukemia.[217] *Cetuximab*, an anti-EGFR monoclonal antibody, caused dyspnea with infusion in 13% of adult colorectal cancer patients.[218] *Trastuzumab*, a humanized monoclonal antibody against the EGFR, has become standard treatment of HER2-expressing breast cancer. Acute interstitial pneumonitis developed after its infusion in a 56-year-old.[219] *Infliximab* (Remicade) is a TNF-α inhibitor used in treatment of rheumatic and inflammatory bowel disease at all ages. Acute interstitial pneumonitis and respiratory failure has been reported in association with infliximab.[220,221] The calcineurin inhibitor *tacrolimus* has been associated with interstitial lung disease in adult rheumatologic patients, where it is often seen in the setting of preexisting chronic lung disease and has a high mortality.[222] Chronic use of *sirolimus* (rapamycin), an immunosuppressive agent used as an alternative to calcineurin inhibitors, has been associated with interstitial pneumonitis or BOOP in adults after renal transplant[223] and children following hematopoietic stem cell transplant.[224] Standard treatment for hepatitis C in children and adults is a combination of *pegylated interferon* and ribavirin. Interstitial pneumonitis with 7% mortality was reported in adult patients treated with peg interferon α-2β for hepatitis C.[225]

AMIODARONE

Amiodarone, a benzofurane derivative with Class III antiarrhythmic activity, is used in the treatment of serious ventricular and supraventricular tachyarrhythmias.[226,227] Pulmonary toxicity is one of the most significant complications of therapy and develops in about 5% of patients.[227–231] Most affected patients have been adults; however, lung toxicity has been reported in at least four children.[232–235] The risk of lung toxicity appears to be dose related; for example, approximately 5%–15% of patients who take ≥500 mg/day and 0.1%–0.5% of those who take up to 200 mg/day develop drug-related lung disease.[230] Onset of symptoms is often insidious, but symptoms can be acute and rapidly progressive with alveolar hemorrhage or the development of ARDS.[236] Risk for ARDS may be increased by exposure to high concentrations of inspired oxygen, cardiothoracic surgery, or iodinated contrast media.

In the more common subacute presentation, patients insidiously develop nonproductive cough, dyspnea on exertion, weight loss, weakness, and in some instances, pleuritic chest pain and fever, usually during the first year of therapy. Approximately one-third of the patients have an acute onset of symptoms more consistent with hypersensitivity pneumonitis. Chest examination reveals tachypnea, crackles and, occasionally, a pleural friction rub. Physiologic abnormalities include hypoxemia, restrictive lung disease, and impaired diffusion. Predominance of cell type on cytology of bronchoalveolar fluid is variable.[237] Diffuse or asymmetrical interstitial or alveolar infiltrates are typically present on chest x-rays. Chest CT shows bilateral involvement with ground-glass or reticular opacities often in the upper lobes or periphery of the lung bases, wedge-shaped consolidations, or nodules and may show pleural effusion or thickening.[227,238]

Amiodarone interferes with movement of phospholipid across intracellular membranes and reduces phospholipid catabolism by inhibition of lysosomal phospholipase.[239] The drug accumulates in structures such as macrophage lysosomes, leading to the recovery of 'foamy' macrophages in BAL fluid that are indicative of "amiodarone effect" (not toxicity) and may accumulate in type II pneumocytes and interstitial cells, interfering with gas exchange and causing a reduction in diffusing capacity that may be asymptomatic in patients with otherwise healthy lungs.[227,240] Among those manifesting subacute symptoms, patterns of abnormalities identified on lung biopsy include eosinophilic pneumonia, nonspecific interstitial pneumonitis with or without fibrosis, chronic organizing pneumonia (BOOP), and rarely nodular lung disease.[230,231,241,242]

Discontinuation of the drug results in gradual symptomatic improvement in most patients and resolution of physiologic and radiographic abnormalities over several months. Clinical evidence supports corticosteroid treatment, particularly for more advanced disease. Recurrence of symptoms was observed in some patients as steroid doses were tapered, potentially related to extended storage of drug in the lung. Alternative approaches for patients who must remain on amiodarone because of life-threatening refractory dysrhythmias are limited. Reinstitution of amiodarone therapy at lower doses after resolution of pulmonary disease, alone or in combination with low-dose corticosteroid therapy, has been successful in a few patients.[243]

Mechanisms that may contribute to lung injury include direct cytotoxic effects on type II pneumocytes and other lung parenchymal cells, immune mediated injury, and injury related to activation of the angiotensin enzyme system leading to apoptosis of alveolar epithelial cells.[227,244-253]

HYDROXYMETHYLGLUTARYL COENZYME A REDUCTASE INHIBITORS

Hydroxymethylglutaryl coenzyme A (HMG-CoA) reductase inhibitors or statins, widely used in the treatment of hypercholesterolemia, have been rarely associated with lung disease heralded by onset of dry cough, dyspnea and bilateral infiltrates, often with ground glass changes on chest CT, after months to years of treatment.[254-258] When measured, lung function has shown a restrictive pattern with reduction in DL_{CO}. In a few cases, BAL fluid or tissue from lung biopsy has been demonstrated to contain "foamy" alveolar macrophages reminiscent of those in the BAL fluid of patients on amiodarone, which is considered indicative of so-called phospholipidosis.[256,258] Discontinuation of the drug and, in some cases, use of corticosteroids have been associated with resolution of symptoms, although mortality of about 25% is described.

Other Agents

A number of other drugs have been implicated sporadically in the development of hypersensitivity/eosinophilic lung disease. Table 59.3 shows a representative list with a focus on medications that may be given to children or adolescents,[259-284] and an extensive compilation has been published by Allen.[259] Eosinophilic granulomatosis with polyangiitis (asthma, eosinophilia, neuropathy, pulmonary infiltrates, and sinus disease) has been linked with *leukotriene antagonists* in a small number of asthma case reports, including some in children.[272-274] *Aspirin* and other nonsteroidal anti-inflammatory drugs (NSAIDs) induce bronchoconstriction via altered leukotriene metabolism in patients with aspirin-exacerbated respiratory disease, a syndrome of chronic sinusitis, nasal polyposis, and often severe asthma.[285-287]

Drugs producing a clinical syndrome consistent with noncardiogenic pulmonary edema are listed in Table 59.4, as reviewed by Lee-Chiong and Matthay and others.[288-304] Some are associated with this clinical syndrome only after an overdose. Pulmonary edema is the pattern of injury most closely associated with heroin overdose.[305] Smoking of *crack cocaine* can be associated with acute respiratory illness including direct thermal injury to airways and air leak syndromes, and it is also associated with subacute syndromes including pulmonary edema, "crack lung" (pleuritic chest pain, dyspnea, hypoxia, diffuse alveolar damage, alveolar

Table 59.3 Additional Drugs Associated With Hypersensitivity/Eosinophilic Lung Disease

Penicillins	Para-aminosalicylic acid	Ranitidine
Erythromycin	Isoniazid	Lansoprazole
Clarithromycin	Cromolyn sodium	Dantrolene
Cephalosporins	Zafirlukast[a]	Chlorpropamide
Imipenem/cilastatin	Montelukast[a]	Hydralazine
Sulfa-containing antibiotics	Methylphenidate	Enalapril
	Imipramine	Captopril
Fluoroquinolones	Duloxetine	Cocaine
Nebulized colistin	NSAIDs[b]	Heroin
Tetracycline	Trazodone[c]	
Daptomycin		

[a]Associated with eosinophilic granulomatosis with polyangiitis syndrome.
[b]Nonsteroidal anti-inflammatory drugs including naproxen, sulindac, piroxicam, fenbufen, diclofenac, ibuprofen.
[c]With overdose.

Table 59.4 Noncytotoxic Drugs Associated With Noncardiogenic Pulmonary Edema

Aspirin[a]	Lidocaine	Tocolytic agents
Ibuprofen	Naloxone	Haloperidol
Propoxyphene[a]	Nitric oxide	Phenothiazines
Calcium channel blockers[a]	Morphine	Tricyclic antidepressants[a]
	Heroin[a]	Hydrochlorothiazide
Propranolol	Methadone[a]	Acetazolamide
Epinephrine	Cocaine	Radiographic contrast media
Phenylephrine		

[a]Pulmonary edema associated with overdose.

hemorrhage), interstitial pneumonitis, or BOOP.[305–308] *Cannabis* smoking can be associated with chronic bronchitis or emphysematous changes with secondary pneumothorax.[309] For both crack cocaine and cannabis, the tendency for air leak is likely related to deep inhalation with Valsalva maneuver to increase drug absorption. Intravenous injection of crushed tablets of methadone, analgesics like acetaminophen/hydrocodone, and other medications has been associated with dyspnea, pulmonary hypertension, and even sudden death related to microembolization of particles of excipients (filler materials used during production of tablets like talc, microcrystalline cellulose, crospovidone, and starch).[310,311] Diffuse nodular changes on chest imaging and angiogranulomatous changes often with demonstration of excipients on lung histology are characteristic. Intravenous injection of crushed methylphenidate has been associated with a distinctive radiographic pattern of predominantly basilar panlobular emphysema.[310,312–314] While the incidence of venous thrombosis and pulmonary embolism is relatively low in childhood, *oral contraceptives*, the antipsychotic drugs *clozapine* and *olanzapine*, and *intravenous immunoglobulins (IVIG)* are used in children and are associated with increased risk.[315–318]

Conclusion

Lung injury caused by pharmacologic agents is recognized increasingly as a significant clinical problem. Lung disease caused by cytotoxic agents is particularly troublesome and survivors of childhood cancer should be followed carefully for chronic pulmonary toxicity. Precise information about risk factors, including genetic predisposition, is required to bolster predictive capabilities for patients using these drugs. Additional information is needed regarding mechanisms of injury to develop more specific interventions. Finally, more sensitive and widely available diagnostic and monitoring approaches are important if early intervention is to be of value.

References

Access the reference list online at ExpertConsult.com.

Suggested Reading

Dimopoulou I, Bamias A, Lyberopoulos P, et al. Pulmonary toxicity from novel antineoplastic agents. *Ann Oncol.* 2006;17:372–379.

Kano Y, Shiohara T. The variable clinical picture of drug-induced hypersensitivity syndrome/drug rash with eosinophilia and systemic symptoms in relation to the eliciting drug. *Immunol Allergy Clin North Am.* 2009;29:481–501.

Kubo K, Azuma A, Kanazawa M, et al. Consensus statement for the diagnosis and treatment of drug-induced lung injuries. *Respir Investig.* 2013; 51:260–277.

Landier W, Armenian SH, Lee J, et al. Yield of screening for long-term complications using the children's oncology group long-term follow-up guidelines. *J Clin Oncol.* 2012;30:4401–4408.

Liles A, Blatt J, Morris D, et al. Monitoring pulmonary complications in long-term childhood cancer survivors: guidelines for the primary care physician. *Cleve Clin J Med.* 2008;75:531–539.

Masson MJ, Collins LA, Pohl LR. The role of cytokines in the mechanism of adverse drug reactions. In: Uetrecht J, ed. *Adverse Drug Reactions, Handbook of Experimental Pharmacology.* Berlin, Heidelberg: Springer-Verlag; 2010:195–231.

Taylor AC, Verma N, Slater R, et al. Bad for breathing: a pictorial of drug-induced pulmonary disease. *Curr Probl Diagn Radiol.* 2016;45:429–432.

Miscellaneous Disorders of the Lung

60 Pulmonary Embolism and Thromboembolic Disease

PETER MICHELSON, MD, MS, and JAMES KEMP, MD

Epidemiology

It is widely appreciated that the timely recognition of pediatric pulmonary thromboembolism (PTE) continues to lag despite recent strong efforts to broaden our understanding of thrombotic complications in children.[1,2] Agreement on standardized treatment algorithms has been delayed by limited prospectively obtained clinical evidence, limited acceptance by some that the incidence is increasing and limited evidence for independent risk factors for PTE among hospitalized patients. These factors, combined with the presumably low incidence of PTE in children compared to adults and the lack of evidence that PTE are preventable,[3] have slowed the development of guidelines on PTE diagnosis and prevention.[4]

A related explanation may be that PTE has been rarely recognized as the primary explanation for death in pediatric patients. An old review of over 46,000 "routine" pediatric autopsies found "fatal" pulmonary emboli in 2.7%, and many of these cases dated from the preantibiotic era when deep and untreated infections were common, resulting in thrombophlebitis and septic emboli.[5]

Occasionally, children dying from other fatal diseases are found to have clots in their lung tissue, but these are rarely assigned a primary role in the child's demise. However, as more children survive with support from an indwelling central venous line (CVL), an understanding of the potential significance of multiple, though smaller, PTEs must be developed. The importance of fatal PTE is beginning to be recognized by forensic pathologists confronted with a child dying suddenly and unexpectedly.[6] In addition, it is now accepted that previously, presumably, healthy children with unrecognized inherited thrombophilia, as well as children and adolescents with systemic lupus erythematosus (SLE) or malignancies are at small but unequivocal risk for PTE.[7,8]

The age distribution of pediatric PTE shows bimodal peaks, in infancy and adolescence.[8,9] The presence of a CVL is consistently recognized to play a critical role in PTE development, most commonly in the upper circulation (superior vena cava [SVC] and right atrium). Among both outpatients and inpatients, PTE is also often associated with clotting dysfunction defined as inherited thrombophilia; among inpatients, acquired and inherited thrombophilia contribute to venous thromboembolism (VTE) in general, especially among children with sepsis and myeloproliferative neoplasms.

In adults, the age-adjusted annual incidence of PTE is 10–20 per 10,000[8]; in pediatrics, the annual incidence is estimated to be 0.14–0.49 per 10,000.[7] Among sick newborns with CVL, the prevalence of deep vein thrombosis may be 80% or higher, but the incidence of clinically significant PTE is unknown.[10–12] The overall incidence cited for PTE among hospitalized pediatric patients is 0.86–5.7 per 10,000 patient years.[10,12] It should be emphasized that these incidence rate estimates are from retrospective reviews of data collected from many centers with variable propensities to consider the diagnosis of PTE. Data on the incidence of PTE in *prospective* studies are scarce, even among high-risk populations.

Adults with chronic thromboembolic disease of the lungs are at risk for pulmonary hypertension from nonlethal emboli showering the pulmonary arterial circulation. Pulmonary hypertension as a manifestation of chronic PTE is not often recognized in pediatric patients, either in published reports or from our personal experience. Perhaps this is because chronic PTE are rare, or, more likely, because more attention is paid to the higher pulmonary vascular resistance that occurs in the context of congenital cardiovascular malformations causing pulmonary overperfusion or to the effects of alveolar hypoxia in children with advanced lung disease who are often also supported with a CVL.

Etiology

One of the dicta regarding PTE in pediatric patients is that there is nearly always an explanation in up to 90% of cases,[10] in contrast with adults where up to 30% of PTE are labeled idiopathic. In children, immobility leading to peripheral DVT is less often invoked than in adults, perhaps because they are less often immobile. After serious trauma involving the spine or lower extremities,[3] and after orthopedic surgery, pediatric patients, particularly adolescents, develop PTE, and advice regarding routine care for these patients often includes, for example, pressure dressings for at-risk lower extremities.[13]

As in adults, DVT and PTE have been linked to estrogen and progesterone use in patients 18 and younger. Injectable medroxyprogesterone and contraceptive patches are associated with an increased risk for eventual DVT.[14]

Adults who are obese (body mass index [BMI] > 30 kg/m²) have a twofold increased risk for having PTE. Since 17% of children in the United States have a BMI greater than 95%,[15] one would expect increased occurrence of PTE in these patients, but limited data exist, linking the obesity epidemic to more PTE in patients less than 18 years old, and the strength of the expected association is not yet clear.[16] Prospective studies are needed in obese pediatric patients evaluating additional antecedent risk factors, such as established deep vein thrombosis or inherited thrombophilia, and these studies would serve to clarify an appropriate index of suspicion, particularly in obese adolescents.

Table 60.1   Risk and Etiologic Factors in the Pathogenesis of Pulmonary Thromboemboli in Childhood and Adolescence

Congenital heart disease	Central intravenous line (CVL)
Contraceptive treatment with estrogen and medroxyprogesterone	Cancer (acute lymphoblastic leukemia, in particular, and treatment with L-asparaginase)
Inherited thrombophilia	Deep soft tissue or bone infection with septic thrombophlebitis
Obesity	Longer hospital stay
Systemic lupus erythematosus	Orthopedic and spinal surgery
Vascular malformations	Trauma with immobilization

AGE-SPECIFIC ETIOLOGIES

Although there are overlaps, the recognized etiologies are somewhat different along the bimodal age distribution of pediatric PTE.

Among *infants*, two etiologic factors in the pathogenesis of PTE are particularly noteworthy, congenital heart disease and the CVL (Table 60.1). With increasing long-term survival of infant born before 28 weeks gestation and of infants with abdominal surgical problems, CVLs reaching into the SVC or right atrium are a mainstay of supportive care. The rate of clinically apparent thrombotic complications from CVL in preterm infants is not clear, however, as it is difficult to make an accurate estimate because of the complexity and acuity of these extremely low gestational age newborns. One review contends that frequent PTE among preterm infants makes them the most commonly affected pediatric age group.[8] It is our impression that there is a wide difference among newborn intensive care units in the practitioners' index of suspicion for PTE.

Adolescents, because they are at risk for serious physical trauma and resultant immobility, are at particular risk among pediatric patients for the same types of DVT leading to PTE as adults. Children older than 2 years, and adolescents in particular, are much more likely to have surgery for scoliosis and other skeletal deformities,[13] with the types of skeletal manipulation and immobility that lead to DVT and PTE in adult patients.

INHERITED AND ACQUIRED THROMBOPHILIA

A variety of clotting abnormalities broadly designated as thrombophilias are particularly important to consider when confronted with a child or adolescent with PTE. While PTE does occur without clotting abnormalities, inherited thrombophilia should be considered as an additional "prothrombotic risk factor," especially when patients have a CVL for treatment of a malignancy.[17] Furthermore, inherited thrombophilias are more commonly found when thrombosis and PTE occur in otherwise healthy children. When studied, genetic thrombophilia traits have usually been shown to be associated with increased risk for VTE, with an adjusted odds ratio of 2.63 for clotting Factor II deficiency and up to 9.44 for antithrombin deficiency among previously healthy children with obvious and severe PTE.[18]

Inherited thrombophilias include genetic mutations altering the amount or function of a protein controlling the coagulation system. Gain-of-function mutations include genes controlling Factor V (Leiden) and prothrombin gene 20210. Relatively frequent loss-of-function mutations causing thrombophilia affect antithrombin, protein C, and protein S. Pulmonologists should be aware that these mutations are not at all rare in the general population. For example, the prevalence of Factor V Leiden gain-of-function mutations is 2%–7% in the general population.[18]

Evaluation for inherited thrombophilias should be undertaken in consort with a specialist in coagulation who is aware of when the testing will or will not be useful and has ready access to a laboratory skilled in this type of testing. In both children and adults with palliative shunts involving the pulmonary circulation, a patient may have a lifetime need for anticoagulation, and the factors contributing to the PTE are less important. However, among otherwise healthy children who present with PTE, without CVL or known malignancy, testing for hereditary thrombophilia is recommended.[7]

Acquired thrombophilia is a part of the antiphospholipid syndrome complicating SLE, but it also occurs during frank sepsis, during treatment with corticosteroids, and as a complication of nephrotic syndrome and myeloproliferative neoplasms.

DISEASE-SPECIFIC ETIOLOGIES

Other diseases with an etiologic link to embolic phenomena and PTE (see Table 60.1) include nephrotic syndrome,[19] inherited thrombophilia,[17] inflammatory bowel disease,[20] sickle cell-related hemoglobinopathies, both solid and lympho-hematogenous malignancies,[21] vascular malformations including the Klippel-Trénaunay-Weber syndrome,[22] and sepsis with vascular endothelial injury due to thrombophlebitis.[23] These diseases, while more common beyond infancy, have a lesser age-dependent association with PTE.

TREATMENT-SPECIFIC ETIOLOGIES

Females receiving estrogens to prevent pregnancy or to address menstrual problems, or ovarian dysfunction also share risks not found in infants. Concern might be directed toward those who are obese and receiving estrogen for the polycystic ovary syndrome, but published reports have not yet quantified risk in these patients.

Pathology/Pathogenesis

When death is attributed to PTE, the gross pathology is that of a clot, often twisted and branched, which **occludes** a large pulmonary artery. Very large clots can cause acute right heart failure. In adults, however, fatal PTE are macroscopic, yet not necessarily critically occlusive, and are believed to cause circulatory collapse, most likely because they elicit release of thromboxane, serotonin, histamine, thrombin, and related vasoactive substances from the vascular endothelium.[24,25]

Very large clots in the pulmonary arterial circulation appear to cause sudden death with inadequate time for lung infarction to develop. The contribution of smaller PTE to nonlethal pulmonary infarction is likely but can only be speculated upon. In children, because deaths are rarely attributed to PTE as a primary cause, it is likely that understanding of the gross "pathology" of PTE in children will depend on imaging studies.[26]

The microscopic picture of a PTE is that of a true thrombus arising in veins elsewhere.[24] The clots are longer and more castlike than the typical arterial thrombus. Thrombi lodging in the pulmonary circulation are composed of platelets in various stages of senescence, red blood cells and white blood cells, in irregular shapes within a fibrin sheath.

In adults, PTE have arisen, most commonly, from thrombi in the venous circulation of the legs and from the pelvic veins during and after pregnancy. In children, trauma and surgery can also give rise to venous thrombi in the lower extremities. More commonly, however, the "upper" circulation is the site of thrombus origin as a complication of a CVL.[1]

Imaging with computed tomography (CT) angiography suggests that segmental pulmonary arteries are the most common final site of PTE in children. In one report, over a third of images diagnostic for a PTE showed it in segmental arteries, followed by lobar and subsegmental arteries. Main pulmonary arteries, the most frequent site of fatal PTE, were the site for nonfatal PTE in only 9% of images.[26]

The classic paradigm for the *pathogenesis of thrombosis* was suggested by Virchow in the 1840s. The causation of thrombi involves (1) *Slowing of blood flow*, (2) *Changes in the vessel wall*, and (3) *"Susceptibilities" arising from the blood itself.*[24] Virchow's triad still seems to be useful, and the venous circulation is a low-velocity system whose blood velocity is very sensitive to diminished cardiac output and the depth of breathing. Veins are relatively easily compressed during times of muscular inactivity. Unlike arterial atheromas, venous thrombi are often associated with demonstrable injury to the vascular intima. Changes in the venous wall can be induced, of course, by in-dwelling CVL, accidental or surgical trauma, and, primarily in the preantibiotic era, deep soft tissue or bone infections leading to septic thromboemboli. In children, developmental changes in the propagation of thrombi[27,28] and inherited or acquired thrombophilias, described above and discovered over the last 30 years, would seem to qualify as "susceptibilities" in the blood itself predicted by Virchow over 150 years ago.

Clinical Features

It is likely that PTE is much more common than currently recognized. In our experience, PTE is rarely considered in pediatrics unless an at-risk patient has a sudden and severe worsening of his/her respiratory status, for example, a patient with lupus erythematosus. Clinicians rarely consider PTE as an explanation for gradual clinical decline. In an era when most patients with severe diseases are surviving, autopsies are less common than in times past. Except in those fatal instances of large, central clots, the absence of standard interpretive criteria undermines our ability to define whether smaller PTE seen at postmortem is incidental or instrumental in contributing to the child's death.

Among adults and older pediatric patients able to articulate their symptoms, clinicians often recognize PTE symptoms retrospectively after diagnostic CT imaging. The symptoms are nonspecific, a "sense of unease," and dyspnea. Pain is relatively late and occurs when the PTE causes significant

ischemia or infarction to lung tissue close to the pleura. Though the pain is most often pleuritic, in adults, it is frequently first attributed to myocardial ischemia. In one series incorporating CT pulmonary angiography for patients aged 4 months to 18 years suspected of having a PTE, 52% described pleuritic pain, but pleuritic pain was equally common among patients suspected of having a PTE but with nondiagnostic CT angiography.[26]

Symptoms eventually linked to PTE in infants and young children are nonspecific, e.g., irritability, poor feeding, and inactivity, and recognized in retrospect in patients with long-standing CVL or solid tumors of the mediastinum.

At all ages, shock, cyanosis, with low SpO$_2$%, and cardiovascular collapse are physical findings consistent with a very large PTE. Other common though nonspecific signs include tachypnea, rapid shallow breathing, and, in small children, chest wall retractions. When pleuritic pain can be described in older patients, physical signs arising from the PTE might include dullness to chest percussion, diminished breath sounds by auscultation, and a pleural friction rub. When diagnosing PTE, two considerations that are of paramount importance in patients of all ages are awareness of the underlying diagnosis and inspection of the patient's extremities for a source of PTE. Finally, although PTE, in general, is rare in children, the prevalence may be as high as 15% among pediatric patients at high risk (see Table 60.1) who also have dyspnea, pleuritic pain, and the other findings of PTE.[26]

Diagnosis and Differential Diagnosis

The differential diagnosis of PTE includes a long list of pulmonary conditions including pneumonia, atelectasis, chest trauma, alveolar hemorrhage, and malignancy. Since all these processes can result in chest pain, dyspnea, hemoptysis, and/or hypoxemia, they all need to be considered as diagnoses.[11] In fact, only relatively large PTEs result in such symptoms, whereas smaller emboli present with more subtle symptoms and less specific clinical features.[7] As a result of the subtlety of the presenting symptoms, a high index of suspicion is critical. In considering PTE, one must also be cognizant of the patient's age, since the recognized occurrence of PTE in childhood is bimodal, as discussed previously.[8]

Infants who present with PTEs have nonspecific symptoms, and the diagnosis is frequently overlooked. As tachypnea and hypoxemia are the primary features of neonatal PTE, the overlap with respiratory distress syndrome, sepsis, birth asphyxia, and congenital heart disease makes confirmation of this diagnosis difficult and affects estimates of incidence rates of PTE in neonates.[29] With younger and more complicated neonates having improved survival, there is an increased use of indwelling catheters that increases the risk of PTE. In addition, increased use of CVL, combined with more awareness, has led to greater recognition of PTE. Central venous catheters and inherited prothrombotic risk factors are the greatest predisposing risk factors for PTE in infants.[30]

In the adolescent age range, the depiction of the presentation and diagnostic criteria of PTE needs revision. Traditionally, presentation with chest pain, dyspnea, and hemoptysis has been described; however, a recent multicenter retrospective review suggests that tachycardia and tachypnea, combined with pleuritic chest pain and dyspnea, are the most common presenting symptoms.[31,32] Additional risk factors identified include obesity, oral contraceptive use, and a history of coagulopathy. Hypercoagulability risk includes rheumatoid disease (e.g., SLE), malignancy and postoperative immobility; nephrotic syndrome and sickle cell anemia were also identified as comorbidities.

In adults presenting with concern for a PTE, clinical prediction rules based on signs, symptoms, and risk factors are frequently used. While these tools are intended to lessen unnecessary testing, no similar tools have been validated for children less than 18 years of age. The Wells criteria[33] were designed to help diagnose PTE in patients with VTE or at risk for VTE; and the revised Geneva score[34] followed to assist in the accuracy of this effort. However, both still have limited sensitivity, especially in children.[35] Neither addresses pediatric-specific concerns, so adult diagnostic criteria are still frequently used, especially in the adolescent age group. Chest radiography, arterial blood gas analysis, and electrocardiography are still encouraged, both to rule out other disorders and to confirm/exclude a PTE.[7] Ultrasonography to assess for deep vein thrombosis is appropriate if suggested by the history or physical examination. Multidetector CT angiography is now the main imaging modality if PTE is suspected.[36]

Imaging

Radiologic imaging is essential in evaluating for PTE in children. Chest radiography alone is of little benefit except to exclude obvious pathology such as pneumonia or a pneumothorax.[8] Nonspecific signs are frequently seen with PTE including parenchymal infiltrates or atelectasis. Multidetector computed tomography pulmonary angiography (CTPA) has become the diagnostic imaging modality of choice with its high sensitivity and specificity, and the apparent sensitivity of this technique yields a truer estimate of childhood PTE incidence rates.[9]

Dual-energy CT scanning shows both anatomical and functional data in a single study. Chest scan times are rapid, sedation is not required except in the youngest patients, and specific techniques can be employed based on age and size to decrease the radiation dosage without compromising the image quality.[26,37] Multiplanar reformatted CT imaging in the sagittal and coronal planes can improve the diagnostic confidence as well as the sensitivity of this technique (Figs. 60.1 and 60.2).[38]

Additional imaging techniques include ventilation-perfusion (V-Q) scanning and magnetic resonance imaging (MRI). While lung ventilation/perfusion scintigraphy was

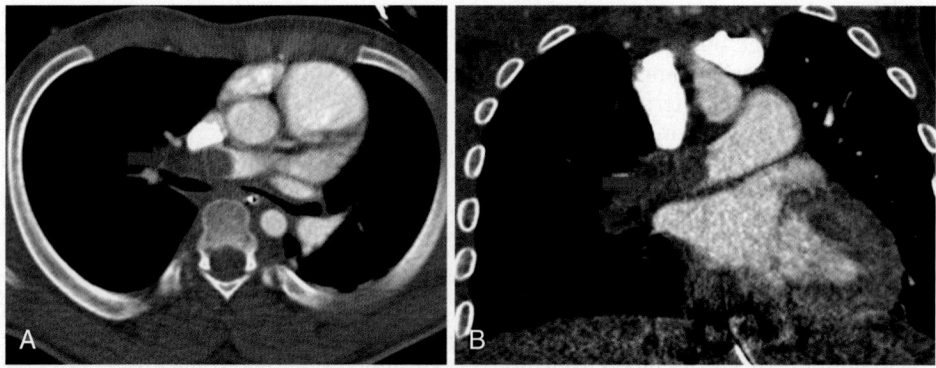

Fig. 60.1 (A) Transaxial computed tomographic pulmonary angiogram image of the chest obtained after administration of intravenous contrast material following a pulmonary embolism protocol. There is a large pulmonary embolism seen within the right main pulmonary artery *(arrow)*. No flow is seen distal to this pulmonary embolism. (B) Coronal computed tomography pulmonary angiogram image of the same area demonstrating a large right main pulmonary artery pulmonary embolism completely occluding the vessel with no contrast distal to the obstruction *(arrow)*.

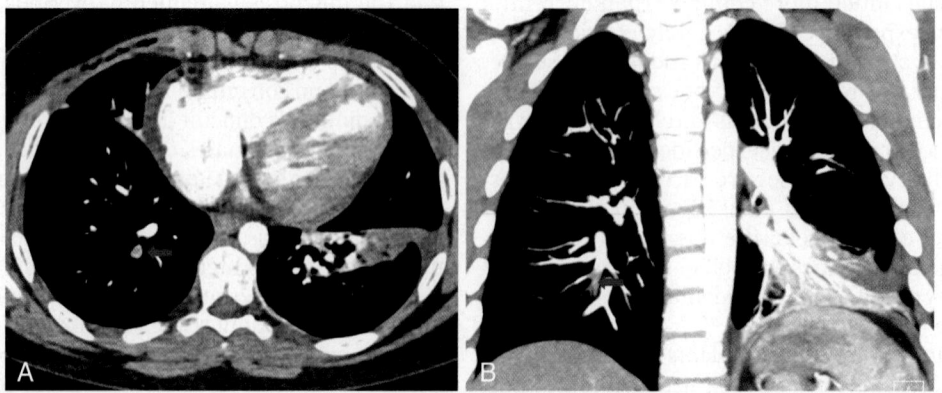

Fig. 60.2 (A) Transaxial computed tomography (CT) image of the chest obtained after administration of intravenous contrast material demonstrating a segmental right lower lobe pulmonary artery embolus *(arrow)*. Additionally, right middle and left lower lobe atelectasis are visualized. (B) Coronal CT image again demonstrating the segmental right lower lobe pulmonary artery embolism *(arrow)* with left lower lobe atelectasis present.

previously the gold standard of imaging,[39] difficulties with image interpretation, often confounded by underlying disease plus reduced specificity, has lowered its usefulness.[40] Although V-Q scanning is easily performed and well tolerated, the limitation of this technique is that most patients will have results that are nondiagnostic.[41] Newer algorithms combining risk factors and V-Q scanning improve the sensitivity; nonetheless, CTPA is still preferred.[42] Limited data, cost, and scanner availability has prevented widespread utilization of MRI in diagnosing PTE. Until more data become available to justify the benefit of MRI, CTPA remain the preferred technique.[43]

Additional Diagnostic Testing

Risk factors for PTE and VTE in children are similar and include venous stasis, endothelial injury, and hypercoagulability. These previously described risk factors are attributed to Virchow (Virchow triad).[44] In children with VTE or PTE, the existence of hypercoagulable states are often not previously established.[17] Although reported rates of inherited prothrombotic disorders vary between neonates and adolescents, a positive family history is associated with an increased odds ratio of a prothrombotic condition.[45] In other studies of VTEs, the prevalence of inheritable prothrombotic conditions were sixfold higher among patients with a spontaneous event compared to children with a known medical condition.[46] Factor V Leiden and prothrombin gene mutations were the most likely causes in those studied.

ULTRASONOGRAPHY

At-risk patients who present with a PTE should have ultrasonographic examination of any affected extremity, as a diagnosis of a deep venous thrombosis (DVT) may indirectly suggest the diagnosis of PTE. While there are many approaches to diagnostic testing, the presence or absence of a DVT via venous ultrasonography does not preclude further examination if clinical evidence is compelling.[47] With limited pediatric data, the prudent clinician should incorporate ultrasonographic examination for DVT if there is a history of central venous access or appropriate clinical context (see Table 60.1).

ECHOCARDIOGRAPHY

There are two clear rationales for echocardiographic evaluation. Echocardiography, either transthoracic or transesophageal, can visualize indirectly associated findings of PTE such as right ventricular dilation, tricuspid regurgitation, or other features of right ventricular dysfunction.[8] Furthermore, imaging of the heart or central pulmonary arteries may directly visualize clots.[7,48] Risk factors associated with poor outcomes in adults that might be identified on echocardiography include free floating right heart thrombi and findings of persistent pulmonary hypertension, right ventricular dilation, and hypokinesis of the septum; and the presence of these findings warrants consideration for embolectomy and/or thrombolysis.[49] Although echocardiography is not sensitive as an imaging modality, it is noninvasive and safe and provides complementary information to assist in the care of the critically ill patient.

PULMONARY ANGIOGRAPHY

Selective percutaneous pulmonary arteriography remains the gold standard for diagnosing PTE. Although not universally available, pulmonary angiography is the most sensitive method for discerning the presence of a PTE. In a large prospective trial of adults with acute PTE, the definitive diagnosis was established with a sensitivity of 96%.[50] Direct signs for PTE include contrast filling defects or nonfilling of pulmonary arteries with abrupt termination of the contrast agent.[11] Even in centers with expertise, bleeding risk and renal insufficiency are relative contraindications. In a large trial, the Prospective Investigation of Pulmonary Embolism Diagnosis (PIOPED), the overall complication rate was 1%, so careful consideration should be associated with a request for pulmonary angiography.[42]

Management

Treatment of PTE in children has followed adult recommendations and has been guided by the child's clinical stability and the relative risks associated with each intervention. Although no severity scoring has been validated in children, therapy is stratified with higher risk patients or symptomatic patients receiving more aggressive care, which is similar to adults. This may include anticoagulation therapy, thrombolysis, inferior vena cava (IVC) filters and/or surgical, or catheter-directed thrombectomy.[40,51] Lower risk patients who demonstrate clinical stability will likely require thrombolytic therapy alone.

Hemodynamically stable patients should receive anticoagulation therapy to prevent extension of the thrombus and the development of recurrence or postthrombotic complications.[11] Before therapy initiation, careful testing for genetic or acquired causes of thrombophilia should be performed. Options for anticoagulation include unfractionated heparin, which is the most frequently used anticoagulant in pediatrics, low-molecular-weight heparin (LMWH), and vitamin K antagonists (warfarin).[8,9] Complications associated with both heparin and LMWH support consideration of early transition to oral therapy with warfarin. Newer anticoagulant drugs, including rivaroxaban, are now available for adult patients with thromboembolic disease, but no pediatric data are available.[52] Although drug level monitoring in children may be difficult, anticoagulant therapy is traditionally recommended for 3 months or longer based on the severity and extent of the lesion.[53] Unfortunately, adherence rates in children are variable with up to one-third of patients being inconsistent with their medication regimen.[54]

In patients with unstable hemodynamics caused by PTE, thrombolytic agents, specifically tissue plasminogen activator (tPA), may be indicated.[8] This may be particularly important in infants in whom plasminogen levels may be reduced. If there are no contraindications (e.g., recent surgery), tPA may be appropriate, especially for catheter-related or localized therapy.[55] Surgical embolectomy or transvenous catheter embolectomy are useful for the unstable individual for whom thrombolysis is unsuccessful or inappropriate. Several techniques are reported including surgical embolectomy on extracorporeal life support (ECLS).[56] Finally, IVC filters may be placed for PTE prevention, but evidence to support their use is limited, and complications and size restrictions have reduced their utilization in children.[57]

Childhood PTE is associated with a mortality of approximately 10% in limited studies,[12,58] but underestimation of incidence rates is likely. Deaths associated with PTE may exceed 10%, but they are most commonly attributed to the underlying diagnosis, where congenital heart disease and malignancy are associated with a worse prognosis. With increasing use of indwelling central venous catheters, the incidence of childhood PTE is likely to increase, as well as consideration of alternative or prophylactic anticoagulant regimens.[8,59]

Prevention

Although VTE prevention and prophylaxis is common in adults, only recently has pediatric VTE prophylaxis become generally recommended.[3] Improved clinical effectiveness has been demonstrated with computerized decision support tools, and these alerts have been shown to sustain their effectiveness over time.[4,60] Utilization of computer-based clinical decision-making systems has been useful both in alerting health care providers of treatment options for acutely symptomatic hospitalized patients and in initiating appropriate preventative care. With a combination of education and electronic medical record (EMR) alerts, a reduction and ultimately prevention of VTE and childhood PTE should be achieved.

References

Access the reference list online at ExpertConsult.com.

Suggested Reading

Antoniou S. Rivaroxaban for the treatment and prevention of thromboembolic disease. *J Pharm Pharmacol.* 2015;67(8):1119–1132.

Mahajerin A, Branchford BR, Amankwah EK, et al. Hospital-associated venous thromboembolism in pediatrics: a systematic review and meta-analysis of risk factors andrisk-assessment models. *Haematologica.* 2015;100(8):1045–1050.

Mahajerin A, Webber EC, Morris J, et al. Development and implementation results of a venous thromboembolism prophylaxis guideline in a tertiary care pediatric hospital. *Hosp Pediatr.* 2015;5(12):630–636.

Shen JH, Chen HL, Chen JR, et al. Comparison of the Wells score with the revised Geneva score for assessing suspected pulmonary embolism: a systematic review and meta-analysis. *J Thromb Thrombolysis.* 2016;41(3):482–492.

Singh RR, Gupte-Singh KR, Wilson JP, et al. Adherence to anticoagulant therapy in pediatric patients hospitalized with pulmonary embolism or deep vein thrombosis: a retrospective cohort study. *Clin Appl Thromb Hemost.* 2016;22(3):260–264.

Stevens SM, Woller SC, Bauer KA, et al. Guidance for the evaluation and treatment of hereditary and acquired thrombophilia. *J Thromb Thrombolysis.* 2016;41(1):154–164.

Tang CX, Schoepf UJ, Chowdhury SM, et al. Multidetector computed tomography pulmonary angiography in childhood acute pulmonary embolism. *Pediatr Radiol.* 2015;45(10):1431–1439.

Thacker PG, Lee EY. Pulmonary embolism in children. *AJR Am J Roentgenol.* 2015;204(6):1278–1288.

Thacker PG, Lee EY. Advances in multidetector CT diagnosis of pediatric pulmonary thromboembolism. *Korean J Radiol.* 2016;17(2):198–208.

Watanabe N, Fettich J, Kucuk NO, et al. Modified PISAPED criteria in combination with ventilation scintigraphic finding for predicting acute pulmonary embolism. *World J Nucl Med.* 2015;14(3):178–183.

Zhang LJ, Lu GM, Meinel FG, et al. Computed tomography of acute pulmonary embolism: state-of-the-art. *Eur Radiol.* 2015;25(9):2547–2557.

61 Diffuse Alveolar Hemorrhage in Children

TIMOTHY J. VECE, MD, MARIETTA MORALES DE GUZMAN, MD, CLAIRE LANGSTON, MD, and LELAND L. FAN, MD

The lungs receive blood from two separate systems: the bronchial circulation and the pulmonary circulation. The bronchial circulation is a high-pressure, low-volume circuit supplied by the bronchial arteries, which vary in number and origin, but most often arise directly from the aorta or one of its branches. These vessels provide blood to the conducting airways from the mainstem bronchi to the terminal bronchioles. Because the bronchial circulation is subject to high pressures, bleeding from this system has the potential to be profuse, sometimes resulting in massive hemoptysis and death.[1-4] In contrast, the pulmonary circulation is a low-pressure, high-capacitance circuit that arises from the right ventricle and provides blood flow to the acinar units involved with gas exchange. Disruption of this system results in alveolar hemorrhage, which is often low-grade, chronic, and diffuse. Although massive hemoptysis is rare, uncontrolled alveolar hemorrhage can be fatal.[3]

Pulmonary hemorrhage arising from either the systemic or pulmonary circulation has multiple etiologies and can be localized or diffuse (Box 61.1). Bleeding from the nasopharynx, oropharynx, or upper digestive tract is common and must be ruled out as a source of "simulated" hemoptysis, or true hemoptysis when the blood is aspirated.[3] Bleeding from the upper airway can occur from intrinsic lesions, such as a subglottic hemangioma or tumor, or from extrinsic causes, such as an inhaled foreign body or intubation.[5-10] Intubation may induce ulceration and granulation tissue formation in the airway wall, which may eventually lead to hemorrhage. More serious iatrogenic causes capable of inducing massive and fatal hemoptysis include erosion of a tracheostomy tube into the aorta or innominate artery, and perforation of the pulmonary artery by a Swan-Ganz catheter.[11-14]

In children with advanced cystic fibrosis, hemoptysis is relatively common because severe, chronic airway inflammation leads to progressive bronchiectasis with increased dilatation and fragility of vessels in the airway walls.[2,9,15,16] Bleeding can also occur with other etiologies of bronchiectasis including primary ciliary dyskinesia and immunodeficiency.[17,18] Infection of the airways or lung parenchyma from viruses, fungi, and bacteria, particularly *Streptococcus pneumoniae* and *Staphylococcus aureus*, is a common cause of hemoptysis in children. In such cases, mechanical trauma from forceful coughing may contribute to bleeding. Finally, factitious hemoptysis should be considered in a child with unusual symptoms and a negative evaluation.

This chapter focuses on diffuse alveolar hemorrhage (DAH) arising from the small vessels of the pulmonary circulation. A cardinal feature of DAH is the presence of hemosiderin-laden macrophages in the acinar units, as macrophages are responsible for clearing free erythrocytes from airspaces. In a simulated alveolar hemorrhage model, hemosiderin-laden macrophages first appeared 3 days following a hemorrhage, peaked at days 7–10 with hemosiderin staining in 60% of macrophages, and continued to be present at 2 months in 10% (Fig. 61.1).[19] The etiology of DAH includes both immune-mediated and nonimmune-mediated disorders (Box 61.2).

Etiology of Diffuse Alveolar Hemorrhage

IMMUNE-MEDIATED ALVEOLAR HEMORRHAGE

A subgroup of children and adolescents with DAH has the pathologic findings of pulmonary capillaritis (PC). Though a histologic diagnosis, PC usually defines an underlying systemic vasculitis or an immune-mediated disease process. PC can occur as an isolated disorder; as part of an antineutrophil cytoplasmic antibody (ANCA)–associated vasculitis; or a systemic disorder, such as systemic lupus erythematosus (SLE). Of the ANCA-associated vasculitides, DAH from PC has been reported in 12%–55% of patients with microscopic polyangiitis[20,21] and in 7%–45% of patients with granulomatosis with polyangiitis (formerly known as Wegener's granulomatosis).[22] In contrast, SLE, a more common disease, has a lower incidence of pulmonary hemorrhage, but the hemorrhage can be life threatening and should be treated aggressively. (See Chapter 58 reviews SLE in detail.) PC also has been reported in Henoch-Schönlein purpura, Behçet's disease, cryoglobulinemic vasculitis, and juvenile idiopathic arthritis.[23,24]

Pathophysiology

ANCA is frequently associated with diseases characterized by the presence of vasculitis, affecting small- and medium-sized vessels. These diseases are associated with circulating autoantibodies directed against the neutrophil granule components, myeloperoxidase (MPO) and proteinase 3 (PR3). In the correct clinical context, the specificity of these autoantibodies for ANCA-associated vasculitides is as high as 98%. This group of disorders includes granulomatosis with polyangiitis, microscopic polyangiitis, and eosinophilic granulomatosis with polyangiitis (formerly Churg-Strauss syndrome). Despite some overlap, PR3-ANCA is particularly associated with granulomatosis with polyangiitis, and MPO-ANCA, with microscopic polyangiitis.[25,26] The primary events in the pathogenesis of these necrotizing vasculitides are not

Box 61.1 Causes of Pulmonary Hemorrhage in Children

Infection
Bronchitis
Bronchiectasis/cystic fibrosis
Primary ciliary dyskinesia
Immunodeficiency
Lung Abscess
Pneumonia
Trauma
Airway laceration
Lung contusion
Artificial airway
Suction catheters
Foreign body
Inhalation injury
Vascular Disorders
Pulmonary embolism/thrombosis
Pulmonary arteriovenous malformation
Pulmonary hemangioma
Coagulopathy
Von Willebrand's disease
Thrombocytopenia
Anticoagulants
Congenital Lung Malformations
Sequestration
Congenital pulmonary airway malformations
Bronchogenic cyst
Miscellaneous
Catamenial
Factitious
Neoplasm
Diffuse Alveolar Hemorrhage Syndromes

Box 61.2 Causes of Diffuse Alveolar Hemorrhage

Immune Mediated

Idiopathic pulmonary capillaritis
Granulomatosis with polyangiitis
Microscopic polyangiitis
Anti-GBM disease
Systemic lupus erythematosus
Henoch-Schönlein purpura
Behçet's disease
Cryoglobulinemic vasculitis
Juvenile idiopathic arthritis
COPA Syndrome

Nonimmune Mediated

Idiopathic pulmonary hemosiderosis
Acute idiopathic pulmonary hemorrhage of infancy
Heiner's syndrome
Asphyxiation/abuse
Cardiovascular causes
Pulmonary vein atresia/stenosis
Total anomalous pulmonary venous return
Pulmonary veno-occlusive disease
Mitral stenosis
Left-sided heart failure
Pulmonary capillary hemangiomatosis
Pulmonary telangiectasia

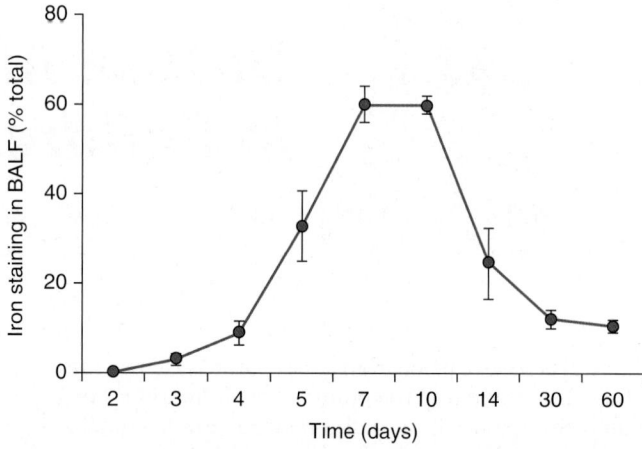

Fig. 61.1 Time course of hemosiderin-laden macrophage production following a single episode of simulated alveolar hemorrhage in mice. *BALF,* Bronchoalveolar lavage fluid. (From Epstein CE, Elidemir O, Colasurdo GN, Fan LL, et al. Time course of hemosiderin production by alveolar macrophages in a murine model. *Chest.* 2001;120:2013-2020, with permission.)

known. Several hypotheses propose that infectious agents trigger and perpetuate such events.[27–30] The presence of these autoantibodies most likely reflects a pathobiological series of events in which neutrophils and monocytes attack the endothelium of small vessels, causing the release of autoantigens with their eventual presentation to the immune system and consequent autoantibody formation. In ANCA-associated vasculitis, it has been shown that autoantibodies to endothelial cell constituents (antiendothelial cell antibodies [AECA]) are commonly produced following the activation and injury of endothelial cells. During this inflammatory attack on the vessel walls, the basal membrane of some vessels also can be damaged and autoantibodies produced to the basement membrane α3 domain of type IV collagen of the pulmonary vessels and glomeruli.[26]

Other autoantibodies have been described in ANCA-associated vasculitis. These autoantibodies are likely related to other factors in the inflammatory cascade and may even be part of an orchestrated attack on the endothelium and basement membrane. They include AECA, antiglomerular basement (GBM) antibodies, antibasal membrane laminin antibodies, and antiphospholipid antibodies (APLA). With the exception of the antibasal membrane laminin antibodies, these autoantibodies are considered to be clinically significant.

Antibodies to constituents of the endothelium are directed to small-vessel endothelial cells, reflecting the typical distribution of such cells in the lungs, nose, and kidneys.[31] An increase in AECA levels has been described in patients with increasing vasculitic activity in idiopathic ANCA-associated and drug-induced vasculitis. An increase of these autoantibodies has been observed in both ANCA-negative and ANCA-positive patients during disease relapse. Levels of ANCA and AECA fluctuate independently as these autoantibodies do not cross-react with the target antigens.[32]

Among patients with anti-GBM disease (also known as Goodpasture syndrome), antibodies to the alpha domain of type IV collagen have been well described. Several groups have found anti-GBM antibodies cooccurring with ANCAs in patients with idiopathic ANCA-associated vasculitis.[33]

Anti-MPO antibodies are the most specific in these patients. Some have proposed that it is essential to test for both types of autoantibodies because the cooccurrence of anti-GBM antibodies and ANCAs may be associated with more severe renal involvement leading to end-stage renal disease and poorer survival.[34]

The presence of APLA, which include anti-beta2 glyco-protein1 antibodies, anticardiolipin antibodies, and the lupus anticoagulant, can be a feature of idiopathic ANCA-associated vasculitis.[35] Several reports have indicated that patients with both ANCA and APLA experience more extensive and more severe disease. In drug-induced vasculitis, APLA of the immunoglobulin M class are more frequently seen. If antihistone antibodies and ANCAs directed to more than one ANCA antigen are found together, a drug-induced condition should be suspected.[36]

Antineutrophil Cytoplasmic Antibody Associated Vasculitis

Granulomatosis With Polyangiitis. Granulomatosis with polyangiitis is a necrotizing vasculitis of the small- and medium-sized blood vessels associated with granulomatous inflammation, which usually affects the respiratory system first and then the kidneys. Upper and lower respiratory manifestations include chronic rhinitis; sinusitis; serous otitis media; nasal cartilage destruction leading to saddle nose deformity; salivary gland swelling, subglottic stenosis, and tracheobronchial ulceration; parenchymal lung nodules or

masses that tend to cavitate; and DAH from PC.[22] Clinically, patients have dyspnea, cough with or without hemoptysis, and hypoxemia. Patients with renal involvement have hematuria and red cell casts. Other affected organs include the eye, heart, gastrointestinal tract, spleen, joints, skin, central nervous system, and pituitary gland.[37–56]

Laboratory evaluation should include a complete blood count (CBC) to identify anemia, erythrocyte sedimentation rate (ESR) and C-reactive protein (CRP) as nonspecific markers of inflammation, and blood chemistries with urinalysis to look for renal disease. Finally, testing for ANCA is essential because the majority of patients will have serum anti-PR3 antibodies (c-ANCA pattern).

Chest radiographs may show impressive nodules or masses with or without cavitation that are disproportionate to respiratory symptoms or pulmonary function studies. Computed tomography (CT) scans of the chest not only better characterize these nodules or cavitary lesions, but also may show diffuse ground glass densities, consolidation related to DAH, or airway abnormalities (Fig. 61.2). Sinus CT is useful in identifying sinus opacification and bony destruction.

Bronchoscopy may identify upper and lower airway lesions including ulceration, granulomata, stenosis, and malacia. In patients with diffuse infiltrates, bronchoalveolar lavage may be overtly bloody and contain red blood cells and hemosiderin-laden macrophages consistent with DAH.

Histopathologic confirmation is still considered the gold standard for the diagnosis of granulomatosis with polyangiitis

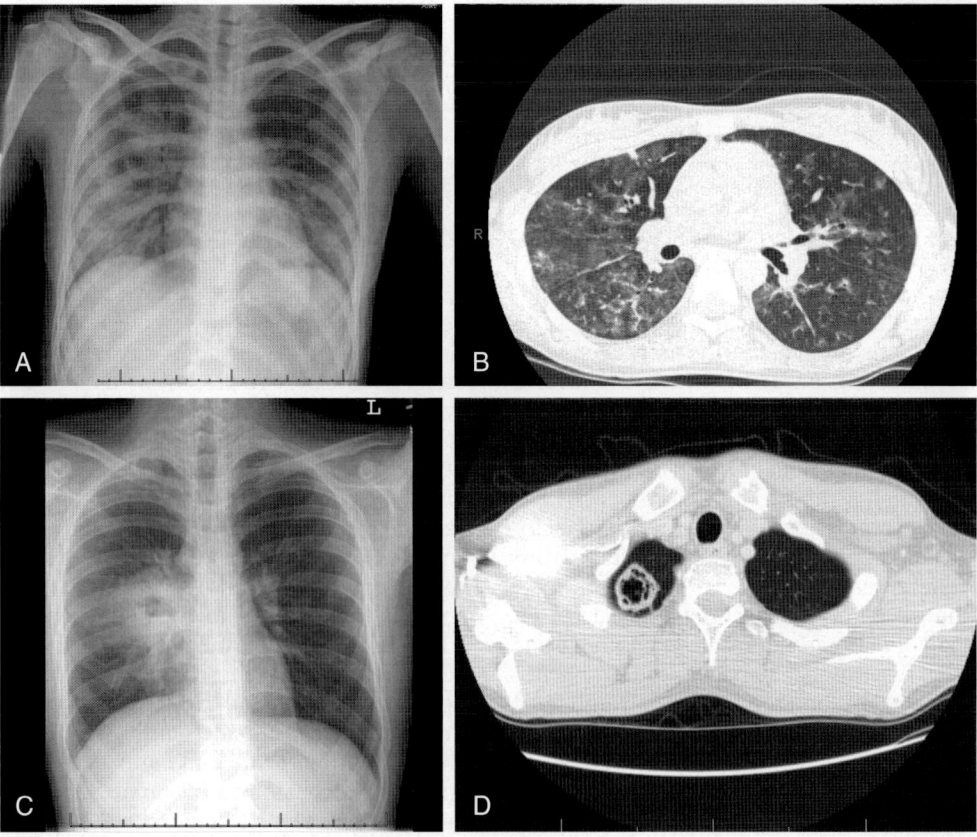

Fig. 61.2 Radiographic findings in granulomatosis with polyangiitis. Radiographic findings in granulomatosis with polyangiitis are variable. Chest x-rays can show diffuse alveolar infiltrates consistent with alveolar hemorrhage (A) with a corresponding chest computed tomography (CT) with diffuse ground glass opacities and septal thickening (B). Alternatively, the chest x-ray can show no evidence of alveolar hemorrhage with cavitary lesions (C). A CT scan in this case will have an absence of ground glass opacities with large cavitary lesions (D).

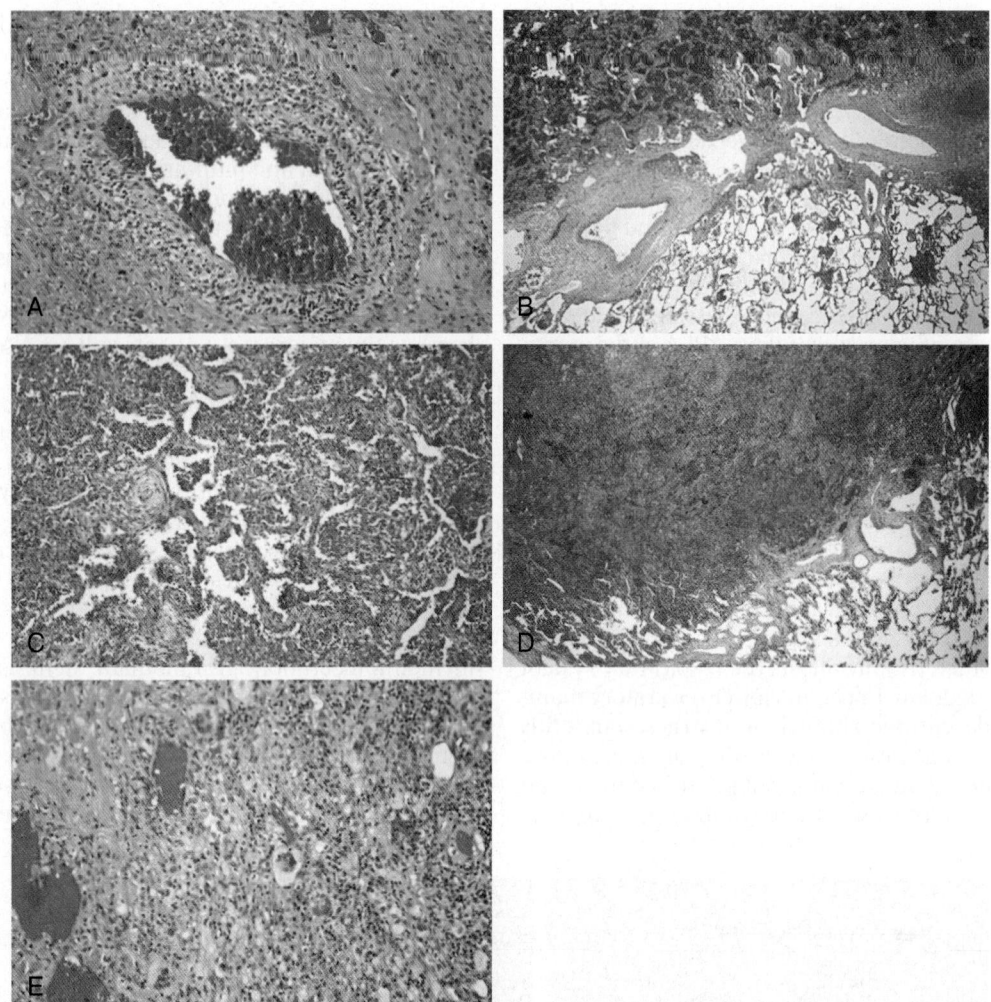

Fig. 61.3 In granulomatosis with polyangiitis, there is vasculitis with parenchymal inflammation and hemorrhage. The vasculitis (A) involves medium-sized and smaller vessels and may be transmural and involve the complete circumference of the vessel as here, or it may involve only a portion of the vessel wall. There may be capillaritis (B) with hemorrhage (C). Necrosis is basophilic due to its neutrophil content, and is geographic (D). There is abundant inflammation with lymphocytes, plasma cells, macrophages, neutrophils, and occasional multinucleate giant cells (E).

in children. Characteristic features include vasculitis of the medium and small vessels and capillaritis associated with necrotizing granulomata (Fig. 61.3). Biopsies from the lung or upper respiratory tract are preferred because of their high sensitivity and specificity. Kidney biopsies typically show segmental necrotizing glomerulonephritis with or without crescent formation, which is nonspecific and can be seen in other immune-mediated renal disorders. However, the paucity of immune complexes is an important characteristic feature of this subset of renal disease.

In 1994, the Chapel Hill Consensus Conference declared that histopathologic documentation of granulomatous involvement of the respiratory tract was not explicitly required to diagnose granulomatosis with polyangiitis.[25] Thus, the diagnosis of granulomatosis with polyangiitis now rests on clinical, serologic, radiographic, and pathologic correlations.

Microscopic Polyangiitis. Microscopic polyangiitis is a small-vessel vasculitis that, in children, appears to be more common than granulomatosis with polyangiitis. The presentation is similar to the other pulmonary-renal syndromes with

hemoptysis, anemia, and new chest x-ray infiltrates in adults. However, hemoptysis is not always present in young children.[4,57] Patients can present with an acute, life-threatening event or with a more indolent course. Hypoxemia, often found at presentation, can be profound and can require intubation and mechanical ventilation. Although renal disease is found in some patients at presentation, its absence does not exclude the diagnosis. Physical exam often reveals diffuse crackles, and imaging studies show characteristic but nonspecific changes of diffuse alveolar infiltrates, sometimes with a tree-in-bud pattern and septal thickening on chest CT (Fig. 61.4). Bronchoscopy and bronchoalveolar lavage reveal evidence of alveolar hemorrhage with blood-tinged lavage and hemosiderin-laden macrophages on cytologic examination. In the absence of renal disease, all of the findings described above are nonspecific and cannot distinguish microscopic polyangiitis from idiopathic pulmonary hemosiderosis (IPH) or any other alveolar hemorrhage syndrome.

A diagnosis of microscopic polyangiitis is suggested by the presence of serum anti-MPO antibodies (p-ANCA pattern). Lung histopathology in microscopic polyangiitis shows PC with neutrophilic infiltration of small arterioles, venules,

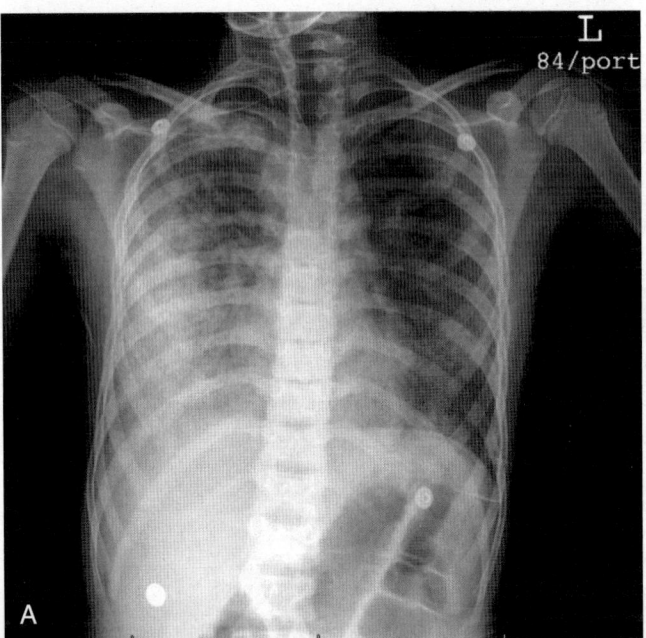

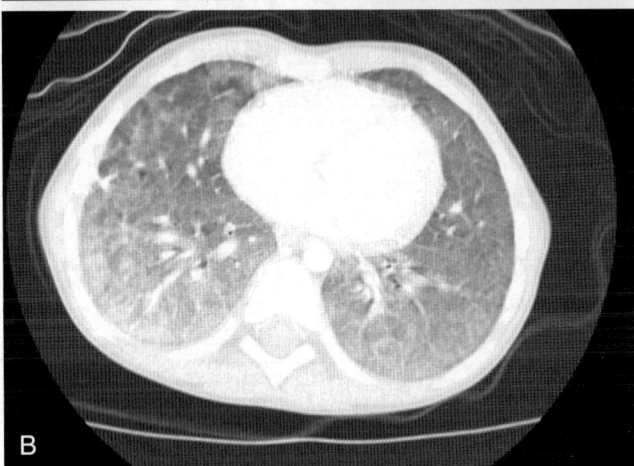

Fig. 61.4 Radiographic findings in microscopic polyangiitis. Chest x-rays in microscopic polyangiitis show diffuse alveolar infiltrates consistent with alveolar hemorrhage (A). Chest computed tomography demonstrates diffuse ground glass opacities with septal thickening that can be subtle (B). These findings are nonspecific and are seen in many causes of alveolar hemorrhage.

and capillaries associated with fibrinoid necrosis (Fig. 61.5). Granulomatous vasculitis, characteristic of granulomatosis with polyangiitis, is not seen. Renal involvement, when present, is typically manifest on biopsy as segmental necrotizing glomerulonephritis.

TREATMENT OF ANCA-ASSOCIATED VASCULITIS

Treatment for ANCA-associated vasculitis in children is broadly similar to the approach used for adult patients based on evidence from a number of clinical trials conducted by the European Vasculitis Study Group.[58] With major concern for the high morbidity and mortality, therapy in ANCA-associated vasculitis is aimed at the preservation of organ function, mainly renal and pulmonary, and maintaining clinical remission.

Induction therapy has traditionally included glucocorticoids and cyclophosphamide. In children, we use both pulse IV methylprednisolone (30 mg/kg, maximum 1 g, for 2–3 days, and then once weekly) and oral prednisone (1–2 mg/kg, daily). Regimens involving oral or IV cyclophosphamide therapy, given over a period of 3–6 months, have demonstrated efficacy in inducing remission, lengthening time to relapse, and reducing adverse events.[59,60] IV pulse cyclophosphamide was shown to be as effective as daily oral cyclophosphamide with a 50% decrease in cumulative cyclophosphamide dose, and therefore fewer adverse effects.[61,62] Despite the efficacy of glucocorticoids and cyclophosphamide in inducing remission, disease relapses occur in as many as 50% of patients, and 20%–53% may develop a relapse within the first 1–2 years following treatment. Disease relapses occur when the drugs are reduced or withdrawn. Given the adverse effects of cyclophosphamide, newer treatment strategies directed at B cell depletion have been developed. In a recent trial, rituximab was as effective as cyclophosphamide in inducing remission with a similar side-effect profile.[63]

Other important components of induction therapy in children include intravenous immunoglobulin (IVIG) and plasmapheresis. In addition to three open studies demonstrating beneficial effect on ANCA-associated vasculitis, a small randomized, placebo-controlled trial of 34 patients showed a significantly higher rate of remission in the IVIG-treated group compared with placebo (15 vs. 6 remissions, $P = .015$).[64] Plasmapheresis has been shown to decrease morbidity in patients with worse renal disease, as part of the induction therapy.[65,66] No controlled trials are available with respect to alveolar hemorrhage and plasmapheresis; however, a retrospective analysis of 20 patients with alveolar hemorrhage who received plasmapheresis reported resolution of hemorrhage in all patients.[65] We believe that plasmapheresis should be considered in the early management of DAH, particularly in an intensive care unit setting due to granulomatosis with polyangiitis, microscopic polyangiitis, macrophage activation syndrome, antiglomerular basement membrane antibody disease, antiphospholipid antibody syndrome, and SLE.

After patients are disease-free for 6 months, maintenance therapy should be initiated with low-dose prednisone and either methotrexate or azathioprine for at least 1–2 years.[67] To date, the optimal duration of maintenance therapy is unknown. A well-defined and structured clinical assessment with urinalysis and basic laboratory testing should be performed regularly to assess for disease activity and relapse, treatment response, and drug adverse effects.

ANTI-GBM DISEASE

Similar to granulomatosis with polyangiitis and microscopic polyangiitis, anti-GBM disease presents with alveolar hemorrhage and renal disease. However, in contrast to the other pulmonary-renal syndromes that may have more systemic involvement, anti-GBM disease is almost exclusively limited to the lung and kidneys. Diagnostic imaging and bronchoalveolar lavage will yield findings consistent with nonspecific DAH. However, the classic distinguishing feature includes the detection of anti-GBM antibodies in serum and by immunofluorescence along the basement membrane in lung and

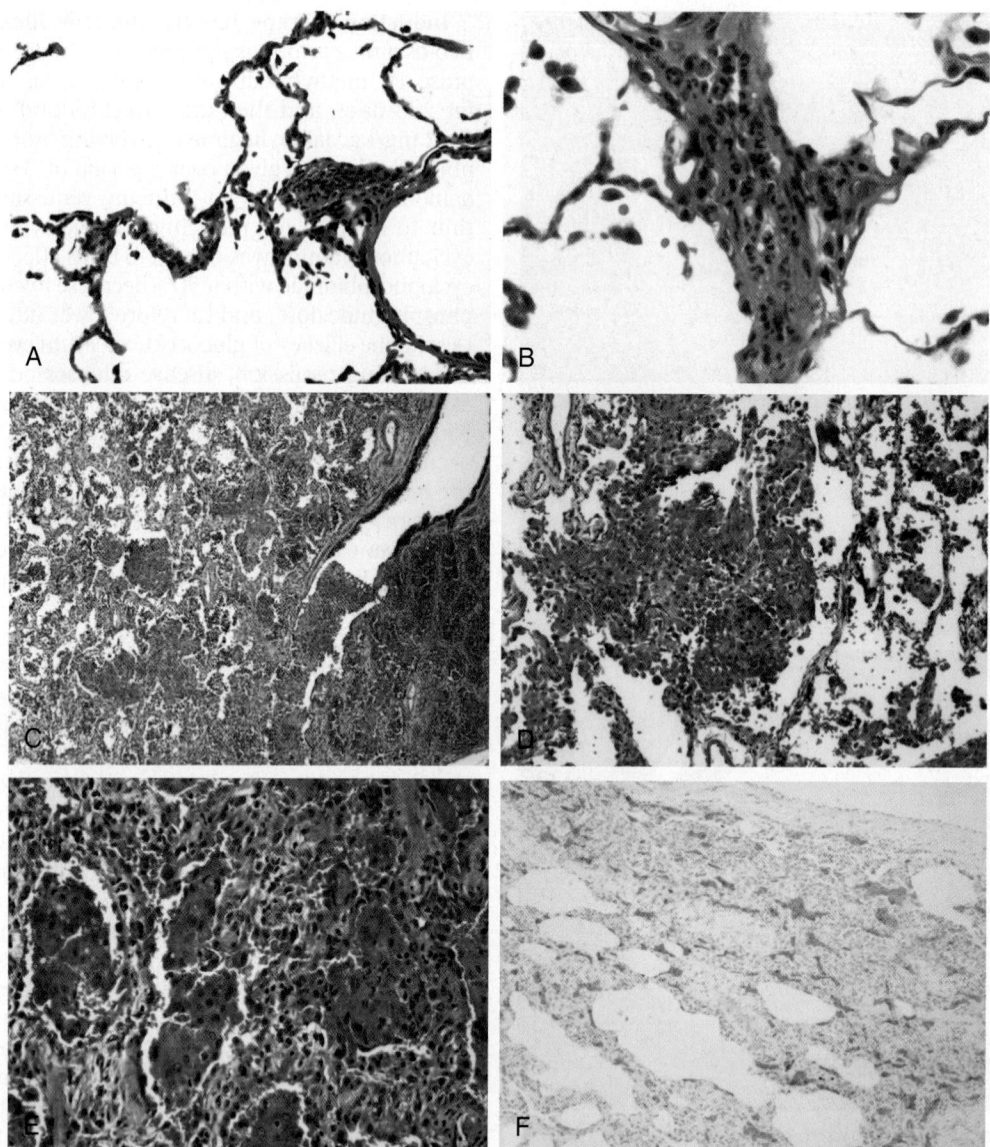

Fig. 61.5 Small-vessel vasculitis is a feature of a number of immune-mediated vasculitic disorders that involve the lung, although in childhood, it is most often related to microscopic polyangiitis, and is often associated with glomerulonephritis (pulmonary-renal syndrome). It is characterized by multiple foci of acute inflammation with clusters of neutrophils widening alveolar walls (A) and infiltrating the walls of small blood vessels within alveolar walls (B). There is often extravasation of erythrocytes with a background of diffuse hemorrhage filling airspaces (C), and there may be evidence of alveolar wall necrosis with fibrinous exudates and neutrophils spilling into airspaces (D), alveolar epithelial hyperplasia, focal organization and more diffuse alveolar wall widening (E), and hemosiderin deposition (F, iron stain).

renal tissue (Fig. 61.6). Treatment of anti-GBM disease is similar to that of ANCA-associated vasculitis, with corticosteroids used as primary treatment, and cyclophosphamide added in severe cases. One important difference is that plasmapheresis is used in all cases of anti-GBM disease to remove the circulating anti-GBM antibodies, limiting the amount of damage in the lungs and kidneys.[68–70]

ISOLATED PULMONARY CAPILLARITIS

In children, isolated PC presents with signs and symptoms of alveolar hemorrhage without renal or other systemic manifestations.[57] Patients have diffuse alveolar opacities on diagnostic imaging studies; low hemoglobin; hemosiderin-laden macrophages on bronchoalveolar lavage cytology; and a normal blood urea nitrogen (BUN), creatinine, and urinalysis. ESR and CRP are often quite elevated. Compared with IPH, PC is associated with a lower hemoglobin and higher ESR.[57] The presence of ANCA, usually MPO but occasionally PR3, is often, but not always, found. In the absence of positive ANCA, lung biopsy is required for diagnosis. Because the neutrophilic capillaritis can be patchy and subtle, an experienced pediatric lung pathologist should review the histopathology.

As with other immune-mediated alveolar hemorrhage, isolated PC can have a fulminate presentation, and aggressive therapy with the same protocol as ANCA-associated vasculitis should be instituted early.

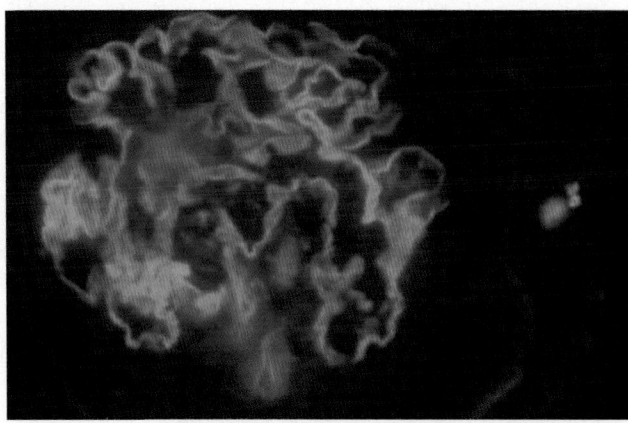

Fig. 61.6 In antiglomerular basement membrane (anti-GBM) disease, diagnosis depends on the detection of antibodies with specificity for the anti-GBM antibodies, either in lung or kidney biopsy tissue. In this case, the kidney shows immunofluorescent staining of the GBM with anti-GBM antibody.

COPA SYNDROME

The recent discovery of a genetic cause of familial pulmonary hemorrhage may shed light on the pathophysiology of alveolar hemorrhage. Watkin et al. described five families with autosomal dominant pulmonary hemorrhage syndrome and variable renal disease.[71] Whole exome sequencing revealed mutations in the cotamer-associated protein alpha (COPA) gene in all affected subjects, leading to the description of this new disease entity now known as COPA syndrome.[72] COPA is part of the coat protein complex I, responsible for retrograde Golgi to endoplasmic reticulum (ER) transport. This process is integral for proper recycling of proteins and lipids necessary for the transport of nascent protein from the ER to the Golgi for further posttranslational processing and trafficking.[73–74] COPA gene mutations lead to increased ER stress and dysfunctional autophagy through unknown mechanisms. The end result is T_H17 skewing in CD4$^+$ cells and immune dysregulation, manifest mainly as pulmonary hemorrhage. Patients often present at a young age with alveolar hemorrhage and have a chronic, relapsing, and remitting course. Chest CT may be important in identifying COPA syndrome as many patients have cystic disease on CT scan.[72] Currently, treatment is similar to other PC disease processes; however, given our understanding of the molecular mechanisms underlying this specific disease, there is hope for more targeted therapies in the near future.

NONIMMUNE-MEDIATED ALVEOLAR HEMORRHAGE

Examples of nonimmune-mediated alveolar hemorrhage include IPH, acute idiopathic pulmonary hemorrhage of infancy (AIPH), Heiner's syndrome, child abuse, and primary cardiovascular disease. Much controversy remains as to whether Heiner's syndrome, alveolar hemorrhage caused by milk allergy, actually exists.[75–77] A diverse group of cardiovascular disorders, including mitral stenosis, veno-occlusive disease, pulmonary capillary hemangiomatosis, and pulmonary telangiectasia, can result in a congestive vasculopathy with resultant hemosiderin-laden macrophages in airspaces (Fig. 61.7). In a recent report of 30 cases of veno-occlusive

disease and five cases of pulmonary hemangiomatosis, Lantuejoul and colleagues[78] found histologic evidence of pulmonary hemosiderosis in 80%. Pulmonary hypertension and pulmonary embolism can both cause hemorrhage with resultant hemosiderin-laden macrophages and should be in the differential diagnosis of pulmonary hemosiderosis.

Idiopathic Pulmonary Hemosiderosis

Previously considered the most common form of DAH, IPH is now a diagnosis of exclusion. Although IPH was reported to have a high mortality in the older literature, more recent studies have suggested a better prognosis.[79–81]

As in any alveolar hemorrhage syndrome, the clinical presentation of IPH is nonspecific with symptoms of malaise, cough, dyspnea, and tachypnea. Hemoptysis may not be present, especially in young children, who swallow their sputum. On physical examination, pallor, crackles, and clubbing, especially in long-standing disease, are present. Previously, the findings of iron-deficiency anemia; diffuse alveolar infiltrates on imaging studies; and hemosiderin-laden macrophages in sputum, gastric aspirate, or bronchoalveolar lavage were considered sufficient for diagnosis, especially when there was no evidence of systemic disease and negative autoimmune serology. Lung biopsy was not deemed necessary in such cases.[3,82]

Recent articles have shown a much higher rate of capillaritis than IPH in children, and many of the patients with capillaritis have negative serology for autoantibodies.[57] Therefore, we recommend that patients with DAH without a cardiovascular cause and negative serology undergo a lung biopsy. In IPH, the biopsy characteristically shows evidence of bland alveolar hemorrhage with multiple hemosiderin-laden macrophages in the airspaces, in the absence of significant inflammation or any evidence of capillaritis or vasculitis (Fig. 61.8). However, we emphasize that the pathologic features of capillaritis can be quite subtle and, on further review, cases with an initial diagnosis of IPH have shown features of PC.

It is important to distinguish between IPH and PC because the treatments are different. In general, PC is much more difficult to treat and requires cytotoxic therapy to induce remission and prevent recurrence. In contrast, many cases of IPH can be successfully treated with corticosteroids alone, with hydroxychloroquine or azathioprine used as steroid-sparing agents when additional therapy is required. However, severe cases may warrant therapy similar to that used for life-threatening immune-mediated DAH and even extracorporeal membrane oxygenation support.[83] In a recent series, 6-mercaptopurine was used successfully as long-term maintenance therapy.[84]

Approach to the Child With Pulmonary Hemorrhage

DIAGNOSIS

A systematic approach to the child with suspected pulmonary hemorrhage is required to determine the specific etiology and institute timely and appropriate therapy. In patients with unexplained hemoptysis, the diagnostic studies to consider include chest CT with contrast to investigate for pulmonary

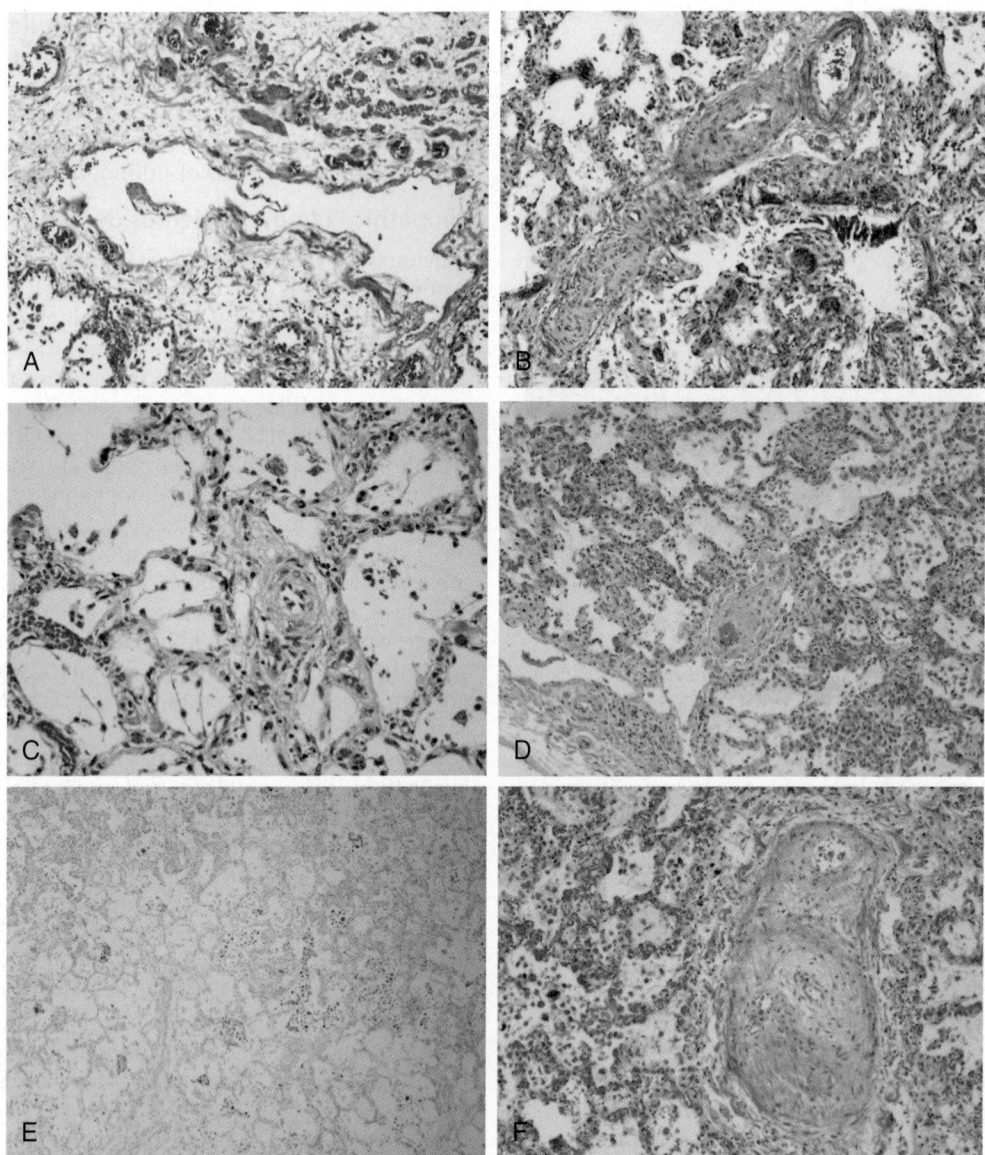

Fig. 61.7 Congestive vasculopathy is a feature of a number of conditions in which there is long-standing elevation of pulmonary venous pressure from a variety of etiologies, including elevated left atrial pressure and pulmonary venous obstruction, which includes pulmonary veno-occlusive disease. Pathologically congestive vasculopathy shows vascular remodeling affecting pulmonary veins with medial hypertrophy, arterialization, and perivenous fibrosis; lymphatics with dilatation and often lymphatic smooth muscle hyperplasia (A); arteries with mild medial hypertrophy and often eccentric intimal fibrosis (B, Movat pentachrome stain); and arterioles with more prominent muscularization (C). There are also parenchymal changes with edema, alveolar wall widening (D), and hemosiderin deposition (E, iron stain). In pulmonary veno-occlusive disease there is also venous intimal fibrosis that may be occlusive (F), and there may be arterial thrombosis and focally prominent alveolar capillary dilatation and congestion resembling foci of pulmonary capillary hemangiomatosis.

embolism and arteriovenous malformations; tests for coagulation defects; and bronchoscopy to detect foreign bodies, airway hemangiomata, or tumors. Children with hemoptysis and bronchiectasis related to cystic fibrosis or other disorders rarely need additional diagnostic evaluation, but they may require intervention with bronchial artery embolization if hemoptysis is severe. In those with possible infectious pneumonia, blood and sputum cultures and a tuberculosis purified protein derivative should be considered, with bronchoscopy and bronchoalveolar lavage reserved for patients who do not respond to conventional therapy.

In any child with diffuse alveolar opacities, cardiovascular causes should be excluded by echocardiogram, CT with contrast, magnetic resonance imaging, or cardiac catheterization as appropriate. In patients with suspected or documented DAH and renal involvement, rash, joint disease, and other systemic manifestations, an immune-mediated vasculitis should be considered, and a pediatric rheumatologist should be consulted. Appropriate diagnostic studies include an antinuclear antibody (ANA) profile, ANCA, CBC, ESR, CRP, urinalysis, metabolic panel, d-dimers, von Willebrand's factor, antiphospholipid antibody, lupus anticoagulant, and other tests as indicated. The cytologic identification of hemosiderin-laden macrophages in sputum, gastric aspirate, or bronchoalveolar lavage may confirm alveolar hemorrhage, but it is not specific as to the cause. Table 61.1 summarizes

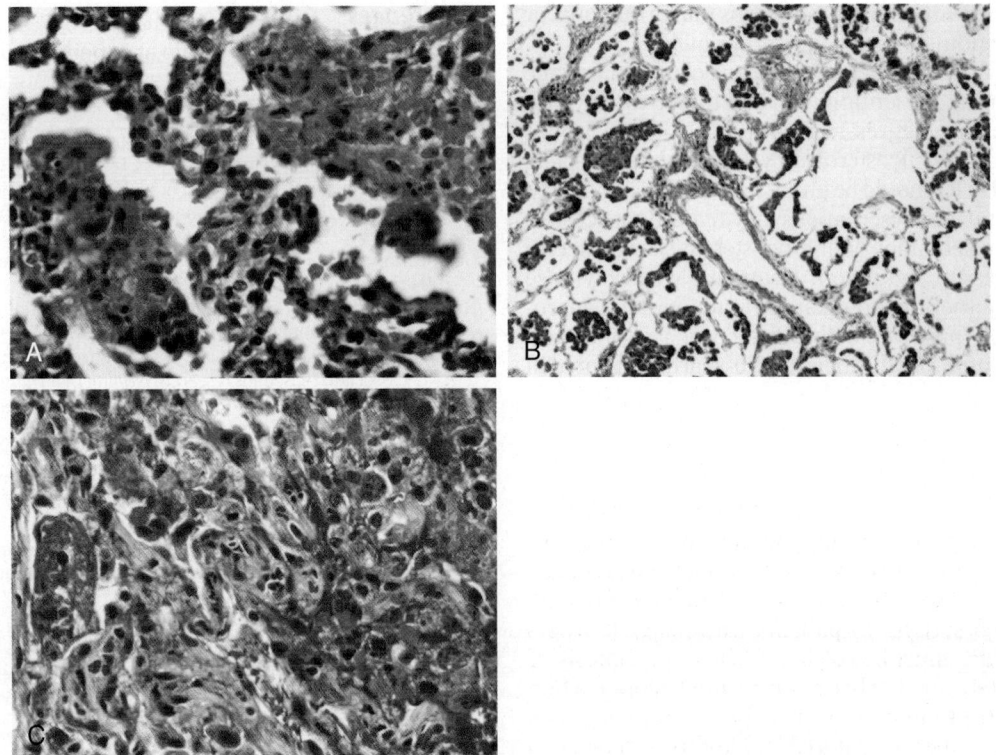

Fig. 61.8 In idiopathic pulmonary hemosiderosis, diffuse alveolar hemorrhage (A) and hemosiderin-laden macrophages (B, iron stain) are present. Although there is mild alveolar wall fibrosis (C, Movat pentachrome stain) and mild alveolar epithelial hyperplasia, there is no alveolar wall or vascular inflammation.

Table 61.1 Clinical Manifestations of Diffuse Alveolar Hemorrhage Syndromes

	GPA	MPA	Anti-GBM	PC	SLE	IPH	COPA Syndrome
Alveolar hemorrhage	++	++++	++++	++++	+	++++	++
Glomerulonephritis	++++	++++	++++	−	++++	−	−
Elevated ESR/CRP	++++	++++	+	++++	++++	+	+
Serologies	PR3	MPO	GBM	PR3, MPO	ANA	−	ANCA, ANA, RF
Extrarenal findings	+++	+++	−	−	++++	−	++++

ANA, Antinuclear antibody; *ANCA,* antineutrophil cytoplasmic antibody; *anti-GBM,* anti-GBM disease; *COPA,* cotamer-assocated protein alpha; *CRP,* C-reactive protein; *ESR,* erythrocyte sedimentation rate; *GBM,* glomerular basement; *GPA,* granulomatosis with polyangiitis; *IPH,* idiopathic pulmonary hemorrhage; *MPA,* microscopic polyangiitis; *MPO,* myeloperoxidase; *PC,* isolated pulmonary capillaritis; *PR3,* proteinase 3; *RF,* rheumatoid factor; *SLE,* systemic lupus erythematosus.

the distinguishing features of the alveolar hemorrhage syndromes.

In patients with DAH who have no cardiac, renal, or other systemic disease and negative ANA, ANCA, and anti-GBM antibodies, we strongly recommend that a transthoracic biopsy be done either through a mini-thoracostomy ("open") or with video-assisted thoracoscopic surgery (VATS). Lung tissue should be processed according to the guidelines set forth by the Children's Interstitial Lung Pathology Cooperative Group.[85] As discussed, histopathology of PC shows intraalveolar and interstitial red blood cells; pauci-immune hemorrhagic, necrotizing alveolar capillaritis with neutrophilic infiltration resulting in fibrinoid necrosis and dissolution of the arteriolar and venular walls; and intraalveolar hemosiderosis. The presence of granulomatous inflammation is consistent with a diagnosis of granulomatosis with polyangiitis. Anti-GBM antibodies along the capillary basement membranes in the lung demonstrated by immunofluorescence

are diagnostic of anti-GBM disease. If bland alveolar hemorrhage with hemosiderin-laden macrophages is found, and capillaritis is excluded, a diagnosis of IPH can be made. It is highly recommended that the biopsy be performed before treatment is initiated as treatment may obscure the histologic picture.

TREATMENT

Treatment of pulmonary hemorrhage is based on the presentation and cause. In cases of massive hemoptysis, intubation and mechanical ventilation with high positive end-expiratory pressures may be necessary. If massive hemorrhage is unilateral, the use of a double-lumen endotracheal tube allowing for airway occlusion of the affected side and ventilation of the unaffected side should be considered. Bronchial artery embolization is the treatment of choice to control bleeding. Underlying etiologies, such as coagulopathy, cystic fibrosis exacerbations, pneumonia, arteriovenous malformations, or foreign bodies, should be treated appropriately.

For patients with immune-mediated alveolar hemorrhage and life-threatening presentation, in addition to airway and ventilatory support, aggressive pharmacologic treatment with pulse and oral corticosteroids, cyclophosphamide, plasmapheresis, and IVIG should be given, as discussed previously. Those with less severe presentations may require corticosteroids and cyclophosphamide or another steroid-sparing agent. Following successful induction, treatment with low-dose prednisone and either methotrexate or azathioprine is appropriate. For most patients with IPH, corticosteroids and hydroxychloroquine or another steroid-sparing agent will control DAH.

Summary

Because of the unique blood supply to the lungs, pulmonary hemorrhage can arise from either the bronchial or pulmonary circulation. Diagnostic considerations and management are different for each system. In patients with DAH, disorders associated with PC must be ruled out before a diagnosis of IPH can be entertained. This requires lung biopsy when serologic markers of immune-mediated disease are negative. Aggressive intervention is required for life-threatening DAH because morbidity and mortality are high.

References

Access the reference list online at ExpertConsult.com.

Suggested Reading

Collins CE, Quismorio FP Jr. Pulmonary involvement in microscopic polyangiitis. *Curr Opin Pulm Med.* 2005;11(5):447–451.

Fullmer JJ, Langston C, Dishop MK, et al. Pulmonary capillaritis in children: a review of eight cases with comparison to other alveolar hemorrhage syndromes. *J Pediatr.* 2005;146(3):376–381.

Godfrey S. Pulmonary hemorrhage/hemoptysis in children. *Pediatr Pulmonol.* 2004;37(6):476–484.

Holle JU, Laudien M, Gross WL. Clinical manifestations and treatment of Wegener's granulomatosis. *Rheum Dis Clin North Am.* 2010;36(3):507–526.

Jayne D, Rasmussen N. Twenty-five years of European Union collaboration in ANCA associated vasculitis research. *Nephrol Dial Transplant.* 2015;30:1–7.

Kiper N, Gocmen A, Ozcelik U, et al. Long-term clinical course of patients with idiopathic pulmonary hemosiderosis (1979-1994): prolonged survival with low-dose corticosteroid therapy. *Pediatr Pulmonol.* 1999;3:180–184.

Pagnoux C, Mahr A, Hamidou MA, et al. Azathioprine or methotrexate maintenance for ANCA-associated vasculitis. *N Engl J Med.* 2008; 359(26):2790–2803.

Pendergraft WF III, Preston GA, Shah RR, et al. Autoimmunity is triggered by cPR-3(105-201), a protein complementary to human autoantigen proteinase-3. *Nat Med.* 2004;10(1):72–79.

Stone JH, Merkel PA, Spiera R, et al. Rituximab versus cyclophosphamide for ANCA associated vasculitis. *N Engl J Med.* 2010;363:211–220.

Vece TJ, Watkin LB, Nicholas SK, et al. Copa syndrome: a novel autosomal dominant immune dysregulatory disease. *J Clin Immunol.* 2016;36(4):377–387.

62 *The Lung in Sickle Cell Disease*

ANNE GREENOUGH, MD (Cantab), MB BS, DCH, FRCP, FRCPCH, and
JENNIFER KNIGHT-MADDEN, MBBS, PhD

Epidemiology

Sickle cell disease (SCD) is the most common inherited disorder affecting African and Caribbean populations. There are more than 200 million carriers of the sickle cell trait, and approximately 250,000 children are born each year with SCD. The sickle cell mutation arose on at least four separate occasions in Africa and as a fifth independent mutation in Saudi Arabia or central India. SCD occurs most commonly in tropical Africa where it affects approximately 1% of all infants, and the sickle cell trait is found in approximately 8% of African Americans and also occurs in the Middle East, Greece, and India. There is a high prevalence of the HbS gene in areas where malaria is common, suggesting that sickle cell trait gives an advantage against severe malaria syndromes. Indeed, although children with sickle cell trait are infected by *Plasmodium falciparum*, the parasite count is low.[1] Individuals with SCD suffer increased respiratory related mortality and morbidity, as discussed in this chapter.

Etiology

Homozygous inheritance of the gene for HbS results in sickle cell anemia (HbSS), the most severe form of SCD. Other clinically important forms of SCD include sickle hemoglobin C disease (HbSC), sickle β^0, and β^+-thalassemia (HbSβthal). The sickle gene results in the substitution of valine for glutamic acid at the sixth position of the amino acid sequence in the beta-globin chain, forming HbS. HbC is produced when the glutamic acid is substituted by lysine at the same position. The β thalassemias have normal structured, but inadequate quantities of hemoglobin A. Coinheritance of various polymorphisms associated with these pathways may explain some of the variation in clinical presentation that occurs in those with identical sickle cell genotypes.

When deoxygenated, partially or fully, HbS undergoes conformational changes, a hydrophobic region surrounding the valine site in the β subunit is left exposed. Polymerization with other hemoglobin tetramers then occurs resulting in the formation of aggregates (crystals) that distort the red blood cell membrane. Neither fully oxygenated HbS nor fetal hemoglobin (HbF) polymerizes. When a "sickle" cell is exposed to a relatively hypoxic/acidic environment, the K^+Cl^- cotransport is activated with loss of potassium from the cell. Deoxygenation also increases intracellular free calcium, and calcium dependent dehydration occurs. HbS molecules form a viscous solution within the erythrocyte. The changes in the membrane stiffen the red blood cell and change it from a biconcave to a sickle shaped cell that is less deformable and subject to hemolysis. In addition, the rigid cells can obstruct small blood vessels, and over time, cells that have sickled repeatedly become irreversibly sickled. Deoxygenation is maximal in the venous circulation, and the sickled cells may cause extensive and progressive damage to the pulmonary vascular bed. The sickle cells occlude vessels especially to organs with sluggish circulation, such as atelectatic areas of the lung.

Pathogenesis

The systemic effects of ongoing hemolysis, the altered adhesion of cellular elements in blood to each other and the endothelium and the elevated activity of inflammatory pathways all interact to cause the morbidity of SCD involving all organ systems, but particularly the lungs.

Intact sickle erythrocytes are deficient in antioxidants (superoxide dismutase, catalase, and glutathione peroxidase) and are excessive producers of oxidant species. This may reflect the greater auto-oxidation of HbS compared to HbA red blood cells, which means that superoxide and hydrogen peroxide are removed less efficiently. Intravascular hemolysis in SCD produces high levels of cell free Hb and extracellular heme, which is a potent proinflammatory agent and oxidant and now classified as a damage-associated molecular pattern molecule (DAMP).[2] Heme and other oxidant species promote the release from activated neutrophils of neutrophil extracellular traps (NET) that are decondensed chromatin decorated by granular enzymes.[3] NET plasma levels increase during painful crises and are particularly elevated during ACS episodes.[4] The scavenging capacity of plasma proteins, particularly haptoglobin and hemopexin, is overwhelmed, leaving them depleted. Hypoxia inhibits nitric oxide (NO) production by decreasing protein levels of constitutive NO synthase in the endothelium, and there is inactivation of NO by free radical species liberated from activated macrophages and leucocytes. Furthermore, extracellular heme scavenges NO resulting in increased cellular adhesion and diminished vasodilation, as NO inhibits endothelin vascular cell adhesion molecule (VCAM-1) upregulation and inhibits endothelin-1 production. The products of hemolysis have been linked to acute lung injury in a murine model of SCD.[5] Toll-like receptor 4 (TLR4) was critical to that model, as TLR4-null mice remained asymptomatic when challenged with hemin, and the TLR4 antagonist TAK-242 was protective in exposed mice.

Enhanced adhesion of sickle erythrocytes to each other and the endothelium is an important part of the pathophysiology of SCD. In addition, neutrophils may adhere both to the endothelium and to the sickled erythrocyte. In murine SCD models, circulating erythrocytes were shown to attach to adherent neutrophils in the postcapillary venules initiating a vaso-occlusive crisis (VOC). Other leukocytes, including monocytes and T-lymphocytes, are involved in this adhesion cascade[6]; and the monocytes are activated by the nuclear factor κB (NF-κB) pathway.[7] Platelet activation, as indicated by circulating platelet-monocyte and platelet-neutrophil aggregates, occurs in VOC, and human platelet alloantigens (HPA) 3 polymorphisms are related to VOC risk.[8]

Monocytes from patients with SCD have elevated tumor necrosis factor-alpha (TNF-α) and interleukin (IL)-1β production.[7] Invariant natural killer T cells (iNKT) cells rapidly produce high levels of cytokines after stimulation by specific antigens,[9] and NF-κB activation in CD4+ iNKT cells may be integral to reperfusion injury after VOC.[10] Platelet activation is elevated at steady state in SCD and further enhanced during VOC. In addition, at least in part through NETs, it may be implicated in the development of pulmonary hypertension (PH) in SCD.[11] Mast cell activation, resulting in the release of bioactive substances such as substance P, has been implicated in the pathophysiology of murine models of SCD[12] and has been found in a proportion of patients who had frequent VOC. Other inflammatory mediators are elevated at SCD steady state or during acute episodes including chemokines, moieties within the coagulation cascade,[13] and high-mobility group box 1 (HMGB1), a chromatin-binding protein that maintains DNA structure.[14] Leukotrienes produced by the 5-lipoxygenase pathway are arachidonic acid derived mediators of inflammation, and leukotriene B4 (LTB4) promotes neutrophil activation and chemotaxis. LTB4 has been shown to be elevated during steady state and VOC.[15]

Clinical Features

SCD is a hemolytic anemia. Newborns, however, are asymptomatic, as they have a high level of HbF in their erythrocytes, but as the levels of HbF decline, the manifestations of SCD become apparent, this may be as early as 10–12 weeks of age. SCD patients have periods of relative stability punctuated with acute episodes such as painful crises or VOCs. They may suffer severe pain, have cerebrovascular accidents, acute splenic sequestration, and acute chest syndrome (ACS). The ongoing inflammatory process leads to chronic end-organ injury.

ACUTE CHEST SYNDROME

The overall incidence of ACS is 10.5 per 100 patient years.[16] ACS episodes occur more commonly in children than adults, and 50% of SCD children will have an ACS episode prior to the age of 10 years.[17] The highest incidence of ACS occurs in children aged between 2 and 4 years of age, and recurrence is common. In addition, the majority of very young children who had an ACS episode were rehospitalized for ACS or severe pain within 1 year.[18] Furthermore, recurrent ACS is the most important risk factor for the development of sickle cell chronic lung disease (SCLD) and increases morbidity.[19]

Risk Factors

There are a number of genetic risk factors for ACS,[17] and the incidence of ACS is most common in those with HbSS and less in those with HbSC. Similarly, the hemoglobin genotype influences the severity of ACS, being more severe in those with HbSS that in those with HbSC.[20] The ACS incidence also varies according to the beta–globin gene cluster haplotype, as indicated by the prevalence and recurrence of ACS episodes being lower in Saudi Arabia than in Africa. This may reflect an interaction between SCD and the "Asian" haplotype,[21] which is associated with a higher HbF level. The risk for ACS is also increased by certain endothelin NO synthase gene polymorphisms.[22] Genetic polymorphisms of heme oxygenase-1(HO-1), an essential enzyme in heme catabolism, have been associated with ACS risk, and a polymorphism enhancing its expression was associated with lower ACS rates.[23] ACS has been associated with rs6141803, a single nucleotide polymorphism (SNP) located 8.2 kilobases upstream of COMMD7, a gene highly expressed in the lung that interacts with NF-κB signaling.[24]

Steady-state hematological profiles impact ACS risk, and the incidence of ACS is inversely proportional to the HbF level[25] and directly proportional to the steady state white blood count. High HbF levels inhibit HbS polymerization, which protects against ACS. An elevated leucocyte count increases the risk as leukocytes release free radicals, elastase, proinflammatory mediators, and cytokines. Children presenting with fever have an increased risk of developing an ACS episode if they have an absolute neutrophil count greater than 9×10^9/L, a hemoglobin level less than 8.6 g/dL, had a previous ACS episode, upper respiratory tract infection symptoms, or noncompliance to penicillin.[26]

Infection is implicated in at least 30% of ACS episodes. In a multicenter study, although 27 different pathogens were identified, *Chlamydia pneumoniae* was the most frequent pathogen, followed by *Mycoplasma pneumoniae* and respiratory syncytial virus. Parvovirus B10 has been associated with marrow necrosis and a particularly severe form of ACS. The causative pathogen in any one area, however, reflects which pathogen is most common locally; and the seasonal variation in ACS episodes in young children reflects the increase in viral infections during the winter months.

In approximately 10% of patients, an ACS is precipitated by a pulmonary fat embolism. Infarction of the bone marrow with embolization of the fatty bone marrow to the lungs results in activation of pulmonary secretory phospholipase A2 (SPLA2). SPLA2 cleaves phospholipids and liberates free fatty acids, which cause acute pulmonary toxicity. Arachidonic acid results in vasoconstriction and oleic acid increases the upregulation of VCAM-1. Infarction of the bony thorax or pain following abdominal surgery may cause splinting, hypoventilation, and atelectasis, leading to hypoxia and intrapulmonary sickling. In addition, opioids prescribed for the pain may suppress respiratory drive compounding the hypoventilation.

Asthma has been reported to be more common in those with ACS and specifically in those who have had recurrent ACS episodes.[27] In the cooperative study for SCD in which children were recruited before 6 months of age and followed beyond 5 years of age, asthma was associated with more frequent ACS episodes.[28] Asthma may, however, have been overdiagnosed in previous studies that used a physician's diagnosis rather than more objective tests such as determination of bronchial responsiveness. It is now apparent that wheezing, without a diagnosis of asthma, is associated with an increase in SCD complications. In a retrospective study, asthma and wheezing were independent risk factors for increased painful episodes, but only wheezing was associated with more ACS episodes.[29] In an observational cohort study, adults who reported recurrent, severe episodes of wheezing, regardless of a diagnosis of asthma, had twice the rates of

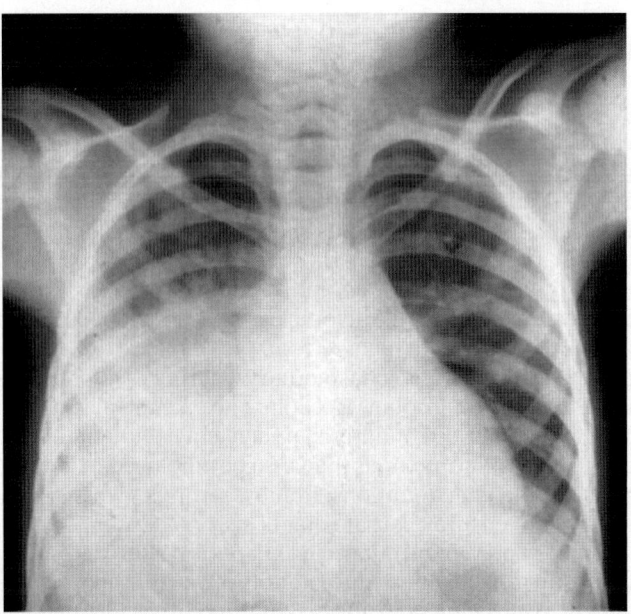

Fig. 62.1 Chest radiograph demonstrating an acute chest syndrome episode, as there is a new pulmonary infiltrate consistent with alveolar consolidation including at least one complete lung segment.

ACS, decreased lung function, and increased risk of death compared with adults without recurrent wheezing.[30] Furthermore, in a cohort of 159 children followed from birth to a median of 14.7 years, an ACS episode prior to 4 years, female gender, wheezing with shortness of breath, and two or more positive skin prick tests were associated with future ACS episodes, but airways obstruction and a bronchodilator response were not.[31]

Clinical Features

ACS episodes are characterized by chest pain, productive cough, and dyspnea; affected individuals are febrile and tachypneic and on auscultation there are crackles and wheezes.[31a] Fever and cough are more common in very young children, whereas chest pain, shortness of breath, and hemoptysis are more prominent with advancing age. Essential to the diagnosis of an ACS is a new pulmonary infiltrate on the chest radiograph (Fig. 62.1), and the lower and middle lobes are more frequently affected than the upper lobes.[31a] Ten to 15% of patients develop severe respiratory failure, necessitating mechanical ventilation and may progress to multiorgan system failure.

If the ACS is precipitated by a fat embolism, the pulmonary signs and symptoms are preceded by bone pain. Affected patients have lower mean oxygen saturation at presentation and have a more severe clinical course.[25] There may be systemic signs of a fat embolism, including changes in their mental state, thrombocytopenia, and petechiae. In addition, they have significant decreases in the hemoglobin and platelet counts and lipid-laden macrophages are found in fluid obtained by bronchoalveolar lavage.

SICKLE CHRONIC LUNG DISEASE

SCLD is a progressive disease with hypoxemia, restrictive lung disease, cor pulmonale, and evidence of diffuse interstitial fibrosis on chest radiography. Recurrent ACS episodes result in damage to the lung parenchyma resulting in restrictive lung disease.

PULMONARY HYPERTENSION

PH in SCD is characterized by progressive obliteration of the pulmonary vasculature. Possible causes include chronic hypoxic stress causing irreversible remodeling of the pulmonary vasculature, recurrent pulmonary thromboembolism, sickle cell related vasculopathy, and pulmonary scarring from recurrent ACS episodes. Sudden death in SCLD patients with PH is common due to pulmonary thromboembolism and cardiac arrhythmia. Adult SCD patients therefore should be screened for PH with echocardiography as, although initially the patients may be asymptomatic, their condition progresses and they suffer worsening hypoxia and chest pain with impaired exercise tolerance.

SLEEP-DISORDERED BREATHING

Children with SCD may be at an elevated risk of sleep-disordered breathing (SDB) including chronic (>6 months) insomnia, restless leg syndrome, habitual snoring, daytime sleepiness evidenced by needing naps, waking up not feeling refreshed, short-term insomnia, and sleep onset latency.[32] The prevalence of obstructive sleep apnea syndrome (OSAS) in children and adolescents with SCD varies from 10.6%[33] to 94% in SCD children who had not undergone adenotonsillectomy.[34] In children investigated for OSAS, although similar sleep architecture was noted, children with SCD had lower median and minimal oxygen saturations than those without SCD. Indeed, children with SCD and OSAS, compared to children with uncomplicated OSAS, had a fourfold risk of a nocturnal oxygen saturation level below 85%.[35]

Risk factors for sleep-related disorders include acute pain and chronic pain syndromes. Functional asplenia leading to compensatory adenotonsillar hypertrophy in younger children and extramedullary hematopoiesis causing alterations in facial bone structure in older children may result in OSAS. An association has been reported between enuresis and SDB in children with SCD.[36] SDB, particularly with nighttime desaturation, has been demonstrated to be associated with increased SCD complications including executive dysfunction,[37] priapism in adults,[38] and possibly painful crisis.[39,40]

LUNG FUNCTION ABNORMALITIES

Obstructive lung abnormalities were reported, in a cross-sectional study, in young children with restrictive abnormalities becoming more prominent with advancing age.[41] Those results have also been demonstrated in two longitudinal studies[42,43] but not in a third.[44] In a cohort of 45 children aged between 5 and 18 measured at baseline and approximately 4 years later, a predominantly obstructive pattern was reported with increased prevalence over time. The occurrence of restrictive abnormalities also increased, but to a lesser extent.[44] In contrast, retrospective analysis of data from 413 SCD children aged between 8 and 18 years demonstrated that the prevalence of restrictive abnormalities increased with increasing age.[42] In two cohorts of SCD children, one of which was followed for 2 years and the other for 10 years, lung function deteriorated in the SCD children compared to contemporaneously studied ethnic and age matched controls.[43] In the cohort followed for 10 years, restrictive abnormalities became more common. The rate of deterioration in lung function was greater in the younger children in whom ACS episodes were more common.[43]

At all ages, obstructive, restrictive, and mixed lung function abnormalities have been documented, as well as normal lung function.[44,44a] Airways hyperresponsiveness (AHR) to methacholine has been reported to be more common in SCD children, but AHR to methacholine has not been related to signs or symptoms of allergy.[45] Overall, the responses to bronchial challenges such as cold air, exercise, or methacholine have been variable, ranging from a positive response rate of 0%[45] to 78%.[46]

Etiology of the Lung Function Abnormalities

The obstructive lung function abnormalities seen in SCD children could be due to asthma. Exhaled NO is elevated in asthma, as there is enhanced expression of inducible NO synthase in inflamed airways. Yet, in a prospective study, the exhaled NO levels were similar in 50 SCD children and 50 controls and airway obstruction in SCD children was not associated with increased methacholine sensitivity or eosinophilic inflammation.[47] An alternative explanation for the airways obstruction in SCD is the hyperdynamic pulmonary circulation due to a raised cardiac output secondary to chronic anemia.[48] SCD children have an increased pulmonary capillary blood volume resulting from their chronic anemia, which has been shown to correlate with the degree of airways obstruction.[49] In a study of 18 SCD children compared to 18 ethnic and age-matched controls, the SCD children had a significantly higher respiratory system resistance, alveolar NO production, and pulmonary blood flow, but not airway NO flux. In addition, there was a significant correlation between the alveolar NO production and pulmonary blood flow, but not between airway NO flux and respiratory system resistance.[50] Furthermore, transfusion in SCD children acutely increased airways obstruction and this was significantly related to an increase in pulmonary capillary blood volume.[51] Those results suggest that the airway obstruction seen, at least in some SCD children, relates to their increased pulmonary capillary blood volume. The clinical implication of those results is that whether a child with SCD and airways obstruction would benefit from bronchodilators should be assessed by comparing lung function assessment results pre and post bronchodilator.

Exercise Capacity

There have been few studies investigating the cardio-respiratory responses to exercise in children with SCD. They have been reported to have more adipose tissue with reduced fitness and exercise performance. Exercise capacity has been reported to be related to the baseline degree of anemia and significantly lower in subjects with a history of recurrent ACS.[52] The metabolic changes imposed by exercise may initiate sickling and vaso-occlusive episodes. Therefore exercise should be started slowly and increased progressively, hydration should be maintained, and sudden changes in temperature should be avoided.[52]

Diagnosis

The sickle test, used in some settings as a screen, includes the HbS solubility test and sodium metabisulfite test.[53] Chemically induced sickling identifies those who have sickle cell trait or SCD but does not distinguish between the two. This test is unreliable in the first 6 months of life due to the predominance of HbF in infants. Other tests separate hemoglobins based on their chemical attributes and include the isoelectric point (isoelectric focusing [IEF]), ionic interaction with absorbent material in a column (high-performance liquid chromatography [HPLC]), and differential movement during electrophoresis in an alkaline environment (cellulose acetate membrane and capillary zone electrophoresis) or acid environment (citrate agar). Molecular methods may also be employed to identify causative genetic mutations. In most settings, two methods are used to ensure accurate diagnosis.

Primary prevention of affected infants is possible by screening adults of childbearing age and providing appropriate genetic counseling, and affected infants can be identified by prenatal testing or neonatal screening. Individuals may also be identified later in life when screened because of suggestive illnesses or the diagnosis of family members.

Management

ACUTE CHEST SYNDROME

Broad-spectrum antibiotics should be given, including macrolides or quinolones to treat atypical organisms. The choice of antibiotics should be guided by the patient's clinical condition and the "local" pathogens. Oxygen therapy should be used to treat any hypoxemia, but there may be a poor correlation of pulse oximetry readings with arterial oxygen tensions; hence, in those with suspected hypoxia, blood gas analysis should be undertaken. Patients should be hydrated but limited to 1.5 times the maintenance fluid rate to avoid further impairment of lung function by aggravating vascular leak in the lungs (Table 62.1). Packed red blood cell or exchange transfusion decreases the fraction of sickle hemoglobin and improves the

Table 62.1   Management of Acute Chest Syndrome

Treatment	Comment
Supplemental oxygen	Maintain oxygen saturation >95%
Antimicrobials	Broad spectrum including a macrolide to cover atypical bacteria
	Antivirals should be considered where appropriate
Blood transfusion	Exchange transfusion when the pretransfusion hemoglobin (Hb) level is close to steady state Hb or where there is rapid progression of the illness
	Simple transfusion when the Hb has fallen
Fluids	Should be titrated replacing insensible losses but to avoid overload
Bronchodilators	In those with evidence of bronchial hyperresponsiveness
Incentive spirometry	Instituted in those with chest pain to prevent atelectasis
Analgesia	Sufficient to prevent splinting

oxygen carrying capacity of the blood. In patients with severe anemia, a "simple" transfusion is used, but if the patient has a relatively high hematocrit, then exchange transfusion should be undertaken to avoid increasing blood viscosity. Predictors of severity include increasing hypoxia, increasing respiratory rate, reduced platelet count, and multilobar disease.[54] Indications for escalation of respiratory support include those with extensive pulmonary involvement, as indicated by increasing hypoxia, dyspnea, and a pH falling below 7.25. In such patients, noninvasive ventilation has been demonstrated to improve oxygenation, but this may be poorly tolerated.[55]

Analgesia should be given to control pain, but the amount limited to avoid respiratory depression. Patient controlled analgesia devices may reduce the risk of narcotic induced hypoventilation. An intercostal nerve block with a long acting local anesthetic can alleviate chest wall pain from rib infarcts and reduce the amount of systemic analgesia, and approximately 25% of patients wheeze during an ACS episode and may benefit from bronchodilator administration. In a small randomized controlled trial (RCT), dexamethasone administered to children with mild to moderately severe ACS was associated with a 40% reduction in the length of hospitalization, a shorter duration of supplementary oxygen requirement, and less need for analgesia. Readmission after an ACS episode, however, was more common in those who reported use of an inhaler or nebulizer at home or had received corticosteroids for the ACS episode.

Inhaled NO (20–80 ppm) in patients with ACS and PH has been reported to result in rapid pulmonary vasodilation. A large prospective trial, however, failed to show any significant differences in the time to resolution of crisis, length of hospitalization, pain scores, cumulative opioid usage, or ACS rate between those who received NO and placebo.[56]

PULMONARY HYPERTENSION

Management of adults with PH consists of anticoagulation for those with thromboembolism, supplementary oxygen for those with low oxygen saturations, treatment of left heart failure, and hydroxyurea or transfusions.[57] The recent guidelines from the American Thoracic Society make only a weak recommendation for either a prostacyclin agonist or an endothelin receptor antagonist but a strong recommendation against phosphodiesterase-5 inhibitor therapy for those with right heart catheterisation-confirmed PH with elevated pulmonary vascular resistance and normal pulmonary capillary wedge pressure.[58]

MONITORING

It is important that children with wheeze are not assumed to have asthma as wheeze in SCD may have other causes. It is therefore important that they undergo assessment for bronchial hyperreactivity according to their lung function, and those with airway function less than 70% of predicted should receive a bronchodilator and those with better airway function better than 70% of predicted should receive either a cold air or exercise challenge. To ensure all children are appropriately diagnosed as having AHR, undertaking both a cold air and exercise challenge should be considered, as some children respond only to one type of challenge.[59] A methacholine challenge should not be used, as this can precipitate an ACS. If there is concern that a bronchial provocation challenge will precipitate an ACS or VOC, then a trial of inhaled steroids could be undertaken, but a detailed diary card and lung function analysis are required to determine if the inhaled steroids have had a positive effect.

The most rapid deterioration in lung function occurs in very young children[43]; thus, annual respiratory monitoring should begin early. Young children, however, have limited ability to perform lung function tests, and detailed lung function testing is not available in all centers. As a consequence, in those less than 5 years of age, impulse oscillometry is recommended, as this does not require volitional input by the child; in older children, spirometry gives additional information.

Certain methods of assessing oxygen saturation in SCD patients may be inaccurate. Pulse oximetry can yield inaccurate results in SCD patients, as the fraction of carboxyhemoglobin (COHb) is increased in some patients because of increased heme catabolism; some modern oximeters, however, can differentiate between COHb and oxyHb. In addition, the patterns of light absorption differ between HbS and HbA and HbA is used to calibrate oximeters.

Given the many reasons for an increased risk of SDB in children with SCD, patients should be screened with questionnaires and, where available, with polysomnography. An ongoing randomized trial may shed light as to whether therapy with overnight supplementary oxygen may ameliorate the impact of SDB on children with SCD.[60]

PH is usually diagnosed by a tricuspid regurgitant jet velocity (TRV) on echocardiography of greater or equal to 2.5 m/s. Echocardiography, however, overestimates the prevalence of PH against the gold standard of cardiac catheterization. An elevated TRV has been reported in 11%–31% of children and adolescents with SCD and associated with a decline in exercise capacity.

Prevention

Agents that increase the HbF level reduce the complications of SCD. Hydroxyurea, a ribonuclease reductase inhibitor, blocks the synthesis of DNA and, because of bone marrow suppression, raises the HbF level. Hydroxyurea is also an NO donor and has been shown to reduce the adhesion of sickle cells to the vascular endothelin in vitro by reducing VCAM-1 production. A systematic review concluded that hydroxyurea is effective and safe in adults severely affected by sickle cell anemia. An RCT in children aged 9–18 months failed to achieve its primary aim, which is whether daily hydroxyurea would reduce spleen and renal damage by at least 50%. There were, however, significantly fewer SCD related events in the hydroxyurea group, including ACS episodes.[61] Hydroxyurea, however, may cause cytopenias and patients must be carefully monitored, especially early in the administration of therapy, and some physicians are reluctant to prescribe it. An evidence-based report by expert panel members gave a recommendation of moderate strength regarding offering treatment with hydroxyurea without regard to the presence of symptoms for infants, children, and adolescents.[62] Chronic transfusion in patients with a history of recurrent or severe ACS episodes has been demonstrated by both a retrospective review[63] and a randomized trial[64] to reduce the frequency of ACS episodes. Routine use of incentive spirometry is recommended in SCD patients admitted to hospital with chest or bone pain, as in an RCT, this was associated with a lower rate of pulmonary complications (atelectasis or infiltrates) on a subsequent chest radiograph.[65] A retrospective review demonstrated that introduction of a guideline initiating mandatory incentive spirometry in children with SCD admitted for nonrespiratory complaints resulted in a reduced number of transfusions and ACS episodes.[66] Stem cell transplantation in adults and children has been associated with no recurrence of painful crisis in those with stable engraftment.[67] The best results are obtained in young children who have human leukocyte antigen (HLA)-identical sibling donors and who are transplanted early in the course of their disease.[68] In certain pediatric populations, the success rate is 85%–90%.[69]

Prognosis

Despite significant improvements in life expectancy in individuals with SCD, the median age of death for women is 48 years and the median age for men is 42 years. Fatal pulmonary complications occur in 20% of adults. The overall mortality for ACS is 3%, but 9% in adults, and the primary cause of death is respiratory failure from pulmonary emboli or bronchopneumonia. Those with SCLD and PH have significantly increased mortality; the median survival for patients diagnosed with PH by catheterization has been reported to be only 25.6 months.

References

Access the reference list online at ExpertConsult.com.

Suggested Reading

Gordeuk VR, Castro OL, Machado RF. Pathophysiology and treatment of pulmonary hypertension in sickle cell disease. *Blood*. 2016;127:820–828.

Howard J, Hart N, Roberts-Harewood M, et al. Guideline on the management of acute chest syndrome in sickle cell disease. *Br J Hematol*. 2015;169:492–505.

Klings ES, Machado RF, Barst RJ, et al. An official American Thoracic Society clinical practice guideline: diagnosis, risk stratification, and management of pulmonary hypertension of sickle cell disease. *Am J Respir Cric Care Med*. 2014;189:727–740.

Klings ES, Wyszynski DF, Nolan VG, et al. Abnormal pulmonary function in adults with sickle cell anemia. *Am J Respir Crit Care Med*. 2006;173: 1264–1269.

Lunt A, McGhee E, Sylvester K, et al. Longitudinal assessment of lung function in children with sickle cell disease. *Pediatr Pulmonol*. 2015;51(7): 717–723.

Parent F, Bachir D, Inamo J, et al. A hemodynamic study of pulmonary hypertension in sickle cell disease. *N Engl J Med*. 2011;365:44–53.

Vichinsky EP, Neumayr LD, Earles AN, et al. Causes and outcomes of the acute chest syndrome in sickle cell disease. National Acute Chest Syndrome Study Group. *N Engl J Med*. 2000;342:1855–1865.

Wang WC, Ware RE, Miller ST, et al. Hydroxycarbamide in very young children with sickle-cell anaemia: a multicentre, randomised, controlled trial (BABY HUG). *Lancet*. 2011;377:1663–1672.

Yawn BP, Buchanan GR, Afenyi-Annan AN, et al. Management of sickle cell disease: summary of the 2014 evidence based report by expert panel members. *JAMA*. 2014;312:1033–1048.

63 *Primary Immunodeficiency and Other Diseases With Immune Dysregulation*

DANIEL R. AMBRUSO, MD, and PIA J. HAUK, MD

Chronic Granulomatous Disease

Chronic granulomatous disease (CGD) of childhood was first described by Berendes and colleagues[1] and by Landing and Shirkey[2] as a distinct clinical entity of unknown cause.[3] This disease is characterized by recurrent infections, usually with low-grade pathogens, formation of abscesses and suppurative granulomas, and normal humoral and cellular immunity. The usual onset of symptoms is early in life (most in the first 2 years of life). The disease is generally chronic, and unless diagnosed and treated, the outcome is commonly death from overwhelming infection.

After the original patients, similar cases were reported using various names.[4–7] CGD is now the generally accepted term for this syndrome. In 1967 Quie and colleagues[8] defined the basic step in pathophysiology as an inability of phagocytic cells to kill ingested bacteria; and Baehner and Nathan[6] reported that CGD neutrophils did not undergo the phagocytosis-associated "respiratory burst" of oxygen consumption and hydrogen peroxide (H_2O_2) production that characterizes phagocytic cells.

Although all of the cases initially documented were in males, later reports described females, suggesting the possibility of autosomal-recessive variants.[9,10] In the 1970s, progress was made in elucidating the nature of the basic biochemical defect, decreased oxidase activity, a process by which oxygen (O_2) is reduced to superoxide anion (O_2^-) using nicotinamide adenine dinucleotide phosphate (NADPH) as the electron source.[11–13] In 1978 Segal and Jones reported the association of a b-type cytochrome and the NADPH oxidase, as well as its deficiency in CGD. Continued studies firmly defined the relationship between X-linked CGD and deficiency of cytochrome b_{558}.[14] In the late 1980s, the gene that is abnormal in X-linked CGD was cloned and subsequently shown to produce the heavy-chain component of the cytochrome b_{558} heterodimer (gp91phox).[15–17] Subsequently, the light chain (p22phox) was described and found to be the basis for the autosomal-recessive form of cytochrome b–deficient CGD.[18]

In the late 1980s and early 1990s, the molecular basis for other forms of autosomal-recessive CGD was defined. Cytosolic components, p47phox and p67phox, were identified, linked to distinct variants of CGD, and sequenced, and their genes were cloned.[19–22] Deficiency of p40phox has been more recently described.[23]

Thus, 84 years after Metchnikoff first posited that phagocytosis is essential in fighting infection (in 1883), studies in patients with CGD demonstrated for the first time clearly that a defect in phagocyte function is a major breach in host defense against severe infections. Since 1967, the biochemistry of the oxidase enzyme system has been elucidated, the major components defined, and the molecular basis for the most common variants of CGD described. Taking advantage of this syndrome as an "experiment of nature" has greatly expanded our knowledge of the role of the phagocyte in host defense.

CLINICAL FEATURES

The hallmark of this disease is the occurrence of purulent inflammation due to catalase-positive, low-grade pyogenic bacteria. This syndrome should be considered in any individual with recurrent catalase-positive bacterial or fungal infections. Table 63.1 summarizes the relative frequencies of the most common clinical findings in patients with CGD in the earliest reported cases, before the general use of prophylactic antimicrobial therapy.[24] A more recent analysis of infections in 368 patients enrolled in a registry for CGD[25,26] shows a general decline in most types of infection, with the notable exception of pneumonia (Table 63.2).

Of the 368 registry patients, 76% had the X-linked recessive form of CGD. The mean age at diagnosis in the registry patients was 3.0 years with the X-linked form and 7.8 years with an autosomal-recessive form.[25] These ages are much higher than they should be for the sake of the patient. In rare instances, the initial diagnosis has been made in adulthood. Reviews have suggested that autosomal-recessive variants generally have clinically milder diseases.[26,27]

Although any organ may be involved with infections, two patterns have been evident in CGD populations across the world.[25–35] Tables 63.1 and 63.2 exemplify data from the United States. First, the inability of phagocytic cells to effect microbicidal activity at the interface between the host and the environment leads to infections such as pneumonitis, infectious dermatitis, and perianal abscesses. With the involvement of the mononuclear phagocyte system, deep-seated infections result in purulent lymphadenitis, hepatomegaly, splenomegaly, and hepatic and perihepatic abscesses. At all sites of infection, microbes may be sequestered and protected from intracellular killing mechanisms and antibiotics. Unable to destroy the microbes, the phagocytes die and release the organisms. Further microbial proliferation and leukocyte accumulation lead to the abscesses and granulomas that characterize the disorder. Septicemia may also occur because of the inability of phagocytes to localize microbial invasion.

Purulent rhinitis and otitis are common clinical features of this disease. With adequate antibiotic therapy, rhinitis

Table 63.1 Clinical Findings in the 168 Earliest Reported Patients With Chronic Granulomatous Disease

Finding	Percentage of Patients Involved
Marked lymphadenopathy	82
Pneumonitis	80
Dermatitis	71
Hepatosplenomegaly	68
Onset by age 1 year	65
Suppuration of nodes	62
Splenomegaly	57
Hepatic-perihepatic abscesses	41
Osteomyelitis	32
Onset with dermatitis	25
Onset with lymphadenitis	23
Facial periorificial dermatitis	21
Persistent diarrhea	20
Septicemia or meningitis	17
Perianal abscess	17
Conjunctivitis	16
Death from pneumonitis	15
Persistent rhinitis	15
Ulcerative stomatitis	15

Modified from Johnston RB Jr, Newman SL. Chronic granulomatous disease. *Pediatr Clin North Am.* 1977;24:365.

Table 63.2 Most Common Infections in 368 Patients Enrolled in a Registry for Chronic Granulomatous Disease

Infection	Percentage of Patients
Pneumonia	79
Abscess (any)	68
Subcutaneous	42
Liver	27
Lung	16
Perirectal	15
Brain	3
Suppurative adenitis	53
Osteomyelitis	25
Bacteremia/fungemia	18
Cellulitis or impetigo	10

Data from Winkelstein JA, Marino MC, Johnston RB Jr, et al. Chronic granulomatous disease. Report on a national registry of 368 patients. *Medicine.* 2000;79:155.

clears slowly, only to recur within a few days after the treatment is discontinued. The oropharynx and gastrointestinal tract are frequently infected, with ulcerative stomatitis, gingivitis, esophagitis, rectal abscesses, perianal abscesses, and fissures being common. Urinary tract infections and glomerulonephritis, renal abscesses, and cystitis have all been reported. Gonadal infections are rare but have been described. Osteomyelitis is common; the most frequent sites include metacarpals, metatarsals, spine, and ribs.

Lymphadenitis, a characteristic clinical feature, occurs in the majority of patients during the course of the disease. It is typically chronic, suppurative, and granulomatous and very often requires surgical drainage. Cervical, axillary, and inguinal nodes are usually involved, but hilar and mesenteric lymph nodes are also commonly enlarged.

Skin lesions include impetiginous eruptions that progress slowly to suppuration. The healing process can be slow, resulting in granulomatous nodules that persist for months. These lesions may be found in any part of the body, the face and neck being the most frequent sites. Sweet's syndrome (acute febrile neutrophilic dermatosis)[36] has been associated with CGD. Furunculosis and subcutaneous abscesses may be chronic problems. Eczematoid dermatitis can be seen early in the diagnosis.

Carriers of X-linked CGD can have discoid lupus, aphthous ulcers, and systemic lupuslike symptoms.[37,38] If X-linked inactivation is skewed so that less than 10% of neutrophils express the normal NADPH oxidase, carrier females can have clinical CGD.[39–42] The progressive skewing of the X chromosome that occurs with age can result in adult-onset CGD in these carriers.[42]

While the major problems of patients with CGD are related to infections, these individuals can also be afflicted with a number of conditions reflecting a vigorous inflammatory response without a clear infectious cause.[27,28] Pyloric stenosis, with associated decrease in gastric emptying, is common, and sterile granulomas can be found in the pyloric antrum. Similar lesions in the small and large bowel may be associated with persistent abdominal pain, diarrhea, malabsorption, or obstruction.[43] Some of the gut lesions have been described as eosinophilic gastroenteritis, gastrointestinal dysmotility, or inflammatory bowel disease. Granulomas in the urinary bladder can result in obstructive uropathy. Pericarditis and pleuritis have been noted. Chorioretinitis was detected in 9 of 30 boys with X-linked CGD and in 3 of 15 related carriers in one clinic.[44] The single patient reported with p40phox deficiency had a partial deficiency in the respiratory burst, no severe infections, but severe and chronic granulomatous colitis.[23] Patients with CGD can also have a typical autoimmune disease, including systemic and discoid lupus, idiopathic thrombocytopenic purpura, juvenile rheumatoid arthritis, IgA nephropathy, or antiphospholipid syndrome.[45] It seems likely that there is a common mechanism for this spectrum of inflammatory conditions, perhaps related to the fact that CGD neutrophils do not undergo normal cell death by apoptosis, are not cleared efficiently by macrophages, and therefore release toxic constituents into the tissues.[46,47] Whatever the mechanism, the response of pyloric and bladder granulomas to steroids is well documented.

PULMONARY COMPLICATIONS

Patient surveys, as exemplified in Tables 63.1 and 63.2, show that pneumonia continues to be one of the most common types of infection, occurring in about 80% of patients with CGD.[25–35] Pulmonary disease has also become a major cause of mortality in this disease.[25] The overall pulmonary infection rate and incidence of fungal infections are increased in adults compared to children.[48] The onset of lower respiratory tract infection may be heralded by the usual clinical presentation of fever, cough, tachypnea, pleuritic pain, and abnormal auscultatory findings. However, in some patients, particularly those with a fungal infection, few if any signs or symptoms have been noted in the presence of marked infiltration on radiography. Chronic granulomatous infiltrations, bronchiolitis obliterans, pulmonary fibrosis, bronchiectasis, interstitial lung disease (ILD), and sarcoidosis have been noted in both pediatric and adult patients.[29,49,50]

The range of microbial agents causing pulmonary infections is shown in Table 63.3. Since the 1970s, the use of daily antimicrobial therapy in CGD has reduced the rate of

Table 63.3 Most Common Infecting Organisms in the 368 Patients in the Chronic Granulomatous Registry

Type of Infection	Organism	Percentage of Patients[a]
Pneumonia	*Aspergillus* species	33
	Staphylococcus species	9
	Burkholderia cepacia	7
	Nocardia species	6
	Serratia species	4
Abscess—subcutaneous, liver, and/or perirectal	*Staphylococcus* species	26
	Serratia species	3
	Aspergillus species	3
Abscess—lung	*Aspergillus* species	4
Abscess—brain	*Aspergillus* species	2
Suppurative adenitis	*Staphylococcus* species	14
	Serratia species	5
Osteomyelitis	*Serratia* species	7
	Aspergillus species	5
Bacteremia/fungemia	*Salmonella* species	3
	Burkholderia cepacia	2
	Candida species	2

[a]Percentage of the 368 patients who had this organism isolated at least once from the infection shown.

Data from Winkelstein JA, Merino MC, Johnston RB Jr, et al. Chronic granulomatous disease. Report on a national registry of 368 patients. *Medicine.* 2000;79:155.

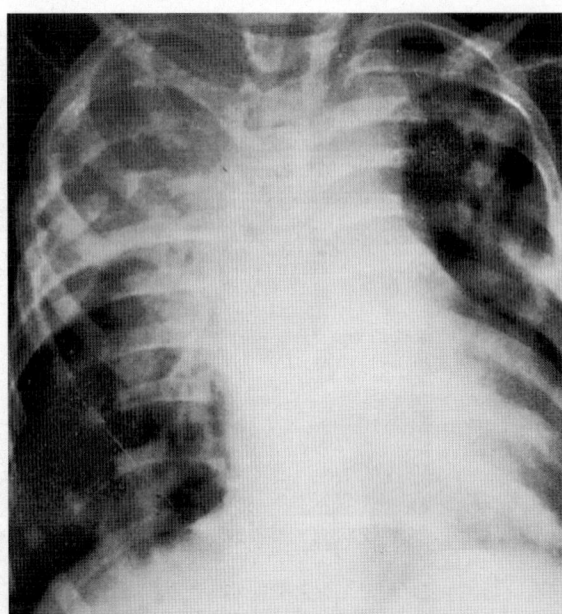

Fig. 63.1 A chest roentgenogram from a patient with chronic granulomatous disease, showing extensive bilateral lung involvement. This patient died of the overwhelming infection.

infections due to *Staphylococcus aureus* and enteric bacteria,[51] but *Aspergillus* species has become a particularly troublesome offender.[25,52] Fungal infection of the lung can present as discreet nodular, miliary, or pan-lobular involvement. Fungi now cause a large percentage of infections in CGD; these typically cause less fever and can be hard to diagnose in early stages. Fungal lung involvement may spread to the pleura and adjacent bone and soft tissues of the chest wall.[48,53,54] Although *Aspergillus* accounts for most of the fungal agents (>80%), other agents such as *Acremonium striatum, Candida albicans, Pneumocystis carinii,* and *Paecilomyces* species may also be isolated from infected lungs.[25,28,52] *Aspergillus* pneumonia, with or without dissemination, was the leading cause of death in the 368 registry patients (23 of 65 total deaths). *Nocardia,* atypical mycobacteria, and the bacillus Calmette-Guérin vaccine strain of mycobacteria can also cause pulmonary disease.[35]

Pulmonary lesions on x-ray include extensive infiltration of the lung parenchyma and prominent hilar adenopathy (Fig. 63.1). Bronchopneumonia, lobar pneumonia, extensive reticulonodular infiltration, pleural effusion, pleural thickening, pulmonary abscess, and atelectasis (especially of the right middle lobe) have been described.

In spite of extensive antibiotic treatment, the various expressions of CGD pulmonary disease often regress slowly over a period of weeks to months, or they can progress to involve an entire lobe. An unusual manifestation of pulmonary involvement observed in these patients is so-called encapsulated pneumonia.[55] This pneumonia is characteristically seen on roentgenography as a homogeneous, discrete, relatively round lesion; it may occur singly or in groups of two to three infiltrates (Fig. 63.2). The size and contour of the lesions may change over days or weeks or remain unchanged. Histologically, they take the form of caseating granulomas (Fig. 63.3). A homogeneous "shotgun" distribution of small granulomatous lesions can occur,

which gives the radiographic appearance of miliary tuberculosis. Discoid atelectasis, thickening of the bronchi, air bronchograms, "honeycombing," loss of lobar volume, and bronchiectasis associated with hemoptysis are occasionally observed.

LABORATORY FINDINGS AND DIAGNOSIS

Except for abnormalities of phagocyte function, clinical laboratory findings reflect acute or chronic infection and inflammation. Leukocytosis with neutrophilia, elevated erythrocyte sedimentation rate and C-reactive protein, and the anemia of chronic inflammation are common. The anemia is usually not due to a deficiency of iron stores but to a decrease in iron release from the mononuclear phagocyte system and diminished utilization by the marrow.[56] It typically does not respond to iron administration but improves with resolution of infection. Evidence of hemolytic anemia with acanthocytosis suggests absence of the K_x antigen on red blood cells, a trait encoded close to the gp91phox gene on the X chromosome.

Screening evaluations of various aspects of immune function are usually normal, including complement, cellular immunity, and antibody production in response to immunization in spite of recent data that the NADPH oxidase may modulate MCH class II antigen presentation by b-cells.[28,57] Polyclonal hypergammaglobulinemia is common. A deficiency of microbicidal activity against catalase-positive bacteria (e.g., staphylococci and *Escherichia coli*) and a diminished or absent respiratory burst by neutrophils and monocytes are the essential functional and biochemical findings of CGD.

Patients with CGD have a predisposition to infections with a broad variety of bacteria and fungi (see Table 63.3). The most common organisms are *S. aureus,* Serratia species and other gram negative organisms, and *Aspergillus,*[24,25,35,52] but unusual and rare pathogenic organisms may cause disease

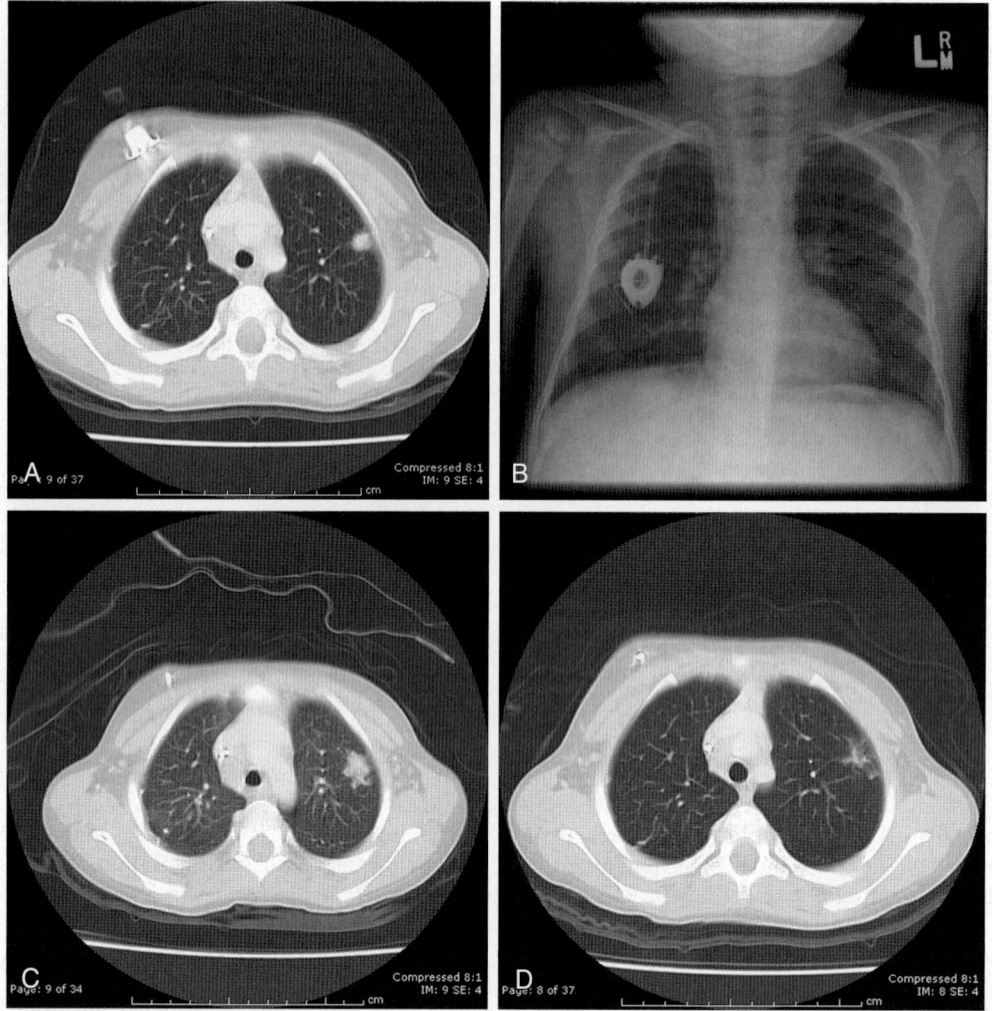

Fig. 63.2 (A) Encapsulated pneumonia in a patient with chronic granulomatous disease. A computed tomography (CT) scan with nodular lesion in left upper lobe. (B) PA chest Roentgenogram for comparison at same time as A does not demonstrate lesion. (C) Progression of lesion on CT scan. (D) Lesion resolving in response to appropriate antifungal therapy. (Images courtesy of Thomas Hay, MD.)

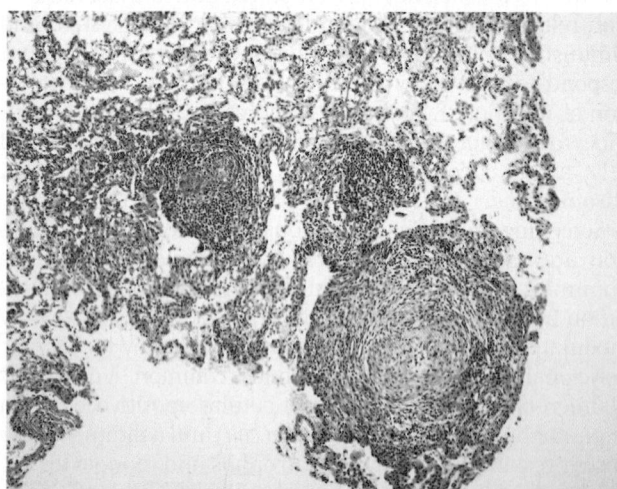

Fig. 63.3 Typical granuloma of lung tissue removed from the patient in Fig. 63.2. (Image courtesy of Kelli Capocelli, MD.)

in patients with CGD. Recent studies have focused on *Burkholderia cepacia* as a significant pathogen, particularly in the lung.[27,58–60] Infection by this organism was the second leading cause of death in patients in the CGD registry. Its propensity to infect patients with either CGD or cystic fibrosis is not understood.

Microbial agents associated with pulmonary infections are the same as those that cause infections in other parts of the body. Fungal pneumonitis is frequent, especially due to *Aspergillus*. Other pulmonary pathogens include *Nocardia* species, *P. carinii*, *Actinomyces*, and mycobacteria. Mycobacterial disease is relatively common in patients with CGD in countries where tuberculosis is endemic, BCG vaccine is mandatory, or both.[61] Infections due to pneumococci, streptococci, and *Haemophilus* species are no more common in children with CGD than in normal children, presumably because these catalase-negative organisms cannot protect against their own H_2O_2 production within the phagocytic vacuole.

Tissue from infected sites shows granulomas like those typically seen with intracellular parasites such as mycobacteria. Granulomas in CGD patients include mononuclear phagocytes that can contain a tan or yellow pigmented material.[2,61] Granulomas in the presence of the pathogens noted above strongly suggest the diagnosis of CGD.

Simple screening tests for CGD are currently available. The histochemical nitroblue tetrazolium (NBT) test[62] remains a reliable screening measure. Stimulation of microbicidal activity and the respiratory burst results in the reduction of O_2 to O_2^-; NBT dye is reduced by the extra electron in O_2^- and converted from a yellow, water-soluble dye to a purple, insoluble substance. In normal individuals, 95% or more of phagocytic cells reduce NBT; the phagocytes from patients with the common variants of CGD do not reduce NBT. Carriers of X-linked CGD exhibit two populations of cells, normal and NBT-negative.

Fluorescence-based screening assays using flow cytometry avoid the subjective element of the NBT test. Dihydrorhodamine-123 can be readily preloaded into neutrophils or monocytes, and it interacts with oxygen metabolites produced during the respiratory burst to generate products with increased fluorescence.[63] Patients' phagocytes do not shift fluorescence after stimulation. X-linked carriers have two populations. Additionally, some CGD variants, e.g., p47phox deficiency and milder variants of X-linked CGD, have very low oxidase activity in all cells, and this activity can be detected with this technique. This assay is more quantitative than the NBT test since it measures oxidase activity of the entire phagocyte population and can quantify partial reduction in the respiratory burst.

A positive screening test should be confirmed with one or more quantitative tests. Bactericidal assays with *E. coli* or *S. aureus* may be diagnostic.[8,64] Quantitative assays of O_2 consumption, O_2^- production, or generation of H_2O_2 can be helpful.[6,32,64,65] Finally, an analysis of the various oxidase components will define the molecular variant of CGD. Cytochrome b_{558} can be quantitated spectroscopically, and the individual oxidase components can be analyzed by Western blot. Several cell-free systems that can reproduce the assembly and activation of the oxidase in intact cells with the use of plasma membrane and cytosol from neutrophils may be helpful in defining the molecular variants of CGD. Identification of the genetic mutation responsible for the protein defect may be helpful for genetic counseling, prenatal studies, and judging prognosis, and a recent review presents a flow diagram for evaluation.[66–68]

Prenatal diagnosis may be achieved with screening tests on fetal neutrophils obtained by percutaneous umbilical blood sampling. The diagnosis for some CGD variants can be made from chorionic villus or amniocyte samples using restriction fragment length polymorphism or gene analysis without the risk of fetal blood sampling.[69]

NADPH OXIDASE

The oxidase enzyme resides in the plasma membrane of stimulated cells, and through the oxidation of NADPH catalyzes the reduction of O_2 to O_2^-, the first step in production of antimicrobial oxygen metabolites. Phagocyte oxidase (phox) activity results from the interaction of several components that form an enzyme complex. In resting cells, these components reside in different compartments. With stimulation of the cell, they assemble in the plasma membrane to express oxidase activity (Fig. 63.4).[28,70–72]

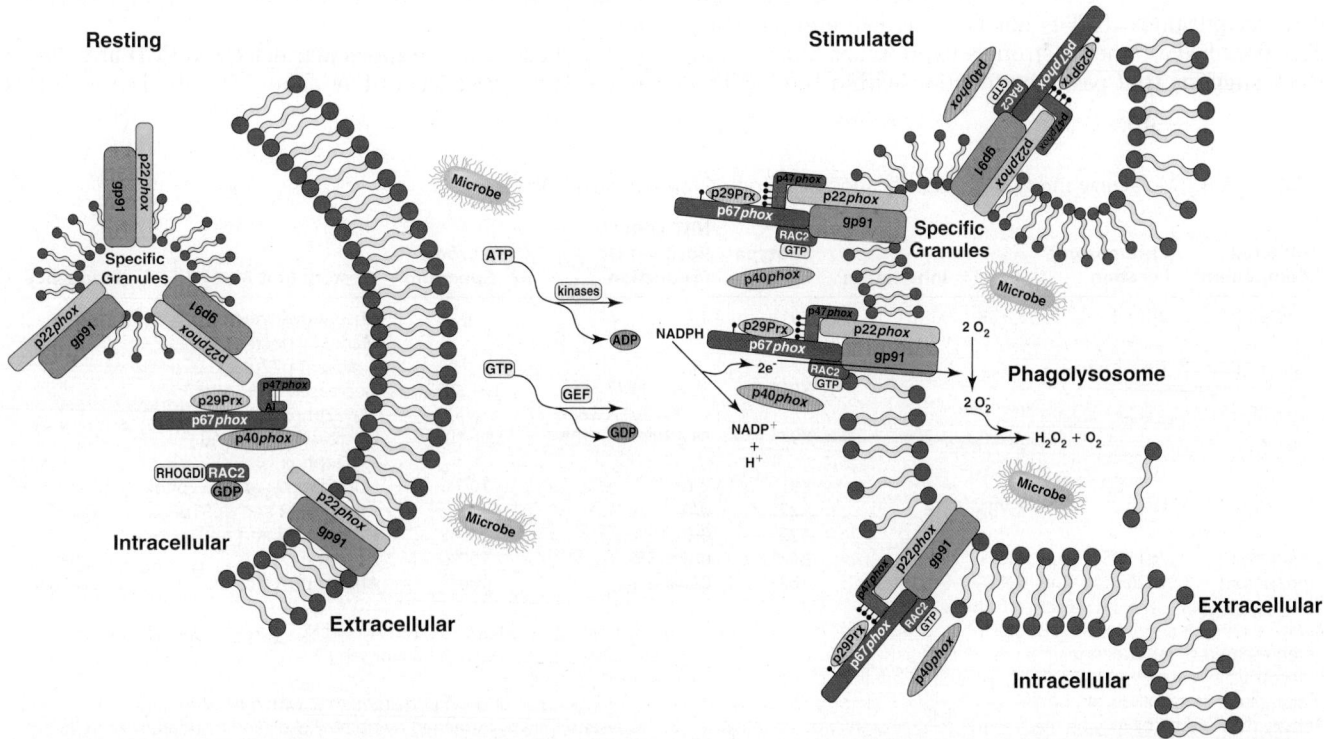

Fig. 63.4 Schematic diagram of the NADPH oxidase enzyme system, its components, and its activation. In resting neutrophils, membrane components (gp91phox and p22phox) reside in plasma membrane and specific granules. With stimulation, degranulation of specific granules expands the amount of cytochrome b558 in plasma membrane and translocation of cytosolic components (rac2, p47phox, p67phox, and p40phox) and p29 peroxiredoxin 6 (Prdx6) to the plasma membrane results in assembly of an active oxidase enzyme system that uses electrons from NADPH to reduce O_2 to form O_2^-.

The main catalytic component of the oxidase is the cytochrome b_{558}. In resting cells, 10%–20% of total cellular cytochrome b_{558} appears to be located in plasma membrane, and 80%–90% is in the membranes of specific granules. This protein is a heterodimer composed of α (p22phox) and β (gp91phox) subunits. Cytochrome b_{558} binds NADPH; its flavin binding site and a heme moiety are critical to shuttling electrons between NADPH and O_2.[73] With stimulation, specific granule membranes fuse with plasma membrane, increasing the amount of cytochrome b_{558} associated with the plasma membrane. The cytosolic oxidase components translocate to the plasma membrane and specific granules, providing an active oxidase complex that is increased in the plasma membrane.[70,71] A low molecular weight G protein, Rap1a, is associated with cytochrome b_{558} and may be important in assembly and activation of the oxidase complex.[28,74]

The cytosolic oxidase components include p47phox, p67phox, and p40phox.[21,22,73] A cytosolic low molecular weight guanosine triphosphate (GTP)–binding protein, p21*rac*2, is also involved, and there may be other proteins that control GTP binding to the *rac*2 protein.[75,76] These latter elements link with receptors on the plasma membrane and help transmit and/or amplify biochemical signals (e.g., from opsonized microbes) that regulate assembly and activation of the oxidase.

p47phox and p67phox appear to exist as a complex in cytosol of resting cells.[73,77] Interactions between this complex, plasma membrane, and the cytoskeletal elements are critical for activation of the oxidase.[72] Precise details of the relevant domains for interactions of phox proteins, changes which occur during cell activation, and the relationship with signaling pathways has been under intense investigation in recent years and is summarized in a recent review.[78] The gene for p40phox (NCF4) has been cloned, and p40phox was identified as binding strongly to p67phox. More recent work suggests that p40phox function within the NADPH oxidase complex depends on its binding to phosphatidylinositol 3-phosphate.[23] An additional protein closely associated with p67phox has been described.[79] This 29-kd protein (termed p29) is categorized as a peroxiredoxin by its sequence and activity. Peroxiredoxins are a class of peroxidases that oxidize H_2O_2 with sulfur groups on cysteine residues.[79] Neutrophil p29 peroxiredoxin enhances O_2^- production in subcellular systems of oxidase activity and in intact cells and translocates to plasma membrane after stimulation of the respiratory burst.[80] The p29 peroxiredoxin stabilizes and enhances the activity of the oxidase enzyme system.[80,81]

MOLECULAR DEFECTS AND INHERITANCE

Genetic testing documenting a patient/family mutation is currently available through commercial or research laboratories. In addition to confirming the correct classification of the patient and his/her prognosis, the specific defect will be important if more aggressive management strategies such as gene therapy and/or hematopoietic stem cell transplantation are considered. With the discovery of the various oxidase components over the past 15 years, the molecular basis of CGD has come into focus. Most patients express genetic or molecular abnormalities in one of the four major components of the oxidase: gp91phox, p22phox, p47phox, or p67phox (Table 63.4).[25,28,66,67] One patient has been reported with a mutation in *rac*2,[82] but no patients have been described with an abnormality of rap-1. p40phox, encoded by the NCF4 gene on chromosome 22 (22a13.1), is reported to be diminished in individuals with p67phox deficiency, and a single patient has been described with an autosomal recessive deficiency in this component, deficiency of the phagocytosis-stimulated respiratory burst, and granulomatous colitis.[23]

The most common molecular defects in CGD are related to gp91phox and account for about 70% of all cases of this

Table 63.4 Molecular and Genetic Classification of Chronic Granulomatous Disease

Affected Component[a]	Chromosome Location	Gene[a]	Inheritance[a]	Subtype Class[a]	NBT/DHR (% Positive)/O_2^- Production	Cytochrome b_{558} Spectrum	Western Blot Analysis[b]	Frequency
gp91phox	Xp21.1	CYBB	XL	X91°	0/0	0	Absent gp91phox Markedly decreased or absent p22phox	70%
				X91⁻	80%–100%/ 3%–30% (weak)	3%–30%	Decreased gp91 and p22phox	
				X91⁻	5%–10%/5%–10%	5%–10%	Decreased gp91 and p22phox	
				X91⁺	0/0	100%	Normal gp91 and p22phox	
p22phox	16p24	CYBA	AR	A22°	0/0	0	Absent p22 and gp91phox	5%–6%
				A22⁺	0/0	100%	Normal p22 and gp91phox	
p47phox	7q11.23	NCF-1	AR	A47°	0/0%–1%	100%	Absent p47phox	20%
p67phox	1q25	NCF-2	AR	A67°	0/1%–1%	100%	Absent p67phox	5%–6%

[a]Oxidase components expressed as gp91phox, p22phox, p47phox, p67phox, and their genes as CYBB, CYBA, NCF-1, and NCF-2, respectively. Subtypes represented by letter designating type of inheritance. The superscripts designate detection of protein in patient samples. *A*, Autosomal; *AR*, autosomal-recessive inheritance; *X*, X-linked; *XL*, X-linked inheritance; *O*, absent, −, diminished, +, present.

[b]For Western blot analysis, abnormalities in specific phox proteins are noted. Other components not described are normal with this technique.

Activity measurements may be made in the cell-free system of activation.[70-71] In this system, activity is defined by both cytosol (and associated components) and membrane. Deficiencies in gp91phox and p22phox exhibit diminished or absent membrane contribution and deficiencies of p47phox and p67phox exhibit diminished or absent cytosol contribution.

Data from Roos D, Kuhns DB, Roesler J, et al. Hematologically important mutations: X-linked chronic granulomatous disease (third update). *Blood Cells Mol Dis*. 2010;45:246; and Roos D, Kuhns DB, Maddalena A, et al. Hematologically important mutations: the autosomal recessive forms of chronic granulomatous disease (second update). *Blood Cells Mol Dis*. 2010;44:29.

syndrome.[26,28–35,66] Located on the short arm of the X chromosome (Xp21.1), defects in the gp91phox gene are inherited as X-linked recessive. In the most common variety, mutations in the gene result in the lack of gp91phox protein due to mRNA or protein instability. NADPH oxidase activity is totally absent, no cytochrome b_{558} is seen spectrophotometrically, and no gp91phox is detected on Western blot. A defect in the membrane contribution to oxidase activity is documented with analysis in cell-free systems. Cytosol and its components are normal. Deletions, insertions, rare duplications and splice site, missense, and nonsense mutations have all been described and reviewed in detail.[66]

Other variants of gp91phox deficiency have been described. Some mutations have resulted in partial loss of protein expression and diminished oxidase activity in proportion to the decrease in protein content. In some, a truncated protein is expressed. Defects are found in exons, introns, intron/exon junctions, and promoters. A few cases have been described with normal gp91phox protein expression but nearly complete absence of oxidase activity. Additional variants have been reported with the inability to interact with NADPH or with p47phox and p67phox or to bind flavin adenine dinucleotide (FAD). Severity of disease in these less common genetic variants correlates with the level of cytochrome b expression and superoxide production.

Patients who lack both the respiratory burst and cytochrome b_{558} and exhibit an autosomal-recessive mode of inheritance have a deficiency in p22phox, the gene for which is found on chromosome 16 (16q24). These patients account for 5%–6% of all cases. In the usual form, the deficiency in membrane contribution of oxidase activity is accompanied by absence of the cytochrome b_{558} spectrum and both gp91phox and p22phox by Western blot. Analysis of cytosolic components is normal. Although fewer genetic analyses have been completed, deletion, insertion, missense, nonsense, and splice site mutations have been described.[67] In one variant, a homozygous missense mutation affects the area of interaction between p22phox and p47phox, resulting in a normal cytochrome b_{558} that cannot form an oxidase complex.

Patients who exhibit an autosomal-recessive mode of inheritance but whose neutrophils contain normal amounts of cytochrome b_{558} may have a deficiency of either p47phox or p67phox. The gene for p47phox falls on chromosome 7 (7q11.23), and that for p67phox on chromosome 1 (1q25). Defects in these genes account for approximately 20% and 5%–6% of CGD cases, respectively. Absent or nearly absent oxidase in whole cells is coupled with deficient cytosol contribution in the cell-free system and deficiency of the protein on Western blot. There appears to be much less heterogeneity in genetic mutations causing deficiency of p47phox than of p67phox.[67] Patients studied to date are either homozygous for a GT dinucleotide (ΔGT) deletion at the start of exon 2 of the NCF-1 gene or are compound heterozygotes with a GT deletion on one allele and a point mutation on the second allele. The reason for the homogeneity is that most normal individuals have p47phox pseudogenes, each of which colocalize with the functional gene at 7q11.23. Recombination events between the functional and pseudogenes lead to incorporation of ΔGT into the NCF-1 gene. In addition to heterozygous GT changes, missense and splice junction changes have been described. In many patients studied, normal amounts of mRNA and complete absence of p47phox are found in neutrophils, suggesting translation of an unstable protein.

Relatively few molecular defects have been characterized in patients with p67phox deficiency. As with p47phox deficiency, mRNA for p67phox is usually present, but in most cases no protein is detected. Nonsense, missense, homozygous point, splice site, insertion, and deletion mutations have been documented, as well as one duplication, suggesting a heterogeneity of genetic abnormalities for p67phox.[28,67]

A patient with rac2 deficiency presented with severe, recurrent perirectal abscesses and pyoderma, omphalitis, and poor wound healing.[82,83] His neutrophils exhibited a unique pattern of functional abnormalities, including markedly diminished random and directed migration, decreased ingestion and bactericidal activity, and absent degranulation of azurophilic granules. Expression of CD11b and degranulation of specific granules were normal. Production of O_2^- in response to N-formyl-methionyl-leucyl-phenylalanine and platelet-activating factor was absent, to opsonized zymosan was decreased, but to phorbol myristate acetate was normal. Rac2 was 30% of control, and all other oxidase components were normal. A mutation in one nucleotide of codon 57 for one rac2 allele resulted in a substitution of asparagine for aspartic acid. Although both the wild-type and mutant alleles were expressed, the mutant protein had a defect in the GTP binding site, could only bind guanosine diphosphate, and had a dominant-negative effect on the wild-type rac2 as well as other low molecular weight GTPases.[82,83] Because of this, the oxidase as well as other neutrophil functions were affected. The patient was cured by a bone marrow transplant from his human leukocyte antigen (HLA)–identical sibling.[84]

Deficiency of glucose-6-phosphate dehydrogenase (G6PD) in leukocytes, which occurs in a small number of patients with erythrocytes deficient in this enzyme, has been considered a variant of CGD.[26,85–87] Patients whose neutrophils contain less than 5% of normal activity suffer from recurrent, sometimes fatal, infections. Their neutrophils do not exhibit a respiratory burst and exhibit a microbicidal defect against catalase-positive organisms. Deficiency of NADPH as the efficient electron donor to the oxidase may explain this disorder.[85]

MANAGEMENT

The key to the successful management of CGD remains early diagnosis, prophylactic antimicrobial therapy, and rapid and vigorous treatment of infections.[28,51,52,88–94] This approach begins with prophylactic daily doses of trimethoprim-sulfamethoxazole (4–5 mg/kg trimethoprim, 20–25 mg/kg sulfamethoxazole, once or divided into two doses daily), which has reduced the incidence of severe bacterial infections by 70%. Ciprofloxacin may be used as an alternative. Interferon (IFN)-γ given at a dose of 1.5 μg/kg (surface area <0.5 m²) or 50 μg/m² (surface area ≥0.5 m²) three times weekly by subcutaneous injection also reduces the incidence and severity of infections.[89,92] Administration before bedtime along with acetaminophen reduces fever and myalgias. Daily itraconazole at 100–200 mg/day (4–5 mg/kg in two doses) taken with food has been advocated as fungal prophylaxis.[51,88] Care should be taken to avoid environmental conditions that present a high risk for exposure to Nocardia and fungi, especially *Aspergillus* (e.g., garden mulch, construction sites, leaves, and marijuana).

When infections develop, aggressive attempts should be made to obtain culture and antibiotic sensitivity of organisms from localized areas. Surgical drainage, including drainage of pulmonary abscesses or empyema, is also critical to treatment, since antibiotics required to resolve infection do not penetrate well into abscesses.[93,94] The infected site should be aggressively débrided with prolonged drainage to prevent loculation and sequestration of infected areas.

In patients with fever and elevated C-reactive protein and sedimentation rate but no definite locus for an infection, an empiric trial of parenteral antibiotics may be necessary. During the initiation of this therapy, definition of the infected area should be sought with routine radiographs, computed tomography, magnetic resonance imaging studies, or radionucleotide scans.

Identification of the infected site may provide clues to initial antibiotic coverage. For example, the vast majority of liver abscesses are caused by staphylococci (see Table 63.3), and vancomycin and levofloxacin might be used initially. *Burkholderia cepacia* is found in a higher incidence in the lung and *Serratia* in soft tissue and bones. For these infections, increasing the trimethoprim-sulfamethoxazole to a full therapeutic dose and adding a cephalosporin, meropenem, or levofloxacin should be considered until antibiotic sensitivities are available. Antibiotic coverage should be reorganized later in response to antibiotic sensitivities of recovered organisms. Initial parenteral treatment and oral antimicrobials for weeks or months may be required to resolve the infection.

If fungus is suspected or defined, vigorous antifungal therapy should be instituted. Although amphotericin has been advocated in the past, other agents may be required, such as itraconazole, voriconazole (6 mg/kg every 12 hours on day 1, then 4 mg/kg every 12 hours), or posaconazole (200 mg 3 times daily; currently approved only for children over 12 years old and adults).[88,95–97] Prednisone may be considered for miliary involvement. Although not proved efficacious, daily granulocyte transfusions (at least 10^{10} granulocytes per transfusion) have been used as a supplement to aggressive surgical and antibiotic therapy,[27,28,98] but these can cause alloimmunization, which could hamper later bone marrow transplantation.

Some patients with CGD inherit, as a closely associated X-linked allele, a deficiency in the K_x antigen affecting both erythrocytes and leukocytes.[28] This results in the lack of Kell antigens on the surface of the red cells, which can be associated with a chronic hemolytic anemia. Transfusion of these patients can result in true isoimmunization for Kell antigens and the risk of immediate or delayed transfusion reactions.

Inflammatory conditions or obstructive lesions of the gastrointestinal tract (seen in up to 50% of the patients) or genitourinary tract (in up to 70% of the patients) usually respond to treatment with steroids.[43,99,100] The response may be prompt, but relapses are common.

HEMATOPOIETIC CELL TRANSPLANTATION AND GENE THERAPY

Hematopoietic cell transplantation has been attempted with mixed results.[101–104] Long-term engraftment and reversal of the defect has been documented. Sources of stem cells include bone marrow, mobilized peripheral blood, and umbilical cord blood. Although unrelated donors have been used, the majority of successful transplants have been completed with HLA-identical siblings.[101,103] In a series from the United Kingdom, transplantation led to resolution of colitis and catch-up growth in children with growth failure.[104] The best predictors of success have been absence of overt preexisting infection at the time of transplantation and transplantation at a relatively early age, before numerous infections and end-organ damage have occurred. A comparison of outcome for children with CGD treated with conservative medical management, compared to those treated with stem cell transplantation, documented fewer infections and better growth after transplantation.[105] However survival was 90% for both transplanted and nontransplanted groups.

Many of the centers transplanting CGD patients have used a myeloablative preparative regimen. While engraftment has occurred in a high percentage of patients, the presence of concurrent infection has presented a significant risk for severe complications, and death has been common. The National Institutes of Health published its experience using a nonmyeloablative preparative regimen with T cell–depleted peripheral blood stem cells from HLA-identical siblings.[103] After a median follow-up of 17 months, 8 of 10 patients had sufficient neutrophils to provide normal host defense and resolution of granulomatous lesions. Another center used marrow from matched unrelated donors; 7 of 9 patients were alive and well 20–79 months after transplantation. Restrictive lung disease was resolved in two of these individuals.

A prospective study from 16 centers in 10 countries worldwide was recently published.[106] Patients with CGD received hematologic stem cell transplantation (HSCT) from matched related or matched, unrelated donors after a reduced intensity conditioning regimen, administration of unmanipulated bone marrow, or peripheral blood stem cells. Fifty-six patients were enrolled of whom 75% were judged to be high risk because of infections or inflammatory complications. With a median follow-up of 21 months, overall survival was 93% and event free survival 89%. Two-year probability of survival was 96% and event free survival 91%.

With results of reduced conditioning regimens, some have suggested that stem cell transplantation should be the preferred choice performed early if a suitable donor is available. However, conventional medical management by many groups does not include IFN-gamma in addition to prophylactic antibiotics and antifungals. A single center U.S. study of 27 patients with CGD was presented of whom which 24 were compliant on the medical management with IFN-gamma, Bactrim, and an azole antifungal.[107] One was lost to follow-up and 23 were alive after 3276 patient months of follow-up with an infection rate of 0.62/patient year. No controlled comparison of medical management with HSCT is available. Although CGD can be cured by successful hematopoietic cell transplantation, the possibility of infections, graft failure and rejection, and graft-versus-host disease remain major impediments, and the risks and benefits must be weighed carefully with each individual patient. Patient selection and timing of bone marrow transplantation are timely areas for developing research.

Since CGD arises from gene defects in a finite group of proteins expressed in myeloid cells, transfer of a normally functioning gene into the pluripotent stem cell would, theoretically, constitute definitive treatment. The groundwork for this approach was laid with experiments in which Epstein-Barr virus–transformed B-lymphocyte or myelomonoblastic cell lines from CGD patients with various molecular defects were transfected with complementary DNA (cDNA) for the missing oxidase component. Partial correction of protein expression and oxidase activity was obtained.[21,108,109] Reconstitution *in vivo*, however, would require transfection of normal genes into pluripotent stem cells. To this end, CD34⁺ peripheral blood hematopoietic progenitor cells were transduced with cDNA for p47phox, p22phox, or gp91phox.[110,111] Murine models of CGD have also provided useful information for successful application of human gene therapy trials.[112,113]

Malech and coworkers developed a model process for CGD gene therapy and employed it in a clinical trial of five patients with p47phox-deficient CGD.[114] CD34⁺ progenitor cells were mobilized by granulocyte colony-stimulating factor infusion, harvested by apheresis, purified, then expanded *ex vivo* in the presence of growth factors. These expanded CD34⁺ cells were transfected with cDNA for normal p47phox in a retroviral vector. The patients received 0.1 to 4.7×10^6 transfected cells/kg. After 3–5 weeks, low levels of blood neutrophils with normal ability to oxidize dihydrorhodamine were detected; but these cells declined to undetectable numbers over 3–6 months. Although the numbers of normal cells were too small to reconstitute the defect and the effect was not long-lasting, the general principles of this approach were demonstrated.

This experience was extended by Ott and colleagues.[115] After nonmyeloablative marrow conditioning with bulsufan, two young adults with X-linked CGD were treated with autologous CD34⁺ stem cells that had been transfected with a retrovirus vector expressing gp91phox. Substantial gene transfer occurred in both individuals, and life-threatening infections resolved within the first few months. However, the level of gene-positive neutrophils subsequently rose as a result of oligoclonal outgrowth of cells in which the vector had inserted at the site of a proto-oncogene.[116] Bone marrow exam showed myelodysplasia with monosomy 7 in both men; one died of sepsis, and the other received an allogeneic hematopoietic stem-cell transplantation.[116,117]

Based on the clearance of severe infections achieved in the otherwise failed trial of Ott et al., Kang, Malech, and colleagues treated 3 adult X-linked CGD patients suffering severe, unresolving infections with a different retroviral vector encoding gp91phox after busulfan marrow conditioning.[118] The three patients had 26%, 5%, and 4% oxidase-normal neutrophils initially, but these normal cells declined over time. One of the patients with a sustained level of 1.1% normal cells cleared treatment-intractable liver abscesses and has been free of infection for 3 years; a second patient with 0.03% sustained normal-cell levels resolved his *Aspergillus* lung infection that had extended to ribs and vertebrae. The patient with no detectable normal cells by 4 weeks died of his *Paecilomyces* lung infection.[118] With improvements in viral vector profiles, stem cell culturing techniques, new sources of stem cells including induced pleuripotent stem cells, and site-specific gene editing platforms, the field of gene therapy continues to progress.[119,120] Although gene therapy has not yet cured a patient, with CGD the field clearly holds out hope for the future.

Common Variable Immunodeficiency Disorders

Common variable immunodeficiency disorders is now the standard term[121] for a group of disorders that is almost always associated with pulmonary complications. The group is characterized clinically by onset in the first 5–10 years of life, or in mid-adolescence to young adulthood, of recurrent bacterial infections, especially sinusitis, pneumonia, and chronic pulmonary disease. Although not common, the disorder can begin in infancy. Autoimmune disease, gastrointestinal disorders, and a predisposition to lymphoma are less commonly associated conditions. The group is characterized immunologically by decreased production of IgG in combination with low levels of IgA and/or IgM, weak or absent antibody response to immunizations, and absence of any other immunodeficiency state.

The condition was once thought of as a single entity and was initially referred to as "late-appearing (or 'acquired') hypogammaglobulinemia." It was diagnosed in males and females and after infancy, and this term differentiated it from the earlier-described congenital X-linked agammaglobulinemia (XLA). As more cases were described, it was given the name "common variable immunodeficiency" (OMIM 240500). The condition is aptly named—it is common, at least among primary immunodeficiency diseases, with an estimated rate in the population of 1 in 25,000–30,000[122–125] and its clinical presentation and underlying immune cellular defects vary widely. It is apparently the expression of several different conditions with multiple underlying single-gene or polygenic defects. Although it is not clear what most of those may be, it is nevertheless appropriate that the new term for the group (used in our title) emphasizes a family of disorders. In describing the *diagnosis* applied to patients within the group, we will use the abbreviation CVID to mean a common variable immunodeficiency disorder.

CLINICAL FEATURES

Major reviews of 248 CVID patients from the United States,[124] 252 patients from France,[126] and 334 patients from the European Common Variable Immunodeficiency Disorders registry,[125] a collaborative analysis by two of the principal authors of these reviews,[127] and a review of CVID in children[128] have greatly expanded understanding of these disorders, recent summaries have broadened our current knowledge of these diseases.

The fundamental feature of CVID is insufficient production of antibodies to pathogens. Thus, almost all patients have a history of serious or recurrent infections (e.g., all but 5 of 248 patients in the U.S. cohort).[124] Table 63.5 summarizes the most common infections that occurred in the American and French cohorts, and the list reflects the experience at other centers (in particular those in references 125 and 127 and citations contained therein).

Recurrent or chronic bronchitis, sinusitis, and/or otitis media occur in almost all patients and are the most common infections at onset of symptoms.[124–130] The microorganisms most commonly cultured before the diagnosis is made and treatment started are those that require antibody for optimal opsonization and phagocytosis, particularly pneumococci,

Table 63.5   Summary of Most Common Infections in Two Large Cohorts of Patients With Common Variable Immunodeficiency Disorder

	Number of Patients of Total 248[124] (%)[a]	Number of Patients of Total 252[126] (%)[a]
Recurrent bronchitis, sinusitis, and/or otitis	243 (98)	
Respiratory and lung infections (total)		240 (95)
Pneumonia	190 (77)	147 (58)
Chronic lung disease, including bronchiectasis	68 (27)	92 (37)
Viral hepatitis	16 (7)	
Severe or recurrent herpes zoster infection	9 (4)	27 (11)
Severe varicella infection		10 (4)
Giardia enteritis	8 (3)	35 (14)
Pneumocystis infection	7 (3)	2 (1)
Mycoplasma pneumonia	6 (2)	
Salmonella or *Campylobacter* enteritis	6 (2)	38 (15)
Osteomyelitis or septic arthritis (2 each)	4 (2)	
Chronic mucocutaneous candidiasis	3 (1)	
Bacteremic sepsis	3 (1)	33 (13)
Bacterial meningitis	2 (<1)	20 (8)

[a]Number of patients (%) with the infection among the total studied. Adapted from references 124 and 126 and their accompanying texts. Reference 124 reports the experience of an academic medical center in New York City, U.S.A. Fifteen percent of the 248 patients developed symptoms between 2 and 10 years old (mean age 23 years for males, 28 years for females). Reference 126 reports the experience of a French national study of adults with primary hypogammaglobulinemia. Fifty-nine percent of the 252 patients developed symptoms between 4 and 10 years of age (median age at onset = 19 years).

Haemophilus influenzae, and streptococci. After treatment has been started with intravenous immunoglobulin (IVIG), infections are more likely to be caused by staphylococci or an enteric pathogen, fungi (e.g., *Candida, Pneumocystis, Nocardia*), a virus (varicella-zoster virus, enteroviruses, hepatitis viruses), protozoa (especially *Giardia*), or *Mycoplasma*.[123–133] In a review of 20 patients diagnosed with CVID and an enteroviral infection, 14 had ECHO or Coxsackievirus infection and 6 had poliomyelitis, particularly due to live polio vaccine.[132]

The clinical findings in 32 children with CVID[130] were very similar to those described in the large reviews of patients of all ages (see Table 63.5). Recurrent or chronic respiratory tract infections (88% of the children), sinusitis (78%), otitis media (78%), pneumonia (78%), bronchiectasis (34%), and intestinal tract infections (34%) were the most common infections. Two children had polio after live poliovirus immunization. An allergic disorder was present in 38% of the children and an autoimmune condition in 31%. The mean time between onset of symptoms and institution of immunoglobulin substitution therapy was 5.8 years.

On physical exam, evidence of complications may include growth retardation (9 of the 32 children)[130] or weight loss (adults), changes associated with chronic otitis or sinusitis, lymphadenopathy, splenomegaly, gingivitis, poor dentition, and signs of chronic pulmonary disease.[123–130]

Gastrointestinal disease occurs in roughly a quarter to a third of patients (15%–47% depending on what conditions are included),[124,126,128,134,135] perhaps especially in those who have an accompanying defect in cell-mediated immunity.[134] These may be caused by infection, cancer, or autoimmune or inflammatory disease. Chronic diarrhea is the most common symptom. The etiology is not always known, but infections with *Giardia, Salmonella* or *Campylobacter* (see Table 63.5, CMV, or *Cryptosporidium* have been reported.[124,126,128,135]

Autoimmune disease develops in 20%–25% of individuals with CVID, most often expressed as autoimmune hemolytic anemia or thrombocytopenic purpura, but also as rheumatoid arthritis, pernicious anemia, immune neutropenia, inflammatory bowel disease, or almost any known autoimmune condition.[124,126,136,137] Patients with CVID are at increased risk for malignancies, with particular susceptibility to non-Hodgkins lymphoma and gastric cancers, but other malignancies have been described.[123–125,128,138,139] Polyclonal lymphocytic infiltration expressed as enteropathy, persistent lymphadenopathy, splenomegaly, organ granulomas, or granulomatous/lymphocytic pulmonary disease, in various combinations, is one of the major phenotypes of CVID.[125]

PULMONARY COMPLICATIONS

Lung disease is the most common serious problem in patients with CVID,[124,128,129,140–143] accounting for disabling morbidity and early mortality. In large clinical studies a quarter to about half of the patients had chronic lung disease including bronchiectasis, or restrictive or obstructive lung disease.[124,139,141,142] Bronchiectasis can be seen in children under 3 years of age as a result of infection and the inflammation it elicits; and it can be the presenting symptom of CVID at almost any age. Some patients have been tested for immunoglobulin levels as an afterthought on their way to resection of a bronchiectatic segment of lung. In children who carry a diagnosis of CVID, the almost universal presence of chronic bronchitis may delay diagnosis of a more serious pulmonary disease.

In one study of B-cell immunodeficiency in subjects over 18 years old, 75% of whom had CVID, bronchiectasis was detected by chest computed tomography (CT) exam, but not by chest radiograph in 8 of 19 patients; the presence of bronchiectasis by CT did not correlate with either the presence of clinical symptoms (cough, sputum, fever) or abnormalities on pulmonary function tests.[144]

Noninfectious pulmonary disease becomes common beginning in adolescence and early adulthood.[136] Granulomatous lung disease, lymphocytic interstitial pneumonia, follicular bronchiolitis, and lymphoid hyperplasia have been grouped in patients with CVID under the term granulomatous-lymphocytic interstitial lung disease (GLILD).[142,143,145–147] An example of radiographic findings from a patient with GLILD is included in Fig. 63.5. This CVID subgroup is at high risk for early mortality and B-cell lymphomas (median survival 14 years versus 29 years in other CVID groups in one careful study).[142] Human herpesvirus 8, a B-cell lymphotrophic virus, was isolated from 6 of 9 CVID patients with GLILD, 1 of 21 CVID patients without GLILD, and no controls; one CVID-GLILD patient later developed a B-cell lymphoma.[147] Granulomatous lung disease in CVID patients has been diagnosed as sarcoidosis.[124,144,146,148]

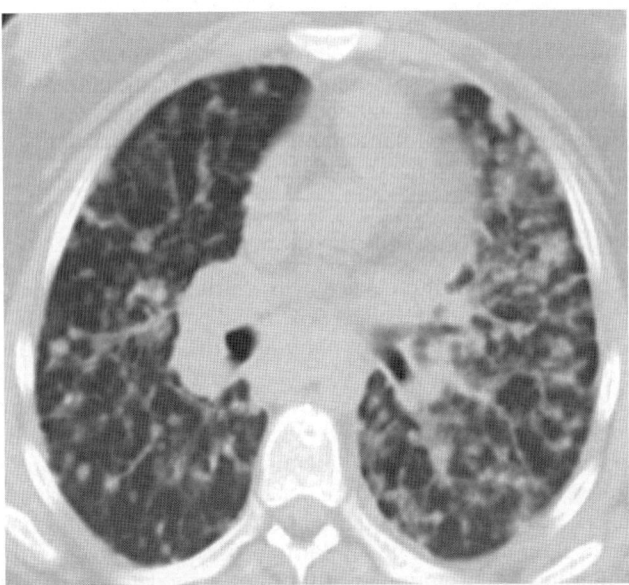

Fig. 63.5 Computed tomography scan of a 16-year-old with biopsy proven granulomatous-lymphocytic interstitial lung disease. Extensive nodular infiltrates throughout both lung fields and interstitial thickening with associated mediastinal and subcarinal adenopathy. (Image courtesy of Robin Deterding, MD.)

LABORATORY FINDINGS AND DIAGNOSIS

The characteristic findings in CVID are levels of IgG that are two standard deviations or more below age-adjusted means[124,128] and decreases in IgM and/or IgA meeting the same criteria. If first-drawn immunoglobulin levels are low, these should be repeated to exclude the possibilities of lab error, and the patient's response to both protein and polysaccharide vaccines should be tested. A normal response should be greater than a two-fold rise from baseline.

Most patients with CVID have normal numbers of circulating B and T lymphocytes, but some patients have decreased levels of circulating phenotypic memory (CD27+) B cells or isotype-switched memory B cells (CD27+ IgD– IgM–).[149–151] Some have mildly abnormal T-lymphocyte function or phenotypic T-cell markers, including T-lymphocyte proliferation in response to standard mitogens and antigens, decreased CD4+ cells and thus CD4/CD8 ratio, reduced numbers of T-regulatory cells, reduced CD19+ B cells, altered expression of interleukin (IL)-2 and other cytokines, defective T-cell receptor signal transduction, and defective Toll-like receptor (TLR) 7 and 9 function in lymphocytes and dendritic cells.[124,125,128,149–158] These phenotypic and functional lymphocyte abnormalities are rarely needed to make the diagnosis of CVID, but they are becoming increasingly important in understanding clinical phenotype and prognosis,[150–154] and they will become even more important as genetic defects are matched with these abnormalities. For example, 9% of 313 CVID patients in the French national registry presented with late-onset combined immunodeficiency associated with opportunistic infections, marked decrease in CD4+ T cells, and increased risk of granulomatous disease, gastrointestinal disease, and lymphoma.[159]

Because CVID is a diagnosis of exclusion, other conditions that may have an almost identical phenotype in some cases must be considered. These include XLA, hyper-IgM

syndromes, and transient hypogammaglobulinemia of infancy. In the last case, cellular immunity (abnormal in about 40% of CVID patients) and response to immunization (abnormal by definition in CVID) are typically normal, and the condition is usually gone by 24 months. XLA results from any of several hundred mutations in the gene *Btk*, and the condition typically presents with absence of B cells and infections within the first 2 years of life. However, hypomorphic *Btk* mutations can allow some B-cell formation and IgG levels that are only moderately depressed or even normal.[42,160,161] As many as 10% of CVID patients may have decreased numbers of B cells, but these are usually well above levels in *Btk* deficiency.

MOLECULAR DEFECTS AND INHERITANCE

It is likely that CVID results from a variety of genetic defects. Most of these probably arise from sporadic mutations, but approximately 10% of patients have family members with CVID or another humoral immune abnormality.[162] Gene defects associated with CVID are beginning to be identified. One of these is the recessive gene for inducible costimulator of activated T-cells (ICOS) on chromosome 2q, which is thought to be important in signaling T-cells for T- and B-cell cooperation.[163–165] One patient with ICOS deficiency presented at 18 months of age, but most developed recurrent sinopulmonary infections in adolescence or young adulthood.[163] Another CVID-associated gene encodes transmembrane activator and calcium-modulator and cyclophilin ligand (TACI) found on chromosome 17p. TACI is expressed on B-cells and CD4+ T-cells and is involved in isotype switching.[166,167] Mutations in this gene are found in 8%–10% of CVID patients and are associated with susceptibility to CVID rather than directly causing it.[167,168] A defect of B-cell activating factor of the tumor necrosis factor family receptor (BAFF-R) encoded on chromosome 22q was described in siblings from one family.[169] Homozygous or compound heterozygous mutations in the gene for CD19 on chromosome 16p can be associated with a CVID phenotype.[170,171] Several other monogenetic defects can result in the phenotypic expression of CVID,[128,129] and it is likely more will be described in the future.

MANAGEMENT

As with other immunodeficiency states, prompt identification of the site of infection and infecting organism and prompt administration of antimicrobial therapy will expedite resolution and reduce the chronic complications. Treatment for an extended period may be required. Administration of prophylactic antibiotics has not been studied and remains controversial. Immunizations may not be useful since these patients have poor responses, but they are still recommended.[172] Although no adverse events have been reported with live vaccines, caution should be used when considering these.

Treatment for infections should be guided by results of cultures. For acute exacerbations of bronchiectasis or sinusitis, both driven by cycles of infection and scarring, options include amoxicillin-clavulanate, cephalosporins, or fluoroquinalones (except ciprofloxacin) for 2–4 weeks. Inhaled glucocorticoids may reduce the cough and dyspnea with bronchiectasis, but they should be used sparingly, and the patient's condition should be monitored with pulmonary function testing and CT scans.

Immunoglobulin replacement has led to major improvement in the management of infections in CVID, preventing acute infections and slowing progression of chronic infections.[173] It may be given intravenously every 3–4 weeks or subcutaneously if venous access is poor, or to circumvent severe reactions to intravenous administration. The usual starting dose is 300–400 mg/kg to keep trough IgG levels (drawn just before administering the next dose) in the middle of the reference range. Higher doses, up to 1 g/kg, may be required,[174] for example, to treat development of central nervous system or systemic (muscle and liver) enteroviral infection, to which CVID patients are predisposed.[132] Immunoglobulin replacement therapy will be needed for the lifetime of the patient, monitored as IgG trough levels and adjusted as indicated. Patients with noninfectious, autoimmune disorders may require immunosuppressive therapy, but this should be undertaken cautiously. Glucocorticoids are first-line treatment for the autoimmune cytopenias; higher doses of IVIG may also be considered.[175,176] Splenectomy should be considered as a last resort, as it may increase the risk for subsequent severe infections.[177] Rituximab has been used successfully in CVID patients with cytopenia.[177,178] CVID patients should be monitored for signs and symptoms of lymphoid malignancy, gastric cancer, and other malignancies and have age-appropriate cancer screening.[124,128]

We are unaware of established treatment guidelines or controlled trials to inform optimal management of GLILD in patients with CVID. Anecdotal experience has shown general improvement in symptoms with corticosteroid treatment.[143] Exercise testing and full pulmonary function testing can be used to monitor the effects of therapy. CT radiographic abnormalities may not resolve though symptoms improve with corticosteroids. Cyclosporin and monoclonal antibody therapy against TNF-α or CD 20 expressed on B cells have been tried, but the experience is limited.[143]

With the advent of immunoglobulin replacement and aggressive management of infections, the risk of death from infection has been reduced dramatically. Nearly two-thirds of patients survive 20 years beyond the diagnosis.[124,128] The highest mortality rates currently are seen in patients with bronchiectasis, GLILD, and noninfectious complications.[125,142]

Other Immunodeficiencies With Pulmonary Manifestations

The estimated worldwide prevalence of primary immunodeficiencies (PIDs) likely exceeds 1 in 1000.[179] They can affect each branch of the immune system with characteristic pulmonary manifestations both infectious and noninfectious. Adaptive immune responses are triggered by binding of microbial antigens to B-cell and T-cell receptors, which have a high degree of antigen specificity. Isolated B-cell or combined B- and T-cell immunodeficiencies develop as a consequence of abnormal B- and T-cell development. Pattern recognition receptors recognize molecular patterns of microbes with less specificity. They are expressed on innate immune cells, neutrophils, macrophages, dendritic cells, and natural killer (NK) and NKT-cells. Complement activation

facilitates elimination of microbes by phagocytes and links innate and adaptive immune responses.[180] Primary immunodeficiencies that also present with characteristic pulmonary manifestations are B-cell deficiencies in general, not only CVID, combined cellular and humoral immunodeficiencies, and deficiencies of the innate immune system.

B-CELL IMMUNODEFICIENCIES

Primary B-cell immunodeficiencies with antibody deficiency are most common and affect 65% of all patients with PID.[181] They include milder forms such as transient hypogammaglobulinemia of infancy (6.8%), selective IgA deficiency (18.7%), IgG subclass deficiency (12%), specific antibody deficiency (1.2%), and more severe forms such as CVID (37.5%) and agammaglobulinemia (10.7%).[182,183] The onset and severity of infections are dependent on the underlying defect. Pulmonary infections and complications that may occur later in life can be similar to those described for CVID. Children with profound or absent antibody deficiency as in XLA usually present with severe bacterial infections after 3–6 months of life when *in-utero* acquired maternal IgG antibodies decline. During infancy, *Pneumocystis jiroveci* pneumonia has been described. In contrast to infants with severe combined immunodeficiency (SCID), infants with XLA show a normal thymic shadow on chest x-ray.[184]

The initial diagnostic workup for all suspected antibody deficiencies includes a complete blood cell count (CBC), lymphocyte phenotyping to determine the number and percentage of CD19 and/or CD20-positive B-cells, measurement of serum immunoglobulins and specific antibody concentrations to protein and polysaccharide vaccines that should be remeasured 4 weeks after revaccination, and IgG subclasses as indicated. In XLA and other antibody deficiencies with profound reduction in all serum immunoglobulin classes, B-cells are severely decreased or absent. The diagnosis of XLA can be confirmed by lack of *BTK* protein expression in monocytes by flow cytometry and gene sequencing. Genetic testing panels for antibody deficiencies are available for clinical use.

The mainstay of treatment for antibody deficiency is intravenous or subcutaneous immunoglobulin G substitution, antibiotic prophylaxis and therapy, and prevention of bronchiectasis and other pulmonary complications.

COMBINED CELLULAR AND HUMORAL IMMUNODEFICIENCIES

Combined cellular and humoral immunodeficiencies include SCID, a medical emergency during infancy, and milder forms such as X-linked hyper-IgM syndrome (CD40-ligand deficiency), DiGeorge syndrome, ataxia telangiectasia (AT), and hyper-IgE syndromes.[185] Unexplained infections with opportunistic pathogens should raise concern for a combined immunodeficiency. When suspected in infancy, live vaccines are contraindicated, and only irradiated, CMV-free blood products should be used for transfusions.

SEVERE COMBINED IMMUNODEFICIENCIES

SCID present early during the first year of life with recurrent infections by bacteria, viruses, fungi, and opportunistic pathogens.[185] The incidence is estimated as 1 in 50,000 newborns. Infants present with lymphopenia and hypogammaglobulinemia. Recurrent pneumonia with *P. jirovecii*, parainfluenza 3 virus, RSV, CMV, adenovirus, or bacteria may occur, at times as simultaneous infection with multiple pathogens. Infants are affected by chronic diarrhea, failure to thrive, oral thrush, and diaper rashes. The thymic shadow on chest x-ray and lymphoid tissue are absent. As of 2014, 14 different genetic mutations causing SCID had been described, with mutations in the *IL-2RG* coding for the common gamma chain of receptors for cytokines IL-2, -4, -7, -9, -15, and -21 causing X-linked SCID being most frequent.[186] Currently, 42 states in the U.S. are conducting newborn screening for SCID by quantifying T cell receptor excision cycles (TRECs) in newborn blood.[187] TRECs are absent or significantly reduced in SCID.

Infants with SCID can present with respiratory distress due to viral and fungal, or bacterial pneumonia. On chest x-ray, a thymus is absent.[184] Hyperinflation, atelectasis, and bilateral, diffuse interstitial changes with nodular opacities may be present in viral pneumonitis.[184] Acute *P. jirovecii* pneumonia and Candida infections can also present with bilateral nodular or granular opacities.[184] Candida infections can be invasive and cause abscess formation.[184] Autosomal-recessive adenosine deaminase (ADA) deficiency is associated with chondro-osseous dysplasia, and flaring of the costochondral junctions can be seen on chest x-ray.[184,188] Interstitial inflammatory infiltrates can occur in ADA deficiency due to the metabolic defect and not related to infection.[189]

The diagnostic workup for suspected SCID includes a CBC, lymphocyte phenotyping to determine the number of T-cells, recent thymic emigrant T-cells (CD4/CD45RA/CD31-positive), naïve (CD4/CD45RA-positive) and memory (CD4/CD45RO-positive) T-cells, lymphocyte function testing with mitogen and antigen stimulation, and measurement of serum immunoglobulins. T-cells are usually low or absent, and B-cells are dysfunctional. The presence or absence of B- and/or NK-cells directs the initial genetic workup. In the absence of T-, B-, and NK-cells and suspected ADA deficiency, one of the most severe forms of SCID, ADA catalytic activity can be measured in hemolysates and peripheral blood mononuclear cells (PBMC), and is usually less than 1% of normal activity. Genetic testing for single gene defects and SCID-gene panels are available to determine the underlying defect. If a diagnosis cannot be confirmed, whole exome or genome sequencing should be considered.[190]

Treatment for SCID includes prevention of viral, fungal, and bacterial infections with antimicrobial therapy, immunoglobulin G replacement, HSCT, and in selected cases, e.g. ADA deficiency, enzyme replacement therapy. Bone marrow transplantation during early infancy without prior infections have resulted in greater than 90% survival of infants with SCID.[191]

ATAXIA TELANGIECTASIA

AT is an autosomal recessive inherited neurodegenerative disease with associated combined immunodeficiency due to mutations in the *ATM* gene, which codes for a protein relevant for DNA repair. Patients present during childhood with progressive loss of motor function and telangiectasias visible on sclerae and skin.

Pulmonary manifestations of AT include recurrent upper and lower respiratory infections complicated by bronchiectasis, ILD, and respiratory symptoms related to neuromuscular and bulbar abnormalities.[192] Often a combination of these phenotypes occurs. The progressive neurodegenerative process contributes to a weak cough and respirations, which decrease effective clearance of respiratory secretions. Coughing and choking during meals increase the risk of aspiration. ILD should be considered in patients with a chronic nonproductive cough, dyspnea, crackles on exam, and fever in the absence of viral or bacterial infections.[192,193] In a retrospective chart review by Schroder et al., ILD was described as a poor prognostic factor.[193] Nineteen of 25 patients with AT and ILD died within 2 years.[193] Eleven of these 25 had developed pneumothoraces as a complication of ILD. Six patients with pneumothoraces refractory to therapy died within 6 months after diagnosis.[193]

The diagnostic workup of cellular and humoral immunity in AT includes a CBC, lymphocyte phenotyping, assessment of lymphocyte function by stimulation of PBMC with mitogens and antigens, serum immunoglobulins and specific antibody titers to vaccines; it may show a varying pattern of cellular and humoral immunodeficiency. Regular lung function testing is advised to follow the restrictive lung disease process. Due to increased radiosensitivity, imaging that exposes patients to ionizing radiation should be minimized. A chest CT can be helpful when concern about bronchiectasis or ILD arise.

Therapy for pulmonary manifestations in AT include oral or intravenous antibiotics for respiratory infections, immunoglobulin G substitution when indicated, airway clearance assistance, speech therapy and other interventions to minimize airway aspiration, supplemental oxygen, and noninvasive respiratory support. A trial of oral corticosteroids may be helpful for ILD.

HYPER-IGE SYNDROMES

Hyper-IgE-syndromes (HIES) share as common features an elevated serum IgE, eosinophilia, eczema, and sinopulmonary infections. Mutations in the genes coding for signal transducer and activator (STAT) 3, dedicator of cytokinesis 8 (DOCK8), and nonreceptor tyrosine-protein kinase 2 (Tyk2) have previously been described to cause HIES phenotypes; more recently mutations in *PGM3* (phosphoglucomutase 3) have been added.[194,195] Autosomal dominant HIES or classical Job syndrome presents in infancy with a pustular rash or later with skeletal, connective tissue, and vascular abnormalities, which include a characteristic facies, retained primary teeth, recurrent fractures, and scoliosis. Characteristic pulmonary manifestations include recurrent bacterial pneumonia with predominantly *Staphylococcus (S.) aureus*, formation of pneumatoceles due to abnormal healing and bronchiectasis, and superinfection with gram-negative bacteria, nontuberculous mycobacteria, and fungal infections after parenchymal damage has occurred. *P. jirovecii* pneumonia may occur in infancy. STAT3 deficiency affects different signaling pathways, which helps explain abnormal healing and a lack of systemic inflammation during bacterial infections.[196] Autosomal recessive DOCK8 deficiency presents with significant cutaneous viral infections and pulmonary infections complicated by bronchiectasis.[197] The rare form of autosomal recessive Tyk2 deficiency is associated with mycobacterial infections due to an associated defect in the IL-12, IFN-γ, STAT1 pathway.[198] Neurologic abnormalities, cytopenias, and pulmonary infections with bronchiectasis are characteristic of PGM3 deficiency.

The diagnostic workup includes a CBC with differential cell count, lymphocyte phenotyping with assessment of memory T and B cells, measurement of serum immunoglobulins, and specific antibody concentrations. Eosinophilia is common, memory T and B cells are decreased with normal lymphocyte numbers, and serum IgE is increased with usually normal IgM, IgG, and IgA; specific antibody concentrations can be low. Genetic testing panels for HIES are available.

Therapy is mainly supportive in autosomal dominant HIES with targeted antimicrobial therapy, antibiotic prophylaxis for *S. aureus* and fungal infections, reduction in *S. aureus* skin colonization with bleach baths, and immunoglobulin G replacement therapy in patients with relevant antibody deficiency. Successful HSCT has been conducted in DOCK8 deficiency.[199]

DEFICIENCIES OF THE INNATE IMMUNE SYSTEM

Rare deficiencies of the complement system, impaired signaling though nuclear factor kappa-light-chain enhancer of activated B cells (NFκB), and Mendelian susceptibility to mycobacterial infections present with characteristic pulmonary infections.

Deficiencies of early complement components (C1–C4) increase susceptibility to pyogenic infections, including recurrent pneumonia similar to antibody deficiency.[200] Decreased total complement activity (CH50) with normal alternative complement pathway activation (AH50) points towards an early complement deficiency. Mannose-binding lectin (MBL) deficiency has also been associated with a predisposition to more severe respiratory tract infections.[201] In patients with recurrent and severe respiratory infections and normal cellular and humoral immunity, a complement screen with CH50 and AH50 should be considered; MBL serum concentrations can also be measured.

Innate immunodeficiencies with impaired signaling through NFκB will decrease the cellular immune response that would otherwise be initiated by engagement of all Toll-like receptors (TLRs; except TLR3) and several other immune receptors including IL-1, T-, and B-cell receptors.[202] Autosomal deficiencies in interleukin-1 receptor-associated kinase 4 (IRAK-4) and myeloid differentiation primary response protein 88 (MyD88), which are essential for TLR signaling, present during early childhood with invasive bacterial infections and bacterial pneumonia with predominantly *Streptococcus pneumoniae*, in the absence of fever or an increase in C-reactive protein. The severity of infections decreases over time as adaptive immunity improves. Patients with immunodeficiency due to mutations in the gene for NFκB, essential modulator

(NEMO; *IKBKG* gene) and deficiency in NFκB inhibitor alpha (IκBα; NF-κBIA gene) present similarly, but are also affected by mycobacterial, opportunistic, and severe viral infections. Anhidrotic ectodermal dysplasia occurs in greater than 90% of patients with NEMO. TLR function can be assessed by measuring cytokine production (e.g. IL-1, IL-6, TNF-α) by PBMC after stimulation with TLR-specific ligands; absent cytokine production raises concern for immunodeficiency related to impaired NFκB signaling. Genetic testing will aid in determining the underlying defect.

Mendelian susceptibility to mycobacterial disease (MSMD) is caused by deficiencies in the IL-12/IL-23/IFN-γ pathway involving macrophages, T-, and NK-cells. Children may present early in life with mycobacterial and Salmonella infections due to inadequate production of IFN-γ or insufficient responses to IFN-γ. Relevant autosomal recessive and dominant mutations have been described in 10 genes, including *IL12B, IL12RB1, IFNGR1, IFNGR2, STAT1, NEMO, CYBB, TYK2, IRF8,* and *ISG15*.[203,204] The diagnostic workup, which is offered in select laboratories, includes measurement of IFN-γ and IL-12 serum concentrations, IFN-γ receptor expression on lymphocytes, IL-12 receptor expression on PBMC after stimulation with phytohemagglutinin (PHA), STAT1 expression in monocytes, and sequencing of respective genes. Depending on the underlying defect, therapeutic options include therapy with recombinant IFN-γ or HSCT.[204]

References

Access the reference list online at ExpertConsult.com.

Suggested Reading

Bonilla F, Barlan I, Chapel H, et al. International Consensus Document (ICON): Common Variable Immunodeficiency Disorders. *J Allergy Clin Immunol Pract.* 2015;4:38.

Cale CM, Jones AM, Goldblatt D. Follow up of patients with chronic granulomatous disease diagnosed since 1990. *Clin Exp Immunol.* 2000;120:351.

Chapel H, Cunningham-Rundles C. Update in understanding common variable immunodeficiency disorders (CVIDs) and the management of patients with these conditions. *Br J Haematol.* 2009;145:709.

Cunningham-Rundles C, Bodian C. Common variable immunodeficiency: clinical and immunological features of 248 patients. *Clin Immunol.* 1999;92:34.

Kang EM, Choi U, Theobald N, et al. Retrovirus gene therapy for X-linked chronic granulomatous disease can achieve stable long-term correction of oxidase activity in peripheral blood neutrophils. *Blood.* 2010;115:783.

Nelson KS, Lewis DB. Adult-onset presentations of genetic immunodeficiencies: genes can throw slow curves. *Curr Opin Infect Dis.* 2010;23:359.

Pogrebniak HW, Gallin JI, Malech HL, et al. Surgical management of pulmonary infections in chronic granulomatous disease of childhood. *Ann Thorac Surg.* 1993;55:844.

Seger RA. Modern management of chronic granulomatous disease. *Br J Haematol.* 2008;140:255.

van den Berg JM, van Koppen E, Ahlin A, et al. Chronic granulomatous disease: the European experience. *PLoS ONE.* 2009;4:e5234.

Winkelstein JA, Marino MC, Johnston RB Jr, et al. Chronic granulomatous disease: report on a national registry of 368 patients. *Medicine (Baltimore).* 2000;79:155.

64 Pulmonary Disease in the Pediatric Patient With Acquired Immunodeficiency States

JONATHAN SPAHR, MD, DANIEL J. WEINER, MD, DENNIS C. STOKES, MD, and GEOFFREY KURLAND, MD

Introduction

Acquired immunodeficiency in children can be the result of a variety of diseases or their treatments. The majority of acquired immunodeficiency states, however, are the result of medical treatments that include pharmacologic, surgical, and radiotherapeutic regimens for the treatment of oncologic diagnoses. In addition, the expanding population of children receiving solid organ transplants is exposed to immunosuppressive medications to prevent graft rejection. Ablation chemotherapy combined with radiation used to prepare patients for hematopoeitic stem cell transplantation (HSCT) can produce direct toxicity to the lungs while rendering these patients temporarily pancytopenic and thus at risk for infectious complications. As a result, pulmonary disease in these patients is relatively common, and often results in significant morbidity and mortality.

This chapter will discuss pulmonary complications of solid organ transplantation, HSCT, and treatment of childhood oncologic disease. Included in these potential complications are pulmonary infections, and this will be the focus of the initial portion of this chapter. In addition, there are important noninfectious complications that will be addressed; some of these are specific to underlying conditions and their treatments.

Pulmonary complications of lung transplantation, human immunodeficiency virus (HIV)–associated acquired immunodeficiency syndrome (AIDS), and congenital immunodeficiencies are discussed in separate chapters (Chapters 67, 66, and 63, respectively). Lung injury caused by pharmacologic agents, including chemotherapeutics, is discussed in Chapter 59.

Pulmonary Infections in the Immunocompromised Pediatric Host

Immunocompromised pediatric patients include patients with congenital defects of innate host defenses including neutrophil abnormalities, defects affecting lymphocyte function, and defects of humoral immunity. The number of entities leading to such defects is rapidly expanding, with improved recognition of the nearly 300 clinical phenotypes associated with single-gene mutations affecting immune function.[1] The major expansion of the population of immunocompromised children, however, has occurred with increased human stem cell and solid-organ transplantation, successful treatment of childhood malignancies, the AIDS epidemic, and the use of biologic agents such as inhibitors of tumor necrosis factor (TNF)-alpha for a variety of autoimmune diseases of childhood. In addition to increasing the at-risk population, these developments have also led to an increase in the number of identifiable pathogens. The term *opportunistic pathogen* is usually reserved for an organism typically infecting a patient with abnormal host defenses. The terms *immunodeficiency* and *compromised host* were first used in the 1960s and 1970s, for patients with primary immunodeficiency and for those patients who survived childhood malignancies.[2] This portion of the chapter will review some of the more common pulmonary infections in this patient population.

Clinical Presentation of Pulmonary Infection in the Immunocompromised Child

The clinical presentations of pulmonary infection in the immunocompromised child are often nonspecific, and a high index of suspicion for atypical or opportunistic pathogens is required. Childhood cancer therapy, HSCT, solid organ transplantation, primary immunodeficiencies, and AIDS are each associated with specific pulmonary pathogens (Table 64.1).

In addition, these patients often have an atypical or more severe course even when infected with a "usual" childhood respiratory pathogen.[3] For example, viruses such as varicella-zoster, influenza, and measles are all capable of leading to devastating pulmonary infections in the immunocompromised host. Although adenovirus (AdV) can cause diffuse pneumonia in any child, it can be particularly common[4] and catastrophic in immunocompromised hosts.[5-7]

The clinical course of opportunistic infections is variable and affected by the type and degree of remaining host defenses. For example, fungal pulmonary infections in patients with chemotherapy-induced neutropenia and defective cell-mediated immunity are often associated with mild clinical symptoms and radiographic findings until the normalization of peripheral blood neutrophil counts leads to significant inflammation, lung destruction, pulmonary cavitation, and clinical deterioration. The interplay of fungal pathogens with the innate and adaptive immune systems is still under investigation. It is clear that fungi can both subvert and exploit the host immune response, allowing for chronic carriage or

Table 64.1   Typical Pulmonary Pathogens Associated With Acquired Immunodeficiency States

	Bacterial	Fungal	Viral/Protozoal/Other
NEUTROPENIA			
Chronic	*Haemophilus influenzae, Streptococcus pneumoniae, Staphylococcus aureus, Klebsiella* spp.	—	—
Acute	*S. aureus*	—	—
Immunosuppressive Therapy	*S. aureus, Listeria* spp., *Mycobacterium tuberculosis*	*Aspergillus* spp., *Mucor* spp., *Histoplasma* spp., *Pneumocystis jirovecii*	Cytomegalovirus (CMV), VZV, *Toxoplasma* spp., Herpes simplex virus, *Cryptococcus* spp.
BONE MARROW TRANSPLANT			
Early (<30 days)	*Pseudomonas* spp., other gram-negative and gram-positive spp.	*Candida* spp.	—
Late (>30 days)	*S. aureus*	*Aspergillus* spp., *P. jirovecii*	CMV, *Toxoplasma* spp., VZV, Epstein-Barr virus, adenovirus
Late (>100 days)	Encapsulated Gram-positive (*H. influenzae, S. pneumoniae*)	—	VZV

pathogenicity. This complex response is likely mediated by various molecular interactions involving cytokines as well as cellular elements.[8–11]

Infectious Risks Shared by Malignancy, Solid Organ Transplantation, and Stem Cell Transplantation

The immune system has multiple components. Disorders of the immune system can be divided into those involving *innate* and *adaptive* components.[1] There are physical barriers to infectious agents, including skin and airway epithelial cells. Humoral components of the immune system include immunoglobulins, complement, and other nonspecific antibacterial molecular species (e.g., defensins) important to innate pulmonary defenses.[12] Cellular components include phagocytic cells, particularly neutrophils, and lymphocytes. A more complete description of the development, interactions, and defects of each of these components is presented in Chapters 8 and 63.

Patients undergoing treatment for malignancy, HSCT, or solid organ transplant have periods of immunosuppression that vary in length and severity. The recovery of the immune system after myeloablative conditioning followed by HSCT, for example, can be divided into three phases. The *preengraftment or early phase,* from day 0 to day 30 or sooner, encompasses the time of marrow recovery leading to normalization of the peripheral neutrophil count; the *postengraftment phase* is considered day 30 to day 100 after HSCT; and the *late phase* follows day 100 post HSCT. For patients with HSCT, each phase is characterized by a susceptibility to certain types of infections correlating with the status of the immune system at that time point.[13] Following solid organ transplantation, many patients initially receive intensive immunosuppressive therapy, leading to a more immunosuppressed state early in the posttransplant period. Patients with malignancies often receive chemotherapy in a cyclic pattern, leading to periods of severe marrow suppression followed by periods of recovery. Fig. 64.1 demonstrates different phases of immunodeficiency in which certain infectious organisms may

predominate. As occurs with individuals who are not immunosuppressed, respiratory viruses and community-acquired bacteria are quite common in the individual who is immunosuppressed. Those who are immunosuppressed, however, have a greater propensity for infection, with a wider variety of organisms (the opportunistic infections). A recent publication reviews radiological findings in children with acquired immunodeficiency states following cancer chemotherapy and is a useful reference for the evaluation of these patients.[14]

Common Pulmonary Infectious Agents in the Immunocompromised Pediatric Host

VIRAL PATHOGENS (See Also Chapter 25)

Cytomegalovirus

Cytomegalovirus (CMV) is a common herpesvirus infection of both neonates and older immunocompromised children.[15,16] Viral carriage does not always lead to disease, however, and the progression from carriage to disease depends on many factors, including the age and the immune status of the infected individual. The organism can be acquired *intrapartum* or from breast milk, saliva, or blood (via infected white cells). CMV infection in the immunocompetent hosts rarely results in overt disease, and humoral and cellular immune mechanisms are important in limiting the infective capabilities of CMV. Such hosts that have latent CMV are seropositive, rendering them at-risk for viral reactivation in the event of immunocompromise. Individuals who are CMV-seronegative prior to either immunosuppression following transplantation or chemotherapy are at increased risk of CMV disease through CMV acquisition from de novo infection, from blood products containing virions, or from transplanted organs from CMV-seropositive individuals.

CMV-infected cells typically contain basophilic nuclear inclusions surrounded by a clear halo, giving an "owl eye" appearance; such inclusions are typically seen in alveolar cells. The pathology of CMV pneumonitis varies from diffuse,

TIMELINE OF INFECTIOUS PULMONARY COMPLICATIONS

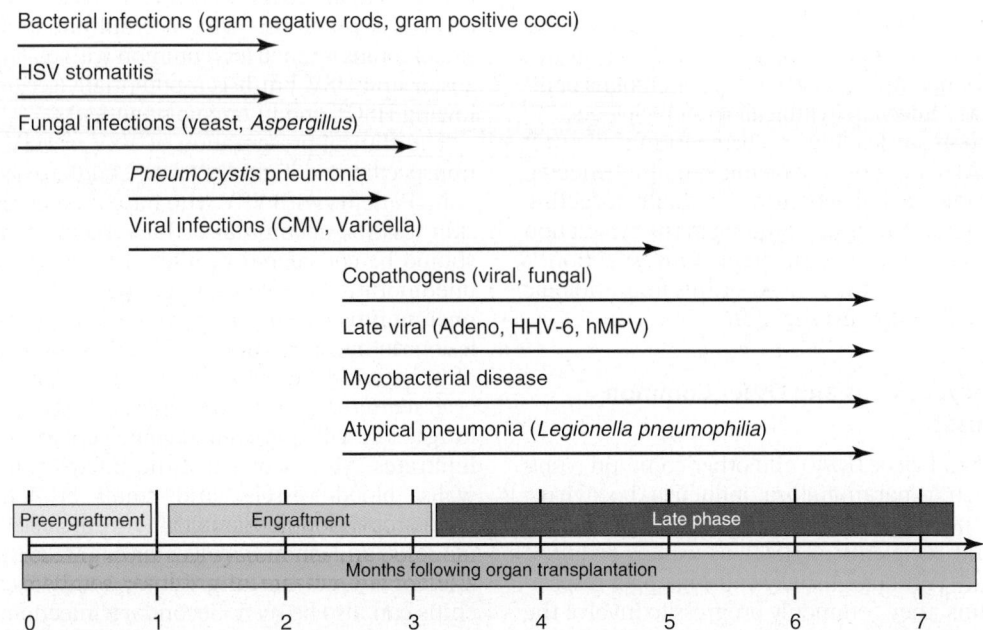

Fig. 64.1 Timeline of infectious pulmonary complications following solid-organ transplantation. *CMV,* Cytomegalovirus; *HHV-6,* human herpesvirus 6; *hMPV,* human metapneumovirus; *HSV,* herpes simples virus.

discrete parenchymal hemorrhagic nodules to diffuse alveolar damage, or chronic interstitial pneumonitis. The radiographic pattern of CMV pneumonia is usually a diffuse reticulonodular pattern that is less "alveolar" than is seen in pneumonia caused by *Pneumocystis jirovecii* (described later). High-resolution computed tomography (CT) of the chest most commonly reveals patchy or diffuse ground-glass attenuation, and more diffuse pulmonary involvement may be predictive of the progression of disease.[17]

Prior to the availability of effective antiviral therapy, approximately 50% of patients with aplastic anemia or hematologic malignancy treated by allogeneic HSCT developed CMV infection and CMV pneumonia,[18] with up to 90% mortality. CMV may also be a copathogen with other opportunistic organisms, including *P. jirovecii,* Epstein-Barr virus (EBV) and *Aspergillus.*

The diagnosis of CMV pneumonia is usually made by demonstration of typical inclusions in lung tissue. Urinary excretion of CMV can be coincident, but not necessarily causally related to disease. The most important methods for the detection of CMV in blood and potentially other fluids such as bronchoalveolar lavage (BAL) are those that estimate the quantity of virus or viral DNA. Of these, determination of CMV DNA using the polymerase chain reaction (PCR) is quite sensitive and widely available.[19] Determination of the presence of the CMV protein pp65 within peripheral white blood cells is also useful to identify those patients harboring the organism. PCR for CMV detection in the blood has become a more commonly used noninvasive test to follow at-risk patients following HSCT, or solid organ transplant recipients, to more accurately predict the development of CMV disease. New standards for measuring the viral load of CMV in body fluids (including BAL) allows for more precision in following the course of the disease.[20] PCR detection of CMV precedes culture isolation of CMV and persists longer than culture-positivity. Other techniques for identifying CMV in BAL include immunofluorescence, DNA hybridization, or microplate culture, combined with CMV antigen detection using monoclonal antibodies. All the techniques described, though highly sensitive, must be interpreted cautiously, since CMV can be a commensal and may be coincidentally present without being the cause of disease. Characteristic pathologic findings as well as a clinical scenario consistent with CMV disease are very important in deciding upon therapy.

The use of CMV-negative blood products has reduced the incidence of CMV pneumonia in seronegative transplant patients. Prophylactic and preemptive strategies for patients at risk utilizing ganciclovir, foscarnet, and high titer anti-CMV IgG have led to a substantial reduction in the incidence and mortality of CMV disease.[13,21,22] Valganciclovir, the L-valyl ester and prodrug of ganciclovir, has improved oral bioavailability compared with ganciclovir, and is now the preferred drug for the prevention and treatment of CMV disease.[23]

"Late" CMV has been observed in HSCT recipients with active graft-versus-host-disease (GVHD) who are receiving high doses of steroids (>1 mg/kg per day of prednisone), with low CD4 counts, and with history of prior CMV reactivation or extended use of anti-CMV treatment or prophylaxis.[24] Reduced intensity conditioning regimens for HSCT, or so-called mini-transplants with fludarabine, single-dose radiation, and posttransplant cyclosporine and mycophenolate mofetil, is an emerging treatment for patients who are not candidates for standard myeloablative conditioning.[25] These patients have shorter periods of neutropenia and lowered risk of CMV disease and viremia during the first 100 days, but may subsequently be faced with a delayed onset of CMV disease. Unlike early-onset disease, which is characterized mainly by interstitial pneumonitis,[26] late

CMV manifestations include retinitis, marrow failure, and encephalitis.[24,27]

The interaction of CMV disease and allograft survival has been of particular interest to the lung transplant community, with reports of an increased incidence of bronchiolitis obliterans following CMV infection in lung allograft recipients.[28–30] The precise mechanism leading to chronic lung allograft dysfunction (CLAD) in lung recipients remains unclear, although immunological mechanisms possibly targeting usually hidden potential antigens resulting in the production of auto-antibodies continue to be a target of investigation.[31] The role played by CMV in the context of this immunologic dysregulation is still under investigation.

Respiratory Syncytial Virus and Other Common Respiratory Viruses

Respiratory syncytial virus (RSV) and other common respiratory viruses such as parainfluenza, influenza, bocavirus, and rhinovirus have long been recognized as important pathogens in adult recipients of HSCT as well as pediatric leukemia patients.[32] Although usually causing upper respiratory tract infections, they commonly progress to involve the lower respiratory tract, carrying significant morbidity and mortality.[33] In addition, RSV and other community-acquired respiratory viruses have been implicated in the subsequent development of CLAD in lung transplant recipients.[34]

With community acquired respiratory viral infections, chest radiographs may have diffuse but nonspecific densities. Nasopharyngeal swabs or washings with cultures or enzyme immunoassays (EIA) are the most commonly used diagnostic tools for most viral pathogens, including RSV. Newer technologies, including reverse-transcriptase PCR (RT-PCR) and direct immunofluorescence assays, may prove to be specific, sensitive, and more rapid for detection,[35] although further clinical studies will be required. Studies of the use of the antiviral agent ribavirin in treating adult recipients with RSV have suggested that early administration of aerosolized ribavirin, before significant lower respiratory disease develops, is superior to treatment with intravenous (IV) ribavirin.[33] However, oral ribavirin, which is much less expensive than aerosolized or IV ribavirin, has been shown to be effective in the treatment of RSV.[36] There is also support for the use of the monoclonal anti-RSV antibody known as palivizumab in patients who develop RSV following HSCT, although the largest study was in adults, and all patients also received inhaled ribavirin.[37] While there is less published data concerning these pathogens in pediatric HSCT recipients, the increased likelihood of childhood exposure in schools and other environments should lead the clinician to consider such pathogens when evaluating an immunosuppressed child with upper or lower respiratory illness of uncertain etiology.

Varicella-Zoster Virus and Herpes Simplex Virus

Varicella-zoster virus (VZV) and herpes simples virus (HSV) are DNA viruses that typically cause infections of the skin and mucous membranes. However, in certain high-risk groups, including neonates, patients with cancer, AIDS, congenital defects of cell-mediated immunity, and recipients of solid organ transplants or HSCT, VZV and HSV can lead to visceral dissemination and pneumonia.[38] Before the availability of specific antiviral therapy, VZV pneumonitis occurred in approximately 85% of cancer patients with visceral dissemination, with a resultant mortality of 85%. Pneumonitis is much less common with reactivation of herpes zoster and HSV, but it is a potentially serious infection following HSCT and in oncology patients.

The clinical presentation of VZV or HSV pneumonitis is nonspecific and includes fever, cough, dyspnea, and chest pain. Patients with VZV who have an increasing number of skin lesions, abdominal or back pain, or persistent fevers should be considered at high risk for dissemination. HSV pneumonitis may be more subtle in its presentation, and pneumonitis can occur in the absence of mucocutaneous lesions in newborns and HSCT recipients. Chest radiographs of herpesvirus pneumonias typically show ill-defined, bilateral, scattered nodular densities, first seen in the peripheral lung fields, with subsequent coalescence into more extensive infiltrates. Microscopically, the infection involves alveolar walls, blood vessels, and small bronchioles. Electron microscopy shows intranuclear viral inclusions. Hemorrhage, necrosis, and extensive alveolar edema are seen in severely affected areas of the lung; hemorrhagic tracheitis and bronchitis can also be seen. Secondary infections with bacterial pathogens were more commonly seen in the preantibiotic era, but with the emergence of resistant organisms such as methicillin-resistant *Staphylococcus aureus*, this remains a worrisome complication. Interstitial lung disease secondary to HSV infection has been reported following HSCT, but this is relatively rare[39] and far less common than CMV-related interstitial lung disease in this population.

Varicella-zoster immune globulin can modify or prevent VZV infection in high-risk hosts exposed to the virus if given within 48–72 hours of exposure. VZV immune globulin, antiviral therapy with acyclovir and related drugs, and routine varicella vaccination have been effective in reducing the incidence of serious VZV pneumonias in immunocompromised hosts. However, a single varicella vaccination given prior to an acquired immunocompromised state may be insufficient to prevent disseminated VZV.[40] In the case of HSV pneumonitis, acyclovir may not always be protective against respiratory complications. *In vitro* testing for antiviral sensitivity and the administration of alternative antiviral treatment may be warranted when proven *HSV* pneumonitis occurs.[41]

Herpesvirus Type 6

Human herpesvirus 6 (HHV-6) is a DNA virus and is the etiologic agent of roseola. It can persist in normal hosts following infection and has been shown to integrate into the host genome in 0.2%–2% of the population.[42,43] Immunosuppression can lead to reactivation of HHV-6, resulting in fever, hepatitis, bone marrow suppression, encephalitis, and interstitial pneumonia.[44,45] HHV-6 may also be associated with coinfection by CMV and other pathogens. Antiviral compounds with activity against CMV, such as ganciclovir, foscarnet, and cidofovir, are also active against HHV-6,[46] although increasing resistance to these agents by HHV-6 and other herpesviruses is becoming increasingly common.[47]

Human Metapneumovirus

Human metapneumovirus (*hMPV*) accounts for a large proportion of cases previously relegated to "undiagnosed" respiratory infections, particularly in young children.[48,49] Its epidemiology is similar to that of *RSV*—that is, winter epidemics—with variation in severity from year to year. Martino and colleagues[50] recently described isolation of *hMPV* as a primary pathogen in 11/177 (6.2%) of nasopharyngeal aspirates from symptomatic adult HSCT recipients. An additional five patients had *hMPV* as a copathogen, one with *Aspergillus,* one with *Aspergillus* and *CMV,* and three with other respiratory viruses (*AdV, RSV,* or *influenza*). Fifty percent of the infections were considered nosocomial; pneumonia complicated *hMPV*-upper respiratory tract infections in four (44%) of nine and one (14%) of seven allo-HSCT and auto-HSCT recipients, respectively. More worrisome, Englund and coworkers[51] reported real-time PCR evidence of metapneumovirus in 5 of 163 (3%) of BAL samples obtained in HSCT recipients experiencing respiratory disease. Of these five patients, four died of respiratory failure and most carried a diagnosis of "idiopathic pneumonia syndrome" (IPS; discussed further in this chapter). Evashuk and colleagues reported metapneumovirus infection leading to severe respiratory failure in an infant recovering from liver transplantation.[52] More recently, an outbreak of *hMPV* affecting 15 immuno-compromised adults with hematologic malignancies that led to respiratory failure in 33% and death in 26.6% was reported, highlighting the potential virulence of this particular pathogen.[53] It is likely that further investigations will underscore the importance of *hMPV* as a viral pathogen in immuno-compromised adults and children.[54]

Adenovirus

AdV is a DNA virus that is a common cause of community-acquired lower respiratory tract disease. Serotypes 3 and 7 are associated with epidemics of bronchiolitis and pneumonia in the general population. In immunocompromised patients such as HSCT recipients, AdV infections can lead to gastro-intestinal, urologic, and pulmonary morbidity with disseminated disease that is associated with a high mortality.[7] AdV typically causes fever, pharyngitis, cough, and conjunctivitis. Pneumonia is usually mild in normal hosts, but rapid progression, with necrotizing bronchitis and bronchiolitis, can occur in immunocompromised patients. The radiographic picture is nonspecific and resembles other causes of diffuse pneumonia. Failure of pneumonia to respond to standard therapy, particularly in the setting of epidemic acute respiratory disease in the community or hospital staff, should raise suspicion of AdV involvement.

The diagnosis is usually made by lung biopsy or brushings demonstrating typical adenoviral inclusions, or by culture, but institution of empiric antibiotic and antifungal therapy leading to delay in invasive procedures may delay the diagnosis. PCR to quantify adenoviral DNA in blood or other fluids[55,56] may be useful as a screening tool. The antiviral agent Cidofovir has been shown to have activity against AdV, but more study is needed before it can be universally recommended.[57] Because very low T-cell counts in HSCT recipients are a major risk factor for disseminated disease in those patients found to harbor AdV, and because PCR is quite sensitive, algorithms have been proposed for determining which patients might benefit from antiviral treatment with agents such as cidofovir.[58,59] Meanwhile, supportive therapy for affected patients includes oxygen, treatment of bacterial superinfections, IV immunoglobulin, and assisted ventilation. A novel approach to treatment of refractory *AdV* (and other

viral) infections in immunocompromised patients involves the production of multivirus-specific T-cells using overlapping peptide libraries incorporating antigens from a variety of pathogenic viruses to stimulate peripheral blood mononuclear cells *in vitro.* While this technology is only recently developed, it may provide a more sustainable treatment in this patient population.[60]

FUNGAL PATHOGENS (See Also Chapter 31)

Pneumocystis jirovecii (Formerly *P. carinii*)

Pneumocystis has been an organism of uncertain taxonomy and was regarded as a parasite because of its resemblance to cystic spore-forming protozoa. DNA sequencing of 16S-like ribosomal RNA of *P. carinii* with phylogenetic analysis demonstrates that it is much more closely related to fungi than to protozoal organisms.[61] There are several animal models for infection with *Pneumocystis,* with no evidence of infection transmission across species. The nomenclature *P. carinii* is now reserved for the organism infecting rats, while *P. jirovecii* is the organism isolated in humans.[62] The term PCP, initially an acronym for *P. carinii* pneumonia, is retained with *P. jirovecii* pneumonia, now indicating *Pneumocystis* pneumonia.

The organism exists in two forms in tissues: the more common trophic, or trophozoite, and the cystic form containing sporozoites.[63] The trophozoites measure 2–5 μm and stain best with Giemsa stains or fluorescein-conjugated monoclonal antibody but are not visible with Grocot-Gomori methenamine-silver nitrate or toluidine blue O stains, which stain the 5–8-μm cyst forms. The cysts are spherical or cup-shaped and often appear to contain up to eight 1–2 μm sporozoites within the cyst wall. The organism cannot be cultured from routine clinical specimens and must be identified in tissue, sputum, or alveolar lavage. The trophozoites appear to attach to type I cells through surface glycoproteins related to lectins and there undergo encystation. This interaction directly or through soluble factors leads to cell injury. The alveoli of lungs infected with *P. jirovecii* are filled with trophozoites and protein-rich debris, and the altered permeability produced by the organism contributes to the development of pulmonary edema and surfactant abnormalities, which lead to decreased pulmonary compliance and altered gas exchange. Latent infection with *P. jirovecii* was thought to be common, since serologic studies indicated that 40% of children had antibodies to the organism, and more recent studies using sensitive PCR assays have found evidence of *P. jirovecii* in the nasopharynx and lungs of normal infants. Colonization appears to be common in immunocompromised patients but less common in normal hosts, and there is some evidence of patient-to-patient transmission. Reactivation of latent infection in the immunocompromised host, previously felt to be the most likely explanation for disease, has been called into question by epidemiologic data, suggesting new acquisition of airborne organisms.[63]

In patients with congenital or acquired immunodeficiency, the clinical features of PCP are nonspecific and include dyspnea, tachypnea, fever, and cough. Cyanosis occurs later, but early hypoxemia with a mild respiratory alkalosis is common. The most common chest radiographic finding is diffuse bilateral infiltrates.

P. jirovecii pneumonia can be treated with several medications, although trimethoprim-sulfamethoxazole (TMP-SMZ) is the preferred agent for both prophylaxis and treatment in children as well as adults.[63] The earliest drug available for PCP was the dihydrofolate reductase inhibitor pentamidine, which was associated with a high rate of immediate adverse reactions including hypotension, tachycardia, and nausea as well as hypoglycemia and nephrotoxicity. Pentamidine may be administered by the aerosol route for treatment or prophylaxis in at-risk patients to prevent PCP, but its effectiveness is highly dependent on the delivery system used. Other "second-line" medications that have activity against *P. jirovecii* include combination therapy of clindamycin and primaquine, dapsone (sometimes combined with trimethoprim), and atovaquone.[63–65] Limited studies and case reports of the use of the antifungal agent caspofungin have shown some promise, but further study is necessary.[66,67] A newer form of combination therapy, reported for patients with AIDS, is trimetrexate-folinic acid,[68] but this will also require further evaluation. For proven PCP infection with moderate to severe hypoxemia, high-dose TMP-SMX with adjuvant glucocorticoid therapy remains the treatment of choice.[63,69]

Patients at known risk for *P. jirovecii* generally receive prophylaxis. For pediatric oncology and immunocompromised patients, oral TMP-SMZ given 3 days per week is effective. However, if patients or parents are noncompliant, there is a risk of breakthrough pneumonias on this schedule. For most patients, TMP-SMZ remains the drug of choice, but other prophylactic regimens have been used, including IV pentamidine.[63,70]

Aspergillus Species

Aspergillus is a group of ubiquitous fungal organisms found in soil and other settings, including the hospital environment. *Aspergillus fumigatus* is the most common species to cause pneumonia in immunocompromised hosts, but other pathogenic species include *A. niger* and *A. flavus*.[71] Invasive *Aspergillus* is most common in pediatric patients with malignancy (especially acute myelocytic leukemia) and HSCT.[72]

In tissues, the organisms are seen as septate hyphae with regular 45-degree dichotomous branching, best seen with methenamine silver staining (Fig. 64.2). Novel PCR-based detection methods for *Aspergillus* (and other fungal pathogens) in BAL samples are being developed but require further testing.[73] *Aspergillus* causes both acute invasive pulmonary aspergillosis and a more chronic necrotizing form. The former occurs most commonly in patients undergoing cancer therapy, as well as other immunocompromised patients, such as those with aplastic anemia. Aspergillosis of the lung is often preceded by or accompanied by invasion of the nose and paranasal sinuses in susceptible hosts. Confirmed risk factors for aspergillosis include prolonged neutropenia, concurrent chemotherapy and steroid therapy, and broad-spectrum antibiotic therapy. Cutaneous aspergillosis is often observed in patients with disseminated disease. The killing and/or clearance of *Aspergillus* by neutrophils and alveolar macrophages are partly dependent on intracellular calcineurin, which itself is a target of widely used antirejection medications. This suggests another reason why transplant recipients are more susceptible to invasive *Aspergillus* infections.[74,75]

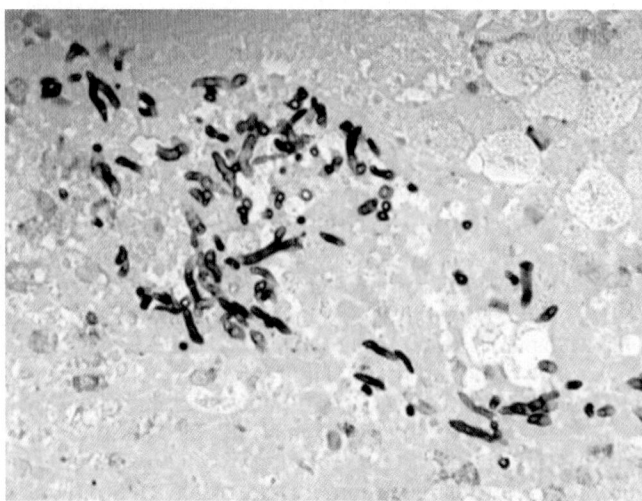

Fig. 64.2 Invasive aspergillosis seen in a patient with pulmonary complications posthuman stem cell transplantation. Methenamine silver stain, 400×.

In the lungs, *Aspergillus* can cause tracheobronchitis, pneumonia, abscesses, cavity formation, and diffuse interstitial pneumonia. The organisms often extend along blood vessels, and nodular lesions of necrosis surrounded by air often develop within an area of pneumonia, leading to the typical air crescent sign, seen on CT scan of the chest. This finding is more common in adults, rather than pediatric, immunocompromised patients,[14] and while strongly suggestive of *Aspergillus* infection, is usually seen early in the disease process, and later it is replaced by nodular infiltrates with or without cavitation. CT scanning of the chest is much more sensitive than plain radiographs and can reveal early evidence of cavitation.

The diagnosis of *Aspergillus* pneumonia is generally made by tissue examination, but this has limitations, as several other fungal species can histologically mimic *Aspergillus* histologically. *Aspergillus* can be isolated from BAL in approximately 50% of cases, and needle aspiration biopsy of peripheral lung lesions can also demonstrate typical fungal lesions.[76] Although direct tissue sampling by needle biopsy or transbronchial biopsy is recommended for diagnosis, the angioinvasive nature of *Aspergillus* increases the risk of bleeding or secondary infection following such procedures.[77] Isolation of *Aspergillus* from a nasal culture in a patient with typical clinical risk features (prolonged neutropenia, progressive nodular infiltrates, cavitary lesion) may be helpful, but negative cultures do not exclude *Aspergillus*.

Galactomannan, a polysaccharide consisting of a mannose backbone linked to galactose side groups, is a component of the cell wall of *Aspergillus* that is released with growth. It can be detected in blood, BAL fluid, and cerebrospinal fluid in patients with invasive aspergillosis.[78] Although most of the studies using galactomannan as a biomarker for invasive fungal disease have been in adult patients, it has gained favor in the pediatric population.[79] *Aspergillus* galactomannan antigen detection in blood and BAL fluid as well as other noninvasive tests such as fungal-specific PCR-based diagnostics under development[80] offer the promise for accurate diagnosis without more invasive procedures such as needle biopsy or transthoracic lung biopsy.[81,82] Further studies to demonstrate utility in clinical practice will be necessary.[82–84]

Although initially amphotericin B was the sole antifungal agent with activity against *Aspergillus*, newer agents are available and include the orally available itraconazole and voriconazole, which have excellent activity against *Aspergillus*; of these, voriconazole is the treatment of choice for invasive aspergillosis.[85–87] Alternative therapies for aspergillosis include lipid formulations of amphotericin B, caspofungin or other echinocandins, or itraconazole. The utility of surgical excision of *Aspergillus* lesions is somewhat controversial. Invasive pulmonary aspergillosis during treatment of hematologic malignancy is generally considered a contraindication to subsequent BMT, but adult patients treated with amphotericin B and surgery have survived free of disease and without reactivation of *Aspergillus* following BMT. The outcome of *Aspergillus* pneumonia depends primarily on host factors, including degree of immunosuppression and recovery of neutrophil counts, as well as early diagnosis and treatment.[88]

Mucor and *Rhizopus*

Mucormycosis includes fungal disease caused by organisms in the order Mucorales, including a variety of species in the genera *Rhizopus, Mucor,* and *Cunninghamella.*[89] In tissues they are differentiated from *Aspergillus* by their broad, nonseptate hyphae that branch at angles up to 90 degrees and have an appearance of "twisted ribbons." *Rhizopus* organisms cause disease only in patients who are immunosuppressed or who have an underlying disease, especially diabetes. In adults, it is associated with chronic or recurrent acidosis, such as uncontrolled diabetes mellitus with ketoacidosis. Most pediatric cases of pneumonia occur in the oncology population, where the organism affects the same risk groups as *Aspergillus*.

Pneumonia due to *Rhizopus* is usually an insidious segmental pneumonia that is slowly progressive despite antifungal therapy. Persistent fever, chest pain, hemoptysis, and weight loss are typical. Cavitation may occur, and dissemination to brain and other sites occurs because of the propensity of the organism to invade blood vessels. Death may occur suddenly with massive pulmonary hemorrhage, mediastinitis, or airway obstruction. The specific diagnosis usually depends on demonstration of the organism in specimens obtained by open, transbronchial, or needle-aspiration biopsy. As with *Aspergillus*, treatment with amphotericin B and possibly surgical resection as early as possible is critical to achieving a cure. Posaconazole has good activity against mucormycosis, which can be aggressive and relatively resistant to voriconazole.[90,91] Correction of chronic acidosis, if present, also appears to be important in some forms of *Rhizopus* disease.

Candida Species

Though important as a cause of fungal sepsis and secondary hematogenous pulmonary involvement, primary *Candida* pneumonia is unusual. *Candida albicans* and *C. tropicalis* are the most important causes of fungal sepsis and secondary pulmonary involvement. Neutropenic children colonized with *C. tropicalis* are at a 10-fold higher risk for dissemination than children colonized with *C. albicans*. Patients with

HIV infection, primary immunodeficiencies, or prolonged neutropenia are at greatest risk, but other predisposing conditions include diabetes, corticosteroid administration, broad-spectrum antibiotic treatment, IV hyperalimentation, and the presence of deep venous access devices (conditions common to the patient with solid organ or HSCT).

In tissue, silver stains show oval budding yeasts 2–6 μm in diameter with pseudohyphae. The prominent histologic features of primary *Candida* pneumonia include bronchopneumonia, intraalveolar exudates, and hemorrhage. Amphotericin B is usually the treatment of choice for invasive *Candida* infections, along with flucytosine if synergism is desired. The imidazole antifungal agents, including ketoconazole, fluconazole, and itraconazole, have activity against *C. albicans* and have been used successfully. Although fluconazole prophylaxis, as well as the use of hematopoietic growth factors, has led to a reduction in the frequency of early *Candida* infections in patients at risk, many institutions have experienced an increase in azole-resistant *nonalbicans Candida* infections.[92–98] In response to this, caspofungin appears to be an excellent alternative, with less toxicity than amphotericin B and improved coverage against systemic *Candida* infections when compared with fluconazole.[99,100] A Cochrane review of various antifungal treatments points out the relative benefits of liposomal Amphotericin as well as the need for further controlled clinical trials to determine the optimal treatment for deep fungal infections in the pediatric host.[101] There is increasing interest in the use of combination therapies to improve the treatment of *Candida*, as well as other fungal pathogens. Such combination therapies take advantage of different therapeutic targets of the various antifungals, possibly reducing the emergence of resistant organisms.[102]

Histoplasmosis and Blastomycosis

Histoplasma capsulatum and *Blastomyces dermatitidis* are ubiquitous soil fungi endemic to the eastern and southeastern United States. Histoplasmosis is especially associated with exposure to bird or bat fecal material[103]; as a result, it is a fairly common infection in immunocompetent children and may be asymptomatic or lead to an acute pneumonia with fever, hilar adenopathy, and pulmonary infiltrates. Blastomycosis is a less common but more serious infection. Both can cause chronic granulomatous pulmonary disease and lead to extrapulmonary dissemination.

In the immunocompromised patient, particularly pediatric oncology patients, histoplasmosis may present as an acute illness with fever, cough, and diarrhea, or in a disseminated form with additional features of hepatosplenomegaly, fevers, and adenopathy.[104] Progressive disseminated histoplasmosis is a rare (<0.1% of cases) complication of primary infection, but it is much more common in immunocompromised patients.[105] Interestingly, neutropenia is not always associated with *H. capsulatum* infections. Chest radiographs or CT scans usually demonstrate hilar adenopathy and nodular parenchymal disease in both forms of the disease. Blastomycosis is much less common in adult or pediatric oncology patients, and may be associated with dermatologic manifestations such as skin ulcers, in addition to diffuse chronic pulmonary infiltrates.[106]

Amphotericin B is indicated for both histoplasmosis and blastomycosis in immunocompromised hosts. Itraconazole is also effective for histoplasmosis and moderate blastomycosis without central nervous system involvement.

Cryptococcus Neoformans

Cryptococcus neoformans is a yeast that causes protean clinical manifestations in immunocompromised patients, often involving the meninges, endocardium, skin, and lymph nodes.[107] The lungs are the portal of entry for *C. neoformans*, and pulmonary involvement may be minimal if dissemination occurs quickly. Pneumonia typically causes chest pain, fever, and cough. The diagnosis of cryptococcosis relies on demonstration of the organism histologically, in biopsy tissue or pleural fluid,[108] or by culture methods.[109] Although controlled trials are lacking, treatment of cryptococcosis in immunosuppressed patients with IV amphotericin B and oral flucytosine followed by fluconazole is recommended.[109,110]

Rarer Fungal Pneumonias

Several recent trends have been noted in fungal infections, among them increased identification of rarer fungal pathogens, including saprophytic fungi such as *Trichosporon beigelii* and *Fusarium* sp. These fungi cause skin and soft tissue infections and occasionally invade the lungs and sinuses. For example, *Scedosporium apiospermum* (formerly *Pseudallescheria boydii*) causes invasive disease in solid-organ transplant patients, with lung involvement in 50%[111]; it is difficult to distinguish histologically from *Aspergillus*.[112,113] These fungi are thus often difficult to diagnose, and unlike *Aspergillus*, their response to therapy with amphotericin B and echinocandins (e.g., Caspofungin) may be very poor.[114] Newer azole agents such as posaconazole and voriconazole have activity against *Fusarium* spp. and *Scedosporium* spp. and should be considered if these species are isolated from immunosuppressed patients. Other rare fungal pathogens seen in immunocompromised patients include filamentous fungi of which there are several species, including *Dactylaria gallopava*, *Cladophialophora bantiana*, and *Exophiala*. Several of these have a proclivity for infecting the CNS, but soft tissues and lungs may also become involved with cavitary lesions.[115]

BACTERIAL PATHOGENS (See Also Chapter 25)

The bacterial pathogens associated with pneumonia in immunocompromised hosts include those pathogens typically associated with pneumonia in children, such as *S. aureus* (particularly methicillin-resistant strains), *H. influenzae*, and *S. pneumoniae*. *Pseudomonas aeruginosa* is an additional important cause of pneumonia and sepsis in hospitalized immunocompromised children. Significant risk factors for bacterial infections include neutropenia, the presence of indwelling venous catheters, and perineal skin lesions. More unusual bacterial causes of pneumonia include *Listeria monocytogenes*, a gram-positive rod that causes primarily septicemia in immunocompromised patients, with subsequent pulmonary involvement. Corynebacteria (commonly called diphtheroids) are gram-positive bacilli or coccobacilli that exist as saprophytes on mucous membranes and skin. *Corynebacterium jeikeium* is a strain from this group that may lead to sepsis and pneumonia in oncology and HSCT patients.[116] *Listeria* can be successfully treated with ampicillin plus an

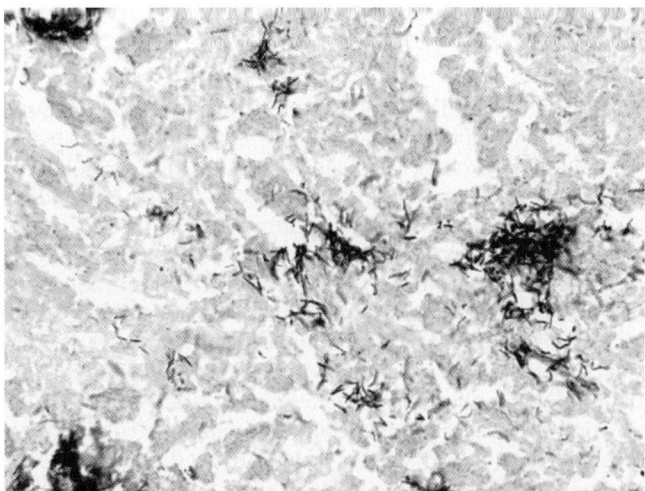

Fig. 64.3 Acid-fast organisms in a patient with end-stage lung disease following human stem cell transplantation. Acid-fast stain, 1000×.

aminoglycoside, but newer cephalosporins are not active against *Listeria*. *C. jeikeium* is resistant to most antibiotics except vancomycin. Other rare Gram-negative organisms that cause pneumonia in the immunocompromised host include *Legionella pneumophila* and *Capnocytophaga* sp. It is important to realize that factors such as geographic location, changes in infection control, prophylactic antimicrobial protocols, and technological advances all have an effect on microbial predominance.[117,118]

Mycobacteria (See Also Chapters 29 and 30)

With the onset of the AIDS epidemic, disease due to both *Mycobacterium tuberculosis* and atypical strains such as *M. avium-intracellulare*, *M. kansasii*, and *M. abscessus* have been increasingly recognized in both AIDS and non-AIDS immunodeficient populations.[119,120]

The development of disseminated *M. tuberculosis* following HSCT is a serious and often fatal complication (Fig. 64.3).[121] Based on data from developed countries, *M. tuberculosis* infections are rare in HSCT recipients.[122–124] However, the incidence of tuberculosis in the HSCT population directly reflects its incidence in the general population. In Turkey, where tuberculosis is endemic (35/100,000 population vs. 7/100,000 in the United States), tuberculosis was 40 times more common in allo-HSCT patients than in the general population.[125] The presence of multidrug-resistant strains of *M. tuberculosis* (indirectly related to treatment of HIV disease) is of great concern[126] and has led some programs to maintain a high index of suspicion for tuberculosis and to treat HSCT recipients with this complication for longer periods of time, often with multidrug regimens.[127]

Nontuberculous mycobacterial (NTM) infections can be either catheter-related or respiratory infections.[127] Mere isolation of NTM on BAL may not be of pathogenic significance, unless there is evidence of tissue invasion or concomitant bacteremia is present. Treatment requires 2–4 antimicrobials guided by in vitro susceptibility testing, and removal of indwelling catheters (if contaminated), as well as surgical debridement of subcutaneous tunnel infection sites.[127]

Legionella Pneumophila

Patients undergoing bone marrow and solid organ transplantation are particularly susceptible to *Legionella* infections due to prolonged neutropenia and abnormalities in cell-mediated immunity. Legionnaires' disease (LD) can be acquired by inhalation of aerosols containing *L. pneumophila*, or by microaspiration of contaminated drinking water.[128] LD should always be in the differential diagnosis of pneumonia among HSCT recipients. Appropriate tests to confirm LD include culturing sputum, BAL, and tissue specimens; testing BAL specimens for *Legionellae* by direct fluorescent antibody (DFA), as well as examining for *L. pneumophila* serogroup 1 antigen in urine and performing testing for 5S rRNA PCR of BAL, urine, or serum samples.[129,130]

PARASITIC AGENTS (See Also Chapter 33)

Toxoplasma Gondii and *Cryptosporidium Parvum*

Toxoplasma gondii infects cats and other animals and secondarily infects humans, causing congenital toxoplasmosis during intrauterine infection. Primary infection later in life usually causes only lymphadenopathy and mild systemic symptoms.[131] *Cryptosporidium parvum* infects a variety of hosts, including immunosuppressed individuals. Its usual routes of transmission are water- or food-borne, but person-to-person transmission is possible.[132] *Toxoplasma* primarily causes central nervous system disease, but disseminated disease with secondary pulmonary involvement can occur, presenting with shortness of breath, cough, fever, and bilateral interstitial infiltrates.[133] *C. parvum* causes severe diarrhea, but disseminated disease with pulmonary involvement can occur. Treatment of *T. gondii* is with pyrimethamine-sulfadiazine, while treatment of *C. parvum* is rapidly evolving, with combination therapy of azithromycin-paramomycin[134] being supplanted by the more effective nitazoxanide in many parts of the developing world.[135]

PULMONARY COINFECTIONS

Late after solid organ transplantation or in the late phase infections following HSCT, it is common to find copathogens—that is, isolation of more than one pathogenic species of bacteria, fungus, or opportunistic virus from BAL or lung biopsy specimens. For example, pulmonary copathogens may be isolated in as many as 53% of patients with *parainfluenza* pneumonia.[136] HSCT recipients with *CMV* disease or respiratory viral infections are more susceptible to invasive fungal infections, especially *Aspergillus*.[137] Alangaden and colleagues described the occurrence of gram-negative bacilli and *Aspergillus* infections among allogeneic BMT recipients with chronic GVHD requiring long-term steroid use.[138] Chronic colonization of the airways of patients with GVHD may be analogous to colonization of the respiratory tract, with *Pseudomonas* and *Aspergillus* species in patients with cystic fibrosis, possibly suggesting an alteration in the homeostasis of the respiratory mucosa, mucociliary clearance, and airway surface liquid. Recovery of bacteria from respiratory secretions in this scenario may represent airway colonization rather than invasive parenchymal disease.

Pulmonary Complications Following Solid-Organ Transplantation

This section will refer mainly to pulmonary complications of nonlung, solid-solid organ transplantation, as lung transplantation and its complications will be discussed in Chapter 67.

PULMONARY EDEMA, PLEURAL EFFUSIONS, AND ACUTE RESPIRATORY DISTRESS SYNDROME

Pulmonary edema can occur posttransplant because of increased hydrostatic pressure (e.g., caused by fluid and blood product administration or poor left ventricular function) or decreased oncotic pressure (e.g., caused by hypoalbuminemia), or because of increased vascular permeability (e.g., caused by immune-mediated transfusion-related acute lung injury [TRALI]).

Pleural effusions may also occur as a result of increased hydrostatic or decreased oncotic pressure. Lymphatic vessels that drain the lungs can be overwhelmed or disrupted in transplantation. Infection or injury in the thoracic, mediastinal, or abdominal cavity can lead to sympathetic effusions or empyema. Finally, abdominal ascites fluid (i.e., in patients with liver or kidney disease) can translocate through pores in the diaphragm and enter the pleural space.

Pleural effusions can occur in up to 40% of children who undergo liver transplantation,[139] are predominantly right-sided, and are thought to occur as a result of disruption of diaphragmatic lymphatic channels.[140] Effusions exclusively in the left pleural space following liver transplantation should prompt evaluation for other causes. Generally, pleural effusions following liver transplantation will enlarge over the first week following transplantation and then resolve over the ensuing 3–4 weeks. Between 14% and 25% of pediatric patients require pleural drainage because of significant respiratory compromise.[141,142] Not surprisingly, pleural effusions significantly increase the duration of mechanical ventilation and ICU days.[142] Persistent pleural effusions may be a sign that acute rejection of the liver allograft is occurring.[143]

Acute respiratory distress syndrome (ARDS) is a devastating complication in up to 15% of liver transplant recipients in the immediate postoperative period. This is primarily caused by sepsis, but in the case of liver and small bowel transplantation, other risk factors should be considered as potential causes (e.g., severe malnutrition of the recipient, the extensive and prolonged abdominal surgery, massive intraoperative blood transfusion, and aspiration in the early posttransplant period).[144]

IMPAIRMENT OF RESPIRATORY MECHANICS

The extensive surgery in the upper abdomen that occurs during orthotopic liver transplantation can have significant effects upon diaphragmatic excursion, especially on the right side. Diaphragmatic dysfunction can also occur in heart, kidney, and small bowel transplantation, but to a lesser degree than after liver transplantation. Poor excursion of the diaphragm can lead to impaired cough and airway clearance, resulting in atelectasis and pneumonia. Diaphragmatic function can be impaired by swelling in the subdiaphragmatic area, as well as phrenic nerve injury when the suprahepatic vena cava is clamped during liver transplantation. Diaphragmatic dysfunction or paralysis can be found in 8%–11% of pediatric liver transplant recipients,[142,143] and with more sensitive techniques, phrenic nerve conduction abnormalities are seen in up to 80% of adult liver transplant recipients.[145] For adults, the injury to the right phrenic nerve does not seem to have significant impact on recovery, as determined by the duration of mechanical ventilation or hospital stay. In infants and small children, compromise of one diaphragm can lead to more respiratory distress, atelectasis, and pneumonia, as well as longer duration of mechanical ventilation and ICU stays.[142]

Recruiting atelectatic lung and performing adequate airway clearance in the postliver transplant period can be challenging because of pain and the "fresh" surgical sites. This is especially true for patients in whom the abdomen is not completely closed in the immediate postoperative period. In this situation, the important abdominal muscles that are needed for cough are impaired. Patients may require noninvasive positive pressure ventilation (NIPPV) after extubation. Airway clearance and the use of a mechanical in-exsufflator (cough assist device) can help clear secretions and prevent atelectasis in the immediate postoperative period. Since physiotherapy to the chest wall may be painful after sternotomy, oscillating positive expiratory pressure devices and incentive spirometry (in patients who can cooperate) and intrapulmonary percussive ventilation (in those that cannot cooperate) can be invaluable in the postoperative period. When diaphragmatic dysfunction or paralysis is present, plication of the diaphragm can be considered (utilized in up to 25% of patients with diaphragm paralysis).[143] However, plication should only be considered if phrenic nerve function has not returned after a period of observation with noninvasive management of at least 90 days, or if the patient develops clinical respiratory deterioration.

MEDICATION TOXICITY

Early infusion of cyclosporine has been reported to cause ARDS in patients receiving liver transplantation.[144] Fortunately, most medications used for immunosuppression in the postorgan transplantation period do not have direct toxicity to the lung. Two exceptions are the mammalian targets of rapamycin (mTOR) inhibitors, sirolimus (rapamycin) and everolimus. Both are potent immunosuppressants that confer less nephrotoxicity than calcineurin inhibitors. They have been increasingly popular because of their overall favorable side-effect profile. However, sirolimus and everolimus cause interstitial pneumonitis at both therapeutic and supratherapeutic drug levels.[146–151] Incidence of this complication ranges from 0.4% to 2.9%.[148,152] Sirolimus-induced interstitial pneumonitis can occur acutely, but the onset is usually insidious. Patients usually present with dyspnea on exertion (66%–90%), dry cough (75%–100%), and fever (60%–87%). Lung function testing may reveal a restrictive defect. Plain films and CT scans of the chest might reveal an interstitial pattern with interstitial infiltrates, consolidation, or ground-glass

opacification with lower lobe predominance. BAL and biopsy specimens can show patterns of lymphocytic alveolitis, pulmonary hemorrhage, or organizing pneumonia.[147,148] Treatment requires discontinuation of the causative medication, and resolution is generally prompt, although radiographic abnormalities may persist. Corticosteroid use should be considered and may be effective, although supportive data are limited.[148]

POSTTRANSPLANT LYMPHOPROLIFERATIVE DISEASE

The immunosuppression required for solid-organ transplant recipients places them at increased risk for developing posttransplant lymphoproliferative disease (PTLD).[153] PTLD typically stems from an immunosuppressive regimen that causes T lymphocyte depletion, which then leads to uncontrolled EBV-driven B cell proliferation. This unregulated growth of B cells can range from benign polyclonal B lymphocyte expansion to aggressive immunoblastic B cell lymphomas.[154] Less frequently, PTLD also can result from T cell or natural killer (NK) cell proliferation.[155,156] PTLD occurs in approximately 3%–9% of heart transplant recipients[155,157,158] and up to 20% of intestinal transplant recipients.[159] PTLD can occur following kidney and liver transplantation as well, but less frequently. PTLD arising in the lung is much more common following heart, lung, and heart-lung transplantation than following transplantation of abdominal organs. The median onset of PTLD is typically within 24 months following solid-organ transplantation.

A significant risk factor for PTLD is seroconversion of an EBV-naïve recipient, either by primary infection in a previously uninfected recipient or by transplantation of a graft from an EBV-seropositive donor. Other risk factors include Rh factor negativity, Rh mismatch, and recipient CMV seronegativity, and a high degree of immunosuppression, although induction immunosuppression does not appear to appreciably increase the risk of PTLD.[157,158,160–162] Shortness of breath, cough, and upper airway obstruction were the most common symptoms in those with pulmonary PTLD. Because many will not have symptoms at presentation, screening of the at-risk patient population with EBV viral load may be the earliest means of detecting the presence of EBV as a marker for PTLD. A retrospective study in liver transplant recipients showed a marked reduction in PTLD and prevention of rejection in patients in the era in which EBV PCR monitoring was available (PTLD incidence decreased from 14.9% to 1.9%).[163] Increasing EBV load may signify a need to adjust the patient's immunosuppressive regimen. Because CMV may be a coinfecting agent in these patients, prophylactic antiviral therapy and CMV PCR monitoring are also recommended. In patients who present with pulmonary disease, nodular abnormalities are the most common finding (Fig. 64.4A and B), although lymphadenopathy, consolidations, or effusions may be seen on chest imaging.[164] Even when PTLD is strongly suggested by the combination of increasing EBV load and typical radiographic findings, biopsy material should be obtained to confirm the diagnosis histologically (see Fig. 64.4C) and assess for the presence or absence of EBV-early RNA (EBER)–staining cells (see Fig. 64.4D). In addition, it is useful to characterize cell surface markers such as CD20, which may guide therapy.

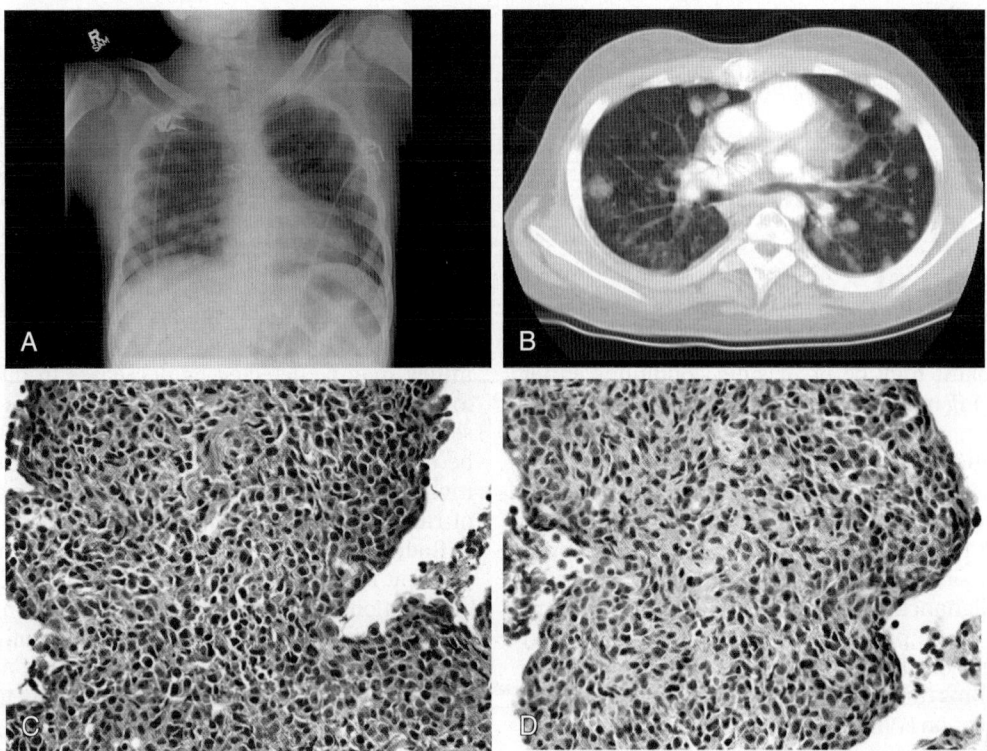

Fig. 64.4 Posttransplant lymphoproliferative disease. (A) Anteroposterior chest radiograph. (B) Computed tomography scan. (C) Histopathology showing monomorphic clonal expansion of lymphocytes that express Epstein-Barr early RNA (D).

Initial therapy for PTLD is the reduction of immunosuppression to reduce the degree of T lymphocyte depletion. This reduction can be associated with further complications (e.g., graft rejection) and still may be insufficient for recovery.[165,166] Thus some have employed novel assays of immune function to monitor the degree of immunosuppression, while at the same time monitoring EBV viral load.[167] Antiviral agents and IV immunoglobulin, including anti–B cell immunotherapy with the monoclonal anti-CD-20 antibody (rituximab), have been attempted with varying degrees of success.[168] The main complication of rituximab therapy is prolonged B cell depletion and hypoimmunoglobulinemia.[169] Anti-CMV therapy should be continued in patients at risk for this coinfection, but it may not decrease the cellular proliferation of PTLD, because there is very little active EBV replication in these lesions.

PTLD following solid-organ transplantation confers an increase in mortality, reflecting the severity of the disease itself or its treatment, specifically the treatment effects upon the transplanted organ.

OTHER NONINFECTIOUS PULMONARY COMPLICATIONS OF SOLID-ORGAN TRANSPLANTATION

Many pulmonary complications that arise pretransplantation may not resolve completely or immediately posttransplantation. Metastatic pulmonary calcifications can occur in patients with kidney or hepatic failure, and while usually benign, can lead to restrictive lung disease. Furthermore, their nodular appearance on chest radiographs can mimic nodules from infection or malignancy (see the previous section).

Pulmonary conditions such as alveolar simplification[170] and primary ciliary dyskinesia (PCD)[171] can be associated with congenital heart disease, including those associated with heterotaxy, and they may not have been recognized before heart transplantation. These conditions should be considered if unexpected pulmonary complications including prolonged hypoxemia and recurrent atelectasis develop in the posttransplant period.

Hepatopulmonary syndrome (HPS) and porto-pulmonary hypertension (PPHTN) are two entities that occur in end-stage liver disease and can significantly improve with liver transplantation. However, improvement is not universal or even expedient. In the case of HPS, significant hypoxemia can occur because of dilation of pulmonary capillaries, and this may persist in the postoperative period, leading to prolonged mechanical ventilation and the use of supplemental oxygen. Typically, resolution of hypoxemia from HPS occurs over the initial 8 months following transplant.[172]

Severe cases of PPHTN may preclude liver transplantation since the operative mortality increases as the severity of pulmonary hypertension increases. Additionally, PPHTN can recur or occur de novo after liver transplantation. Posttransplant pulmonary hypertension (PHTN) can occur in those with pretransplant HPS, those with recurrent liver disease, and those with no apparent liver disease and isolated PHTN. Severe PHTN in either the pretransplant or the posttransplant period increases the risk of mortality.[173,174] Continuous infusion of prostaglandins can serve to lower pulmonary pressures, acting as a bridge to transplant and attenuating surgical risk.

Venous thromboemboli (VTE) can occur in the posttransplant period, thus leading to respiratory distress and hypoxemia, but they are uncommon in pediatric patients. Renal transplant patients may be at higher risk because of manipulation of pelvic veins, although this has mainly been reported in adult patients.[175]

Pulmonary Complications of Childhood Tumors and Their Treatment

Pulmonary complications of solid organ and hematopoietic stem cell transplant may be preexisting conditions either from the underlying malignancy or from the initial treatment for malignancy.

Childhood cancers are treated with a combination of surgery (primarily for solid tumors), chemotherapy, and radiotherapy. See Chapter 59 for a further discussion of pulmonary toxicity from chemotherapy. Radiation therapy is an integral component of curative treatment for a variety of oncologic malignancies, both for the treatment of primary tumors and for those patients with distant metastases. A common site for metastases is the lung, particularly in diseases such as Wilms tumor, sarcomas, and hepatoblastoma. Whole lung irradiation (WLI) is often used as adjuvant therapy for patients with distant lung metastases. Unfortunately, lung tissue is particularly sensitive to the effects of radiation, and the untoward effects of WLI are a concern, both during and well beyond the end of therapy. In addition, total body irradiation (TBI) is commonly used as part of pretransplant conditioning regimens.

Therapeutic doses of radiation can cause acute (radiation pneumonitis) and chronic (radiation fibrosis) lung injury. The incidence of acute radiation pneumonitis is up to 15% of adults treated for breast and lung cancers and Hodgkin disease, but the incidence in pediatric patients is less well described.[176] The incidence may be dependent on the radiation dose, fractionation, and volume of lung exposed,[177] as well as concurrent chemotherapy.[178] At thoracic radiation doses approximating 1000 cGy or more, total lung capacity and diffusing capacity may be significantly impaired.[179–181] Some chemotherapeutic agents (bleomycin, dactinomycin) have additive toxicity with radiation, and others (actinomycin

D and Adriamycin) can result in a "radiation recall" effect, with delayed presentation of toxicity, up to 6 weeks later.[182,183]

Acutely, radiation injury results in the release of a number of proinflammatory cytokines that can cause subendothelial and perivascular damage. Over time, this causes type II pneumocyte hypertrophy and infiltration of inflammatory cells.[184] Radiation pneumonitis typically presents 30–90 days after radiation therapy, with symptoms of cough, dyspnea, hypoxemia, and pleuritic pain. Examination may reveal crackles or a pleural friction rub, and chest radiography may show diffuse haziness or ground-glass densities. Early injury may be detected by decreases in diffusing capacity for carbon monoxide. The differential diagnosis for this presentation includes infections and other etiologies that must be excluded. Treatment of radiation pneumonitis usually involves systemic corticosteroids, based on a murine model of radiation toxicity.[185]

Radiation fibrosis may appear 6–24 months after radiation therapy. It is usually but not always preceded by symptoms of radiation pneumonitis, and itself most commonly presents with progressive dyspnea. Radiographically, there may be streaky densities, decreased lung volume or atelectasis, or pleural thickening. Pulmonary function findings include hypoxemia, a restrictive defect, and decreased diffusing capacity. Histologic findings include pleural and subpleural fibroses, interstitial fibrosis, interstitial pneumonitis, interlobular septal fibrosis, and obliteration of pulmonary vessels (Fig. 64.5). Unfortunately, there is no useful treatment for radiation fibrosis. Some patients with severe lung disease because of radiation fibrosis have undergone lung transplantation. As such, efforts should be focused on prevention (with considerations of shielding, dose, and effects of other agents) and close monitoring for patients at high risk.

Analysis of self-report data from the Childhood Cancer Survivor Study[186,187] cohort showed that in survivors who were more than 5 years from diagnosis and received radiation to the chest or TBI, there was a statistically significant increase in the relative risk of developing late pulmonary complications. These included lung fibrosis, emphysema, recurrent pneumonia, chronic cough, persistent shortness of breath, and abnormal chest wall development. As more children survive cancer and live well into adulthood, it is

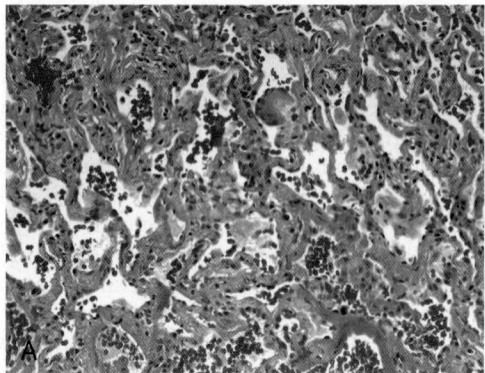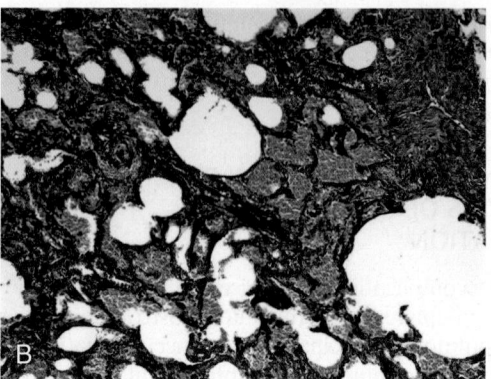

Fig. 64.5 Radiation fibrosis. (A) Hematoxylin and eosin (H&E) stain, 20×, showing pleural, subpleural, and interstitial fibrosis; foci of chronic interstitial pneumonitis; and irregular scars within the parenchyma. The interlobular septa are fibrotic and thickened with obliteration of some of the pulmonary vasculature. (B) Trichrome stain showing significant collagen deposition.

important to consider the late effects associated with WLI.[178] Beyond the lung parenchyma itself, radiation can also impair the growth of the muscle, cartilage, and bone of the thorax. Studies in adults receiving WLI suggest that mild restrictive disease usually resolves over a period of 2–4 years. However, the ongoing development of the chest wall and the lung in children makes the impact of such toxic therapy quite different. Continued alveolar multiplication occurs until 2–4 years of age, and alveolar enlargement continues for some time after that.[188] The growing chest wall may also be impacted by radiation treatment. Weiner and colleagues reported a retrospective review of pulmonary function in 30 children who had received WLI[189] for treatment of malignancy. At a median of almost 3 years post radiation, 20% of subjects had moderate or severe reduction in FEV_1, 43% had moderate or severe reduction in TLC, and 43% had moderate or severe reduction in diffusing capacity. At least two patients demonstrated a clear progressive decline over time. These authors suggested that recognition of early abnormalities might allow for earlier intervention for radiation pneumonitis (e.g., corticosteroid therapy) and that it cannot be presumed (as in adults) that loss of lung function after radiation is transient.

Benoist and coworkers[180] followed 48 children treated with WLI for Wilms tumor for 2–17 years following treatment. Two subjects had clinical evidence of radiation pneumonitis shortly after treatment, which resolved within 3–8 weeks. In this study, the percentage of patients with abnormal TLC or lung compliance increased over time, with reduced TLC observed in 50% at 6 months and greater than 90% at 6 years. These authors posit that early lung function abnormalities are caused by parenchymal lung injury, while later effects result from impaired chest wall growth. These findings argue for continued pulmonary follow-up of children treated with thoracic irradiation.

Pulmonary Complications of Hematopoietic Stem Cell Transplantation

Significant advances in transplantation immunology as well as innovations in chemotherapy and irradiation have allowed HSCT to become a more viable therapy for the treatment of hematologic diseases. The science of bone marrow transplantation, which began as the allogeneic transplantation of whole bone marrow, has progressed to include allogeneic altered marrow (e.g., T cell depleted), autologous marrow, and HSCT. Despite many advances, even the most experienced transplant centers encounter significant posttransplantation morbidity and mortality. Infectious and noninfectious pulmonary complications remain common following marrow transplantation in both adults[190–192] and children.[193–196] While most studies of HSCT recipients deal with adults rather than children, many important principles apply across age barriers. Although different sources of stem cells for transplantation (e.g., allogeneic or autologous) portend different risks of particular complications, we will describe potential complications in a more general fashion and will refer to relative incidences when appropriate. In addition, we will refer to these procedures collectively as HSCT.

Table 64.2 Recommendations for Pulmonology Evaluation Prior to Hematopoietic Cell Transplantation

History/physical examination
Chest radiograph
High-resolution, thin cut, computed tomography (CT) scan of chest
Pulmonary function testing[a]: Spirometry
Lung volumes
Transfer factor (diffusing capacity)
Maximal inspiratory/expiratory pressure
Six-minute walk test

[a]Pulmonary function testing will depend on patient age and cooperativity.

PRETRANSPLANT FACTORS

Some preexisting diseases that themselves are treated with HSCT may have significant pretransplant pulmonary complications. For example, sickle cell disease (SCD) can be complicated by previous acute chest syndrome and pulmonary infarction,[197] and patients with underlying malignancies may have been treated with irradiation targeting the lung or with pulmonary toxic chemotherapy including bleomycin, busulfan, or cyclophosphamide. These all may affect lung function prior to HSCT.

It is critical that patients previously exposed to treatments that are potentially "pneumotoxic" have pre-HSCT pulmonary screening (Table 64.2), including the determination of lung volumes, flows, diffusing capacity, and respiratory muscle strength. The monitoring of PFTs remains useful during the posttransplantation period and can be especially important as adjuncts to radiographic evaluation of intercurrent illness affecting the lung. Recent reports suggest that pre-HSCT pulmonary function can predict post-HSCT pulmonary complications as well as survival.[198,199] Musculoskeletal weakness is both a common preexisting condition and a known complication of HSCT[200]; several relatively simple tests (6-minute walk test and respiratory muscle strength test) are useful in identifying patients at risk,[201] allowing for musculoskeletal rehabilitation and nutritional support in both the pre- and post-HSCT period.

Spirometry, plethysmographic lung volumes, and even diffusing capacity have been performed in infants and toddlers unable to cooperate with traditional testing. See Chapter 11 for a further discussion of these techniques. Whether infant lung function testing can be used to predict risk for pulmonary complications of HSCT has not been studied but is an area that requires further investigation.

The impact of some conditioning regimens on post-HSCT pulmonary complications has led to alterations in the intensity of these regimens. This approach may lead to improved survival with diminished toxicity in selected circumstances, such as in recipients with primary immunodeficiencies who are to receive HSCT from an HLA-matched unrelated donor[202] or in patients with SCD.[202,203]

There is a variety of other pre-HSCT factors that may adversely affect post-HSCT pulmonary status and complications. These consist of pulmonary infections, including viral illnesses, thoracic surgical procedures, chronic aspiration, and gastroesophageal reflux. Several lower respiratory infections, particularly invasive fungal disease, can increase the risk of both recurrent infection and pulmonary debilitation post-HSCT. The increased risk of recurrent fungal infection in patients undergoing intensive chemotherapy[204] led to more widespread use of antifungal prophylaxis to prevent recurrence following HSCT.[205] This practice has allowed consideration of HSCT in these high-risk patients.[206,207] Thoracic surgical procedures prior to HSCT may include lobectomy or wedge resection of pulmonary metastatic disease or for surgical diagnosis of localized fungal infections. The added risk of HSCT closely following thoracic surgery is unknown, but reduced lung function from surgery undoubtedly contributes to the additional risks of low pretransplant lung function.

Cytoreductive therapy and irradiation alter host defenses and disturb mucosal integrity, potentially leading to colonization with potential pathogens. Potential HSCT recipients with dysphagia or odynophagia should be evaluated for esophagitis, as the damaged esophageal mucosa, aided by neutropenia, increases the risk of esophageal colonization with organisms, including *Candida* and *Herpes simplex*. Esophagoscopy may help direct therapy for such patients.[208] In addition, gastroparesis and delayed gastric emptying resulting in nausea, gastroesophageal reflux, or decreased oral intake may be seen following HSCT.[209,210]

Malnutrition is common in pediatric patients being considered for HSCT, and accurate determination of the degree of malnutrition is important.[211] Because myeloablative and irradiative conditioning regimens can lead to mucositis affecting oral intake and because malnutrition is felt to be an independent risk factor for mortality following HSCT,[212] the use of enteral or parenteral feeding is common following HSCT.[213,214]

EARLY NONINFECTIOUS POSTTRANSPLANT COMPLICATIONS (Fig. 64.6)

Oral and Perioral Complications

Oral mucositis affects the majority of patients undergoing HSCT[215] and can lead to dysphagia, as well as laryngeal or epiglottic edema, resulting in upper airway obstruction. It is recognized to increase the risk of infection, lengthen hospital stay, and increase the cost of care.[216] Although oral mucositis likely represents the sequelae of intensive chemotherapy and irradiation,[217] other important factors (e.g., bacterial colonization of the mucosal surface, upregulation of proinflammatory cytokines, and oxidative radical production) play an important role.[215,218,219] It is usually seen within the first week of irradiation and reaches its peak 1–2 weeks following HSCT.[220] Impaired mucociliary clearance in the nasopharynx, along with oropharyngeal mucositis, can lead to both upper and lower airway complications, including sinusitis, oropharyngeal bleeding, upper airway obstruction, stridor, and aspiration pneumonia. Advances in the understanding of the pathophysiology of oral mucositis have led to newer treatments, including dietary manipulation, mucosal administration of monochromatic light, and the administration of cytokines, such as keratinocyte growth factor.[215,221,222]

Pulmonary Edema and Capillary Leak Syndrome

Pulmonary edema in the posttransplant period is relatively common[195,223,224] and is characterized by a rapid onset, usually within the 2–3 weeks following HSCT. Potential etiologies include increased hydrostatic pressure from either overly vigorous rehydration or fluid overload via parenteral nutrition, cardiac dysfunction following the use of anthracyclines, and renal toxicity following cyclophosphamide. Other causes of increased pulmonary capillary permeability may include sepsis and direct pulmonary toxicity secondary to irradiation and chemotherapy. Clinical features may include dyspnea, tachypnea, weight gain, hypoxemia, and basilar crackles on chest auscultation. Chest radiographs often show bilateral infiltrates, and pleural effusions may be present. Treatment usually involves vigorous diuresis.

Peri-Engraftment Respiratory Distress Syndrome

This entity has a low incidence (~5%), and it occurs within the first 14 days following HSCT, at a time coinciding with

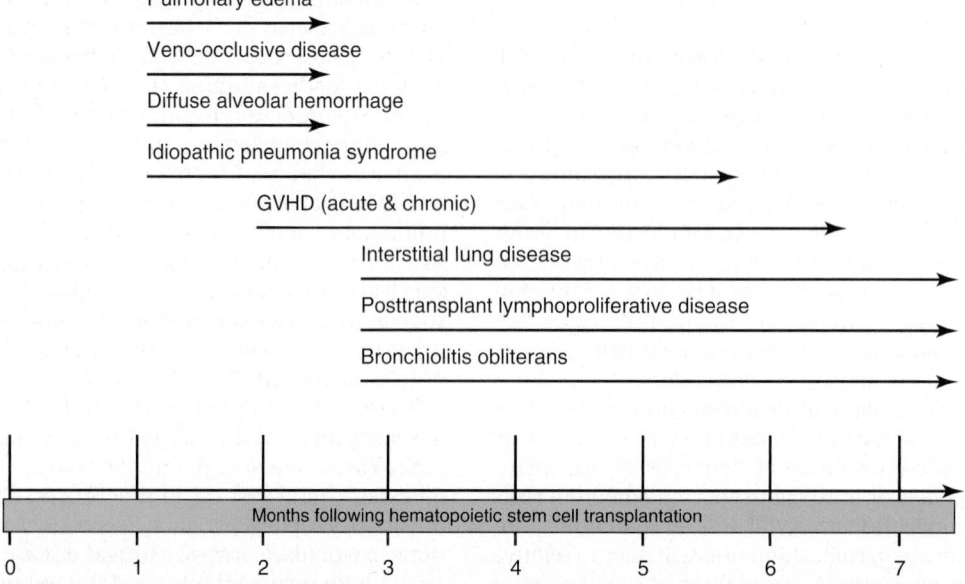

Fig. 64.6 Timeline of noninfectious pulmonary complications following hematopoietic stem cell transplantation. *GVHD,* Graft-versus-host-disease.

neutrophil engraftment.[225,226] The characteristic clinical and radiographic features include hypoxemia and respiratory distress. Chest radiographic findings include diffuse edema and pulmonary infiltrates, and in some cases pleural effusions.[227] BAL and other invasive studies are consistently negative for pathogens. While its name and timing might suggest a specific pathology, there are no biochemical markers or pathognomonic histopathologic findings to distinguish it from other forms of respiratory distress in the period closely following HSCT. Therapy is supportive, and although steroids have often been utilized for treatment, their efficacy is unproven.

Idiopathic Pneumonia Syndrome

IPS (also known as *idiopathic interstitial pneumonitis*) has a reported incidence of 5%–10% in adult HSCT recipients,[228,229] although the incidence in pediatric recipients is more difficult to assess. A National Heart, Lung, and Blood Institute Workshop[230] refined the definition of IPS and established clinical and diagnostic criteria for it. Accordingly, the clinical manifestations of IPS include dyspnea, nonproductive cough, hypoxemia, and crackles on auscultation; pulmonary function testing (PFT) reveals a restrictive pulmonary physiology, and diffuse or nonlobar infiltrates are seen on chest radiograph. In order to confirm this diagnosis, BAL cultures must be negative for bacterial, viral, and fungal pathogens; a second negative BAL is recommended 2–14 days following the initial negative BAL. Open lung biopsy is not specifically suggested, although transbronchial biopsy may be considered if the patient's condition will allow it. Pathologically, IPS can have two distinct histopathologic types: interstitial pneumonia and diffuse alveolar damage. IPS is typically an early complication of HSCT. Previous reports of IPS incidence described a bimodal pattern, with an initial peak approximately 2 weeks and a later peak 6–7 weeks post-HSCT.[230] While an entity essentially identical to IPS can be seen greater than 100 days following HSCT, the incidence of this much later complication is unknown. A review of more than 1000 HSCT recipients[229] indicated that the overall incidence of IPS was 7.3%, with no significant difference in incidence between recipients of autologous and allogeneic HSCT. Pediatric patients (<20 years of age) had a slightly lower incidence of IPS. The median time between HSCT and onset of symptoms of IPS was 21 days; the hospital mortality was 74%, and multiorgan failure rather than isolated respiratory failure was associated with mortality. Potential causes for IPS have included direct pulmonary toxicity resulting from pre-HSCT conditioning, as well as immunologically mediated factors resulting from alloreactivity.[231–234]

Treatment for IPS remains supportive; steroids, although often used, have not been shown to have a beneficial effect. The need for mechanical ventilation in these patients is associated with a poor prognosis.

Diffuse Alveolar Hemorrhage

Robbins and colleagues are generally credited with the description of what is known as diffuse alveolar hemorrhage (DAH) in recipients of HSCT, although the syndrome has been recognized for more than 30 years.[235,236] This entity appears to be much more common in adult than in pediatric recipients of HSCT.[236,237] It usually appears within 30 days post-HSCT and coincides with marrow recovery. Of interest is the finding of relative BAL neutrophilia, despite peripheral leucopenia.[235] A retrospective analysis of pediatric HSCT recipients suggests that the incidence of DAH is approximately 5%, with allogeneic recipients being at higher risk.[238] The clinical onset is often relatively sudden and rapidly progressive, with dyspnea, hypoxemia, and crackles on auscultation. On BAL, the characteristic feature is that with each successive aliquot instilled, the effluent becomes more hemorrhagic[236]; however, the specificity and sensitivity of the findings are not completely clear. Agusti and coworkers reported on four of eight HSCT recipients who had DAH on postmortem and nonhemorrhagic BALs, while 7 of 13 patients without pathologically proven DAH had hemorrhagic BALs.[239] Thus clinical correlation, timely performance of BAL, and sampling of multiple sites may be important in establishing the presence or absence of DAH.

Pulmonary and Hepatic Veno-Occlusive Disease

First reported by Troussard and colleagues, this entity presents as a form of pulmonary hypertension, with dyspnea, signs of right-sided heart failure, and pulmonary infiltrates on chest radiograph.[240] Children compose the most significant proportion of HSCT recipients affected by veno-occlusive disease (VOD).[241,242] Hepatic VOD, another vascular complication of HSCT, is often associated with pulmonary VOD and interstitial pneumonitis.[243] In both, small veins and venules are partially or completely occluded by intimal fibrosis. The explanation of the relatively common coexistence of hepatic and pulmonary VOD is unknown. Possibilities include coexistent underlying toxicities or genetic factors. The diagnosis of pulmonary VOD requires a high index of clinical suspicion, as many cases reported in the literature are diagnosed postmortem.[240] Some recent reports suggest that serum levels of vascular endothelial growth factor or plasma protein C activity may be useful surrogate markers for the development of VOD,[244,245] but larger controlled studies will be needed before their routine use can be recommended. Echocardiography, cardiac catheterization, BAL to rule out intercurrent infection, and transbronchial or transthoracic lung biopsy are potential clinical investigations that should be tailored to the patient's condition and the clinical circumstances. Treatment options for pulmonary VOD are few, although reports demonstrate that defibrotide, a polydisperse oligonucleotide with fibrinolytic and antithrombotic properties,[246,247] may be effective therapy for hepatic VOD.[248] There are also reports of its utility in preventing VOD in HSCT recipients at increased risk for this complication.[249]

PULMONARY FUNCTION FOLLOWING HUMAN STEM CELL TRANSPLANTATION

A significant proportion of children who undergo HSCT have abnormalities in PFT both soon after HSCT and later after engraftment has taken place.[196,198,250] Ginsberg and coworkers[198] reported a retrospective analysis of serial pulmonary function test subjects; 273 had at least one pretransplant PFT. The majority of patients had normal or mildly reduced spirometry (FVC and FEV_1) and lung volumes prior to transplant. In addition, the majority had a decreased diffusing capacity, with 25% having moderately or severely reduced diffusion. Following HSCT, FVC and FEV_1 decreased significantly over the first 6 months, improved slightly between 6 and 12 months, and remained stable at 1–2, 2–5, and more than 5 years. Diffusing capacity also decreased 6 months post-HSCT, with gradual but incomplete improvement by 5 years posttransplant. In a multivariate analysis, patient age, underlying diagnosis, and transplant type (autologous vs. allogeneic) all had independent predictive value for decline in DLCO following HSCT. Similar reports describe pulmonary function abnormalities in those who have received HSCT with TBI conditioning.[251–253] Other studies have shown that older age at HSCT,[254] female sex,[254,255] busulfan,[254] TBI,[256,257] chronic GVHD,[258] and peripheral blood stem cell graft[254] are also associated with risk for pulmonary function decline.

LATE NONINFECTIOUS POSTTRANSPLANT COMPLICATIONS

The differential diagnosis of late-onset pulmonary complications extends from the complications listed in the early non-infectious group to include obliterative bronchiolitis (OB), also known as bronchiolitis obliterans, possibly associated with underlying chronic GVHD, cryptogenic organizing pneumonia (COP, formerly *bronchiolitis obliterans organizing pneumonia*, or BOOP) and posttransplant lymphoproliferative disorder (PTLD).[133] In addition, persistent post-HSCT pulmonary findings of VOD and IPS continue to occasionally complicate the late posttransplant course.

Obliterative Bronchiolitis ("Bronchiolitis Obliterans Syndrome")

Development of chronic lower airways obstruction is a common late pulmonary complication following HSCT and is most commonly associated with pathologic changes of OB.[192,259,260] Bronchiolitis obliterans syndrome (BOS) refers to the finding of progressive obstruction, even when pathologic evidence of OB has not been demonstrated on open lung biopsy and is most commonly associated with evidence of chronic GVHD, and is much more common following allogeneic, as opposed to autologous, marrow transplantation. Additional risk factors include early posttransplant viral infection and advanced age of the recipient.[192,261] Symptoms are generally seen 12–24 months after HSCT but have been described as early as 90 days after transplantation. The primary symptoms reported at clinical presentation include dyspnea, wheezing, and nonproductive cough; fever is not common.

The chest radiograph is usually normal although hyperinflation and increased linear markings may be present. High-resolution lung CT scans performed on inspiration (TLC) and expiration (RV) in cooperative individuals or using passive lung maneuvers in pediatric patients demonstrate characteristic abnormalities and have become the standard diagnostic technique. The most common chest CT findings in BOS is a heterogeneous pattern with areas of patchy hyperaeration, areas with bronchial dilatation, and other areas characterized by hypoattenuation or increased density.[262,263] This combination of findings is often referred to as *mosaic perfusion or attenuation* and is highly suggestive for BOS (Fig. 64.7A).

PFT demonstrates airflow obstruction, as shown by a decrease in FEV_1 and a reduction of the FEV_1/FVC ratio without significant reversiblity.[228] The degree of air trapping

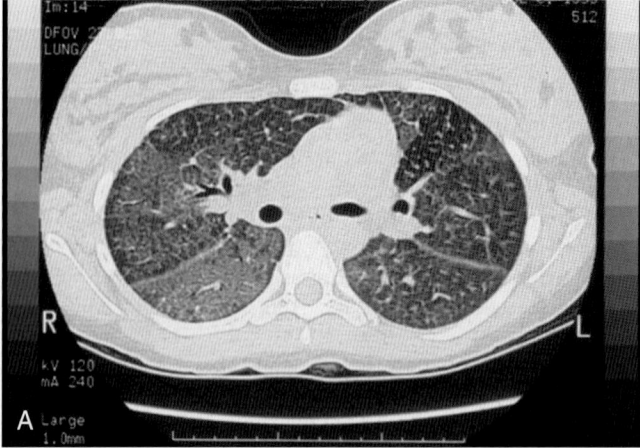

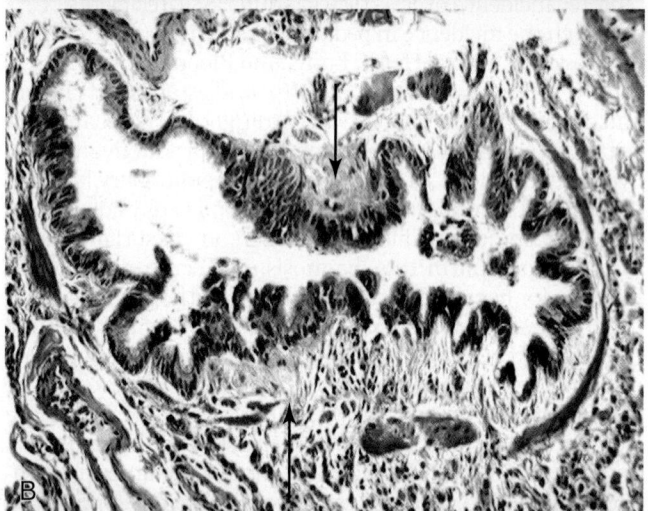

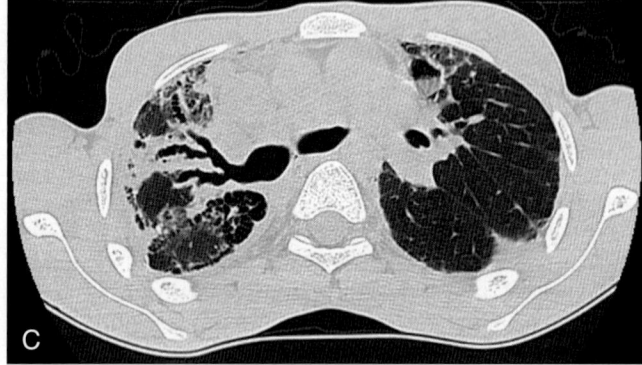

Fig. 64.7 Bronchiolitis obliterans. (A) Early changes of bronchiolitis obliterans are seen on this chest high-resolution computed tomography (CT) scan. Note the changes consistent with mosaic perfusion *(arrows)*, characterized by areas of varying attenuation. (B) A photomicrograph of an airway demonstrating subepithelial fibrosis *(arrows)*. Trichrome stain, 100×. (C) Severe lung disease following human stem cell transplantation seen on chest high-resolution CT scan. Note bronchomegaly and bronchiectasis, seen best in the right upper lobe. Additional findings included widespread fibrosis of the right upper lobe and lingula, with relative sparing of the left lower lobe, and bilateral pleural thickening.

seen on CT images may correlate with the pulmonary function abnormality. Confirmatory biopsy to make the diagnosis of BOS is now rarely indicated based on the sensitivity of imaging studies.[192,264] The diagnosis of post-HSCT BOS is often made based on the clinical presentation of cough or dyspnea, and there may be changes in lung function testing when screening asymptomatic patients.[265] Overall, up to 10% of allogeneic transplant recipients will have some degree of BOS and chronic air flow obstruction.[266] If lung biopsy is performed for confirmation of the diagnosis and to exclude other causes, this will demonstrate subepithelial fibrotic changes in the airways, a common pathologic finding in OB (see Fig. 64.7B). The insidious nature of this process, together with continuing inflammatory changes involving the airways and parenchyma, can result in end-stage lung disease with diffuse areas of traction bronchiectasis and fibrosis (see Fig. 64.7C).[267]

The incidence is variable, with reports ranging from 2% to 20%.[261] The lack of direct evidence of small airway inflammation resulting in BOS leads to the implication that donor T helper cell alloreactivity causes distal airway epithelial cell injury, which in turn leads to the pathologic changes seen.[263] Patients undergoing aggressive treatment for chronic GVHD, as well as those who had specific conditioning regimens utilizing busulfan and irradiation,[266] are at most risk for BOS; however, these simply remain recognized associations, resulting in an increased incidence of airways obstruction without a defined mechanism.

Therapy for post-HSCT BOS remains controversial and has generally centered on augmenting immunosuppression. Calcineurin-inhibitors and azathioprine, as well as steroids, have reduced the decline in lung function and have shown improvement in a small proportion of subjects.[268] Azithromycin, a macrolide antimicrobial, may improve lung function in patients suffering from BO post-HSCT,[269] and has been combined with leukotriene-receptor antagonists, and combination inhalers with long-acting bronchodilators and high-dose inhaled steroids in adults with new onset BOS with modest benefit.[270] Cycled high-dose corticosteroids have been shown to increase oxyhemoglobin saturation and improve FEV_1 in a small cohort of pediatric patients following transplant.[271] Additional multicenter clinical trials of these and other innovative therapies for BOS in pediatric HSCT patients are clearly needed.

Interstitial Lung Diseases

Interstitial lung disease, which presents with a restrictive pattern and diffusion impairment on PFT, has also been reported as a late posttransplant complication. Here the typical presentation is that of an asymptomatic subject, who on posttransplant monitoring is found to have a progressive decline in the vital capacity and/or diffusion capacity for carbon monoxide.[265] Whereas IPS may be the etiology for these changes, irradiation, chemotherapy, infectious pneumonitis, and BOOP could all contribute to these PFT alterations. Despite efforts to develop a good predictive model, these authors were unable to demonstrate any specific covariates that might predict development of restrictive change. This may be similar to an entity seen in adult HSCT recipients and termed *delayed pulmonary toxicity syndrome.*[272]

Although the diagnosis is often delayed if based on lung function testing alone, certain predisposing conditions should raise awareness of the potential for developing this restrictive pattern. Some of these may extend from the early posttransplant period and include infection and VOD. However, the most common cause remains pre-HSCT exposure to cytotoxic drugs or irradiation.[273,274] Although steroids may result in clinical improvement,[271] full diagnostic studies should be undertaken to rule out deterioration related to known pretransplant pulmonary causes, as well as to rule out infectious etiologies.

Cryptogenic Organizing Pneumonia

COP, formerly known as *bronchiolitis obliterans with organizing pneumonia* or *BOOP,* differs from OB histologically, physiologically, and most significantly in its response to treatment. It is histologically distinguished by patchy areas of consolidation with polypoid plugs of loose organizing connective tissue in the respiratory bronchioles and alveolar ducts.[267,275,276] Associated inflammation may be mild to moderate, but the proliferative bronchiolitis is manifest by patchy infiltrates on chest radiograph and by restriction on PFT.[192,276] Unlike many other post-HSCT complications, COP/BOOP often improves with corticosteroid therapy. However, it is critical to rule out other post-HSCT complications, particularly infections that may cause similar symptoms and pulmonary radiographic changes. For this reason, bronchoscopies with BAL as well as open lung biopsy are often required to seek potential infectious causes as well as to document the histopathology of the lung.[264] In addition, a response to steroids will help differentiate between OB and COP/BOOP if the diagnosis is obscure, despite studies such as bronchoscopy and open lung biopsy.[277]

Posttransplant Lymphoproliferative Disorder

PTLD can occur after HSCT, as it does after solid-organ transplantation (described earlier in the chapter). In this population, allogeneic transplants, human leukocyte antigen (HLA) mismatched transplants, T cell-depleted grafts, and Epstein-Barr virus (EBV) seronegative recipients who receive transplants from EBV seropositive donors are at increased risk.[278] The pathogenesis, monitoring, and treatment of PTLD in the HSCT recipient are similar to those described previously for the solid-organ transplant recipient. The presentation is usually within the first year following HSCT, with the peak incidence 1–5 months after transplant.

Pulmonary Alveolar Proteinosis

Pulmonary alveolar proteinosis (PAP) has rarely been described in conditions associated with immune impairment including post-HSCT.[192,279] This condition is associated with the excessive accumulation of surfactant lipoprotein in the alveolar space and results in defective air exchange and hypoxemia. The diagnosis can be suggested on CT and is easily made on BAL, where the distinctive finding is the lipoproteinaceous milky white fluid recovered from the lower airway. This finding can be subsequently confirmed via laboratory analysis.[192] The treatment for PAP requires the physical removal of this excessive surfactant material, usually by sequential lavage.[280]

Respiratory Failure

Chronic respiratory complications following HSCT, particularly BOS and interstitial lung disease, can lead to respiratory insufficiency and, ultimately, respiratory failure. Because of this, monitoring the pulmonary and cardiac status of HSCT recipients who have these complications will allow the clinician to intervene appropriately with treatment when possible. Unfortunately, the treatments for BOS and interstitial lung disease are often unsuccessful. For such conditions with end-stage lung disease, lung transplantation may be a treatment option.[281] As in the case of other chronic lung diseases, such as cystic fibrosis,[282,283] the use of noninvasive ventilatory support will likely play an increasingly important role in allowing patients to be "bridged" to lung transplantation. Whether a HSCT patient is a candidate for lung transplantation may depend upon the time from remission from the primary malignancy and varies from 2 to 5 years. One review of lung transplantation in HSCT patients reported that outcome of HSCT patients after lung transplantation was comparable to other transplant recipient populations.[284]

Approach to Pulmonary Disease in the Immunocompromised Pediatric Host

RADIOGRAPHIC TESTING

In pediatric patients with either oncologic disease or other states of significant immunosuppression, radiographic evaluation including chest radiographs or, in selected cases, CT scans will help define pulmonary abnormalities before proceeding to further treatment such as ablative chemotherapy and HSCT. These preliminary studies will be useful, should post-HSCT pulmonary complications such as pulmonary edema, pulmonary hemorrhage, pneumonia, or BO develop.[133]

The common causes of general radiographic patterns in the immunocompromised patient are shown in Table 64.3, but it must be emphasized that findings on plain chest radiograph are often nonspecific and may underestimate the extent of disease. CT scans may demonstrate other findings such as early cavitation or visceral fungal lesions and, in addition, can better demonstrate pulmonary anatomy, directing other interventions such as bronchoscopy or biopsy.

Common radiographic findings include air-space consolidation, ground-glass opacities, nodules, and air trapping. Nodular opacities are common, ranging from relatively large and discrete lesions, to smaller nodules that appear to run along bronchovascular bundles (tree-in-bud pattern). Consideration of factors such as medication exposures, the duration of patient symptoms, and the underlying patient immune status can help narrow the differential diagnosis and guide treatment or further diagnostic testing.

Noninvasive Diagnostic Studies

PFT can be a useful adjunct to other noninvasive studies when evaluating a patient with acute pulmonary complications. PFTs alone will rarely provide strong evidence of a specific diagnosis, but there are important exceptions to this. The first is the chronic and progressive decrease in diffusing capacity, coupled with a decrease in TLC, which is commonly seen secondary to interstitial disease from radiation pneumonitis. The second is the progressive development of airflow obstruction and air trapping, as is seen with BO. PFTs

Table 64.3 Differential Diagnosis of Radiographic Abnormalities

Airspace consolidation	Hospital/community acquired pneumonia Fungal pneumonia Aspiration pneumonitis/pneumonia Idiopathic pneumonia syndrome Tuberculosis/nontuberculous mycobacteria DAH ARDS Pulmonary edema TRALI
Nodule	Discrete nodule Fungal infection Nocardia infection Metastatic calcification PTLD Malignancy Septic emboli Tree-in-bud Viral pneumonia Bacterial pneumonia BOS
Ground-glass opacities	Pulmonary edema TRALI ARDS DAH Cytomegalovirus *Pneumocystis jirovecii* Common viruses (e.g., influenza, RSV, parainfluenza) Drug toxicity
Mosaic attenuation	Air trapping BOS Viral infection Vascular disease Pulmonary hypertension/porto-pulmonary hypertension Venous thromboembolism

ARDS, Acute respiratory distress syndrome; *BOS*, bronchiolitis obliterans syndrome; *DAH*, diffuse alveolar hemorrhage; *PTLD*, posttransplant lymphoproliferative disease; *RSV*, respiratory syncytial virus; *TRALI*, transfusion-related acute lung injury.

otherwise, however, must be viewed in the context of other factors, including the patient's degree of immunodeficiency, the type of pulmonary symptoms and signs, and the timing of symptoms relative to previous therapy. More important is the utility of following PFTs longitudinally in patients with acquired immunosuppression, as this may alert the clinician to the development of more chronic complications, especially BO. In addition, tests of small airway dysfunction (e.g., multiple breath washout) may be useful for detection of chronic graft versus host disease.[285]

The majority of the data on post-HSCT pulmonary function is from adults, although several pediatric case series have been described.[196,198,250,255,286,287] Pre-HSCT therapy, including chemotherapy and preparative myeloablative therapy, is an important risk factor for pulmonary sequelae. In addition, patient age is important, as the continuing lung development of pediatric patients may mitigate the risk of pulmonary toxicity from chemotherapeutic or myeloablative regimens, lung irradiation, or immunosuppressive medications posttransplantation. Specific agents that may cause pulmonary injury include busulfan, cyclophosphamide, methotrexate, BCNU, and radiation.[288] See Chapter 59 for a further discussion of these agents.

Analysis of sputum produced by cough induced with inhalation of hypertonic saline aerosols has been useful in older immunocompromised children with suspected PCP. Gastric aspirates can be used in the younger child with suspected atypical infections (e.g., tuberculosis). If the child requires endotracheal intubation for respiratory failure, endotracheal aspirates are easy to obtain.

The ability to detect capsular polysaccharide antigens of bacterial pathogens, even after antimicrobials have been administered, is occasionally helpful in hospitalized patients. A number of tests for direct detection of fungal antigens have been described (e.g., the serum galactomannan assay for *Aspergillus*), although its sensitivity and specificity in children may be lower than in adult patients.[81] Direct immunofluorescence can be used to detect *Legionella* sp. with high sensitivity and specificity.[130] Enzyme-linked immunosorbent assays or direct immunofluorescence tests of blood or BAL are now available for the rapid diagnosis of RSV, influenza A virus, parainfluenza viruses, *Chlamydia,* and mycobacterial infections.[289] Viral cultures are generally available, and the shell vial technique for rapid identification of CMV is very useful.

Genetic probes for detecting respiratory viruses, *P. jirovecii, Legionella, Mycobacterium,* and *Mycoplasma pneumoniae,* are now commercially available, and the ability of the PCR to amplify specific regions of genomic DNA or RNA should allow a broader application of these sensitive diagnostic approaches in the immunocompromised patient, particularly when combined with BAL to obtain specimens. Diagnostic tests for the rapid detection of potential respiratory pathogens is an area of expanding importance, and a recent review summarized several technologies, including nucleic acid amplification tests (NAATs).[290]

Invasive Diagnostic Studies

Unfortunately, radiography and other noninvasive diagnostic studies rarely result in a specific diagnosis in the immunocompromised child with pulmonary disease. The clinician is often faced with either continuing empiric antimicrobial therapy or performing a more invasive diagnostic study to make a specific diagnosis. Fortunately, the safety and availability of these studies have improved significantly over the last decade.

FLEXIBLE BRONCHOSCOPY AND BRONCHOALVEOLAR LAVAGE

Flexible bronchoscopy is safe in experienced hands and provides excellent diagnostic material in the immunocompromised child with pneumonia (see Chapter 9 for a detailed discussion).[291–293] Indications for bronchoscopy in children with pneumonia generally include (1) failure of pneumonia or fever to improve with empiric antimicrobial therapy, (2) suspicion of endobronchial obstruction by infection or tumor, (3) recurrent pneumonia in a lobe or segment, and (4) suspicion of unusual organisms. Although the yield of gastric aspiration or BAL is probably superior to bronchoscopy for suspected tuberculosis,[294] bronchoscopy has the added value of allowing evaluation for endobronchial disease or bronchial compression.[295] Simple cytology

brushing obtained through the pediatric bronchoscope can be used for cytological examination and viral cultures, but the yield is usually low. The bronchoscope suction channel may become contaminated by upper airway organisms during the procedure, and simple washings obtained through the bronchoscope channel are generally less useful than quantitative cultures of BAL. Nonetheless, BAL is the most useful bronchoscopic technique in the immunocompromised host, and a variety of infectious and noninfectious diagnoses can be made this way.[296] Further, BAL is generally safe, even in patients with thrombocytopenia.[297]

Although bronchoscopy with BAL may provide useful diagnostic information and is generally well tolerated, its limitations should also be appreciated. In immunocompromised patients who have received empiric broad-spectrum antimicrobial therapy for some period of time, the yield of BAL in isolating a new bacterial pathogen is likely to be low.[298] In oncology patients and other non-AIDS immunocompromised patients, the number of *P. jirovecii* organisms is usually low compared with AIDS patients, and BAL may be falsely negative.[299] In populations receiving prophylaxis for this infection, the yield for PCP will also probably be low. CMV can also be diagnosed rapidly by assays on BAL, but CMV may be a commensal rather than an infecting organism. In addition, patients may have copathogens that are the predominating organism, rather than CMV. *Aspergillus* and other fungi are often difficult to diagnose by bronchoscopy, particularly early in the infection when therapy is most likely to be effective. In pediatric HSCT recipients, fungal infections were the most common infection diagnosed by BAL, but the yield was only 17% in the early conditioning (pre-HSCT) period (where broad-spectrum antimicrobial coverage was common), compared with 82% following transplant.[300]

Transbronchial biopsies can also be taken via the flexible bronchoscope. Though safe in older patients, transbronchial lung biopsies may yield an unacceptable number of false-negative results in immunosuppressed patients and are most useful when organisms such as *P. jirovecii* or granulomatous lesions are probable. The standard pediatric bronchoscopes, 2.8 or 3.6 mm in diameter, have suction/biopsy channels of only 1.2 mm diameter, accommodating biopsy forceps of only 1 mm diameter. The resultant biopsies from such forceps are quite small, leading to the risk of false-negative results in infants. Older children are more likely to tolerate larger bronchoscopes with 2 mm (or larger) channels, allowing for the passage of 1.8-mm forceps and larger biopsy samples. Reported experience with transbronchial biopsies in pediatric patients is limited,[300] but transbronchial biopsy has a significant role in monitoring acute rejection and infections in the pediatric lung transplant patient and in skilled hands can be done with conscious sedation and a transnasal approach in the older child.[301] Transbronchial biopsy for the diagnosis of BO complicating HSCT is not recommended, as it is difficult to obtain adequate specimens using this technique.

TRANSTHORACIC NEEDLE ASPIRATION BIOPSY

Needle aspiration of the lung has been used for the diagnosis of PCP in pediatric cancer patients and for the diagnosis of localized infections in other immunosuppressed patients.

Pneumothorax has been reported as a relatively frequent complication of needle aspirates done for PCP,[302] and this risk must be considered even with more modern "thin"-needle techniques. The use of CT guidance greatly improves the yield and safety of transthoracic needle aspiration biopsy, particularly in the presence of peripheral nodular disease. As a result, it is the procedure of choice for children with peripheral lesions that are difficult to reach with a flexible bronchoscope, as they can safely be sampled, avoiding an open biopsy.[303]

OPEN-LUNG BIOPSY

Open-lung biopsy (OLB) is the gold standard by which other pulmonary diagnostic modalities are judged. Its advantages include the larger amount of lung tissue sampled and the ability to sample different lobes. Using current surgical techniques, OLB is generally a procedure with a low morbidity[304] that can be done rapidly and allows the surgeon to select optimal tissue for culture and microscopic examination. "Mini-thoracotomy" for lingular biopsy may provide sufficient tissue for the diagnosis of diffuse pulmonary processes, significantly reducing the morbidity of the procedure.

Biopsy using video-assisted thoracoscopy (VATS) is now supplanting OLB in many centers, as it can be performed safely in very small infants[305] and does not require chest tube placement following biopsy.[306] Mechanical ventilation is no longer considered a contraindication to VATS.[307] Complications such as respiratory failure, thrombocytopenia, or coagulopathies, and prior antimicrobial/antifungal therapy, increase the risk of VATS as well as OLB and may also reduce the diagnostic yield.

Some studies have questioned how often lung biopsy results will lead to a change in therapy, if one excludes patients with organisms covered by empiric therapy such as *P. jirovecii* and nonspecific histologic findings without specific therapies such as fibrosis or nonspecific lung injury. Published results on OLB and VATS in immunocompromised pediatric patients have indicated yields that range from 36% to 94% for a specific diagnosis and generally support the utility of either procedure.[264,304,308-310]

Although OLB or VATS are considered the procedures most likely to yield definitive diagnostic information in immunosuppressed patients with pulmonary infiltrates, other invasive procedures (e.g., bronchoscopy with BAL as well as CT-guided needle biopsy) may be useful. In addition, choice and timing of procedures in immunocompromised patients requires consideration of the patient's history and response to therapy. If the patient is improving with empiric therapy, any invasive procedure may not be warranted. On the other hand, if a patient is deteriorating despite therapy, then moving expeditiously to a more definitive diagnostic procedure is advised. Early bronchoscopy is relatively safe and may provide a diagnosis without the need for a more invasive procedure. Limitations of bronchoscopy with BAL, however, must be acknowledged. For example, CT-guided needle biopsy has a higher diagnostic yield for isolated peripheral nodular disease. If a more extensive biopsy is deemed necessary, the choice of OLB or VATS will depend on the condition of the patient and the available surgical and anesthetic expertise. In most centers with experienced surgical and anesthetic staff, either procedure is relatively safe, especially when performed before

respiratory failure ensues. Even in this situation, OLB or VATS may be indicated in order to establish a specific diagnosis.

Prevention Strategies

Prevention of infections in immunocompromised patients starts with good hand hygiene and avoidance of exposure to sick contacts (including use of contact precautions, where appropriate).

Antiviral medications (ganciclovir, valganciclovir) may be used to prevent reactivation of CMV. Palivizumab may be used to prevent severe lower respiratory tract infection from RSV in profoundly immunocompromised children less than 2 years of age.[311] Antifungal agents (voriconazole, posaconazole) are often used to prevent infection with *Aspergillus* species. Prophylaxis for *Pneumocystis* in neutropenic patients is usually accomplished with thrice weekly TMP-SMX, pentamidine (inhaled or intravenously), or dapsone. One should consider isoniazid prophylaxis for patients who are immune suppressed in endemic areas of *M. tuberculosis*. This must be balanced, however, with the potential hepatotoxicity of isoniazid; especially in liver transplant recipients.

Ideally, patients should be fully immunized prior to undergoing immunosuppression, as once immunosuppressed they cannot receive live attenuated vaccines. Patients should receive annual inactivated influenza vaccination, although the antibody response may be attenuated[312] with standard dosing. Patients with increased risk for pneumococcal infection (those undergoing splenectomy or stem cell transplant) should receive pneumococcal vaccination at least 2 weeks prior to therapy.[313]

References

Access the reference list online at ExpertConsult.com.

Suggested Reading

Catherinot E, Lanternier F, Bougnoux M-E, et al. *Pneumocystis jirovecii* pneumonia. *Infect Dis Clin North Am.* 2010;24:107–138.

Centers for Disease Control and Prevention, Infectious Disease Society of America, American Society of Blood and Marrow Transplantation. Guidelines for preventing opportunistic infections among hematopoietic stem cell transplant recipients. *MMWR Recomm Rep.* 2000;49(RR–10):1–125 CE1-7.

Frey NV, Tsai DE. The management of posttransplant lymphoproliferative disorder. *Med Oncol.* 2007;24:125–136.

George MP, Masur H, Norris KA, et al. Infections in the immunosuppressed host. *Ann Am Thorac Soc.* 2014;11:S211–S220.

Ginsberg JP, Aplenc R, McDonough J, et al. Pre-transplant lung function is predictive of survival following pediatric bone marrow transplantation. *Pediatr Blood Cancer.* 2010;54:454–460.

Gower WA, Collaco JM, Mogayzel PJ Jr. Lung function and late pulmonary complications among survivors of hematopoietic stem cell transplantation during childhood. *Paediatr Respir Rev.* 2010;11:115–122.

Gower WA, Collaco JM, Mogayzel PJ Jr. Pulmonary dysfunction in pediatric hematopoietic stem cell transplant patients: non-infectious and long-term complications. *Pediatr Blood Cancer.* 2007;49:225–233.

Huang TT, Hudson MM, Stokes DC, et al. Pulmonary outcomes in survivors of childhood cancer: a systematic review. *Chest.* 2011;140(4):881–901.

Kotloff RM, Ahya VN, Crawford SW. Pulmonary complications of solid organ and hematopoietic stem cell transplantation. *Am J Respir Crit Care Med.* 2004;170:22–48.

Kumar D. Emerging viruses in transplantation. *Curr Opin Infect Dis.* 2010;23:374–378.

Kurland G, Michelson P. Bronchiolitis obliterans in children. *Pediatr Pulmonol.* 2005;39:193–208.

Lee B, Michaels MG. Prophylactic antimicrobials in solid organ transplant. *Curr Opin Crit Care*. 2014;20(4):420–425.

Mertens AC, Yasui Y, Liu Y, et al. Pulmonary complications in survivors of childhood and adolescent cancer. A report from the Childhood Cancer Survivor Study. *Cancer*. 2002;95:2431–2441.

Steinbach WJ. Invasive aspergillosis in pediatric patients. *Curr Med Res Opin*. 2010;26:1779–1787.

Wistinghausen B, Gross TG, Bollard C. Post-transplant lymphoproliferative disease in pediatric solid organ transplant recipients. *Pediatr Hematol Oncol*. 2013;30(6):520–531.

Yen KT, Lee AS, Krowka MJ, et al. Pulmonary complications in bone marrow transplantation: a practical approach to diagnosis and treatment. *Clin Chest Med*. 2004;25:189–201.

Yoshihara S, Yanik G, Cooke KR, et al. Bronchiolitis obliterans syndrome (BOS), bronchiolitis obliterans organizing pneumonia (BOOP), and other late-onset noninfectious pulmonary complications following allogeneic hematopoietic stem cell transplantation. *Biol Blood Marrow Transplant*. 2007;13:749–759.

65 Hypersensitivity Pneumonitis and Eosinophilic Lung Diseases

ALAN PAUL KNUTSEN, MD, JAMES TEMPRANO, MD, DEEPIKA BHATLA, MD, and RAYMOND G. SLAVIN, MD

Hypersensitivity Pneumonitis

EPIDEMIOLOGY

Hypersensitivity pneumonitis (HP), also known as extrinsic allergic alveolitis, is an immune mediated lung disease occurring in response to repeated inhalation of an antigen.[1-6] It appears to be an underdiagnosed condition, often masquerading as a recurrent pneumonia, idiopathic pulmonary fibrosis, Hamman-Rich disease, or interstitial pneumonia. Extrinsic allergic alveolitis seems particularly appropriate as terminology, because it describes the disease in graphic terms: "extrinsic," meaning it comes from an outside source; "allergic," denoting a hypersensitivity basis; and "alveolitis," referring to that part of the lung most affected by the disease. Whatever term is used, HP is a hypersensitivity reaction of the lung in response to inhalation of an antigen—most often an organic dust. The prevalence and incidence of HP is difficult to estimate. Among individuals exposed to a known antigen(s), the prevalence of pigeon breeder's disease HP is 6%–20% and the prevalence of farmer's lung is 0.5%–19% among farmers.[1,2] The incidence rate of HP at a Danish referral center was 2 cases per year over a 12-year period during a national cohort study on interstitial lung disease.[7]

ETIOLOGY

There are more than 200 antigens known to cause HP (Table 65.1). The etiology of HP differs between adults and children and is due to differences in exposure. The majority of adult cases of HP are due to various occupational exposures. In children, most cases are due to household exposures, with avian antigens being the most common etiology, followed by molds.[6,8] There are multiple categories of antigenic sources, including fungal, bacterial and amoebal proteins, animal proteins, and chemicals and medications (see Table 65.1). In addition, there are a number of factors that determine how one will respond to inhalation of an organic dust. First, what is the basic immunologic reactivity of the host? An atopic individual will characteristically respond with production of IgE antibody. A nonatopic person will more likely produce IgG. Second, what is the nature and source of the antigen? Is it small enough to reach the distal part of the lung? Is it temperature-required such that it will grow in the respiratory tract, such as Aspergillus? Finally, consider the nature and circumstances of the exposure: Is it intense and intermittent or is it low-grade and chronic? An intermittent short-term intensive exposure such as that experienced by a pigeon breeder while cleaning out the coops will manifest acute reversible disease. A pet-store employee who has intermittent, lower grade but long-term exposure will develop a subacute form that is usually reversible. Finally, a long-term low-grade exposure experienced by a parakeet owner may result in chronic irreversible disease.[3]

The first example of HP described was farmer's lung due to a thermophilic organism. These are unicellular branching organisms that resemble true bacteria. A previously common occupational form of HP was bagassosis or Louisiana sugarcane workers' disease.[4] Mold can also be a cause of HP, with two examples being maple bark strippers disease, developing in loggers who strip the bark and are exposed to *Cryptostroma corticale* underneath the bark and malt workers lung, developing in brewery workers exposed to *Aspergillus clavatus* present in the moldy barley on brewery floors.[4] Probably the most common cause of HP today is avian antigen. Birds are becoming an increasingly popular pet and serve as a potent source of antigens responsible for HP.[5] Finally, an example of a chemical source is toluene diisocyanate, which may cause disease in bathtub refinishers.[6]

Bird Fancier's Lung

Avian antigens are the most commonly reported cause of HP in children.[9,10] Proteins derived from the bloom, serum, or excrement of several avian species have been demonstrated to cause HP. Bloom, a dust coating the feathers composed of keratin covered with IgA, is produced in large quantities by flying birds. While pigeons are the principal source of avian antigen in HP, several other birds have been implicated, such as parakeets, parrots, doves, and cockatiels.[11-17] Although bird fancier's lung is the commonest form of HP seen in children, it is still a rare disease.[10] Most pediatric reports note that children were initially treated for pulmonary infections or had multiple health care encounters before a diagnosis was made.[10,17-19] The diagnosis should be considered in any child with persistent, unexplained respiratory symptoms. The mainstay of therapy is bird avoidance, and therapy with corticosteroids is frequently required. Importantly, bird antigens have been found to persist at high levels as long as 18 months after bird elimination from the home.[20,21] As is the case with other forms of HP, patients with acute forms of the disease have the best prognosis, while those with chronic disease have higher morbidity.[22]

Table 65.1   Common Etiologic Antigens and Sources in Hypersensitivity Pneumonitis

Disease	Source	Antigen
BACTERIA		
Farmer's lung	Moldy hay, moldy plant materials	*Faeni rectivirgula*
		Saccharopolyspora rectivirgula,
		Thermoactinomyces vulgaris
		Thermoactinomyces actinomycetes
		Thermoactinomyces sacchari
		Aspergillus spp
Bagassosis	Moldy sugar cane	*Thermoactinomyces sacchari*
		Thermoactinomyces vulgaris
Ventilation pneumonitis	Contaminated air conditioners	*Thermoactinomyces candidus*
		Thermoactinomyces actinomycetes
		Thermoactinomyces sacchari
		Naegleria gruberi
		Acanthamoeba polyphagia
		Acanthamoeba castellano
Humidifier lung	Ultrasonic cool mist humidifiers	*Bacillus subtilis*
		Klebsiella oxytoca
Mushroom worker's lung	Moldy compost and mushrooms	*Thermoactinomyces sacchari*
Machine operator's lung	Contaminated/aerosolized metal working fluid	Nontuberculous mycobacteria
		Aspergillus fumigatus
		Mycobacterium immunogenum
Floor finisher's lung	Moldy wood	*Cephalosporium acremonium*
Hot tub lung	Hot tub mists, tub water, mold on ceiling	*Mycobacterium avium* complex
Swimming pool lung	Mist from pool water, sprays, fountains	*Mycobacterium avium* complex
FUNGI		
Enoki mushroom worker's lung (Japan)	Moldy mushroom compost	*Penicillium citrinum*
Composter's lung	Compost	*Aspergillus* spp
		Thermoactinomyces vulgaris
Peat moss HP	Contaminated peat moss	*Monocillium* spp
		Penicillium citreonigum
Suberosis	Moldy cork	*Thermoactinomyces viridis*
		Aspergillus fumigatus
		Penicillium spp
Malt worker's lung disease	Moldy or contaminated barley	*Aspergillus clavatus*
		Aspergillus fumigatus
Sequoiosis	Mold redwood dust	*Aureobasidium pullulans*
		Pullularia spp
		Graphium spp
		Trichoderma spp
Maple bark stripper's lung	Contaminated maple logs	*Cryptostroma corticale*
Winemaker's lung	Mold on grapes	*Botrytis cinerea*
Tobacco grower's lung	Mold on tobacco, tobacco plants	*Aspergillus* spp
Woodman's disease	Mold on oak and maple trees	*Penicillium* spp
Potato riddler's lung	Moldy hay around potatoes	*Thermoactinomyces actinomycetes*
		Faeni rectivirgula
		Thermoactinomyces vulgaris
		Aspergillus spp
Cheese washer's lung	Moldy cheese casing	*Penicillium casei*
		Aspergillus clavatus
Thatched roof lung	Dead/dried grasses and leaves	*Saccharomonospora viridis*
		Thermoactinomyces vulgaris
		Aspergillus spp
Wood worker's lung	Contaminated wood pulp or dust	*Alternaria* spp
		Wood dust
Hardwood worker's lung	Kiln-dried wood	*Paecilomyces*
Wood trimmer's lung	Contaminated wood trimmings	*Rhizous* spp
		Mucor spp
Dry rot lung	Rotten wood	*Merulius lacrimans*
Familial HP	Contaminated wood dust in walls	*Bacillus subtilis*
Paprika slicer's lung	Moldy paprika	*Mucor stolonifer*
Stipatosis	Esparto dust	*Thermoactinomyces actinomycetes*
		Aspergillus fumigatus
		Pseudomonas spp
Basement shower HP	Mold or unventilated shower	*Epicoccum nigrum*
Basement lung	Contaminated basement	*Cephalosporium* spp
		Penicillium spp
Wind instrument lung	Contaminated saxophones, trombones	Mold
		Bacteria
Steam iron HP	Contaminated water reservoir	*Sphingobacterium spiritivorum*
Summer-type HP	Japanese house dust	*Trichosporon cutaneum*
Lycoperdonosis	Lycoperdon puffballs	Puffball spores
Chiropodist's lung	Foot skin and nail dust	Fungi

Continued

Table 65.1   Common Etiologic Antigens and Sources in Hypersensitivity Pneumonitis—cont'd

Disease	Source	Antigen
ANIMAL PROTEINS		
Pigeon-breeder's disease	Pigeons, parakeets, parrots, doves, cockatiels	Avian proteins from bird excreta, feathers or bloom
Bird fancier's lung		
Feather duvet lung	Feather beds, pillows, duvets	*Avian proteins*
Laboratory worker's lung	Rat or gerbil urine	Rodent urinary, serum, pelt protein
Animal handler's lung		
Furrier's lung	Animal pelts	*Animal fur dust*
Miller's lung	Infested wheat flour	*Sitophilus granaries*
Wheat weevil disease		
Pearl oyster shellfish HP	Oyster/mollusk shell protein	Pearl oyster proteins. shell dust
Mollusk shellfish HP	Sea snail shell dust	Sea snail shell proteins
Silk producer HP	Dust from silkworm larvae and cocoons	Silkworm proteins
Pituitary snuff taker's lung	Bovine and porcine pituitary powder	Pituitary proteins, snuff
Fish meal worker's lung	Fish meal dust	Fish meal
Bat lung	Bat droppings	Bat serum proteins
CHEMICAL AND DRUGS		
Chemical worker's lung	Polyurethane foams, paints, elastomers, glues	Diisocyanates
		Isocyanate
		Trimellitic anhydride
Epoxy resin lung	Heated epoxy resin	Phthalic anhydride
Dental technician's lung	Polishing and grinding prostheses	Methyl methacrylate
Paint refinisher's disease,	Varnishes, lacquer, foundry casting, polyurethane foam	Toluene diisocyanate
Bathtub refinisher's lung		
Pauli's reagent alveolitis	Laboratory reagent	Sodium diazobenzene sulfate
Pyrethrum lung	Insecticide	Pyrethrum
Bible printer's lung	Moldy typesetting water	Unknown
Coptic lung	Cloth wrapping of mummies	Unknown
Grain measurer's lung	Cereal grain	Unknown
Coffee worker's lung	Coffee bean dust	Unknown
Drug Induced HP	Medications	Amiodarone
		Closporine
		Gold
		Minocycline
		Chlorambucil
		Sulfasalazine
		Nitrofurantoin
		Methotrexate
		Beta blockers
		Mesalamine

HP, Hypersensitivity pneumonitis.

Modified from Selman M, and Buendía-Roldán I. Immunopathology, diagnosis, and management of hypersensitivity pneumonitis. *Semin Respir Crit Care Med.* 2012;33(5):543-554 and Costabel U, Bonella F, Guzman J. Chronic hypersensitivity pneumonitis. *Clin Chest Med.* 2012; 33(1):151-163.

Other Environmental Exposures

HP may also result from exposure to various fungal or bacterial antigens. *Thermophilic actinomycetes, Neurospora,* and *Candida albicans* have been reported as causes of HP in patients that used covered swimming pools.[23,24] Residential mold contamination with *Aureobasidium pullulans* has been reported to cause HP in an adult and in child siblings.[25–28] This same species has been implicated as the etiologic agent causing HP in a child exposed to indoor hydroponics.[27] Household exposure to a fungus, *Trichosporon cutaneum,* causes summer-type HP, a common form of HP in Japan.[29] Contamination of the home with the fungus *Bjerkandera adusta* was found to cause HP in an elderly male.[29] A report of two children with HP secondary to exposure from an unventilated basement shower identified *Epicoccum nigrum* as the causative mold.[30] *Fusarium napiforme* was also found to be the etiologic agent in a 17-year-old with HP due to residential mold exposure.[31] Exposure to mold or various bacteria through ultrasonic humidifiers and saunas has also been demonstrated

to cause HP.[32–34] *Aspergillus fumigatus* was found to be the causative agent in a child with HP who had repeated exposure to organic compost on a playground.[35] There are also numerous reports of "hot tub lung," caused by *Mycobacterium avium* complex, a nontuberculous mycobacteria.[36–41] This disease typically occurs after exposure to hot water aerosols from hot tubs, showers, and swimming pools.[39] Most reports note that poor hot tub maintenance or poor personal hygiene practices contribute to the development of the disease. Some controversy does exist on whether this disease is a true representation of HP or has an infectious etiology. Patients with hot tub lung have well-formed, sometimes necrotic, granulomas, obstructive lung disease, and usually lack serum precipitating antibodies to the offending antigen, all supporting an infectious nature of the illness.[38,39] However, the clinical presentation, bronchoalveolar lavage (BAL) lymphocytosis, high-resolution computed tomography (HRCT) findings, and therapeutic response to cessation of exposure and treatment with corticosteroids are consistent with HP.[37–41] *Cladosporium* has also been implicated as a cause of HP in

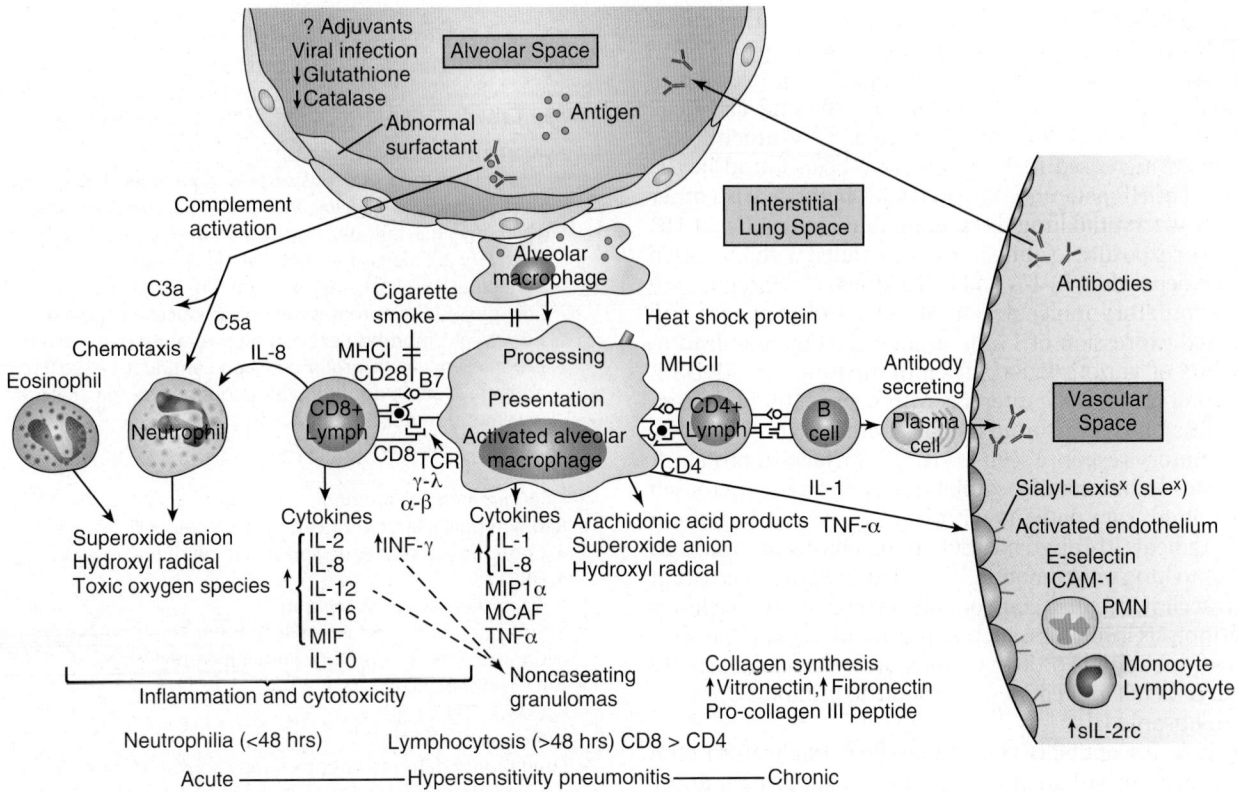

Fig. 65.1 Pathogenesis of hypersensitivity pneumonitis. Small molecular weight antigen that enters the alveoli is engulfed by alveolar macrophages, which become activated and interact with both CD4+ and CD8+ T cells. Other cell types are attracted through chemokines and release a variety of inflammatory mediators typical of T helper cell type 1 (Th1) profile. Many factors, including adjuvants, environmental influences, surfactant composition, and balance of cytokines, influence the inflammatory responses. This response eventually leads to a lymphocytic infiltration and granuloma formation of the interstitial lung spaces and alveoli. (Used with permission from Dr. Jordan Fink and Elsevier Publishing.)

an enclosed hot tub area.[42] Finally, "lifeguard lung," a granulomatous pneumonitis from indoor swimming pool exposure, was reported in several lifeguards exposed to water spray features at an indoor pool.[43]

PATHOLOGY/PATHOGENESIS

The pathogenesis of HP is incompletely understood. The initial event involves sensitization to an inhaled antigen in the distal airway, but the level and duration of antigen exposure that is required for sensitization is unknown (Fig. 65.1). After antigen exposure in a sensitized individual, an acute alveolitis develops with an increase in neutrophils.[44–50] This typically peaks at 48 hours and is followed by an increase in the number of macrophages and lymphocytes.[50–54] Typically CD8+ T cells predominate, but CD4+ T cells can also be found distinguishing HP from sarcoidosis.[52] In 2009, Ye et al.[53] identified interleukin (IL) 12, IL-18, and tumor necrosis factor alpha (TNF-α) synthesis by BAL macrophages from patients with acute and chronic HP. Spontaneous and lipopolysaccharide stimulated BAL cell culture revealed higher IL-12, IL-18, and TNF-α secretion compared with controls, indicating a TH1-macrophage axis pathogenesis. Another study by Bellanger et al.[54] revealed significantly higher IL-8, IL-6, TNFα, IL-17, and IL-23 levels in BAL fluid samples from HP patients compared with patients with other forms of interstitial lung disease.

Type III and Type IV Hypersensitivity Responses

It appears that both type III antigen-antibody complex and type IV cell-mediated responses are involved (see Fig. 65.1). Antigen-specific precipitating antibodies are found in patients with HP in response to the offending antigen supporting a type III reaction[55]; however, precipitating antibodies can also be found in exposed subjects without evidence of clinical disease.[56] In addition, there is no immune complex deposition in the lungs. Inhaled soluble antigens can bind to immunoglobulin and cause complement activation, leading to increased vascular permeability and an influx of neutrophils and macrophages.[57,58] This leads to the production of IL-1, IL-8, TNF-α, monocyte chemoattractant protein (MCP)-1, macrophage inflammatory protein (MIP)-1α, RANTES (regulated on activation, normal T cell expressed and secreted), and CCL18, with resultant migration of leukocytes into the alveolar interstitium.[59,60] Several studies illustrate the role of T cell mediated immunity in the pathogenesis of HP.[57–61] A variety of factors, such as MIP-1α, MCP-1, CCL18, and IL-2, lead to an influx and proliferation of lymphocytes in the lung of patients with HP.[62–65] Secretion of IL-12 and MIP-1α by alveolar macrophages promotes the polarization of CD4+ Th0 lymphocytes to Th1 cells (T helper type 1), which produce interferon (IFN)-γ and are essential for granulomatous inflammation and the development of HP.[66,67]

Several other factors may play a role in the pathogenesis of HP. Natural killer (NK) cells are increased in the BAL and lung tissue of patients with HP and appear to provide a protective effect.[61,62] Aberrant regulatory T cell and Th17 cell function may also play a pathologic role.[63-68] As mentioned previously, increased IL-17 levels have been found in the BAL fluid of HP patients compared with patients with other forms of interstitial lung disease. In a murine model of HP, long-term exposure to antigen was associated with increased collagen deposition, IL-17, and IL-1α levels.[54,69] Upregulation of costimulatory molecules on alveolar macrophages and increased expression of L-, E-, and P-selectins may lead to the influx of various leukocytes into the lung.[70-74] MyD88, an adapter protein that interacts with several Toll-like receptors (TLRs), has been found to play an important role in the inflammatory response seen in HP.[74,75] Surfactant protein A stimulates inflammatory cytokine release and is increased in BAL fluid from patients with HP.[76] Increased formation of free radicals, through a variety of mechanisms, also contributes to lung inflammation.[55,77-79] Excessive accumulation of extracellular matrix components through increased levels of fibrinolysis inhibitors, such as thrombin-activatable fibrinolysis inhibitor and protein C inhibitor, or decreased activity of matrix metalloproteinases, contribute to the fibrotic process seen in chronic HP.[80,81]

Multiple susceptibility factors have been implicated in the pathogenesis of HP, such as cigarette smoking, viral infections, endotoxin, and genetic predisposition. Several studies have observed a negative relationship between cigarette smoking and the development of HP in similarly exposed individuals.[82-88] Many patients with HP report a viral type illness or flulike symptoms during the initial stage of disease. An acute viral infection could enhance the antigenic response in HP by increasing the ability of alveolar macrophages to present antigen, decreasing the clearance of antigens and inducing the release of proinflammatory cytokines.[88] Endotoxin coexposure with antigen has been shown to augment lung pathology in a murine model of HP, and may act through TLRs on macrophages, leading to a Th1 T cell response, or play an indirect role in the pathogenesis of HP as an adjuvant.[62,89] Finally, various HLA haplotypes and genetic polymorphisms, such as those of the *TNFA* promoter and *IL6* gene, encoding TNF-α and IL-6, respectively, have been associated with susceptibility to HP.[90-100] Familial cases of HP have also been reported.[25,101]

CLINICAL FEATURES

Symptoms and Physical Findings

Schuyler and Cormier[56] proposed criteria for the diagnosis of HP (Box 65.1). Major criteria included symptoms compatible with HP, evidence of antigen exposure, radiographic abnormalities consistent with HP, lymphocytosis on bronchoalveolar lavage fluid (BALF), lung biopsy demonstrating histologic changes consistent with HP, and reproduction of symptoms of HP upon antigen exposure. Minor criteria included bibasilar rales, decreased diffusion capacity for carbon monoxide (DLCO), and hypoxemia. The clinical manifestations of HP depend on the nature and circumstances of exposure and are divided into three stages: acute, subacute, and chronic.

Box 65.1 Diagnostic Criteria for Hypersensitivity Pneumonitis

Major Criteria (Four Major Criteria Need to Be Present)

- Symptoms compatible with HP
  - Acute: High level of exposure to antigen over short period of time. Symptoms develop within 4–8 h and include fever, chills, myalgia, fatigue, dyspnea, nonproductive cough. Recovery 2–5 days after removal of exposure.
  - Subacute: Low-level, intermittent, repeated exposure. Low-grade fever, progressive nonproductive cough, dyspnea over weeks-months. Recovery after removal of exposure.
  - Chronic: Low-level, prolonged, and continuous exposure of antigen. Chronic nonproductive cough, dyspnea, malaise, weakness, anorexia, weight loss.
- Evidence of exposure to antigen
  - History
  - IgG antibody to antigen
- Radiographic characteristics consistent with HP
  - Chest radiograph: Reticulonodular infiltrates, linear opacities
  - HRCT:
  - Acute: Ground-glass infiltrates
  - Subacute: Micronodules, air-trapping
  - Chronic: Fibrosis ± honeycombing, emphysema
- BALF lymphocytosis
  - CD8 > CD4 T cells
  - Increased NK cells
- Lung biopsy demonstrates histology consistent with HP
  - Alveolitis, noncaseating granulomas, giant cells, foamy alveolar macrophages or fibrosis
- Positive natural challenge that produces symptoms and objective abnormalities after reexposure to the offending antigen

Minor Criteria (Two Minor Criteria Need to Be Present)

- Bibasilar rales
- Decreased DLCO
- Hypoxemia, either at rest or with exertion

Clinical Prediction

- Exposure to known offending antigen
- Positive IgG antibody to offending antigen
- Recurrent episodes of symptoms
- Respiratory crackles
- Symptoms occurring between 4 and 8 h after exposure
- Weight loss

DLCO, Diffusing capacity carbon monoxide; *HP,* hypersensitivity pneumonitis; *HRCT,* high-resolution computed tomography.
Modified from Schuyler M, Cormier Y. The diagnosis of hypersensitivity pneumonitis. Chest. *1997;111(3):534-536.*

Acute Stage

In the acute form such as seen in pigeon breeders, chills, fever up to 40°C, cough, and shortness of breath are seen within 4–6 hours after exposure. Symptoms may persist for up to 18 hours. Patients usually recover within 2–5 days, with episodes occurring after each subsequent exposure. Physical examination reveals only crackling rales in the lower lung fields. HP is an example of an interstitial pneumonia in which there is a disparity between the symptoms of the patient and the physical findings. Wheezing is uncommon, as most patients exposed to organic dusts do not develop HP and asthma.

Subacute Stage

This form occurs as a result of an intermittent low grade but continuous long-term exposure, such as seen in a pet-store employee. The symptoms are milder and include malaise, low-grade fever, cough, chills, and progressive dyspnea, often associated with anorexia and weight loss. This form is usually reversible.[102]

Chronic Stage

A long-term low-grade exposure experienced by a parakeet owner or a contaminated home humidifier may result in chronic irreversible disease. These patients present with dyspnea, chronic cough, fatigue, anorexia, and weight loss.[103]

Immunologic Studies

Laboratory evaluation generally reveals a marked leukocytosis with prominent neutrophilia during the acute phase of HP.[104] Elevation of markers of inflammation such as erythrocyte sedimentation rate and C-reactive protein may be seen. Elevated rheumatoid factor is found in 50% of patients, along with elevation in serum IgG, IgA, and IgM. Skin testing has limited value in the workup of HP. A high percentage of patients without HP have positive skin tests reactions, and there is a lack of commercially available standardized extracts. A diagnostic hallmark of HP is an IgG precipitating antibody seen on a double gel diffusion plate (Fig. 65.2). However, the presence of a precipitating antibody is only a marker of exposure and sensitization and does not correlate with disease activity. Approximately 40%–50% of asymptomatic exposed individuals will have precipitating antibody to the offending antigen.[105] Reports from commercial laboratories are sometimes inaccurate, and the selection of a laboratory experienced in assays for the diagnosis of HP is important. Methods more sensitive than gel diffusion are available, including counterimmunoelectrophoresis (CIE), enzyme-linked immunosorbent assays (ELISA), and radioimmunoassay (RIA). Lymphocyte proliferation assays to the offending antigen are usually positive in patients with HP.[106] In one study, alveolar macrophages from patients with HP enhanced the lymphoproliferative response, while the response was inhibited in normal patients. This suggests that a defect in the ability of alveolar macrophages to suppress the lymphoproliferative response leads to the development of the observed lymphocytic alveolitis seen in patients with HP.[106] It should be emphasized that these studies are available only in research laboratories.

Radiologic Findings

Radiologic findings in HP correlate with stage of disease. In acute HP, chest radiography usually demonstrates poorly defined, nodular infiltrates, but patchy ground-glass opacities or diffuse infiltrates may also occur.[62,104,107,108] It is important to note that patients with acute HP may have a normal chest radiograph after cessation of exposure and resolution of the acute episode. HRCT of the chest typically demonstrates ground-glass opacities in acute HP, but the presence of ground-glass opacities is generally a nonspecific finding.[109–111] Ground-glass opacification represents cellular interstitial infiltration, small granulomas within the alveolar septa, or both. These opacities may be found either centrally or peripherally, but are predominantly in the lower lung zones with sparing of the apices in acute HP.[1–3,9,59] In subacute HP, a reticulonodular appearance with fine linear shadows and small nodules is typically present on chest radiograph, although the chest radiograph may also be normal as seen in acute HP.[1–3,9,59] The infiltrates in subacute HP usually predominate in the mid to upper lung zones. HRCT of the chest in subacute HP typically demonstrates centrilobular nodules associated with larger areas of ground-glass opacity, as well as air trapping and mosaic perfusion (Fig. 65.3).[110] Centrilobular nodules correspond to the presence of poorly marginated granulomas and active alveolitis, while mosaic perfusion indicates the redistribution of blood flow, and air trapping denotes obstructive bronchiolitis. The presence of ground-glass opacities, air trapping, mosaic perfusion, and areas of normal lung attenuation on the same film yields

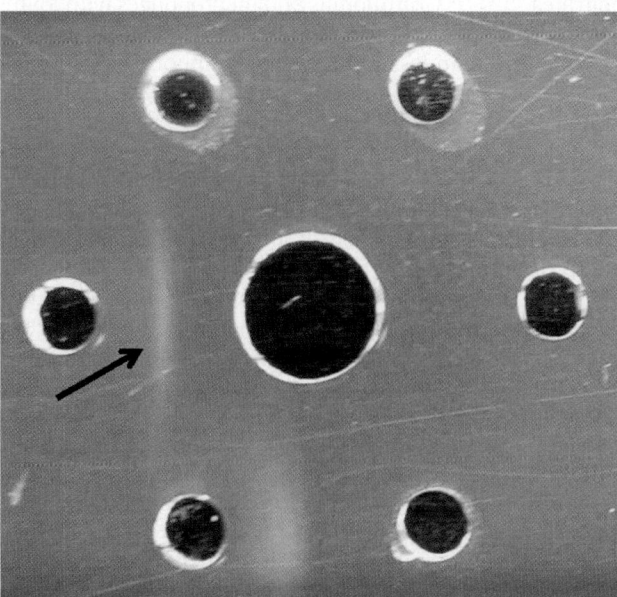

Fig. 65.2 Ouchterlony double immunodiffusion (agar gel immunodiffusion). The center well contains patient serum and the outer wells contain different antigens. Note the strong line of precipitation between the patient's serum and the antigen (arrow).

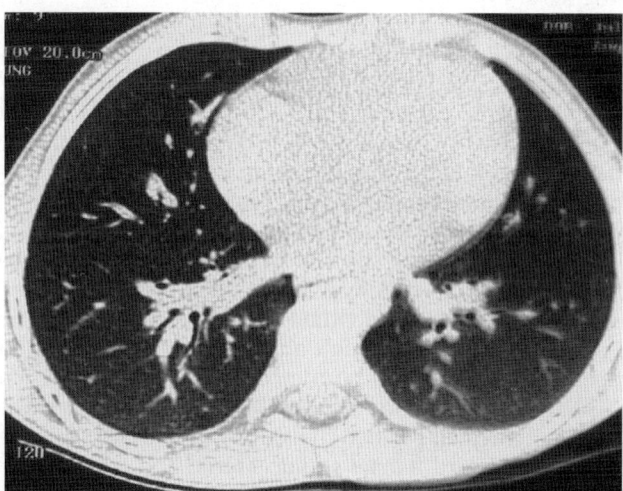

Fig. 65.3 High-resolution computed tomography scan of the chest in a child with hypersensitivity pneumonitis demonstrating ground glass opacities.

an appearance on HRCT known as the headcheese sign.[110] This is characteristic for subacute HP. Chronic HP is characterized by diffuse reticulonodular infiltrates, volume loss, and coarse linear opacities on chest radiography.[1-3,9,110,111] The findings in chronic HP appear to be more severe in the mid to upper zones of the lung. HRCT often demonstrates fibrotic changes that include irregular linear opacities, honeycombing, and traction bronchiectasis. These changes can also be found in several other disorders, such as sarcoidosis, interstitial pulmonary fibrosis, and collagen vascular diseases. Centrilobular nodules are often found in chronic HP when ongoing antigen exposure is occurring. The radiographic findings in chronic HP, unlike acute HP, are unlikely to resolve when antigen exposure ceases. There are several findings that are not characteristically found and may be helpful in differentiating HP from other disorders. Pleural effusions or pleural thickening, as well as cavitation, calcification, or atelectasis, are usually absent in HP. Hilar adenopathy, commonly seen in sarcoidosis, is rarely seen in HP.[104]

Pulmonary Function Testing and Bronchial Challenge

Pulmonary function testing typically reveals restriction with a reduction in lung volumes and a decrease in DLCO; however, obstructive, mixed obstructive and restrictive, or normal pulmonary function tests can be seen.[1-3,9,59,104,108,109] A decrease in airway compliance is often seen with a shift in the pressure-volume curve down and to the right. A decrease in arterial oxygen tension (PaO$_2$) on arterial blood gas analysis is most commonly seen in chronic HP, but can be found in both acute and subacute forms of the disease.[55] The hypoxemia and decreased diffusion capacity may be accounted for by filling of the alveolar space with fluid and inflammatory cells. In a cross-sectional longitudinal study of children diagnosed with HP, the forced expiratory volume 1 second (FEV1) was abnormal in only 9.1% of patients, but DLCO and total lung capacity (TLC) were abnormal in 40.9% and 13.6%, respectively. DLCO/alveolar volume (VA) was within the normal range, and peak oxygen uptake was normal in nearly 90% of subjects, suggesting a favorable long-term prognosis.[112]

Oxygen desaturation with exercise or with sleep is not an uncommon finding.[1-3] Twenty percent to 40% display nonspecific airway reactivity, and 5%–10% have asthma.[25,108,113,114] In addition, in patients with farmer's lung, Karjalainen et al.[115] showed an increased risk in developing asthma after their diagnosis of HP. The concomitant or future development of asthma after HP has also been shown in HP caused by diisocyanates, after summer-type HP or after residential mold exposure.[25,29,115-118] Bronchial challenge has been studied in adults but is infrequently used in children.[9,119] These challenges can be performed either through reexposure to the suspected setting or through a controlled challenge in an experienced laboratory. In a review by Fan,[9] 20 of 86 children with HP underwent bronchial challenge, and only 55% of these patients had positive challenges. In a large cohort of patients with bird fancier's lung, Morell and colleagues[55] reported a sensitivity of 92% and specificity of 100% using bronchial challenge to avian extracts. As the authors note in their study, bronchial challenge testing should be performed in a hospital setting with experienced staff and high-quality antigenic extracts.[55] Some difficulties that may be encountered in bronchial provocation are poor standardization of the antigen dose used for the challenge, difficulties in objectively defining a positive test, as well as the difficulty that many young children have in performing routine pulmonary function testing.[119]

Bronchoalveolar Lavage and Lung Biopsy

The BAL from normal individuals typically reveals a preponderance of alveolar macrophages, with approximately 10% lymphocytes that have a CD4+/CD8+ ratio of 1.8.[1-3,119] Following acute antigen exposure, patients with HP reveal a predominance of neutrophils, which is then followed by a lymphocytic alveolitis and usually comprises 60% or greater of the white blood cell differential in BAL.[1-3,44,46,49,58,103,120] Historically, a low CD4+/CD8+ ratio has been associated with HP, while a CD4+/CD8+ ratio of more than 3.5 : 1 has been associated with sarcoidosis.[58,62,103,120-123] More recent studies, however, have disputed this finding with the demonstration of HP cases with higher CD4+/CD8+ ratios.[58,100,123] A study by Ando and colleagues[124] also suggested that the CD4+/CD8+ ratio may differ by the causative antigen and the smoking status of the patient. The BAL findings in HP may also differ based on the age of the patient. Ratjen et al.[62] evaluated BAL findings in children with HP. Nine subjects, aged 6–15 years, with acute HP were included in this study. The BAL uniformly revealed an increase in the percentage of lymphocytes and foamy macrophages in children with HP. All patients were found to either have an increased expression of human leukocyte antigen (HLA)-DR (7 of 8 children) on BAL lymphocytes or an increase in NK cells (5 of 8 children) in BAL fluid. Importantly, there were no significant differences between normal controls and patients with HP with respect to the CD4+/CD8+ T cell ratio. Histologic findings in HP vary based on the stage of disease.[57,59,125,126] There are few reports on the pathology associated with acute HP, but most note the presence of interstitial mononuclear cell infiltrates.[57,125,126] Granulomas and macrophages with foamy cytoplasm have also been reported.[126] The classic triad of subacute HP includes an interstitial lymphocytic-histiocytic cell infiltrate, bronchiolitis obliterans, and scattered, poorly formed, nonnecrotizing granulomas.[55,57] In a large series of patients with bird fancier's lung, this triad was only seen in 9% of cases that underwent transbronchial lung biopsy, but at least one of the findings was present in 69% of cases.[55] An example of a lung biopsy of an 11-year-old boy with HP due to pigeon sensitivity is shown in Fig. 65.4. There was interstitial pneumonia with inflammation composed of predominantly lymphocytes, macrophages, and plasma cells. Macrophages with foamy cytoplasm surrounded by large numbers of mononuclear cells are unique to HP. Lymphocytes stained for CD3+ T cells and CD56+ NK cells. Typically there is a predominance of CD8+ T cells. CD20+ B cells were also in the center of a lymphoid follicle. Other findings commonly seen in HP include interstitial giant cells, interstitial noncaseating granulomas, or Schaumann bodies.[127] In a pathologic review of 25 cases with chronic HP, giant cells, granulomas, or Schaumann bodies were seen in 88% of cases, and 72% of cases exhibited a usual interstitial pneumonia (UIP)–like pattern.[127] A nonspecific interstitial pneumonia (NSIP)–like pattern or a bronchiolitis obliterans organizing pneumonia-like disease can also be seen in chronic HP.[128-130] Multiple

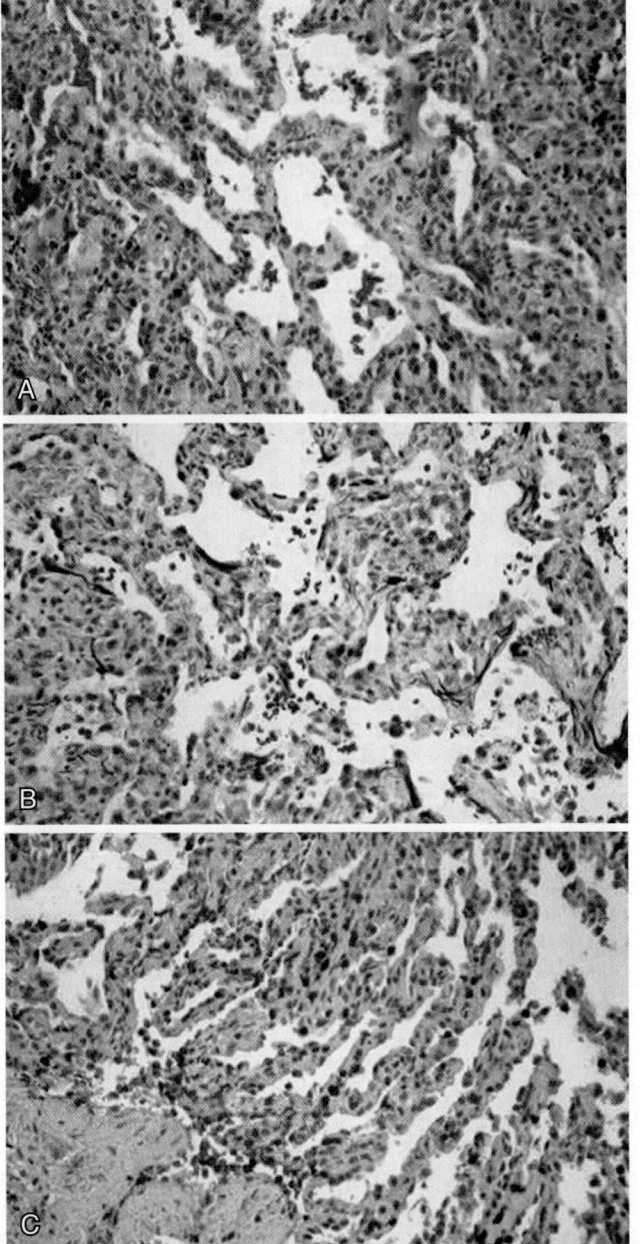

Fig. 65.4 Transbronchial lung biopsy of an 11-year-old boy at the onset of his illness with hypersensitivity pneumonitis due to sensitivity to pigeon droppings. (A) H&E staining, demonstrates alveolar and interstitial inflammation composed predominantly of lymphocytes, macrophages, and plasma. Macrophages with foamy cytoplasm surrounded by large numbers of mononuclear cells are unique to hypersensitivity pneumonitis. (B) Anti-CD3 immunoperoxide staining, demonstrates the presence of numerous CD3+ T cells in the interstitium. (C) Anti-CD56 immunoperoxide staining, demonstrates the presence of numerous NK cells in the interstitium.

studies have demonstrated decreased survival rates in patients with UIP-like or NSIP-like patterns of fibrosis.[127,131,132] The usefulness of biopsy for the diagnosis of HP has been questioned.[59,132,133] Although the aforementioned findings are commonly seen in various stages of HP, none of the findings are pathognomonic for the disease, as they can be found in other lung disorders. Most patients with HP can be diagnosed based on signs, symptoms, exposure history, radiographic,

laboratory, and BAL findings, obviating the need for lung biopsy. When a biopsy is performed, a surgical lung biopsy is the preferred method, as it has greater diagnostic yield.[59] A study in patients with farmer's lung found limited usefulness of transbronchial biopsies as a diagnostic tool in HP.[134] Since the utility of transbronchial biopsies in HP is questioned and the majority of cases can be diagnosed without biopsy, surgical lung biopsy is usually reserved for cases when other studies do not yield a definitive diagnosis.

MANAGEMENT AND TREATMENT

In the acute form, simple removal from the offending environment generally suffices. If symptoms are severe, the patient should be started on a tapering dose of prednisone, beginning with 60 mg per day. Supportive measures would include oxygen (O_2), antitussives, and antipyretics. For repeated, acute, or subacute form, exposures should be decreased as much as possible, with administration of long-term corticosteroids emphasizing alternate day therapy. The chronic form can be treated with long-term corticosteroids, but only if radiographic findings and physiologic changes indicate a response. Clinical follow-up should include spirometry with lung volume and diffusion capacity and chest radiograph. It is vital that the antigen responsible for HP be determined so that appropriate environmental control measures can be carried out. Several initiatives can decrease the antigenic burden. Chemicals can be used to prevent the growth of organisms. A good example is propionic acid, which, when added to sugarcane, eliminates the growth of the thermophilic organism responsible for bagassosis. Water should be changed frequently in humidification or air conditioning units. Storage dryers will decrease the growth of mold and thermophilic organism in hay and straw. Finally, crops should be harvested when the moisture content is low. There are many ways to decrease exposure to organic dust. Dusty materials within closed spaces should be mechanically handled. Effective ventilation will remove dust from the ambient air. In some instances, personal respirators or masks may be used. Finally, when the previous measures have failed, the worker should be removed from the disease-producing environment.

PREVENTION

The incidence of HP may be reduced by decreasing exposure to responsible antigens. This may be accomplished by decreasing contact with potential agents, reducing microbial contamination, or using protective equipment.

PROGNOSIS

The prognosis for patients with HP is generally good if the offending antigen is detected and avoidance measures are enforced during the acute and subacute stages. In a review of HP in children by Fan (9), 97% of reported pediatric cases of HP had a favorable outcome when exposure was eliminated. A study in patients with farmer's lung demonstrated a recovery in DLCO up to 2 years from initial diagnosis.[135] In chronic HP, the prognosis is not as good, especially in patients with continued antigen exposure.[22] The presence of fibrosis seems to be the most important factor in prognosis, as antigen class, symptom duration, and pulmonary function

---

Box 65.2 Pulmonary Diseases With Eosinophilia

1. Allergy bronchopulmonary aspergillosis and mycosis
2. Drug and toxin induced eosinophilic disease
3. Acute eosinophilic pneumonia
4. Chronic eosinophilic pneumonia
5. Eosinophilic granuloma (formerly Histiocytosis X)
6. Helminth associated eosinophilic lung disease
7. Churg-Strauss syndrome (allergic angiitis and granulomatosis)
8. Hypereosinophilic syndrome

Box 65.3 Diagnostic Criteria of Allergic Bronchopulmonary Aspergillosis in Asthma and Cystic Fibrosis[a]

Minimum Criteria

Patients with asthma or cystic fibrosis
Worsening lung function not attributable to another etiology
Positive skin prick test with *Aspergillus* species
Total serum IgE ≥1000 ng/mL (416 IU/mL)
[b]In CF, total serum IgE levels:

- ≥1000 IU/mL, classic
- ≥500 IU/mL, minimum
- 200–500 IU/mL. If ABPA is suspected, repeat in 1–3 months. If patient is taking steroids, repeat when steroid treatment is discontinued.

Increased *Aspergillus* species-specific IgE and IgG antibodies
New or recent abnormalities on chest radiography or chest CT that have not cleared with antibiotics and standard physiotherapy

Additional Criteria

Increase in blood eosinophilia ≥400 eosinophils/µL when patient is not on corticosteroids
Aspergillus species-specific precipitating antibodies
Central bronchiectasis
Aspergillus species-specific containing mucus plugs

[a]Adapted from Agarwal R, Chakrabarti A, Shah A, Gupta D, Meis JF, Guleria R, Moss R, Denning DW. ABPA complicating asthma ISHAM working group. Allergic bronchopulmonary aspergillosis: review of literature and proposal of new diagnostic and classification criteria. *Clin Exp Allergy.* 2013;43(8):850-873.
[b]Stevens DA, Moss R, Kurup VP, Knutsen AP, Greenberger P, Judson MA, Denning DW, Crameri R, Body A, Light M, Skov M, Maish W, Mastella G, and the Cystic Fibrosis Foundation Consensus Conference. Allergic bronchopulmonary aspergillosis in cystic fibrosis: Cystic Fibrosis Foundation Consensus Conference. *Clin Infect Dis.* 2003;37(suppl 3):S225-S264.

---

did not appear to be significant predictors for survival in patient with HP.[136] Fortunately, with early identification and treatment, progression to the chronic stage of HP can be avoided.

Eosinophilic Pulmonary Diseases

ETIOLOGY

The eosinophilic lung diseases include a group of disorders that are characterized by increased peripheral blood and/or pulmonary eosinophilia.[137–140] As seen in Box 65.2, there are diverse causes of eosinophilic pulmonary diseases, including allergic bronchopulmonary aspergillosis (ABPA) and mycosis, drug and toxin induced eosinophilic disease, helminth associated eosinophilic lung disease, acute eosinophilic pneumonia, chronic eosinophilic pneumonia (CEP), eosinophilic granuloma, Churg-Strauss syndrome (CSS; eosinophilic granulomatosis with polyangiitis), and hypereosinophilic syndrome (HES). The clinical presentation of pulmonary eosinophilia consists of pulmonary symptoms, abnormal chest radiographs, and blood and sputum eosinophilia.

Allergic Bronchopulmonary Aspergillosis

ETIOLOGY

Hinson et al.[141] first described ABPA in adults in 1952 in England, and Slavin et al.[142] described the first case in a child in 1970 in the United States. ABPA is a Th2 hypersensitivity lung disease caused by bronchial colonization with *Aspergillus fumigatus* that affects asthmatic and cystic fibrosis (CF) subjects.[143–147] As seen in Box 65.3, ABPA is characterized by exacerbations of asthma, recurrent transient chest radiographic infiltrates, peripheral and sputum eosinophilia, IgE and IgG sensitization to *A. fumigatus*, and elevated total serum IgE level. *A. fumigatus* hyphae are generally found in the sputum at the time of acute exacerbations of ABPA. ABPA may lead to corticosteroid-dependent asthma, bronchiectasis, and/or pulmonary fibrosis. ABPA is most commonly caused by *A. fumigatus*; however, other fungi species such as *Candida*, *Penicillium*, and *Curvularia* have been identified as causing symptoms similar to ABPA.[148,149] Those patients who have symptoms of ABPA with identification of a fungus other than *Aspergillus fumigatus* are classified with allergic bronchopulmonary mycoses or ABPM.[148–150] Chowdhary et al.[151] reviewed 143 cases worldwide of ABPM and found that

Candida albicans is the most common fungi causing ABPM seen in 60% of cases. Of note, 70% of the cases from the review of ABPM did not have asthma, which is a clear distinction from ABPA. ABPA is relatively uncommon in childhood, although it has been reported in children with CF from England and the United States. *A. fumigatus* is a ubiquitous mold that is commonly encountered around farm buildings, barns, stables, silos, and compost heaps. Human disease has been reported from most countries of the world. ABPA should be distinguished from other lung diseases caused by *A. fumigatus*, such as invasive aspergillosis, aspergilloma, IgE-mediated asthma from *A. fumigatus* sensitivity, and HP due to *A. fumigatus* or *A. clavus* (malt worker's disease).

EPIDEMIOLOGY

The prevalence of ABPA is estimated to be 1%–2% in asthmatic patients and 7%–9% (up to 15%) of patients with CF.[143–147] Denning et al.[152] estimated that the global prevalence of ABPA may be 0.7%–3.5% of patients with asthma.

PATHOLOGY/PATHOGENESIS

The pathology of ABPA demonstrates cylindrical bronchiectasis of the central airways, particularly the upper lobes.[143-147] These airways may be occluded by "mucoid impaction," a condition in which large airways are occluded by impacted mucus and hyphae. Airway occlusion may lead to atelectasis of a segment or lobe, and if the atelectasis is long-standing, saccular bronchiectasis may result. Typically, ABPA is worse in the upper lobes than in the lower lobes. Microscopic examination of the airways shows infiltration of the airway wall with eosinophils, lymphocytes, and plasma cells. The airway lumen may be occluded by mucus containing hyphal elements and inflammatory cells, especially eosinophils. Squamous metaplasia of the bronchial mucosa develops commonly, and sometimes granulomas form. Rarely, bronchiolitis obliterans or bronchocentric granulomatosis develops.

Biology of Eosinophils

In ABPA and the other eosinophilic pulmonary diseases discussed later in this chapter, eosinophilic inflammation is prominent. In the pathogenesis of ABPA, there is extensive eosinophilic infiltration and inflammation in the bronchial airways and in the lung parenchyma (Fig. 65.5). Furthermore, there is extensive degranulation of eosinophil mediators, such as major basic protein (MBP) in the lung interstitium.[153] Eosinophils are inflammatory granulocytes

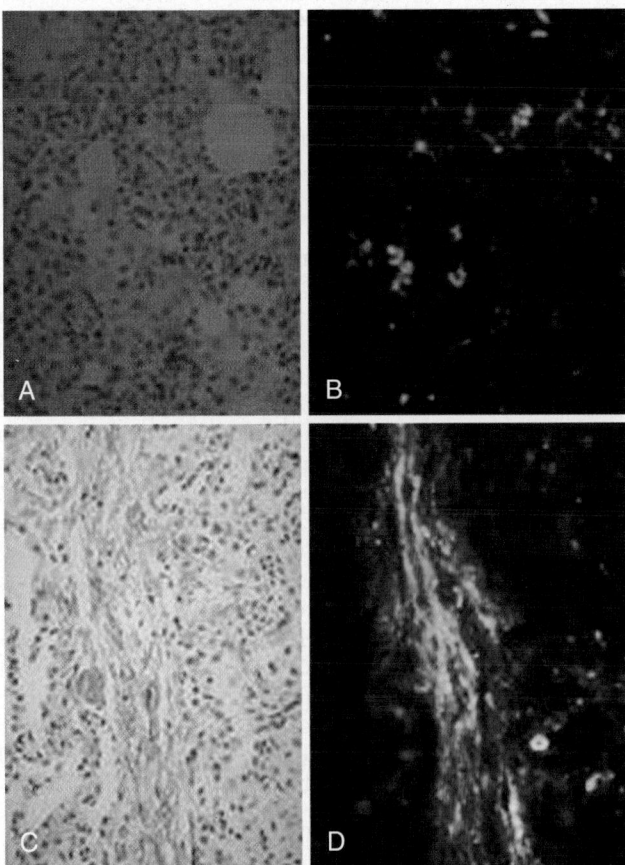

Fig. 65.5 Lung biopsy of a CF patient with ABPA. (A) H&E stain and (B) major basic protein (MBP) of intact eosinophils in same section as (A); (C) H&E stain and (D) MBP fluorescent staining demonstrating extensive deposits of MBP in the interlobar septum. (Used with permission from Slavin RG, Bedrossian CW, Hutcheson PS, Pittman S, Salinas-Madrigal L, Tsai CC, Gleich GJ. A pathologic study of allergic bronchopulmonary aspergillosis. *J Allergy Clin Immunol.* 1988;81(4):718-725.)

important in host defense principally against helminth parasites.[141] They also play an important inflammatory role in a variety of diseases, including asthma, allergic diseases, eosinophilic esophagitis, and HESs. Eosinophils are bone-marrow derived granulocytes.[141] The key cytokines that are critical for bone production of eosinophils are IL-3, IL-5, and granulocyte-monocyte-colony stimulating factor (GM-CSF), produced by CD4+ T cells. The activation of eosinophils is principally by IL-5 stimulation, which also increases tissue eosinophil survival. Tissue recruitment of eosinophils from the vascular system is stimulated by the chemokines platelet activating factor (PAF), leukotriene (LT)-D4, C5a, CCL11/eotaxin, and CCL5/RANTES (regulated on activation normal T cells expressed and secreted). Stimulation by eotaxin is selective for only eosinophils.

Eosinophils possess a number of preformed granule-derived proteins (MBP, eosinophil peroxidase, eosinophil cationic protein, eosinophil-derived neurotoxin, and Charcot-Leyden crystal protein), de novo synthesized lipid mediators (LTC4, PGE1, PGE2, TXB2, 15-HETE, and PAF), and reactive oxygen species that are released upon stimulation and result in inflammation. Eosinophils synthesize a number of Th2 cytokines (IL-4 and IL-5), Th1 cytokines (IFN-γ), and chemokines (eotaxin, RANTES). Eosinophils also have Fc receptors for principally IgA, which may regulate antibody-dependent cellular cytotoxicity (ADCC) eosinophil degranulation. Thus eosinophils are principally Th2-driven granulocytes that have potent inflammatory and tissue destructive properties.

In the pathogenesis of ABPA, *A. fumigatus* spores 3–5 μm in size are inhaled and germinate into hyphae deep within the bronchi (Fig. 65.6).[143-147] In addition, fragments of the hyphae can be identified within the interstitium of the pulmonary parenchyma (see Fig. 65.6). The implication is that there is the potential for high concentrations of *A. fumigatus* allergens to be exposed to the respiratory epithelium and immune system. *A. fumigatus* releases a variety of proteins, including superoxide dismutases, catalases, proteases, ribotoxin, phospholipases, hemolysin, gliotoxin, phthioic acid, and other toxins. The first line of defense against *Aspergillus* colonization in the lungs is macrophage and neutrophil killing of the conidia and the hyphae. In the development of ABPA, Kauffman's group proposed that *Aspergillus* proteins have a direct effect on the pulmonary epithelia and macrophage inflammation.[154-157] They demonstrated that *Aspergillus* proteases induce epithelial cell detachment. In addition, protease-containing culture filtrates of *Aspergillus* induce human bronchial cell lines to produce proinflammatory chemokines and cytokines, such as IL-8, IL-6, and MCP-1. Thus various *Aspergillus* proteins have significant biologic activity that disrupts the epithelial integrity and induces a monokine inflammatory response. This protease activity allows for enhanced allergen exposure to the bronchoalveolar lymphoid tissue immune system. This is evident by the bronchoalveolar lymphoid tissue synthesis of *Aspergillus*-specific IgE and IgA antibodies.

Genetic susceptibility factors have been proposed in the development of ABPA (Box 65.4). Chauhan and colleagues[158-160] observed that asthmatic and CF patients who expressed HLA-DR2 and/or DR5 and lacked HLA-DQ2 were at increased risk to develop ABPA after exposure to *A. fumigatus*. Furthermore, within *HLA-DR2* and *HLA-DR5*, there are restricted genotypes. In particular, *HLA-DRB1*1501* and

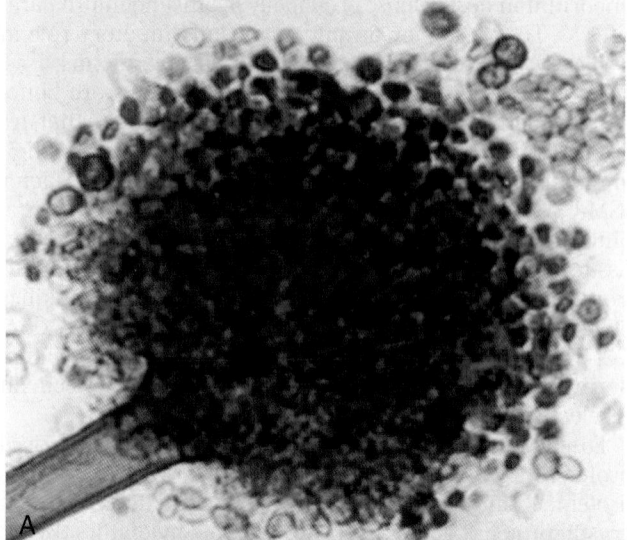

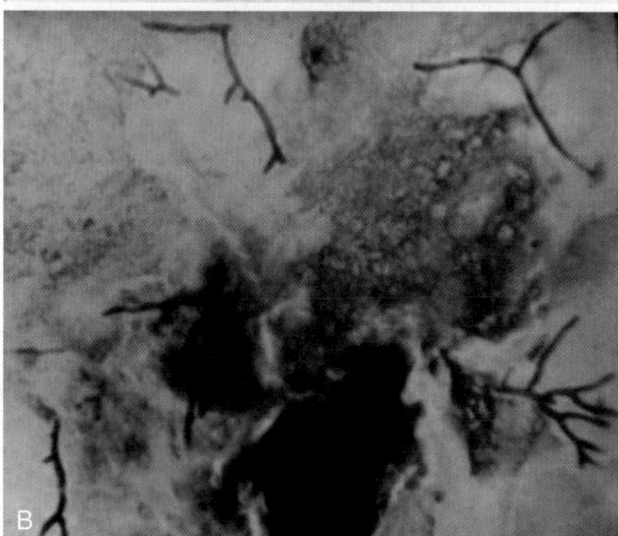

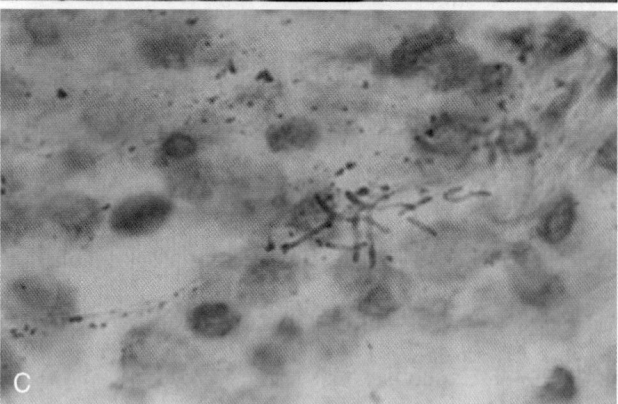

Fig. 65.6 *Aspergillus fumigatus* conidia (A). *Aspergillus fumigatus* hyphae in sputum (B) and a fragment of hyphae in the pulmonary interstitum (C) from a patient with allergic bronchopulmonary aspergillosis.

Box 65.4   Genetic Risk Factors in the Development of Allergic Bronchopulmonary Aspergillosis

HLA-DR restriction and HLA-DQ protection
  HLA-DR2: HLA-DRB1*1501 and *HLA-DRB1*1503
  HLA-DR5: HLA-DRB1*1101 and HLA-DRGB1*1104
  HLA-DQ2 protective, decreased in ABPA
    DQB1*0201
IL-4RA polymorphisms
  IL-4RA ile75val
IL-10 polymorphisms
  Promoter *-1082 GG* genotype
Surfactant protein A2 (SP-A2) polymorphisms
  SP-A2 ala91pro
Cystic fibrosis transmembrane conductance regulator (CFTR) mutations
  Heterozygous *CFTR* mutations in asthmatic patients with ABPA
Toll-like receptor (TLR) polymorphisms
  TLR9 T-1237C

HLA, Human leukocyte antigen; *IL,* interleukin.

from the development of ABPA. Recently, increased sensitivity to *in vitro* IL-4 stimulation, as measured by enhanced expression of the low-affinity IgE receptor (CD23) on B cells, was observed in ABPA patients. This was associated with single-nucleotide polymorphisms of the IL-4 receptor alpha chain *(IL4RA)* in 92% of ABPA subjects, principally the IL-4-binding single-nucleotide polymorphism ile75val.[143,145,147]

This increased sensitivity to IL-4 is demonstrated by increased expression of CD23 and CD86 on B cells of ABPA subjects and increased CD23 expression during flares of ABPA.[143,147] CD23 is expressed on a variety of cells, including B cells, NK cells, subpopulations of T cells, and a subpopulation of dendritic cells. T-cell CD23 and B-cell CD21 form a costimulatory pathway. T-cell CD28 and B-cells CD80 and CD86 costimulatory pathways activate both T and B cells, and CD28:CD86 is important in IgE synthesis. CD86 is also found on dendritic cells that have the histamine receptor 2, which skews antigen-specific T cells to a Th2 response. In a murine model of ABPA, Kurup and colleagues have found that CD86 expression is upregulated in the lung tissue (V.P. Kurup, Medical College of Wisconsin, personal communication). Recently, we have also observed increased CD86 expression on monocyte-derived dendritic cells of ABPA subjects. Thus antigen-presenting cells such as monocytes and dendritic cells bearing HLA-DR2 and/or HLA-DR5 and increased sensitivity to IL-4 stimulation probably play a critical role in skewing *A. fumigatus*-specific Th2 responses in ABPA.

Brouard and coworkers[161] recently reported a third genetic risk, the association of the *-1082GG* genotype of the IL-10 promoter with colonization with *A. fumigatus* and the development of ABPA in CF. The *-1082GG* polymorphism has been associated with increased IL-10 synthesis, whereas the *-1082A* allele has lower IL-10 synthesis. Thus dendritic cells expressing HLA-DR2/DR5 that have an HR2 phenotype, increased IL-10 synthesis, and increased sensitivity to IL-4 stimulation due to *IL-4RA* polymorphisms may be responsible for skewing *Aspergillus*-specific Th2 responses in ABPA.

Studies in asthma have implicated the role of bronchial epithelia and mesenchymal cells forming the

*HLA-DRB1*1503* were reported to produce high relative risk. On the other hand, 40%–44% of non-ABPA atopic *Aspergillus*-sensitive individuals have the *HLA-DR2* and/or *HLA-DR5* genotype. Additional studies indicated that the presence of *HLA-DQ2* (especially *HLA-DQB1*0201*) provided protection

epithelial-mesenchymal trophic unit (EMTU) with a profibrotic response when stimulated with proteases such as Der p1 and with IL-4 and IL-13.[162] In ABPA subjects, *Aspergillus* proteases and allergen stimulation of the EMTU in conjunction with increased sensitivity to IL-4 due *IL-4RA* SNPs may result in increased bronchial epithelial secretion of IL-8, GM-CSF, and transforming growth factor (TGF-α), the ligand for epidermal growth factor leading to bronchial destruction and fibrosis.

CLINICAL FEATURES

Symptoms and Physical Findings

Clinical symptoms of ABPA include increased coughing, episodes of wheezing, anorexia, malaise, fever, and expectoration of brown plugs (see Box 65.3). ABPA can present acutely with acute symptoms and signs associated with transient pulmonary infiltrates and eosinophilia or with mucoid impaction; it may also present an exacerbation of a chronic disease characterized by proximal bronchiectasis. It is thought that the chronic form of the disease develops following the acute process and that it can be prevented by effective therapy. In chronic ABPA, the acute episodes are superimposed on a background of chronic cough and sputum production. In adults, ABPA usually affects the younger age group of adult asthmatics, and most cases occur before 40 years of age. In pediatrics, ABPA rarely affects children with asthma, and it is usually seen in children with CF, who may simply appear to have a worsening of their pulmonary status or an acute pulmonary exacerbation of CF. ABPA does sometimes affect children with asthma, and there is a report of three children who developed it before 2 years of age. Physical examination shows the signs of chronic lung disease from CF or asthma, such as hyperaeration of the lungs, expiratory wheezing, a chronic productive cough, and crackles or wheezes. The chronically ill patient with bronchiectasis may have coarse crackles, weight loss, and digital clubbing.

The criteria for the diagnosis of ABPA are shown in Box 65.5.[144,163] The minimal criteria are worsening of lung function not attributed to another cause in asthmatic or CF patients, new pulmonary infiltrates and/or high-attenuation mucus (HAM) impaction, IgE to *A. fumigatus* demonstrated by either allergy prick skin test or *in vitro* specific IgE to *A. fumigatus*, elevated IgG to *A. fumigatus* demonstrated either

by *Aspergillus* specific precipitins or *in vitro* IgG to *A. fumigatus*, elevated serum IgE ≥1000 ng/ml (≥416 IU/ml), and blood eosinophilia ≥400/mL. When central bronchiectasis is also present, ABPA is classified as ABPA central bronchiectasis (ABPA-CB) and when absent classified as ABPA serologic (ABPA-S). In CF, the Cystic Fibrosis Foundation Consensus Conference recommended different criteria for total serum IgE levels.[144] In the diagnosis of ABPA in CF, elevated serum IgE was defined as a level ≥1000 IU/ml. Minimum IgE level was defined as ≥500 IU/mL. If ABPA is suspected and the total level is 200–500 IU/mL, it is recommended to repeat testing in 1–3 months. A problem with applying the criteria in children is that usually ABPA occurs in children with CF in whom many of the criteria could be due to the underlying disease. Some children with CF appear to have a clinical variant of ABPA without having all the typical criteria, and they may respond clinically to corticosteroids. Patients being considered for this diagnosis should have skin testing with *A. fumigatus* antigen.

Aspergillosis in Cystic Fibrosis

In 2013, Denning's group proposed a novel immunologic classification of aspergillosis in adult CF patients.[164] Four classification of aspergillosis were identified by examinations of sputum *Aspergillus* colonization using RT-PCR and *Aspergillus* hyphae by galactomannan (GM), total IgE level, and *Aspergillus* specific IgE and IgG level. Class 1 (nondisease) represented ± RT-PCR, negative GM, negative IgE, and IgG *Aspergillus* serology; class 2 (serologic ABPA), positive RT-PCR, positive GM, elevated total IgE, and *Aspergillus* specific IgE/IgG; and class 3 (*Aspergillus* sensitized), ± RT-PCR, negative GM, elevated *Aspergillus* IgE, but not *Aspergillus* IgG; and class 4 (*Aspergillus* bronchitis), positive RT-PCR, positive GM, elevated *Aspergillus* IgG, but not IgE.

In 2016, Mirković et al.[165] reported using *Aspergillus* stimulated basophil activation test (BAT) measuring surface marker CD203c expression to identify ABPA in CF patients. Three groups were identified. In Group 1 (nonsensitized), decreased BAT CD203c, decreased total IgE, and decreased *Aspergillus* specific IgE; Group 2 (*Aspergillus* sensitized), decreased BAT CD203c, decreased total IgE, and decreased *Aspergillus* specific IgE; and Group 3 (ABPA), elevated BAT CD203c, elevated total IgE, and elevated *Aspergillus* specific IgE.

Clinical Staging

The spectrum of ABPA varies widely, from individuals with mild asthma and occasional episodes of pulmonary eosinophilia (with no long-term sequelae), to patients with fibrosis, honeycomb lung, and respiratory failure. Patterson and colleagues[166] have suggested a clinical classification with five clinical stages, as shown in Table 65.2. Stage I is the acute stage of ABPA, with many of the typical features of the disease. If this stage goes into remission, the infiltrates clear, symptoms reduce, and the serum IgE value will decline by up to 35% within 6 weeks. Stage II is remission. Stage III is an exacerbation associated with the recurrence of the initial symptoms and a twofold increase in serum IgE level. Stage IV is reached when patients need continuous corticosteroids either to control their asthma or to prevent a recurrence of ABPA. Stage V is the fibrotic stage, which is present when there is severe upper lobe fibrosis present on the chest radiograph, and it may be associated with honeycombing. The

---

Box 65.5 Helminth-Associated Eosinophilic Lung Diseases

1. Transpulmonary passage of helminth larvae (Loeffler's syndrome)
   - Ascaris lumbricoides, Ancylostoma duodenale, Necator americanus, Strongyloides stercoralis
2. Hematogenous seeding with helminth larvae
   - Cutaneous larva migrans—nonhuman ascarids and hookworms, Trichinella spiralis, Schistosoma
   - Visceral larva migrans—aberrant infection—Toxocara canis
   - Disseminated Strongyloides
3. Pulmonary parenchymal invasion with helminthes
   - Parogonimus westermani lung flukes
4. Tropical pulmonary eosinophilia—Filaria
   - Wucheria bancrofti, Brugia malayi

Table 65.2   Staging of Allergic Bronchopulmonary Aspergillosis

Stage	IgE Level	Precipitins	Eosinophilia	IgE-Af	IgG-Af	Pulmonary Infiltrates
(I) Acute	+++	+	+	+	+	+
(II) Remission	+	±	—	±	±	—
(III) Exacerbation	+++	+	+	+	+	+
(IV) Corticosteroid-dependent	++	±	±	±	±	—
(V) Fibrotic	+	±	—	±	±	—

IgE, Immunoglobulin E; *IgE-Af*, IgE antibody to *Aspergillus fumigatus*; *IgG-Af*, IgG antibody to *Aspergillus fumigatus*.
Reprinted with permission from Knutsen AP, Slavin RG. Allergic bronchopulmonary aspergillosis in asthma and cystic fibrosis. *Clin Dev Immunol.*
2011;2011:843763.

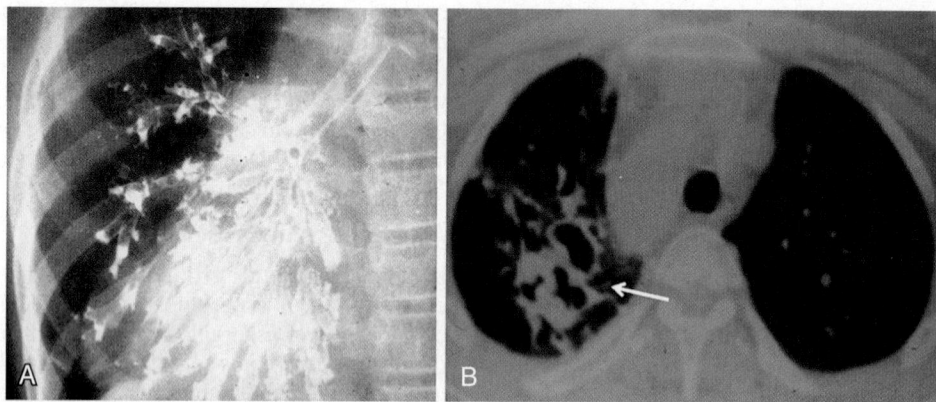

Fig. 65.7 Central bronchiectasis in allergic bronchopulmonary aspergillosis demonstrated by (A) radiocontrast bronchography and (B) chest scan *(arrow)*. (Used with permission from Dr. Raymond G. Slavin.)

stage V lesions may not respond to corticosteroids, although steroids are often necessary to maintain a bronchodilator response, and severe wheezing may develop if steroids are discontinued. Pulmonary fibrosis is an advanced complication that can lead to pulmonary hypertension and cor pulmonale.

Radiographic Findings

There are several characteristic radiographic abnormalities associated with ABPA.[144,166–170] The most common lesion is a large, homogeneous shadow in one of the upper lobes with no change in volume. The shadow may be triangular, lobar, or patchy, and it frequently moves to another site. "Tram line" shadows are fine parallel lines radiating from the hila that represent inflammation of airway walls. Mucoid impaction causes toothpaste shadows or gloved-finger shadows. Several adult patients have been reported with normal chest radiographs, so radiographic abnormalities are not invariably present. In these individuals, cylindrical bronchiectasis was demonstrated by high-resolution computerized tomography (HRCT) scan (Fig. 65.7).

HAM has been proposed by Agarwal et al.[167–170] to be evaluated with HRCT. Based on multiple studies, Agarwal et al.[170] found that the presence of HAM is pathognomonic of ABPA. They have also investigated the immunologic severity of these patients with HAM. They, along with International Society for Human and Animal Mycology (ISHAM), have proposed a change in severity and classification based on radiographic studies as follows: mild ABPA-serologic (ABPA-S), moderate ABPA-central bronchiectasis (ABPA-CB), and severe ABPA-CB-HAM.[170] In a study of 234 patients, Agarwal et al. found 25% normal HRCT, 76.5% with CB, 20.9% with HAM,

and 11.5% with other radiologic findings.[168] It was noted that patients with CB or HAM had frequent relapses; however, those with HAM had significantly elevated immunologic markers compared with the other groups, which was correlated with more severe cases of ABPA. Of note, failure to achieve remission was associated with CB, not with HAM. HAM has been shown to be 100% specific in the diagnosis of ABPA.[169]

Laboratory Findings

Laboratory tests that support the diagnosis of ABPA are those that demonstrate allergy to the mold, such as a positive specific IgE test and positive *Aspergillus* precipitins.[143–147] The precipitins are only weakly positive compared with the strong reactions seen in patients with mycetomas. Culture of *A. fumigatus* from the sputum is only a secondary criterion for the diagnosis of ABPA, because a large proportion of individuals with CF without ABPA have *Aspergillus* on sputum cultures. Some normal individuals and many individuals with lung diseases have small numbers of spores in their sputum; these are probably present because of passive inhalation. The presence of hyphae is more specific, and the presence of eosinophils in association with hyphal elements is suggestive of the diagnosis. The presence of eosinophilia in sputum or blood is suggestive of ABPA and is a primary diagnostic criterion. The peripheral blood eosinophil count is usually greater than 1000/mm³, and values greater than 3000/mm³ are common.

An increased serum IgE value is very characteristic of ABPA, and values may reach as high as 30,000 IU/mL. Usually, the value is greater than 1000 IU/mL. Much of the IgE is not specific to *Aspergillus* but is the result of polyclonal

B-cell activation. The IgE level is a very useful marker of disease activity, and it can be used to follow outpatients for "flares." The simple skin-prick test is a useful screening test, as ABPA is very unlikely in patients with a negative reaction. A dual-reaction of intradermal *Aspergillus* skin test with an immediate (10–15 minutes) and a late (4–8 hours) reaction occurs in one-third of patients with ABPA. Alternatively, serum may be measured for the presence of specific IgE and IgG antibodies. Patients with ABPA and *Aspergillus*-sensitive asthma will have *Aspergillus* specific IgE antibody, but patients with ABPA will have quantitatively increased *Aspergillus*-specific IgE levels. Crameri's group[171] has reported that ABPA and *Aspergillus*-sensitive patients have elevated IgE antibodies to recombinant *Aspergillus* Asp f1, Asp f3, Asp f4, and Asp f6 allergens, and that IgE levels to Asp f4 and Asp f6 are highly specific for ABPA.

The usual pattern of serum precipitins is that immunoelectrophoresis shows one to three precipitin lines, often to only one extract.[153,166] Patients with aspergilloma will have multiple precipitin lines to all antigen extracts. Extracts of *A. fumigatus* contain a complex mixture of proteins that are mainly derived from the hyphae. Antigenic composition varies between batches according to the culture conditions, even within the same laboratory. Thus there is a lack of standardization that makes it difficult to compare results between laboratories. However, there has been some success with purification of the major antigenic components that may lead eventually to improved diagnosis. We find it best to send all our testing to one central laboratory that has well-established methods for the characterization of the serologic responses to *A. fumigatus*.

DIFFERENTIAL DIAGNOSIS

Several diseases cause pulmonary infiltrates in children with asthma or CF. The differential diagnosis of ABPA should include the following: viral or bacterial pneumonia, poorly controlled asthma with mucoid impaction or atelectasis, inhaled foreign body, CF (with or without ABPA), immotile cilia syndrome, tuberculosis with eosinophilia, sarcoidosis, pulmonary infiltrates with eosinophilia, HP, and pulmonary neoplasm.

MANAGEMENT AND TREATMENT

Treatment is designed first to control the acute episodes and then to limit the development of chronic lung disease.[154,166] Most cases of ABPA require treatment with systemic corticosteroids, and the treatment of choice is prednisone. Steroid therapy rapidly clears the eosinophilic infiltrates and the associated symptoms, although it is less effective at treating mucus impaction. The usual starting dose is 0.5 mg/kg per day, taken each morning, and this dose is maintained for 2–4 weeks while following the patient clinically and checking the chest radiograph for resolution of the acute process. After this induction treatment, the dose of prednisone should be reduced to 0.5 mg/kg given on alternate days. If mucus impaction persists and is associated with atelectasis, bronchoscopy should be performed to confirm the diagnosis and to attempt to remove the mucus plugs.

Following resolution of the acute process, the dose of prednisone should be reduced over 1–3 months. Chronic treatment with corticosteroids is controversial, especially in adults, because a minority of patients with ABPA are at risk of chronic lung disease. The relationship between acute episodes and lung damage is unclear, and the precise dose of prednisone is not certain, since acute exacerbations may continue while the patients are on low doses of steroids. However, children with ABPA usually have CF and may need treatment with long-term corticosteroids to prevent progressive lung damage. Therefore we usually maintain therapy with a dose of 0.5 mg/kg on alternate days for 3 months, and then, after 3 months, the dose of prednisone is tapered over an additional 3 months while checking the chest radiograph and the serum IgE level for evidence of relapse. Initially the serum IgE level should be checked at every visit and, if the level increases by twofold or more, the steroid dose should be increased. We recommend that patients are followed with serum IgE levels and chest radiographs every 6 months for the first 1–2 years, and then, if the patient remains in remission, it should be possible to reduce the frequency of these studies.

The antifungal agent itraconazole has been used to reduce the doses of steroids that are required.[172,173] Initially there were only open nonrandomized studies indicating that itraconazole is a useful adjunct to systemic corticosteroid therapy. Two recent randomized controlled trials have also favored itraconazole use. A double-blind, randomized, placebo-controlled trial of itraconazole 200 mg twice daily dose resulted in decreased IgE levels and an increase in pulmonary function and exercise tolerance. Another randomized, controlled trial showed that treatment of stable ABPA in adults with 400 mg/day itraconazole resulted in a significant reduction in sputum eosinophil count, sputum eosinophilic cationic protein levels, serum IgE concentrations, and *Aspergillus*-specific IgG. There was also a reduction in episodes of exacerbation, requiring treatment with systemic steroids. In the treatment of children with ABPA, we have used a dose of 10 mg/kg per day of itraconazole.

Omalizumab, a humanized monoclonal antibody that binds free IgE, has been used in patients with refractory ABPA.[174] Current dosing of omalizumab is based on total serum IgE levels. However, patients with ABPA can have IgE levels that far exceed the upper limit of omalizumab dosing, as part of their disease process. Therefore they should be treated with the maximum recommended weight-based dose of omalizumab. Collins et al.[175] performed a retrospective chart review of 21 patients who had received omalizumab for refractory ABPA. This group of patients overall had decrease in steroid use, decrease in levels of total serum IgE, and improved symptoms which were noted with an increase in Asthma Control Test (ACT) scores.[131] In France, Tillie-Leblond et al.[176] evaluated 16 patients with ABPA who received omalizumab for 1 year. This group of patients had decreased exacerbations and the need for oral steroids during this time. In 2016, Voskamp et al.[177] reported a randomized, double-blind, placebo-controlled, cross-over trial with 2 treatment phases of 4-month duration. Thirteen patients with asthma and ABPA were identified and underwent the active treatment phase with omalizumab 375 mg every 2 weeks for 4 months with a washout period of 3 months, and crossover arm. ABPA exacerbations occurred less frequently during omalizumab treatment compared with the placebo period, 2 versus 12 events. Mean fractional exhaled nitric oxide (FeNO) decreased from 30.5 to 17.1 ppb during omalizumab treatment. In addition, omalizumab treatment resulted in decreased basophil reactivity to *A. fumigatus* and FcεR1 and surface-bound IgE levels. These recent studies and many case reports show the benefit this additional treatment option offers patients with ABPA.

Recent studies have shown utility in inhaled amphotericin B to provide localized treatment of ABPA and thereby decrease side effects.[178–180] In addition, hypertonic saline has been used to help clear mucus from the airways in patients with bronchiectasis, though patients must be monitored carefully with their first dose, as it can induce bronchoconstriction.[181,182] Macrolide antibiotics have been used for antiinflammatory effects in patients with bronchiectasis, though no studies have been done in patients with ABPA or to compare macrolide versus itraconazole therapy.

There is no place for immunotherapy in children with ABPA, since it is ineffective and potentially dangerous. Inhaled antiinflammatory agents, such as cromoglycate and beclomethasone, are not generally thought to be effective. The role of inhaled spores in the pathogenesis of ABPA is unclear, but there is a seasonal incidence of ABPA that is probably related to seasonal changes in mold spore counts. Therefore it is reasonable to advise patients with ABPA to avoid exposure to places with high spore counts, such as damp basements, barns, and compost heaps.

PROGNOSIS

The prognosis for children with ABPA is good if the disease is detected early and treatment started promptly.[183] It is important that the diagnosis is made and treatment commenced before there is permanent lung damage from bronchiectasis. In such patients, there should be no progression of the disease, although relapses can occur many years later, and long-term follow-up is recommended. In patients with CF, the relapses seem to be more frequent than in asthma, and careful surveillance is necessary to ensure resolution of the disease process. In some CF patients, it is difficult to wean the steroids without an increase in symptoms, such as dyspnea and wheezing; whether this is due to the underlying CF lung disease or due to patients going from stage II to stage III ABPA on withdrawal of steroids is unclear. Symptoms are not a reliable guide to therapy; therefore it is important to reevaluate the chest radiograph and the serum IgE at regular intervals until a long-term remission is established.

Drug-Induced Eosinophilia

ETIOLOGY

Many drugs have been associated with the development of pulmonary eosinophilia (Table 65.3).[184–191] In fact, drug reactions are one of the most commonly reported causes of pulmonary infiltrates with blood or pulmonary eosinophilia. Sulfonamides, including sulfasalazine, were the first recognized cause of this reaction, but more recently it has been described with the structurally similar drugs, sulfonylurea and chlorpropamide, and the antituberculous drug *p*-aminosalicyclic acid. The tricyclic compounds imipramine

Table 65.3 Drugs That Cause Eosinophilic Lung Disease

Ampicillin	L-Tryptophan
Aspirin	Mephenesin carbamate
Beclomethasone dipropionate (inhaled)	Methotrexate
Bleomycin	Minocycline
Captopril	Naproxen
Carbamazepine	Nickel
Chlorpromazine	Nitrofurantoin
Clarithromycin	*p*-Aminosalicyclic acid
Chlorpropamide	Penicillamine
Clofibrate	Penicillin
Cocaine (inhaled)	Pentamidine (inhaled)
Cromolyn (inhaled)	Phenytoin
Desipramine	Pyrimethamine
Diclofenac	Rapeseed oil
Febarbamate	Sulfadimethoxine
Fenbufen	Sulfadoxine
Glafenine	Sulfasalazine
GM-CSF	Sulindac
Gold	Tamoxifen
Ibuprofen	Tetracycline
Imipramine	Tolazamide
IL-2	Tolfenamic acid
IL-3	Vaginal sulfonamide cream
Iodinated contrast dye	

and carbamazepine may also cause pulmonary eosinophilia. Of the hydantoins (nitrofurantoin, dantrolene, and phenytoin), nitrofurantoin is most likely to cause an adverse pulmonary reaction. The reaction may be seen within days of starting treatment.

Other drugs that have been implicated in pulmonary eosinophilia are listed in Table 65.3. In addition, toxins from occupational exposures, such as rubber workers exposed to aluminum silicate and particulate metals, sulfite-exposed grape workers, and Scotchguard® inhalation, should be considered. Loeffler's-like syndrome has been seen in crack cocaine users. Drug reactions may be associated with the simple form of pulmonary eosinophilia-like syndrome, a fulminant acute eosinophilic pneumonia-like syndrome, or may follow a more chronic source. Symptoms normally start within a month of starting the drug and include cough, dyspnea, and fever. Histologically, there is pulmonary interstitial edema with a lymphocytic and eosinophilic infiltrate, and the alveoli contain eosinophils and histiocytes. Peripheral eosinophilia, though common, is not an invariable finding. Chest radiographs show interstitial or alveolar infiltrates and often demonstrate Kerley B lines. High-resolution CT chest scans demonstrate areas of ground-glass attenuation, airspace consolidation, nodules, irregular lines, and sometimes hilar adenopathy or pleural effusion.[192,193]

Drug-induced eosinophilic lung disease resembles other eosinophilic lung diseases, such as Loeffler's syndrome. Thus other causes need to be considered. Confirmation of the adverse reactions may be carried out by challenging the patient with a single dose of the drug. Skin testing with either patch or prick tests is usually negative. In vitro lymphocyte transformation tests have been positive with some drugs, such as nitrofurantoin and carbamazepine. When the offending drug is discontinued, there is usually resolution of the symptoms and the eosinophilia, together with clearing of the chest radiograph. When resolution is slow,

Table 65.4 Characteristics of Acute and Chronic Eosinophilic Pneumonitis

Characteristic	Acute	Chronic
Ages	Children and adults 20–40 years	Adults 40–50 years peak, rare in children
Sex	Male preponderance	Female preponderance 2:1
Smoking risk	Yes	No
Underlying asthma	None	50%
Symptoms	Acute febrile illness 1–5 days	Insidious over 7.7 months
	Fever, dyspnea, cough, myalgias, pleuritic chest pain, hypoxemia	Fever, night sweats, weight loss, cough, wheezing, anorexia
PE	High fever, basilar rales, wheezing	Fever, wheezing, lymphadenopathy, hepatomegaly
Chest radiograph, HRCT scan	Diffuse bilateral ground glass and/or reticular opacities involving alveolar or mixed interstitial/alveolar infiltrates, pleural effusions	Dense peripheral infiltrates (negative image of pulmonary edema)
PFT	Restrictive pattern	Restrictive pattern
DLCO	Decreased	
Lung biopsy	Diffuse acute organizing alveolar damage, eosinophilic infiltration of alveoli, interstitium, bronchial epithelium	Eosinophils and lymphocytes in alveoli and interstitium, thickened alveolar walls. Interstitial fibrosis in 50%; BO in 25%
BALF	45 ± 11% eosinophils, 20 ± 11% lymphocytes	>25% eosinophils, lymphocytes
Blood eosinophilia	Normal	Elevated
IgE level	Elevated in some	Elevated in most
Corticosteroids	Prompt response. No relapse of tapered corticosteroids over 8 weeks	Prompt response. Relapse if corticosteroids discontinued within 6 months
Omalizumab	ND	Responsive in case report

Exclusion of drug-induced eosinophilia, helminth infection, fungal associated eosinophilic lung diseases.
BALF, Bronchoalveolar lavage fluid; *BO*, bronchiolitis obliterans; *DLCO*, diffusing capacity carbon monoxide; *HRCT*, high resolution computed tomography; *ND*, not done; *PE*, physical examination; *PFT*, pulmonary function testing.

corticosteroid drugs may hasten the recover, though not invariably.

Acute Eosinophilic Pneumonia

EPIDEMIOLOGY/ETIOLOGY

The cause of acute eosinophilic pneumonia is unknown (Table 65.4). It is hypothesized that acute eosinophilic pneumonia is caused by an acute hypersensitivity reaction to an unidentified inhaled antigen.[194,195] However, other causes of eosinophilic lung diseases, such as parasitic, drug-induced, and fungal hypersensitivities, do need to be excluded. It affects predominantly males twice as often as females, and though it may affect individuals at any age, it occurs most often between 20 and 40 years. It has been reported that acute eosinophilic pneumonia developed in individuals who recently started smoking or resumed smoking after a period of cessation.[196] It has also been suggested that home environmental factor exposure may play a role. Provocative home challenges were performed in stable patients who had recovered from acute eosinophilic pneumonia and resulted in the development of acute symptoms of fever, cough, fatigue, and dyspnea.[197] Since leaving the house, the symptoms did not recur.

PATHOLOGY/PATHOGENESIS

Tazelaar et al.[198] reported on the histopathology from lung biopsies of nine adult patients with acute eosinophilic pneumonia. They reported acute and organizing diffuse alveolar damage (DAD) involving 75% of the surface area of the lung. The main finding was the presence of acute and organizing

DAD with marked infiltration of eosinophils in the interstitium and alveoli. Hyaline membranes were seen in seven of the nine patients. There was interstitial widening due to edema, fibroblast proliferation, and in the organizing phase of DAD, eosinophilic inflammation. Type II pneumocyte hyperplasia, interstitial lymphocytes, and organizing intraalveolar fibrinous exudate were also observed. However, granulomata were absent.

CLINICAL FEATURES

Symptoms and Physical Findings

Acute eosinophilic pneumonia is a distinct clinical entity that occurs in both children and adults with a male preponderance (see Table 65.4).[197–204] The clinical manifestations include acute onset of fever, cough, and dyspnea for 1–5 days. There may be associated pleuritic chest pain and myalgias. Patients then develop hypoxemia and respiratory failure, often requiring a mechanical ventilator. Physical examination reveals high fever, respiratory distress, and basilar rales, sometimes with fever. Initial chest radiographs reveal interstitial infiltrates.[199,200] These may progress to diffuse alveolar infiltrates. Chest CT scans demonstrate diffuse alveolar infiltrates, pleural effusions, pronounced septal markings, and normal lymph nodes.

Laboratory Findings

At the onset of disease, chest radiographs demonstrate reticular and/or ground-glass opacities.[194–196] As the disease progresses, there are bilateral diffuse mixed ground-glass and reticular opacities. Pleural effusions are common, which contain up to 42% eosinophils. Chest HRCT demonstrates bilateral ground-glass and/or reticular opacities. Pulmonary function testing demonstrates a restrictive pattern with decreased diffusing capacity (DLCO). BAL fluid reveals eosinophilia ($45\% \pm 11\%$) and lymphocytosis ($20\% \pm 11\%$). There is evidence of eosinophil degranulation in the pleural fluid with an elevated pH. Lung biopsy specimens demonstrate eosinophil infiltration of the interstitium, alveoli, and epithelium. Other findings include type II pneumocyte hyperplasia, interstitial lymphocytes, organizing intraalveolar fibrinous exudate, and perivascular and intramural inflammation without necrosis. Peripheral blood eosinophilia is typically absent; however, serum IgE levels may be elevated in some patients.

TREATMENT AND MANAGEMENT

Though the etiology of acute eosinophilic pneumonia is unknown, there is a dramatic response to high-dose corticosteroids, typically within 24–48 hours. Steroids are then tapered over an 8-week course.[194,197–201] Relapses or recurrences are unusual.

PROGNOSIS

Acute eosinophilic pneumonia has a very favorable outcome.[196] After initiation of corticosteroids, there is rapid clinical, radiographic, and pulmonary function testing improvement over a 1–2 months treatment period. Relapse may recur, especially with resumption of cigarette smoking.

Chronic Eosinophilic Pneumonia

EPIDEMIOLOGY/ETIOLOGY

Idiopathic CEP is a rare disorder, with an incidence of 0.23 cases/100,000 in Iceland,[205] and accounts for 2.5% of interstitial lung disease in Europe.[206] CEP is a disorder that affects primarily middle-age adults (peak 40–50 years), with a 2 : 1 female preponderance (see Table 65.4).[207–212] CEP is rare in childhood. In contrast to acute eosinophilic pneumonia, the majority of patients are nonsmokers. The cause of CEP is unknown, and other conditions that cause eosinophilic lung diseases need to be excluded. A risk factor may be asthma, which occurs in 50% of patients.

PATHOLOGY/PATHOGENESIS

The inflammatory response is similar to asthma, though the pathogenesis is unknown. Indeed, an underlying risk factor is asthma seen in 50% of the patients with CEP. There is accumulation of eosinophils, which may be the result of a stimulus triggering release of T helper 2 cells and IL-5. Lung biopsy specimens of patients with CEP demonstrate interstitial and alveolar septa infiltration of eosinophils, lymphocytes, histiocytes, and the presence of multinucleated giant cells.[207] In addition, there are alveolar luminal eosinophil and macrophage infiltration. Organizing pneumonia is a common finding, and eosinophilic abscesses may also be seen. There is also prominent intraluminal fibrosis.

CLINICAL FEATURES

Symptoms and Physical Findings

The symptoms of CEP are insidious developing over a 6–8 months period (see Box 65.8).[207–212] They include fever, night sweats, weight loss, cough, and wheezing. The cough is typically nonproductive. Some patients may also experience hemoptysis, lymphadenopathy, and hepatomegaly.

Laboratory Findings

Chest radiographs reveal extensive, bilateral, peripheral infiltrates, so-called "negative image of pulmonary edema," which is diagnostic of CEP. Chest HRCT scans show peripheral airspace disease and may show hilar adenopathy. Peripheral blood eosinophilia is prominent. BALF examination reveals increased eosinophils greater than 25% and increased lymphocytes. IgE levels are also frequently elevated.

Lung biopsy specimens display moderate to extensive accumulation of eosinophils and lymphocytes in the alveoli and the interstitium with thickened alveolar walls. Sometimes multinucleated histiocytic giant cells, lymphocytes, and plasma cells are found in the alveoli, a noncaseating granuloma reaction. There is also mild perivascular cuffing of venules with eosinophils and lymphocytes. Interstitial fibrosis has been reported in 50% of patients and bronchiolitis obliterans in 25% of patients.

TREATMENT AND MANAGEMENT

Response to high-dose corticosteroids is dramatic, with resolution of symptoms within 24–48 hours. Radiographically, pulmonary infiltrates resolve over 10–21 days. Taper of corticosteroids needs to be prolonged typically more than 6 months to prevent relapse. The mean duration of corticosteroid treatment is approximately 19 months. Recurrent attacks have occurred in 34% patients, especially in those with asthma. The outcome for most patients with CEP is excellent despite the risk of recurrences. Some patients have subsequently developed CSS (eosinophilic granulomatosis with polyangiitis), raising the possibility of overlap of the two diseases. Inhaled corticosteroids have been reported to be effective. Nonetheless, long-term prognosis is excellent for most patients. In case reports, omalizumab has been reported to be successful in patients with both atopic asthmatic and CEP who have prolonged dependence on systemic glucocorticoids.[213]

PROGNOSIS

CEP is responsive to corticosteroid treatment, and the prognosis of CEP is excellent with few relapses.[211] Naughton et al.[212] reported on the long-term follow-up, mean of 10.2 years (range 4–12 years), of 12 patients with CEP. All 12 patients were well on long-term follow-up. Two patients (17%) were tapered off corticosteroids without relapse, 9 patients (58%) had a relapse on corticosteroid withdrawal but responded to increased doses, and 3 patients (25%) have required long-term low-dose corticosteroids. Omalizumab treatment may have a therapeutic role in those patients with corticosteroid dependency.[213] Development of asthma in follow-up of CEP patients is common, and it has been suggested that inhaled corticosteroids may be beneficial.

Eosinophilic Granuloma (Pulmonary Langerhans Cell Histiocytosis)

EPIDEMIOLOGY/ETIOLOGY

Eosinophilic granuloma, also known as pulmonary Langerhans cell histiocytosis (PLCH), is a rare histiocytic disorder in which the incidence is unknown (Table 65.5).[214,215] PLCH is the nonmalignant form of the three forms of Langerhans cell histiocytosis: Letterer-Siwe disease, Hand-Schuller-Christian disease, and eosinophilic granuloma. The incidence appears to be 3–5 cases per million children. Eosinophilic granuloma affects children from 1 to 3 years old and particularly young adult males 20–40 years.[208] Males and females are equally affected. The etiology and pathogenesis of pulmonary eosinophilic granuloma is unknown. PLCH is strongly associated with cigarette smoking.

PATHOLOGY/PATHOGENESIS

The Langerhans cell is a differentiated cell of the monocyte-macrophage lineage and is the pathologic cell in pulmonary eosinophilic granuloma.[214–216] Langerhans cells are identified by pale staining cytoplasm, a large nucleus and nucleoli, and classic pentilaminar cytoplasmic inclusions or Birbeck granules seen on electron microscopy. Langerhans cells also demonstrate positive immunohistochemical staining for S100

protein CD1a on the cell surface. In PLCH, the Langerhans cells are typically found in clusters and are nonmalignant. Cigarette smoking has been linked to pulmonary eosinophilic granuloma, but not to extrapulmonary Langerhans cell histiocytosis.[215–218] It has been hypothesized that cigarette smoke induces bombesin-like peptide synthesis, a neuropeptide produced by neuroendocrine cells.[219–222] Bombesin-like peptides are increased in the lungs of smokers and are chemotactic for monocytes, stimulate epithelial cells and fibroblasts, and stimulate cytokine synthesis. Several abnormalities in immune function have been identified, including increased IgA in BALF, increased immune complexes, and abnormal T cell function.[219,223] Although these factors may be important in the pathophysiology of pulmonary PLCH, they may also represent nonspecific generalized activation of immune effector cells.

CLINICAL FEATURES

Symptoms and Physical Findings

Patients with eosinophilic granuloma present with pulmonary and/or extrapulmonary symptoms (see Table 65.5).[214,215] In PLCH, there is typically only a solitary lesion, but there may be multiple lesions, which may be asymptomatic or may cause pain. The most common presenting symptoms are nonproductive cough, dyspnea, pleuritic chest pain, hemoptysis, pneumothorax, fatigue, weight loss, and fever. Extrapulmonary symptoms include bone lesions and diabetes insipidus. Cystic bone lesions are present in 4%–20% of patients and may produce localized pain and/or a pathologic bone fracture. Any bone may be involved, with the calvarium, ribs, and femur being the most common sites, and the lesions are usually solitary. Histologically, they are composed of foamy vacuolated histiocytes with variable numbers of eosinophils, neutrophils, lymphocytes, and plasma cells. Diabetes insipidus is seen approximately 15% of patients and is due to hypothalamic infiltration. Diabetes insipidus is associated with a worse prognosis.

Laboratory Findings

Pulmonary interstitial lung disease occurs in approximately 20% of patients with eosinophilic granuloma. Chest radiographs demonstrate an alveolar pattern in an early state. This may be followed by 3–10 mm nodular shadows or a reticulonodular pattern with a predilection for the apices. Fibrosis and honeycombing may also ensue. Chest HRCT reveals multiple nodules and/or cysts. Honeycombing is seen in advanced disease. Histologically, eosinophils are present in the lesions; however, they are not present in BALF specimens. Pulmonary function tests in patients with PLCH are variable, with the most common finding being decreased DLCO. Lung volumes are typically normal or increased and demonstrate a restrictive, obstructive, or mixed pattern.

Table 65.5 Characteristics of Eosinophilic Granuloma (Pulmonary Langerhans Cell Histiocytosis)

Characteristic	Eosinophilic Granuloma
Ages	Children and adults 20–40 years
Sex	Male:Female equal
Smoking risk	Yes
Pulmonary symptoms	Nonproductive cough, dyspnea, chest pain, hemoptysis, pneumothorax, fatigue, weight loss, fever
Extrapulmonary symptoms	Cystic bone lesion 4%–20% of patients. Localized pain, pathologic bone fracture Diabetes insipidus 15% of patients
PE	Typically unremarkable. Rales and digital clubbing may be present
Chest radiograph HRCT scan	Alveolar pattern, 3–10 mm nodular/ reticulonodular pattern affecting apices, fibrosis, honeycombing
PFT	Variable
DLCO	Decreased
Lung biopsy	Eosinophils present in lesions
BALF	Eosinophils absent
Blood eosinophilia	Normal
IgE level	Elevated in some
Treatment	Smoking cessation Curettage single lesion corticosteroids ± vinblastine, mercaptopurine, etoposide, methotrexate

BALF, Bronchoalveolar lavage fluid; *DLCO*, diffusing capacity carbon monoxide; *HRCT*, high-resolution computed tomography; *PE*, physical examination; *PFT*, pulmonary function testing.

TREATMENT AND MANAGEMENT

In the context of Langerhans cell histiocytosis, the intensity of treatment depends on whether the patient has single-system or multisystem disease.[214] In single-system disease, there is unifocal or multifocal involvement of one organ, such as skin, lymph node(s), or bone. The Histiocyte

Society has initiated treatment protocols of LCH. Treatment options include single-agent corticosteroids, combination of corticosteroids plus vinblastine, or curettage of bone lesions, and topical therapy such as nitrogen mustard or PUVA for skin lesions. In multisystem disease, ≥2 organs or systems are involved with or without the involvement of "risk organs." Risk organs include the bone marrow, liver, spleen, and central nervous system, which denote a worse prognosis. Chemotherapy is the treatment of multisystem disease, using chemotherapeutic medications, such as prednisone, vinblastine, mercaptopurine, etoposide, and methotrexate. Other treatments include monoclonal antibodies that target CD1a or CD207, cytokine inhibitors, and 2-chlorodeoxyadenosine. In addition, there are new treatment protocols in clinical trials.

In the treatment of isolated pulmonary eosinophilic granuloma, smoking cessation is recommended. Immunosuppressive treatment with corticosteroids and cytotoxic drugs, such as cladribine (2-chlorodeoxyadenosine), a chemotherapeutic agent cytotoxic for lymphocyte and monocyte cells, are used.

PROGNOSIS

The overall prognosis for patients with pulmonary eosinophilic granuloma is good, with a 5-year survival greater than 75%.[215,224,225] However, the natural history is variable with some patients progressing to end-stage pulmonary fibrosis. The major causes of death in PLCH are respiratory failure from progressive disease and malignancy.

Helminth Associated Eosinophilic Lung Disease

Helminth associated eosinophilic lung diseases can be characterized based on their natural life cycle or history of the parasites (see Box 65.5).[226–233] Infection in humans may occur by ingestion of eggs or larvae, penetration of skin by larvae, or inoculation of larvae by biting insects. Eosinophilic inflammation is a host response mechanism to resist these infections. Helminth infections may also lead to elevated serum IgE levels and a dominant Th2 cytokine profile. In developing countries, this Th2 response to parasites may decrease expression of asthma and allergic diseases. The lungs may be affected by transpulmonary passage of helminth larvae, hematogenous seeding with helminth larvae, and pulmonary parenchymal invasion with helminthes. Hematogenous seeding with helminth larvae may be further divided into cutaneous visceral migrans, visceral larva migrans, and disseminated disease.

In transpulmonary passage, the helminth larvae have as part of their life-cycle infecting larvae that pass through the lungs entering via the blood stream. The larvae penetrate into the alveoli and then the ascending airway to transit down the esophagus into the small intestines. In the intestines, the larvae mature and become adult worms. The nematodes that cause Löffler syndrome are *Ascaris lumbricoides,* the hookworms *Ancylostoma duodenale* and *Necator americanus,* and *Strongyloide stercoralis.*[227,228] In hematogenous seeding, there is heavy hematogenous infection by helminth larvae or eggs causing eosinophilic pneumonitis. The etiologic

helminths include nonhuman *Ascaris* and hookworms, which cause cutaneous larva migrans; *Toxocara canis,* which causes visceral larva migrans; *Trichinella spiralis; Schistosoma;* and disseminated *Strongyloides.*[229,233] In pulmonary parenchymal invasion, human infection is acquired by eating freshwater crab or crawfish. The larvae penetrate the wall of the intestine and migrate through the diaphragm to reach the lungs. Pulmonary infection may be asymptomatic or cause a chronic cough producing blood-streaked sputum. Eosinophilia is common. Pulmonary paragonimiasis is diagnosed by identification of eggs in the stool or sputum specimens. In tropical pulmonary eosinophilia, infection is acquired through insect bites, during which larvae are transmitted. Migration of microfilariae to the lungs causes eosinophilic pneumonitis manifested by wheezing, cough, chest pain, pulmonary infiltrates, and eosinophilia. Diagnosis is established by identification of microfilaria in blood or urine specimens. Tropical pulmonary eosinophilia is caused by *Wucheria bancrofti* and *Brugia malayi.*[227,228] This is described in greater detail in Chapter 33.

Churg-Strauss Syndrome (Eosinophilic Granulomatosis With Polyangiitis)

ETIOLOGY

CSS is also called eosinophilic granulomatosis with polyangiitis and allergic angiitis and granulomatosis because of its association in patients with asthma, allergic rhinitis and sinusitis, and with its findings of eosinophilic vasculitis and granulomatous lesions (Box 65.6).[234–246] Nearly all patients have allergic rhinitis and pansinusitis. Three phases have been described in CSS. The first phase involves development of asthma with variable severity, typically in adults. Tapering of systemic corticosteroid treatment of asthma may unmask CSS.[238,239] This has been reported as a risk in asthmatic patients treated with omalizumab when prednisone is decreased or discontinued. The second phase is characterized by the development of peripheral blood eosinophilia and eosinophilic tissue infiltrates. The third phase involves eosinophilic vasculitis of extrapulmonary organs, typically skin, gastrointestinal tract, heart, and nervous system.

EPIDEMIOLOGY

In a population-based study of asthma, the incidence of CSS was 34.6 per million person-years.[247] This was based on identification of 21 cases of CSS from medical records of 184,667 adult asthmatics being treated with ≥3 asthma medications in three managed care organizations.

CLINICAL FEATURES

Symptoms and Physical Findings

CSS may involve multiple organ systems, including pulmonary, cutaneous, cardiac, gastrointestinal, hematologic, and peripheral and central nervous system (see Box 65.6). Pulmonary symptoms are present in nearly all patients.[234–242]

Box 65.6   Characteristics of Churg-Strauss Syndrome (Eosinophilic Granulomatosis With Polyangiitis)

Findings

- History of asthma
- Pulmonary
  - Patchy, transient infiltrates
  - Eosinophilic infiltration of alveoli, interstitium, blood vessels
  - Necrotizing and nonnecrotizing granuloma
  - Eosinophilic angiitis
- Systemic vasculitis involving ≥2 extrapulmonary organs
  - Eosinophilic vasculitis of small and medium-size arteries and veins
  - Eosinophilic granulomas
- Nasal symptoms
  - Allergic rhinitis
  - Pansinusitis
- Cutaneous
  - Maculopapular rash
  - Petechiae, purpura, ecchymosis
  - Cutaneous and subcutaneous nodules on scalp and extremities
  - Cardiac
  - Hypertension
  - Pericarditis
  - Heart failure
- Gastrointestinal
  - Abdominal pain
  - Diarrhea
  - Bleeding
  - Obstruction
- Peripheral neuropathy
  - Mononeuritis multiplex
  - Polyneuropathy
- Central nervous system
  - Cerebral infarction
- Hematologic
  - >1500 eosinophils/μL
- Radiologic
  - Chest X-ray: Transient pulmonary infiltrates
  - HRCT: Airspace consolidation or ground-glass appearance, septal lines, bronchial wall thickening

HRCT, High-resolution computed tomography.

This is manifested by worsening of asthma and poorly controlled asthma. Recurrent sinusitis with nasal polyposis is commonly seen. Pulmonary function tests demonstrate primarily an obstructive pattern consistent with the underlying asthma. With lung parenchymal involvement of CSS, a restrictive pattern coincides with airflow obstruction, decreased pulse oximetry, and decreased DLCO. Cutaneous lesions are common, occurring in 70% of patients, variably manifesting as maculopapular rashes, petechiae, purpura and/or ecchymoses, and cutaneous and subcutaneous nodules of the scalp or extremities.[242] Peripheral neuropathies occur in up to 75% of CSS patients, including mononeuritis multiplex and polyneuropathies.[241] Cerebral infarctions may occur and can be a cause of death. Eosinophilic lymphadenopathy has been noted in 30%–40% of patients. Cardiac involvement is a common cause of death and occurs in a third of patients. Gastrointestinal problems include abdominal

pain (59%), diarrhea (33%), bleeding (18%), obstruction, and colitis, and may precede or coincide with the vasculitic phase of CSS.[234-238]

Laboratory Findings

Eosinophilia ≥1500 cells/mm^3 is uniformly present.[234-238] Patchy and transient pulmonary infiltrates are seen on chest radiographs.[245] Chest HRCT reveals a variety of findings, which include airspace consolidation or interstitial ground-glass opacities, septal lines, and bronchial wall thickening.[244] Lung biopsy specimens demonstrate extensive eosinophil infiltration present in the interstitium, air spaces, and perivascular spaces.[234,235,244-246] In addition, both necrotizing and nonnecrotizing granulomas may be present, involving blood vessels. The angiitis varies from eosinophilic infiltration of blood vessels to necrotizing vasculitis of small- and medium-sized vessels. Biopsies of the cutaneous nodules reveal eosinophilic infiltration. Antineutrophil cytoplasmic antibodies (ANCA) are found in 40–60% of patients with CSS. The majority of ANCA-positivity is directed against myeloperoxidase (MPO), with a perinuclear staining pattern (MPO-ANCA or P-ANCA). ANCA positivity is associated typically with renal involvement, peripheral neuropathy, and systemic vasculitis.

MANAGEMENT AND TREATMENT

The treatment of CSS is divided into induction of remission and maintenance of remission.[234-238] Induction of remission is achieved with a combination of high-dose glucocorticoids, prednisone 1 mg/kg per day (maximum 60 mg), and cyclophosphamide 2 mg/kg per day (maximum 200 mg/day) for patients with generalized disease, such as renal or other life-threatening disease. For localized disease, prednisone alone may suffice. For patients with nonlife-threatening systemic involvement from pANC-associated vasculitis, methotrexate may be substituted for cyclophosphamide. Treatment with a combination of low-dose prednisone plus azathioprine or methotrexate for ≥18 months is used to maintain remission. If left untreated, the mortality is significant, as high as 50% in the first 3 months after the onset of vasculitis. In treated patients, the mean survival is 9 years.

In 2010, Kim et al.[248] reported the results of an open-label pilot study treating seven CSS patients with mepolizumab, anti-IL-5 monoclonal antibody. The patients received 4 monthly doses of mepolizumab 750 mg intravenously. Mepolizumab resulted in reduced eosinophilia, and allowed for reduction of corticosteroid dosages. CSS symptoms recurred on cessation of mepolizumab, necessitating corticosteroid bursts. However, as a proof of concept, mepolizumab was safe and effective in the treatment of CSS. Further studies of prolonged use of mepolizumab should be performed.

PROGNOSIS

Prognosis of CSS depends upon recognition of the disease, initiation of early treatment, and the presence or absence of extrapulmonary organ involvement, such as cardiac failure, myocardial infarction, cerebral hemorrhage, renal failure, or gastrointestinal bleeding. Samson et al.[249] reported on the long-term outcome of 118 patients with CSS. Seventy-four patients had only pulmonary involvement and were treated with corticosteroids alone, while 44 patients had extrapulmonary involvement as well and were treated with corticosteroids plus cyclophosphamide. Overall survival was 90% at 7 years, regardless of extrapulmonary involvement. In the future, mepolizumab treatment may improve on the prognosis.

Hypereosinophilic Syndrome

EPIDEMIOLOGY

The term *hypereosinophilic syndrome (HES)* encompasses a group of rare disorders characterized by increased eosinophil count in peripheral blood and end-organ damage caused by eosinophilic inflammation. The incidence and prevalence are not well characterized. The Surveillance, Epidemiology, and End Results (SEER) database estimated the age-adjusted incidence from 2001 to 2005 to be approximately 0.036 per 100,000.[250]

ETIOLOGY

HES was first defined by Chusid et al.[251] in 1975 and specified the following three criteria for diagnosis: (1) absolute eosinophil count ≥1500/mm³ in peripheral blood for greater than 6 months; (2) lack of evidence for parasitic, allergic, and other recognized causes of eosinophilia; and (3) end-organ dysfunction due to eosinophilic infiltration. Tissue hypereosinophilia is defined as greater than 20% eosinophils of all nucleated cells on bone marrow examination or eosinophil tissue infiltration that is extensive, or marked deposition of eosinophil granule proteins in tissue. It is now recognized that HES represents a spectrum of disorders that includes not only the previously described idiopathic HES (IHES) but also disorders characterized by eosinophilic organ infiltration that may or may not be accompanied by peripheral blood eosinophilia, such as eosinophilic pneumonia, eosinophil-associated gastrointestinal disorders (EGID), CSS, and eosinophilic dermatitis (Wells syndrome).[252–254] A revised classification of HES was presented in 2006 by Klion et al.[255] This classification system was the culmination of a workshop conducted by the Hypereosinophilic Diseases Working Group of the International Eosinophil Society, with the intent of allowing accurate identification of the causes of hypereosinophilia, which in turn guides the clinical management of these patients.

In 2011, the Working Conference on Eosinophil Disorders and Syndromes proposed a new terminology for eosinophilic syndrome.[256] The panel recommended the term "hypereosinophilia" (HE) for persistent and marked eosinophilia (absolute eosinophil count >1500/mm³). HE subtypes were further divided into hereditary variant, HE of undetermined significance (in place of idiopathic hypereosinophilia), primary (clonal/neoplastic) HE produced by clonal/neoplastic eosinophils, and secondary or reactive HE. Any HE associated with organ damage is referred to as HES with specific subscripts in each category.

The classification of eosinophilic diseases was revised in the 2008 World Health Organization scheme of myeloid neoplasms (Box 65.7).[257] In recognition of the growing list of recurrent, molecularly defined primary eosinophilia

---

Box 65.7 World Health Organization Classification of Myeloid Malignancies

Acute Myeloid Leukemia and Related Disorders

Myeloproliferative Neoplasms

- Chronic myelogenous leukemia, BCR-ABL1 positive
- Chronic neutrophilic leukemia
- Polycythemia vera
- Primary myelofibrosis
- Essential thrombocythemia
- Chronic eosinophilic leukemia, not otherwise specified
- Mastocytosis
- Myeloproliferative neoplasms, unclassifiable

Myelodysplastic Syndromes

- Refractory cytopenia with uni-lineage dysplasia
- Refractory anemia
- Refractory neutropenia
- Refractory thrombocytopenia
- Refractory anemia with ring sideroblasts
- Refractory cytopenia with multilineage dysplasia
- RAEB
- RAEB-1
- RAEB-2
- Myelodysplastic syndrome with isolated del(5q)
- Myelodysplastic syndrome, unclassifiable

Myelodysplastic Syndromes/Myeloproliferative Neoplasms

- CMML
- CMML-1
- CMML-2
- Atypical chronic myeloid leukemia, BCR-ABL1 negative
- Juvenile myelomonocytic leukemia
- MDS/MPN, unclassifiable
- RARS-T

Myeloid and Lymphoid Neoplasms Associated With Eosinophilia and Abnormalities of Platelet-Derived Growth Factor Receptor, Alpha Polypeptide, Platelet-Derived Growth Factor Receptor, Beta Polypeptide, or Fibroblast Growth Factor Receptor 1

- Myeloid and lymphoid neoplasms associated with PDGFRA rearrangement
- Myeloid neoplasms associated with PDGFRB rearrangement
- Myeloid and lymphoid neoplasms associated with FGFR1 abnormalities

CMML, Chronic myelomonocytic leukemia; *FGFR1,* fibroblast growth factor receptor 1; *MDS,* myelodysplastic syndromes; *MPN,* myeloproliferative neoplasms; *PDGFRA,* platelet-derived growth factor receptor, alpha polypeptide; *PDGFRB,* platelet-derived growth factor receptor, beta polypeptide; *RAEB,* Refractory anemia with excess blasts; *RARS-T,* refractory anemia with ring sideroblasts and thrombocytosis.

Modified from Bain BJ. The idiopathic hypereosinophilic syndrome and eosinophilic leukemias. Haematologica. 2004;89(2):133-137.

---

disorders, a new major category was created: myeloid and lymphoid neoplasms with eosinophilia and abnormalities of platelet-derived growth factor receptor alpha (PDGFRA), platelet-derived growth factor receptor beta (PDGFRB), or fibroblast growth factor receptor 1 (FGFR1). Chronic eosinophilic leukemia—not otherwise specified (CEL-NOS) is one of eight disease entities within the group of myeloproliferative neoplasms (MPN), as classified in the 2008 WHO

Box 65.8 Criteria for Chronic Eosinophilic Leukemia, Not Otherwise Specified

Eosinophilia (eosinophil count >1.5×10^9/L)

No Philadelphia chromosome or BCR-ABL fusion gene or other myeloproliferative neoplasms (PV, ET, PMF, systemic mastocytosis) or MDS/MPN (CMML or atypical CML)

No t(5;12)(q31_q35;p13) or other rearrangement of PDGFRB

No FIP1L1-PDGFRA fusion gene or other rearrangement of PDGFRA

No rearrangement of FGFR1

Blast cell count in the peripheral blood and bone marrow is <20% and there is no inv(16)(p13q22) or t(16;16)(p13;q22) or other feature diagnostic of AML

Clonal cytogenetic or molecular genetic abnormality, or blast cells are >2% in the peripheral blood or >5% in the bone marrow

AML, Acute myeloid leukemia; *BCR-ABL fusion gene,* Abelson (Abl) tyrosine kinase gene at chromosome 9 and the break point cluster (Bcr); *CEL-NOS,* chronic eosinophilic leukemia, not otherwise specified; *CML,* chronic myeloid leukemia; *CMML,* chronic myelomonocytic leukemia; *FIP1L1,* factor interacting with PAPOLA and CPSF1.; *PDGFRA,* platelet-derived growth factor receptor, alpha polypeptide; *PDGFRB,* platelet-derived growth factor receptor, beta polypeptide.

Classification. CEL-NOS is defined by the absence of the Philadelphia chromosome or a rearrangement involving PDGFRA/B and FGFR1, and the exclusion of other acute or chronic primary marrow neoplasms associated with eosinophilia, such as acute myeloid leukemia (AML), myelodysplastic syndrome (MDS), systemic mastocytosis (SM), the classic MPNs (chronic myeloid leukemia, polycythemia vera, essential thrombocythemia, and primary myelofibrosis), and MDS/MPN overlap disorders (e.g., chronic myelomonocytic leukemia, CMML; Box 65.8). CEL-NOS is characterized histologically by an increase in blasts in the bone marrow or blood (but fewer than 20% to exclude acute leukemia as a diagnosis), and/or evidence for clonality in the eosinophil lineage.[258] A diagnosis of idiopathic HES requires exclusion of all primary and secondary causes of hypereosinophilia, as well as lymphocyte-variant hypereosinophilia, with persistence of elevated absolute eosinophil count (AEC) greater than 1500/mm³ and tissue damage from eosinophil infiltration.[256] For the purposes of clinical management, it remains useful to think of HES in the following clinical categories: myeloproliferative (now classified as chronic eosinophilic leukemia NOS in the 2008 WHO classification), lymphocytic, familial, idiopathic, overlap (blood eosinophilia ≥1500/mm³ with single organ involvement), and associated (blood eosinophilia ≥1500/mm³ in association with a distinct second diagnosis, such as inflammatory bowel disease; Box 65.9).

PATHOLOGY/PATHOGENESIS

There appear to be two mechanisms that account for the hypereosinophilia seen in HES: (1) clonal eosinophilic proliferation as a result of a primary molecular defect(s) involving hematopoietic stem cells or defects in signal transduction from the receptors that mediate bone marrow eosinophil differentiation, and (2) reactive processes, which often involve overproduction of eosinophil activation cytokines, such as IL-5.[259]

CLINICAL FEATURES

Symptoms and Physical Findings

Overall HES is more common in males, mainly due to the fact that the majority of patients with the FIP1L1-PDGFRA myeloproliferative variant are males. In the SEER database, incidence was noted to increase with age with a peak noted between 65 and 74 years.[259] HES is uncommon but has been reported in the pediatric age group.

The clinical presentation of HES can be variable and is influenced by the underlying pathophysiology. The onset of symptoms of HES is often insidious. Common presenting symptoms include fatigue, cough, dyspnea, myalgia, rash, and retinal lesions. HES may affect and damage many organs, including cardiac, cutaneous, neurologic, pulmonary, splenic, hepatic, ocular, and gastrointestinal. Cardiac involvement is the major cause of mortality in patients with HES. Eosinophilic granules and mediators are deposited on the endocardium, resulting in myocardial degeneration and fibrosis.[260] Cardiac disease is characterized by eosinophilic endocardial myelofibrosis, cardiomyopathy, valvular disease, or mural thrombus formation. Serum tryptase levels are often elevated and splenomegaly present. Pulmonary disease affects up to 49% of patients with HES, and typical symptoms are a chronic nonproductive cough. Asthma is not usually present. Pulmonary infiltrates may develop and may be focal or diffuse. Pulmonary fibrosis may develop. CSS may also occur as an associated variant of HES.

The myeloproliferative variant or "classic" HES presents with features of myeloproliferative disease (i.e., hepatosplenomegaly, cytopenias, circulating myeloid precursors, as well as increased bone marrow cellularity).[261] Elevated serum vitamin B12 or tryptase levels may be seen. There is a strong adult male preponderance, though children can also be affected. Eosinophilic endomyocardial disease and mucosal ulcers are common. Eosinophilic granules and mediators are deposited on the endocardium, resulting in myocardial degeneration and fibrosis.[262–265] This form of HES is thought to arise from a mutation in the hematopoietic stem cell that results in clonal expansion, predominantly of eosinophils. The majority of these patients have a cryptic interstitial deletion on chromosome 4q12 that results in the formation of a fusion protein FIP1L1-PDGFRA that brings together the FIP1L1 and the gene for the cytoplasmic domains of the PDGFRα receptor. This gene fusion results in the formation of a constitutively active tyrosine kinase that is responsible for clonal expansion of eosinophils.[266–268] Other cytogenetic abnormalities that involve PDGFRB and fibroblast growth factor receptor have been reported in patients presenting with the myeloproliferative form of HES. This category also includes HES with features of myeloproliferative disease without proof of clonality as well as chronic eosinophilic leukemia, as defined in the WHO classification.[258]

The lymphoproliferative subtype of HES is characterized by polyclonal expansion of eosinophils, usually in response to chemokines like IL-5 produced by dysregulated T-cells. These cells have a characteristic immunophenotype (CD4+CD3– or CD3+CD4–CD8–) and may show monoclonal or polyclonal expansion. Cutaneous manifestations are common in this group of patients. Some may progress to an overt T-cell lymphoma. The undefined subtype comprises asymptomatic eosinophilia, necrotizing eosinophilic vasculitis, episodic

Box 65.9 Hypereosinophilic Syndromes

Myeloproliferative Variants (M-HES)

- Myoproliferative HES, etiology unknown
  - Features of myeloproliferative disease without proof of clonality
  - FIP1L1-PDGFRA fusion negative
  - Dysplastic eosinophils on peripheral smear
  - Serum vitamin B12 >1000 pg/ml
  - Serum tryptase >12
  - Anemia and/or thrombocytopenia
  - Hepatosplenomegaly
  - Bone marrow cellularity >80%
  - Spindle shaped mast cells
  - Myelofibrosis
  - PDGFRA associated HES
  - Deletion on 4q12 leading to FIP1L1-PDGFRA fusion
- Chronic eosinophilic leukemia (CEL) HES
  - CEL with cytogenetic abnormalities and/or blasts on peripheral smear
- Other gene mutations
  - PDGFRA or PDGFRB rearrangements
  - PDGFRB and FGFR1 rearrangements
  - JAK2 point mutation and translocation

T Lymphocytic Variant (L-HES)

- Usually a benign lymphoproliferative disorder, but may progress to T cell lymphoma
  - Polyclonal hypergammaglobulinemia
  - Prominent skin findings (including plaques, erythroderma, urticaria)
  - Aberrant IL-5 producing T cells
  - Increased serum TARC levels

Familial HES

- Asymptomatic eosinophilia from birth, autosomal dominant
  - Progression may occur
  - Mapped to chromosome 5q 31-33

Undefined HES

- Benign
  - Asymptomatic with no evidence of organ involvement
- Complex
  - Organ dysfunction, but does not meet criteria for myeloproliferative or lymphocytic variants
- Episodic (Gleich syndrome)
  - Cyclical angioedema, urticarial, fever, weight gain, oliguria, and eosinophilia
  - Increased serum IgM
  - Increased serum IL-5

Overlap HES (Organ-Restricted HES)

- Eosinophilia associated with eosinophilic infiltration and associated signs/symptoms in a single organ
  - Eosinophil-associated gastrointestinal disease
  - Eosinophilic pneumonia
  - Eosinophilia myalgia syndrome
  - Other organ restricted eosinophilic disorders

Associated HES

- Marked eosinophilia in the setting of an underlying disorder associated with eosinophilia:
  - Churg-Strauss syndrome
  - Systemic mastocytosis
  - Inflammatory bowel disease
  - Sarcoidosis
  - HIV
  - Other disorders

FGFR1, Fibroblast growth factor receptor 1; *FIP1L1*, Fip1-like1; *HES*, hypereosinophilic syndromes; *IL-5*, interleukin-5; *JAK2*, Janus kinase 2; *L-HES*, lymphocytic variant HES; *PDGFRA*, platelet-derived growth factor receptor alpha; *PDGFRB*, platelet-derived growth factor receptor beta; *TARC*, thymus and activation-regulated chemokine.
Adapted from Simon HU, Rothenberg ME, Bochner BS, Weller PF, Wardlaw AJ, Wechsler ME, Rosenwasser LJ, Roufosse F, Gleich GJ, Klion AD. Refining the definition of hypereosinophilic syndrome. J Allergy Clin Immunol. 2010;126(1):45-49.

angioedema with eosinophilia, and other symptomatic forms of eosinophilia that do not have features of the myeloproliferative or lymphocytic forms.[254,255] It is possible that patients with these forms of HES, as well as those with the overlapping or associated HES, have dysregulated IL-5 producing T-lymphocytes as well.

Laboratory Findings

The evaluation of patients with hypereosinophilia should begin with a meticulous search for triggering factors—drug history, travel history and habitat, history of allergies, and exclusion of underlying malignancy or collagen vascular disease. Careful assessment of organ function to evaluate eosinophil mediated organ damage is critical.[259] In the absence of underlying disease or if features of myeloproliferative disease are present, patients with HES should be referred to hematology/oncology for complete evaluation to exclude malignancies, which includes bone marrow examination, radiological imaging to exclude lymphoma, as well as

exclusion of a cytogenetic abnormality by TCR gene rearrangement and RT-PCR or FISH for FIP1L1-PDGFRA. Plasma cytokine levels, especially IL-5, should be measured as should serum tryptase, though these may be elevated in both the myeloproliferative and lymphocytic forms of HES.[269]

MANAGEMENT AND TREATMENT

Control of the eosinophilia is important to prevent organ damage from deposition of eosinophilic mediators. Corticosteroids have been the mainstay of treatment and remain the first-line treatment for FIP1L1-PDGFRA negative HES. Imatinib mesylate (Gleevec 100–400 mg/day) is a tyrosine kinase inhibitor that targets the fusion protein FIP1L1-PDGFRA[266–268] and now constitutes the treatment of choice for the FIP1L1-PDGFRA positive myeloproliferative variant of HES. Dramatic clinical responses to imatinib are described in FIP1L1-PDGFRA-positive HES, with eosinophilia resolving within a 1 week period and reversal of organ dysfunction as early as

1 month. Other myeloproliferative variants that are negative for the FIP1L1-PDGFRA fusion protein may also respond to imatinib.[268] Other drugs, including azathioprine, cyclosporine A, and hydroxyurea, have been used in conjunction with corticosteroids or as steroid sparing agents, particularly for the lymphocytic variant of HES.[268] These patients need careful monitoring for development of a lymphoid malignancy. Immunomodulatory therapy with IFN-α and monoclonal antibody to IL-5 (mepolizumab) has also been described. In two recent reports, patients with HES were treated with three doses of antibody to IL-5.[269,270] Blood eosinophils declined by 10-fold and were sustained for 12 weeks after the last dose of antibody to IL-5. The anti-CD52 monoclonal antibody alemtuzumab has been used to successfully treat patients with HES, with complete hematologic responses seen in up to 80% of patients.[271-273] Allogeneic stem cell transplant has been used for patients with aggressive disease, with disease-free survival ranging from 8 months to 5 years.[273,274]

PROGNOSIS

The prognosis of HES or HE depends on the underlying pathophysiology as well as the extent of organ damage. With greater understanding of the cellular and molecular basis of eosinophilia, the treatment of hypereosinophilic disorders is no longer limited to corticosteroids alone. The identification of clonal cytogenetic abnormalities identifies a subset of patients who respond dramatically to imatinib.[266-268] Elucidation of the drivers of eosinophil proliferation may help identify patients who respond to other targeted therapies, including monoclonal antibodies. The overall aim of treatment remains to limit end organ damage from persistent eosinophilia.

References

Access the reference list online at ExpertConsult.com.

Suggested Reading

Agarwal R, Chakrabarti A, Shah A, et al. ABPA complicating asthma ISHAM working group. Allergic bronchopulmonary aspergillosis: review of literature and proposal of new diagnostic and classification criteria. *Clin Exp Allergy*. 2013;43(8):850–873.

Agarwal R, Gupta D, Aggarwal AN, et al. Clinical significance of hyperattenuating mucoid impaction in allergic bronchopulmonary aspergillosis: an analysis of 155 patients. *Chest*. 2007;132(4):1183–1190.

Agarwal R, Khan A, Gupta D, et al. An alternate method of classifying allergic bronchopulmonary aspergillosis based on high-attenuation mucus. *PLoS ONE*. 2010;5(12):e15346.

Allen JN. Drug-induced eosinophilic lung disease. *Clin Chest Med*. 2004;25(1):77–88.

Allen JN, Pacht ER, Gadek JE, et al. Acute eosinophilic pneumonia as a reversible cause of noninfectious respiratory failure. *N Engl J Med*. 1989;321(9):569–574.

Bain B. The idiopathic hypereosinophilic syndrome and eosinophilic leukemias. *Haematologica*. 2004;89(2):133–137.

Baxter CG, Dunn G, Jones AM, et al. Novel immunologic classification of aspergillosis in adult cystic fibrosis. *J Allergy Clin Immunol*. 2013;132(3):560–566.

Crane MM, Chang CM, Kobayashi MG, et al. Incidence of myeloproliferative hypereosinophilic syndrome in the United States and an estimate of all hypereosinophilic syndrome incidence. *J Allergy Clin Immunol*. 2010;126(1):179–181.

Garcia LS. Classification and nomenclature of human parasites. In: Mandell GL, Bennett JE, Dolin R, eds. *Mandell, Douglas, and Bennett's Principles and Practice of Infectious Diseases*. 7th ed. Philadelphia: Churchill Livingstone; 2010:2654–2660.

Gleich GJ, Leiferman KM. The hypereosinophilic syndromes: still more heterogeneity. *Curr Opin Immunol*. 2005;17(6):679–684.

Greenberger Lacy P, Adamko DJ, Odemuyiwas SO. Biology of eosinophils. In: Adkinson NF Jr, Yunginger JW, Busse WW, et al, eds. *Allergic Bronchopulmonary Aspergillosis*. J Allergy Clin Immunol Pract 2014;2(6):703–708.

Katzenstein AL. Diagnostic features and differential diagnosis of Churg-Strauss syndrome in the lung. A review. *Am J Clin Pathol*. 2000;114(5):767–772.

Klion AD. Recent advances in the diagnosis and treatment of hypereosinophilic syndromes. *Hematology*. 2005;209–214.

Klion AD, Bochner BS, Gleich GJ, et al. Approaches to the treatment of hypereosinophilic syndromes: a workshop summary report. *J Allergy Clin Immunol*. 2006;117(6):1292–1302.

Knutsen AP, Bush RK, Demain JG, et al. Fungi and allergic lower respiratory tract disease. *J Allergy Clin Immunol*. 2012;129(2):280–291.

Knutsen AP, Slavin RG. Allergic bronchopulmonary aspergillosis in asthma and cystic fibrosis. *Clin Dev Immunol*. 2011;2011:843763.

Mirković B, Lavelle GM, Azim AA. The basophil surface marker CD203c identifies Aspergillus species sensitization in patients with cystic fibrosis. *J Allergy Clin Immunol*. 2016;137(2):436–443.

Mochimaru H, Kawamoto M, Fukuda Y, et al. Clinicopathological differences between acute and chronic eosinophilic pneumonia. *Respirology*. 2005;10(1):76–85.

Moqbel R. *Allergy: Principles & Practice*. 7th ed. Philadelphia: Mosby, Inc.; 2009:295–310.

Philit F, Etienne-Mastroïanni B, Parrot A, et al. Idiopathic acute eosinophilic pneumonia: a study of 22 patients. *Am J Respir Crit Care Med*. 2002;166(9):1235–1239.

Satter EK, High WA. Langerhans cell histiocytosis: a review of the current recommendations of the Histiocyte Society. *Pediatr Dermatol*. 2008;25(3):291–295.

Selman M, Buendía-Roldán I. Immunopathology, diagnosis, and management of hypersensitivity pneumonitis. *Semin Respir Crit Care Med*. 2012;33(5):543–554.

Spagnolo P, Rossi G, Cavazza A, et al. Hypersensitivity pneumonitis: a comprehensive review. *J Invest Allergol Clin Immunol*. 2015;25(4):237–250.

Valent P, Klion AD, Horny HP, et al. Contemporary consensus proposal on criteria and classification of eosinophilic disorders and related syndromes. *J Allergy Clin Immunol*. 2012;130(3):607–612.

66 Respiratory Disorders in Human Immunodeficiency Virus–Infected Children and Adolescents

HEATHER J. ZAR, MBBCh, FCPaeds, FRCP (Edinburgh), PhD, and
DIANE GRAY, MBChB, FRACP, PhD

Respiratory disease is the most common complication occurring in human immunodeficiency virus (HIV)-infected children. Prior to widespread use of antiretroviral therapy (ART), acute respiratory infection was a major cause of mortality and morbidity in HIV-infected children with chronic lung disease, a common sequelae.[1] Revised World Health Organization (WHO) guidelines now recommend ART initiation early in all children and adolescents, with a particular focus on infants.[2] The use of ART early after birth or as soon as a child is diagnosed with HIV, improved diagnostics for infant HIV and better preventative and management strategies have reduced HIV-associated mortality substantially. Furthermore, with improved ART formulations for children and strengthened management strategies, pediatric HIV has evolved to become a chronic disease with long-term survival of children through adolescence and adulthood. Nevertheless, respiratory illness remains the commonest cause of morbidity in HIV-infected children and adolescents on ART.

The epidemiology of pediatric HIV has changed as access to mother to child preventative strategies has strengthened and with the increasing availability of ART. Pediatric HIV infection is predominantly a disease of sub-Saharan Africa, with most HIV-infected children currently residing in this geographical area. In 2015, there were approximately 1.8 million children under 15 years old living with HIV, of whom 89% lived in sub-Saharan Africa, and there were 150,000 new infections and 110,000 deaths among HIV-infected children.[3] Since 2000, there has been a 60% decline in new pediatric HIV infections and a 42% decline in HIV-related deaths, but scale-up of ART has been inadequate with only a third of HIV-infected children who need treatment receiving ART.[4] Many children are still diagnosed with HIV late and have limited access to therapy; among these children, acute severe respiratory infection and chronic respiratory disease are common.[5,6] Furthermore, as pediatric HIV infection has become a chronic disease, increased numbers of HIV-infected children are reaching adolescence and adulthood. Adolescent HIV has become a global health priority, with a trebling in HIV related adolescent deaths since 2000, making HIV/acquired immunodeficiency disease (AIDS) the leading cause of death among adolescents in sub-Saharan Africa and the second leading cause of death among adolescents globally. Forty percent of new adolescent infections occurred outside sub-Saharan Africa, highlighting the imperative of HIV preventive efforts.[3] Chronic lung disease in perinatally infected HIV-infected adolescents is also common.[7,8]

In areas with strong prevention of mother-to-child HIV transmission programs, the prevalence of pediatric HIV infection has fallen dramatically; however, HIV-exposed children (who are HIV-negative but born to an HIV-infected mother) have an increased risk of respiratory morbidity compared to unexposed children.[9–12] As prevention and treatment programs in underresourced areas are strengthened and become more available, this group of children will be increasingly important in considering the burden of respiratory disease.

Spectrum of Respiratory Disease

The spectrum of respiratory disorders ranges from acute infection to chronic disease (Box 66.1). A pulmonary problem may frequently be the presenting manifestation of HIV infection. Among children known to be HIV-infected, including those on ART, acute pulmonary infections are among the most common causes of poor health. Bacterial pneumonia and tuberculosis (TB) are the most common respiratory infections in both ART-naïve and ART-exposed children.

Acute Respiratory Disease

LOWER RESPIRATORY TRACT INFECTION OR PNEUMONIA

HIV-infected children have a much higher risk of developing pneumonia and of severe disease or mortality compared to HIV-uninfected children, with a sixfold higher rate of hospitalization or death.[13] The most common respiratory infections in ART-naïve children are episodes of bacterial pneumonia (which comprise approximately 25% of all opportunistic infections [OIs] in such children) or pulmonary tuberculosis (PTB) comprising around 10% of all OIs.[14] Extrapulmonary TB (EPTB) also occurs commonly in around 7% of OIs; pneumocystis pneumonia (PCP) occurs in 4% of OIs. In children on ART, OIs due to bacterial pneumonia, PTB, EPTB, or PCP were reported to comprise 22%, 4%, 1%, and 2.5%, respectively, of all OIs. The effect of ART in reducing these infections is most marked for EPTB (85% reduction), PTB (60% reduction), and PCP (30% reduction); however, for bacterial pneumonia, the impact is more modest with a 15% reduction.[14]

Box 66.1 Pulmonary Complications of Human Immunodeficiency Virus Infection

Acute Lung Disease

Infections
  Viral
  Bacterial
  Mycobacterial
  Fungal
  Mixed infections

Chronic Lung Disease

Chronic infection
Interstitial pneumonia
  Lymphoid interstitial pneumonia
  Nonspecific interstitial pneumonitis
  Desquamative interstitial pneumonia
Malignancies
  Kaposi sarcoma
  Lymphoma
Immune reconstitution inflammatory syndrome
Bronchiectasis
Bronchiolitis obliterans
Aspiration pneumonitis
Airway hyperresponsiveness/asthma
Pulmonary hypertension

Furthermore, HIV-exposed infants are at higher risk of developing pneumonia or other respiratory diseases compared to HIV-unexposed children.[10–12,15] Exposure in utero to HIV viral proteins, a maternal proinflammatory and/or immune compromised state, exposure to ART and other drugs both in utero and in breast milk, reduced levels of protective maternal antibodies or increased exposure to infections in a HIV-household may contribute to this susceptibility.[12,16,17] In addition, HIV-exposed or infected children living in sub-Saharan Africa often have exposure to several other risk factors for pneumonia or severe disease such as poor birth outcomes (preterm birth or low birth weight), suboptimal or no breastfeeding, compromised growth and nutrition, maternal ill health or death, and poverty.[12]

The highest incidence of pneumonia occurs in infancy, especially in the first 6 months of life. HIV-infected children are more susceptible to developing pneumonia from a broader spectrum of pathogens, including opportunistic pathogens such as *Pneumocystis jirovecii*, *Mycobacterium tuberculosis*, or cytomegalovirus (CMV). Coinfections with bacterial, viral, mycobacterial, or fungal pathogens may be common, with increasing numbers of pathogens associated with more severe disease.[18] However, attributing etiology may be especially difficult, as obtaining a representative specimen from the lower respiratory tract can be challenging, and sensitive diagnostic assays may not distinguish colonizing from pathogenic organisms.[19]

BACTERIAL PNEUMONIA

Bacterial pneumonia is the most common lower respiratory tract infection in both ART-naïve and ART-exposed children.[14] Bacterial pneumonia occurs more frequently and with greater severity in HIV-infected than uninfected children because of defects in both cellular and humoral immunity.[18] HIV-exposed or infected children also have a higher risk of developing severe pneumonia, with a poorer outcome than HIV-negative children.

The use of newer conjugate vaccines including pneumococcal conjugate vaccine (PCV) and *Haemophilus influenzae* b (Hib) vaccine has reduced the burden of bacterial pneumonia and bacteremia in HIV-infected and uninfected children. Prior to PCV, *Streptococcus pneumoniae* was the most commonly reported bacterial pathogen causing pneumonia and bacteremic illness, with an incidence of pneumococcal bacteremia or invasive disease that was 9 to 43-fold greater in HIV-infected compared to uninfected children.[20] *Staphylococcus aureus* has also been reported to have a higher incidence in HIV-infected children.[21] Other bacterial pathogens include *Haemophilus influenzae*, *Escherichia coli*, and *Salmonella* spp. A postmortem study of Zambian children found that bacterial pneumonia was the predominant cause of death in both HIV-infected and uninfected children; TB occurring in 8% had not been diagnosed in 90% prior to death.[22] Pneumonia associated with *Bordetella pertussis* has increasingly been reported in young infants; a study of infants hospitalized with pneumonia or apnea reported that HIV-infected infants had the highest incidence followed by HIV-exposed infants.[23] The risk of pertussis also decreased with each extra dose of vaccine received, with the lowest risk after completion of a primary three-dose schedule.

The high incidence of antimicrobial-resistant bacteria that colonize the nasopharynx may potentially cause pneumonia in HIV-infected children.[24]

The clinical symptoms or signs and radiological features of bacterial pneumonia are similar to those in HIV-negative children. Bacteremic illness occurs in a minority of cases, and induced sputum induction (obtained through nebulization of hypertonic saline) may be useful for diagnosis of *B. pertussis* by polymerase chain reaction (PCR), with a higher yield than nasopharyngeal samples.[10,23]

Treatment of bacterial pneumonia should be with broad-spectrum antimicrobials and supportive therapy including oxygen as required, which is similar to immunocompetent patients.[25] The use of case management guidelines for treatment of pneumonia, as contained in the WHO Integrated Management of Childhood Illness (IMCI) program, are effective for reducing pneumonia and all-cause mortality,[26] but these require adaptation for use in high HIV prevalence areas.[18,27] Modified IMCI guidelines for use in high HIV prevalence settings include ampicillin and gentamicin or ceftriaxone as first-line therapy for pneumonia, while cotrimoxazole (CTX) should be added for infants (Table 66.1).[25]

Immunization with PCV and Hib provides protection against specific bacterial infections, but long-term immune responses may be impaired with a shorter duration of seroprotection in HIV-infected compared to uninfected individuals even with use of ART.[28–30] Generally, children on ART have lower levels of immunity to vaccines given before treatment, but most respond to revaccination.[30] Although the efficacy of PCV for prevention of invasive pneumococcal disease and pneumonia is lower in HIV-infected children compared to uninfected children, the overall burden of disease prevented is much greater among HIV-infected children because of the higher burden of pneumococcal disease.[28] Thus, the overall vaccine-attributable reduction in invasive

Table 66.1   Antibiotic Treatment of Pneumonia in Human Immunodeficiency Virus Infected Children

Infection	First Line Therapy	Dose	Regimen
Bacterial pneumonia	If severe pneumonia, broad spectrum antibiotic β-lactam plus aminoglycoside **or** second or third generation cephalosporin	Amoxicillin 45 mg/kg per dose Ampicillin 50 mg/kg per dose Gentamicin 7.5 mg/kg Ceftriaxone 50–75 mg/kg per dose Cefotaxime 50 mg/kg per dose	Orally, twice daily for 5 days IV, 4 times daily IV, daily, for 5 days IV or IM daily IV, 3 times daily
	If *S. aureus* suspected: Cloxacillin	Cloxacillin 25 mg/kg per dose or 50 mg/kg per dose	Orally, 4 times a day IV, 4 times a day
	If methicillin resistant *S. aureus* suspected: vancomycin	Vancomycin 10–15 mg/kg	IV, 3 times daily
Cytomegalovirus	Ganciclovir for CMV	*Induction* 5 mg/kg per dose *Maintenance* Valganciclovir	Daily, 14–21 days Oral, daily
Influenza A or B	Neuraminidase inhibitor influenza A or B	Oseltamivir <9 months: 3 mg/kg 9–12 months: 3.5 mg/kg 1–12 years: <15 kg: 30 mg; 15.1–23 kg: 45 mg; 23.1–40 kg: 60 mg; >40 kg: 75 mg	Orally, 2 times daily, for 5 days
Pneumocystis jirovecii	Trimethoprim-sulfamethoxazole (TMP-SMX) Corticosteroids if hypoxic	6–12 mg of TMP Prednisone 1 mg/kg per day	IV or orally four times a day Daily for 5 days, taper dose over 10–14 days

pneumococcal disease was almost 60 times higher in HIV-infected children compared to uninfected children, while the reduction in pneumonia was 15-fold greater following PCV.[31] As most pneumococcal serotypes associated with antimicrobial resistance are included in PCV, vaccination has also been associated with a reduction in infections with antimicrobial-resistant pneumococci.[28] Pneumococcal vaccination is indicated for HIV-infected children according to the regular immunization schedule.[32] The long-term efficacy of PCV wanes in HIV-infected children who are not on ART; vaccine efficacy against invasive disease declined from 65% by 2 years post vaccination to 39% by 6 years in HIV-infected children in the absence of a booster dose, while efficacy was maintained in HIV-uninfected individuals. Reimmunization after 3–5 years is therefore recommended in children not on ART.[33] Quantitative and qualitative antibody responses to PCV in HIV-infected infants are enhanced when vaccination occurs on ART and if vaccination occurs when the CD4+ cell percentage is ≥25% and if the nadir CD4+ is greater than 15%.[34]

The Hib conjugate vaccine also has reduced efficacy in HIV-infected ART-naïve children compared to uninfected children.[29,35] However, similar to PCV, a substantial proportion of immunized children will be protected from Hib-related pneumonia or invasive disease because of the increased disease burden in HIV-infected children, with an almost sixfold higher risk of invasive disease.[29] HIV-infected children should therefore be immunized with Hib vaccine according to the routine childhood immunization schedule.

Continuing CTX prophylaxis in older children after at least 2 years on ART has been shown to reduce hospitalization in African children due to pneumonia, malaria, sepsis, or meningitis.[36] This occurred in children of all ages irrespective of CD4 count. Long-term CTX prophylaxis is therefore recommended as a strategy to prevent infections in settings with a high burden of infectious diseases. Strategies for the prevention of lower respiratory tract infections in HIV infected children are summarized in Box 66.2.

TUBERCULOSIS

The incidence of TB has increased in parallel with the HIV epidemic. Epidemiologically, both TB and HIV have the highest prevalence in sub-Saharan Africa; HIV predisposes to TB disease, while infection with *M. tuberculosis* worsens immunosuppression and hastens progression to AIDS. Children living in a household with an HIV-infected adult are more likely to be exposed to TB.[37,38] Moreover, HIV-infected children progress more rapidly to disease or disseminated illness following infection. Mortality from TB is also higher in HIV-infected children than uninfected children, with coinfected children having a poorer clinical and radiologic response to treatment.[39,40] The use of ART has reduced the incidence of EPTB and PTB by around 85% and 60%, respectively.[14] However, HIV-infected children on ART still have a higher risk of TB disease than immunocompetent children.[41] Because of the association of TB and HIV, children presenting with TB disease should be tested for HIV infection. Conversely, screening for TB should be done in HIV-infected children with respiratory symptoms or weight loss.

The clinical manifestations of TB in HIV-infected children are similar to those in uninfected children. However, disease in HIV-infected children may be more severe, and extrapulmonary disease (e.g., miliary disease or TB meningitis) may occur more commonly.[42] The clinical presentation of PTB includes chronic cough and failure to thrive, but may also frequently present as acute pneumonia.[43] The use of clinical scoring systems for diagnosis of PTB performs poorly with wide interobserver variability especially in HIV-infected children.[44] Chest radiographic changes may be nonspecific, and interpretation, particularly of hilar lymphadenopathy, is subject to wide interobserver variation; a cavity, pleural effusion, expansile pneumonia with airway compression or a miliary pattern may suggest PTB in the appropriate epidemiological context (Fig. 66.1).[45]

Annual screening of HIV-infected children for *M. tuberculosis* infection is recommended using the tuberculin skin

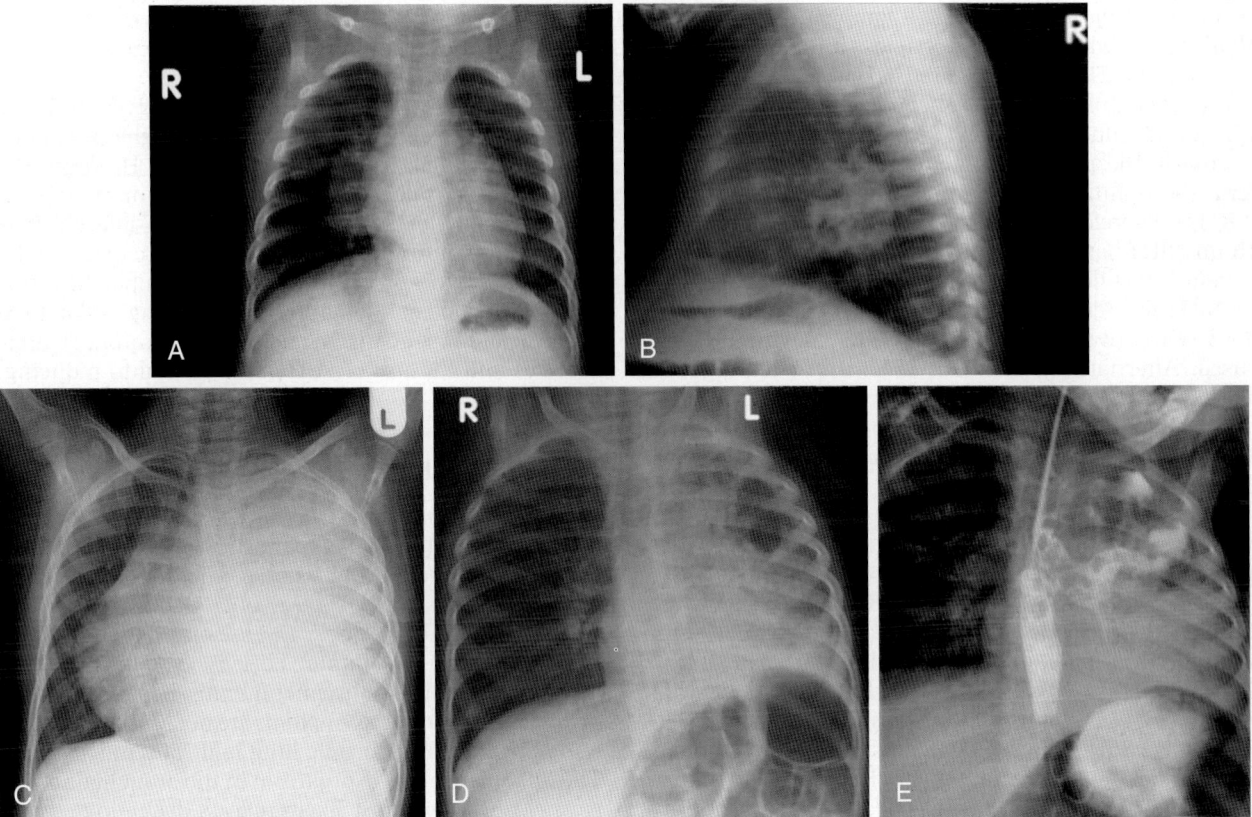

Fig. 66.1 Chest radiographs of tuberculosis (TB) in human immunodeficiency virus (HIV) infected children. (A) Chest radiograph of an HIV-infected child with culture confirmed TB. Note the right parahilar nodal mass, marked right and left bronchial compression by lymphadenopathy and, on the lateral view (B), the classical parahilar nodal mass. (C) Chest radiograph of an HIV-infected child with large left sided TB pleural effusion with mediastinal shift towards the right. (D–E) Bronchogenic TB in an HIV infected child with complication of a bronchoesophageal fistula secondary to lymph node erosion. (D) Chest radiographic showing parahilar adenopathy, extensive left sided bronchogenic TB with dense left lower lobe consolidation. (E) Contrast swallow outlining the bronchoesophageal fistula.

test in children who have a negative test. A reaction greater than 5 mm is considered positive. However, the sensitivity of skin testing is reduced in HIV-infected children compared to uninfected children because of anergy; a blood interferon (IFN) gamma assay has a higher sensitivity and specificity for diagnosis of *M. tuberculosis* infection in HIV-infected children.[46] However, discordance between skin test and IFN gamma results occurs, and neither can distinguish infection from disease.[47]

If PTB is suspected, respiratory specimens for microbiologic confirmation, using molecular methods and liquid culture, should be obtained. The availability of rapid PCR-based molecular methods (Xpert *mycobacterium tuberculosis* [MTB]/ Rifampicin [RIF] [Xpert]) enables rapid diagnosis of TB and detection of Rifampicin resistance. Bacteriologic confirmation of PTB in infants and children is underutilized, especially in hospitalized children. Expectorated sputum is the recommended initial specimen for testing to diagnose TB in the older child who can produce sputum. In children who cannot expectorate, sputum induction using 3%–5% hypertonic saline is effective and safe, even in infants, with a yield that is higher than gastric lavage for culture confirmation.[48] In addition, use of induced sputum has been shown to be useful and effective for microbiologic confirmation of TB in young children in community-based studies.[49] At least two specimens should be obtained, as a second specimen increases the yield from Xpert by 25%–30% and from culture by approximately 20%.[48] Xpert has a reported sensitivity of approximately 66% in children, with a specificity of approximately 99%.[50] The WHO has endorsed Xpert as the first-line investigation to replace smear microscopy as the initial diagnostic test for suspected HIV-associated TB or multidrug-resistant (MDR) PTB in children and adults (http:// www.who.int) on respiratory specimens. The potential to rapidly make a microbiologic diagnosis at the point of care including rapid identification of Rifampicin resistance makes use of sputum induction in children even more important. The organism can also be identified from bronchoalveolar lavage (BAL), from fine needle aspirate of an enlarged node, from fluid from a discharging ear, or from lung tissue obtained by biopsy.

Empiric therapy for PTB in HIV-infected children should include four drugs (isoniazid, rifampicin, pyrazinamide, ethambutol) daily for a 2-month induction period followed by 4 months of daily isoniazid and rifampin.[51] Modification of therapy should be made based on susceptibility testing. The minimum duration of treatment is 6 months, with some recommending up to 9 months, especially in severely immunocompromised children who are at increased risk of relapse.[32,52] Adjunctive corticosteroids are recommended for endobronchial disease with bronchial obstruction at 1–2 mg/kg per day tapered over 6–8 weeks.

For children on ART, the antiretroviral regimen should provide optimal TB and HIV therapy and minimize potential toxicity and drug interactions.[51] Rifampicin is compatible with all nucleoside reverse transcriptase inhibitors (NRTIs); therefore two NRTIs should be used as the backbone of ART. However, rifampicin induces hepatic Cytochrome P450 enzymes and reduces the levels of some antiretroviral agents, particularly the protease inhibitors (PIs) and, to a lesser extent, the nonnucleoside reverse transcriptase inhibitors (NNRTIs). Therefore rifampicin should preferably be used with an NRTI-based regimen rather than with a PI-based regimen. For children older than 3 years, two NRTIs with the NNRTI efavirenz are recommended. For children younger than 3 years, two NRTIs with the NNRTI nevirapine may be used. Alternatively, if a PI is used, a boosted regimen (additional ritonavir boosting with lopinavir/ritonavir) is recommended.[53] Adding ritonavir to lopinavir/ritonavir sufficient to achieve milligram-for-milligram parity may achieve adequate lopinavir levels, but doubling the dose of lopinavir/ritonavir is ineffective.[53,54] Rifabutin is a less potent inducer of the P450 enzymes and is therefore a suitable alternative to rifampicin, but there is limited pediatric experience with its use. For a child who is not yet on ART, the decision when to initiate ART depends on the child's age and clinical and/or immunologic condition. ART should be started in all children less than 5 years within 8 weeks. In children with CD4 less than 750 cells/mm³ or less than 25% or with WHO clinical stage 3 or 4 disease, ART must be started within 2 weeks of starting TB treatment. In children older than 5 years, ART should be started for all children and as a priority if CD4 is less than 350 cells/mm³ or there is clinical stage 3 or 4 disease.[2] ART may be deferred for 2 weeks in children with mild immunosuppression, which reduces the risk of immune reconstitution inflammatory syndrome (IRIS).

For MDR TB, a minimum of three drugs to which the organism is susceptible should be given. Streptomycin, cycloserine, or ethionamide may be substituted for ethambutol (see Chapter 29); regimens should be individualized based on the resistance pattern of the organism from the child or source case. Daily therapy should be given for at least 12 months, and second-line drugs include clarithromycin, azithromycin, and ciprofloxacin. Directly observed therapy should be used when possible to ensure adherence.[55]

Primary isoniazid (INH) prophylaxis for HIV-infected children living in a high TB prevalence area has been reported to reduce mortality by approximately 50% and to reduce TB incidence by approximately 70% in the setting of limited access to ART.[56] However, in a study of infants who were initiated on ART early and who were carefully followed with initiation of prophylaxis on exposure to a TB contact, no effect of primary INH prophylaxis was shown.[41] The impact in older children established on ART is less clear, but further study suggests that INH prophylaxis may reduce TB incidence in such children, even when they are taking ART.[57] The WHO revised policy for primary INH prophylaxis in HIV-infected children advises use in high TB prevalence areas in children who are older than 1 year. The optimal duration of prophylaxis is unknown, but extended use appears safe and effective: WHO policy now recommends prophylaxis for up to 3 years in high TB prevalence areas.[58,59]

Secondary prophylaxis should be given to all HIV-infected children (irrespective of the tuberculin skin test or IFN gamma test) for 6–9 months following exposure to a close contact with TB once TB disease has been excluded in the child. If the source case has an INH-resistant strain, rifampicin should be used. If the strain is MDR, then two drugs to which the strain is susceptible should be used.[32,44]

Bacillus Calmette–Guérin (BCG) vaccine is contraindicated in HIV-infected children because of the high risk of developing disseminated disease and of death.[60] However, BCG is given at birth as part of the routine immunization program in many high incidence TB areas; thus HIV-infected children may receive immunization before they are diagnosed with HIV. The key to TB control is adequate public health measures with good contact and source tracing and adherence to medication regimens. In addition, integrating TB and HIV services and the use of ART are essential to reducing the TB caseload.

NONTUBERCULOSIS MYCOBACTERIA

Nontuberculosis mycobacteria (NTM), of which Mycobacterium avium complex (MAC) is the most common, are ubiquitous in the environment. MAC was a common OI in HIV-infected children in the pre-ART era, but ART has substantially reduced the risk of disease.[14] Disease may manifest as a localized infection or disseminated disease, and localized disease includes cervical adenitis, pneumonitis, hepatic dysfunction, or abscess. Respiratory symptoms are not a prominent feature, but tachypnea and chronic lung infiltrates may be present. The importance of the organism in the bronchial secretions is unclear, but it most likely reflects disseminated disease rather than localized pulmonary infection. Symptoms caused by disseminated MAC infection are nonspecific, including fever, weight loss, night sweats, cachexia, and diarrhea.[61] Patients with disseminated MAC have a poor prognosis[62]; for example, of children who died in one report, 42% had disseminated MAC, and it was the underlying cause of death in 24%.[63]

Recommendations for prophylaxis and therapy for disseminated MAC in patients with HIV[32] are to use a minimum of two agents to minimize the development of resistant strains. Treatment should include either azithromycin or clarithromycin with ethambutol as a second drug. For disseminated disease, a third or fourth drug (clofazimine, rifabutin, rifampin, ciprofloxacin, or amikacin) may be added. Improved immunologic status is essential to controlling MAC infection; ART should be initiated in children who are not on therapy. The optimal timing of ART is unclear; at least 2 weeks of antimycobacterial therapy is recommended prior to starting ART to minimize the potential for IRIS.[32,44]

Primary prophylaxis with clarithromycin or azithromycin is recommended for severely immunosuppressed children with CD4+ cell counts less than 50/μL if older than 6 years of age, less than 75/μL if 2–6 years of age, less than 500/μL if 1–2 years of age, and less than 750/μL if younger than 1 year of age.[32] Prophylaxis may be discontinued in children older than 2 years of age who are stable on ART for 6 months or longer and who have sustained immune recovery.

VIRAL INFECTION

Viruses are increasingly reported as a cause of pneumonia in the context of high immunization coverage with PCV and Hib.[64,65] Among viral pathogens, respiratory syncytial virus (RSV) predominates; other common viruses include influenza,

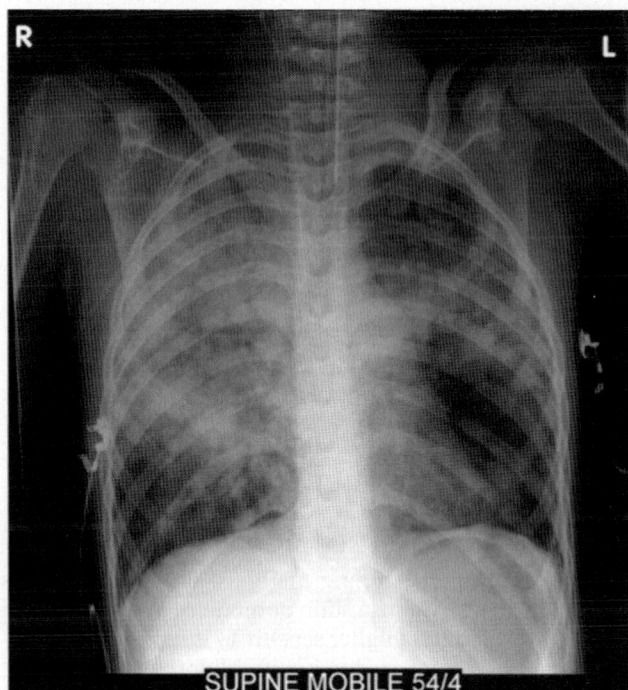

Fig. 66.2 Chest radiograph of varicella zoster pneumonia in a human immunodeficiency virus-infected child showing bilateral diffuse infiltrates and consolidation.

parainfluenza, human metapneumovirus, and adenovirus.[10,66] Multiple infections may occur including viral-viral, viral-bacterial, viral-mycobacterial, or viral-fungal pathogens. HIV-infected children with viral lower respiratory tract infection have more severe disease compared to uninfected children and are likely to develop pneumonia rather than bronchiolitis.[21,64] Prolonged RSV antigen shedding for up to 90 days may occur in HIV–infected children.

In HIV-infected children, measles virus and varicella-zoster virus may cause severe pulmonary disease (Fig. 66.2).[67] Acyclovir or valacyclovir are the agents of choice for varicella infection. HIV-infected children with influenza should be treated with a neuraminidase inhibitor such as oseltamivir for 5 days (ideally within 72 hours) of symptom onset, as this may reduce severity of disease and complications. High-dose vitamin A should be given to children with measles.

CMV has been reported to commonly cause pneumonia in HIV-infected children who are ART-naïve. In postmortem studies, CMV has been reported to be a common pathogen, since it has been found in around 9% of HIV-infected children dying from pneumonia, similar to that in HIV-uninfected children.[22] However, CMV may coexist with other pathogens such as pneumocystis, so defining the contribution of CMV to severity of disease may be difficult. Antemortem diagnosis of CMV pneumonitis is difficult, as isolation of CMV from respiratory secretions may represent infection but not disease; consequently, definitive diagnosis requires a lung biopsy. A study of HIV-infected South African infants hospitalized with severe pneumonia reported that approximately 70% of children had CMV viremia as detected by PCR, while 36% also had CMV identified in BAL fluid or induced sputum, which was more common than PCP.[68] Children with CMV-associated pneumonia had a 2.5-fold higher

mortality than those without CMV pneumonia despite treatment with ganciclovir in most. However, this association was not evident when adjusting for severe immunosuppression, indicating that CMV pneumonia may be a marker of severe immunosuppression.

Histologically, alveolar macrophages, type II pneumocytes, bronchial and bronchiolar epithelial cells, and capillary endothelial cells may manifest cytomegaly and nuclear and cytoplasmic inclusions. Infection with CMV stimulates HIV replication, leading to more rapid HIV disease progression. ART has substantially reduced the incidence of CMV disease reflected in a reduction in the prevalence of CMV retinitis.[14,69–71]

Ganciclovir should be used for treatment of CMV pneumonia, switching to oral valganciclovir once clinical improvement has occurred, for a total of 6–8 weeks of therapy. To prevent recurrence, prophylactic valganciclovir should be given to children with severe immunosuppression. Initiation of ART is crucial to contain CMV infection and prevent recurrence of disease, and prophylaxis may be discontinued once sustained immune reconstitution has been achieved with ART.

Strategies to prevent other viral infections are available; for example, yearly inactivated influenza vaccine is recommended for children 6 months of age and older. However, a randomized controlled study of two doses of inactivated influenza vaccination in HIV-infected children (median age 2 years; 92% on ART) reported an efficacy of only 18%, possibly due to poor immunogenicity or mismatch between circulating strains and vaccine strains.[72] Immunization of pregnant women has an efficacy of around 50% in HIV-infected women, but a much lower efficacy in their HIV-exposed infants.[73] HIV-infected children mount antibody responses to influenza vaccination, but antibody titers are lower than in HIV-negative controls. Varicella and measles vaccines are recommended for children who are not severely immunocompromised. Passive immunization should be given to children who are exposed to measles with intramuscular immunoglobulin within 6 days of exposure. Postexposure prophylaxis with human varicella immune globulin (VariZIG) or varicella-zoster immune globulin (VZIG) should be given to unvaccinated children or those who are moderate or severely immunosuppressed within 96 hours of a close contact with chickenpox.

FUNGAL INFECTION

Pneumocystis jirovecii Pneumonia

P. jirovecii is a fungus that attaches to the alveolar epithelium, leading to a diffuse desquamative alveolitis, and filling of the alveoli with a foamy exudate of alveolar macrophages and cysts containing sporozoites with accompanying interstitial inflammation.

P. jirovecii is the most common pathogen identified in HIV-infected infants with pneumonia who are not taking prophylaxis or ART.[74,75] Postmortem studies report P. jirovecii to be one of the most common pathogens, occurring in around 33% of children dying from pneumonia, with a 10-fold higher incidence in HIV-infected than uninfected infants.[22,27] The incidence during the first year of life in the pre-ART era was estimated to range from 10% to 42% in antemortem

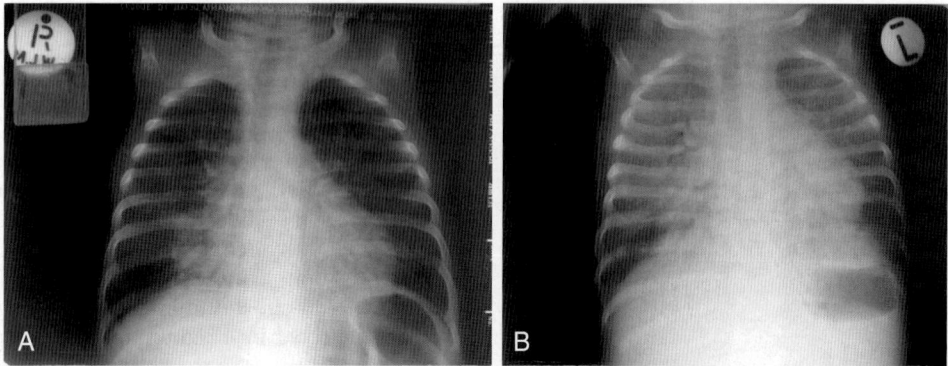

Fig. 66.3 Chest radiograph of a 3-month-old infant presenting with *Pneumocystis jirovecii* pneumonia. (A) The initial radiograph shows a bilateral infiltrate most prominent in the perihilar region. (B) A chest radiograph taken 72 hours later shows progression of disease with opacification of both lung fields.

studies[74,76,77] and up to 52% in postmortem studies.[78–80] The incidence is highest in the first year of life, peaking at 3–6 months of age, and use of ART and CTX prophylaxis has substantially reduced the incidence of disease.[14]

Clinical features include acute onset of cough, fever, tachypnea, and hypoxia. Normal, decreased breath sounds or crackles may be present, while hypoxia may be severe. A high plasma HIV RNA load strongly predicts PCP; CD4+ measures may be less useful, especially in young children. Approximately one-quarter of infants had CD4+ counts greater than 1500 cells/mm³ at the time of PCP diagnosis.[81,82] However, a rapid rate of decline in CD4+ is associated with the development of PCP, and low CD4+ counts in older children are associated with PCP.

There is a high rate of respiratory failure and need for mechanical ventilation. Early reports indicated a mortality rate exceeding 40% with the initial episode and the majority surviving less than a year thereafter.[75,83]

Laboratory findings include a normal white blood cell count, elevated lactic dehydrogenase (LDH), and normal immunoglobulin G (IgG). LDH levels greater than 1000 IU/L are associated with PCP but are nonspecific. The most common changes on chest radiographs are hyperinflation, diffuse bilateral opacification, and reticulonodular infiltrates most prominent in the perihilar region and extending peripherally (see Fig. 66.3).[84] Air bronchograms, focal infiltrates, a normal radiograph, pneumothorax, pulmonary interstitial emphysema, or pneumatoceles have also been described.[84]

Microbiologic diagnosis relies on identification of the organism from bronchial washings, sputum, or lung tissue. BAL with fiberoptic bronchoscopy is a reliable method for diagnosis.[85] Sputum induction with 3% saline can be useful for diagnosis,[86,87] but the diagnostic yield is variable and dependent upon expertise for specimen collection and the diagnostic test. Nasopharyngeal aspirates have been used to identify *P. jirovecii*; the yield is lower than with induced sputum using staining methods,[75,86] but it is similar to lower respiratory secretions (BAL or induced sputum) when PCR based diagnosis is used.[88]

Methenamine silver, toluidine blue O, and fluorescein-conjugated monoclonal antibody are stains that identify the thick-walled cysts of *P. jirovecii*. Fluorescein staining is more sensitive than other staining methods. Trophozoite forms are identified with Giemsa stain or modified Wright-Giemsa stain. However, much higher sensitivity is reported for PCR-based diagnosis compared to immunofluorescence.[88,89]

High-dose intravenous CTX (trimethoprim-sulfamethoxazole [TMP-SMX]) is the treatment of choice for PCP. The conventional dose is 6–12 mg/kg per day TMP and 30–60 mg/kg per day SMX for 21 days. In addition, oral treatment can be given to complete the 21-day course when there is clinical improvement or if the disease is mild. Revised WHO management guidelines recommend empiric therapy with TMP-SMX in HIV-infected or exposed infants with pneumonia (Table 66.2).[90]

A clinical response is usually observed in 5–7 days, although deterioration may occur in the first days of therapy; and side effects to TMP-SMX include a rash and thrombocytopenia. An alternative treatment is pentamidine administered intravenously or intramuscularly (4 mg/kg per dose once daily) if TMP-SMX is poorly tolerated or no response occurs after 1 week of treatment. The intramuscular route is painful and can cause sterile abscesses, so it should be avoided if possible. Side effects from pentamidine include pancreatitis, renal dysfunction, and both hyperglycemia and hypoglycemia. Other alternatives include atovaquone, dapsone with trimethoprim, trimetrexate glucuronate with leucovorin, and clindamycin with primaquine.[32]

A National Institutes of Health consensus panel recommended that corticosteroids be used as adjunctive therapy in hypoxic adults with PCP based on studies showing improved survival and decreased incidence of respiratory failure.[91] Moderate to severe infection has been defined for this purpose as partial pressure of oxygen in arterial blood (PaO₂) less than 70 mm Hg in room air or an alveolar-arterial oxygen gradient more than 35 mm Hg. Controlled clinical trials using corticosteroids in children with PCP have not been conducted, but uncontrolled data suggest that corticosteroids are beneficial[92] at a dose of 1 mg/kg per dose twice daily 1 mg/kg per dose twice daily for 5 days; 0.5 mg/kg, twice daily, day 6–10; 0.5 mg/kg, once daily, for day 11 through 21.[93]

Because of the high mortality and morbidity associated with PCP, prevention should be the primary objective. Guidelines for prophylaxis for PCP prophylaxis for children

Table 66.2 Recommended Cotrimoxazole Prophylaxis in Human Immunodeficiency Virus Infected Children

Age	Prophylaxis
Birth to 4–6 weeks	No
4–6 weeks to 12 months	Yes, all
1–5 years	CD4+ count < 500 cells/µL or CD4% < 15%
≥5 years	CD4+ count < 200 cell/µL or CD4% < 15%

Box 66.2 Strategies for Prevention of Pneumonia in Human Immunodeficiency Virus Infected Children

Early antiretroviral therapy
Immunization
    Pneumococcal conjugate vaccine[a]
    Haemophilus influenzae type b vaccine
    Pertussis
    Measles
    Influenza
Antibiotic prophylaxis
    Cotrimoxazole prophylaxis
    Isoniazid prophylaxis
Optimizing nutrition
Decreasing indoor air pollution

[a]Consider reimmunization after 3–5 years in children not on antiretroviral therapy.

infected with HIV are shown in Table 66.2, and prophylaxis for PCP is recommended in all infants born to HIV-infected mothers beginning at 4–6 weeks of age. Prophylaxis can be stopped once HIV-infection in the infant has been excluded and infants are no longer breastfeeding. For HIV-infected children, prophylaxis should continue throughout the first year of life. Discontinuation of PCP prophylaxis should be considered for HIV-infected children when, after receiving ART for at least 6 months, the CD4+ percentage is ≥15% or the CD4+ count is ≥200 cells/µL for those older than 6 years of age and the CD4+ percentage is ≥15% or the CD4+ percentage is ≥500 cells/µL for children 1–5 years of age for more than 3 consecutive months.[94] However, an African randomized controlled trial of stopping or continuing CTX prophylaxis in older children on ART for at least 2 years demonstrated benefit in children continuing CTX prophylaxis irrespective of CD4 count, with a substantial reduction in hospitalization.[36]

CTX is the drug of choice for prophylaxis. The recommended regimen is 150 mg TMP/m^2 per day with 750 mg SMX/m^2 per day administered orally once or divided twice daily dose, three times a week on consecutive or alternate days. Alternatively, prophylaxis can be given 7 days a week. TMP-SMX prophylaxis may also be effective for reducing bacterial infections, and daily therapy is associated with a lower incidence of bacteremia than thrice-weekly therapy.[95] If TMP-SMX is not tolerated, alternative prophylactic regimens include dapsone 4 mg/kg (not to exceed 200 mg), orally, once a week; or atovaquone 30 mg/kg once daily for children 1–3 months of age and older than 24 months of age and 45 mg/kg for infants 4–24 months of age. In children older than 5 years of age who cannot take TMP-SMX, dapsone, or atovaquone, aerosolized pentamidine 300 mg administered via inhaler once monthly is recommended.

Other Fungal Infections

Opportunistic fungal infections can cause severe pulmonary disease, but the number of reported cases is small. The most common infections are with *Candida* spp., *Cryptococcus neoformans*, *Histoplasma capsulatum*, *Coccidioides immitis*, *Aspergillus*. Dissemination of infection is common, and treatment is difficult. Constitutional symptoms (e.g., weight loss and fever) may reflect extrapulmonary involvement.

Cryptococcus usually presents as meningitis, but this can involve the lungs and cause interstitial pneumonia.[96] *Histoplasma capsulatum* most commonly affects the lungs and is likely to become disseminated in HIV-infected patients.[97,98] Standard serologic tests can be positive for both coccidioidomycosis and histoplasmosis, but false-negative results occur in the most profoundly immunocompromised patients.[99] In addition, skin testing is not useful because of problems with anergy and lack of standardization of most fungal skin test

preparations. Cultures of bone marrow, cerebrospinal fluid, and lymph node or lung biopsy can be diagnostic. *Candida* spp. is often found in the oropharynx and esophagus in HIV-infected children, and tracheobronchial candidiasis or pulmonary infection is less common. Isolation of *Candida* from BAL fluid most likely represents an oropharyngeal contaminant, because pulmonary infection is rarely confirmed on lung biopsy. Tissue invasion should be demonstrated on bronchial or lung biopsy to confirm the diagnosis.

Aspergillus infection has been reported in HIV-infected patients, late in the course of disease, or following corticosteroid use or neutropenia.[100] Aspergilloma and invasive cavitary aspergillosis have been described[101,102]; *Aspergillus* infection can cause formation of a fungal pseudomembrane, resulting in severe airway obstruction.[103] Transmural and peribronchial extension of the infection may occur, and the most prominent symptoms are cough, fever, and dyspnea.

Amphotericin-B is the drug of choice for most life-threatening fungal infections (see Chapter 31). Alternative regimens include fluconazole and itraconazole. However, even with treatment, relapse and mortality is high. Chronic suppressive therapy is required following infection.

Chronic Lung Disease

Chronic lung disease is common in HIV-infected children as they survive longer.[1,7,104,105] The spectrum of chronic lung disease includes lymphocytic interstitial pneumonitis (LIP), chronic infection, IRIS, malignancies bronchiectasis, bronchiolitis obliterans, and asthma (see Box 66.1). In HIV-infected adults, chronic obstructive pulmonary disease, pulmonary hypertension, and lung cancer are increasingly recognized.[106]

Factors contributing to chronic lung disease in perinatally infected children and adolescents are multifactorial and include direct influences of HIV, immune dysregulation with increased inflammation, recurrent or severe infections, ART and is compounded by environmental exposures such as microorganisms, diet, poverty, tobacco smoke, or environmental pollution (Fig. 66.4). Delayed access to ART, pneumonia, particularly TB, and extent of preexisting immunosuppression

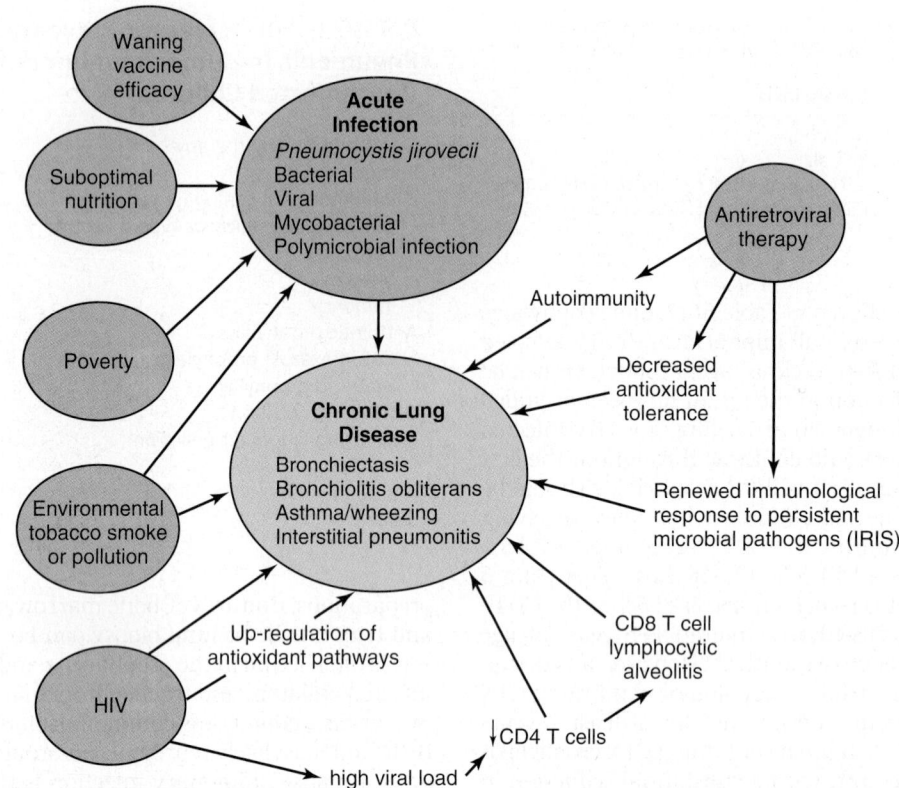

Fig. 66.4 Factors associated with chronic lung disease in human immunodeficiency virus (HIV) infected children.

impact the severity or extent of chronic lung disease. Although ART may halt progression of lung damage, it will not reverse established chronic disease. Improvement of lung disease on ART is suggested by radiological improvement[105]; a study of lung function in perinatally infected adolescents on ART showed relatively mild lung function impairments despite children only being started on ART at 5 years.[8]

In the absence of ART, chronic lung disease was dominated by LIP, chronic or recurrent infections with bronchiectasis, bronchiolitis obliterans, and decreased lung function.[7,104] Use of early ART prevents lung damage[107] but even when ART is only started in the early childhood years, it may provide substantial protection from development of severe chronic lung disease. For example, among African HIV-infected adolescents started on ART at 5 years of age, only a minority (<10%) had evidence of severe lung function abnormalities at adolescence.[8] Further use of ART can lead to chest radiographic improvement and prevent radiological progression even when started in late childhood.[105]

The Pediatric Pulmonary and Cardiovascular Complications of Vertically Transmitted HIV followed 287 HIV-infected US children (some of whom were receiving one or two antiretroviral therapies [ARVs]), for 4 years.[104] Chronic lung disease was defined as persistent bronchovascular or reticular markings for 6 months or longer, or consolidation or nodules present for 3 months or longer. The cumulative prevalence of chronic radiographic changes was 29%, of which 23% were severe radiological abnormalities, either persistent consolidation or nodules. Chronic changes were associated with

lower CD4 counts and higher viral loads. Radiographic changes were associated with an increased frequency of clubbing, crackles, tachypnea, and decreased oxygen saturation. LIP was diagnosed in 19%, chronic PCP in 6% and TB in 2%. Among those with no defined cause for the chronic chest x-ray (CXR) abnormality, an increase in bronchovascular markings was the most common finding, followed by focal consolidation and pulmonary nodules.[104] Mortality in HIV-infected children with chronic radiographic changes was not different from that in HIV-infected children without these changes.

In a South African study of 330 HIV-infected children (median age 24 months), mostly with advanced clinical disease and moderate or severe immunosuppression, almost 85% had an abnormal chest x-ray.[108] Only 23% of children were on ART, as the study predated the availability of ART. In addition, bronchial wall thickening occurring in 70% and was the most common radiographic abnormality. A third had increased bronchovascular markings, while around 50% of x-rays had extensive diffuse or multifocal changes either opacification, reticulonodular infiltrates, or a combination of these.[108] Atelectasis (12%), bronchiectasis (4%), or isolated thin-walled pulmonary cysts (2%) were also reported in association with diffuse changes. More extensive radiological disease was associated with advanced clinical disease, CD4 count less than 20%, and age greater than 2 years. Children were followed for a median of 24 months, with chest radiology performed every 6 months; during this time, almost 80% of participants went onto ART (median ART duration was 16 months). In the first 6 months, the proportion with severe radiological abnormality increased slightly from 50% to 54%

remaining mostly unchanged at 12 months.[105] Subsequently, slow but sustained radiological improvement occurred, with 40%, 28%, 19%, and 16% showing severe abnormality at 24, 36, 48, and 54 months, respectively. The cumulative prevalence of persistent, severe abnormality was 60% (almost 3 times that in American children) and lasted a median of 18 months. LIP (45%) and pulmonary TB (31%) were the leading causes of persistent, severe abnormality, accounting for over three-quarters of cases. The use of ART was associated with an improvement in radiological findings and less deterioration, within 6 months of use including for LIP and TB.[105]

LYMPHOID INTERSTITIAL PNEUMONITIS

Prior to availability of ART, LIP was common, with chronic nodular densities observed in 8% of patients by 5 years of age in a North American study.[104] In 25 studies of 128 children with biopsy proven LIP, almost all reported chest x-ray findings as diffuse, bilateral, nodular, or reticulonodular (Fig. 66.5A).[109] In HIV-infected children under 5 years of age who died at home in Zimbabwe, 9% had LIP on autopsy.[110] However, the prevalence of LIP has reduced dramatically with use of ART.

LIP is characterized by diffuse infiltration of lymphocytes into the interstitium and scattered nodules of mononuclear cells; the etiology of the abnormal lymphoproliferative response is unclear. The principal hypotheses are that lymphoproliferation is a response to the HIV (Fig. 66.5B) alone or coinfection with another virus. Epstein-Barr viral DNA has been found in lung biopsies of children with LIP, and HIV RNA has been identified in the lungs of infants with LIP.[111]

The onset of LIP is insidious and the course slowly progressive. The median age of onset is 2.5–3 years of age. However, reticulonodular changes on x-ray may be observed before 12 months of age.[104] Cough or tachypnea may be present. Auscultation of the chest may be normal or reveal crackles and wheezes. Generalized lymphadenopathy, hepatosplenomegaly, clubbing, and parotid gland enlargement are commonly associated physical findings. The chest radiograph typically shows a bilateral diffuse interstitial reticulonodular pattern with or without hilar adenopathy.[104,109] Elevated serum immunoglobulin levels are associated with LIP and IgG levels greater than 2500 mg/dL are strongly

associated with LIP. Lung biopsy establishes the diagnosis. However, a presumptive diagnosis of LIP can be made based on the clinical findings and the typical reticulonodular radiographic pattern lasting more than 2 months without another cause. In a longitudinal study of African children, LIP was the leading causes of persistent, severe abnormality on chest x-rays, accounting for 45% of cases.[105] Chest x-ray findings may resolve with steroid treatment or with ART.[112]

Treatment of LIP is nonspecific. Inhaled bronchodilators may provide symptomatic relief, and oxygen is administered for hypoxemia. Although treatment of LIP with corticosteroids has been reported to improve hypoxemia in a small number of patients, there are no controlled clinical trials.[112]

Some cases of LIP may progress to a lymphoproliferative disorder characterized by polyclonal, polymorphic B-cell content with extranodal systemic and prominent pulmonary involvement, or to malignant lymphoma.

CHRONIC INFECTION

Chronic lung disease may result from recurrent or persistent infection from bacterial, mycobacterial, viral, fungal, or mixed infections. Although ameliorated by ART, susceptibility to recurrent and severe bacterial or viral infection persists even with use of ART. TB is one of the most common causes of chronic lung disease and of chronic chest radiological abnormalities in African children.[1,105,113]

Localized or disseminated disease from *Mycobacterium bovis* or the NTM (particularly *M. avium-intracellulare* complex) may also result in chronic disease. Chest x-ray features include mediastinal adenopathy, diffuse pulmonary nodules, cavitation, or bronchiectasis.

Case reports of chronic PCP in children have been described with focal opacification, cysts, pneumothorax, pneumatoceles, or diffuse interstitial disease.[114–116]

PULMONARY TUMORS

Children with HIV have an increased risk of malignancy, occurring in 2.5% of children with AIDS in the United States.[117] Non-Hodgkin lymphoma (NHL) is most common, followed by Kaposi sarcoma (KS), leiomyosarcoma, and Hodgkin lymphoma.[117] Although the ART reduces the risk of AIDS-defining malignancies, HIV-infected children remain at increased risk of malignancies compared to HIV-uninfected

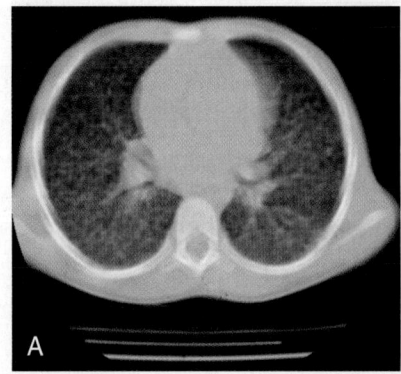
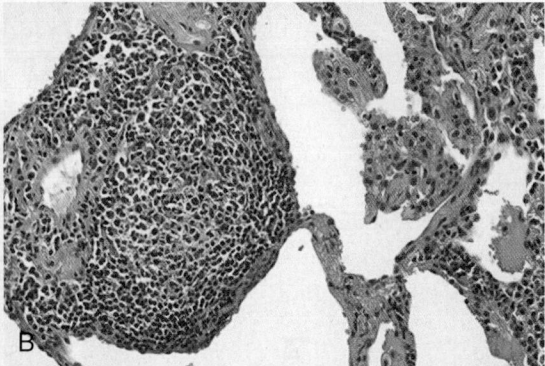

Fig. 66.5 (A) Computed tomography scan of a child with lymphocytic interstitial pneumonitis (LIP). Diffuse nodular infiltrates are present bilaterally with perihilar prominence. (B) Lung biopsy from a child with LIP. Note the interstitial and peribronchiolar lymphoid infiltration.

children.[118] Primary NHL may arise in a lymph node or be extranodal. AIDS-related NHL may occur in almost any extranodal site including the lungs. In addition, pulmonary disease may result from dissemination from a primary focus. In African HIV-infected children, KS is the most common AIDS-defining malignancy probably due to the prevalence of Kaposi sarcoma-associated herpes virus (KSHV).[118–120] In high-income settings, most cases of KS in the pediatric age group have occurred in adolescents, and KS lesions may produce upper airway obstruction. Pulmonary dissemination may result in chronic progressive dyspnea, cough, and fever; hemoptysis may occur with endobronchial lesions.[122] Chest radiograph abnormalities include multifocal homogeneous opacification, a diffuse reticular or nodular pattern, pleural effusion, mediastinal adenopathy, or a combination of these.[114]

A single case of a child with a tumor of the trachea (leiomyoma) and of the left main bronchus (leiomyosarcoma), presenting as tracheal narrowing and left lower lobe collapse respectively has been described.[123] Pseudolymphomas and lymphomas have also been reported.

Aspiration Pneumonitis

Esophagitis, related to candida, herpes simplex virus (HSV), and CMV infections may occur in HIV infected children, particularly those with severe immunosuppression, and can be associated with swallowing difficulties and risk of pulmonary aspiration.[124,125] Neurological impairment secondary to HIV encephalopathy can also increase risk of pulmonary aspiration and recurrent lower respiratory tract infections or aspiration pneumonitis. Pulmonary aspiration should be considered in HIV infected children with clinical or radiological concerns of aspiration and recurrent lower respiratory tract infection (LRTI).

Bronchiectasis

Bronchiectasis is an important cause of chronic infiltrates and atelectasis on chest radiographs and may be focal or bilateral. Bronchiectasis may be associated with LIP or lower respiratory tract infection. Development of bronchiectasis is associated with the severity of immunosuppression. A retrospective review of 749 HIV-infected children (mostly before the availability of ART) found that all 19 who developed bronchiectasis were Centers for Disease Control and Prevention (CDC) immunological category stage 3.[126] In Zimbabwean adolescents with vertically transmitted HIV and delayed access to ART, 43% had bronchiectasis on chest computed tomography (CT) scans and 66% had a chronic productive cough.[7] Diagnosis may be suspected in a child with a recurrent productive cough and chest radiographs that show persistent abnormalities for more than 6 months. Diagnosis is confirmed with a CT scan of the chest. Therapy includes optimizing ART, physiotherapy to improve lung clearance, and aggressive treatment of intercurrent infections. The efficacy and safety of long-term azithromycin has not been evaluated in HIV-infected children with bronchiectasis.

Bronchiolitis Obliterans

In vertically infected Zimbabwean adolescents, chronic respiratory symptoms, hypoxia, reduced lung function, and high resolution CT scan findings suggestive of postinfective bronchiolitis obliterans (BO) have been described.[7] Over half (55%) had areas of decreased attenuation on chest CT scan in keeping with small airway disease. Coexisting bronchiectasis was common as is typical of postinfectious BO, and BO may be a sequel of acute lower respiratory tract infection or of repeated infections (Fig. 66.6).[127,128] The extent of mosaic attenuation on CT scan was inversely correlated with lung function as measured by forced expiratory volume in 1 second (FEV1). Management includes lung protective strategies (optimizing ART therapy, vaccinations against respiratory pathogens, nutritional support, regular screening, and prophylaxis for TB in endemic areas) and pulmonary rehabilitation as appropriate. Bronchodilators may be used for those who are bronchodilator responsive. The role of inhaled corticosteroids or azithromycin has not been evaluated in HIV infected children with BO.

IMMUNE RECONSTITUTION INFLAMMATORY SYNDROME

With increasing use of ART, an IRIS associated with mycobacterial infection or with other OIs (e.g., CMV) has been

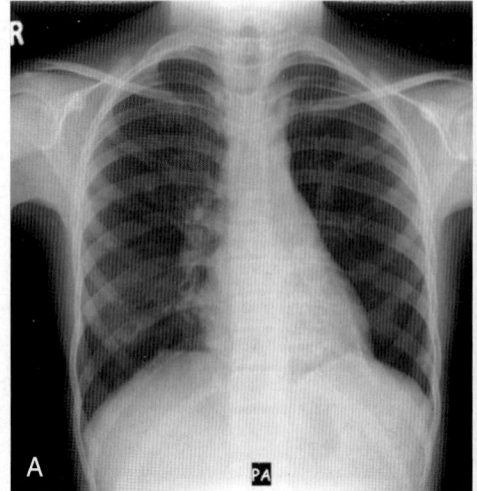
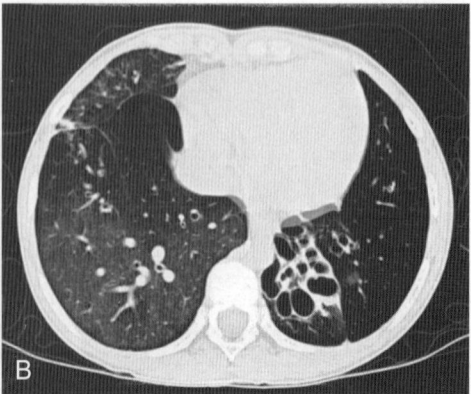

Fig. 66.6 (A) Chest radiograph of a human immunodeficiency virus infected adolescent showing hyperinflation and left lower lobe bronchiectasis. (B) Computed tomography scan, note the mosaic perfusion and bronchiectasis.

reported.[129] TB IRIS may occur weeks to months after initiation of ART therapy and may result either from unrecognized mycobacterial infection or from a florid immune response directed against a mycobacterial antigen in those already on therapy.[130] IRIS has been described with different mycobacterial species including *M. tuberculosis, M. bovis,* or MAC infection.[131–134] Clinically, IRIS is characterized by a paradoxical worsening in signs with increasing lymphadenopathy and new clinical and radiological respiratory signs.[131,132,134] The tuberculin skin test may become positive, and chest radiographs may show development of lymphadenopathy or new infiltrates. IRIS must be distinguished from other infections, drug resistant TB, or nonresponse to TB therapy caused by nonadherence. To minimize the risk of IRIS, HIV-infected children with confirmed or probable TB should be treated with anti-TB drugs when possible for 2 weeks before commencing ART.[51,131] When IRIS develops in a child who was unknown to have TB, therapy for TB should be initiated without stopping the ART. If lymphadenopathy or respiratory signs are severe, oral corticosteroids may be beneficial, although there are no controlled trials in children.

AIRWAY HYPERREACTIVITY/ASTHMA

The prevalence of asthma has been reported to be higher in cohorts of HIV infected children on ART compared to uninfected children, but the data are limited.[135–137] A study comparing use of asthma medications in HIV infected children on ART with HIV infected children not on ART, suggested that immune reconstitution may increase asthma risk.[135] However, asthma diagnosis was based on use of asthma medication and confounding factors associated with ART usage, such as severe immune suppression, were not accounted for. Some studies have reported HIV infected children to have a higher incidence of asthma and atopic dermatitis compared to uninfected children, although only use of asthma medication was significantly different.[137] A recent study investigating clinical asthma and lung function in HIV-infected and HEU youth found that, compared to HEU youth, HIV-infected youth had decreased bronchodilator reversibility of obstructive lung disease. This suggests that much of the clinically diagnosed asthma may indeed reflect early chronic obstructive lung disease rather than airway hyperresponsiveness.

Lung Function as a Measurement of Chronic Lung Disease

Lung function may be useful to describe the functional impairment of respiratory disease, understand the underlying mechanisms of disease, and track progression or regression. In HIV-infected children and adolescents, there is a paucity of lung function data. Most data are from small cross-sectional studies, with heterogeneous patient groups and minimal longitudinal data. It is likely that lung involvement begins in early life or in utero. In a birth cohort study investigating respiratory and cardiovascular disease in infants born to HIV infected mothers,[139] HIV infected children had higher respiratory rates and more respiratory symptoms compared to HIV exposed but uninfected infants.[140] To assess if early potentially serious pulmonary disease could be detected before onset of clinical symptoms, infants born to HIV infected mothers were screened with technetium 99m diethyltriaminepentacetic acid (^{99m}Tc DTPA) radioaerosol inhalation-clearance scintigraphy from 3 months onwards and repeated every 6 months.[141] HIV infected infants had a higher ^{99m}Tc DTPA radioaerosol clearance compared to HIV exposed but uninfected infants, suggesting early alveolar interstitial inflammation. Another infant study measuring airflow resistance using the interrupter technique found HIV-infected children (aged 9–113 months) to have higher airway resistance compared to age matched HIV uninfected infants. Airway resistance was similar between symptomatic and asymptomatic HIV-infected infants.[142] Resistance measured after 1 year was significantly higher than initial measurement in HIV infected children, in contrast to the growth associated decline in airway resistance that was seen in healthy HIV uninfected children.[142] These studies suggest that lung involvement occurs early, that clinical symptoms are insensitive measures of early lung damage, and that in the absence of ART these changes are progressive.

In older HIV-infected children and adolescents, abnormal spirometry is common, with restrictive, obstructive, or mixed spirometric patterns described. Reduced FEV1 has been reported in small African[7,143,144] and Italian[142] cross-sectional studies of HIV-infected children. In a Zimbabwean study of 116 children (70% on ART but diagnosed with HIV late at a median of 12 years), 45% had a reduced FEV1.[7] The group had a 71% incidence of physician diagnosed chronic lung disease with exercise intolerance in 21%, dyspnea and/or hypoxia at rest in 35%, and desaturation following a walk test in 29%. Despite the limitations of these studies, they suggest that delayed treatment with ART in HIV infected children results in severe debilitating lung disease with low lung function in those who survive infancy. However, a South African study in which children were started on ART at around 5 years of age found that, although mildly reduced lung function was common 7 years after ART initiation, severe lung function abnormalities were rare.[8]

Impairment of diffusion capacity and airway hyperreactivity has been described in HIV-infected adults, but HIV-infected children or adolescents have not been tested. Obstructive lung disease in HIV-infected adults on ART has been reported, but whether this is mediated by direct viral factors, ART related immune preservation or restoration, lifestyle issues (most notably tobacco smoking), or inflammation related to recurrent OIs is unclear.[145,146] The impact of early ART and immune reconstitution or preservation on lung function has not been assessed in HIV infected children.

Human Immunodeficiency Virus-Associated Cardiomyopathy and Pulmonary Hypertension

Ventricular dysfunction and cardiomyopathy may occur frequently in HIV-infected children in the absence of ART.[147] In the pre-ART era, up to 25% of HIV-infected children manifested significant cardiac abnormalities, such as dilated cardiomyopathy, left ventricular hypertrophy, or pericardial disease.[148] However, the prevalence of severe cardiovascular impairment has decreased substantially with ART. The Pediatric Pulmonary and Cardiovascular Complications of Vertically

Transmitted HIV study showed that inadequate or reduced left ventricular wall thickness was an independent predictor of morbidity and mortality, while even small decreases in fractional shortening were associated with marked increases in 5-year mortality.[149] It is therefore important to consider cardiac disease with congestive heart failure in HIV-infected children presenting with respiratory symptoms.

Pulmonary hypertension was reported in 7% of Zimbabwean HIV-infected adolescents, who were only diagnosed with HIV at 12 years.[7] Primary pulmonary hypertension has been increasingly reported in HIV-infected adults, but there are very limited data in children.[106]

Upper Airway Disease

Recurrent upper airways infections including otitis media or sinusitis may occur. Lymphoid proliferation with tonsillar and adenoidal hypertrophy, and pharyngeal infiltration may lead to upper airway obstruction.[150] Lymphoid infiltration of the epiglottis has also been described with gradual onset of drooling and dysphagia.[151] *Candida* epiglottitis has been described in HIV-infected children and highlights the importance of considering uncommon pathogens in immune-compromised children presenting with supraglottic inflammation.[152] Airway obstruction requiring tracheostomy was most commonly due to severe laryngotracheobronchitis in HIV-infected children in a South African cohort. The majority of children in this study were not on ART at time of tracheostomy and subsequently did well after treatment initiation.[153]

Summary

Respiratory diseases cause major morbidity and mortality in HIV-infected children, particularly in sub-Saharan Africa. The spectrum of illness encompasses acute and chronic disease. HIV-exposed, uninfected children have a higher risk of respiratory infections early in life compared to unexposed children. General and specific preventive strategies are effective for reducing respiratory morbidity and mortality, while early use of ART is highly effective for reducing the incidence of OIs, pulmonary morbidity, and mortality. Preventive interventions including immunization and use of long-term CTX prophylaxis reduce the incidence of specific respiratory infections and improve survival. With long-term survival, chronic lung disease in perinatally HIV-infected adolescents is an important cause of morbidity that may be ameliorated by the use of ART.

References
Access the reference list online at ExpertConsult.com.

67 Pediatric Lung Transplantation

JOSHUA A. BLATTER, MD, BLAKESLEE NOYES, MD, and
STUART CHARLES SWEET, MD, PhD

Introduction

With reports of successful heart-lung and lung transplantation in adults in the early 1980s,[1,2] the application of lung transplantation to the pediatric population became an appealing prospect. Early reports of success in children undergoing lung transplantation[3-5] led to a marked increase in such procedures beginning in the early 1990s. Between January 1986 and June 2014, more than 2000 lung and almost 700 heart-lung transplantations in patients less than 18 years old have been reported to the Registry for the International Society for Heart and Lung Transplantation (ISHLT).[6] The number of lung transplant procedures performed annually from 2006 to 2015 has varied between approximately 95 and 140. Historically, heart-lung transplant was considered for patients with end-stage lung disease, with the relatively healthy native recipient heart considered for use in a "domino" transplant. Heart-lung transplant was also considered in patients with right ventricular failure associated with severe pulmonary hypertension. However, in the current era, heart-lung transplant is typically reserved for cases associated with left ventricular failure or congenital heart disease not amenable to surgical repair. Thus the number of heart-lung transplants performed has dropped to approximately 10 per year worldwide.

Typically, 40–45 centers report pediatric lung transplants, yielding a statistical average of 2–3 transplants per center annually. In reality, a few centers perform the majority of these procedures, and most centers perform very few.[6] The number of lung transplants performed yearly is far below the number of other solid-organ transplants such as heart, liver, and kidney transplantation. This relative paucity is likely due to multiple factors, including lower prevalence of end-stage pulmonary diseases in children, improved therapies for cystic fibrosis (CF) and pulmonary hypertension, the significantly lower procurement rate of donor lungs compared with other organs, and the small number of pediatric lung transplant centers in the United States and worldwide.[7] Notwithstanding changes in the allocation of lung allografts (discussed later), the mortality rate for pediatric candidates aged 1–11 years awaiting lung transplantation remains higher than that in adults, underscoring the need to expand the potential donor pool and perhaps the number of centers performing this procedure.[8]

Indications and Timing

Indications for lung transplantation in children have undergone considerable change in the past three decades as experience with this procedure has grown. Lung transplantation has been performed successfully even in young infants with distinctly uncommon problems such as surfactant protein B deficiency and alveolar capillary dysplasia.[9,10] The most common diagnoses for which children are transplanted are listed in Fig. 67.1 according to the age in years at time of transplantation. In children younger than 1 year, the most common indications are pulmonary hypertension, usually associated with congenital heart disease, other pulmonary vascular diseases, primarily pulmonary vein stenosis, and rarely alveolar capillary dysplasia; disorders of surfactant metabolism, including surfactant protein B and C deficiencies and ABCA3 transporter mutations; and a spectrum of "fibrotic" lung diseases. Less common indications include interstitial lung disease, bronchopulmonary dysplasia,[4] and pulmonary hypoplasia. In patients 6–17 years of age, CF is the most common indication, and in the 12- to 17-year group, nearly 70% of pediatric lung transplants are performed in CF patients. In the 1- to 5-year age group, disorders leading to pulmonary hypertension remain a common indication. The relative percentage of children with primary pulmonary hypertension coming to lung transplant has diminished significantly during the past two decades, largely because of the introduction of effective medical therapies, including prostaglandins (epoprostenol), phosphodiesterase (PDE) inhibitors (bosentan), and sildenafil (see Chapter 35).[6] Surprisingly, despite a steady increase in the median survival for CF, the relative percentage of children with CF receiving lung transplants has not changed appreciably in recent years. Historically, timing of referral for lung transplant has been predicated on matching predictions of mortality with the anticipated waiting time for donor lungs. For example, studies in CF led to recommendations for referral for lung transplantation once the forced expiratory volume in 1 second (FEV_1) declined below 30% predicted.[11] Although more recent studies have attempted to add to these criteria,[12,13] none have improved significantly on the ability to predict waiting list mortality. Even in the best model, the positive predictive value is less than 50%.[12] In other diseases leading to lung transplant, criteria are less clear. Given absent or imperfect disease-specific criteria, before committing a child to lung transplant, most pediatric centers carefully consider multiple factors beyond lung function, including growth and nutritional status, frequency of hospitalizations, and potential for improvement in overall quality of life.

During the past 10 years, listing practices for children >12 years of age and adults have been affected by the adoption in 2005 of the "Lung Allocation System" (LAS) in the United States by the Organ Procurement and Transplantation Network (OPTN).[14] Based on models of waiting list mortality and posttransplant survival, this new system attempts to allocate donor lungs to maximize the 1-year transplant survival benefit. The survival models are based on diagnosis and other factors including age, height and weight, need for supplemental oxygen, pulmonary artery pressures, 6-minute

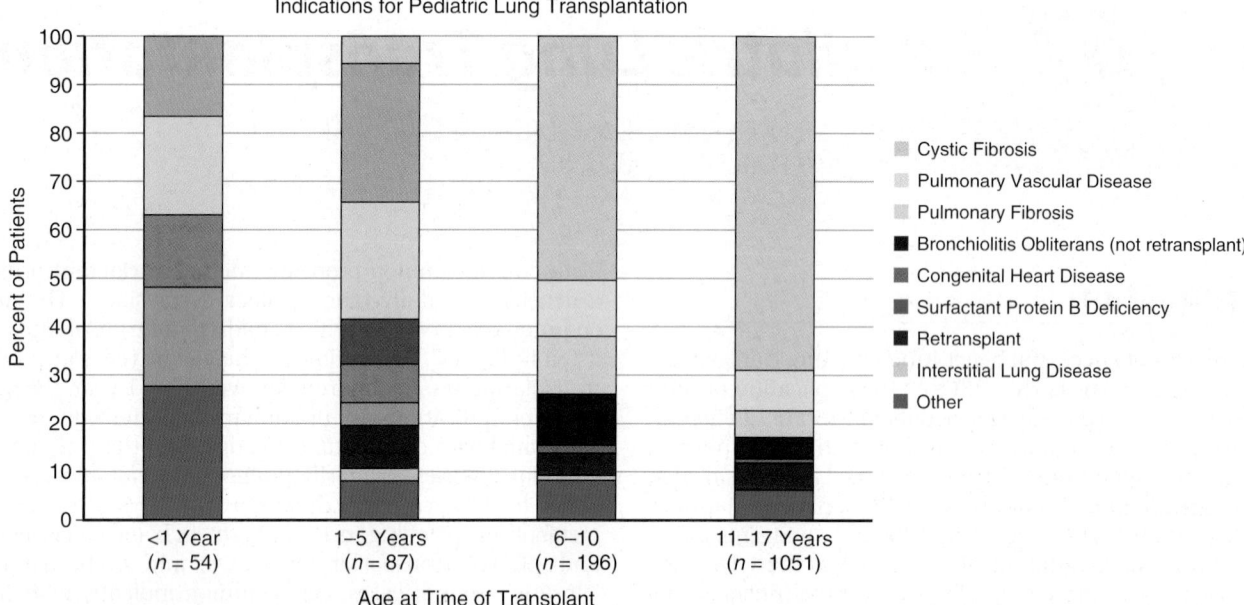

Fig. 67.1 Indications for pediatric lung transplant, January 2000–June 2014. (Data modified from Goldfarb SB, Benden C, Edwards LB, et al. The Registry of the International Society for Heart and Lung Transplantation: Eighteenth Official Pediatric Lung and Heart-Lung Transplantation Report—2015; Focus Theme: Early Graft Failure. *J Heart Lung Transplant*. 2015;34(10):1255-1263.)

walk distance, and lung function. Since adoption of the LAS, waiting time and waiting list mortality have decreased in the United States.[8] Nevertheless, an increased number of sicker patients are undergoing transplant—and a significant proportion of those patients (primarily those requiring mechanical ventilation) have had poorer overall survival than historical lung transplant cohorts—because the contribution of the waiting list mortality to the LAS is twice that of posttransplant survival[15]:

LAS = posttransplant survival − 2 × waiting list survival, normalized to a 0–100 scale.

An important aspect of the LAS is the potential for serially collected data from patients listed for lung transplant to be used for refinement of the underlying models that generate the priority score. For children younger than 12 years of age, in an effort to reduce waiting list mortality for these candidates, lung allocation was modified in the fall of 2010 to create two urgency tiers, similar to the status 1 and 2 in heart transplant allocation. Current changes in allocation involve the broader geographic sharing of pediatric donor lungs with pediatric recipients, which has been predicted to improve access for pediatric patients without adversely affecting adult ones.[16] It is difficult to predict the long-term benefits of these policy modifications.

There are numerous unsolved challenges in pediatric lung allocation, and a root problem is the relative scarcity of organs. Some usable organs are probably not being transplanted: among children whose families have agreed to donate at least one organ, less than 5% of 11-year-old-and-younger donors are providing lungs.[17] Extending pretransplant survival with lung bypass technologies, as well as salvaging suboptimal lung allografts (e.g., with *ex vivo* lung perfusion, [EVLP] discussed later in this chapter), have the potential to marginally increase the numbers of available donor lungs at a given time.[18]

Contraindications

As experience with pediatric lung transplant has grown, the number of absolute contraindications has declined, with most considered *relative* contraindications based on each transplant center's experience and expertise (Table 67.1).[19] Common absolute contraindications to pediatric lung transplantation include systemic disease affecting other organ systems, such as malignancy, HIV, hepatitis B or C, tuberculosis, and liver, renal, or left ventricular failure. However, in some transplant centers, multiorgan transplantation (e.g., liver-lung transplantation) may be an option in selected patients with failure of an organ other than the lung. In CF patients, *Burkholderia cepacia* complex (BCC) organisms are often a concern. Initially, all BCC organisms were thought to lead to poor outcome after lung transplantation, but more recent analyses have suggested that only colonization with *B. cenocepacia* (formerly BCC, Genomovar III), and a related organism, *B. gladioli*, carries significant risk.[20–22] *B. cenocepacia* colonization remains an absolute contraindication to lung transplant at a significant percentage of pediatric centers. Infection or colonization with Aspergillus, atypical mycobacteria (particularly *Mycobacterium abscessus*), or multiresistant organisms is a relative but not absolute contraindication in patients with CF.[23–26] It is not uncommon for lung transplant candidates to present unique and complex challenges to the transplant center, including malnutrition, diabetes, osteoporosis or osteopenia, vertebral compression fractures, and the use of systemic corticosteroids. These are considered relative, but not absolute, contraindications. Prior pleurodesis, either chemical or surgical, although not a contraindication to transplant, may prolong the ischemic time because of excessive bleeding from the parietal pleura, particularly when cardiopulmonary bypass and attendant heparinization are used, and is associated with higher mortality.[27]

Table 67.1 Contraindications to Pediatric Lung Transplantation

Absolute	Relative
Active malignancy within 2 years[a]	Pleurodesis
Sepsis	Renal insufficiency
Active tuberculosis	Markedly abnormal body mass index
Severe neuromuscular disease	Mechanical ventilation
Documented, refractory nonadherence	Scoliosis
Multiple organ dysfunction[b]	Poorly controlled diabetes mellitus
Acquired Immunodeficiency Syndrome	Osteoporosis
Hepatitis C with histologic liver disease	Chronic airway infection with multiply resistant organisms[c]
—	Fungal infection/colonization
—	Hepatitis B surface antigen positive

[a]Some centers prefer a disease-free interval of 5 years.

[b]Consider heart-lung transplant with concomitant left ventricular insufficiency or irreparable congenital heart disease, liver-lung transplant with concomitant hepatic failure.

[c]For some transplant centers, infection with *Burkholderia cepacia* complex organisms, particularly genomovar III (*B. cenocepacia*), is an absolute contraindication.

Modified from Faro A, Mallory GB, Visner GA, et al. American Society of Transplantation executive summary on pediatric lung transplantation. *Am J Transplant*. 2007;7(2):285-292.

Finally, psychosocial concerns for children, particularly nonadherence, can be particularly challenging, especially when the responsibility for adherence is shared between separated parents. Decisions about how to handle such cases—without creating the perception that the parent's misbehavior led to the child being denied the opportunity for transplant—must be an individualized, shared responsibility of both the referring and transplant centers. In families where nonadherence to a recommended treatment regimen is recognized, some centers recommend formulation of a contract between the referring physician and family that outlines the need for strict adherence to a treatment program over a 3- to 6-month period prior to evaluation/listing for lung transplant. In general, adherence concerns become an absolute contraindication only in combination with other medical risk factors or after persistent failure on the part of the child and family to meet a set of agreed upon expectations for care and follow-up. In contrast, a significant psychiatric or mental health disorder in either the primary caregiver or the patient is considered an absolute contraindication to transplant.

Surgical Technique

Potential donor lungs are evaluated using arterial blood gases, chest radiographs, airway cultures, and airway examination by bronchoscopy. The donor history is reviewed for signs/symptoms of acute viral infection. In addition, the donor is routinely screened for hepatitis A, B, and C, HIV, varicella-zoster, cytomegalovirus (CMV), Epstein-Barr virus (EBV), and herpes virus.[28]

One response to organ scarcity has been to explore the feasibility of longer-term lung bypass technologies. Extracorporeal membrane oxygenation (ECMO) is now being used as a "bridge to transplant" in some patients with end-stage disease. Patients who undergo short pretransplant ECMO runs may spend a longer intraoperative period on cardiopulmonary bypass, but they do not have worse survival.[29] This approach to bridging is now being extended to include "ambulatory ECMO," which allows for intensive physical rehabilitation for patients on the waiting list. Most pediatric patients undergoing ambulatory ECMO have had only short ECMO courses,[30] but an evaluation of outcomes in these cases will help to determine whether extended courses of ECMO could be used to augment the quality and quantity of pretransplant survival. Paracorporeal lung assist devices, which remove and oxygenate blood from the pulmonary artery, subsequently returning it to the left atrium, have been used as a longer-term bridge (e.g., greater than 2 months).[31] Nevertheless, these bypass technologies put patients at elevated risk of bleeding or infectious complications.

Another promising perioperative approach to organ scarcity is EVLP, which entails organ procurement followed by *ex vivo* diagnostics and organ reconditioning. Antibiotics can be used to perfuse the organ, thereby reducing bacterial load,[32] and clots can be washed from the pulmonary circulation.[33] Outcomes to date with EVLP lungs have been similar to non-EVLP lungs, and there is hope that this technology could be used to capture "marginal donor lungs" that would otherwise go unused.[34]

In most pediatric transplant procedures, cardiopulmonary bypass with heparinization has traditionally been used for the implantation procedure, but ECMO has become an increasingly common alternative.[35] The surgical approach is via a bilateral anterolateral transsternal incision (the "clamshell" incision), which optimizes visualization and access to both pleural spaces. The clear majority of children undergo bilateral sequential lung transplantation with telescoped bronchial-to-bronchial anastomoses. Pericardial or peribronchial lymphatic tissue from the donor and recipient is used to cover the anastomosis. This improves the blood supply to the anastomosis and may reduce the exposure of adjacent vascular structures to infection, in the event of airway infection and subsequent dehiscence.[36] In patients with CF, careful attention to maintaining sterility of the donor allograft requires vigorous washing of the recipient trachea and bronchial stumps with an antibiotic solution prior to implantation.

Heart-lung transplantation is rarely used in children in the United States at this time.[6] Even in the presence of marked right ventricular hypertrophy associated with pulmonary hypertension, successful bilateral lung transplantation is generally associated with resolution of right ventricular dysfunction.[37,38] In patients with pulmonary hypertension caused by a congenital heart defect, intracardiac repair of the anatomic defect may take place at the time of bilateral lung transplant, obviating the need for heart-lung transplantation.[39] Single lung transplantation is used infrequently among children, and much less than in adults.[6]

Success with living donor lobar lung transplantation was first reported by Starnes in 1994.[40] In this procedure, a right lower lobe from one healthy donor and a left lower lobe from another (generally family members) are implanted in the recipient. Typically, this technique has been used in both adults and children in the setting of rapidly progressive respiratory failure where cadaveric lung allografts were judged unlikely to be available or where further deterioration in clinical status would make the patient ineligible for deceased donor transplantation. Although living donor lung transplant has virtually disappeared in the United States since the introduction of the LAS, it is still used in Japan, where access to donor organs suitable for children has been restricted. Other strategies for increased availability of organs for children and other smaller recipients include donor downsizing using linear stapling devices or lobectomy and lobar transplant.[41]

Posttransplant Management

IMMUNOSUPPRESSIVE REGIMEN

In the immediate preoperative period, triple drug immunosuppression and directed antimicrobial therapy is begun. In virtually all circumstances, immunosuppression consists of a calcineurin inhibitor (CNI; either tacrolimus or cyclosporine A [CSA]), a cell cycle inhibitor (azathioprine or mycophenolate mofetil [MMF]), and corticosteroids. Based on studies suggesting marginally better efficacy, there has been a trend in recent years toward the use of tacrolimus and MMF over CSA and azathioprine.[42,43] Nearly all pediatric lung transplant recipients are on tacrolimus and more than 80% are on MMF at the end of the first year.[6] Because lung transplant recipients have a higher risk for rejection episodes than other solid organ transplant recipients, more intense immunosuppression regimens have been developed.[44] For example, the initial targets for trough levels for tacrolimus and CSA are typically maintained in a range of 10–20 mg/mL and 300–500 mg/mL, respectively. Initial dosing for prednisone is typically 0.5–1.0 mg/kg per day with the goal of 0.25–0.5 mg/kg per day by 3–4 months after transplant, depending on the clinical course. Nearly all patients remain on prednisone at 1 and 5 years posttransplant.[6] In addition, the use of induction immunotherapy at the time of transplant remains widely used in pediatric lung transplantation; recent data indicate that almost 70% of patients receive either a polyclonal agent (antilymphocyte or antithrombocyte globulin) or, more commonly, an interleukin-2 (IL-2) receptor antagonist (daclizumab or basiliximab).[6]

ANTIMICROBIAL REGIMEN

Most patients receive intravenous (IV) antibiotics before and after lung transplantation, based on the most likely potential infecting organisms. Cultures from the donor may allow precise choices of antibiotics. In patients without CF, a single antibiotic with broad gram-positive and gram-negative coverage is typically used for 7–10 days posttransplant. In recipients with CF, their pretransplant sputum cultures help guide therapy; typically, such antimicrobial therapy is directed against gram-negative organisms, commonly *Pseudomonas aeruginosa* and occasionally *Achromobacter* spp. Vancomycin is often included to cover methicillin-resistant *Staphylococcus aureus* (MRSA), which is being found increasingly in children with CF and advanced lung disease. In CF patients in whom *Aspergillus fumigatus* has been found, many transplant centers use voriconazole or anidulofungin postoperatively and, in

some circumstances, aerosolized amphotericin, oral itraconazole, or oral voriconazole.[7] Prophylaxis against *Pneumocystis jiroveci* is begun shortly after transplant with trimethoprim/sulfamethoxazole (TMP/SMX) administered three times weekly. In patients unable to tolerate TMP/SMX, nebulized pentamidine, oral atovaquone, or dapsone are alternatives. Oral nystatin is begun in the early posttransplant period to reduce the likelihood of candida infection.

Although the availability of ganciclovir has reduced the significance of CMV in lung transplant recipients, CMV remains a serious potential complication associated with an increased risk of mortality.[45,46] The approach to CMV prophylaxis in the pediatric lung transplant recipient is controversial, varying considerably among transplant centers. In most instances, CMV prophylaxis is not administered when both recipient and donor are CMV seronegative.[47] If either the donor or recipient is seropositive for CMV, ganciclovir or valganciclovir are administered for 4–12 weeks posttransplant. More recent studies have suggested a potential benefit to extending the duration of prophylaxis (with IV ganciclovir or oral valganciclovir) to 6 months or longer.[48,49] Some pediatric centers administer CMV hyperimmune globulin (CMVIg) in conjunction with ganciclovir based on reports of improved outcomes with CMV disease in adult patients.[50] However, the long-term benefit of CMVIg remains unclear.[51]

Management Issues Unique to Pediatrics

Although guided by the strategies used in adult lung transplant recipients, several significant differences exist in therapy and monitoring for pediatric lung transplant recipients, most importantly related to the ability to diagnose chronic lung allograft dysfunction (CLAD; defined later in this chapter).

Although spirometry is essential for the clinical diagnosis of CLAD, it is generally not reliable until children reach 6 years old. Using thoracoabdominal compression techniques, infant pulmonary function testing (PFT) can identify the presence of airflow obstruction, but this testing requires specialized equipment and experience.[52,53] Moreover, such tests cannot be performed as frequently as conventional spirometry because they require sedation or anesthesia. Infant PFT has not been used in recent chronic allograft dysfunction diagnostic criteria.[54]

An additional limitation for infants and toddlers relates to transbronchial biopsies (TBBx). Although TBBx forceps small enough to fit through the suction channels of endoscopes used for bronchoscopy in young children became available in the 1990s, the smaller forceps typically yield much smaller pieces of tissue. Therefore obtaining tissue for the diagnosis of rejection in infants may be technically challenging.

Therapeutic challenges also exist. Newer immunosuppressant and antiinfective agents often are not available in the liquid forms required for young children. Management of liquid forms can be difficult for patients and families, as they usually must be compounded by local pharmacies and may have a short shelf life. In addition, the use of liquid forms may be problematic for transplant centers because dosing decisions must often be made when appropriate absorption and pharmacokinetic data for infants and children are not available.

Complications

Complications following lung transplantation occur in predictable timelines: a few weeks after transplant, when the most common complications are related to the condition of the donor organs and the surgical procedure; an early phase, 1–6 months after transplant, when infectious and acute immunologic complications become more prevalent; and a late phase, >6 months after transplantation when chronic immunologic complications such as bronchiolitis obliterans (BO) and malignancies are observed more frequently (Fig. 67.2).

IMMEDIATE POSTTRANSPLANT PHASE

Because pediatric lung transplant procedures are performed with cardiopulmonary bypass or ECMO, postoperative bleeding, particularly in the pleural space or at the site of the vascular anastomoses, is a common concern.[4] Other complications of the surgical procedure include injury of the phrenic or recurrent laryngeal nerve, causing diaphragmatic or vocal cord dysfunction. Dehiscence at either the vascular or the bronchial anastomoses may require prompt surgical attention and an early return to the operating room. Most transplant centers perform flexible bronchoscopy within 24–48 hours of transplantation to obtain cultures from the lower airways and to assess the integrity of the airway anastomosis. Fortunately, dehiscence of the airway anastomosis has become rare since the development of techniques to cover the anastomosis with vascularized tissue.[36,55] However, other airway complications occur at a frequency comparable to that seen in adult lung transplant recipients, including fibrotic strictures, excessive granulation tissue, and airway collapse at the site of the anastomosis.[56,57] In the event of the development of stenosis of the airway lumen, balloon dilatation or stent placement by bronchoscopy may be necessary. Mechanisms invoked to explain the development of anastomotic narrowing include donor airway ischemia, impaired airway healing, and barotrauma if prolonged ventilation is needed after transplantation.[56]

Rejection

Lung allograft rejection remains problematic, representing an important obstacle to long-term success of transplantation, particularly in comparison to other solid organ transplant procedures. A variety of mechanisms have been proposed to explain this discrepancy, including the richness of immune effector cells resident in the pulmonary vasculature and lymphatic system, the ongoing daily exposure of the vast epithelial surface of the lung allograft to potential environmental irritants, toxins, and pathogens, and the fact that the lungs are exposed to the entire cardiac output.[58]

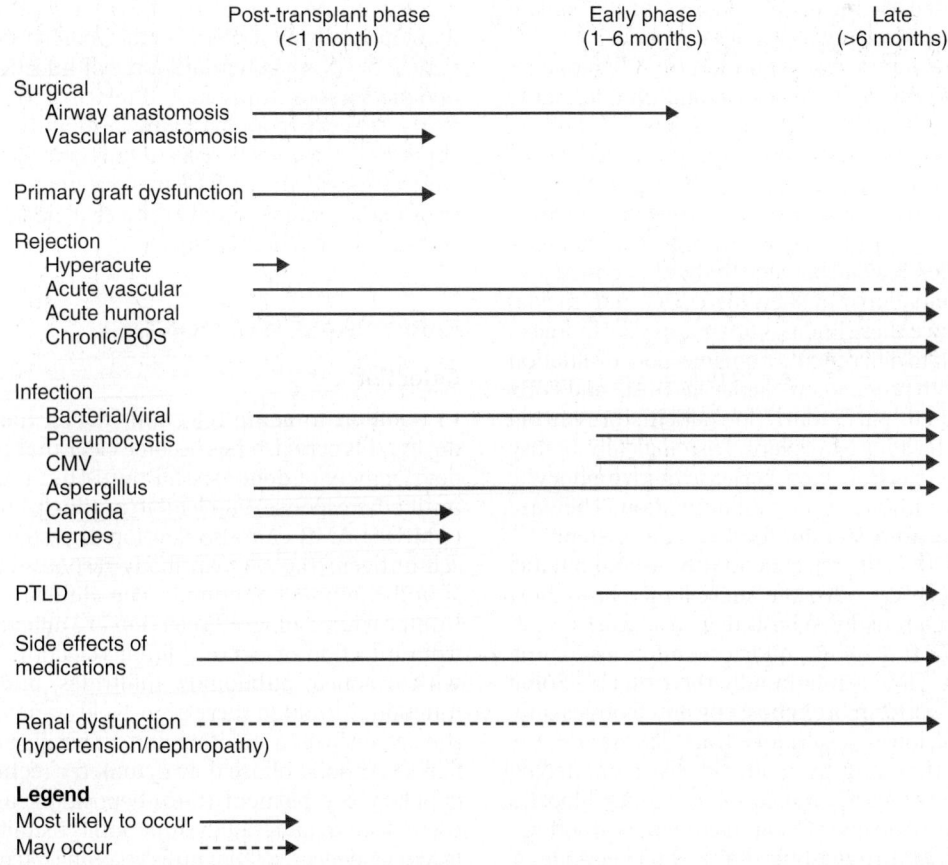

Fig. 67.2 Timing of complications after lung transplantation. *BOS,* Bronchiolitis obliterans syndrome; *CMV,* cytomegalovirus; *PTLD,* posttransplant lymphoproliferative disease.

Hyperacute rejection within hours of transplant is a rare, potentially catastrophic complication in the immediate post-transplant period associated with circulating recipient antibodies that bind to donor human leukocyte antigen (HLA) molecules on vascular endothelium, leading to significant graft ischemia.[4] It can be prevented by screening the recipient for anti-HLA antibodies and avoiding donors with related antigens. However, because the logistics of organ allocation often preclude HLA information being available at the time of organ offer, this approach is typically reserved for patients with antibodies to a significant percentage of HLA types. Alternatively, patients with a low percentage of antibodies reactive to the spectrum of HLA antigens undergo cross-matching at the time of transplant. Patients with positive cross-matches are usually treated with plasmapheresis to prevent hyperacute rejection, and even highly sensitized patients can undergo transplant.[59]

The most frequent problem that occurs in the first post-transplant week is primary graft dysfunction (PGD) related to reimplantation lung injury.[60,61] PGD is associated with the procurement procedure and duration of ischemia prior to implantation; the generation of hydroxyl radicals and proinflammatory cytokines during ischemia may be causative factors.[62–64] Complications related to graft dysfunction vary from mild, noncardiogenic pulmonary edema to a picture of acute respiratory distress syndrome histologically characterized as diffuse alveolar damage. Patients generally have marked hypoxemia and diffuse infiltrates. Treatment is supportive with careful fluid management and ventilatory support[65]; ECMO support has also been used in selected cases.[66,67] Although early retransplantation may be considered, outcomes in this setting are generally poor.[68]

Acute rejection is much more common than hyperacute rejection: most patients undergo at least one episode. Acute rejection can occur as early as 1 week after transplantation or as long as 2–3 years later. Most commonly, episodes of acute rejection occur 2–12 weeks after transplantation.[58] Nonspecific signs and symptoms of acute rejection include cough, fever, dyspnea, hypoxemia, and radiographic changes. Lung function studies, if available, tend to show an obstructive pattern. Chest examination may show tachypnea and crackles on auscultation. Since these findings are not specific for rejection and are difficult to differentiate from infection, evaluation by bronchoscopy with bronchoalveolar lavage (BAL) and TBBx is generally indicated, particularly for patients presenting in the first 3 months after transplant. Histologically, biopsy specimens in acute rejection show perivascular lymphocytic infiltrates with or without airway inflammation. They are classified according to a standardized scoring system.[69,70] Because patients with acute rejection may be asymptomatic, many transplant centers advocate surveillance bronchoscopy with TBBx on a scheduled basis (e.g., at 2 weeks, 1, 2, and 3 months after transplant, quarterly intervals for the rest of the first year, and semiannually thereafter).[19] Some transplant centers perform bronchoscopy and biopsies only when symptoms of lower respiratory tract disease become manifest, arguing that long-term outcomes are unaffected with this approach.[71] Performance of screening biopsies during the first posttransplant year has increased following publication of data suggesting that a single episode of minimal acute rejection is an independent risk factor for chronic rejection.[72,73] However, this finding was not confirmed

in a multicenter analysis of pediatric lung transplant recipients.[74]

Treatment of acute rejection consists of 10 mg/kg of IV methylprednisolone daily for 3 days. For persistent or recurrent acute rejection, lympholytic therapy with, for example, antithymocyte globulin may be initiated or the daily immunosuppressive regimen may be altered or enhanced. Although episodes of acute rejection are common after lung transplantation (perhaps even expected), there are data suggesting that younger transplant recipients (<3 years of age) have fewer episodes of acute rejection than older children or adults.[75–77]

Infection

Sources of increased risk of infection in the immediate post-transplant period and beyond are multifactorial. These include organisms present in the donor at the time of procurement, the intensity of immunosuppression, the loss of a normal cough reflex because of postoperative pain and the disruption of afferent and efferent nerves responsible for coordinating the cough response, impairment of mucociliary transport, and alteration in trafficking of immune effector cells to regional lymph nodes.[78] Despite the use of prophylactic antibiotics in the perioperative period, recipient factors (particularly in patients with CF) and donor factors (e.g., active viral infection) may lead to significant infectious complications early in the postoperative period. Younger children appear to be at greatest risk for early viral infections, perhaps because they are less likely to have developed immunity.[9] In CF transplant recipients, the chronically infected lungs may cause seeding of the blood or mediastinum with recipient airway flora during explantation. Furthermore, chronic sinus disease typical of CF is a potential source of infection to the allograft and has led some transplant centers to advocate pretransplant sinus surgery coupled with antibiotic washing of the sinuses.[79,80] However, a recent retrospective analysis of sinus surgery in patients with CF undergoing transplant at a major transplant center showed no survival benefit associated with pretransplant sinus surgery.[81]

EARLY PHASE (1–6 MONTHS)

Rejection

In addition to acute rejection, which has peak incidence during this period, it has become clear that the posttransplant development of donor specific anti-HLA antibodies (i.e., *allo*antibody response) can lead to antibody-mediated rejection (AMR).[82] AMR can also develop in response to circulating self-antigens (i.e., *auto*antibody response) such as collagen V and K-alpha 1 tubulin.[83] The clinical manifestations of humoral lung allograft rejection are difficult to differentiate from infection or acute cellular rejection. Patients present with dyspnea, pulmonary infiltrates, and decreased lung function. Although there is no "gold standard" for diagnosis, the presence of circulating donor specific antibodies (identified using solid phase flow cytometry techniques), alveolar capillary complement (C4d) deposition, and capillaritis in the setting of allograft dysfunction is usually considered sufficient evidence.[84,85] Diagnosis is complicated by disagreement regarding the meaning of laboratory testing: many laboratories report a mean fluorescence intensity (MFI) value, which—although it represents some amount of bound antibody to a single antigen bead—cannot be interpreted as a true titer.[86] Treatment of humoral rejection is also controversial. Most centers use some combination of steroids, plasmapheresis, IV immunoglobulin, and B-cell reduction (Cytoxan or rituximab).[87,88] The role of newer agents such as bortezomib, a proteosome inhibitor targeted at plasma cells, or complement inhibitors such as eculizumab remains to be elucidated.[89,90]

Infection

During this period, the risk of infectious complications is typically highest, especially in patients who have received an induction agent. The initial concern is for organisms carried with the donor organs during implantation or (primarily in the case of CF) harbored in the upper airways of the recipient. Subsequently, community and nosocomial organisms may cause infection, as may opportunistic (pneumocystis, candida) pathogens. Patients who are seropositive for CMV or who are seronegative and receive lungs from a CMV-positive donor are at risk for CMV disease during this early phase because most prophylactic regimens against CMV are completed during this period.

Clinical manifestations of CMV infection vary from a febrile, viral syndrome associated with leukopenia to invasive disease with viremia affecting, most commonly, the lung but also other organs, particularly the gastrointestinal (GI) tract. In CMV pneumonitis, patients may develop a constellation of signs and symptoms, including cough, fever, chills, respiratory distress, crackles, and diffuse interstitial infiltrates. Isolation of CMV by BAL or TBBx in the setting of a typical clinical picture is strongly suggestive of CMV pneumonia, although it is worth noting that asymptomatic shedding of CMV occurs. Treatment for CMV includes IV ganciclovir for 2–6 weeks and, in some centers, adjunctive therapy with CMV hyperimmune globulin. Oral valganciclovir may be administered for 2–3 months after completion of the IV ganciclovir course.

In the preganciclovir era the incidence of CMV disease in mismatched recipients reached 75% or higher in the first 6 months after transplant,[91] and CMV pneumonitis was a risk factor for the subsequent development of BO.[92] With the availability of ganciclovir for prophylaxis and treatment, the frequency of CMV pneumonitis has decreased and the significance of CMV disease in the lung transplant population has been reduced.[93,94]

P. jiroveci was a frequent problem in lung transplant recipients in the early phase after transplant before routine administration of TMP/SMX began in the late 1980s. As with other solid organ recipients, TMP/SMX prophylaxis has resulted in a marked decline in disease attributable to this fungus in lung transplant recipients. Patients ill with *Pneumocystis* present with acute onset of fever, respiratory distress, hypoxemia, and interstitial infiltrates. Silver or fluorescent staining of BAL specimens will demonstrate organisms with a typical morphology and is diagnostic of disease. IV TMP/SMX is the treatment of choice.

Viral infections can be particularly problematic during this period. Adenovirus[95] and paramyxoviruses including parainfluenza and respiratory syncytial virus (RSV) can cause significant lung injury or mortality.[96,97] Many centers treat these viruses aggressively with cidofovir and ribavirin,

respectively.[97–99] Moreover, fungal infections also pose significant risk.[100]

Medication Side Effects

Triple drug immunosuppressive therapy has offered a therapeutic approach that allows long-term success in solid organ transplantation. However, the side effects of these medications can be troublesome enough in some patients to ultimately affect functional outcome and quality of life. The degree of immunosuppression is a delicate balance between too much, with risks for the development of opportunistic infections, and too little, with its attendant risks of allograft rejection.

CSA and tacrolimus are both associated with hypertension and nephropathy, although these may be less severe with tacrolimus.[101] The risks of renal dysfunction with CSA or tacrolimus are compounded by the frequent use of other nephrotoxic drugs, such as aminoglycosides, ganciclovir, or amphotericin. One year after lung transplantation, 41% of patients have hypertension and 9% have renal dysfunction; this rises to 68% and 30%, respectively, 5 years after transplant.[6] Hirsutism and gingival hyperplasia appear to occur more frequently in CSA-based immunosuppression.[101] CNIs also cause neurologic toxicity, and seizures, headache, and sleep disturbance are common problems in the first months after transplant.[102] In patients with CF, inconsistent and erratic metabolism and absorption of CNI can occur and underscores the need for close monitoring of blood levels. Routine blood counts are necessary for patients receiving azathioprine or MMF because of their effects on white blood cell counts. Systemic and oral corticosteroids have the potential to cause a host of well-known side effects. For example, daily use of oral corticosteroids may lead to glucose intolerance and diabetes, particularly in patients with CF, with prevalence rates of more than 35% in long-term survivors of lung transplantation.[6] Patients receiving tacrolimus have a higher risk of developing diabetes than those receiving CSA.[42]

LATE PHASE (>6 MONTHS)

Ongoing complications in the late phase include those related to infection, drug toxicity, acute cellular and humoral rejection, and airway anastomotic narrowing. Posttransplant lymphoproliferative disease (PTLD) and CLAD, two very serious complications, also become apparent.

Posttransplant Lymphoproliferative Disease

The incidence of malignancy after lung transplantation in children is 5% 1 year after transplant and rises to 10% at 5 years; PTLD is by far the most common malignancy.[6] PTLD is generally an EBV-driven lymphoma in an immunosuppressed patient[104,105] and appears to occur more commonly in lung transplant recipients (as compared with other solid organ transplant recipients), in patients with CF, and in children as compared with adults.[106] These findings are probably explained by the intensity of immunosuppression in lung transplant recipients and the fact that many pediatric patients are EBV seronegative at the time of transplantation.[105]

Manifestations of PTLD are protean, often vague, and often confusing. A high index of suspicion is required because early diagnosis and treatment improves the likelihood of resolution of disease. In the first posttransplant year, the most common site of PTLD involvement in lung transplant patients is the allograft.[107] Although PTLD can be asymptomatic, symptoms of cough, fever, and dyspnea are typical. The typical radiographic finding is single or multiple round or ovoid pulmonary nodules.[108] Involvement of lymph nodes draining the chest is not uncommon. After the first year, the incidence of extrapulmonary PTLD increases. Other sites of involvement in PTLD include the GI tract, the skin, and other lymphatic tissue including lymph nodes and the nasopharynx.[109,110] Elevated quantitative measurement of EBV by polymerase chain reaction (PCR) has been shown to be a sensitive and somewhat specific marker for PTLD; most centers monitor this test on a regular basis.[111] In addition, positron emission tomography can be a sensitive and specific test that is often performed when EBV PCR or other clinical indicators raise suspicion for PTLD.[112] After a suspicious lesion is identified, histologic diagnosis is important for prognostic purposes. CD20-positive tumors may be more amenable to antibody therapy. A monomorphous histologic pattern has a worse prognosis.[113]

If PTLD is identified early, the mainstay of treatment is reduction in immunosuppression alone. Although some adult centers reduce immunosuppression based only on the presence of elevated EBV PCR,[114] a study suggests caution should be taken with this approach in children.[115] Although reduced immunosuppression can be successful in some patients, in many cases additional therapy is needed. Most centers now use therapy modeled after a Children's Oncology Group protocol that includes rituximab, an anti-CD20 monoclonal antibody shown to be effective in non-Hodgkin's lymphoma, low-dose cyclophosphamide, and prednisone. This approach has been promising in pediatric solid organ transplant recipients with PTLD.[116]

Chronic Lung Allograft Dysfunction

Chronic allograft dysfunction, most commonly BO, is the greatest obstacle to long-term success of adult and pediatric lung transplantation. By 6 years after lung transplantation in children, only 40% of survivors are free of BO, a worrisome figure because BO is the leading cause of death after the first year posttransplant.[6] Histologic analyses of lesions of BO show progressive and irreversible stenosis of the bronchiolar lumen, eventually resulting in fibrosis and near occlusion of the airway lumen with collagen.[94]

BO is generally equated with chronic lung allograft rejection, although the immunologic basis of BO remains poorly understood. As diagnosis of BO from tissue obtained by TBBx may be difficult because of the patchy and uneven distribution of the disease, a clinical correlate, bronchiolitis obliterans syndrome (BOS) was described. Among the criteria used to establish a diagnosis of BOS is an otherwise unexplained fall in FEV_1 of greater than 20% from the best previous baseline studies.[117] BOS was previously considered the clinical manifestation of BO, but it is now known that BOS is not specific for BO[118] and that chronic rejection can occur without evident changes in tissue pathology. Due to the variety of disease presentations of chronic rejection, the term "chronic lung allograft dysfunction" is now used to describe persistent lung function decline in transplant patients. Although BOS is associated with obstructive PFTs (i.e., FEV_1 decline), it is now recognized that some patients with chronic rejection develop progressively restrictive PFT changes (i.e., decline in

total lung capacity) and have a worse prognosis—a clinical entity that has come to be known as "restrictive allograft syndrome" (RAS).[119]

A variety of risk factors for the development of CLAD have been proposed, most based on single-center studies. A comprehensive review of these reports identified acute rejection as the only consistent risk factor with acute rejection episodes occurring more than 3 months posttransplant carrying the greatest significance.[92] The presence of lymphocytic bronchitis or bronchiolitis ("B-grade" rejection) was also significant, particularly when observed beyond 6 months after transplant. The role of CMV (based on donor or recipient serology, CMV "infection," or CMV pneumonitis) as a risk factor was deemed inconclusive, likely due in part to the use of ganciclovir prophylaxis and treatment.[93,94] More recently the presence of anti-HLA antibodies,[120,121] as well as autoantibodies to structural proteins such as K-alpha 1 tubulin and collagen V, have been identified as risk factors.[122,123] In addition, gastroesophageal reflux has been identified as a risk factor, with some evidence that fundoplication can reduce the incidence of BO.[124,125] An association between community-acquired respiratory viruses (paramyxoviruses, influenza, and adenovirus) has been suggested.[126,127] Finally, nonadherence with the immunosuppressive regimen can also result in BO.[128] In contrast, there are center-specific data showing that younger children[77] and patients receiving living related lobar transplantation[129,130] are at lower risk for developing BOS. Currently, the most prevalent hypothesis is that CLAD represents a final common pathway resulting from the immune response to an airway injury induced by one or more of these above risk factors leading to chronic airway epithelial damage and eventually severe airway obstruction.[131] The consistent identification of acute rejection as a risk factor for BO reinforces the importance of routine surveillance bronchoscopy to detect and treat subclinical acute rejection. As noted previously, this issue is further complicated by reports that episodes of minimal acute rejection (grade A1) were a risk factor for early-onset BO.[72,73] Although the consensus approach to grade A1 rejection in asymptomatic patients has been observation, to reduce the risk for early development of BO, the possibility of altering or enhancing immunosuppression in this setting has been entertained.

Treatment of CLAD is problematic at best, with augmented immunosuppression the general recommendation. Some transplant centers have endorsed changing the immunosuppressive regimen from CSA to tacrolimus, with anecdotal reports of success (though most pediatric centers no longer use CSA as their primary CNI).[132] The use of azithromycin 3 times weekly as an antiinflammatory agent appears to benefit a subset of patients, typically those with airway neutrophilia, leading to the suggestion that BO has at least one phenotype based on azithromycin responsiveness.[133] Treatment is complicated by the phenotypic variability of what is known as chronic rejection. Antilymphocyte agents such as antithymocyte globulin or OKT3 may be effective adjunctive therapy in some patients.[134] Recently, treatment with photopheresis has shown some benefit,[135,136] although not all CLAD patients will show equal response to therapy.[137] As with PTLD, early identification and treatment is most likely to be effective. However, in many patients, progression of disease is inexorable and often complicated by infection with bacterial or viral pathogens. The goal of therapy is to ameliorate the chronic rejection, reduce the risk of infectious complications, and prevent further deterioration in lung function. Many centers consider retransplantation as an option in patients with progressive decline in lung function.

Outcomes

SURVIVAL

Survival after pediatric lung transplantation for patients transplanted between January 1990 and June 2013 is depicted in Fig. 67.3.[6] There is no statistical difference in survival rates among the different age groups shown, with a 50% survival rate of 5.3 years collectively. When analyzed by era, median survival has improved significantly, from 3.3 years in the era between 1988 and 1999 to 5.8 years in the recent era (2000–2007). This improvement mostly reflects better early outcomes, not late outcomes[6]—with CLAD providing the primary barrier to longer-term survival. However, there has not been an improvement in survival between the eras 2000–2007 and 2008–2013. In addition, these results do not compare favorably with pediatric patients undergoing heart transplantation, in whom the median survival is more than 14 years.[138] In the most recent ISHLT report,[6] analyses of risk factors for 1-year mortality also demonstrated increased mortality in patients requiring ventilation at the time of transplant (hazard ratio [HR], 2.8) and in retransplant patients (HR, 2.8). Risk factors for 5-year mortality include retransplant (HR, 1.6) again. The hazard of 5-year mortality has a U-shaped distribution, with HR approximately 1 at age 1 that decreases to 0.85 at age 7, then rises to 1.4 by age 17,[6] with this significant rise typically attributed to issues with patient adherence.[139]

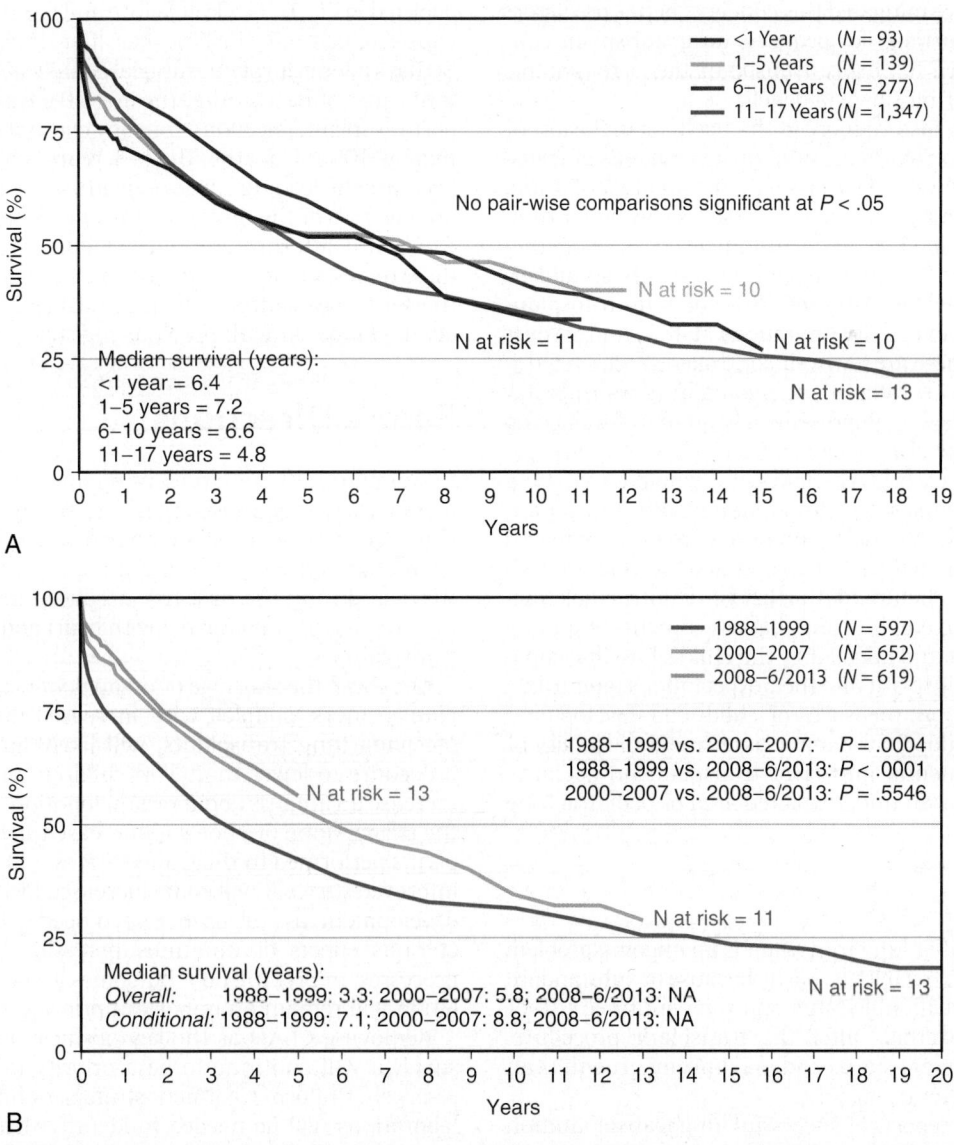

Fig. 67.3 (A) Survival after pediatric lung transplant, stratified by age (transplants January 1990–June 2013). (B) Survival after pediatric lung transplant, stratified by transplant era ("conditional" survival is contingent on patient surviving 1 year). (Reprinted from Goldfarb SB, Benden C, Edwards LB, et al. The Registry of the International Society for Heart and Lung Transplantation: Eighteenth Official Pediatric Lung and Heart-Lung Transplantation Report—2015; Focus Theme: Early Graft Failure. *J Heart Lung Transplant.* 2015;34(10):1255-1263.)

TRANSPLANT BENEFIT, FUNCTIONAL OUTCOME, AND QUALITY OF LIFE

Although transplant is generally viewed as a means for prolonging life, a provocative paper by Liou and colleagues[140] challenged the concept that pediatric lung transplant in the United States has achieved that goal. This was in contrast to an earlier report indicating a survival benefit from a group in the United Kingdom.[141] The validity of the recent study was challenged based on the fact that the dataset was biased against transplantation because covariates were obtained well before the time of transplant and estimates of benefit were based on factors that could change between listing and transplant.[142] Nonetheless, an important finding was that 57% of the children listed for lung transplant in the United States had a predicted survival of 5 years or greater,[140] suggesting that the waiting time–based system in the United States may have led to patients being listed well before transplant would have provided a survival benefit. Although the new LAS may have mitigated this concern, better predictors of waiting list mortality for pediatric lung transplant candidates are needed to ensure transplant has a reasonable chance of conferring survival benefit.

The Liou study also reinforced the need for inclusion of objective evaluation of quality of life in assessments of transplant benefit. Perhaps not surprisingly, the quality of life and survival in adult lung transplant recipients was better than candidates who remained on the waiting list.[143–145] Nonetheless, extrapolation to children and adolescents should be approached cautiously. Although 80% of lung transplant survivors report no activity limitations at 1, 3, and 5 years posttransplant, there are few well-controlled studies regarding quality of life in children undergoing lung transplantation. Nixon found a 24% improvement in quality of well-being in a small number of recipients after transplantation.[146] A group of 47 thoracic organ recipients (of whom 6 were lung transplant recipients) scored lower on a health status questionnaire administered to the parent or caregiver compared with a normal population but was similar to children with asthma, juvenile rheumatoid arthritis, or intractable epilepsy.[147] It is worth emphasizing that assessments of quality of life are difficult and affected by the child's baseline capabilities prior to transplant and their expectations after transplant.[146] In addition, measures of childhood development must also be included. Systematic assessment of quality of life and developmental impact of transplant on pediatric recipients remains an underexplored area of pediatric lung transplantation.

GROWTH

Somatic growth after lung transplant is an ongoing problem for most transplant recipients, partly because of substandard pretransplant nutritional status and the continued use of systemic corticosteroids after the transplant procedure. Improving nutritional status and maximizing growth is an important goal after transplant.

Since the early reports of successful lung transplantation in young children, concerns have been raised concerning the potential for lung allograft growth.[3] Animal data indicate that allogeneic lung transplantation is associated with an increase in lung volumes and airway size with age.[148]

Although spirometry and lung volume measurements following lung transplant have been reported to be normal in infants[149] and older children,[75] these measurements may reflect increased volume of each alveolar unit rather than alveolar tissue growth or increased surface area for gas exchange. Serial CT scan data to support growth of intrathoracic airways over time comes from Ro and colleagues.[150] However, the diffusing capacity of the lungs for carbon monoxide (DLCO) did not show an appreciable increase in a single-center study of pediatric recipients of cadaveric and living donor transplants.[151] Although DLCO provides a better estimate of gas exchange surface area, it is not easily measurable in infants. Thus further study is required to determine whether surface area for gas exchange increases as lung volumes increase in pediatric lung transplant recipients.

CAUSES OF DEATH

Causes of death after pediatric lung transplantation are depicted in Fig. 67.4. Graft failure and infection are important causes of death in the first year after transplant. In the first 30 days after transplant, surgical complications are an important cause of death. After the first 30 days and before a year posttransplant, infections from any cause account for approximately 30% of deaths. By 1–3 years after transplant, BO becomes the leading cause of death, accounting for approximately 35% of the mortality. Infection remains a significant cause of death throughout the follow-up period. Although these represent the most recent data available from the ISHLT, there has been little shift in the distribution of causes of death compared with previous registry data.[6]

Future Directions

In summary, although presenting unique challenges related to pediatrics, lung transplant is a life-saving option for infants, children, and adolescents with end-stage pulmonary parenchymal and vascular disease. In spite of improvements in survival during the past two decades,[6] long-term survival rates remain poor compared with heart and other solid organ transplants.

Moreover, the shortage of organ donors and of lung transplant centers, coupled with increased numbers of adults receiving lung transplants, will likely limit access to this procedure to fewer than 100 children annually. Efforts to increase awareness about organ donation will likely remain the cornerstone of efforts to increase the number of transplants performed in the United States and worldwide. With improved survival will come increased focus on growth and development, as well as increased need to minimize the deleterious effects of immunosuppression on these critical processes. Improving poor outcomes in the adolescent population will remain an important priority.

Removing CLAD as the key obstacle limiting long-term survival will continue to be a priority in lung transplant research. Uniform treatment strategies and multicenter collaborations will be needed to identify strategies for earlier diagnosis and determine treatment efficacy as few centers perform enough transplants each year to power such studies adequately. A key research opportunity would include identifying environmental factors, such as the lung microbiome,

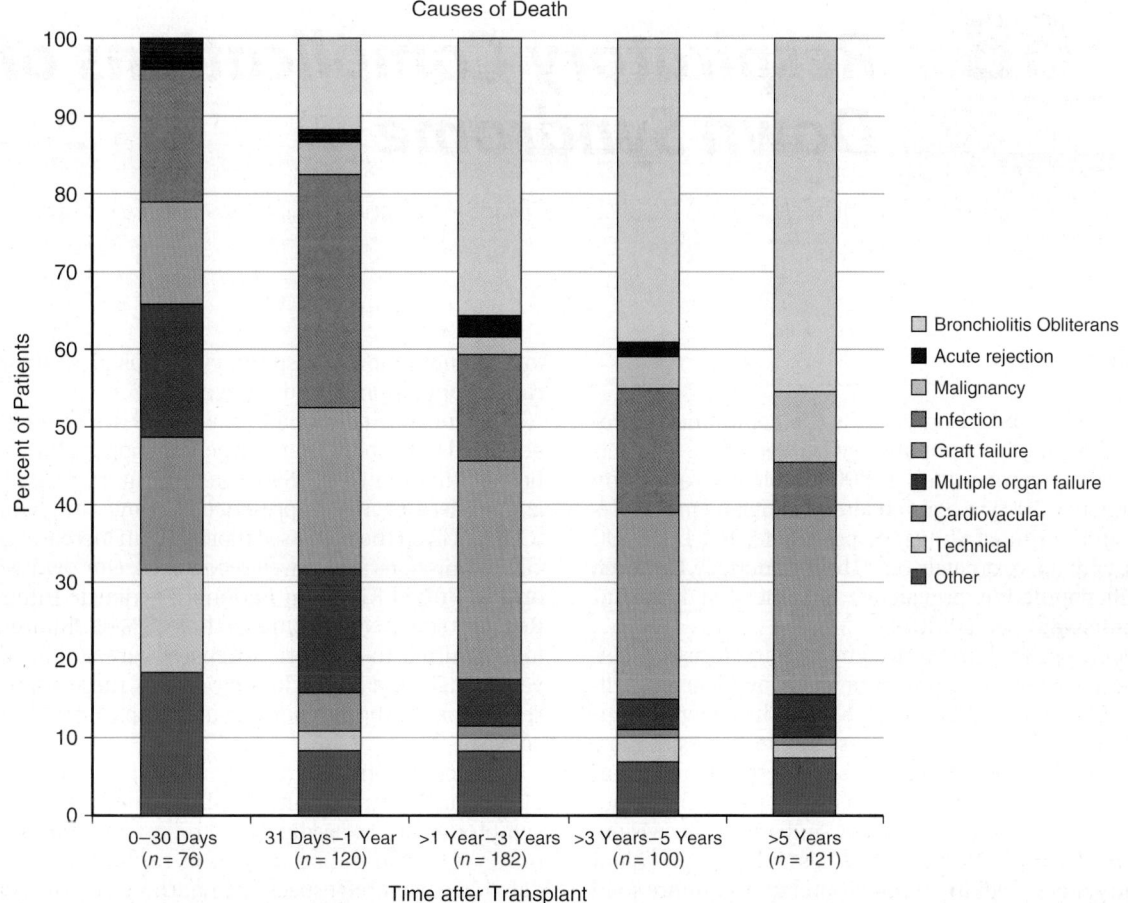

Fig. 67.4 Causes of death after pediatric lung transplant, January 2000–June 2014. (Data modified from Goldfarb SB, Benden C, Edwards LB, et al. The Registry of the International Society for Heart and Lung Transplantation: Eighteenth Official Pediatric Lung and Heart-Lung Transplantation Report—2015; Focus Theme: Early Graft Failure. *J Heart Lung Transplant*. 2015;34(10):1255-1263.)

that might directly contribute to—or be used as a biomarker that predicts—allograft failure.[152]

Despite these obstacles, more than 2000 children in the past three decades have been given a chance for long-term survival because of the success of lung and heart-lung transplantation. Although recent improvements in outcome for children with CF and pulmonary hypertension will hopefully reduce the number of children needing lung transplants, those who do should continue to benefit.

References

Access the reference list online at ExpertConsult.com.

68 Respiratory Complications of Down Syndrome

ANDREW P. PRAYLE, BMedSci, BMBS, PhD, and HARISH G. VYAS, DM, FRCP, FRCPCH

Introduction

Down syndrome (DS; trisomy 21) is the commonest chromosomal abnormality compatible with live birth. There is an incidence of approximately 1/800 live births, translating to approximately 700 live born children in England and Wales per year.[1] In the United States the prevalence is 14/10,000 live births, with approximately 6000 births annually. However, the overall population prevalence is somewhat lower, at approximately 8.3 per 10,000.[2]

The phenotype is characterized by a characteristic facies and stature, variable developmental delay and learning difficulties, and an increased incidence (over the general population) of multiple specific diseases, including respiratory disease, congenital heart defects, gastrointestinal malformations, autoimmunity, endocrine disease (in particular hypothyroidism), hematologic malignancy, and orthopedic, vision, and hearing disorders. Respiratory illness is highly prevalent within the general pediatric population but even more so in children with DS. Within this chapter we discuss the pertinent complications of DS for the respiratory pediatrician.

The lifespan of individuals with DS is gradually improving (Fig. 68.1). In 1983 median age at death was 25 years, significant progress was made in the 1990s, and by 1997 it was 49 years.[3] More recent estimates suggest that a child born in 2000 in Australia with DS had a life expectancy of 60 years.[4] Part of this improved survival is likely related to improved access to care, accompanied by a shift in public, professional, and parental attitudes to care of children with DS in the past few decades.[5]

Within this context of improving life expectancy, efforts should be made to understand and improve the pulmonary health of children with DS. Although some children with DS will unfortunately have devastating illness in childhood (often a combination of cardiac and respiratory disease), much of the respiratory disease either improves with maturity or is amenable to treatment. Therefore respiratory pediatricians need to be vigilant for symptoms of respiratory disease, judicious in investigation, and mindful that the consultation involves careful explanation in a way that the patient and carers can understand.

Children with DS are more likely to develop respiratory disease than their peers without DS, and mortality from respiratory disease in childhood in DS is higher than the general population. Respiratory disease is the second leading cause of death in children with DS, after cardiac disease.[3] The rate of death of children with DS can be compared with the general population with the standard mortality odds ratio (SMOR). The SMOR in children under 10 with DS (compared with children without DS) is 14 for cardiac disease, and 3.0 for a combination of respiratory pathologies including aspiration, pneumonia, and influenza.

Not unexpectedly, children with DS are more likely to be admitted to hospital than the general population. More than half of children with DS have a respiratory related hospitalization, irrespective of presence of congenital heart disease (CHD).[6] Given the increased mortality, an increase in intensive care admissions is also well recognized. Our own work based on the United Kingdom national Paediatric Intensive Care Registry (PICANet) estimates that 25% of children with DS are admitted to pediatric intensive care units (ICUs) by 1 year of age, and approximately half of these admissions are respiratory, although cardiac and respiratory disease often coexist.

The common clinical manifestations of respiratory disease in DS are summarized in Table 68.1. Respiratory symptoms are exceedingly common in infants with DS; however, because most studies of respiratory symptoms to date have been retrospective in nature, the true scale of the problem has not yet been fully characterized. A prospective web-based parent-reported observational study is ongoing in the Netherlands, which seeks to characterize the relationship between respiratory symptoms, health care use, and comorbidities.[7] This study will provide useful information for clinicians.

Given the multiple manifestations of respiratory disease in DS, in this chapter we will elaborate on respiratory disease in DS using an anatomically structured approach and categorize disease into that of the upper and lower airways. However, it should be noted that frequently patients with DS may have multiple disease processes of both the upper and lower airways, and there is considerable overlap between symptoms and disease. Therefore it is appropriate to take a holistic "whole respiratory tract" approach to diagnosis and management. In addition, it is important to note that disease of other organ systems (chiefly cardiac, gastrointestinal, immunologic, and neurologic) and obesity in DS can increase the severity of respiratory disease (Table 68.2).

Upper Airway Disease and the Trachea

ANATOMY OF THE UPPER AIRWAY IN DOWN SYNDROME

In DS the upper airway is narrowed both above and below the vocal folds. Narrowing above the trachea is due to relative macroglossia, midface hypoplasia, narrowed nasopharynx, choanal stenosis, enlarged tonsils and adenoids, lingual

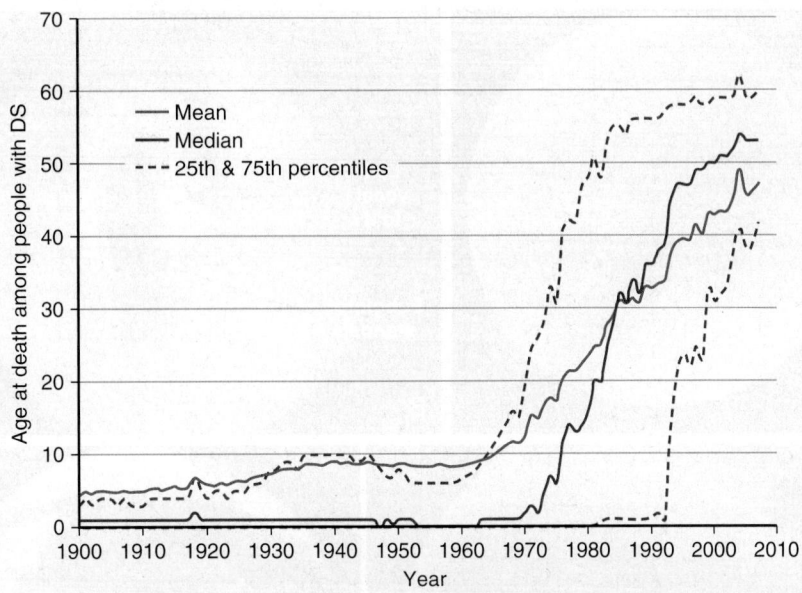

Fig. 68.1 Improvement in survival in people with Down syndrome (DS) in the United States. Presson and colleagues combined data from live births of infants with DS from 1907 to 2007, published birth prevalence estimates of DS, and mortality data from death certificates to inform a Monte Carlo model of survival over the past century. The improvement in survival commencing in the 1970s is striking. (Presson AP, Partyka G, Jensen KM. Current estimate of Down syndrome population prevalence in the United States. *J Pediatr.* 2013;163(4):1163-1168.)

Table 68.1 Respiratory Disease Patterns in Down Syndrome

Symptom	Etiology
Upper airway obstruction	Stridor
	Obstructive sleep apnea/sleep-disordered breathing.
	Postextubation stridor
Recurrent respiratory infections	Viral upper respiratory tract infections
	Lower respiratory tract infections (viral/ bacterial)
	Lobar pneumonia
	Aspiration pneumonia
Wheeze	Pulmonary edema/pulmonary hypertension
	Asthma

Table 68.3 Upper Airway Anomalies in Down Syndrome

Smaller midface and lower face skeleton	Shorter hard palate length
	Smaller mandible volume
	Shorter mental spine–clivus distance
Soft tissues	Smaller tonsils
	Smaller adenoids
	Smaller tongue
Relative impact of skeletal size upon soft tissue to airway size ratio	Higher tongue to skeletal size ratio
	Reduced upper airway size due to soft tissue crowding

Modified from Uong EC, McDonough JM, Tayag-Kier CE, et al. Magnetic resonance imaging of the upper airway in children with Down syndrome. *Am J Respir Crit Care Med.* 2001;163(3 Pt 1):731-736 and Guimaraes CV, Donnelly LF, Shott SR, et al. Relative rather than absolute macroglossia in patients with Down syndrome: implications for treatment of obstructive sleep apnea. *Pediatr Radiol.* 2008;38(10):1062-1067.

Table 68.2 Disease Complicating Respiratory Illness in Down Syndrome

Organ System	Manifestation
Cardiovascular	Airway compression secondary to congenital heart disease
	Pulmonary hypertension
	Pulmonary edema (including high altitude related)
	Complications of cardiac surgery
Gastrointestinal	Swallowing dysfunction
	Gastroesophageal reflux disease
	Respiratory complications following repair of esophageal atresia
Immune system	Recurrent respiratory tract infections
	Increased severity of respiratory tract infections
Neurologic	Hypotonia
Other	Obesity

tonsils, and a short palate (Table 68.3). Below the vocal folds, the trachea itself is considerably narrowed, with an internal diameter approximately 2 mm narrower than the general population in the pediatric age range.[8] This narrowing likely contributes to the increased incidence of postintubation stridor historically observed in children with DS.[9]

TRACHEOMALACIA AND LARYNGOMALACIA

Airway abnormalities contribute significantly to symptoms in DS (Fig. 68.2), but this information is largely based on case series naturally representing groups of patients who have particularly serious symptoms. Without background population data, case series can produce incorrectly elevated prevalence of diseases. In addition, case series are usually limited to small numbers of children, and so estimates of prevalence of rarer conditions vary widely between series.

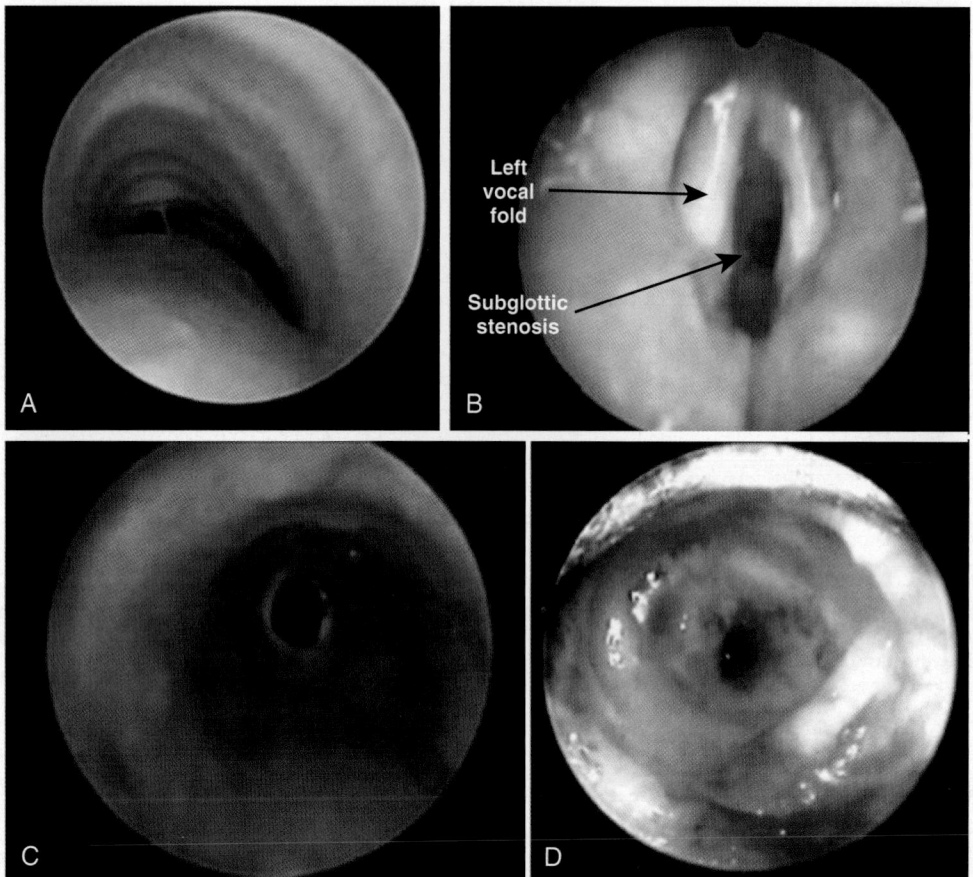

Fig. 68.2 Airway endoscopy abnormalities in Down syndrome. (A) Lower trachea appearance under general anesthesia, showing severe airway malacia. (B) Appearance of subglottic stenosis immediately below the vocal fold. (C) Midtracheal stenosis due to previous intubation. (D) "Pinpoint" severe tracheal stenosis. ([A–C] From Hamilton J, Yaneza MM, Clement WA, et al. The prevalence of airway problems in children with Down's syndrome. *Int J Pediatr Otorhinolaryngol.* 2016;81:1-4. [D] From Shapiro NL, Huang RY, Sangwan S, Willner A, Laks H. Tracheal stenosis and congenital heart disease in patients with Down syndrome: diagnostic approach and surgical options. *Int J Pediatr Otorhinolaryngol.* 2000;54(2-3):137-142.)

Table 68.4   Endoscopic Findings in Down Syndrome

Series	Hamilton[10]	Bertrand[11]	Estimated Down Syndrome Population Prevalence (%) (From Hamilton[10])
Number studies	39	24	
Subglottic stenosis	14	1	5.9
Laryngeal cleft	2	0	0.8
Laryngomalacia	2	12	0.8
Tracheomalacia	14	8	5.9
Bronchomalacia	10	5	4.2
Tracheal stenosis	2	1	0.8

Data from Hamilton J, Yaneza MM, Clement WA, et al. The prevalence of airway problems in children with Down's syndrome. *Int J Pediatr Otorhinolaryngol.* 2016;81:1-4 and Bertrand P, Navarro H, Caussade S, et al. Airway anomalies in children with Down syndrome: endoscopic findings. *Pediatr Pulmonol.* 2003;36(2):137-141.

In a series of 239 children with DS of whom 39 (16%) underwent endoscopy for airway symptoms,[10] the most common finding was tracheobronchomalacia (Table 68.4). In approximately half of patient with tracheobronchomalacia, this affected both the trachea and bronchi.[11] Laryngomalacia is common in children with DS and usually presents in the first months of life. Supraglottoplasty is uncommonly performed for laryngomalacia and is reserved for complications such as feeding failure, respiratory distress, and sleep-related symptoms or apnea, often in the context of subglottic stenosis and cardiac surgery. However, surgical failure can occur in up to a third of patients, and in some patients tracheostomy may be required.[12] When undertaking surgery for laryngomalacia, the possibility of further surgical intervention should be considered and discussed with families.

Tracheal bronchus (wherein the right upper lobe bronchus originates directly from the trachea rather than the right main bronchus) can predispose to lower respiratory tract infection (LRTI).[13] In a report on bronchoscopy findings in children, 2 of 18 patients with a tracheal bronchus had DS, which would suggest that the incidence in children with DS is elevated. Where recurrent right upper lobe pneumonia occurs in DS, a tracheal bronchus should be considered. When associated with other airway anomalies such as stenosis, tracheal bronchus can cause significant management challenges. This is especially so in the critical care setting where distortion of the usual anatomy can lead to significant hypoxic events in association with changes in the position of the head and neck.[14]

SUBGLOTTIC AND TRACHEAL STENOSIS

Narrowing can occur at any point in the airways in DS. However, subglottic stenosis deserves particular discussion. The overall prevalence of congenital subglottic stenosis in DS is approximately 1.3%.[10,11] Most subglottic stenosis occurs in the context of previous intubation, although this is not always the case. Laryngotracheoplasty has a good success rate and is presumably undertaken for patients on the more severe end of the spectrum, of whom most have preen previously intubated.[15]

Despite the prevalence of subglottic stenosis, the diagnosis should not be presumed in all cases of postoperative stridor. In children with DS ventilated for cardiac surgery, up to 25% develop postoperative stridor in the absence of subglottic stenosis.[16] These children tended to be less than the 10th centile for weight and younger (with a mean age of 8 months, compared with a mean age of 30 months in those without postoperative stridor).

Tracheal stenosis (narrowing below the subglottic space extending a varying length along the trachea) can be challenging to evaluate in DS. Tracheal stenosis in DS is associated with vascular rings and hypoplasia of the aortic arch. At induction of general anesthetic, it may be that the extent of the stenosis prevents the admission of even a narrow fiberoptic bronchoscope, especially if one or more complete tracheal rings are present. When this occurs, a nonionic tracheobronchogram or thin cut computerized tomography (CT) scan can be used to delineate the extent of the narrowing.[17]

CLINICAL PRESENTATION OF UPPER RESPIRATORY TRACT DISEASE IN DOWN SYNDROME

The clinical features of upper respiratory tract disease in DS include cough and parental report of noisy breathing and snoring. Sleep-disordered breathing in DS is discussed later. Parents and carers describe a wide range of breathing-associated sounds, with varying diagnostic utility. Snoring should be specifically asked for because a history of snoring is not always spontaneously volunteered. In more severe disease, upper airway abnormalities can lead to increased work of breathing and failure to thrive. Symptoms often worsen with self-limiting (presumed viral) upper respiratory tract infections and in LRTIs where the increased respiratory rate unmasks previously asymptomatic upper airway disease. A history of stridor, croup, chronic aspiration, and difficulty in extubation should motivate careful assessment and investigation.

Sleep-Related Breathing Disorders

Sleep-disordered breathing, including obstructive sleep apnea (OSA), is common in DS. There are multiple structural and functional factors contributing to disordered and disturbed sleep in DS, including midfacial hypoplasia, relatively large tongue, small upper airway with superficial tonsils, increased secretions, obesity, and hypotonia (Fig. 68.3).[18] It is worth noting that the tongue in DS is actually smaller than in

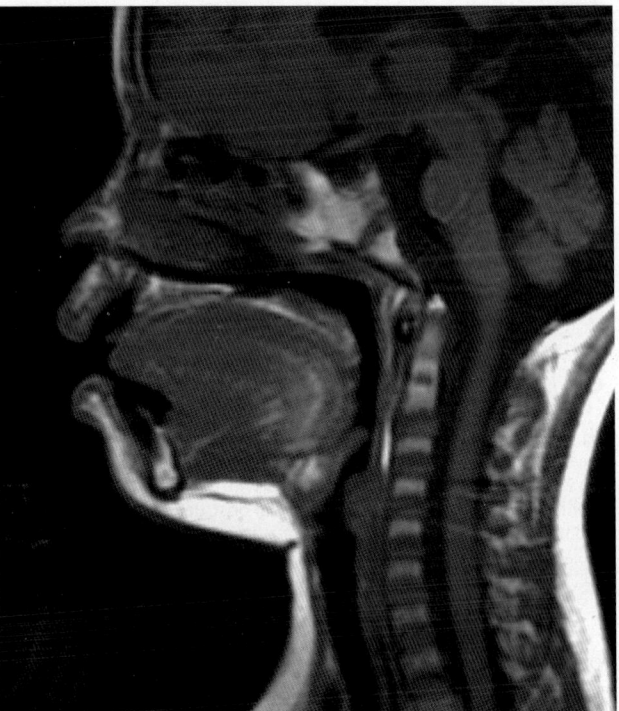

Fig. 68.3 Sagittal magnetic resonance imaging of the head in Down syndrome. Note the apparent macroglossia caused by the small midface. The tongue is in fact normal in size, and the midface is small. (Courtesy Prof. Lane F. Donnelly MD, Texas Children's Hospital, Baylor College of Medicine Texas Children's Hospital.)

age- and sex-matched controls on magnetic resonance imaging (MRI) scans. The apparent macroglossia is actually due to small craniofacial parameters, leading to relative macroglossia for the size of the oral cavity.[19] Similarly, adenoid and tonsil volume is actually smaller in children with DS without symptoms of OSA, but there is soft tissue crowding within a smaller midface.[20]

Disturbed sleep behavior is frequently reported in DS. Snoring occurs in half of school-age patients and is accompanied by parental report of restlessness, frequent waking, bedwetting, delay in becoming alert after waking, and challenging sleep behavior. However, there is little correlation between polysomnography findings and parental report.[21]

Sleep-disordered breathing is associated with neurocognitive difficulties, including developmental delay, challenging behavior, tiredness, pulmonary hypertension, and faltering growth. Unfortunately, these are all also associated with DS, and therefore the impact of sleep-disordered breathing may be unrecognized.[22] Sleep disturbance can be assessed with a respiratory disturbance index; in children with DS, there is a significantly higher respiratory disturbance index than in controls (Fig. 68.4).[23] In addition to OSA, the sleep of children with DS demonstrates increased fragmentation, numerous awakenings and arousals, and periodic leg movements. These characteristics are to a certain extent independent of the respiratory system and occur in the presence or absence of OSA.

The reported incidence of OSA in DS depends to a certain extent on the definition used and how aggressively patients are investigated. In unselected consecutive patients with DS

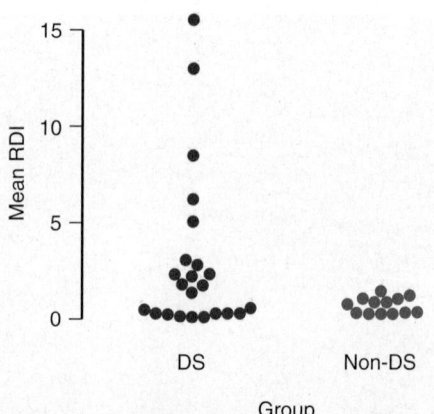

Fig. 68.4 Respiratory disturbance index (RDI) in children with and without Down syndrome (DS). Comparison of RDI in children with and without DS. 23 children with DS were compared with 13 children with primary snoring. RDI, calculated as the number of obstructive or mixed apneas and hypopneas per hour of sleep. (Data from Levanon A, Tarasiuk A, Tal A. Sleep characteristics in children with Down syndrome. *J Pediatr.* 1999; 134(6):755-760.)

prospectively evaluated with polysomnography, there is evidence of a high background rate of OSA, up to 80%. An increased apnea index and elevated arousal index is found in individuals with a high body mass index (BMI). This is not always associated with snoring.[24,25]

Adenotonsillectomy is usually the first-line treatment for OSA. However, the success rate of adenotonsillectomy is lower in DS than in the general population,[26] with only partial improvement in polysomnogram parameters such as the apnea-hypoxia index. Importantly, OSA is prevalent even after surgery.[27] Thus adenotonsillectomy may not be effective alone in treating OSA in DS.

In addition to surgical management of OSA being less effective in DS, tonsillectomy and adenoidectomy in DS are associated with an increased risk of postoperative complications,[28] and therefore careful postoperative monitoring is required for these patients. For patients with severe OSA it may be prudent that postoperative care takes place on the ICU. In all DS cases, we advocate an inpatient (rather than day case) procedure, to allow for monitoring on the night after the surgery. If adenotonsillectomy is unsuccessful, further therapeutic options can include home oxygen, continuous positive airway pressure (CPAP), further surgery, and tracheotomy in extreme cases.

Central hypoventilation can occur in the absence of upper airway anomalies, and higher rates of central apnea are seen compared with other syndromes of developmental delay such as fragile X.[29] Sleep apnea in DS is multifactorial in origin, and both airway abnormalities and a central mechanism may play a role.

Lower Respiratory Tract

ETIOLOGY

Like the upper respiratory tract, the lower respiratory tract has multiple recognized malformations in DS. Within this context, even minor superimposed infection becomes more severe than would be anticipated in a child without DS.

Pulmonary infection is multifactorial in origin, with contributing factors including decreased pulmonary reserve due to morphologic differences, poor immunologic function, gastroesophageal reflux disease and aspiration, interactions with CHD, and thoracic cage malformations.

HISTOPATHOLOGY OF THE LOWER RESPIRATORY TRACT IN DOWN SYNDROME

A number of morphologic differences in lung parenchyma contribute to reduced functional reserve in children with DS. The changes can be so severe that an experienced pediatric pathologist may recognize that a sample of lung tissue is from a patient with DS on external macroscopic evaluation alone.

In DS the lung has a diffuse uniform porous pattern, with increased size of alveoli and alveolar ducts.[30] This pattern occurs postnatally; the lung tissue has a more normal appearance in prenatal life. These features are due to a failure of alveolar multiplication within the acinus. The enlarged alveoli and acinar hypoplasia (deficient alveolar multiplication) can be formally characterized by radial count. In late gestation fetuses the radial count in DS is higher than controls. However, postnatally the radial count drops, and this reduction is present throughout life (Fig. 68.5). This causes a reduction in the number of alveoli and the overall lung surface area. This acinar hypoplasia has been suggested to be due in part to the complex interaction of the heart and lungs in patients with severe CHD who undergo mechanical ventilation, because radial counts are known to be low in CHD in the absence of DS. However, acinar hypoplasia appears to occur independently of CHD in children with DS.

Subpleural cysts are well recognized in DS (Fig. 68.6), although the relevance of these to pulmonary disease has not yet been fully elucidated.[31,32] These cysts are approximately 1–2 mm in diameter and are lined by cuboidal epithelium. Up to 20% of patients with DS have them at postmortem, and they have been found in 36% of chest CT scans.[33] They are underrecognized and usually not apparent on chest radiographs. Their development has been suggested to occur secondary to reduced postnatal production of peripheral small airways and alveoli, which likely occurs in early postnatal life.

EPIDEMIOLOGY OF LOWER RESPIRATORY TRACT INFECTION IN DOWN SYNDROME

Children with DS are at high risk of early hospitalization in the preschool age due to respiratory disease.[6,34] In a cohort of children with DS who survived to discharge from hospital after birth, half were admitted again at least once in their first 3 years of life, with a median number of two further admissions. The most common reasons for admission (in order of frequency) are CHD, pneumonia, acute bronchitis, and bronchiolitis, with respiratory disease occurring in approximately 50%. The length of stay for children with DS is often 2–3 times longer than that of children without DS, and respiratory support is more likely to be required.

The importance of even apparently mild respiratory tract infections in DS should not be underestimated. Recurrent respiratory tract infections can have implications for neurodevelopment in DS.[35] Children with DS whose parents report

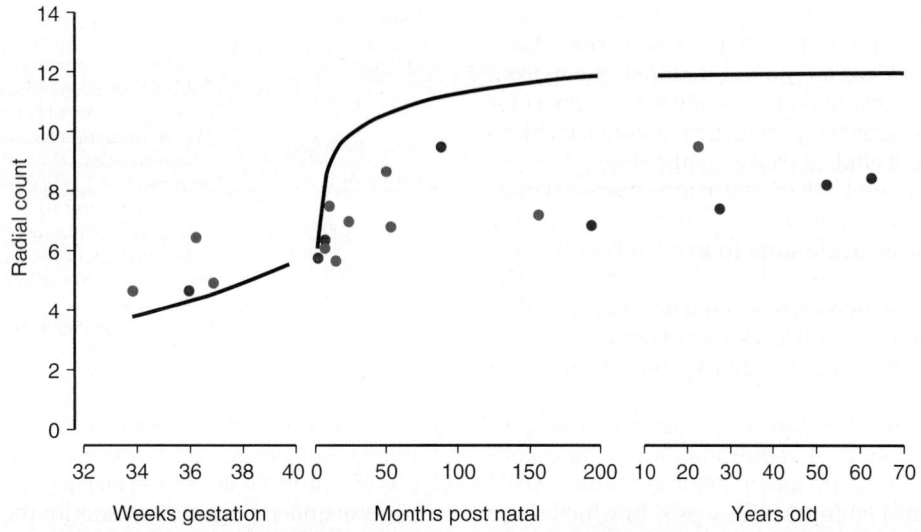

Fig. 68.5 Comparison of radial count in Down syndrome (DS), cardiac disease, and normal individuals. Points represent individuals with DS *(solid circles)* or cardiac disease *(hollow circles)*. Solid line indicates expected values for people without DS. (Modified from Cooney TP, Wentworth PJ, Thurlbeck WM. Diminished radial count is found only postnatally in Down's syndrome. *Pediatr Pulmonol.* 1988;5(4):204-209.)

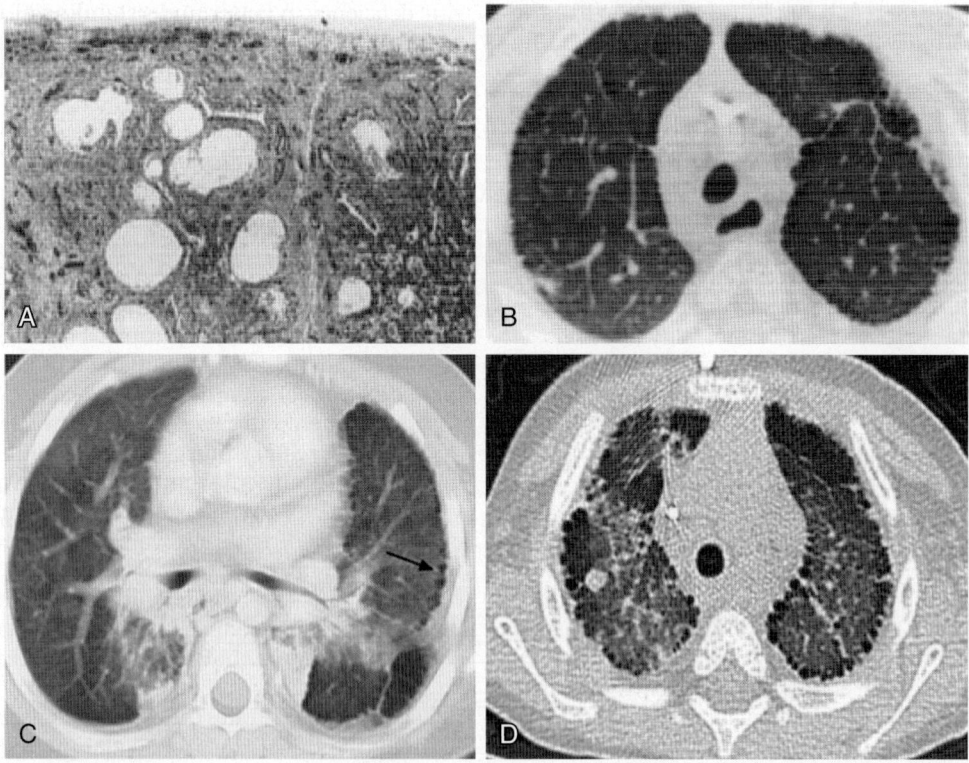

Fig. 68.6 Subpleural cysts in Down syndrome. (A) Histopathology sample showing cysts lined by a cuboidal epithelium along the pulmonary surface. (B) Computerized tomography appearance of subpleural cysts, of approximately 3–5 mm in diameter. (C) Subpleural cysts can be unilaterally distributed, in this case in only the left hemithorax, and associated with pleural thickening. (D) Cysts can be diffusely spread over both hemithoraces in the subpleural region.

frequent LRTI have lower developmental scores translating to a 5-month drop in abilities when measured at 8 years of age.

Viral infection is an important cause of respiratory disease in DS, and respiratory syncytial virus (RSV) is particularly troublesome. Between 10% and 15% of children with DS without significant comorbidity are hospitalized due to RSV.[36,37] The odds of a child with DS being admitted with RSV are 6 times higher than the general population, and of those hospitalized approximately 10% require mechanical ventilation. Children with DS and RSV are more likely to have fever and consolidation on chest radiograph and more frequently receive bronchodilators (implying an increased rate of wheeze) compared with children without DS.

Guidelines regarding the use of palivizumab in children with DS vary, and this remains a controversial area.[38] Randomized trials are lacking, but nonrandomized studies from Canada and the Netherlands demonstrate some support for the notion that palivizumab may be beneficial for all children with DS[39]; however, a clinical trial is required.

In addition to increased risk of severe lung disease requiring respiratory support, when receiving intensive care, there is an increased risk of acute lung injury (ALI) and acute respiratory distress syndrome (ARDS)[40]; surprisingly, the overall mortality is not increased. It could be speculated that ALI and ARDS occur in DS with less severe underlying disease, and that it is the underlying disease that ultimately drives mortality.

Overall mortality in DS is low in the pediatric intensive care unit (PICU), with rates of approximately 6%[41] and standardized mortality rates similar to children without DS.[42] However, the scenario changes with sepsis, in which there is an increased risk of mortality.[43] Our interpretation of these results is that respiratory infection in DS, even in critically ill children, does not necessarily confer an increased risk of mortality, although ALI and ARDS are more likely to occur. However, if infection progresses to sepsis, this confers a much poorer prognosis. We therefore aim to treat infection as early as possible in respiratory disease, with the aim of preventing sepsis.

Where standard intensive care is insufficient to rescue patients from severe respiratory failure, extracorporeal membrane oxygenation (ECMO) is an option. Cashen and colleagues report on results from the international Extracorporeal Life Support Organization Registry, which collects data from more than 200 ECMO centers worldwide.[44] They presented data from 623 patients with DS who received ECMO. In keeping with studies on ICU management of respiratory failure in DS, they found no increased risk of mortality for children with DS who received ECMO when compared with children without. Over time the use of ECMO in DS has increased.

IMMUNE DYSFUNCTION AND SEVERITY OF LOWER RESPIRATORY TRACT INFECTION

Children with DS are at an increased risk of infection. Often this will present as more frequent upper respiratory tract infections, although in general all respiratory infections (including LRTIs) are increased. Mechanical factors, such as the airway abnormalities and gastroesophageal reflux, clearly play a part in this. In addition, there are well-described abnormalities of immune cell function in DS, which are summarized in Table 68.5.[45-49] Research to characterize the immune deficit is ongoing, but the deficit includes reduction of multiple immune cell lines and antibody levels. A maturational component of the immunodeficiency can normalize with age. Studies investigating the correlation between the immune deficit and rates of admission have given conflicting results that appear to depend on which components of the immune system are investigated.

After immunization, the specific antibody response for a wide range of antigens in DS is reduced, including immunization against important respiratory pathogens such as pertussis and pneumococcus. In general, immunization does induce a specific antibody response, albeit with reduced titers. In addition to defects in adaptive immunity, children with DS have abnormalities of innate immunity. These include

Table 68.5 Immune Function in Down Syndrome

Cell numbers	Mild to moderate reduced T-cell counts
	Mild to moderate reduced B-cell counts
	Absence of normal lymphocyte expansion
	Mild to moderate reduced naïve T-cell percentages
Anatomic	Reduced thymus size compared to age-matched controls
Antibody production	Suboptimal antibody response to immunization
	Decreased total and specific immunoglobulin A in saliva
Innate immunity	Decreased neutrophil chemotaxis

reduced neutrophil chemotaxis,[50] and reduced killing of Candida, but normal oxidative burst. In addition, absolute levels of natural killer (NK) cells are reduced.[51]

Several underlying mechanisms for the immunodeficiency in DS have been postulated, but a clear unifying genetic mechanism has yet to be defined.[45] Hypotheses that have been considered include overexpression of genes on chromosome 21 (including SOD1, ITGB2, and RCAN1) and a secondary immunodeficiency caused by accelerated aging and zinc deficiency. A better understanding of the immunodeficiency in DS may be useful in the future in stratifying patients according to risk of infectious disease and could help guide therapy.

CLINICAL PRESENTATION OF LOWER RESPIRATORY TRACT INFECTION IN DOWN SYNDROME

Infections of the lower respiratory tract present in a similar manner to those without DS. However, in our experience, the onset of disease can be rapid. The hallmark symptoms of cough and fever are accompanied by a varying degree of increased work of breathing—elevated respiratory rate, subcostal and intercostal recession, with tracheal tug, grunting, and use of accessory muscles in older children or head bob in younger infants. Asymmetric chest expansion may be visible. There are crackles sometimes accompanied by bronchial (tubular) breathing over the affected lobes, with or without increased tactile vocal fremitus. Left untreated, respiratory muscle fatigue will lead to respiratory failure. Sputum may be produced or swallowed and vomiting is common; it may be the most prominent feature. Fever may be cyclic, especially in complicated pneumonia. The chest radiograph demonstrates the expected consolidation, although it should be noted that consolidation is common in viral respiratory infections such as RSV. A key role of the chest radiograph is in excluding complicated pneumonia.

WHEEZE IN DOWN SYNDROME APPEARS INDEPENDENT FROM ATOPY

Children with DS are frequently reported to be "noisy breathers," and this may often be reported by their caregivers as a wheeze. The parental report of wheeze can of course indicate a wide variety of respiratory noises. It may well be the case that many children reported to wheeze do not have asthma.

Wheeze is diagnosed in up to 30% of children with DS and appears independent from RSV infection, which is a major risk factor in children without DS.[52] If asthma-related wheezing is highly prevalent in DS, one might suspect that markers of atopy such as positive skin prick testing would be highly prevalent. However, this is not the case—the rates of atopy are low in children with DS.[53,54] Lung function tests (especially spirometry) can be difficult to perform in DS, preventing the accurate diagnosis of reversible bronchospasm. However, these data on the discrepancy between the rates of atopy, and rates of wheeze in DS raise the question of whether this wheeze is in fact a manifestation of asthma, or whether there are alternate explanations in many children with DS. Therefore when given a history of wheeze, alternate explanations other than asthma should be considered, including intrathoracic airway malacia, muscle hypotonia with upper airway collapse, and vascular malformations.

EFFUSIONS IN DOWN SYNDROME

Effusions (both pleural and pericardial) are frequently seen in DS and can be pleural (chylous or nonchylous) or pericardial. Fetal pleural effusion is a recognized sign of DS. It is worth noting that pericardial and pleural effusions can be presenting features of hematologic malignancy, which have increased incidence in children with DS.[55]

Chylothorax has been associated with DS in several case reports. It can occur spontaneously,[56,57] after cardiac surgery,[58] and in association with congenital pulmonary lymphangiectasia (see later). Chylothorax often presents in the newborn period or in infancy with signs of respiratory distress in the absence of overt infection. Typical features are stony dullness on percussion with reduced breath sounds and a pleural effusion on the chest radiograph. Chylothoraces can be significant and several hundred milliliters of fluid can be produced per day, even in relatively young children. Nonchylous congenital pleural effusions are also described in DS but appear to be uncommon.[59,60]

Cardiac effusions are well recognized in the context of DS and can be clinically significant and cause tamponade. They typically present with dyspnea, respiratory failure, and cyanosis and therefore should be included in the differential diagnosis of respiratory failure in DS.[61,62] The association between effusion and hypothyroidism is described, and some cases respond to thyroxine replacement therapy.[63]

RARE DISEASES OF THE LOWER RESPIRATORY TRACT IN DOWN SYNDROME

DS is a common variant, and so there are numerous case reports of rare diseases in patients who also have DS. When a child with DS has an unusual respiratory presentation and disease progression does not proceed as normal, this should lead to consideration of a second diagnosis in addition to DS. There are case reports of DS coexisting with idiopathic pulmonary hemosiderosis (where the clue to diagnosis may be recurrent anemia requiring transfusion coincident with presumed pneumonia—Fig. 68.7),[64] cystic fibrosis,[65] primary ciliary dyskinesia,[66] and several interstitial lung diseases.

Childhood interstitial lung disease (ChILD) appears to be more common in children with DS, although the increased risk is difficult to quantify. Alveolar capillary dysplasia (ACD) or congenital alveolar dysplasia (CAD) has been described in a case series, but the overall frequency in DS is unknown.[67] Given that lung alveolarization is known to be abnormal in DS and that CAD and ACD are primary disorders of lung development, it is tempting to speculate that the lung development in DS is on a continuum with the developmental disorder category of ChILD. Indeed, in their classification scheme, Deutsch and colleagues categorized 46 cases as "growth abnormalities reflecting deficient alveolarization," of which 15 were related to chromosomal disorders.[68] Other entities such as pulmonary interstitial glycogenosis (PIG) (Fig. 68.8)[69–71] and congenital pulmonary lymphangiectasia (Fig. 68.9) are rare in children with DS.[69]

Imaging of the Lower Respiratory Tract in Down Syndrome

Chest radiograph findings of pneumonia are similar to those in children without DS, including lobar consolidation and collapse. In RSV bronchiolitis, findings include the typical

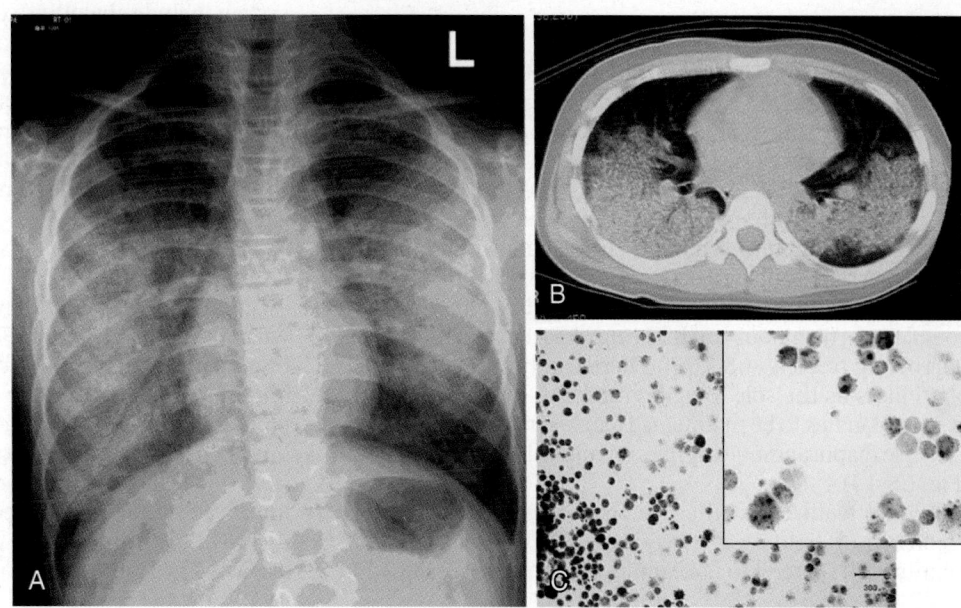

Fig. 68.7 Pulmonary Hemosiderosis in Down Syndrome. (A) Chest radiograph of a 9-year-old girl with Down syndrome showing bilateral diffuse infiltrates. (B) The computed tomography scan of the chest demonstrated bilateral diffuse infiltrates in the posterior aspects of the lungs. (C) A cytospin of bronchoalveolar lavage fluid stained with Prussian blue revealed many hemosiderin laden macrophages. (From Hirofumi Watanabe, Mamoru Ayusawa et al., Idiopathic pulmonary hemosiderosis complicated by Down syndrome, *Japan Pediatric Society*, Volume 57, Issue 5 October 2015, Pages 1009–1012.)

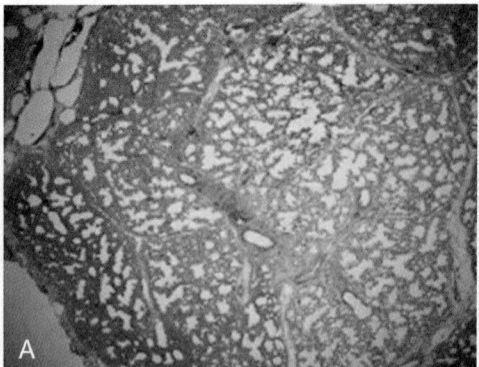
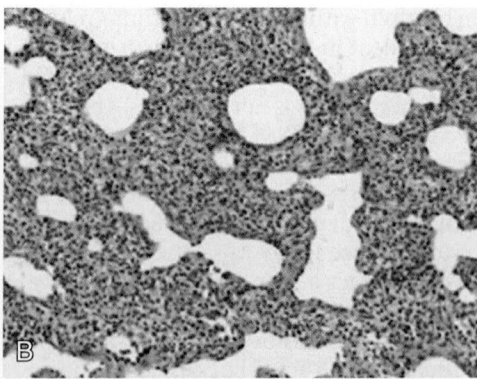

Fig. 68.8 Histopathology of pulmonary interstitial glycogenosis (PIG). PIG is a recently described manifestation of childhood interstitial lung disease. There is interstitial widening due to increased mesenchyme. (A) Hematoxylin and eosin (H&E) stain showing alveolar simplification and enlarged and poorly septated airspaces. (B) Higher power H&E showing oval nuclei with clear cytoplasm in the interstitium typical of PIG. (From Popler J, Lesnick B, Dishop MK, et al. New coding in the International Classification of Diseases, Ninth Revision, for children's interstitial lung disease. *Chest.* 2012; 142(3):774-780.)

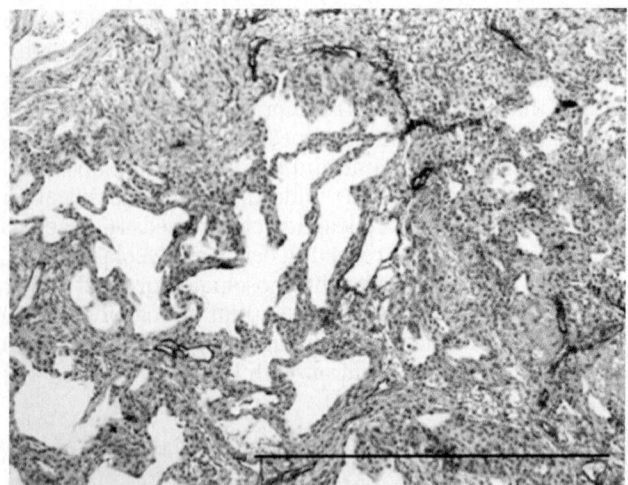

Fig. 68.9 Histopathology in congenital pulmonary lymphangiectasia. Immunohistochemistry (antibodies against podoplanin) highlighting dilated lymphatic vessels in a child with trisomy 21 and congenital pulmonary lymphangiectasia. (From Reiterer F, Grossauer K, Morris N, et al. Congenital pulmonary lymphangiectasis. *Paediatr Respir Rev.* 2014; 15(3):275-280.)

hyperinflated lungs, bronchial cuffing, and streaky perihilar regions (Fig. 68.10A). However, in DS, RSV bronchiolitis is more likely to cause lobar consolidation. In patients with chronic pulmonary disease, the radiograph can show changes of diffuse disease. CT scans may show subpleural cysts, which are typically less than 4 mm in diameter. In addition, CT scans can delineate vascular and lung malformations, such as an aberrant subclavian artery (Fig. 68.11) or a tracheal bronchus (Fig. 68.12). A CT scan can also demonstrate a complete cartilaginous tracheal ring, associated with tracheal narrowing (see Fig. 68.10C). There can be pitfalls in using plain films as the sole imaging modality, and a high index of suspicion has to be maintained for alternate diagnoses—for example diaphragmatic hernia can mimic lung consolidation (Fig. 68.13).

Several features on the newborn chest radiograph are predictive of trisomy 21 (see Fig. 68.10B). In particular, infants with DS tend to have multiple manubrial ossification centers, 11 pairs of ribs, and a bell-shaped chest.[70] If all three of these are present, the probability of the infant having DS approaches 60%.

Cardiorespiratory Interactions and Pulmonary Vasculature

CONGENITAL HEART DISEASE IN DOWN SYNDROME

Cardiovascular abnormalities occur in approximately 40% of children born with DS. Overall mortality for CHD has improved significantly over the past decades, and much of the improvement appears to be due to a reduction in mortality in the first 2 years of life.

Within this context of better survival after significant cardiac disease, many patients who are seen in the respiratory clinic have current or a past history of significant cardiac morbidity. Thus care must be taken to consider both primary lung disease and lung disease secondary to cardiac disease. Cardiac surgery complications impacting the respiratory system include chylothorax, recurrent laryngeal nerve palsy, diaphragmatic paralysis, and subglottic stenosis. Patients with DS appear particularly susceptible to pulmonary hypertension. Secondary lung disease in patients following cardiac surgery can result from airway compression, for example from vascular anomalies, atrial enlargement, enlarged pulmonary arteries, or cardiomegaly (see Upper Airway Disease earlier).

The impact of cardiac surgery and postoperative ventilation on the lungs should not be underestimated. Histologic findings of patients with DS, compared with patients without DS, showed that 92% (22/24) of the patients with DS had interstitial emphysema and 96% had overdistension of peripheral air spaces. In contrast, the majority of control patients (who had undergone cardiac surgery but did not have DS) did not have interstitial emphysema or overdistension.[71] Although ventilator technology and strategies have improved significantly since this report, these data speak to the fragility of the lungs in children with DS. Cardiovascular disease can lead to pulmonary edema with a subsequent

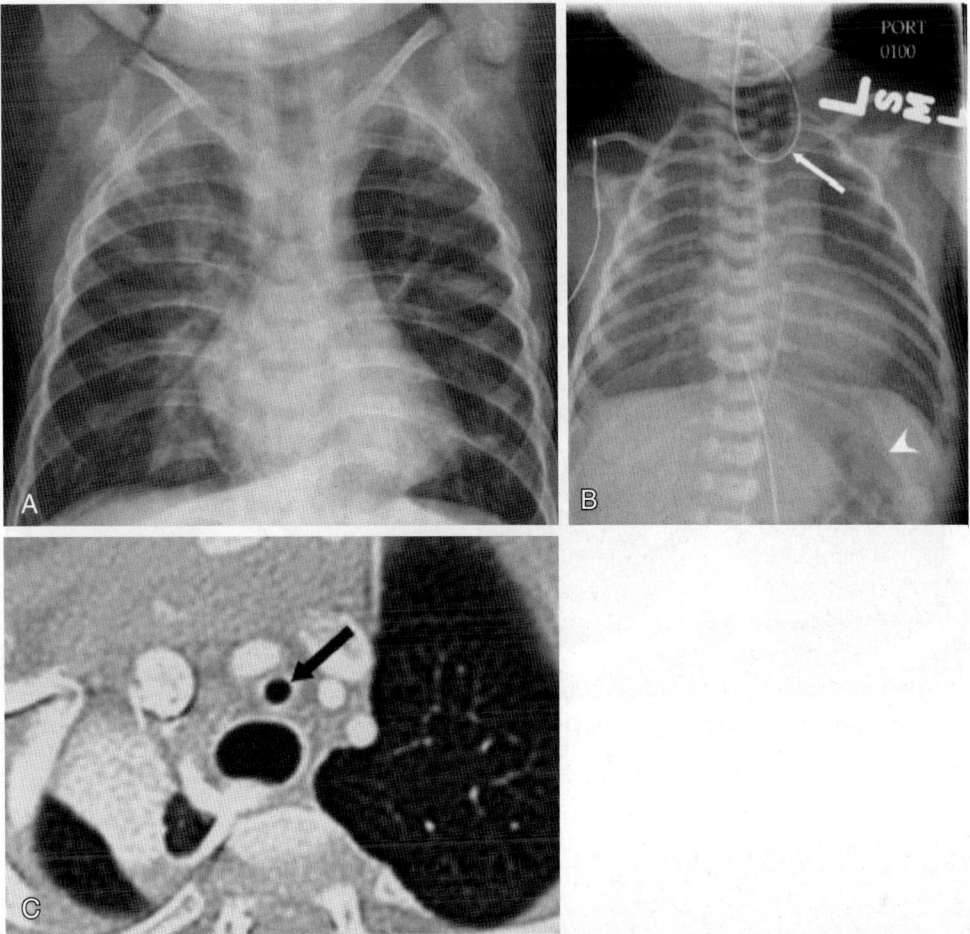

Fig. 68.10 Imaging abnormalities in Down syndrome (DS). (A) Respiratory syncytial virus bronchiolitis in an infant with DS. (B) Chest radiograph that is highly suggestive of an underlying diagnosis of DS due to abnormal heart shape (tetralogy of Fallot), esophageal atresia (note the coiled nasogastric tube), and bowel gas in the abdomen *(arrowhead)* (indicating a tracheoesophageal fistula). Note also that there are 13 pairs of ribs. (C) Complete tracheal ring *(arrow)* in a child with DS on computerized tomography. (From Radhakrishnan R, Towbin AJ. Imaging findings in Down syndrome. *Pediatr Radiol.* 2014;44(5):506-521.)

impact upon pulmonary function, causing a restrictive defect.[72] Numerous cardiovascular diseases can lead to pulmonary edema (Table 68.6).

Cardiac surgery can result in trauma to the respiratory system, causing chylothorax (due to direct injury to the thoracic duct, high central venous pressure, or central vein thrombosis) and recurrent laryngeal nerve injury (from direct trauma, stretching of the nerve or disruption of the blood supply) leading to diaphragmatic paralysis, and subglottic stenosis (Table 68.7).

THE PULMONARY VASCULATURE AND RESPIRATORY DISEASE IN DOWN SYNDROME

In tandem with the alveolar growth disruption seen in DS, there is also disturbance of the pulmonary vasculature. Infants with DS who died in the first year of life demonstrated persistence of the double capillary layer from fetal development and thickened pulmonary arteries. All of these patients had intrapulmonary bronchopulmonary anastomoses.[73]

Given the developmental anomalies of the pulmonary vasculature, it is not surprising that there is a predisposition for pulmonary hypertension in DS. Weijerman and colleagues

Table 68.6 Cardiac Disease Leading to Pulmonary Edema in Down Syndrome

Pulmonary venous hypertension	Pulmonary veno-occlusive disease
	Pulmonary vein stenosis
	Cor triatriatum
	Supramitral ring
	Left ventricular dysfunction
	Transposition of the great arteries
	Hypoplastic left heart (with intact atrial septum)
Decreased lymphatic flow	Lymphangiectasia
	Superior venacaval syndrome
	Single ventricle physiology
	Tricuspid valve stenosis
	Failing right ventricle
	Right ventricular outflow tract obstruction
Left-to-right heart shunts	Ventricular septal defect
	Atrial septal defect
	Patent ductus arteriosus
	Partial anomalous pulmonary venous connection
	Systemic arteriovenous malformations
	Aortopulmonary connections including surgical shunts

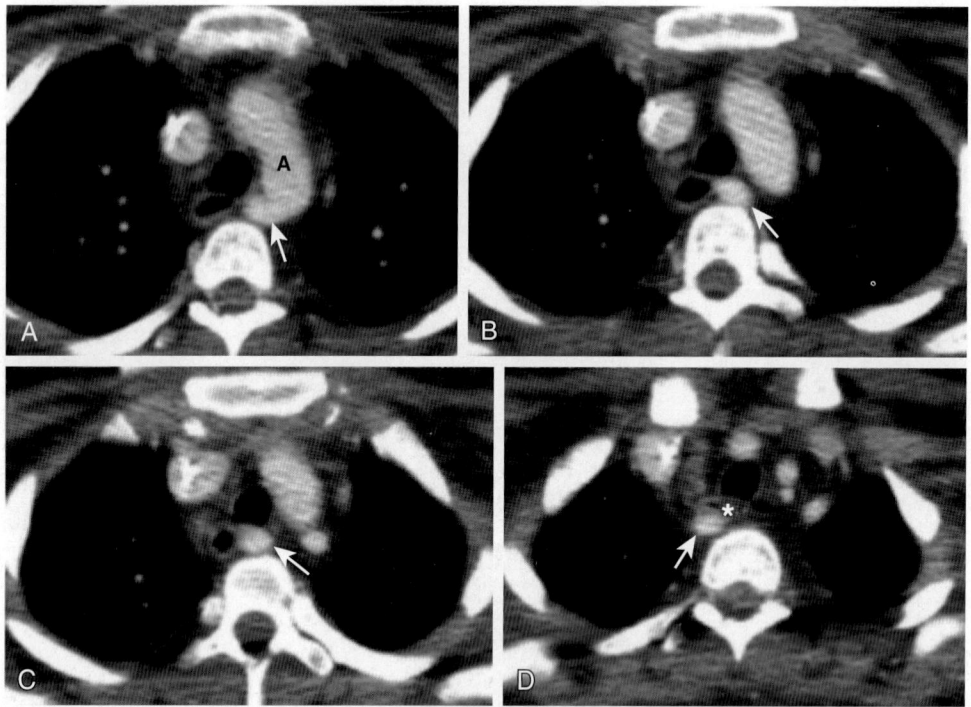

Fig. 68.11 Aberrant right subclavian artery in Down syndrome. Chest computerized tomography series (proceeding caudally to cranially from panels A–D) demonstrating an aberrant right subclavian artery. The artery traverses posteriorly behind the esophagus (indicated by the * in panel D). (From Radhakrishnan R, Towbin AJ. Imaging findings in Down syndrome. *Pediatr Radiol.* 2014;44(5):506-521.)

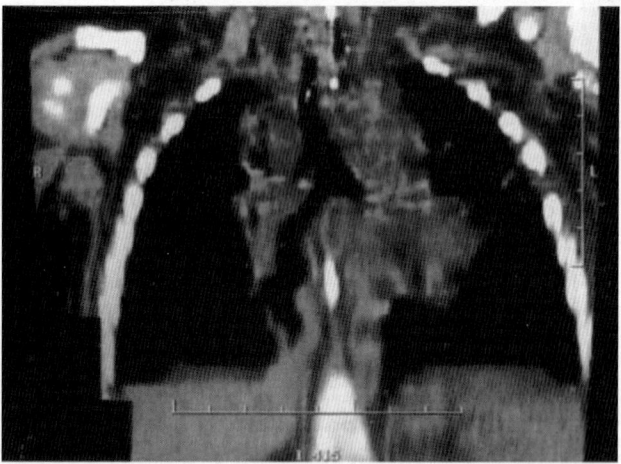

Fig. 68.12 Tracheal bronchus. Coronal images from a chest computerized tomography in Down syndrome demonstrating a tracheal bronchus. (From O'Sullivan BP, Frassica JJ, Rayder SM. Tracheal bronchus: a cause of prolonged atelectasis in intubated children. *Chest.* 1998;113(2):537-540.)

Table 68.7 Pulmonary Complications of Cardiac Surgery

Pulmonary Complication	Etiology
Chylothorax	Direct injury to the thoracic duct or smaller vessels
	High central venous pressure
	Central vein thrombosis
Recurrent laryngeal nerve palsy	Surgery involving the ductus arteriosus, descending aortal, or left pulmonary artery
	Manipulation of right common carotid artery or internal jugular vein for extracorporeal membrane oxygenation
Diaphragmatic paralysis	Direct trauma to the phrenic nerve
	Stretching of the phrenic nerve
	Disruption of blood supply to the phrenic nerve
Subglottic stenosis	Compression of the trachea by the endotracheal tube, in particular given the small size of the trachea in Down syndrome

Modified from Healy F, Hanna BD, Zinman R. Pulmonary complications of congenital heart disease. Paediatr Respir Rev. 2012;13(1):10-15.

reported a recent series from the Dutch Paediatric Surveillance Unit (DPSU). The overall population rate of CHD in DS is 43%, within which the incidence of persistent pulmonary hypertension of the newborn (PPHN) was 5.2%, compared with 0.1% in the general population.[74] Atrioventricular septal defect is recognized to be particularly associated with pulmonary hypertension.[75]

In DS, even in the absence of CHD, there is increased risk of PPHN, which is present in up to 10% of admissions to the neonatal ICU.[76] Reassuringly, the majority of patients demonstrate resolution of pulmonary hypertension. We advocate treating comorbidities such left-to-right shunts,

upper airway obstruction, and hypoxia to prevent the establishment of pulmonary hypertension. Treating upper airway abnormalities is particularly helpful because adenotonsillectomy can reduce the prevalence of pulmonary hypertension from 85% preoperatively to 5% postoperatively.[77]

It is speculated that the reduced alveolar count, the abnormal fetal capillary network, and the reduced pulmonary vascular bed seen in DS significantly increase the risk of pulmonary hypertension.

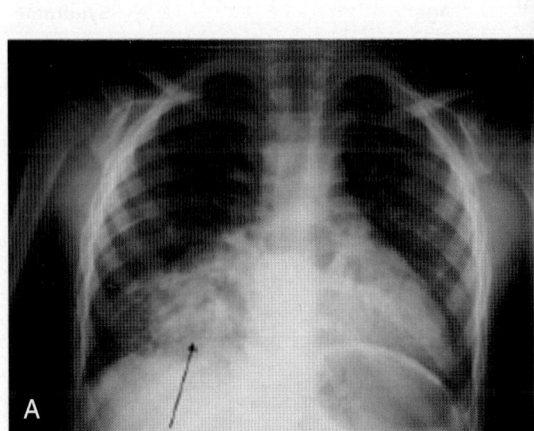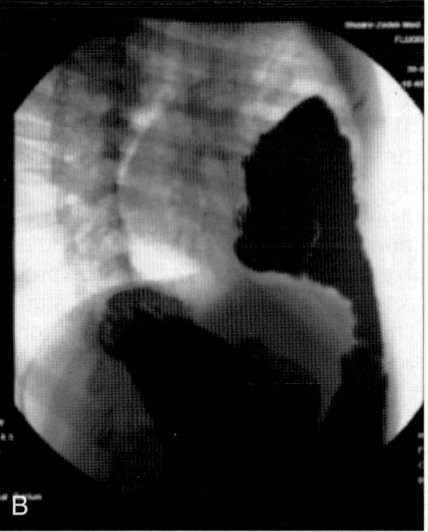

Fig. 68.13 Unusual pathology in the lung masquerading as pneumonia in Down syndrome. (A) Chest radiograph shows apparent right lower zone consolidation. (B) Barium swallow demonstrating a right-sided anterior diaphragmatic hernia. (From Picard E, Ben Nun A, Fisher D, et al. Morgagni hernia mimicking pneumonia in Down syndrome. *J Pediatr Surg.* 2007;42(9):1608-1611.)

High-altitude pulmonary edema (HAPE) at moderate altitudes appears more common in children with DS compared with normal children.[78] Intriguingly, it has been suggested that HAPE could be an initial sign of developing pulmonary hypertension.[79]

Gastrointestinal–Respiratory Interactions in Down Syndrome

Gastrointestinal–respiratory interactions are particularly important in DS. Within this, it is common to distinguish between functional (dysmotility, reflux, and swallowing dysfunction) and structural (e.g., esophageal atresia) abnormalities, recognizing that these often coexist. As research progresses, the underlying pathogenesis of functional disorders is gradually being elucidated. The role of the respiratory pediatrician is to minimize this impact on the pulmonary health; so much of the work done in this domain is aimed at assessing and treating functional disorders irrespective of antecedent structural defects.

Congenital gastrointestinal defects are common in DS. In a large US study of 1892 children with DS, gastrointestinal malformations occurred in 6.7%.[80] The most common malformations were duodenal stenosis or atresia (3.9%), anal stenosis or atresia (1.0%), Hirschsprung disease (0.8%), esophageal atresia with or without tracheoesophageal fistula (0.4%), and pyloric stenosis (0.3%).

Esophageal atresia is particularly associated with increased respiratory problems long term postsurgery, even in children without DS.[81] Respiratory disease is multifactorial from tracheomalacia, aspiration, gastroesophageal reflux disease, tracheoesophageal fistula recurrence, and chest wall deformities. Large case series of outcomes in children with DS are lacking.

Functional disorders of gastrointestinal motility are particularly important in DS. DS is associated with disordered development of the enteric nervous system, which is thought to underlie the spectrum of functional disorders of the gastrointestinal tract that are prevalent in DS.[82] Animal models of DS have shown evidence of disordered neuronal migration and dendritic development. In people with DS, there are reduced numbers of esophageal plexus ganglia neurons, and this decreased ganglion cell population likely extends over the complete length of the gut. In addition to reduced neuronal cell numbers, there is also evidence of altered physiology—differences in action potential and ion channel kinetics have been identified.

Gastroesophageal dysmotility and reflux disease (GERD) is common in the DS population.[83] Approximately 50% patients with DS are asymptomatic, but the other 50% have symptoms such as dysphagia, regurgitation, and chest pain. We suspect that GERD also occurs without reported symptoms, where the patient may not recognize the symptoms, or it may be truly asymptomatic. Approximately 25% have dysmotility and retention of food in the esophagus. In children following major cardiac surgery, such as a VSD repair, medical management of GERD has a high readmission rate due to aspiration, failure to thrive, and poor feeding. However, the outcomes of surgical management of GERD are also unsatisfactory, with a significant rate of revision of fundoplication due to bloating. The choice of medical versus surgical therapy is difficult and requires balancing the risk of inadequate medical therapy versus operative risk and the chances of requiring further surgical procedures.

Swallowing dysfunction occurs in DS and causes aspiration pneumonia.[84,85] Pharyngeal dysfunction occurs commonly and is associated with cardiac surgery and failure to thrive; it often requires a gastrostomy.

Obesity and Its Impact on the Lung in Down Syndrome

Obesity is increasingly present in the general population. A recent US series of 303 children with DS found that up to 50% of children have a BMI greater than the 95th percentile for age and sex,[86] whereas a Dutch study, which used different definitions, found a prevalence of overweight of 25%–32% and of obesity of 4%–5%.[87] Obesity is not solely due to changing demographics and increased obesity in the general population, because in both studies children with DS had higher BMI than the general population. In DS the BMI is increased most in children over the age of 12 years, and high BMI is a risk factor for OSA. Although obesity prevalence varies from country to country, children with DS are consistently more obese than the general population. Both inactivity and overeating may contribute to this problem. Overeating or hyperphagia can be assessed with standard questionnaires such as those used in Prader-Willi syndrome. When formally assessed, children with DS have hyperphagia scores somewhat between children with lifestyle-related obesity and children with Prader-Willi syndrome.[88]

In general, obesity has a negative impact on health, and this is particularly the case for respiratory health in DS. In children, obesity has a negative effect on pulmonary mechanics, prevalence of asthma, and sleep-disordered breathing.[89] In obesity, increased abdominal volume pushes the diaphragm upward, reducing the functional residual capacity, and this is made worse in DS by the effect of hypotonia on the chest wall. Thus the combination of DS and obesity has a significant impact on lung function, and obesity exacerbates the already high rates of sleep-disordered breathing.

TREATMENT OF THE RESPIRATORY COMPLICATIONS OF DOWN SYNDROME

Children with DS are frequently seen within the context of pediatric respiratory/pulmonology clinics. The approach to the history includes a focus on current and past symptoms, including cough, wheeze, upper airway noises, and snoring. The impact of current and previous comorbidities on pulmonary health should be considered, along with the limitations that respiratory disease causes to the patient's lifestyle. Specific points to consider include hospital admissions, respiratory tract infections, daytime somnolence, and missed school or other life opportunities. Growth should be monitored carefully, with attention to faltering growth in infancy, and obesity in later life. Multiple clinicians are often involved in patients with DS, and it should be clear where responsibility lies for routine surveillance, such as for thyroid disease. With respect to respiratory symptoms, there is a fine line between overinvestigating children and missing important symptoms of treatable conditions such as airway malformation, sleep-disordered breathing, and GERD. In particular, it is important to carefully consider alternative diagnoses before making a diagnosis of asthma. Success in being able to perform lung function testing is variable. Many treatments for children with DS are extrapolated from treatment of the same condition in children without DS, and this may not always be the best approach.

CONSIDERATIONS WHEN TREATING UPPER RESPIRATORY TRACT DISEASE IN DOWN SYNDROME

Treatment of upper airway disease requires a close liaison between the respiratory pediatrician, otolaryngologist, anesthesiologist, and intensive care team. One approach is to undertake joint bronchoscopies (as rigid bronchoscopies are

Table 68.8   Size of Endotracheal Tube Diameter in Down Syndrome

Age	Down Syndrome	Non-Down Syndrome
Premature	2.0–2.5	2.5–3.0
Full-term newborn to 9 months	2.5–3.0	3.5–4.0
9–18 months	3.0–3.5	4.0–4.5
1.5–3 years	3.5–4.0	4.5–5.0
4–5 years	4.0–4.5	5.0–5.5
6–7 years	5.0	5.5–6.0
8–10 years	5.5	6.0–6.5
10–11 years	5.5	6.5–7.0
12–13 years	6.0	7.0–7.5
14 years and older	6.5	7.5–8.0

From Shott SR. Down syndrome: analysis of airway size and a guide for appropriate intubation. *Laryngoscope.* 2000;110(4):585-592.

more frequently in the domain of the otolaryngologist and flexible in the domain of the respiratory physician). The surgical, ICU, and respiratory management of patients with upper airway disease can be challenging.[90]

In intensive care and anesthetic practice, care must be taken to use an endotracheal tube of appropriate diameter (Table 68.8). Care should also be taken to ensure that after intubation there is a leak around the endotracheal tube. The presence of subglottic stenosis or a narrowed trachea also has implications for the appropriate size of the pediatric flexible bronchoscope if this is undertaken via an endotracheal tube. Anecdotally, if severe airway anomalies are anticipated (such as in children with DS who have noisy breathing, or those who have previously had long periods of intubation), it may be sensible to undertake flexible endoscopy prior to intubation to look for airway anomalies such as subglottic stenosis and to allow informed decisions regarding the size of the endotracheal tube to use.[90]

AN APPROACH TO PREVENTION AND TREATMENT OF LOWER RESPIRATORY TRACT INFECTION IN DOWN SYNDROME

Much of the treatment of respiratory disease in DS is centered on the treatment and prevention of LRTI. Frequent LRTIs are an important source of morbidity and may well impact developmental progress. Although LRTI does not usually progress to sepsis, given the serious nature of sepsis when it occurs, we advocate a general position of aiming to reduce the risk of LRTI. The general approach consists of immunization, parent and patient education for early signs of infection, careful surveillance for modifiable risk factors, and early treatment.

It should be ensured that patients are up to date with the current immunization schedule at each clinic visit. Consideration should be given to checking immunoglobulin levels, functional antibodies, and lymphocyte subsets either as a routine or for DS patients with frequent respiratory tract infections. These should be checked in individuals who have had an episode of sepsis or a history of four or more infections over 6 months, even if the patient was managed in the community. Consultation with an immunologist is often useful for individuals with specific functional antibody deficiency, especially with respect to repeating the relevant immunizations and consideration of further immunologic workup. Yearly influenza immunization is recommended unless contraindicated. Due to the increased risk of pneumococcus, in addition to administering the pneumococcal conjugate vaccine in infancy, we recommend the administration of pneumococcal polysaccharide vaccine after the second year of life. Functional antibodies (such as pneumococcal and *Haemophilus*) should be undertaken, with reimmunization considered where necessary.

For children with frequent infections, we consider prophylactic antibiotics. Strategies include administering them throughout the year or for the winter months only. One approach is to use the frequency of symptomatic infections to guide when to stop, and we generally consider a trial off antibiotics in the late spring.

There is an extensive differential diagnosis of respiratory disease in DS, especially when the patient's course is unusual. Treatment of gastroesophageal reflux disease (see Gastrointestinal–Respiratory Interactions in Down Syndrome), and swallowing disorders leading to aspiration can lead to a resolution of respiratory symptoms. Where respiratory symptoms are chronic or recurrent, consider pulmonary and airway malformations, external compression of the airway, and rarer parenchymal disorders and organize appropriate radiologic investigation and bronchoscopy.

Liaison between the respiratory clinic and emergency department (ED) is useful. Some institutions are able to put an "alert" on patient's case notes informing the ED of the diagnosis of DS and emphasizing the need for prompt and aggressive therapy on arrival to the ED. One approach to an episode of infection is to increase (usually double) the duration of the course of antibiotics. For individuals who present with respiratory failure or sepsis, early consultation with pediatric intensive care is essential, especially given the overall excellent prognosis from respiratory failure but poor prognosis in sepsis.

TREATMENT OF GASTROINTESTINAL DISORDERS IN DOWN SYNDROME—THE PULMONOLOGISTS VIEW

Given the increased prevalence of swallowing dysfunction, dysmotility, and GERD, careful assessment for functional gastrointestinal disorders should be undertaken. Involvement of speech and language therapists is often helpful. Initial treatment of reflux disease is usually medical, proceeding to surgical management if there is failure of medical management.

Careful counseling of parents with regard to the risks of surgical management is important but should be put into the context of the risks of untreated chronic aspiration. Treatment of gastroesophageal reflux is undertaken with the expectation that this will prevent episodes of pulmonary infection and reduce the chance of significant pulmonary hypertension.

At present there are no clinical trials to guide the best approach to management of GERD in DS. In young infants, milk thickeners are a first step, with elevation of the thorax as much as possible during and after feeds. Pharmacologic therapies include antacids, prokinetics, H2 blockers, and proton pump inhibitors. Surgical management includes Nissen fundoplication (positioning the distal esophagus intraabdominally, hiatus hernia repair, and a fundal wrap). It can be undertaken with varying degrees of fundal wrap and can be performed laparoscopically. Alternatives to fundoplication include gastrojejunal tube feeding and jejunostomy; these procedures reduce food reflux but do not prevent reflux of swallowed saliva and stomach contents.

Conclusions

Providing respiratory care for children with DS requires a long-term approach to lung disease throughout the pediatric period, with different pathologies presenting at different ages. Given the intellectual impairment that is often present, there are challenges throughout in terms of managing disease, in ensuring that children are able to understand and adhere to a treatment program, and that parents are supported in undertaking this treatment.

Other Genetic Anomalies

Several other genetic disorders can be associated with significant pulmonary manifestations, and these are mostly associated with pulmonary hypoplasia. Table 68.9 lists selected genetic syndrome known to be associated with pulmonary hypoplasia. The chromosomal abnormalities Edwards (trisomy 18) and Patau syndrome (trisomy 13) are recognized to have pulmonary hypoplasia. Page reported on a series of more than 700 postmortem examinations and

Table 68.9 Rare Syndromes Associated With Alveolar Simplification

Syndrome	Cause	Survival	Reference
Patau	Trisomy 13	Death in neonatal period early infancy	91
Edwards	Trisomy 18	Death in neonatal period and early infancy	91
Arthrogryposis multiplex congenital	AMCN (5q35) OMIM %208100 (though is genetically heterogeneous)	Heterogeneous prognosis survival to adulthood has been described for those without significant pulmonary or cardiac involvement.	91
Spondyloepiphyseal dysplasia congenital	COL2A1 (12q13.11) OMIM #183900 Autosomal dominant	Wide clinical variability, survives to adulthood	91
Larsen syndrome	FNLB Mutation (3p14) Autosomal dominant OMIM #150250	Variable severity—adult cases reported.	92

Continued

Table 68.9 Rare Syndromes Associated With Alveolar Simplification—cont'd

Syndrome	Cause	Survival	Reference
Lethal pterygium syndrome	Autosomal recessive CHRNG, CHRND, CHRNA1 (2q) OMIM 253290	Lethal in the fetal stage of development	93
Roberts syndrome/SC phocomelia syndrome	Autosomal recessive ESCO2 (8p21.1) OMIM #269000	Survival poor after the neonatal period.	94
Pulmonary hypoplasia associated with oligohydramnios	Preterm rupture of membranes, or renal agenesis.	Survival depends on extent of hypoplasia.	95
Fetal akinesia deformation sequence (FADS), Pena Shokeir syndrome	Autosomal recessive DOK7 (4p16.3) MUSK (9q31.3) RAPSN (11p11.2)	Lethal congenital syndrome	95
Asphyxiating thoracic dystrophy/short-rib thoracic dysplasia 11 (SRTD)/Jeune syndrome	WDR34 (9q34.11) Autosomal recessive	Lethal in neonatal period. The SRTD of which Jeune syndrome is a well-known member of the group, are a group of autosomal recessive skeletal dysplasias, and within this group there is phenotypic variability. Some forms are less severe with survival to later life.	95
Thanatophoric dysplasia	FGFR3 (4p16.3) Autosomal dominant OMIM #187600	Fatal in early infancy	95
Spondylocostal dysotosis 1	The spondylocostal dysostoses are a group of usually autosomal recessive disorders which include Jarco-Levin syndrome. Rib abnormalities are common leading to pulmonary hypoplasia. Autosomal recessive Mutation in Notch signaling gene DLL3 at 19q13.1	The prognosis is variable within the group, with some forms having normal lifespan, and others dying early in infancy.	95
Cerebrocostomandibular syndrome	Autosomal dominant, autosomal recessive SNRPB (20p13) OMIM #117650	Rib gaps are associated with pulmonary hypoplasia.	96
Pulmonary agenesis/dysgenesis/hypoplasia, micropthalmia/anopthalmia and diaphragmatic defect (PDAC) syndrome (also termed *Spear syndrome* and *Matthew-Wood syndrome*	Autosomal recessive STRA6 (15q24.1) OMIM #601186 There is genetic heterogeneity.	Usually die shortly after delivery, although some survival to early childhood occurs. Not all cases show pulmonary hypoplasia.	97

AMCN, Arthrogryposis multiplex congenita; *CHRNA1*, cholinergic receptor, nicotinic, alpha polypeptide1; *CHRND*, cholinergic receptor, nicotinic, delta polypeptide; *CHRNG*, cholinergic receptor, nicotinic, gamma polypeptide; *COL2A1*, collagen Type II; Alpha-1; *DLL3*, delta-like 3; *DOK7*, downstream of tyrosine kinase 7; *ESCO2*, establishment of cohesion 1, S. Cerevisiae, Homolog of, 2; *FGFR3*, fibroblast growth factor receptor 3; *FNLB*, filamin B; *MUSK*, muscle, skeletal, receptor tyrosine kinase; *OMIM*, online mendelian inheritance in man; *RAPSN*, receptor-associated protein of the synapse; *SNRPB*, small nuclear ribonucleoprotein polypeptides B and B1; *STRA6*, stimulated by retinoic acid 6; *WDR34*, WD repeat-containing protein 34.
The reader is directed onwards to the references within the table.

identified multiple cases of pulmonary hypoplasia on histopathologic grounds, of which three had trisomy 13, one trisomy 18, and one deletion of the long arm of chromosome 13.[91] In this series of pulmonary hypoplasia, there were also cases of arthrogryposis multiplex, osteogenesis imperfecta, thanatophoric dysplasia, and spondyloepiphyseal dysplasia congenita. Pulmonary hypoplasia is also recognized to occur in Larsen syndrome,[92] lethal pterygium syndrome,[93] and Roberts-SC phocomelia syndrome.[94] Unfortunately, the outcome of major syndromic malformations associated with pulmonary hypoplasia is very poor, with death occurring either in utero, in the neonatal period, or in early infancy.

References

Access the reference list online at ExpertConsult.com.

Suggested Reading

Gupta P, Rettiganti M. Association between Down syndrome and mortality in young children with critical illness: a propensity-matched analysis. *Acta Paediatr.* 2015;104(11):e506–e511.

Hilton JM, Fitzgerald DA, Cooper DM. Respiratory morbidity of hospitalized children with Trisomy 21. *J Paediatr Child Health.* 1999;35(4):383–386.

Ram G, Chinen J. Infections and immunodeficiency in Down syndrome. *Clin Exp Immunol.* 2011;164(1):9–16.

Radhakrishnan R, Towbin AJ. Imaging findings in Down syndrome. *Pediatr Radiol.* 2014;44(5):506–521.

Shott SR. Down syndrome: analysis of airway size and a guide for appropriate intubation. *Laryngoscope.* 2000;110(4):585–592.

Verstegen RH, et al. Significant impact of recurrent respiratory tract infections in children with Down syndrome. *Child Care Health Dev.* 2013;39(6):801–809.

69 Air and Fluid in the Pleural Space

BERNADETTE PRENTICE, BSc, MB BS, MPH, and
ADAM JAFFÉ, BSc(Hons), MBBS, MD, FRCPCH, FRCP, FRACP, FThorSoc

The pleural space plays an essential role in the normal physiology of respiration. It consists of a layer of lubricated fluid that prevents friction between the two pleural layers and creates a negative pressure gradient to allow alveolar expansion and gas transfer. The balance of fluid, air, and pressure forces within the pleural space is very delicate, and when this is disrupted by the accumulation of air or fluid, there may be a significant impact on the cardiorespiratory system. Disorders of the pleura cause significant morbidity and mortality in children.

Embryology and Anatomy

In the developing fetus, by the fourth week of gestation a primordial intraembryonic body cavity has developed in the shape of a horseshoe. This cavity develops from the lateral plate mesoderm and is termed the *intraembryonic coelom* (embryonic body cavity).[1] It is lined by simple squamous epithelium, or *mesothelium*, made up of two layers. The outermost parietal layer is derived from somatic mesoderm, and the inner visceral layer of mesothelium is derived from splanchnic mesoderm (Fig. 69.1).[1] Eventually this horseshoe-shaped cavity elongates, forming the bilateral pericardioperitoneal canals, which are then subdivided into pleural, pericardial, and peritoneal spaces. External to the developing cavities, the laryngotracheal diverticulum develops a "bud" that pushes into the pleural cavity and continues to branch 22 times to form the segments of the bronchial airway. The numerous branches deliver an increased surface area throughout which gas exchange can occur.[2] The preceding formation of the pleural cavities provides a space in which the lung parenchyma can grow.

In the second month of development, lymphatic channels begin to form, first in the shape of lymphatic "sacs" throughout the upper and lower regions of the body. These sacs are joined by lymphatic vessels, which form from vascular precursor cells and ultimately drain into the venous circulation. The early lymphatic system consists of two lymphatic channels (right and left thoracic duct precursors), which drain the jugular, iliac, retroperitoneal, and the cisterna chlyi lymphatic sacs and are connected by an anastomosis.[1] The two major lymphatic channels then undergo significant remodeling and partial obliteration such that the resulting thoracic duct is derived from the primordial right caudal lymphatic vessel, the cranial left lymphatic vessel, and the anastomosis between the original channels (Fig. 69.2).[3] If the thoracic duct is damaged—for example, during cardiothoracic surgery—the side of the chest in which a chylothorax develops will depend on whether or not damage has occurred

in the lower portion of the duct (the original right-sided channel) or the upper portion of the duct (the original left-sided channel). Given the significant remodeling that the lymphatic system undergoes, there are numerous anatomic variations in the origin, termination, and passage of the thoracic duct. This variability may contribute to the difficulty often found in attempting to surgically identify the exact site of thoracic duct injury.

The embryonic pleural space is formed by two layers: the visceral pleura attached to the lung parenchyma and interlobar fissures and the parietal pleura attached to the chest wall and the superior aspect of the diaphragm. The visceral pleura is a tightly adherent membrane made up of a single layer of flattened cuboidal mesothelial cells.[4] The superior surfaces of these mesothelial cells are lined with apical microvilli, which play a key role in fluid movement across the visceral surface.[5,6] The apical portion of the visceral pleura is relatively thin, with flattened mesothelial cells. This thinner pleura is also the site of potential bleb and bullae formation. If these blebs and bullae rupture, a spontaneous pneumothorax ensues, as discussed later in this chapter.[7] Basal areas of the lung demonstrate greater movement with chest expansion than more apical areas and exhibit thicker visceral pleura and a higher density of mesothelial cell microvilli to assist with lubrication.[7] The visceral pleura is predominantly supplied by bronchial arteries, with only a minor contribution from the pulmonary circulation. There is no somatic sensory innervation of the visceral pleural layer, and this is often reflected clinically when pain is detected only once disease processes involve the parietal pleura.[8] Underlying the mesothelial layer of the visceral pleura is a fibrous supportive structure that is contiguous with the fibrous ultrastructure of the lung parenchyma. This fibrous tissue, which extends into the lung parenchyma, forms septae.[4] The normal lymphatic fluid filtration from the alveolar or pulmonary interstitial space drains via lymphatic capillaries that coalesce into lymphatic vessels along the lobular and lobar fibrous septae of the lung or superficial surface of the visceral pleura. These vessels drain toward the hilar region of the lung. In physiologic conditions, filtration across the visceral pleura toward the pleural space is essentially nonexistent, limited by the presence of "tight junctions" between the visceral mesothelial cells. However, in disease states, the endothelial and mesothelial barriers are disrupted and may result in the abnormal accumulation of fluid in the pleural space as either a transudate or an exudate.[7]

The parietal pleura is also formed by a single layer of mesothelial cells overlying a connective tissue support structure.[5] There are small voids, each called a *stoma* (from the Greek meaning "mouth"), in the cellular layer of the parietal pleura,

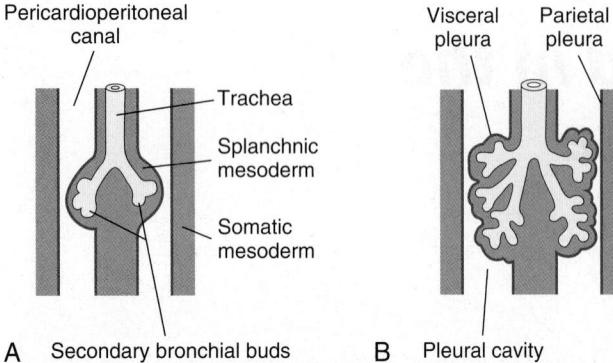

Fig. 69.1 The developing lungs. (A) Bronchial buds are seen forming within the splanchnic mesoderm. Somatic mesoderm forms the external boundary of the pericardioperitoneal canals (primordial pleural cavity). (B) Development of the pleural layers. (Reproduced with permission from Moore K, Persaud T, Torchia M. *The Developing Human: Clinically Oriented Embryology.* 10th ed. London: Elsevier Health Sciences; 2015:F10-F18.)

which provide a direct connection to the parietal lymphatic drainage network via small lymphatic spaces, *lacunae*, in the submesothelial connective tissue layer.[6] The majority of physiologic pleural fluid drains from the pleural space via these stomata and lacunae.[9] Maximum filtration into the pleural space occurs from the parietal pleura in the apical region of the lung and maximum drainage occurs in dependent regions of the parietal pleura, particularly diaphragmatic and mediastinal surfaces.[9] The increased drainage achieved in the lower regions of the pleural space occurs because of the greater density of stomata on the diaphragmatic and mediastinal surface of the parietal pleura.[9] There are so many stomata on the mediastinal portion of the pleura that it is called the *cribriform membrane* (from the Latin *cribrum* meaning "sieve"). The stomata of the parietal pleura vary in size with respiration; they increase in size with inspiration, which creates a negative pressure gradient drawing fluid and particles from the stoma to within the draining lacunae. This process, combined with positive pressure from the expanding lung, allows pleural drainage into the lymphatic circulation to occur with each respiratory cycle. On expiration, the parietal pleural stomata decrease in size as the chest wall contracts, thus expelling the lacunar contents into the draining lymphatic system.[7] Once fluid is within the lymphatic channels, retrograde flow is prevented by intravascular valves. The key role in pleural space drainage played by the parietal pleura is illustrated in patients with mesothelioma. On autopsy, "black spot" asbestos fibers, too large to be drained, are found lining the inner parietal layer around the stomata.[9] The parietal pleura is supplied by the intercostal and internal mammary arteries and is innervated by the intercostal and phrenic nerves.

The two pleural layers form a closed sac on either side of the chest, with each layer contiguous at the hilum.[5] The internal space formed by the "sac" is called the *pleural cavity.* This cavity is filled with a small amount of pleural fluid, the volume of which is maintained by specific hydrostatic and oncotic pressures; this keeps the pleural layers separated and provides a lubricated surface on which the lung can move.[10] Ventilatory movements allow for the constant redistribution of fluid to further minimize contact between the pleural layers.[11]

Physiology

In physiologic conditions, the amount of fluid in the thorax is preserved by a very precise balance: the parietal pleura lymphatic system manages pleural space fluid, and the intraparenchymal lymphatic drainage system ensures that excess intrapulmonary interstitial fluid does not restrict the surface area of gas exchange.[9] Several key forces are required to maintain this balance and allow the mechanics of respiration to occur. During normal tidal breathing, alveolar pressure is more negative than atmospheric pressure in order to create a gradient that allows airflow in the direction of the lower pressure (i.e., toward the airways and alveoli). This gradient is called the *transpulmonary pressure.* The negative pressure gradient is created by contraction of the muscles of inspiration, thus increasing the volume of the alveoli and lowering alveolar pressure.[12]

The pleural fluid is constantly under negative pressure, estimated to be approximately -3 to -5 cm of water[12]; the transmural gradient is the difference in pressures across the alveolar wall. This negative pressure gradient is a consequence of the inward alveolar elastic recoil and pressure to collapse, acting in concert with the passive elastic recoil of the chest wall forcing chest expansion. The resulting negative pressure in the pleural space, often termed *negative intrathoracic pressure,* persists even when inspiratory muscles are resting and then increases with inspiratory effort, thus increasing the transmural gradient.[13] The negative pressure in the pleural space creates an increasingly negative airway pressure, thus increasing airflow into the airways.

Normal pleural fluid is alkaline and has low protein levels, approximately 1–2 g/dL.[7,14] In normal physiologic states it contains a small number of cells, predominantly mesothelial cells, macrophages and lymphocytes. The cellular balance varies in different pleural diseases, and this may be a useful diagnostic clinical tool in some conditions such as lymphangiectasia and empyema. The depth of the pleural fluid layer is up to 30 μm in an adult when well; however, the negative pressure in the pleural space and the depth of pleural fluid within the cavity vary, demonstrating a gravity-dependent distribution.[9]

Pleural fluid is sterile, colorless and approximately 0.1–0.3 mL/kg in volume.[14] It is a microvascular filtrate with solute contents similar to that of interstitial fluid in other areas of the body.[7] The fluid is filtered from the apical regions of the parietal pleura, where parietal vessels lie closer to the mesothelial surface as compared with more dependent regions.[7] The pleural filtrate is governed by Starling's forces, namely tissue and capillary pressure, in addition to plasma and tissue colloidal osmotic pressure[7]; as a result, fluid drains according to the net hydrostatic and oncotic pressure gradient from the high-pressure systemic parietal pleural capillaries into the negative-pressure pleural space.[7] Pleural fluid turnover is approximately 0.2 mL/kg per hour, and complete fluid renewal is estimated to occur every hour in healthy adults.[9] The main control mechanism maintaining volume of the pleural space is the pleural lymphatic drainage system, which increases in response to increased filtration and provides an efficient negative feedback regulation system.[9] The lymphatic system is adaptive and can increase flow by up to 30 times; but when normal filtration from the parietal pleura increases

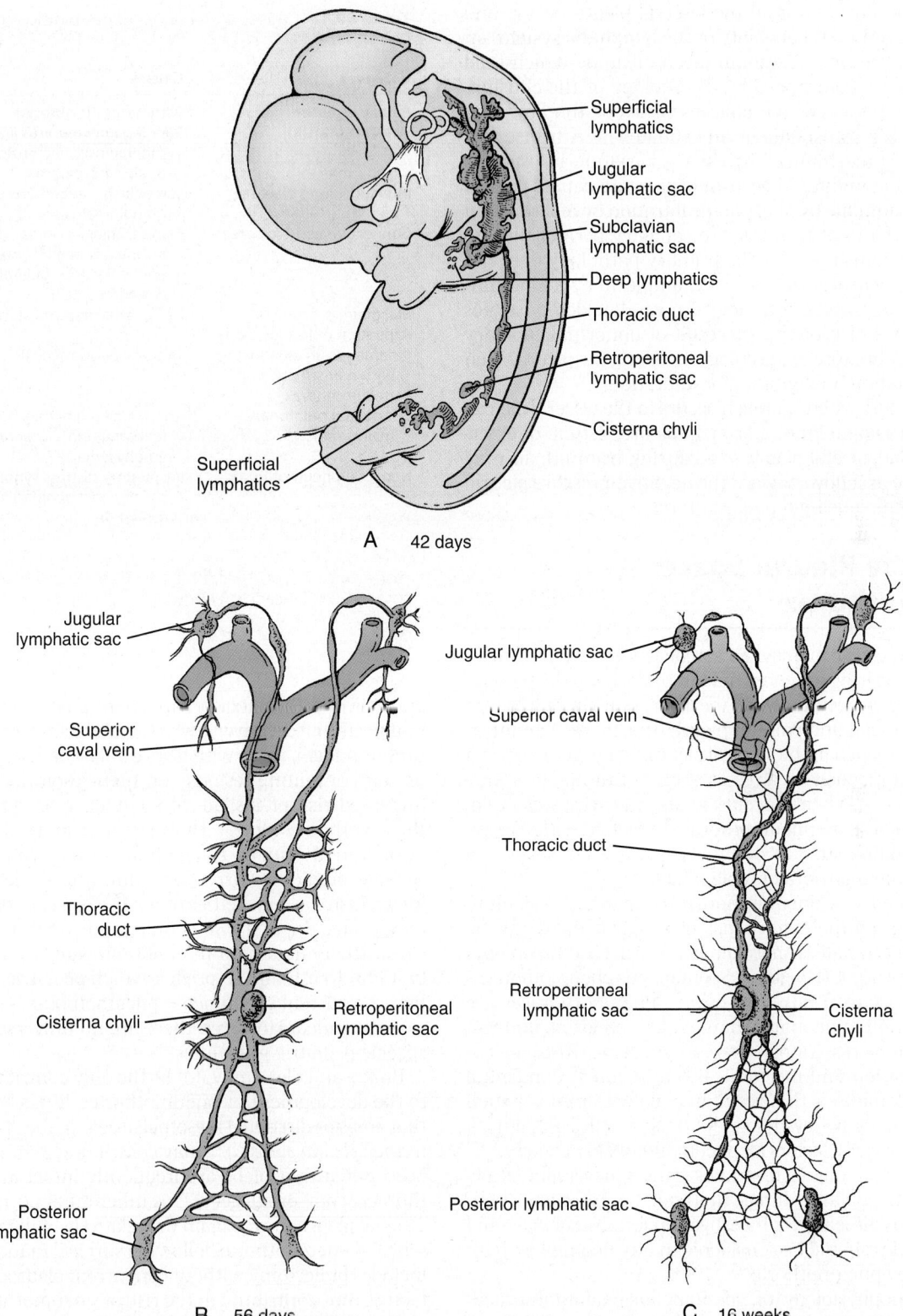

Fig. 69.2 Development of the lymphatic system. The lymphatic sacs and ducts in the process of development (A). (B and C) The significant remodeling that occurs within the lymphatic drainage system. (Reproduced with permission from Schoenwolf GC, Bleyl SB, Brauer PR, Francis-West PH, Philippa H. *Larsen's Human Embryology.* 5th ed. New York; Edinburgh: Churchill Livingstone; 2015:F13-F27.)

or abnormal filtration from the visceral pleura occurs and exceeds the drainage capability of the lymphatic system, an effusion will result.[7] The main mechanism by which fluid accumulates is determined by the etiology of the effusion, which also influences the characteristics of the fluid and whether it is a transudate or an exudate.[15,16] A transudate occurs when mechanical forces or a variation in osmotic, systemic or pulmonary hydrostatic pressure causes pleural fluid to accumulate by altering the filtration or reabsorption capability of the pleura, but the capillary permeability to proteins remains normal. The primary pathology does not involve the pleural surfaces—for example, in hypoalbuminemic states or cardiac pathology. An exudate demonstrates a higher level of protein as a result of abnormal capillary permeability because of pathology involving the pleura, such as inflammation, malignancy, or infarction.[17]

In the setting where a breach occurs in the visceral pleura, as in the development of a bronchopleural fistula, or externally via the parietal pleura (e.g., during trauma), air may accumulate as it flows toward the negative-pressure pleural environment, causing a pneumothorax.

Air in the Pleural Space: Pneumothorax

A pneumothorax occurs when air collects in the chest cavity outside of the lung parenchyma but underlying the parietal pleura. Air may accumulate in the pleural cavity via a breach in the chest wall and parietal pleura or if there is an intrapulmonary breach in the visceral pleura. Pneumothorax can occur spontaneously, as a result of chest trauma, or it may be iatrogenic.[18] When it occurs in an otherwise well child, it is called a *primary* pneumothorax. In a child with a respiratory condition such as cystic fibrosis, it is classified as a *secondary* pneumothorax (Table 69.1).[18]

The incidence of pneumothorax in children is difficult to ascertain, given the relative lack of available data, but the most recent estimate is approximately 4 per 100,000 in boys and 1.1 per 100,000 in girls.[19] Spontaneous pneumothoraces classically occur in tall, thin boys.[20] Pneumothoraces are more common in neonates than in older children, and risk factors include respiratory distress syndrome (RDS), meconium aspiration and mechanical ventilation.[21] Congenital renal malformations that result in oligohydramnios—such as renal agenesis, polycystic kidneys, or obstructive uropathy—are also known risk factors for pneumothorax in neonates.[22,23] It is likely that oligohydramnios causes developmentally abnormal hypoplastic lungs that can be associated with spontaneous air leak.[22,23] Investigation for obstructive renal abnormalities should be considered in any neonate with an unexplained pneumothorax.

The pathophysiology of spontaneous pneumothoraces remains controversial. Pulmonary "blebs" or larger "bullae" (Fig. 69.3) are developmentally abnormal enlarged airspaces and have historically been cited as risk factors for pneumothorax in children. They do not appear to occur in pediatric healthy controls but are found relatively frequently in children who have undergone computed tomography (CT) after a primary spontaneous pneumothorax (PSP).[24,25] However, in healthy adult controls, these bullae are found in about 15% of those who have undergone chests CT.[26] In a retrospective

Table 69.1 Causes of Secondary Pneumothorax in Children

Category	Causes
Airway disease	Asthma, cystic fibrosis
Postinfectious	Measles, *Pneumocystis jirovecii*, tuberculosis, necrotizing pneumonia or abscess, parasitic
Interstitial lung disease	Sarcoidosis, Langerhans cell granulomatosis
Connective tissue disease	Marfan, Ehlers–Danlos, rheumatoid arthritis, systemic lupus erythematosus, polymyositis, dermatomyositis
Malignancy	Lymphoma, metastasis, sarcoma
Aspiration of foreign body	
Catamenial (in conjunction with menstruation) pneumothorax	Thoracic endometriosis
Congenital pulmonary malformations	Congenital pulmonary adenomatoid malformation, congenital lobar emphysema
Neonatal pneumothorax	Respiratory distress syndrome, pulmonary hypoplasia, meconium aspiration

Modified from Robinson PD, Cooper P, Ranganathan SC. Evidence-based management of paediatric primary spontaneous pneumothorax. *Paediatr Respir Rev.* 2009;10(3):110-117; quiz 7.

analysis of 114 children with spontaneous pneumothorax managed conservatively (with supplemental oxygen or chest tube drainage), those with visible bullae on chest x-ray (CXR) or "air-containing lesions" on high-resolution CT, had an increased risk of ipsilateral recurrence as compared with those without bullae.[27] However, in a study of 70 episodes of pneumothorax in 46 children, CT abnormalities did not reliably predict recurrence[28]; thus the evidence remains inconclusive as to whether or not the presence of blebs found on CT after the first PSP should guide treatment decisions. Given the limited data in children, routine chest CTs after first PSP to attempt to predict which pediatric patients will have a recurrent spontaneous pneumothorax is not currently recommended. However, there are no universally accepted specific pediatric guidelines.[18]

Bullae and blebs may not be the only contributing factors to the development of pneumothorax. It has been reported that areas of disrupted mesothelial cells in the visceral pleura, termed *pleural porosity*,[29] may contribute to the risk, as it has been noted that blebs are frequently intact at the time of thoracoscopy or surgery. This inherent abnormality of the visceral pleura may explain the relatively high rates of recurrence of pneumothorax following surgical management that includes bullectomy without concurrent pleurodesis.[29] Other factors that contribute to the risk of pneumothorax include genetic connective tissue disorders such as Marfan syndrome,[30] Birt-Hogg-Dubé[31] or other folliculin gene mutations[19] as well as environmental factors such as exposure to tobacco smoke.[32]

When a pneumothorax occurs, air accumulates under the parietal pleura external to the lung parenchyma, causing direct compression of the lung. PSP classically occurs at rest but may be precipitated by a maneuver that increases intrathoracic pressure, such as the Valsalva maneuver or by lifting

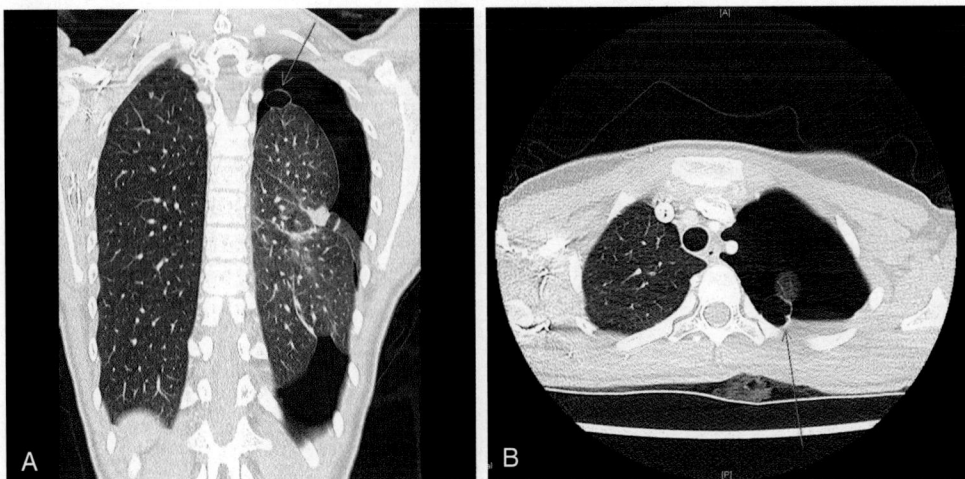

Fig. 69.3 Computed tomography scan of a 14-year-old female patient demonstrating left-sided pneumothorax with a 17-mm apical bleb. Axial (A) coronal (B) sections of the same patient for comparison. Blebs are identified by *green arrows*. (B) Abnormal pleural reaction at the site of a previous chest drain (placed 4 weeks earlier) for ipsilateral pneumothorax.

and straining.[19] Typically, pneumothorax presents as chest or back pain, dyspnea, or shortness of breath. Initial pain is often pleuritic in nature but may change to become a dull or a constant ache and may resolve after a few days, even without intervention.[19] Examination findings will vary depending on the size of the pneumothorax and may include tachypnea, tachycardia, low oxygen saturations, tracheal shift away from the side of the pneumothorax, hyperresonance on percussion and decreased air entry of the side of the pneumothorax. Small pneumothoraces may be difficult to detect clinically.

On rare occasions, air leaks into the pleural space and if it is unable to drain, a "ball and valve" effect develops. In this circumstance air will accumulate with each inspiratory effort and collect under "tension," forming a tension pneumothorax. This process may also occur with trauma to the chest wall and is a medical emergency, requiring immediate intervention, as it may ultimately result in decreased cardiac output and cardiorespiratory arrest. The patient will have the classic symptoms of pneumothorax but may also develop significant cardiorespiratory compromise manifest as progressive tachypnea, tachycardia, and eventually mediastinal shift with tracheal deviation away from the side of the pneumothorax.

In patients with a pneumothorax that is not under tension, CXRs demonstrate lung collapse and hyperlucency of air in the pleural space. This will often be more obvious on the expiratory film, but general recommendations are to quantify the size of the pneumothorax on an inspiratory film (Fig. 69.4).[18] More recent studies have demonstrated that ultrasonography may be a useful tool to diagnose pneumothorax.[33] A meta-analysis by Ding and coworkers indicates that, when performed by skilled operators on adult patients, ultrasonography had a higher sensitivity and similar specificity compared with CXR.[34] It may be a particularly useful technique in cases of trauma, where a supine CXR would otherwise be performed,[35] or in neonates with respiratory distress.[36] A CXR should never be performed when a tension pneumothorax has developed because it delays intervention, with potentially catastrophic consequences.

Table 69.2	Methods Used to Quantify Pneumothorax
	Method of Calculation
Light method	Volume (%) = 100 − [(average diameter lung)^3/ (average diameter hemithorax)^3 × 100]
Rhea method	Average of interpleural distances (cm) at three points on erect chest x-ray: 1. Apex 2. Midpoint upper half of lung 3. Midpoint lower half of lung Use nomogram to convert into volume
Collins Method	Size (%) = 4.2 + 4.7 [sum of interpleural distances at apex, midpoint upper half of collapsed lung, and midpoint lower half of collapsed lung]

From Robinson PD, Cooper P, Ranganathan SC. Evidence-based management of paediatric primary spontaneous pneumothorax. *Paediatr Respir Rev.* 2009;10(3):110-117; quiz 7.

The treatment of pneumothorax depends on the clinical status of the patient, whether it is primary, secondary, or under tension and its size. A tension pneumothorax should be treated immediately with needle thoracentesis to the affected side.[37] In cases of pneumothoraces not under tension, quantifying the size in order to select the optimal course of management may be helpful. However, the size of the pneumothorax does not always correlate with clinical manifestations.[38] Several methods may be used to quantify the size of the pneumothorax, including measuring the distance to the cupola or apical dome of the lung (considered large if greater than 3 cm to the apex),[39] distance to the lateral edge (considered large if >2 cm) (Fig. 69.5)[38] or complete dehiscence.[40] Other methods used to quantify size include the Light method, Rhea method or the Collins method (Table 69.2).[18] However, there is often variation in the results of these calculations, as the shape of the pneumothorax can affect accuracy.[18] The British Thoracic Society (BTS) guidelines recommend that large pneumothoraces be identified "by the presence of a visible rim of >2 cm between the lung margin and chest wall at the level of the hilum."[38]

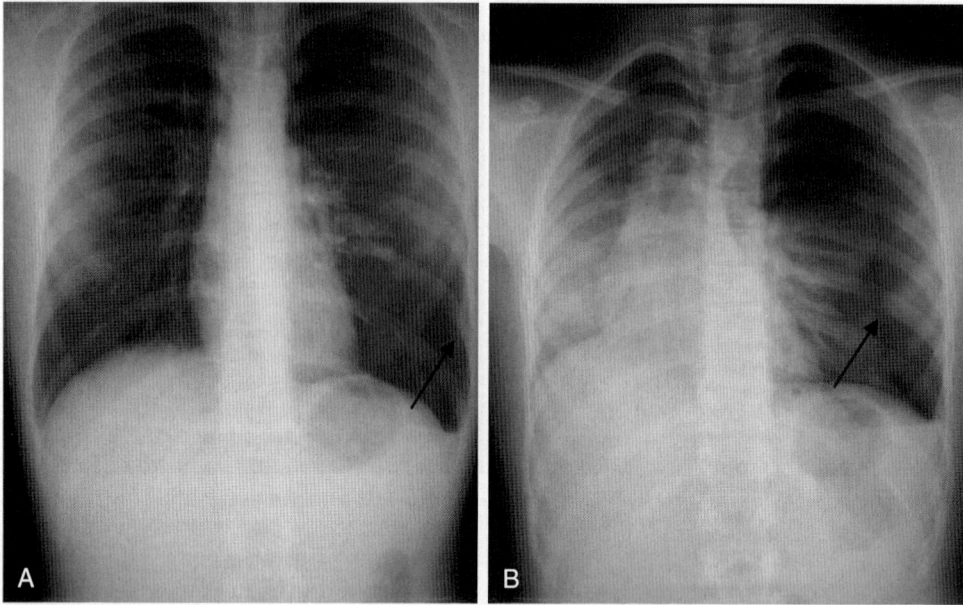

Fig. 69.4 Chest x-ray (CXR) images of pneumothorax in a 12-year-old child. CXR images of primary spontaneous pneumothorax taken at the same time. (A) Inspiratory view. (B) Expiratory view. The two images demonstrate the significant change in the size of the pneumothorax with respiration. Despite the mediastinal shift seen in (B), this pneumothorax was not under tension. (Reused with permission from Robinson PD, Cooper P, Ranganathan SC. Evidence-based management of paediatric primary spontaneous pneumothorax. *Paediatr Respir Rev*. 2009;10(3):110–117, quiz 7.)

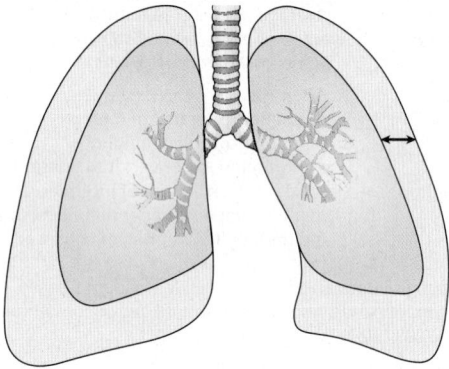

Fig. 69.5 Measurement of the pneumothorax by the interpleural distance at the level of the hilum as described in the British Thoracic Society Pleural Disease Guideline.[38]

The treatment of a small primary pneumothorax may be conservative, including high-flow oxygen and observation in an emergency department. Normal oxygen saturations do not preclude the use of oxygen therapy. Concurrent oxygen therapy may decrease the length of time taken for a pneumothorax to reinflate after intervention and may hasten the reinflation process by up to four times in the case of larger pneumothoraces.[41] The mechanism by which oxygen helps resolve a pneumothorax is thought to be by decreasing the partial pressure of nitrogen in the pleural space to hasten the reexpansion on the lung. However, the evidence for this recommendation comes from animal studies, and limited evidence is available to support this theory in humans. Although current guidelines still recommend the use of oxygen even if the patient is not hypoxic, the recommendation is derived from weak evidence and may not be appropriate in all cases.[42]

The treatment for a large nontension PSP may include a trial needle aspiration prior to proceeding to an intercostal drain, but universal agreement among guidelines is lacking.[39] The BTS guidelines[38] propose this intervention as first-line therapy for PSPs greater than 2 cm requiring intervention; however, needle aspiration in children is not commonly undertaken and is not yet considered the standard of care universally. There is an increasing body of evidence in adult patients with pneumothorax suggesting that needle aspiration may be just as effective, less invasive, and associated with a lower rate of complications and length of stay in hospital compared with thoracentesis[43,44]; however, care should be taken in extrapolating this evidence to children. Recent studies suggest that needle aspiration success rates in children are lower than those for adult patients with pneumothorax, and failure rates of up to 50% have been reported.[45,46] Needle aspiration is painful and, because of a significant risk of failure in children who would require a second intervention, it may not be appropriate in this population.

The treatment of a secondary pneumothorax generally requires insertion of a drain[47] because of the additional impact on respiratory function of the underlying disease. The recommended technique may depend on the area of collection but will generally be via the axillary or "safe triangle"[48] to avoid the internal mammary artery or anteriorly above the second rib on the ipsilateral side of the air accumulation. Small-bore chest drains (<14F) have been found to be just as successful as large-bore catheters, with less pain, and as such should be used routinely.[38] Catheter insertion should be done by an experienced clinician and may be helped by ultrasound guidance (Fig. 69.6).[38] Chest drains may be inserted by a blunt dissection technique or by the less traumatic Seldinger approach using small percutaneous drains. In inserting a chest drain, care must be taken to avoid the neurovascular bundle that runs on the inferior aspect of the ribs. Children will require analgesia, and conscious sedation

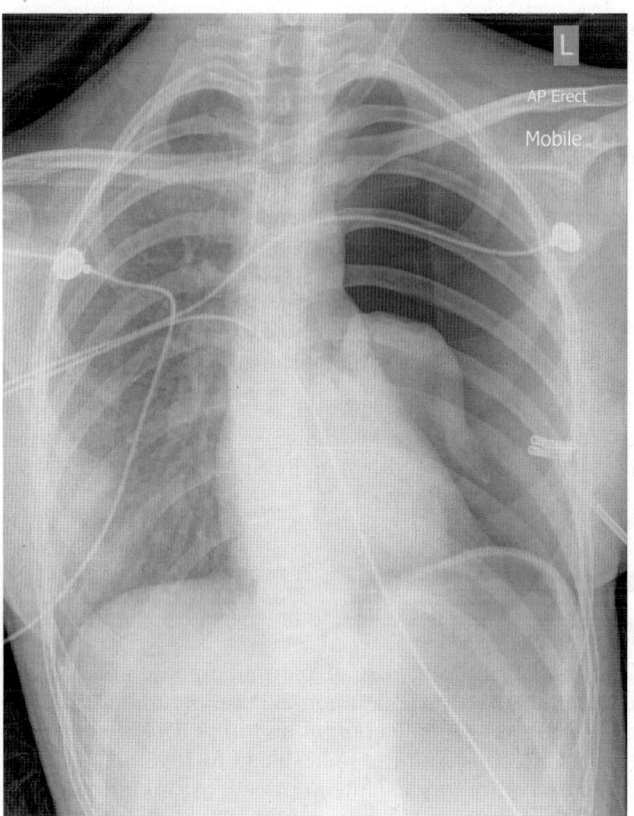

Fig. 69.6 Chest x ray of a 15 year old male patient with left sided primary spontaneous pneumothorax. The image demonstrates a large left-sided pneumothorax and an inserted pigtail chest tube. The lung remained deflated despite the pigtail catheter and suction was required to reinflate the lung.

should be considered. Nitrous oxide should be avoided owing to the risk of nitrous gas entering the pleural space and increasing the size of pneumothorax. Once a chest catheter is in place, it should not be put on immediate suction because of the increased risk of persistent air leak and the theoretical risk of reexpansion pulmonary edema (RPE), which has been seen in younger adults (20–40 years) with large pneumothoraces.[18] There is a paucity of evidence regarding the risk of RPE in children, but in adult patients it appears to correlate with the duration of lung collapse and size of the pneumothorax.[49] If there is minimal improvement with conservative management after 48 hours, high-volume, low-pressure suction may be considered.[38] Pressures of −10 to −20 cm H_2O are recommended in the BTS adult pneumothorax guidelines.[38]

In adults, the risk of recurrence after the first episode of pneumothorax averages 30%[50] and increases with each subsequent recurrence. In children, the risk of recurrence after a single spontaneous pneumothorax appears to be greater than that in adults, possibly closer to 60%,[20,51] although Seguier-Lipszyc and coworkers found that the risk after the first and second episodes of pneumothorax in children remained unchanged at about 50%.[28] If the pneumothorax is treated conservatively, the risk of recurrence does not appear to be altered by the method of treatment: oxygen alone or with a chest drain.[28]

Definitive treatment for a spontaneous pneumothorax may include bullectomy with pleurodesis, which has been shown to decrease the recurrence rate; but surgical intervention is associated with significant pain and morbidity. Methods of pleurodesis include those using a chemical (such as talc, minocycline, or glue) or mechanical pleurodesis, which is done by abrading the pleural surfaces to create an inflammatory process, causing the two pleural membranes to adhere.[52] Pleurodesis with mechanical abrasion appears to involve less morbidity and lower recurrent rates.[28] Video-assisted thoracoscopic surgery (VATS), as an alternative to open thoracotomy, is becoming more popular in children, as it is minimally invasive and has been shown to have good outcomes in those with PSP; however, it does rely on the availability of local expertise.[28,51,53] Ideally a definitive surgical intervention would occur at the time of presentation to avoid multiple procedures. But until patients with the highest risk of treatment failure or recurrent pneumothorax can be reliably identified, VATS cannot be recommended as routine first-line therapy.[54,55]

Flying and Diving After Pneumothorax

Patients who have had a spontaneous pneumothorax must be cautioned against scuba diving. Adult pneumothorax guidelines recommend avoiding scuba diving unless a definitive surgical procedure, such as a bilateral pleurectomy, has been undertaken[38] and normal lung function and chest CT have been confirmed postoperatively. This recommendation is made because of the risk of contralateral pneumothorax, and patients who have had a spontaneous pneumothorax are at risk of a recurrent pneumothorax during a dive.[56] There is a risk that if a pneumothorax occurs while the diver is under water, it will enlarge during the ascent in accordance with Boyle's law, and the diver may develop a rapidly enlarging pneumothorax—a potentially life-threatening situation.

Patients with a closed pneumothorax should not fly owing to low cabin atmospheric pressure. There should be no increased risk of developing a recurrent pneumothorax with flying after a PSP; however, the pneumothorax must be entirely resolved, with radiologic confirmation.[47] There is no consensus regarding travel postpneumothorax in children; adult pneumothorax guidelines recommend delaying flying anywhere between 7 days and 6 weeks postresolution.[47] The BTS air travel guidelines recommend that complete resolution of the pneumothorax be confirmed on CXR and that then a minimum 7 days should elapse prior to flying, with a longer delay if the pneumothorax was traumatic or if the patient has underlying lung disease.[57] Without a definitive surgical procedure, the risk of recurrence from pneumothorax may remain elevated for at least a year, particularly in patients with secondary pneumothorax, and such patients should be advised of the risk of recurrence.[38]

Fluid in the Plural Space

EFFUSIONS

As discussed earlier, in the healthy state, a small amount of fluid lies between the parietal and visceral pleural layers. The fluid continues to be filtered and reabsorbed by the lymphatic system within a very delicate balance of hydrostatic and oncotic pressure forces. When an imbalance occurs, fluid will accumulate at a rate faster than the lymphatic system is capable of draining. The etiology of the fluid accumulation will determine the nature of fluid. A transudate results from a change in the transpleural pressure balance,[6] and the resulting fluid will have a relatively low leukocyte count, lower levels of protein and be relatively alkalotic[58] as is seen in hypoalbuminemic states and cardiac failure. Alternatively, an exudative accumulation results from either increased vascular permeability of pleural capillary beds or impaired lymphatic drainage, such as seen in infection.[6] The resulting exudate will be more acidic, high in white blood cells (neutrophils, lymphocytes, eosinophils), protein, and lactate dehydrogenase (LDH) but relatively low in glucose[59] (see Table 69.3 for causes of pleural effusions). Light's appear to be the most robust criteria applied to differentiate a transudate from an exudate, and they are used to guide treatment in adult patients. Although useful, these criteria are not 100% specific (Table 69.4).[17,60] Criteria such as these are not routinely used in the management of children, partly because children rarely undergo a "diagnostic" tap, as the causes of pleural effusion are generally fewer than adults; by far the most common type of pleural effusion in children is a parapneumonic effusion.[59] This occurs when the equilibrium between pleural fluid secretion and pleural lymphatic drainage is disrupted because of an underlying pneumonia. It classically presents as a syndrome of progressive pneumonia

not responding to treatment and can be divided into three stages[61]:

1. Exudative stage—simple parapneumonic effusion with low leukocyte count.
2. Fibrinopurulent stage—deposition of fibrin resulting in septations and loculations (Fig. 69.7). An increase in leukocytes occurs and microorganisms invade the pleural space, resulting in purulent material filling the pleural cavity. A parapneumonic effusion that contains pus is defined as an empyema.
3. Organizational stage—fibroblasts enter the pleural cavity, forming tight fibrous membranes.

Nonparapneumonic pleural effusions in children can occur as a result of congenital heart disease, renal and liver disease, connective tissue disorders, malignancy, or as postoperative surgical complications.[59]

EMPYEMA

Etiology

The most common cause of parapneumonic effusion and empyema is bacterial pneumonia. Parapneumonic effusions can occur as a complication of a viral or *Mycoplasma pneumoniae* infection and are more likely to be simple and less likely to require surgical intervention.[62] Although empyema is relatively rare in children, up to 28% of those requiring hospitalization for pneumonia may have an associated effusion.[63] The process of pleural fluid accumulation is mediated by increased vascular permeability secondary to mesothelial cell cytokines including interleukin (IL)-1, IL-6, IL-8, tumor necrosis factor (TNF)-α, and platelet activating factor.[64] Initially the fluid accumulating in the pleural space is an exudate resulting from the inflammatory process involving the pleura in response to an underlying pneumonia. The pleura leaks proteins and fluid and eventually leukocytes. As the disease progresses, the number of leukocytes increases, and eventually the pleural cavity is infiltrated by organisms. When the fluid becomes purulent, it is called an empyema (from the

Table 69.3 Common Causes of Pleural Effusions

Transudate	Exudate
Cardiac disease (e.g., congestive heart failure, congenital heart disease, pericarditis)	Infectious
	Malignancy (e.g., leukemia, lymphoma)
Renal disease (e.g., nephrotic syndrome)	Lymphatic abnormalities and chylothorax
Hypoalbuminemia (e.g., secondary to liver failure)	Postoperative surgical complications (e.g., scoliosis surgery)
Superior vena cava obstruction	Pulmonary infarction
Hepatic cirrhosis	Connective tissue and vasculitic disorders (e.g., rheumatoid pleurisy, Churg-Strauss, sarcoidosis)
	Abdominal pathology (e.g., pancreatitis, viral hepatitis, subphrenic abscess)
	Endocrine (e.g., hypothyroidism)

Modified from Light RW, Macgregor MI, Luchsinger PC, Ball JWC. Pleural effusions: the diagnostic separation of transudates and exudates. *Ann Int Med.* 1972;77(4):507-513.

Table 69.4 Lights Criteria: Pleural Fluid Is an Exudate if the Following Criteria Are Met

Pleural fluid protein/serum protein	>0.5
Pleural fluid LDH/serum LDH	>0.6
Pleural fluid LDH	>2/3 upper limit normal serum LDH

LDH, Lactate dehydrogenase.
From Light RW, Macgregor MI, Luchsinger PC, Ball JWC. Pleural effusions: the diagnostic separation of transudates and exudates. *Ann Int Med.* 1972;77(4):507-513.

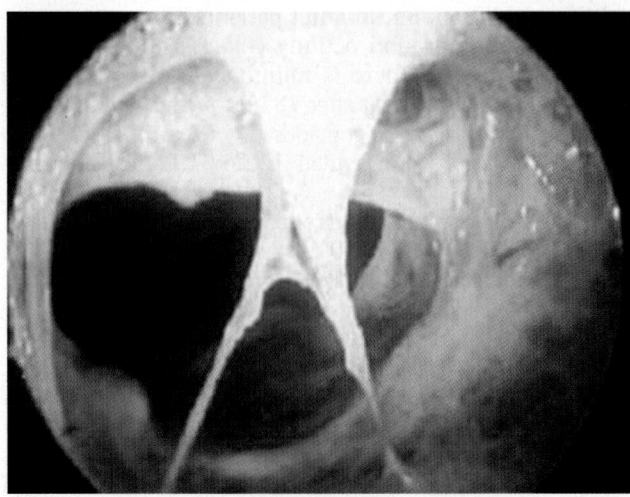

Fig. 69.7 Thoracoscopic image of fibrinous septations taken in a child with empyema. (Image reprinted with permission from Professor Gordon Cohen.)

Greek *empuein,* meaning "to suppurate"). As the disease progresses, there is increasing deposition of fibrinous material, which leads to septation and the formation of loculations. This fibrinous material can obstruct the free flow of fluid and block the draining lymphatic stomata, thus preventing spontaneous resolution of normal lymphatic draining and often requiring an intervention to drain the fluid (Video 69.1). In the later "organizational" stage in the disease process, fibroblasts penetrate the pleural cavity and can form a membrane called a *peel.* This peel is made of firm fibrous material that can impair lung function by "trapping" the lung and limiting recovery if not identified. Although lung trapping is often seen in adult patients, it rarely occurs in children with empyema.[65]

Epidemiology

The incidence of parapneumonic effusions and empyema has been reported to be up to 10 per 100,000 children in the United States[66] and appears to have increased, particularly in the younger age groups,[67] following the introduction of pneumococcal conjugate vaccine (PCV7)[66,68–70] against serotypes 4, 6B, 9V, 14, 18C, and 19F[71] despite a reduction in invasive pneumococcal disease.[72] Similarly, one study in Australia found that the overall hospitalization rate for pneumonia had decreased after the introduction of the 7-valent vaccine, but the percentage of empyema as a proportion of pneumonia increased from 0.27% to 0.7% of hospitalizations.[73] The reason for the increase is unknown but may reflect replacement of serotypes by those that are particularly virulent with a predilection for the pleural space, such as serotype 1, 3 and 19A.[72] Following the recent introduction of PCV13 into national vaccination schedules, which includes six additional serotypes (1, 3, 5, 6A, 7F and 19A),[71] the rates of invasive pneumococcal disease have further decreased.[74] More recent studies after the introduction of the 13-valent pneumococcal vaccine have described a decrease in the rates of pediatric empyema, with the greatest reduction in children below 4 years of age.[75] Ongoing enhanced surveillance is required to ensure that serotype replacement does not occur in the future.

Empyema occurs more commonly in boys, infants, and younger children[76] and is seen more frequently in the spring and winter months, given that this is when bacterial pneumonia is more likely to occur. Mortality, more common in the adult population, is uncommon in children but still occurs rarely.[68,77] Children with certain risk factors—including immunodeficiency, malignancy, genetic conditions such as Down syndrome, congenital heart disease, and cystic fibrosis—are at an increased risk of empyema[76,78,79]; the presence of comorbid conditions increases the risk of death.[79] Although it is unknown why empyema occurs in healthy children, evidence from adult studies suggests that there may be a genetic predisposition. Transcription factor nuclear factor (NF-κB) plays a key role in host innate and adaptive immune responses and may play a role in the development of empyema.[80] Inhibitors of NF-κB (IκB) control the nuclear factor activity, and rare mutations in IκB are known to cause immunodeficiency syndromes complicated by severe infections.[81] Chapman and coworkers demonstrated that more common IκB polymorphisms are associated with invasive pneumococcal disease, which may determine why invasive pneumococcal disease does not occur in all patients when

pneumococcal colonization in the nasopharynx is known to be relatively widespread.[81] Alternatively, bacterial virulence and load may be a factor that results in invasive disease. Esposito and coworkers demonstrated that in their cohort of 72 otherwise well children less than 5 years old with *Streptococcus pneumoniae* community-acquired pneumonia, those with high bacterial loads were more likely to have an associated parapneumonic effusion.[82] Furthermore, Munoz-Almago and coworkers were able to show that bacterial load correlated with serum inflammatory markers (c-reactive protein [CRP]), hospital length of stay, and number of hours of pleural drainage.[83] Another factor implicated in why some healthy children develop an empyema may be a delay in accessing appropriate antibiotic therapy.[84] However, empyema can complicate pneumonia even if the children have been appropriately treated with antibiotics. Empyema as a result of delayed initiation of treatment is reflected in the greater burden of empyema in communities that have poorer access to antibiotics, and it is an ongoing cause of pediatric morbidity worldwide as well as of potential mortality, particularly in the low- and middle-income settings.[85] In one study, use of ibuprofen was noted to be a potential risk factor for the development of empyema.[86]

Another factor that may contribute to the development of empyema is a precipitating viral respiratory tract infection.[87] During influenza pandemics an increase in hospitalizations has been noted, with children suffering respiratory complications including bacterial pneumonia and empyema.[88] One U.S. center noted that, although rare, 2% of the children hospitalized with influenza also had positive bacterial cultures, most commonly *S. pneumoniae* and *Staphylococcus aureus,* and several eventually developed lung abscesses or empyema.[89] The exact mechanism by which a preceding viral infection potentially increases the risk of empyema is not yet clear, but the viral infection with associated increased secretions may create an environment in which bacterial coinfection can occur.

As the incidence of childhood empyema has increased, a concurrent increase in the rates of pneumococcus-associated hemolytic uremic syndrome (P-HUS) has been described. P-HUS causes hemolytic anemia, thrombocytopenia, and acute renal failure. P-HUS has been associated with considerable morbidity and prolonged hospital stay[90] in addition to high rates of mortality.[91] A retrospective review undertaken in the United Kingdom reported P-HUS to have occurred in 7.5% of patients with pneumococcal empyema, and children less than 2 years of age were particularly at risk.[90]

Microbiology

The bacterial cause of empyema depends on several patient-specific and environmental factors. These include the health status of the child, risk of immunocompromise, immunization history, geographical location and the local prevalence of bacteria. *S. pneumoniae* (and to a lesser extent *S. aureus*) has historically been the primary causative organism. The development of newer antibiotics and the introduction of newer vaccinations in recent decades have changed the profile of bacteria causing empyema. There also appears to be a significant increase in the number of cases caused by penicillin- and cephalosporin-resistant *S. pneumoniae,*[92] which may have led to an increasing number of complicated cases of necrotizing pneumonia. As already described, following the introduction of the 7-valent pneumococcal conjugate vaccine, several studies have demonstrated an increase in the prevalence of *S. pneumoniae* serotypes 1, 3, 7F and 19A, causing empyema. These serotypes were not included in the 7-valent vaccine but are now included in the 13-valent conjugate vaccine, which has been introduced into the national vaccination schedules of many countries.[71] Other than the streptococcal species, *S. aureus* is an important cause of empyema in children.[93] Methicillin-resistant *S. aureus* (MRSA) has also been described in empyema, and rates of occurrence appear to be increasing.[92,94] In some cases, the cause of chronic empyema is pulmonary tuberculosis, which should be considered along with parasitic causes if the empyema is bilateral.[95] Other causes of empyema include *Streptococcus pyogenes* and other streptococcal species, including *S. viridans* and *S. milleri*. Other parapneumonic effusion–causing organisms include *Haemophilus influenzae*, *M. pneumoniae*, and *Pseudomonas aeruginosa*. The Australian Research Network in Empyema (ARNiE) prospectively described the bacterial causes of empyema in Australia between 2007 and 2009 and confirmed that the streptococcal and staphylococcal species continue to be the most common causes of empyema in children (Box 69.1).[96] Gram-negative anaerobic organisms and specific fungi[59] are known to cause empyema in rare cases but usually represent complications of risk factors such as aspiration, immunocompromise or nosocomial infection.

The prevalence of the microbiologic causes of pediatric empyema is difficult to ascertain accurately because there is extensive variation in the ability to identify the infectious organism.[59,97] This is further complicated by treatment with antibiotics, which may sterilize the fluid prior to sampling.[59] With the advent of molecular techniques such as polymerase chain reaction (PCR), the identification of a causative organism in sterile fluid is enhanced,[98–101] and this technique is more sensitive than traditional culture methods.[100] Strachan and coworkers were able to culture streptococcal species in

---

Box 69.1 **Bacterial Causes of Empyema: Bacteria Isolated by Culture of Blood, Pleural Fluid Samples, and Polymerase Chain Reaction of Pleural Fluid Samples From Children With Empyema, Australia, 2007–2009, in Order of Frequency**

Streptococcus pneumoniae
Streptococcus pyogenes
Streptococcus milleri
MSSA
MRSA
Coagulase-negative staphylococci
Haemophilus influenzae
Mycobacterium tuberculosis
Pseudomonas aeruginosa
Mycoplasma pneumoniae
Chlamydia pneumoniae

MRSA, Methicillin-resistant *S. aureus*; *MSSA*, methicillin-sensitive *S. aureus*.
Modified from Strachan RE, Snelling TL, Jaffé A. Increased paediatric hospitalizations for empyema in Australia after introduction of the 7-valent pneumococcal conjugate vaccine. Bull World Health Organ. 2013;91(3):167-173.

---

only 5.9% of pleural fluid samples from children with empyema, but PCR identified streptococcus as the causative organism in 54.4%.[101] In the case of *S. pneumoniae*, latex agglutination appears to be the most sensitive and specific test that can identify pneumococcal antigen in pleural fluid and is more sensitive than PCR.[102] However, unlike culturing the organism, a limitation of PCR or pneumococcal antigen detection is the lack of information regarding antibiotic resistance.

Clinical Manifestations of Empyema

Empyema classically presents as a clinical syndrome including fevers, lethargy, productive cough, respiratory distress, and toxicity resulting from the underlying pneumonia. Examination reveals a febrile child in respiratory distress, possibly requiring oxygen or ventilatory support.[59] The child may be tachypneic, with shallow breaths to minimize the pleuritic pain caused by deep inspiration. Infection in the lower lobes may present as abdominal pain and must be considered as part of the differential diagnosis in children presenting with acute abdominal pain. Empyema typically causes pleuritic pain in the chest and back. The child may splint the painful side by lying on the affected side or by refusing to move and change position. Chest examination reveals decreased chest expansion, dullness to percussion, classically described as "stony dullness," and decreased or absent breath sounds over the affected side. Depending on the size of the effusion, the child may exhibit scoliosis, often confirmed on CXR, which resolves spontaneously when the empyema resolves.[103] In children who present with pneumonia and a scarlatiniform rash, who appear toxic, and who have signs of circulatory failure or low leukocyte levels, consideration should be given to the possibility that the infective organism may be group A streptococcus (GAS), resulting in streptococcal toxic shock syndrome (STSS).[104] Risk factors for GAS empyema include recent corticosteroid usage and varicella infection.[104] The treatment in this instance is to use an antitoxin antibiotic such as clindamycin, as this is a particularly aggressive, potentially fatal disease that causes severe sepsis and hypotension, often requiring inotropic support.

Investigations

The first-line treatment of bacterial pneumonia includes antibiotics and respiratory support. Empyema should be considered in children who do not respond to appropriate antibiotics within 48 hours, as evident by ongoing fevers, toxicity, and respiratory distress. In this scenario a CXR should be undertaken to assess for progression of the pneumonia or pleural fluid collection. Fluid will collect in dependent regions, so an erect or lateral decubitus film may allow easier identification of a dependent opacification, loss of the costophrenic angle or a meniscus suggestive of fluid (Fig. 69.8). An effusion on CXR that is performed in the supine position may show a more subtle increase in generalized opacification, reflecting the underlying layer of fluid behind the lungs or showing opacification throughout the pleural space (Fig. 69.9). A routine lateral chest film is not required and is associated with unnecessary exposure to ionizing radiation.[105] In the setting of infrapulmonary effusion, where the effusion collects between the inferior surface of the lung and the dome of the diaphragm, an elevated lateral hemidiaphragm

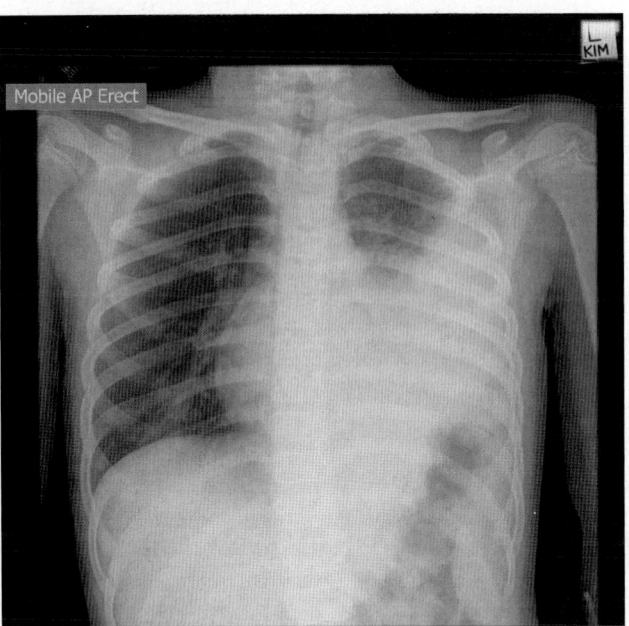

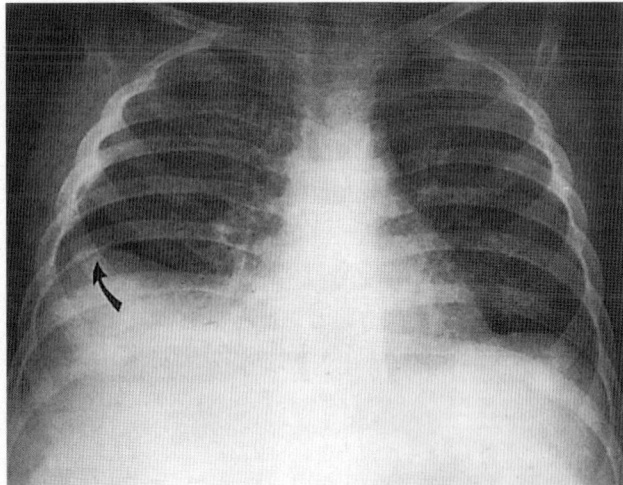

Fig. 69.10 Chest x-ray demonstrating infrapulmonary/subpulmonary effusion. The right hemidiaphragm has a lateral peak with relative lucency of the costophrenic angle.

Fig. 69.8 Chest x-ray (CXR) of empyema, erect image. CXR of a 7-year-old female with left-sided empyema. There is extensive opacity in the left middle and lower zones consistent with a combination of left-lower-lobe consolidation with collapse and a moderate to large pleural effusion, which was confirmed on ultrasound.

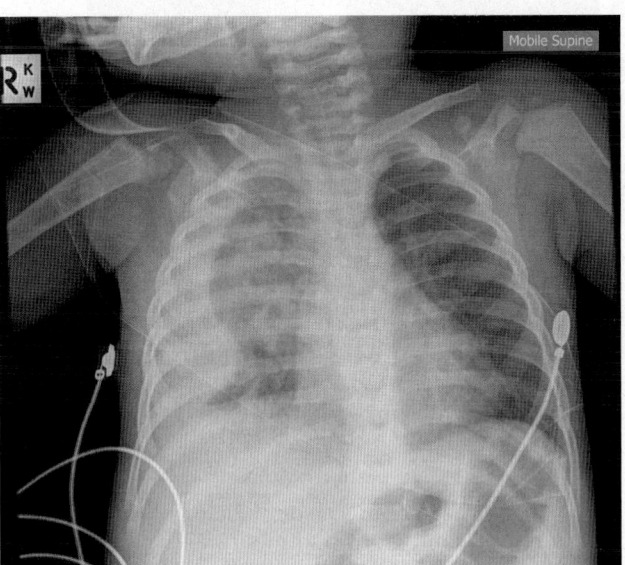

Fig. 69.9 Chest x-ray (CXR) of empyema, supine image. CXR of a 22-month-old female with empyema. There is a large, dense, right-sided pleural collection extending up the lateral chest wall with an associated reduction in the volume of the right lung. There is patchy consolidation within the aerated right lung and collapse consolidation of the right lung base.

may be demonstrated on CXR (Fig. 69.10). Ultrasound is the investigation of choice,[106] but if unavailable, a CXR may be helpful in identifying whether a pleural effusion has become loculated. In this situation, when an erect CXR is compared with a decubitus film, failure of the fluid to shift with a change in position is suggestive of loculated fluid (Fig. 69.11). Given the additional radiation with repeat CXRs and the poor sensitivity of x-ray as compared with ultrasound, multiple CXRs

in different positions should not be routinely undertaken. Within the context of pneumonia, any air in the pleural space suggests a complicated effusion that may involve a bronchopleural fistula or perforated viscus.

Children who are not clinically improving or who have a CXR suggestive of an effusion should undergo a chest ultrasound. This will allow a more accurate assessment of pleural fluid volume and will also better characterize the fluid (Fig. 69.12). Ultrasound will enable grading of the empyema.[107] Jaffe and coworkers developed an ultrasound scoring system for children with empyema based on complexity. Grades 1 and 2 effusions did not have septations; grade 1 fluid was defined as anechoic and grade 2 defined as echoic fluid without septation. Grade 3 and 4 empyemas were more complex, grade 3 defined as having thick septations and grade 4 had greater than one-third of the effusion comprising solid components.[107] These ultrasound findings are clinically relevant and may help determine which effusions need further intervention, including those that are less likely to resolve with antibiotics alone. If the fluid is found to be complex and loculated, further interventions such as insertion of a chest drain or surgical intervention should be considered.[107,108] Furthermore, ultrasound allows fluid volume to be estimated and enables the identification of optimal sites for chest drain insertion[105]; it is also more sensitive than CT in detecting early loculations and septations.[108] Ultrasound can be performed without sedation, which is required in some young children undergoing a CT scan. Importantly, ultrasound does not expose the child to radiation.

During a clinical trial comparing VATS versus chest drain with fibrinolytics,[107] Jaffe and coworkers assessed the utility of routine CT scans in children with empyema; all subjects underwent a CT of the chest. Unsurprisingly, CT scans were able to demonstrate more parenchymal changes with greater sensitivity, such as cavitary necrosis and pneumatoceles, than CXRs. However, no abnormality detected on CT led to a change in management. Thus, although CT scans demonstrate greater detail of the underlying lung pathology, the performance of routine CT of the chest in empyema does not alter management; therefore this should not be performed

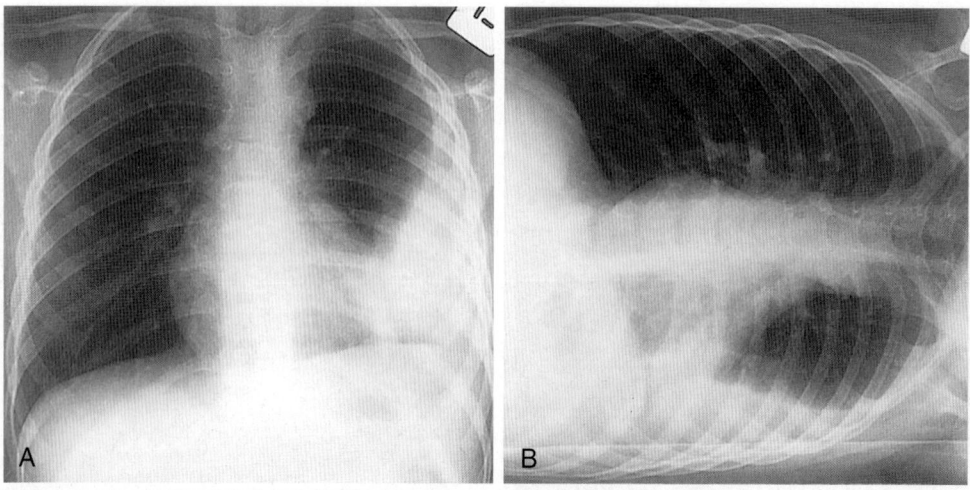

Fig. 69.11 Comparison of chest x-ray (CXR) of empyema taken in erect and left lateral decubitus positions. (A) Posteroanterior erect CXR of a large left empyema and adjacent atelectasis. (B) Left lateral decubitus CXR demonstrating no change in the configuration of the effusion, suggesting a loculated empyema.

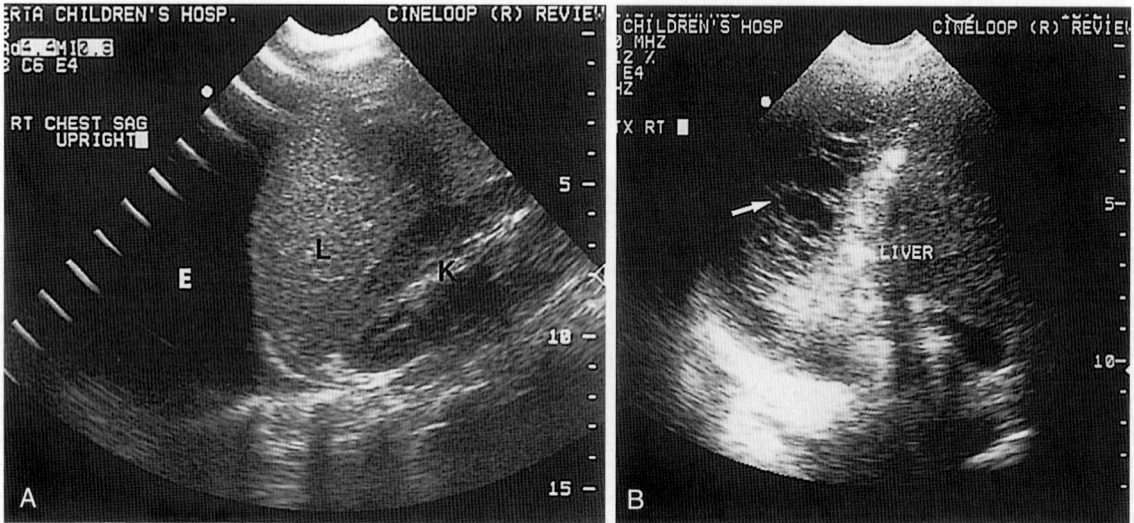

Fig. 69.12 Ultrasound images of lower right hemithorax and upper quadrant of abdomen. (A) A large anechoic right pleural effusion *(E)* with liver *(L)* and kidney *(K)* identified. (B) Repeat sonogram 6 days later with mixed echogenicity consistent with an empyema *(arrow)*.

routinely.[59,105] However, there are a few circumstances in which CT of the chest may be useful; these include specific evaluation of parenchymal disease,[107] cases involving concerns about an underlying malignancy and assessment for abscess formation. Neither ultrasound nor CT, nor a combination of the two, is reliably able to predict length of hospital stay for children with empyema.[107]

Initial blood investigations often demonstrate raised white cell count, inflammatory markers such as CRP, erythrocyte sedimentation rate (ESR), or procalcitonin. Secondary hypo-albuminemia from loss of protein into the pleural space or malnutrition may occur with large effusions.[109] Reactive thrombocytosis is also very common and resolves after approximately 3 weeks; it does not require any treatment.[59] Blood cultures should be drawn and may be positive in up to 22% of cases of empyema in children.[110] An antistreptolysin O titer (ASOT) may also be helpful to guide rationalizing antibiotics. The role of routine repeat blood investigations is limited and they are not recommended in empyema. If a child is not responding to treatment, repeat inflammatory markers may play a role in guiding the clinician in further management of the disease process, but these cannot differentiate bacterial from nonbacterial causes.[59] In older children who are able to expectorate, sputum samples may help with organism identification; however, there is no indication for routine bronchoscopy in empyema unless there is a specific concern about an inhaled foreign body.[59]

The BTS and Australian guidelines for pleural infection in children do not recommend that all otherwise healthy children routinely undergo immunologic testing in the setting of a single empyema.[59,105] However, the guidelines acknowledge that immune deficiency syndromes have been diagnosed in this way, and investigations should certainly be undertaken in the setting of a child with a history of repeated infections, unusual infections or a family history of immune deficiency. Guidelines recommend that if *S. aureus* or *P. aeruginosa* is identified as the causative organism, a sweat test to exclude cystic fibrosis should be arranged.[59]

Thoracentesis is rarely undertaken for diagnostic purposes in children with empyema; if it is performed, the simultaneous placement of a chest drain should be considered to minimize the number of invasive procedures.[105] Mitri and coworkers have demonstrated that children undergoing thoracentesis had significantly higher reintervention rates as compared with children who had chest catheters inserted.[111] If a drain is inserted for clinical reasons, pleural fluid should be sent for analysis, including Gram stain and culture, cytology and molecular testing such as PCR (if available). Pleural fluid is often sterile owing to prior administration of antibiotics; however, the use of PCR significantly improves the identification of bacteria.[101] A differential cell count may help in differentiating between bacterial, mycobacterial, or noninfectious causes, as lymphocytes rather than neutrophils may predominate in the last two conditions.[112] There is currently no role for biochemical analysis of pleural fluid in the setting of empyema to guide management in children, although this is the norm in adults.[59,105]

Management

The aim of empyema treatment is to treat the microbial cause, sterilize the pleural fluid, and allow reexpansion of the lung to support the return to normal lung function. This occurs either through gradual reabsorption of excess pleural fluid over time or by active drainage by tube thoracostomy or surgery.[59] All children with empyema should be admitted to the hospital and treated with high-dose intravenous (IV) antibiotics and respiratory support (as required).[59,105] Ideally this should occur in a tertiary pediatric center with care by respiratory physicians in conjunction with pediatric surgeons, or at least with their consultation. The choice of antibiotics will depend on the severity of the clinical presentation, local incidence of microorganisms, and whether or not the child has any specific risk factors such as immunocompromise, aspiration, or hospital-acquired infection. Ideally the choice of antibiotic should be guided by microorganism identification from sputum, blood, or pleural fluid. As discussed earlier, diagnostic pleural aspiration for biochemical or microbiologic examination is not routinely undertaken.

In the absence of an identified causative organism, the choice of antibiotic should be determined by local community-acquired pneumonia guidelines and should include coverage for *S. pneumoniae*, *S. pyogenes*, and *S. aureus*.[59,105] Some communities have a high incidence of MRSA; this should be taken into consideration in choosing the appropriate antibiotic regimen. A macrolide should be added if there is high suspicion or confirmation of *M. pneumonia*.[59] If pneumatoceles are seen on CXR, the antibiotic chosen should specifically include cover for *S. aureus*.[113]

IV antibiotics are given until the child is afebrile; failure to respond to antibiotics should warrant consideration of an alternative regimen. There are few data regarding the duration of IV antibiotics required after defervescence, but the BTS guidelines note that IV therapy is generally given until the patient has been afebrile for at least 24 hours and that it should continue until the chest drain is removed.[59] Ongoing oral antibiotics are recommended for

a minimum of 1 week, with some guidelines advocating up to 6 weeks of oral antibiotics.[59,65,105] The choice of oral antibiotic should be determined on the basis of the organism identified or the class of IV antibiotic that led to clinical improvement.[105]

Other aspects of management of empyema in children include management of hydration with IV fluids as required, analgesia, and antipyretics for comfort. The analgesic regimen should be optimized to encourage early mobility and maximize opportunities for lung reexpansion.[59] The patient will require titration of oxygen therapy and ventilatory support. Supplemental oxygen should be given if saturations fall below 93% in room air.[105] Chest physiotherapy does not play a role in the management of empyema,[59,105] but physiotherapy support—with early mobilization, deep breathing and coughing—is important.

Most cases of empyema will respond to conservative management, defined as antibiotics alone or with chest drain insertion, particularly for patients with small effusions and no respiratory compromise.[59] The rates of response to conservative management are varied; in one case series Gocmen and coworkers reported a 92% success rate in treating empyema with antibiotics and simple tube drainage.[114] However, most centers do not report success rates this high. Even if conservative management is successful, this approach results in a more prolonged stay in hospital compared with treatment by surgery or with fibrinolytics.

In a child with an empyema, the decision on when to intervene actively with pleural fluid drainage is often difficult, as some children, even with large effusions, improve spontaneously without chest drain insertion. Children who are acutely unwell, with severe respiratory distress, who are hypoxic or have moderate to large empyemas should not be managed with antibiotics alone; surgical intervention should be considered early.[59,113] Carter and coworkers performed a retrospective review of 180 otherwise healthy children with empyemas and found that the strongest predictors of a requirement for pleural drainage was admission to an intensive care unit or having a large effusion (comprising more than half of the thorax) or a mediastinal shift.[115] It was possible to treat half of these children with empyemas with antibiotics alone and they had shorter lengths of stay in hospital if they did not have the mentioned risk factors.[115] The specific intervention performed will depend on the level of service and clinical experience of the treating staff. The most commonly performed interventions include insertion of a chest drain (Figs. 69.13 and 69.14) or thoracoscopic VATS. Open thoracotomy has essentially been superseded by VATS but may be required in centers with limited access to thoracoscopic equipment or experienced staff.[105]

There is sufficient evidence to suggest that a smaller chest tube (<14F or pigtail) is sufficient to drain an empyema.[59] Smaller percutaneous drains have the advantage that they can be inserted easily under sedation by the Seldinger technique and are less painful than large-bore drains, allowing earlier mobilization. Furthermore, they can be inserted under ultrasound guidance by experienced staff such as emergency physicians or radiologists. The initial drainage rate should be monitored, as rapid rates of drainage have been known to cause RPE in adults[116]; however, this is rare in children. All chest drains should be connected to an underwater drainage system, which must be kept below

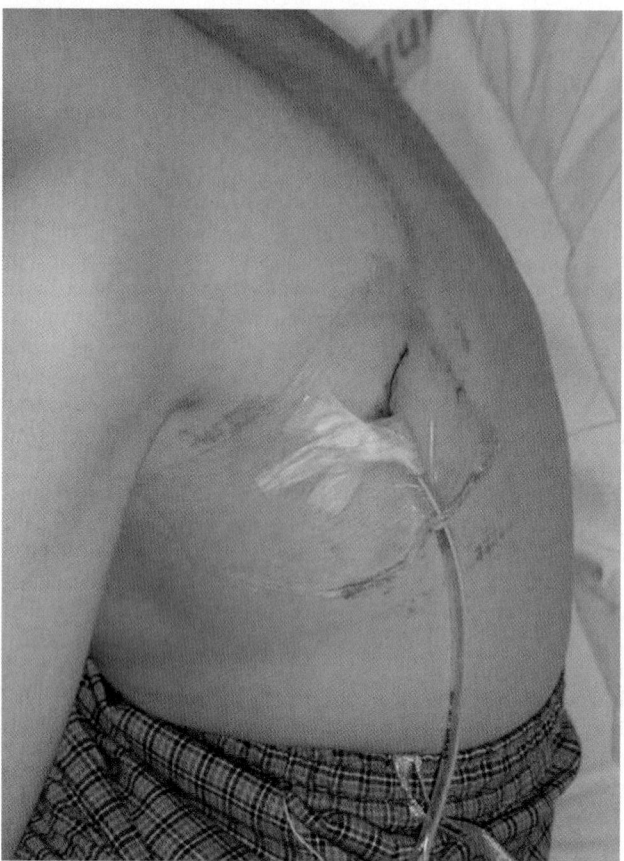

Fig. 69.13 Pediatric patient with chest drain inserted.

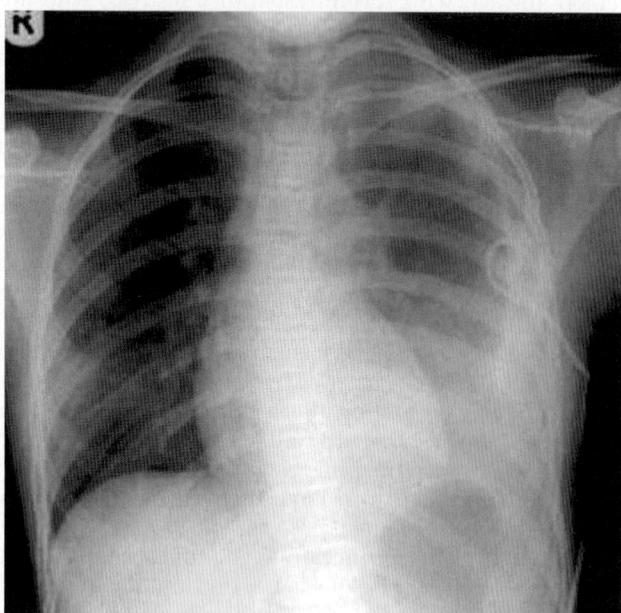

Fig. 69.14 Chest x-ray (CXR) image of empyema with visible chest drain catheter. CXR image of left sided empyema with increased opacification and loss of costophrenic angle. Chest drain catheter in situ.

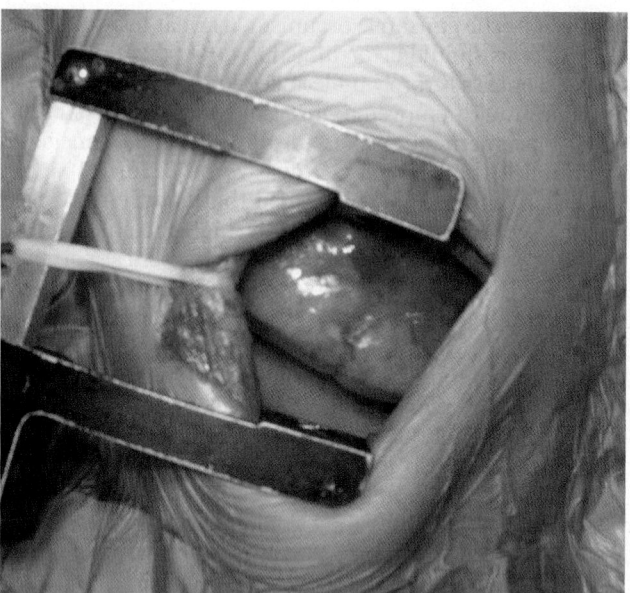

Fig. 69.15 Photograph of open thoracotomy. Note the size of the incision made and the visible underlying lung. (Image reproduced with permission from Professor Gordon Cohen.)

If a chest drain is inserted, intrapleural fibrinolytics are recommended, as they have been shown to shorten the hospital stay compared with standard chest drainage.[59] Fibrinolytics are infused via the chest catheter into the pleural space to allow lysis of pleural septations and fibrinous strands and to clear lymphatic stomata so as to reestablish physiologic drainage from the pleural space.[113] Of the fibrinolytics used in adults with empyema, urokinase, streptokinase, tissue plasminogen activator, and alteplase have all undergone randomized controlled trials in children and were proven to be safe.[117–121] The use of recombinant human DNase with tissue plasminogen activator has proven successful in adults,[122] but there are no data for children. The BTS guidelines recommend urokinase twice daily for 3 days.[59]

Historically, surgical intervention was recommended only once conservative management with antibiotics alone had failed, or in the case of chest tube drainage and fibinolytics with disease progression or if there was ongoing clinical toxicity. This is still the recommended approach in the BTS guidelines as there are no evidence-based criteria for the timing of surgical intervention. There is no difference in clinical outcome between children who are treated with chest catheter drainage and fibrinolytics and VATS,[123,124] but fibrinolytic usage is significantly cheaper.[125,126] A VATS procedure enables the surgeon to drain the purulent material and debride fibrinous septations and loculations under direct vision using a thoracoscopic minimally invasive approach. This approach is preferred to a minithoracotomy approach or open posterolateral thoracotomy (Fig. 69.15) as it involves fewer complications, such as scarring, pain and infection. Early VATs may be the preferred option in some children, if they can be identified, who are at greatest risk for failed fibrinolytic treatment. Livingston and coworkers have reported that children with a positive blood culture, requirement for immediate intensive care admission, and those without complex

the level of the patient's chest.[59] The drain should only be removed if there is clinical resolution and should never be clamped if bubbling, as this is an indication of air leak and clamping of the drain will precipitate the development of a pneumothorax.

septations on ultrasound may be at greater risk of fibrinolytic treatment failure.[127] Inflammatory markers such as CRP and necrosis on initial CXR have little prognostic value.

Monitoring Progress

Routine daily imaging such as chest CXR is not recommended for monitoring the progress of empyema, as it does not alter management.[105] CXR findings lag behind clinical improvement and may point to significant abnormalities that are not manifest clinically. More useful indications of improvement include defervescence, decreased respiratory distress, and decreasing oxygen requirements and respiratory support. Clinical findings may be supported by improving inflammatory markers such as CRP, ESR, or procalcitonin but should not be performed routinely.[59]

Complications of Empyema

Empyema is commonly associated with cavitary pneumonia—up to 20% in some series.[128] Less commonly, empyema may be complicated by the development of a bronchopleural fistula and pneumothorax, lung abscess (particularly with organisms such as *S. aureus*) and rarer still, empyema necessitans when purulent material perforates through the chest wall.[59] If the empyema is diagnosed late, the effusion may have become increasingly organized, so that the underlying lung becomes "trapped," which warrants surgical intervention to clear the loculations and fibrinous peel from the lung pleura and allow complete reexpansion. Fortunately, this development is rare in children.[65]

Follow-Up of Empyema

Unlike the case with adult cohorts, where mortality rates can be as high as 30%,[129] the outlook for children with empyema is usually excellent.[113,130] CXRs will usually be abnormal at the time of discharge and do not alter management, so they should not be routinely performed.[59] A delayed CXR should be performed in all children approximately 6 weeks after the event to ensure that the condition is resolving (Fig. 69.16).[105] Most CXRs will have returned to near normal by 6 months[114,131] and nearly all by 12 months.[130] Complications of empyema can still occur if not treated appropriately; they include the recurrence of empyema, osteomyelitis of the rib, bronchopleural fistulas, and death.[132] However, these are all exceedingly rare in children.

Healthy children managed with appropriate antibiotic courses are unlikely to have a repeat episode or any long-term consequences from empyema. Parents should be reassured that their child will have an excellent long-term outcome. After the follow-up CXR, unless there are concerns about secondary complications, no further imaging is required if the child is asymptomatic.[105] A recent study using chest MRI performed many years after empyema demonstrated persistent pleural abnormalities including pleural scarring, thickening, and subpleural nodules; the clinical significance of these findings is unknown (Fig. 69.17).[133] Spirometry performed after empyema is usually normal; however, some asymptomatic children do demonstrate abnormal lung function on subsequent testing.[134] There are insufficient data on cardiopulmonary exercise testing in children postempyema to determine if there are any effects at high levels of activity, but there does not appear to be a significant difference in exercise tolerance.[135]

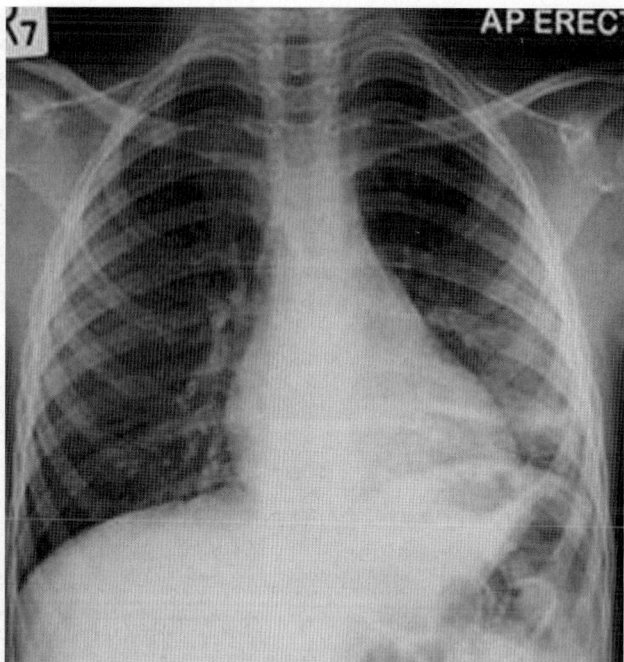

Fig. 69.16 Chest x-ray (CXR) image taken 4 weeks after treatment of a left-sided empyema. This patient underwent insertion of a pigtail chest drain and fibrinolysis with urokinase. The empyema is resolving on CXR but is not completely back to normal after 4 weeks, as expected.

Box 69.2   Physical and Chemical Characteristics of Chyle

Sterile
Ingested lipophilic dyes stain the effusion
Cells are predominantly lymphocytes
Sudan stain shows fat globules
Total fat content exceeds that of plasma
Electrolytes same as in plasma
Blood urea nitrogen same as in plasma
Glucose level same as in plasma

OTHER CAUSES OF EFFUSIONS—CHYLOTHORAX

The Lymphatic System

The function of the lymphatic system is to transport lipids and lipid-soluble vitamins from the gastrointestinal system into the systemic circulation, to circulate lymphocytes and to allow fluid and protein in the interstitial space to be returned to the systemic circulation.[136] Chyle fluid is lymphatic fluid that contains chylomicrons drained from the intestinal lacteal system. Chlyomicrons are formed from long-chain triglycerides, cholesterol, phospholipids, and protein to enable water-insoluble long-chain-fatty-acid triglycerides to be absorbed from the gastrointestinal tract. The chyle fluid also contains lipid-soluble vitamins, electrolytes, protein, glucose, and numerous lymphocytes[137] (see Box 69.2), with smaller amounts of other cell types including erythrocytes. Chylomicrons give chyle fluid a "milky" appearance (Fig. 69.18), but this classical appearance may occur

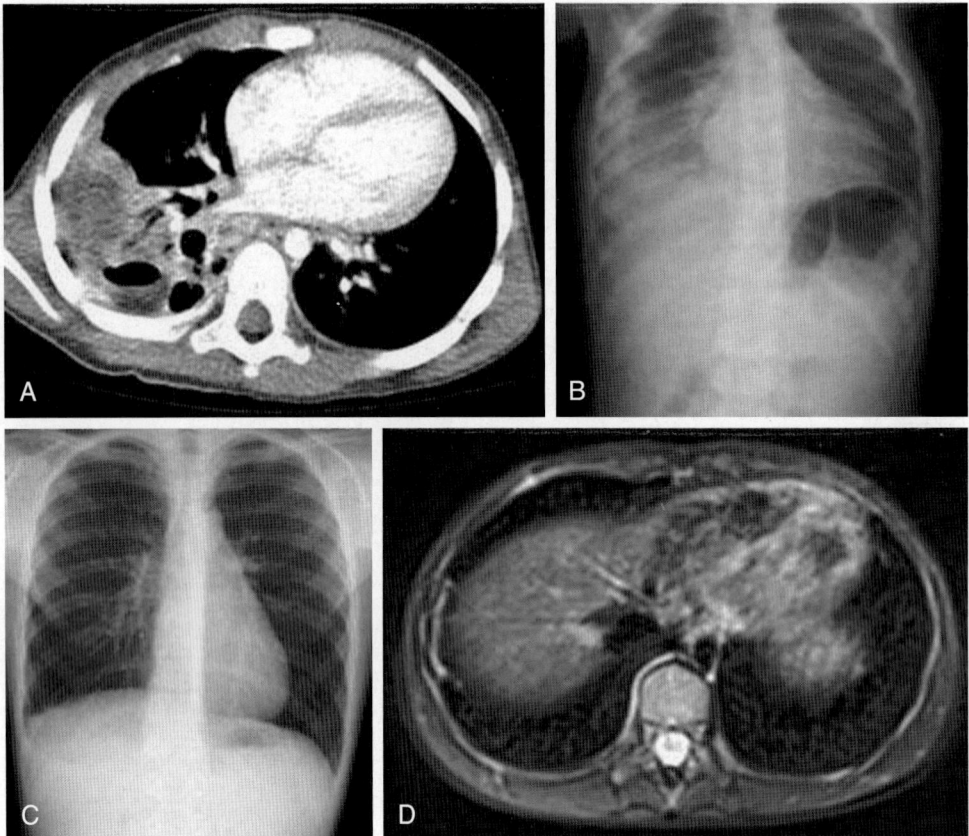

Fig. 69.17 Images demonstrating the radiologic course of empyema in a 2-year-old boy. Pneumonia complicated by *Streptococcus pneumoniae* empyema in a 2-year-old boy treated with antibiotics and surgery. (A) Initial chest computed tomography demonstrating pleural fluid in the right hemithorax. (B) The initial chest x-ray (CXR) shows increased opacification of the right thoracic infiltrate with pleural thickening. (C) 6 ½ years later, CXR demonstrates pleural scarring in the right lateral recess. (D) The follow-up lung magnetic resonance image shows pleural thickening (5 mm × 30 mm × 20 mm) in the right lung, pleural scarring (30 mm × 4 mm × 10 mm) in the right lateral recess, and a subpleural micronodule (<5 mm) in the left-upper-lobe lingula. (Reused with permission from Honkinen M, Lahti E, Svedström E, et al. Long-term recovery after parapneumonic empyema in children. *Pediatr Pulmonol.* 2014;49(10):1020-1027.)

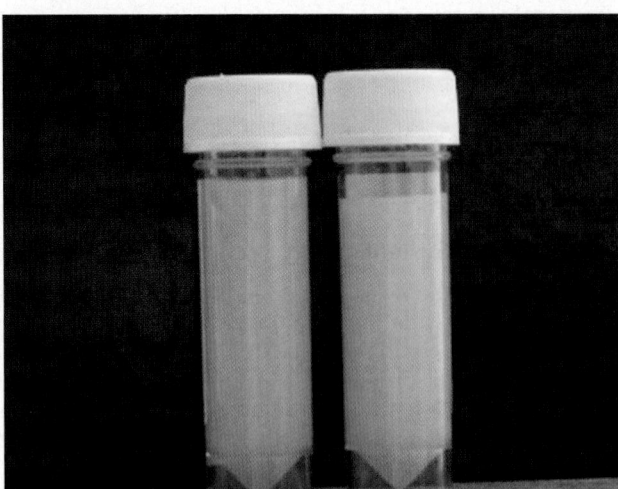

Fig. 69.18 Image of chyle sample. Classic "milky" appearance of chylous fluid. (Used with permission from McGrath EE, Blades Z, Anderson PB. Chylothorax: aetiology, diagnosis and therapeutic options. *Respir Med.* 2010;104(1):1–8.)

in only 50% of cases with chylothorax.[138] The thoracic duct is the main conduit by which the chyle fluid is transported from the gastrointestinal system via the lymphatic drainage system into the systemic circulation. There is significant day-to-day variability in the lipid content (and color) and flow through the thoracic duct, as it changes with food intake.[138] During periods of fasting, the lipid content will be lower, and after meals and water the flow will increase.

As described earlier, the thoracic duct has many normal anatomic variations, but typically it arises from the coalescing lumbar and intestinal lymphatics and proceeds superiorly in the posterior mediastinum up to the level of the cervical vertebrae, eventually terminating between the left jugular and subclavian veins.[136] Numerous collaterals are often present. The right lymphatic duct, which drains the right upper limb, liver surface and the right side of the head, neck, and thorax, does not contain chyle.[137] The thoracic duct drains all the other regions of the body.

Etiology

A chylothorax is defined as an accumulation of lymphatic fluid (chyle) in the pleural space,[136] which accumulates if the thoracic duct is disrupted by a congenital anatomic abnormality, a change in pressures within the duct or trauma (e.g., during cardiothoracic surgery). The level at which the duct is damaged will determine at which side of the thoracic cavity the chylothorax will occur or if bilateral chlyothoraces will form. The chylothorax occurs on the left if the thoracic duct is damaged above the level of the fifth thoracic vertebra and on the right if the damage is lower, between the fifth thoracic vertebra and the diaphragm.[137]

Chylothorax is a rare cause of fluid in the pleural space except during the neonatal period, when it is the most common cause of pleural effusion.[136] The etiology is varied and the incidence in children unknown, but the most common presentations of chylothorax in children are postoperative complications, congenital forms secondary to birth trauma, or in association with genetic syndromes such as Noonan or Down syndrome.[138-140] Congenital abnormalities such as lymphatic malformations, including lymphangiectasia and lymphangiomas, can result in a chylothorax.[140] The incidence varies with age and is more common in neonates than older children because of the association with congenital malformations and birth trauma.[138,141]

There are many causes of chylothorax (Table 69.5).[136] In the antenatal setting, if the chylothorax occupies a significant proportion of the pleural space, it may also result in pulmonary hypoplasia.[137] Chylothorax can occur secondary to direct or indirect trauma to the thoracic duct, and iatrogenic causes include thoracic surgery, particularly cardiac surgery (classically post-Fontan procedures),[142] scoliosis surgery, and repair of congenital diaphragmatic hernia.[143] Chylothorax also results from high central venous pressure, as in the case of superior vena cava obstruction and thrombosis[144] or severe vomiting.[145] Chylothorax can be associated with cancer, most commonly lymphoma in children, as thoracic lymphadenopathy can place significant pressure on the thoracic duct, causing disruption and leakage of contents. There are also several case reports of chylothorax occurring with child abuse, in some cases related to rib fractures.[146-148] Lymphadenopathy from nonmalignancy causes that obstruct the thoracic duct can also present as chylothorax.

Clinical Manifestations of Chylothorax

Chylothorax may have a similar presentation to other causes of pleural effusions in children, but without signs of infection or toxicity unless the chyle is secondarily infected. The presentation is varied and may reflect the size and clinical effects of the chylothorax, or it may be a manifestation of the underlying etiology. Classically children present with dyspnea and cough, but many children are asymptomatic. The degree of respiratory distress is determined by the size and rate of fluid accumulation; in cases of large and rapid accumulation, chylothoraces can lead to significant cardiorespiratory complications.

In traumatic chylothorax, there is often a significant delay between damage to the thoracic duct and clinical symptoms, which may not develop for up to a week.[138] Once the duct is damaged, fluid will leak directly into the posterior mediastinum, with eventual breach of the pleura and a gradual accumulation of fluid in the pleural space.

As in the case of clinical findings with other causes of pleural effusion, examination of the child reveals a dull percussion note on the affected side and reduced breath sounds on auscultation. The patient may be hypoxic, tachypneic, and have increased work of breathing. There may be other signs that indicate the cause or complications of chylothorax; malnutrition and immune dysfunction can cause opportunistic infections owing to the failure to recirculate lipids, chylomicrons, or lymphocytes.[136,138]

Investigations

Investigations will include those that confirm the presence of a chylothorax and those used to determine the underlying etiology (Fig. 69.19). The pleural fluid is identified on a CXR, which demonstrates the size and location of the fluid (Fig. 69.20).[149] An ultrasound helps to delineate the nature of the fluid. Thoracentesis is necessary to determine if the effusion is chylous. The fluid is generally described as "milky" but cannot be differentiated from empyema on sight alone. The physical and chemical characteristics of chyle are listed in Box 69.2. A chylothorax is confirmed on biochemical analysis of pleural fluid which, when stained with Sudan III,[138] will confirm the presence of chylomicrons. In a setting where this analysis is not possible, surrogate measurements may be helpful, such as the triglyceride concentration (diagnostic if >1.1 mmol/L)[150] or finding other products in chyle such as a high T-lymphocyte count or immunoglobulins.[138]

Once a chylothorax is confirmed, a search for the etiology should be undertaken. In some cases this will be obvious from the history, as in a postoperative case or after trauma. In other cases it is important to exclude malignancy, granulomatous conditions, and congenital malformations and to perform a thorough examination to exclude nonaccidental injury.

Identification of the specific site of the chylous leak is important. Lymphangiography, lymphoscintigraphy and CT scans may be helpful but are generally available only at specialist centers.[137,138] Lymphangiography requires a skilled

Table 69.5	Etiology of Chylothorax in Children
Congenital	*Congenital lymphatic malformations:* Lymphangiomatosis, lymphangiectasia, atresia of the thoracic duct
	Associated with various syndromes: Down Syndrome, Noonan Syndrome, Turner Syndrome
	Hydrops fetalis
Traumatic	*Surgical:* Cervical surgery (e.g., lymph node excision), thoracic surgery (e.g., congenital heart disease or lung malformations)
	Subclavian vein catheterisation
	Hyperextension of chest wall or thoracic spine
	Forceful coughing or vomiting
	Childbirth
High central venous pressure	Thrombosis of the superior vena cava or subclavian vein
	Post-Fontan surgery
Malignancies	Lymphoma
	Teratoma
	Sarcoma
	Neuroblastoma
Other	Benign tumors
	Tuberculosis or histoplasmosis
	Sarcoidosis
	Transdiaphragmatic movement of chylous ascites

Modified from Soto-Martinez M, Massie J. Chylothorax: diagnosis and management in children. *Paediatr Respir Rev.* 2009;10(4):199-207.

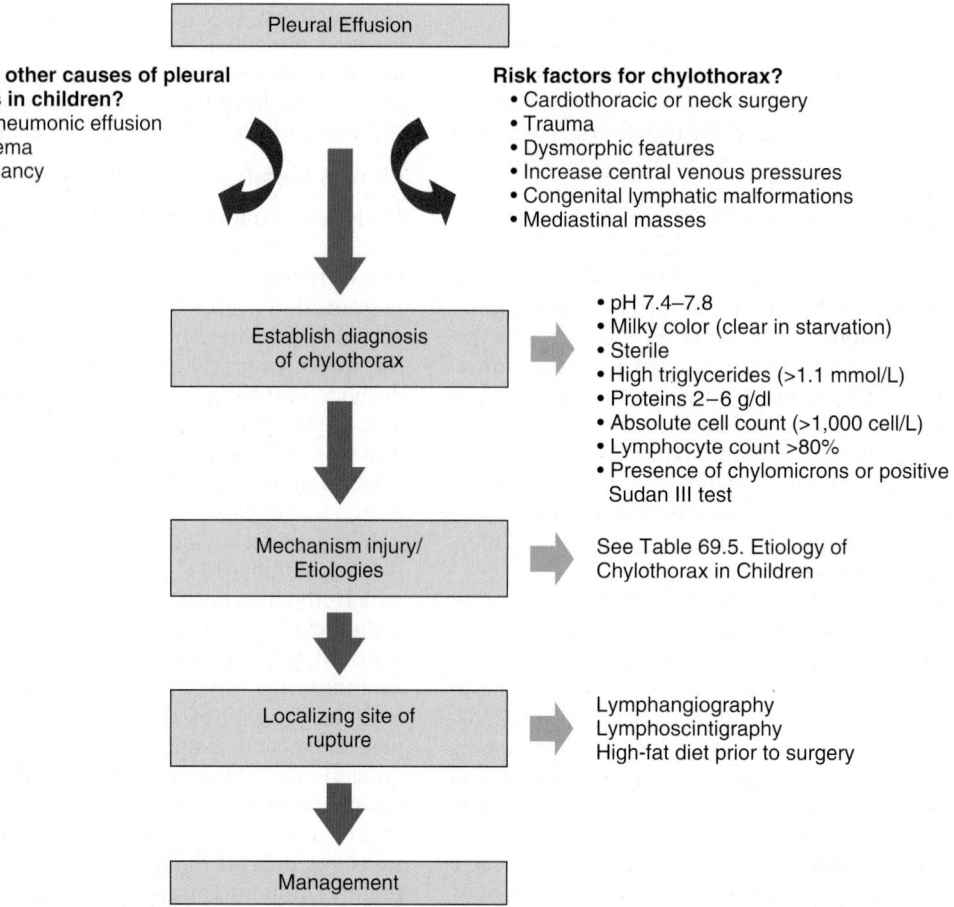

Consider other causes of pleural effusions in children?
- Parapneumonic effusion
- Empyema
- Malignancy

Risk factors for chylothorax?
- Cardiothoracic or neck surgery
- Trauma
- Dysmorphic features
- Increase central venous pressures
- Congenital lymphatic malformations
- Mediastinal masses

Pleural Effusion

Establish diagnosis of chylothorax
- pH 7.4–7.8
- Milky color (clear in starvation)
- Sterile
- High triglycerides (>1.1 mmol/L)
- Proteins 2–6 g/dl
- Absolute cell count (>1,000 cell/L)
- Lymphocyte count >80%
- Presence of chylomicrons or positive Sudan III test

Mechanism injury/ Etiologies
See Table 69.5. Etiology of Chylothorax in Children

Localizing site of rupture
Lymphangiography
Lymphoscintigraphy
High-fat diet prior to surgery

Management

Fig. 69.19 Diagnostic algorithm for chylothorax. (Reproduced with permission from Soto-Martinez M, Massie J. Chylothorax: diagnosis and management in children. *Paediatr Respir Rev.* 2009;10(4):199-207.)

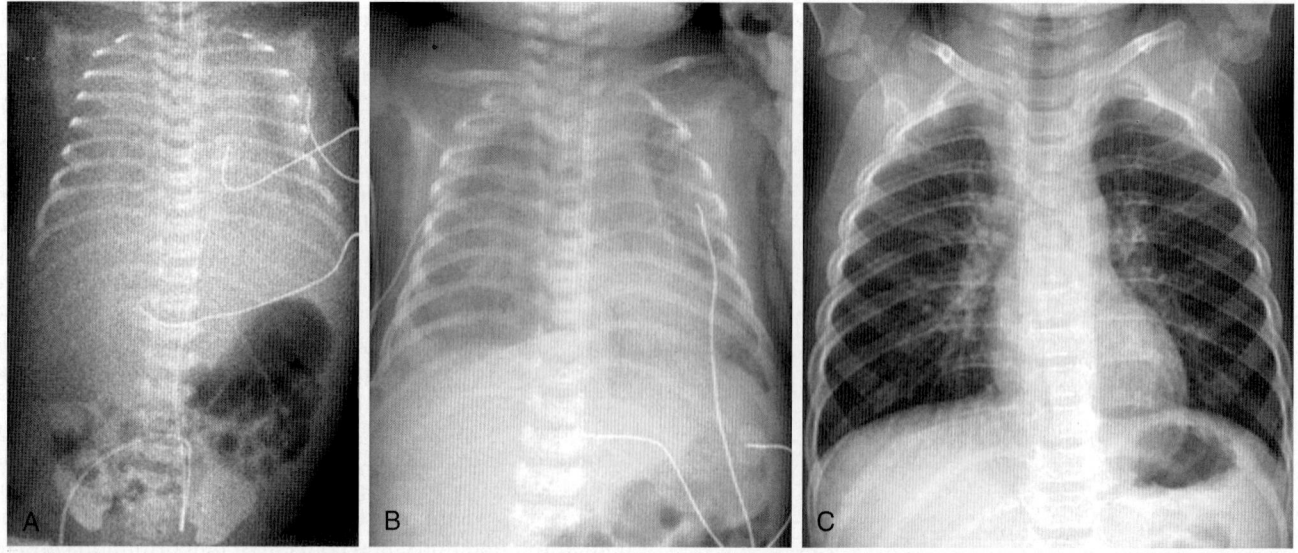

Fig. 69.20 Serial chest x-rays of a neonate with chylothorax. (A) Male newborn with congenital bilateral chylothorax. (B) 12 days later, with improvement in the bilateral pleural effusions. (C) 12 months later, normal thorax. (Reproduced with permission from Lopez-Gutierrez JC, Tovar JA, Chylothorax and chylous ascites: management and pitfalls. Semin Pediatr Surg; 2014; 23(5):298-302.)

clinician to cannulate the lymphatic vessel and inject contrast to perform a radiologic scan (CT or MRI) to outline the course of the vessel, identify any breaches, and demonstrate contrast in the pleural space. Lymphoscintigraphy is the injection of radionuclides into the dermis or subcutaneous tissue; it utilizes nuclear medicine techniques to demonstrate the lymphatic draining system.

In some cases the patient may need to undergo a surgical procedure to identify the source of the chyle leak; this can often be done thoracoscopically and may be part of a definitive intervention.

Management

The management of a chylothorax will include identification and treatment of the cause, appropriate management of any complications, such as malnutrition and immune deficiency, and prevention of ongoing leak. The management approach will be determined by the size and clinical effects of the chylothorax, but it generally includes a period of conservative "medical" management before surgical intervention. The latter is recommended after 4 weeks of failed medical treatment[136,137] or if there is significant nutritional decline or chylothorax progression during conservative medical management. Medical therapeutic options are aimed at decreasing the flow through the thoracic duct and "switching off" the chylous leak to allow the damaged surfaces of the duct to oppose and to enable spontaneous healing. This is done by limiting the consumption of long-chain fatty acids and their conversion to chylomicrons absorbed via the intestinal lymphatics.[136] In order to maintain nutrition in a patient who may already be suffering consequences of malnourishment, the patient is placed on a diet of medium-chain fatty acids.[137] Medium-chain triglycerides are absorbed directly into the portal system and thus bypass the intestinal lymphatics. In cases where dietary management fails, the patient may be trialed on total parenteral nutrition with complete enteric rest.[137] If children are going to respond to enteral or total parenteral nutrition, most will have done so by 3 weeks.[151]

Somatostatin is an endogenous hormone, and octreotide (its synthetic analogue) has been used in the medical management of chylothorax.[152] The mechanism of action remains unclear but is presumed to be the result of vasoconstriction of the splanchnic circulation, causing a decrease in intestinal blood flow, and by decreasing gastrointestinal secretions, thus ultimately diminishing lymph production.[137] As a result, the decreasing lymph flow allows time for the thoracic duct breach to heal. In up to 80% of cases,[153] medical therapy will allow the chylothorax to resolve, but this may take several weeks. The timing and duration of therapy remains uncertain.

If pharmacologic therapy of chylothorax fails, surgical options may be considered. Ideally the site of the chyle leak is identified with preoperative or intraoperative techniques that highlight the lymphatic flow. These options include injection of dye or having the patient drink a mixture of milk and cream a few hours prior to surgery to enable visualization of the site of leakage intraoperatively[136]; the identified breach is then ligated surgically. Unfortunately, the exact site may not always be easily identified, and ligation of the duct and surrounding tributaries may have to be considered. Surgical access may be open or thoracoscopic, and VATS has proven successful.[142] Alternatively, should the thoracic duct not be amenable to ligation, pleurodesis has enabled

resolution of the chylothorax in some cases.[137,142] There are some small neonatal case series of intrapleural injection of povidone-iodine via chest drains for chemical pleurodesis.[154] The procedure appears to be well tolerated, but the risk of hypothyroidism must be considered. A particular clinical challenge in neonates with bilateral chylothoraces requiring pleurodesis is deciding whether to treat only one side in the first instance in the hope that the second side will resolve spontaneously. However, with this approach there is the potential risk that the contralateral effusion may worsen.

Fluoroscopically guided embolization of the thoracic duct has been successful in some patients[155,156] but requires specialized techniques that are not available in all centers. Radiotherapy may be an option for patients with chylothorax secondary to lymphatic malformations such as lymphangiomatosis,[157] where radiation impairs the function of the lymphatic tissue function and inhibits further excess drainage.

As a last resort, if the chylothorax is not corrected with the mentioned interventions or there is significant hemodynamic compromise, a pleuroperitoneal shunt may be considered,[149] which allows recirculation of chyle contents and prevents further respiratory compromise secondary to fluid accumulation in the pleural space.

HEMOTHORAX IN CHILDREN

Hemothorax in children is a rare occurrence but is a relatively common complication of serious thoracic trauma and is associated with a high mortality rate.[158,159] Children have more compliant thoracic cages than adults because of ligamentous laxity and developing bones; as a result, significant intrathoracic trauma can occur with minimal external signs of injury[160]. Therefore hemothorax should be considered in all cases of blunt and penetrating chest trauma in children. Hemothoraces can also be iatrogenic, occurring after chest drain insertion,[161] intrathoracic surgery, or with inappropriate placement of central lines.[162] Hemothoraces can cause significant cardiorespiratory effects, including cardiac arrest, and can be complicated by secondary infection and fibrosis, causing "trapped lung," although these complications appear to be less frequent than the rates seen in adult patients with hemothorax.[160] Hemothorax can be diagnosed on CXR or in the setting of trauma. A focused assessment with sonography for trauma (FAST) ultrasound scan may be considered and may be more sensitive than CXR.[163] Treatment will depend on the nature of the injury (either penetrating or blunt force), size of the hemothorax, and clinical status of the patient. Some pediatric patients with hemothorax can be managed conservatively with close observation. Others, particularly those with penetrating chest injuries or large hemothoraces, will require tube thoracostomies or open thoracic surgery to stop the bleeding.[160] The hemothorax may develop from blood draining into the pleural space from the lung, airway, esophagus, heart, or chest wall[159] and may occur in conjunction with a pneumothorax.

Conclusion

Pleural diseases in children are not common, but they cause significant morbidity and may require prolonged hospital admissions, often with significant interventions. Evidence to guide therapy is still lacking in some areas and will require significant collaboration between pediatric centers to provide the best evidence-based clinical guidelines.

References

Access the reference list online at ExpertConsult.com.

Suggested Reading

Balfour-Lynn IM, Abrahamson E, Cohen G, et al. BTS guidelines for the management of pleural infection in children. *Thorax.* 2005;60(suppl 1):i1–i21.

Islam S, Calkins CM, Goldin AB, et al. The diagnosis and management of empyema in children: a comprehensive review from the APSA Outcomes and Clinical Trials Committee. *J Pediatr Surg.* 2012;47(11):2101–2110.

Miserocchi G. Physiology and pathophysiology of pleural fluid turnover. *Eur Respir J.* 1997;10(1):219–225.

Robinson PD, Cooper P, Ranganathan SC. Evidence-based management of paediatric primary spontaneous pneumothorax. *Paediatr Respir Rev.* 2009;10(3):110–117.

Soto-Martinez M, Massie J. Chylothorax: diagnosis and management in children. *Paediatr Respir Rev.* 2009;10(4):199–207.

Strachan RE, Jaffe A, Thoracic Society of A, New Z. Recommendations for managing paediatric empyema thoracis. *Med J Aust.* 2011;195(2):95.

Strachan RE, Snelling TL, Jaffé A. Increased paediatric hospitalizations for empyema in Australia after introduction of the 7-valent pneumococcal conjugate vaccine. *Bull World Health Organ.* 2013;91(3):167–173.

Tutor JD. Chylothorax in infants and children. *Pediatrics.* 2014;133(4): 722–733.

70 *Atelectasis*

KAI HÅKON CARLSEN, MD, PhD, SUZANNE CROWLEY, DM, and BJARNE SMEVIK, MD

The word *atelectasis* stems from two Greek words: *ateles*, meaning "imperfect," and *ektasiz*, meaning "expansion." Atelectasis thus means imperfect expansion, and the word is used to describe incomplete expansion of a lung or lung tissue. After inventing the stethoscope in 1816, René Laennec was the first to describe atelectasis as a finding during an autopsy in 1819.[1] There are many causes of atelectasis, which is a common complication of both acute and chronic lung disease affecting patients of all ages. It may be congenital or acquired. Congenital atelectasis is usually due to incomplete expansion of the lungs, including primary and secondary congenital atelectasis. The most common cause of atelectasis is loss of air in lung tissue that was previously expanded, thus resulting in the collapse of a lung or lung tissue.

Etiology and Pathogenesis

Several mechanisms associated with a variety of pulmonary and extrapulmonary diseases may cause atelectasis. Pulmonary causes include obstruction of the bronchial lumen (the most common cause) and increased surface tension of the fluid lining the respiratory tract and alveoli. Extrapulmonary causes include compression of airways and lung tissue from outside the lung and weakness of respiratory muscles in neuromuscular disease. Obstruction of the bronchial lumen by mucus may have several causes, such as airway inflammation and impaired clearance of airway mucus caused by increased mucous viscosity (cystic fibrosis), reduced ciliary function, or a weak cough reflex secondary to neuromuscular disease. Box 70.1 shows the causes of atelectasis.

Pathogenic Mechanisms

Congenital pulmonary airway malformations may prevent the normal aeration of parts of the lungs at birth due to lack of communication of the main bronchial tree with the affected parts of the lungs that have never been inflated, thus causing primary atelectasis. However, a secondary atelectasis may develop shortly after birth if a congenital malformation occludes or narrows the bronchial lumen, thus presenting as a differential diagnosis to primary atelectasis.[2]

Secondary atelectasis is most often caused by collapse of normal lung tissue due to obstruction or alternatively due to compression of the bronchial lumen. The pores of Kohn form at 3–4 years of age[3] and function as collateral communications between neighboring alveoli; they ensure a more even ventilation/perfusion ratio in the lung, thereby playing a role in preventing atelectasis. At more proximal levels no such collateral communications exist, and occlusion of the bronchial lumen initially leads to air trapping in lung tissue peripheral to the occluded bronchus. The trapped air is gradually absorbed, leading to atelectasis. Causes of obstruction

or compression of the bronchial lumen are shown in Box 70.1.

The solubility of the trapped gases determines their absorption rate. The absorption of atmospheric air will take place within hours, whereas oxygen is absorbed within minutes.[4] Atelectasis therefore occurs more rapidly during ventilation with an increased inspired oxygen fraction and especially with 100% oxygen, compared with breathing normal air. This may partly explain the increased risk of atelectasis during anesthesia.[4] The ventilation/perfusion ratio of the atelectatic tissue is regulated through the increased vascular resistance resulting from hypoxic vasoconstriction of the pulmonary vessels secondary to occlusion of the bronchial lumen.[5]

Atelectasis may be caused by any process or procedure that occludes the bronchial lumen. Foreign bodies in the lower respiratory tract may lead to partial or complete occlusion of a bronchus, and complete occlusion will cause atelectasis. With an initial incomplete occlusion, the foreign body may cause inflammation of the mucous membranes, with resulting mucosal swelling and increased respiratory secretions causing complete obstruction of the bronchial lumen and the development of atelectasis.

Misplaced endotracheal intubation may cause total collapse of one lung when the distal part of the tracheal tube is located in a main bronchus (most often the right one).

Inflammatory processes within the bronchial tree are among the most common causes of obstruction of the bronchial lumen, including bronchial asthma (often eosinophilic inflammation)[6] and acute bronchiolitis due to respiratory syncytial virus infections.[7] In asthma and bronchiolitis, the right middle lobe and the lingula are the most common locations of atelectasis, so common that this is given the name of middle-lobe syndrome.[6,8] The finding of positive bacterial cultures from the respiratory tract in children with asthma and bronchiolitis with atelectasis and middle-lobe syndrome has led to a suggested role for bacterial infection in long-standing atelectasis of asthma and bronchiolitis.[7,9]

Airway inflammation due to asthma, bronchiolitis, and other respiratory infections may cause increased bronchial secretions, mucosal edema, bronchial smooth muscle contraction, and destruction of bronchial epithelium with reduced ciliary function, leading to the retention of mucus within the bronchial lumen. Destruction of the bronchial epithelium may alter the airway surface liquid, with an effect on surfactant function; it may thus enhance the tendency for bronchial collapse. In both bronchopulmonary dysplasia and respiratory distress syndrome of prematurity, abnormal surfactant function may contribute to the formation and persistence of atelectasis.[10] Aspiration of meconium, acids, alkali and amniotic fluid also has this effect.

Many diseases increase the susceptibility of the respiratory tract to infection and lead to the accumulation of mucus, which predisposes to the development of atelectasis. These

Box 70.1 Causes of Atelectasis

Intraluminal Causes

Airways inflammation with increased bronchial mucus and
  formation of mucus plug due to
  Bronchial asthma
  Respiratory tract infection
    Bronchiolitis, Pneumonia
  Bronchopulmonary dysplasia
  Cystic fibrosis (increased viscosity of the mucus)
  Primary and secondary ciliary dyskinesia (impaired mucociliary
    clearance)
  Immunodeficiency
  Tracheoesophageal fistula or esophageal atresia
Foreign body in the lower respiratory tract
  Nuts, plastics, other foreign bodies, misplaced tracheal tube

Compression of the Airways

Lobar emphysema
Lymph node enlargement
Vascular ring
Complex congenital heart disease (e.g., enlargement of left
  atrium compressing left main bronchus)

Bronchial Wall Involvement

Airway stenosis
  After aspiration or inhalation injury
  After intubation
  Complete cartilaginous rings
Bronchiectasis
Tracheobronchomalacia
Bronchial tumor

Compression of Lung Tissue

Pneumothorax
Congestive heart failure with cardiac enlargement
Hemothorax
Chylothorax
Lung tumor

Surfactant Dysfunction

Respiratory distress syndrome of the newborn
Adult respiratory distress syndrome
Other

Primary Atelectasis

Congenital malformation

---

include immunodeficiency, primary ciliary dyskinesia (PCD),[11] and cystic fibrosis.[12]

Bronchial wall processes that narrow the bronchial lumen, including tracheobronchomalacia, vascular rings,[13] tumors such as polyps, papillomas, and (rarely) bronchocentric carcinoma,[14] may cause atelectasis in children. Bronchiectasis, usually caused by recurrent or long-standing airway inflammation, is often complicated by atelectasis.[12]

Extrapulmonary processes may compress normal lung tissue and cause atelectasis without affecting the bronchi, as seen in some patients with congenital heart defects and also with pneumothorax or hemothorax. Rounded atelectasis, seen more often in adults than children, is mostly asymptomatic and associated with chronic pleural disease, lung fibrosis, or pleural effusions. It consists of infolding of

atelectatic lung tissue with blood vessels, pleura, and sometimes bronchi.[15]

Atelectasis is common in neuromuscular diseases. Muscular hypotonia impairs ventilation because of reduced movement of respiratory muscles and causes difficulty in clearing bronchial secretions, thus increasing the individual's susceptibility to respiratory infections and atelectasis.[16] Hypoventilation may also contribute to the development of atelectasis that is seen in children during anesthesia.[4]

Clinical Manifestations

The symptoms and signs of atelectasis will depend on whether single or multiple lobes are involved, the underlying cause, and the age of the patient. In full-term newborn infants with respiratory distress, the presence of atelectasis when accompanied by situs inversus and the need for prolonged supplemental oxygen is highly predictive of a PCD diagnosis (see Chapter 71).[11] In this instance, atelectasis caused by mucous plugging secondary to poor mucociliary clearance is most prevalent in the upper (75%) and middle (25%) lobes. Infants with bronchiolitis who develop lobar atelectasis are more likely to have severe disease and require admission to the intensive care unit,[17] while exhaustion and sudden severe deterioration may indicate the development of massive atelectasis affecting a whole lung. Preterm infants with bronchiolitis are at higher risk of developing atelectasis,[17] and younger children in general are more at risk of developing atelectasis than older children and adults owing to less well developed collateral ventilation effected by the pores of Kohn and the canals of Lambert.[3] In children with asthma, acute deterioration of symptom control may be due to the development of atelectasis affecting the right middle lobe, so-called right-middle-lobe syndrome (Fig. 70.1). Similarly, an exacerbation of symptoms in children with cystic fibrosis or PCD may be due to the development of atelectasis secondary to bacterial infection in the lower airways, causing increased production of mucus and cellular debris with subsequent mucus plugging.[12]

An episode of sudden paroxysmal coughing with or without subsequent respiratory distress in a previously healthy young child accompanied by x-ray features of atelectasis may indicate the need for bronchoscopy to exclude an inhaled foreign body. Atelectasis may not cause detectable abnormalities on clinical examination; thus the diagnosis must be made radiologically. But generally clinical signs relate to the size of the atelectasis. There may be impaired oxygen saturation, decreased expansion of the chest on the affected side, dullness to percussion, and diminished or absent breath sounds. If the atelectasis is partial or airway obstruction is not complete, crackles may be heard during inspiration and expiration. In some cases of significant or even whole-lung atelectasis, oxygen saturation may be normal, since alveolar hypoxia can induce reflex vasoconstriction and thus minimize ventilation/perfusion mismatch. Paradoxically, intubation and mechanical ventilation of such patients with supplemental oxygen may cause a temporary deterioration in oxygen saturation due the abolition of the protective vasoconstrictive reflex, thus inducing intrapulmonary shunting and the perfusion of unventilated, atelectatic lung tissue that does not take part in gas exchange.[4] Lung function in patients with atelectasis

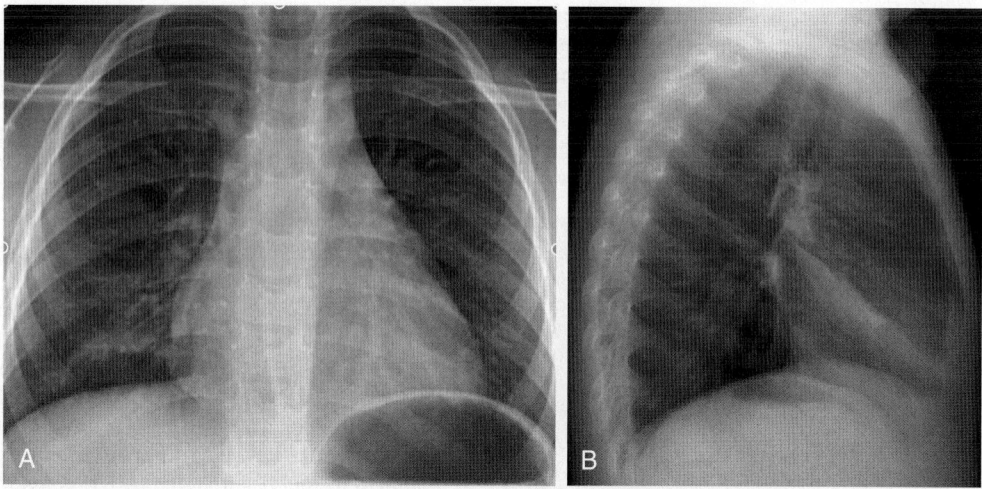

Fig. 70.1 Three-year-old girl with repeated episodes of atelectasis of the middle lobe. Chest radiograph. (A) Frontal projection shows slight blurring of right heart contour. (B) Lateral projection shows triangular opacity with apex toward the hilum.

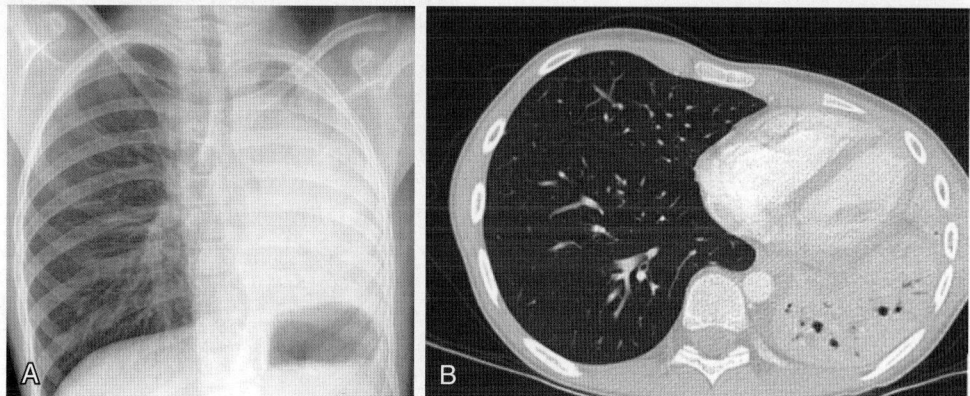

Fig. 70.2 Eleven-year-old girl with asthma and idiopathic eosinophilic pneumonitis and subtotal atelectasis of the left lung. She had coughed up a bronchial cast. (A) Chest radiograph shows opacification and volume reduction of left hemithorax and shift of trachea/mediastinum toward the affected side, as well as elevation of the contour of the left diaphragm. It also shows reduced left intercostal spaces. (B) Computed tomography shows volume reduction and reduced intercostal spaces on the left side; the heart is shifted to the left, and there is atelectasis of the left lung and some hyperinflation of the right lung (Video 70.1).

may be normal if the atelectasis is small or demonstrate a restrictive pattern with a reduced FEV_1 and FVC, and a normal FEV_1/FVC.

Diagnosis

The prompt diagnosis of atelectasis in children is important, since early detection and subsequent treatment may lead to an improved outcome.[18] Diagnosis is aided by an understanding of situations in which atelectasis is more likely to occur and the underlying pathophysiologic mechanisms. For example, postoperative atelectasis is not uncommon, particularly in children undergoing cardiac surgery.[19] However, since atelectasis is not always detectable clinically, it may be discovered unexpectedly, for example, during routine chest x-ray in a child with a chronic underlying condition such as asthma or PCD. Flexible bronchoscopy has a role in the diagnosis of atelectasis when there is suspected airway obstruction due to, for example, foreign-body inhalation, mucous plugging, endobronchial tuberculosis, airway malacia, external

compression from a vascular ring, enlarged lymph nodes, or an enlarged heart. It may also be therapeutic in cases of intraluminal obstruction.

The most frequently used modality for the diagnosis of atelectasis is *chest radiography*. Frontal projection is always included, but sometimes lateral views are better suited, as in atelectasis of the right middle lobe and the lower lobes. Oblique views may be of particular value in segmental atelectasis. Sometimes *fluoroscopy* is also used to delineate difficult locations of increased opacification. Fluoroscopy may also be used to diagnose air trapping and mediastinal shift when a foreign body is suspected. In older children, however, an x-ray at end-inspiration followed by another at end-expiration will suffice. Because atelectasis results in volume reduction of the affected part of the lung, this may lead to general signs such as elevation of the diaphragm and narrowing of ipsilateral intercostal spaces (Fig. 70.2). Shift of the mediastinum and tracheal contours toward the affected side is quite common, but these general signs may be absent if emphysema develops in the ipsilateral lung or if the atelectasis occurs together with ipsilateral pleural effusion.

Atelectasis of the right upper lobe is seen as a combination of increased opacity and volume reduction leading to elevation of the interlobar fissure (Fig. 70.3). A summary of major findings on chest radiography related to extent and location of the atelectasis is presented in Table 70.1.

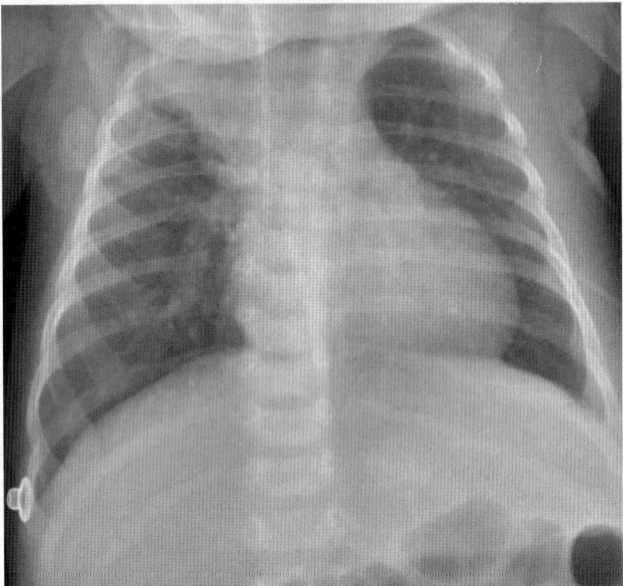

Fig. 70.3 Two-month-old girl with cystic fibrosis. Chest radiograph shows atelectasis of the right upper lobe and elevation of the interlobar fissure.

Table 70.1 Chest Radiographic Signs of Atelectasis Related to Location

Location	Chest Radiographic Signs
Complete atelectasis of lung	Opacification of one hemithorax
	Shift of mediastinum and heart to ipsilateral side
	Narrowed intercostal spaces
	On lateral view: blurring of cardiac silhouette, one diaphragmatic contour and one hilum
Right upper lobe	Opacification of volume-reduced upper lobe and elevation of interlobar fissure
Right middle lobe	Indistinct right cardiac contour
	On lateral view: triangular density with apex toward hilum
Right lower lobe	Visible major fissure shifts downward as lower lobe retracts
	On lateral view: posterior third of right diaphragm indistinct
Left upper lobe	Opacity in upper left hilar region
	Shift of mediastinal structures to the left; elevation of left diaphragm
Left lower lobe	Opacity in retrocardiac space
	Indistinct vessels in the left lower lobe, visible air bronchogram in lower lobe
	Left hilum displaced caudally
	Indistinct medial diaphragmatic contour
Segmental atelectasis	Affects parts of a lobe; oblique projections may be helpful
Focal atelectasis	Density usually located in the basal lung fields as a thin line
Rounded atelectasis	Rounded density adjacent to the pleural surface
Alveolar atelectasis	Decreased aeration, generally bilateral

Computed tomography (CT) and multislice CT with reconstruction may reveal atelectasis not visible on chest x-ray, but the use of general anesthesia, often required in very young children, may induce atelectasis in up to 70% of cases (Fig. 70.4).[20] CT is of particular value with lesions located close to the chest wall or at the periphery of the lung and close to the spine. The use of a controlled ventilation protocol reduces the frequency of atelectasis in these children.[21] Segmental atelectasis affecting a part of a lobe may be more clearly seen with CT (Fig. 70.5).

CT may also offer a better understanding of the whole lesion when atelectasis occurs in combination with bronchiectasis (Fig. 70.6). Rounded atelectasis is also best depicted with CT: a rounded mass at the periphery of the lung adjacent to a pleural thickening and with blurred contours toward the hilum where vessels and bronchi enter the lesion.

Magnetic resonance imaging (MRI) is also very well suited for the diagnosis and follow-up of atelectasis.[22] Because the

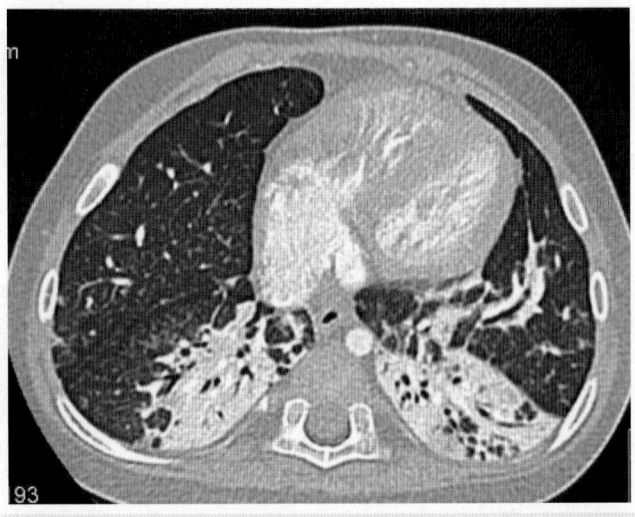

Fig. 70.4 Two-year-old boy born prematurely. He has bronchopulmonary dysplasia and pulmonary hypertension. Computed tomography after sedation shows extensive dependent atelectases in both lungs (Video 70.2).

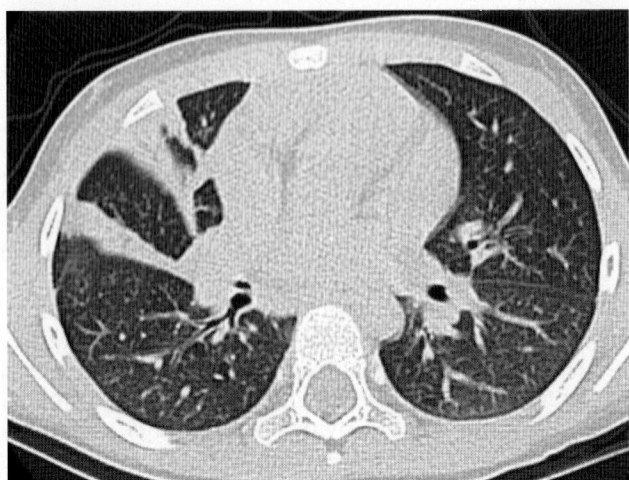

Fig. 70.5 Four-year-old girl with subsegmental atelectasis in the right lung. Bronchoscopy for suspicion of foreign body was negative.

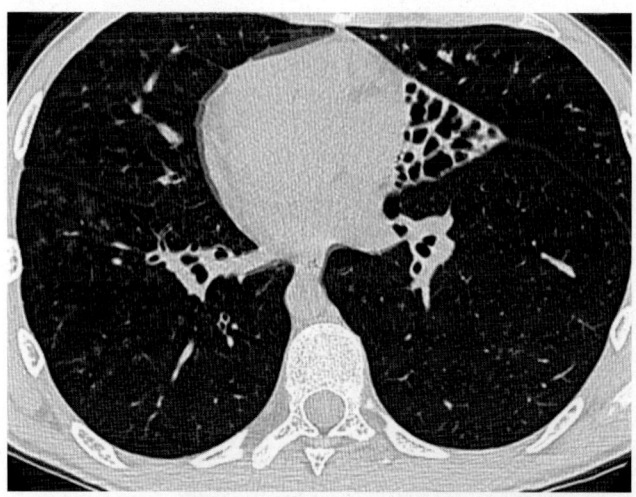

Fig. 70.6 Sixteen-year-old boy with Kartagener syndrome. Bronchiectasis is most pronounced in the atelectatic left-sided middle lobe (Video 70.3).

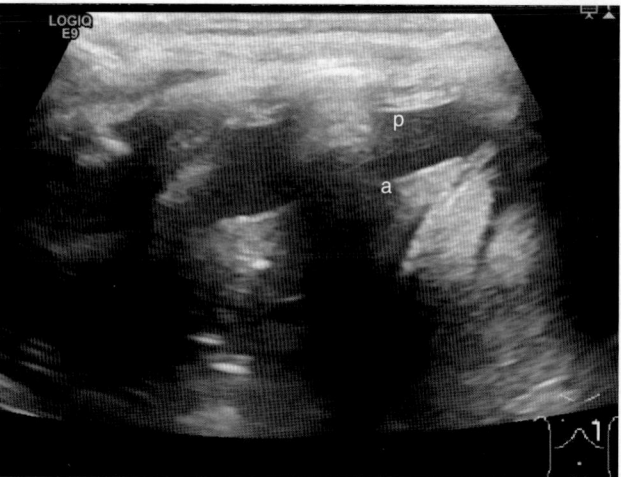

Fig. 70.8 Two-year-old girl treated with extracorporeal membranous oxygenation because of pneumonia. Ultrasound shows atelectasis of the left lung (a), which is clearly seen next to pleural effusion (p) (Video 70.5).

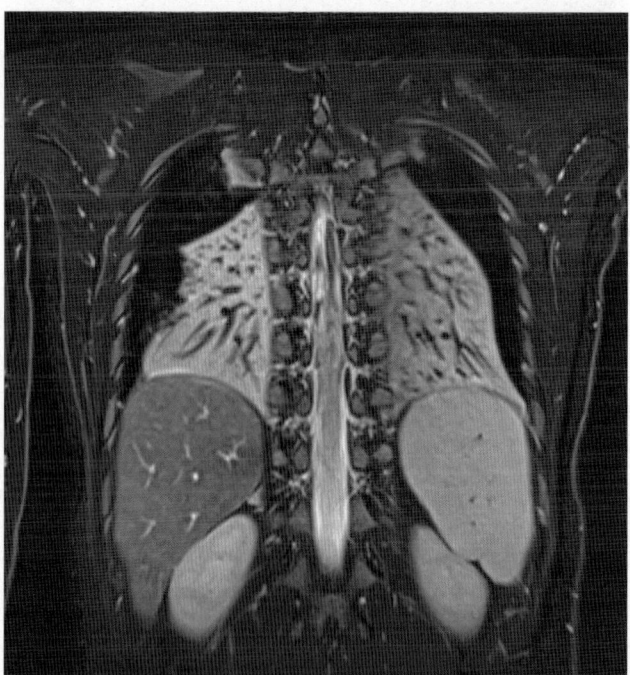

Fig. 70.7 Ten-year-old girl who underwent heart transplantation at 9 years of age. Magnetic resonance imaging shows extensive atelectasis of both lower lobes (Video 70.4).

Bronchography is rarely used but may be combined with diagnostic and therapeutic bronchoscopy in selected cases to show short segments of localized stenosis or bronchomalacia. Difficult postoperative situations with repeated episodes of atelectasis may be better understood when bronchography is combined with monitoring of ventilation pressure (Fig. 70.9).

Treatment and Management

The cause of the atelectasis and the presence of any preexisting condition will determine the type of treatment and the need for future prophylactic measures. Schindler in 2005 asked "Treatment of atelectasis: Where is the evidence?"[23] Today it remains elusive. Chest physiotherapy is often used as a first-line approach, but proof of its efficacy is not firmly established. In a prospective controlled study of 46 mechanically ventilated preschool children with atelectasis, children who were randomized to intrapulmonary percussive ventilation comprising ventilation at 180–220 cycles per minute at pressures of 15–30 cm H_2O for 10–15 minutes 4 times daily following instillation of 0.9% saline had clinically important and significant improvement in their atelectasis scores, while children receiving conventional physiotherapy in the form of clapping and vibration showed no improvement.[24] Transient atelectasis, often affecting the right upper lobe, is frequently observed in children hospitalized for acute bronchiolitis and is associated with more severe illness.[17] In the only prospective but uncontrolled study of prognostic factors relating to right-middle-lobe atelectasis in children with acute asthma admitted to hospital, atelectasis resolved in 13 of 27 children after 6 days, at which point chest physiotherapy was initiated. Children who were using controller medications at the time of admission had a higher rate of resolution of atelectasis at 14 days,[6] suggesting a therapeutic advantage of antiinflammatory treatment with inhaled or oral steroids.

Bacterial colonization and infection is common in children with atelectasis[7] and long-standing right middle-lobe

modality produces pictures of excellent quality in any plane, it is a very good alternative to CT in children who are able to cooperate during the study (Fig. 70.7). For MRI studies, smaller children will often need general anesthesia, and fast multislice CT with an unsedated child may be a better option.

When the atelectasis is located near the thoracic cage, and especially when it is combined with pleural effusion (as is often the case after cardiac surgery or pleural empyema), *ultrasonography* is a quick and reliable bedside method.[21] The collapsed lung is easily differentiated from surrounding pleural effusion (Fig. 70.8). Ultrasonography and MRI can both be used without considering the burden of ionizing radiation.

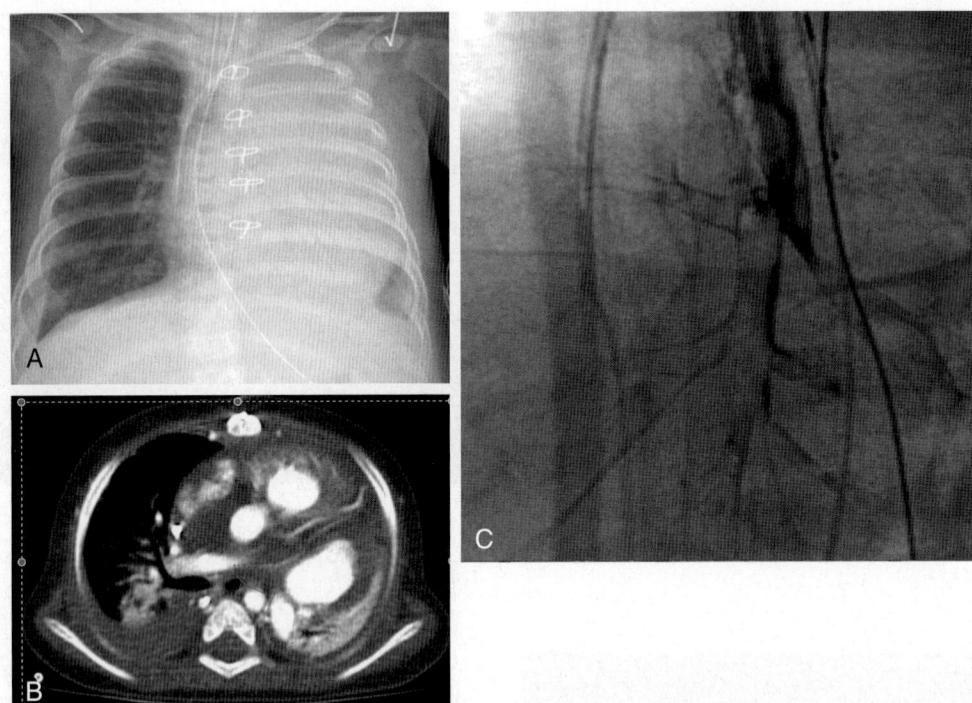

Fig. 70.9 Seven-month-old boy with complex congenital heart disease. Repeated episodes of atelectasis of the left lung occurred after corrective surgery. (A) Chest radiograph shows atelectasis of the left lung and air bronchogram. (B) Computed tomography shows a compressed left main bronchus 12 mm in length between the enlarged heart and the left pulmonary artery anteriorly and the descending aorta posteriorly. (C) Bronchography performed with monitoring of ventilation pressure shows constant collapse of the left main bronchus at pressures less than 5 cm H_2O, partly opening between 5 and 10 cm H_2O, and no collapse above 10 cm H_2O (Video 70.6).

syndrome[9]; thus, in tandem with chest physiotherapy and optimization of asthma control, treatment with broad-spectrum antibiotics should be started. Administration of dornase alfa (Pulmozyme), either via nebulizer or direct instillation in intubated patients, may lead to a rapid improvement in atelectasis in children severely ill with respiratory syncytial virus bronchiolitis[25] and after cardiac surgery.[19] There are anecdotal reports of the successful use of dornase alfa in children with plastic bronchitis causing massive atelectasis,[26] but inhaled tissue plasminogen activator, particularly in children following cardiac palliation with a Fontan operation, may represent a better therapeutic option.[27] Fiberoptic bronchoscopy has a clear role in both the diagnosis and treatment of right-middle-lobe syndrome and may prevent the subsequent development of bronchiectasis.[18] The timing of bronchoscopy will depend on the likely cause and preexisting disease. In children with atelectasis due to suspected inhalation of a foreign body, flexible bronchoscopy to confirm the diagnosis is performed urgently in the case of severe respiratory compromise or electively within the next 24 hours in the majority of cases.[28] Rigid bronchoscopy should be available to retrieve the foreign body if necessary. The absence of an air bronchogram on chest x-ray in lobar atelectasis is suggestive of proximal airway occlusion and, in this case, bronchoalveolar saline lavage or the direct instillation of dornase alfa may be useful. Bronchoscopic insufflation can also be useful in acute total lung atelectasis.[29]

In some patients with atelectasis, operative intervention may be indicated. Diaphragmatic eventration and paralysis can cause lobar collapse that responds to plication of the diaphragm.[30] Lobectomy has been advocated in symptomatic

children with persistent right-middle-lobe[31] and left-lower-lobe[32] syndrome that has not responded to intensive medical therapy, but this is controversial and rarely indicated. In children with tracheobronchial obstruction secondary to adjacent vascular structures or an enlarged heart, tumor, lymphadenopathy or severe airway malacia, silicone or wire mesh stents have been used to relieve airway obstruction. However, these approaches have been complicated by stent migration, infection, granulation tissue formation, stent fracture, and catastrophic pulmonary hemorrhage, giving rise to considerable concern over their safety and effectiveness.[33,34] That said, stent placement may be appropriate in carefully selected patients,[35] and new biodegradable stents currently undergoing assessment may offer a safer alternative.[36]

Pulmonary tuberculous lymphadenopathy in children occurs most frequently in the subcarinal lymph nodes. In one large series, this caused airway compression in all patients, with more severe compression in infants.[37] The use of systemic steroid therapy for this indication is controversial,[38] with at least one-third of children requiring surgical decompression of their airway obstruction after 1 month of antituberculous and steroid treatment.[39]

Prevention of Atelectasis

Based on a systematic review, the use of routine prophylactic airway clearance techniques including incentive spirometry was not recommended in hospitalized noncystic fibrosis patients except for those with neuromuscular illness and weak cough.[40] When cough is weak, cough assist devices may be useful. Children undergoing lung resection may benefit from early postoperative physiotherapy, including intermittent positive end expiratory pressure by mask.[41] Although this study was retrospective, the use of physiotherapy was associated with a significantly lower rate of postoperative atelectasis and bronchoscopic intervention. Ventilation strategies in severely ill children requiring assisted ventilation may play a role in the prevention of atelectasis. In a large study of 691 intubated children with inhalation injury, ventilation with a high tidal volume (15 mL/kg) significantly decreased ventilator days and prevented the development of atelectasis and acute respiratory distress syndrome compared with low tidal volume (9 mL/kg).[42] There was a slightly higher rate of pneumothorax in the high-tidal-volume group, but the authors concluded that the use of a high-volume strategy may interrupt sequences, leading to lung injury in this group of patients. In view of the morbidity associated with atelectasis, there is a clear need for prospective randomized controlled studies of the effectiveness of physiotherapy techniques, including the use of mucolytic agents and ventilation strategies in preventing the development of atelectasis in children hospitalized with bronchiolitis, inhalational injury, pulmonary infection, and postcardiac and pulmonary surgery.

References

Access the reference list online at ExpertConsult.com.

Suggested Reading

Hedenstierna G, Edmark L. Effects of anesthesia on the respiratory system. *Best Pract Res Clin Anaesthesiol.* 2015;29(3):273–284.

Mullowney T, Manson D, Kim R, et al. Primary ciliary dyskinesia and neonatal respiratory distress. *Pediatrics.* 2014;134(6):1160–1166.

Priftis KN, Mermiri D, Papadopoulou A, et al. The role of timely intervention in middle lobe syndrome in children. *Chest.* 2005;128(4):2504–2510.

Ring-Mrozik E, Hecker WC, Nerlich A, et al. Clinical findings in middle lobe syndrome and other processes of pulmonary shrinkage in children (atelectasis syndrome). *Eur J Pediatr Surg.* 1991;1(5):266–272.

Serio P, Fainardi V, Leone R, et al. Tracheobronchial obstruction: follow-up study of 100 children treated with airway stenting. *Eur J Cardiothorac Surg.* 2014;45(4):e100–e109.

Soyer O, Ozen C, Cavkaytar O, et al. Right middle lobe atelectasis in children with asthma and prognostic factors. *Allergol Int.* 2016;65(3):253–258.

71 *Primary Ciliary Dyskinesia*

THOMAS FERKOL, MD, and MARGARET W. LEIGH, MD

Epidemiology

Eighty years ago, Kartagener described a clinical syndrome characterized by the triad *of situs inversus totalis*, chronic sinusitis, and bronchiectasis[1] that later was defined as Kartagener syndrome. Alfzelius and colleagues later found that individuals with Kartagener syndrome, as well as others with chronic sinusitis and bronchiectasis, have defects in the ultrastructural organization of motor cilia.[2-4] Initially, the term "immotile cilia syndrome" was used to describe this disorder, but subsequent studies showed that cilia are often motile but their beat uncoordinated and ineffective. Thus the name was changed to "primary ciliary dyskinesia" (PCD) to more appropriately describe the spectrum of ciliary dysfunction and to distinguish "primary" or genetic ciliary defects from "secondary" or acquired defects associated with epithelial injury.

PCD is an inherited disorder characterized by impaired motor ciliary function leading to diverse clinical manifestations. The frequency of PCD is approximately between 1 in 12,000 and 20,000 live births, based on the prevalence of *situs inversus totalis* and bronchiectasis in population surveys, but these values likely underestimate its incidence in the general population.[5,6] Although PCD is considered a rare lung disease, its prevalence in children with repeated respiratory infections has been estimated to be as high as 5%.[7]

Our understanding of the epidemiology, genetics, pathophysiology, and clinical manifestations of PCD has rapidly advanced over the four decades since the disease was linked to ultrastructural defects of the ciliary axoneme. Advances in cilia genetics and biology have provided new insights into genotype-phenotype relationships and may yield potential therapeutic targets to restore ciliary structure and function.

Etiology

PCD is a heterogeneous genetic disorder, usually autosomal recessive, of motile ciliary structure function and biogenesis. A wide spectrum of clinical features may be seen, reflecting the numerous organs where cilia are important for maintaining health. The large airways and contiguous structures, such as the nasopharynx, paranasal sinuses, and middle ear, are lined by a ciliated, pseudostratified columnar epithelium that is important for mucociliary clearance. The cells on the lumenal surface of this epithelium are predominantly ciliated cells with interspersed goblet cells. Other epithelia containing motile ciliated cells are found in the ependyma of the brain and the fallopian tubes. Spermatozoa flagella have a core structure similar to that of cilia with the same fundamental motility characteristics.

NORMAL MOTILE CILIARY STRUCTURE AND FUNCTION

Mature respiratory ciliated cells contain approximately 200 cilia of uniform size, with an average length of 6 μm. Each normal cilium contains an array of longitudinal microtubules, consisting of nine doublets arranged in an outer circle around a central pair (Fig. 71.1). The microtubules are anchored by a basal body in the apical cytoplasm of the cell. Several different proteins contribute to ciliary structure and function. Tubulin, a dimeric molecule with α- and β-subunits, forms long microtubules that extend the entire length of the cilium. These microtubules are arranged in a distinct 9+2 pattern, with 9 microtubule doublets arranged in a circular array around a central pair of microtubules. The protein nexin links the outer microtubular doublets, creating a circumferential network, and radial spokes connect the outer microtubular doublets with a central sheath of protein that surrounds the central tubules. Dynein is attached to the microtubules as distinct inner and outer "arms," recognizable on electron micrographs of axonemal cross-sections, and is thought to participate in the provision of energy for microtubule sliding through adenosine triphosphatase (ATPase) activity. Inner and outer dynein arms are attached to each microtubule doublet at precise, repeated intervals—24 nm for outer dynein arms and 96 nm for inner dynein arms. The outer dynein arms are longer and form a hook, whereas the inner dynein arms are straight and linked to radial spokes. Each dynein arm is a multimer of two or three heavy chains (400–500 kd), two or four intermediate chains (45–110 kd), and at least eight light chains (8–55 kd),[8,9] with each chain protein encoded by a distinct gene. The dynein heavy chains contain the ATPase that provides the energy for ciliary movement.

Dynein arms extend from the A tubule and interact with the B tubule of the neighboring outer pair, and the force generated translates to a sliding motion of two neighboring tubules, while the inner dynein arms are central for controlling the rhythmic motion of cilia. The inner dynein arm is also part of a complex referred to as the dynein regulatory complex, a key regulator of motor activity.[10] Located within the nexin link, an elastic element that limits sliding between microtubules. The dynein regulatory complex consists of several closely associated proteins that coordinate the activity of the multiple dyneins. The radial spokes also regulate dynein arm activity, sending signals from the central apparatus to the dynein arms.[11] All these structures work in a coordinated fashion to produce a synchronized ciliary beat and maintain alignment of the doublet microtubules (Fig. 71.2).[12]

Ciliary motion takes place within an aqueous layer of airway surface liquids and is divided into two phases: an effective stroke phase that sweeps forward; and a recovery phase during which the cilia bend "backward" and extend

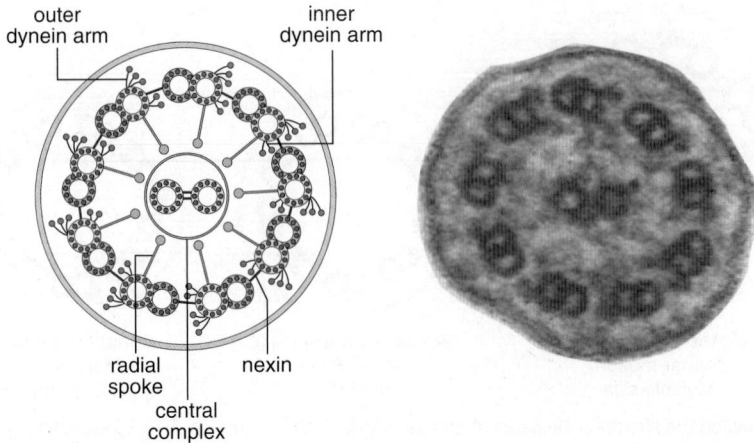

Fig. 71.1 Schematic diagram *(left)* and transmission electron photomicrograph *(right)* of a normal motor cilium in cross-section showing the ultrastructural features of the ciliary axoneme.

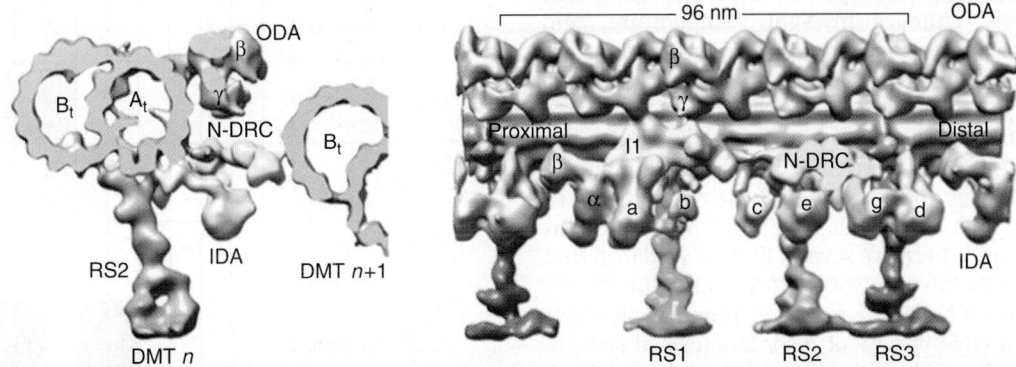

Fig. 71.2 Isosurface renderings show cross-sectional and longitudinal-front views of the averaged 96-nm repeat in a normal cilium created from axonemal tomograms. *DMT,* Doublet microtubule; *IDA,* inner dynein arm; *N-DRC,* nexin-dynein regulatory complex; *ODA,* outer dynein arm; *RS,* radial spoke. (Adapted from Lin J, Yin W, Smith MC, et al. Cryo-electron tomography reveals ciliary defects underlying human RSPH1 primary ciliary dyskinesia. *Nat Commun.* 2014;5:5727.)

into the starting position for the stroke phase. Typically, the tips of cilia contact the overlying mucus during the stroke phase to propel mucus forward, but during the recovery phase, cilia lose contact with the mucus. Normal human cilia bend in a rhythmic, wavelike motion within a single plane. The normal beat frequency of human cilia ranges between 8 and 14 Hertz, which can vary with testing conditions.[13] Cila beat quicker in the proximal airways than in more distal airways and faster in young children (13 beats/s) than in adults (11.5 beats/s).[14] In healthy epithelium, cilia are aligned spatially with parallel orientation of the central pair of tubules in adjacent cilia; therefore ciliary motility is maintained in the same general orientation along the length of airways. Normal mucociliary transport rates may be as rapid as 20–30 mm/min. Although the intracellular and intercellular regulation of ciliary actions is complex and not fully understood, several signaling mechanisms including intracellular calcium, cyclic adenosine monophosphate (cAMP), extracellular adenosine triphosphate (ATP), and airway nitric oxide (NO) play key roles in regulating ciliary beat frequency.[15–18] Ciliary motion is synchronized along the respiratory epithelium by calcium signaling through gap junctions. Motile cilia also respond to external stimuli, such as infectious agents and airborne pollutants, suggesting that motile cilia can sense their environment like primary cilia.[19–21]

There are other types of cilia in the body (Fig. 71.3). Nodal cilia exist transiently in the ventral node of the gastrula during embryonic development. The ultrastructure of embryonic nodal cilia has many features of epithelial motile cilia, including the circular array of 9 microtubule doublets with inner and outer dynein arms; however, there is no central pair of microtubules, hence a 9+0 array. This structure allows the organelle to rotate in a whirling motion that generates unidirectional flow of fluid critical for directing left-right asymmetry in the developing embryo.[22] The node includes two populations of cilia: motile and sensory[23]—the motile nodal cilia generate leftward flow of extracellular fluid across the surface that is detected by peripheral sensory cilia, which activates a cascade of transcription and growth factors to establish body sidedness.[24] In the absence of leftward flow, left-right laterality becomes a random event.

Primary (sensory) cilia are solitary structures present on the surface of many nondividing cells, as well as epithelia-lined sensory organs, biliary ductules, renal tubules, chondrocytes, and astrocytes.[9,25] These structures were long considered vestigial remnants of no physiologic significance but are now recognized as vital signaling organelles that

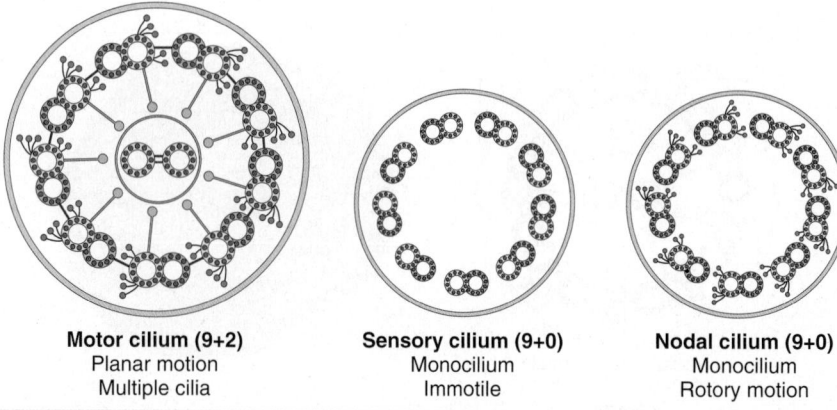

Fig. 71.3 Schematic diagram showing the structural elements of normal motile "9+2," nonmotile "9+0," and motile "9+0" ciliary axonemes. (Adapted from Ferkol T, Leigh M. Pediatric ciliopathies: the central role of cilia in a spectrum of pediatric disorders. *J Pediatr.* 2012;160:366-371.)

sense the extracellular environment. Primary cilia serve as chemoreceptors, mechanoreceptors, osmoreceptors, and, in specialized cases, changes in light, temperature, and gravity.[26,27] Development, growth, and repair functions are also mediated by primary cilia through surface receptors, and genetic defects are associated with clinically diverse pediatric conditions, collectively known as ciliopathies.[28,29] Primary cilia have a 9+0 structure like nodal cilia but do not have dynein arms and consequently are not motile. Otherwise, primary cilia and motile cilia share many proteins and structures, and there are several lines of evidence that suggest motile cilia have sensory and signaling functions. Defects in the assembly and function of primary cilia have been linked to a wide variety of disorders termed *primary ciliopathies*, including polycystic kidney disease, Bardet-Biedl syndrome, Joubert syndrome, and retinitis pigmintosa (Fig. 71.4).[9,25,30] New insights into the molecular basis for primary ciliopathies has raised interest in potential overlap between sensory and motor ciliopathies.

Pathology and Pathogenesis

GENETICS

PCD has been reported in diverse ethnic groups without apparent racial or gender predilection. In most families, PCD appears to be transmitted by an autosomal-recessive pattern of inheritance; however, rare instances of autosomal-dominant or X-linked inheritance patterns have been reported.[31,32] Parents of affected children are normal and have no evidence of impaired ciliary structure or function.

Genetic heterogeneity of PCD is suggested by its various ultrastructural phenotypes.[33,34] The conservation of cilia and flagellar structures along the phylogenetic tree, from algae (*Chlamydomonas reinhardtii*) to flies (*Drosophila melanogaster*) to fish (*Danio rerio*) to mammals, has provided insights into the genetics of the human cilium. For instance, *C. reinhardtii*, a biflagellated single-cell organism,[35] has been a widely used as a powerful model to study motile cilia. The entire genome for Chlamydomonas has been sequenced, and genetic analyses in dysmotile mutant strains of *Chlamydomonas* have identified numerous orthologous human genes that are mutated[9] in PCD. Indeed, most of the mammalian

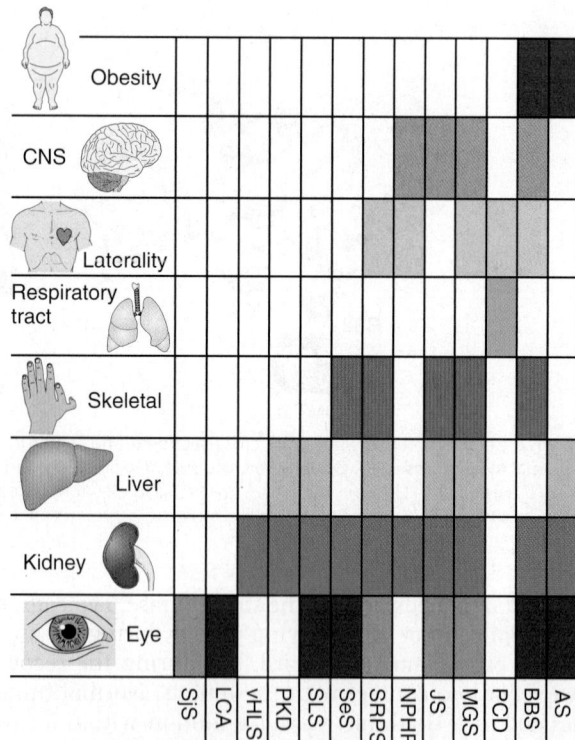

Fig. 71.4 Diagram showing the varied clinical manifestations and organ involvement of genetic ciliopathies. *AS,* Alstrom syndrome; *BBS,* Bardet-Biedel syndrome; *CNS,* central nervous system; *JS,* Joubert syndrome; *LCA,* Leber congenital amaurosis; *MGS,* Meckel-Gruber syndrome; *NPHP,* nephronophthisis; *PCD,* primary ciliary dyskinesia; *PKD,* polycystic kidney disease; *SeS,* Sensenbrunner syndrome; *SjS,* Sjögren syndrome; *SLS,* Senior-Löken syndrome; *SRPS,* short rib-polydactyly syndrome; *vHLS,* von Hippel-Lindau syndrome. (Adapted from Albee AJ, Dutcher SK. Cilia and human disease. *Encyclopedia of Life Sciences (eLS).* Chichester, England: John Wiley and Sons Ltd; 2012. http://www.els.net.)

genes linked to PCD have *Chlamydomonas* orthologs. The identification of PCD-associated genes has relied on a combination of experimental models, creation of cilia-related transcriptomes and proteomes, and powerful sequencing techniques of candidate genes. Massive parallel sequencing has permitted rapid identification of new mutations in PCD subjects without previous knowledge of candidate genes.[36]

Table 71.1   Genes Mutated in Primary Ciliary Dyskinesia

Human Gene	Encoded Protein	Protein Location	Ultrastructural Defect
DNAH5	Dynein heavy chain 5	ODA-HC	Absent or truncated ODA
DNAH11	Dynein heavy chain 11	ODA-HC	Normal ultrastructure
DNAI1	Dynein Intermediate chain 1	ODA IC	Absent or truncated ODA
DNAI2	Dynein intermediate chain 2	ODA IC	Absent or truncated ODA
DNAL1	Dynein light chain 1	ODA-LC	Absent or truncated ODA
TXNDC3	Thioredoxin domain–containing protein 3	ODA LC/IC	Absent or truncated ODA
CCDC103	Coiled-coil domain–containing protein 103	ODA docking	Absent or truncated ODA
CCDC114	Coiled-coil domain–containing protein 114	ODA docking	Absent or truncated ODA
DNAAF1	Dynein (axonemal) assembly factor 1	Cytoplasm	Absent ODA and IDA
DNAAF2	Dynein (axonemal) assembly factor 2	Cytoplasm	Absent ODA and IDA
DNAAF3	Dynein (axonemal) assembly factor 3	Cytoplasm	Absent ODA and IDA
HEATR2	HEAT repeat–containing protein 2	Cytoplasm	Absent ODA and IDA
LRRC6	Leucine-rich repeat–containing protein 6	Cytoplasm	Absent ODA and IDA
SPAG1	Sperm-associated antigen-1	Cytoplasm	Absent ODA and IDA
ZMYND10	Zinc finger, MYND-type containing 10	Cytoplasm	Absent ODA and IDA
DYX1C1	Dyslexia susceptibility 1 candidate 1	Cytoplasm	Absent ODA and IDA
CCNO	Cyclin O	Cytoplasm	Reduced numbers of cilia
MICDAS	Multicilin	Cytoplasm	Reduced numbers of cilia
CCDC39	Coiled-coil domain–containing protein 39	DRC	Absent IDA with axonemal disorganization in some cilia
CCDC40	Coiled-coil domain–containing protein 40	DRC	Absent IDA with axonemal disorganization in some cilia
CCDC65	Coiled-coil domain–containing protein 65	DRC	Normal ultrastructure
CCDC164	Coiled-coil domain–containing protein 164	DRC	Normal ultrastructure
RSPH1	Radial spoke head protein 1	RS	Normal ultrastructure
RSPH4A	Radial spoke head protein 4A	RS	Central apparatus defect
RSPH9	Radial spoke head protein 9	RS	Central apparatus defect
HYDIN	Hydrocephalus-inducing protein homolog	CA	Central apparatus defect

CA, Central apparatus; *DRC,* dynein regulatory complex; *HC,* heavy chain; *IC,* intermediate chain; *IDA,* inner-dynein arm; *LC,* light chain; *ODA,* outer-dynein arm; *RSH,* radial spoke.

Initial genetic studies focused on genes encoding dynein arm proteins but more recently expanded to include other proteins in ciliated cells. Through a collaborative, international research effort, great progress has been made in identification of PCD genes.[37–40] To date, more than 35 genes have been liked to PCD (Table 71.1), and approximately 70% of all patients tested have biallelic mutations of these genes. As gene discovery continues, that number will continue to rise. Many of the gene mutations have been linked to specific ultrastructural defects and ciliary dysmotility, including genes that encode outer dynein arm components: *DNAH5* (MIM 603335), *DNAI1* (MIM 604366), *DNAL1* (MIM 610062), *DNAI2* (MIM 605483), *TXNDC3* (MIM 607421), and *CCDC114* (MIM 615038); inner dynein arm, dynein regulatory complex, and nexin components: *CCDC39* (MIM 613798) and *CCDC40* (MIM 613799); or the radial spokes and central apparatus: *RSPH9* (MIM 612648), *RSPH4A* (MIM 612647), and *HYDIN* (MIM 610812). More recently, mutations in genes coding for several cytoplasmic proteins not integral to the cilia axoneme have been reported. These genes encode proteins that presumably have roles in cilia assembly or protein transport, including: *HEATR2* (MIM 614864), *DNAAF1* (MIM 613190), *DNAAF2* (MIM 612517), *DNAAF3* (MIM 614566), *CCDC103* (MIM 614677), *LRRC6* (MIM 614930), *DYX1C1* (MIM 608706), *CCDC114* (MIM 615038), *SPAG1* (MIM 603395), and *ZYMND10* (607070) (Fig. 71.5).[41–62]

The genetics of PCD has provided unexpected and sometimes surprising insights into ultrastructural phenotypes. For instance, mutations in the dynein axonemal heavy chain 11 *(DNAH11)* gene (MIM 603339) encodes an outer dynein arm protein and, unlike the genes listed previously, is not associated with an ultrastructural defect and cilia have normal

(or more rapid) beat frequency. It is likely that an abnormal waveform leads to inefficient mucociliary clearance.[54,63,64] Mutations in *CCDC39* (MIM 613798) and *CCDC40* (MIM 613799), genes that are essential to assembly of the nexin-dynein regulatory complex and inner dynein arms, yield inconsistent ultrastructural abnormalities characterized by absent inner dynein arms in all axonemes and misplaced radial spokes, and microtubular disorganization in only 10%–20% of cilia.[65,66] Investigations have shown that CCDC39 and CCDC40 serve as "rulers" and are critical for the construction of the ciliary scaffold and accurate spacing of the radial spokes along the axoneme.[67]

More recently, several patients who have mutations in genes encoding cyclin O *(CCNO)* and multiciliate differentiation and DNA synthesis–associated cell cycle protein *(MCIDAS)* were found to have symptoms consistent with PCD and markedly reduced motor cilia on the epithelial surface. CCNO is required for centriole production, and mutations cause mislocalization of basal bodies, consistent with defective basal body replication and migration to the cell surface.[68,69] MCIDAS controls centriole replication required for normal ciliated cell formation.[70] Thus, although the absence of epithelial cilia frequently can be sequelae of infectious insults, it may also have a genetic etiology.

Although the genetic testing holds considerable promise as a diagnostic tool for PCD, it has limitations. First, because PCD is an autosomal recessive condition, presence of a single mutation (or single mutations in different genes) is insufficient to make the diagnosis. Whole exome or genome sequencing is a powerful tool that has allowed more rapid identification of sequence variants,[71] but it is not always clear whether these variants are disease causing. Polymorphisms are fairly common, especially in larger PCD-associated genes, like the

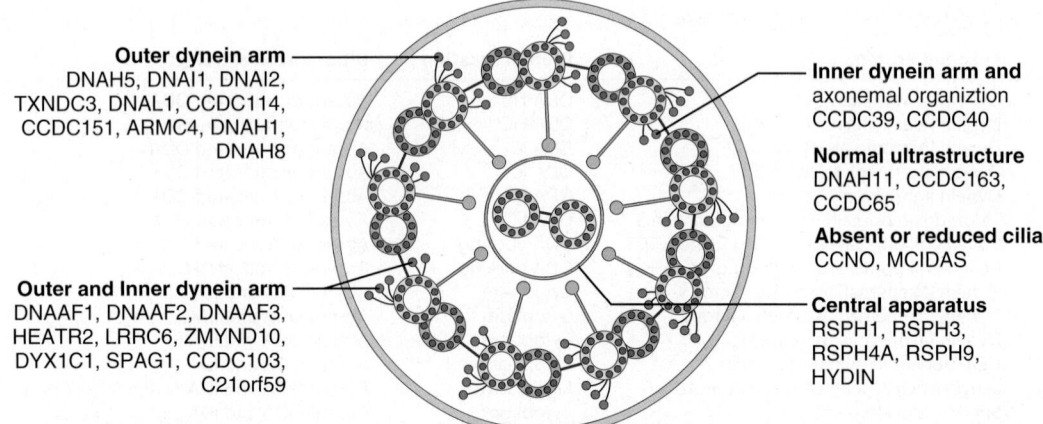

Fig. 71.5 Classification of proteins mutated in primary ciliary dyskinesia segregated based on ultrastructural defects of the ciliary axoneme. (Adapted from Horani A, Ferkol TW. Molecular genetics of primary ciliary dyskinesia. *Encyclopedia of Life Sciences (eLS)*. Chichester, England: John Wiley and Sons Ltd; 2013. http://www.els.net.)

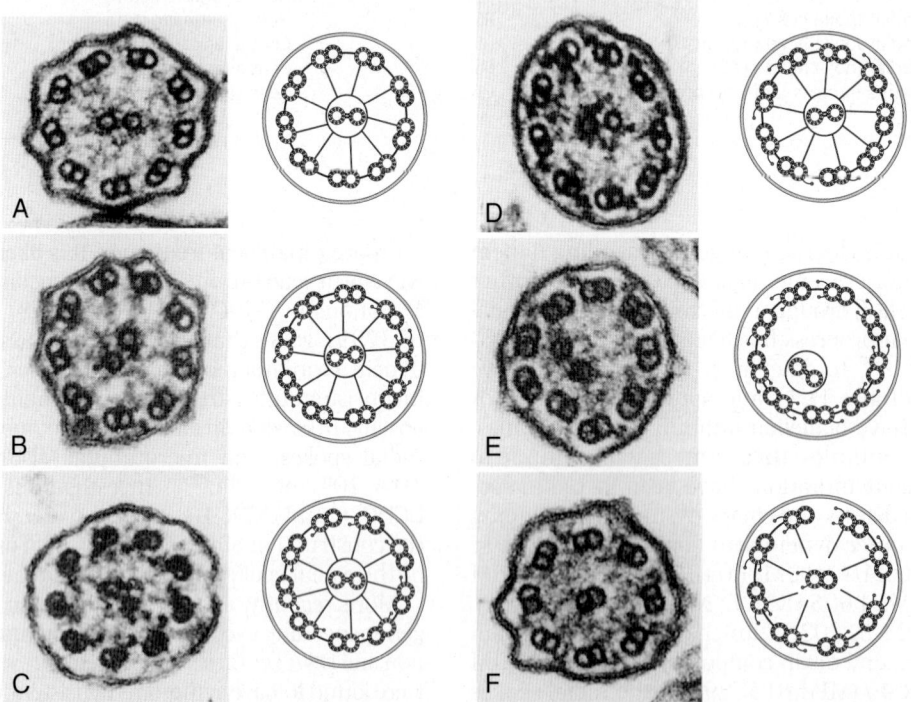

Fig. 71.6 Specific ciliary defects that cause primary ciliary dyskinesia. Each panel shows transmission photomicrograph of ciliary cross-section *(left)* with corresponding diagrammatic representations *(right)*. (A) Dynein arm defect: total absence of outer and inner dynein arms. (B) Dynein arm defect: partial absence of outer and inner dynein arms (~60% of dynein arms are absent). (C) Dynein arm defect: absence of outer dynein arms. (D) Dynein arm defect: absence of inner dynein arms. (E) Radial spoke defect: absence of radial spokes with eccentric central core. (F) Microtubular transposition defect: absence of central tubules with transposition of one doublet to the central axis of the cilium. (A, B, and D, original magnification ×106,000; C, original magnification ×104,000; E, original magnification ×140,000; F, original magnification ×110,000.) (Photomicrographs courtesy of J.M. Sturgess and J.A.P. Turner.)

heavy chain dyneins. Irrespective of the gene affected, nonsense mutations or deletions result in a truncated protein and loss of function and are likely pathogenic. However, rare sequence variants and missense mutations that change a single amino acid are more difficult to link to disease. In addition, it is possible that some biallelic variants may not cause classic PCD but result in mildly reduced cilia function and more subtle clinical manifestations.

ULTRASTRUCTURAL CILIARY DEFECTS

The ciliated epithelium of patients with PCD may appear normal, but distinct ultrastructural defects of the ciliary axoneme have been identified of cilia using transmission electron microscopy, including abnormalities in the dynein arms, radial spokes, nexin links, and microtubular organization (Fig. 71.6, Table 71.2). These distinct ultrastructural defects are generally apparent in cilia throughout the airways, middle ear, and oviduct, as well as in sperm flagella, demonstrating that PCD is a generalized disorder of genetic origin.

Dynein abnormalities occur in approximately 80% of PCD patients who have ultrastructural defects and include complete absence of both inner and outer dynein arms,[2,72] complete or partial absence of outer dynein arms alone, and in rare cases absence of inner dynein arms alone.[73,74] Outer dynein arms are readily identifiable, but inner dynein arm analyses can be difficult because these structures are often obscured by abundant overlying electron-dense material. Computer-assisted image analysis has been used to improve visualization of inner dynein arms, thereby enhancing the ability to detect inner arm defects.[75,76] Because inner dynein arms abnormalities may be observed in normal subjects with recent respiratory infections or other epithelial insults, the diagnosis of PCD in individuals with only inner dynein arm defects can be challenging and repeat confirmatory testing is recommended.[74,77]

Table 71.2 Axonemal Ultrastructural Defects That Have Been Associated With Primary Ciliary Dyskinesia

DYNEIN ARM DEFECTS

Total or partial absence of inner and outer dynein arms
Total or partial absence of inner dynein arms
Total or partial absence of outer dynein arms
Shortening of dynein arms

RADIAL SPOKE DEFECTS

Total absence of radial spokes
Absence of radial spoke heads

MICROTUBULAR TRANSPOSITION DEFECTS

Absent central pair of tubules with transposition of outer doublet(s)

OTHER

Ciliary aplasia
Absence of nexin links
Basal body anomalies
Central microtubular agenesis
Normal ultrastructure but impaired function

A number of defects in radial spokes have been associated with ciliary dysmotility, including total absence of radial spokes and absence of radial spoke heads.[78] These defects are recognized by an eccentric position of the central pair of microtubules that are normally stabilized in a central position by the radial spokes. Central displacement of one of the outer microtubular doublets may also occur. A characteristic alteration in the 9+2 configuration of axonemal microtubules has been described in some families with PCD. Typically, the central pair of tubules is missing, and one of the outer microtubular doublets is transposed to the center in both cilia and flagellae.[79]

Acquired ultrastructural defects have been described that are likely secondary to epithelial insults, such as viral infections. Indeed, ciliary disorientation was initially described as an ultrastructural phenotype of PCD,[80] but this defect is more likely related to airway injury than a genetic defect.[81] One approach to discern whether defects are acquired or congenital is to examine ciliary ultrastructure in epithelial cell cultures grown at air-liquid interface, which allows cells to polarize and redifferentiate.

It is important to note that approximately 30% of patients who have typical clinical manifestations of PCD and ciliary dysmotility will have normal ciliary ultrastructure, indicating that some defects affect function but not structure.[82] As mentioned previously, some ciliary abnormalities in PCD are not found in every axoneme and the changes are often attributed to an acquired defect, further complicating the use ciliary ultrastructural analyses as a diagnostic tool.

FUNCTIONAL CILIARY DEFECTS

In contrast to cystic fibrosis, in which abnormal apical channels result in obstruction and persistent infection, the ineffective cilia beat leads to impaired mucociliary clearance and chronic infections in the PCD airway (Fig. 71.7). Advances in high-speed, high-resolution videomicroscopy have led to its development as a diagnostic tool for PCD, mainly in Europe.[83–85] Digital imaging of ciliary motion in multiple

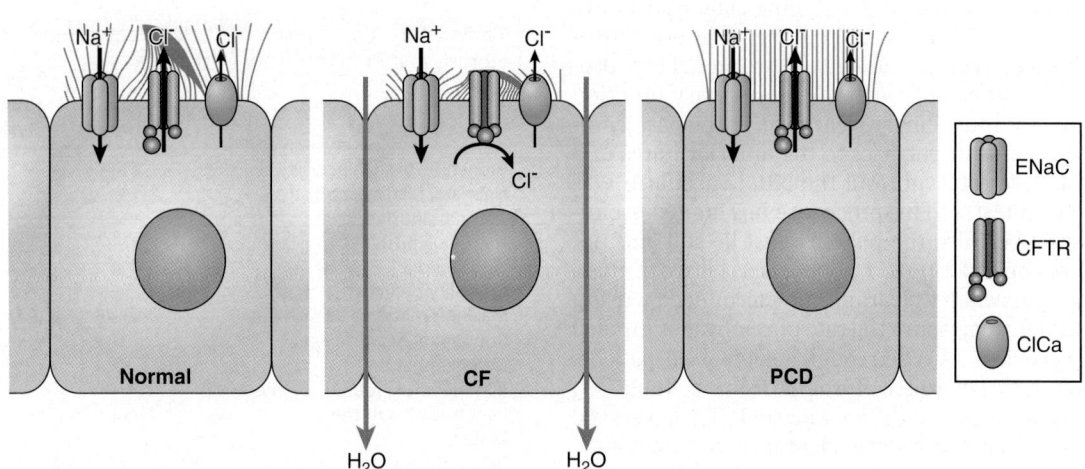

Fig. 71.7 Schematic diagram showing the pathophysiology of two inherited motor ciliopathies, cystic fibrosis (CF) and primary ciliary dyskinesia (PCD). *CFTR,* Cystic fibrosis transmembrane conductance regulator; *ClCa,* alternative chloride channel; *ENaC,* epithelium sodium channel.

planes has permitted comprehensive analysis of abnormal beat patterns. Ciliary motion may be assessed by videomicroscopy of freshly excised ciliated epithelium obtained by scrape or brush biopsy of the inferior surface of the nasal turbinate, or by bronchial brush biopsy. Freshly collected ciliated cells maintain ciliary beating for several hours if placed in appropriate culture media. In PCD the cilia may be immotile or dyskinetic. High-speed videomicroscopy has shown that certain beat patterns are associated with specific ultrastructural defects; specifically, absence of outer dynein arms is associated with immotility or a slightly flickering beat pattern; isolated inner dynein arm defects or radial spoke defects are associated with a slow, stiff motion; and ciliary transposition defects are associated with a circular beat pattern that may have a normal beat frequency but lacks the directional bend.[86] Representative high-speed videomicroscopy videos of ciliary motility (provided by Amelia Shoemark at National Heart & Lung Institute, Imperial College, London, recorded at 500 frames per second and playback at 60 frames per second, magnification 100×, temperature 37°C) are available online for healthy control (Videos 71.1A and 71.1B) and individuals with PCD confirmed by genetic mutations in *DNAH5* (Video 71.2), and *DNAH11* (Video 71.3).

Other disorders, including viral infections and asthma, can cause acquired ciliary dysfunction,[87] which can complicate analyses. To address this limitation, several European sites grow airway epithelial cells in primary culture at an air-liquid interface. The cells redifferentiate and undergo ciliogenesis, and acquired ciliary defects can be reduced.[87] Assessment of ciliary beat pattern and frequency as a diagnostic tool should be performed at specialized PCD centers. This approach requires considerable experience, because some forms of PCD characterized by subtle changes in ciliary waveform can be missed. To address these limitations, investigators are developing computational methods that quantitatively analyze elemental components of ciliary motion that could be refined as a diagnostic tool in the future.[88]

Ciliary beat frequency measurements that use conventional microscopic techniques have been used as a screen, but this method alone is insufficient[84] and will miss cases of PCD. Cilia inspection using standard brightfield light microscopy should not be used to support or exclude the diagnosis.

Other tests have been used to examine ciliary structure and function. Some PCD research centers use fluorescence-labeled antibodies to confirm absence of marker ciliary proteins.[55,56,89–91] Another approach to assess ciliary function is measurement of mucociliary clearance. In the past, clinicians applied saccharin particles to the anterior nares and measured the time interval until the bitter saccharin was tasted (saccharin test).[92] This procedure has limited usefulness in children because the patient must lie still and not sneeze, sniff, or cough for up to 1 hour. In specialized centers, nasal or lung mucociliary clearance is determined by using a gamma counter to measure the rate of removal of inhaled radiolabeled particles.[93,94] When cough is suppressed, patients with PCD have little clearance of isotope from the lung.[93–97] Unlike in cystic fibrosis, cough clearance in PCD is preserved and serves as a compensatory clearance mechanism.[97] This approach is largely used as a research tool, and few centers are using mucociliary clearance as a diagnostic tool for PCD.[98]

NASAL NITRIC OXIDE

Nasal nitric oxide (NO) measurement has been adopted by many PCD centers in Europe and North America as a screening or diagnostic tool for PCD. First described more than 2 decades ago, children with PCD produce very little nasal NO.[99] Subsequent studies have demonstrated that nasal NO is extremely low (5%–15% of normal) in most but not all PCD patients.[100–104] NO is formed by the nitric oxide synthase (NOS) enzyme system in the presence of appropriate substrate (L-arginine and oxygen) and cofactors, including tetrahydrobiopterin. Although NOS is localized to the proximal cilia, the actual relationship between motile cilia and NO levels still needs to be defined. Indeed, the mechanism for altered nasal NO production in PCD is still unknown.[105]

In normal adults, production of NO from the nasopharynx and primarily from paranasal sinuses is 10- to 50-fold greater than from the lower airways. Accurate assessment of nasal NO production requires maneuvers for palate closure, breath-holding, or intubation to exclude contaminating gases from the lower airway that have much lower NO concentrations. Preschool children cannot cooperate with palate closure or breath-holding maneuvers, which have limited the use of nasal NO measurement in young children.[104] Interestingly, some patients with cystic fibrosis also have reduced nasal NO but not as low as in PCD.[104] Thus cystic fibrosis must be excluded from consideration as part of the diagnostic evaluation for PCD.[104] In addition, nasal NO levels may be lower in individuals heterozygous with PCD-associated mutations.[103]

Clinical Features

SYMPTOMS AND PHYSICAL FINDINGS

Clinical symptoms in PCD affect the entire respiratory tract and are distinctive from cystic fibrosis (Table 71.3). The majority of respiratory symptoms occur daily and begin soon after birth.[106] Neonatal respiratory distress is a common feature, and infants typically develop symptoms 12–24 hours of life with increased work of breathing, tachypnea, and upper

Table 71.3   Comparison of Clinical Features in Cystic Fibrosis and Primary Ciliary Dyskinesia

Clinical Features	Cystic Fibrosis	Primary Ciliary Dyskinesia
Bronchitis/bronchiectasis	++++	++++
Neonatal respiratory distress	–	++++
Chronic sinusitis	++++	++++
Nasal polyposis	++	++
Otitis media	+	++++
Laterality defects	–	+++
Male infertility	++++	++++
Congenital heart defects	–	++
Hydrocephalus	–	+
Blindness (i.e., retinitis pigmentosa)	–	+
Pancreatic insufficiency	++++	–
Diabetes	++	–
Biliary cirrhosis	++	+

Prevalence range: ++++, >75%; +++, 31%–74%; ++, 11%–30%; +, 2%–10%; –, <2%.

and middle lobe atelectasis on chest radiographs.[107] Often diagnosed with transient tachypnea of the newborn or pneumonia, PCD infants frequently require supplemental oxygen flow for days to weeks and are more likely to have lobar consolidation. When neonatal respiratory distress occurs in infants with situs anomalies, PCD is highly likely.

Children with PCD have a history of chronic and recurrent respiratory infections, beginning early in life, including rhinitis, sinusitis, otitis media, bronchitis, and pneumonia.[103–106,108,109] Daily, year-round productive (wet) cough that begins in infancy is a distinctive feature of PCD.[110] Sputum may be mucoid or purulent that clears with antibiotic therapy, but the cough persists. In many children, exercise tolerance is normal but can become impaired with advancing obstructive airways disease in older children and young adults. Findings on chest examination are variable. Some patients have localized crackles that may or may not clear following forceful cough, and some may have hyperinflation of the chest. Wheezing is relatively uncommon. Digital clubbing may be apparent in the older patients with bronchiectasis. Bacterial cultures of sputum and bronchoalveolar lavage yield a number of organisms, such as nontypable *Haemophilus influenzae*, *Staphylococcus aureus*, *Streptococcus pneumoniae*, and *Pseudomonas aeruginosa*.[103] Older patients with long-standing disease may be chronically infected with *P. aeruginosa*, although young children with PCD may be infected with this organism, at least transiently. Nontuberculous mycobacteria, particularly *Mycobacterium avium* complex and *Mycobacterium abscessus* have been recovered in respiratory cultures from older children and adults with PCD.[103]

Early studies identified chest radiographic findings in children with PCD, including lung hyperinflation, bronchial wall thickening, segmental atelectasis/consolidation, situs inversus, and bronchiectasis.[111] Computed x-ray tomography (CT) findings suggest that bronchial wall thickening and mucus plugging are more prevalent than hyperinflation and air-trapping.[112–114] Bronchiectasis can occur in early childhood and becomes more prevalent with age such that close to 100% of adults with PCD have bronchiectasis,[112–115] frequently involving the middle lobe, lingual, and lower lobes. With the exception of situs inversus, these radiographic features may be apparent in other chronic disorders, including cystic fibrosis, immunodeficiency, and chronic aspiration.

Pulmonary function tests may be normal during early childhood but more typically demonstrate obstructive airway disease that becomes more severe in adulthood. Typical findings include reduced forced expiratory flow between 25% and 75% of vital capacity ($FEF_{25\%-75\%}$) and forced expiratory volume in 1 second (FEV_1), increased residual volume (RV), and elevated ratio of residual volume to total lung capacity (RV/TLC). Bronchodilator responsiveness is variable. Longitudinal analyses of children with PCD suggest that lung function may remain stable over relatively long periods of time; however, there is a wide variation in course of lung function in PCD.[116–118] Genotype-phenotype relationships are emerging. A cross-sectional study of subjects with ultrastructural defects showed that individuals who had inner dynein arm defects associated with microtubular disorganization, primarily due to biallelic mutations in *CCDC39* or *CCDC40*, had more severe lung disease.[119] Conversely, patients with biallelic mutations in *RSPH1* have milder respiratory phenotypes.[120]

Daily, persistent nasal congestion and rhinitis is a common feature, typically present since early infancy, with little to no seasonal variation.[110] Most patients describe chronic mucopurulent nasal drainage. Typically, sinus radiographs or computed x-ray tomograms demonstrate mucosal thickening and/or opacification of all paranasal sinuses, even in the absence of sinus symptoms. Anosmia, hyponasal speech, and halitosis are more apparent in severely affected patients.

Situs inversus totalis occurs in nearly 50% of patients with PCD. Typically, all viscera in the chest and abdomen are transposed (i.e., situs inversus totalis). The underlying basis for situs inversus totalis in PCD is attributed to dysfunction of the embryonic nodal cilia that play a key role in directing normal rotation of viscera.[22–24,46,121,122] Without functional nodal cilia, thoracoabdominal laterality becomes random, which has been demonstrated in genetically identical twins with PCD: one with situs solitus and one with situs inversus totalis,[123] as well as in mouse models.[46,121,122,124,125] Studies have demonstrated that heterotaxy (situs ambiguus or organ laterality defects other than situs inversus totalis) occurs in at least 6%–12% of individuals with PCD.[126,127] Heterotaxia is often associated with complex congenital heart disease and includes a wide array of laterality defects such as abdominal situs inversus, polysplenia (left isomerism), and asplenia (right isomerism and Ivemark) syndromes.[128] More than 100 genes have been linked to laterality defects, including PCD genes, which has led to greater focus on the overlap between PCD and the full spectrum of laterality defects between situs solitus and situs inversus totalis.[129] Respiratory ciliary dysfunction is frequently found in patients with heterotaxy and congenital heart disease, which demonstrates the importance of cilia function in normal cardiac development.[130] Indeed, these findings have led to searches for ciliary anomalies in children with congenital heart disease to uncover the genetic cause of these defects.[131] Mutations in some PCD genes, such as those encoding radial spoke proteins, CCNO and MCICAS, do not alter nodal cilia and hence are not associated with laterality defects.[51,68,70,120]

The presence or absence of the clinical manifestations listed previously should assist the clinician in determining whether further testing is needed. They may not be seen in all affected individuals, but most patients with PCD have at least two or three of these features. The combination of these clinical features markedly increases the likelihood of diagnosis (see Table 71.3).[110]

Chronic otitis media of variable severity is present in almost all patients with PCD. At the time of diagnosis, many patients older than 2 years have a history of either chronic tympanic membrane perforations or have had tympanostomies with insertion of ventilation tubes in the tympanic membranes. Many have conductive hearing loss at least intermittently during early childhood, which improves by during adolescence.[132–135] While recurrent or chronic otitis media is not predictive of PCD, middle ear findings may be most helpful in distinguishing PCD from cystic fibrosis or other causes of chronic lung disease.

Male infertility is common and attributable to impaired sperm motility. The ultrastructural and functional defects in cilia are mirrored in sperm flagellae in some but not all

PCD patients.[72,136–138] The occurrence of ultrastructural ciliary defects in ciliated cells lining fallopian tubes[139–141] has led to speculation that subfertility and ectopic pregnancies could be increased in women with primary ciliary defects, but this association has not been examined systematically.

Although common in mouse models, hydrocephalus is rare in PCD.[142–145] Ultrastructural and functional defects in ventricular ependymal cilia provide a theoretical basis for this association. Defective leukocyte migration has been reported in a few PCD patients, suggesting that the cytoplasmic microtubules of leukocytes may be altered, but specific defects in neutrophil chemotaxis have not been defined.[146,147]

OVERLAPPING CILIOPATHIES

Advances in our understanding of the genetics and molecular abnormalities in sensory cilia has helped to define a diverse group of diseases or primary ciliopathies. Primary cilia are found in almost all cells at some time in development and play key roles in sensation and signaling; therefore primary ciliopathies include a wide range of disorders. Some primary ciliopathies are manifested primarily in one organ (e.g., retinitis pigmentosa, polycystic kidney disease, or nephronophthisis), whereas others are manifested as complex syndromes (e.g., Bardet-Biedl syndrome, Joubert syndrome, Leber congenital amaurosis).[148] Rare case reports have demonstrated features of PCD and primary ciliopathies in the same patient, which has heightened interest in potential overlapping ciliopathies. Retinitis pigmentosa leads to progressive blindness due to mutations in the retinitis pigmentosa guanosine triphosphatase (GTPase) regulator gene *(RPGR)*, but these individuals can develop progressive respiratory symptoms due to motile cilia dysfunction.[32,149–153] There are also case reports that suggest respiratory disease secondary to motile cilia dysfunction in Usher syndrome, a rare genetic condition that affects the retinal photoreceptors and cochlear cilia.[154,155] Similarly, a family with mutations in *OFD1* (linked to the primary ciliopathy syndrome, oral-facial-digital syndrome, type 1) had clinical features and functional respiratory ciliary studies consistent with PCD.[156] Finally, adults with autosomal dominant polycystic kidney disease, which is caused by mechanoreceptor polycystin 1 or polycystin 2 mutations, have increased risk of respiratory disease and radiographic evidence of bronchiectasis[157–159] Finally, there are growing associations between ciliary defects (involving motile and sensory cilia) with congenital heart disease, which may provide further insights into pathogenesis of this birth defect.[160] The mechanistic link between sensory and motor functions is largely unknown, and further investigation into the function of motile cilia in primary ciliopathies is needed.

Diagnosis

The diagnosis of PCD requires clinical phenotypic features in conjunction with diagnostic testing. Definitive diagnosis can be challenging and requires involvement of specialized centers with expertise in clinical features of PCD, as well as the different tests to assess ciliary motility, ciliary ultrastructure, high-speed videomicroscopy, nasal NO measurement, and genetic testing. Suitable samples for examination of ciliary motility and ultrastructure include nasal biopsy obtained by brushing or curettage of the inferior surface of the nasal turbinates, or bronchial brush biopsy. Identification of impaired motility and one of the specific ultrastructural defects in a patient with clinical characteristics, including daily productive cough, nonseasonal rhinosinusitis, left-right laterality defects, or neonatal respiratory distress, provides solid evidence for the diagnosis. Airway insults such as exposure to pollutants and respiratory viral infections may be accompanied by nonspecific ultrastructural changes in cilia that impair motility. Therefore analysis of ciliary ultrastructure should be performed by an electron microscopist who has extensive experience examining ciliated cells. Despite expert review, the ultrastructural analysis may be inconclusive in some cases because of uncertainty in distinguishing primary from secondary ciliary defects; repeat biopsies may be needed before a conclusive diagnosis can be made. Nasal NO measurement has become a useful adjunctive test for PCD in individuals older than 5 years.[100–104] However, few studies in younger children have been reported, and the accuracy of nasal NO measurements in infants has not been established. With recent advances in identification of PCD genes, genetic testing has increasingly become a viable diagnostic tool.

Management and Treatment

At present, no specific therapies are available to correct ciliary dysfunction, and to date there have not been large randomized controlled trials of any treatment for PCD. Management should include aggressive measures to enhance clearance of mucus, prevent respiratory infections, and treat bacterial superinfections.[106,108]

Approaches to enhance mucus clearance in PCD are similar to those used in the management of cystic fibrosis. Chest percussion and postural drainage facilitate clearance of distal airways. Because cough is an effective clearance mechanism, patients are encouraged to cough and to engage in activities such as vigorous exercise that stimulate cough. All patients and families should be counseled about the importance of cough and instructed to avoid cough suppressants. Bronchodilators such as albuterol may aid mucus clearance in patients who have airway hyperreactivity. As in cystic fibrosis, antiinflammatory agents, deoxyribonuclease, nebulized hypertonic saline, and other measures to facilitate airway clearance may be beneficial; however, specific indications and utility in PCD have not been defined.

A number of measures to prevent respiratory tract infection and irritation should be considered. PCD patients should receive routine immunizations that provide protection against a number of respiratory pathogens, including pertussis, measles, *H. influenzae* type b, S. pneumoniae, and influenza. Preventive counseling should include avoidance of exposure to respiratory pathogens, tobacco smoke, and other pollutants and irritants that may damage airway mucosa and stimulate mucus secretion.

Prompt institution of antibiotic therapy for bacterial superinfections (bronchitis, sinusitis, and otitis media) is crucial for preventing irreversible damage. Sputum Gram stain and culture results may be used to direct appropriate choice of antimicrobial therapy. In some patients, symptoms recur within days to weeks after completing a course of antibiotics. This subgroup may benefit from extended use of a broad-spectrum antibiotic such as trimethoprim-sulfamethoxazole.

Surgical intervention may be indicated for specific complications. Tympanostomy with ventilation tube placement have been used to control chronic serous otitis media that persists despite antibiotic therapy. Tympanostomy placement may improve hearing but is often complicated by offensive otorrhea; therefore there is ongoing debate about indications and utility of this intervention in PCD.[134,135] Sinus drainage may benefit patients with severe sinusitis that does not respond to antibiotic therapy. Lobectomy may be considered in patients with localized bronchiectasis or atelectasis that is thought to be a nidus for chronic infection. However, lobectomy should be approached cautiously, recognizing that removal of any functioning lung tissue in patients with progressive lung disease could have long-term adverse consequences. Lung transplantation (including heart-lung, bilateral lung, and living related bilateral lung transplantation) has been performed successfully in PCD patients with end-stage lung disease, with surgical modifications for patients with situs inversus.

Prognosis

Chronic lung disease with bronchiectasis and some degree of pulmonary disability has been the usual outcome and has a negative impact on overall quality of life for individuals with PCD. Progression of lung disease is variable, with some individuals experiencing normal or near-normal life span while others develop advanced lung disease progressing to respiratory failure in early adulthood. Several longitudinal studies suggest that aggressive approaches to airway clearance and controlling lung function can slow progression of lung disease.[117,118]

References

Access the reference list online at ExpertConsult.com.

Suggested Reading

Afzelius BA. A human syndrome caused by immotile cilia. *Science*. 1976;193:317–319.

Davis SD, Ferkol TW, Rosenfeld M, et al. Clinical features of childhood primary ciliary dyskinesia by genotype and ultrastructural phenotype. *Am J Respir Crit Care Med*. 2015;191:316–324.

Horani A, Brody SL, Ferkol T. Picking up speed: advances in the genetics of primary ciliary dyskinesia. *Pediatr Res*. 2014;75:158–164.

Ibanez-Tallon I, Heintz N, Omran H. To beat or not to beat. Roles of cilia in development and disease. *Hum Mol Genet*. 2003;12:R27–R35.

Knowles MR, Daniels LA, Davis SD, et al. Primary ciliary dyskinesia. Recent advances in diagnostics, genetics, and characterization of clinical disease. *Am J Respir Crit Care Med*. 2013;188:913–922.

Leigh MW, Ferkol TW, Davis SD, et al. Clinical features and associated likelihood of primary ciliary dyskinesia in children and adolescents. *Ann Am Thorac Soc*. 2016;13:1305–1313.

Shapiro AJ, Zariwala MA, Ferkol T, et al. Diagnosis, monitoring, and treatment of primary ciliary dyskinesia: PCD Foundation consensus recommendations based on state of the art review. *Pediatr Pulmonol*. 2016;51:115–132.

72 Chest Wall and Respiratory Muscle Disorders

JEAN-PAUL PRAUD, MD, PhD, and GREGORY J. REDDING, MD

Introduction

Since Lavoisier's stipulation in 1791 that respiration is essentially a phenomenon of oxygen (O_2) consumption and carbon dioxide (CO_2) production, the chest wall has been recognized as the vital pump responsible for the movement of gases between the atmosphere and the lungs. Today, much is known regarding the adaptability of this vital pump to satisfy the changing metabolic needs under various physiological and pathological conditions (e.g., rest, exercise, and hyperthermia). Patients must overcome adverse conditions affecting chest wall function: conditions ranging from the cartilaginous, pliable rib cage of the preterm infant to the scoliotic thorax of the adolescent, and from the weak chest wall in neuromuscular disease to the stiff rib cage in asphyxiating thoracic dystrophy or obesity. The vital pump also participates in numerous functions, such as singing, talking, wind instrument playing, coughing, sneezing, load lifting, parturition, and hiccupping, all of which can interfere with lung ventilation.

In normal resting conditions, the diaphragm is the principal muscle used for inspiration while the accessory inspiratory muscles mainly stabilize the rib cage. When the inspiratory workload is increased, additional diaphragmatic motor units and accessory inspiratory muscles are recruited, the latter producing an upward motion of the ribs resulting in a more pronounced thoracic expansion. In normal resting conditions, expiratory muscles are inactive. During increased demands for air pumping, the expiratory muscles become activated during the second phase of expiration and decrease the end expiratory volume below functional residual capacity (FRC). Any decrease in the force of the expiratory muscles leads to an increased residual volume and decreased vital capacity.

Sleep is responsible for significant modifications in lung mechanics and respiratory muscle control. Assuming the supine position leads to a decrease in FRC, mainly due to the cephalad movement of the abdominal contents. Sleep also leads to a decrease in tonic activity of intercostal muscles and upper airway muscles, a phenomenon further pronounced in rapid-eye-movement (REM) sleep. These changes are responsible for paradoxical inward rib cage movement during inspiration in infants due to their compliant rib cage and in patients with neuromuscular disorders. Nocturnal hypoventilation with alteration of blood gases is often the first sign of chronic respiratory failure in progressive neuromuscular disorders, such as Duchenne muscular dystrophy. In addition to nocturnal hypoventilation, obstructive and/or central sleep-disordered breathing have been reported in a number of neuromuscular diseases, including Duchenne muscular dystrophy, myotonic dystrophy, congenital myopathies, metabolic myopathies, myasthenia gravis, and spinal muscular atrophy.[1]

THE CHEST WALL IN THE NEWBORN

The features of the chest wall and respiratory muscles in the newborn period predispose to pump failure during illness (Fig. 72.1). The very compliant chest wall of the premature and to a lesser extent the full-term infant results in chest wall distortion rather than efficient ventilation when inspiratory muscles contract against high mechanical loads, such as during lower respiratory infections. Ossification of the ribs is responsible for stiffening of the chest wall, so that chest wall compliance is up to seven-fold greater than lung compliance at birth, and reduced by half by the age of 3. The ribs are aligned perpendicular to the spine, rendering intercostal muscles unable to add volume with the "bucket handle" motion present in adults. This spine-rib angle approaches adult values by 2–3 years of age. The insertion of the diaphragm to the rib cage is also more perpendicular, which favors inward displacement of the lower ribs with any forceful diaphragmatic contraction. Therefore excessive diaphragm contraction has to be used to produce an adequate tidal volume. In addition, respiratory muscle mass and the proportion of fatigue-resistant fibers in the diaphragm are lower, resulting in less resistance to fatigue. This can be further amplified by nutritional difficulties and hypoglycemia, hypocalcemia, hypophosphatemia, or acidosis. To cope with all of this, the newborn in resting conditions breathes rapidly, with limited excursion of the diaphragm. In disease conditions, rather than increasing the depth of each breath, the newborn further increases the respiratory rate, thereby preventing diaphragmatic fatigue by decreasing the duration of inspiratory contraction. Functional residual capacity is actively maintained in the newborn by increasing the respiratory rate, hence decreasing the time devoted to lung deflation, or by breaking the expiratory flow through active glottal closure. Extremely prematurely born infants are particularly at risk of respiratory pump failure. Respiratory muscle fatigue is more often the cause of respiratory failure in the newborn than at any other time in life.

RESPIRATORY MUSCLE DISORDERS— GENERAL CONSIDERATIONS

Diaphragm dysfunction can be due to a wide variety of disorders. Disorders of the diaphragm produce abnormalities in its position within the chest, excursion with inspiratory efforts, weakness and fatigability. These features often coexist. Hyperinflation due to intrathoracic airway obstruction

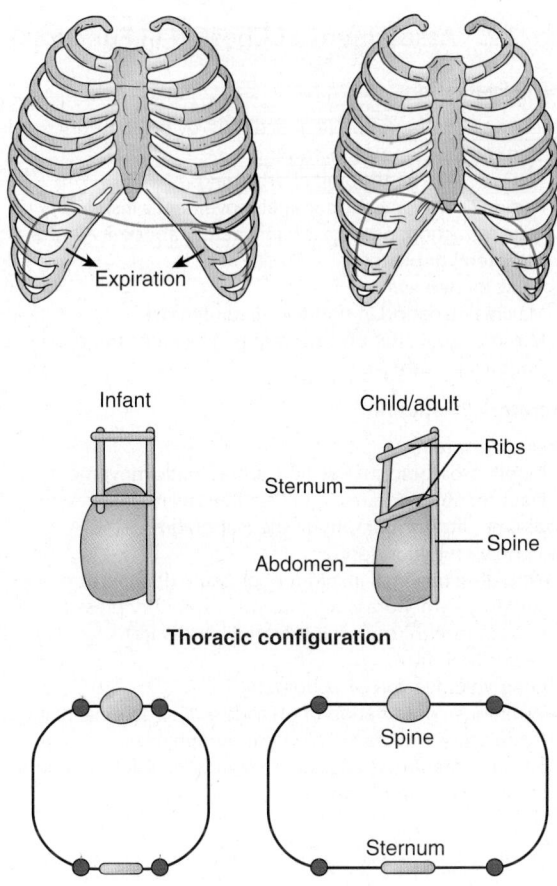

Thoracic configuration

Infant   Child/adult

Ribs
Sternum
Spine
Abdomen

Spine

Sternum

Thoracic cross section

Fig. 72.1 Peculiar features of the chest wall in the newborn. The features of the rib cage predisposes the newborn to diaphragmatic fatigue and respiratory failure: (1) the rib cage is very compliant due to nonossification of the ribs; (2) intercostal muscles are unable to add volume with the "bucket handle" motion present later in life, due to the perpendicular alignment of the ribs to the spine; (3) the insertion of the diaphragm to the rib cage is perpendicular, which favors inward displacement of the lower ribs with any forceful diaphragmatic contraction. (From Taussig, Landau, Pediatric Respiratory Medicine, 2nd edition, 2008, Mosby, Elsevier.)

a less nutrient substrate is delivered to the respiratory muscles. Hypoxemia, as experienced at high altitude, reduces endurance time among healthy individuals breathing against large inspiratory resistive loads. Acute hypercapnia also produces inspiratory muscle fatigue in healthy adults breathing against increased mechanical loads.

In addition, certain therapies can lead to respiratory muscle dysfunction as a result of injury and atrophy. The use of paralytics, corticosteroids, and controlled mechanical ventilation leads to muscle atrophy remarkably quickly. Ventilator-induced diaphragm dysfunction can occur as quickly as 18 hours in patients without respiratory efforts receiving controlled mechanical ventilation. Diaphragmatic atrophy develops in proportion to the degree of muscle inactivity during controlled ventilator support, and the duration of that support. Promoting patient-initiated breaths while administering ventilator support prevents this effect. Aside from ventilator-induced diaphragmatic dysfunction, sepsis appears to result in very early onset muscle injury and loss of contractility before the occurrence of atrophy (i.e., independently of mechanical ventilation).[3]

Clinically, these conditions can be present concurrently, such as controlled ventilation for paralyzed septic patients. Similarly, babies with bronchopulmonary dysplasia who are poorly nourished and who receive corticosteroids to treat acute viral lower respiratory tract infections have multiple etiologies for respiratory muscle dysfunction and failure. The relative importance of each factor when their combined risks occur clinically is unclear, although all etiologies for respiratory muscle dysfunction should be addressed.

RESPIRATORY MUSCLE FATIGUE

Respiratory muscle fatigue develops when there is a reduction in the force-generating capacity of the neuromuscular respiratory apparatus. This occurs when the energy supply to the respiratory muscles is reduced in the presence of increased work demands. It is also present when respiratory work requirements exceed the work capacity of normal respiratory muscles. In normal adults, inspiratory work that is less than 40% of maximal inspiratory force can be maintained indefinitely. The closer the workload approaches 100% of maximal inspiratory force, the faster respiratory muscle fatigue develops.

When a superimposed inspiratory mechanical load occurs, several mechanisms are called into play to meet muscle work requirements. There is an increase in respiratory drive and phrenic nerve output, which leads to the recruitment of diaphragm motor units. There is an increased recruitment of fast-twitch muscle fibers, which are more capable of generating force than slow-twitch (fatigue-resistant) fibers. There is also recruitment of accessory respiratory muscles of the chest wall and neck and a change in respiratory patterns to reduce the inspiratory time per breath. Despite these responses, mechanical loads imposed on the respiratory system can be of sufficient degree and duration to produce respiratory muscle fatigue and lead to hypoventilation and hypercapnia. Clinical features of impending acute respiratory failure are listed in Box 72.1.

Chronic respiratory muscle fatigue is less easily identifiable, and respiratory symptoms may not correlate well with the degree of respiratory muscle fatigue. General fatigue and

flattens the diaphragm contour and reduces the surface area of the zone of apposition of the diaphragm, and hence inspiratory force. The higher the lung volume above FRC, the greater the reduction in maximal inspiratory force. Muscle weakness due to phrenic nerve injury leads to an elevated diaphragm on the affected side. Distortion of the diaphragm, as occurs with scoliosis, also causes a reduction in inspiratory force generation and excursion.[2] Primary inspiratory muscle weakness predisposes these muscles to fatigue in the presence of mechanical loads due to disease processes.

Disorders that alter functional properties of the diaphragm and the other respiratory muscles include neuropathic processes, such as quadriplegia, or myopathic processes (e.g., muscular dystrophies). In addition, conditions producing primary respiratory disease can also affect the respiratory muscles secondarily. Examples include hyperinflation in asthma, cystic fibrosis, and bronchopulmonary dysplasia, as well as malnutrition, as observed with cystic fibrosis. Conditions that reduce blood flow to the diaphragm, such as heart failure and sepsis, predispose to diaphragm fatigue, as

---

Box 72.1   Clinical Signs of Impeding Acute Respiratory Muscle Failure

Inability to Perform Nonventilatory Functions

- Inability to eat/drink/cry
- Reluctance to pause breathing voluntarily

Major Use of Accessory Muscles

- Sternocleidomastoid muscles, pectoral

Increase in Respiratory Rate to Critical Level

- Adolescents: 55 breaths/min
- Children, 4–10 years: 70–75 breaths/min
- Infants, 1–3 years: 90 breaths/min
- Neonates: 120 breaths/min

Signs Reflecting Options Taken to Relieve Fatigue

- Shallow breathing
- Deep breaths with a brief pause to rest the muscles
- Respiratory alternans

Signs Indicating Pending Respiratory Arrest

- Cyanotic spells
- Cyanosis with brief cough or brief pause
- Recurrent apnea
- Sustained paradoxical thoracic/abdominal movement
- Drooling in absence of airway obstruction (cannot pause to swallow)
- Central nervous system signs (confusion)

Box 72.2   Assessment of Chest Wall Function

Clinical Evaluation

- Chest wall configuration (e.g., scoliosis, overdistention)
- Pattern of spontaneous breathing
  - Thoracic and/or abdominal breathing
  - Paradoxical thoracoabdominal movements: inspiratory rib cage retraction, paradoxical inspiratory abdominal retraction (unilateral or bilateral)
- Specific maneuvers:
  - Maximal variation in thoracic circumference
  - Maximal excursion of diaphragm (inspection and percussion)
  - Cough strength?

Laboratory Evaluation

- Roentgenograms:
  - Cinefluoroscopic studies of diaphragmatic movements
  - Plain roentgenograms in full expiration and inspiration
- Real-time ultrasonography of the diaphragm
- Pulmonary function tests:
  - Pressures: maximal inspiratory pressure (PI max) at mouth, sniff inspiratory pressure, maximal expiratory pressure (PE max) at mouth (transdiaphragmatic pressure)
  - Peak cough flow
  - Lung volumes, forced spirometry
  - Variations/coordination of rib cage and abdominal diameter (respiratory inductance plethysmography)
- Electromyographic studies of respiratory muscles (magnetic stimulation of phrenic nerve)

---

dyspnea on exertion can be the first symptoms of chronic respiratory pump impairment. Additional manifestations of chronic respiratory muscle impairment include sleep hypoventilation, nocturnal parasomnias, enuresis, increased sweating, and daytime symptoms, such as morning headaches, hypersomnolence, chronic fatigue, and decreased attention span. New onset of unexplained symptoms of right heart failure due to unsuspected pulmonary hypertension may also reflect chronic sleep-related hypoxemia and hypoventilation. Serial assessment of chest wall function is necessary to predict or recognize the first signs of chronic respiratory muscle fatigue in patients with neuromuscular disorders (Box 72.2).

Etiologies

Chest wall movements should be envisioned as the result of a chain of effectors that successively transmit the drive to breathe from the respiratory centers to the upper motor neurons of the central nervous system, the lower motor neurons, and finally the respiratory muscle fibers. The central drive to breathe is transformed into a mechanical force resulting from contractions of respiratory muscles, which move the chest wall and generate inspiratory and expiratory pressures responsible for air movement into and out of the lungs. Table 72.1 illustrates the systemic conditions that cause disturbances at these various levels. *Neurological diseases* at the level of the central nervous system (upper motor neurons) or at the level of peripheral innervation of the chest wall (lower motor neurons) may lead to secondary dysfunction of the muscular components of the chest wall. The best examples of these entities are hemiplegia,

quadriplegia, infantile spinal muscular atrophies, and polyradiculitis (Guillain-Barré syndrome). *Myopathies* from various types of muscular dystrophy or from metabolic origin, as well as disorders of the neuromuscular junction, result in failure of the respiratory muscles to produce an adequate contraction. In addition, systemic diseases associated with severe malnutrition may lead to a loss in respiratory muscle mass and force. *Disorders involving the bony structures of the chest wall,* such as scoliosis and asphyxiating thoracic dystrophy, are responsible for restrictive lung disease and impair the transformation of respiratory muscle contraction into adequate pressure, due to the malposition of these muscles. Finally, *obesity* causes an additional mechanical load on both the thoracic and abdominal components of the chest wall and limits its performance capacity.

Despite their differences in pathogenesis, the various entities that cause chest wall dysfunction share some clinical and physiological features. Chest wall dysfunction leads to restrictive pulmonary disease with reduced lung volume, reduced absolute flow rate values, normal forced expiratory volume in 1 second/forced vital capacity (FEV_1/FVC) ratio, reduced strength of respiratory muscles and decreased ventilatory performance in response to exercise. Residual volume can be normal or augmented, depending on normal or decreased strength of the expiratory muscles, respectively. With respiratory muscle strength at less than 50% predicted, the decrease in vital capacity is generally greater than expected, due to the decreased compliance of the lung (atelectasis) and the rib cage (costovertebral and costosternal joint ankylosis). Hypercapnia is usually present during wakefulness when respiratory muscle strength is less than 25% predicted, but it can occur when weakness is less profound

Table 72.1 Classification of Disorders Responsible for Chest Wall Dysfunction

Site of Defect	Causes
Central drive of breathing	Congenital or acquired
Upper motor neuron	Hemiplegia
	Cerebral palsy
	Quadriplegia
Lower motor neuron	Poliomyelitis
	Spinal muscular atrophies
	Guillain-Barré syndrome
	Tetanus
	Traumatic nerve lesions
	Phrenic nerve paralysis
Neuromuscular junction	Myasthenia gravis
	Congenital myasthenic syndromes
	Botulism
	Drugs
Respiratory muscles	Muscular dystrophies
	Congenital myopathies
	Metabolic myopathies
	Steroid myopathy
	Connective tissue disease
	Diaphragmatic malformation
Nonmuscular, chest wall structures	Scoliosis
	Congenital rib cage abnormality
	Overinflated rib cage in chronic obstructive pulmonary disease
	Connective tissue disease
	Thoracic burns
	Obesity
	Giant exomphalos, Prune-belly syndrome

in the presence of coexisting mechanical loads due to additional respiratory disorders. With less severe disease, hypercapnia may be present during sleep, and patients are at risk of ventilatory failure during critical periods of their lives, such as in the neonatal period, during respiratory infections, following general anesthesia, and during the last trimester of pregnancy.

Pathogenesis

DIAPHRAGM PARALYSIS

Diaphragm paralysis generally results from injury to the phrenic nerve during thoracic or neck surgery. Tumors of the mediastinum, peripheral neuropathy, and agenesis of the phrenic nerve are less likely causes. In the newborn, stretching of the root C3–C5 during breech delivery is a frequent cause, most often in association with brachial plexus injuries (Erb's paralysis). Most diaphragm paralyses are on the right side, with bilateral paralysis occurring in only 10% of cases. Bilateral diaphragm paralysis can be responsible for a severe restrictive syndrome, with total lung capacity often below 50% of predicted value. Elevation of the paralyzed diaphragm is greater in the supine position, due to pressure from the abdominal content, and can be responsible for orthopnea.

SPINAL MUSCULAR ATROPHIES

Childhood spinal muscular atrophies (SMA) are a group of autosomal recessive neurodegenerative disorders with onset from birth to adulthood. Spinal muscular atrophies are due to a deficient survival motor neuron (SMN) protein, which is encoded by two adjacent and nearly homologous genes, *SMN1* and *SMN2*, located on chromosome 5. *SMN1* is the only gene able to produce the full-length SMN protein that is essential to the survival of motor neurons. Although the *SMN2* gene differs by only a few nucleotides from the *SMN1* gene, it mainly produces a truncated, rapidly degraded SMN protein. Spinal muscular atrophies are due to a mutation of the *SMN1* gene, which results in the degeneration of the anterior horn cells of the spinal cord and often of the bulbar motor nuclei, leading, in turn, to skeletal muscle weakness and atrophy.

NEUROMUSCULAR JUNCTION DISEASES

Myasthenia Gravis

Juvenile Myasthenia Gravis. Similar to the adult form, juvenile myasthenia gravis is an acquired autoimmune disorder of neuromuscular transmission associated with circulating autoantibodies against acetylcholine receptors (AChR) in 80%–90% of cases. The juvenile form accounts for 10% of all cases of myasthenia gravis.

Neonatal Myasthenia Gravis. Neonatal myasthenia is a transient disorder, which affects 10%–30% of infants born to mothers with autoimmune myasthenia gravis. It results, at least partly, from passively transmitted maternal AChR autoantibodies, even if the mother has shown no clinical symptoms.

Congenital Myasthenic Syndromes

Congenital myasthenic syndromes refer to a group of various inherited disorders resulting from mutations of genes crucial for neuromuscular transmission. At least 24 different genes are known to cause congenital myasthenic syndromes.[4]

MYOPATHIES

Duchenne Muscular Dystrophy

Duchenne muscular dystrophy (DMD) is the most common and severe form of muscular dystrophy afflicting humans. Inherited as an X-linked recessive trait, it has an incidence of approximately 1:3500 male births. Almost one-third of cases result from new mutations. The gene responsible has been localized within the dystrophin gene located on the short arm of the X chromosome (Xp21). Dystrophin links the normal contractile apparatus to the sarcolemma in skeletal muscle. Dystrophin gene mutations result in either a lack of dystrophin (usually DMD) or the expression of mutant forms of dystrophin (usually Becker muscular dystrophy).

Other Myopathies

Aside from DMD, myotonic dystrophy is the other muscular dystrophy which commonly leads to respiratory failure before adulthood. Myotonic dystrophy type I (Steinert disease) is a multisystem disease, which includes anomalies of the skeletal and smooth muscle as well as of the eye, central nervous system, heart, and endocrine system. Myotonic dystrophy type I follows a pattern of autosomal dominant inheritance and has a worldwide prevalence of 1:8000. The culprit mutation is an expansion of the cytosine-thymine-guanine (CTG) trinucleotide in the nontranslating region of the dystrophia myotonica protein kinase *(DMPK)* gene on chromosome 19. The highly variable phenotype, with an age of onset spanning from the prenatal period to adulthood, is closely related to the size of the CTG expansion, so that a longer expansion is responsible for a more severe phenotype.[5]

In addition, pulmonary function abnormalities and respiratory failure have been reported in metabolic myopathies as well as in the childhood form of limb girdle muscle dystrophy, facioscapulohumeral dystrophy, and Emery-Dreifuss syndrome.

DISORDERS INVOLVING THE BONY STRUCTURE OF THE CHEST WALL

Pectus Excavatum

Pectus excavatum is characterized by a symmetric or asymmetric depression of the sternum and anterior chest deemed to be due to defects in the sternum cartilage or overgrowth of the costal cartilage of the ribs. It is accompanied by an abnormally shallow chest in the anterior-posterior dimension in 60% of cases, described as a pectus gracilis.[6] Severity of the pectus excavatum is directly correlated with the severity of the pectus gracilis, raising the question as to whether the pectus excavatum is a thoracic as well as a sternal deformity. It occurs predominantly in white males, with an estimated incidence of 1 in every 300–400 live births and represents more than 90% of all congenital chest wall abnormalities. Its etiology remains unclear, although a genetic base is suggested by the observation that about one-fourth of patients have an affected family member. Pectus excavatum appears to be polygenetic, following various patterns of inheritance.[7] It is frequently associated with idiopathic scoliosis, and is a component of a number of connective tissue disorders, especially Marfan syndrome. Severe pectus excavatum can induce mild restrictive syndrome and can be associated with limitation in exercise tolerance.

Kyphoscoliosis

Scoliosis is the result of underlying pathological processes leading to lateral displacement in the coronal plane of the spine. Kyphosis describes the curvature of the spine in the sagittal plane, which curves the spine forward. There are children with major scoliosis and minor kyphosis and children with major kyphosis and minor scoliosis. Kyphoscoliosis is also associated with rotation of the spine, which contributes to spine deformity and distorts the thoracic cage. Kyphoscoliosis distorts the ribs, sternum, and respiratory muscles, as well as intrathoracic organ orientation.

Classification of Kyphoscoliosis. The age of onset and etiology are most often used to classify kyphoscoliosis in children. The most common form of scoliosis has its onset at the time of adolescence in otherwise healthy children. Less than 10% of spine deformities are those first diagnosed before 10 years of age, known as early onset scoliosis. The specific ages of different idiopathic scoliosis and the categories of etiologies that are nonidiopathic are listed in Box 72.3.

Box 72.3 Classification of Scoliosis

Idiopathic (85% of All Scoliosis)

- Infantile (<3 years old)
- Juvenile (3–9 years old)
- Adolescent (10 years old to skeletal maturity)

Congenital (5% of All Scoliosis)

- Failure of formation (hemivertebra(e))
- Failure of segmentation
- Mixed

Neuromuscular (5% of All Scoliosis)

- Neuropathic
- Lower motor neuron (e.g., poliomyelitis)
- Upper motor neuron (e.g., cerebral palsy)
- Other (e.g., syringomyelia)
- Myopathic
- Progressive (e.g., muscular dystrophy)
- Static (e.g., amyotonia)
- Others (e.g., Friedreich's ataxia)

Associated With Neurofibromatosis (Von Recklinghausen Disease)

Mesenchymal

- Congenital (e.g., Marfan syndrome)
- Acquired (e.g., rheumatoid disease)
- Others (e.g., juvenile apophysitis)

Traumatic

- Vertebral (e.g., fracture, radiation, surgery)
- Extravertebral (e.g., burns, thoracoplasty)
- Secondary to irritative phenomenon (e.g., spinal cord tumor)

Idiopathic Kyphoscoliosis. Idiopathic kyphoscoliosis is defined as a spine deformity without any overt malformations of the vertebral bodies or predisposing conditions leading to secondary spine deformity. Autosomal dominant, X-linked and multifactorial patterns of inheritance have been reported to account for the hereditary factors of the disease. Idiopathic scoliosis, which accounts for 80%–85% of cases, is further categorized into infantile, juvenile, and adolescent idiopathic scoliosis, depending on the age of onset.

Congenital Scoliosis. Congenital scoliosis is due to the presence of vertebral anomalies with or without associated rib deformities. Common malformations include single or multiple hemivertebrae and segmentation defects, which produce block vertebrae of variable length. Congenital scoliosis can be present at birth with associated pulmonary hypoplasia, or can be mild and diagnosed later in childhood. Congenital scoliosis is often accompanied by other congenital anomalies and represents one component of a multiorgan syndrome (e.g., VACTERL syndrome).

Respiratory Effects of Kyphoscoliosis. The respiratory effects of kyphoscoliosis vary with age of onset, initial severity, and progression of deformity over time. The degree of respiratory impairment is primarily due to the constraint of the lung by a relatively rigid thoracic cage related to the severity of the three-dimensional deformity of the spine. In addition, kyphoscoliosis can be responsible for a decrease in inspiratory muscle strength, as well as impaired lung growth.

The consequences of scoliosis on lung growth remain unclear. Postmortem quantitative studies among adolescents who died of severe kyphoscoliosis suggest that alveolar number and complexity are decreased in congenital or infantile scoliosis, whereas the alveoli may not enlarge normally in idiopathic juvenile or adolescent scoliosis. The number of pulmonary vessels in scoliotic children is also reduced in proportion to alveolar hypoplasia. Lung function studies have demonstrated a greater reduction in vital capacity for the same Cobb angle among children with early onset scoliosis compared to adolescent onset, raising the question of associated pulmonary hypoplasia in those with early onset spine disease. Pulmonary hypoplasia has recently been produced in rabbits that undergo iatrogenic scoliosis with postnatal rib tethering.[8] Pulmonary hypertension and cor pulmonale have been described in a small minority of children with spine and chest deformities, and this number may be even less when sleep-related breathing abnormalities are treated with oxygen or noninvasive positive pressure ventilation.

The term *"thoracic insufficiency syndrome"* has been used to identify those children with spine and chest wall disorders that impair lung function, or postnatal lung growth with skeletal immaturity and future bone growth.[9] The syndrome includes children with early onset scoliosis, regardless of etiology, which is sufficiently severe to impair lung function. Early onset scoliosis may become thoracic insufficiency syndrome as it progresses and as respiratory function becomes compromised over time. Clinical and/or objective measurements of lung function are needed to make this diagnosis.

Hypoplastic Thorax Syndromes

A variety of syndromes are associated with small thoraces leading to secondary respiratory failure in the first year of life and high mortality rates. These conditions represent a separate category of thoracic insufficiency syndrome. Hypoplasia can occur due to a reduced circumference or due to reduced thoracic vertebral height. There is a continuum of hypoplasia in most of these syndromes, so some patients live to adulthood without respiratory support.

Asphyxiating Thoracic Dystrophy. The most common hypoplastic thorax syndrome is asphyxiating thoracic dystrophy, also known as Jeune syndrome or thoracic-pelvic-phalangeal dystrophy. This autosomal recessive disorder is part of the ciliary chondrodysplasias, a group of inherited conditions resulting from cilia malfunction affecting skeletal development in mammals.[10] It is characterized by a narrow, hypoplastic rib cage, and generalized chondrodystrophy with short limb dwarfism. Pelvic and phalangeal abnormalities, polydactyly, renal, and hepatic disorders, thrombocytopenia as well as Shwachman syndrome have also been reported in conjunction with asphyxiating thoracic dystrophy, with renal disease emerging later in life as a serious concern. Estimates suggest that up to 600 patients per year are born with this disease worldwide.

Jarcho-Levin Syndrome. An alternative type of chest wall hypoplasia is illustrated by patients with Jarcho-Levin syndrome. This syndrome includes two distinct genetic disorders, spondylocostal dysostosis and spondylothoracic dysplasia, which present with multiple vertebral and costal anomalies. The vertebral anomalies result in a shortened spinal height

and increased anterior–posterior dimension albeit with a reduced intrathoracic volume.

Spondylocostal dysostosis is associated with mutations in the *DLL3* (delta-like canonical Notch ligand 3) gene, which is involved with the Notch pathway in separating future vertebrae from one another during early development (somite segmentation). It has both autosomal dominant and recessive inheritance patterns. *Spondylothoracic dysplasia* is associated with mutations in the *MESP2* (mesoderm posterior bHLH transcription factor 2) gene, which is of Puerto Rican heritage and controls activity of genes in the Notch pathway. It is inherited in an autosomal recessive manner.

Clinical Features

DIAPHRAGM PARALYSIS

Unilateral diaphragm paralysis is usually asymptomatic, but can lead to exercise limitation in some patients. When bilateral, the prominent clinical features include unexplained tachypnea, hypoxia, or respiratory distress, which usually worsen in the supine position. Respiratory failure or difficult weaning from ventilatory support after surgery can occur, especially in the neonate or when underlying pulmonary disease is present. In chronic cases, respiratory insufficiency, recurrent atelectasis and infections can be observed, as well as failure to thrive.

SPINAL MUSCULAR ATROPHIES

While there is no clear delineation of SMA subtypes, the clinical classification by age of onset and maximum function achieved is useful for prognosis and management.[11]

Spinal Muscular Atrophy Type I

In infants with SMA I (incidence ~1:10,000 live births), poor muscle tone and muscle weakness begin at age 0–6 months and are associated with a lack of motor development and an inability to sit without support. There is minimal or absent facial weakness, but fasciculation of the tongue is observed in most children. Tendon reflexes are absent. There is no sensory loss and cerebral function is normal, including intellect. A prenatal subtype with overt manifestations at birth occurs. Infants with prenatal SMA and SMA I have impaired head control, with a weak cry and cough. Intercostal muscle weakness is responsible for paradoxical inward rib cage movement with each inspiration, the diaphragm being relatively spared. Chest x-rays show a reduced intrathoracic volume and a bell-shaped thorax. Affected patients suffer from swallowing disorders and aspiration, and are at risk of recurrent respiratory failure with viral respiratory infections. The prognosis is poor, with 95% of infants dying from respiratory failure by the age of 18 months without intensive respiratory intervention.

Spinal Muscular Atrophy Type II

In children with SMA II, muscle weakness usually begins after the age of 6 months. The child can sit independently when placed in a sitting position, but cannot walk. Low muscle tone is present and tendon reflexes are absent in about two-thirds of children. They have average intellectual skills

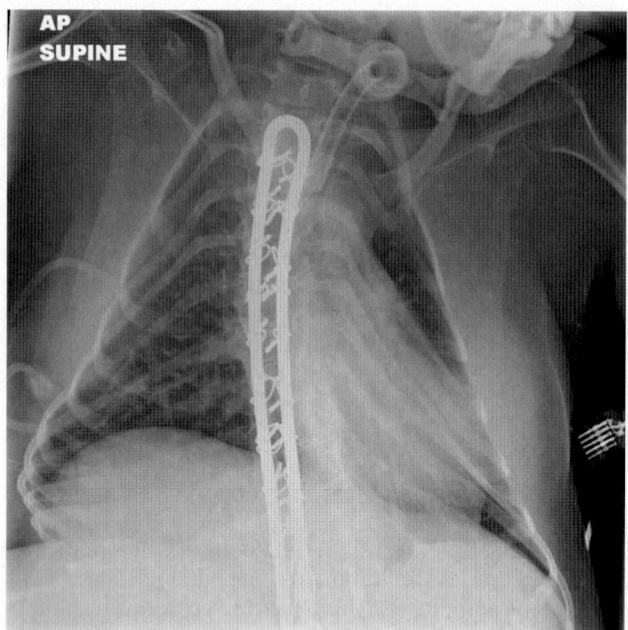

Fig. 72.2 "Closing parasol" appearance of the thorax in an SMA 2 patient with continuing chest wall collapse despite spinal surgery.

during the formative years and above average by adolescence. Swallowing disorders, gastric reflux, recurrent atelectasis, and respiratory infections vary in their degree of severity and carry the risk of respiratory failure. In the majority of older children, thoracic and thoracolumbar scoliosis further aggravates respiratory function. Even after the spine is fused and stabilized, the chest wall can continue to collapse, producing the appearance of a closing parasol (Fig. 72.2). Typically, recurrent pulmonary infections precede nocturnal hypoxemia, nocturnal hypoventilation, and then daytime hypoventilation. With adequate respiratory management tailored to respiratory involvement, including noninvasive ventilation, mechanical in-exsufflation, and the prevention of respiratory infections, a good quality of life and lifespan into adulthood is expected for most patients.[11]

Spinal Muscular Atrophy Type III

Patients with SMA III usually present with proximal limb weakness after the age of 10 months. The legs are more severely affected than the arms; they are able to walk at least 25 meters, but frequently fall or have trouble walking up and down stairs at the age of 2–3 years. Respiratory involvement is usually minimal, and a normal lifespan is expected.

NEUROMUSCULAR JUNCTION DISEASES

Pediatric myasthenia is a group of rare disorders due to anomalies of the neuromuscular junction. Three subtypes are generally recognized: juvenile myasthenia gravis, congenital myasthenia gravis, and congenital myasthenic syndromes.[12]

Juvenile Myasthenia Gravis

Juvenile myasthenia gravis (JMG) may present at any age during childhood, even as early as 6 months. It is characterized by fatigable muscle weakness, which improves with rest.

While ocular JMG mainly presents with ptosis, ophthalmoplegia or diplopia, JMG can present with swallowing difficulties and dysphonia, or as a more generalized form consisting of generalized progressive weakness in all muscles, and abnormal fatigability on exertion, which improves with rest. Severe generalized disease can cause a progressive decrease in respiratory muscle strength, leading to a restrictive lung pattern. Myasthenia gravis crisis with life-threatening respiratory involvement can also be triggered by infections, stress, or certain drugs.

Neonatal Myasthenia Gravis

Neonatal myasthenia gravis usually presents within hours of birth with feeding and respiratory difficulties, hypotonia, weak cry, facial weakness, and ptosis. Respiratory difficulties are related to feeding problems causing aspiration pneumonia, upper airway obstruction due to the inability to handle pharyngeal secretions, plus respiratory muscle weakness and fatigability.

Congenital Myasthenic Syndromes

Congenital myasthenic syndromes are characterized by a wide spectrum in terms of age of onset. With early neonatal onset, clinical features can mimic neonatal myasthenia gravis and lead to respiratory failure with sudden apnea, or patients may present with bilateral vocal cord paralysis. Other types beginning after the neonatal period are characterized not only by usually mild symptoms but also by sudden exacerbations of muscle weakness and respiratory failure, which can be triggered by infections or stress. Some cases have been reported to mimic congenital myopathies, muscular dystrophies, or metabolic myopathies.

MYOPATHIES

Duchenne Muscular Dystrophy

DMD presents in boys with proximal muscle weakness at 2–4 years of age. The progression is fairly rapid, with the patient becoming confined to a wheelchair at around 10–12 years of age, requiring spine fusion for scoliosis in early adolescence. In the early phases of the disease, when the gait is still preserved, respiratory function is essentially normal, although a loss in the strength of the respiratory muscles can be readily shown. Impairment of respiratory function is accelerated by the loss of ambulation. Every patient with DMD experiences a maximum plateau in absolute vital capacity between the ages of 10 and 12 years, and a progressive decrease thereafter. Patients with DMD present a restrictive syndrome due to muscle weakness and contractures, spinal deformity, vertebro-costal joint ankylosis, and frequent obesity. The first sign of chronic respiratory failure is nocturnal hypoventilation, which can be aggravated by obstructive sleep-disordered breathing, a frequent occurrence in patients with DMD, even in the first decade.[13] Premature death has been reported at a median age of 19 years or a mean age of 17.7 years (range 11.6–27.5) in patients without ventilatory support. The use of ventilatory support, together with early, aggressive management of respiratory infections, has been shown to prolong life. A median age of 27.0 years and a mean age of 27.9 years (range 23–38.6) for death have been reported in patients with ventilator support.[14,15] Given that prolonged survival to adult age in patients with DMD is mainly due to better respiratory care, pediatric pulmonologists must be aware of how quality of life is affected by this chronic disease. While there is agreement on decreased physical aspects of health-related quality of life, conclusions of recent studies are conflicting with regard to psychosocial areas, ranging from preservation[16] and satisfaction with overall quality of life[17] to poor health-related and global quality of life.[18] Cultural differences may explain part of this discrepancy. However, the fact that patients with DMD are heterogeneous in relation to neuropsychosocial and neurobehavioral functioning, due to the lack of dystrophin normally present in a number of brain areas,[19] likely explains part of the literature discrepancy on quality of life.

Myotonic Dystrophy

Myotonia and muscle weakness are the prominent clinical features of myotonic dystrophy, although a number of other organ systems can be affected (cataracts, cardiac dysrhythmias, sleep disorders and hypersomnia, cognitive deficit, frontal balding and endocrine disorders). Involvement of the respiratory system contributes substantially to morbidity and mortality.

Congenital Myotonic Dystrophy. Congenital myotonic dystrophy has a prevalence of ~1/47,000.[5] Newborns with this severe phenotype typically present with generalized hypotonia and immobility, contractures, bilateral talipes, facial dysmorphia, and weak cry, along with respiratory and feeding difficulties. Myotonia is absent. Thin ribs and right diaphragmatic elevation can be observed on chest x-ray. Diagnostic suspicion is increased by examining the mother, who often presents mild weakness of eyelid closure and more or less overt grip myotonia. Genetic testing confirms the diagnosis. Polyhydramnios, prematurity, hydrops fetalis with pleural effusions and pulmonary hypoplasia can increase respiratory difficulties due to diaphragmatic weakness at birth. Important respiratory difficulties with a need for ventilatory support are present in 50% of cases and are responsible for neonatal death in approximately 30% of patients. The condition usually improves in early childhood, although features of the classic disease gradually appear in late childhood or adolescence. If ventilatory support is needed beyond 4 weeks of life in the neonatal period, the prognosis is poor, with the risk of sudden death in survivors, even without apparent respiratory exacerbation.

Childhood-Onset Myotonic Dystrophy. Childhood-onset myotonic dystrophy begins between ages of 1 and 10 years and mainly affects cognition, muscle strength, and respiratory, central nervous, and gastrointestinal systems. *Juvenile myotonic dystrophy type I* begins between 10 and 20 years.[5] Although expiratory muscle weakness has been shown in children and adolescents, a true restrictive syndrome is commonly reported in adult patients only and chronic respiratory failure is rare before late adulthood. However, weakness of the respiratory and swallowing muscle renders patients with myotonic dystrophy type I prone to repeated aspiration pneumonias and pulmonary infections as well as postanesthetic failure. Sleep disorders often represent a significant issue, with 50% of children and adolescents complaining of excessive daytime sleepiness. The latter has been blamed on sleep

fragmentation secondary to central hypoventilation and/or obstructive apneas that have been reported in 30% of children with myotonic dystrophy type I, and can occur concurrently with periodic leg movement disorder and REM sleep dysregulation.[15] Obesity or adenotonsillar hypertrophy can act as aggravating factors.

RESPIRATORY FUNCTION TESTING IN NEUROMUSCULAR DISEASES

Respiratory function must be assessed annually in children with neuromuscular disorders. Routine measurements of lung function usually include spirometry, static lung volumes, maximal inspiratory pressure (or sniff inspiratory pressure) and maximal expiratory pressure, peak cough flow, and gas exchange. Although advocated by some teams, the measurement of esophageal pressure is not commonly used in clinical practice. When below 80% in the sitting position, vital capacity should also be measured in the supine position, to investigate for diaphragm weakness (defined by a decrease in vital capacity >20% from the sitting position). Peak cough flow values under 160–200 L/min in adolescents and adults indicate that cough is ineffective and could place patients at risk of recurrent respiratory infections and respiratory failure. Corresponding reference values in younger children are now available.[20,21]

Overnight polysomnography or combined pulse oximetry and transcutaneous/end tidal arterial pressure of carbon dioxide (PCO_2) should be performed annually in children, especially when vital capacity is less than 60%. The relevance of performing polysomnography, when available, stems from the recognition that sleep-disordered breathing is frequent, even before the loss of ambulation, and includes not only diaphragm weakness-related alveolar hypoventilation but also obstructive apneas.[13,22–24] In DMD patients, an inspiratory vital capacity of less than 60% or 40% has been found to be both sensitive and specific for sleep-disordered breathing and nocturnal hypoventilation, respectively.[13]

DISORDERS INVOLVING THE BONY STRUCTURE OF THE CHEST WALL

Pectus Excavatum

Most patients with pectus excavatum (PEx) do not present any symptoms at rest. Although they frequently complain of a limited ability to exercise due to dyspnea or chest pain, studies on the association between pulmonary function and PEx have yielded conflicting results. A multicenter study of 310 patients aged between 6 and 21 years reported that pulmonary function was related to the depth of the depression, so that patients with severe PEx with a Haller score (ratio of the transverse to the anteroposterior diameter of the thorax measured on a computed tomography [CT] scan) greater than 5 were more likely to display a mild restrictive defect on lung function.[25] In addition, severe PEx is responsible for causing compression and displacement of the heart, resulting in distortion of normal cardiac geometry, which, in turn, restricts right ventricular filling during diastole. Some patients with PEx also demonstrate reduced systolic contractility, which can be segmental or global.[26] Although there is a lack of definitive evidence that the mild impairments in lung and cardiac function reported in PEx patients are responsible for the frequent complaint of exercise limitation, a recent communication has reported decreased cardiopulmonary adaptation to exercise, which was proportional to the severity of PEx.[27]

Kyphoscoliosis

Although the natural history of scoliosis is one of curve progression, cardiopulmonary impairment, back pain, cosmetic deformity, poor balance, and neurological compromise, the condition varies greatly, depending on specific etiology, the age of onset, the genetic background, and the curve pattern. Adults whose scoliosis is first diagnosed before 8 years of age have a higher mortality rate than the general population after the age of 40 years.

Radiographic measurements of the structural severity of spine curves include the angle of displacement on an anterior–posterior spine radiograph, known as the Cobb angle, and the degree of kyphosis and lordosis of the spine in the lateral projection. Each curve can vary according to the site of the curve's apex (cervical, high thoracic, thoracic, thoracolumbar, lumbar) and the number of curves (single or double) as well as the number of vertebrae involved. In addition, the spine rotates with the angle of rotation greatest at the apex of the Cobb angle. Given that kyphoscoliosis is a three-dimensional deformity, two-dimensional structural descriptors, such as the Cobb angle, do not correlate well with respiratory functional measurements at any age.[28]

Adolescent Idiopathic Scoliosis.
In the general school population, the prevalence of adolescent idiopathic scoliosis with a curve greater than 10 degrees is 2%–3%, dropping to 0.5% and 0.2% for curves greater than 20 degrees and 30 degrees, respectively. Untreated adolescents with severe idiopathic scoliosis followed over a 50-year period have been shown to have a mortality rate 2.2 times greater than controls. These deaths generally occur in the fourth or fifth decade of life, due to cardiopulmonary insufficiency. Most of the survivors show significant physical disability characterized by dyspnea, back pain, and exercise limitation.

Infantile Idiopathic Scoliosis.
Infantile idiopathic scoliosis in untreated children followed to maturity may progress to become a severe and crippling deformity, with a Cobb angle that can exceed 70 degrees. Spontaneous regression of idiopathic scoliosis is uncommon, although progression does not always occur. The greatest risks for progression occur during rapid somatic growth (e.g., the adolescent growth spurt).

Congenital Scoliosis.
Congenital scoliosis is usually progressive and, if untreated, results in severe spinal deformity. The ultimate severity of the curve depends on both the type of anomaly and the site at which it occurs. The most progressive of all anomalies is a unilateral unsegmented bar combined with single or multiple convex hemi-vertebrae on the contralateral side with or without associated fused ribs. At an early stage of the disease, scoliosis is generally painless and asymptomatic. While restrictive lung disease is detectable when the Cobb angle is greater than 50–60 degrees, a Cobb angle greater than 90 degrees greatly predisposes the patient to cardiorespiratory failure.

Respiratory Function Testing in Kyphoscoliosis.
The degree of restrictive lung disease in a child with kyphoscoliosis is related to the severity of the three-dimensional deformity of the spine. In adolescent idiopathic scoliosis, multiple structural features of the spine, when used in combination, account for 14%–18% of the variation in lung function in populations of affected children.[29] Reduction in chest wall compliance, and thus, lack of chest wall excursion, impaired lung growth, and decreased inspiratory muscle strength due to chest deformity, also account for reductions in vital capacity and other lung volumes. In addition, most imaging is static and does not measure motion over time. Dynamic magnetic resonance imaging (MRI) methods are currently being developed for motion imaging.

FVC is most sensitive to reductions in both thoracic cage size and chest wall compliance as well as inspiratory and expiratory respiratory muscle dysfunction. Residual volume (RV) is reduced less (as a percent of predicted value) than vital capacity. This may explain the elevated residual volume (RV)/total lung capacity (TLC) ratio reported in patients with scoliosis. Airway resistance may be normal or slightly increased, due to main stem bronchial distortion associated with chest deformity. This occurs in up to 10% of patients with adolescent idiopathic scoliosis and up to 30% of children with early onset scoliosis.[30] In children with obstructive lung disease and scoliosis, more common etiologies for airway obstruction (e.g., asthma) should be investigated. Absolute values of spirometric lung functions are normalized as a percentage of predicted values based on arm spans or length of specific bones (e.g., ulnar length), since height is directly influenced by spine curvature. Nutritional values, such as body mass index, must also be corrected using these surrogates for height. Ventilation and lung perfusion scans demonstrate right–left lung functional imbalance in up to 50% of children with early onset scoliosis (EOS). However, the side that is least functional cannot be determined by an antero-posterior chest film. Ventilation and perfusion usually match well in the absence of additional pulmonary diseases. There is seldom significant alteration of blood gases in patients with kyphoscoliosis and a Cobb angle of less than 60 degrees. Nocturnal alveolar hypoventilation has been observed in patients with a Cobb angle greater than 60 degrees, and cardiorespiratory failure can be present in the most severe patients with a Cobb angle greater than 90 degrees. The Apnea-Hypopnea Index is usually increased in children with EOS irrespective of CO_2 elevation due to recurrent oxyhemoglobin desaturation associated with hypopneas.[28] Apnea *per se* is a rare event and should signal other etiologies (e.g., tonsillar and adenoidal enlargement) in children with spine and chest wall deformities. Patients with moderate to severe scoliosis, and obesity or neuromuscular weakness in particular, should therefore be evaluated with nocturnal polysomnography or, if not available, at least with oximetry and PCO_2 recorded during sleep.

Hypoplastic Thorax Syndromes

Asphyxiating Thoracic Dystrophy.
Asphyxiating thoracic dystrophy is usually diagnosed immediately after birth when the thoracic circumference is found to be less than 75% of head circumference and the infant is tachypneic. If untreated,

most infants with asphyxiating thoracic dystrophy die within the first year of life due to respiratory failure. Less severe variants have been reported with clinical courses that vary from respiratory failure in infancy to few or no respiratory symptoms at all. In those patients who survive the neonatal period, respiratory failure may occur later during infancy and childhood because of chest constriction, impaired lung growth, and superimposed pneumonia. Improvement in bone abnormalities may occur with age, thereby justifying life-support procedures in early life, such as long-term mechanical ventilation.

Jarcho-Levin Syndrome. Clinical features of both spondylocostal dysostosis and spondylothoracic dysplasia include a shortened thoracic height due to vertebral anomalies; however, congenital scoliosis is present (in spondylocostal dysostosis only). Spondylothoracic dysplasia is more severe and can present with respiratory distress in the neonatal period, with up to one-third of children dying of respiratory failure in the first year of life.[31] Lung function in adults with either form of Jarcho-Levin syndrome reflects severe restrictive changes, including tachypnea and a vital capacity of less than 30% predicted values.

Diagnosis

DIAPHRAGM PARALYSIS

On chest x-ray, unilateral paralysis of the right hemidiaphragm should be suspected if it is more than two rib spaces higher than the left hemidiaphragm; on the left side, it results in an elevation of the hemidiaphragm of at least one rib space above the right hemidiaphragm. Contralateral mediastinal shift also can be observed in severe cases. Fluoroscopy with a sniff test and ultrasonography in a spontaneously breathing patient show a paradoxical inspiratory upward motion of the paralyzed hemidiaphragm compared to the contralateral side. Electromyography in association with percutaneous stimulation of the phrenic nerve can confirm the paralysis. *Repeated* evaluations by fluoroscopy, ultrasonography, or electromyography can aid in assessing diaphragmatic function.

SPINAL MUSCULAR ATROPHIES

The diagnosis of SMA is established in children with motor difficulties, physical signs of motor unit disease and mutations in the *SMN1* gene.[11]

In addition to the clinical classification of SMA subtypes, the diagnosis of SMA is based on molecular genetic testing. About 95%–98% of individuals with SMA are homozygous for a deletion (lack of exon 7 in both copies of *SMN1* genes) or gene conversion of *SMN1* to *SMN2*. A number of *SMN2* copies of three or more is associated with a milder phenotype.

If molecular genetic testing of *SMN1* does not identify mutations, additional tests can be used. Electromyography reveals denervation and diminished motor action potential amplitude. Motor and sensory nerve conduction velocities are normal. Muscle biopsy reveals group atrophy of type 1 and type 2 muscle fibers.

NEUROMUSCULAR JUNCTION DISEASES

Juvenile Myasthenia Gravis

Diagnosis of JMG relies on the following: clinical symptoms, a transient improvement upon administration of the anticholinesterase medication edrophonium chloride (Tensilon), abnormal electrophysiological studies (including an abnormal response to repetitive stimulation during nerve conduction study), anomalies of single fiber electromyography, and a positive test for circulating AChR autoantibodies.

Neonatal Myasthenia Gravis

The diagnosis of neonatal myasthenia gravis is made on the presence of myasthenia gravis in the mother, a transient improvement in clinical symptoms after the administration of edrophonium chloride or neostigmine, and the presence of circulating antibodies against acetylcholine receptors.

Congenital Myasthenic Syndromes

Diagnosis relies on family history, clinical myasthenic findings, the absence of circulating AChR antibodies, the stimulation single fiber electromyography, and a positive response to pyridostigmine or the detection of one of the known mutations.

MYOPATHIES

Duchenne Muscular Dystrophy

The frequent findings of delayed muscle function, speech delay, and elevated serum CK concentration (most often 50–100 times the reference range) in a young boy are highly suggestive of DMD. Molecular genetic testing from peripheral blood samples can establish the diagnosis of dystrophinopathy in nearly all individuals with DMD or Becker muscular dystrophy. The correct genetic diagnosis is crucial for DMD patients in order to provide both the optimal care to the patient and genetic counseling to the family, according to published guidelines.[32] In addition, with mutation-specific therapies under development for DMD, a specific genetic diagnosis is also important for assessing whether patients are eligible for treatments.

A stepwise approach for genetic analysis is currently recommended, searching first for large deletions and duplications in the *DMD* gene, which are present in ~70% of the patients; the multiplex ligation-dependent probe amplification technique is the most reliable method for this purpose. If a whole exon mutation or deletion is not found, the next step is to perform exon sequencing to search for a smaller mutation on 1 of the 79 exons of the *DMD* gene (~20% of cases). Lastly, if no mutations are found, next-generation sequencing approaches, such as whole exome sequencing, are needed to complete the genetic testing. Finally, in the exceptional cases where genetic testing is negative, dystrophin protein analysis may be necessary to make the diagnosis from muscle biopsy.

Myotonic Dystrophy

The diagnosis is established by identification of a heterozygous pathogenic variant in the *DMPK* gene on chromosome 19, using a targeted analysis for an expansion of the CTG trinucleotide repeat in *DMPK*.

DISORDERS INVOLVING THE BONY STRUCTURE OF THE CHEST WALL

Kyphoscoliosis

Kyphoscoliosis is diagnosed initially by physical features of a posterior rib hump, uneven shoulder height, or abnormal posture. Delineation of the type of scoliosis and the vertebrae and ribs involved requires imaging, initially with an anterior-posterior and lateral view of the entire spine. Further imaging, such as a MRI, of the spine is needed to detect spinal cord and canal disorders, such as syringomyelia and tethered spinal cord. A CT scan of the spine and thorax with three-dimensional reconstruction may help to develop surgical strategies. Of note, diagnosing the structural deformity does not describe respiratory function. Functional severity of kyphoscoliosis should be performed in concert with the structural assessment.

Hypoplastic Thorax Syndromes

Hypoplastic thoraces may be obvious or subtle at birth. Severe abnormalities are apparent on physical examination. Imaging of the chest wall will reveal abnormal contours. The heart may look abnormally large in a small chest. Lung volumes may be low due to pulmonary hypoplasia. CT imaging of the spine and thorax is helpful where primary vertebral and costo-vertebral abnormalities (i.e., Jarcho-Levin syndrome) are suspected. Abnormal rib structure, including fused ribs, is also identified with CT scanning and three-dimensional image reconstruction. Recently, gender-specific correlations between pelvic dimensions, spine height, and chest wall dimensions have been made, and norms have been published.[33]

Asphyxiating Thoracic Dystrophy. Characteristic chest x-ray findings reveal a narrow chest cage, with high-positioned clavicles, short horizontal ribs, and flaring of the costochondral junctions (Fig. 72.3A). The CT scan is characteristic with a four-leaf clover appearance due to foreshortened ribs (see Fig. 72.3B). The lungs are constrained by the chest and are elongated in the process.

Jarcho-Levin Syndrome. The diagnosis is made from characteristic spine and rib abnormalities on spine films and CT scan of the thorax. In spondylocostal dysostosis, broadening, bifurcation, and fusion of the ribs, as well as congenital scoliosis, are seen (Fig. 72.4). In spondylothoracic dysplasia, ribs are symmetrically fused bilaterally at the costo-vertebral junctions, producing a crablike appearance to the thoracic skeleton (see Fig. 72.5).[34]

Management

GENERAL MANAGEMENT OF CHILDREN WITH CHEST WALL DYSFUNCTION

Adequate nutrition is essential for ensuring adequate functioning of the respiratory muscles. Patients with a chronic condition, such as severe DMD, are commonly malnourished, a state that can lead to muscle atrophy and loss of respiratory muscle capacity to perform the work of breathing. An adequate O_2 supply and the correction of electrolytic imbalance (hypophosphatemia, hypocalcemia, hypokalemia, acidosis) are also needed for muscles to perform their work.

Associated nonrelated respiratory problems, such as asthma, allergic rhinitis, enlarged adenoids, and tonsils causing sleep-disordered breathing, must be carefully investigated and treated. Prevention of respiratory infections must be implemented by ensuring an optimal environment (e.g.,

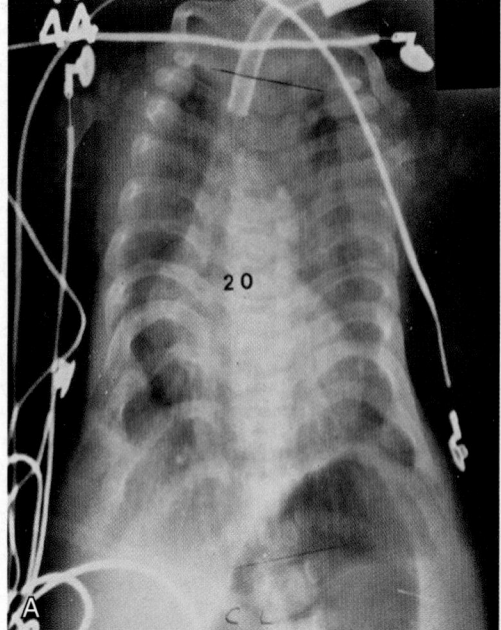
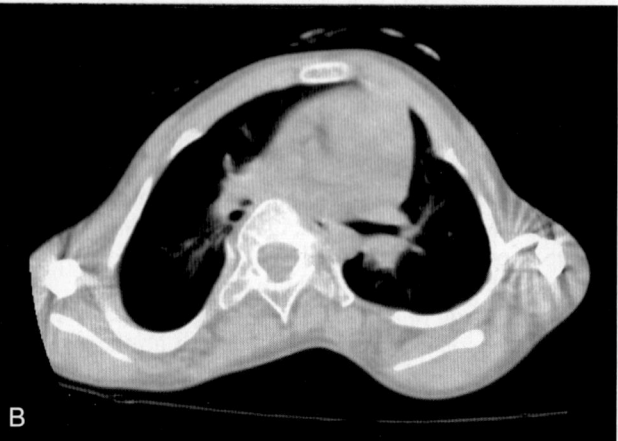

Fig. 72.3 Imaging features of asphyxiating thoracic dystrophy. (A) Chest radiograph of an intubated infant with asphyxiating thoracic dystrophy showing the narrow chest cage with high-positioned-clavicles, short horizontal ribs and flaring of the costochondral junctions. (B) Features of shortened ribs that curve inward toward the cardiac borders in a "four-leaf clover" appearance on computerized tomography of a child with asphyxiating thoracic dystrophy.

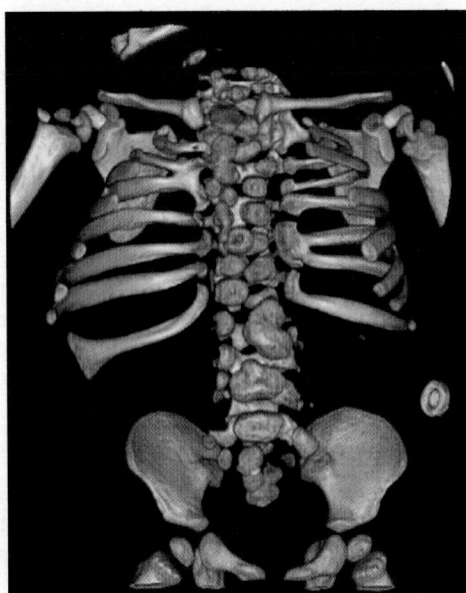

Fig. 72.4 Reconstructive computed tomography scan of a child with Jarcho-Levin syndrome—subset spondylocostal dysostosis. Vertebral and asymmetric rib anomalies are seen. The thorax is foreshortened with few normal thoracic vertebrae.

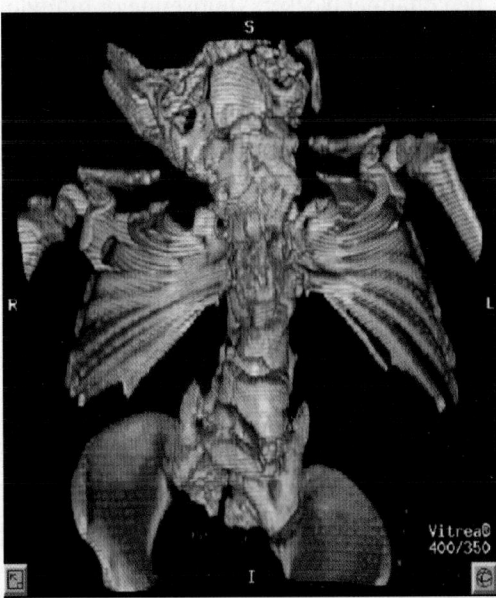

Fig. 72.5 Reconstructive computed tomography scan of a 2-year-old patient with spondylothoracic dysplasia—subset spondylothoracic dysplasia. Note the symmetrically fused ribs at the costo-vertebral angle, producing the characteristic "fan" or "crab" appearance. (Reproduced with permission from Cornier AS, Ramirez N, Carlo S, et al. Controversies surrounding Jarcho-Levin syndrome. *Curr Opin Pediatr.* 2003;15:614–620.)

avoidance of passive smoking and large daycare centers) and by providing pneumococcal and annual flu vaccination.

Respiratory muscle training is clearly beneficial in specific conditions where respiratory muscles are intact, such as in quadriplegic patients, following spinal cord injury. However, it must be used with caution in myopathies in order to avoid further muscle injury; in such cases, swimming and aquatic sports can be recommended without reaching fatigue threshold, as long as it is physically possible.

The daily use of assisted cough with lung recruitment techniques, either manually or through the use of an insufflation-exsufflation device, is of paramount importance in the management of patients with severe neuromuscular problems, especially during respiratory infections. In addition, ventilatory support has become an essential tool for increasing quality of life and prolonging life in severely affected patients with neuromuscular disorders by resting weakened respiratory muscles.[35] The development of noninvasive intermittent positive pressure using BiPAP ventilation *via* nasal mask during nocturnal sleep has been especially instrumental in this regard. Current consensus suggests that noninvasive nocturnal ventilatory support is indicated for patients with alveolar hypoventilation,[36] and should be discussed in the presence of failure to thrive or recurrent chest infections (more than three per year). In addition, nocturnal ventilatory support can be indicated in the presence of obstructive sleep-disordered breathing.[13] While most experts state that noninvasive mask ventilation is generally preferred, tracheostomy for ventilatory support should be considered in patients with bulbar involvement and severe retention of secretions despite assisted cough techniques, and those with extreme ventilator dependency or ineffective noninvasive ventilation.[36] Of note, however, the use of tracheostomy poses ethical dilemmas in patients with very severe disease and short life expectancy, as in SMA type I, where treatment burden must not outweigh the benefits.[37]

DIAPHRAGM PARALYSIS

Treatment of diaphragmatic paralysis caused by phrenic nerve impairment primarily depends on the presence of respiratory symptoms. Asymptomatic diaphragmatic paralysis does not require any therapy. Treatment for symptomatic cases first consists of ventilatory support, when needed. Surgical plication is generally indicated in the presence of persistent or recurrent respiratory symptoms, and is more often needed in infants than in older children. The optimal timing for surgery in the neonate or child with diaphragmatic paralysis is controversial. Waiting for spontaneous recovery in symptomatic patients can be associated with significant morbidity, especially in high-risk patients on ventilatory support. Recommendations for such patients vary from immediate repair to waiting 2–4 weeks for signs of spontaneous recovery. The use of video-assisted thoracoscopic surgery for diaphragm plication decreases the morbidity associated with traditional open thoracotomy. Long-term intermittent positive pressure ventilation, usually using BiPAP via a nasal mask, is useful in the most severe cases of bilateral diaphragmatic paralysis.

SPINAL MUSCULAR ATROPHIES

Spinal Muscular Atrophy Type I

Respiratory management for patients with SMA I raises important and unresolved ethical concerns and varies between countries and institutions. Any therapeutic intervention must aim at increasing the quality of life of the child and must be preceded by information to the family on both the burden of treatment and the grim prognosis. According to the Consensus Statement for Standard of Care in SMA,[11] palliative care or proactive respiratory interventions, which include noninvasive ventilation and insufflation-exsufflation, are usually offered and determined by parental choice in North America. Infants treated by noninvasive ventilation have been shown to survive longer (over half were alive at 4 years of age), albeit at the expense of hospitalizations and a burden of respiratory care that increases with time.[38] A growing number of publications, especially from Europe, defend that it is usually more in the interest of the child to include him/her in a palliative care program that includes aspiration of secretions, nasogastric feeding, nasal oxygen, and morphine/sedation to alleviate dyspnea, without noninvasive ventilation, aside from transient ventilation if needed to facilitate extubation.[39,40] If proactive respiratory support is offered, most experts will recommend noninvasive ventilation over tracheotomy in patients with SMA I, due to the complete loss of spontaneous breathing capability and the impossibility of language development usually associated with tracheotomy. Importantly, a written care plan must be decided in advance with the parents with regard to resuscitation and intubation/ventilation in case of a reversible acute event, such as a respiratory infection.

Spinal Muscular Atrophy Type II

Spinal muscular atrophy type II requires adequate respiratory management tailored to respiratory involvement, including noninvasive ventilation, mechanical in-exsufflation, and prevention of respiratory infections. A good quality of life and lifespan into adulthood is expected for most patients.[11]

Spinal Muscular Atrophy Type III

Patients with SMA III usually have minimal respiratory involvement, which does not require ventilatory support, or only in adult life.

Perspectives for Drug Therapy in Patients With Spinal Muscular Atrophy

The availability of new animal models of SMA (particularly mouse models) has significantly contributed to our understanding of the basic mechanisms, which has translated into several phase 1 and 2 clinical trials. While all patients with SMA have a mutated, unproductive *SMN1* gene, they also retain one to four copies of the *SMN2* gene, which mainly encodes a truncated SMN protein that cannot ensure motor neuron survival. Two promising strategies are currently being tested in clinical trials, aiming at SMN upregulation through either gene therapy or the modulation of SMN2 preRNA splicing. With regard to gene therapy, adeno-associated virus serotype 9 (*AAV9*)-mediated *SMN* gene delivery to motor neurons via systemic injection is currently being tested in a phase 1 clinical trial in patients with SMA I. Modulation of SMN2 splicing is obtained by using antisense oligonucleotides designed to allow the expression of the normally silenced exon 7 in *SMN2*. Two phase 3, randomized, double-blind studies are currently under way to assess efficacy and safety of intrathecal injection of an antisense oligonucleotide in infants with early onset, as well as in children with later-onset, SMA. In addition, further phase 1 clinical trials are currently using small molecules to modify SMN2 splicing.[41]

MANAGEMENT OF NEUROMUSCULAR JUNCTION DISEASES

Juvenile Myasthenia Gravis

The management of JMG is primarily based on anticholinesterase medication (pyridostigmine bromide). However, improvement with such medication is usually incomplete and most patients require further therapeutic measures, such as prednisone and consideration of thymectomy. During acute exacerbations of the disease, or in the course of respiratory complications, respiratory support may be required for various lengths of time (a few days to several weeks), in association with short-term immunotherapy, including intravenous immunoglobulins and plasmapheresis.

Neonatal Myasthenia Gravis

Management relies on pyridostigmine as well as adequate feeding and respiratory support until spontaneous remittance of muscle weakness occurs. Total and definitive resolution occurs within 2–8 weeks.

Congenital Myasthenic Syndromes

Depending on the subtype, treatment for congenital myasthenic syndromes includes cholinesterase inhibitors, such as pyridostigmine, the potassium channel blocker 3,4-DAP, AChR open channel blockers (fluoxetine or quinidine) and beta-2-adrenergic receptor agonists (ephedrine and salbutamol). Importantly, salbutamol or ephedrine, alone or combined with other drugs, is increasingly reported as beneficial for many subtypes of congenital myasthenic syndromes.[4]

MANAGEMENT OF MYOPATHIES

Duchenne Muscular Dystrophy

The natural history of DMD has been profoundly altered by treatment, particularly respiratory care, and more recently by the use of corticosteroids.

Long-Term Management of Respiratory Disability. Given that death is most often related to respiratory insufficiency, a key component of the management of patients with DMD is directed at slowing down the progression of respiratory insufficiency, while ensuring good quality of life. In the first decade, prevention of respiratory infections, undertaking regular submaximal exercise, and the treatment of any associated respiratory problems (e.g., asthma or obstructive sleep apnea due to adenotonsillar hypertrophy) are mandatory and sufficient. Loss of ambulation coincides with the onset of progressively increasing respiratory problems. At some time during the second decade, loss of respiratory muscle strength will lead to recommending the use of lung volume recruitment maneuvers (either by a self-inflating bag or mechanical in-exsufflation)[42] and "respiratory aids," namely assisted cough techniques (either manually or by mechanical in-exsufflation) and noninvasive ventilation. Consensus recommendations on when to use these techniques in patients with DMD are detailed in Box 72.4. While nasal mask ventilation with BiPAP is most often used for nocturnal ventilation, an oral interface with a volume-cycled ventilator is usually the most appropriate device for providing, on demand, daytime assisted ventilation. Many patients with

Box 72.4   Consensus on Respiratory Care in Duchenne Muscular Dystrophy

Step 1: Volume Recruitment/Deep Lung Inflation Technique

- Volume recruitment/deep lung inflation technique (by self-inflating manual ventilation bag or mechanical in-/ex-sufflation) when FVC < 40% predicted

Step 2: Manual and Mechanically Assisted Cough Techniques

Necessary when:
- Respiratory infection present and baseline peak cough flow <270 lpm[a]
- Baseline peak cough flow <160 lpm or max expiratory pressure <40 cm water
- Baseline FVC < 40% predicted OR < 1.25 L in older teen/adult

Step 3: Nocturnal Ventilation[b]

Nocturnal ventilation[c] is indicated in patients who have any of the following:
- Signs or symptoms of hypoventilation (patients with FVC < 30% predicted are at especially high risk)
- A baseline SpO_2 < 95% and/or blood or end-tidal pCO_2 > 45 mm Hg while awake
- An apnea-hypnea index >10/h on polysomnography OR four or more episodes of SpO_2 < 92% OR drops in SpO_2 of at least 4%/h of sleep

Step 4: Daytime Ventilation

In patients already using nocturnally assisted ventilation, daytime ventilation[d] is indicated for:

- Self-extension of nocturnal ventilation into waking hours
- Abnormal deglutition due to dyspnea, which is relieved by ventilatory assistance
- Inability to speak a full sentence without breathlessness, and/or
- Symptoms of hypoventilation with baseline SpO_2 < 95% and/or blood or end-tidal pCO_2 > 45 mm Hg while awake.

Continuous noninvasive assisted ventilation (along with mechanically assisted cough) can facilitate endotracheal extubation for patients who were intubated during acute illness or during anesthesia, followed by weaning to nocturnal noninvasive assisted ventilation, if applicable

Step 5: Tracheostomy

Indications for tracheostomy include:
- Patient and clinician preference[e]
- Patient cannot successfully use noninvasive ventilation
- Inability of the local medical infrastructure to support noninvasive ventilation
- Three failures to achieve extubation during critical illness despite optimal use of noninvasive ventilation and mechanically assisted cough
- The failure of noninvasive methods of cough assistance to prevent aspiration of secretions into the lung and drops in oxygen saturation below 95% or the patient's baseline, necessitating frequent direct tracheal suctioning via tracheostomy

[a]All specified threshold values of peak cough flow and maximum expiratory pressure apply to older teenage and adult parents.
[b]Note: Optimally, use of lung volume recruitment and assisted cough techniques should always precede initiation of noninvasive ventilation.
[c]Recommended for nocturnal use: noninvasive ventilation with pressure cycled bi-level devices or volume cycled ventilators or combination volume pressure ventilators. In bi-level or pressure support modes of ventilation, add a back-up rate of breathing. Recommended interfaces include: a nasal mask or a nasal pillow. Other interfaces can be used and each has its own potential benefits.
[d]Recommended for day use: noninvasive ventilation with portable volume cycled or volume-pressure ventilators; bi-level devices are an alternative. A mouthpiece interface is strongly recommended during day use of portable volume-cycled or volume-pressure ventilators, but other ventilator-interface combinations can be used based on clinician preference and patient comfort.
[e]Note, however, that the panel advocates for the long-term use of noninvasive ventilation up to and including 24 h/day in eligible patients.
Birnkrant DJ, Bushby KM, Amin RS, et al. The respiratory management of patients with Duchenne muscular dystrophy: a DMD care considerations working group specialty article. *Pediatr Pulmonol.* 2010;45:739-748.

DMD are successfully managed with noninvasive ventilation 24 hours a day.[43] Most experts now reserve tracheostomy for patients who cannot use noninvasive ventilation successfully or prefer tracheostomy, when noninvasive cough assistance techniques are not able to avoid lung aspiration of secretions with repeated SaO_2 drops < 95%, or those with multiple failed attempts at extubation after acute respiratory failure despite "optimal" use of mechanical in-exsufflation and noninvasive ventilation.[36] However, of note, a recent retrospective study by one team using hourly mechanical in-exsufflation reported successful extubation to noninvasive ventilation in 97/98 neuromuscular patients who were deemed unweanable by other teams.[44]

Early surgical correction of DMD-related scoliosis is considered the treatment of choice, since spinal bracing is not effective in patients with DMD, and may further reduce vital capacity. Surgery has been recommended in patients with DMD with a progressing Cobb angle of 20 degrees and a vital capacity of at least 40% of predicted values, in an attempt to avoid postoperative respiratory failure. However, several reports have shown that scoliosis surgery can be performed successfully in patients with DMD with very severe respiratory disability (FVC < 30% predicted), with careful preoperative and postoperative care.[45] Of note, a recent Cochrane systematic review was unable to find any randomized, clinical trial assessing the effectiveness of scoliosis surgery in patients with DMD; therefore there are no evidence-based results for more accurately guiding clinical practice.[46]

Obesity is frequent in patients with DMD after loss of ambulation, especially when treated with corticosteroids. Obesity in these patients increases the work of breathing, further compromises chest wall function, and favors obstructive sleep apnea-hypopnea syndrome. All obese patients should undergo a controlled weight reduction program. Conversely, patients with end-stage disease may suffer from severe weight loss with muscle wasting and bedsores, secondary to bulbar weakness (mastication and swallowing difficulties) and an inability to feed themselves. Recommendations on specialized dietary management in patients with DMD have recently been published,[47] as well as an algorithm to manage dysphagia.[48] If necessary, the use of gastrostomy for enteral feeding should be discussed with patients and their families.

Management of Acute Respiratory Deteriorations.
Respiratory infection is a serious complication in patients with DMD, since muscle weakness impairs both the ability to breathe and to clear airway secretions. Affected children should avoid contact with individuals with respiratory infections, and preventive immunization (influenza, pneumococcal pneumonia) should be performed. During respiratory infections, patients with DMD must increase their use of assisted cough techniques and noninvasive ventilatory support to maintain $SaO_2 \geq 95\%$. Oxygen therapy must be used with great caution and only in conjunction with respiratory aids to avoid masking and aggravating alveolar hypoventilation. Early appropriate antibiotic treatment is recommended when a lower respiratory tract infection is diagnosed by culture or with $SaO_2 < 95\%$. The inability to maintain $SaO_2 \geq 95\%$ in room air is an indication for hospitalization. Again, when endotracheal intubation is necessary, extubation to noninvasive ventilation has been reported to be nearly always successful by using an "aggressive" in-exsufflation device.[44] An action plan for respiratory infections should be given to all patients with DMD with significant respiratory involvement.

When using nocturnal and daytime noninvasive respiratory aids, together with early, aggressive, and adapted management of respiratory infections, patients with DMD can often live beyond 30 years, while usually ensuring an appreciable quality of life. However, even despite preventive treatment including angiotensin-converting enzyme inhibitors with β blockers, intractable cardiac insufficiency claims the life of some patients much earlier, sometimes as early as adolescence.

Corticosteroid Therapy. Glucocorticoid treatment has been repeatedly shown to improve the course of DMD. While the cellular and molecular mechanisms of action are largely unknown, recent evidence suggests that in addition to their antiinflammatory effect, glucocorticoids may delay the depletion of muscle progenitor cells.[49] A practice guideline on the use of corticosteroids in patients with DMD has recently been updated by the American Academy of Neurology and endorsed by the American Academy of Pediatrics. Prednisone (0.75 mg/kg per day) or deflazacort (0.9 mg/kg per day) improves strength and pulmonary function and should be offered to patients. Both prednisone and deflazacort are effective in improving motor function, decreasing the need for scoliosis surgery, and delaying the onset of cardiomyopathy. Patients and families must be informed of the potential beneficial effects and adverse events from corticosteroid treatment. Among others, adverse events include increased weight gain (especially with prednisone), cataracts (especially with deflazacort), behavioral changes, and fractures. Over a period of 1 year, a weekly dose of prednisone 10 mg/kg has been shown to be as effective as a daily dose of 0.75 mg/kg. Unfortunately, evidence is still lacking with regard to making recommendations on the age to initiate treatment with corticosteroids, as well as on the duration of treatment.[50]

Future Perspectives on Duchenne Muscular Dystrophy Treatment. While DMD still remains an untreatable disease in humans, encouraging results have been obtained nevertheless, and several therapeutic approaches are currently being tested. Early phase clinical trials on a drug to upregulate utrophin, a protein analogous to dystrophin, are ongoing.

Mutation-specific therapies have been tested in animal models of DMD for several years, with some currently being tested in clinical trials. In 2014, the European Medicines Agency issued a conditional marketing authorization for the drug Ataluren, which is able to read through premature stop-codon mutations. Clinical trials are also ongoing with antisense oligonucleotides being used to skip an exon close to a deleted gene, bringing the genetic code back into frame and allowing the expression of a functional dystrophin. Despite some encouraging results, substantial work remains to be done before these oligonucleotides can be used to effectively treat patients with DMD. Finally, adenoviral-based gene therapy and stem cell therapy are also under investigation.

Myotonic Dystrophy

Regular surveillance dictates treatment that is mainly supportive, especially with modification of food consistency and physiotherapy to enhance swallowing, as well as respiratory support as needed. Sleep-disordered breathing, often present in myotonic dystrophy patients, merits appropriate treatment tailored to obstructive apneas/hypopneas (adenotonsillectomy, continuous positive airway pressure [CPAP]) or central hypoventilation (bilevel positive airway pressure [BiPAP]).

DISORDERS INVOLVING THE BONY STRUCTURE OF THE CHEST WALL

Pectus Excavatum

Surgical repair of PEx is considered in the presence of exercise limitation or poor self-image responsible for adverse psychological symptoms and decreased quality of life. The Ravitch procedure (costochondral osteotomy) and, more recently, the minimally invasive Nuss procedure (retrosternal placement of a curved metal bar via videoscopy without sternal osteotomy or costal resection) are both in use. Recent reviews comparing the two procedures do not favor one over the other.[7,51] A small improvement in exercise tolerance has been reported after PEx repair.[25,26]

Kyphoscoliosis

Management of scoliosis depends on the age of the child, the degree of scoliosis, the degree of respiratory impairment, the rate of progression of structural deformities, and the underlying condition that led to the scoliosis (e.g., neuromuscular weakness disorders).

Adolescent Idiopathic Scoliosis. Management of adolescent scoliosis should start with early detection before onset of the adolescent growth spurt. In skeletally immature patients with curves of less than 25 degrees, the risk of progression is low and close follow-up may be sufficient. In patients with progressive curves greater than 25 degrees and those that progress, bracing is used first to control spinal curve progression. Bracing efficacy is dependent on the number of hours per day of use with greatest effect when used more than 20 hours/day. However, the Charleston brace is used at nighttime only. Brace therapy continues until spine growth stops. Uncontrolled curve progression despite orthotic treatment and curves with Cobb angles greater than 50 degrees require spinal fusion with pedicle screw instrumentation to correct for the three-dimensional deformation.[52]

In younger adolescents with Cobb angles of less than 30 degrees, a new surgical treatment has been proposed using staples between the vertebrae along the convex side of the scoliotic curve at the apex in order to promote unilateral vertebral growth on the concave side and maintain spinal flexibility. In addition, unilateral vertebral tethers are under study as a less invasive means to control curve progression. Postoperative follow-up of lung function using these newer methods has yet to be reported.

Juvenile Scoliosis. Children with nonprogressive spinal curves of less than 20 degrees usually require no additional intervention other than close follow-up, especially at the time of the adolescent growth spurt. Children with a progressive spinal curve should be treated with a brace individualized to minimize further respiratory impairment[53] with selective cut-outs. Those whose curve progression has not stopped or who have spinal curves greater than 40 degrees at the time of diagnosis will likely require surgical treatment. Since 2002, a variety of "growth friendly" and "growth modulating" devices have been developed that are expandable over years of spine growth. Recently, these have been classified according to their effect on the spine and are listed in Box 72.5.[54] These techniques have replaced spine fusion in skeletally immature children in order to maximize potential vertebral, and hence thoracic cage, volumetric growth. Patients with nonprogressive juvenile scoliosis should be followed closely until skeletal maturity is attained.

Congenital and Infantile Scoliosis. Both congenital and infantile scoliosis are potentially very serious conditions. Most cases of congenital scoliosis are progressive and do not respond to bracing. Although spine fusion was once considered as first-line therapy, long-term follow-up studies on children fused while growing have demonstrated significant restrictive chest wall disease proportional to the length of spine that was fused and the location of the apex prior to surgery.[55] As with juvenile and infantile idiopathic scoliosis, congenital scoliosis is treated with expandable distraction devices to prevent further spine curvature and preserve lung function. In addition, with fused ribs, an expansion thoracoplasty with rib lysis and separation by means of a vertical expandable titanium prosthetic rib has been approved for use on a case-by-case basis for congenital scoliosis (Fig. 72.6).[9] Growth-friendly distraction devices are placed rib to rib, spine to rib, spine to spine, and pelvis to rib or spine, all meant to distract the spine in the cephalad-caudad direction.[56] Expansion of the devices performed operatively every 6 months increases vertebral height significantly more than expansions on an as-needed basis. Recently, a growth-friendly device that can be advanced noninvasively using a magnetically driven mechanism has been approved for clinical use, dramatically reducing the number of operative expansion procedures for each growing child. Ideal noninvasive rod lengthening intervals have yet to be determined. This device has reduced the cumulative complication rate for repeated surgeries as well. Depending on the duration and amount of growth remaining, each of these devices must be replaced with a larger version after several years. Preliminary results obtained a few years after surgery suggest that this procedure promotes continued spine growth even for abnormal vertebrae, with no increase in curve amplitude. Postoperative studies with serial measurements of vital capacity under anesthesia over 3 years demonstrated an improvement in absolute lung volume but no change or slight loss of lung function expressed as a percentage of predicted norms.[57] Another study of 53 older children undergoing vertical expandable prosthetic titanium rib insertion found no change in vital capacity, but a small increase in residual volume, suggesting that the lung had been stretched as the thorax was expanded.[58] The longest follow-up period for children with scoliosis undergoing growth-friendly device implantation and expansion has been 6 years. Over this longer interval, serial measurements of vital capacity fell by 28% of predicted normal values, suggesting that current surgical treatments do not maintain normal lung growth despite some degree of spine curve correction.[59]

Active treatment is mandatory for progressive scoliosis. There is some suggestion that lung function may be better preserved when children undergo nonfusion surgical correction of the scoliosis when they are less than 6 years of age. However, to reduce surgical complications, several spine centers resort to serial casting in children less than 5 years of age, followed by surgical intervention in those who do not improve. The effect of serial casting on pulmonary function over time has not been reported. The surgical strategy for an individual child is developed on a case-by-case basis, and varies among spine centers according to local experience and expertise. Preoperative halo traction has been used to minimize the severity of the spine curvature prior to surgery, particularly when the spine is flexible.

Spine Deformities in Neuromuscular Diseases. The issues in patients with neuromuscular diseases are more complex (severity of deformity, pelvic obliquity, associated nutritional, neurological, and cardiopulmonary problems). Although surgery provides significant benefit with regard to quality of life, the consequences on long-term pulmonary function depend on the underlying disease and the nature of the spine deformity. New surgical devices are now being proposed to improve the severe lordosis that occurs in children with spina bifida. Of note, early treatment with corticosteroids largely prevents scoliosis development in patients with DMD.

Postoperative Pulmonary Function in Scoliosis. Pulmonary complications are a principal cause of morbidity

---

Box 72.5 Classification of Growth-Friendly Spine Implants for Early-Onset Scoliosis

Distraction-Based Systems

- Vertical expandable prosthetic titanium ribs (VEPTR)
- Growing rods (spine to spine)
- Hybrid growing rods (spine to ribs)

Compression-Based Systems

- Vertebral staples
- Vertebral tethers

Growth Guidance Systems

- Shilla device
- Luque trolley

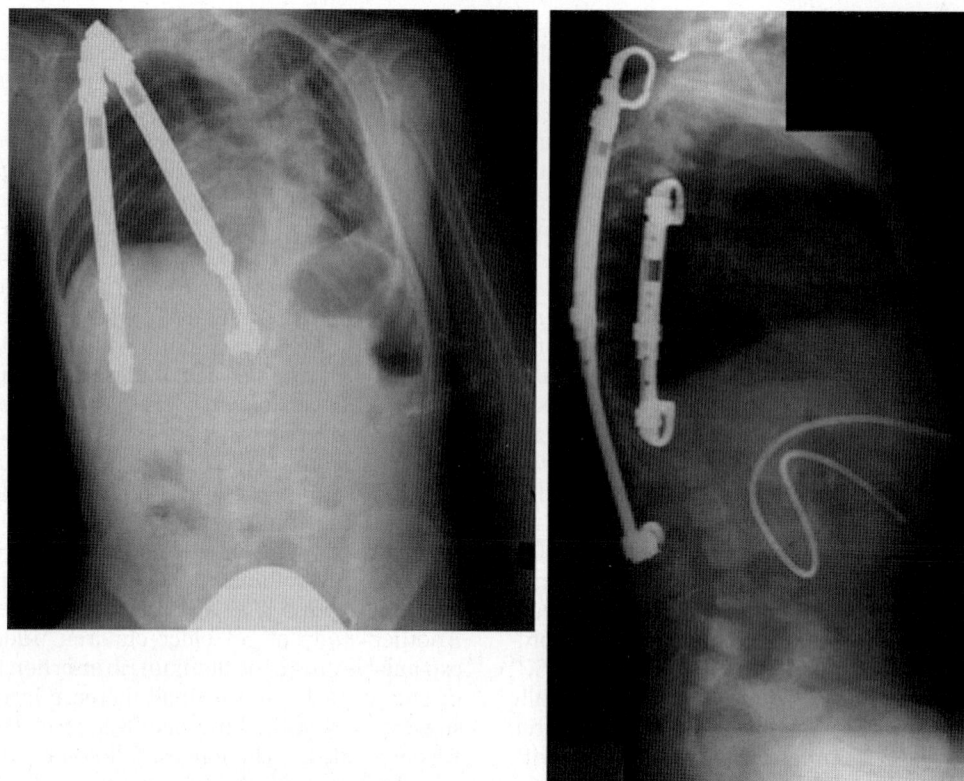

Fig. 72.6 A pair of vertical expandable titanium prosthetic ribs (VEPTRs) in a child with early onset thoracic scoliosis. The slide mechanism for expansion is located in the middle of each VEPTR. One device is attached from rib to rib (shorter device on the lateral film) and one is attached from ribs to the spine.

and mortality in the immediate period following surgery for scoliosis. Therefore preoperative assessment of pulmonary function, including overnight oximetry and the assessment of hypercapnia, should be performed as a guide to prevent and treat postoperative complications. Children with skeletal dysplasia and those with cervical vertebral involvement often have upper airway obstruction and pose intubation challenges at the time of surgery. The most frequent respiratory problems reported in the immediate postoperative course of surgery for scoliosis include atelectasis, pneumonia, pulmonary edema, pulmonary fat emboli, and respiratory failure. Immediate pulmonary complications result from multiple factors such as the surgical procedure itself, the degree of preoperative pulmonary disability, the intraoperative fluid management, the transient limitation of chest wall expansion as a result of pain, and the effects of anesthetics and analgesics. In neuromuscular diseases, respiratory muscle weakness, cough impairment, and swallowing disorders increase the risk of immediate postoperative pulmonary complications. Children with adolescent idiopathic scoliosis whose vital capacities are less than 40% predicted have a three-fold increase in pulmonary complication rate following spine fusion compared to those with better preoperative lung function.[60] Children with underlying neuromuscular weakness who undergo spine fusion have longer postoperative hospitalizations than children with other conditions. Noninvasive ventilation and mechanical in-exsufflation devices can be of invaluable help in patients with and without neuromuscular weakness in the immediate postoperative period.

Spine fusion reduces the spinal curvature, but improvements in lung volume and arterial oxygenation only become apparent late after surgery. The decrease in vital capacity usually lasts for 6 weeks to 3 months after fusion but can persist for up to 1 year. By 1–2 years after spine fusion, vital capacity returns to preoperative values. Combined anterior fusion and posterior spine fusion is more likely than posterior fusion alone to impair lung function postoperatively for longer periods; the combined fusion approach also reduces the likelihood of further scoliosis postoperatively. Patients with severe scoliosis and marginal lung function who undergo fusion may require outpatient BiPAP support indefinitely following surgery.

Management of Hypoplastic Thorax Syndromes

The recent development of expandable titanium devices has led to novel interventions with short-term respiratory improvements over several years, although the long-term outlook—even with these new surgical interventions—remains unclear.

Asphyxiating Thoracic Dystrophy. Several surgical procedures have been proposed and used clinically to increase thoracic cage size. These include the interposition of adjacent ribs with titanium connectors to make the existing ribs longer. Alternatively, customized curved VEPTR expandable devices have been used in conjunction with osteotomies of the ribs to enlarge the thoracic cavity. The latter can then be regularly expanded to increase the thorax as the child grows. Lung functions have not been reported following these surgical treatments, although mortality has been reduced to 50% in the first year of life in uncontrolled case series.[61]

Jarcho-Levin Syndrome. Children with Jarcho-Levin syndrome have received growth-friendly spine distraction devices to further increase thoracic height and width, although lung function following surgical interventions has not been reported.

References
Access the reference list online at ExpertConsult.com.

73 Disorders of the Respiratory Tract Caused by Trauma

CHAD M. THORSON, MD, MSPH, and MATIAS BRUZONI, MD, FACS

General Considerations

Traumatic thoracic injury in infants and children is uncommon; it is usually secondary to blunt mechanisms and is often managed nonoperatively. Penetrating injuries, such as stab and gunshot wounds are, fortunately, rare, but they usually require some sort of operative intervention, and result in increased morbidity and mortality.[1-5]

More than 75% of pediatric blunt chest trauma is due to automobile accidents, with the remainder resulting from sports injuries, nonaccidental trauma, and falls from heights.[6] Children involved in automobile accidents tend to be pedestrians rather than occupants of vehicles. The complete spectrum of chest trauma includes pneumothorax, hemothorax, destruction of the integrity of the chest wall and diaphragm, thoracic visceral damage, and combined thoracoabdominal injuries. The mortality rate from thoracic trauma has been reported to be approximately 26%, and can be as high as 33% when penetrating injuries are involved.[3,7,8] Overall, recent literature suggests that the mortality rate for childhood thoracic trauma has decreased.[9] Thoracic trauma is frequently associated with head, abdominal, and spine trauma, making the mortality rate higher in this combined scenario.

Pediatric deaths may occur in the prehospital setting and are usually secondary to hemorrhagic shock or cardiopulmonary arrest related to a tension pneumothorax or cardiac tamponade. The mortality and morbidity rate can be improved if the patient is transferred to a tertiary level pediatric trauma center and managed within "the golden hour" described by the Advanced Trauma Life Support (ATLS) guidelines.

Most blunt thoracic injuries in children can be managed without operative intervention. This often involves significant respiratory support, including analgesia, assisted ventilation, and aggressive physiotherapy. As in adults, the significance of thoracic trauma results from the concomitant pulmonary, cardiac, and systemic dysfunction that follows. In the pediatric age group, because of chest wall plasticity, profound physiologic aberrations can occur in the absence of fractures. Respiratory and circulatory dysfunction secondary to chest injury is frequently complicated by blood loss and hypotension. Hypotension from hemorrhage can usually be managed through volume replacement; algorithmic therapy is monitored and refined by serial determination of blood pressures, hematocrit, central venous pressure, blood gases, and, if necessary, blood volume. Restoration of the normal cardiopulmonary function fundamentally depends on a clean airway, intact chest and diaphragm,

and unrestricted cardiopulmonary dynamics. The primary and secondary surveys recommended by the ATLS guidelines are mandatory in pediatric trauma as well. If the patient is hemodynamically stable with a significant mechanism of injury, computed tomography (CT) of the chest should be considered to search for undetected injuries if felt that they would alter the clinical approach. Otherwise, chest radiography is typically adequate and avoids the radiation risk.[10]

The long-term outcome of thoracic trauma in children has not been well studied. A single European study addressed the 5-year outcome of thoracic trauma in children; they concluded that most injuries resolve without significant late sequelae.[11]

Features of the Pediatric Thorax

The thorax of a child is different from that of an adult from both an anatomic and a physiologic point of view. The pediatric chest is typically more rounded with less developed musculature. This characteristic, together with a more flexible and elastic rib cage, results in a very compliant chest. The ribs and sternum of a child can thus support a significant amount of blunt force without fracture. Deformability is such that the anterior and posterior curvatures of the ribs can contact each other without fracture. Therefore, blunt injury to the chest presents a diagnostic challenge since obvious external signs of injury may be minor, chest radiographs may be normal, and yet the visceral structures may still have sustained serious injury.

Additionally, the mediastinum is relatively mobile and thus less susceptible to the rapid acceleration and deceleration forces commonly experienced in blunt trauma. Increased mediastinal mobility, together with the absence of preexisting vascular disease in children, make injuries to the mediastinum and great vessels less frequent than in adults. On the other hand, conditions such as tension pneumothorax or hemothorax are very poorly tolerated and must be recognized and addressed emergently.

Physiological compensation to trauma is different in children when compared with adults; the cardiovascular and pulmonary reserves are much less in children. Tachycardia may be the only compensatory mechanism in children who present with hypovolemic shock, even with 30% loss of estimated blood volume. Hypotension will only occur in the very late stage, just before cardiac arrest. The pulmonary reserve can be seriously affected by massive gastric distention, a very common finding in pediatric trauma. Prompt insertion of a nasogastric tube is recommended since many children will develop gastric distention due to aerophagia following any type of trauma.

Sternal Fractures

Fractures of the sternum in infancy and childhood follow high-compression crush injuries and are usually associated with other thoracic and orthopedic injuries. Interestingly, one series has reported sternal fractures as the result of surprisingly minor trauma. The most common injury identified in this report was an isolated anterior cortical fracture.[12]

On physical examination, there is local tenderness, ecchymosis, and sometimes a concavity or paradoxical respiratory movement. The sternal segments are typically well aligned without much displacement. Dyspnea, cyanosis, arrhythmias (most commonly sinus tachycardia), and hypotension may be evidence of an underlying cardiac contusion. Radiographic demonstration of fractures is most commonly by chest x-ray or CT scan, although ultrasound is being used more frequently with high sensitivity/specificity.[13]

Children with traumatic injury of the sternum should be admitted to the intensive care unit given the increased risk for arrhythmias. Cardiac tamponade and blunt myocardial damage must be ruled out by various studies, including serial electrocardiography, echocardiography, and careful monitoring of vital signs. Although cardiac enzymes were once used as a screening tool, their use has been abandoned due to low sensitivity and specificity.[14]

If the bony deformity is minimal, there is no specific treatment indicated. Markedly displaced fragments are reduced under general anesthesia by a closed or open technique in order to prevent a traumatic pectus excavatum. Violent paradoxical respirations can be controlled by assisted mechanical respiration through an endotracheal tube, or rarely by operative fixation of rib fragments.

Rib Fractures and Flail Chest

Rib fractures are unusual in children because of the extreme flexibility of the osseous and cartilaginous framework of the thorax. The upper ribs are protected by the scapula and related muscles, and the lower ones are quite resilient. As such, rib fractures are present in only about 3% of all children

admitted with thoracic injury.[15] Predictably, children with more than one rib fracture are more likely to have sustained multisystem trauma; crush and direct-blow injuries are the usual etiologic factors.[16] Multiple fractures of the middle ribs are almost diagnostic of nonaccidental trauma.

Multiple rib fractures resulting in the destruction of the integrity of the thoracic skeleton can cause the paradoxical motion of the "flail chest" (Fig. 73.1). The unsupported area of the chest moves inward with inspiration and outward with expiration; these paradoxical respiratory excursions inexorably lead to dyspnea (Fig. 73.2). The explosive expiration of coughing is dissipated and made ineffectual by the paradoxical movement and intercostal pain. In effect, the ideal preparation for acute respiratory distress syndrome—airway obstruction, atelectasis, and pneumonia—has been established.

The clinical picture includes local pain that is aggravated by motion. Tenderness is elicited by pressure applied directly over the fracture or elsewhere on the same rib. The fracture site may be edematous and ecchymotic. The clinical

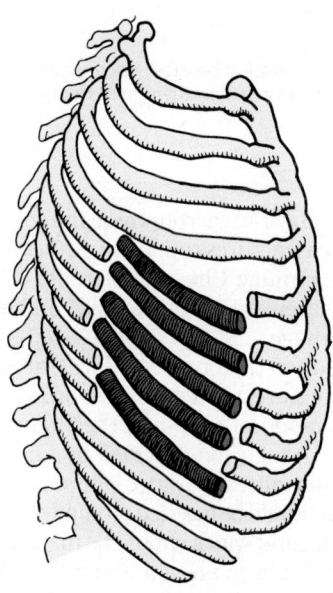

Fractured ribs

Fig. 73.1 An illustration of five ribs broken in two places, with loss of chest wall stability and resultant paradoxical or "flail chest" wall.

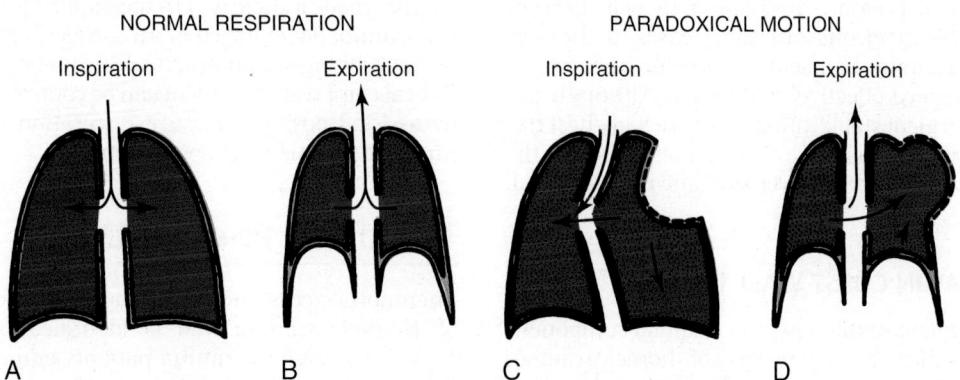

NORMAL RESPIRATION

Inspiration   Expiration

PARADOXICAL MOTION

Inspiration   Expiration

A   B   C   D

Fig. 73.2 (A–D) A diagram of the action of a normal chest compared with that of a "flail chest" during phases of the respiratory cycle.

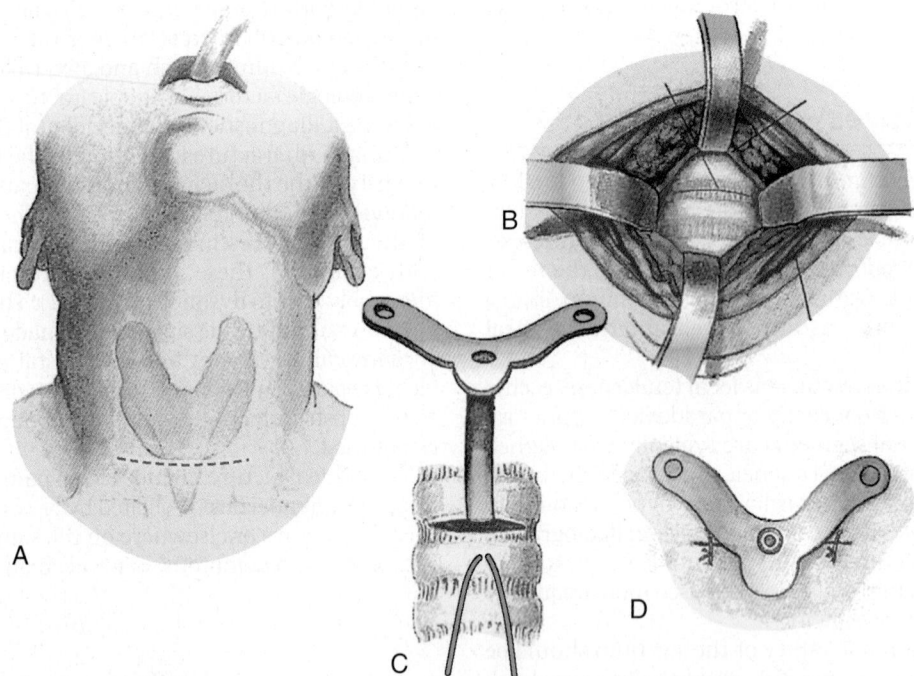

Fig. 73.3 Techniques of tracheostomy performed over an oral endotracheal tube. Note the transverse skin incision (A) and the suture on the lower tracheal flaps to facilitate subsequent tube changes (C). (B) The anatomy of the area. (D) The tube in place.

manifestations may range from these minimal findings with simple, restricted fractures to severe ventilatory distress with underlying lung injury. Chest radiographs demonstrate the extent and displacement of the fractures and hint at underlying visceral damage.

The treatment of uncomplicated fractures requires pain control to allow unrestricted respiration. With severe fractures, the alleviation of pain and the restoration of cough are important and can be provided by analgesics, physiotherapy, and intermittent positive-pressure breathing. Thoracostomy tubes should be inserted promptly for pneumothorax and hemothorax, and shock should be managed by appropriate resuscitation. There are a few small studies to suggest that surgical fixation results in a reduction in pneumonia, chest deformity, tracheostomy, duration of mechanical ventilation, and length of intensive care unit (ICU) stay.[17]

Paradoxical respiratory excursions with flail chest must be promptly brought under control, sometimes requiring mechanical positive pressure ventilation to help prevent respiratory distress syndrome. In some cases, a thoracic epidural anesthetic may be useful to provide appropriate analgesia and achieve effective ventilation. Although not routinely used, surgical stabilization in severe flail chest has been shown to lower the incidence of pneumonia, shorten the ICU stay, reduce ventilatory requirement, and reduce overall hospital cost.[18,19]

TRACHEOSTOMY IN CHEST WALL INJURY

Controlled mechanical ventilation is an essential component for respiratory insufficiency in the setting of thoracic trauma. Despite vigorous therapy, secretions may be troublesome, and are managed using intermittent tracheal suctioning or bronchoscopy. There is evidence that tracheostomy in children can be avoided by long-term intubation in many cases.[20,21] However, prolonged intubation has become the most important indication for tracheostomy, since it allows an avenue for the control of secretions, diminishes ventilatory dead space, and obtains control of an obstructed airway (Fig. 73.3).

During the first year of life, tracheostomy is a particularly morbid operation.[20] Common complications are pneumomediastinum, pneumothorax, tracheal stenosis, and tracheomalacia. Secretions may be difficult to aspirate, as the small tracheostomy tube easily becomes plugged. Distal infection, often with staphylococci, is poorly handled by such young patients. In addition, withdrawal of the tracheostomy tube is a precarious and unpredictable endeavor. Nevertheless, even in this age group, tracheostomy can be lifesaving in specific instances of chest trauma.

The decision for tracheostomy in cases of chest injury can often be made if there is (1) a mechanically obstructed airway that cannot be managed more conservatively, (2) flail chest, or (3) prolonged endotracheal intubation. Unstable, paradoxical chest wall movement can be controlled for long periods by assisted positive pressure respiration through a short, uncuffed Silastic tracheostomy tube.

Traumatic Pneumothorax

Pneumothorax is one of the most common consequences of thoracic trauma and is identified in approximately 12%–50% of chest trauma patients admitted to hospital.[7] Pneumothorax is potentially fatal and requires specific maneuvers to prevent or reverse a malignant chain of events.

The creation of a tension pneumothorax requires a valvular mechanism through which the amount of air entering the pleural space exceeds the amount escaping it. The positive intrapleural pressure is initially dissipated by a mediastinal shift, which compresses the opposite lung and can result in ipsilateral pulmonary collapse and angulation of the great vessels entering and leaving the heart. Intrapleural tension can be increased by traumatic hemothorax, and respiratory exchange and cardiac output are thus critically diminished.

The etiologic possibilities, in addition to chest wall and lung trauma, include rupture of the esophagus, pulmonary cyst, emphysematous lobe, and postoperative bronchial fistula. These latter sources of tension pneumothorax almost always require thoracotomy for control.

The clinical findings may include external evidence of a wound, tachypnea, dyspnea, cyanosis with hyperresonance, the absence or transmission of breath sounds, and displacement of the trachea and apical cardiac impulse. The hemithoraces may be asymmetric, with the involved side appearing larger and hyperresonant.

A confirmatory radiograph is comforting but often cannot be afforded in this thoracic emergency. Chest tube insertion is indicated for a tension pneumothorax or simple pneumothorax associated with respiratory distress or shock. Prompt relief and pulmonary expansion can be anticipated if the source of the intrapleural air has been controlled. A traumatic valvular defect in the chest wall can be occluded. If the pulmonary air leak persists or recurs, the possibility of tension pneumothorax is circumvented by the insertion of one or more intercostal tubes connected to water-seal drainage with low-pressure suction. Most instances of traumatic tension pneumothorax require tube drainage for permanent decompression, although needle aspiration is indispensable for emergency management. Stubborn bronchopleural fistulas that continue to remain widely patent despite adequate intercostal tube drainage may need thoracotomy and repair or resection of the affected lung segment.

An open pneumothorax ("sucking" chest wound) in which atmospheric air has direct, unimpeded entrance into and exit from the pleural space is a second, equally urgent, thoracic emergency. This pathology is almost always due to a large traumatic wound. Ingress of air during inspiration and egress during expiration produce an extreme degree of paradoxical respiration and mediastinal flutter, which is partially regulated by the size of the chest wall defect in comparison with the circumference of the trachea. If a considerable segment of chest wall is open, more air is exchanged at this site than through the trachea, because the pressures are similar. Inspiration collapses the ipsilateral lung and drives its alveolar air into the opposite side. During expiration, the air returns across the carina. In addition, the mediastinum becomes a widely swinging pendulum compressing the uninjured lung on inspiration and the lung on the injured side during expiration (Fig. 73.4). Obviously, under these circumstances, little effective ventilation is taking place because of the tremendous increase in the pulmonary dead space and the decrease in tidal volumes. A totally ineffective cough completes the clinical picture. The diagnosis is readily made by inspection of the thoracic wound and the peculiar sound of air rushing in and coming out of the wound.

Emergency management of this critical situation includes prompt occlusion of the chest wall defect by sterile dressings (Fig. 73.5) and measures to prevent conversion of this open pneumothorax into an equally threatening tension pneumothorax, which can occur if the underlying visceral pleura has been injured. Pleural decompression by closed intercostal tube drainage is essential. When immediate chest tube is not available (i.e., in the prehospital setting), closure of the wound with an occlusive dressing sealed on three sides is appropriate. This acts as a one-way valve allowing air to escape from the pleural space on expiration but sealing and preventing further air entry on inspiration. After systemic stabilization, more formal surgical débridement, reconstruction, and closure of the chest wound can be done in the operating room.

Hemothorax

Blood in the pleural cavity is perhaps the most common sequel of thoracic trauma, regardless of type. Depending on the speed of the hemorrhage, it can be life threatening. Bleeding sources are abundant, with either systemic (high pressure) or pulmonary (low pressure) sources. Systemic bleeding usually originates in the chest wall from the intercostal vessels.

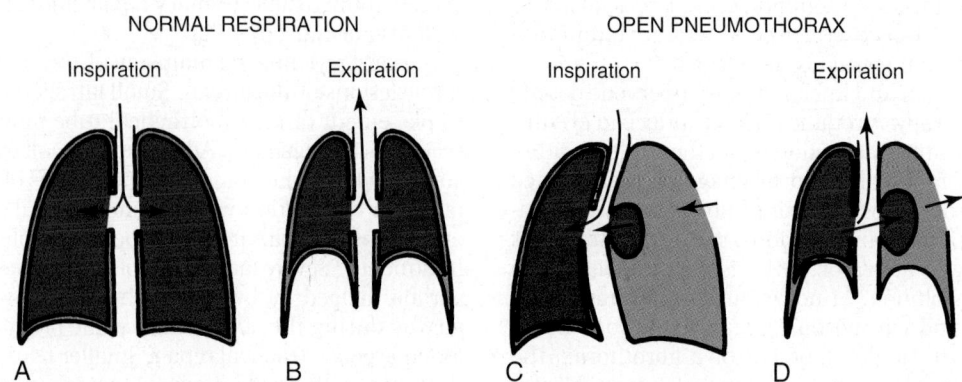

NORMAL RESPIRATION

Inspiration   Expiration

OPEN PNEUMOTHORAX

Inspiration   Expiration

A   B   C   D

Fig. 73.4 (A–D) Changes in the normal respiratory pattern brought about by an open, sucking thoracic wall injury.

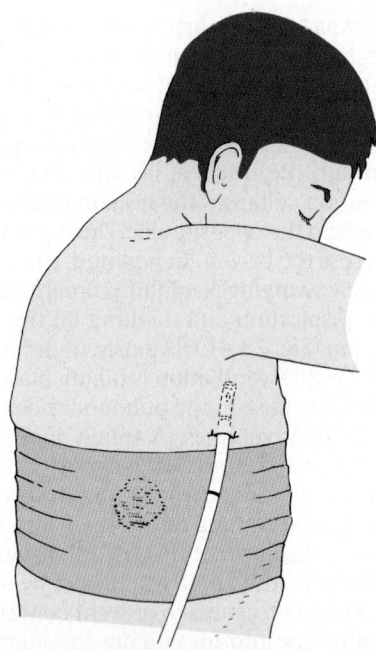

Fig. 73.5 A temporary occlusive chest wall dressing applied to a sucking wound with underwater intercostal chest tube drainage. Once the period of emergency is over, operative debridement and closure of the chest wound is necessary.

Hemorrhage from pulmonary vessels is usually self-limiting unless major tributaries have been transected. It is important to note that a child can accumulate about 40% of his/her blood volume in the chest.

The immediate findings are those of blood loss compounded by respiratory distress. The trachea and apical impulse may be dislocated, the percussion note is flat, and the breath sounds are indistinct. The actual diagnosis is confirmed by thoracentesis if time allows after adequate radiographic studies.

Management of hemothorax is accomplished by total evacuation of air and blood with a large-bore chest tube. Most often, the evacuation of blood will obliterate the pleural space, and pleural apposition will tamponade parenchymal bleeding. Small-volume hemothorax may be safely observed as long as cardiorespiratory mechanics are not altered.[22] A simple formula to define the need for urgent thoracotomy is a bloody chest tube output of more than 1 mL/kg per minute with associated hemodynamic instability despite rigorous resuscitation. The surgeon's common sense is crucial in this setting, and if one suspects either persistent or voluminous bleeding, an operation should be performed.

Clotting, loculation, and infection may supervene despite vigorous initial therapy. A retained hemothorax can eventually result in empyema. Publications from the adult literature support early thoracoscopy and drainage of the retained hemothorax in order to avoid late infections.[23] As with management of parapneumonic effusions, use of thrombolytics (tissue plasminogen activator [tPA]) is well established to assist with clot dissolution.[24] Unevacuated intrapleural blood eventually clots and can become organized fibrous tissue (fibrothorax). With the development of a fibrothorax, the lung becomes incarcerated and the chest wall is immobilized, chronically altering cardiorespiratory dynamics. Empyema

from secondary contamination is always a threat when the pleural space is filled with blood. Patients rarely eventually require thoracotomy and decortication.

Tracheobronchial Trauma

Rupture of the trachea or bronchus in infants and children is usually preceded by a sharp blow to the anterior part of the neck (clothes-line injury), by penetrating injuries, or severe compression injury of the chest against a closed glottis.[25,26] These injuries represent a diagnostic and therapeutic challenge. Discontinuity of a major airway is characterized by intrathoracic tension phenomena. When the leak is massive, unilateral or even bilateral pneumothorax is present compromising not only the respiratory function, but also cardiac venous return.

Proximal upper airway lesions often present with pneumomediastinum and subcutaneous emphysema, followed by bilateral pneumothorax. This is due to the intramediastinal location of the trachea, directing any air leak to this space, which is in continuity with the neck compartments. When the distal airway is involved, the air leak opens easily into the pleural space causing tension pneumothorax and a persistent air leak. Hemoptysis may also be present.

Conventional chest radiographs may show pneumomediastinum, pneumothorax, and subcutaneous emphysema. Air tracheobronchogram can suggest the diagnosis in the presence of a compatible clinical picture. Spiral CT of the thorax and the neck may allow better visualization of complete or major disruptions, but bronchoscopic demonstration of the rupture is diagnostic.[27–29] The diagnosis may not be suspected in the acute phase of smaller bronchial transections, but becomes obvious when late stricture with distal atelectasis and chronic pneumonitis is related retrospectively to a history of fairly severe chest trauma.

The initial management of bronchial rupture consists of maintenance of a patent airway and decompression of the pleura and mediastinum by thoracostomy tubes connected to closed drainage with suction. Occasionally, multiple tubes may be necessary for control of the associated air leak. Tracheobronchial transection with massive air leak resulting in the inability to ventilate is the rare indication to clamp a thoracostomy tube. This should be followed by emergent, expeditious transport to the operating room for bronchoscopy and immediate repair of the defect, as this maneuver may result in tension pneumothorax. Operative repair requires thoracotomy, usually primary repair, and reinforcement with a pleural or muscular flap.[25]

Surgery remains the mainstay of treatment for posttraumatic lesions of the airway. Small iatrogenic injuries related to placement of an endotracheal tube may heal with conservative management. Additionally, small traumatic injuries confirmed by bronchoscopy without signs of sepsis, evidence of major connection with the mediastinal space, or associated esophageal injuries may be amenable to nonsurgical treatment.[30] Severe lacerations of the trachea can be immeasurably helped by bypassing the glottis with an artificial airway during the acute phase while preparing the patient for emergency tracheal repair. Smaller tears may heal spontaneously with tracheostomy alone; others result in stricture and require selective operative repair.

Pulmonary Compression Injury (Traumatic Asphyxia)

Explosive blasts compress a child's flexible ribs, sternum, and cartilages against the lungs with a sudden, violent increase in intraalveolar pressure. These injuries are associated not only with pulmonary, but also with hepatic and cardiac contusions.[31] Alveolar disruption, interstitial emphysema, and pneumothorax may follow if the glottis is closed when the compression occurs. Distribution of this force to the great veins of the mediastinum and jugular system leads to venous distention. Extravasation of blood, purplish edema of the head, neck, and upper extremities, and possible central nervous system changes due to intracerebral edema and petechial hemorrhages may also occur with traumatic asphyxia. The pulmonary contusion is represented pathologically by edema, hemorrhage, and atelectasis.

Clinically, there may be dyspnea, cough, chest pain, hemoptysis, hypoxia, hypercarbia, and mental confusion. The face and the neck can be grotesquely swollen, with crepitus and submucosal/subconjunctival hemorrhage. There is no need for evidence of external trauma or fractured ribs in a child, and accordingly, the indication for chest radiograph is merely the possible history of a blast, acceleration (fall), or deceleration (automobile) injury. Pulmonary contusions, hemothorax, pneumothorax, and pneumomediastinum may all be encountered.[32]

There is a high risk of airway compromise associated with these types of injuries; therefore, rapid establishment of a definitive airway is vital. With mild injuries, the subcutaneous emphysema and purplish hue gradually and spontaneously disappear over several days. Patients with more serious blast injuries are initially treated for anoxia and hypotension, and attention is then directed to atelectasis, pulmonary edema, and pleural complications. Rapid progression of the mediastinal and subcutaneous emphysema indicates a serious disruption of the trachea, bronchi, or lungs, and may require intercostal tube drainage or even thoracotomy.[32]

Posttraumatic Atelectasis

With pulmonary contusion from any source, the production of tracheobronchial secretions is stimulated, but elimination may be simultaneously impeded by airway obstruction, pain, and depression of cough. The addition of hemorrhage to these accumulated secretions produce atelectasis in the damaged lung and inevitable infection—a syndrome aptly called "wet lung."[33] The clinical findings are dyspnea and cyanosis, an incessant, unproductive cough with wheezing and audible rattling, and gross rhonchi or rales. Chest radiographs show varying degrees of unilateral and bilateral atelectasis.

The syndrome demands vigorous treatment—frequent postural changes, insistence on coughing, humidified oxygen, antibiotics, mechanical ventilation, diuretics, and cautious hydration are all useful. If a child with chest trauma will not cough, tracheal suctioning is instituted. Failure of this step should be followed in quick succession by endotracheal tube insertion or tracheostomy.

The adult respiratory distress syndrome (ARDS) that occurs after critical illness with congestion, edema, hemorrhage, pneumonia, and pulmonary fibrosis is rarely encountered in pediatric practice (see Chapter 38). It is often a related sequel to an infectious process and severe hypotension. The mortality rate for pediatric ARDS is between 22% and 35%.[34]

Cardiac Trauma

Though rare, cardiac wounds should be suspected after penetration of any part of the chest, the lower part of the neck, or the upper part of the abdomen. The possibility of injury to the heart also exists in the presence of blunt trauma to the anterior hemithorax, laceration from fractured sternum or ribs, or severe compression between the sternum and the vertebral column. The most common mechanism is blunt trauma, which is most often sustained by adolescent patients in motor vehicle collisions.[35]

The spectrum of blunt cardiac injury ranges from myocardial contusion to anatomic disruption, such as valve dysfunction or myocardial rupture. The clinical manifestations of a myocardial contusion are arrhythmia, hypotension and, in severe cases, aneurysms from myocardial wall weakness. Blood loss with perforation varies from exsanguination, to cardiac tamponade, to minimal bleeding. Tamponade usually follows trauma to the myocardium when both pleura are intact; the hemopericardium cannot decompress. The resulting increase in intrapericardial pressure constricts the heart and great veins, and venous return and cardiac output are critically impaired. By contrast, delayed diagnosis of myocardial injury may occur in the presence of a left-sided hemothorax, as the blood preferentially decompresses into the left chest without the development of tamponade.[36]

The physical findings with acute tamponade are often archetypal. The veins of the neck and upper extremity may be distended. The heart sounds are distant and perhaps inaudible. The systolic pressure is depressed, the pulse pressure is narrow, and the venous pressure is elevated. However, the classic symptoms of distended neck veins, a raised central venous pressure, and pulsus paradoxus are not often evident in children with tamponade. The diagnosis is confirmed during the Focused Assessment with Sonography in Trauma (FAST) exam or with formal echocardiogram. As stated before in the sternal trauma section, there is no utility in serial cardiac enzyme measurements, although the degree of elevation may indicate increasing severity of the injury.[14,37]

Cardiac tamponade is imminently life threatening and requires emergent intervention. With a suggestive clinical picture, emergency needle aspiration of the pericardial sac through a subxiphoid approach should be performed in addition to systemic resuscitation while the operating room is being prepared. Aspiration of small amounts of blood can restore cardiopulmonary dynamics (Fig. 73.6). If an immediate adjacent operating room is available, a subxiphoid pericardial window can also be diagnostic and therapeutic.[38]

Blunt trauma can produce various degrees of myocardial contusions ranging from a small area of edema to a ruptured chamber. The chest pain and tachycardia may be difficult to evaluate without evidence of cardiac failure. Serial electrocardiograms are recommended to monitor these patients. In cases where persistent arrhythmias or hypotension occur,

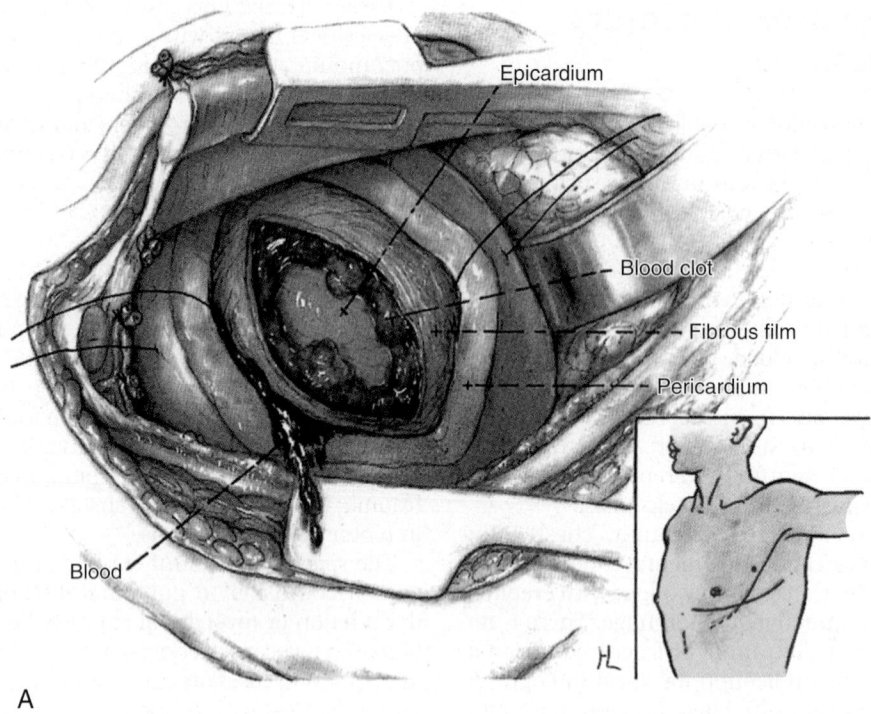

A

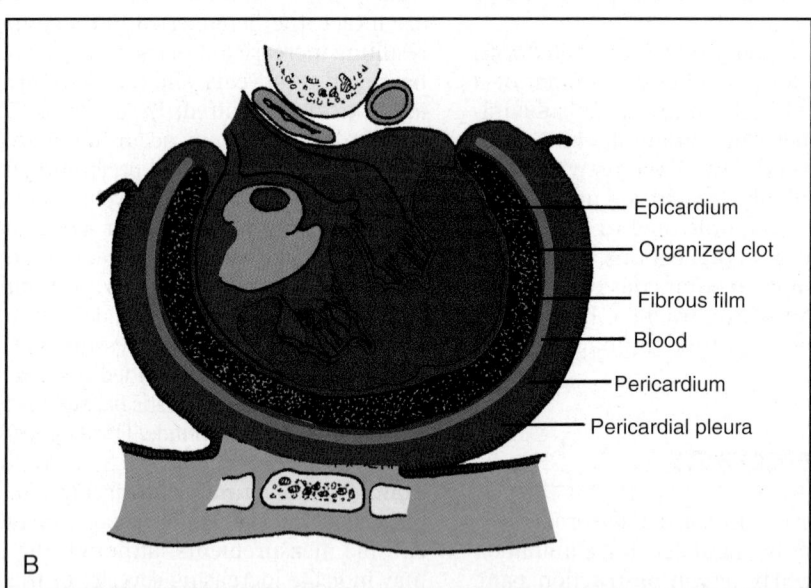

B

Fig. 73.6 (A and B) A traumatic cardiac tamponade relieved by an open thoracotomy 5 days following trauma and after two partially relieving pericardiocenteses.

an echocardiogram should be obtained for further work-up.[39] Physicians attending to an acutely injured child must be prepared to institute prompt external cardiac massage (Fig. 73.7), internal cardiac massage (Figs. 73.8 and 73.9), or cardiac defibrillation (Fig. 73.10).

Penetrating trauma may injure myocardial chambers or coronary arteries, and may require closure of the myocardial chambers or even coronary revascularization. In patients presenting *in extremis,* resuscitative thoracotomy in the emergency department may be lifesaving, with reported results

similar to adult literature (survival ~10% in penetrating trauma).[40]

Traumatic Rupture of the Thoracic Aorta

Thoracic aorta rupture is very uncommon. In a series published at Children's National Medical Center in Washington DC, only 0.14% of the pediatric traumas treated over a period of 6 years presented with thoracic aorta injuries.[41] Aortic transection typically occurs at the level of the ligamentum arteriosum, near the take-off of the left subclavian artery, and usually results from strong deceleration forces. Mediastinal widening on routine chest radiography with a distorted aortic contour is the most significant initial diagnostic study.

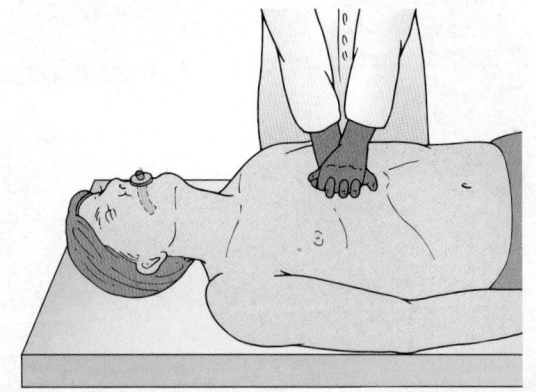

Fig. 73.7 External cardiac massage: rhythmic compression of the chest and heart in an effort to restore and maintain circulation after cardiac arrest.

Even though thoracic aortography is the procedure of choice in hemodynamically stable patients, CT angiogram is becoming widely accepted in many trauma centers as the gold standard.[42] Many injuries of this type are associated with life-threatening injuries in other organs such as the abdomen and head. Treatment consists of aortic repair, usually requiring cardiopulmonary bypass, although endovascular techniques are showing promising results in both the adult and pediatric populations.[43,44] There are case reports and some small series in children with good short-term outcomes.[44-47] Long-term results of this approach are not yet available.

Injuries to the Esophagus

Esophageal injury is more commonly associated with penetrating trauma. In this scenario, the cervical esophagus is commonly injured, and is usually associated with upper airway or vascular injuries. Blunt abdominal trauma or violent, forceful vomiting, may cause a sudden increase in gastric pressure, and thus create a tear in the wall of the distal esophagus. However, the most common cause of esophageal injury is iatrogenic during instrumentation of the esophagus, such as that seen in dilatations for esophageal strictures, or during endoscopic removal of foreign bodies. Esophageal rupture can also follow the ingestion of caustic agents. Perforation of the esophagus in the pediatric age group can also occur in the delivery room from extreme positive pressure resuscitation or aspiration with a stiff

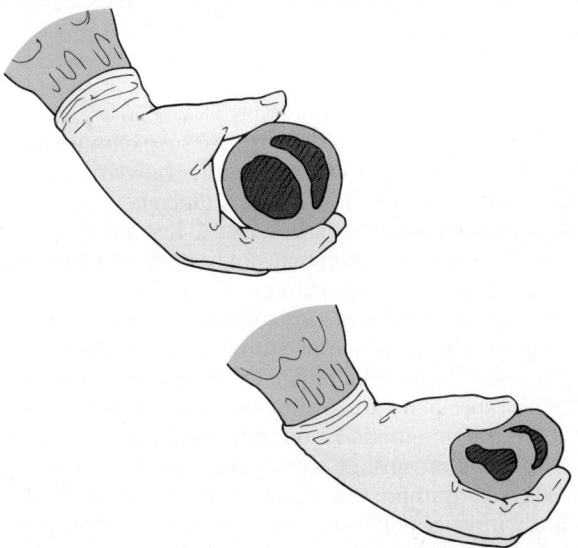

Fig. 73.8 Internal cardiac massage: one-handed technique for neonates and infants.

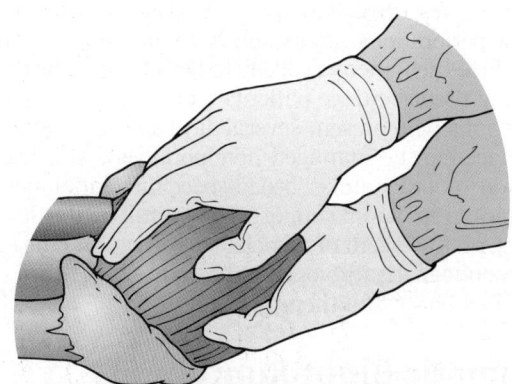

Fig. 73.9 Internal cardiac massage: bimanual technique for older children and adults.

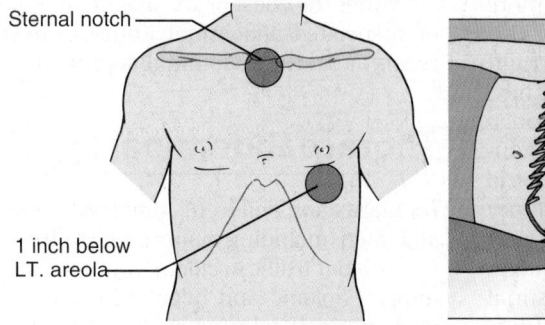

Sternal notch

1 inch below
LT. areola

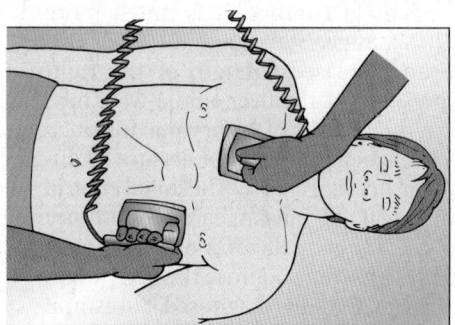

Fig. 73.10 Electrode application for external cardiac defibrillation.

catheter. Finally, spontaneous rupture proximal to an esophageal web has been described.

Clinically, fever, hypotension, and chest and neck pain reflect the presence of mediastinitis. Pneumomediastinum, tension pneumothorax, subcutaneous emphysema, and hematemesis may be encountered.

Plain chest radiographs followed by a contrast esophagram will usually demonstrate the esophageal defect. Sometimes, CT of the chest with a water-soluble, oral contrast study will help in the diagnosis as well as localize the site and size of the leak.

The fundamental principles of management in esophageal perforation include adequate pleural space drainage, intravenous antibiotics, and maintenance of adequate nutrition.[48] The operative therapy varies with the cause, the location of the perforation, and the time interval between the perforation and presentation. Many surgical maneuvers have been described. Given its anatomic location, the mid esophagus is approached via the right chest, whereas the lower esophagus is approached via the left chest. Thoracic esophageal perforation that is recognized early (<48 hours) can be treated with primary repair and muscle or pleural flap reinforcement. If the tissues are very inflamed and cannot hold sutures, resection with proximal diversion and staged reconstruction is recommended. Alternatively, placement of an esophageal T-tube to create a controlled fistula is a viable option and avoids the high morbidity of resection and diversion.[49]

Modern technology and improvements in thoracoscopic and endoscopic techniques have allowed minimally invasive approaches to these lesions. Primary thoracoscopic repair and placement of esophageal stents or endoscopic clipping have been described with good short-term outcomes.[50,51] Cervical perforations can usually be managed with drainage alone since they are more likely to be contained by the surrounding tissues. Stable patients with thoracic esophageal perforations who present several days after the perforation took place can be managed nonoperatively. This includes cessation of oral intake, broad-spectrum antibiotics, and parenteral nutritional support. The overall health status of the patient, the extent of associated injuries, and the underlying esophageal pathologic findings are the critical determinants of successful therapy.

Traumatic Blunt Rupture of the Diaphragm

Traumatic injury of the diaphragm is often due to penetrating thoracic or abdominal trauma; however, severe thoracic blunt force can also result in rupture. It is much more common on the left (90%). Suggested explanations for this phenomenon include an increased strength of the right hemidiaphragm, the presence of the liver, and a weakness of the left hemidiaphragm at points of embryonic fusion.[52] Most of these injuries are small and will not declare themselves until later during the hospital course. The initial clinical presentation is very nonspecific. Significant cardiorespiratory dysfunction may complicate the early stages. Many significant injuries in other organ systems may confuse the early diagnosis. If the rupture is not initially diagnosed, intestinal obstruction may be the leading symptom at the time of late diagnosis.

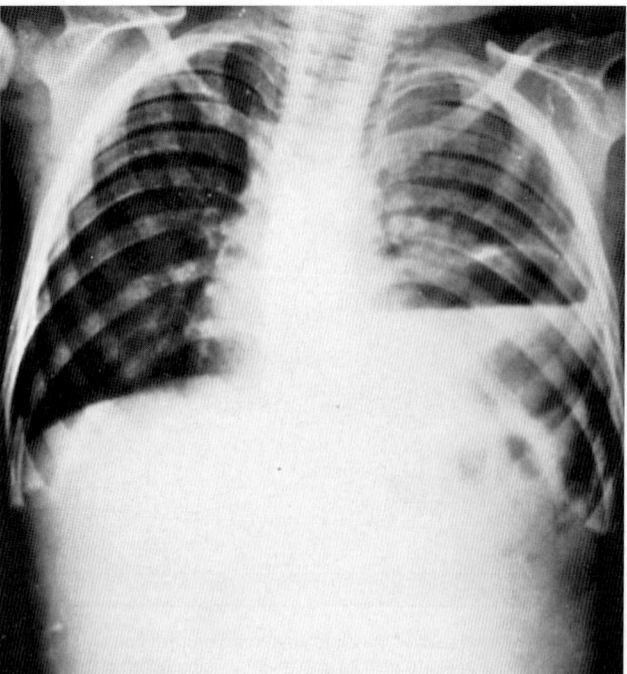

Fig. 73.11 A blunt traumatic rupture of the left hemidiaphragm that went unrecognized. Death occurred 1 hour later from acute gastric dilation of the intrathoracic stomach (same physiologic effects as tension pneumothorax).

The most significant study to arouse suspicion is routine chest radiography, which will frequently show an abnormal diaphragmatic contour (Fig. 73.11). Placement of a nasogastric tube can sometimes show gastric herniation into the chest. Initially, the herniation may not be present or suspected. Serial radiographs are important to determine later herniation. A contrast swallow of Gastrografin or thin barium will help confirm the presence of stomach or intestine in the hemithorax. CT can be helpful in the diagnosis, but the sensitivity and specificity are low for small diaphragmatic injuries.[53,54] While magnetic resonance imaging (MRI) shows exquisite detail of most of the diaphragm, it is not recommended given its impracticality in the acute setting. In those patients with high suspicion for traumatic diaphragmatic rupture, exploratory laparoscopy or thoracoscopy plays an important role and should be strongly considered.[55,56]

Acute traumatic diaphragmatic injuries are treated with surgical reduction of the herniated organs and closure of the diaphragmatic defect (Fig. 73.12). It can be approached via either the chest or the abdomen, but given the high rate of associated abdominal injuries, most trauma surgeons recommend the abdominal approach.

Thoracoabdominal Injuries

In infants and children, combined injury to the thorax and abdomen, including diaphragm rupture, is usually preceded by a violent traffic accident or other forms of sudden, jolting impact. Splenic and hepatic lacerations commonly occur with minimal external evidence of injury and need not be associated with fractured ribs or soft tissue mutilation.

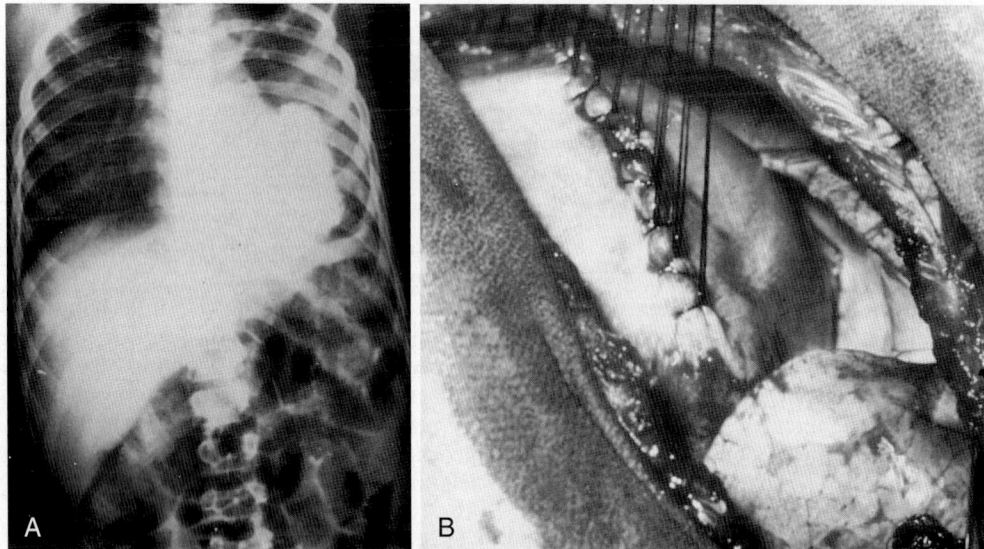

Fig. 73.12 A blunt traumatic rupture of the left hemidiaphragm, with barium swallow confirmation (A) and final closure at operation (B).

The clinical signs of upper abdominal tenderness, rigidity, and rebound tenderness almost uniformly accompany lower chest trauma and are explained by the abdominal distribution of the intercostal nerves. Therefore, peritoneal irritation, of itself, is not conclusive evidence of a combined or abdominal injury.

Diaphragm rupture can occur with minimal soft tissue injury, and there may be chest pain, dyspnea, and hypotension. On inspection, the involved chest wall lags during inspiration, and percussion can be dull or hyperresonant. Chest radiographs may not show fractured ribs, but almost invariably demonstrate abnormality or absence of the diaphragmatic shadow on the affected side. There is usually mediastinal shift to the right, because in 90% of cases the posterolateral left leaf of the diaphragm is torn in a radial manner. At times a spontaneous pneumoperitoneum is seen. The presence of blood alone (lacerations of spleen/liver) typically does not result in peritonitis in the absence of hollow viscous injuries (stomach, small bowel, colon).[57] Therefore, careful repeated examinations correlated with laboratory data are necessary for the diagnosis of intraabdominal hemorrhage and perforation in the presence of chest trauma.

The preliminary management of combined thoracoabdominal injuries must provide an adequate airway and circulation, gastric decompression, and evaluation and control of other injuries. Intraabdominal hemorrhage and perforation with thoracic and abdominal soiling is an obvious indication for immediate exploration. Ideally, exploration should be undertaken as soon as systemic stabilization has been achieved.

References

Access the reference list online at ExpertConsult.com.

74 Tumors of the Chest

JEONG S. HYUN, MD, and STEPHANIE D. CHAO, MD

Epidemiology

Tumors of the chest in the pediatric population represent many pathologies. They can differ in location from the chest wall, to the mediastinum, to the lung itself. They can be benign or malignant, primary or metastatic. Therefore, depending on the etiology, the incidence and epidemiology differ widely. All forms of primary neoplasms of the lung in the pediatric population are rare. A lung mass in the pediatric population is 10 times more likely to be a benign process than a malignant one.[1] Chest wall tumors account for only 1.8%[2] of all pediatric solid tumors, but tend to be malignant. The most common location of chest tumors is the mediastinum, and mediastinal masses can be further divided by their location into three compartments: anterior, middle, and posterior mediastinum. Mediastinal masses tend to occur early in the pediatric population, with around 40% of mediastinal masses occurring before the age of 2.[3] A case series of 120 patients showed that roughly 30% of these masses occur in the anterior mediastinum, around 25% in the middle mediastinum, and 40% in the posterior mediastinum.[4]

Etiology

The etiology of tumors of the chest ranges widely, depending on the location of the tumor. In terms of primary pulmonary lesions, tumors can arise from both the tracheobronchial tree and the pulmonary parenchyma itself, and they can accompany a wide variety of subtypes, from benign (inflammatory pseudotumor and hamartomas) to malignant (bronchial adenoma, bronchogenic carcinoma, pleuropulmonary blastoma).[5]

Benign Primary Pulmonary Lesions

PLASMA CELL GRANULOMA

Plasma cell granulomas have also been known as inflammatory pseudotumor, histiocytoma, inflammatory myofibroblastic tumor, and fibrohistiocytoma. These lesions are typically seen in patients less than 40 years old, with the majority in the pediatric population occurring in the age group between 8 and 12 years old. They are the most common benign lung tumors in the pediatric population, making up more than 50% of benign lesions and 20% of all primary lung lesions.[6] They usually present as a solitary peripherally based pulmonary nodule, but can also become locally invasive, causing symptoms such as fever, cough, pain, and hemoptysis, which require resection. In a cases series of 28 patients, there was predominance toward male patients,

and up to 85% of the diagnosed cases required surgical intervention.[7]

It is unclear whether the underlying etiology is that of a primary inflammatory process or a low-grade malignant process with an inflammatory component. There have been reports that plasma cell granulomas are usually preceded by respiratory infections. Most of these lesions are slow growing, although in some rare cases they can spread quickly, leading to airway compromise.

HAMARTOMAS

Hamartomas were first described by Eugen Albrecht in 1904.[8] They are benign malformations composed of disorganized components of normal lung tissue, including cartilage, epithelium, fat, and muscle. The lesions are usually located peripherally in the parenchyma of the lung but have also been noted, rarely, to be located centrally, as well as within the chest wall.[9] Hamartomas are the most common benign lesion in the adult population and the second most common benign pulmonary lesion in the pediatric population (18%–23%).[5] Unlike in adults, where they tend to be asymptomatic, hamartomas can grow to be large and symptomatic in children, causing respiratory distress and requiring surgical excision.[1] Popcorn-like calcifications are considered pathognomonic and they can be part of a triad (Carney) consisting of pulmonary hamartomas, extraadrenal paraganglioma, and gastric smooth muscle tumors.

Malignant Primary Pulmonary Lesions

BRONCHIAL ADENOMAS

Bronchial adenomas are tumors that derive from the mucous gland of the bronchi or the cells that line the excretory ducts of these glands. While the name *adenoma* suggests a benign process, bronchial adenomas can become malignant. There are three histologic types of bronchial adenomas: carcinoid, cylindroma, and mucoepidermoid. Around 80%–85% of bronchial adenomas in children are the carcinoid type, and they are similar in resemblance to carcinoid tumors of the small bowel. Bronchial carcinoids are thought to derive from neuroendocrine Kulitchsky cells. They are low-grade tumors, which can metastasize, but most are slow-growing tumors that can grow into the bronchial wall. Carcinoid syndrome itself is rare, although it has been reported in the pediatric population.[10] Cylindromas make up around 10%–15% of bronchial adenomas, and they consist of cuboidal or flattened epithelial cells that derive from the mucous secreting cells of the larynx and tracheobronchial tree. They are also low-grade, slow-growing malignancies, but they are considered the most aggressive of all three histologic types and can metastasize. Mucoepidermoid tumors originate in the larger airways and are the rarest subtype, comprising only 1%–5% of bronchial adenomas.

Bronchial adenomas usually present with vague pulmonary symptoms such as fever, cough, chest pain, recurrent pneumonitis, and hemoptysis as the tumor slowly grows into the airway and causes incomplete obstruction. These symptoms can cause children to be treated for asthma. The rarity of these disorders commonly causes a delay in diagnosis, often for years. The tumors usually involve the right main bronchus and are 5 times more likely to be seen in boys.

Treatment consists primarily of resection of a segment, lobe, or complete lung, according to the degree of involvement, which may be done thoracoscopically or via thoracotomy, depending on the location and extent of the lesion. Luminal excision by bronchoscopy should not be done because it does not permit complete removal of the tumor. Rarely a bronchial adenoma can be removed by bronchial or sleeve resection, followed by airway reconstruction.

BRONCHOGENIC CARCINOMA

Bronchogenic carcinomas are exceedingly rare in the pediatric population, with only 60 reported cases in children,[11] and they represent approximately 20% of primary malignant lung tumors. Most present during adolescence. Most pediatric bronchogenic carcinomas are undifferentiated adenocarcinomas, with squamous cell carcinomas being much less common in the pediatric population, in contrast to the adult population. Usually asymptomatic, the majority of cases present late in the course of the disease leading to a poor prognosis; the mortality is more than 90%, with a mean duration of survival of only 7 months. Localized lesions can be resected with postoperative chemotherapy, but this applies to only a small subset of patients. The presenting symptoms are vague, including cough, hemoptysis, and weight loss. The tumor presents as a central pulmonary mass with endobronchial growth.

PLEUROPULMONARY BLASTOMA

Pleuropulmonary blastomas (PPB) are rare malignant tumors that arise from the primitive interstitial mesenchyme of the lung. These typically occur in younger children prior to the age of 6 years and can behave aggressively with high rates of metastasis. There are three pathologic types of PPBs. Type I is purely cystic and is diagnosed around the age of 10 months, with a survival rate of 80%–85%.[12] Type II is a combination of cystic and solid, and type III is a purely solid lesion. There is evidence that all three types may develop on a continuum, where type II and III types present later, with type II presenting around 34 months and type III around 44 months. There have been reports linking congenital pulmonary airway malformations (CPAM) to PPB. Specifically, type IV CPAMs are highly suspicious for malignancy and may be cystic PPB. With CPAMs, the presence of symptoms, lack of a systemic feeding vessel, and hyperinflated lung lead toward a higher suspicion of possible malignancy.[13] There appears to be a familial component to PPB in up to 25% of cases. The DICER 1 gene has been implicated as an important genetic factor in the development of familial pleuropulmonary

blastoma.[14] Often, PPBs occur in the right chest with metastasis to the liver, brain, and spinal cord. Surgical excision of cystic PPBs, with or without adjuvant chemotherapy, offers cure rates exceeding 85%. However, cure rates drop significantly if PPBs present later to care, when they have evolved into mixed cystic/solid or solid phases.[15]

Chest Wall Tumors

Chest wall tumors are rare, and they encompass a wide variety of disease processes based on tumor types, tissue of origin, and behavior, so it is difficult to characterize them. They can be primary or secondary to invasion from adjacent structures. They are primarily mesenchymal tumors and are divided into benign and malignant disease, with up to 60% being malignant.[16] The majority of chest wall tumors come from skeletal structures (55%), with the remainder originating in the soft tissues of the chest wall (45%).

Chest wall masses often present as seemingly innocuous lumps that are noticed on the chest, which may demonstrate growth. They are typically slow-growing and asymptomatic, but pain can be a presenting symptom that raises the concern for a malignant process. A small percentage of these tumors can have effects on respiratory mechanics, depending on their location and size.

Benign tumors of the chest wall are less common than malignant ones and have a wide variety of etiologies. Lipomas of the chest wall are rare in the pediatric population. The most common soft tissue benign lesion of the chest wall derives from the myofibroblast,[17] including infantile myofibromatosis and desmoid fibromatosis tumor. Infantile myofibromatosis typically presents at birth or early in life and usually undergoes spontaneous regression. In contrast, desmoid fibromatosis can be more challenging to deal with, as they originate as overgrowths of fibrous tissue that can extend through muscle and fascial planes. Full excision can be challenging, and these patients often undergo multiple surgeries.

BENIGN TUMORS

Mesenchymal hamartomas are benign lesions typically found at birth that may present as a deforming chest mass, or they may be found incidentally on chest radiograph. These lesions tend to grow intrathoracically, causing respiratory symptoms. They have a characteristic appearance on radiograph with large calcifications arising from one or more ribs causing distortion of the osseous thorax. Although this description suggests an aggressive, possibly malignant process, mesenchymal hamartomas are benign, with no reports of malignant degeneration, recurrence, or metastasis after resection. Resection should only be undertaken to relieve respiratory symptoms related to mass effect from the lesion.

The most common benign skeletal neoplasms are osteochondromas, and they account for almost half of all tumors arising from the ribs.[18] These tumors consist of bony and cartilaginous components occurring near the end of long bones. They present during puberty, with an almost 3 : 1 predominance in males. They are frequently asymptomatic, but they can present with pain, can grow into adjacent nerves, may cause pathologic fractures, and can cause physical asymmetry of the chest, which is often cosmetically distressing. There is a characteristic "cartilage cap" seen on plain radiograph, and if the cap is greater than 1 cm, there is concern for the risk of chondrosarcoma.

Chondromas are benign tumors that arise in the costal cartilage and are composed of mature hyaline cartilage, usually at the sternocostal junction. They are typically slow-growing, painless masses that are not aggressive in nature. While benign, they are very similar in clinical course and in terms of imaging features to chondrosarcomas. Therefore they often have to be treated with wide local excision.

MALIGNANT TUMORS

In contrast, chondrosarcomas are rare malignant tumors in the pediatric population, typically peaking in adult males in their thirties. However, given their similar appearance to chondromas, they are important to distinguish. They are slow-growing lesions that can start to cause pain, and they have a risk of late metastasis. The direction of growth appears to be entirely internal, thus stimulating the radiologic appearance of a primary pleural or mediastinal tumor. However, there is usually an externally visible and palpable mass. Chemotherapy and radiotherapy are not effective against chondrosarcomas. Thus they require a wide resection, as there is a high risk for local recurrence.

Of malignant chest wall lesions, primitive neuroectodermal tumors (PNET), often referred to as Ewing's sarcoma or Askin's tumors, are the most common in the pediatric population. They were first described by Askin and colleagues[19] in a series of 20 children. These tumors originate from embryonal neural crest cells and behave aggressively. It should be assumed that there is micrometastasis present at the time of diagnosis. PNETs of the chest typically present in the early teenage years, with a 2:1 male to female ratio. Symptoms include the development of a painful mass, dyspnea, weight loss, and, in some cases, Horner syndrome. Radiographs show lytic destruction, with an accompanying pleural effusion. Often computed tomography (CT) scan and magnetic resonance imaging (MRI) are needed to define the extent of the lesion and to determine presence of pulmonary metastasis, which can occur in up to 25% of cases at the time of presentation. Cytogenetic studies have shown that PNETs have a characteristic balanced translocation between chromosome 11 and 22 (t11:22 [q24:q21]). Treatment of PNETs is multimodal including chemotherapy, wide excision, and radiotherapy due to their high local recurrence rate. Prognosis for these tumors can be quite dismal, with 2- and 6-year survival rates being reported at 38% and 14%, respectively.[20]

Mediastinal Tumors

The mediastinum is the portion of the body that lies between the lungs and contains all the structures within the thoracic cavity except the lung. It is bounded anteriorly by the sternum and posteriorly by the vertebrae and extends superiorly from the suprasternal notch to terminate inferiorly at the diaphragm. Cysts or tumors that arise within the mediastinum may originate from any of the structures contained therein or may be the result of developmental abnormalities.

For ease of definition of sites of disease, the mediastinum may be thought of as divided into three compartments: (1) the anterior mediastinum—the portion of the mediastinum that lies anterior to the anterior plane of the trachea; (2) the middle mediastinum—the portion containing the heart and pericardium, the ascending aorta, the lower segment of the superior vena cava, bifurcation of the pulmonary artery, the trachea, the two main bronchi, and the bronchial lymph nodes; and (3) the posterior mediastinum—the portion that lies posterior to the anterior plane of the trachea.

LYMPHOMAS

The most common mediastinal masses in children are lymphomas. Any lymph node enlargement in a child should be viewed with suspicion, since lymphatic tumors are one of the more frequently observed malignant growths in childhood. Lymphoma is the third most common malignancy in children overall and represents almost half of all mediastinal malignancies. Hodgkin disease, lymphosarcoma, and reticulum cell sarcoma are found primarily in children older than 3 years of age, with a peak incidence between 8 and 14 years of age. Lymphomas can occur in any of the compartments of the mediastinum, but in children, they most frequently are in the anterior and middle mediastinum. One-third of the lymphomas are Hodgkin lymphoma and two-thirds are non-Hodgkin lymphoma. Non-Hodgkin lymphoma is more likely to occur in younger children, while Hodgkin lymphoma tends to present in adolescent populations.

More than 95% of children with primary lymphatic malignancy have lymph node enlargement as the presenting sign. Tonsillar hypertrophy and adenoidal hyperplasia, pulmonary hilar enlargement, splenomegaly, bone pain, unexplained fever, anemia, infiltrative skin lesions, and rarely central nervous system symptoms may also be present.

The diagnosis should be sought through the study of peripheral blood smears, lymph node biopsy, pleural fluid examination, and bone marrow examination.

If all other diagnostic studies are negative, the mediastinal node can be biopsied. Fine-needle aspiration is usually not satisfactory; thus core needle biopsy (directly or via mediastinoscopy, thoracoscopy, or anterior thoracotomy) is frequently required. Importantly, anesthetic management is complicated if there is greater than 50% tracheal luminal compression or significant preoperative dyspnea. Surgery is rarely required in the treatment of lymphomas, although the diagnosis is often made via surgical biopsy. Biopsy of mediastinal lymph nodes requires careful, multidisciplinary preoperative planning. Often there are palpable cervical or axillary nodes, which may be amenable to biopsy and may pose less risk in establishing the diagnosis.

HYPERPLASIA OF THE THYMUS

Hyperplasia of the thymus is the most frequent of the thymic lesions. Because the normal thymus varies greatly in size and with age, *thymic hyperplasia* is a relative term. Steroids, infection, androgens, and irradiation may cause involution; the stimuli that cause hyperplasia are not well understood. As in other ductless glands, variations in size are probably related to patient individuality.

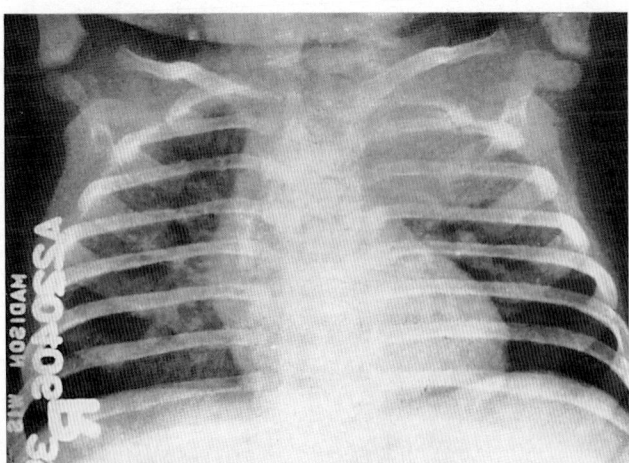

Fig. 74.1 Mild respiratory distress in an infant with an enlarged thymus. Gradual improvement occurred with age and no specific therapy.

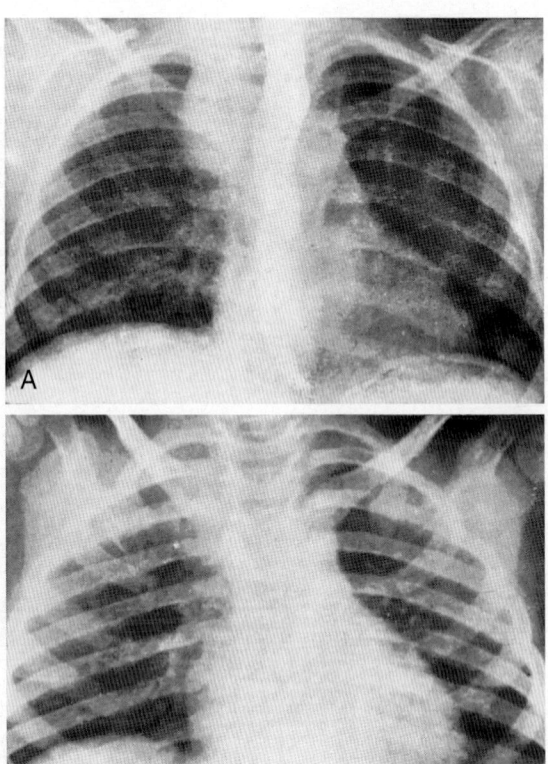

Fig. 74.2 (A) An enlarged thymus in an infant. (B) A reduction in size can be seen after 7 days of steroid therapy.

On the chest radiograph of normal infants, a thymic shadow of variable size and shape is typically present during the first month of life. The mediastinal shadow in young infants is proportionally wider than in older children and adults, because of the proportionally larger heart and thymic shadow. The thymic shadow typically disappears by 1 year of age. Among children older than 4 years of age, 2% still have a recognizable thymus on radiographic examination. Cervical extension of the thymus gland is common. If the thymus is in the superior thoracic inlet, its enlargement may cause tracheal compression (Fig. 74.1).

In the unusual situation in which an enlarged thymus causes respiratory obstruction, treatment may be carried out in one of three ways. While the thymus does respond rapidly to small doses of irradiation (70–150 cGy), the concern of a carcinogenic effect has caused this method of treatment to be abandoned. Corticosteroids cause a rapid decrease in the size of the thymus, usually within 5–7 days. However, after cessation of corticosteroid therapy, the gland may reach a size greater than that before treatment was instituted. Such a response may also be used in distinguishing between a physiologic enlargement of the thymus and a neoplasm (Fig. 74.2). Excision may be indicated both for the treatment of respiratory obstruction and for diagnosis.

NEOPLASMS OF THE THYMUS

Malignant thymic tumors in children are quite rare. Lymphosarcoma is more frequent, and primary Hodgkin's disease of the thymus and carcinoma have both been described. In only one 19-year-old patient has there been an associated myasthenia gravis syndrome. An ectopic parathyroid carcinoma located in the thymus has also been documented.[21]

Benign Thymoma

Rarely benign thymic tumors have been reported in children, accounting for only 1%–2% of mediastinal masses (Fig. 74.3). Roughly one-third of patients with thymomas will have symptoms of local invasion. They are classified as invasive or noninvasive, depending on whether they extend past their fibrous capsule.

Thymic Cysts

Thymic cysts are rare, cystic remnants of the thymopharyngeal duct. Multiple small cysts of the thymus are frequently observed in necropsy material, but large thymic cysts are rare (Fig. 74.4). While they are typically asymptomatic, manifesting after 2 years of age, there have been reports of cysts causing respiratory failure in infants, as they can be located anywhere between the pyriform sinus and the anterior mediastinum.[22] Techniques and operative approaches are site-specific. Thymic cysts have been resected from a cervical approach (Fig. 74.5).

Teratoma of the Thymus

Several cases of thymic teratoma have been reported. Patients typically have a good prognosis after resection.[23]

TERATOID MEDIASTINAL TUMORS

Teratoid tumors of the mediastinum may be classified as: (1) benign cystic teratomas, (2) benign teratoids (solid), or (3) teratoids (carcinoma). They make up 10%–12% of all teratomas and 20% of all mediastinal pediatric neoplasms.[24]

Benign Cystic Teratoma

Teratoma of the anterior mediastinum probably results from faulty embryogenesis of the thymus or from local dislocation during embryogenesis. Benign cystic teratomas (mediastinal dermoid cyst) contain such elements of ectodermal tissue as hair, sweat glands, sebaceous cysts, and teeth. Other elements, including mesodermal and endodermal tissue, may also be found when benign cystic teratoid lesions are subjected

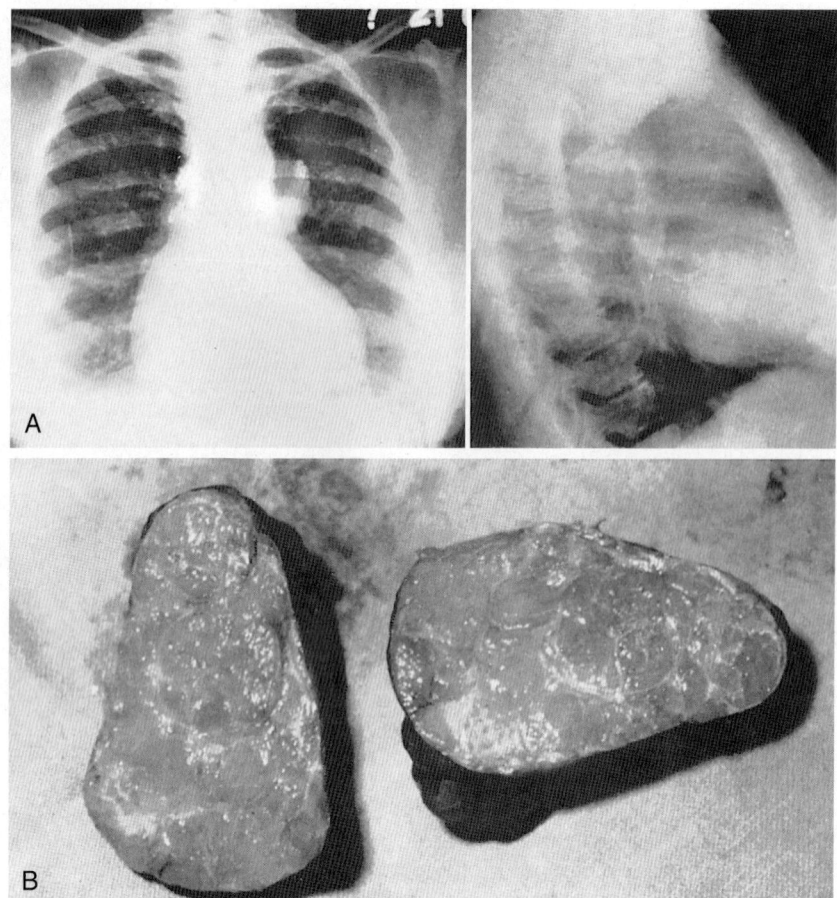

Fig. 74.3 Benign thymoma located in the anterior superior mediastinum. (A) Posteroanterior and lateral radiographs before surgery. (B) Photograph of thymoma after excision.

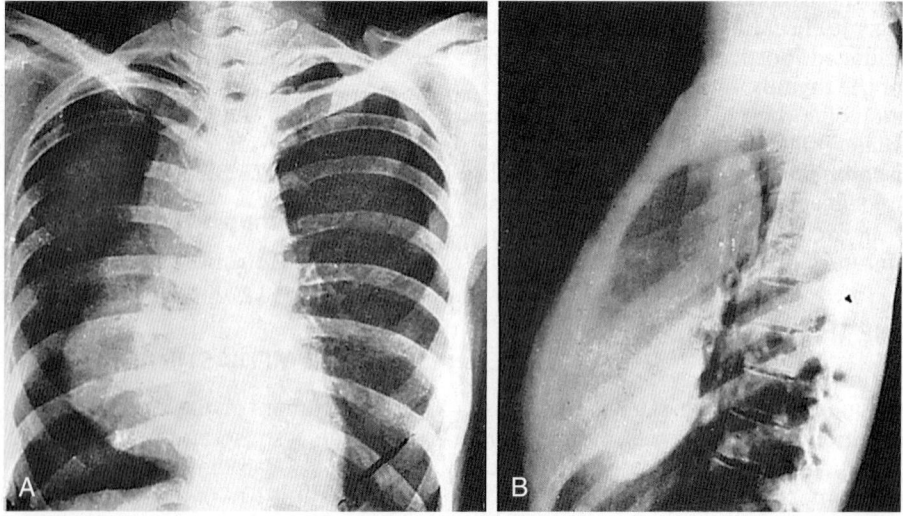

Fig. 74.4 Large thymic cyst located near the diaphragm in an adult. Posteroanterior (A) and left lateral (B) radiographs.

to comprehensive examination; thus such tumors are more properly classified as teratoid than dermoid cysts.

Cystic teratomas are more common than solid ones. These lesions are predominantly located in the anterior mediastinum and may project into either hemithorax, more commonly

the right. In children, females are affected more often than males. Malignant degeneration is less common than in the solid form of teratoid tumor.

These cystic masses usually cause symptoms because of pressure on, or erosion into, the adjacent respiratory

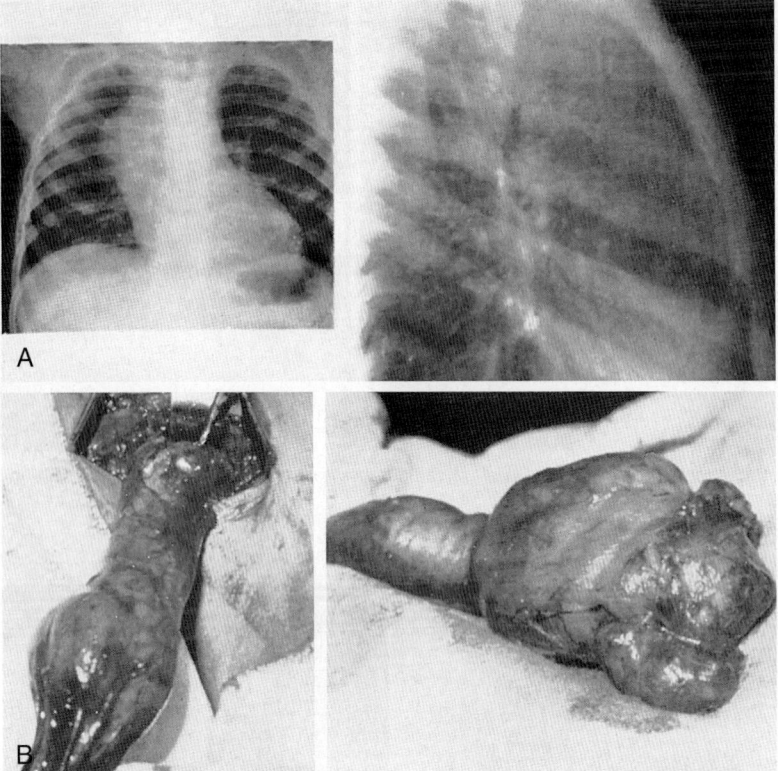

Fig. 74.5 (A) Large thymic cyst in a 4-year-old boy that was evident as a mass in the right side of the neck clinically as well as on a chest x-ray. Removal required a thoracotomy and a supraclavicular incision. (B) Thymic cyst as seen after a thoracotomy and at the time of removal through a neck incision.

structures. Symptoms usually include vague chest discomfort associated with cough, dyspnea, and pneumonitis. Infection may cause a sudden exacerbation of symptoms, and rupture of the mass into the lung may occur with expectoration of hair and other materials; rupture into the pleura or pericardium may also occur.

On radiography, the lesion is well outlined, with sharp borders; definite diagnosis on plain radiograph is not possible unless teeth can be demonstrated in the mass. Calcification, which is not unusual, appears as scattered masses rather than as diffuse stippling. Cystic swelling in the suprasternal notch may be visible.

Benign cystic teratomas should be removed. In cases in which infection, perforation, intracystic hemorrhage, or malignant degeneration has occurred, complete removal may be difficult or impossible, owing to adherence to surrounding vital structures.

Benign Solid Teratoid Tumors and Malignant Teratoid Tumors

Teratomas are the most common tumor occurring in the anterior mediastinum of infants and children (Fig. 74.6), and the mediastinum is the second most common location for these masses. The solid tumors in the teratoid group are much more complex and have a greater propensity for malignant change (Fig. 74.7). The incidence of malignancy has been reported as 10%–25%. In addition to standard imaging studies, preoperative serum studies should include serum α-fetoprotein, carcinoembryonic antigen, and β-human chorionic gonadotropin, both as diagnostic markers and as baseline values to monitor disease burden.

Patients present with chest pain, cough, dyspnea, and rarely hemoptysis.[25] Most mediastinal teratomas are present at birth, and many are now detected prenatally. However, there are multiple reports of large masses discovered only in adulthood.[26]

Benign solid teratoid tumors have well-differentiated structures that are rarely observed in malignant tumors. They contain tissue from one or more of the three germ cell layers. The connective tissue stroma of malignant teratomas is usually poorly arranged, but that of benign teratomas is dense and of the adult type. In the benign type, nerve tissue, skin, and teeth may be found. Skin and its appendages are usually present and remarkably well formed. Hair follicles preserve their normal slightly oblique position relative to the free surface and are always accompanied by well-developed sebaceous glands. Sweat glands, often of the apocrine type, are frequently located near the sebaceous glands. Smooth muscle closely resembling *arrectores pilorum* is occasionally encountered.

Mesodermal derivatives, such as connective tissue, bone, cartilage, and muscle arranged in organoid patterns, are frequently found. When present, hematopoietic tissue is found only in association with cancellous bone. Smooth muscle is most often observed as longitudinal or circular bundles in organoid alimentary structures. Occasionally it is also seen in bronchial walls. Endodermal derivatives representing such structures as intestine and respiratory and pancreatic tissue are also present.

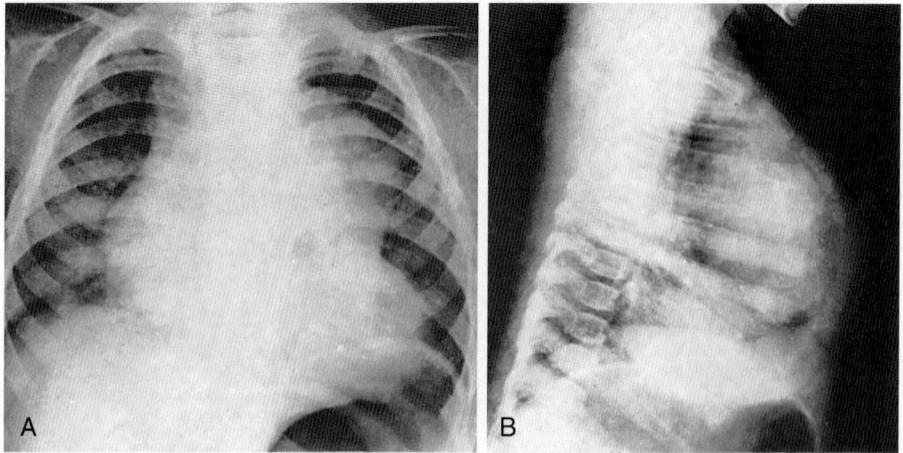

Fig. 74.6 (A) Large, solid, benign teratoma in an infant. (B) On lateral radiograph, note the anterior mediastinal position and the forward displacement of the sternum.

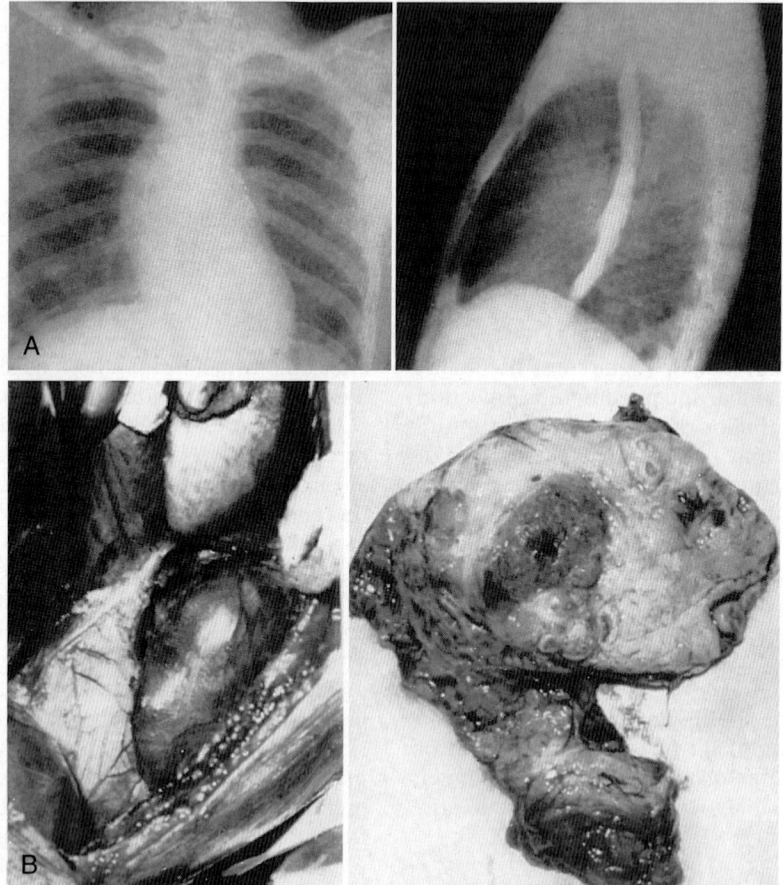

Fig. 74.7 (A) Posteroanterior and lateral radiographs of an anterior malignant teratoma in an older child. (B) Note the anterior mediastinal position, with the teratoma wedged between the heart and the sternum.

The final diagnosis of malignancy can be determined only after removal and histologic study of the tumor. Malignant degeneration is typically rare and generally only involves one of the cellular components. In general, the outcome is poor with malignant teratomas, chemotherapy and radiotherapy notwithstanding, which usually consists of etoposide, bleomycin, and cisplatin.

Nonseminomatous Germ Cell Tumors

The nonseminomatous germ cell tumors or embryonal tumors consist of a wide variety of diseases such as seminomas, yolk-sac carcinomas, choriocarcinomas, and embryonal carcinomas. These tumors are all malignant and require multimodal therapy, including resection and chemotherapy. Standard workup should always include cross-sectional imaging, and preoperative serum studies should include serum α-fetoprotein, carcinoembryonic antigen, and β-human chorionic gonadotropin.

VASCULAR-LYMPHATIC ABNORMALITIES OF THE MEDIASTINUM

Vascular-lymphatic abnormalities of the mediastinum may be classified as (1) cavernous hemangioma, (2) hemangiopericytoma, (3) angiosarcoma, or (4) lymphangioma (cystic hygroma).

Vascular tumors isolated to the mediastinum in children are rare, and they may occur at any level in the mediastinum but are more frequent in the upper portion of the thorax and in the anterior mediastinum. They are uniformly rounded in appearance and are moderately dense. There are two major subtypes of hemangiomas: rapidly involuting and nonrapidly involuting. If hemangiomas do not cause respiratory symptoms, they are left untreated as they tend to disappear over time.

Though rare, *isolated* mediastinal lymphangiomas occur more often in infants and children than in adults. These tumors consist of masses of dilated lymphatic channels that contain lymph; they are lined with flat endothelium and are usually multilocular. They may appear to be isolated in the mediastinum (Fig. 74.8) but usually have an associated cervical component. They may be rather large and unilateral, with lateral masses in the superior mediastinum.

Diagnosis of a cervicomediastinal lymphangioma is aided by physical examination of cervical swelling and radiographic examination of the chest. Periodic fluctuation in size frequently occurs in the cervical location. Radiographic and fluoroscopic examination may show descent of the mass into the mediastinum on inspiration, with prominence in the neck during expiration.

Cystic hygroma confined to the mediastinum is usually discovered as an unanticipated finding on radiographic examination. The soft and yielding nature of the cysts allows them to attain considerable size without producing symptoms.

On radiograph, there is a somewhat lobulated, smoothly outlined mass; however, it is usually not possible to distinguish lymphangiomas from other benign tumors or cysts of the mediastinum by imaging.

When respiratory infections occur, lymphangiomas may become infected. Such infections are usually controlled with antibiotics or drainage. Infection may be followed by local fibrosis and disappearance of the mass. Spontaneous or posttraumatic hemorrhage into a cyst may result in extension of the cyst; this may cause sudden tracheal compression, which is a surgical emergency. Malignant change in lymphangiomas has not been reported.[27]

Surgical excision is the treatment of choice for localized lesions, although it may be challenging due to their tendency to grow around other structures. Incomplete resection ensures almost certain recurrence. Extensive disease remains an unsolved problem; for macrocystic variants, intralesional sclerotherapy has had some utility. Chylothorax may result when there is involvement of the thoracic duct. Antiangiogenesis therapy has shown some promise in treating angiosarcoma, although further investigation is needed.[28] Sclerotherapy has gained favor in complex cervical lymphangiomas; the same principles should apply to thoracic locations.

MEDIASTINAL LIPOMA, LIP SARCOMA, AND LIPOBLASTOMA

Intrathoracic lipoma is rare in children. Lipomas of the mediastinum have been divided into three groups according to their location and form: (1) tumors confined within the thoracic cage, (2) intrathoracic lipomas that extend upward into the neck, and (3) intrathoracic lipomas, with an extrathoracic extension forming a dumbbell configuration. Lipomas tend to be soft, so most of these lesions tend to be asymptomatic.

Of the mediastinal lipomas reported in the world literature, 76% were intrathoracic, 10% were cervicomediastinal, and 14% were of the dumbbell type. Only 15 occurred in the

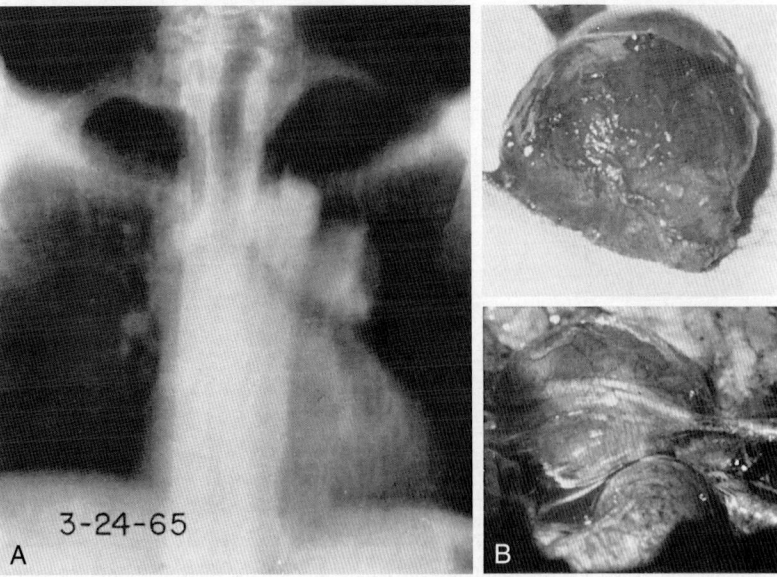

Fig. 74.8 Large lymphatic cyst in the anterior mediastinum. (A) Posteroanterior radiograph. (B) Photographs.

pediatric age group, and these were intrathoracic. They may grow to very large size; a mass weighing 7.9 kg has been reported.[29] Seven cases of liposarcoma of the mediastinum in children have been reported.[30] Although these tumors usually do not metastasize, their invasiveness and tendency to recur locally place them in the malignant group.

Lipoblastoma is a rare benign tumor that occurs in children and arises from fetal embryonal fat. Thirty-five cases have been reported in the world literature, only 1 of which was in the mediastinum. Nearly 90% of the tumors are detected in children younger than 3 years of age.[31] At surgery, the lipoblastoma appears as a soft, yellow-gray or white-gray mass that can be easily removed. Histologically they may be confused with liposarcomas.

Complete surgical excision is the procedure of choice. Repeated surgical excisions may serve as a method of extended control, and radiation therapy may be added for palliative purposes.

NEUROGENIC MEDIASTINAL TUMORS

Neurogenic tumors, by far the most common tumors with posterior mediastinal origin, make up 25%–35% of all mediastinal tumors. More than 50% present before the age of two, and they account for around 10% of pediatric tumors. They have highly variable behavior, sometimes regressing spontaneously, undergoing differentiation, or proliferating to malignant disease. They may be classified as follows:

1. Neurofibroma and neurilemoma
   - Malignant schwannoma
2. Tumors of sympathetic origin
   - Neuroblastoma
   - Ganglioneuroma
   - Ganglioneuroblastoma
   - Pheochromocytoma
3. Chemodectoma

Benign neurofibromas, neurilemomas, and malignant schwannomas are extremely unusual in the pediatric age group, and when present they are most often asymptomatic (Fig. 74.9).

A neuroblastoma is a malignant tumor arising from a neural crest origin; the usual site is the adrenal medulla, but it may occur anywhere along the ganglia of the sympathetic chain from the neck to the pelvis. Although a primary neuroblastoma may cause the first clinical signs or symptoms (such as Horner's syndrome or respiratory distress), metastases in the bone, skin, or lymph nodes can also be the first indication of its presence. While most other childhood cancers have shown marked improvement in survival over the last 3 decades, neuroblastoma has not. Infants younger than 1 year of age do have a better prognosis and respond better to chemotherapy. The International Neuroblastoma Staging System, adopted in 1988, relies on complete surgical resection along with lymph node and distal metastases to dictate treatment.[32] The ganglioneuroma is a benign tumor made

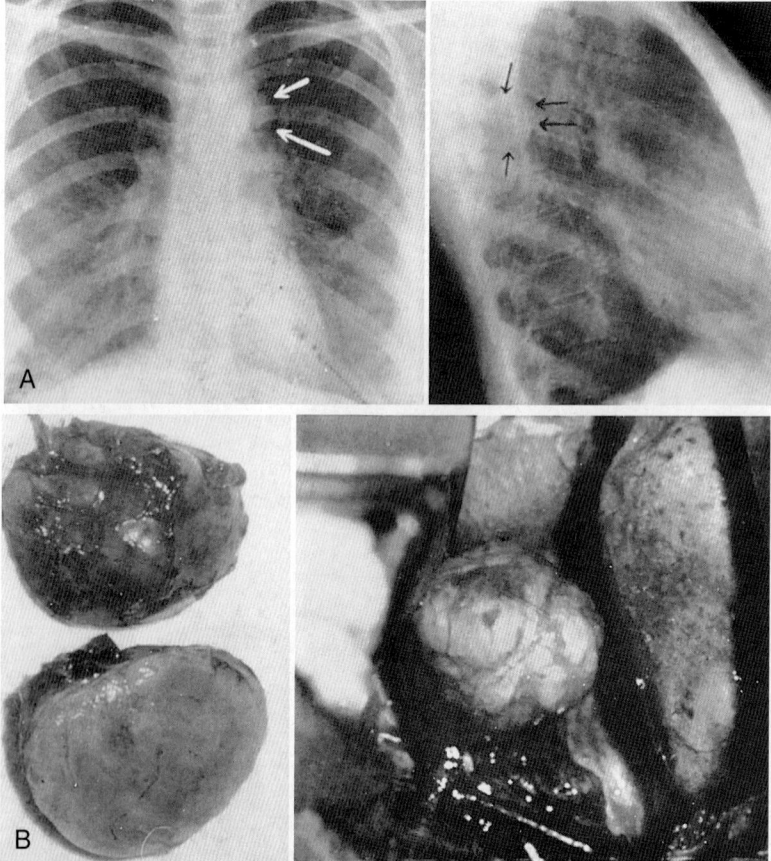

Fig. 74.9 (A) Neurofibroma seen posteriorly located in posteroanterior and lateral radiographs. (B) Note the solid nature of the lesion, its round smooth outline, and its attachment to the intercostal nerve.

up of mature ganglion cells, few or many, in a stroma of nerve fibers. Ganglioneuroblastoma is a tumor composed of various proportions of neuroblastoma and ganglioneuroma.

Ganglioneuroma and ganglioneuroblastoma are more likely to present after 2 years of age. The more malignant forms, such as neuroblastoma, frequently manifest before the age of 2 years. Ganglioneuroma is more common in children than in adults; respiratory symptoms are rare.

Most of these tumors usually occur in the upper two-thirds of the hemithorax and tend to extend locally. They may grow into the lower part of the neck, across the midline through the posterior mediastinum to the opposite hemithorax, descend through the diaphragm into the upper part of the abdomen or into the intercostal spaces posteriorly, and involve one or several of the vertebral foramina.

While some such tumors are discovered incidentally, symptoms such as radicular pain, paraplegia, motor disturbances, and Horner syndrome may be the presenting complaint. Upper respiratory tract infections, dyspnea, fever, and weight loss may occur. Neurogenic tumors of the neuroblastoma group usually occur in younger children, and respiratory symptoms, thoracic pain, and fever are more common (Fig. 74.10).

On radiographic examination, neurogenic tumors are round, oval, or spindle-shaped and are characteristically located posteriorly in the paravertebral gutter. On thoracic radiographs, a ganglioneuroma appears as an elongated lesion and may extend over several vertebrae. Typically a neurofibroma tends to be more rounded in outline. Calcifications within the tumor may be seen, more commonly in the malignant forms. Even though not demonstrated on radiographic examination, calcification may be found at the time of histologic examination. Bone lesions, such as intercostal space widening, costal deformation, vertebral involvement, and metastatic bone disease, are common. Staging with CT or MRI scans is routine and well prescribed in oncologic protocols.

The primary therapy for localized thoracic neurogenic tumors is surgical excision. Ganglioneuroma (benign) are generally amenable to resection. In malignant neurogenic tumors, principles and timing of surgical resection depend on the degree of extension at presentation. The extent of tumor resection and postoperative irradiation therapy also depend on tumor grade and histology. Radiotherapy must be given judiciously, because growth disturbances, pulmonary fibrosis, and other sequelae may develop.

Mediastinal chemodectomas are usually located anteriorly; they are likely to be associated with similar tumors in the carotid body and elsewhere. There is a tendency for these tumors to be multiple. Mediastinal pheochromocytomas make up less than 1% of all mediastinal tumors; extra-adrenal pheochromocytomas are more common in children than in adults. The tumor may be a cause of refractory hypertension in children as in adults.[33]

PRIMARY MEDIASTINAL CYSTS

Lesions occurring within the mediastinum may be predominantly cystic or predominantly solid. Cystic lesions are usually benign; solid lesions have higher malignant potential. Primary mediastinal cysts likely represent abnormalities in embryologic development at the site of the foregut just when separation of esophageal and lung buds occurs (Fig. 74.11).

Structures that arise from the foregut are the pharynx, thyroid, parathyroid, thymus, respiratory tract, esophagus, stomach, upper part of the duodenum, liver, and pancreas; thus abnormal development at this stage may give rise to bronchogenic cysts, esophageal duplication cysts, and gastroenteric cysts.

Bronchogenic Cysts

Maier[34] classified bronchogenic cysts according to location as tracheal, hilar (Fig. 74.12), carinal (Fig. 74.13), esophageal, and miscellaneous (Fig. 74.14). This classification remains useful. Modern nomenclature also uses the term *foregut duplication cysts*, which is a correct embryologic description of their developmental origin.

Bronchogenic cysts are usually located in the middle mediastinum, but have been described in all mediastinal locations. Under microscopic examination, bronchogenic cysts may contain any or all the tissues normally present in the trachea and bronchi (fibrous connective tissue, mucous glands, cartilage, smooth muscle, and a lining formed by ciliated pseudostratified columnar epithelium or stratified squamous epithelium). The fluid inside the cyst is either clear waterlike liquid or viscous gelatinous material.

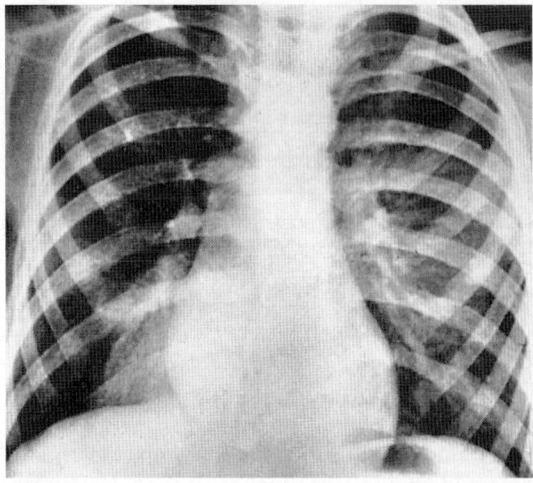

Fig. 74.10 Chest X-ray of a neuroblastoma in a 6-year-old boy.

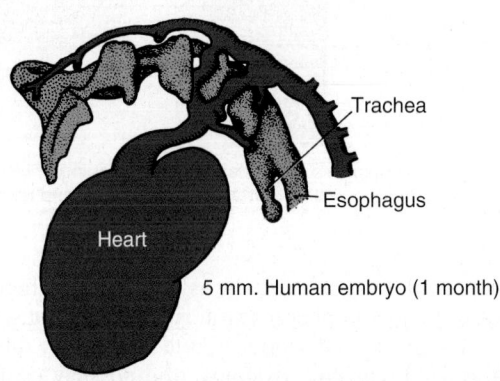

Fig. 74.11 The foregut, which lies between the tracheal and esophageal buds, is the probable site of embryologic maldevelopment, which gives rise to the growth of foregut cysts.

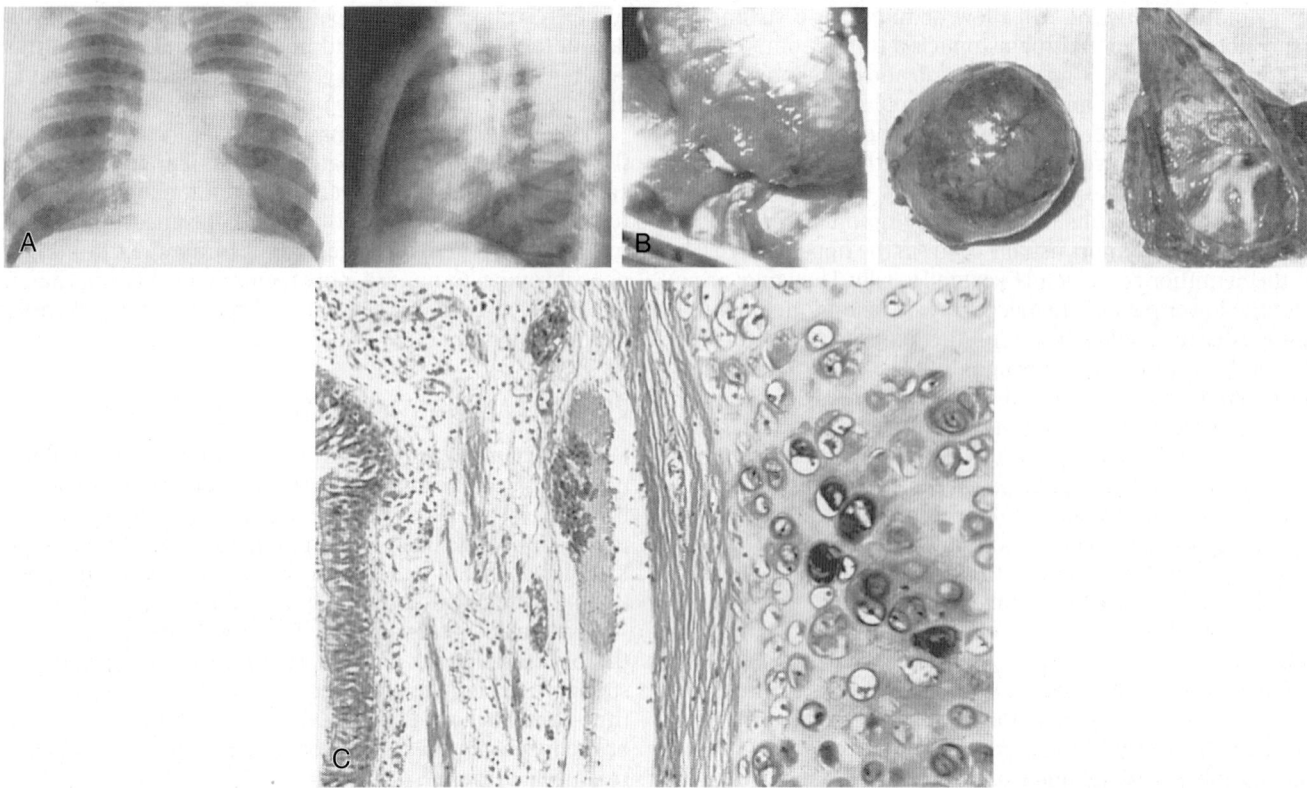

Fig. 74.12 (A) Typical left hilar bronchogenic cyst with a rounded, smooth border and a density similar to cardiac density. (B) At the time of thoracotomy, a solid stalk was found attached to the left main bronchus. The cyst was unilocular and contained thick, yellowish mucoid material. The wall was thin with typical trabeculations. (C) Microscopic study revealed cartilage, smooth muscle, and pseudostratified, ciliated, columnar epithelium.

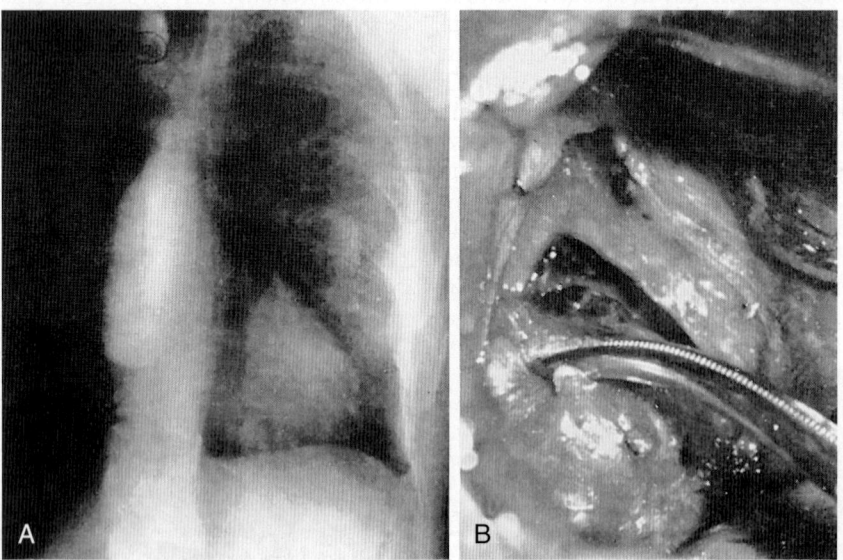

Fig. 74.13 (A) Overexposed posteroanterior chest radiograph shows a carinal bronchogenic cyst. (B) At the operation, the location is clearly seen at the carina. A solid fibrous stalk is attached at the carina and is separated just beneath the instrument dissector.

Bronchogenic cysts are usually asymptomatic. There may, however, be frequent upper respiratory tract infections, vague feelings of substernal discomfort, and respiratory difficulty (cough, noisy breathing, dyspnea, and possibly cyanosis). Bronchogenic cysts may communicate with the tracheobronchial tree and show varying air-fluid levels accompanied by the expectoration of purulent material. If communication

with the tracheobronchial tree is present, it may be visualized by bronchoscopy.

On radiographic examination, the bronchogenic cyst is usually a single, smooth-bordered, spherical mass (Fig. 74.15). It has a uniform density similar to that of the cardiac shadow. Calcification is unusual. Fluoroscopic examination of the cyst may demonstrate that it moves

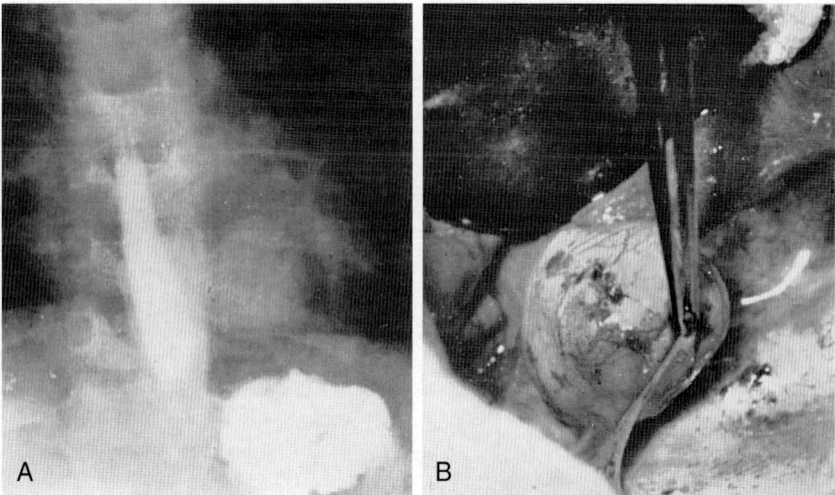

Fig. 74.14 Bronchogenic cyst in a child. (A) Radiograph. (B) Photograph at surgery. The cyst is located retropleurally, overlying the distal thoracic aorta, and is not attached to the respiratory tract or esophagus.

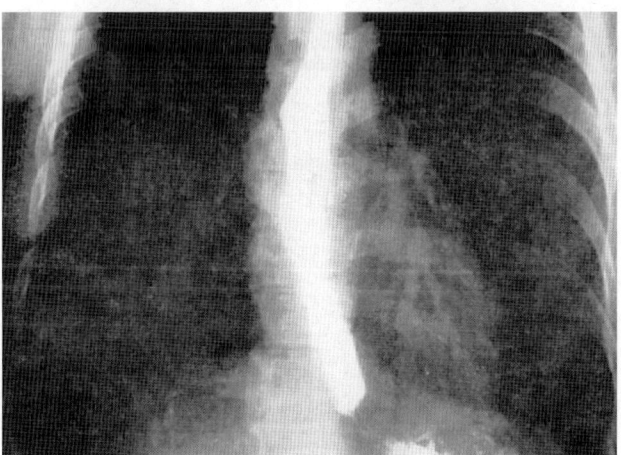

Fig. 74.15 Esophogram of a hilar bronchogenic cyst with an esophageal indentation.

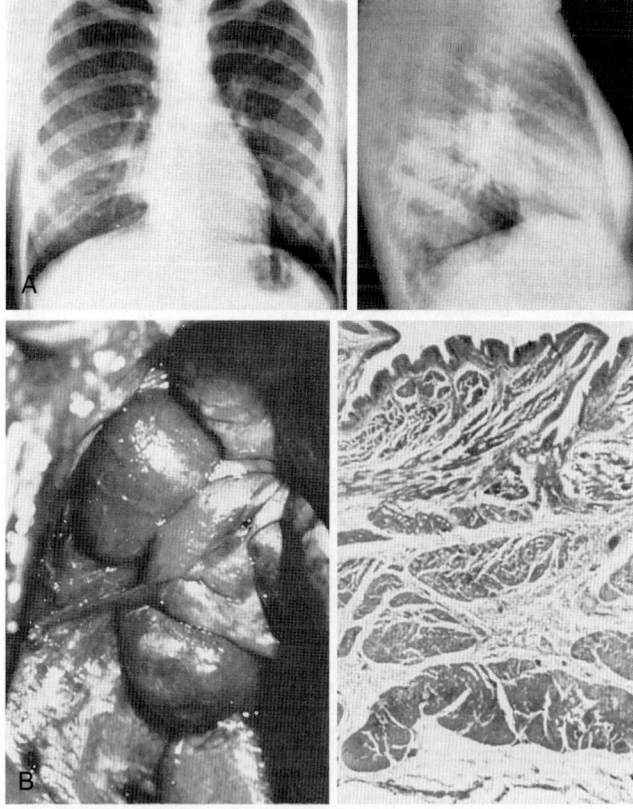

Fig. 74.16 (A) Bronchogenic cyst in a child whose mother had tuberculosis. The child was treated with antituberculosis drugs for 1 year without change. (B) A dumbbell-shaped bronchogenic cyst was found in the region of the inferior pulmonary vein during an operation. The microscopic section shows a wall with ciliated epithelium, no cartilage, and a smooth muscle wall of two layers.

with respiration (due to attachment to the tracheobronchial tree) and its shape may alter during the cycles of respiration. These lesions are occasionally identified on prenatal ultrasound.

When the bronchogenic cyst is located just below the carina, it may cause severe respiratory distress due to compression of either one or both major bronchi (Fig. 74.16). Early diagnosis and prompt removal are necessary.

There are no meticulous population-based studies of bronchogenic cysts, so its incidence is conjecture. Phillipart and Farmer assembled perhaps the best composite review of all mediastinal masses; some 7% of mediastinal tumors were bronchogenic cysts.[35]

Bronchogenic cysts should be treated by surgical removal. Like most discrete lesions, most of these can be handled with thoracoscopic techniques. Regardless of approach, care must be taken when these lesions share a common wall with either the airway or the esophagus. If there has been antecedent infection, resection is complicated, as normal tissue planes may be obliterated.

Esophageal Cysts (Duplication)

Esophageal cysts are located in the posterior mediastinum; they are usually on the right side and are intimately associated in the wall of the esophagus (Fig. 74.17). They occur more frequently in males than in females.

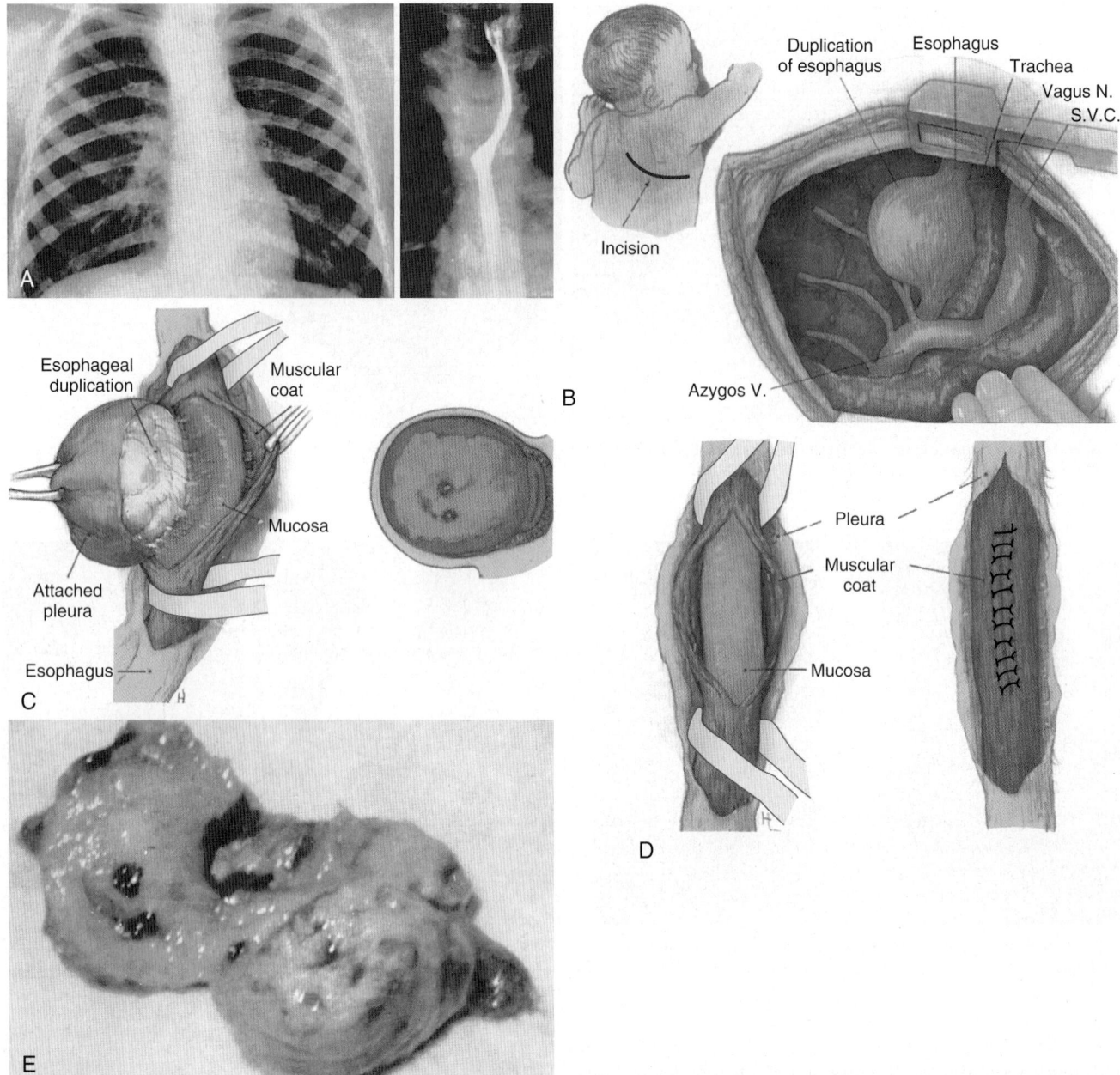

Fig. 74.17 (A) Posteroanterior chest radiograph taken of a child with an upper respiratory tract infection. A mass is seen in the posterior superior mediastinum presenting into the right hemithorax. At the time of an esophogram, the esophagus is seen displaced toward the left by a smooth mass. (B–D) Drawings of findings at the operation. Note the plane of separation from the mucosa of the esophagus and the lack of communication with the esophageal lumen. (E) An opened operative specimen, the cavity of which was filled with mucoid fluid. The lining of the duplication was typical squamous epithelium.

There are two types of esophageal cyst; the more characteristic type resembles adult esophagus with the cyst lined by noncornified stratified squamous epithelium having a well-defined muscularis mucosae and striated muscle in the wall. Intimate association in the muscular wall of the esophagus is not, however, accompanied by communication with the lumen of the esophagus. A review of 36 patients suggests that early resection between the ages of 6 and 12 months leads to better conservation of normal pulmonary parenchyma and a reduction in complications.[36] Ciliated mucosa lines the second type, thus resembling the fetal esophagus.

Esophageal cysts may be associated with mild dysphagia and regurgitation but are usually asymptomatic. Barium esophagram shows smooth indentation of the esophagus. On esophagoscopy, there is indentation of the normal mucosa by a pliable, movable, soft extramucosal mass. Removal is indicated for the same reasons as bronchogenic cysts and thoracoscopic techniques are similar. Technically these lesions may be more difficult to excise, especially if they are extensive or cross the diaphragm.

Gastroenteric Cysts

The third type of cyst arising from the foregut is the gastroenteric cyst, which typically lies in the posterior mediastinum against the vertebrae. Such cysts are typically posterior or lateral to and free of the esophagus, with attachments posteriorly. The normal fetal esophagus is lined by columnar epithelium, much of which is ciliated, which only gradually converts to the stratified epithelium of the mature organ. The change is generally complete, or almost complete, at birth. Thus if a cyst arises from the embryonic esophagus, it has a ciliated lining.

The enteric nature of a posterior mediastinal cyst is moderately certain if microscopic examination reveals a frank gastric or intestinal type of epithelium, but a better indication of the nature and origin is the presence of well-developed muscularis mucosae, and two or even three main muscle coats. Gastric glands are common, but esophageal, duodenal, or small-intestinal glands may also be found. At operation, the cyst sometimes seems grossly "stomach-like" or "bowel-like." Cysts encountered in the posterior mediastinum show a highly developed mesodermal wall and even the presence of Meissner's and Auerbach's plexuses, whereas the lining epithelium varies from columnar ciliated to typical small intestinal. Two types of gastroenteric cysts have been described: (1) acid-secreting cysts, which are functionally active; and (2) cysts in which the mucosa has no functional activity.

Males are predominantly affected with this abnormality. Unlike other foregut cysts, posterior gastroenteric cysts are usually symptomatic. The symptoms are usually due to pressure on thoracic structures or rupture into bronchi with massive hemoptysis and death. Actual peptic perforation of the lung with hemorrhage has been reported.

Hemoptysis in young infants is difficult to distinguish from hematemesis; it may follow ulceration of a gastroenteric cyst (with gastric lining) of the mediastinum, with subsequent erosion into the lung. Gastric epithelium associated with intestinal or respiratory epithelium is apparently less secretory. Many functional cysts may lose their functional activity when the secretory areas of the mucosa are destroyed. Renin, pepsin, chlorides, and free hydrochloric acid have been demonstrated in the contents of some of the cysts.

Posterior gastroenteric foregut cysts of the mediastinum are frequently associated with two other types of congenital anomalies: mesenteric abnormalities and vertebral abnormalities. When these are suspected, MRI is the preferred diagnostic test. Both types may occur in the same case. In the embryo, the notochord and the endoderm are in intimate contact at one time; thus this combined developmental anomaly may result from abnormal embryonic development.

Penetration of the diaphragm by a cyst arising primarily from the thorax may occur; conversely, penetration of the diaphragm by the free end of an intramesenteric intestinal duplication is also possible.

A survey of the literature confirms that as many as two-thirds of patients with mediastinal cysts have vertebral anomalies, including hemivertebrae, spina bifida anterior, or infantile scoliosis. Most of these vertebral lesions involve the upper thoracic and lower cervical vertebrae, and the cyst tends to be caudal to the vertebral lesion. MRI may be helpful in demonstrating these lesions. The presence of spina bifida anterior, congenital scoliosis, Klippel-Feil syndrome, or similar but less well-defined lesions in the cervical or dorsal vertebrae suggests enteric cysts in the mediastinum or abdomen.

Pericardial Coelomic Cysts

These mesothelial cysts are developmental in origin, and persistence is related to the pericardial coelom. The primitive pericardial cavity forms by the fusion of coelomic spaces on each side of the embryo. During the process, dorsal and ventral parietal recesses are formed. Dorsal recesses communicate with the pleuroperitoneal coelom, and the ventral recesses end blindly at the septum transversum. The persistence of segments of the ventral parietal recess accounts for most pericardial coelomic cysts.

The cysts are usually located anteriorly in the cardiophrenic angles, more frequently on the right, and occasionally on or in the diaphragm (Fig. 74.18). They are usually asymptomatic and are discovered on routine chest radiography. Rarely do they reach sufficient size to cause displacement of the heart or to produce pressure on the pulmonary tissue. Infection is unusual.

Pericardial cysts are usually unilocular. The walls are thin, and the intersurfaces are smooth and glistening, lined by a single layer of flat mesothelial cells. The mesothelium is supported by fibrous tissue with attached adipose tissue.

These cysts are very rare; only two have been reported in children. Because they are benign, observation may be warranted. Alternatively, thoracoscopic excision can be undertaken.

Intrathoracic Meningoceles

Intrathoracic meningoceles are not true mediastinal tumors or cysts; they are diverticuli of the spinal meninges that protrude through the neuroforamen adjacent to an intercostal nerve and manifest beneath the pleura in the posterior medial thoracic gutter. The wall represents an extension of the leptomeninges, and the content is cerebrospinal fluid. Enlargement of the intervertebral foramen is common; vertebral or rib anomalies adjacent to the meningocele are also frequent. The most commonly associated anomalies are kyphosis, scoliosis, and bone erosion or destruction. The walls of these cysts are formed by two distinct components, the dura mater and the arachnoidea spinalis, with small nerve trunks and ganglia occasionally incorporated.

A syndrome of generalized neurofibromatosis (von Recklinghausen disease), kyphoscoliosis, and intrathoracic meningocele may occur, but thoracic meningocele as an isolated defect is much less frequent; only four pediatric cases have been reported. This lesion is usually asymptomatic; it occurs on the right side approximately 3 times more often than on the left. Rarely the lesion may be bilateral. In patients with neurofibromatosis, posterior sulcus tumors are usually meningoceles and rarely neurofibromas.

On radiographic examination, the lesion is a regular, well-demarcated intrathoracic density located in the posterior sulcus; associated congenital anomalies of the spine and thorax may be noted. On fluoroscopic examination, pulsations

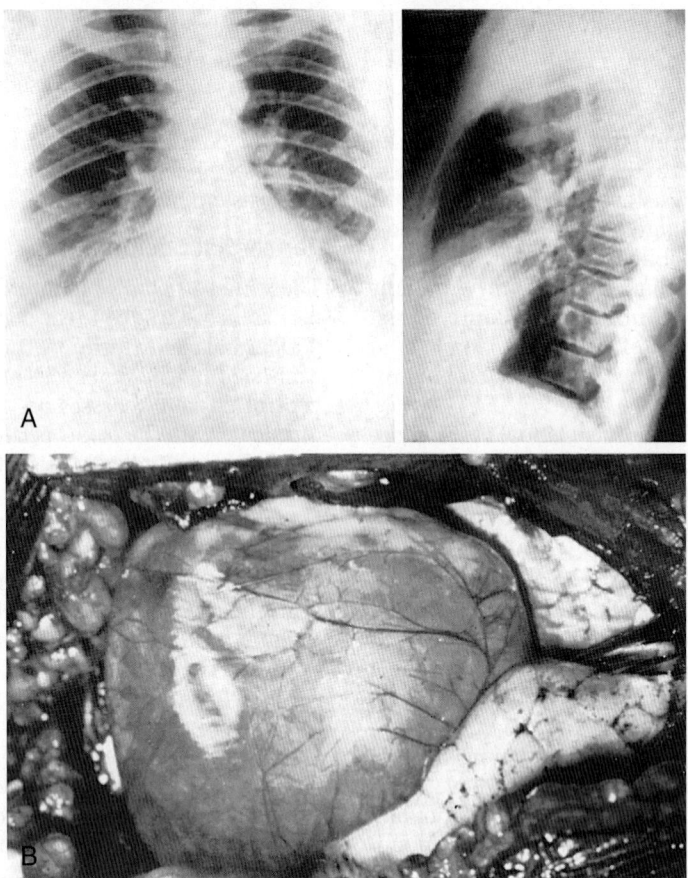

Fig. 74.18 (A) Typical location of a pericardial cyst in posteroanterior and lateral chest radiographs at the right cardiophrenic angle. (B) A large cyst seen at the time of a thoracotomy.

may be noted in the sac; diagnosis may be confirmed by myelography or MRI.

When diagnosis is securely established, no therapy is indicated unless the lesion is symptomatic. Operative complications such as empyema, meningitis, and spinal fluid fistula have been greatly reduced with appropriate antibiotic therapy.

Primary Cardiac and Pericardial Tumors

Primary tumors of the heart in infants may cause cardiac enlargement or enlargement of the cardiac silhouette, giving rise to symptoms in the lungs or esophagus. Usually the signs and symptoms of congestive heart failure are much more prominent than those of tumors of the respiratory system or esophagus.

Rhabdomyoma appears to be the only cardiac tumor showing a definite predilection for the younger age groups. This is particularly true of children with tuberous sclerosis, in whom rhabdomyoma of the heart is prone to occur. Such tumors are not considered true neoplasms and probably represent an area of developmental arrest in the fetal myocardium. It is not unusual for rhabdomyoma to regress spontaneously without having caused any appreciable impairment of cardiac function.

Myxoma is by far the most common primary tumor of the heart, accounting for slightly more than half of all primary cardiac tumors. It may be encountered at almost any age. The signs and symptoms vary widely but ultimately lead to cardiac failure that does not respond to the usual medical management. Most myxomas are in the atria, more frequently on the left than on the right. They tend to proliferate and project into the chambers of the heart, preventing normal cardiac filling by obstruction to the mitral or tricuspid valve. The origin appears to be in the atrial septum. Excision on cardiopulmonary bypass is curative.

Primary sarcoma of the heart is less common than myxoma but may occur at any age. As a rule, it does not proliferate into the chambers of the heart; it infiltrates the wall of the myocardium and frequently extends into the pericardial cavity.

An aggressive surgical approach is advised in the management of these cardiac tumors, using a variety of surgical techniques ranging from hypothermic circulatory arrest, on pump excision, and even cardiac autotransplantation.

Primary neoplasms of the pericardium are rare. On histologic examination, the predominant tumors are mesotheliomas (endotheliomas) and sarcomas, but leiomyomas, hemangiomas, and lipomas occasionally occur. Several case reports of pericardial hemangiomas have been reported in the literature, occurring in any age group. Cavernous hemangiomas are the most common type to present in this location, usually arising from the visceral pericardium.[37,38]

Tumors of the Diaphragm

Tumors involving the diaphragm may cause chest pain and discomfort or pulmonary compression; thus they may simulate mediastinal or primary pulmonary neoplasms. Primary tumors of the diaphragm are extremely rare in the pediatric age group, with 41 cases reported in the world literature.[39]

Benign tumors of the diaphragm that have been reported, though not necessarily in children, are lymphangioma, hemangioma, lipoma, fibroma, chondroma, angiofibroma, neurofibroma, rhabdomyofibroma, fibromyoma, and primary diaphragmatic cysts.

Malignant tumors of the diaphragm that have been reported are rhabdomyosarcoma, fibrosarcoma, myosarcoma, leiomyosarcoma, and fibromyosarcoma. None of these tumors appear to have been reported in children.

General Approach to Evaluation of Children With Suspected Tumors of the Chest

Infants or children presenting with respiratory symptoms should be first worked up in the usual manner for common respiratory illnesses. Those who do not recover promptly when treated appropriately, with the use of therapies such as expectorants, bronchodilators, and antibiotics, should be suspected of having a space-occupying lesion. The location, tissue type, and rate of growth will all affect whether a chest mass will produce symptoms and will also determine the rapidity of onset. A slow-growing space-occupying lesion may have a long indolent course that does not produce symptoms until it reaches a sufficient size. Typical symptoms include shortness of breath, wheezing, repeated infections not amenable to usual treatment, fevers, cough, and hemoptysis. Depending on the location of the lesion, a patient may present with cardiac dysfunction, esophageal involvement causing dysphagia, or growth into the sympathetic chain causing Horner syndrome, for example. The wide differential involving tumors of the chest requires a keen clinical eye to be able to correlate symptom development and progression with the possible location of a chest lesion.

When symptoms persist, a posteroanterior and lateral chest radiograph should be included in the initial workup. Prenatal ultrasound, now routine, has led to a greater understanding of the natural history of lesions presenting in the fetus.

Previously undiagnosed lesions are now seen with increasing frequency. When symptoms present after birth, chest radiographs should be the first step in the diagnostic workup. Only by such techniques can obstructive emphysema (Fig. 74.19), atelectasis (Fig. 74.20), and actual solid masses be seen at a stage of development when a resection may offer some hope of cure (Figs. 74.21–74.25).

In addition to undergoing an exhaustive history and physical examination, children with persistent symptoms and radiographic lesions should have other studies to rule out infections (e.g., mycobacterial or fungal) and genetic lung disorders. Examination of the bone marrow may give diagnostic evidence of a blood dyscrasia (e.g., leukemia or myeloma) or even metastatic malignancy, such as neuroblastoma.

Radiographic examination of the chest with special views such as apical lordotic and right and left oblique may be required. In addition, other imaging techniques such as ultrasound, CT, or MRI may be necessary for final definition. Ultrasonography is useful in locating and assisting in the needle aspiration of pleural fluid collections (Fig. 74.26). Mediastinal, pulmonary, and diaphragmatic densities are best detailed with axial CT of the thorax, which has added greatly to accuracy in study of all these areas (Figs. 74.27–74.29). MRI has had a substantial impact on thoracic diagnostic workup in the last decade. It can distinguish masses in the mediastinum from vascular structures and is more sensitive than CT in detecting intraspinal extension. The two studies may be complementary, since CT demonstrates calcifications and bronchial abnormalities that are not seen on MRI.

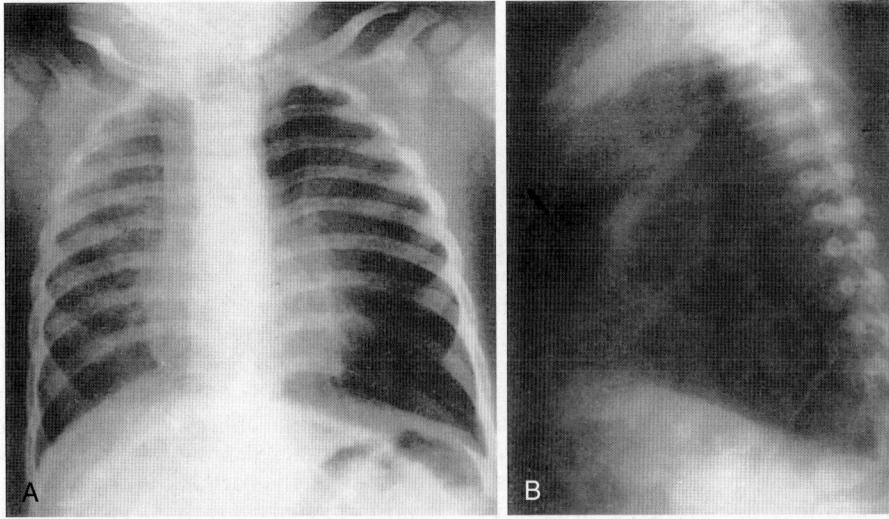

Fig. 74.19 Chest radiograph revealing obstructive emphysema of the left lower lobe bronchus caused by partial occlusion of the lumen. (A) Posteroanterior view. (B) Lateral view. The left diaphragm is flattened, mediastinal and cardiac shadows are displaced toward the right, the left upper lobe is compressed, and there is increased radiolucency of the left lower lobe.

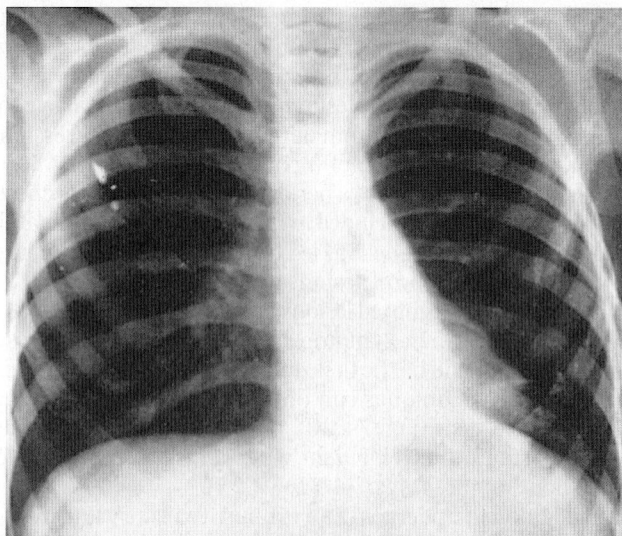

Fig. 74.20 Chest radiograph revealing total atelectasis of the left lower lobe secondary to an inflammatory stricture of the left lower lobe bronchus. A retrocardiac position tends to confuse diagnosis in some cases.

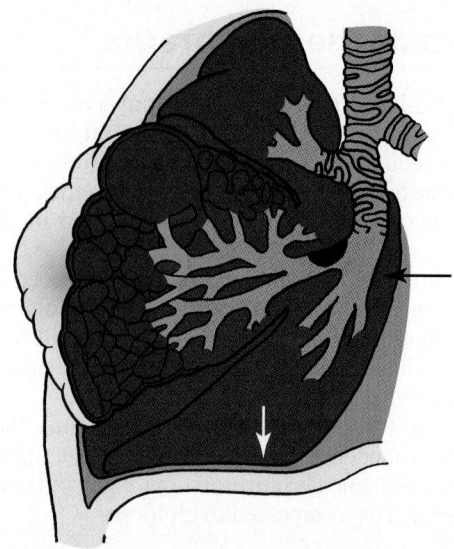

Fig. 74.22 Diagram illustrating obstructive emphysema. A partial obstruction leads to the retention of air in the pulmonary parenchyma distal to the obstructed bronchus. Retention of air will cause an ipsilateral compression of the adjacent normally aerated lung tissue, widening of intercostal spaces, descent of the diaphragm, a shift of the mediastinum away from the lung with the partially obstructing lesion, and a wheeze accompanied by decreased breath sounds over the affected lung.

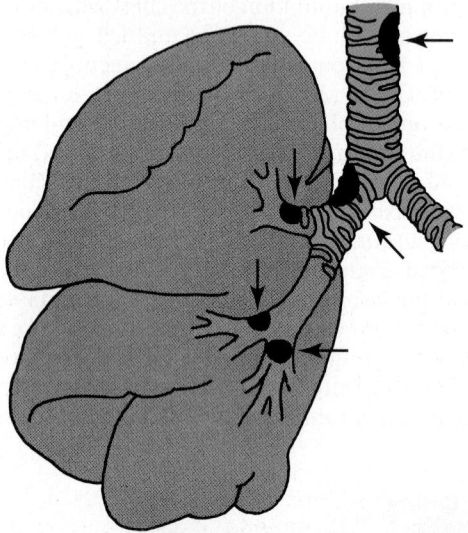

Fig. 74.21 Diagram illustrating locations of lesions within the lumens of the major bronchi. The location of such lesions dictates the area of pulmonary involvement, unilaterality or bilaterality, and the extent of signs and symptoms.

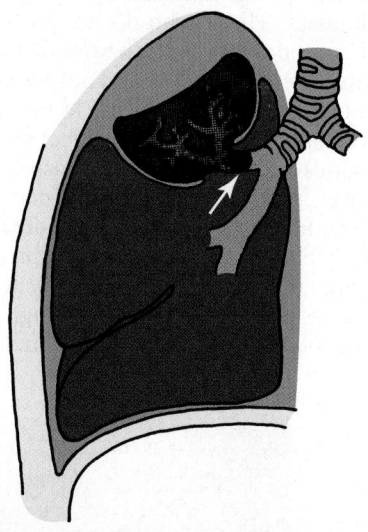

Fig. 74.23 Diagram illustrating that persistence of a lesion with ultimate total obstruction gives rise to atelectasis, an absence of breath sounds over the affected lung tissue, an overexpansion of the surrounding lung tissue, and a shift of the diaphragm to a more normal position, with a return of the mediastinum to midline. Bronchial secretions may actually decrease in amount.

Thoughtful use and sequencing of these studies should be based on the location of the abnormality and a provisional working diagnosis, given the risk of radiation dose with different imaging modalities.

Echocardiography and occasionally cardiac catheterization demonstrate any displacement of the heart due to masses in the lung, mediastinum, or pericardium. Esophagrams are used to identify vascular rings, along with CT angiograms or magnetic resonance angiograms (MRA) of the chest. Aortograms may be used to define bronchial arteries in patients with massive hemoptysis and can assist with the diagnosis of congenital vascular malformations of the pulmonary tree and congenital sequestration.

Bronchoscopy is an essential procedure for the study of the tracheobronchial tree. This procedure permits visual study of the vocal cords, larynx, trachea, and major bronchi, and their segmental orifices. Congenital anatomic abnormalities may be visualized; prognosis in extensive lesions is evaluated by study of the carina and trachea. Bronchoscopy-guided transbronchial biopsy has been described in children for the diagnosis of chronic bronchiolitis, sarcoidosis, interstitial lung disease, and acute rejection in transplant recipients.[40,41] There are reports of resecting mass lesions bronchoscopically

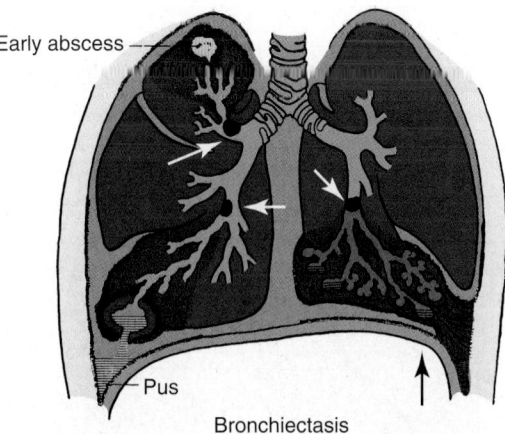

Fig. 74.24 Diagram illustrating that persistence of an obstructing lesion leads to permanent destructive changes in the pulmonary parenchyma distal to the lesion, such as abscess formation, chronic pneumonitis with fibrosis, pleurisy, empyema, and bronchiectasis, with parenchymal contracture secondary to fibrosis.

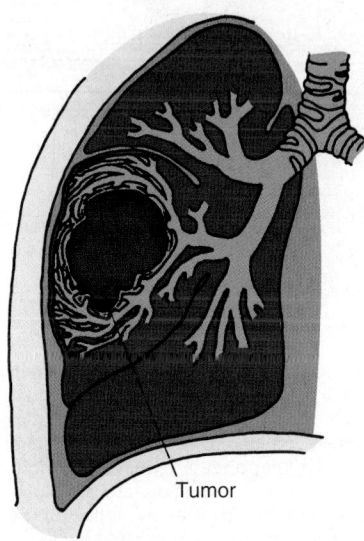

Fig. 74.25 Diagram illustrating that if a tumor is within the pulmonary parenchyma, pressure on the adjacent lung and bronchi will give rise to a surrounding zone of pneumonitis that may actually show incomplete, temporary improvement with antimicrobial therapy.

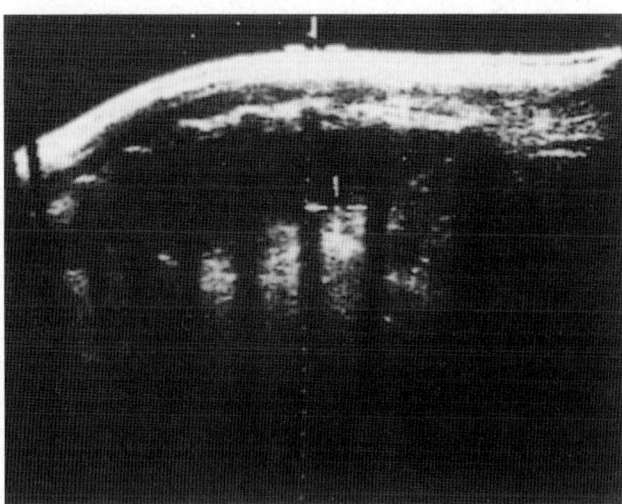

Fig. 74.26 Typical ultrasonogram of pleural fluid. With such accurate localization, needle aspiration is easily carried out.

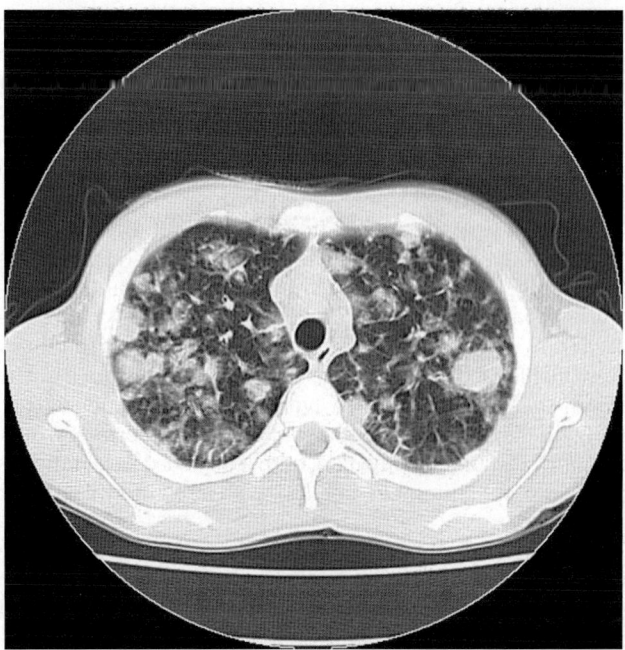

Fig. 74.27 Computed tomography study of the chest showing metastatic pulmonary disease in a 14-year-old boy with testicular rhabdomyosarcoma.

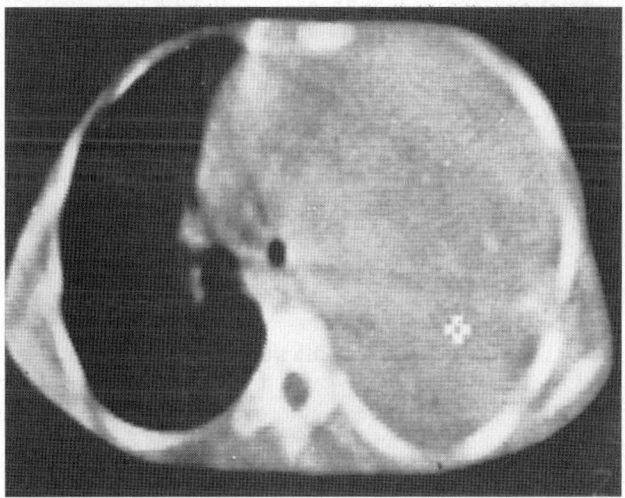

Fig. 74.28 Computed tomography scan of a child with small-cell carcinoma.

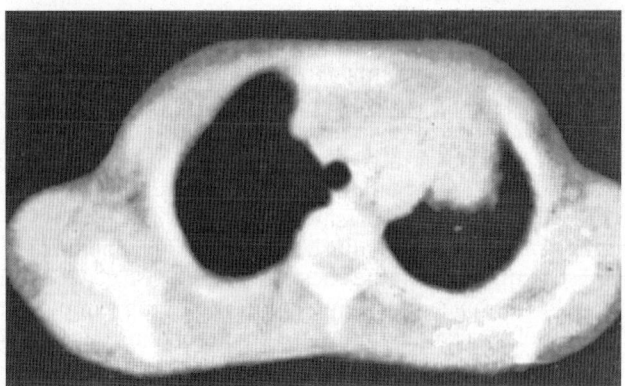

Fig. 74.29 Computed tomography scan of the mediastinum and lung in a child with Hodgkin disease.

with the aid of energy hemostasis (usually laser). Aspiration of secretions is another potential therapeutic contribution from bronchoscopy. Bronchoalveolar lavage (BAL) allows sampling from distal airways and alveoli; investigation must include cytologic studies for malignant cells, routine bacterial smear, culture and sensitivity studies, acid-fast smear and cultures, and fungal smear and cultures.

Biopsy of palpable lymph nodes may aid in the diagnosis of abnormal processes in the lung. The scalene lymph nodes are usually the primary target because they drain the pulmonary parenchyma. Scalene lymph node biopsy, mediastinoscopy, or, now more directly, thoracoscopy with biopsy of available mediastinal nodes are of great assistance in the diagnosis of sarcoidosis, in lymphatic malignancies (e.g., Hodgkin disease) and lymphosarcoma, and in primary neoplasms of the lung and mediastinum. CT-guided percutaneous biopsy is now common in children, with a reported diagnostic rate of 85%.[42]

Lymph nodes obtained at the time of biopsy should be subjected to histologic study, and a portion must be sent to the bacteriology laboratory for routine bacterial smear and culture, studies for sensitivity of the organism to antimicrobials, acid-fast smear and culture, and fungal smear and culture (Fig. 74.30).

When all other methods have failed to produce a definitive diagnosis, thoracoscopy or thoracotomy should be considered. The use of single-lung ventilation (selective bronchial intubation or the use of balloon occlusion catheters) and preoperative placement of a radiologically guided blood patch can greatly facilitate the pursuit of tiny lesions. If the situation seems to present an inoperable problem, biopsy may still afford useful information (Fig. 74.31).

While thoracoscopy has been in use for a century, its use in children is a little over 3 decades old. Today it is the *primary mode of treatment* for not only limited procedures such as biopsy, decortication, and bleb resection but also for more extensive operations such as lobectomy, pneumonectomy, thymectomy, and repair of tracheoesophageal fistula.[43] Its rise has been facilitated by several technological improvements, including improved optics and light sources, and the development of specially designed instrumentation including hemostatic energy sources. Endoscopic linear staplers have made wedge biopsies and resections safe and simple procedures, leading many physicians to aggressively treat tumors that they may have just observed in the past.[44]

Management and Treatment of Thoracic Tumors

Due to the wide differential diagnosis involving potential masses in the chest, prompt diagnosis is essential in determining the correct course of treatment. Lesion-specific treatments have already been previously discussed in their respective sections. In general, a good starting point is to determine whether a lesion is benign or malignant, to decide if the potential morbidity and possible mortality of a surgical resection is warranted, particularly given the preponderance of vital structures within the chest. Treatment also depends on whether the space-occupying lesion is causing symptoms. In cases of clear malignancy, treatment options have often been clearly delineated. However, as discussed previously,

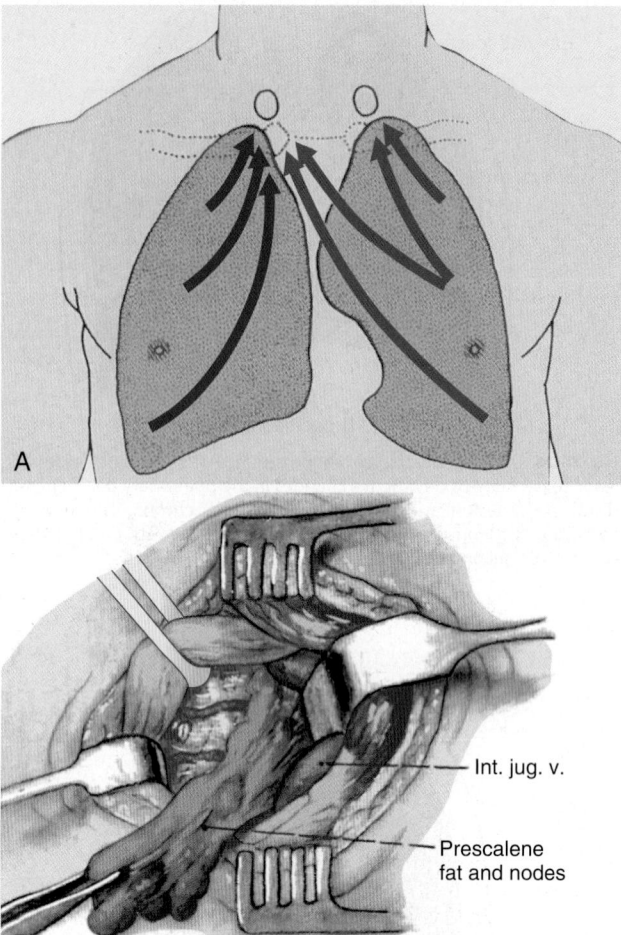

Fig. 74.30 (A) Disease within the right lung usually drains into the right scalene lymph node group. Disease within the left lung may drain to either scalene node group in a pattern similar to that indicated on the illustration. Generally, left lung disease requires bilateral scalene node biopsy, whereas right lung disease requires only right scalene node biopsy. Regardless of the side of lung disease, all palpable nodes in the scalene node area should be examined by biopsy. (B) The scalene group of nodes is contained in the fat pad bounded medially by the internal jugular vein, inferiorly by the subclavian vein, and superiorly by the posterior belly of the omohyoid muscle. The base of the triangle is formed by the anterior scalene muscle. Retraction of the internal jugular vein is essential to obtain access to all nodes in this group.

with lesions such as plasma cell granulomas and lipomas, a sizable percentage of these masses can be completely asymptomatic and discovered incidentally. In such cases, where lesions appear benign, not enlarging, and not producing any symptoms, there can be benefit in watchful waiting without aggressive therapy that may potentially result in undue harm. Another important consideration in the pediatric population is whether the lesion will regress over time like a hemangioma.

Ultimately masses in the chest often require a multidisciplinary approach, given the wide differential diagnosis of chest tumors in the pediatric population. Management, including whether surgical biopsy or resection is indicated, should include consultation from a broad range of subspecialties, which may include pulmonology, anesthesia, oncology,

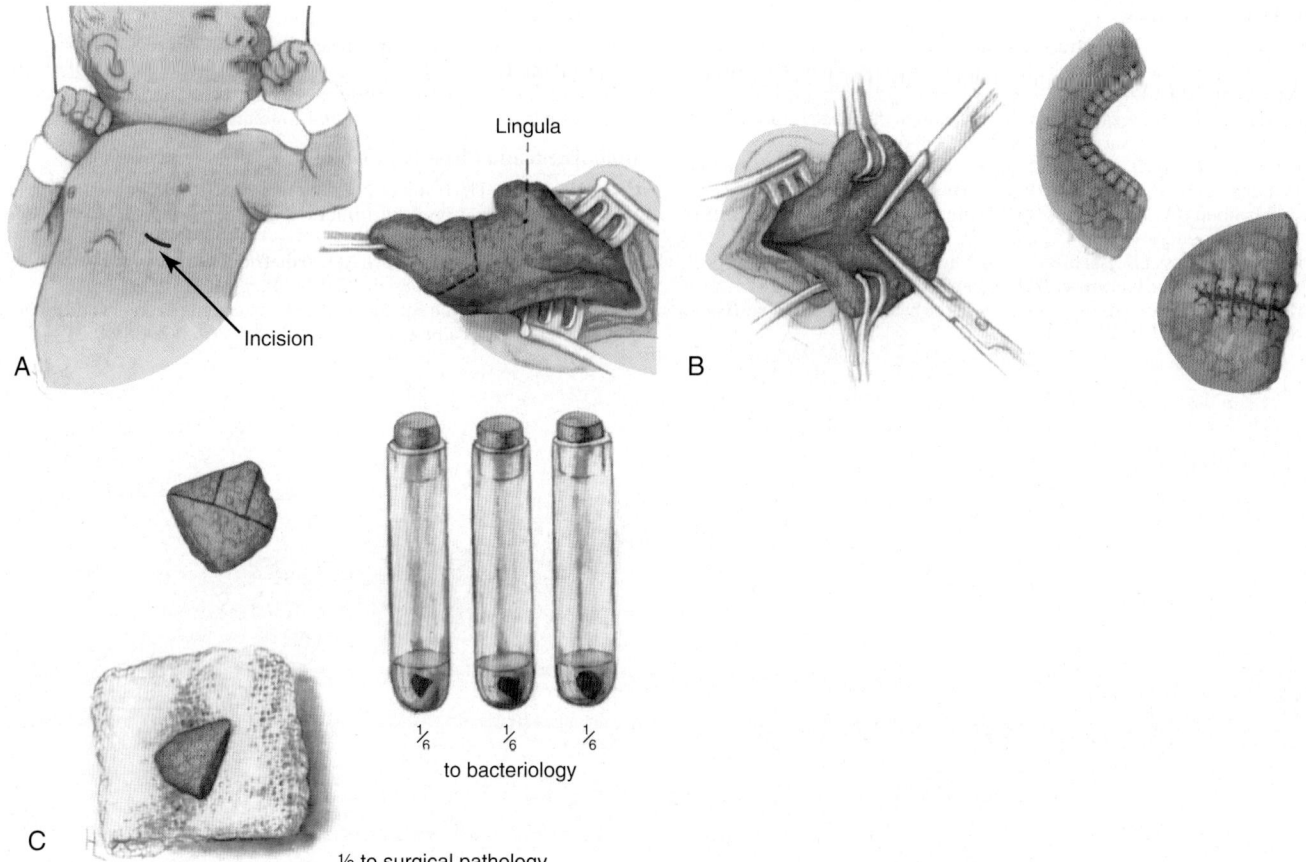

Fig. 74.31 (A–C) An adequate lung biopsy with specimens for bacteriology and pathology laboratories is essential. In general, a small open thoracotomy has many advantages over the blind needle biopsy technique.

pediatric general surgery, cardiothoracic surgery, and neurosurgery. This may require transfer to a tertiary care center that specializes in treatment of these, often rare entities. While the scope of the differential diagnosis can be large, a careful, studied approach can ascertain the correct diagnosis and a multidisciplinary approach can lead to an effective approach that brings maximum benefit to the patient.

Acknowledgments

We would like to acknowledge Dr. Thomas M. Krummel and Dr. Timothy A. Plerhoples for their significant contributions to this chapter.

References

Access the reference list online at ExpertConsult.com.

Suggested Reading

General

Adzick NS, Flake AW, Crombleholme TM. Management of congenital lung lesions. *Semin Pediatr Surg.* 2003;12:10.

Gushiken BD, Filly RA. Sonography for fetal thoracic intervention. In: Harrison MR, Evans MI, Adzick NS, et al, eds. *The Unborn Patient.* Philadelphia: Saunders; 2001:95.

Harrison MR, Evans MI, Adzick NS, et al, eds. *The Unborn Patient.* Philadelphia: Saunders; 2001.

Hebra A, Othersen HD, Tagge EP. Bronchopulmonary malformations. In: Ashcroft KW, ed. *Pediatric Surgery.* 3rd ed. New York: Saunders; 2000:273.

Rodgers BM, McGahren ED. Laryngoscopy, bronchoscopy, and thoracoscopy. In: Grosfeld JL, O'Neil JA, eds. *Pediatric Surgery.* 6th ed. Philadelphia: Mosby; 2006:971–982.

Rothenberg SS. Experience with thoracoscopic lobectomy in infants and children. *J Pediatr Surg.* 2003;38:102.

Shochat SJ. Tumors of the lung. In: Grosfeld JL, O'Neil JA, eds. *Pediatric Surgery.* 6th ed. Philadelphia: Mosby; 2006:640–648.

Sylvester KG, Albanese CT. Bronchopulmonary malformation. In: Ashcraft K, Murphy P, Holcomb GW, eds. *Pediatric Surgery.* 4th ed. Philadelphia: Saunders; 2004.

Tsao K, Albanese CT, Harrison MR. Prenatal therapy for thoracic and mediastinal lesions. *World J Surg.* 2003;27:77.

Benign Pulmonary Tumors

Adzick NS, Farmer DL. Cysts of the lungs and mediastinum. In: Grosfeld JL, O'Neil JA, eds. *Pediatric Surgery.* 6th ed. Philadelphia: Mosby; 2006:955–970.

Morini F, Quattrucci S, Cozzi DA, et al. Bronchial adenoma: an unusual cause of recurrent pneumonia in childhood. *Ann Thorac Surg.* 2003;76:2085–2087.

Rutter MJ. Evaluation and management of upper airway disorders in children. *Semin Pediatr Surg.* 2006;15:116–123.

Weldon CB, Shamberger RC. Pediatric pulmonary tumors: primary and metastatic. *Semin Pediatr Surg.* 2008;17:17–29.

Primary and Metastatic Malignant Pulmonary Tumors

Dishop MK, Kuruvilla S. Primary and metastatic lung tumors in the pediatric population: a review and 25-year experience at a large children's hospital. *Arch Pathol Lab Med.* 2008;132:1079–1103.

Kayton ML. Pulmonary metastasectomy in pediatric patients. *Thorac Surg Clin.* 2006;16:167–183, vi.

Mediastinal Tumors

Agrawal D, Suri A, Mahapatra AK, et al. Intramedullary neurenteric cyst presenting as infantile paraplegia. A case and review [Comment]. *Pediatr Neurosurg.* 2002;37:93.

Franco A, Mody NS, Meza MP. Imaging evaluation of pediatric mediastinal masses. *Radiol Clin North Am.* 2005;43:325–353.

Laberge J, Puligandla P, Flageole H. Asymptomatic congenital lung malformations. *Semin Pediatr Surg.* 2005;14:16–33.

Rizk T, Lahoud GA, Maarrawi J, et al. Acute paraplegia revealing an intraspinal neurenteric cyst in a child. *Childs Nerv Syst.* 2001;17:754.

Rothstein DH, Voss SD, Isakoff M, et al. Thymoma in a child: case report and review of the literature. *Pediatr Surg Int.* 2005;21:548–551.

Wright CD. Mediastinal tumors and cysts in the pediatric population. *Thorac Surg Clin.* 2009;19:47–61, vi.

Cardiac Tumors

Burke A, Virmani R. Pediatric heart tumors. *Cardiovasc Pathol.* 2008; 17:193–198.

DeBusatmante TD, Azpeitia J, Mirailes M, et al. Prenatal sonographic detection of pericardial teratoma. *J Clin Ultrasound.* 2000;28:194.

Diaphragm and Chest Wall Tumors

Cada M, Gerstle JT, Traubici J, et al. Approach to diagnosis and treatment of pediatric primary tumors of the diaphragm. *J Pediatr Surg.* 2006;41:1722–1726.

van Aalst JA, Phillips JD, Sadove AM. Pediatric chest wall and breast deformities. *Plast Reconstr Surg.* 2009;124(suppl 1):38e–49e.

van den Berg H, van Rijn RR, Merks JH. Management of tumors of the chest wall in childhood: a review. *J Pediatr Hematol Oncol.* 2008;30:214–221.

The Aerodigestive Model

The Aerodigestive Model: Improving Health Care Value for Complex Patients Through Coordinated Care

ROBIN T. COTTON, MD, FACS, FRCS(C), and
KARTHIK BALAKRISHNAN, MD, MPH, FAAP, FACS

Historical Perspective

While multidisciplinary coordinated care is rapidly becoming the norm for complex patients and diseases, the Cincinnati Children's Hospital Medical Center aerodigestive model was a pioneering example of this approach. The development of the Cincinnati aerodigestive program was an outgrowth of advances made in the care of premature and critically ill infants, in which significantly increased survival rates led to children presenting with subsequent problems arising from either their underlying conditions or their management. Many children, particularly those with a history of prolonged endotracheal intubation or pulmonary disease, were tracheotomy-dependent and in need of airway reconstruction. Other patients required the care of multiple subspecialists in fields, including otolaryngology, pulmonary medicine, gastroenterology, and surgery. Beyond their anatomic and physiologic problems, many of these children also had functional problems such as oral aversion, feeding difficulty, and aspiration. As a result, these patients presented multiple challenges: complex diagnostic and therapeutic needs, associated social and financial health care burdens placed on their families, and the need for ongoing care across a range of specialties.

In this context, it was essential for involved pediatric subspecialties to develop a model for the delivery of efficient, unfragmented care built on constant communication between specialists and families, longitudinal tracking and follow-up of patients, and coordinated scheduling of appointments, diagnostic tests, and procedures. Since the development of this model at the Cincinnati Children's Hospital Medical Center, it has spread across the country and around the world, with other leading pediatric and adult hospitals adopting very similar approaches to children with complex aerodigestive disorders.

In view of this success, the objective of this section is to provide the reader with more detail regarding the structure of the coordinated aerodigestive care model. We also describe criteria by which we select children who might benefit from this horizontally integrated approach to medical and surgical care.

Patient Selection

Selection criteria for inclusion of patients in an aerodigestive care program vary between centers. Some centers, particularly those with patients traveling long distances frequently for visits, have developed specific criteria to assist pediatricians and other referring providers in deciding whether a patient might benefit from referrals that could involve significant travel and financial costs. This approach allows patients to avoid visits that may not provide benefit and allows involved specialists to focus on those patients to whom they might offer the most benefit. Other centers have elected to use less specific criteria, improving access for many patients but increasing the number of referrals that may not lead to a comprehensive treatment plan.

Regardless of the specifics of each aerodigestive program, certain characteristics and diseases serve to define "typical" aerodigestive patients (Table 75.1). The reader will notice that these components cover a wide spectrum of patients with interrelated symptoms and pathologies. The pathologies may be congenital, acquired, or a combination of the two.

Screening and Evaluating Potential Patients

Potential patients from either within or outside the institution are initially screened via a detailed telephone intake interview by a registered nurse or nurse practitioner who will remain the patient's main contact point throughout their aerodigestive care cycle. Information obtained at this stage provides a basis for a preliminary evaluation and management plan. After a thorough review of the patient's medical history, a lead physician is chosen based on the patient's primary presenting problem. At weekly interdisciplinary meetings involving all participating specialties, the patient's lead physician and designated nurse practitioner discuss ongoing clinical issues with other team members and finalize a diagnostic plan. The recommended tests and procedures are then scheduled in a coordinated fashion so as to minimize

procedure, maintaining the tracheal tube and temporarily placing a suprastomal laryngeal stent above the tracheal tube. Alternatively, in selective cases a single-stage procedure may be performed, with removal of the tracheal tube on the day of surgery and with the child requiring intubation for 1–14 days.[26,27] Higher decannulation rates have been achieved with cricotracheal resection than with laryngotracheal reconstruction in the management of severe SGS.[28,29] However, cricotracheal resection is a technically demanding procedure that carries a significant risk of complications.

VASCULAR COMPRESSION

Although vascular compression of the airway is not uncommon, most affected children are either asymptomatic or only minimally symptomatic. Forms of vascular compression affecting the trachea include innominate artery compression (most common), double aortic arch, and pulmonary artery sling. Although symptomatic vascular compression of the trachea or bronchi is rare, it is associated with marked symptoms, including biphasic stridor, retractions, a brassy cough, and "dying spells." Symptoms tend to become worse when the child is distressed. Vascular rings that result from a retroesophageal subclavian artery and a ligamentum arteriosum are less likely to be associated with airway compromise. Bronchial compression by either the pulmonary arteries or aorta may be significant, but in the absence of associated major cardiac anomalies, it is typically a unilateral problem.

The diagnosis of airway compression is best established with rigid or flexible bronchoscopy or both procedures. Thoracic imaging is then useful in assessing the intrathoracic vasculature. Imaging modalities generally include high-resolution computed tomography (CT) with contrast enhancement and three-dimensional reconstruction, magnetic resonance imaging (MRI), magnetic resonance angiography (MRA), and echocardiography. In some cases, angiography is required.

In a neonate with acute airway compromise, intubation may be required to maintain the airway prior to definitive treatment. In some cases, CPAP offers a degree of temporary improvement because segmental tracheomalacia may be present in the region of the vascular compression. Prolonged intubation should be avoided because of the risk of forming an arterial fistula from erosion of an endotracheal tube into the area of compression. Similarly, although tracheotomy will establish an unobstructed airway, there is also an increased risk of an arterial fistula into the airway.

The surgical management of symptomatic vascular compression varies, depending on individual pathology. Strategies for managing innominate artery compression include thymectomy and aortopexy; however, if little thymus is present, an alternative procedure is reimplantation of the innominate artery more proximately on the aortic arch. A double aortic arch requires ligation of the smaller of the two arches, which is usually the left one. A pulmonary artery sling is transected at its origin, dissected free, and reimplanted into the pulmonary trunk anterior to the trachea. There is a high incidence of complete tracheal rings in children with a pulmonary artery sling, and these should be repaired at the same time.

Although alleviating vascular compression improves the airway, it takes time for the airway to completely normalize. This is a consequence of long-standing vascular compression having adversely affected the normal cartilaginous development of the compressed segment of trachea, with resultant cartilaginous malacia or stenosis. Until the airway normalizes, children who are persistently symptomatic may require stabilization with a tracheotomy. Tracheal stabilization with the use of intratracheal stents is alluring, but the incidence of complications is high. Placement of a temporary tracheotomy is therefore a more desirable alternative.[30]

POSTERIOR LARYNGEAL CLEFTS

Posterior laryngeal clefts result from a failure of the laryngotracheal groove to fuse during embryogenesis. In a widely used anatomic classification system, these clefts are divided into four subtypes associated with varying levels of severity; type I cleft is the least and type IV cleft the most severe.[31] Other associated anomalies are common and may be divided into those that affect the airway and those that do not. Associated airway anomalies include tracheomalacia (>80%) and TEF formation (20%). Nonairway associations include anogenital anomalies and GER. The most common syndrome in which posterior laryngeal clefting occurs is Opitz-Frias syndrome; hypertelorism and anogenital anomalies are other features of this syndrome.

Although aspiration is the hallmark clinical feature of this disorder, signs and symptoms may be nonspecific, making the diagnosis elusive. Symptoms may also include apnea, recurrent pneumonia, feeding difficulties, and airway obstruction.

VSS and FEES may suggest the risk of aspiration in children with clefts; however, definitive diagnosis requires rigid laryngoscopy and bronchoscopy, with the interarytenoid area being specifically probed to determine if a posterior laryngeal cleft is present.

Initial management decisions should consider whether the infant requires tracheotomy placement, gastrostomy tube placement, or Nissen fundoplication. Although none of these procedures is essential, each increases the likelihood of a successful cleft repair. Protection against aspiration is also crucial, and nasojejunal feeding may be a useful preventative measure. Surgical repair may be performed endoscopically for most type I and type II clefts, and some type III clefts; however, longer clefts that extend into the cervical or thoracic trachea require open repair. The transtracheal approach is advocated in that it provides unparalleled exposure of the cleft while protecting the recurrent laryngeal nerves. A two-layer closure is recommended, with the option of performing an interposition graft if warranted; a useful interposition graft is a free transfer of clavicular or tibial periosteum, or costal cartilage. Because all clefts are prone to anastomotic breakdown, repeat endoscopy and postoperative swallowing studies should be performed to evaluate for aspiration and to confirm a successful repair.[32,33] Despite successful repair, patients may experience continued problems with dysphagia.[34]

Recently there has been an increasing emphasis placed on type I clefts and associated deep interarytenoid notches. Endoscopic repair of minor clefts has become far more common in children who are diagnosed because of a high index of suspicion or evidence of recurrent or chronic aspiration.[35,36] This suggests that in such patients, type I clefts may be more of a functional diagnosis than an anatomic diagnosis.

TRACHEOMALACIA

Tracheomalacia is the most common congenital tracheal anomaly. Most children are either asymptomatic or minimally symptomatic, and most cases involve posterior malacia of the trachealis, with associated broad tracheal rings. Commonly associated abnormalities include laryngeal clefts, TEF, and bronchomalacia. Presenting symptoms include a brassy cough, wheezing, respiratory distress when agitated, and "dying spells." Diagnosis is established with rigid or flexible bronchoscopy, while maintaining spontaneous respiration. The key diagnostic elements include: (1) ascertaining the severity of the malacia; (2) ascertaining the location of the malacia, particularly the possible presence of associated bronchomalacia; and (3) determining whether positive pressure support improves the malacia.

Although mild tracheomalacia is watched expectantly and anticipated to improve with time, more severe symptoms warrant intervention.[37] The most common intervention is tracheotomy placement, with the tip of the tracheotomy tube bypassing the malacic segment. Positive pressure support delivered through the tracheotomy tube assists with the management of associated bronchomalacia. Although there is currently no definitive surgical approach to repair tracheomalacia, this is an area of active research.

COMPLETE TRACHEAL RINGS

Complete tracheal rings are a rare but life-threatening anomaly that presents with progressive worsening of respiratory function over the first few months of life, stridor, retractions, and marked exacerbation of symptoms during intercurrent upper respiratory tract infections. Children with distal tracheal stenosis usually have a characteristic biphasic wet-sounding breathing pattern that transiently clears with coughing; this pattern is referred to as "washing machine breathing." The risk of respiratory failure increases with age.

An initial high-kilovolt airway film may indicate tracheal narrowing; however, the diagnosis is established with rigid bronchoscopy. This should be performed with utmost caution, using the smallest possible telescopes, as any airway edema in the region of the stenosis may turn a narrow airway into an extremely critical airway. If the stenosis is severe, the stenotic airway should not be instrumented, even with the smallest telescope. The initial bronchoscopic view is often sufficient to establish the diagnosis, thereby avoiding the risk of airway edema. Because 50% of children have a tracheal inner diameter of approximately 2 mm at the time of diagnosis, the standard interventions for managing a compromised airway are not applicable. More specifically, the smallest endotracheal tube has an outer diameter of 2.9 mm, and the smallest tracheotomy tube has an outer diameter of 3.9 mm; hence the stenotic segment cannot be intubated. This may leave extracorporeal membrane oxygenation (ECMO) as the only viable alternative for stabilizing the child. This situation is best avoided by performing bronchoscopy with the highest level of care. More than 80% of children with complete tracheal rings have other congenital anomalies, which are generally cardiovascular. As such, investigation should include a contrast-enhanced high-resolution CT scan of the chest and an echocardiogram. Specifically, a pulmonary artery sling should be excluded because this is a common association and, if present, should be repaired concurrent with the tracheal repair. Most children with complete tracheal rings require tracheal reconstruction.[38] The recommended surgical technique is the slide tracheoplasty.[39–41] This approach yields significantly better results than any other form of tracheal reconstruction and is applicable to all anatomic variants of complete tracheal rings.

References

Access the reference list online at ExpertConsult.com.

80 Sudden Infant Death Syndrome and Apparent Life-Threatening Events

ANDREA COVERSTONE, MD, and JAMES KEMP, MD

Infants experiencing an apparent life-threatening event (ALTE) and premature infants with apnea may later die suddenly and unexpectedly, with a diagnosis of sudden infant death syndrome (SIDS). However, because about 80% of victims who died suddenly and unexpectedly were born at term and were never known to be apneic until they died, discussing ALTE, apnea of prematurity (AOP), and SIDS together has become controversial, particularly when the issue of apnea monitoring is raised.

The American Academy of Pediatrics has recently promulgated a new category for this discussion—BRUE, Brief Resolved Unexplained Event. This new designation attempts to address the appropriate clinical approach to young infants coming to emergency departments with a history of events that, far more often than not, prove to be benign, and may be properly managed by reassuring parents and caregivers.

Acute Life-Threatening Events (ALTE) and BRUE

EPIDEMIOLOGY

The term apparent life-threatening event (ALTE) was first coined following the 1986 National Institute of Health Consensus Conference on Infant Apnea. The intention at the time was to replace the term "near-miss sudden infant death syndrome." ALTE is defined as "an episode that is frightening to the observer that is characterized by some combination of apnea (central or occasionally obstructive), color change (usually cyanotic or pallid but occasionally erythematous or plethoric), marked change in muscle tone (usually marked limpness), or choking or gagging."[1]

In 2016, the American Academy of Pediatrics (AAP) released a clinical practice guideline with the objective of replacing the term ALTE with a new term: BRUE.[2] This guideline was published to allow the clinician a practical approach to the evaluation of a child with the features of an ALTE who is considered low risk. BRUE was specifically defined as an "event occurring in an infant younger than 1 year" who is reported to have a "sudden, brief, and now resolved episode of one or more of the following: (1) cyanosis or pallor; (2) absent, decreased, or irregular breathing; (3) marked change in tone (hypertonia or hypotonia); and (4) altered level of responsiveness." A BRUE is distinguished from an ALTE in that it is defined as both brief and resolved (Table 80.1). Therefore children who have not returned to their baseline state of health would not fit into this category. By providing a more specific definition of these events, it is anticipated

that clinicians will avoid overuse of medical interventions and testing in the group that is considered low risk. In addition to clarifying what an event entails, the term BRUE is favored by the AAP over ALTE, because the term "life-threatening" is often misleading and has the potential to reinforce caregivers' perceptions that the event was, in fact, life-threatening, making it more challenging to provide reassurance when often that is all that is needed.

The incidence of ALTE in the population worldwide is estimated between 0.6 and 4.1 per 1000 live births[3-5]; however, the true incidence of ALTEs is unknown, especially given that the International Classification of Disease (ICD) code for ALTE was not introduced until 2012.[3] It is estimated that ALTE accounts for 0.6%–1.7% of emergency department visits for children younger than 1 year.[6,7] The usefulness of the BRUE designation and its impact on ALTE statistics remains to be seen.

DIAGNOSIS AND DIFFERENTIAL DIAGNOSIS

As described above, BRUE refers to an event (Table 80.1) with specific parameters.[2] BRUE should be diagnosed only when there is no explanation for a qualifying event after conducting an appropriate history and physical examination.

When evaluating the child who presents for medical attention following an event, a thorough physical examination and history is required to determine the risk of severe sequelae, as management guidelines for BRUE pertain only to those individuals who meet lower risk criteria, which are as follows:

- Age more than 60 days
- Prematurity: gestational age ≥32 weeks and postconceptional age ≥45 weeks
- First BRUE (no previous BRUE ever and not occurring in clusters)
- Duration of event less than 1 minute
- No cardiopulmonary resuscitation (CPR) required by trained medical provider
- No concerning historical features
- No concerning physical examination findings

The differential diagnosis for a child presenting with an apparent life-threatening event is shown in Box 80.1.

Etiology and Pathology/ Pathogenesis

We will now discuss potential explanations for ALTE as that term is currently used. Box 80.1 outlines considerations when

Table 80.1   BRUE Definition and Factors for Inclusion and Exclusion

	Includes	Excludes

Brief Resolved	Duration <1 min; typically 20–30 s
	Patient returned to his or her baseline state of health after the event
	Normal vital signs
	Normal appearance
		Duration ≥1 min
		At the time of medical evaluation:
		  Fever or recent fever
		  Tachypnea, bradypnea, apnea
		  Tachycardia or bradycardia
		  Hypotension, hypertension, or hemodynamic instability
		  Mental status changes, somnolence, lethargy
		  Hypotonia or hypertonia
		  Vomiting
		  Bruising, petechiae, or other signs of injury/trauma
		  Abnormal weight, growth, or head circumference
		  Noisy breathing (stridor, stertor, wheezing)
		  Repeat event(s)

Unexplained	Not explained by an identifiable medical condition	Event consistent with GER, swallow dysfunction, nasal congestion, etc. History or physical examination concerning for child abuse, congenital airway abnormality, etc.
Event Characterization		
Cyanosis or pallor	Central cyanosis: blue or purple coloration of face, gums, trunk Central pallor: pale coloration of face or trunk	Acrocyanosis or perioral cyanosis Rubor
Absent, decreased, or irregular breathing	Central apnea Obstructive apnea Mixed obstructive apnea	Periodic breathing of the newborn Breath-holding spell
Marked change in tone (hypertonia or hypotonia)	Hypertonia Hypotonia	Hypertonia associated with crying, choking, or gagging due to GER or feeding problems Tone changes associated with breath holding spell Tonic eye deviation or nystagmus Tonic-clonic seizure activity Infantile spasms
Altered responsiveness	Loss of consciousness Mental status change Lethargy Somnolence Postictal phase	Loss of consciousness associated with breath holding spell

From Tieder JS, Bonkowsky JL, Etzel RA, et al. Clinical practice guideline: Brief Resolved Unexplained Events (Formerly Apparent Life-Threatening Events) and Evaluation of Lower-Risk Infants. *Pediatrics*. 2016;137(5):e20160590.

Box 80.1   Selected Causes in the Differential Diagnosis of an Apparent Life-Threatening Event

Respiratory syncytial virus, pertussis
Sepsis with apnea
Syndromes compromising the upper airway (e.g., Pierre Robin sequence)
Breath-holding spells
Seizures
Intracranial hemorrhages (e.g., caused by vascular malformations, child abuse, vitamin K deficiency)
Exaggerated laryngeal chemoreflex with or without gastroesophageal reflux
Drugs (e.g., phenothiazines, over-the-counter cold remedies)*
Tachyarrhythmias (e.g., Wolfe-Parkinson-White syndrome, prolonged QT syndrome)
Inborn errors of metabolism (e.g., MCAD deficiencies)
Hypoventilation during bed sharing or because nose and mouth become covered with bedding

From Pitetti RD, Whitman E, Zaylor A. Accidental and non-accidental poisonings as a cause of apparent life-threatening events in infants. *Pediatrics*. 2008;122:e359-e362.

the findings of hypotonia, cyanosis, and possible apnea persist or recur, thus exceeding the criteria for a BRUE.

It is our experience, and the published experience of others linking GER to ALTE,[8] that the history in ALTE infants often suggests apnea after choking. It seems likely that infants whose ALTE resembles apnea after choking have an exaggerated laryngeal chemoreflex. For this reason, we will discuss Laryngeal ChemoReflex Apnea (LCRA) in detail (Fig. 80.1).

The larynx is a complex structure enriched with hundreds of nonmyelinated sensory nerve endings, including chemoreceptors and mechanoreceptors involved in maintaining upper airway patency. Laryngeal mucosal chemoreceptors function as irritant receptors, water receptors, and C fiber endings.[9] These nerve endings are most numerous in the mucosal epithelium of the epiglottis, aryepiglottic folds, and interarytenoid space.[10] Water receptors respond to either reduced osmolarity or reduced chloride ion concentration. C fibers are stimulated by noxious agents, such as temperature, ammonium, capsaicin, and H^+ ions. Stimulation of these unmyelinated nerve fibers arising in the laryngeal epithelium and traveling in the superior laryngeal nerve cause prolonged apnea, bradycardia, and marked increases in central venous and arterial blood pressure in experimental animals. Thus, both animals and humans can develop laryngeal chemoreflex apnea.

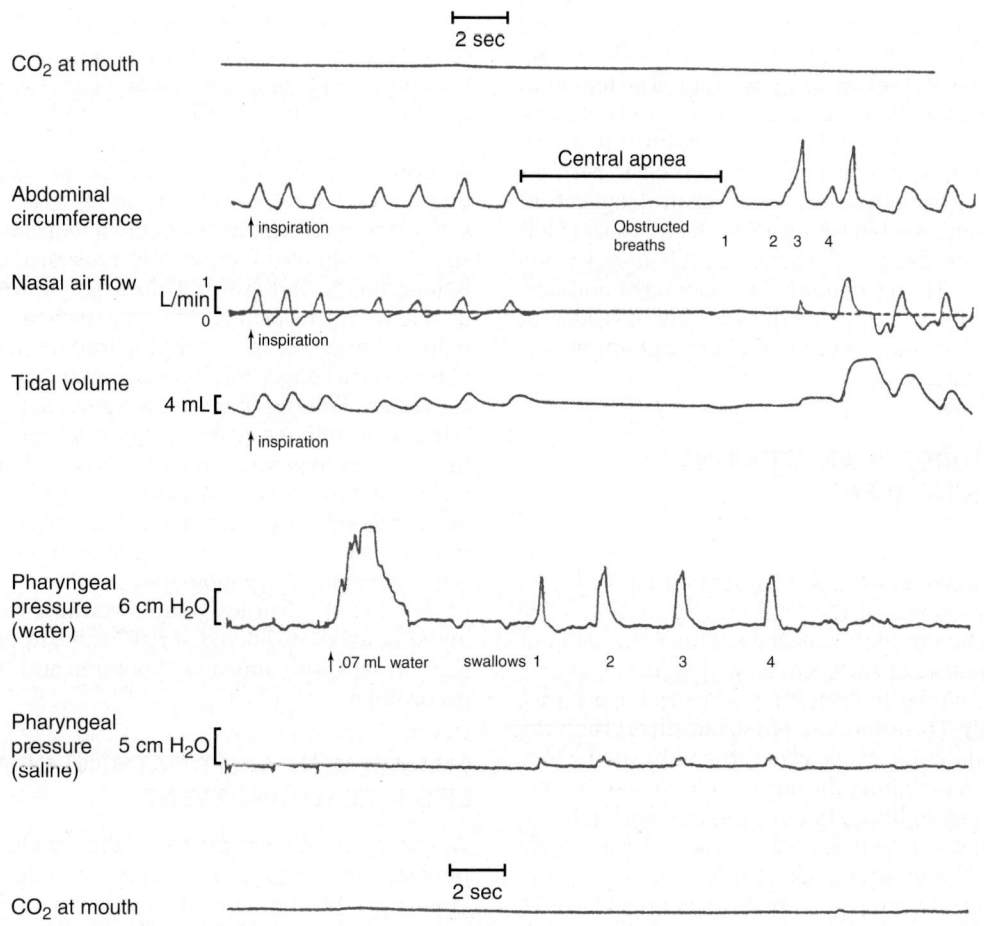

Fig. 80.1 Sequence of response representing laryngeal chemoreflex apnea in an infant. Upward deflections on pharyngeal pressure tracing reflect swallows. Application of less than 0.1 mL of water onto the larynx leads to swallows and central apnea, followed by obstructive apnea and restoration of eupnea after water has been cleared by swallows. (From Davies AM, Koenig JS, Thach BT. Upper airway chemoreflex responses to saline and water in preterm infants. *J Appl Physiol.* 1988;64:1412-1420.)

Any liquid in contact with the laryngeal mucosa will trigger a more or less brisk LCRA. The sequence of response after single-fiber stimulation of these nerves is dramatic and is most marked in younger animals (e.g., piglets, lambs, and puppies). Apnea beginning within 0.25 seconds of the stimulus may last 20–90 seconds and may be fatal in the laboratory.[11,12] Saline elicits little or no response, whereas water and cow's milk elicit a dramatic LCRA.[11-13]

As in experimental animals, among human preterm infants, water is more potent than normal saline in eliciting severe LCRA.[13,14] In infants, should swallowing be delayed or fail to occur, the apneic phase of the laryngeal chemoreflex can be prolonged, extending over 20 seconds and causing hypoxemia. The duration of the apneic phase of the laryngeal chemoreflex (LCR) seems to be inversely proportional to postnatal age.[12] Taken together, these findings suggest that in immature subjects, airway protection from aspiration takes precedence over ventilation in some circumstances when even small quantities of fluids (~0.1 mL), including water, come in contact with the larynx.

Human infants attempt to clear fluid that elicits LCRA by laryngeal closure and swallowing during a central apnea (see Fig. 80.1).[13] After the central apnea, any breaths attempted are obstructed so long as upper airway closure persists. When swallowing clears the fluid, the upper airway

is opened with a return to eupneic breathing. The LCR sequence in more mature infants and experimental animals does not involve prolonged apnea, and is as follows: cough, swallowing, and arousal if asleep.[15] The cough-swallow-arousal sequence is much less common when elicited during sleep in immature subjects.[10]

With maturation in older infants and older experimental animals, apnea occurs as part of the laryngeal chemoreflex, but it is shorter than in preterm infants and newborn animals. Maturation is associated with reduction in central respiratory inhibition. Cough and arousal from sleep are also more likely to occur among mature subjects when water, acid, or milk come in contact with the larynx.[10] Nevertheless, in susceptible infants, delays in maturational influences could put them at risk for prolonged apnea as part of the laryngeal chemoreflex.[16]

The role of gastroesophageal reflux (GER) in eliciting apnea through the LCR and therefore as a cause of ALTE or BRUE is controversial. Indeed, the new guidelines defining BRUE explicitly state that any event consistent with GER is *not* a BRUE, perhaps because GER in and of itself may be associated with a changed respiratory pattern.[2] As noted above, in animals and infants, milk and water can have a profound response from LCR. Stimulation need not be acidic to elicit a LCRA.[9] There are no distal esophageal receptors known to elicit apnea; therefore reflux must be to the level of the pharynx to stimulate LCRA. Reflux to the level of the larynx may occur in 60%–70% of episodes of GER.[17] The temporal sequence of GER eliciting a subsequent apnea and potential pathogenesis in term infants has been demonstrated, but the association among preterm infants is less clear, perhaps because the high background rate of central apneas in preterm infants makes establishing a link to antecedent GER events more challenging.[17–20] Therefore GER may be one explanation for ALTE, particularly in select term and premature infants, however, proving the association is difficult and, moreover, reflux may occur in the absence of any abnormal respiratory patterns.

CLINICAL FEATURES OF AN APPARENT LIFE-THREATENING EVENT

Symptoms

Most infants who come to medical attention following an ALTE are asymptomatic at the time of presentation.[7] The history should attempt to provide a clear understanding of the timing and nature of the event as well as pertinent past medical history, family history, environmental exposures, and social history. The attending physician supervising the evaluation should make every effort to obtain the history himself or herself, including the duration of the event, time of day, adequacy of lighting, infant's position within his or her surroundings, and whether the episode began while awake or asleep. The infant's color, tone, activity, and movements at the time of event (e.g., repetitive motions) must be noted. Was blood or pink froth coming from the infant's mouth or nose, for instance, or did the caregiver notice any other unusual findings? Were any measures taken to stop the event (stimulating the infant through touching or blowing on the face) and did the infant require resuscitation (i.e., CPR)? Who was present and witnessed the event and who was the responsible caregiver at the time that this occurred? The appropriateness of the caregivers' concern should be noted. Any glaring inconsistencies in the history should raise suspicion for nonaccidental trauma or attention-seeking behavior. Beyond the event itself, a thorough medical and family history should be obtained. Has the infant been growing and developing normally? Is there a history of prematurity, prior hospitalization, GE reflux, prior injury, snoring, or noisy breathing? Was the infant in the early stages of a respiratory illness, or was he or she having coughing paroxysms? Family history of seizures, arrhythmias, sudden death, or serious illness with coma among young people must be ascertained. A thorough list of pertinent questions to ask when taking a history for an ALTE or BRUE is available in the BRUE guidelines.[2]

Physical Findings

Just as the majority of infants are asymptomatic at presentation, physical exam findings are often normal. Nevertheless, a thorough physical examination is essential in detecting a possible etiology for the event, and suggesting specific needs for further diagnostic evaluation. As with any disease presentation, accurate vital signs are an essential initial assessment. Fever, tachypnea, hypotension, or hypoxemia should clue the clinician into an underlying illness such as focal infection, generalized sepsis, or underlying cardiovascular or respiratory disease. Growth parameters can also be clues, with poor weight gain since birth suggestive of chronic underlying disease, and large head circumference suggesting a neurological disorder or bleeding related to head trauma. A thorough neurological examination should consider the infant's level of responsiveness and alertness as well as tone, symmetry of reflexes and movement, pupillary responses, and size; it should also include a funduscopic exam for retinal hemorrhages. A limb that does not move spontaneously or one that is deformed, bruised, swollen, or painful when palpated suggests an underlying fracture and possible child abuse. Nasal congestion, coryza, cough, and other abnormal respiratory findings (crackles, wheezes, tachypnea, stridor, or retractions) might suggest an upper or lower respiratory tract infection. A hyperdynamic precordium, cardiac murmurs, gallop rhythms, or heart rhythm irregularities warrant further investigation for an underlying congenital or infectious cardiac disorder such as cardiomyopathy or myocarditis. Abdominal distension or organomegaly could be clues to infection or a metabolic disorder. Infants younger than 2 months of age should be considered at risk for bacteremic sepsis when they present with apnea or hypotonia and should be treated accordingly.

MANAGEMENT AND TREATMENT OF APPARENT LIFE-THREATENING EVENT

A systematic review for the management of ALTEs was published in 2013 that attempted to address some of the challenges of the clinical management of patients who experience such an event.[21] The challenges increase when trying to address the patient who is asymptomatic by the time of presentation to the medical team. While events called ALTE are ultimately benign, they may be an initial presentation of a significant underlying disorder. Trying to determine which child deserves a more extensive evaluation and what that evaluation may entail, including diagnostic testing and need for hospitalization, is not only challenging but fraught with controversy. Indeed, some institutions have developed clinical decision rules to determine which infants may be safely discharged home from the ER following an ALTE.[22,23] The newer BRUE guidelines attempt to further address these issues and outline management recommendations based on available research to apply to those infants deemed low risk. The guidelines were developed by a multidisciplinary subcommittee of the AAP composed of a group of experts from various fields of medicine, epidemiologists, methodologists, and parent representatives. They performed an extensive review of the literature related to ALTEs from 1970 through 2014 to develop their definition and recommendations.[2] The authors recognized that the strength of their recommendations for low-risk infants is moderate to weak because of lack of high-quality evidence and studies. It is essential to understand that the guidelines for BRUE only apply to low-risk infants who have returned to baseline and any abnormal physical examination findings or history should warrant further investigation.

Management guidelines for higher risk infants have not yet been established but the available studies to date would recommend a tailored approach based on the findings from the history and physical examination (for further reading, we recommend reviewing the tables within Tieder et al., *Pediatrics* 2016 outlining the historical features to be considered in the evaluation of a potential BRUE). That is, while there are many laboratory studies and diagnostic tests that could be performed to determine the etiology of the event, only certain tests may be necessary or appropriate in individual cases.

IMAGING AND LABORATORY FINDINGS

The 2016 guidelines for BRUE suggest minimal testing for those infants who meet the criteria for low risk. These recommendations advise against the routine use of chest radiographs, blood gases, polysomnograms, echocardiograms, neuroimaging, and blood evaluations for culture, white blood cell count, or metabolic disorders. They do recommend that caregivers be offered resources for CPR training and given education on BRUEs. Furthermore, recommendations and testing should be done through a shared decision-making platform between medical provider and caregiver.[2]

The following tests may be informative when the criteria for a BRUE are exceeded, for example, recurrent events over a short period of time, abnormal physical findings, or worrisome history. Initial laboratory evaluation may include measurement of hemoglobin and white blood cell count with differential cell count; culture of blood and urine; nasal swabs for respiratory syncytial virus (RSV) and pertussis; a chest radiograph; and serum glucose, sodium, potassium, chloride, and bicarbonate. The child who has a concerning history and is not back to baseline should be admitted to a unit where cardiorespiratory monitoring is available so that abnormalities in cardiac or respiratory rate can be recorded. If the infant continues to be limp, or if apnea recurs, one should measure arterial blood gases, serum lactate, and ammonia, and screen the urine for abnormal levels of amino and organic acids, and drugs.[24] In children who continue to appear ill or who have altered mental status with no other cause detected, video electroencephalography (EEG) should be conducted and imaging of the central nervous system by computed tomography or, preferably, magnetic resonance imaging, should be performed.[25]

The clinical approach to an ALTE should, of course, be based on one's assessment of the validity of the caregivers' observations: "benign physiological events in babies may sometimes cause an overreaction by parents, particularly those who are anxious, are attention-seeking, or suffer a personality disorder."[26,27] On the other hand, one's approach should also be informed by the knowledge that 89% of infants with documented prolonged apnea, bradycardia, and marked hypoxemia when subsequently hospitalized for an ALTE had appeared well in the emergency department (Fig. 80.2).[7]

PREVENTION: HOME APNEA MONITORS AND FEEDING INFANTS WITH EXAGGERATED LARYNGEAL CHEMOREFLEX APNEA

Because the pathophysiology and underlying causes of ALTEs or BRUEs are usually difficult to identify, how to prevent these events is not known. That said, much concern regarding BRUE and ALTE arises from the worry that they are a signal of an

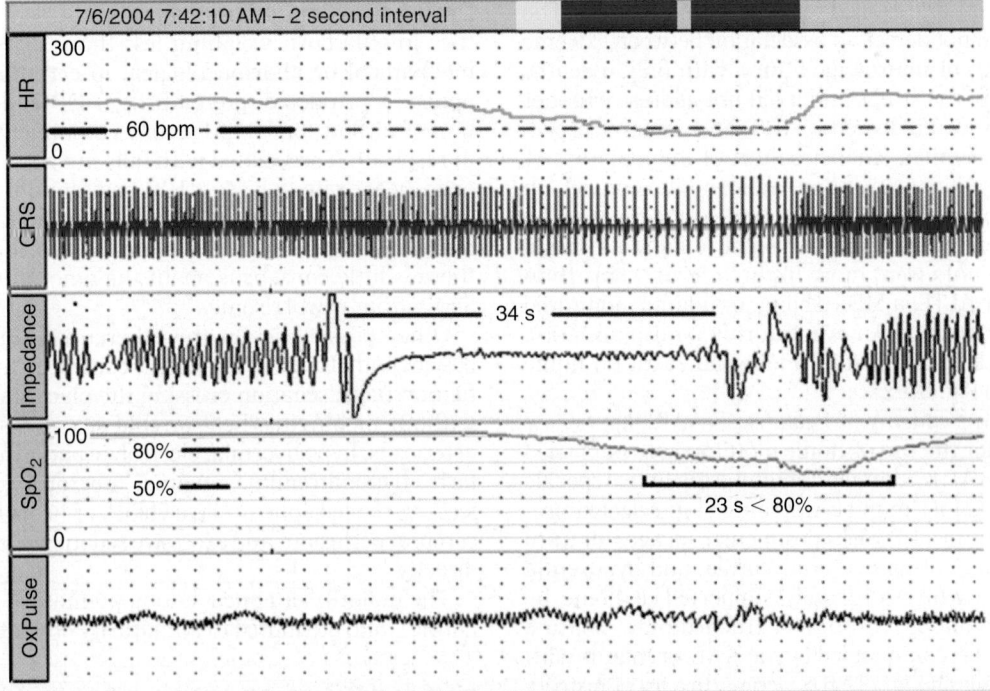

Fig. 80.2 Recording from an infant hospitalized with an apparent life-threatening event. Representative example of the most common event classified as an extreme event. Note the 34-second central apnea with the associated desaturation below the level of 80%. The apparent small respiratory movements on the impedance channel during the apnea correspond to cardiogenic artifacts. *HR,* Heart rate; *QRS,* QRS wave of the electrocardiogram; *impedance,* respiratory movements detected by transthoracic impedance; *oxpulse,* plethysmographic wave obtained from the pulse oximeter. (From Al-Kindy HA, Gelinas J, Hatsakis G, Cote A. Risk factors for extreme events in infants hospitalized for apparent life-threatening events. *J Pediatr.* 2009;154:322-327.)

underlying condition or an indication of risk for a future SIDS event. Therefore these children are often discharged home with apnea monitors in the hope of preventing SIDS. Home monitors are often prescribed by practicing physicians when a child is deemed at risk for a cardiorespiratory event. In a retrospective review of 88 infants prescribed home monitors at a tertiary hospital, indications for monitoring included family history of SIDS in 21%, apnea of prematurity in 25%, history of previous ALTE in 21% and a choking episode in 15%.[28]

The CHIME (Collaborative Home Infant Monitoring Evaluation) study was an NIH-funded study developed in order to determine whether home monitors were effective in identifying episodes of apnea or bradycardia that were potentially threatening to an infant's health.[29] It enrolled a total of 1079 infants between 1994 and 1998, and included a group of healthy term infants, preterm infants, infants who had experienced an ALTE, and infants whose siblings died from SIDS. Extreme and conventional events were determined based on degree and duration of bradycardia and apnea. The CHIME monitor included both EKG and pulse oximetry recordings as well as Respiratory Inductance Plethysmography (RIP) bands. The RIP bands allowed the researchers to evaluate episodes of apnea as obstructive or not and found that 70% of "extreme" events and 50% of "conventional events" were associated with obstructed breaths. By using RIP bands, they were able to show that apnea identified by impedance cardiorespiratory monitoring was concordant with that found by RIP. The authors concluded that events, in general, were common, including in the healthy term infants. Extreme events, defined as apneas ≥30 seconds and heart rate less than 50 bpm (≥44 weeks PCA) or 60 bpm (<44 weeks PCA) for at least 10 seconds were more likely in preterm infants, and tended to recur within 6 weeks. The CHIME study did not detect an association between extreme events and death or neurologic injury, with only 6 deaths occurring during the study, and it did not address whether use of monitors would decrease SIDS rates. In a retrospective review of a similar, smaller cohort of infants, 36% of infants had a significant event on home monitoring, which occurred most often within the first month, and more so the first week, of monitoring.[30] This retrospective study also found that preterm infants were more likely to have events than those with prior ALTE, a SIDS sibling, or infants monitored due to parental anxiety. An event during a hospitalization also increased the likelihood of finding an event on home monitoring (see Fig. 80.2).

The American Academy of Pediatrics' (AAP) last review and guidelines for the use of home monitors was published in 2003.[31] The AAP recommends monitoring in two specific circumstances: (1) it "may be warranted" in selected premature infants until "43 weeks postmenstrual age," or until "extreme episodes" of apnea, bradycardia, and hypoxemia stop; (2) infants who are usually supported at home by mechanical ventilation through a tracheotomy. Routine monitoring is not recommended by the AAP for infants with an ALTE or among siblings of SIDS victims. In a list of instructions, the AAP states: (1) "Home cardiorespiratory monitoring should not be prescribed to prevent SIDS"; (2) "Parents should be advised that...monitoring has not been proven to prevent sudden unexpected deaths..."[31] The AAP's recommendations reflect an accurate interpretation of published reports but also reflect compromises that are believed by some to be too generous toward or too restrictive of monitoring.[32]

A 2011 systematic review of the reduced rates of SIDS identified 11 prospective studies, but only one provided high-level evidence.[33] The majority of studies reviewed were cohort studies from the 1980s. Many of these studies were flawed in their methodology or description of study design, and the type of home monitoring device varied among the studies and even within a single study. A total of 2210 infants had been studied over an average of 5.5 months with a rate of SIDS deaths of 5.0 deaths per 1000 (95% CI 1.4–11.0). While the review concludes that there is little evidence that home monitoring may prevent SIDS, the authors go on to say that "the lack of high-level evidence of effectiveness of home monitoring does not prove that it is ineffective. Indeed, the lack of evidence may be more of a reflection of the difficulty in designing an appropriate and rigorous study in this sensitive area, where the well-being of any child enrolled must be given much higher priority than the more abstract needs of researchers."

In our opinion, approaches to monitoring that are dogmatic, either pro or con, and not sympathetic to parents' concerns, should not be the norm. Thus, although it is the official recommendation of the AAP that ALTE patients not be monitored, this recommendation remains controversial, and home monitoring appears to be a common practice.

Apnea in Premature Infants

DIAGNOSIS AND DIFFERENTIAL DIAGNOSIS

During their initial hospitalization, 50%–100% of premature infants born weighing less than 1500 g will require mechanical or pharmacological interventions because of apnea.[34,35] Apnea of prematurity (AOP) is defined as cessation of airflow for 10–20 seconds or longer. Shorter pauses in respiration associated with falls in SpO_2% (e.g., to <90%) or in heart rate (e.g., to <100 beats/min) are also seen as important episodes of apnea in most neonatal intensive care units (NICUs). However, if apnea is less than 10 seconds, there is little consensus about the amount of reduction in SpO_2% that is worrisome.[34,36–38]

Other possibilities in the differential diagnosis of AOP besides immaturity of ventilatory control include: intracranial hemorrhage, sedation crossing the placenta, sepsis with or without meningitis, heat or cold stress,[39] a patent ductus arteriosus, hypoglycemia, electrolyte abnormalities (particularly hyponatremia), anemia, necrotizing enterocolitis, feeding-related apnea,[40] heart block or heart failure lowering cerebral perfusion, and excessive sedation given to the infant directly.

The majority of apnea among premature infants is "idiopathic," and attributed to immaturity of ventilatory control.

PATHOGENESIS OF APNEA OF PREMATURITY

Ventilatory control among premature infants is sufficiently unstable that apnea, even prolonged, is provoked by problems (e.g., hyponatremia, heart failure) that would not be sufficient explanations beyond term postmenstrual age (PMA). Thus, the primary instability of ventilatory pattern and drive among premature infants, even when they are "well," is important.[38]

It is simplistic to state that most apnea among premature infants is central, although most episodes can be prevented with stimulants whose primary action is central. Indeed, it is probable that the majority of apneic events in premature infants have both obstructive and central components (i.e., they are mixed).[41] Furthermore, it seems likely that all three types of apnea described in preterm infants—central, obstructive, and mixed—occur when the frequency of output from the respiratory controller is at a low ebb, "suggesting that all 3 patterns had one common underlying mechanism."[38]

There is little recent published work that describes the prevalence of the various types of apnea (central, obstructive, or mixed) or the impact of sleep state, or that explores critically the continued relevance of what has become "cribside" dogma.[42] Moreover, clinical rules have often been based on few observations; for example, the dogma that apnea is much more common in active than in quiet sleep is based on studies done on nine term infants.[43] With many smaller and more premature infants surviving, since the introduction of artificial surfactant over 25 years ago, these dicta should be reexplored.

It was observed in the 1980s that the majority of central apneic episodes were either preceded or followed by evidence of upper airway obstruction.[44,45] During apnea in premature infants, respiratory effort often continues, or resumes, before airflow returns, with phasic contraction of the diaphragm (electromyogram) associated with generation of progressively more negative intrathoracic pressures (P_{esoph}). Near the end of a typical mixed apnea, genioglossus contraction (submental electromyogram) opens the airway and flow resumes.[46] It was thus recognized that apneic episodes in premature neonates could also appear on recordings to be bradycardia with desaturation, because impedance chest movement monitors would correctly indicate that respiratory efforts continued.[47]

During quiet sleep, premature neonates with frequent apnea are less able than nonapneic controls to compensate for progressive increases in upper airway resistance. Neonates with apnea have much shorter and weaker inspiratory efforts in response to end-expiratory occlusion. Premature neonates with apnea also have a higher $PaCO_2$ (~9 mm Hg higher) and a much flatter ventilatory response to breathing 4% CO_2 (V_E/min/kg) compared to controls.[48,49] In addition, infants, in general, have a flatter CO_2 response when breathing progressively more hypoxic gas mixtures.[50]

A series of explanations for the most common type of apnea among premature infants—mixed apnea—can be constructed from these classic studies:

1. Upper airway obstruction, for which the infant has shorter and weaker "load compensation," is preceded by brief central apnea, or leads to longer central apnea.
2. Infants with a lower minute volume response to increasing CO_2 become progressively more hypercarbic and hypoxemic.
3. The development of hypoxemia further blunts CO_2 response, and the increasing CO_2 makes the activities of the diaphragm and genioglossus asynchronous,[51] perpetuating the cycle of obstructive and central (i.e., mixed) apneas.

Other "classic" studies from the mid-1980s suggested additional physiologic mechanisms to explain why premature infants might be more at risk for mixed apnea and its complications during active sleep:

1. The inspiratory "load" for which premature infants are unable to "compensate" is due to upper airway narrowing,[42,43] which usually occurs at the pharynx.[41]
2. Loss of intercostal tone[52] during active sleep would increase wasted "distortional" work[53] during the paradoxical breathing caused by pharyngeal airway narrowing.[41,54]
3. Loss of intercostal tone would also diminish functional residual capacity and thus worsen hypoxemia during compromised breathing.[52,55]

Furthermore, the LCRA, described above, may also play a role in AOP. Swallowing interrupts LCRA. Premature infants swallow more frequently during apnea than during eupneic breathing. This suggests that exaggerated LCRA, such as that caused by spontaneous pooling of saliva, may explain some apneic episodes.[56] LCRA is, in fact, mixed apnea, and similar to the most frequent type of AOP.

Although it may be simplistic to describe AOP as "primarily central," inadequate responses to upper airway obstruction do reflect a significant "central immaturity" among premature infants. Other evidence of the "central immaturity" of younger infants is the marked increase in periodic breathing particularly during active sleep.[43] After the onset of periodic breathing, transient upper airway obstruction at the pharynx is common during the first inspiratory effort after the apneic pause. Thus, excessive periodic breathing, which is considered pathognomonic for "central immaturity" of respiratory control, frequently has both central and obstructive (i.e., mixed) apnea components.

During epochs of periodic breathing, preterm infants have falls in SpO_2% and are widely believed to be more susceptible to prolonged apneas (Fig. 80.3). A recent longitudinal study of 24 infants born between 27 and 36 weeks gestation showed that all but one had periodic breathing during 2–3 hour recordings during naps.[57] The infants were 2, 4, and 6 months postterm corrected age. For most infants, the periodic breathing runs were short and benign, though falls in SpO_2% and cerebral tissue oxygenation index were often statistically significant. Three infants had large and sustained falls in heart rate, SpO_2% (to <80%), and cerebral oxygenation index.[57] Their susceptibility to periodic breathing may be enhanced by the fact that their $PaCO_2$ during eupneic breathing may be only 1.3 mm Hg above their apneic threshold.[58] Thus any ventilatory overshoot after a periodic apnea makes preterms particularly vulnerable to resuming apnea. In this regard, evidence from lambs induced to have periodic breathing suggests that increases in lung volume from adding CPAP served to reduce the overshoot, or "loop gain," after a periodic apnea, followed by shortened epochs of periodic breathing.[59]

Premature infants also have more active sleep than quiet sleep, with the attendant irregularity in tidal volume (V_T) and ventilatory frequency (V_f), and increases in both prolonged apnea and periodic apnea/breathing. In the episodes of apnea when obstruction is not found (<50%), irregularities in respiratory pattern (V_f, V_T, periodic breathing) often explain a propensity for apnea that is "primarily central."

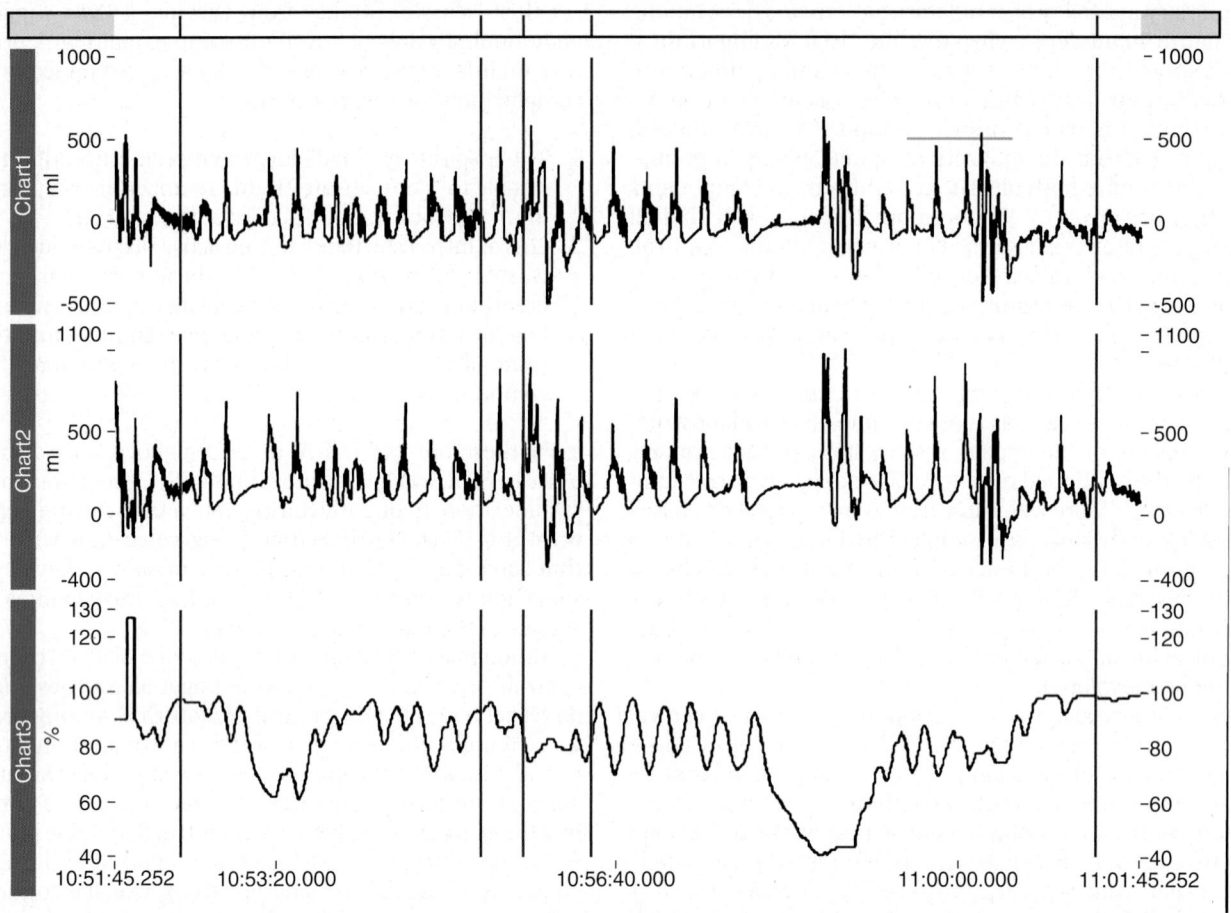

Fig. 80.3 A 10-minute recording in a 26-week premature infant at 36 weeks postmenstrual age. Upper two tracings are respiratory inductance plethysmography (RIP) from rib cage and abdominal belts. The pattern seen during the first 6 minutes is typical for periodic breathing. Lower tracing shows oscillations in SpO₂% with periodic breathing/periodic apnea. Fall in SpO₂% to 46% is associated with a 38-second central apnea recorded by the RIP belts. (Data from the Prematurity and Respiratory Outcomes Program (PROP) Study.)

PROGNOSIS OF APNEA OF PREMATURITY

The natural history of AOP is unclear because interventions to treat it, and thus alter its natural history, have been tried ever since it was first described.

Apneic pauses longer than 5 seconds are common on the first day of life among premature infants without respiratory distress syndrome and can increase to 25 per day by the third day.[60] During a 5-year period (1989–1994), one NICU discharged 457 infants born at 24–28 weeks PMA.[35] All infants enrolled in the study had been treated because all had apnea lasting longer than 20 seconds. In general, infants born earlier had apnea and bradycardia events that persisted until an older PMA. In the study by Eichenwald and coworkers,[35] apnea was diagnosed when chest wall movement was not detected by impedance monitoring. The last events to disappear with maturation were bradycardia episodes without associated central apnea. As noted earlier and as recognized by the Eichenwald et al., the explanation may be that obstructive apneic episodes with bradycardia continued until the age that the bradycardia episodes ceased. Another study using transthoracic impedance but incorporating motion-artifact resistant oximetry has led to similarly plausible speculation.[61] Finally, evidence for persistent propensity for undetected mixed apneas is also suggested by detailed

descriptions of maturation of upper airway–stabilizing mechanisms.[62] There seems to be a growth- and age-dependent threshold for improvement in upper airway stability beginning at about 36 weeks PMA.

One group of preterm infants whose ventilatory and general "autonomic instability" may not be appreciated are so-called late preterm infants, born at 33 or 34–37 weeks PMA. The majority (75%) of preterm births in the United States each year are in this group, and over 400,000 infants are born at 33–37 weeks annually.[63] Most attention in diagnosing and treating apnea of prematurity is directed to infants born less than 32 or less than 28 weeks PMA.[35,64,65] However, compared to term infants in the CHIME study (Collaborative Home Infant Monitoring Evaluation),[29] late preterm infants had a relative risk less than 5 for "extreme" apnea lasting longer than 30 seconds, or bradycardia (see Fig. 80.2). Further, in our experience, late preterm infants not infrequently return to hospital with, for example, excessive periodic breathing, hypoxemia, and apnea at 40 weeks PMA or older, and clinicians seem surprised at the severity of their ventilatory instability. It is clear that postnatal maturation of ventilatory control among very preterm infants is not the same as infants of the same PMA but born at term.[65] Whether and how much this delay in maturation occurs in late preterm infants is not clear. But concerns are growing about respiratory morbidity and about neurodevelopmental milestones in late preterms, particularly with regards to mathematics and reading skills.[66] This has led to trials of interventions such as betamethasone[67] during late preterm labor (34–37 weeks) to begin to address a series of problems that are common and that were underappreciated until recently. Studies are also needed to clarify whether the ventilatory control problems of some late preterm infants, as in the CHIME study, contribute to neurodevelopmental complications.

MANAGEMENT AND TREATMENT FOR APNEA OF PREMATURITY

The first-line treatment for AOP remains methylxanthines,[68] with approximately 75% of premature infants responding. Caffeine has replaced theophylline as the methylxanthine of choice because it is as effective and less likely than theophylline to cause tachycardia or poor feeding.[69] Caffeine is thought to act by blocking brainstem inhibitory adenosine A_1 receptors, leading to increased respiratory neural output.[47]

Pulmonologists should also know that much enthusiasm has developed recently for the early introduction of caffeine for prematures weighing 500–1250 g, even before apnea of prematurity necessitates increased ventilatory support. It is not clear why, but subjects started on caffeine within the first 10 days of life in a randomized, controlled trial involving 2006 infants had: (1) shorter need for supplemental O_2 and CPAP[70]; and (2) less neurodevelopmental disability at 18–21 months postterm corrected age.[71] Caffeine was begun before chronic lung disease had developed, and continued until apnea, if it developed, had resolved. How caffeine given more or less prophylactically might reduce the incidence of chronic lung disease is not clear.[72,73] Studies in animal models suggest that its effect may be through adenosine

receptors both on lung inflammatory cells and on airway smooth muscle that determine the responses to inflammation[74] or through prevention of the functional, structural, and inflammatory changes induced by hyperoxia.[75] Furthermore, although it reduces apnea frequency and, presumably, the associated hypoxemia, whether these effects on ventilatory stability provide the explanation for caffeine's apparent impact on neurodevelopmental outcome was not addressed in the large randomized trial.[72] The longer-term effects of caffeine on oxygenation are suggested by a study showing that earlier cessation of caffeine treatment according to nursery protocol was associated with longer periods of intermittent hypoxemia at 35 and 36 weeks PMA than if caffeine was continued longer until clinical concerns regarding apnea had resolved.[76]

Infants who fail to respond to methylxanthines will often respond to nasal continuous positive airway pressure (NCPAP) or nasal intermittent positive pressure ventilation.[77] However, concerns about toxicity from high-dose methylxanthines and mucosal injury from NCPAP have led to widespread enthusiasm for early use of high-flow nasal cannulas. High-flow nasal cannulas use adequately warmed and humidified air to deliver distending pressures that are presumably comparable to NCPAP, and are often used at flow rates of 2.5 L/min, or more.[78] These catheters have been shown to be as effective as NCPAP in reducing apnea, bradycardia, and episodes of desaturation. High-flow cannulas appear to stave off intubation both by stabilizing respiratory mechanics and treating AOP.[79] Potential explanations for the efficacy of high-flow therapy in treating AOP have not been tested empirically, despite its frequent use for this purpose.[80] However, it seems plausible that distending pressures from the high-flow catheters might mitigate the obstructive component of a typical preterm's mixed apnea (Fig. 80.4). Also, continued

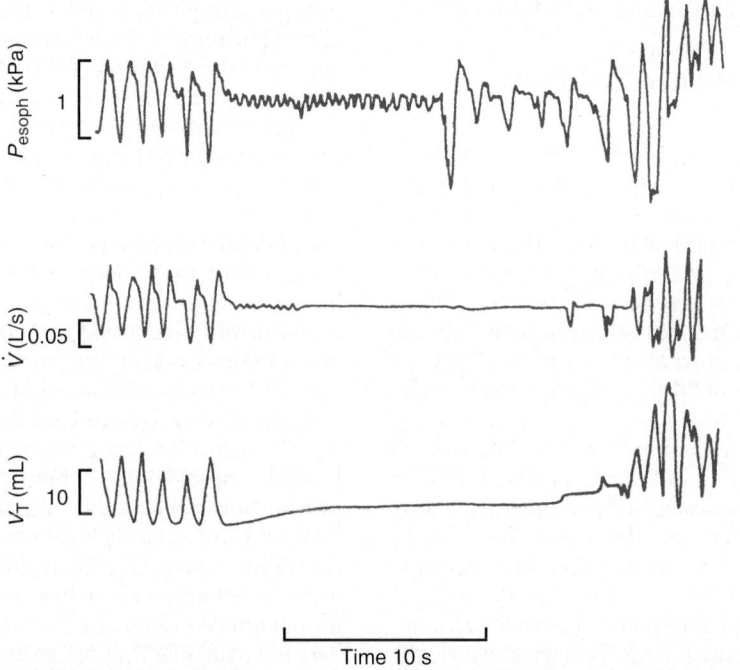

Fig. 80.4 Spontaneous apnea in a premature infant. Esophageal pressure tracing, with cardiogenic artifact, demonstrates first central apnea, then respiratory efforts. Flow and volume tracings show that the first four or five efforts after central apnea are obstructed. Such mixed apneas are the most common type of apnea of prematurity. P_{esoph}, Intrathoracic pressure; V_T, tidal volume; $\dot{V}$, airflow. (From Milner AD, Greenough A. The role of the upper airway in neonatal apnea. *Semin Neonatol.* 2004;9:213-220.)

flow *per se* might stimulate laryngeal flow receptors[9] and, in effect, feed forward to stimulate continued respiratory effort.[81]

Another older intervention for apnea, blood transfusion, remains controversial.[82] The long-term effect of transfusion therapy on reducing AOP is not clear. However, it has recently been shown that infants have more apnea when their hematocrit is lower, and apnea is less frequent for 3 days after a transfusion.[83]

Pediatric pulmonologists who are not based in NICUs should be reminded that premature infants are at much greater risk for serious apnea after general anesthesia.[84] After anesthesia, increased frequency of apnea and bradycardia can continue to beyond 46 weeks PMA, particularly among infants who required prolonged ventilatory support just after birth, or who have significant residual lung injury. Pulmonologists should be aware of the policies of local pediatric anesthesiologists with respect to perioperative monitoring, even for semielective surgery such as herniorrhaphy. A systematic review from Copenhagen emphasized that "Grade 1 evidence (randomized, controlled trial) exists for recommending regional versus general anesthesia when possible, and for the efficacy of prophylactic caffeine (10 mg/kg IV) on the day of surgery for preterms less than 44 weeks PMA."[85] The Danish authors recommend at least 12 hours of nurse-supervised, postanesthesia monitoring using ECG and oximetry for: (1) all preterms less than 46 weeks PMA; (2) for infants 46–60 weeks PMA with a hematocrit less than 30%; and, (3) those 46–60 weeks PMA with "co-morbidities" including chronic lung disease, a history of apnea, or CNS abnormalities. Six hours of recovery room monitoring is otherwise recommended for preterms 46–60 weeks PMA.[85] A recent study by the Pediatric Sedation Research Consortium involving over 57,000 patients receiving sedation showed that former preterm infants are at a small but significant risk for airway obstruction, lower SpO$_2$%, and other complications, and that risk that can extend into adulthood.[86]

Monitoring Premature Infants at Home

Studies evaluating compliance with apnea monitor use suggest high rates of compliance among infants with AOP, particularly during the first month at home.[87] Abuses because of self-interest among those prescribing monitors notwithstanding,[32,88] the promise or potential of monitors, when used to prevent deaths among "nursery graduates," should not be discounted. Infants born at 24–36 weeks PMA are 2.1–3.3 times as likely to die of SIDS as infants born at greater than 37 weeks.[89]

The issue of monitor use is quite complex, however. In their review of more than 37,000 deaths and 3.8 million linked births, Malloy and Hoffman showed that, depending on the estimated gestational age, the age of SIDS deaths among premature infants was, on average, 44.2 weeks to 47.8 weeks PMA (range, 32–85 weeks).[89] On the basis of these data and those of the CHIME study,[29] wherein "extreme" apneic spells among premature infants "disappeared once the infants were 43 weeks postconceptional age," one editorial writer declared that the usefulness of prescribing monitors to detect extreme apneic spells and to prevent sudden death among premature infants and the "physiological basis for

such a practice are more in doubt than ever."[32] However, because infants who have died were certainly apneic at least once, another possible scenario is that the time course of dangerous apnea activity among those premature infants dying is different from those having apnea and not dying. The vexing problem remains whether it is possible to select candidates who will benefit most from monitoring. Monitoring for apnea in preterm infants must continue to be part of this discussion. Malloy has shown that the adjusted odds ratio for deaths called SIDS for infants born between 24 and 28 weeks was 2.57, even given the propensity for attributing their deaths to causes related to complications of prematurity.[90]

For the time being, we are in agreement with the AAP recommendations for monitoring premature infants having apnea until they are 43 weeks PMA.[32,91] Because the average time course until cessation of apnea among those infants dying must be different from that for the premature infants in the CHIME study, monitoring infants past 43 weeks PMA who have frequent apnea lasting longer than 20 seconds, especially with reductions in heart rate, also seems prudent.

Sudden Infant Death Syndrome

PATHOGENESIS: TRIPLE RISK MODEL

The definition for SIDS during the first 20 years after the syndrome was recognized was "the sudden death of an infant or young child, which is unexpected by history, and in which a thorough postmortem examination fails to demonstrate an adequate cause of death."[92] Because of the recognition of risk factors related to sleep practices, the definition was broadened in 1991 to "the sudden death of an infant under one year of age which remains unexplained after a thorough case investigation, including performance of a complete autopsy, *examination of the death scene*, and review of the clinical history."[93,94] For a complete discussion of issues surrounding the definition of SIDS,[95] categorization when investigations are incomplete, and the importance of alternative definitions with subtle changes in emphasis, the reader can refer to reviews by Rognum and by Krous and coworkers.[94,96]

In this regard, it is important to recall that the "SIDS era" arose from the recognition in the late 1960s that most sudden infant deaths occurred without sufficient pathologic findings to explain them.[97,98] Explanations were lacking beyond otitis media, or mild interstitial pneumonia, found at autopsy. This fundamental insight led to much research into reflexes, ventilatory control, and brainstem neurochemistry to clarify what was defined as "unexplained" by conventional histopathology.

While serving to stimulate new thinking about why infants die, the definition just cited requiring a scene investigation has led to nosologic uncertainty, and much controversy, with one author decrying the "disappearance" of deaths labeled SIDS as a large step backward in studies of unexpected infant mortality.[99] Accepting an explanation for some deaths from a group defined because they "remain unexplained" presents an obvious conundrum. For example, once empirical data became available that suggested how infants diagnosed as having died from SIDS might have subtly suffocated while face down on soft bedding,[100–104] it was claimed that these deaths were not due to SIDS (a mystery) as they were originally diagnosed, but, in fact, due to suffocation (Fig. 80.5).[105]

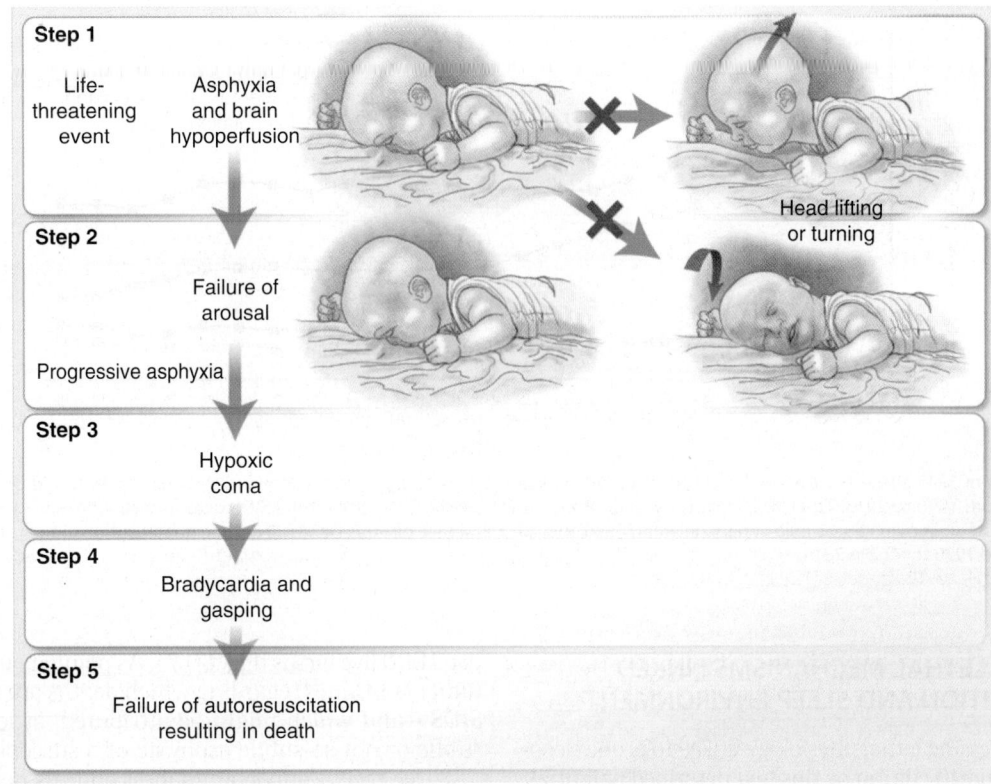

Fig. 80.5 Five steps in the putative terminal respiratory pathway associated with the sudden infant death syndrome. Death results from one or more failures in protective mechanisms against a life-threatening event during sleep in the vulnerable infant during a critical period. In particular, infants unaccustomed to prone sleep are at an 18-fold increased risk for sudden death when placed prone. (Reprinted from Kinney HC, Thach BT. The sudden infant death syndrome. *N Engl J Med*. 2009;361:795-805, Copyright Massachusetts Medical Society.)

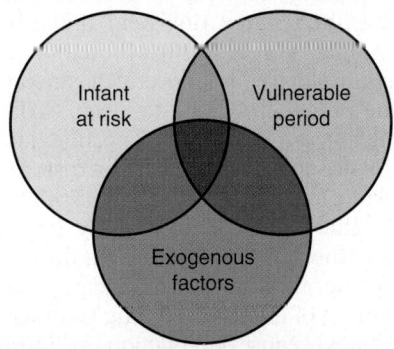

Fig. 80.6 The triple-risk model, developed to address the problem of SIDS. It emphasizes the likelihood that most deaths have several partial explanations, within a causal sequence. It remains relevant when death scene investigations have caused diagnostic shifting among the diagnoses of SIDS, unexpected suffocation, and cause of death undetermined. (From Filiano JJ, Kinney HC. A perspective on neuropathologic findings in victims of the sudden infant death syndrome. The triple risk model. *Biol Neonate*. 1994;65:194-197.)

The diagnostic shifting described[106] is understandable in the context of a definition that, while useful in stimulating research, assured a nosologic conundrum if progress was made and some of the deaths became explicable.

A framework that, in our opinion, has stood the test of time as a way to study sudden unexpected infant deaths is the triple-risk model (Fig. 80.6).[107] Susceptible infants at a vulnerable physiologic and developmental stage are exposed to more-or-less potent environmental stressors that lead to death. In a given infant or group of infants the relative importance of each influence may vary. Investigations into sleep practices over the past 20 years have increased the understanding of exogenous stressors.[108,109] Some would argue that these deaths should not be categorized as SIDS because they have had partial, new explanations,[102] even though the triple-risk model for SIDS encompasses them perfectly.

Although theoretically problematic, practical approaches to understanding related types of sudden unexpected infant deaths are possible under the rubric of SIDS. It is essential, however, to realize that there is little to be gained by an exclusionary definition of "true SIDS."[94,96]

Within the triple-risk model, for a given infant it is more helpful to think of a causal sequence. For example, we might consider a hypothetical infant with a sluggish arousal response to sleep environment threats while prone[107,110] who comes to lie prone on bedding that covers the nose and mouth.[111-113] The infant also has a respiratory infection[114] and is at a vulnerable age when the skills at gaining access to fresh air are poor.[110] Perhaps the infant has come to lie in the prone position for the first time, without the requisite learned skills to be safe prone.[110,111,115,116] In a given infant, each of these variables could be critical antecedents before autoresuscitation failure and sudden death. Moreover, amelioration of one or more of the risk factors present in this example would reduce the risk for death. The success of supine sleep interventions in many countries suggests that the prone position is critical at several junctures in a hypothetical causal sequence, at least among infants sleeping alone.[113,117-119]

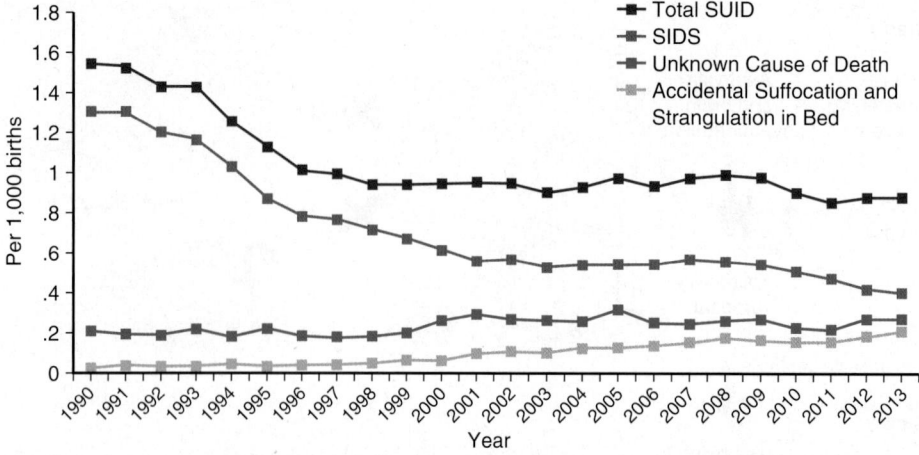

Fig. 80.7 US rates of SIDS and other sleep-related causes of infant death (1990–2013). A graph showing the rates of SIDS and other sleep-related causes of death from 1990 to 2013. Total SUID deaths declined from ~1.5 in 1990 to 1 in 2013. Total SIDS deaths declined from ~1.3 in 1990 to ~0.5 in 2013. Deaths from unknown causes held steady between 1990 and 2013 at a rate of ~0.2. Deaths from accidental suffocation and strangulation in bed rose from ~0 in 1990 to ~0.2 in 2014. (From Fast Facts about SIDS. NIH Child Health and Human Development Safe to Sleep Public Education Campaign. https://www.nichd.nih.gov/sts/about/SIDS/Pages/fastfacts.aspx.)

POTENTIALLY LETHAL MECHANISMS LINKED TO SLEEP POSITION AND SLEEP ENVIRONMENT

The section addressing lethal physiology linked to prone sleep position in the eighth edition of this text described potential rebreathing of air exhaled by the infant and thermal stress in much detail. It summarized the epidemiologic and physiologic research supporting an interaction between sleep position and a sleep environment containing loose blankets and soft sleep surfaces leading to rebreathing that can be lethal and to thermal stress. If an infant's nose and mouth are encumbered at all, rebreathing of air depleted of O_2 and polluted with CO_2 will occur. Whether this is lethal depends on the severity of limitation of access to room air imposed by the sleep environment and the infant's susceptibilities.[106,107] When rebreathing occurs, which it does when an infant's airway is at all encumbered, the challenge is to understand when rebreathing can be or is likely to be lethal.[103]

The physiology of the mechanism(s) of death remains somewhat obscure when infants are exposed to putative thermal stress that does not cause cellular injury akin to that occurring with heat stroke.[120] Infants have been shown to thermoregulate effectively and predictably when exposed to sleep environments predicted to cause dangerous thermal stress and linked to increased risk of death.[121] Relative thermal stress, compared to sleeping alone, occurs when infants bed-share,[120] but infants dying while bed sharing do not have postmortem changes of heat injury, nor has the impact of comparable levels of thermal stress on ventilatory pattern and other homeostatic mechanisms been established.

EPIDEMIOLOGY

The 50% fall in the number of deaths attributed to SIDS from the early 1990s through 2004 has been justly labeled "a success story for epidemiology."[122] Interventions in many countries motivated by the apparent causal association between prone sleep and SIDS seemed highly successful. After 2004, however, though deaths called SIDS were fewer, total sudden unexpected deaths have continued at a rate near 1.0

per 1000 live births (Fig. 80.7). As pointed out above, uncertainty continues regarding which deaths are unexplained—SIDS—and which might be attributed, at least in part, to subtle or not-so-subtle asphyxia of a susceptible infant.

Three recent important papers address newer issues pertinent to the apparent but sometimes confusing decline in unexpected infant deaths in the 1990s and early in this century. The first considers the decline in SIDS deaths over the last 25 years.[123] Causes for postneonatal infant mortality between 1983 and 2012 were analyzed for over 947,000 deaths in the United States. Goldstein et al. make the case that falls in numbers of deaths attributed to SIDS must be understood relative to trends for overall postneonatal mortality. Before the practice of Back-to-Sleep, SIDS rates were already falling at a rate similar to all postneonatal mortality (Fig. 80.8). Deaths labeled SIDS fell at a faster rate than all postneonatal mortality from 1994 to 1996, 1998 to 2001, and in 2012—that is, for only 8 of nearly 20 years of Back-to-Sleep. The authors argue that though Back-to-Sleep was successful, the success should be more completely described within populations of infants becoming less likely to die from all causes, perhaps because of reductions in "intrinsic factors" for SIDS and for deaths from other causes. Among reductions they cite are less smoking during pregnancy and fewer mothers never breastfeeding.

The second paper describes attempts to circumvent confusion arising from diagnostic shifting among SIDS, cause of death undetermined, and subtle asphyxia.[124] A system for evaluating cases within a standardized registry at the Centers for Disease Control and Prevention was applied to 436 infant deaths occurring in 9 participating states in 2011 (~13% of all sudden unexpected deaths in the United States).[125] The authors tabulated whether the deaths were believed to be unexplained (SIDS, cause undetermined) or possibly explained by asphyxia, whether thorough postmortem investigations including an investigation of the death were done, and whether unsafe sleep practices and obvious compromise of the infants' external airway were described.[124] This recently developed centralized case registry from the CDC, at first glance, would suggest a bias in favor of the idea that most

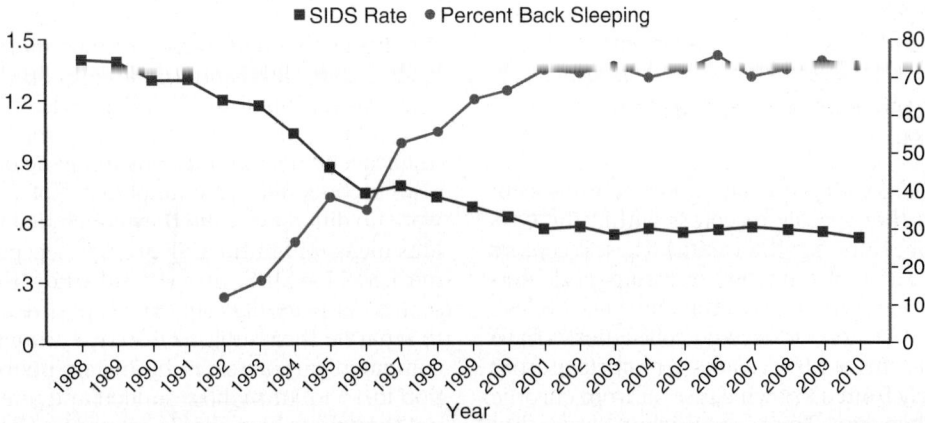

Fig. 80.8 US SIDS rate and sleep position, 1988–2010 (deaths per 1000 live births). A line graph showing the US SIDS rates and the percent of infants on the back sleep position from 1988 to 2010. The SIDS rate decreased steadily from a rate of approximately 1.4 in 1988 to approximately 0.5 in 2010. The percent of infants being put to sleep in the back sleeping position increased from approximately 15% in 1998 to approximately 72% in 2010. (From Progress in Reducing SIDS. NIH Child Health and Human Development Safe to Sleep Public Education Campaign. https://www.nichd.nih.gov/sts/about/SIDS/Pages/progress.aspx.)

infant deaths can be explained by some degree of asphyxia. However, as the authors claim, they want to quantify how frequently this occurs and recognize "...how suffocation or asphyxiation may contribute to death..." by better describing the completeness of the information on which these decisions are or should be based.

The third recent important paper reviews the well-known impact of being born prematurely on rates of SIDS and related sudden unexpected infant deaths,[90] taking into consideration diagnostic shifting due to scene investigations and interventions to promote nonprone, safe sleep. The focus was on comparing very preterm infants (24–28 weeks PMA) to those born at term. For the years 2005–2007, the SIDS mortality rate for preterm infants was higher than for term infants (1.23 vs. 0.37 per 1000 live births). The odds ratio for SIDS among preterm infants was 2.57 when adjusted for age. The postnatal age of preterm victims was greater (17.9 vs. 12.8 weeks), but the postconception age was younger (44.2 vs. 52.7 weeks). This suggests that the developmental processes leading to vulnerability occurred earlier in preterm infants.

NEWER APPROACHES TO THE PATHOLOGY AND PHYSIOLOGY OF SUDDEN INFANT DEATH SYNDROME

By definition, conventional gross or microscopic necropsy materials do not explain a SIDS death. Consequently, studies of its pathology have usually described subtle quantitative abnormalities in groups of SIDS victims that distinguish them from controls dying of identified causes.[96,126] Alternatively, investigations relying on novel techniques that have been developed since SIDS was defined have been used to begin to understand lethal mechanisms that work quickly and do not yield abnormalities visible with light microscopy (e.g., autoradiography of neuroligands or markers for apoptosis, or analysis of gene polymorphisms seen more frequently among some children dying suddenly and unexpectedly). Studies of specimens from SIDS victims using the newest techniques have attempted to piece together its pathophysiology, rather than attempting to describe findings that are, by consensus, sufficient to explain death.

Thus, in general, when infants die suddenly and unexpectedly, perhaps 1 in 6 of the deaths will be explained by postmortem findings or tests done on autopsy specimens.[127] However, when infants die without forewarning in the first week of life—SUEND, or sudden, unexpected early neonatal death—conventional postmortem investigations may more often yield diagnostic findings. In a study from London, UK, there were 55 SUEND from 1996 to 2005. Over half (58%) were explained by autopsy, primarily by congenital heart disease, acute infections, and fatty acid oxidation deficiencies.[128]

Epidemiologic findings have always influenced studies of SIDS pathology. In particular, it has been recognized for the past 25 years that many deaths diagnosed as SIDS have involved sleep practices that increase risk for death (see Fig. 80.8).[117] For this reason, pathogenetic models based on dysfunctional responses to stressors arising from sleep practices will be the focus of our review of newer approaches to pathology. In these models, the ultrastructural uniqueness of SIDS victims could cause abnormalities of ventilation, ventilatory control, or airway protection.

PROGRAMMED CELL DEATH WITHIN THE CENTRAL NERVOUS SYSTEM

In earlier studies, markers of apoptosis, triggered presumably by CNS hypoxia within the previous 48 hours, have been demonstrated in 80% of 29 SIDS victims, and 0 controls.[129] A detailed review of this topic has recently been published.[130] It outlines how "pathologic apoptotic activity" might lead to abnormalities in the dorsal motor nuclei of the vagus, which are believed to play an important role in the "efferent autonomic control of cardiorespiratory mechanisms." The model asserts that intermittent hypoxia and, in particular, intermittent hypercapnic hypoxia, causes apoptosis of neurons trafficking in important neurotransmitters (described below), and that the changes in neurotransmitter function are secondary to apoptosis induced by hypercapnic hypoxia. Thus, although most research into the role of neurotransmitters in sudden unexpected infant death has focused on ventral nuclei, apoptosis in victims has been more prominent in dorsal sites. The model outlined[130] may be particularly relevant to increased risk for death linked to nicotine exposure.

NEURAL RECEPTORS AND SUDDEN INFANT DEATH SYNDROME

Extensive investigations using carefully chosen controls seem to have established that specific receptors within the CNS are reduced in number among SIDS victims. These receptors are needed for the excitatory function of serotonergic networks within the brainstem, across sleep and wake cycles.

During the past 30 years, Kinney and colleagues[107] have compared the brainstems of SIDS victims to brainstems from infants dying acutely from a known cause, or from chronic diseases causing hypoxia. Their approaches show that attempts to explain abnormal function, rather than only histologic neuropathology, are critical to understanding SIDS. Highlights of their work, for our purposes, can be summarized as follows:

1. These authors believe that structures in the human brainstem are "anatomically homologous" to chemosensitive areas in animals,[131] and two SIDS victims they studied had hypoplasia of the arcuate nucleus, a prime "candidate" site for human brainstem chemosensitivity.
2. SIDS victims have less functional activity of receptors binding radiolabeled cholinergic transmitters within the arcuate nucleus in vitro, compared with acute and chronic controls.[132]
3. Serotonin binding by serotonin receptors in the brainstems of SIDS victims compared with controls is reduced not only in the arcuate nucleus but also in four other brainstem structures derived from the embryonic "rhombic lip" and the intermediate reticular zone.[133] In SIDS, it appears that the abnormal receptor binding patterns in the arcuate nucleus and other nuclei of the medullary serotonergic system are different than in infants who died of hypoxia of known etiology. This suggests that hypoxia alone does not cause the aberrant serotonin binding patterns in SIDS infants, but that other genetic or environmental exposures during development unique to SIDS are responsible for the aberrant patterns.[134]
4. The differences they describe occur within a serotonergic neural network involved with arousal, respiratory patterns, thermoregulation, chemoreception, and upper airway patency.[135] These findings are particularly relevant to asphyxia and hypercarbia that might occur but not be sensed by infants dying prone or supine with their nose and mouth covered.
5. There is a growing body of evidence that the medullary serotonergic system has neurons that are present as early as 7 weeks postconception, and that the nuclei comprising the system are fully developed by 20 weeks.[134] The activity of receptors binding serotonin seems to be developmentally regulated, at least between 35 and 70 weeks after conception.[133]
6. The serotonergic neurons and receptors of this system are vulnerable to in utero exposure to nicotine and alcohol, with markedly decreased serotonin binding in the arcuate nucleus in babies who were exposed.[136]

Two recent publications by Kinney and colleagues have explored the potential forensic applications of their findings regarding serotonergic networks. The first was based on the theory that a deficiency of medullary serotonin (5-HT) leads to 5-HT level abnormalities in SIDS cases and the fact that extrasynaptic 5-HT is deposited in the cerebrospinal fluid (CSF).[137] They measured 5-HT metabolites (5-hydroxy indoleacetic acid and homovanillic acid) in the CSF of 59 SIDS victims and 29 infants dying of other causes. There were no differences and they concluded that 5-HT metabolites measured in the CSF are not acceptable "forensic biomarkers" for SIDS. In a second study, they used a scoring system for potential asphyxial exposure at the time of death to separate their subjects into two primary groups.[138] They compared parameters of brainstem neurotransmitter function in 15 infants whose sudden and unexpected death was not thought to be asphyxia-related to 35 for whom asphyxia was at least implicated because of prone sleep on an unsafe sleep surface or sharing a sleep surface. Methods were those used by Kinney et al. between 1998 and 2008, and included autoradiography, high-performance liquid chromatography, and Western blots. Among other results, they quantified GABA receptor density, serotonin and its receptors, and a key protein regulating serotonin synthesis (14-3-3 isoform). The results from the two groups were not different in these four parameters, suggesting that the difference among SIDS victims in serotonergic network function is primary, and not an epiphenomenon of asphyxial exposure just before death.

In any event, it seems apparent, with respect to key receptor networks, that SIDS victims have the substrate for underlying susceptibilities that change with development. Taken together, these findings complete a triple-risk model (see Fig. 80.6) that might include exogenous stressors within the sleep environment.

FATTY ACID OXIDATION DEFICIENCIES AND THE CONTRIBUTION OF GENETIC DISEASES OF METABOLISM TO SUDDEN INFANT DEATH SYNDROME

The last two topics in our discussion of new pathology do not primarily involve respiration. However, a pulmonologist dealing with the sudden death of an infant will need a working familiarity with them.

Under the wide umbrella of SIDS and related causes of death, there has been much interest in heritable diseases affecting energy metabolism.[94] It is not clear whether the diseases are similar to SIDS in that they can be lethal in 2 hours or less in previously healthy infants, or whether the age of death from inherited metabolic disease overlaps classic SIDS ages (peak rate at 3 months, 95% of deaths by age 6 months).[139]

The epidemiologic features of sudden deaths due to inborn errors of energy metabolism are not well established. Furthermore, although techniques such as tandem mass spectroscopy can be used on neonatal blood spots to screen for many inborn errors, the ratios of false positive to true positive may be 8 : 1 or greater. It is unclear whether the public health resources exist to address with new parents the problems of false-positive tests, or unpredictable prognosis of many diseases.[140] Nevertheless, it is certain that some deaths once called SIDS, or attributed to parental neglect, can be explained by deranged energy metabolism. We will discuss two important examples.

During significant fasting, beta oxidation of fatty acids occurs in mitochondria to provide energy substrates as alternatives to dietary sources of energy. There are 11 proteins controlling the 20 steps leading to beta oxidation, and, ultimately, the tricarboxylic acid cycle and flavoprotein electron transport cycle.[141] Disorders may disrupt any step in the process, from substrate uptake to actual beta oxidation, and have their primary effects on the liver, the CNS, or the heart. The disorders are manifest during fasting, either very shortly after birth, or, in particular, associated with anorexia caused by a viral illness.

The most well-known defects are those causing pediatric cardiomyopathies. Newborns need the relevant enzyme, VLCAD (very long chain acyl-CoA dehydrogenase) to meet the extreme demands on their heart during the transition to extrauterine life. Infants with VLCAD deficiency may die suddenly but usually present in heart failure with a cardiomyopathy that is often familial and that responds to low-fat diets and avoidance of fasting.[142]

Altogether, recognized disorders of fatty acid beta oxidation are more common (1 : 10,000 live births) than phenylketonuria (1 : 15,000). The most common inborn error of beta oxidation is a deficiency in medium-chain acyl-CoA dehydrogenase (MCAD). After periods of inadequate oral intake, infants present with hypoglycemia, neonatal apnea, and, in as many as one-third of cases, sudden death.[143] However, their most frequent presentation is profound encephalopathy with cerebral edema, hypoketotic hypoglycemia, elevation of liver transaminases, and hyperammonemia. Because MCAD deficiency was not recognized until the early 1980s, it is probable, in retrospect, that some cases of Reye syndrome were crises occurring in children with MCAD deficiency.[141,144]

In a recent investigation of the potential importance of abnormalities of energy metabolism, tandem mass spectroscopy was performed on blood and bile samples from 410 autopsies on children dying suddenly and unexpectedly at younger than 1 year of age.[145] The autopsies were done at Great Ormond Street Hospital, between 1996 and 2009, and included autopsies done on behalf of the coroner. The authors concluded, reasonably, that about 2% of deaths had an underlying metabolic cause, a percentage consistent with earlier studies from the United States. The most common abnormalities based on acylcarnitine profiles were MCAD and VLCAD deficiencies.

Details about age at death, sleep practices, and prevalence of other SIDS risk factors have not been provided in the largest published series of infants with beta-oxidation defects, although there may be some age overlap with SIDS. Two of three infants with MCAD or VLCAD deficiencies from Oregon died within the first 48 hours of life, and two of three were sharing a bed when found dead.[146]

PROLONGED ELECTROCARDIOGRAM QT INTERVALS AND LETHAL CARDIAC ARRHYTHMIAS

Schwartz and coworkers in Italy have been the most consistent proponents of the theory that cardiac arrhythmias can be lethal in SIDS victims with normal cardiac autopsy results. Arguments against this theory were as difficult to envision as were even partial proofs in empirical, population-based studies. Nevertheless, by recording more than 33,000 electrocardiograms on days 3 or 4 of life, Schwartz and coworkers reported that the mean corrected QT (QT_C) interval was longer in the 24 infants eventually dying of SIDS (435 ± 45 vs. 400 ± 20 ms) than in survivors.[147] None of the thousands of survivors had QT_C intervals greater than 440 ms, but 12 of 24 SIDS victims did. The prolonged QT_C interval is believed to be fatal because of an associated malignant arrhythmia (torsade de pointes).

In 2001, Ackerman and coworkers showed that 2 of 93 infants diagnosed as SIDS in Arkansas had mutations causing cardiac sodium channel dysfunction, as compared with none of 400 controls.[148] The mutation in the SCN5A sodium channel they studied is estimated to cause up to 10% of cases of long QT_C interval syndrome.

A recent review summarized current understanding of the importance of "inheritable monogenic arrhythmia syndromes" as causes of sudden unexpected deaths in infancy.[149] The review considered children younger than 1 year and older than 1 year of age separately. The review asserted that Na^+ and K^+ channel malfunctions, and related channelopathies may have been present in as many as 14% of deaths called SIDS between 2006 and 2014. The authors suggest that fever, or overheating, may be the environmental triggers within the familiar Triple Risk Model context that proves lethal for an infant genetically vulnerable to fatal arrhythmias.

The theories of Schwartz and coworkers, and the findings of subsequent investigators now seem well established as causes for a percentage (~2%–5%) of deaths that might meet the criteria for SIDS. The impact of potent SIDS risk factors (e.g., prone sleep, maternal smoking) on the risk for lethal outcomes in infants who are homozygous, or even heterozygous for mutations in, for example, cardiac sodium channels, has not been calculated,[150] so it is not yet possible to use this information to understand how it fits into the classic epidemiology of sudden death in infancy.

Also, it is becoming less clear where the pathologic investigation of SIDS or other sudden unexpected infant deaths should stop,[94,151] as more causes for sudden death are discovered that were not known when SIDS was defined. Should molecular genetic mechanisms be pursued in all deaths? Alternatively, should they only be considered when there is a family history of SIDS, or only when sleep practices are not clearly implicated?[152,153] Or might, for example, exposure to hypoxia, described below and arising from the sleep environment, place infants with mutations causing channelopathies at even greater risk for lethal dysrhythmias, according to the Triple Risk Model?

THE USE OF INVESTIGATIONS OF THE SCENE AND CIRCUMSTANCES OF SUDDEN INFANT DEATH

One type of sudden unexpected death for which scene investigations have always been crucial is infanticide. The perceived importance of infanticide as a frequent cause of death has waxed and waned. Dramatic series of cases[88] remind us that infanticide, with or without antecedent Munchausen syndrome by proxy, cannot be ignored. Gross and, occasionally, microscopic autopsy findings are of obvious importance when diagnosing nonaccidental trauma as a cause of death;

however, it is less clear by autopsy how to prove intentional but subtle suffocation (e.g., using a pillow).[154] Southall and coworkers used covert video surveillance in the hospital to document that 30 of 39 very high-risk infants were subjected to intentional suffocation.[155] Twelve had siblings who had died suddenly and unexpectedly. Although bloody froth from the nose and mouth is common among SIDS victims, 11 of 38 subjects in Southall's study had a history of an ALTE associated with frank bleeding from the nose and mouth, compared with none of 46 controls.

Two studies compared the presence of alveolar hemosiderin-laden macrophages (AHLM) as evidence for pulmonary hemorrhage in cases of SIDS, suffocation,[156] and sudden unexpected infant deaths when nonaccidental injuries were suspected. AHLM were more likely to be present in deaths associated with direct or circumstantial evidence for nonaccidental injuries.[157] Nevertheless, in this study, two-thirds of infants with significant numbers of AHLM had no historical or postmortem evidence to suggest nonaccidental injury.

It seems probable that the percentage of sudden unexpected infant deaths that will be proven to be intentional will increase as the overall number of sudden deaths declines.[158] Before the Back-to-Sleep campaign in the United States, based on serial cross-checks of data from social and law enforcement agencies, it was estimated that about 5% of SIDS deaths were likely to be due to maltreatment.[159] Certainly, both multiple deaths within families after genetic causes have been ruled out, and simultaneous deaths of twins should raise cautious suspicion. Nevertheless, the best evidence suggests that foul play is unlikely in the vast majority of second-infant deaths within a family.

The addition of scene data and the appreciation of the potential for thermal stress and lethal rebreathing have led to diagnostic shifting: very similar deaths that had been called unexplained (SIDS) before death scene data became available are increasingly diagnosed as accidental suffocation or positional asphyxia, or undetermined.[106,160,161] This evolution in designation of manner and cause of death reflects the increase in information available to forensics teams. The prevalence of risks created within the sleep environment, especially for prone infants, is also more broadly realized.

Thus, it seems likely though still controversial that, compared to the early 1990s, fewer deaths will be designated as unexplained and SIDS, not because of arbitrary decisions, but because "previously unsuspected sleeping accidents are now being detected."[106]

PHYSIOLOGY RELATED TO THE SLEEP ENVIRONMENT THAT MAY MAKE INFANTS MORE VULNERABLE TO SIDS

Infants at increased risk for SIDS have been postulated and shown to have abnormal arousal, hypoxic drive, and airway protective reflexes, among other physiologic aberrations.[162,163] These abnormalities are reviewed below, and in light of the risk associated with prone sleep position.

Arousal and Prone Positioning

Arousal during sleep is defined as full awakenings with eyes opened, or as a change to a different sleep stage by electroencephalogram (EEG) criteria, or by a constellation of EEG, electromyographic, and airflow changes. Arousal may be cortical as evidenced by obvious changes in EEG frequency, or imputed (subcortical arousal) from changes in autonomic measurements (e.g., changes in heart rate) or suppression of EEG sleep spindles.[164,165] Arousal has been assessed experimentally in response to airway obstruction[165–167] and central apnea,[166] breathing hypercarbic[168] or hypoxic gas mixtures,[169] laryngeal stimulation with fluid,[15,170] sound,[171] and jets of air hitting the face.[172] Changes in sleep state or awakening "may produce a fundamental change in the nature of the ventilatory response to a respiratory stimulus."[170] Arousal is often associated with the termination of obstructive apnea[167] and is the probable cause, at some level, of sleep fragmentation leading to daytime sleepiness with obstructive sleep apnea.

Although arousal may be essential to ending some threats to ventilation during sleep (see Fig. 80.5) in infants, the reliability of arousal from sleep in interrupting threats to sleep in risky environments is uncertain. For example, infants dying beneath bedclothes have often pulled them over their face, or moved beneath them.[173] Although these infants died while unobserved, it is conceivable that they suffocated while awake and not asleep, and that arousal played little role, except possibly to cause the awakening that got them into trouble in the first place. It has also been shown that the normal arousal sequence after having the nose and mouth covered—sigh, startle, arm thrashing, head lift, and turn—can actually worsen the infant's predicament within the sleep microenvironment, by pulling bedclothes farther over the head or by placing the infant face down into soft bedding.[100,174]

Arousal deficits also do not appear to explain gender differences in susceptibility to SIDS. Male infants are at greater risk for dying suddenly and unexpectedly, but their arousal thresholds to air jets are the same as females at 2–3 months of age, and actually lower at 2–4 weeks.[175] Thus, a consistent finding when infants die suddenly and unexpectedly, male preponderance, seems not to be explained by deficient arousal but may be explained by too brisk arousal. In this regard, it should be pointed out that arousal may foster excessive ventilatory compensation for transient underventilation. An "increased loop gain" in response to airway obstruction has been shown to increase respiratory pattern instability, and sustain rather than interrupt obstructive events.[59,176,177] Finally, as discussed above, infants may gain access to fresh air and end the threat to effective ventilation by subtle head (nose and mouth) repositioning without apparent awakening or EEG changes.[178]

In any event, whether or not an infant arouses to compromised ventilation, and how much ventilation is improved, or further compromised, as a result of movements or changes in breathing pattern during an arousal, may together define a developmental vulnerability for specific infants exposed to threats within their sleep environment.

SOFT BEDDING AND LEARNED INFANT BEHAVIORS AS EFFECT MODIFIERS

Arousal and ventilatory responses to challenges may be less in prone than in supine sleeping infants. What gives rise to the "challenge" that must be responded to is suggested by studies of factors within the sleep environment that increase risk in the prone position. The epidemiologic findings and physiologic studies implicating rebreathing of exhaled air from near an infant's face have been spelled out in detail in the eighth edition of this text. It has been possible to show with mechanical and animal models and human infants that assuming the prone and face-down position on items of soft bedding can markedly increase CO_2 concentration and decrease O_2 concentration near the face of an infant so positioned.[103,109]

Waters and coworkers have also shown that this scenario occurs spontaneously.[100] In a study done using home recordings of SpO_2%, transcutaneous (PCO_2), respiratory effort, and videos, they showed that an infant sleeping prone, without adults present, assumed the face-down position on a mattress pad. Although the infant escaped this position, her $PtcCO_2$ rose from 50 to 87 mm Hg. The danger of such a scenario would be obvious for an otherwise healthy infant with blunted responses to hypoxemia or CO_2 concentration, or inefficient airway-protective behaviors.

It is also interesting to speculate about neurodevelopmental mechanisms for the very high risk of dying when infants who usually sleep supine are placed prone for the first time (see Fig. 80.5).[111] It is possible that infants who are usually placed prone learn to lift and turn their heads in order to gain access to fresh air. The cerebellum may have a role in learning this unconscious motor choreography. Some neurons in the cerebellum are known to respond to changes between real and anticipated sensory input and to modulate motor activity to respond to a changed environment with an unconscious change in motor activity.[116] Delayed cerebellar "motor learning" might be explained by brainstem findings implicating the medullary serotonergic system, which has multiple links to the cerebellum, including the inferior olivary nucleus.

In addition to preventing the ingress of fresh air, soft bedding, particularly comforters (duvets), provides much thermal insulation and has the potential to cause thermal stress.[179,180] What the mechanism or resultant cardiorespiratory abnormality due to thermal stress is, particularly beyond the first month of life, remains unknown. Infants do seem to be able to thermoregulate when exposed to environments that had been presumed to cause thermal stress,[120,121] and success with Back-to-Sleep occurred without reduction in thermal stress.[179,181,182] Furthermore, analysis of data from New Zealand, based on hypothetical models of SIDS infants' thermal environment, has shown that "Too little thermal insulation for the lower critical temperature was associated with an increased risk of SIDS..."[183]

BED SHARING AND RACIAL DISPARITIES

The epidemiologic evidence linking bed sharing to sudden unexpected infant death (SUID) is consistent and quite strong. Carpenter et al.[184] have outlined an argument for a causal association between bed sharing and SUID, using classic epidemiologic constructs.[185] The increased risk remains even when maternal smoking and alcohol use have been accounted for. Avoiding prone or side sleeping does not reduce SIDS risk when infants are bed sharing.[186,187] Higher rates of bed sharing and higher rates of SUID occur among both African Americans and Maori people from New Zealand. The most recent data from the United States National Infant Sleep Position Study, covering 1993–2000 and 2001–2010, show that the rates of bed sharing among white respondents increased during the earlier years but stayed the same for 2001–2010.[188] In contrast, rates of bed sharing among black and Hispanic respondents increased over both time periods. For whites, the rates rose from 4.9% in 1993 to 9.1% in 2010; for blacks, from 21.2% to 38.7%; and for Hispanics, from 12.5% to 20.5%. The impact of increased rates of bed sharing on the leveling off of the rates of all SUIDS is plausible but has not been quantified (see Fig. 80.7).

In a recent historical review based on over 60 years combined years of work on SIDS and SUID, Mitchell, from New Zealand, and Krous, from the United States, have concluded that the major risk factors for SUID are "maternal smoking and bed sharing and the major challenge is to implement effective strategies that will reduce the exposure to such risks as was done with prone sleeping position."[189]

In this regard, there are encouraging findings from New Zealand, where the decline in postneonatal mortality associated with nonprone sleeping had "plateaued" after 2000, as it had in the United States. A 2009 modification of their decades-old safe sleep program emphasized use among Maoris of a "wahakura, a bassinet-like portable infant Safe Sleeping Device, hand-woven from native flax that was designed to increase safety in the bed sharing environment," and, later, widespread use of a plastic infant sleeping surface (Pepi-Pod).[190] From 2009 through 2015, there was a 29% fall in postneonatal mortality in New Zealand that was most dramatic among the Maori people.

With respect to why babies die while bed sharing, in addition to increased risk for suffocation,[191] there is other evidence that might explain increased risk for sudden and unexpected death among infants sharing an adult bed. Careful studies of infants in their homes[120] comparing bed-sharing infants to those room sharing but in a separate crib ("cot") have shown that infants sharing a bed are exposed to an increased relative thermal stress, "requiring more vasodilatation to maintain core temperature." Baddock and colleagues also found that bed-sharing infants were more likely to sleep on their sides and less likely to be found supine, and much more likely to have their heads covered,[120,192] both factors that increase SIDS risk dramatically. Infants who bed shared also awoke more often. If they also had more spontaneous arousals, particularly with their heads covered, they might be more likely to experience the ventilatory instability discussed above, associated with desaturations and a dysfunctional arousal that did not gain access to fresh air.

Summary

It was estimated in 1967, that in industrialized countries, 25,000 infants per year died suddenly and unexpectedly.[97] Most children who died suddenly and unexpectedly then and now did not have pathologic findings to explain their demise and, after 1967, their deaths were diagnosed as SIDS.[193] A triple-risk model can be used to explore explanations for sudden death: infant susceptibility, developmental vulnerability, and exogenous stressors of varying magnitude. Abnormalities in ventilatory control or reflexes and in behavioral or minute volume responses can usually be implicated. These abnormalities may be nonlethal when most infants sleep supine on their own sleep surface. Newer approaches to the pathology of cardiorespiratory control, lethal inherited dysrhythmias and energy metabolism, and continued emphasis on safe sleeping practices should lead to further reductions in the number of infants dying suddenly and unexpectedly each year.[194,195]

Acknowledgments

The authors would like to acknowledge the substantial contribution to the science and understanding of sudden infant death syndrome provided by Dr. Bradley Thach, an author on previous versions of this chapter.

References

Access the reference list online at ExpertConsult.com.

Suggested Reading

Darnall RA, Ariagno RL, Kinney HC. The late preterm infant and the control of breathing, sleep, and brainstem development. *Clin Perinatol.* 2006;33:883–914.

Dwyer T, Ponsonby A-L. Sudden infant death syndrome and prone sleep position. *Ann Epidemiol.* 2009;19:245–249.

Kemp JS, Thach BT. Rebreathing of exhaled air. In: Byard RW, Krous HF, eds. *Sudden Infant Death Syndrome—Problems, Progress and Possibilities.* London: Arnold; 2001:138–155.

Kinney HC, Thach BT. The sudden infant death syndrome. *N Engl J Med.* 2009;361:795–805.

Poets CF. Apnea of prematurity: what can observational studies tell us about pathophysiology? *Sleep Medicine.* 2010;11:701–707.

Reix P, St. Hilaire M, Praud JP. Laryngeal sensitivity in the neonatal period: from bench to bedside. *Pediatr Pulmonol.* 2007;42:674–682.

Tester DJ, Ackerman MJ. Cardiomyopathic and channelopathic causes of sudden unexplained death in infants and children. *Annu Rev Med.* 2009;60:69–84.

Tieder JS, Bonkowsky JL, Etzel RA, et al. Clinical practice guideline: Brief Resolved Unexplained Events (Formerly Apparent Life-Threatening Events) and Evaluation of Lower-Risk Infants. *Pediatrics.* 2016;137(5):e20160590.

81 Disorders of Breathing During Sleep

DAVID GOZAL, MD, MBA, and LEILA KHEIRANDISH-GOZAL, MD, MSc

Basic Mechanisms and Architecture of Normal Sleep

NEURAL CIRCUITRY OF SLEEP AND WAKING

Sleep is a global and dynamically regulated life-sustaining state, the control mechanisms of which are manifested at every level of biologic organization, from genes and intracellular mechanisms to networks of cell populations, and to all central neuronal systems at the organismal level, including those that control movement, arousal, autonomic functions, behavior, and cognition.[1-4] In mammals, sleep states can be readily differentiated into two major types, namely rapid eye movement (REM) and nonrapid eye movement (NREM) sleep. These two distinctive sleep states are defined in terms of their electroencephalographic (EEG) and electromyographic (EMG) characteristics. NREM sleep involves high-voltage, low-frequency "synchronized" wave activity with relatively preserved skeletal muscle tonic activity, whereas REM sleep is characterized by wakelike high-frequency, low-amplitude "desynchronized" activity in the EEG along with a typical attenuation of skeletal muscle tonic activity (i.e., REM atonia). Bursts of 12- to 14-Hz sleep spindles are characteristic of NREM sleep in adults and children, although such bursts may also occur during REM sleep; maximal development of phasic spindle activity emerges after approximately 16 weeks postnatally.

The neural sites underlying the onset, maintenance, and function of NREM and REM sleep continue to be the object of intensive research; however, sufficient insights are now available to link certain breathing patterns with the neural properties and activity patterns of state-related regulatory structures. Areas within the basal forebrain, including regions within the preoptic region, have long been implicated in initiating NREM sleep, with local stimulation eliciting the typical NREM sleep state and lesion studies resulting in pronounced loss of sleep. Single-cell studies assessing the discharge patterns of neurons within these neural regions conclusively demonstrate the existence of neurons that selectively fire with the onset of NREM sleep in this area. Certain features of NREM sleep, such as the large synchronous slow waves (delta waves) and bursts of 12- to 14-Hz sleep spindles, are critically dependent on the integrity of the thalamocortical circuitry, even if these characteristic neural activity patterns can be generated under certain pharmacologic conditions, such as subsequent to atropine administration during waking states. Furthermore, recent work has implicated adenosine and its cognate receptors as an important mechanism of NREM sleep regulation, such that this neurotransmitter is currently believed to regulate metabolic and recovery aspects of NREM sleep within the basal forebrain and thalamocortical regions.[5,6] It should also be stressed that thermoregulatory areas of the anterior hypothalamus closely interact with sleep-associated regions in the brain and dictate the generation of close relationships between warming, discharge of thermoregulatory neurons, and induction of sleep. Indeed, higher temperatures, whether externally applied or through localized warming of hypothalamic structures, will lead to increased sleepiness and NREM sleep duration.

Since the principal physiologic characteristics of REM sleep persist even after separation of the forebrain from the pons, it has been suggested that mechanisms underlying this unique sleep state lie caudal to the diencephalon within specific and spatially restricted brain stem regions such as the locus coeruleus and several pontine nuclei; notably, areas within the dorsal lateral pons have been particularly implicated in eliciting some of the characteristics of REM sleep state. For example, the atonia of REM sleep can be abolished by lesions in the dorsal pons, ventral to the locus coeruleus, and phasic somatic events can be terminated by lesions in the pedunculopontine tegmentum. Certain phasic elements, such as the variation of sympathetic and parasympathetic outflow during REM sleep, are dependent on the integrity of vestibular nuclei, while phasic eye movements, a hallmark of REM sleep, will persist even in the presence of lesions in the vestibular sites. A number of brain stem regions, namely the dorsal and caudal raphe, locus coeruleus, and ventral medullary surface, show declines in neural activity during REM sleep[7,8]; however, most of the brain will manifest substantial increases in neural cell activity and glucose consumption during REM sleep, sometimes exceeding levels seen during wakefulness. Brain regions that decrease their discharge patterns during REM sleep play important roles in blood pressure regulation; however, it is unclear whether the state-related cell patterns in these regions bear a relationship to blood pressure control (and indirectly to breathing patterns) during REM sleep.

Developmental Aspects of Sleep

Sleep state organization undergoes rapid development during the first 6 months of life.[9,10] Neonates and young infants spend a disproportionate amount of time in REM sleep; indeed infants exhibit REM sleep at sleep onset, an event that is considered abnormal in the adult. NREM sleep (also termed quiet sleep) is poorly developed in newborns, since the slow oscillatory EEG patterns that define this state are not as readily apparent during early postnatal life and may manifest as intermittent slow and faster EEG patterns (e.g., tracé alternans). However, the relative amount of quiet sleep increases over the first 3 months of life, with K-complexes and sleep spindles becoming increasingly evident. Therefore scoring of sleep using adult criteria is not applicable before 3–6 months of age, and a more simplistic categorization of sleep states into awake, quiet sleep, active sleep (equivalent to REM sleep), and indeterminate sleep is usually used during the first year of life.[11-17] The total duration of sleep decreases relative to the 24-hour period, the relative proportion of NREM sleep increases, and that of REM sleep decreases with advancing age. At the age of 1 year, children will typically require 12–13 hours of sleep, primarily during the night, with one or two naps during the day.[18,19] At this age, well-defined NREM sleep alternates with REM sleep, the latter accounting for 30% of total sleep time in recurring 90-minute cycles very similar to those found in the adult. At approximately 2 years of age, the relative proportion of REM sleep will stabilize at approximately 20%–25% of total sleep time and will remain somewhat constant until old age, despite gradual reductions in total sleep duration with advancing age. NREM sleep acquires its maximal expression in duration and depth during the first decade of life. Indeed, the depth of sleep in childhood is quite remarkable considering how difficult it is to arouse a child during the first cycle of slow-wave sleep. During the second decade of life, slow-wave sleep gradually decreases by approximately 40%, continuing its gradual decline until old age. It is during slow-wave sleep that growth hormone is secreted in large amounts, and thus either sleep deprivation or disorders of sleep may interfere with the secretion and regulation of growth hormone, with potential and rather immediate clinical consequences.[20]

Respiratory Control Mechanisms

Our understanding of respiratory control has undergone multiple evolutionary waves in the last century. Obviously, breathing is an important and vital function. Nevertheless, despite the critical functions of respiration, it is undeniable that the respiratory control system undergoes substantial maturation during the first few years of life. There is no doubt that the relative uncertainty about the anatomic and functional aspects pertaining to the neural respiratory pathways, the complexities of neuronal firing activities, the multitude of neurotransmitters within each brain stem nucleus, and the frequently nucleus-dependent opposing roles played by these neurotransmitters in respiratory function can be quite overwhelming and difficult to comprehend. Despite such problems, the field of respiratory control has evolved tremendously in recent years, and we are now witnessing the initial discovery of several of the genes that control the development and maturation of multiple neurally controlled respiratory functions.[21]

THE RESPIRATORY RHYTHM GENERATOR

The putative neural center responsible for generation of respiratory rhythmic activity has now been identified,[22] and specific markers such as neurokinin and opioid receptors in these neurons have yielded estimates that this uniquely important neural center is a cluster of 150–200 neurons in the brain stem region designated as Pre-Botzinger complex.[23] This small number of rhythmically firing neurons appears both necessary and sufficient to generate most of the complex

normal respiratory behaviors that we know such as eupnea, sigh, and gasping.[24-26] The development of several elegant models ranging from highly reductionistic (brain stem slice) to less reductionistic approaches (whole brain stem–heart-lung preparation) will undoubtedly permit extensive characterization of the network configuration responses, the functional neurotransmitters involved in generation of respiratory rhythm, and permit a thorough understanding of the electrophysiologic properties of these unique cells both during development as well as during disease. Several genes, such as PHOX2A, HOX paralogs, and HOX-regulating genes MAFB (formerly "Kreisler [mouse] maf-related leucine zipper homolog") and EGR2 (formerly Krox20), have been identified as important players in the embryonic generation of respiratory centers and their intrinsic connectivities.[27,28] These and other yet unknown genes that regulate the ontogeny of brain stem development may provide initial insights into the regulation of the initial phases involved in the normal and abnormal formation of the respiratory network.

SLEEP AND BREATHING DURING DEVELOPMENT

The cyclic activity of respiratory rhythm generation is further modulated by suprapontine sites that include important efferent projections to areas mediating the sleep-wake cycle, thermoregulation, and circadian rhythm rhythmicity. Respiratory control areas also receive afferent inputs from central and peripheral chemoreceptors and from other receptors within the respiratory pump (upper airways, chest wall, and lungs). During fetal life, breathing is discontinuous and coincides with REM-like sleep. After birth, respiratory rhythm is established as a continuous activity to maintain cellular O_2 and CO_2 homeostasis. Respiratory pattern instability during sleep is typically present during early life such that short apneic episodes lasting less than 5 seconds are extremely common in preterm neonates, and their frequency is reduced in full-term newborns. These episodes occur predominantly during REM sleep as a result of the greater respiratory instability in this state. Several developmental differences between the neonate and the adult respiratory systems may further account for the emergence of sleep-associated disruption of normal gas exchange in early postnatal life, and include the following:

- Neonates have greater difficulty switching from the nasal to the oral route of breathing, and the majority of younger neonates can be considered as obligatory or near-obligatory nasal breathers.
- In neonates, reflexes originating in the upper airway (laryngeal chemoreflex) are potentiated and can induce profound apnea and bradycardia. This respiratory depressant component of the laryngeal chemoreflex decreases with maturation, such that prolonged apnea induced by stimulation of the laryngeal chemoreflex is more prominent in preterm than in full-term neonates.[29]
- The chest wall compliance is increased in neonates, thereby requiring dynamic, rather than passive, maintenance of the functional residual capacity of the lungs. Furthermore, neonates have "barrel-shaped" rib cages, and the rib cage contribution to tidal breathing is smaller than in older children and adults. Thus, any condition whereby the ability

to maintain functional residual capacity is compromised, as in REM sleep, will lead to increased susceptibility.

- Paradoxical breathing (i.e., asynchronous or out-of-phase motion of the chest and abdomen), especially during REM sleep, is common in newborns because of uncoordinated interactions between chest and abdominal respiratory musculature. The duration of paradoxical breathing during sleep decreases as postnatal age increases. Paradoxical breathing is rare or absent after 3 years of age.[30]

- The respiratory rate is high in the neonatal period and decreases during infancy and early childhood. Respiratory rate decreases exponentially with increasing body weight and parallels changes in overall metabolic rates. Notably, respiratory rate is higher during REM sleep than it is in NREM sleep.

- Apneas of short duration (less than 10 seconds) are extremely common during the early period of life. Apneic episodes are more frequent in REM sleep than during NREM sleep. Apneic episodes are mostly central and will decrease in number with advancing postnatal age. Obstructive and mixed apneic episodes are more frequently seen in preterm than in full-term neonates, possibly reflecting developmental changes in pharyngeal, laryngeal, and central airway collapsibility.

- Periodic breathing, defined as three episodes of apnea lasting longer than 3 seconds and separated by continued respiration over a period of 20 seconds or less, is a common respiratory pattern in preterm neonates, and may also be highly prevalent in full-term newborns.[31,32] However, periodic breathing decreases in frequency during the first year of life and is usually not considered to be of any specific pathologic significance. Notwithstanding such considerations, environmental variables such as sleep state transitions, arousals, hypoxia, and hyperthermia can enhance the frequency and magnitude of periodic breathing in newborns, and ultimately lead to destabilization of cardiorespiratory homeostasis.

- Apneic episodes during sleep in neonates are associated with a fall in heart rate, particularly during NREM sleep. The presence of hypoxemia will enhance this reflex bradycardia during apnea.

- Arousal from sleep is thought to be a major determinant for termination of apnea, and therefore arousal deficits have been implicated in the pathophysiology of the sudden infant death syndrome (SIDS). However, fewer than 10% of apneic episodes will be terminated by a full-fledged EEG arousal in neonates. Autonomic arousals are nevertheless quite frequent during the period surrounding the termination of an apneic event. Moreover, while hypercapnia is a potent stimulus of arousal, hypoxia, and particularly rapidly developing hypoxia, is much less effective in inducing arousal. Finally, prone position, sleep deprivation, and prenatal-postnatal exposure to cigarette smoking are all accompanied by decreased arousability in neonates.

- Healthy full-term newborns will usually maintain oxyhemoglobin saturation values of 92%–100% during sleep in the first 4 weeks of life. Arterial blood O_2 levels are lowest during the first week of life and increase over the next 1–3 months, such that all newborns will have values of 97%–100% after the age of 2 months. Basal values for arterial CO_2 tension during sleep are generally between 36 and 42 mm Hg in newborns and infants.

As delineated earlier, the implications of REM sleep on breathing are substantial, and as discussed later, the loss of muscle tone during REM sleep is particularly important to the upper airway muscles and airway patency. An important aspect of breathing control is the close interaction of breathing and blood pressure regulation. The respiratory system, using primarily somatic musculature, exerts substantial influence on moment-to-moment blood pressure; conversely, transient elevation of blood pressure can inhibit breathing efforts, while lowering of blood pressure can increase them. The interactions between the systems can be observed readily in breathing influences on heart rate (a classic example being respiratory sinus arrhythmia). Inspiratory efforts normally are associated with accelerated heart rate and expiratory efforts with deceleration, the result of reflex activity from pulmonary afferents and vagal outflow; the resulting coupling between breathing and heart rate is particularly prominent during NREM sleep, and measures of the interaction can provide a useful indication of state.[33] In addition, phasic activity during REM sleep induces substantial parasympathetic and sympathetic outflow, resulting in larger but typically slower variation in heart rate. Plots of cardiac beat-to-beat intervals demonstrate the substantial influences exerted normally during each state, with NREM sleep exerting a highly cyclic effect on heart-rate variation and REM sleep showing less modulation by breathing but larger slower sources of variation. Waking shows a large variation in heart-rate changes; typically very active periods are accompanied by high heart rates with little variation. The cyclic nature of cardiac rate variation has led to a variety of procedures to measure the sympathetic and parasympathetic influences. Particular syndromes exert unique patterns of respiration-related variation; for example, children with congenital central hypoventilation syndrome (CCHS) show a relative absence of variation of respiratory modulation of heart rate, and infants who later succumb to SIDS also show reduced variation to breathing.

CENTRAL CHEMORECEPTORS AND THEIR DEVELOPMENT

The chemoreflexes exert powerful influences over breathing as well as cardiac and vascular control. Chemoreflex physiology is complex, and the exact molecular mechanisms by which the chemoreflexes are activated remain unclear. The traditional and classic theory formulated during the late 1950s proposed that the central chemoreceptors were located in the ventrolateral medullary surface of the brain stem and responded to hypercapnia and pH changes, whereas the peripheral chemoreceptors were located in the carotid bodies and primarily responded to changes in blood O_2 tension. While this concept has now evolved (see later), it is worthwhile to mention that hypercapnia (particularly transient changes in CO_2 tension above the apneic threshold) can also activate the peripheral chemoreceptors, and may account for as much as one-third of peripheral chemoreceptor activity. Activation of either central or peripheral chemoreflexes exerts powerful effects on sympathetic activity in both health and disease and may be an important contributor to pathophysiology of obstructive sleep apnea (OSA)-induced morbidities.

Multiplicity of Central Chemosensitive Centers

A critically important advance in the field of respiratory control involved discarding the classic concept of central chemosensitive sites as being located in restricted areas of the ventral medullary surface. Indeed, several lines of evidence have now clearly established that neurons showing intrinsic chemosensitive properties (i.e., the ability to sense changes in extracellular pH and contribute to the ventilatory response) are diffusely located in the central nervous system, and that regions such as the posterior hypothalamus, cerebellum, locus coeruleus, raphé, and multiple nuclei within the brain stem all contribute to the well-characterized hypercapnic ventilatory response.[34–36] Why is this important? One reason is that the phenotypic manifestations of conditions such as central alveolar hypoventilation, particularly when occurring secondary to other disorders (e.g., myelomeningocele, tumors, stroke) are not adequately explained by either the location or the magnitude of the brain lesions in these patients. Second, it is very possible that the normal developmental processes of the ventilatory response to elevations of CO_2 are not only important to long-term stability of the homeostatic system but may be even more important to the preservation of respiratory stability during respiratory transients, particularly during sleep. Conditions such as apparent life-threatening events or even SIDS may originate from dysfunctional development of either the respiratory rhythm controllers or, alternatively, that of the neural networks underlying hypoxic and hypercapnic chemosensitivities as well as those mediating arousal from sleep.[37,38]

The neurotransmitters involved in the intrinsic sensory pathways associated with central chemoreception are currently incompletely defined, although serotoninergic pathways are clearly involved.[39–42] The presence of cholinergic muscarinic receptors in those brain stem areas traditionally associated with CO_2 chemosensitivity appears to play a major role in the neuronal excitation associated with the enhanced ventilatory response to hypercapnia, although additional neurotransmitters are also clearly involved. It must be emphasized that the central CO_2 chemosensory mechanisms may not be fully functional or mature at birth. Indeed, animal models in various species show that hypercapnic ventilatory responses will increase with advancing age. Hypercapnia elicits a relatively sustained ventilatory increase in term infants that is almost entirely due to an increase in tidal volume without consistent change in respiratory frequency. In contrast, the ventilatory response to hypercapnia in premature infants is attenuated and can even become inhibitory at higher concentrations of inhaled CO_2, with CO_2 overall respiratory responses increasing with postconceptional age. In preterm neonates, the ventilatory increase to hypercapnia is accompanied by a progressive increase in expiratory duration and a consequent reduction in frequency over time, both of which appear to be associated with diaphragmatic recruitment during expiration (respiratory braking or grunting). This unique mechanism appears to preserve a high-end expiratory lung volume such as to optimize gas exchange and promote respiratory stability. Little is known about the development of central chemoreceptor function beyond infancy. In awake prepubertal children there appears to be an enhanced ventilatory response to hypercapnia compared with adults, and these differences may underlie differences in metabolic rate.[43] Similarly, significant developmental differences in CO_2 responses emerge when the CO_2 stimulus is presented in either a step (sudden increase) or ramp (slow progressive increase) fashion.[44] These findings in older children suggest that at some time during transition from infancy to childhood and on to adulthood, major changes occur in the relative contributions and integration of peripheral and central chemoreceptor activity. The cascades of genes, receptors, and neurotransmitters that mediate these developmental changes are unknown at the present time. Similarly, the elements involved in the integrated coordination of the developmental changes at the level of the carotid body, neural transmission, or central nervous system remain unclear.

PERIPHERAL CHEMOREFLEXES

The ventilatory responses related to changes in blood O_2 levels are a complex interaction of a variety of peripheral and central responses. Nevertheless, the rapidity of the peripheral chemoreceptor responses to blood oxygenation changes allows for assessment of the initial stimulatory effect elicited by activation of these peripherally located chemosensory cells, of which the most important are glomus cells within the carotid bodies.[45] Peripheral chemoreceptor activity is typically assessed by monitoring the fast transient increase in minute ventilation after inhalation of gases containing low concentrations of O_2. Isocapnic hypoxic responses (over a period of 2–3 minutes) or five tidal breaths of pure N_2 are among the strategies that have been used.[46–48] Alternatively, the ventilatory decline subsequent to inhalation of 100% O_2 is also considered as a reliable indicator of peripheral chemoreceptor gain (Dejours test). However, it is important to indicate that the ventilatory decrease to acute hyperoxia is ultimately followed by an increase in ventilation that is centrally mediated.[49] More sophisticated paradigms using random alternations of N_2 and O_2 in a computerized setting have recently permitted the development of reproducible and consistent findings in infants and children suspected to be at risk for chemoreceptor dysfunction.[50–53] Independent of the test selected, substantial attention to sleep state is required when assessing respiratory chemoreceptor drive in infants and in the interpretation of such tests, so these tests are best reserved for specialized laboratories, in which specific normative values have been developed, and therefore allow for more reliable clinical assessment of individual patients presenting with symptoms suggestive of chemosensory dysfunction.

A typical phenomenon associated with more sustained exposure to hypoxic gas mixtures is the emergence of a relative ventilatory decline after 5–6 minutes of hypoxic exposure. This hypoxic ventilatory decline has also been termed hypoxic ventilatory roll-off. The phenomenon is particularly prominent during infancy, such that with sustained hypoxia in neonates there is a well-characterized increase in breathing followed by a reduction in ventilation that will usually reach levels below normoxic breathing. In more mature children and in adults, the reduction in ventilation will usually reach levels that are below peak but still higher than the ventilation measured during baseline, room-air breathing. A study of premature neonates showed that this biphasic response will persist into the second month of postnatal life, but this only represented a postconceptional age of about 35 weeks.[54]

Even term neonates may retain the biphasic response for at least 2 months when tested with normal bedding at room temperature of 24°C during NREM sleep. In addition, very small preterm neonates may show only a decrease in ventilation with hypoxia. The apparent differences between preterm and term neonates may be partially accounted for by developmental status in relation to postnatal age; indeed, premature but not term lambs or piglets also exhibit an attenuated hypercapnic response. Thus, prematurity and factors delaying normal maturation emerge as important contributors to the attenuated hypercapnic and hypoxic responses in newborns.

Studies suggest that a relatively high ventilatory drive exists during wakefulness in children, and that this drive decreases during adolescence and stabilizes during adulthood; the reason for this transition is currently unknown. Marcus and colleagues[43] studied hypercapnic and hypoxic ventilatory responses in a group of subjects aged 4–49 years and found significant correlations between both the awake hypercapnic and hypoxic ventilatory responses when corrected for age and body size.

The Upper Airway

UPPER AIRWAY CONTROL

Since both snoring and OSA are opposite ends of a spectrum of increased upper airway resistance, it is important to review the anatomic and physiologic mechanisms that underlie the maintenance of upper airway patency during sleep.[55] The upper airway comprises the nose, pharynx, larynx, and extrathoracic trachea, and is designed for vocalization, ingestion, airway protection, and respiration. Maintenance of a rigid and patent upper airway is mandatory for achieving adequate respiration and is the result of a balance between forces that promote airway closure and dilatation. Thus, the inherent collapsibility of the pharynx predisposes to impaired respiration when the regulation of the pharyngeal muscles is impaired, such as may occur during sleep.

Anatomically, it is clear that a smaller cross-sectional area of the upper airway is associated with decreased ability to maintain upper-airway patency, and in adults the upper airway behaves as predicted by the Starling resistor model, a model that has been well-characterized in biologic systems. This model describes the major determinants of airflow in terms of the mechanical properties of collapsible tubes and predicts that, under conditions of flow limitation, maximal inspiratory flow will be determined by the pressure changes upstream (nasal) to a collapsible site of the upper airway, and flow will be independent of downstream (tracheal) pressure generated by the diaphragm. Collapse occurs when the pressure surrounding the collapsible segment of the upper airway becomes greater than the pressure within the collapsible segment of the airway. Pressures at which collapse of the airway occurs have been termed critical closing pressure (P_{crit}).[56,57] In normal subjects with low upstream resistance, pressures downstream never approach P_{crit} and airflow is not limited. This model explains why snoring and obstructive apnea worsen during a common cold (increased nasal upstream resistance). Marcus and colleagues[58] further demonstrated the validity of this model in children and found

that the upper airway collapsibility in children is reduced compared with the adult. Notably, and as predicted by the Starling model, the collapsible segment of the upper airway in children displayed less negative (higher and thus more collapsible) pressures in children with OSA. It follows that components that affect the upstream segment pressures or increase P_{crit} will be of major consequence to the ability to maintain airway patency. Generally speaking, the smaller the cross-sectional area of the upper airway, the higher the upper airway collapsibility will be, because the upper airway behaves as a collapsible tube, such that increased inspiratory efforts may induce enhanced collapse of the airway rather than generate the desired increases in inspiratory flow.[58] Accordingly, it is not surprising that both snoring and obstructive apnea may worsen during a common cold (i.e., increased nasal upstream resistance), which provokes more inspiratory effort. In addition, tube law dictates that the longer the airway is, the more collapsible it is.[59,60] The contribution of the various anatomic nasopharyngeal structures to P_{crit} and the interactions between these structures that will lead to upper airway patency or obstruction during sleep are thus of clear importance in increasing our understanding of the pathophysiology of childhood OSA.

Although the overall ventilatory drive appears to be normal in children with OSA, it is possible that central augmentation of upper airway neuromotor function is abnormal. During sleep, upper airway tone is diminished even though the same structural factors are present during wake and sleep, and OSA occurs only during sleep. It is unknown whether children with OSA become obstructed because of a relatively larger decrease in airway tone during sleep in comparison to controls, or whether the decrease in tone is similar but subjects with OSA have an increased structural load. The upper airway muscles are accessory muscles of respiration and, as such, are activated by stimuli such as hypoxemia, hypercapnia, and upper airway subatmospheric pressure. Previous studies have shown that, when upper airway muscle function is decreased or absent, as in postmortem preparations, the airway is prone to collapse.[61] Conversely, stimulation of the upper airway muscles with hypercapnia[62,63] or electrical stimulation[64] results in decreased collapsibility. These studies confirm that the tendency of the upper airway to collapse is inversely related to the level of activity of the upper airway dilator muscles. Therefore increased upper airway neuromotor tone may be one way that patients can compensate for a narrow upper airway. Indeed, this has been shown in adults. Mezzanotte and colleagues demonstrated that adult patients with OSA compensated for their narrow upper airway during wakefulness by increasing their upper airway muscle tone.[65] This compensatory mechanism was lost during sleep.[66] Recent studies in children have shown that children with OSA have greater genioglossal EMG activity during the awake state than control children and a greater decline in EMG activity during sleep onset.[66] Furthermore, upper airway dynamic responses are decreased in children with OSA but appear to recover after treatment.[67,68] Thus, pharyngeal airway neuromotor responses are present in normal children and serve as a compensatory response for a relatively narrow upper airway compared with adults. However, this compensatory neuromotor response is reduced or even lacking in children with OSA, probably as a result of habituation to chronic respiratory abnormalities during sleep, mechanical damage to the upper airway, or genetically determined differences in these upper airway protective reflexes.[69-72]

Ventilatory control in patients with OSA is the subject of intense study. In adults with OSA, it is suggested that there is a high-gain ventilatory control system that results in ventilatory instability and apnea.[73] However, studies in children have shown overall normal ventilatory responses to hypoxia and hypercapnia during wakefulness and during sleep when using standard tests.[43,44,74] Indeed, ventilatory responses to rebreathing hyperoxic hypercapnia were measured in 20 children and adolescents with OSA, and the mean slopes of the hypercapnic response were similar to those measured in age- and sex-matched controls.[75] Furthermore, no differences were found in the slopes calculated from plotting minute ventilation against O_2 saturation during isocapnic hypoxia. Nevertheless, other investigators have found some degree of blunting in central chemosensitivity of children with OSA undergoing surgery.[76,77] Despite such findings, central chemosensitivity during sleep was similar in children with OSA and matched controls. However, arousal to acutely induced hypercapnia was blunted during sleep in children with OSA, suggesting that subtle alterations in the central chemosensitive-arousal network have occurred in these patients. These subtle changes have been further substantiated by examination of the ventilatory responses to repetitive hypercapnic challenges during wakefulness, whereby reciprocal changes in respiratory frequency and tidal volume do occur.[78] In the study by Gozal and colleagues,[79] repeated CO_2 challenges were given in the early morning to children with OSA who were hypercapnic (as a result of obstructive alveolar hypoventilation) during sleep. These children showed a respiratory response to the CO_2 challenge but did not show the same adaptive changes in respiratory pattern that would be anticipated over the course of several CO_2 challenges as elicited from children without OSA. However, when children with OSA were studied later in the day (i.e., a few hours after awakening and resolution of sleep-associated alveolar hypoventilation) or after treatment of OSA, a similar respiratory pattern to that seen in controls emerged, suggesting that such deficits may be related to habituation to nocturnal episodic hypercapnia. Additional evidence in support of this comes from Marcus and colleagues,[43] who found an inverse correlation between the duration of hypercapnia during the night and the awake hypercapnic ventilatory responses. In addition, children with OSA demonstrate impaired arousal responses to inspiratory loads during REM and non-REM sleep compared with control children.[61] This arousal threshold was particularly high during REM sleep, a time when most obstructive apneic events occur, and suggests that neuromotor influences play a key role. The absence or delayed arousal in children during an obstructive respiratory event and the presumed lack of ventilatory compensation to upper airway loading may contribute to the development of the prolonged periods of obstructive alveolar hypoventilation that uniquely characterize OSA in children. Furthermore, diminished laryngeal reflexes to mechanoreceptor and chemoreceptor stimulation with reduced afferent inputs into central neural regions underlying inspiratory inputs could be present. For example, chemoreceptor stimuli such as increased $Paco_2$ or decreased Pao_2 stimulate the airway dilating muscles in a preferential mode; that is, upper airway musculature is more stimulated than the diaphragm.[80,81] This preferential recruitment tends to correct an imbalance of forces acting on the airway and therefore maintain airway patency. Similarly, stimuli resulting from suction pressures in the nose, pharynx, or larynx rapidly stimulate the activity of upper airway dilators, and this effect is also preferential to the upper airway, causing some degree of diaphragmatic inhibition and thus compensating for increase in upstream resistance. The function of these upper airway receptors in children with adenotonsillar hypertrophy with and without OSA is currently unknown.

While dynamic factors such as those just discussed have been implicated in the pathophysiology of upper airway obstruction during sleep in children, we should not omit the contribution of either anatomic elements or genetic factors to this complex equation. In otherwise normal children, Arens and colleagues have shown that the mandibular dimensions of children with OSA are similar to those of controls.[82] However, regional analysis of the upper airway using magnetic resonance imaging techniques further suggested that the upper airway in children with OSA is most restricted where adenoids and tonsils overlap. Furthermore, the upper airway is narrowed throughout the initial two-thirds of its length in pediatric patients with OSA, and this narrowing is not in a discrete region adjacent to either the adenoids or tonsils, but rather emerges in a continuous fashion along both lymphadenoid structures.[83,84] It should be emphasized that, contrary to the previous conceptual framework whereby the higher prevalence of OSA in children during the age period from 2 to 8 years was attributed to the increased growth rate of lymphadenoid tissue within the upper airway compared with other upper airway structures,[85,86] recent evidence refutes this concept. It shows that all tissues within the upper airway including adenoids and tonsils grow proportionally and thus that stimuli leading to enhanced proliferation of lymphadenoid tissues within the airway are probably implicated in the pathophysiology of OSA.[87,88] In fact, recent evidence has further indicated that the extent of lymphadenoid proliferation is not confined to the adenoids and tonsils, and in fact encompasses the full length of the upper airway including the nose and sinuses, suggesting that OSA is a diffuse disease of the upper airway.[89] Recent exploration of upper airway characteristics in obese children provided further confirmation on the integrated roles of the upper airway structures and their estimated contributions to the upper airway flow characteristics, thereby enabling prediction of risk for OSA when applying computational fluid dynamic approaches to MRI or CT images of the airways.[90-94]

Upper Airway Dysfunction

In infancy, abnormalities that reduce the patency of the upper airway are frequently associated with OSA. The upper airway has decreased muscle tone, there is high nasal resistance, and the chest wall is highly compliant. The exact prevalence of OSA in infants is not well documented, since most epidemiologic studies have thus far concentrated on older children. However, OSA has been shown to occur in as many as 10% of infants, is more frequent in preterm infants, and is associated with hypoxemia. OSA may occur more frequently in male infants than in females, and this may be attributable to sex-related differences in the anatomy of the upper airway than to a protective role of female hormones.[95] The main risk factors for OSA in this age group include: (1) craniofacial abnormalities (e.g., micrognathia, cleft palate, Pierre Robin syndrome, Treacher Collins syndrome, choanal atresia, muco-polysaccharidoses, Down syndrome); (2) soft tissue infiltration, which may result from infection, inflammation, laryngomalacia, subglottic stenosis, and adenotonsillar hypertrophy. Indeed, adenotonsillar hyperplasia or hypertrophy has been found to contribute significantly to the generation of OSA in infants younger than 1 year old[96,97]; (3) neurologic disorders that induce pharyngeal hypotonia, such as Arnold-Chiari malformation, cerebral palsy, and poliomyelitis, are also associated with an increased risk for obstructed breathing. Although the anatomic site of obstruction in infants is widely believed to be the retroglossal region,[98] evidence using magnetic resonance imaging and airway manometry suggests that upper airway obstruction with clinically significant OSA occurs in the retropalatal region 80% of the time and only 20% of the time in the retroglossal region.[99] Other influences may alter breathing characteristics and predispose infants to OSA, including upper airway reflexes such as the laryngeal chemoreflex. This unique defense reflex that aims to prevent aspiration of food is enhanced by upper airway infection, and indeed, respiratory syncytial virus infection, which potentiates the laryngeal chemoreflex, has also been shown to facilitate the occurrence of both central and obstructive apneic episodes.[100] Similarly, prenatal exposure to maternal smoking, which potentiates the laryngeal chemoreflex, also increases the frequency of OSA in infants.[101,102]

To determine the region of maximal airway narrowing in children with OSA, the static pressure/area relationships of the passive pharynx were endoscopically measured in 14 children with OSA and 13 normal children under general anesthesia with complete paralysis.[103,104] The minimum cross-sectional area was found to be at the level of the adenoid and the soft palate. Thus, children with OSA closed their airways at the level of enlarged tonsils and adenoids at low positive pressures, whereas normal children required sub-atmospheric pressures to induce upper airway closure. The cross-sectional area of the narrowest segment was significantly smaller in children with OSA, and particularly involved the retropalatal and retroglossal segments, such that it becomes clear that anatomic factors, both congenital and acquired, play a significant role in the pathogenesis of pediatric OSA.[105,106] For these reasons, use of endoscopic approaches is increasingly being adopted in the clinical evaluation of OSA or residual OSA after treatment.[107-110] Furthermore, as mentioned earlier, airway narrowing in children with OSA occurs along the upper two-thirds of the airway and is maximal where the adenoids and tonsils overlap.[83,111]

In summary, several potential mechanisms have been identified in the maintenance of upper airway patency during sleep and wakefulness. Each of these mechanisms or a combination thereof probably plays a role in the causation of respiratory compromise in the normal child during sleep and in children with clinical problems that predispose to OSA. A systematic approach to identification and modification of these mechanisms should lead to improved therapeutic approaches and reduction of unnecessary morbidities in these patients.

Apnea

CENTRAL APNEA OR HYPOVENTILATION SYNDROMES

Unrelated to upper airway obstruction, insufficient central respiratory drive can also be a cause of hypoventilation. The presence of a hypoventilation syndrome is suggested by the medical history as well as examination of the patient during wakefulness and sleep. All disorders that could explain the hypoventilation must be excluded, and to confirm the diagnosis, a polysomnographic evaluation, including measurements of tidal volume, should be conducted. The measurement of spontaneous resting tidal volumes and noninvasive blood gas values across all sleep states should be sufficient to establish the presence and severity of alveolar hypoventilation. The most important objective finding is the inability to increase respiratory frequency, tidal volume, or both, regardless of the severity of the progressive asphyxia that occurs.

Congenital Central Hypoventilation Syndrome

Central hypoventilation syndromes can be primary (congenital CHS [CCHS] and late-onset CHS) or secondary (Box 81.1). Primary CCHS is a relatively rare genetic disorder, yet it is being increasingly recognized around the world. It was originally described in 1970 by Mellins and colleagues[112] and is traditionally defined as the idiopathic failure of automatic control of breathing.[113,114] The classic presentation of CCHS is a life-threatening disorder primarily manifesting as sleep-associated respiratory insufficiency and markedly impaired ventilatory responses to hypercapnia and hypoxemia very shortly after birth.[115] Ventilation is most severely affected during quiet sleep, a state during which automatic neural control is predominant. Abnormal respiratory patterns also occur during active sleep and even during wakefulness, though to a milder degree. The spectrum of disease in CCHS cases is wide, ranging from relatively mild hypoventilation during quiet sleep with fairly good alveolar ventilation during wakefulness to complete apnea during sleep with severe hypoventilation when awake. Progress in the recognition and clinical management of CCHS patients has revealed the

---

Box 81.1   Causes of Central Hypoventilation in Children

Primary

- Congenital (CCHS/Ondine's curse)
- Late-onset CHS
- Idiopathic hypothalamic dysfunction
- Arnold-Chiari malformation

Secondary

- Trauma
- Infection
- Tumor
- Central nervous system infarct
- Asphyxia
- Increased intracranial pressure
- Metabolic

CCHS, Congenital central hypoventilation syndrome.

presence of broader structural and functional impairments of the autonomic nervous system.[116–118] In particular, Hirschsprung disease[116] and tumors of autonomic neural crest derivatives such as neuroblastoma, ganglioneuroblastoma, and ganglioneuroma[118,119] are noted in 20% and in 5%–10% of CCHS patients, respectively. Several major clinically relevant advances have undoubtedly advanced our understanding of the pathophysiology and treatment of CCHS: (1) the identification of the putative gene underlying CCHS; (2) the functional assessment of neural structures in patients with CCHS to provide insights into the respiratory and autonomic disturbances that characterize the syndrome[120]; (3) the successful transition of many patients to noninvasive ventilatory support; and (4) the publication of a consensus statement on the diagnosis and management of this condition.[121]

A genetic origin was originally hypothesized for CCHS because of (1) its manifestation in the newborn period; (2) published reports of familial recurrence of CCHS, including cases of monozygotic female twins, female siblings, and male-female half-siblings[122,123]; and (3) its association with Hirschsprung disease, an autosomal-recessive disorder of neural crest origin.[124] Furthermore, a genetic segregation analysis among families of 50 probands with CCHS also indicated that CCHS was consistent with familial transmission.[125] Importantly, vertical transmission of CCHS was also reported, and among infants born to women with CCHS without Hirschsprung disease.[126,127] The association of CCHS and Hirschsprung disease suggested that both disorders may be related to abnormal development or migration of the neural crest cells; indeed, mutations of genes (e.g., the RET proto-oncogene) that are involved in neural crest development and migration have been found in patients with Hirschsprung disease.[127–129] The putative gene, pairedlike homeobox 2B (PHOX2B), underlying CCHS was ultimately discovered in 2003 by Amiel and colleagues in France.[130] The PHOX2B gene mutation, consisting primarily of increased polyalanine expansions, manifests an autosomal-dominant mode of inheritance and de novo mutations at the first generation. This gene is critical for embryologic development of the autonomic nervous system, and Phox2b$^{-/-}$ mice die in utero with absent autonomic nervous system circuits, since neurons either fail to form or degenerate.[131–134] Furthermore, selective stimulation of Phox2b neurons in specific regions of the brainstem elicits the anticipated respiratory and cardiovascular responses,[135–137] and targeted disruption of Phox2b in brainstem neurons leads to alterations in Task2 potassium channels, which are believed to be the main effectors in central chemoception.[138] Accordingly, heterozygous mutations of PHOX2B may account for several combined or isolated disorders of autonomic nervous system development, namely late-onset CHS,[139] Hirschsprung disease,[140] and tumors of the sympathetic nervous system such as neuroblastoma.[141] The identification of PHOX2B mutations in most patients with CCHS is an important landmark in the pursuit of the pathophysiologic mechanisms of this condition. Furthermore, the finding of de novo PHOX2B polyalanine expansions in the majority of patients with CCHS along with improved delineation of other mutations allows for accurate genetic counseling in a disease with an unexpected autosomal-dominant mode of inheritance.[142] The prevalence of SIDS is high in CCHS families, suggesting that these two disorders

may share developmental breathing control abnormalities in a subset of SIDS cases.[143]

Taken together, the genetic data strongly suggest a diffuse alteration in autonomic nervous system function in patients with CCHS. This concept includes major disruption of multiple brain regions underlying autonomic functions, in particular those sites mediating respiratory, cardiovascular, and thermal regulation,[144] as evidenced from recent studies using functional magnetic resonance imaging.[145–151] Decreased heart rate beat-to-beat variability is consistently found in Holter recordings, and the circadian patterning of such variability further suggests an imbalance in sympathetic/parasympathetic regulation in patients with CCHS.[152–155] As additional testament to such an assumption, alterations in blood pressure regulation during simple daily maneuvers or during sleep further support the presence of predominantly vagal dysfunction with signs of vagal withdrawal and baroreflex failure, and relative preservation of the cardiac and vascular sympathetic function.[156–158] In addition, the frequent neuro-ocular findings in children with CCHS[159] and the marked reduction in the size of arterial chemoreceptors, carotid bodies, and neuroepithelial bodies with decreased staining for tyrosine hydroxylase and serotonin[160] can all be construed as evidence for a more diffuse autonomic nervous system involvement. Putative models aiming to dissect the specific contributions of the various components of cardiorespiratory control have been recently proposed and provide a comprehensive and structured approach to the evaluation of patients with CCHS.[161]

Diagnosis and Clinical Management

The clinical presentation of CCHS varies greatly depending on the severity of the disorder. Some infants will not breathe at birth and will require assisted ventilation in the newborn nursery. Such infants may mature to a pattern of adequate breathing during wakefulness over time. However, apnea or hypoventilation will persist during sleep. The apparent improvement over the first few months of life most likely results from normal maturation of the respiratory system and does not represent a true change in the severity of the disorder.[162] Other infants may present at a later age with cyanosis, edema, and signs of right-sided heart failure and may be mistaken for patients with cyanotic congenital heart disease (Box 81.2). However, cardiac catheterization reveals only pulmonary hypertension. Infants with even less severe CCHS may present with tachycardia, diaphoresis, and/or cyanosis during sleep, and others may present with unexplained apnea or an apparent life-threatening event. Thus, the wide spectrum of severity in clinical manifestations determines the age at which recognition of CCHS takes place. Increased awareness of this unusual clinical entity and a comprehensive evaluation of every patient are critical for early diagnosis and appropriate intervention.

Although other symptoms indicative of brain stem or autonomic nervous system dysfunction may be present, the criteria for diagnosis of CCHS usually include: (1) persistent evidence of sleep hypoventilation (Paco$_2$ >60 mm Hg), particularly during quiet sleep (best achieved by overnight polysomnography); (2) presentation of symptoms during the first year of life; and (3) absence of cardiac, pulmonary, or neuromuscular dysfunction that could explain the hypoventilation.[121] Hypercapnic ventilatory challenges are an important

Box 81.2 Conditions Associated With Apnea in Infants

- Prematurity
- Infection
- Impaired oxygenation
- Central nervous system problems (intracranial hemorrhage, asphyxic episode, malformation of the brain)
- Gastroesophageal reflux
- Metabolic disorders (hypoglycemia, electrolyte imbalance, fatty acid disorders, metabolic acidosis)
- Temperature instability (hyperthermia, hypothermia)
- Drugs (e.g., narcotics, anticonvulsants)

component for the diagnosis of CCHS. Steady-state or rebreathing incremental CO_2 challenges are similarly valid and will usually reveal an absent or near-absent response.[163] Confounding issues, including asphyxia, infection, trauma, tumor, and infarction, must be distinguished from CCHS by appropriate assessments. Specific guidelines regarding the use of genetic testing for CCHS and other diagnostic considerations have now become available, and should be implemented.[121] Identification of mutations in genes such as RET, HASH, BDNF, GDNF, and the endothelin gene family may be helpful when the phenotype is atypical, but assessment of PHOX2B gene mutations in the context of clinical manifestations supporting central alveolar hypoventilation should be carried out to support the diagnosis of CCHS.[121,164,165]

Congenital CHS is a lifelong condition and, depending on the severity of clinical manifestations, patients may require ventilatory support while asleep or as much as 24 hours a day. As such, a multidisciplinary approach to provide for comprehensive care and support of the child is needed. The treatment of CCHS should aim to ensure adequate ventilation when the patient is unable to achieve adequate gas exchange while breathing spontaneously. Since CCHS does not resolve spontaneously, chronic ventilatory support is required, such as positive pressure ventilation, bilevel positive airway pressure, or negative pressure ventilation. The majority of children with CCHS use positive pressure ventilation through a permanent tracheotomy, although successful transition to noninvasive ventilation has now been extensively reported,[113] with a trend toward earlier intervention (sometimes even during infancy) and more widespread transition to noninvasive ventilation (typically mask ventilation).[166–172] Several families have opted to use negative pressure ventilation. Daytime diaphragm pacing in children with CCHS who exhibit 24-hour mechanical ventilation dependency provides greater mobility compared with mechanical ventilation. Thus, potential candidates for diaphragm pacing will be ambulatory patients who require ventilatory support 24 hours per day by means of tracheotomy and do not exhibit significant ventilator-related lung damage. Diaphragm pacer settings must provide adequate alveolar ventilation and oxygenation during rest as well as during daily activities such as exercise. Major disadvantages of diaphragm pacing include cost, discomfort associated with surgical implantation, and potential need for repeated surgical revisions due to pacer malfunction.[173,174] Despite such potential limitations, parental reports of their experience are favorable in the vast majority. Recent development of a quadripolar electrode offers several

advantages, which primarily include greater durations of pacer support at diminished risk of phrenic nerve damage and diaphragmatic fatigue, and optimization of pacing requirements during exercise.[175,176] Neurocognitive deficits are a disappointing outcome that may be detected in early preschool ages, and were initially attributed to unrecognized hypoxic events during infancy.[177] However, the possibility is now being invoked that such cognitive deficits may reflect dysmaturation of neural pathways in cortical regions.

Secondary Central Hypoventilation Syndromes

Patients with myelomeningocele or Arnold-Chiari type I or type II malformation frequently exhibit sleep-disordered breathing, and such respiratory control disturbances are frequently suspected as causative mechanisms in the sudden unexpected deaths that occur in this population. Moderate or severe breathing disturbances occur in approximately 20% of cases.[178–183] The largest proportion of patients exhibit central apnea, while others show obstructed breathing; patients with obstruction are seldom helped by surgical intervention for tonsillectomy, suggesting that the primary dysfunction is of neural origin. The possible damage to vermis cerebelli structures from foramen magnum herniation in Chiari type II malformation has the potential to interfere with both blood pressure and breathing regulation, particularly under extreme challenges of hypotension or prolonged apnea. Compression of ventral neural surfaces is also a concern. The presence of thoracic or thoracolumbar myelomeningocele or the addition of severe brain stem malformations has been shown to enhance the potential for sleep-disordered breathing. Support for affected patients with either Chiari I or II must consider the need for recovery from pronounced hypotension during sleep, the overall respiratory disturbances that are present, and the surgical interventions required for decompression of neural structures. As such, a multidisciplinary approach is necessary to yield optimal outcomes.[184]

Patients with Prader-Willi syndrome (PWS) present a unique combination of sleep- and breathing-related manifestations. Excessive daytime sleepiness and increased frequency of REM sleep periods is pervasively present in PWS patients, while others show disturbances in circadian rhythmicity with a tendency for multiple microsleep periods. In addition, the combination of obesity and hypotonia favors the occurrence of OSA. Patients with PWS also display significant alterations in central and peripheral elements of respiratory control that, though not immediately related to the obesity, can be severely affected by the mechanical consequences of increased adiposity and that ultimately lead to ventilatory failure. A unique and almost universal feature of these patients is the absence of ventilatory responses to peripheral chemoreceptor stimulation; this deficiency leads to abnormal arousal patterns during sleep.[185–187] When untreated, obesity progressively reduces central chemosensitivity as well, with the latter being ameliorated by growth hormone therapy and increased muscle mass.[188,189] However, it is important to emphasize that sudden death cases have been reported worldwide in children with PWS receiving growth hormone therapy, and that the mechanisms of such adverse outcomes remain unclear.[190–192] Accordingly, overnight sleep studies have been advocated as part of the evaluation routine before initiation of growth hormone therapy and additional monitoring after implementation of growth hormone is also recommended, usually within a few weeks and subsequently on a yearly basis.[193–200]

A condition termed late-onset central hypoventilation has been observed in some children. Although an underlying congenital brain stem abnormality is probable, significant hypoventilation becomes evident only as a consequence of an intercurrent illness such as pneumonia, with the development of severe obesity, or as a consequence of cor pulmonale.[201–205] In addition, a recognizable entity consisting of hypothalamic dysfunction and late onset of central hypoventilation is now well established, has been termed Rapid-onset Obesity with Hypothalamic dysfunction, Hypoventilation, and Autonomic Dysregulation (ROHHAD) and does not appear to be associated with Phox2B mutations.[206–208] Alveolar hypoventilation can also develop in a child with previously normal control of breathing subsequent to an event resulting in brain stem injury, such as severe asphyxia, encephalitis, and infectious encephalopathies.

OBSTRUCTIVE SLEEP APNEA

The spectrum of sleep-disordered breathing, which includes OSA and upper airway resistance syndrome, occurs in children of all ages, from neonates to adolescents. OSA is characterized by repeated events of partial or complete upper airway obstruction during sleep, resulting in disruption of normal gas exchange and sleep patterns (Figs. 81.1–81.5).[209] Nighttime symptoms and signs include snoring, paradoxical chest and abdomen motion, retractions, witnessed apnea, snoring episodes, difficulty breathing, cyanosis, sweating, and disturbed sleep. Daytime symptoms can include mouth breathing, difficulty in waking, moodiness, nasal obstruction, daytime sleepiness, hyperactivity, and cognitive problems, with severe cases of OSA associated with cor pulmonale, failure-to-thrive, developmental delay, or even death. This complex and relatively frequent disorder is only now being recognized as a major public health problem, despite being initially described more than a century ago[210] and rediscovered in children in 1976 by Guilleminault and colleagues.[211] It is clear that the classic clinical syndrome of OSA in children is a distinct disorder from the condition that occurs in adults, in particular with respect to gender distribution, clinical manifestations, polysomnographic findings, and treatment approaches.[212,213] As discussed before, childhood OSA is frequently diagnosed in association with adenotonsillar hypertrophy, and is also common in children with obesity, craniofacial abnormalities, and neurologic disorders affecting upper airway patency.

Epidemiology

Obstructive sleep apnea occurs in all pediatric age groups including infancy. Accurate prevalence information is only now emerging in infants, and suggests that habitual snoring and mild sleep-disordered breathing are frequent even during infancy, and that the risk for OSA is exacerbated by tobacco smoke exposure and reduced by breastfeeding.[214–216] OSA is particularly common in young children (preschool and early

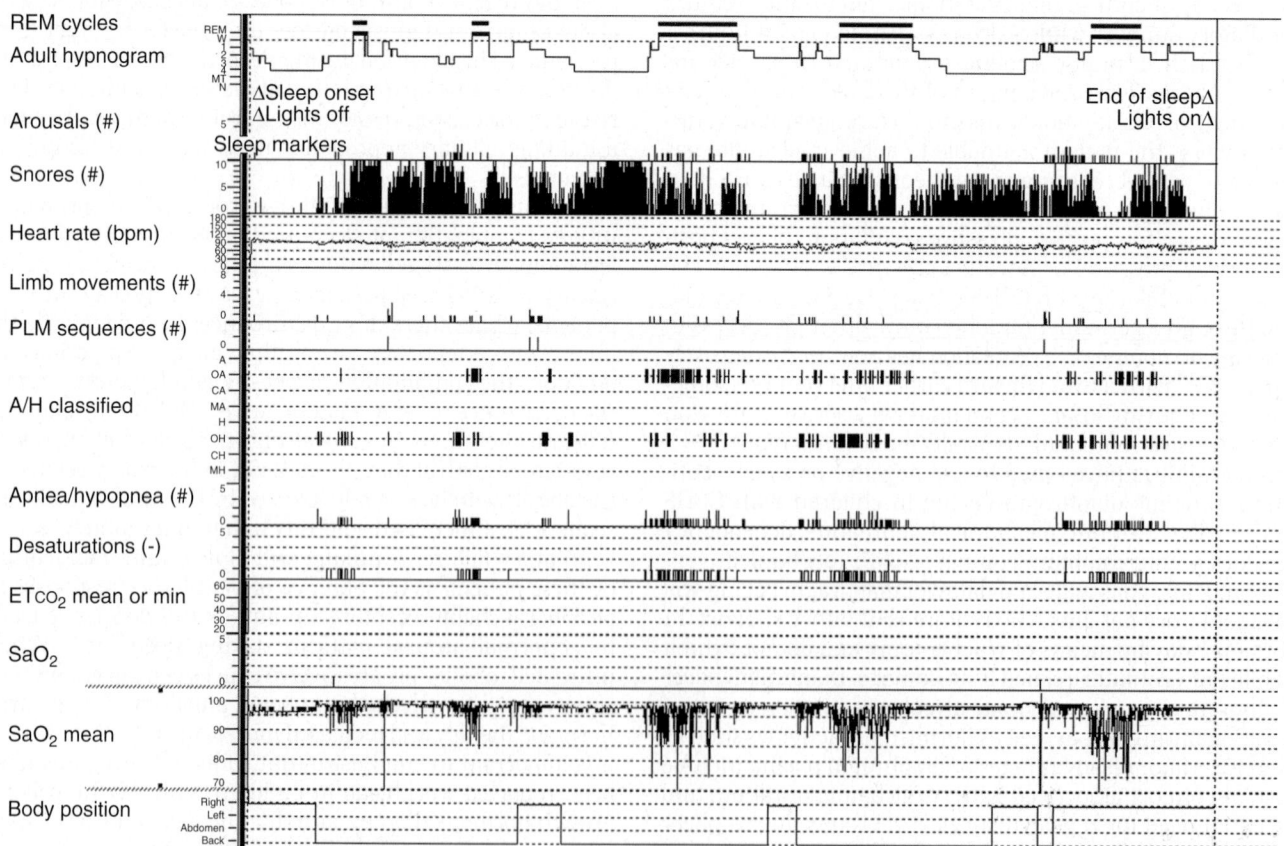

Fig. 81.1 Overnight trends in several polysomnographic measures in a 7-year-old child with moderately severe OSA. Note REM sleep clustering of respiratory events. *A*, Apnea; *ET*, end-tidal; *H*, hypopnea; *OSA*, obstructive sleep apnea; *PLM*, periodic leg movement; *REM*, rapid eye movement.

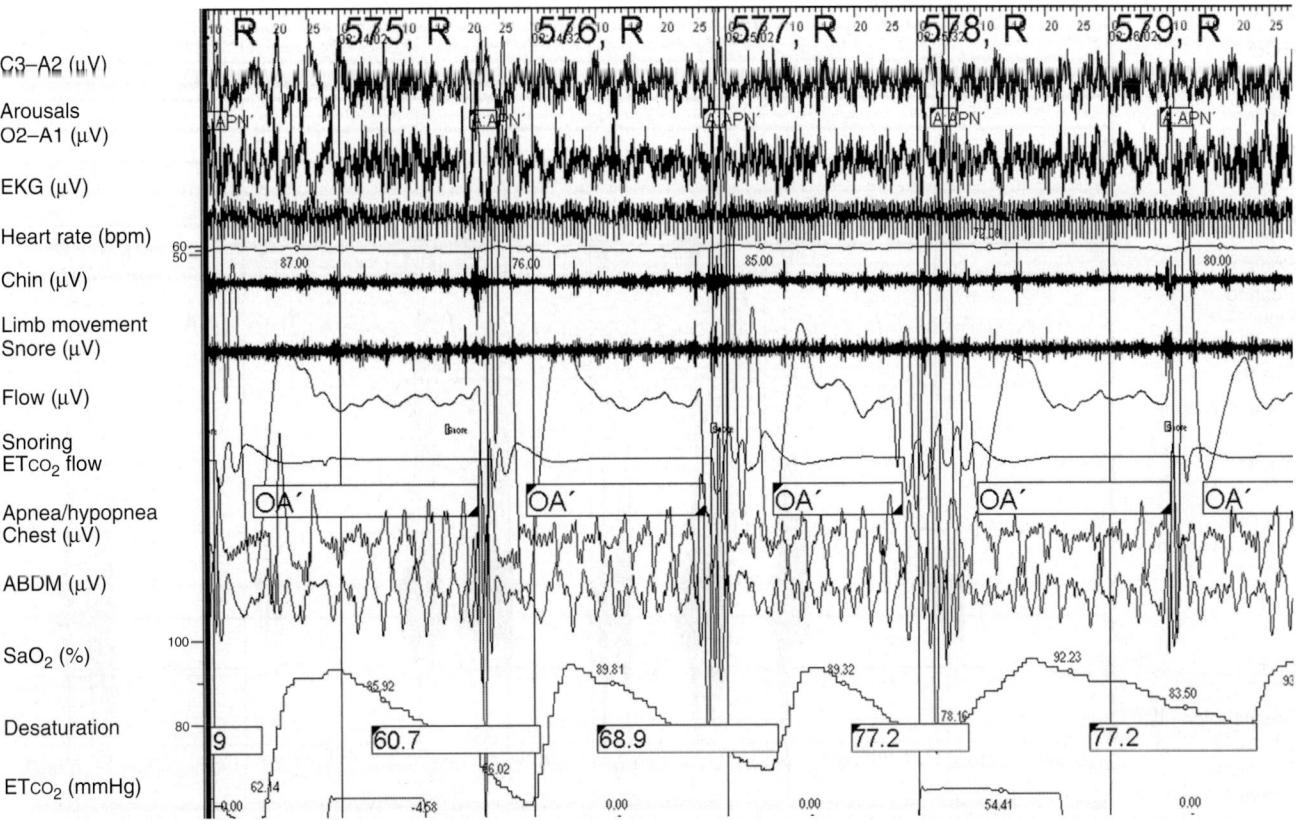

Fig. 81.2 Polygraphic tracing in a child with rapid eye movement–associated obstructive apneic events. *ABDM,* Abdominal excursion; *EKG,* electrocardiogram; *ET,* end-tidal.

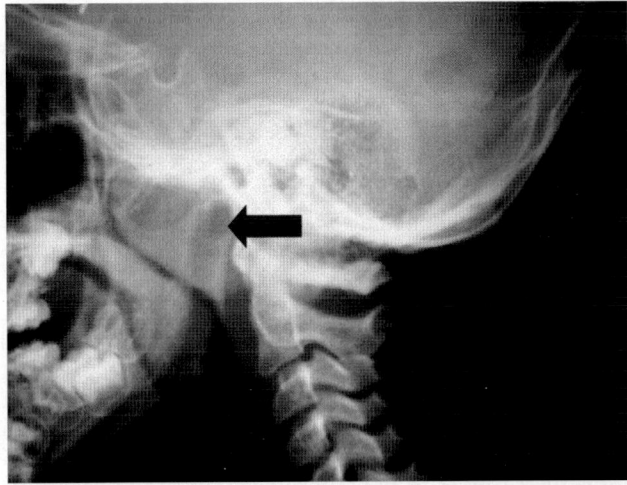

Fig. 81.3 Lateral roentgenogram of the neck in a child with enlarged adenoid tissue *(arrow)* and OSA.

school years), with a peak prevalence around 2–8 years, and it subsequently declines in frequency,[217] possibly related to reductions in viral loads associated with adenotonsillar lymphoid tissue proliferation.[218–221] Habitual snoring during sleep, the hallmark indicator of increased upper airway resistance, is an extremely frequent occurrence and affects as many as 27% of children.[222–229] While the exact clinical polysomnographically defined thresholds associated with morbidity in snoring children are still being defined, the diagnosis of OSA based on consensus criteria[230] is currently estimated to affect approximately 2%–4% of young children.[231] Thus, the ratio of habitual snoring to OSA is between 4:1 and 6:1, and accurate identification of habitually snoring children who have OSA is particularly challenging, considering that clinical history and physical examination are poor predictors of the presence or absence of disease.[232] Although simple questionnaire-based,[233–236] overnight oxymetry,[237–240] multichannel recordings,[241] or biologically based[242–244] screening tools are being developed, they are either unreliable,[233] have not been extensively validated,[240] or are not yet available for widespread use.[241,244] Thus, despite the objections to its widespread implementation and current prominent underuse,[245–248] the overnight polysomnographic recording remains the only currently accepted approach to unequivocally establishing whether a snoring child has OSA or not.[249–251]

Pathophysiology

The pathophysiology of childhood OSA remains relatively poorly understood. As discussed earlier, OSA occurs when the upper airway collapses during inspiration. Such collapse is a dynamic process that involves interaction between sleep state, pressure-flow airway mechanics, and respiratory drive. When resistance to inspiratory flow increases or when activation of the pharyngeal dilator muscles decreases, negative inspiratory pressure may collapse the airway.[61] Both functional and anatomic variables may tilt the balance toward airway collapse. Indeed, it has been determined that the site of upper airway closure in children with OSA is at the level of the tonsils and adenoids, whereas in normal children it is at the level of the soft palate.[103] The size of the tonsils and adenoids

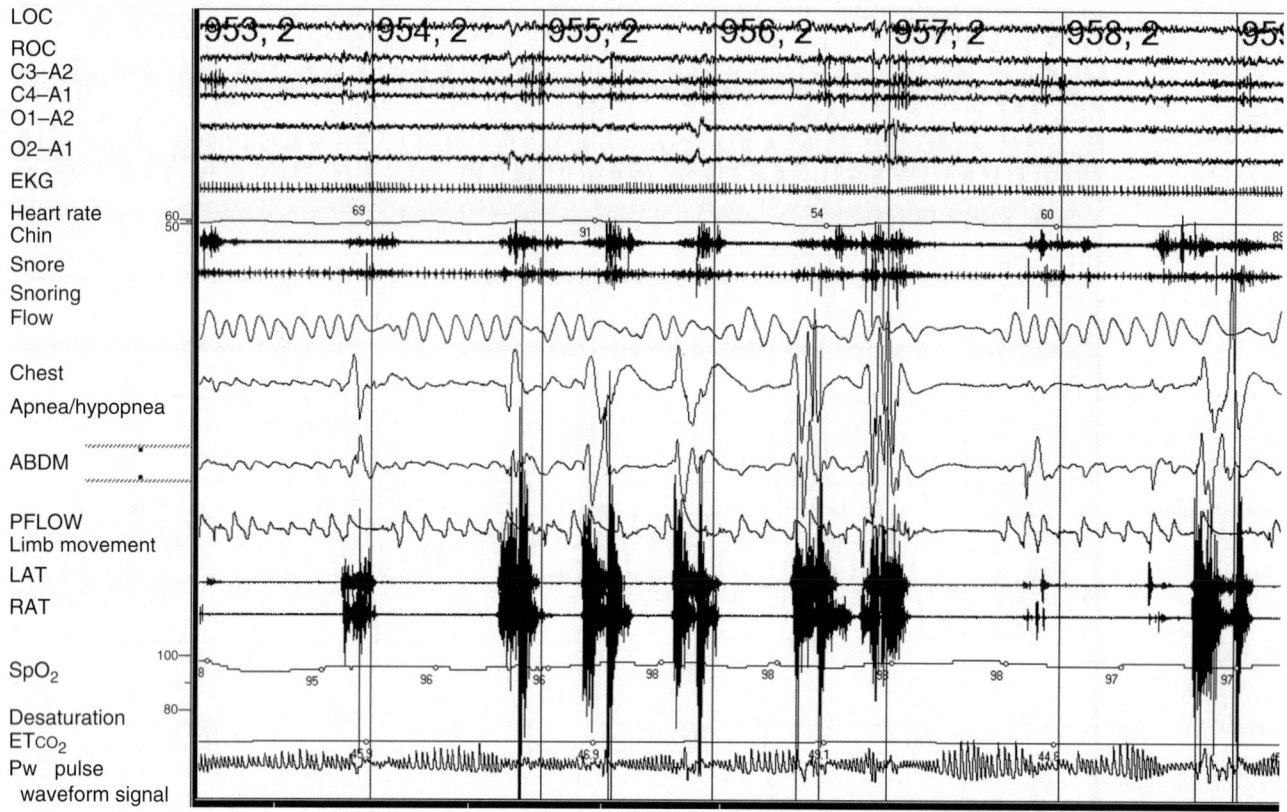

Fig. 81.4 Bruxism in a child with mild sleep-disordered breathing. *ABDM,* Abdominal excursion; *EKG,* electrocardiogram; *ET,* end-tidal; *LAT,* left anterior tibialis electromyogram (EMG); *LOC,* left oculogram; *PFLOW,* nasal pressure–derived flow; *RAT,* right anterior tibialis EMG; *ROC,* right oculogram.

increases from birth to approximately 12 years of age, with the greatest increase being in the first few years of life, albeit proportionately to the growth of other upper airway structures.[55] However, lymphadenoid tissue will grow especially large in children exposed to cigarette smoking,[252,253] children with allergic rhinitis,[254,255] children with asthma,[256–259] and obviously children exposed to a variety of upper airway respiratory infections, particularly viruses.[219,220]

Although childhood OSA is associated with adenotonsillar hypertrophy, it is not caused by large tonsils and adenoids alone. Several lines of evidence suggest that OSA is the combined result of structural and neuromuscular variables within the upper airway. Indeed, patients with OSA do not obstruct their upper airway during wakefulness, and thus structural factors alone cannot be fully responsible for this condition. In addition, several studies have failed to show a definitive and robust correlation between upper airway adenotonsillar size and OSA, even if it accounts for a great proportion of the variance in the prediction of upper airway dysfunction during sleep. Furthermore, a small percentage of nonobese children with adenotonsillar hypertrophy but no other known risk factors for OSA are not cured by surgical removal of tonsils and adenoids. Finally, Guilleminault and colleagues reported a cohort of children whose OSA temporarily resolved after surgery but in whom OSA recurred during adolescence.[260,261] Thus, it appears that childhood OSA is a dynamic process resulting from a combination of structural and neuromotor abnormalities rather than from structural abnormalities alone. These predisposing factors occur as part of a spectrum: In some children (e.g., those with craniofacial anomalies), structural abnormalities predominate, whereas in others (e.g., those with cerebral palsy), neuromuscular factors predominate. In otherwise healthy children with adenotonsillar hypertrophy, neuromuscular abnormalities are probably subtle.

Conditions Associated With OSA

Obstructive sleep apnea also occurs in children with upper airway narrowing due to craniofacial anomalies, or those with neuromuscular abnormalities such as hypotonia (e.g., muscular dystrophy) or muscular lack of coordination (e.g., cerebral palsy). In addition to craniofacial anomalies and abnormalities of the central nervous system, altered soft tissue size may result from infection of the airways, allergy, supraglottic edema, adenotonsillar hypertrophy, mucopolysaccharide storage disease, laryngomalacia, subglottic stenosis, neck tumor, or hypothyroidism. In recent years, the epidemic increase in obesity seems to be leading to substantial changes in the cross-sectional demographic and anthropometric characteristics of the children being referred for evaluation of OSA. Indeed, while fewer than 15% of all children were obese (i.e., >95th percentile for body mass index adjusted for age and gender) in the early 1990s, more than 50% met the criteria for obesity in the last 2 years in our Sleep Center.[262] Genetic factors also play a role in the pathophysiology of OSA, as demonstrated by studies of family cohorts.[263,264] It is unclear whether the influence stems from modulating effects of genetic factors on ventilatory drive, anatomic features, or both. Ethnicity is also important, with OSA occurring more commonly in African Americans. Finally, asthmatic

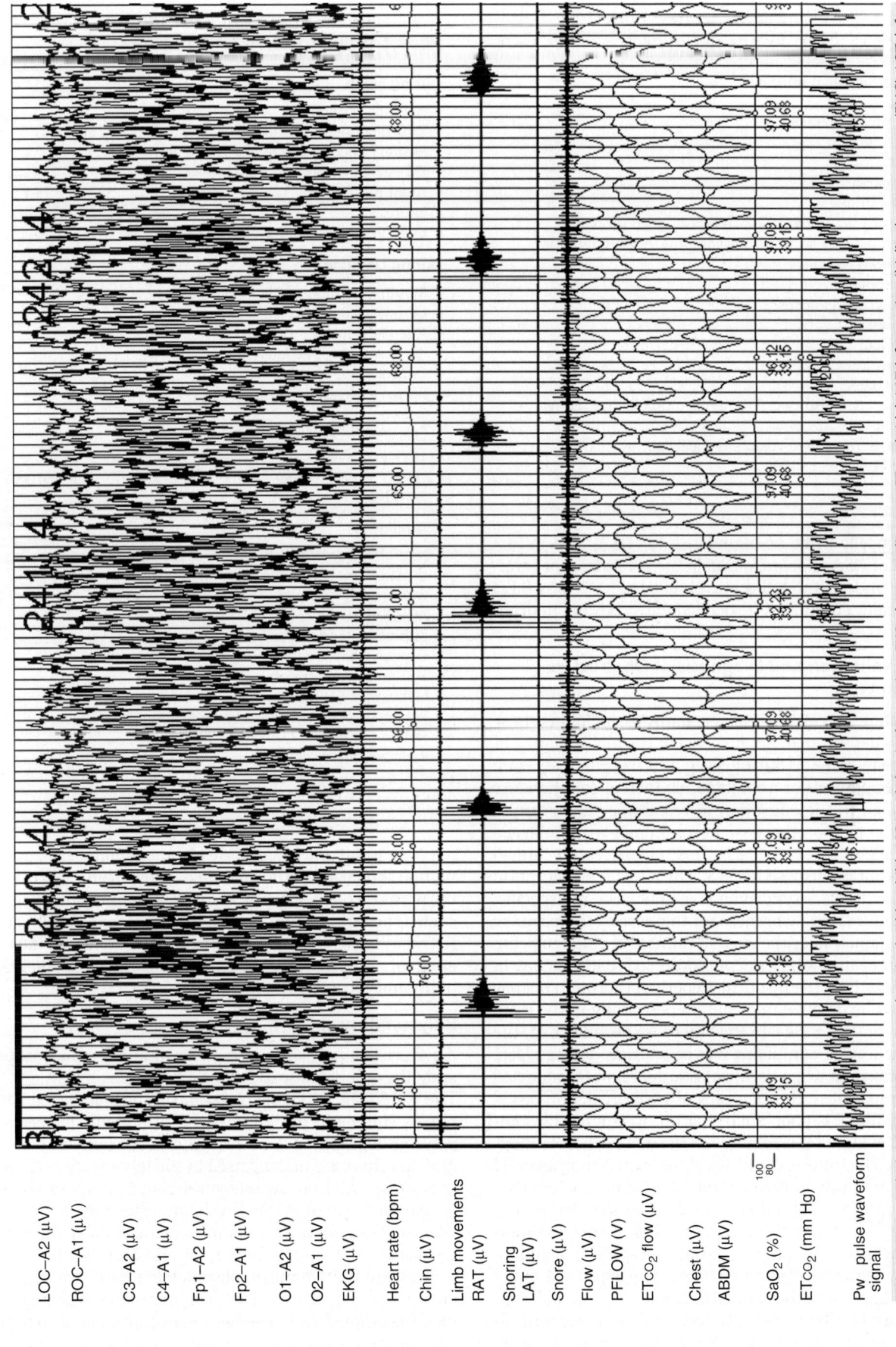

Fig. 81.5 Periodic leg movements in an otherwise healthy child. *ABDM,* Abdominal excursion; *EKG,* electrocardiogram; *ET,* end-tidal; *LAT,* left anterior tibialis electromyogram (EMG); *LOC,* left oculogram; *PFLOW,* nasal pressure–derived flow; *RAT,* right anterior tibialis EMG; *ROC,* right oculogram.

Box 81.3   Conditions Associated With Obstructive Sleep Apnea in Children

- Adenotonsillar hypertrophy
- Obesity
- African American race
- Allergic rhinitis
- Asthma
- Micrognathia
- Down syndrome
- Craniofacial syndromes (e.g., Treacher Collins syndrome, midfacial hypoplasia, Crouzon syndrome, Apert syndrome, Pierre Robin sequence)
- Achondroplasia
- Mucopolysaccharidoses
- Macroglossia
- Sickle cell disease
- Myelomeningocele
- Cerebral palsy
- Neuromuscular disorders (Duchenne muscular dystrophy, spinal muscular atrophy)
- Cleft palate repair and velopharyngeal flap
- Foreign body

Box 81.4   Pertinent Clinical Findings in Pediatric Obstructive Sleep Apnea

During Sleep

- Habitual snoring
- Difficulty breathing during sleep with snorting episodes
- Restless sleep and frequent awakenings
- Excessive sweating
- Night terrors
- Enuresis
- Breathing pauses reported by parents

During Daytime

- Mouth breathing and limited nasal airflow
- Chronic rhinorrhea
- Adenoidal facies
- Recurrent ear infections
- Difficulty swallowing
- Pectus excavatum
- Retrognathia
- Enlarged neck circumference
- Truncal obesity
- Frequent visits to primary care physician for respiratory-related symptoms

Sequelae

- Neurobehavioral deficits (poor school performance, learning deficits, aggressive behavior, moodiness, shyness, and social withdrawal)
- ADHD-like behaviors
- Depression and low self-esteem
- Excessive daytime sleepiness
- Systemic hypertension
- Left ventricular hypertrophy
- Pulmonary hypertension and *cor pulmonale*
- Failure to thrive
- Reduced quality of life

ADHD, Attention deficit–hyperactivity disorder.

children appear to be at higher risk for OSA, and in fact treatment of OSA appears to benefit the persistence or severity of the underlying asthmatic condition.[265–268] Box 81.3 lists the major conditions associated with OSA in children.

Clinical Evaluation and Diagnosis of Obstructive Sleep Apnea

It is clear that several potential mechanisms, including those genetically determined, are involved in the maintenance of upper airway patency during sleep and wakefulness. Each of these mechanisms or a combination thereof can therefore be implicated in the causation of respiratory compromise during sleep in the otherwise normal child with enlarged tonsils or adenoids, as well as in those children with clinical problems that predispose to OSA. The clinical presentation of a child with OSA syndrome is usually very nonspecific, requiring increased awareness on the part of the primary care professional, since the current number of children being referred for evaluation of sleep-disordered breathing may in fact represent only the tip of the iceberg. A thorough history should include detailed information pertaining to the sleep environment (Box 81.4). In the otherwise normal child, the principal parental complaint will be snoring during sleep. Nevertheless, even when the diagnostic interview is conducted by a sleep specialist, the accuracy of OSA prediction based on history alone is poor, such that an overnight polysomnographic evaluation is required as the more definitive diagnostic tool. The routine clinical evaluation of a snoring child is usually not likely to demonstrate significant and obvious findings. Attention should be directed to the size of the tonsils,[269,270] with careful documentation of their position and relative intrusion into the retropalatal space. In addition, nasopharyngoscopic evaluation or imaging approaches may be helpful in guiding the clinical decision.[271–273] In addition, the presence of allergic rhinitis, nasal polyps, nasal septum deviation, or any other condition likely to increase nasal airflow resistance should be evaluated. The relative size (i.e.,

micrognathia) and positioning of the mandible (e.g., retrognathia) should also be documented. Body habitus, particularly the presence of obesity, and associated signs of complications such as acanthosis nigricans should be noted. Finally, attention should be paid to blood pressure values and to the presence of auscultatory findings suggestive of increased pulmonary artery pressures.

Polysomnography

An overnight polysomnographic evaluation is, at least presently, the only definitive diagnostic approach for OSA.[249,274,275] The American Academy of Pediatrics has published a consensus statement outlining the requirements for pediatric polysomnography.[249] Box 81.5 shows the currently recommended channels usually used in the laboratory evaluation of snoring children. Available reference values in children are clearly lower than the thresholds defined for adults.[276–284] While the reasons are not completely understood, the relative resistance of the upper airway of children to collapse may underscore that complete obstructive events are less likely and that prolonged periods of heightened upper airway resistance associated with alveolar hypoventilation (also termed obstructive hypoventilation) are more readily apparent in children.[285] It should also be mentioned that, unlike adults,

Box 81.5 Usual Polysomnographic Montage in Children Evaluated for Suspected Sleep-Disordered Breathing[a]

- Electroencephalogram: minimum two channels (central and occipital leads); usually four to eight channels
- Chin EMG
- Anterior tibial EMG, left and right
- Electro-oculogram, left and right
- Electrocardiogram
- Pulse oximeter and pulse waveform
- Oronasal airflow thermistor
- Nasal pressure catheter[b]
- End-tidal capnography and waveform
- Chest and abdominal respiratory inductance plethysmography
- Body position sensor
- Tracheal sound sensor or microphone
- Time-synchronized video

[a]In younger children, consider transcutaneous CO_2 tension measurements.

[b]Esophageal catheters are used in some laboratories instead of nasal pressure catheters to assess respiratory effort.

EMG, Electromyogram.

children with OSA often will not develop obvious EEG arousals following obstructive apneas,[286,287] and as a result, sleep architecture is relatively preserved in many children with OSA.[288] This reduced propensity to manifest arousals (based on the 3-second EEG criteria developed for adults) has led to the assumption that excessive daytime sleepiness, the cardinal symptom of OSA syndrome in adults, is an uncommon feature in children with OSA. Indeed, in initial parental surveys only 7% of parents indicated that excessive sleepiness was a problem.[232] Furthermore, more objective measurement of excessive daytime sleepiness using the multiple sleep latency test in snoring children revealed that, although linear relationships existed between the severity of OSA (as measured by the obstructive apnea-hypopnea index) and the mean sleep latency measured during the multiple sleep latency test, manifest excessive daytime sleepiness occurred in only 13% of children.[289] However, excessive daytime sleepiness is very likely to occur in obese children with OSA,[290] and has prompted the delineation of 2 distinct phenotypes in pediatric OSA.[291] More elaborate examination of the patterns of arousal among snoring children further showed that as respiratory-related arousals increase in frequency with increasing OSA disease severity, the opposite phenomenon (i.e., decreases in spontaneous arousal index) occurs,[292] suggesting a very powerful attempt by these children to preserve sleep homeostasis. On the basis of the mutual interdependencies of these two types of arousal, a model was developed that allows for sensitive assessment of the resulting sleep pressure derived from disrupted sleep using polysomnographic data.[293] This approach has thus far permitted assessment of the independent contribution of sleep fragmentation to neurobehavioral morbidity in snoring children.[294] Thus, more subtle manifestations of arousal may be present in children, even if apnea-related EEG arousals are less common than in adults. For example, subcortical arousals, as demonstrated by movement, or autonomic changes, occur frequently in children.[295] It is also possible that subtle disturbances in sleep architecture

are present that go undetected by routine polysomnography but are detectable through spectral analysis of EEG frequency domains[296] and may contribute to neurobehavioral and autonomic complications of OSA (see later). Treatment of OSA has resulted in improved reports of sleepiness by parents.[297]

As mentioned earlier, the role of ambulatory sleep studies, whether abbreviated (home video, sound recordings, or nocturnal oximetry) is now being intensively explored, along with exploration of biomarkers.[237–244,298–303]

Short-Term and Long-Term Morbidity of Obstructive Sleep Apnea

One of the major drives to treat any medical condition is the prevention of morbidity and mortality. Indeed, the consequences of untreated OSA in young children can be serious. Early reports of children with severe OSA were often associated with failure to thrive, although currently only a minority of children with OSA will present with this problem, most probably because of earlier recognition and referral for evaluation and treatment. The mechanisms mediating reductions in growth velocity most likely represent a combination of increased energy expenditure during sleep,[304,305] and disruption of the growth hormone and insulin-like growth factor and binding proteins.[306,307] Tonsillectomy and adenoidectomy (T&A) and complete resolution of OSA in children with failure to thrive will result in catch-up growth and will also increase the height and weight velocities even in children with normal growth and OSA. Interestingly, even obese children with OSA will demonstrate weight gain following surgery.[308]

Frequent O_2 desaturations during sleep are common in children with OSA. Elevation of pulmonary artery pressure due to hypoxia-induced pulmonary vasoconstriction is a serious consequence of OSA in children, and can lead to cor pulmonale. While pulmonary hypertension is probably more frequent than predicted from clinical assessment, the exact prevalence of this complication is unknown.[309–312] In addition, while treatment of OSA will result in normalization of pulmonary artery pressures,[313] it remains unclear whether untreated OSA will result in persistent vascular remodeling of the pulmonary circulation. Indeed, evidence from animal models exposed to hypoxia for a short period of time during early postnatal life reveals that pulmonary hypertension is increased when exposed to hypoxia later in infancy, suggesting that some remodeling may have occurred.[314] Furthermore, intermittent hypoxia may also affect left ventricular function through both direct and indirect effects on myocardial contractility.[315] In the context of OSA, systemic hypertension has emerged as a major cardiovascular consequence in adult patients. Although the pathophysiologic mechanisms of such elevation in arterial tension are still under intense investigation, it appears that intermittent hypoxemia is the major contributor to this serious consequence of OSA, with lesser roles being played by sleep fragmentation and episodic hypercapnia. It is now thought that intermittent hypoxia during the night will lead to increased sympathetic neural activity, and that the latter will be sustained and induce changes in baroreceptor function leading to hypertension.[316] While the data pertaining to pediatric patients are still scant, increased surges in sympathetic activity have been reported in children with OSA,[317,318] and elevation of arterial blood pressure will occur.[319–321] It is also probable that episodic nocturnal hypoxia will induce changes in the physical properties of resistance vessels and contribute to the overall elevation of blood pressure.[322,323] Furthermore, preliminary evidence suggests that OSA-induced disruption of baroreceptor function may not resolve after treatment and in fact may be lifelong.[324–326] Thus, early childhood perturbations may lead to lifelong consequences, or in other words, certain types of adult cardiovascular disease may represent, at least in part, sequelae from *a priori* "unrelated events" during childhood. Therefore early identification of children with alterations of baroreceptor and autonomic nervous system function in the context of pediatric OSA may lead to detection of a population potentially at risk for ultimate development of hypertension and its cardiovascular-associated morbidity. More recent studies have further uncovered that pediatric OSA is associated with a systemic inflammatory response; leads to excessive catecholaminergic release, indicative of increased sympathetic activity; and promotes the occurrence of endothelial dysfunction, the latter being palliated by the intrinsic recruitment of endothelial progenitor cells.[327–340] However, accurate assessment of the long-term implications of the cardiovascular morbidity found in pediatric OSA has yet to be systematically pursued.

It is likely that similar mechanisms induced by OSA, particularly in the presence of concurrent obesity, will promote the development of dyslipidemia and insulin resistance, and also potentiate hepatic injury.[341–344]

Another potentially very serious consequence of intermittent hypoxia may involve its long-term deleterious effects on neuronal and intellectual functions. Reports of decreased intellectual function in children with tonsillar and adenoidal hypertrophy date back to 1889, when Hill reported on "some causes of backwardness and stupidity in children."[345] Schooling problems have been repeatedly reported in case series of children with OSA, and in fact may underlie more extensive behavioral disturbances such as restlessness, aggressive behavior, excessive daytime sleepiness, and poor test performances.[346–359] Moreover, habitual snoring in the absence of OSA has also been demonstrated to be associated with neurocognitive deficits, and therefore even mild disturbances in breathing patterns during sleep may change regional brain responses during attention tasks.[360,361]

There is increasing evidence to support an association between OSA and attention-deficit/hyperactivity disorder (ADHD) in children, particularly with the hyperactive-impulsive subtype.[362] Several subjective studies have documented that children with habitual snoring and with OSA often have problems with attention and behavior similar to those observed in children with ADHD. In addition, several survey studies encompassing almost 8000 children have documented daytime sleepiness, hyperactivity, and aggressive behavior in children who snored. In a recent study from our laboratory, both subjective and objective sleep measures were obtained, and showed that objectively measured sleep and respiratory disturbances are relatively frequent among children with ADHD, albeit not as frequent as anticipated from parental reports. In this study, the prevalence of OSA in a cohort of children with ADHD, verified by neuropsychologic testing, did not seem to differ from the prevalence found in the general population. However, an unusually high frequency of OSA was found among children with mild-to-moderate increases in hyperactivity, as opposed to those children with

true ADHD. This suggests that while OSA can induce significant behavioral effects manifesting as increased hyperactivity and inattention, it will not overlap with true clinical ADHD when the latter is assessed by more objective tools than just parental perception.[224] Therefore in a child presenting with parental complaints of hyperactivity and who does not meet the diagnostic criteria of ADHD after undergoing a thorough evaluation, a careful sleep history should be taken and if snoring is present, an overnight polysomnographic evaluation should be performed.

The mechanism(s) by which OSA may contribute to hyperactivity remain unknown. It is possible that both the sleep fragmentation and episodic hypoxia that characterize OSA will lead to alterations within the neurochemical substrate of the prefrontal cortex, with resultant executive dysfunction.[362,363] Notwithstanding these considerations, sleep disturbances are frequently reported by parents of ADHD children, even when snoring is excluded. According to the available literature, the comorbidity of OSA and ADHD could be shared by a substantial number of hyperactive children, and in fact, it has been suggested that as many as 25% of children with a diagnosis of ADHD may actually have OSA.[361] However, such rather extensive overlap may be less prominent than previously estimated if medication status and psychiatric comorbidity are accounted for in the analysis.

Inverse relationships between memory, learning, and OSA have also been documented. In addition, improvements in learning and behavior have been reported subsequent to treatment for OSA in children,[364–366] suggesting that the neurocognitive deficits are at least partially reversible. In a large cohort of first graders whose academic performance was in the lowest (10th) percentile of their class, a six- to nine-fold increase in the expected incidence of OSA was found. More importantly, however, a significant improvement in school grades following T&A and resolution of OSA occurred in these children.[347] Since the optimal learning potential for these children is unknown, it is possible that long-term residual deficits may occur even after treatment. Indeed, children who snored frequently and loudly during their early childhood were at greater risk for poor academic performance in later years, well after snoring had resolved.[367] These findings suggest therefore that even if a component of the OSA-induced learning deficits is reversible, there may be a long-lasting residual deficit in learning capability, and that the latter may represent a "learning debt"; in other words, the decreased learning capacity during OSA may have led to such a delay in learned skills that recuperation is only possible with additional teaching assistance. Alternatively, the processes underlying the learning deficit during OSA may have irreversibly altered the performance characteristics of the neuronal circuitry responsible for learning particular skills. Another important observation is that at any level of severity, not all children suffering from OSA manifest evidence of cognitive or behavioral pathology, even if a dose-dependent relationship is detectable.[368,369] Of note, such severity-dependent relationship is applicable only to cognition and not to behavioral functioning, whereby the more severe behavioral perturbations appear at the milder levels of sleep-disordered breathing.[370] This conundrum has been further exacerbated by the inability to detect major improvements in cognitive function in children randomized to be treated with either T&A or watchful waiting,[371] even if a posthoc secondary analysis revealed some degree of improvements in a subset of the neurocognitive tests.[372]

As mentioned before, overt excessive daytime sleepiness is not immediately apparent in children with OSA, yet morbidity that could be construed as related to sleepiness is indeed detectable. Recent studies clearly support a role for sleepiness (measured as sleep pressure) in the cognitive and behavioral disturbances occurring in children with OSA.[373]

In animal models, we found that intermittent hypoxia during sleep is associated with significant increases in neuronal cell loss and adverse effects on spatial memory tasks in the absence of significant sleep fragmentation or deprivation. Furthermore, when this model was applied to developing rodents, a unique period of neuronal susceptibility to episodic hypoxia during sleep emerged and corresponded to ages at which OSA prevalence peaks in children.[374-376] Since this age coincides with that of a critical period for brain development, it is possible that, during a critical time for brain development, delayed diagnosis and treatment of OSA will impose a greater burden on vulnerable brain structures and ultimately hamper the overall neurocognitive potential of children with OSA. Adverse effects of sleep-disordered breathing on quality of life,[377-379] mood,[379] enuresis,[380-382] and health-related costs[383,384] further buttress the extensive and multifactorial impact of this condition.

In summary, it is becoming increasingly clear that OSA in children can have adverse effects on somatic growth, induce cardiovascular and metabolic alterations such as pulmonary hypertension, systemic hypertension, endothelial dysfunction and atherosclerosis,[385,386] insulin resistance,[387-389] and hyperlipidemia, and lead to substantial neurobehavioral deficits, some of which may not be reversible if treatment is delayed. Based on our current understanding of the morbidity affecting pediatric OSA, it is imperative to direct future efforts toward an improved definition of the spectrum of OSA-induced syndrome, so as to provide more accurate guidelines for treatment.

Treatment of Obstructive Sleep Apnea

Tonsillectomy and adenoidectomy is usually the first line of treatment for pediatric OSA, and a meta-analysis on the efficacy of T&A suggested a relatively high immediate curative rate of surgery for OSA in children.[390] Since OSA is the conglomerate result of the relative size and structure of the upper airway components, rather than the absolute size of the adenotonsillar tissue, both tonsils and adenoids should be removed, even when one or the other seems to be the primary culprit. Although the majority of children will have improvement in the severity of OSA, cure may actually occur in a smaller proportion than previously estimated, particularly in children with more severe OSA, in those who are obese, and in those with a positive family history of OSA or asthma.[371,391-395]

Children with OSA are at risk for respiratory compromise postoperatively, as a result of upper airway edema, increased secretions, respiratory depression secondary to analgesic and anesthetic agents, and postobstructive pulmonary edema. A high risk for such complications is particularly encountered among children younger than 3 years of age, those with severe OSA, and those with additional medical conditions such as craniofacial syndromes; these patients should not undergo outpatient surgery, and cardiorespiratory monitoring should be performed for at least 24 hours postoperatively to ensure their stability.[396-400] Postoperative polysomnographic evaluation 10–12 weeks after surgery is probably needed in most patients.[395] However, it should definitely be recommended for those patients with additional risk factors, and thus ensure that additional interventions are not required.[395]

Additional treatment options are available for the management of OSA in children either before T&A, for those children who do not respond to T&A, or for the small minority in whom T&A is contraindicated. Nasal CPAP has been reported to be both effective and well tolerated in hundreds of infants and older children, with only minor side effects (similar to those seen in adults), such as nasal symptoms and skin breakdown.[401-409] However, adherence is routinely low, and the implementation of behavioral modification programs and family supportive services aimed at improving adherence results in relatively high health care costs that are unlikely to be assumed by third-party payers.[410] Younger children may develop central apneas or alveolar hypoventilation at higher pressure levels, presumably due to activation of the Hering-Breuer reflex by stimulating pulmonary stretch receptors. However, this can be remedied by the use of bilevel positive airway pressure ventilation with a backup rate. Supplemental O_2 results in improved arterial O_2 saturation in children with OSA without worsening the degree of obstruction. However, since O_2 does not address many of the pathophysiologic features associated with the symptoms of OSA, it should be reserved as a temporary palliative measure preceding T&A, and it clearly should not be used as a first-line treatment. Furthermore, supplemental O_2 should never be used without monitoring the potential resultant changes in Pco_2, since some patients with OSA can develop unpredictable and potentially life-threatening hypercapnia when breathing supplemental O_2.[411,412]

Uvulopharyngopalatoplasty has not been systematically evaluated in children. It has been found to be useful in patients with upper airway hypotonia; in other words, those with Down syndrome or cerebral palsy. Craniofacial reconstructive procedures are reserved for some children with craniofacial anomalies. Other procedures such as tongue wedge resection, epiglottoplasty, mandibular advancement, and lingual tonsillectomy occasionally may be indicated. Additionally, the role of intraoral appliances and myofunctional therapy remains unclear, even if favorable outcomes have been reported in recent clinical series.[413-415] With the advent of CPAP, tracheostomy is now rarely required. Although pharmacologic agents are not usually useful in frank OSA, recent work has demonstrated that intranasal steroids and oral leukotriene receptor modifiers may have a role in the clinical management of symptomatic children with either primary or secondary (after T&A) upper-airway-resistance syndrome.[416-426]

Finally, the use of high-flow oxygen via a nasal cannula has recently been proposed as an alternative to CPAP in selected cases. Further studies, however, will be necessary to validate this approach and appraise its limitations.[427,428]

References

Access the reference list online at ExpertConsult.com.

Index

Note: Page numbers followed by *b* indicate boxes; *f*, figures; and *t*, tables.